Pediatric Kidney Disease

Pediatric Kidney Disease

SECOND EDITION

VOLUME I — The Kidney and Urinary Tract:
Development, Morphology, and Physiology
in Health and Disease

Editor   **Chester M. Edelmann, Jr., M.D.**
Senior Associate Dean and Professor of Pediatrics, Albert
Einstein College of Medicine of Yeshiva University;
Attending Physician, Department of Pediatrics, Bronx
Municipal Hospital Center and Montefiore Medical
Center, Bronx, New York

Associate Editors   **Jay Bernstein, M.D.**
William Beaumont Hospital, Royal Oak, Michigan
S. Roy Meadow, M.B.
Leeds University, Leeds, England
Adrian Spitzer, M.D.
Albert Einstein College of Medicine of Yeshiva University,
Bronx, New York
Luther B. Travis, M.D.
University of Texas Medical School at Galveston, Galveston,
Texas

Little, Brown and Company
Boston/Toronto/London

Library of Congress Cataloging-in-Publication Data

Pediatric kidney disease / Chester M. Edelmann, Jr.
   editor, associate editors, S. Roy Meadow . . . [et al.]:
   with 151 contributors. —2nd ed.
        p.   cm.
     Includes bibliographical references and index.
     ISBN 0-316-21072-2
     1. Pediatric nephrology.   I. Edelmann, Chester M.,
   1930-
   II. Meadow, S. R.
     [DNLM: 1. Kidney Disease—in infancy &
     childhood.   WS 320 P369]
   RJ476.K5P43   1992
   618.92'61—dc20
   DNLM/DLC
   for Library of Congress   91-43804
                                                    CIP

Printed in the United States of America

RRD-VA

To Norma

VOLUME II — Diseases of the Kidney and Urinary Tract

VI. Neonatal, Congenital, and Heritable Disorders

VII. Glomerular Diseases

Preface

In his first Porter lecture, Homer Smith concluded with a statement written in 1804 by a French chemist named Fourcroy:

The urine of man is one of the animal matters that have been the most examined by chemists and of which the examination has at the same time furnished the most singular discoveries to chemistry, and the most useful applications to physiology, as well as the art of healing. This liquid, which commonly inspires men only with contempt and disgust, which is generally ranked amongst vile and repulsive matters, has become, in the hands of the chemists, a source of important discoveries and is an object in the history of which we find the most singular disparity between the ideas which are generally formed of it in the world, and the valuable notion which the study of it affords to the physiologist, the physician and the philosopher.

One might conclude that Fourcroy had the scientific prescience to anticipate Claude Bernard's formulation of the concept of the internal environment, the maintenance of which we now recognize to be the main task of the kidneys. Even more remarkable than the ability of the kidneys to regulate the *milieu interieur*, however, is their capacity to adapt to the homeostatic needs of the fetus, the transition from intrauterine to extrauterine existence, and the continuously changing requirements for growth.

The undertaking of the first edition of *Pediatric Kidney Disease*, published in 1978, was prompted by the need for a comprehensive treatment of renal and renal-related disorders in infants, children, and adolescents, since these subjects are dealt with at a superficial level in texts of nephrology that are written by internists. The purpose of *Pediatric Kidney Disease*, as stated in the first edition, was ". . . to provide as complete a compendium as possible of all aspects of nephrology that relate to infants and children. The goal is to introduce nephrology to the student and to provide a source book for the experienced physician, including internists, pediatricians, family physicians, urologists, and nephrologists."

The goal, organization, and format of the second edition of *Pediatric Kidney Disease* are basically unchanged from the first edition. It emphasizes that developmental nephrology must provide the foundation for the training and practice of the pediatric nephrologist, particularly, although by no means exclusively, with regard to the care of low-birthweight and young infants. Ontogeny, the central theme of pediatric nephrology, is, therefore, the subject of the greatly expanded first section, now comprising 12 chapters. Since the mechanisms of renal injury, the evaluation for disease, the manifestations of renal disease and renal insufficiency, and general principles of treatment are common to all renal disorders, they are considered collectively in Volume I, avoiding unnecessary repetition in subsequent chapters.

In Volume II, which deals with specific disorders, greater emphasis has been placed on neonatal, congenital, and heritable disorders, conditions that in many instances are unique to pediatrics. Sections on primary glomerular diseases, renal abnormalities that occur in the setting of systemic disease, other nephropathies, disorders that affect tubular function, and circulatory disorders follow. The final section considers disorders of the urinary tract, including infection, trauma, urolithiasis, enuresis, and urologic conditions that come at least in part under the purview of the pediatrician or pediatric nephrologist. Finally, not to be overlooked, is the unfortunate occurrence of factitious renal disease, which is discussed in this section.

It was amazing to me and the associate editors that so much new information had become available since production of the first edition. Every attempt has been made to critically evaluate the extensive nephrologic literature and to include all essential elements. The results are reflected in the expanded length of the second edition. This undertaking has required the enormous effort of numerous experts, a labor of love for most of us that has extended over a period of years. I must express my deepest and sincerest thanks and gratitude to the associate editors and to all the hard-working contributors. In addition, many individuals at Little, Brown provided essential help, encouragement, and assistance. Finally, I must acknowledge the invaluable and irreplaceable participation of Jean Massaro, who continues to provide the secretarial and editorial assistance that is needed to bring a work such as this to completion.

Many colleagues have commented that the first edition

Kenneth I. Glassberg, M.D.
Associate Professor of Urology, State University of New York Health Science Center at Brooklyn; Director, Division of Pediatric Urology, University Hospital of Brooklyn, Brooklyn, New York

David I. Goldsmith, M.D.
Corporate Medical Director and Director of Product Safety Surveillance, Sterling Drug Inc., New York, New York

Robin S. Goldstein, Ph.D.
Assistant Director, Department of Investigative Toxicology, SmithKline Beecham Pharmaceuticals, King of Prussia, Pennsylvania

Gregory A. Grabowski, M.D.
Associate Professor of Pediatrics and Genetics, Mount Sinai School of Medicine of the City University of New York; Associate Professor, The Mount Sinai Hospital, New York, New York

Donald Gribetz, M.D.
Professor of Pediatrics, Mount Sinai School of Medicine of the City University of New York; Attending Pediatrician, The Mount Sinai Hospital, New York, New York

Paul C. Grimm, M.D.
Research Fellow, University of California at Los Angeles, UCLA School of Medicine; Attending Physician, Department of Pediatric Nephrology, UCLA Medical Center, Los Angeles, California

Warren E. Grupe, M.D.
Vice President, Medical Education, Project HOPE Health Sciences Education Foundation, Inc., Millwood, Virginia

Alan B. Gruskin, M.D.
Professor and Chairman, Department of Pediatrics, Wayne State University School of Medicine; Pediatrician-in-Chief, Children's Hospital of Michigan, Detroit, Michigan

Niilo Hallman, M.D.
Professor Emeritus of Pediatrics, Helsinki University; Researcher, Foundation of Pediatric Research, Helsinki, Finland

C. Keith Hayden, Jr., M.D.
Deputy Director of Pediatric Radiology, Cook–Fort Worth Children's Medical Center, Fort Worth, Texas

Jerry B. Hook, Ph.D.
Vice President of Development, SmithKline Beecham Pharmaceuticals, King of Prussia, Pennsylvania

Ian B. Houston, M.D.
Professor and Head, Child Health Department, University of Manchester; Honorary Consultant, Royal Manchester Children's Hospital, Manchester, England

Niilo-Pekka Huttunen, M.D.
Senior Lecturer, Department of Pediatrics, University of Oulu; Head, Pediatrics Unit, Central Hospital of Central Finland, Jyväskylä, Finland

Julie R. Ingelfinger, M.D.
Associate Professor of Pediatrics, Harvard Medical School; Co-chief, Pediatric Nephrology, Massachusetts General Hospital, Boston, Massachusetts

Robert A. Jodorkovsky, M.D.
Assistant Professor of Pediatrics, University of Maryland School of Medicine; Director, Division of Pediatric Nephrology, University of Maryland Hospital, Baltimore, Maryland

K. Verrier Jones, M.B., B.Ch.
Laura Ashley Senior Lecturer in Pediatric Nephrology, University of Wales College of Medicine; Consultant Pediatrician and Pediatric Nephrologist, Department of Child Health, Cardiff, Wales

Pedro A. Jose, M.D., Ph.D.
Professor of Pediatrics, Georgetown University School of Medicine; Attending Physician, Georgetown University Hospital, Washington, D.C.

Stephanie D. Kafonek, M.D.
Instructor of Medicine, Johns Hopkins University School of Medicine, Baltimore, Maryland

Alok Kalia, M.B., B.S.
Associate Professor of Pediatrics, University of Texas Medical School at Galveston, Galveston, Texas

Bernard S. Kaplan, M.B., B.Ch.
Professor of Pediatrics, University of Pennsylvania School of Medicine; Director, Division of Nephrology, Children's Hospital of Philadelphia, Philadelphia, Pennsylvania

George W. Kaplan, M.D.
Professor of Surgery and Pediatrics, University of California, San Diego, School of Medicine; Chief of Urology, Children's Hospital and Health Center, San Diego, California

Leslie M. Kaplan, M.D.
Adjunct Assistant Professor, University of California, Los Angeles, UCLA School of Medicine; Chief Resident, Department of Surgery and Urology, UCLA Medical Center, Los Angeles, California

Frederick J. Kaskel, M.D., Ph.D.
Associate Professor, Director of Pediatric Nephrology, State University of New York at Stony Brook, Health Sciences Center School of Medicine; Director of Pediatric Nephrology, The University Hospital at Stony Brook, Stony Brook, New York

Evan J. Kass, M.D.
Chief of Pediatric Urology, William Beaumont Hospital, Royal Oak, Michigan

Thomas L. Kennedy III, M.D.
Associate Professor, Department of Pediatrics, Yale University School of Medicine, New Haven; Chairman, Department of Pediatrics, Bridgeport Hospital, Bridgeport, Connecticut

Melanie S. Kim, M.D.
Instructor of Pediatrics, Harvard Medical School; Director of General Renal Service, Division of Nephrology, Children's Hospital, Boston, Massachusetts

Youngki Kim, M.D.
Professor, Departments of Pediatrics, and Laboratory Medicine and Pathology, University of Minnesota Medical School, Minneapolis, Minnesota

John M. Kissane, M.D.
Professor of Pathology and Pathology in Pediatrics, Washington University School of Medicine; Pathologist, Barnes and Affiliated Hospitals and Saint Louis Children's Hospital, Saint Louis, Missouri

Claire Kleinknecht, M.D.
Director of Research, Institut National de la Santé et de la Recherche Medical, Hôpital des Enfants Malades, Paris, France

Leonard I. Kleinman, M.D.
Professor of Pediatrics, State University of New York at Stony Brook, Health Sciences Center School of Medicine; Attending Neonatal Physician, and Director, Newborn Division, The University Hospital at Stony Brook, Stony Brook, New York

Peter O. Kwiterovich, Jr., M.D.
Professor of Pediatrics and Medicine, Johns Hopkins University School of Medicine, Baltimore, Maryland

Craig B. Langman, M.D.
Associate Chair of Pediatrics, Northwestern University Medical School; Director, Mineral Metabolism Department, Children's Memorial Hospital, Chicago, Illinois

D. Laouari, M.D.
Chargé de Recherches, Institut National de la Sante et de la Recherche Medicale, Hopital des Enfants Malades, Paris, France

Jill A. Largent, M.D.
Pediatric Nephrologist, Geisinger Medical Center, Danville, Pennsylvania

Lars Larsson, M.D., Ph.D.
Professor, Karolinska Institute, Stockholm; Director, Pediatric Outpatient Clinic, Eksjö County Hospital, Eksjö, Sweden

Joseph Laufer, M.D.
Lecturer in Pediatrics, Sackler School of Medicine, Tel Aviv; Attending Pediatric Nephrologist, Department of Pediatrics, Pediatric Nephrology Unit, Chaim Sheba Medical Center, Tel Hashomer, Israel

Michael Levin, M.B.
Senior Lecturer in Pediatric Infectious Diseases, Institute of Child Health; Consultant in Infectious Diseases, Hospital for Sick Children, London, England

Sherman D. Levine, M.D.
Professor of Medicine, and Physiology and Biophysics, Albert Einstein College of Medicine of Yeshiva University; Attending Physician, Bronx Municipal Hospital Center and Jack D. Weiler Hospital of the Albert Einstein College of Medicine, Bronx, New York

Micheline Lévy, M.D.
Director of Research, Unité de Génètique Epidemiologique, Paris, France

Edmund J. Lewis, M.D.
Professor of Medicine, Rush Medical College of Rush University; Director of Nephrology, Presbyterian–St. Luke's Hospital, Chicago, Illinois

Kenneth V. Lieberman, M.D.
Assistant Professor of Pediatrics, Mount Sinai School of Medicine of the City University of New York; Chief of Pediatric Nephrology, The Mount Sinai Hospital, New York, New York

Michael A. Linshaw, M.D.
Professor of Pediatrics, Tufts University School of Medicine; Staff Pediatrician and Chief, Division of Pediatric Nephrology, Department of Pediatrics, Boston Floating Hospital, Boston, Massachusetts

William Scott Long, M.D.
Postdoctoral Fellow, Department of Internal Medicine, Yale University School of Medicine, New Haven, Connecticut

Mark D. Ludman, M.D.
Assistant Professor of Pediatrics and Genetics, Mount Sinai School of Medicine of the City University of New York; Attending Physician, The Mount Sinai Hospital, New York, New York

A. Madrazo, M.D.
Associate Clinical Professor of Pathology, Mount Sinai School of Medicine of the City University of New York, New York, New York; Director of Laboratory Pathology, Palisades General Hospital, North Bergen, New Jersey

Walter C. Martinez, M.D.
Chief of Neurology, St. Mary's Hospital, West Palm Beach, Florida

S. Michael Mauer, M.D.
Professor of Pediatrics, University of Minnesota Medical School; Attending Physician, Variety Club Children's Hospital, Minneapolis, Minnesota

S. Roy Meadow, M.B.
Professor and Head, Department of Pediatrics and Child Health, Leeds University; Consultant Pediatrician, St. James's University Hospital, Leeds, England

Alfred F. Michael, M.D.
Regents' Professor of Pediatrics, Laboratory Medicine, and Pathology, and Chairman, Department of Pediatrics, University of Minnesota Medical School; Chief of Pediatric Services, Variety Club Children's Hospital, Minneapolis, Minnesota

Dawn S. Milliner, M.D.
Assistant Professor of Medicine and Pediatrics, Mayo Medical School; Consultant, Division of Nephrology and Internal Medicine, and Consultant, Section of General Pediatrics and Pediatric Nephrology, Mayo Clinic and Mayo Foundation, Rochester, Minnesota

Eddie S. Moore, M.D.
Professor and Chairman of Pediatrics, University of Tennessee Medical Center at Knoxville; Attending Physician, University of Tennessee Memorial Hospital, Knoxville, Tennessee

A. Vishnu Moorthy, M.D.
Associate Professor, Departments of Medicine and Pathology, University of Wisconsin Medical School; Chief, Renal Section, William S. Middleton Veterans Administration Hospital, Madison, Wisconsin

Martin A. Nash, M.D.
Associate Professor of Clinical Pediatrics, Columbia University College of Physicians and Surgeons; Director of Nephrology, Pediatrics Department, Babies Hospital, Columbia-Presbyterian Medical Center, New York, New York

Thomas E. Nevins, M.D.
Associate Professor of Pediatrics, University of Minnesota Medical School; Attending Pediatrician, Variety Club Children's Hospital, Minneapolis, Minnesota

Antonia C. Novello, M.D., M.P.H.
Clinical Professor of Pediatrics, Georgetown University School of Medicine; Surgeon General of the United States Public Health Service, Department of Health and Human Services, Washington, D.C.

Robert F. O'Dea, M.D., Ph.D.
Associate Professor of Pediatrics and Pharmacology, University of Minnesota Medical School; Attending Physician, University of Minnesota Hospital and Clinic of the University of Minnesota Health Sciences Center, Minneapolis, Minnesota

Donald E. Oken, M.D.
Professor of Medicine, Virginia Commonwealth University Medical College of Virginia School of Medicine, Richmond, Virginia

John M. Opitz, M.D.
Chairman, Department of Medical Genetics, Shoclair Children's Hospital, Helena, Montana

Bernard Pollara, M.D., Ph.D.
Professor and Chairman, Department of Pediatrics, Albany Medical College; Pediatrician-in-Chief, Albany Medical Center Hospital

Mordechai Pras, M.D.
Professor of Medicine, Sackler School of Medicine, Tel Aviv; Director, Department of Medicine, Chaim Sheba Medical Center, Tel Hashomer, Israel

Isabelle Rapin, M.D.
Professor of Neurology and Pediatrics, Albert Einstein College of Medicine of Yeshiva University; Attending Neurologist and Child Neurologist, Einstein Affiliated Hospitals, Bronx, New York

Juhani Rapola, M.D.
Professor of Pathology, University of Helsinki; Head of the Pathology Unit, Children's Hospital, University of Helsinki, Helsinki, Finland

Jean E. Robillard, M.D.
Professor of Pediatrics, University of Iowa College of Medicine; Director, Renal Division, Department of Pediatrics, University of Iowa Hospitals and Clinics, Iowa City, Iowa

Alan M. Robson, M.D.
Professor of Pediatrics, Tulane University School of Medicine; Medical Director, Children's Hospital of New Orleans, New Orleans, Louisiana

Juan Rodriguez-Soriano, M.D.
Professor of Pediatrics, Basque University School of Medicine; Director of Pediatrics, Hospital Infantil de Cruces, Bilbao, Spain

H. Gil Rushton, M.D.
Associate Professor of Urology and Pediatrics, George Washington University School of Medicine and Health Sciences; Vice Chairman, Department of Pediatric Urology, Children's Hospital National Medical Center, Washington, D.C.

Paul Saenger, M.D.
Professor of Pediatrics, Albert Einstein College of Medicine of Yeshiva University; Attending Physician, Montefiore Medical Center, Bronx, New York

Lisa M. Satlin, M.D.
Assistant Professor of Pediatrics, Albert Einstein College of Medicine of Yeshiva University, Bronx, New York

Karl Schärer, M.D.
Professor of Pediatrics, University of Heidelberg; Head, Division of Pediatric Nephrology, University Children's Hospital, Heidelberg, Germany

George J. Schwartz, M.D.
Professor of Pediatrics, Albert Einstein College of Medicine of Yeshiva University; Attending Physician, Bronx Municipal Hospital Center, and Jack D. Weiler Hospital of Albert Einstein College of Medicine, Bronx, New York

Stanton Segal, M.D.
Professor of Pediatrics and Medicine, University of Pennsylvania School of Medicine; Director, Division of Biochemical Development and Molecular Diseases, Children's Hospital of Philadelphia, Philadelphia, Pennsylvania

Norman J. Siegel, M.D.
Professor of Pediatrics and Medicine, Yale University School of Medicine; Vice Chairman, Department of Pe-

Jean E. Robillard
Francine G. Smith
Fred G. Smith, Jr.

1

Developmental Aspects of Renal Function During Fetal Life

Knowledge of fetal renal physiology, once mainly of theoretical value, is now essential for clinical care of premature babies and the detection and management of fetal renal abnormalities. It is now generally accepted that, at least in late gestation, amniotic fluid is regulated largely through the production of urine by the fetal kidneys. Although the placenta is the major regulatory organ of the fetus, the fetal kidney also influences fetal growth, absence of fetal kidneys leading to marked intrauterine growth retardation and anomalies of bone formation [219]. The fetal kidney also produces a number of growth factors and hormones. In addition, the kidney contributes to the maintenance of fetal cardiovascular integrity, fluid and electrolyte homeostasis, and acid–base balance. This chapter summarizes our current understanding of the developmental aspects of renal function during fetal life.

Renal Development

The renal excretory system of the human passes through a series of successive and interdependent stages of morphogenic and physiologic development. This first stage is characterized by the emergence of paired tubules that arise from the cephalic end of the nephrotomes to form the pronephros, a rudimentary, nonfunctional organ that appears about the third week of gestation and undergoes complete involution within two weeks. Its only role is to give rise to the mesonephric duct. The mesonephros develops more caudally along the nephrotome and consists of approximately 20 pairs of glomeruli and thick-walled tubules. By the fifth week of gestation, the mesonephric kidneys are able to form urine [60,209]. The mesonephros degenerates by the eleventh to twelfth week of gestation as the metanephros begins to function. The most important role of the mesonephros is to induce the formation of the ureteric bud, which is required for the formation of the metanephros. In addition, it supplies tubules that become the

ducts of the epididymis, the *ductus deferens,* and the ejaculatory duct in males. In females, the entire system regresses at the beginning of the third month of gestation to become nonfunctional vestigial ducts. A failure of mesonephric differentiation may lead to renal agenesis, renal hypoplasia, or congenital cysts, as well as to the anomalous development of the gonads and adrenal glands [198]. The definitive nephrons arise from the metanephros, which is dependent for its development on the interaction between the ureteric bud and the undifferentiated mesenchymal cell mass containing the contiguous nephrogenic ridges (nephrogenic blastema).

Renal tubular function begins in the human metanephric kidney by the ninth week of gestation. By the fourteenth week of gestation, the loop of Henle is functional, and tubular reabsorption occurs. Nephron formation ceases by the thirty-sixth week of gestation, the term kidneys containing about one million nephrons.

Prior to the development of the chronic fetal sheep preparation [67,149], the study of renal function in utero was limited to the analysis of fetal amniotic fluids [85,114] and to the determination of fetal renal clearances in acute animal experiments [5,6,9,10,39,201]. The chronic fetal sheep model has permitted investigators to study the ontogeny of the fetal kidney in its normal environment and in the absence of stresses imposed by surgery and anesthesia.

Renal Blood Flow

Whereas the kidneys of the newborn receive 15% to 18% of the cardiac output, the fetal kidneys receive only 2% to 4% of the combined ventricular output during the last trimester of gestation [17,141,179,180,191]. This relatively low rate of renal blood flow (RBF) is associated with a high renal vascular resistance (RVR) and low filtration fraction (FF) when compared with newborn animals [11,171] (Fig. 1-1).

In lambs, there is no immediate increase in RBF at birth [11]. There is, however, a redistribution of intrarenal blood flow to the superficial cortex so that the ratio of inner

A portion of the work presented in this chapter has been supported by the Public Health Service Grants. HD 11466, HD 14388, HL 35600 and HD 20576, and Iowa Heart Association Grants 83-G-32 and 85-G-21.

3

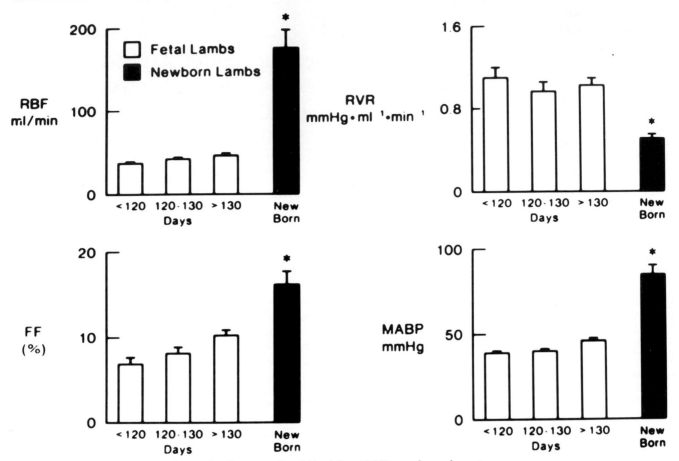

FIG. 1-1. Renal hemodynamics during development. *Renal blood flow (RBF), renal vascular resistance (RVR), filtration fraction (FF), and mean arterial blood pressure (MABP) in fetal sheep (term 145 days) and newborn lambs (5–19 days of age). Values are mean ± SEM. *P < 0.05 when fetal values are compared with newborn values. (Data adapted from Robillard JE, Weismann DN, Herin P: Ontogeny of single glomerular perfusion rate in fetal and newborn lambs. Pediatr Res 15:1248, 1981, with permission.)*

cortical to outer cortical flow is less than in the fetus [11]. In the weeks following birth, RBF increases in puppies [91], in piglets [69], and in lambs [171], the result probably of a greater decrease in RVR than that of other organs and an increase in arterial pressure (Fig. 1-1). Since the increase in arterial pressure is often of lesser magnitude than the rise in RBF, factors other than pressure alone are probably responsible for the postnatal changes in renal hemodynamics.

The intrarenal distribution of glomerular blood flow in the fetus is quantitatively different from that measured in the newborn [11,171]. Glomerular perfusion rate (GPR) is similar throughout the cortex during the last third of gestation [171], but the quotient between inner and outer cortical glomerular blood flow decreases significantly at birth [11], reflecting a shift of blood toward the superficial cortex. After birth, values of GPR continue to increase in the outer zone of the cortex, whereas no changes are observed in the inner cortex [11,171].

Factors Influencing Fetal Renal Hemodynamics

RENIN-ANGIOTENSIN SYSTEM

The vasopressor response [156] and the renal vasoconstrictor response [154] to infusion of angiotensin II (AII) are less in fetal than in adult sheep, possibly the result of a high receptor occupancy by endogenous AII [154]. Administration of AII to fetal sheep also results in an increase in arterial pressure, a decrease in umbilical flow [79,81,156], a decrease in RBF, and an increase in FF. Glomerular filtration rate (GFR) remains unchanged [156], suggesting that AII acts primarily by increasing the tone of the efferent arteriole, as shown previously in adults [100].

Controversy exists with respect to the role of the renin-angiotensin system in modulating fetal renal hemodynamics during stressful conditions, including hypoxemia and hemorrhage [23,64,65,82,129,155]. Inhibition of AII synthesis using captopril, an angiotensin-converting enzyme inhibitor, or saralasin, an AII antagonist, does not protect against the decrease in RBF and the rise in RVR associated with fetal hypoxemia [129]. On the other hand, the decrease in RBF in fetal sheep associated with removal of about 20% of fetoplacental blood volume is abolished by the administration of captopril [64,65] but not by infusion of saralasin [82]. These differences may be due to the fact that captopril, but not saralasin, inhibits the degradation of bradykinin. The subsequent rise in circulating bradykinin may blunt the effect of hemorrhage on RBF [198].

It is important to note, however, that maternally administered captopril is a fetotoxic agent in sheep and rabbits [27,28] through its prolonged depressor effects and low fetal tissue perfusion that results from a decreased uterine blood flow. It is also associated with decreased prostaglandin (PG) production, disruption of the normal preparturient increase in cortisol, and inhibition of increased oxytocin levels induced by AII [28]. In humans there are a number of documented instances of fetal and neonatal morbidity resulting from captopril treatment of pregnant women [177]. These observations suggest that the fetal renin-angiotensin system may play an important role in fetal survival and in the onset of events associated with parturition.

ARGININE VASOPRESSIN

Arginine vasopressin (AVP) increases blood pressure and decreases heart rate when infused intravenously to fetal sheep during the last trimester of gestation [3,84,172,181]. A rise in fetal plasma AVP concentration also produces a redistribution of blood flow from the gastrointestinal tract and peripheral organs to the umbilical–placental unit, myocardium, and central nervous system. RBF and RVR are not affected. Furthermore, the specific vascular AVP inhibitor [d(CH$_2$)$_5$Tyr(Me) AVP] does not alter the fetal renal hemodynamic response to hypoxemia [14]. Thus, AVP does not appear to affect fetal renal hemodynamics either at rest or during stressful conditions.

ATRIAL NATRIURETIC FACTOR

The renal hemodynamic response to systemic infusion of atrial natriuretic factor (ANF) is different when fetal, newborn, and adult sheep are compared [163]. Infusion of ANF to chronically instrumented fetal and newborn sheep produces a decrease in RBF and a rise in RVR, whereas no significant changes are observed in nonpregnant adult ewes [163]. It is possible that this decrease in RBF observed in fetal and newborn sheep may be secondary to either a decrease in cardiac output, as previously shown in adult animals; an increase in renal sympathetic tone and circulating catecholamines; and/or a direct vasoconstrictor action of ANF on fetal and neonatal renal vasculature [200]. On the contrary, intrarenal infusion of ANF to fetal and newborn sheep causes renal vasodilation [224]. Thus, the renal vasoconstriction previously observed during systemic infusion of ANF [163] is probably secondary to activation of compensatory mechanisms.

The role of ANF in influencing intrarenal blood flow

distribution during renal maturation and during the transition from fetal to newborn life remains to be investigated.

PROSTAGLANDINS

The presence of high concentrations of the prostaglandin (PG) PGE$_2$, PGF$_{2\alpha}$, and metabolites of postacyclin and thromboxane in urine of fetal sheep [116,226,227] confirms previous findings that the fetal kidney has the ability to synthesize PGs [139,140]. Terragno et al. [217] suggested that PGs produced by the fetal kidney may be involved in the regulation of renal hemodynamics and function, because, at least in the pig, fetal renal vessels have a higher capacity to produce and to release PGE$_2$ and PGI$_2$ than those of the adult.

Millard et al. [123] observed a transient reduction in fetal RBF following administration of the PG inhibitor meclofenamate or indomethacin to chronically catheterized fetal sheep. Matson et al. [116] demonstrated that this reduction in fetal RBF following inhibition of PG synthesis was larger in the inner than in the outer renal cortex. Because this reduction in RBF was associated with a significant increase in FF in the absence of any appreciable change in GFR, the authors suggested that PGs produced by the fetal kidney affected mainly efferent arteriolar tone.

Renal PGs also blunt the renal vasoconstriction associated with chronic fetal hypoxemia [161], whereas inhibitors of PG synthesis block the renal vasodilation seen during the acute phase of fetal hypoxemia [123].

KALLIKREIN-KININ

Urinary kallikrein excretion rate, expressed in absolute values or corrected for kidney weight or GFR, increases significantly during fetal life and after birth. This increase in urinary kallikrein excretion rate correlates closely with the increase in RBF. Inhibition of kininase II is also associated with a decrease in RVR in near-term fetal sheep, whereas administration of [sar^1],[gly^8]-AII, a competitive antagonist of AII, does not alter RVR [170].

SYMPATHETIC NERVOUS SYSTEM

Studies in puppies [119] and rats [68] have revealed that, at birth, adrenergic fibers enter the kidney with the renal artery and follow the arterial supply into the inner cortex. The outer cortex, which in these animal species undergoes nephrogenesis up to two weeks postnatally, contains only single adrenergic fibers. Unlike the cortex, the outer medulla does not contain nerve fibers at birth, although the *vasa recta* are present. Nerve fibers begin to join the *vasa recta* by about 3 weeks of age.

The fetal convoluted tubules of 13- to 16-week-old human fetuses contain nerve endings [237]. Furthermore, the renal circulation of 113 to 120 day old fetal sheep (term 145 days) responds to exogenous norepinephrine [131] but not to tyramine [238], suggesting that adrenergic innervation of the kidney is not complete at this stage.

Denervation of the ovine fetal kidney has no effect on resting RBF [161] but partially inhibits the renal vasoconstriction associated with fetal hypoxemia [161]. Direct stimulation of renal sympathetic nerves produces a decrease in RBF and an increase in RVR in fetal sheep and newborn lambs, but the changes are less pronounced in the fetus [164]. Similarly, Buckley et al. [31] demonstrated that the renal vasculature of newborn piglets was less responsive to renal nerve stimulation than that of mature swine. Contrary to previous findings in adult animals [44], renal nerve stimulation is associated with renal vasodilation in fetal sheep during α-adrenoceptor blockade [164]. This renal vasodilation, limited to the developmental period, is independent of cholinergic or dopaminergic receptors but is completely inhibited by propranolol, a nonselective β-adrenoceptor blocker, and with ICI [118,551], a selective β_2-adrenoceptor antagonist [164]. Thus, neuronally released norepinephrine probably activates β_2-adrenoceptors to produce renal vasodilation of the fetal renal vasculature. Similar results have been observed during intrarenal infusion of norepinephrine in the presence of α-adrenoceptor blockade [131].

One can speculate that maturation of the renal adrenergic system may be associated with down-regulation of β-adrenoceptors in renal vessels [160], as has been described for other vascular beds.

Autoregulation of Renal Blood Flow During Fetal Life

The mature kidney is capable of maintaining the rate of RBF relatively constant when major changes in perfusion pressure occur, a phenomenon known as autoregulation [178]. Limited data are available on the renal autoregulatory phenomenon of the fetus. During infusion of AVP [172] or AII [156] to chronically catheterized fetal sheep, there is no change in RBF, despite a moderate increase in arterial blood pressure. These data suggest that the fetus may autoregulate RBF during modest increases in renal perfusion pressure [198].

Glomerular Filtration

Glomerular filtration rate (GFR) is low during fetal life and increases in relation to gestational age [67,107, 111,121,157,167,171]. In fetal sheep, GFR increases 2.5 times during the last trimester of gestation (from 1.24 ml/min at 100 days to 3.25 ml/min at term) and correlates closely with both fetal age and fetal body weight (Table 1-1, Fig. 1-2). When expressed as a function of fetal body weight, however, there is no significant change in GFR during the latter period of gestation [111,157].

During the first 24 hours after birth, GFR measured in preterm infants reflects the stage of intrauterine development. GFR also correlates closely with gestational age in newborn infants delivered between 27 and 43 weeks' gestation [70,95]. Interestingly, GFR per kilogram of body weight of premature infants (1.07 ± 0.12 ml/min/kg) measured during the first 24 hours after birth is similar to that of near-term fetal sheep (1.14 ± 0.08 ml/min/kg). Beyond 24 hours of life, the increase in GFR exceeds the increase in body weight in both premature and full term infants [95].

The maturation of GFR during fetal life is probably the result of a combination of events affecting both the factors that promote and those that oppose filtration: (1) active nephrogenesis; (2) changes in RVR; (3) increasing function of the superficial nephrons; and (4) modification of forces involved in the process of ultrafiltration [198]. The observation that the increase in GFR during fetal life correlates with the increase in kidney weight, however, makes it reasonable to assume that the main factor influencing

TABLE 1-1. *Renal function and hemodynamics in fetal and newborn sheep*

	Fetus		Newborn	
	<120 days	>130 days	24 h	3–21 days
MABP (mm Hg)	39 ±	55 ± 1	56 ± 2	85 ± 6
RBF (ml/min)	37 ± 2	46 ± 4	—	176 ± 26
RVR (mm Hg·ml^{-1}·min^{-1})	1.1 ± 0.1	1.0 ± 0.1	—	0.5 ± 0.1
GFR (ml/min)	1.8 ± 0.1	3.1 ± 0.2	10.1 ± 1.2	21.9 ± 4.5
FF (%)	6.9 ± 0.9	10.2 ± 0.7	—	16.1 ± 1.7
$U_{Na}V$ (μeq/min)	30 ± 8	36 ± 7	13 ± 4	5 ± 1
FE_{Na} (%)	8 ± 2	8 ± 1	1.1 ± 0.3	0.6 ± 0.1
U_KV (μeq/min)	2.2 ± 0.9	11 ± 3	15 ± 3	11 ± 2
FE_K (%)	19 ± 5	90 ± 26	40 ± 8	42 ± 5
U_{Osm} (mOsm/kg H_2O)	111 ± 10	194 ± 38	150 ± 20	524 ± 46
C_{H_2O} (ml/min)	0.4 ± 0.1	0.3 ± 0.1	0.3 ± 0.1	−0.1 ± 0.1

Values are mean ± SEM. MABP, mean arterial blood pressure; RBF, renal blood flow; RVR, renal vascular resistance; GFR, glomerular filtration rate; FF, filtration fraction; $U_{Na}V$ and U_KV, urinary excretion of sodium (Na) and potassium (K), respectively; FE_{Na} and FE_K, fractional excretion of Na and K, respectively; U_{Osm}, urine osmolality; C_{H_2O}, free water clearance. (*From* Nakamura KT, Matherne GP, McWeeny OJ, et al: Renal hemodynamics and functional changes during the transition from fetal to newborn life in sheep. *Pediatr Res* 21:229, 1987; Robillard JE, Weismann DN, Herin P: Ontogeny of single glomerular perfusion rate in fetal and newborn lambs. *Pediatr Res* 15:1248, 1981; Smith FG: *Factors Influencing Fetal and Neonatal Fluid Balance*. Sydney, Australia, University of New South Wales, 1987.)

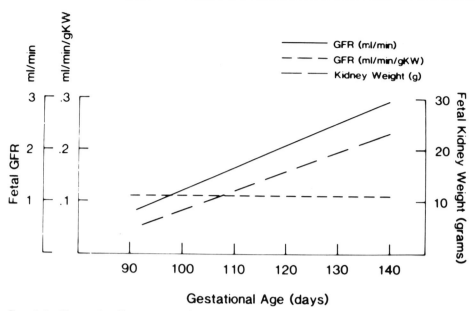

FIG. 1-2. Glomerular filtration rate during development. *Glomerular filtration rate (GFR) is expressed in milliliters per minute (___) and per gram of kidney weight (KW) (- - -). KW is expressed in grams (—). (From Robillard JE, Kulvinskas C, Sessions C, et al: Maturational changes in the fetal glomerular filtration. rate. Am J Obstet Gynecol 122:601, 1975, with permission.)*

GFR prior to birth is the addition of new nephron units [157].

GFR increases in the weeks following birth in guinea pigs [121,122], puppies [92], and lambs [171]. This rise in GFR in lambs ocurs within the first few hours of postnatal life [132,195] (Fig. 1-3) and continues during the first week of postnatal life [132,197]. Such a rapid increase in GFR indicates the occurrence of a functional rather than a morphologic change [132,195] and is consistent with increased glomerular perfusion resulting from recruitment of superficial cortical nephrons [11,171].

Tubular Handling of Sodium and Glomerulotubular Balance

In the adult, more than 99% of the filtered sodium load is reabsorbed by the renal tubules. During fetal life, sodium reabsorption is comparatively low, so a greater proportion of sodium is excreted, than later in life [73,107,162, 165,167] (Table 1-1). In the ovine fetus, sodium reabsorption is between 85% and 95% and increases with gestational age [107,165]. Fractional excretion of sodium (FE_{Na}) decreases from 11% at 130 days of gestation to 5% near term [167]. A similar pattern has been observed in other animal species [121,122], including the human [12,49]. In infants of less than 30 weeks of gestation, FE_{Na} may exceed 5% during the first 3 days of life, whereas it is only about 0.2% in term newborns [49].

The relatively large extracellular fluid volume of the fetus may influence renal reabsorption of sodium. In fetal sheep,

contraction of extracellular fluid space by peritoneal dialysis results in a decrease in FE_{Na} from 10% to 6% [166]. The fetal kidney does, however, respond appropriately to volume expansion [24,78,183,199], an infusion of isotonic saline [78] or dextran [199] producing a natriuretic response.

Based on morphologic evidence [53], it has been postulated that a functional glomerulotubular imbalance may be partly responsible for the high FE_{Na} seen prior to birth. Merlet-Benichou et al. [122] noted that in fetal guinea pigs there is a phase of functional glomerular preponderance associated with an augmentation in the number of glomeruli during the early stages of superficial nephron maturation. This phase is followed by a tubular "catch-up" phase associated with a large increase in proximal tubular length. On the other hand, functional glomerulotubular balance of superficial nephrons was observed in the canine puppy [207] as early as collections of tubular fluid by micropuncture techniques were possible, even though nephrogenesis continues after birth in this species. Furthermore, in the guinea pig (an animal born like the human with a full complement of nephrons), functional glomerulotubular balance was documented immediately after birth [208].

There is also a direct correlation between GFR and proximal sodium reabsorption in fetal sheep [108], demonstrating again the existence of glomerulotubular balance. At birth, there is a transient disruption in this glomerulotubular balance: A natriuresis occurs within 2 hours of delivery of the lamb by caesarean section despite an increase in GFR (Fig. 1-4) [194,195]. By 24 hours after delivery, FE_{Na} increases to adult levels [132,194,197], re-

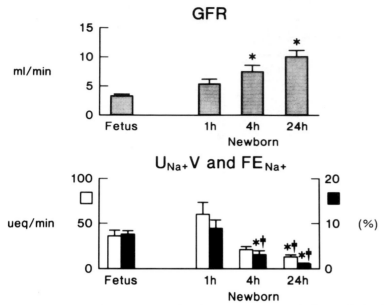

FIG. 1-3. Glomerular filtration and sodium excretion rates before and after birth. *Glomerular filtration rate (GFR), sodium excretion ($U_{Na}V$), and fractional excretion of sodium ($FE_{Na}+$) before and after delivery of the lamb by cesarean section. Values are mean $\pm$ SEM. *P < 0.05 fetal values compared with newborn values. †P < 0.05 newborn values at 1 hour compared with values at 4 and 24 hours. (From Nakamura KT, Mathern GP, McWeeny OJ, et al: Renal hemodynamics and functional changes during the transition from fetal to newborn life in sheep. Pediatr Res 21:229, 1987, with permission.)*

flecting a rapid adaptation by the term kidney to extrauterine life.

It is possible that these rapid changes associated with birth at term cannot occur before term because of renal tubular immaturity, which may also explain the inappropriate excretion of salt by the premature infant [198].

Factors Influencing Tubular Handling of Sodium

The adrenal gland of the fetus has the ability to synthesize and secrete aldosterone *in vitro* following stimulation by AII, adrenocorticotrophin (ACTH), or high serum potassium concentration [233,234]. Elevation of plasma AII also stimulates aldosterone secretion in fetal sheep during the last trimester of gestation, although to a lesser degree than in the adult ewe [155,156,190]. In vivo attempts to stimulate aldosterone secretion by infusing ACTH [4,29] or potassium [233,234] have remained unsuccessful. The high rate of FE_{Na} during fetal life may therefore reflect a relative tubular insensitivity to circulating aldosterone [91,198, 207].

An additional factor may be the differences in the distribution of sodium reabsorption between proximal and distal portions of the nephron in the immature as opposed to the mature kidney. Recent studies have shown that in fetal sheep, a greater fraction of the filtered sodium load is reabsorbed in distal portions of the nephron compared with the adult kidney (see Fig. 1-4) [108]. Furthermore, distal reabsorption constitutes a greater percentage of total sodium reabsorption in younger than in older fetuses [108].

Another explanation for the greater FE_{Na} observed during fetal life is the elevated PGs seen during this time, because some PGs (PGE_2 and PGI_2) have potent natriuretic properties [46]. This is probably not the case, however, since inhibition of PG synthesis in the fetus produces an increase in electrolyte excretion despite a decrease in RBF [116].

Finally, a limited delivery of oxygen to the fetal kidney and, hence, a lower renal oxygen consumption, may also contribute to the greater FE_{Na} of the fetus. In support of this hypothesis is the observation that sodium excretion increases during fetal hypoxemia [173] but not during fetal hemorrhage [64].

Other factors contributing to the elevated FE_{Na} during fetal life include the natriuretic influence of cortisol and ANF. Systemic infusion of ANF to fetal sheep increases the excretion of potassium, chloride, and calcium, as well as free water clearance [163,200], and enhances sodium excretion [163,188] by depressing proximal sodium reabsorption [188]. Cortisol, when infused to near-term fetal sheep [74], also causes proximal sodium reabsorption to be depressed and distal reabsorption to be enhanced, so that, overall, there is no change in total fractional sodium reabsorption. On the other hand, Wintour et al. [235] showed that a natriuresis did occur following infusion of cortisol to younger fetal sheep (aged 111 to 120 days). Interestingly,

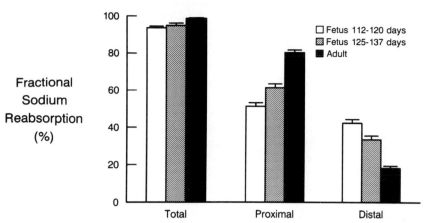

FIG. 1-4. Fractional sodium reabsorption during development. *Fractional sodium reabsorption in nonpregnant ewes and in two groups of fetal sheep. The percentage of total sodium reabsorbed proximally, measured using the clearance of lithium, increases with age. Values are mean ± SEM. (Data adapted from Lumbers ER, Hill KJ, Bennett VJ: Proximal and distal tubular activity in chronically catheterized fetal sheep compared with the adult. Can J Physiol Pharmacol 66:697, 1988, with permission.)*

glucocorticoid hormones appear to be an endogenous driving force for the maturation of the sodium pump near term [45].

Potassium Excretion

Based on the results of acute studies, Alexander et al. [9] reported that the fractional excretion of potassium (FE_K) of the ovine fetus was about 20% by 61 days of gestation and remained unchanged until term. However, in chronically catheterized fetal sheep [165], an increase in FE_K occurs as the fetus matures (Table 1-1). Moreover, net secretion of potassium is low in early gestation and increases towards term [108]. A few of the factors that could explain the rise in the rate of potassium secretion as the fetus approaches term include an increase in flow through the distal nephron, larger tubular surface area available for potassium secretion relative to body size, an increase in Na-K-adenosinetriphosphatase (ATPase) activity [59], and an increase in the sensitivity of the fetal nephron to aldosterone [165].

Tubular Transport of Calcium, Phosphate, and Magnesium

CALCIUM

In humans, sheep, and guinea pigs, the concentrations of total, ultrafilterable, and ionized calcium are higher in fetal than in maternal plasma [43,187,231]. These levels appear to be generated and maintained by the placenta, which transports calcium actively from the mother to the fetus [148,223,228]. Calcium-binding protein has been isolated from the placenta of the rat [30,115] and a calcium-stimulated ATPase has been found in the placenta of the guinea

pig [186]. In fetal sheep, there is an increase in plasma parathyroid hormone levels after intravenous infusion of EDTA [58,202], indicating that the fetal parathyroid glands can respond to a hypocalcemic stimulus. The fetal kidney contributes to the transplacental transfer of calcium by the synthesis of 1,25-dihydroxycholecalciferol [126]. Fetal nephrectomy abolishes the transplacental calcium gradient, which can be restored by intravenous injection of parathyroid hormone [33]. However, the excretion of AMP in response to parathyroid hormone and calcitonin is attenuated in fetal rats [218] and newborn infants [103], suggesting that the decreased sensitivity of the kidney to parathyroid hormone may contribute to the hypocalcemia of the neonate.

PHOSPHATE

Like calcium, the concentration of inorganic phosphate (P_i) in fetal plasma is greater than that in maternal plasma [15], indicating active transport across the placenta [47]. On the other hand, P_i is low in fetal urine [118], suggesting that the fetal kidney has the ability to reabsorb larger amounts of phosphate. Hill and Lumbers [73] reported that fractional phosphate reabsorption varied between 60% and 100%. The fetal kidney also responds to parathyroid extract with an increase in urinary excretion of phosphate and a rise in urinary excretion of AMP [8,205]. A similar response also occurs after an endogenous rise in plasma parathyroid hormone levels induced by EDTA [125,202]. In addition, acute expansion of the extracellular volume of fetal sheep produces a significant increase in urinary phosphate excretion, independent of plasma calcium concentration and parathyroid hormone but related to renal sodium excretion [125]. Phosphate excretion also increases during metabolic acidosis [90] and following the administration of cortisol to the fetus [74]. Because phosphate is the major urinary buffer and is responsible for the excretion of titratable acid, an increased phosphate excretion enables the fetal kidney to excrete protons and generate new bicarbonate. These results indicate that, at least in some animal species, the fetal kidney responds appropriately to stimuli known to affect P_i reabsorption. The mechanism that accounts for the high rate of tubular reabsorption of P_i by the fetus remains unexplained.

MAGNESIUM

Magnesium transfer across the placenta is thought to be active [1,34] and similar to that of calcium, the human fetus receiving 3 to 4 mg/kg body weight of magnesium daily from the mother [113]. Severe maternal deprivation of magnesium results in a reduction in total body magnesium of the fetus [41]. Regulation of magnesium balance by the fetal kidney has not been investigated. It is known, however, that the urinary excretion of magnesium is low immediately after birth [98].

Tubular Reabsorption of Glucose

The fetal kidney of several animal species has the ability to reabsorb glucose, a process that is inhibited by phlorhizin [7,97,185]. Alexander and Nixon [7] suggested that before the midpoint of gestation, the ovine fetal kidney has the capacity to reabsorb most of the filtered glucose, confirming a previous study on the mesonephros of fetal pigs [142]. The reabsorptive capacity for glucose is high during fetal life [7], the tubular maxima being greater per unit GFR in fetal than in adult sheep [168]. The renal threshold for glucose increases with fetal body weight during the last trimester of gestation, fetal and adult blood glucose values at threshold being 200 ± 13 mg/dl and 177 ± 3.8 mg/dl, respectively [168].

Lelievre-Pegorier and Geloso [97] have demonstrated that the transport of the non-metabolizable sugar α-methyl-D-glucopyranoside by kidney slices of near-term rat fetuses occurs mainly through a sodium-dependent, low-affinity, high-capacity transport system that is inhibited by phlorhizin. This transport system is also present in the kidney of adult animals. In addition, these investigators reported the existence of a high-affinity, low-capacity system that is specific to fetal and newborn rats. They speculated that the presence of this high-affinity system may explain the ability of immature newborn kidneys to reabsorb the entire load of filtered glucose, resulting in the absence of glucose from the urine. Smith and Lumbers [196] investigated the fetal renal response to maternal and subsequently fetal hyperglycemia in sheep. Glycosuria occurred in all fetuses and was associated with a diuresis and natriuresis. An increase in the fraction of the glomerular ultrafiltrate excreted indicated that the diuresis was the direct result of nonreabsorbed glucose acting as an osmotic diuretic. Thus, glucose causes an osmotic diuresis in the fetal kidney as it does in the adult when the tubular maxima is exceeded.

Beck et al. [16] provided further evidence that the fetal transport system for glucose is qualitatively similar to that of the adult by demonstrating the development of a sodium-dependent glucose transport system in proximal tubular cells of the near-term fetal rabbit. Like that of the adult, this transport system was shown to be stereospecific, electrogenic, cation-specific, and pH-sensitive [16].

Organic Acids and Bases

Plasma clearance of the organic acid para-aminohippurate is low in the fetus and in the neonate [6,32], suggesting that, during development, tubular secretory pathways are immature. This finding may also reflect the fact that the juxtamedullary circulation shunts blood through the *vasa recta*, decreasing the peritubular circulation perfusing the secretory cells. On the other hand, evidence suggests that the fetal kidney can secrete organic bases, although at very much lower levels than seen in the adult [48].

Acid–Base Homeostasis

The regulation of acid–base homeostasis by the kidney involves the reabsorption of filtered bicarbonate and the excretion of hydrogen ions as titratable acid and ammonium. During fetal life the placenta plays a major role in modulating the fetal response to acidosis. The fetal kidney is, however, also involved in the regulation of acid–base balance.

Urinary pH is always less than plasma pH [89,166]. There is an age-dependent increase in the excretion rates of titratable acid and ammonium [73] and hence, net acid excretion. Thus, there is an increasing contribution by the fetal kidney to the regulation of acid–base homeostasis. Fetal sheep reabsorb between 80% and 100% of the filtered bicarbonate load [73,89,166], the renal threshold for bicarbonate being lower in fetal than in adult sheep (17.7 ± 1.4 mmol/L in fetuses; 28.7 ± 1.7 in nonpregnant adult ewes) [166]. This may result from the relatively large extracellular fluid volume normally found in the fetus, because bicarbonate reabsorption increases during fetal volume depletion [166]. These data suggest that the low threshold for bicarbonate is not solely due to a limited reabsorptive capacity.

In the ovine fetus, bicarbonate and subsequently chloride reabsorption increases with gestational age [73,89]. This probably reflects an increase in carbonic anhydrase activity, because inhibition of carbonic anhydrase with acetazolamide produces a significant increase in bicarbonate excretion and in urinary pH [169]. Carbonic anhydrase is also known to be present in the human fetal kidney in late gestation [105].

The renal response to metabolic acidosis is limited in the fetus compared with the adult [204], primarily because of a low-rate excretion of phosphate, but also because of a limited capacity to synthesize ammonia [89]. Prolonged and severe metabolic acidosis results in an increase in hydrogen ion excretion [90], indicating that the distal segments of the fetal renal tubule are able to generate a pH gradient. However, metabolic acidosis induced by fetal hyperglycemia [196] causes no change in urinary pH or in the excretion rates of the urinary buffers. Thus, under a moderate acidosis, the placental regulation of fetal acid–base balance is probably sufficient so that no increase in the buffering capacity of the fetal kidney is necessary [198].

Concentrating Capacity of the Fetal Kidney

Urine produced by the mammalian fetal kidney is hypotonic with respect to fetal plasma [5,10,22,32, 118,121,159]. Urinary osmolality in fetal sheep increases after 130 days of gestation [159], the result probably of an increase in free water reabsorption rather than in the amount of solute excreted in the urine, because free water clearance decreases (Table 1-1).

The fetal kidney is able to produce either a concentrated or dilute urine depending upon the state of maternal and hence fetal hydration. Infusion of hypertonic mannitol to the ewe [112,210] or maternal water deprivation [18,175,211] leads to a decrease in fetal urinary flow rate and free water clearance. A similar decrease in fetal free water clearance is seen after intravenous infusion of AVP to fetal sheep [104,172,236] or during fetal hypoxemia [42,173] or hemorrhage [64,181]. There is also a direct correlation between fetal free water clearance and net fluid transfer across the placenta [110,194]. Thus, a decrease in net transplacental fluid transfer to the fetus results in a decreased fetal urine production. Hence, the observation has been made that an increased urinary osmolality and decreased urine flow in utero is a reflection of fetal stress [232]. This is supported by the finding that maternal water restriction over 10 days can result in anuria and fetal death [210].

The ability of the kidney to concentrate the urine to adult levels is not reached until after birth [153,207]. The structural immaturity of the medulla, characterized by short loops of Henle [206], and the relatively high blood flow through the vasa recta [13,137,171] may limit the build-up of an osmotic gradient by the fetal kidney.

ARGININE VASOPRESSIN

AVP is present in the posterior pituitary of fetal animals [57,184,225] and as early as the 11th week of gestation in humans [101]. The AVP content of the fetal pituitary and hypothalamus increases with fetal age [193]. Furthermore, both volume and osmoreceptor controls of AVP secretion are functional during the last trimester of gestation, at least in the ovine fetus [96,174,230]. Nevertheless, the increase in urinary osmolality that follows infusion of AVP is three times lower in the fetus than in the adult animal at the same plasma concentration of AVP, suggesting an end-organ hyporesponsiveness to AVP during fetal life [172]. This may be accounted for by the relative inability of the renal cells to generate AMP in response to stimulation by AVP [86,147]. In addition, PGE_2 found in high concentration in the urine of fetal sheep [226,227] may blunt the action of AVP on the collecting duct.

The neuropeptide arginine vasotocin (AVT) is also present in fetal plasma, urine, and amniotic fluid [50]. The physiological significance of circulating AVT has not been defined, although it has been shown that infusion of AVT

to fetal sheep increases urinary osmolality from 160 ± 30 to 292 ± 19 mOsm/kg H_2O [51].

Hormones of Renal Origin

In addition to its excretory function, the fetal kidney is able to synthesize various hormones. Components of the renin-angiotensin, prostaglandin, and kallikrein-kinin systems, as well as the enzymatic machinery necessary for vitamin D metabolism, have been identified in the fetal kidney of mammals.

THE RENIN-ANGIOTENSIN SYSTEM

Kaplan and Friedman [87] first described renin activity in the fetal hog kidney. Since than, renin-like granules have been identified in the juxtaglomerular apparatuses of fetal kidneys of humans [20,124,143] and animals [203,213, 222]. Plasma renin activity (PRA) is high during fetal life [25,26,77,220], the levels being substantially above those present in the maternal circulation [37,128]. Removal [26] or absence [214] of fetal kidneys is associated with low PRA, indicating that the major source of fetal renin is the fetal kidney. In contrast, the major sources of aminotic fluid renin [192,215,216], which is mainly in an inactive form [106,146], are the trophoblastic cells of chorionic laeve [144,145].

Fetal PRA and plasma AII levels increase after stimulation by furosemide [54,189,220], blood volume reduction [174], fetal hypotension [109,150], and hypoxemia [173]. Conversely, expansion of fetal blood volume [127], inhibition of PG synthesis by indomethacin [116], AVP infusion [172], and hypertension [109] are associated with significant decreases in fetal PRA.

Intravenous infusion of the β-adrenoceptor agonist, isoproterenol, also promotes renin release [152] in near-term fetal sheep, suggesting that, as in the adult, β-adrenoceptors are involved in promoting the secretion of renin.

Recently, Nakamura et al. [130,133] have measured the secretion rate of active and inactive renin from renal cortical slices during development in sheep. From 110 days of gestation, the kidney can secrete renin in both active and inactive forms [130], following β-adrenoceptor stimulation. Rawashdeh et al. [151] recently confirmed these findings in near-term fetal sheep and also demonstrated that renin secretion cannot be promoted from renal cortical slides of very young fetuses (90–110 days). Incubation of renal cortical slices with veratridine, a substance known to promote neuronal release of norepinephrine, promotes release of active renin in fetal and newborn animals [133] as in the adult. This veratridine-stimulated release of renin was also found to be dependent upon activation of β-adrenoceptors [133]. Interestingly, the newborn has the greatest absolute response to β-adrenoceptor stimulation, secreting more active renin per milligram of renal cortex than that by fetal or adult sheep [130]. This may be explained by the fact that in the newborn there are more renin-secreting cells and that these cells may be more responsive to norepinephrine release. In favor of this hypothesis, Gomez et al. [61], using immunocytochemistry in WKY fetal, newborn, and adult rats, observed renin in arcuate and interlobular arteries early during fetal life, with the localization shifting to a classical juxtaglomerular localization in the adult rat, suggesting that the renin gene is subject to developmental regulation. They later confirmed these results by measuring renin mRNA distribution using Northern and dot blot techniques [62] and in situ hybridization [63].

Hence, these data suggest that the higher activity of the renin-angiotensin system during fetal and early postnatal life is the result of an increased renal renin gene expression, along with a more remote arteriolar localization. These findings suggest that the renin-angiotensin system may play an important regulatory role early during development.

PROSTAGLANDINS

Synthesis and catabolism of PGs occur early during gestation in fetal animals [138–140] and humans [55]. In the ovine fetus, PGF is present in renal homogenates by 40 days of gestation; PGE$_2$ is first formed by 77 days of gestation and is predominant by 116 days of gestation [140]. PG catabolism via the PG 15-hydroxydehydrogenase pathway is present at 40 days of gestation [140], while catabolism through the PG 13-reductase pathway occurs by about 116 days of gestation, persisting until term [140]. Terragno et al. [217] found that renal cortical slices from fetal pig kidneys can convert arachidonic acid to PGs and that the fetal renal cortex possesses higher biosynthetic activity than that of the adult. They also found that an inhibitor of PG synthesis, which is released by cortical slices of adult kidneys, is apparently absent in fetal kidneys [217].

Inhibition of PG synthesis by indomethacin [116,123] produces a decrease in fetal RBF. Unlike the adult, indomethacin administration also results in a natriuresis and chloruresis with no change in potassium excretion [116]. Indomethacin administration also decreases PRA in the fetus [116], indicating that, as in adults [56,94], PGs stimulate renin secretion.

In view of the fact that PGs are involved in the process of parturition [136], one may speculate that the fetal kidney plays a role in this process. In support of this hypothesis, a substance has been found in the urine of human fetuses that stimulates PG biosynthesis by the fetal membranes [38,212].

THE KALLIKREIN-KININ SYSTEM

Kallikreins are serine proteases that generate kinins from kininogen substrates by limited proteolysis [35,36,102, 117,134]. Factors regulating the activity of the kallikrein-kinin system during development are not understood. It has been suggested, however, that during the latter part of gestation in the ovine fetus, urinary kallikrein excretion is dependent on both age and plasma aldosterone concentration [158]. There is also an inverse relationship between urinary kallikrein excretion and sodium excretion. Furthermore, a rapid rise in fetal arterial PO$_2$, produced by hyperbaric oxygenation of the ewe, activates the bradykinin-generating system and produces both a fall in plasma kininogen concentration and a rise in the fetal plasma concentration of bradykinin [72]. In human newborn infants, Melmon et al. [120] found that an increase in arterial PO$_2$ and a decrease in ambient temperature resulted in activation of plasma or tissue kallikrein and, hence, kinin generation. Finally, a recent study by Betkerur et al. [19] revealed that urinary kallikrein excretion decreased by 50% after inhibition of PG synthetase by indomethacin in premature infants with patent ductus arteriosus. This suggests that PGs modulate renal kallikrein release soon after birth. Kinins may also mediate circulatory changes during the transition from fetal to newborn life [120].

VITAMIN D METABOLISM

Vitamin D, 25-hydroxyvitamin D [25(OH)D], and 24,25-dihydroxyvitamin D$_3$[24,25(OH)$_2$D] are transferred across the placenta of the rat from mother to fetus [71,75,76,135]. There appears to be little maternal fetal crossover of 1,25-dihydroxyvitamin D[1,25(OH)$_2$D] or 25(OH)D in the rat [135], but in the monkey [182] and the sheep [176] placental transfer does occur.

The fetus also participates in the synthesis of 1,25(OH)$_2$D [21,52,176,229], fetal plasma levels of 1,25(OH)$_2$D being greater than in adult sheep [221]. In human fetuses, 1,25(OH)$_2$D levels are also greater in arterial than in umbilical venous blood [231]. In fetal sheep the renal conversion of ^{3}H-25(OH)D to ^{3}H-1,25(OH)D was reported to be about 20%, whereas the conversion rate to ^{3}H-24,25(OH)$_2$D was only 4% [221]. Kidney homogenates from fetal rats, guinea pigs, chicks, and rabbits are also capable of hydroxylating 25(OH)D to 1,25(OH)$_2$D [21,229].

Akiba et al. [2] have found significant production of 1,25(OH)$_2$D in proximal convoluted tubules and pars recta of the rabbit kidney, whereas very little 1,25(OH)$_2$D was produced in the remaining parts of the nephron. In young rats, 1-α-hydroxylase activity was localized exclusively to the proximal tubules [88].

It is important to stress that the finding of 1,25(OH)$_2$D production by the fetal kidney in vitro does not prove that this situation pertains in vivo. Kooh and Vieth [93], using radiolabeled ^{3}H-25(OH)D, failed to find evidence for the hydroxylation of 25(OH)D to 1,25(OH)$_2$D in fetal sheep after infusion of parathyroid hormone. Moreover, the predominant metabolite present in fetal rat plasma after maternal administration of ^{3}H-vitamin D is ^{3}H-24-25(OH)$_2$D rather than ^{3}H-1-25(OH)$_2$D [229]. On the other hand, the fact that 1,25^{3}H-24-25(OH)$_2$D concentration in the fetal plasma falls markedly following fetal bilateral nephrectomy [66,99] suggests that the fetal kidney is able to synthesize 1,25(OH)$_2$D.

Energy Metabolism

Most of the energy produced by the kidney through aerobic oxidative metabolism supports energy-dependent tubular transport, substrate interconversion, intrarenal synthesis of hormones, and catabolism of low molecular weight proteins. In the adult, renal O$_2$ consumption accounts for about 7% of total-body O$_2$ uptake, whereas kidney mass is only 0.5% of total body weight [40]. During fetal life, renal

O_2 consumption is about half (1.23 ± 0.16 mol/g/min) that of the adult and accounts for 3% to 4% of total O_2 uptake [80].

Iwamoto et al. [80] observed that half of the O_2 consumption rate of the fetal kidney can be accounted for by the oxidation of lactate to carbon dioxide and water. Other possible substrates include amino acids, glycerol, pyruvate, and ketone bodies. During fetal hypoxemia, renal O_2 consumption is maintained within the normal range because of an increase in renal O_2 extraction from 25 to 45% [83]. In addition, fetal hypoxemia alters renal metabolism from net lactate uptake to net lactate release and from net glucose release to net glucose uptake [83]. After birth, renal O_2 consumption increases rapidly, becoming six times higher than that of the fetus [80] and twice as high as that found in the adult [40]. This increase probably reflects the increased tubular reabsorptive capacity after birth [198].

In summary, the fetal kidney plays an active role in the genesis of a number of hormones important for growth and for influencing cardiovascular and electrolyte homeostasis. As in the adult, the fetal kidney is responsive to a number of natriuretic stimuli and responds appropriately to pertubations in blood volume and to in utero stress. Despite the fact that much of our knowledge of fetal renal physiology has been gained through animal studies over the last 20 years, we are only just beginning to understand the mechanisms controlling renal function and renal hemodynamics prior to birth.

References

1. Aikawa JK, Bruns PD: Placental transfer and fetal tissue uptake of Mg28 in the rabbit. *Proc Soc Exp Biol Med* 105:95, 1960.
2. Akiba T, Endou H, Koseki C, et al: Localization of 25-hydroxyvitamin D3-1 alpha-hydroxylase activity in the mammalian kidney. *Biochem Biophys Res Commun* 94:313, 1980.
3. Alexander DP, Bashore RA, Britton HG, et al: Antidiuretic hormones and oxytocin release and antidiuretic hormone turnover in the fetus, lamb and ewe. *Biol Neonate* 30:80, 1976.
4. Alexander DP, Britton HG, James VHT, et al: Steroid secretion by the adrenal gland of foetal and neonatal sheep. *J Endocrinol* 40:1, 1968.
5. Alexander DP, Nixon DA: The foetal kidney. *Br Med Bull* 17:112, 1961.
6. Alexander DP, Nixon DA: Plasma clearance of p-amino-hippuric acid by the kidneys of foetal, neonatal and adult sheep. *Nature* 194:483, 1962.
7. Alexander DP, Nixon DA: Reabsorption of glucose, fructose and meso-inositol by the foetal and post-natal sheep kidney. *J Physiol* 167:480, 1963.
8. Alexander DP, Nixon DA: Effect of parathyroid extract in foetal sheep. *Biol Neonate* 14:117, 1969.
9. Alexander DP, Nixon DA, Widdas WF, et al: Renal function in the sheep foetus. *J Physiol* 140:14, 1958.
10. Alexander DP, Nixon DA, Widdas WF, et al: Gestational variations in the composition of foetal fluids and foetal urine in sheep. *J Physiol* 140:1, 1958.
11. Aperia A, Broberger O, Herin P, et al: Renal hemodynamics in the perinatal period: A study in lambs. *Acta Physiol Scand* 99:261, 1977.
12. Arant BS Jr: Developmental patterns of renal functional maturation compared in the human neonate. *J Physiol* 92:705, 1978.
13. Aschinberg LC, Goldsmith DI, Olbing H, et al: Neonatal changes in renal blood flow distribution in puppies. *Am J Physiol* 228:1453, 1975.
14. Ayres NA, McWeeny OJ, Robillard JE: The role of arginine vasopressin in modulating the cardiovascular response in hypoxemic fetal lambs (abstr). *Pediatr Res* 18:134A, 1984.
15. Barlet JP, Davicco MJ, Lefaivre J, et al: Endocrine regulation of plasma phosphate in sheep fetuses with catheters implanted in utero. In Massry SG (ed): *Homeostasis of Phosphate and Other Minerals*. New York, Plenum Press, 1978, p 243.
16. Beck JC, Lipkowitz MS, Abramson RG: Characterisation of the fetal glucose transporter in rabbit kidney. Comparison with the adult brush border electrogenic Na + - glucose symporter. *J Clin Invest* 82:379, 1988.
17. Behrman RE, Lees MH, Peterson EN, et al: Distribution of the circulation in the normal and asphyxiated fetal primate. *Am J Obstet Gynecol* 108:956, 1970.
18. Bell RJ, Congui M, Hardy KG, et al: Gestation-dependent aspects of the response of the ovine fetus to the osmotic stress induced by maternal water deprivation. *Q J Exp Physiol* 69:187, 1984.
19. Betkerur MV, Yeh TF, Miller K, et al: Indomethacin and its effects on renal function and urinary kallikrein excretion in premature infants with patent ductus arteriosus. *Pediatrics* 68:99, 1981.
20. Biava CG, West M: Fine structure of normal human juxtaglomerular cells. II. Specific and nonspecific cytoplasmic granules. *Am J Pathol* 49:955, 1966.
21. Bishop JE, Norman AW: Studies on calciferol metabolism. Metabolism of 25-hydroxyvitamin D3 by the chicken embryo. *Arch Biochem Biophys* 167:769, 1975.
22. Boylan JW, Colbourn EP, McCance RA: Renal function in the foetal and newborn guinea-pig. *J Physiol* 141:323, 1958.
23. Brace RA, Cheung CY: Fetal cardiovascular and endocrine response to prolonged fetal hemorrhage. *Am J Physiol* 251:R417, 1986.
24. Brace RA, Miner LK, Siderowf AD, et al: Fetal and adult urine flow and ANF responses to vascular volume expansion. *Am J Physiol* 255:R846, 1988.
25. Broughton-Pipkin F, Kirkpatrick SM, Lumbers ER, et al: Renin and angiotensin-like levels in foetal, newborn and adult sheep. *J Physiol* 241:575, 1974.
26. Broughton-Pipkin F, Lumbers ER, Mott JC: Factors influencing plasma renin and angiotensin II in the conscious pregnant ewe and its foetus. *J Physiol* 243:619, 1974.
27. Broughton-Pipkin F, Symonds EM, Turner SR: The effect of captopril (SQ14,225) upon mother and fetus in the chronically cannulated ewe and in the pregnant rabbit. *J Physiol* 323:415, 1982.
28. Broughton-Pipkin F, Turner SR, Symonds EM: Possible risks with captopril in pregnancy. Some animal data. *Lancet* 1:1256, 1980.
29. Brown EH, Coghlan JP, Hardy KJ, et al: Aldosterone, corticosterone, cortisol, 11-deoxycortisol and 11-deoxycorticosterone concentrations in the blood of chronically cannulated ovine foetuses: Effect of ACTH. *Acta Endocrinol* 88:364, 1978.
30. Burns MEH, Fausto A, Avioli LV: Placental calcium binding proteins in rats. Apparent identity with vitamin D dependent calcium binding protein from rat intestine. *J Biol Chem* 253:3186, 1978.

31. Buckley NM, Brazeau P, Gootman PM, et al: Renal circulatory effects of adrenergic stimuli in anesthetized piglets and mature swine. *Am J Physiol* 237:H690, 1979.

32. Buddingh F, Parker HR, Ishizaki G, et al: Long-term studies of the functional development of the fetal kidney in sheep. *Am J Vet Res* 32:1993, 1971.

33. Care AD: Calcium homeostasis in the fetus. *J Dev Physiol* 2:85, 1980.

34. Care AD, Pickard DW, Weatherly AJ, et al: The measurement of transplacental magnesium fluxes in the sheep. *Res Vet Sci* 27:121, 1979.

35. Carretero OA, Scicli AG: The renal kallikrein-kinin system. *Am J Physiol* 238:F247, 1980.

36. Carretero OA, Scicli AG: Possible role of kinins in circulatory homeostasis: State of the art review. *Hypertension* 3:I4, 1981.

37. Carver JG, Mott JC: Renin substrate in plasma of unanaesthetized pregnant ewes and their foetal lambs. *J Physiol* 276:395, 1978.

38. Casey ML, Cutrer SI, Mitchell MD: Origin of prostanoids in human amniotic fluid: The fetal kidney as a source of amniotic fluid prostanoids. *Am J Obstet Gynecol* 147:547, 1983.

39. Chez RA, Smith FG Jr, Hutchinson DL: Renal function in the intrauterine primate fetus. I. Experimental technique; rate of formation and chemical composition of urine. *Am J Obstet Gynecol* 90:128, 1964.

40. Cohen JJ, Kamm DE: Renal metabolism: Relation to renal function. *In* Brenner BM (ed): *The Kidney.* New York, WB Saunders, 1976, p 126.

41. Dancis J, Springer D, Coglan SQ: Fetal homeostasis in maternal malnutrition. II. Magnesium deprivation. *Pediatr Res* 5:131, 1971.

42. Daniel SS, Stark RI, Husain MK, et al: Excretion of vasopressin in the hypoxic lamb: Comparison between fetus and newborn. *Pediatr Res* 18:227, 1984.

43. Delivoria-Papadopoulos M, Meschia G, Battaglia FC, et al: Total protein-bound and ultrafiltrable calcium in maternal and fetal plasmas. *Am J Physiol* 213:363, 1967.

44. DiBona GF: The functions of the renal nerves. *Rev Physiol Biochem Pharmacol* 94:76, 1982.

45. Dobrovic-Jenik D, Milkovic S: Regulation of fetal Na+/K+-ATPase in rat kidney by corticosteroids. *Biochim Biophys Acta* 942:227, 1988.

46. Dunn MJ: Renal prostaglandins: influences on excretion of sodium and water, the renin angiotensin system, renal blood flow, and hypertension. *In* Brenner BM (ed): *Hormonal Function and the Kidney.* New York, Churchill-Livingstone, 1979, p 89.

47. Economou-Mavrou C, McCance RA: Calcium, magnesium and phosphorus in foetal tissues. *Biochem J* 68:573, 1958.

48. Elbourne I, Lumbers ER: Organic acid and base excretion by the fetal kidney (abstr). *Proc Aust Phys Pharm Soc* 18:15P, 1987.

49. Engelke SC, Shah BV, Vasan V, et al: Sodium balance in very low birth-weight infants. *J Physiol* 93:837, 1978.

50. Ervin MG, Leake RD, Ross MG, et al: Arginine vasotocin in ovine fetal blood, urine and amniotic fluid. *J Clin Invest* 75:1696, 1985.

51. Ervin MG, Ross MG, Leake RD, et al: Changes in steady state plasma arginine vasotocin levels affect ovine fetal renal and cardiovascular function. *Endocrinology* 118:759, 1986.

52. Fenton E, Britton HG: 25-hydroxycholecalciferol 1 alpha-hydroxylase activity in the kidney of the fetal, neonatal and adult guinea pig. *Biol Neonate* 37:254, 1980.

53. Fetterman GH, Shuplock NA, Philipp FJ, et al: The growth and maturation of human glomeruli and proximal convolutions from term to adulthood: Studies by microdissection. *Pediatrics* 35:601, 1965.

54. Fleischman AR, Oakes GK, Epstein MF, et al: Plasma renin activity during ovine pregnancy. *Am J Physiol* 228:901, 1975.

55. Friedman Z, Demers LM: Prostaglandin synthetase in the human neonatal kidney. *Pediatr Res* 14:190, 1980.

56. Froelich JC, Hollifield JW, Dormois JC, et al: Suppression of plasma renin activity by indomethacin in man. *Circ Res* 39:447, 1976.

57. Froger JL, Aminot A, Blouquit-Debray MF, et al: Antidiuretic activity in the fetal and newborn rabbit hypophysis. *Biol Neonate* 30:224, 1976.

58. Garel JM, Barlet JP: Calcitonin in the mother, fetus and newborn. *Ann Biol Anim Biochim Biophys* 18:53, 1978.

59. Geloso JP, Basset JC: Role of adrenal glands in development of foetal rat kidney Na-K-ATPase. *Pflugers Arch* 348:105, 1974.

60. Gersh I: The correlation of structure and function in the developing mesonephros and metanephros. *Contrib Embryol* 26:35, 1937.

61. Gomez RA, Chevalier RL, Sturgill BC, et al: Maturation of the intrarenal reinin distribution in Wistar-Kyoto rats. *J Hypertens* 4:S31, 1986.

62. Gomez RA, Lynch KR, Chevalier RL, et al: Renin and angiotensinogen gene expression in maturing rat kidney. *Am J Physiol* 254:F582, 1988.

63. Gomez RA, Lynch KR, Sturgill BC, et al: Distribution of renin mRNA and its protein in the developing kidney. *Am J Physiol* 257:F850, 1989.

64. Gomez RA, Meernik JG, Kuehl WD, et al: Developmental aspects of the renal response to hemorrhage during fetal life. *Pediatr Res* 18:40, 1984.

65. Gomez RA, Robillard JE: Developmental aspects of the renal response to hemorrhage during converting-enzyme inhibition in fetal lambs. *Circ Res* 54:301, 1984.

66. Gray TK, Lester GE, Lorenc RS: Evidence for extra-renal 1 alpha-hydroxylation of 25-hydroxyvitamin D3 in pregnancy. *Pediatr Res* 18:40, 1984.

67. Gresham EL, Rankin JHG, Makowski EL, et al: An evaluation of fetal renal function in a chronic sheep preparation. *J Clin Invest* 51:149, 1972.

68. Grignolo A, Seidler J, Bartolome M, et al: Norepinephrine content of the rat kidney during development: Alterations induced by perinatal methadone. *Life Sci* 31:3009, 1982.

69. Gruskin AB, Edelmann CM Jr, Yuan S: Maturational changes in renal blood flow in piglets. *Pediatr Res* 4:7, 1970.

70. Guignard JP, Torrado A, DaCunha O, et al: Glomerular filtration rate in the first three weeks of life. *J Pediatr* 87:268, 1975.

71. Haddad JG Jr, Biosseau V, Avioli LV: Placental transfer of vitamin D3 and 25-hydroxycholecalciferol in the rat. *J Lab Clin Med* 77:908, 1971.

72. Heymann MA, Rudolph AM, Nies AS, et al: Bradykinin production associated with oxygenation of fetal lamb. *Circ Res* 25:521, 1969.

73. Hill KJ, Lumbers ER: Renal function in adult and fetal sheep. *J Dev Physiol* 10:149, 1988.

74. Hill KJ, Lumbers ER, Elbourne I: The actions of cortisol on fetal renal function. *J Dev Physiol* 10:85, 1988.

75. Hillman LS, Haddad JG: Human perinatal vitamin D metabolism 1,25-hydroxyvitamin D in maternal and cord blood. *J Pediatr* 84:742, 1974.

76. Hillman LS, Slatopolsky E, Haddad JG: Perinatal vitamin D metabolism. IV. Maternal and cord serum 24,25-dihydroxyvitamin D concentrations. *J Clin Endocrinol Metab* 47:1073, 1978.

77. Hodari AA, Hodgkinson CP: Fetal kidney as a source of renin in the pregnant dog. *Am J Obstet Gynecol* 102:691, 1968.
78. Hurley JK, Kirkpatrick SE, Pitlick PT, et al: Renal responses of the fetal lamb to fetal or maternal volume expansion. *Circ Res* 40:557, 1977.
79. Ismay MJA, Lumbers ER, Stevens AD: The action of angiotensin II on the baroreflex response of the conscious ewe and the conscious fetus. *J Physiol* 288:467, 1979.
80. Iwamoto HS, Oh W, Rudolph AM: Renal metabolism in fetal and newborn sheep. *In* Jones CT and Nathanielsz PW, (eds): *The Physiological Development of the Fetus and Newborn.* Orlando, Academic Press, 1985, p 37.
81. Iwamoto HS, Rudolph AM: Effects of endogenous AII on the fetal circulation. *J Dev Physiol* 1:283, 1979.
82. Iwamoto HS, Rudolph AM: Role of renin-angiotensin system in response to hemorrhage in fetal sheep. *Am J Physiol* 240:H848, 1981.
83. Iwamoto HS, Rudolph AM: Metabolic responses of the kidney in fetal sheep: Effect of acute and spontaneous hypoxemia. *Am J Physiol* 249:F836, 1985.
84. Iwamoto HS, Rudolph AM, Keil LC, et al: Hemodynamic responses of the sheep fetus to vasopressin infusion. *Circ Res* 44:430, 1979.
85. Jacque L: De la genese des liquides amniotique et allanto-idin: Cryoscopie et analyses chimiques. *Arch Int Physiol* 3:463, 1905.
86. Joppich R, Schrader J, Haberle DA: Effect of antidiuretic hormone and dibutyryl cAMP upon the urinary concentrating capacity in neonatal piglets. *Pediatr Res* 14:1234, 1980.
87. Kaplan A, Friedman M: Studies concerning the site of renin formation in kidney; apparent site of renin formation in tubules of mesonephros and metanephros of hog fetus. *J Exp Med* 76:307, 1942.
88. Kawashima H, Torikai S, Kurokawa K: Localization of 25-hydroxyvitamin D3-1 alpha-hydroxylase and 24-hydroxylase along the rat nephron. *Proc Natl Acad Sci USA* 78:1199, 1981.
89. Kesby GJ, Lumbers ER: Factors affecting renal handling of sodium hydrogen ions, and bicarbonate by the fetus. *Am J Physiol* 251:F226, 1986.
90. Kesby GJ, Lumbers ER: The effects of metabolic acidosis on renal function of fetal sheep. *J Physiol* 396:65, 1988.
91. Kleinman LI: Developmental renal physiology. *Physiologist* 25:104, 1982.
92. Kleinman LI, Lubbe RJ: Factors affecting the maturation of glomerular filtration rate and renal plasma flow in the newborn dog. *J Physiol* 223:395, 1972.
93. Kooh SW, Vieth R: 25-hydroxyvitamin D metabolism in the sheep fetus and lamb. *Pediatr Res* 14:360, 1980.
94. Larsson C, Weber P, Anggard E: Arachidonic acid increases and indomethacin decreases plasma renin activity in the rabbit. *Eur J Pharmacol* 28:391, 1974.
95. Leake RD, Trygstad CW, Oh W: Insulin clearance in the newborn infant: Relationship to gestational and postnatal age. *Pediatr Res* 10:759, 1976.
96. Leake RD, Weitzman RE, Effros RM, et al: Maternal fetal osmolar homeostasis: Fetal posterior pituitary autonomy. *Pediatr Res* 13:841, 1979.
97. Lelievre-Pegorier M, Geloso JP: Ontogeny of sugar transport in fetal rat kidney. *Biol Neonate* 38:16, 1980.
98. Lelievre-Pegorier M, Merlet-Benichou C, Roinel N, et al: Developmental pattern of water and electrolyte transport in rat superficial nephrons. *Am J Physiol* 254:F15, 1983.
99. Lester GE, Gray TK, Lorenc RS: Evidence for maternal and fetal differences in vitamin D metabolism. *Proc Soc Exp Biol Med* 159:303, 1978.
100. Levens NR, Peach MJ, Garey RM: Role of the intrarenal renin-angiotensin system in the control of renal function. *Circ Res* 48:157, 1981.
101. Levina SE: Endocrine features in development of human hypothalamus, hypophysis and placenta. *Gen Comp Endocrinol* 11:151, 1968.
102. Levinsky NG: The renal kallikrein-kinin system. *Circ Res* 44:441, 1979.
103. Linarelli LG: Newborn urinary cyclic AMP and developmental renal responsiveness to parathyroid hormone. *Pediatrics* 50:14, 1972.
104. Lingwood B, Hardy KJ, Horacek I, et al: The effects of antidiuretic hormone on urine flow and composition in the chronically cannulated ovine fetus. *Q J Exp Physiol* 63:315, 1978.
105. Lonnerholm G, Wistrand PJ: Carbonic anhydrase in the human fetal kidney. *Pediatr Res* 17:390, 1983.
106. Lumbers ER: Activation of renin in human amniotic fluid by low pH. *Enzymologia* 40:329, 1971.
107. Lumbers ER: A brief review of fetal renal function. *J Dev Physiol* 6:1, 1983.
108. Lumbers ER, Hill KJ, Bennett VJ: Proximal and distal tubular activity in chronically catheterized fetal sheep compared with the adult. *Can J Physiol Pharmacol* 66:697, 1988.
109. Lumbers ER, Lewes JL: The actions of vasoactive drugs on fetal and maternal plasma renin activity. *Biol Neonate* 35:23, 1979.
110. Lumbers ER, Smith FG, Stevens AD: Measurement of net transplacental transfer of fluid to the fetal sheep. *J Physiol* 364:289, 1985.
111. Lumbers ER, Stevens AD: Factors influencing glomerular filtration rate in the fetal lamb. *J Physiol* 298:28, 1979.
112. Lumbers ER, Stevens AD: Changes in fetal renal function in response to infusions of a hyperosmotic solution of mannitol to the ewe. *J Physiol* 343:439, 1983.
113. Macy IG, Hunscher HA: Evaluation of maternal nitrogen and mineral needs during embryonic and infant development. *Am J Obstet Gynecol* 27:878, 1934.
114. Makepeace AW, Fremont-Smith F, Dailey ME, et al: Nature of the amniotic fluid. A comparative study of human amniotic fluid and maternal serum. *Surg Gynecol Obstetr* 53:635, 1931.
115. Marche P, Delorme A, Cuisinier-Gleizes P: Intestinal and placental calcium-binding proteins in vitamin D deprived or supplemented rats. *Life Sci* 23:2555, 1978.
116. Matson JR, Stokes JB, Robillard JE: The effects of inhibition of prostaglandin synthesis on fetal renal function. *Kidney Int* 20:621, 1981.
117. Mayfield RK, Margolius HS: Renal kallikrein-kinin system. Relation to renal function and blood pressure. *Am J Nephrol* 3:145, 1983.
118. McCance RA, Widdowson EM: Renal function before birth. *Proc Roy Soc Bull* 141:488, 1953.
119. McKenna OC, Angelakos ET: Development of adrenergic innervation in the puppy kidney. *Anat Rec* 167:115, 1970.
120. Melmon KL, Cline MJ, Hughes T, et al: Kinins: Possible mediators of neonatal circulatory changes in man. *J Clin Invest* 57:1295, 1968.
121. Merlet-Benichou C, deRouffignac C: Renal clearance studies in fetal and young guinea pigs: Effect of salt loading. *Am J Physiol* 232:F178, 1977.
122. Merlet-Benichou C, Pegorier M, Muffat-Joly M, et al: Functional and morphologic patterns of renal maturation in the developing guinea pig. *Am J Physiol* 241:F618, 1981.
123. Millard RW, Baig H, Vatner SF: Prostaglandin control of the renal circulation in response to hypoxemia in the fetal lamb in utero. *Circ Res* 45:172, 1979.

124. Molteni A, Rahill WJ, Koo J-H: Evidence for a vasopressor substance (renin) in human fetal kidneys. *Lab Invest* 30:115, 1974.
125. Moore ES, Chung EE, Cevallos EE, et al: Renal phosphate clearance in fetal lambs. *Pediatr Res* 12:1066, 1978.
126. Moore ES, Langman CB, Loghman-Adham M, et al: Divalent mineral metabolism in utero (abstr). *Pediatr Res* 16:326A, 1982.
127. Mott JC: The place of the renin-angiotensin system before and after birth. *Br Med Bull* 31:44, 1975.
128. Mott JC: The renin-angiotensin-aldosterone system in pregnancy and its relation to that of the fetus and newborn. *In* Nitzau M (ed): *The Influence of Maternal Hormones on the Fetus and Newborn.* Basel, Karger, 1979, p 126.
129. Nakamura KT, Ayres NA, Gomez RA, et al: Renal responses to hypoxemia during renin-angiotensin system inhibition in fetal lambs. *Am J Physiol* 249:R116, 1985.
130. Nakamura KT, Klinkefus JM, Smith FG, et al: Ontogeny of neuronally released norepinephrine on renin secretion in sheep. *Am J Physiol* 257:R765, 1989.
131. Nakamura KT, Matherne GP, Jose PA, et al: Ontogeny of renal beta-adrenoceptor mediated vasodilation in sheep: Comparison between endogenous catecholamines. *Pediatr Res* 22:465, 1987.
132. Nakamura KT, Matherne GP, McWeeny OJ, et al: Renal hemodynamics and functional changes during the transition from fetal to newborn life in sheep. *Pediatr Res* 21:229, 1987.
133. Nakamura KT, Page WV, Klinkefus JM, et al: Ontogeny of isoproterenol-stimulated renin secretion from sheep renal cortical slices. *Am J Physiol* 256:R1258, 1989.
134. Nasjletti A, Malik KU: The renal kallikrein-kinin and prostaglandin systems interaction. *Annu Rev Physiol* 43:597, 1981.
135. Noff D, Edelstein S: Vitamin D and its hydroxylated metabolites in the rat: Placental and lacteal transport, subsequent metabolic pathways and tissue distribution. *Horm Res* 9:292, 1978.
136. Novy MJ, Liggins GC: Role of prostaglandins, prostacyclin, and thromboxanes in the physiologic control of the uterus and in parturition. *Perinatology* 4:45, 1980.
137. Olbing H, Blaufox MD, Aschinberg LC, et al: Postnatal changes in renal glomerular blood flow distribution in puppies. *J Clin Invest* 52:2885, 1973.
138. Pace-Asciak CR: Activity profiles of prostaglandin 15 and 9 hydroxydehydrogenase and 13-reductase in the developing rat kidney. *J Biol Chem* 250:2795, 1975.
139. Pace-Asciak CR: Biosynthesis and catabolism of prostaglandins during animal development. *Adv Prostaglandin Thromboxane Res* 1:35, 1976.
140. Pace-Asciak CR: Prostaglandin biosynthesis and catabolism in the developing fetal sheep kidney. *Prostaglandins* 13:661, 1977.
141. Paton JB, Fisher DE, Peterson EN, et al: Cardiac output and organ blood flows in the baboon fetus. *Biol Neonate* 22:50, 1973.
142. Perry JS, Stanier MW: The rate of flow of urine of foetal pigs. *J Physiol* 161:344, 1962.
143. Phat VN, Camilleri JP, Bariety J, et al: Immunohistochemical characterization of renin-containing cells in the human juxtaglomerular apparatus during embryonal and fetal development. *Lab Invest* 45:387, 1981.
144. Poisner AM, Wood GW, Poisner R: Release of inactive renin from human fetal membranes and isolated trophoblasts. *Clin Exp Hypertens [A]* 4:2007, 1982.
145. Poisner AM, Wood GW, Poisner R, et al: Localization of renin in trophoblasts in human chorion leave at term pregnancy. *Endocrinology* 109:1150, 1981.
146. Poisner AM, Wood GW, Poisner R, et al: Renin and inactive renin in human amnion at term pregnancy. *Proc Soc Exp Biol Med* 169:4, 1982.
147. Rajerison RM, Butlen D, Jard S: Ontogenetic development of antidiuretic hormone receptors in rat kidney: Comparison of hormonal binding and adenylate cyclase activation. *Mol Cell Endocrinol* 4:271, 1976.
148. Ramberg CF, Delivoria-Papadopoulos M, Crandall ED, et al: Kinetic analysis of calcium transport across the placenta. *J Appl Physiol* 35:682, 1973.
149. Rankin JHG, Gresham EL, Battaglia FC, et al: Measurement of fetal renal inulin clearance in a chronic sheep preparation. *J Appl Physiol* 32:129, 1972.
150. Rawashdeh NM, Ray ND, Sundberg DK, et al: Comparison of hormonal responses to hypotension in mature and immature fetal lambs. *Am J Physiol* 255:67, 1988.
151. Rawashdeh NM, Rose JC, Kerr DR: Renin secretion by fetal lamb kidneys in vitro. *Am J Physiol* 258:R388, 1990.
152. Rawashdeh NM, Rose JC, Ray ND: Differential maturation of beta-adrenoceptor mediated responses in the lamb fetus. *Am J Physiol* 255(24):R794, 1988.
153. Rees L, Brook CGD, Forsling ML: Continuous urine collection in the study of vasopressin in the newborn. *Horm Res* 17:134, 1983.
154. Robillard JE: Changes in renal vascular reactivity to angiotensin II during development in fetal, newborn and adult sheep: Role of AII vascular receptors occupancy (abstr). *Pediatr Res* 17:355A, 1983.
155. Robillard JE, Gomez RA, Meernik JG, et al: Role of angiotensin II on the adrenal and vascular responses to hemorrhage during development in fetal lambs. *Circ Res* 50:645, 1982.
156. Robillard JE, Gomez RA, VanOrden D, et al: Comparison of the adrenal and renal responses to angiotensin II in fetal lambs and adult sheep. *Circ Res* 50:140, 1982.
157. Robillard JE, Kulvinskas C, Sessions C, et al: Maturational changes in the fetal glomerular filtration rate. *Am J Obstet Gynecol* 122:601, 1975.
158. Robillard JE, Lawton WJ, Weismann DN, et al: Developmental aspects of the renal kallikrein-kinin activity in fetal and newborn lambs. *Kidney Int* 22:594, 1982.
159. Robillard JE, Matson JR, Sessions C, et al: Developmental aspects of renal tubular reabsorption of water in the lamb fetus. *Pediatr Res* 13:1172, 1979.
160. Robillard JE, Nakamura KT: Neurohormonal regulation of renal function during development. *Am J Physiol* 254:F771, 1988.
161. Robillard JE, Nakamura KT, DiBona GF: Effects of renal denervation on renal responses to hypoxemia in fetal lambs. *Am J Physiol* 250:F294, 1986.
162. Robillard JE, Nakamura KT, Matherne GP, et al: Renal hemodynamics and functional adjustments to postnatal life. *Semin Perinatol* 12:143, 1988.
163. Robillard JE, Nakamura KT, Varille VA, et al: Ontogeny of the renal response to natriuretic peptide in sheep. *Am J Physiol* 254:F634, 1988.
164. Robillard JE, Nakamura KT, Wilkin MK, et al: Ontogeny of renal hemodynamic response to renal nerve stimulation in sheep. *Am J Physiol* 252:F605, 1987.
165. Robillard JE, Ramberg E, Sessions C, et al: Role of aldosterone on renal sodium and potassium excretion during fetal life and newborn period. *Dev Pharmacol Ther* 1:201, 1980.
166. Robillard JE, Sessions C, Burmeister L, et al: Influence of fetal extracellular volume contraction on renal reabsorption of bicarbonate in fetal lambs. *Pediatr Res* 11:649, 1977.
167. Robillard JE, Sessions C, Kennedy RL, et al: Interrelationship between glomerular filtration rate and renal transport

of sodium and chloride during fetal life. *Am J Obstet Gynecol* 128:727, 1977.

168. Robillard JE, Sessions C, Kennedy RL, et al: Maturation of the glucose transport process by the fetal kidney. *Pediatr Res* 12:680, 1978.

169. Robillard JE, Sessions C, Smith FG Jr: In vivo demonstration of renal carbonic anhydrase activity in the fetal lamb. *Biol Neonate* 34:253, 1978.

170. Robillard JE, Weismann DN, Gomez RA, et al: Renal and adrenal responses to converting-enzyme inhibition in fetal and newborn life. *Am J Physiol* 244:R249, 1983.

171. Robillard JE, Weismann DN, Herin P: Ontogeny of single glomerular perfusion rate in fetal and newborn lambs. *Pediatr Res* 15:1248, 1981.

172. Robillard JE, Weitzman RE: Developmental aspects of the fetal renal response to exogenous arginine vasopressin. *Am J Physiol* 238:F407, 1980.

173. Robillard JE, Weitzman RE, Burmeister L, et al: Developmental aspects of the renal response to hypoxemia in the lamb fetus. *Circ Res* 48:128, 1981.

174. Robillard JE, Weitzman RE, Fisher DA, et al: The dynamics of vasopressin release and blood volume regulation during fetal hemorrhage in the lamb fetus. *Pediatr Res* 13:606, 1979.

175. Ross MG, Sherman DJ, Ervin MG, et al: Maternal dehydration-rehydration: Fetal plasma and urinary responses. *Am J Physiol* 255:E674, 1988.

176. Ross R, Care AD, Taylor CM, et al: The transplacental movement of metabolites of vitamin D in the sheep. *In* Norman AW (ed): *Vitamin D: Basic Research and its Clinical Application.* Berlin, deGruyter, 1979, p 341.

177. Rothberg AD, Lorenz R: Can captopril cause fetal and neonatal renal failure? *Pediatr Pharmacol* 4:189, 1984.

178. Rothe CF, Nash FD, Thompson DE: Patterns in autoregulation of renal blood flow in the dog. *Am J Physiol* 220:1621, 2971.

179. Rudolph AM, Heymann MA: Circulatory changes during growth in the fetal lamb. *Circ Res* 26:289, 1970.

180. Rudolph AM, Heymann MA, Teramo KAW, et al: Studies on the circulation of the previable human fetus. *Pediatr Res* 5:452, 1971.

181. Rurak DW: Plasma vasopressin in foetal lambs. *J Physiol* 256:36P, 1976.

182. Schedewie H, Slikker W, Hill D, et al: Placental crossover and fetal tissue distribution of 1,25(OH)₂ vitamin D in rhesus monkey (abstr). *Pediatr. Res.* 14:580A, 1980.

183. Schroeder H, Gilbert RD, Power GG: Urinary and hemodynamic responses to blood volume changes in fetal sheep. *J Dev Physiol* 6:131, 1984.

184. Schubert F, George JM, Rao MB: Vasopressin and oxytocin content of human fetal brain at different stages of gestation. *Brain Res* 213:111, 1981.

185. Segal S, Rea C, Smith I: Separate transport systems for sugars and amino acids in developing rat kidney cortex. *Proc Natl Acad Sci USA* 68:372, 1971.

186. Shami Y, Radde IC: Calcium stimulated ATPase of guinea pig placenta. *Biochim Biophys Acta* 249:345, 1971.

187. Shauberger CW, Pitkin RM: Maternal perinatal calcium relationships. *Obstet Gynecol* 53:74, 1979.

188. Shine P, McDougall JG, Towstoless MK, et al: Action of atrial natriuretic peptide in the immature ovine kidney. *Pediatr Res* 22:11, 1987.

189. Siegel SR, Leake RD, Weitzman RE, et al: Effects of furosemide and acute salt loading on vasopressin and renin secretion in the fetal lamb. *Pediatr Res* 14:869, 1980.

190. Siegel SR, Oakes GK, Palmer S: Effects of angiotensin II on blood pressure, plasma renin activity and aldosterone in the fetal lamb. *Dev Pharmacol Ther* 3:144, 1981.

191. Siimes ASI, Creasy RK, Heymann MA, et al: Cardiac output and its distribution and organ blood flow in the fetal lamb during ritodrine administration. *Am J Obstet Gynecol* 132:42, 1978.

192. Skinner SL, Lumbers ER, Symonds EM: Renin concentration in human fetal and maternal tissues. *Am J Obstet Gynecol* 101:529, 1968.

193. Skowsky WR, Fisher DA: Fetal neurohypophyseal argine vasopressin and arginine vasotocin in man and sheep. *Pediatr Res* 11:627, 1977.

194. Smith FG: *Factors Influencing Fetal and Neonatal Fluid Balance.* Sydney, Australia, University of New South Wales, Doctoral Dissertation, 1987.

195. Smith FG, Lumbers ER: Effects of maternal hyperglycemia on fetal renal function in sheep. *Am J Physiol* 255:F11, 1988.

196. Smith FG, Lumbers ER: Changes in renal function following delivery of the lamb by caesarian section. *J Dev Physiol* 10:145, 1988.

197. Smith FG, Lumbers ER: Comparison of renal function in term fetal sheep and newborn lambs. *Biol Neonate* 55:309, 1989.

198. Smith FG, Robillard JE: Pathophysiology of fetal renal disease. *Semin Perinatol* 13:305, 1989.

199. Smith FG, Sato T, McWeeny OJ, et al: Role of renal sympathetic nerves in the response of the ovine fetus to volume expansion. *Am J Physiol* 259:R1050, 1990.

200. Smith FG, Sato T, Varille VA, et al: Atrial natriuretic factor during fetal and postnatal life: A review. *J Dev Physiol* 12:55, 1989.

201. Smith FG Jr, Adams FH, Borden M, et al: Studies of renal function in the intact fetal lamb. *Am J Obstet Gynecol* 96:240, 1966.

202. Smith FG Jr, Alexander DP, Buckle RM, et al: Parathyroid hormone in foetal and adult sheep: The effect of hypocalcemia. *J Endocrinol* 53:339, 1972.

203. Smith FG Jr, Lupu AN, Barajas L, et al: The renin angiotensin system in the fetal lamb. *Pediatr Res* 8:611, 1974.

204. Smith FG Jr, Schwartz A: Response to the intact lamb fetus to acidosis. *Am J Obstet Gynecol* 106:52, 1970.

205. Smith FG Jr, Tinglof BO, Meuli J, et al: Fetal response to parathyroid hormone in sheep. *J Appl Physiol* 27:276, 1969.

206. Speller AM, Moffat DB: Tubulo-vascular relationships in the developing kidney. *J Anat* 123:487, 1977.

207. Spitzer A: The developing kidney and the process of growth. *In* Seldin DW and Giebisch G, (eds): *The Kidney: Physiology and Pathophysiology.* New York, Raven, 1985, p 1979.

208. Spitzer A, Brandis M: Functional and morphologic maturation of the superficial nephrons: Relationship to total kidney function. *J Clin Invest* 53:279, 1974.

209. Stanier MW: The function of the mammalian mesonephros. *J Physiol* 151:472, 1960.

210. Stevens AD: *Factors Affecting Renal Function and the Renin Angiotensin System in the Sheep Fetus.* Sydney, Australia, University of New South Wales, 1987.

211. Stevens AD, Lumbers ER: The effect of maternal fluid intake on the volume and composition of fetal urine. *J Dev Physiol* 7:161, 1985.

212. Strickland DM, Saeed SA, Casey ML, et al: Stimulation of prostaglandin biosynthesis by urine of the human fetus may serve as a trigger for parturition. *Science* 220:521, 1982.

213. Sutherland LE, Hartroft PM: Juxtaglomerular cells are present in early metanephros of the hog embryo (abstr). *Anat Rec* 148:342A, 1964.

214. Symonds EM, Furler I: Plasma renin levels in the normal and anephric fetus at birth. *Biol Neonate* 23:133, 1973.

215. Symonds EM, Skinner SL, Stanley MA, et al: An investi-

gation of the cellular source of renin in human chorion. *J Obstet Gynaec Brit Common* 77:885, 1970.

216. Symonds EM, Stanley MA, Skinner SL: Production of renin by in vitro cultures of human chorion and uterine muscles. *Nature* 217:1152, 1968.

217. Terragno NA, McGiff JC, Terragno A: Prostacyclin (PGI2) production by renal blood vessels: Relationship to an endogenous prostaglandin synthesis inhibitor (EPSI) (abstr). *Clin Res* 26:545A, 1978.

218. Thomas ML, Anast CS, Forte LR: Regulation of calcium homeostasis in the fetal and neonatal rat. *Am J Physiol* 240:E367, 1981.

219. Thorburn GD: The role of the thyroid gland and kidneys in fetal growth. *In* Elliot K, et al (eds): *Size at Birth. Ciba Foundation Symposium No. 27.* Amsterdam, Elsevier/North Holland Biomedical Press, North Holland, 1974, p 185.

220. Trimper CE, Lumbers ER: The renin-angiotensin system in foetal lambs. *Pfluegers Arch* 336:1, 1972.

221. Tsang RC, Greer F, Steichen JJ: Perinatal metabolism of vitamin D: Transition from fetal to neonatal life. *Clin Perinatol* 8:287, 1981.

222. Tsuda N, Nickerson PA, Molteni A: Ultrastructural study of developing juxtaglomerular cells in the rat. *Lab Invest* 25:644, 1971.

223. Twardock AR, Austin MK: Calcium transfer in perfused guinea pig placenta. *Am J Physiol* 219:540, 1970.

224. Varille VA, Nakamura KT, McWeeny OJ, et al: Renal hemodynamic response to atrial natriuretic factor in fetal and newborn sheep. *Pediatr Res* 25:291, 1989.

225. Vizosolyi E, Perks AM: New neurohypophyseal principle in foetal mammals. *Nature* 223:1169, 1969.

226. Walker DW, Mitchell MD: Prostaglandins in urine of foetal lambs. *Nature* 271:161, 1978.

227. Walker DW, Mitchell MD: Presence of thromboxane beta-2 and 6-ketoprostaglandin F1 alpha in the urine of fetal sheep. *Prostaglandins Med* 3:249, 1979.

228. Wasserman RH, Comar CL, Nold MM, et al: Placental transfer of calcium and strontium in the rat and rabbit. *Am J Physiol* 189:91, 1957.

229. Weisman Y, Sapir R, Harell A, et al: Maternal-perinatal interrelationships of vitamin D metabolism in rats. *Biochim Biophys Acta* 428:388, 1976.

230. Weitzman RE, Fisher DA, Robillard JE, et al: Arginine vasopressin response to an osmotic stimulus in the fetal sheep. *Pediatr Res* 12:35, 1978.

231. Wieland P, Fisher JA, Trechsel U, et al: Perinatal parathyroid hormone, vitamin D metabolites and calcitonin in man. *Am J Physiol* 239:E385, 1980.

232. Wintour EM, Bell RJ, Congui M, et al: The value of urine osmolality as an index of stress in the ovine fetus. *J Dev Physiol* 7:347, 1985.

233. Wintour EM, Brown EH, Denton DA, et al: The ontogeny and regulation of corticosteroid secretion by the ovine foetal adrenal. *Acta Endocrinol* 79:301, 1975.

234. Wintour EM, Brown EH, Denton DA, et al: In vitro and in vivo adrenal cortical steroid production by fetal sheep: Effect of angiotensin II, sodium deficiency and ACTH. *In* Vermeulen A, et al (eds): *Research on Steroids. Vol VII. Transaction of the Seventh Meeting of the International Study Group for Steroid Hormones.* Amsterdam, Elsevier, North Holland, 1977, p 475.

235. Wintour EM, Coghlan JP, Towstoless MK: Cortisol is natriuretic in the immature ovine fetus. *J Endocrinol* 106:R13, 1985.

236. Woods LL, Cheung CY, Power GG, et al: Role of arginine vasopressin in fetal renal response to hypertonicity. *Am J Physiol* 251:F156, 1986.

237. Zimmermann HD: Electronenmikroskopiche befunde zur Innervation des Nephron nach Untersuchungen an der Fetal nachmere des Menschen. *Z Zellforsch* 129:65, 1972.

238. Zink J, VanPetten GR: Noradrenergic control of blood vessels in the premature lamb fetus. *Biol Neonate* 39:61, 1981

ANDREW P. EVAN
LARS LARSSON

2
Morphologic Development of the Nephron

Mammals develop three kidneys in the course of intra-uterine life. The kidneys are, in order of their appearance, the pronephros, the mesonephros, and the metanephros (Fig. 2-1). The first two organs regress in utero, and the third becomes the permanent kidney.

Embryologically, the uriniferous tubules of all three kidneys develop from the intermediate mesoderm. As the notochord and neural tube form, the intraembryonic mesoderm on either side of these structures differentiates into three regions: paraxial (somite), intermediate, and lateral mesoderm (Fig. 2-2A). As the embryo undergoes transverse folding, the intermediate mesoderm loses its attachment to the paraxial mesoderm and migrates ventrally toward the intraembryonic coelom (Fig. 2-2B). There is also progressive craniocaudal development of the intermediate mesoderm to form bilateral longitudinal mesodermal masses, termed the *nephrogenic cord*. With time, each cord with its ventral covering of splanchnopleure is seen bulging from the posterior wall of the coelomic cavity, producing the urogenital ridge (Fig. 2-3).

Pronephros

The human pronephros is a transitory, nonfunctional kidney (Fig. 2-4); however, it is as well developed as those of other amniote embryos. The first evidence of its formation in humans is seen in the VIIth to Xth somite embryo (middle to late third week), and it is completely degenerated by the start of the fifth week. The pronephros develops in the region of the future neck and thorax. At the level of the first to sixth somites, the nephrogenic cord segments into separate blocks of mesoderm called *nephrotomes*. Each nephrotome hollows to form a vesicle that rapidly degenerates. No tubule is generated [198].

Caudal to the VIIth somite, distinct segmentation of the nephrogenic cord into nephrotomes is gradually lost. From the VIIth to approximately the XIVth somite, the nephrogenic cord develops a longitudinal cleft dividing it into a narrow dorsolateral portion and a larger medial section. The lateral division forms the nephric duct, while the medial side differentiates into nephrons.

Rudimentary nephrons of the pronephros are found between the VIIth and IXth/Xth somites. One end of each convoluted tubule has a funnel-shaped opening, termed the *nephrostome*, which communicates with the coelomic cavities. A glomerulus is seen close to the nephrostome but is not part of the tubule. The opposite end of the nephron joins the nephric duct, called the *pronephric duct* at this level, which is developing in the lateral portion of the nephrogenic cord. Development of the pronephric tubules and duct occurs first at the cranial end of the nephrogenic cord and progresses caudally. As each tubule reaches maturation, it immediately begins to degenerate. In addition, that segment of the nephric duct to which the tubule was attached also degenerates. At the time that the pronephric system is degenerating, the mesonephric tubules and duct are developing. Thus, it is important to understand that the development of the pronephros and mesonephros represents only a sequential process of a single morphogenetic event (Fig. 2-1).

Mesonephros

The second kidney, the mesonephros, is also transient, but serves as an excretory organ for the embryo while the metanephros begins its development (Fig. 2-5). An abrupt change is not seen in the morphology of the tubules from the pronephric to the mesonephric kidneys. Instead, there is a gradual transition that occurs at about the IXth to Xth somite level. Both the mesonephric tubules and duct arise from the nephrogenic cord.

Development of the mesonephric duct precedes the development of the tubules. The duct can be seen between the IXth and XIIIth somites in the 20-somite embryo, developing from the dorsolateral portion of the nephrogenic cord. Caudal to the level of the XIVth somite, the distal blind end of the duct grows freely toward the cloaca and communicates with it in the 29-somite (4-mm) human embryo. Soon after the appearance of the mesonephric duct at the beginning of the fourth week, vesicles begin to differentiate. Initially, several spherical masses of cells are found along the medial side of the nephrogenic cord at the

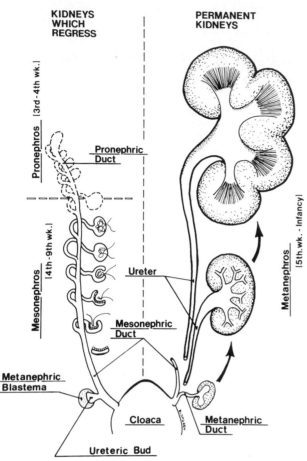

FIG. 2-1. *This drawing schematically represents the development of the three paired kidneys during intrauterine life of most mammals. The kidneys represented on the left are the pronephros (without glomeruli) and mesonephros (possessing glomeruli and tubules), which regress in utero. As the mesonephric duct extends caudally, a diverticulum termed the ureteric bud evaginates from this duct and grows into the nearby mesodermal tissue. The right side of the drawing illustrates development of the metanephros or permanent kidney.*

teriole leaves to empty into a subcardinal sinus. The resulting glomerular corpuscle closely resembles that of the metanephric kidney. The mature mesonephric tubule is composed of a convoluted proximal segment, followed by a poorly differentiated distal segment that attaches to the nephric duct. No loop of Henle is present. Gersh [55] determined that the mesonephric tubules were functional as soon as they had acquired a mature morphology and that they were able to eliminate phenol red and Prussian blue.

Certain elements of the mesonephros are retained in the urogenital system of the male and female. In the male, some of the cranially placed mesonephric tubules become the efferent ductules of the testis. The epididymis and ductus deferens are formed from the mesonephric duct. In the female, remnants of cranial and caudal mesonephric

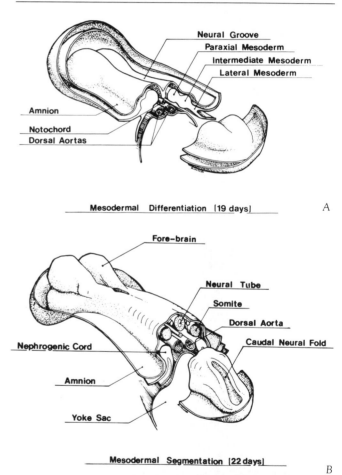

FIG. 2-2. *Figure 2-2A illustrates selected features of a 19-day-old human embryo. The embryonic mesoderm differentiates into three regions, thereby forming paraxial, intermediate, and lateral mesoderm. It is the intermediate mesoderm that gives rise to all three kidneys. Figure 2-2B shows the progression of mesodermal differentiation that occurs by day 22. The intermediate mesoderm has lost its attachment to the paraxial (somite) mesoderm and migrates in a ventral direction. Further differentiation of the intermediate mesoderm forms the nephrogenic cords.*

more cranial somite levels. This differentiation progresses caudally and results in the formation of 40 to 42 pairs of tubules; however, only 30 to 32 pairs are seen at any one time, because the cranially placed tubules start to degenerate during the fifth week. By the fourth month, the human mesonephros has almost completely disappeared, leaving a few elements that persist into maturity.

Shortly after the cell clusters are formed, they develop lumens and take the shape of vesicles. As the vesicle elongates, each end curves in an opposite direction to form an **S**-shaped tubule. The lateral end forms a bud that grows forward and connects with the mesonephric duct. The medial end also lengthens and enlarges to form a double-walled, cup-shaped structure, the future glomerular (Bowman's) capsule and glomerular epithelial cells. A tuft of capillaries originating from a branch of the dorsal aorta invades the developing glomerulus, while an efferent ar-

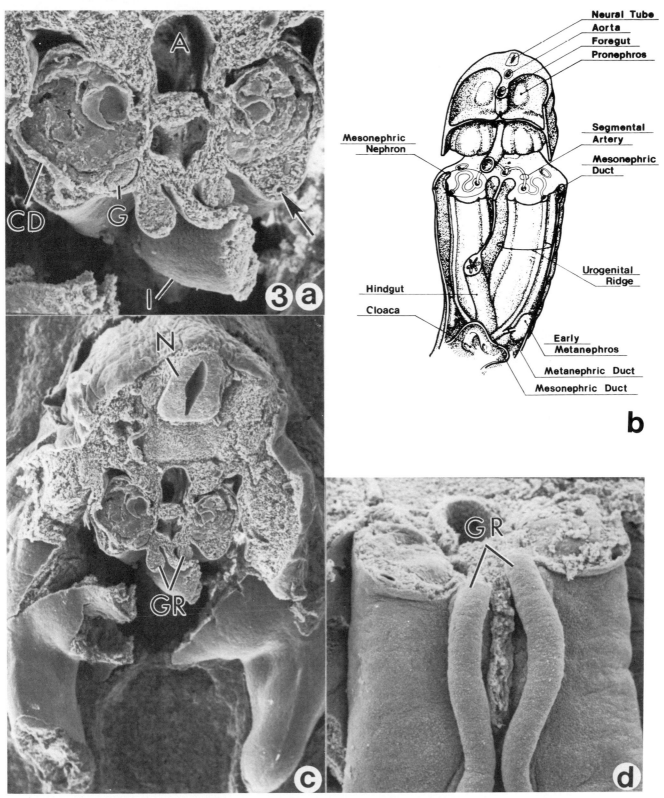

FIG. 2-3. *The scanning electron micrographs of Fig. 2-3A and C are transverse sections through the abdominal cavity of a 29-day-old dog embryo. At this stage each urogenital ridge is divided into a gonadal ridge (GR) and a nephrogenic cord, where the mesonephric duct (arrow) and components [glomerulus (G) and collecting tubule (CT)] of the mesonephric tubules are present. Note the developing notochord (N), aorta (A), and small intestine (I). Figure 2-3D is a ventral view of the urogenital ridge of the 29-day-old dog embryo, and Fig. 2-3B is a composite drawing showing features of the developing nephrogenic cord. (Reproduced from Evan AP: SEM I:455, 1984, with permission from SEM, Inc.)*

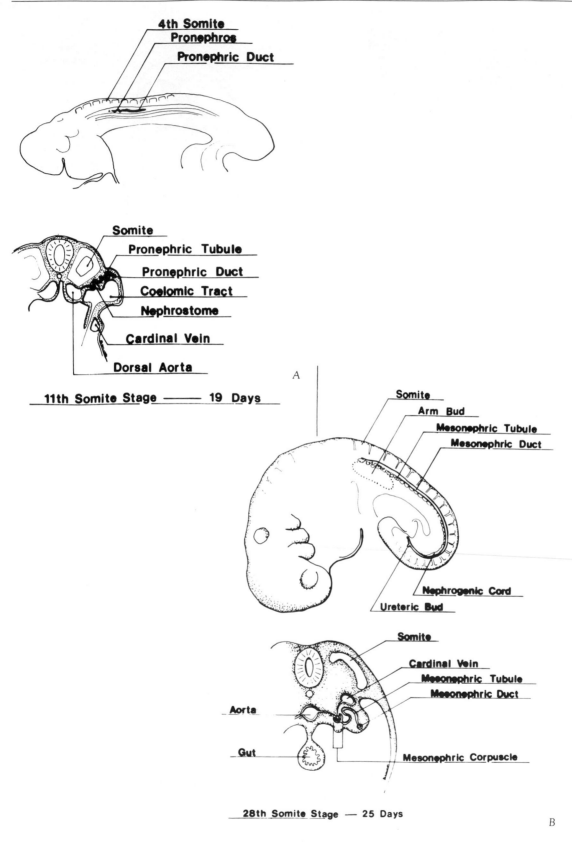

FIG. 2-4. *Human embryo at the eleventh and twenty-eighth somite stages. Figure 2-4A illustrates development of the pronephros in a 19-day-old human embryo. This nonfunctioning kidney develops at the level of the future neck and thorax. On cross-section, the pronephric tubule and duct are positioned between a somite and the coelomic tract. Figure 2-4B illustrates development of the mesonephros in a 25-day-old human embryo. The pronephros and mesonephros do not appear as two distinct kidneys but as a continuum. The cranial end of the mesonephros is located at the ninth and tenth somite level.*

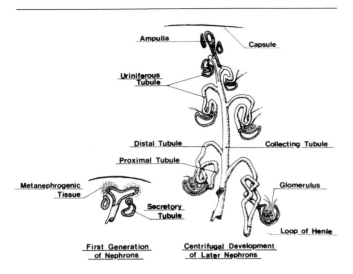

Fig. 2-5. *Schematic representation of metanephric nephrogenesis. As the ampulla of the developing collecting duct extends into the surrounding mesoderm, a condensation of cells forms the metanephric blastema. An inductive process within this condensation of mesoderm cells forms a small, tear-drop vesicle lined with epithelium. This vesicle undergoes elongation into an S-shaped structure. The inner third of this vesicle will form a glomerulus and Bowman's capsule, whereas the outer two-thirds will form most of the tubular components of the nephron, including the proximal tubule, the loop of Henle, and the distal tubule. Meanwhile, the outer end of the S-shaped vesicle connects to the collecting duct. The ampullar end of the collecting duct continues to grow toward and to divide near the kidney capsule. This process of nephron formation creates a centrifugal pattern of development, with the youngest nephrons always near the kidney capsule and the oldest tubules toward the corticomedullary junction.*

tubules form minute, nonfunctional mesosalpingeal structures called the *epoophoron* and the *paroophoron*.

Metanephros

The final mammalian kidney (metanephros) undergoes a series of complex changes during its differentiation to maturity. Our knowledge of these processes is based on several detailed light microscopic [76] and microdissection studies [137,141,142,143,144,154]. The normal development of the kidney requires an outgrowth of the ureteric bud from the mesonephric duct. The ureteric bud grows in a cranial direction toward the mesodermal tissue of the nephrogenic cord. As the ureteric bud grows into the mesodermal tissue, which is now called the *metanephrogenic tissue* or *metanephric blastema*, the tip of the bud divides dichotomously (Fig. 2-5). The first divisions of the ureteric bud give rise to the renal pelvis, calyces, and collecting ducts [141,142] (Fig. 2-1). Thereafter, the first generations of collecting tubules are formed. The tip of the ureteric bud, also named the *ampulla*, is thought to induce formation of the future nephrons in the metanephric blastema [173]. Saxén suggests that these mesenchymal cells respond in three main

ways to the inductive stimulus. First, there is stumulation of DNA synthesis in the target cells by a dual control mechanism. Initially, the target cells must remain in contact with the inductor, which is probably released by a mitogen. Thereafter, the target cells become responsive to organismal growth factors such as transferrin, resulting in aggregation of the mesenchymal cells and growth of the anlage. The second type of response involves the disappearance of interstitial proteins. These changes occur concomitantly with increased DNA synthesis. It has been suggested that several proteolytic enzymes are activated to digest components of the extacellular matrix. This event is thought to bring the mesenchymal cells of the blastema closer together. One matrix component, laminin, remains within and around the blastema and is thought to aid in cell-to-cell attachment. All these changes lead to aggregation of the mesenchymal cells. The third response is the enhanced synthesis of epithelial proteins. These proteins include components of the basement membrane, cell membranes, epithelial cells, cytoskeleton, and enzymes.

In principle, all nephrons are formed in the same way and can be classified into fairly well defined developmental stages [105] (Fig. 2-5). The first identifiable precursors of the nephron are cells of metanephric blastema that have formed a vesicle completely separated from the ureteric bud or ampulla [76,83,92,105]. Cells of the renal vesicle or stage I of nephron development are tall columnar in shape and measure about 15 μm in height. They face a narrow lumen and are surrounded by a basement membrane (Fig. 2-6). The cells of the vesicle become stabilized by their attachments to the newly formed basement membrane and by the development of lateral membrane junctions. The vesicle or stage I nephron differentiates to an S-shaped tubule or stage II nephron (Fig. 2-7) that connects to the dividing ureteric bud. At this stage, the first anlage of the glomerular capsule is recognized in the lowest limb of the S-shaped tubule, and the glomerular capsule is cup-shaped as demonstrated in serial sections. The rest of the S develops into the proximal tubule, the loop of Henle, and the distal tubule. When the cup-shaped glomerular capsule at stage II has matured to an oval structure (Figs. 2-8, 2-10), the nephron has passed into stage III of development. Now the nephron can be divided into an identifiable proximal tubule and a more primitive distal tubule, even though their appearances at both the light and electron microscopic levels markedly differ from those in the adult [105]. The stage IV nephron is characterized by a round to oval glomerulus (Figs. 2-9, 2-11) that closely resembles the mature renal corpuscle; however, it is smaller and the epithelial cells occupy a larger portion of the corpuscle than in the adult. Furthermore, the morphology of the proximal tubular portions of the nephron resembles that of the mature proximal tubule, despite differences at the subcellular level [105], whereas the distal segments are still primitive [37]. In most species the most mature nephrons of the newborn belongs to stage IV. In some species, e.g., the rat and mouse, all stages of nephron development are present at birth, whereas in others, e.g., the human and guinea pig, all nephrons at term are in varying steps of stage IV development. In all species examined, the juxtamedullary nephrons are those tubules that have formed

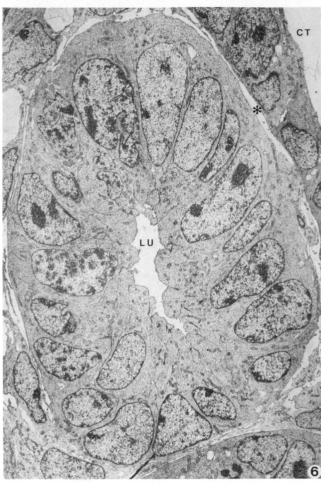

FIG. 2-6. *Survey picture of Stage I (renal vesicle). The cells are tall with large nuclei. The renal vesicle is separated from the collecting-tubule (CT) by a narrow zone with low electron density (*). Lumen (LU). Magnification ×4000 before a 43% reduction. (Reproduced from Larsson L: J Ultrastruct Res 51:119, 1975, with permission from Academic Press.)*

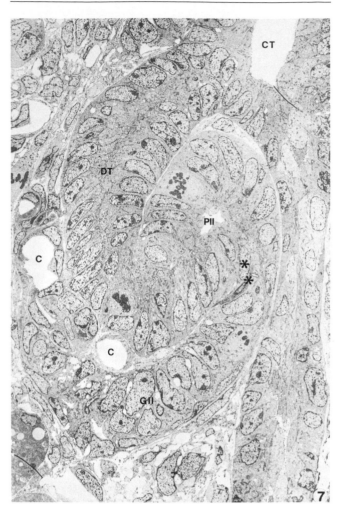

FIG. 2-7. *Survey picture of stage II (**S**-shaped body). This micrograph illustrates the level of nephron development at stage II. Note the proximal tubule anlage (PII); the distal tubule anlage (DT) is connected to the collecting tubule (CT). There are capillaries (C) in close proximity to the glomerular anlage (GII). Cells in the transitional zone between the proximal tubule anlage are marked with asterisks. Magnification ×2000 before a 40% reduction. (Reproduced from Larsson L: J Ultrastruct Res 51:119, 1975, with permission from Academic Press.)*

first and the superficial nephrons are the ones that have developed last, a pattern of development that results in a gradient of developmental stages throughout the kidney cortex. This feature of the developing kidney makes it difficult for one to perform functional studies on the whole kidney and then attempt to correlate structural and functional maturation [71].

Number and Size of Glomeruli

The number of nephrons in adult animals differs among species. The rat kidney contains about 30,000 nephrons [9,96,110,170,207]; the mouse kidney 12,000 [15,20]; the guinea pig kidney 75,000 to 100,000 [15,20] (a single study reports 42,000 [191]); the rabbit kidney 200,000 [100,170]; and the dog kidney 400,000 to 600,000 [51,72,100, 140,170,179,207]. The human kidney has been thought to contain approximately 1,000,000 [40,92,207], although a recent estimate* places the number at about 600,000. The number of nephrons in the developing kidney increases as long as the nephrogenic zone (e.g., the zone of stages I and II nephrons) persists. In man, the nephrogenic zone disappears at about the 32nd to 34th gestational week [154], in the rat at about the fifth postnatal day [105,110]. The complement of nephrons in man and guinea pig [191] is complete at birth. Several authors have shown that the number of the glomeruli remains constant in different species after the cessation of nephrogenesis [72,110,191]. There are also reports of renewed nephrogenesis postnatally

---

* by R. Osterby (unpublished data)

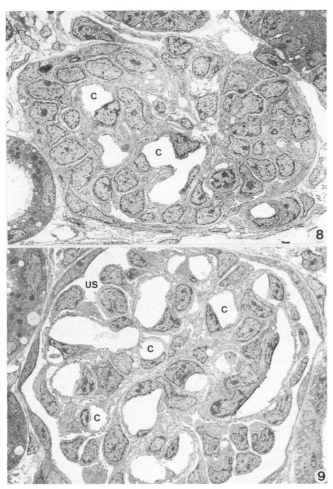

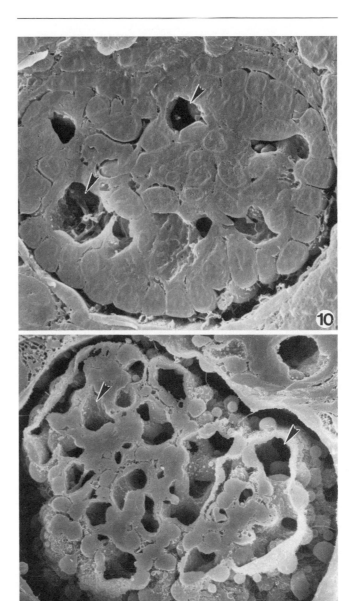

FIGS. 2-8 and 2-9. *Figure 2.8. Survey picture of a glomerulus in stage III. There are few capillaries (C) and the intercellular spaces of the glomerular epithelial cells are narrow. Magnification ×2200. (Reproduced from Larsson L: J Ultstruct Res 51:119, 1975, with permission from Academic Press.) Figure 2-9. Survey picture of a glomerulus in stage IV. At this stage there are many capillaries (C) in comparison to stage III, and the glomerular visceral epithelial cells at stage IV are separated to form in a larger urinary space (US) than in stage III (compare with Fig. 2-8). Magnification ×1300 before a 43% reduction. (Reproduced from Larsson L: J Ultrastruct Res 51:119, 1975, with permission from Academic Press.)*

FIGS. 2-10 and 2-11. *Scanning electron micrographs of developing glomeruli. Figure 2-10 shows a cryofractured stage III glomerulus. There are only a few capillary loops (arrowhead). Figure 2-11 shows a stage IV glomerulus that is characterized by a larger number of capillary loops than shown in Fig. 2-10. Magnification: Fig. 2-10 ×2500; Fig. 2-11 ×1500 before a 26% reduction.*

[20,28,81], but the studies may be flawed, as Chevalier [32] has recently shown that the technique of injection and maceration, as used in the studies, results in an underestimation of the number of glomeruli in a developing animal because the immature glomeruli are insufficiently vascularized.

Glomerular size increases during development in all species examined so far (Figs. 2-12–2-15). The diameter of a stage III rat glomerulus, the earliest developmental stage at which glomerular filtration takes place [108], is about 50 μm and that of a stage IV glomerulus in a three-day-old rat about 80 μm. Estimations of the diameters of superficial glomeruli in the adult rat vary between 110-140

μm [9,96,111,139]. In man, mature glomerular diameter is about 200 μm [193; see also 206 for references].

The size of the juxtamedullary nephron is of particular interest because there is evidence that these nephrons have a larger glomerular filtration (GFR) rate than do superficial nephrons [159]. At least among physiologists, it has been considered a fact that the juxtamedullary glomeruli are larger than the superficial ones. The reported results of studies are indeed conflicting. The most widely cited paper

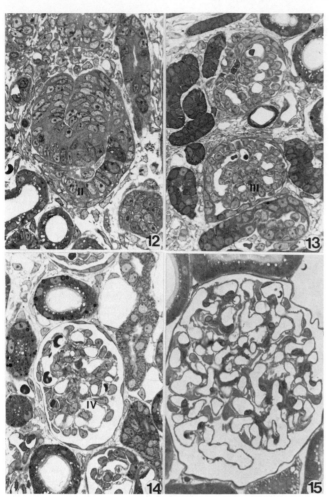

FIGS. 2-12, 2-13, 2-14, and 2-15. *Light micrographs from renal cortex of a 3-day-old and adult rat. The micrographs illustrate the histological appearance of different stages of the glomerular development. Figure 2-12 shows stage II, the **S**-shaped body (II); Fig. 2-13, stage III (III); Fig. 2-14, stage IV (IV), and Fig. 2-15, and mature superficial glomerulus. The glomerular diameter and number of capillary profiles increases during development. Magnification ×610 before 33% reduction. (Reproduced from Larsson L, Maunsbach AB: J Ultrastruct Res 72:392, 1980, with permission from Academic Press.)*

development. Particularly convincing is the study of human kidneys performed by Fetterman et al. [50], showing that the juxtamedullary and superficial glomeruli equalize at about five months. There are studies in other species showing the same pattern of maturation [96,111]; however, a recent study by Olivetti et al. [138] seems to show unequivocally that there is a significant difference between justamedullary (164 μm) and the superficial (114 μm) rat glomeruli, a difference that persists during maturation. The reason for these differing results is not clear, and systematic studies still need to be done over a wide range of ages and in different species.

Origin of Glomerular Capillaries

Initially, a vessel grows into the cleft between the lower and middle portion of the S-shaped tubule and quickly branches by a poorly understood process into a portal system. In the early 1900s, Huber [76] showed in his classical studies of renal development such a sequence of capillary development. Early electron microscopic [61,62,101, 102,116,194] and light microscopic studies [118], however, claimed an in situ development of the glomerular capillaries. These discrepancies are probably related to several major technical difficulties that were present in the early days of electron microscopy. First, it was extremely difficult to obtain ultrathin sections for analysis, and it was not possible to obtain serial sections. Thus, one could not obtain detailed three-dimensional reconstructions of the developing glomerulus. Second, it was not recognized that developing tissue is more difficult to preserve than mature tissue [105], and suboptimal cell preservation made ultrastructural analysis difficult. A more detailed discussion of this question appears elsewhere [153]. No doubt remains today that the glomerular capillaries arise from an ingrowth of capillaries into the glomerular anlage. This has been convincingly shown by light microscopy [76,154,218], electron microscopy [83], and microdissection studies [144]. It is also quite clear from the studies by Potter [153] and Osathanondh et al. [144] that there is always a connection between the afferent and efferent arterioles, which had previously been questioned [42,120].

Glomerular Development

The following description of glomerular development will follow the developmental stages already described. It is necessary to mention that Reeves et al. [156] used different terminology to describe the same developmental events: their vesicle stage corresponds to stage I, S-shaped stage to stage II, developing capillary loop stage to stage III, and maturing glomerulus stage to stage IV.

A crosssection of the cup-shaped glomerular anlage of stage II nephrons shows one to four capillaries (Figs. 2-7, 2-10, 2-12). Stage III glomeruli are oval in shape and, when sectioned through their equators, have five capillaries per cross-section (Figs. 2-8, 2-13). Then the number of capillary loops in the developing glomeruli appears to in-

describing a difference in size between juxtamedullary and superficial nephrons is that of Arataki [9]. Careful examination of his results, however, shows that the diameter of the juxtamedullary glomeruli in the albino rat was 129 μm, while that of the superficial glomeruli, was 119 μm. These values are probably not significantly different. There are some studies that clearly show a difference in size [63,64,139,221], but other reports, both older [96] and more recent [111,188], show no differences. During early maturation of the cortex the juxtamedullary glomeruli are undoubtedly larger than the superficial ones. Several studies indicate that the difference disappears during postnatal

crease gradually during maturation [105,111] (Figs. 2-9, 2-11, 2-14, 2-15).

Parietal Glomerular Epithelial Cells (Bowman's Capsule)

The transition between the stage I (renal vesicle) and stage II (S-shaped tubule) nephron is marked by the beginning of a cleft in the lateral wall of the stage I nephron. At this point, the presumptive cells of the Bowman's capsule change in shape from tall pyramidal to flattened (Figs. 2-6, 2-7, 2-13, 2-15). The cells develop different types of junctional complexes between each other, the most common being intermediate junctions and desmosomes [169]. Gap junctions and tight junctions have so far not been clearly shown in this epithelium. The paucity of tight junctions during development, as in the adult glomerulus [210], may indicate that this epithelium is highly permeable to small and large molecules [211], although some tight junctions are clearly present (Fig. 2-16). Permeability to large molecules [211] suggests that the tight junctions are not continuous. The parietal epithelial cells contain a large number of both free ribosomes and membrane-bound ribosomes, although little rough endoplasmic reticulum is seen. Scattered mitochondria, lysosomes, and vesicles are also observed. Bundles of microfilaments (Fig. 2-17) run parallel to the capsule in an arrangement suggesting that the parietal epithelial cells have a contractile function and can influence the hydrostatic pressure in the urinary space. The parietal cells change little during maturation, except for the alteration in cell shape.

Endothelial Cells

The question of whether the increase in glomerular size during maturation is accompanied by an increase in the number of endothelial cells (hyperplasia) or an increase in size of cells (hypertrophy) has been debated, because these cells are seldom seen in division. Olivetti et al. [138] have shown by morphometry that the size of rat glomerular endothelial cells remains unchanged, whereas the number of cells increases during the postnatal period between 15 and 50 days. Perhaps gradual endothelial cell enlargement occurs during earlier development.

The characteristic fenestrations or pores of the adult glomerular endothelial cells are rarely observed in stage II glomeruli [111,156,157,158] (Fig. 2-18). The endothelial wall is continuous and rather thick. During stage III, fenestrations are still few (Figs. 2-19, 2-21), although more abundant than at stage II. Then the number of endothelial fenestrations appears to increase gradually during development (Figs. 2-20, 2-22). The pores, as observed in grazing sections, are round, about 10 nm in diameter, and sometimes covered by one or two diaphragms (see Fig. 2-25) [111,112].* The shape and size of the fenestrations remain unchanged during glomerular maturation, but they are always unevenly distributed. During glomerular development the number of fenestrae in the free glomerular capillary wall, where the endothelial cells face the glomerular epithelial cells, is 6 to 10 times higher than in the portion of endothelium facing the mesangium [111].

* Also supported by Larsson L, Aperia A, Maunsbach AB: Unpublished observation.

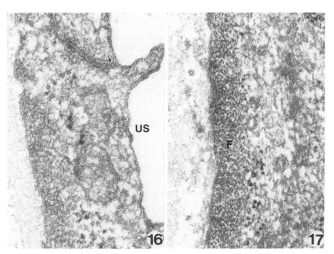

FIGS. 2-16 and 2-17. *Figure 2-16. Parts of two adjacent glomerular parietal epithelial cells in a superficial glomerulus, showing the appearance of a five-layered junctional complex, tight junction (arrow). Urinary space (US). Magnification ×10,000 before a 33% reduction. Figure 2-17. Part of a glomerular parietal epithelial cell of an adult superficial glomerulus showing many cross-sectioned fibrils (F). Magnification ×76,000 before a 33% reduction.*

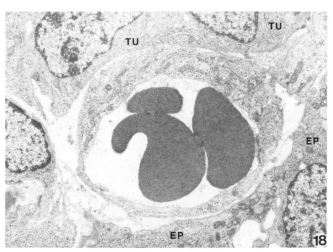

FIG. 2-18. *Cross-sectioned capillary from stage II glomerular anlage (S-shaped) body. At this stage, there are no endothelial fenestrae observed in the developing glomerulus. Epithelial cells (EP); tubular cells (TU). Magnification ×9500 before a 38% reduction. (Reproduced from Larsson L, Maunsbach AB: J Ultrastruct Res 72:392, 1980, with permission from Academic Press.)*

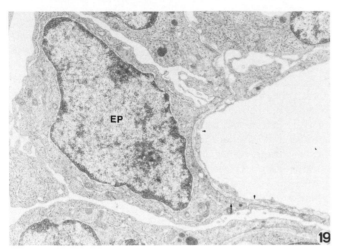

FIG. 2-19. *Part of a glomerular capillary from a stage III glomerulus. At this stage of glomerular development, only a few endothelial fenestrae are seen (arrow heads). Note that the endothelium in this stage is thinner than in stage II (see Fig. 2-18). One foot process is seen (arrow). Epithelial cell (EP). Magnification ×9500 before a 38% reduction. (Reproduced from Larsson L, Maunsbach AB: J Ultrastruct Res 72:392, 1980, with permission from Academic Press.)*

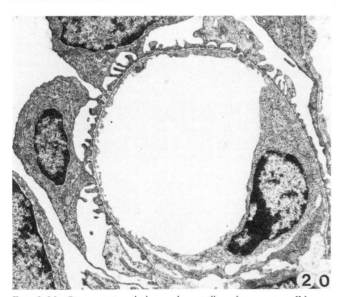

FIG. 2-20. *Cross-sectioned glomerular capillary from a stage IV glomerulus. The number of endothelial fenestrae and epithelial foot processes are increased in comparison to previous developmental stages (compare with Figs. 2-18 and 2-19). Magnification ×11500 before a 27% reduction. (Reproduced from Larsson L, Maunsbach AB: J Ultrastruct Res 72:392, 1980, with permission from Academic Press.)*

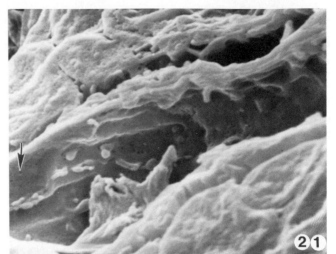

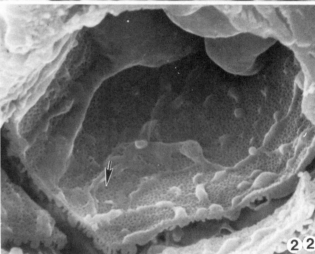

FIGS. 2-21 and 2-22. *Scanning electron micrograph of developing glomerular endothelium. Stage III glomeruli (Fig. 2-21) have few endothelial fenestrae (arrow), while stage IV glomeruli (Fig. 2-22) possess numerous endothelial fenestrae (arrow). Magnification: Fig. 2-21 ×16,500; Fig. 2-22 ×15,000 before a 35% reduction.*

With the increase in number of fenestrae occurring from stage III to adulthood (Figs. 2-23–2-25), there is a sixfold enlargement in the total fenestral surface area. The total fenestral area for one adult glomerulus is about 2×10^4 μm^2 [111]. Little is known about the process by which these pores are formed.

The increase in endothelial pore area during maturation of the nephron may have at least two functional implications. First, it is very probable that this change alters the hydraulic conductivity of the glomerular capillary wall and thereby alters also the GFR. Second, it is also possible that this morphologic change increases endothelial cell permeability to larger molecules, such as proteins. The marked increase in endothelial pore number during development parallels changes in the glomerular basement membrane (GBM; see the next section), which is initially thin and then thicker. Reeves et al. showed that anionic sites are

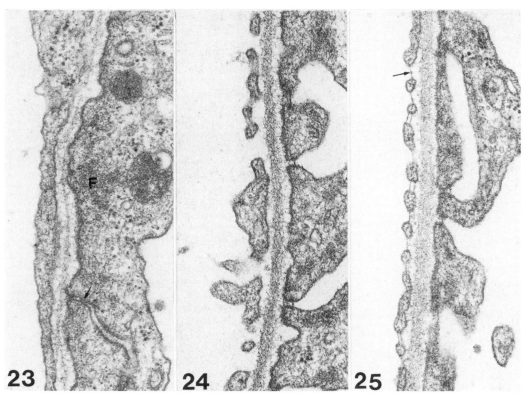

Figs. 2-23, 2-24, and 2-25. *Fig. 2-23. Part of glomerular capillary at stage III of development. At this stage of glomerular development, the endothelium is continuous and the GBM and its three layers are thin. Adjacent cells are sometimes connected by five-layered occluding membrane complexes (arrow). The epithelial cells contain bundles of filaments (F). Magnification ×57,000. Fig. 2-24. Part of glomerular capillary at stage IV of development. At stage IV there are several endothelial fenestrae and in particular the lamina densa of the GBM is thicker than in stage III (compare with Fig. 2-23). Magnification ×57,600. Fig. 2-25. Part of a superficial glomerular capillary from an adult rat. The endothelial fenestrae are numerous and covered by one or two diaphragms. The diaphragms sometimes exhibit a central knob-like structure (arrow). Magnification ×57,600. (Reproduced from Larsson L, Maunsbach AB: J Ultrastruc Res 72:392, 1980, with permission from Academic Press.)*

present on endothelial cell surfaces during glomerular capillary development but not in later stages [157,158]. These sites disappear from the endothelial cell coat as the cells become more fenestrated. Conversely, the GBM concurrently acquires anionic sites that probably act as barriers to the passage of anionic proteins [29,48]. Thus, the immature thick endothelium, with its small endothelial pore area, protects the body from losing proteins such as albumin during the period when the GBM is immature and lacks anionic sites. The tracer experiments of Webber and Blackbourn showed that ferritin did pass the immature endothelial cell layer of the glomerular capillaries but to a much lesser degree than in the mature glomerulus [211].

Glomerular Basement Membrane

The GBM is composed of three layers, a central thick electron dense layer, called the *lamina densa*, and two outer, thinner, less dense layers called the *lamina rara*

interna and the *lamina rara externa*. The thickness of the GBM varies among species. The thickness in adult humans is about 300 nm [84,113,145,197], in the mouse about 120 nm [160], and in the rat 115 nm [111,115]. The lamina densa is the thickest of the three layers and is about 65 nm in the rat. At the ultrastructural level, the GBM contains filaments of variable thickness in all three layers [113,164,197]. The major components are collagen type IV, laminin, fibronectin, and proteoglycans rich in heparan sulfate [87,95,197]. Several morphologic changes in the GBM are apparent during development of the glomerulus. During stage II, when the capillaries are first growing into the cleft of the nephron anlage, there are separate endothelial and epithelial basement membranes (see Fig. 2-18) that fuse into a single glomerular basement membrane in stage III (see Fig. 2-19). Thus, from a morphologic point of view, it seems quite clear that at least the initial GBM has dual origin from both endothelial and epithelial cells. Sariola et al. used a hybrid glomerulus developed in vitro from murine nephrogenic cells and chick or quail chorioal-

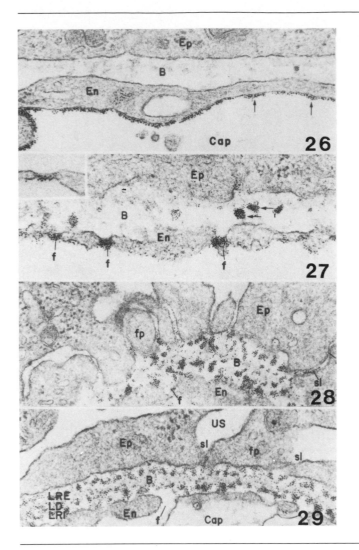

Figs. 2-26, 2-27, 2-28, and 2-29. *Distribution of cationized ferritin (CF) in developing early, middle, and late stage III glomeruli. The terminology used in these micrographs to describe capillary loop stage was established by Reeves et al: (J Cell Biol 85:735, 1980). Figure 2-26 shows that before the development of endothelial fenestrae CF binds in a patchy distribution (arrows) to the luminal side of the endothelium (En) and does not reach the GBM (B) or epithelium (Ep). A capillary lumen is marked (Cap). In Fig. 2-27, endothelial fenestrae (f) have appeared and CF binds in large amounts to the diaphragms that close these early fenestrae. Small amounts of CF are also found in the GBM (B), binding in clumps to large proteoglycan particles (arrows). CF gains entry to the GBM either through open fenestrae (lacking diaphragms) or through open junctions between endothelial cells located outside the plane of the section. The inset (upper left) shows another fenestra with bound CF in which the diaphragm is clearly visible. In Fig. 2-28, open fenestrae are present (f), and CF has gained access to the GBM (B) and the intercellular spaces between developing foot processes (fp). Considerable CF is bound to anionic sites in the GBM. At this stage, many of the epithelial sites are sealed by focal occluding junctions (j) that are located at some distance from the GBM. A filtration slit is marked (sl). In Fig. 2-29, open fenestrae (f) are more frequent, and the GBM has organized into its three characteristic layers. CF binds to anionic sites concentrated in the lamina rara interna (LRI) and externa (LRE). Epithelial foot processes (fp) and filtration slits (sl) are present at this stage. Note that no CF is seen within the urinary space (US) or binding to the epithelial (Ep) surfaces. Binding to the endothelium (En) is minimal, compared to previous stages. Cap, capillary lumen; LD, lamina densa. Magnification: Figs. 2-26, 2-27, and 2-28 ×75,000; Fig. 2-29 ×54,000; inset ×110,000 before a 13% reduction. (Reproduced from Reeves WH, Kanwar YS, Farquhar M: J Cell Biol 85:735, 1980, with permission from the authors and The Rockefeller University Press.)*

lantoic capillaries to demonstrate by immunohistochemistry that the GBM consisted of components derived from both endothelial and epithelial cells [171]. Both cell types probably contribute throughout life to the synthesis of the GBM, and mesangial cells may also be involved.

Increasing thickness of the GBM during development is mainly due to an increased thickness of the lamina densa (Figs. 2-23–2-25). As the number of capillary loops in the glomerulus increases during development, the area of the GBM increases [82,98,111]. Larsson and Maunsbach [111] measured the GBM area facing endothelial cells at different developmental stages and found the surface area of GBM to increase 54 times between stage II and adult glomeruli. The total area of the GBM in two kidneys of a three-day-old rat was 5.6 cm² and in an adult animal 157 cm² [111]. The latter value corresponds well with 168 cm² obtained by Østerby et al. [148]. Furthermore, the estimation of relative GBM area [111] (0.164 $\mu m^2/\mu m^3$ glomerular volume) is close to that reported by Olivetti et al. (0.177 $\mu m^2/\mu m^3$ glomerular volume) [139]. Other studies, however, indicate a higher relative GBM area (area/glomerular volume) in the adult rat. Shea and Morrison reported 0.229 $\mu m^2/\mu m^3$ [180] and Pinto and Brewer 0.232 $\mu m^2/\mu m^3$ [150]. The different results may be due to technical differences and to the use of different strains of rats.

Obviously the increase in GBM area during development affects the glomerular filtration rate. Reeves et al. [157,158] have shown an increase in the number of GBM anionic sites during development of the glomerulus from stage II to stage IV (Figs. 2-26–2-29). These anionic sites correspond to heparan sulphate [87,88,89]. Other biochemical changes in the GBM take place during development [103,184]. These maturational changes probably affect the permeability of the GBM.

Visceral Glomerular Epithelial Cells (Podocytes)

The development of the visceral glomerular epithelial cells has been described by transmission electron microscopy in mouse [33,160], rat [32,61,62,83,92,111,112,138,139,

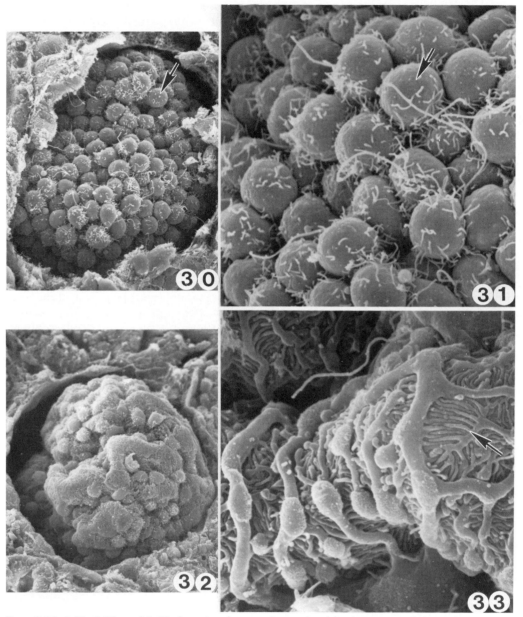

FIGS. 2-30, 2-31, 2-32, and 2-33. *Scanning electron micrographs of developing visceral glomerular epithelium. Figures 2-30 and 2-31 show the visceral epithelium (arrow) of a stage III glomerulus as seen by scanning electron microscopy. The cells are cuboidal to columnar in shape and are densely positioned around the capillaries' loops like bunches of grapes. They also lack primary processes and terminal pedicels. Figures 2-32 and 2-33 show the degree of visceral epithelial development characteristic of stage IV. These cells are flattened and possess numerous large and small foot processes, but still lack the number and preciseness of the pedicels (arrow) that mark the adult glomerulus. Magnification: Fig. 2-30 ×1350; Fig. 2-31 ×5000; Fig. 2-32 ×800; Fig. 2-33 ×7200 before a 14% reduction.*

156,174,194, 196,211,216,217],[*] rabbit [116], puppy [65], pig [16,53], cow [27], and human [1,3,101,102,204,205] and by scanning electron microscopy in rat [25,67,

[*] Also supported by Larsson L, Aperia A, Maunsbach AB: Unpublished observation.

93,94,189] and dog [46,54]. Work performed before 1971 has previously been reviewed [39,92,203,206] and will not be included here. The development of the glomerular visceral epithelial cell is characterized by a gradual increase in the frequency of foot processes (Figs. 2-30–2-33; see also Figs. 2-19–2-25), resulting in a separation of adjacent cell bodies that were initially closely apposed (see Figs. 2-13, 2-14). The relative volume of epithelial cells per glomerulus simultaneously decreases [138]. During late postnatal development in the rat (about 15–50 days), the number of visceral epithelial cells seems to be constant, while the size of the cells significantly increases [138]. The increase in the number of epithelial foot processes naturally results in an increase in the number of epithelial slits (see Figs. 2-23–2-25) and enlarges the surface area possessed by the epithelial slits. From stage III to stage IV there is a 50-fold increase in total epithelial slit area and a further tenfold increase from stage IV to the adult rat glomerulus. We have determined that the total epithelial slit surface area is 2.5×10^4 μm^2/glomerulus and 15.3 cm^2/animal, a figure close to the value of 11.4 cm^2 observed by Shea and Morrison [180]. The development of the epithelial slits precedes that of the endothelial pores. Thus, the area of the epithelial slits/GBM area in stage IV has reached 80% of that in the adult glomerulus, whereas the endothelial pore area/glomerulus only is about 45% of that in the adult. It seems reasonable to assume that the differentiation of both the endothelial pores and the epithelial slit areas are important for the maturation of GBM permeability and hydraulic conductivity.

The cells of the glomerular anlage in stage II nephrons resemble very much the cells of stage I (see Fig. 2-7). They are columnar in shape and possess large nuclei, few mitochondria, numerous free ribosomes, some membrane-bound ribosomes, a Golgi apparatus, and some lysosomes and vesicles.

At stage I, adjacent cells are connected by tight junctions located close to their luminal surfaces [106]. However, the cell contacts seen at stage II appear to have migrated from their original apical positions toward the capillary side of the epithelium. Thus, the cell junctions are found at varying distances from the glomerular capillaries [3,77,156]. These tight junctions in stages III and IV glomeruli are found between epithelial foot processes only where a slit diaphragm is not present (see Fig. 2-23). By stage IV and later, the tight junction-like cell contacts are infrequent, having been replaced by slit diaphragms (see Figs. 2-24, 2-25). During the migration of the cell contacts, the cell coats on the lateral surfaces of these epithelial cells become stainable with colloidal iron, indicating the appearance of polyanions (sialoproteins). At stage IV, the stain becomes more concentrated at the level of the slits [156,157]. The appearance of the polyanions at the slits suggests an involvement of these polyanions in regulating the passage of molecules through the epithelial slits (see Fig. 2-23). Moreover, the polyanions may function in maintaining the shape of the foot processes [128], because it has been shown that neutralization of these sites with polycations (protamine sulphate and poly-L-lysine) reduces the number of foot processes [178].

The studies by Rodewald and Karnovsky [164] in tissue treated with tannic acid showed a porous structure to the epithelial slit region in the adult glomerulus, an observation confirmed in stage IV rat glomeruli [111]. Thus, the structural organization of the epithelial slit area appears to have matured by stage IV. The visceral epithelial cells of stage III glomeruli contain a large number of microfilaments preferentially located in the foot processes, suggesting that the cells have contractile properties. There seems to be no dramatic change in number and location of these filaments during development.

Mesangial Cells

The mesangium and mesangial cells were first described by Zimmermann in 1933 [220], but the cells were not generally accepted as a separate line until 1960, when they were studied in detail by electron microscopy [49,114,115]. Mesangial cells are located at the centers of glomerular capillary clusters, and they lie in close proximity to endothelial cells and the GBM. They are iregular in shape, possessing many cytoplasmic processes that can extend between the GBM and the endothelial cells (Fig. 2-34). Under normal conditions mesangial cells never form a continous layer between the endothelial cells and the GBM. It is not possible to derive a specific function for the mesangial cell from simply an appreciation of the number and distribution of the cell organelles. These cells in the rat [49,113] and human fetus [205] have been shown to have the capacity of phagocytizing macromolecules. The presence of microfilaments suggests a contractile function, and cultured cells of probable mesangial origin contract in the presence of angiotensin II [11]. Mesangial cell contraction is believed to regulate the diameters of glomerular capillaries and thereby the area of filtering surface. A decreased filtration coefficient in glomeruli exposed to angiotensin II has been attributed to mesangial cell contraction [79], but results of scanning electron microscopy [69] are difficult to interpret. Mesangial cells are also capable of producing cytokines and prostaglandins, and they participate in glomerular inflammatory reactions.

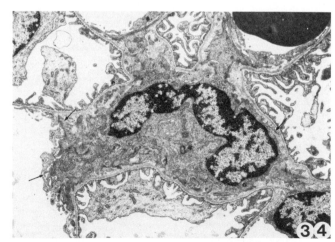

FIG. 2-34. *A glomerular mesangial cell from an adult superficial glomerulus. There are many cytoplasmic protrusions of the cell (arrows). Magnification* ×8000 *before a 27% reduction.*

Mesangial cells do not originate from the metanephrogenic cells [17]. It is not known whether they originate from the glomerular capillaries as smooth muscle–like cells or from undifferentiated mesenchymal cells. By stage II both mesangial cells and glomerular capillaries are seen in the cleft of the nephron anlage, but no smooth muscle cells are present [83,92]. Perhaps, therefore, the mesangial cell originates from undifferentiated mesenchymal cells rather than from vascular smooth muscle cells. During late postnatal development in the rat (around 15–50 days), mesangial cells increase both in number and size [138]; however, similar studies have not been performed for the earlier stages of glomerular development.

Recent immunohistochemical data suggest that there may be two types of mesangial cells in the adult glomerulus [176]. So far similar studies have not been performed during development of the kidney.

Juxtaglomerular Apparatus

The juxtaglomerular apparatus is composed of both granular and agranular juxtaglomerular cells. These cells are found between the afferent and efferent arterioles and within the walls of these arterioles [14,113] (Fig. 2-35). Recently, another group of granulated cells, called the peripolar cells, have been found in sheep as cuffs around the vascular poles [168]; they also belong to the juxtaglomerular apparatus.

The development of the juxtaglomerular apparatus has not been studied as extensively as have other aspects of glomerular development. Kazimierczak [92] found, in studying the early development of the juxtaglomerular apparatus in the pig, rat, and human that it was not possible by either light or electron microscopy to recognize the juxtaglomerular apparatus before stage III. Granulated cells

can be recognized by stage III in the walls of the afferent and efferent arterioles, and cells of the future macula densa are recognizable. At the same time, cells similar in shape to future mesangial cells appear in the region between afferent and efferent arterioles at the vascular pole. The granular cells acquire increased numbers of granules as cells of the macula densa acquire a mature appearance (Fig. 2-36). Kazimierczak's observations have been repeatedly confirmed in a variety of species [22,26,43,45,90,91,123 125,128,129,131,165,175,185,193,201]. It is of interest that renin first appears in the developing fetal mouse kidney in interlobular arteries and later in the afferent arterioles [130].

Although renin has been suspected for a long time to be localized in granules [56] of the juxtaglomerular cells, it has been confirmed by direct evidence only recently [195]. Renin content is low during fetal life in most species, but increases prior to delivery and reaches its maximal concentration during the first days of postnatal life [12, 21,57,68,99,132,147,151,181,183,200,209]. The only exception is seen in the rabbit, in which renin continuously increases during maturation; however, there seems to be no correlation between plasma renin activity and the number of granules in the cells. Therefore, during nephron development the juxtaglomerular granular index is not a good measure of renin activity. Peripolar cells appear to contain more granules during nephron maturation than in the adult condition, but the content of these granules is not known [167]. The high renin content in the developing animal may be responsible for the high renal vascular resistance present in the immature kidney.

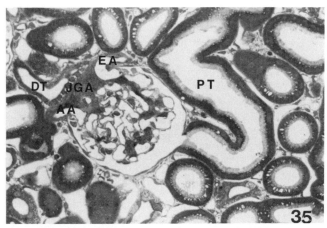

FIG. 2-35. This low-magnification light micrograph shows a glomerulus with its juxtaglomerular apparatus (JGA). Proximal tubule (PT), distal tubule (DT), afferent arteriole (AA), efferent arteriole (EA). Magnification ×500 before a 20% reduction.

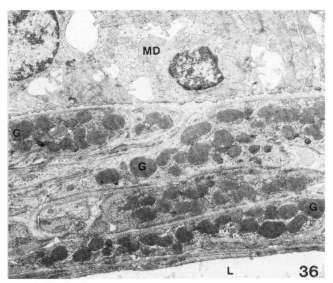

FIG. 2-36. Part of the juxtaglomerular apparatus in an adult rat showing the macula densa (MD) of the distal tubule and granular cells containing a large number of granules (G) in the wall of the afferent arteriole lumen (L). Magnification ×9000 before a 30% reduction.

Structural and Functional Correlations

Both whole kidney and single nephron GFR increase during maturation. This change has been shown during the postnatal period in the rat [3,7,13,35,36,44,74,78,80,117, 152,155,186,187,202], the dog [8,70,75,86], the guinea pig [127,191,192], the pig [23,52,146], and humans [4,5,59,60,166,182], and in the sheep during both the fetal [24,161,162] and the postnatal periods [6,163]. The maturation of the GFR has previously been summarized [41,123,126,133,190,217].

The direct determinant of GFR is the effective filtration pressure, i.e., the glomerular capillary oncotic pressure and proximal tubular hydrostatic pressure. Furthermore, GFR is proportional to the glomerular filtration coefficient (K_f), which is the product of the hydraulic conductivity of the glomerular capillary per unit area and the effective area used for filtration. Indirectly, the GFR depends on the glomerular plasma flow, which determines the glomerular capillary oncotic pressure and thereby affects the effective filtration pressure.

Before discussing the individual factors that affect the development of the GFR it is appropriate to make some comments on the anatomy of the filtration area. The filtration area has usually been considered to be the area of the GBM facing both the endothelial and epithelial cells. Recent studies by Bohman et al., however, suggest that the epithelial (podocyte) slit area is the actual filtering area [19]. They determined the GFR in children with minimal change nephrotic syndrome and analyzed renal biopsies from the same children by morphometry. They found a direct correlation between the frequency of glomerular epithelial foot processes and GFR. The frequency of epithelial foot processes can be considered to represent the epithelial slit areas because an increase in the number of foot processes results in an increased number and a larger area of epithelial slits.

It is also necessary to consider whether the filtration process is in a state of equilibrium or disequilibrium. If filtration equilibrium is present during maturation, K_f cannot be determined. If, on the other hand, filtration disequilibrium is the case, it is possible to assess K_f and thereby to estimate the influence on the GFR by changes in filtration area and hydraulic permeability (see Chap. 3).

During the development of the kidney, several changes of the physiologic parameters just discussed take place and affect the GFR. The increases seen in both glomerular capillary hydrostatic pressure [44,192] and renal plasma flow [6,7,10,58,97,197] increase the GFR during development.

It is difficult to evaluate the importance to increasing GFR of changes in K_f, i.e., filtering area and hydraulic permeability, during glomerular maturation because it is not completely known when and if the process of glomerular filtration is in a state of disequilibrium in different species. The 24-day-old Sprague-Dawley rat is in a state of filtration equilibrium, whereas the mature animal (40 days old) is in disequilibrium [214]. Therefore, it is reasonable to suggest that filtration equilibrium in these animals is present up to an age of 24 days. It is not possible before that age to estimate the influence on GFR by changes in

K_f because it is not possible to determine the proportion of available filtering area that is used. Indirect evidence suggests, however, that the glomerular filtration ceases well before the end of the glomerular capillary, because the increase in total surface area of GBM is far less than the increase in GFR during the first three weeks of postnatal development [109,112]. This conclusion seems to be valid also if one considers the filtration area to be the epithelial slit area, because the epithelial slit area per GBM area increases very little during the same period [111]. This is further supported by the observation that young Sprague-Dawley rats in filtration equilibrium increase their GFR more than can adult rats in filtration disequilibrium when subjected to volume expansion after hydropenia [44,214]. Thus, it is possible at filtration equilibrium to use an increased proportion of the available filtration area by increasing the renal plasma flow, thereby slowing the rise in glomerular capillary oncotic pressure and increasing effective filtration. Therefore, an increase in renal plasma flow causes a larger increase in GFR at filtration equilibrium than at disequilibrium. In order for us to link a developmental increase in GFR of the magnitude observed to an increase in renal plasma flow, however, there must be an increase in the total available filtering surface area. Otherwise, glomerular filtration should turn from equilibrium to disequilibrium rather quickly during development, and the GFR would not increase to the same degree because changes in glomerular plasma flow are not as effective at filtration disequilibrium in elevating the GFR as they are during filtration equilibrium.

Filtration equilibrium in the Spraque-Dawley rat turns to disequilibrium somewhere between the twenty-fourth and fortieth day of age [214]. Thus, K_f can be theoretically estimated within this period, and its possible influence on the development of the GFR can be determined. During this period there is only a minor increase in hydrostatic pressure (25%) along the glomerular capillary [44], whereas the renal plasma flow increases by a factor of two [7]. Futhermore, the total GBM area per glomerulus increases by a factor of 1.6 [109]. Because the single nephron GFR increases by a factor of six [214,218], it seems very likely that the hydraulic permeability is changing and thereby increasing K_f and GFR. A postnatal increase in hydraulic permeability might be structurally related to the increase seen in both the endothelial pores and the filtration slit area [111]. Other factors, such as the chemical composition of the GBM (i.e., number of anionic sites) [156,157,158], may affect the hydraulic permeability. It is also likely that changes in hydraulic permeability may take place without accompanying ultrastructural changes, because it has been shown that the hydraulic permeability can change during different experimental conditions in the same animal. The work of Wolgast et al. [214] has shown that in the Sprague-Dawley rats, in which filtration disequilibrium is apparent, the conditions of volume expansion did not increase single nephron GFR as one would have predicted from changes in renal plasma flow and effective filtration pressure, thus indicating a decreased hydraulic permeability. The possibility exists, however, that during filtration disequilibrium there is a change in the filtering area as a result of mesangial contraction, which would reduce the diameter of the glomerular capillaries. There is, however, still no direct evidence for such a mechanism other than the observation that mesangial cells cultured in vitro have contractile properties.

It is possible that vascular shunts, which have been demonstrated in the mature glomerulus between the afferent and efferent arteriole [30,121], may also be important for the development of the GFR. Shunts have not, however, been unequivocally shown to be present during the development of the glomerulus.

In summary, we believe that increased vascular resistance during the early phases of glomerular development gives rise to a low glomerular plasma flow. This condition results in filtration equilibrium and probably a low degree of utilization of the available filtration area, thereby explaining the initially low GFR. As vascular resistance decreases during the development of the glomerulus, the resulting increase in glomerular plasma flow allows plasma to be filtered through a larger proportion of the glomerular filtration area. Increments in effective filtration pressure, as well as in hydraulic permeability, can partially explain the developmental increase in GFR. The relative importance of the increased filtration surface area as a determinant of the GFR is difficult to quantify because glomerular filtration equilibrium is present during the early period of glomerular development, at least in the Sprague-Dawley rat [82,111,112].

Development of the Proximal Tubule

The proximal tubule develops through a series of predictable stages (Figs. 2-37, 2-38). An anlage of the future proximal tubule is first identifiable in the stage II S-shaped body [83,92] (see Figs. 2-6, 2-7, 2-12). The upper end of the S has joined an ampulla of the collecting duct, and the lower blind end of the S has thinned to form the two layers of the developing glomerulus. Between these two ends of the S-shaped body, three separate regions or limbs (upper, middle, and lower) are arbitrarily identified. It is the lower limb that becomes the proximal tubule.

The cells of the proximal tubular anlage at stage II are characteristically columnar in shape (15 μm in height), with narrow intercelluar spaces (see Figs. 2-7, 2-12) [105]. The apical cell surfaces each possess a solitary cilium, while the lateral cell membranes run parallel to each other. The ovoid nucleus with its many infoldings is located toward the base of the cell. These cells possess few organelles, and they are greatly reduced in number and volume when compared to adult cells. Only a few profiles of the rough and smooth endoplasmic reticulum are present. Lysosomes are also few in number and small (0.5 μm in diameter). These cells contain numerous microtubules (24 nm in diameter), however, singly or in bundles. Most microtubules are located in the apical half of the cell and are oriented perpendicular to the basement membrane. A thin basement membrane (0.4 μm in thickness) surrounds all cells that constitute the S-shaped body. The entire length of the tubule possesses a lumen that is continuous with a cortical collecting duct (see Fig. 2-50). Tracer studies suggest that the cells that form this early anlage are highly permeable and therefore possess "open tight junctions" [106].

By stage III, a distinct proximal tubule has developed (Figs. 2-39–2-41). It is extremely short, and all the proximal tubular cells appear morphologically similar. In comparison with the proximal tubular cells of stage II, the proximal tubular cells of stage III have a decreased height,

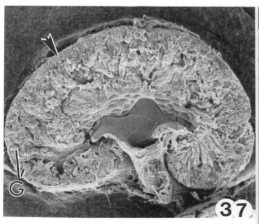
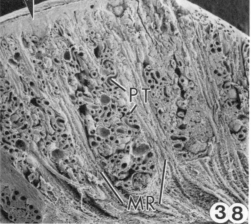

FIGS. 2-37 and 2-38. *Developing renal cortex. Figure 2-37 shows the primitive cortex and medulla of a kidney from a 44-day-old dog fetus. A prominent nephrogenic zone (arrowhead) is present at the kidney capsule, while the thickness of the entire cortex is occupied by only glomeruli (G). By birth, Fig. 2-38, multiple layers of glomeruli and numerous profiles of the proximal tubule are seen (PT); however, a nephrogenic zone (arrowhead) is still present. At this time, the medullary rays (MR) are distinct. Magnification: Fig. 2-37 ×23; Fig. 2-38 ×80 before a 14% reduction.*

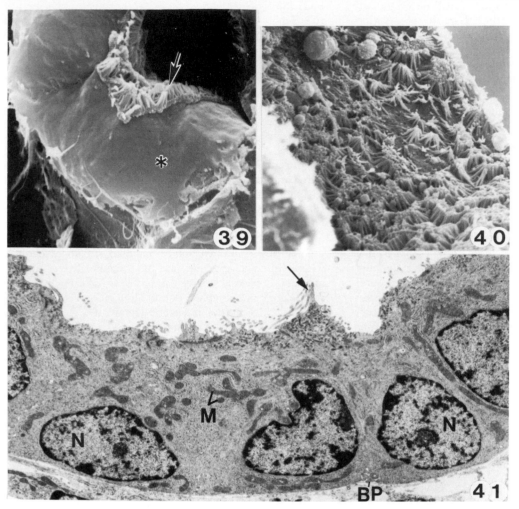

FIGS. 2-39, 2-40, and 2-41. *Stage III proximal tubule development. Figure 2-39 shows morphological features of several stage III proximal tubular cells. The apical surface has a few short microvilli (arrow), while the lateral cell surface is smooth (*). Figure 2-40 shows the paucity of apical microvilli. By transmission electron microscopy (Fig. 2-41), these cells are characterized by a simple shape with few apical microvilli (arrow), small mitochondria (M), large nucleus (N) and limited basolateral processes (BP). Magnification: Fig. 2-39 ×6300; Fig. 2-40 ×3750; Fig. 2-41 ×6500 before a 14% reduction.*

whereas the tubular lumen is increased. Ultrastructurally, these cells characteristically have (1) a simple cuboidal shape, (2) few short apical microvilli, (3) round to elongated mitochondria, (4) irregularly shaped basal processes, (5) elaborate cisternae of rough endoplasmic reticulum, (6) a prominent Golgi apparatus, (7) few lateral interdigitating processes, (8) moderate numbers of small and large endocytic vacuoles, and (9) lysosomes of about 1 μm in diameter (Fig. 2-41) [105,109]. Several lysosomal enzymes (acid phosphatase, acid beta-galactosidase, N-acetylglucosaminidase, and dipeptidylaminopeptidase) are already present [136]. Concomitant with the appearance of apical microvilli are brush border enzymes such as alkaline phosphatase, alpha-glutamyltranspeptidase, and dipeptidylaminopeptidase [136]. There appears to be a reduction in the number of microtubules. Morphometric analysis of the proximal

tubular cells shows a significant increase in mitochondrial volume percent (6.9%) and apical cell area (0.18 μm^2/μm^3) when compared with stage II cells. These changes may indicate an increased energy requirement for cellular processes, such as electrolyte transport.

By stage III, tracer studies show the region of the tight junctions of the developing proximal tubular cells to be less permeable to macromolecules than at stages I and II [106]. In addition, Horster and Larsson [73] suggested that these tubules have a hydraulic conductivity sevenfold higher than that of mature proximal tubules. They also noted that net fluid transport increased when the immature proximal tubules were exposed to an increased protein-osmotic peritubular environment. These data suggest "open tight junctions" but also indicate decreased dominance of paracellular pathway flow relative to transcellular pathway flow [119]. Linshaw and Welling [119] have also considered changes in basolateral membrane hydraulic conductivity with maturation of the proximal tubular cells. They noted that estimations of basolateral membrane hydraulic conductivity did not change when basolateral membrane surface area for immature and mature proximal tubular cells was expressed per unit length of tubule. They concluded that maturation of the proximal tubule from the postnephrogenic period to adulthood was the result of an increase in basolateral membrane surface area and that the intrinsic property of hydraulic conductivity per unit membrane remained constant.

By stage IV, the developing proximal tubule can be divided into the three segments, S1, S2, and S3, characteristic of the adult tubule [47,66,105] (Figs. 2-42–2-44). The cells of the immature S1 segment have (1) an elaborate brush border that is about 1.1 μm in height, (2) elongated mitochondria that occupy 13.5% of cell volume and are aligned parallel to the lateral cell processes, (3) many endocytic vacuoles, (4) prominent basal villi, (5) basolateral processes that extend half the cell height, and (6) numerous lysosomes and microbodies. There is more than a 20% increase in the apical membrane area as a result of increased length and density of the apical microvilli. Cell membrane area has increased threefold.

The S2 segment appears as a short connecting piece between S1 and S3 and is characterized by cells that have (1) an elaborate brush border, (2) limited basolateral interdigitations, (3) distinct basal villi, (4) irregularly shaped mitochondria, and (5) many lysosomes. The cells of the S3 segment are ultrastructurally similar to the cells described at stage III, discussed earlier.

We stated earlier in this chapter that nephron growth follows a centrifugal pattern and that the oldest nephrons are located in the inner cortex, the youngest beneath the kidney capsule. In order to determine the level of development of the various nephron populations in newborn rabbits, Evan et al. [47] examined the morphologic maturation of the proximal tubules obtained from precise cortical levels (outer, middle, and inner). These tubules were identified by microdissection and whole tissue section analyses. At one week, a nephrogenic zone was still present in the outer cortex, with nephrons at stages I and II of development, and only the inner cortical proximal tubules showed structural evidence of segmentation (beyond stage IV). The middle cortical proximal tubules had undergone segmentation by the second postnatal week, whereas the outer cortical tubules did not show morphologic evidence of segmentation until the third week. These data lead one to predict that each nephron will mature during the newborn period at a rate consistent with the chronological age of the animal and that the inner cortical nephrons will reach maturity many weeks ahead of the outer cortical nephrons. In this same study, morphometric analysis showed the inner cortical proximal tubules to be morphologically mature by the third to fourth postnatal week. The middle cortical proximal tubules reached maturity by 34 to 40 days postnatally, however, and the outer cortical proximal tubules by 40 to 48 days. These data strongly support the concept of centrifugal development and maturation,

the inner cortical proximal tubules reaching the adult level well before the outer cortical tubules.

In contrast, however, is the recent thesis of Welling and Linshaw [213], who collected structural and functional data suggesting that developing proximal tubules may not mature at a steady rate but that they enter a quiescent phase after reaching a moderate level of maturity. In other words, despite centrifugal development, nephrons mature to their adult level only after all tubules have been formed, suggesting the existence of some stimulus that directs tubular maturation once nephrogenesis is complete. The study by Evan et al. [47] did show that maturation of both the outer cortical and inner cortical proximal tubules was delayed until completion of nephrogenesis, suggesting that the maturational process does not simply continue along a straight pathway toward the adult state. The observations of Schwartz and Evan [177] that bicarbonate, glucose, and volume reabsorption by juxtamedullary proximal tubules of the rabbit remains approximately constant until a marked increase occurs in the fifth postnatal week also support the idea of delayed maturation. It has not been established, however, whether tubules from all levels of the renal cortex reach some level of structural/functional maturation and then all proceed together to an adult level. Definitive conclusions about the validity of centrifugal versus synchronized tubular maturation require the examination of nephrons positioned throughout the developing cortex at multiple time points.

In order to determine the role that changes in apical and basolateral membrane surface areas might have on proximal tubular reabsorptive rates, Welling et al. [212] studied the development of proximal tubules in the guinea pig, in which nephrogenesis is completed before birth. They found the apical and basolateral membrane densities to approximate each other throughout the period of tubular maturation. Total membrane area increased as tubular volume and length increased, and the product of membrane area multiplied by tubular length correlated with increasing resorptive function of the tubule as a function of age.

Development of the Loop of Henle

As stated earlier in this chapter, the proximal tubular cells are easily identified by the presence of apical microvilli at stage III, while the more distal segments of the nephron show limited development. The only hint of the prospective loop of Henle cells is diminished basophilia in cells located at the distal end of the proximal limb [135]. The cells of the future loop of Henle are cuboidal in shape and possess large nuclei and limited cytoplasm [199]. The anlage of the ascending limb is positioned near the vascular pole of the glomerulus and oriented in a horizontal plane [135], where it forms the macula densa.

By stage IV, both the descending and ascending limbs of the loop of Henle are identifiable. The descending limb in the human kidney is approximately 60 μm in length, the ascending limb about 110 μm. The transition from proximal tubule to descending limb is initially subtle, with

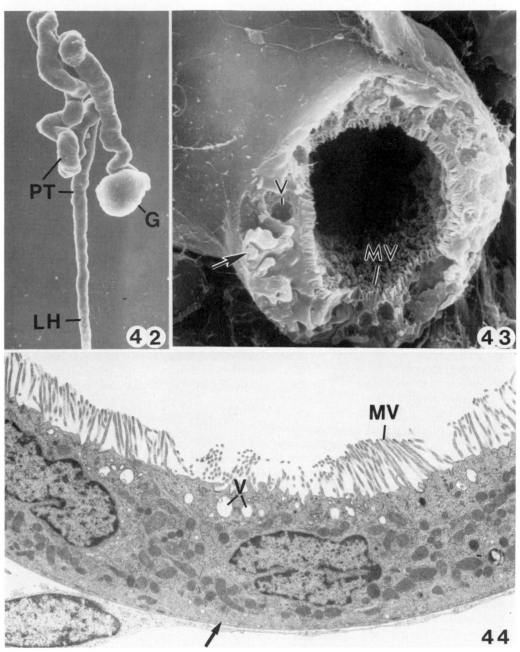

Figs. 2-42, 2-43, and 2-44. *Proximal tubule development beyond stage IV. Figure 2-42 shows a microdissected nephron with the glomerulus (G), proximal tubule (PT), and loop of Henle (LH) intact. The transition between the proximal tubule and loop of Henle is noted by a gradual decrease in tubular diameter. Figure 2-43 shows the cells of a stage IV proximal tubule that has been cryofractured, while Fig. 2-44 reveals ultrastructural features of these cells. The proximal tubular cells are characterized by numerous apical microvilli (MV), numerous apical vacuoles (V), and a few basolateral processes (arrow). Magnification: Fig. 2-42 ×275; Fig. 2-43 ×4800; Fig. 2-44 ×7200 before an 11% reduction.*

a gradual change in tubular diameter (Fig. 2-45), a gradual decrease in cell height, a loss of apical microvilli (Fig. 2-46), and an absence of lysosomes and basolateral interdigitations [37]. The bend of the loop is now located within a medullary ray or the outer medulla and is surrounded by numerous mescenchymal cells. The ascending limb arises from the distal tubule and is easily distinguished from the descending limb by its lighter staining properties and close positioning to collecting ducts (Figs. 2-46, 2-47). These loop cells are characterized by smooth apical surfaces, few

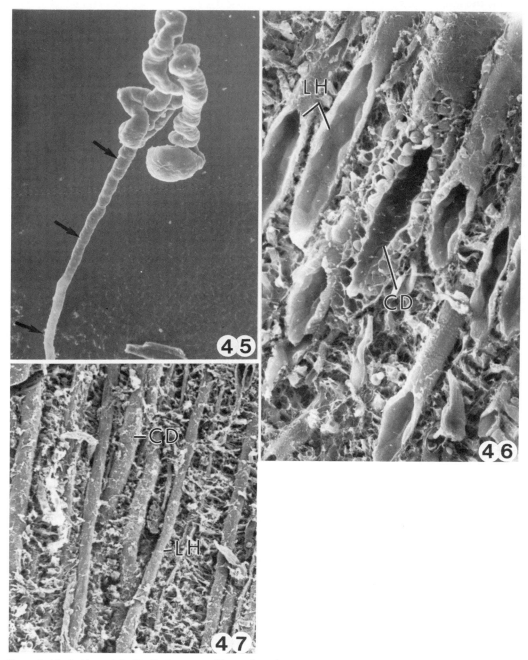

Figs. 2-45, 2-46, and 2-47. *Early stages of loop of Henle. Figure 2-45 shows the gradual transition (arrows) that exists between the proximal tubule and loop of Henle in the immature nephron (stage IV). Within the outer medulla, loops of Henle (LH) are embedded in a loose undifferentiated network of mesenchymal cells (Figs. 2-46 and 2-47) surrounded by collecting ducts (CD) and capillaries. The cells lining the immature loops of Henle have a simple cuboidal shape and an apical cilium (Fig. 2-46). Magnification: Fig. 2-45 ×300; Fig. 2-46 ×6000; Fig. 2-47 ×220 before a 12% reduction.*

mitochondria, and an absence of basolateral interdigitations.

Further maturation of the loop of Henle occurs in three concurrent steps: (1) the pars recta (S3 segment) of the proximal tubule elongates, and (2) the thin descending and (3) thin ascending limbs undergo differentiation [134]. Development of the short-looped nephrons is complete when the pars recta of the proximal tubule and the thin descending limb have reached an adult level. In these nephrons, the entire ascending limb is formed from the distal tubular epithelium. However, the long-looped nephrons show progressive transformation of the distal tubular epithelium into thin ascending limb cells.

Proximal tubular cell differentiation in the mature tubule ceases distally at the borderline between outer and inner medullary stripes. As a result, a sharp transition point occurs between cells of the proximal tubule and those of the descending limb, and this sharp transition is a sign of maturity. Maturation of the descending limb is marked by a gradual decrease in cell height until these cells are squamous in appearance, their nuclei bulging toward the tubular lumen. Although cells of the descending limb possess only a few short apical microvilli, their cell surfaces display alpha-glutamyl transpeptidase and dipeptidylaminopeptidase enzyme activity [134].

Formation of the thin ascending limb requires transformation of the thick distal tubular epithelium into a flattened cell type. The immature thick distal tubular cells possess numerous large autophagosomes that display high activity for acid phosphatase and acid beta-galactosidase [134]. There is a gradual maturation of these cells into a cell type that is sequamous in shape with little cytoplasm. This transformation terminates abruptly for all long-looped nephrons at the boundary of the outer and inner medulla.

Development of the Distal Tubule

While a tubular and glomerular anlage are identifiable at stage II (S-shaped body), it is not until stage III that the more distal segments of the nephron can be clearly differentiated from the proximal tubule (see Fig. 2-7). Stage III distal tubule cells have a flatter nucleus and more small apical vacuoles than do the tubular cells noted at stage II [107].

By stage IV, the human distal tubular segment can be divided into an ascending limb of the loop of Henle, the macula densa, the convoluted distal tubule, and a connecting tubule [37]. Tubular cell height is significantly greater in the macula densa than in other divisions of the distal tubule. The inner tubular diameter decreases significantly, however, from the ascending limb (12.0 μm) to the connecting segment (7.7 μm). Consequently, the ratio of tubular wall volume to tubular length also declines from the ascending limb to the connecting segment.

In both the rat and human kidney, the ultrastructural features of tubular cells at stage IV include large basally located nuclei, few basolateral interdigitations, some lysosome-like bodies, adult-like apical microvilli, a limited number of mitochondrial profiles with no particular orientation to the plasma membranes, and a reduced number of small apical vacuoles (Fig. 2-48) [37,107,134]. A transition zone between the distal convoluted tubule and the connecting segment contains a few cells showing the characteristics of intercalated cells. These cells possess dark-staining cytoplasmic ground substance, apical vesicles, and irregular apical cell surfaces [134].

Maturation of the distal tubule from stage IV to the adult level includes doubling of mitochondrial profiles and basolateral cell membranes [107]. The mitochondria become elongated and positioned parallel to the basolateral

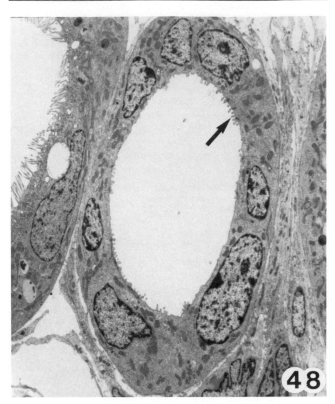

FIG. 2-48. *Early distal tubule. The cells of a stage IV distal tubule are characterized by large nuclei, small mitochondria, apical microvilli (arrow), few apical vacuoles, and a limited number of basolateral interdigitations. Magnifications ×3100 reproduced at 108%.*

interdigitations (Fig. 2-49). Larsson [107] noted that surface densities of the basal and lateral cell membranes in superficial distal convoluted tubules are reached two weeks ahead of the nearby developing proximal tubules. He has concluded that the morphologic maturation of superficial distal convoluted tubules occurs at a more rapid rate than in proximal tubules.

The connecting segment, the link between the developing nephron and the collecting duct, is considered in the adult kidney to be part of the collecting duct. In the developing kidney, however, the anlage of this segment is formed from the S-shaped body and not the ampulla of the collecting duct [83,92,135,137,142].

The arcades of cortical collecting tubules, however, are derived from the ureteric bud [149]. During stage II, the future distal tubule joins a terminal ampulla, and continuity of the lumens is established [83,92,137]. As long as new ampullae are being formed [142], one nephron usually connects to one ampulla. In the human kidney, however, between weeks 14 to 15 and 20 to 22, the ampullae no longer actively divide but still induce new nephron formation. As successive generations of nephrons are formed, the connecting segments of several nephrons of different ages open into the same terminal ampulla. The oldest nephrons reach the more peripheral ampulla by way of a

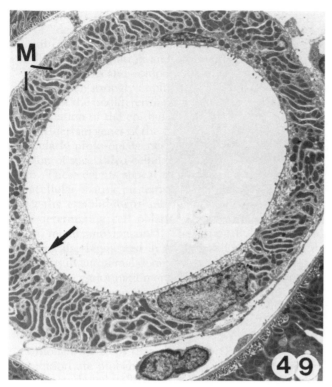

FIG. 2-49. *Adult distal tubule. These cells possess numerous elongate mitochondria (M) positioned between elaborate basolateral interdigitations, apical vacuoles, and apical microvilli (arrow). Magnifications ×3100 reproduced at 108%.*

common tubular segment termed an *arcade*. By gradual lengthening of this tubular segment, several nephrons drain into a single collecting duct. After 20 to 22 weeks in the human kidney, the collecting ducts advance beyond the arcades, and new nephrons attach directly to a terminal ampulla. The ampulla advances four to six times without dividing and then stops, and the outer cortical nephrons attach directly to a straight cortical collecting duct. Nephrogenesis lasts until 33 to 36 weeks.

Development of the Collecting Duct

At about the fourth week of gestation in humans, the ureteric bud advances toward the metanephric blastema and divides dichotomously. The ducts that form the first several divisions of the ureteric bud remodel to become the renal pelvis and major calyces. As the ureteric bud continues to divide, the next several divisions form the minor calyces. At about the fifth week of gestation, approximately 40 papillary ducts empty into about 15 renal papillae. Each of these papillary ducts elongates and divides another seven or eight times, resulting in as many as 156 collecting ducts per papillary duct and about 100,000 collecting ducts per kidney.

The cells of the ampulla of the collecting ducts have a uniform ultrastructure suggestive of an undifferentiated cell type. The cells are tall, with few organelles, and possess a smooth apical surface except for a solitary cilium (Figs. 2-50–2-52) [37,46]. There is no evidence of either principal or intercalated cells, which normally line the adult cortical and medullary collecting ducts. The cells of the early papillary collecting duct are also columnar in shape and possess few organelles. The cytoplasm contains a few scattered mitochondria; large number of ribosomes, free and attached; and glycogen granules [208]. Wade et al. [208] found both that when a 14-day-old rat was injected with ADH the glycogen granules were completely depleted from the collecting ducts cells within 3½ hours.

Once the cortical collecting ducts are established, further differentiation of cells lining the outer medullary collecting ducts is marked by the appearance of intercalated cells. These cells are characterized by apical microplicae and an increased number of mitochondria. With maturation, these cells increase in number and size [46].

As the ampulla continues to advance toward the kidney capsule, it is lined with undifferentiated cells. The cortical collecting tubule just distal to the ampulla is also lined with an undifferentiated cell. Immature intercalated cells are present along the rest of the developing cortical collecting ducts, however. Clark [33] did not find dark cells lining the cortical collecting ducts of the newborn mouse but did see cells possessing a large number of cytoplasmic vesicles and apical microvilli. Evan et al. [46] used scanning electron microscopy to detect immature intercalated cells along the entire cortical and outer stripe collecting ducts of the developing rabbit kidney. When present, intercalated cells were easily identified by their apical microvilli or microplicae (Figs. 2-50, 2-52). Transmission electron microscopy showed these cells to be enriched in mitochondria and to possess numerous apical vesicles (Fig. 2-53). They found no intercalated cells along the outer cortical collecting ducts of the one-week-old rabbit; however, there was a gradual increase in the number of intercalated cells along the middle and inner collecting ducts.

In a separate study, Satlin et al. [172] followed the postnatal maturation of the rabbit cortical collecting ducts. The cortical collecting ducts increased 60% in tubular diameter and dry weight from birth to one month of age. Concomitant with the increase in tubular size, total cell number per millimeter of tubular length rose by 30%. The increase in tubular size was related to both cellular hypertrophy and hyperplasia, each accounting for approximately 50% of the tubular growth. The most peripheral ends (ampullae) of the cortical collecting ducts had a tenfold higher mitotic rate than the midcortical collecting ducts (midcortical mitotic frequency was 3/1000 cells). The total number of intercalated cells did not increase significantly from birth to four weeks of age. However, the number of intercalated cells doubled after the fourth postnatal week.

An unanswered question relates to the origin of the intercalated cells that line the connecting tubules, the cortical straight, and the medullary collecting ducts. Neiss [135] suggested that the intercalated cells of the connecting tubules arise from stem cells that line the immature connecting segments and not from cells of the developing collecting ducts. He detected intercalated cells in a ma-

27. Canfield PJ: Electron microscopic examination of the developing bovine glomerular filtration barrier. *Zbl Vet Med C Anat Histol Embryol* 10:46, 1981.

28. Canter CE, Gross RJ: Induction of extra nephrons in unilaterally nephrectomized immature rats (38525). *Proc Soc Exp Biol Med* 148:294, 1975.

29. Caulfield JP, Farquhar MG: Distribution of anionic sites in glomerular basement membranes. Their possible role in filtration and attachment. *Proc Natl Acad Sci USA* 73:1646, 1976.

30. Casselas B, Mimran A: Shunting in renal microvasculature of the rat: A scanning electron microscopic study of corrosion casts. *Anat Rec* 201:237, 1981.

31. Cheignon M, Schaeverbere J, Gelsos-Meyer A, et al: Differentiation of glomerular selective permeability to protein in fetal rat kidney. *Biol Cell* 42:35, 1981.

32. Chevalier RL: Glomerular number and perfusion during normal and compensatory renal growth in the guinea pig. *Pediatr Res* 16:436, 1982.

33. Clark SL, Jr: Cellular differentiation in the kidney of newborn mice studied with the electron microscope. *J Biophys Biochem Cytol* 3:349, 1957.

34. De Rouffignac C, Monnens L: Functional and morphologic maturation of superficial and juxtamedullary nephrons in the rat. *J Physiol* 262:119, 1976.

35. Dlouha H: A micropuncture study of the development of renal function in the young rat. *Biol Neonate* 29:117, 1976.

36. Dlouha H, Bibr B, Jezek J, et al: Single nephron glomerular filtration rate ratios of superficial, intercortical and juxtamedullary nephrons in rat during development. *Pflugers Arch* 366:277, 1976.

37. Dorup J, Maunsbach AB: The ultrastructural development of distal nephron segments in the human fetal kidney. *Anat Embryol* 164:19, 1982.

38. Drukker A, Donoso VS, Linshaw M, et al: Intrarenal distribution of renin in the developing rabbit. *Pediatr Res* 17:762, 1983.

39. Du Bois AM: The embryonic kidney. *In* Rouiller C, Muller AF (eds): *The Kidney.* Vol 1, New York, Academic Press, 1969, p 1.

40. Dunnill MS, Halley W: Some observations on the quantitative anatomy of the kidney. *J Pathol* 110:113, 1972.

41. Edelmann CM, Jr: Glomerulo-tubular balance in the developing kidney. *Proceedings of the 4th International Congress of Nephrology* 1:22, 1970.

42. Edwards JG: Development of efferent arterioli in human metanephros. *Anat Rec* 109:495, 1951.

43. Eguchi Y, Yamakawa M, Morikawa Y, et al: Granular cells in the juxtaglomerular apparatus in prenatal rats. *Anat Rec* 181:627, 1975.

44. Elinder G, Aperia A, Herin P, et al: Effect of isotonic volume expansion on glomerular filtration rate and renal hemodynamics in the developing rat kidney. *Acta Physiol Scand* 108:411, 1980.

45. Ertl N: Zur Entwichlung des juxtaglomeerularen Apparates in Nieren von Nanschembryonen. *Zeits Anat Entwichlungsges* 126:132, 1967.

46. Evan AP, Satlin LM, Gattone VH, II et al: Postnatal maturation of rabbit renal collecting duct II. Morphological observations. *Am J Physiol* 261:F91, 1991.

47. Evan AP, Gattone VH, Schwartz GJ: Development of solute transport in rabbit proximal tubule. II. Morphologic segmentation. *Am J Physiol* 245:F391, 1983.

48. Farquhar MG, Palade GE: Functional evidence on the existence of a third cell type in the renal glomerulus. Phagocytosis of filtration residues by a distinctive "third" cell. *J Cell Biol* 13:55, 1962.

49. Farquhar MG, Kanwar YS: Functional organization of the glomerulus: Presence of glycosaminoglycans (proteoglycans) in the glomerular basement membrane. *In* Cummings NB, Michael AF, Wilson CB (eds): *Immune Mechanism in Renal Disease.* New York, Plenum Medical Book Co., 1983, p 1.

50. Fetterman GH, Shuplock NA, Philipp FJ, et al: The growth and maturation of human glomeruli and proximal convolutions from term to adulthood. *Pediatrics* 35:601, 1965.

51. Finco DR, Duncan JR: Relationship of glomerular number and diameter to body size of the dog. *Am J Vet Res* 33:2447, 1972.

52. Friis C: Postnatal development of renal function in piglets: Glomerular filtration rate, clearance of PAH and PAH extraction. *Biol Neonate* 35:180, 1979.

53. Friis C: Postnatal development of the pig kidney: Ultrastructure of the glomerular and the proximal tubule. *J Anat* 130:513, 1980.

54. Gattone VH, Johnsson ML, Morse DE: A scanning electron microscopic study of developing mesonephric and metanephric renal glomeruli. *Micron* 10:210, 1979.

55. Gersh I: The correlation of structure and function in the developing mesonephros and metanephros. *Contrib Embryol Carnegie Inst Wash* 26:35, 1937.

56. Goormaghtigh N: Existence of an endocrine gland in the media of the renal arterioles. *Proc Soc Exp Biol Med* 42:688, 1939.

57. Granger P, Rojo-Ortega JM, Casado Perez S, et al: The renin-angiotensin system in newborn dogs. *Can J Physiol Pharmacol* 49:134, 1971.

58. Gruskin AB, Edelmann CM Jr, Yuan S: Maturational changes in renal blood flow in piglets. *Pediat Res* 4:7, 1970.

59. Guignard JP, Torredo A, Da Cunha O, et al: Glomerular filtration role in the first three weeks of life. *J Pediatr* 87:268, 1975.

60. Guignard JP: Renal function in the newborn infant. *Pediatr Clin North Am* 29:777, 1982.

61. Hall BV: Further studies of normal structure of renal glomerulus. *In* Metcoff J (ed): *Proceedings of Sixth Annual Conference on Nephrotic Syndrome.* National Nephrosis Foundation, 1955.

62. Hall BV, Roth LE: Preliminary studies on development and differentiation of cells and structures of renal corpuscles. *In Proceedings of Stockholm Conference on Electron Microscopy.* Almqvist and Wiksells International Booksellers, 1956.

63. Hanberg-Sorensen F: Quantitative studies of the renal corpuscle. I. Intraglomerular, interglomerular and interfocal variation in the normal kidney. *Acta Pathol Microbiol Immunol Scand* 80:115, 1972.

64. Hanberg-Sorensen F, Ledel T: Quantitive studies of the renal corpuscles. II. A methodological study. *Acta Pathol Microbiol Immunol Scand* 80:721, 1972.

65. Hay DA, Evan AP: Observations on the development of glomerular capillaries of the puppy kidney. *Scanning Electron Microsc* 1:455, 1984.

66. Hay DA, Evan AP: Maturation of the glomerular visceral epithelium and capillary endothelium in the puppy kidney. *Anat Rec* 193:1, 1979.

67. Hay DA, Evan AP: Maturation of the proximal tubule in the puppy kidney: A comparison to the adult. *Anat Rec* 195:273, 1979.

68. Hodari AA, Hodgkinson CP: Fetal kidney as a source of renin in the pregnant dog. *Am J Obstet Gynecol* 102:691, 1968.

69. Hornych H, Beaufils M, Richet G: The effects of exoge-

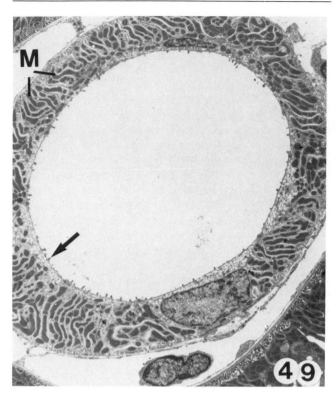

Fig. 2-49. *Adult distal tubule. These cells possess numerous elongate mitochondria (M) positioned between elaborate basolateral interdigitations, apical vacuoles, and apical microvilli (arrow). Magnifications ×3100 reproduced at 108%.*

common tubular segment termed an *arcade.* By gradual lengthening of this tubular segment, several nephrons drain into a single collecting duct. After 20 to 22 weeks in the human kidney, the collecting ducts advance beyond the arcades, and new nephrons attach directly to a terminal ampulla. The ampulla advances four to six times without dividing and then stops, and the outer cortical nephrons attach directly to a straight cortical collecting duct. Nephrogenesis lasts until 33 to 36 weeks.

Development of the Collecting Duct

At about the fourth week of gestation in humans, the ureteric bud advances toward the metanephric blastema and divides dichotomously. The ducts that form the first several divisions of the ureteric bud remodel to become the renal pelvis and major calyces. As the ureteric bud continues to divide, the next several divisions form the minor calyces. At about the fifth week of gestation, approximately 40 papillary ducts empty into about 15 renal papillae. Each of these papillary ducts elongates and divides another seven or eight times, resulting in as many as 156 collecting ducts per papillary duct and about 100,000 collecting ducts per kidney.

The cells of the ampulla of the collecting ducts have a

uniform ultrastructure suggestive of an undifferentiated cell type. The cells are tall, with few organelles, and possess a smooth apical surface except for a solitary cilium (Figs. 2-50–2-52) [37,46]. There is no evidence of either principal or intercalated cells, which normally line the adult cortical and medullary collecting ducts. The cells of the early papillary collecting duct are also columnar in shape and possess few organelles. The cytoplasm contains a few scattered mitochondria; large number of ribosomes, free and attached; and glycogen granules [208]. Wade et al. [208] found both that when a 14-day-old rat was injected with ADH the glycogen granules were completely depleted from the collecting ducts cells within 3½ hours.

Once the cortical collecting ducts are established, further differentiation of cells lining the outer medullary collecting ducts is marked by the appearance of intercalated cells. These cells are characterized by apical microplicae and an increased number of mitochondria. With maturation, these cells increase in number and size [46].

As the ampulla continues to advance toward the kidney capsule, it is lined with undifferentiated cells. The cortical collecting tubule just distal to the ampulla is also lined with an undifferentiated cell. Immature intercalated cells are present along the rest of the developing cortical collecting ducts, however. Clark [33] did not find dark cells lining the cortical collecting ducts of the newborn mouse but did see cells possessing a large number of cytoplasmic vesicles and apical microvilli. Evan et al. [46] used scanning electron microscopy to detect immature intercalated cells along the entire cortical and outer stripe collecting ducts of the developing rabbit kidney. When present, intercalated cells were easily identified by their apical microvilli or microplicae (Figs. 2-50, 2-52). Transmission electron microscopy showed these cells to be enriched in mitochondria and to possess numerous apical vesicles (Fig. 2-53). They found no intercalated cells along the outer cortical collecting ducts of the one-week-old rabbit; however, there was a gradual increase in the number of intercalated cells along the middle and inner collecting ducts.

In a separate study, Satlin et al. [172] followed the postnatal maturation of the rabbit cortical collecting ducts. The cortical collecting ducts increased 60% in tubular diameter and dry weight from birth to one month of age. Concomitant with the increase in tubular size, total cell number per millimeter of tubular length rose by 30%. The increase in tubular size was related to both cellular hypertrophy and hyperplasia, each accounting for approximately 50% of the tubular growth. The most peripheral ends (ampullae) of the cortical collecting ducts had a tenfold higher mitotic rate than the midcortical collecting ducts (midcortical mitotic frequency was 3/1000 cells). The total number of intercalated cells did not increase significantly from birth to four weeks of age. However, the number of intercalated cells doubled after the fourth postnatal week.

An unanswered question relates to the origin of the intercalated cells that line the connecting tubules, the cortical straight, and the medullary collecting ducts. Neiss [135] suggested that the intercalated cells of the connecting tubules arise from stem cells that line the immature connecting segments and not from cells of the developing collecting ducts. He detected intercalated cells in a ma-

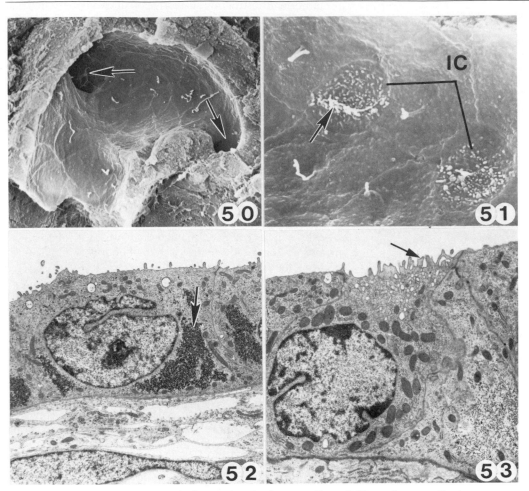

FIGS. 2-50, 2-51, 2-52, and 2-53. Collecting duct development. Figure 2-50 is a low-magnification SEM showing the ampulla of the collecting duct located at the kidney capsule. The ampulla has already divided into two tubules (arrows). The cells that line this part of the developing collecting duct are characterized by a smooth apical surface and a cilium indicative of an undifferentiated cell. Principal nor intercalated cells are noted. Immature intercalated cells (IC) are seen in regions of the mid and inner cortex (Fig. 2-51). These cells are recognized by their apical microvilli (arrows) or microplicae. Figure 2-52 reveals only one cell type lining the ampulla. These cells possess few organelles, large glycogen deposits (arrow), irregularly shaped nucleus, and smooth apical and basal cell surfaces. The developing intercalated cells show apical microplicae or microvilli (arrow), numerous apical vesicles, and many mitochondria. Magnification: Fig. 2-50 ×2000; Fig. 2-51 ×4500; Fig. 2-52 ×5000; Fig. 2-53 ×11,000 before an 11% reduction.

turing segment of an arcade and in a shaft of a maturing cortical collecting duct at a time when these two segments were still separated by an immature neck piece of a connecting tubule, a terminal ampulla, or an immature segment of collecting duct in a growth zone. No intercalated cells were found in the three interposed segments. From these observations he concluded that the intercalated cells of the connecting tubules arose from the nephrogenic blastema, whereas the intercalated cells of the collecting ducts arose from the ureteric bud. In addition, he suggested that a progenitor cell located along the immature connecting tubule gave rise to intercalated and connecting tubular cells, while another progenitor cell located along the col-

lecting ducts formed both principal and intercalated cells. How this process of differentiation occurs is not known.

Future Directions

Renal epithelial differentiation normally takes place in a temporally and spatially tight and synchronized manner. While this process is clearly complex, our understanding of nephron development has progressed significantly through studies of the morphologic events of nephron formation. Saxén [173] has used biochemical probes to investigate morphogenetic interactions during the transformation of undifferentiated mesenchymal cells into several types of highly specialized epithelial cells. An initial process of "determination" commits undifferentiated mesenchymal cells to an epithelial lineage and opens the door to cellular differentiation and proliferation.

Growth factors and components of the exracellular matrix have been strongly implicated in directing the cellular behavior of the undifferentiated mesenchymal cells and the differentiation of the epithelial cells [11a]. Growth factors activate certain genes of the differentiating cell population, particularly proto-oncogenes, thereby controlling the expression of specialized cellular features and cellular metabolism. These events appear to stimulate the production of extracellular matrix proteins, which in turn initiate and direct the establishment and maintenance of specific features determining cell polarity (i.e., cytoskeletal organization, membrane domains). The extracellular matrix proteins are also implicated in abnormal development of the kidney, as in autosomal dominant polycystic kidney disease [125]. Both cyst formation and cyst growth may be directed in part by the components of the extracellular matrix. Precisely how the components of the extracellular matrix regulate cellular function and structure remains to be identified.

Although the steps that control cell differentiation and polarization are probably small and incremental, the specializing epithelial cells must also go through the process of tubulogenesis at the same time that angiogenesis molds the microvascular system of the kidney. These events occur as the early nephron progresses from the vesicle stage to the S-shaped body. It appears that the extracellular matrix proteins are also involved in both of these events.

Future success in studying developmental biology of the kidney will depend upon the use of highly controlled experimental protocols that can correlate the morphogenetic interactions occurring at the molecular, cellular, and tissue levels. These experiments need to be performed both in vivo and in vitro to delineate the mechanisms by which an undifferentiated cell population acquires such highly specialized structural and functions characteristics.

References

1. Accini L, De Martino C: Development and morphologic differentiation of podocytes in human embryo metanephron. *J Submicrosc Cytol* 4:101, 1972.
2. Alcorn D, Cheshire CR, Coghlan JP, et al: Peripolar cell hypertrophy in the renal juxtaglomerular region of newborn sheep. *Cell Tissue Res* 236:197, 1984.
3. Aoki A: Temporary cell junctions in the developing human renal glomerulus. *Dev Biol* 15:156, 1967.
4. Aperia A, Broberger O, Herin P: Maturational changes in glomerular perfusion rate and glomerular filtration rate in lambs. *Pediatr Res* 8:758, 1974.
5. Aperia A, Herin P: Development of glomerular prefusion rate and nephron filtration rate in rats 17–60 days old. *Am J Physiol* 228:1319, 1975.
6. Aperia A, Broberger O, Elinder G, et al: Postnatal development of renal function in pre-term and full-term infants. *Acta Paediatr Scand* 70:183, 1981.
7. Aperia A, Broberger O, Elinder G, et al: Postnatal changes in glomerular filtration rate in pre-term and full-term infants. *In* Spitzer A (ed): *The Kidney during Development, Morphology and Function.* New York, Masson Publ. Co. Inc., 1982, p 133.
8. Arant BS, Jr: Glomerulotubular balance following saline loading in the developing kidney. *Am J Physiol* 235:F417, 1978.
9. Arataki M: On the postnatal growth of the kidney, with special reference to the number and size of the glomeruli (albino rat). *Am J Anat* 36:399, 1926.
10. Aschinberg LC, Goldsmith DE, Olbing H, et al: Neonatal change in renal blood flow distribution in puppies. *Am J Physiol* 228:1453, 1975.
11. Ausiello DA, Kreisberg JI, Roy C, et al: Contraction of cultural rat glomerular cells of apparent mesangial origin after stimulation with angiotensin II and arginine vasopressin. *J Clin Invest* 65:754, 1980.
11a. Bacallao R, Fine LG: Molecular events in the organization of renal tubular epithelium: From nephrogenesis to regeneration. *Am J Physiol* 257:F913, 1989.
12. Bailie MD, Derkex FHM, Schalekamp MADH: Release of active and inactive renin by the pig kidney during development. *Dev Pharmacol Ther* 1:47, 1980.
13. Baker JT, Solomon, S: Maturation of the renal response to hypertonic chloride loading in rats: Micropuncture and clearance studies. *J Physiol* 258:83, 1976.
14. Barajas L, Latta H: A three-dimensional study of the juxtaglomerular apparatus in the rat. Light and electron microscopic observations. *Lab Invest* 12:257, 1963.
15. Bengele H, Solomon S: Development of the renal response to blood volume expansion in normal and fast-growing rats. *Am J Physiol* 231:832, 1976.
16. Bergelin, ISS, Karlsson, BW: Functional structure of the glomerular filtration barrier and the proximal tubuli in the developing fetal and neonatal pig kidney. *Anat Embryol* (Berl) 148:223, 1975.
17. Bernstein J, Cheng F, Roszka BS: Glomerular differentiation in metanephric culture. *Lab Invest* 45:183, 1981.
18. Bloom PM, Hartmann JF, Venier RL: An electron microscopic evaluation of the width of normal glomerular basement membrane in man at various ages. *Anat Rec* 133:251, 1959.
19. Bohman SO, Jaremko G, Bohlin AB, et al: Foot process fusion and glomerular filtration rate in minimal change nephrotic syndrome. *Kidney Int* 25:47, 1984.
20. Bonvalet JP, Champion M, Courtalon A, et al: Number of glomeruli in normal and hypertrophied kidneys of mice and guinea pigs. *J Physiol* 269:627, 1977.
21. Broughton Pipkin F, Kirkpatrick SML, Lumbers ER, et al: Renin and angiotensin-like levels in fetal, newborn and adult sheep. *J Physiol* 241:575, 1974.
22. Bruhl V, Taugner R, Forssmann WG: Studies on the juxtaglomerular apparatus. 1. Prenatal development in the rat. *Cell Tissue Res* 151:433, 1974.
23. Buchley NM, Charney AN, Bragean P, et al: Changes in cardiovascular and renal function during catecholamine infusions in developing swine. *Am J Physiol* 240:F276, 1981.
24. Buddingh F, Parker HR, Ishizaki G, et al: Long-term studies of the functional development of the fetal kidney in sheep. *Am J Vet Res* 32:1993, 1971.
25. Buss H: Development of podocytes in the rat glomerulus. A scanning electron microscopic study. *Proc VII Internat Congr Electron Microscopy Grenoble* III:605, 1970.
26. Cain H, Krans B: Der juxtaglomerulare Apparat der Rattensniere in Verlauf von Wachtum, Reifung und Alterung. *Virchows Arch Abt B Zellpath* 9:164, 1971.

27. Canfield PJ: Electron microscopic examination of the developing bovine glomerular filtration barrier. *Zbl Vet Med C Anat Histol Embryol* 10:46, 1981.

28. Canter CE, Gross RJ: Induction of extra nephrons in unilaterally nephrectomized immature rats (38525). *Proc Soc Exp Biol Med* 148:294, 1975.

29. Caulfield JP, Farquhar MG: Distribution of anionic sites in glomerular basement membranes. Their possible role in filtration and attachment. *Proc Natl Acad Sci USA* 73:1646, 1976.

30. Casselas B, Mimran A: Shunting in renal microvasculature of the rat: A scanning electron microscopic study of corrosion casts. *Anat Rec* 201:237, 1981.

31. Cheignon M, Schaeverbere J, Gelsos-Meyer A, et al: Differentiation of glomerular selective permeability to protein in fetal rat kidney. *Biol Cell* 42:35, 1981.

32. Chevalier RL: Glomerular number and perfusion during normal and compensatory renal growth in the guinea pig. *Pediatr Res* 16:436, 1982.

33. Clark SL, Jr: Cellular differentiation in the kidney of newborn mice studied with the electron microscope. *J Biophys Biochem Cytol* 3:349, 1957.

34. De Rouffignac C, Monnens L: Functional and morphologic maturation of superficial and juxtamedullary nephrons in the rat. *J Physiol* 262:119, 1976.

35. Dlouha H: A micropuncture study of the development of renal function in the young rat. *Biol Neonate* 29:117, 1976.

36. Dlouha H, Bibr B, Jezek J, et al: Single nephron glomerular filtration rate ratios of superficial, intercortical and juxtamedullary nephrons in rat during development. *Pflugers Arch* 366:277, 1976.

37. Dorup J, Maunsbach AB: The ultrastructural development of distal nephron segments in the human fetal kidney. *Anat Embryol* 164:19, 1982.

38. Drukker A, Donoso VS, Linshaw M, et al: Intrarenal distribution of renin in the developing rabbit. *Pediatr Res* 17:762, 1983.

39. Du Bois AM: The embryonic kidney. *In* Rouiller C, Muller AF (eds): *The Kidney.* Vol 1, New York, Academic Press, 1969, p 1.

40. Dunnill MS, Halley W: Some observations on the quantitative anatomy of the kidney. *J Pathol* 110:113, 1972.

41. Edelmann CM, Jr: Glomerulo-tubular balance in the developing kidney. *Proceedings of the 4th International Congress of Nephrology* 1:22, 1970.

42. Edwards JG: Development of efferent arterioli in human metanephros. *Anat Rec* 109:495, 1951.

43. Eguchi Y, Yamakawa M, Morikawa Y, et al: Granular cells in the juxtaglomerular apparatus in prenatal rats. *Anat Rec* 181:627, 1975.

44. Elinder G, Aperia A, Herin P, et al: Effect of isotonic volume expansion on glomerular filtration rate and renal hemodynamics in the developing rat kidney. *Acta Physiol Scand* 108:411, 1980.

45. Ertl N: Zur Entwichlung des juxtaglomeerularen Apparates in Nieren von Nanschembryonen. *Zeits Anat Entwichlungsges* 126:132, 1967.

46. Evan AP, Satlin LM, Gattone VH, II et al: Postnatal maturation of rabbit renal collecting duct II. Morphological observations. *Am J Physiol* 261:F91, 1991.

47. Evan AP, Gattone VH, Schwartz GJ: Development of solute transport in rabbit proximal tubule. II. Morphologic segmentation. *Am J Physiol* 245:F391, 1983.

48. Farquhar MG, Palade GE: Functional evidence on the existence of a third cell type in the renal glomerulus. Phagocytosis of filtration residues by a distinctive "third" cell. *J Cell Biol* 13:55, 1962.

49. Farquhar MG, Kanwar YS: Functional organization of the glomerulus: Presence of glycosaminoglycans (proteoglycans) in the glomerular basement membrane. *In* Cummings NB, Michael AF, Wilson CB (eds): *Immune Mechanism in Renal Disease.* New York, Plenum Medical Book Co., 1983, p 1.

50. Fetterman GH, Shuplock NA, Philipp FJ, et al: The growth and maturation of human glomeruli and proximal convolutions from term to adulthood. *Pediatrics* 35:601, 1965.

51. Finco DR, Duncan JR: Relationship of glomerular number and diameter to body size of the dog. *Am J Vet Res* 33:2447, 1972.

52. Friis C: Postnatal development of renal function in piglets: Glomerular filtration rate, clearance of PAH and PAH extraction. *Biol Neonate* 35:180, 1979.

53. Friis C: Postnatal development of the pig kidney: Ultrastructure of the glomerular and the proximal tubule. *J Anat* 130:513, 1980.

54. Gattone VH, Johnsson ML, Morse DE: A scanning electron microscopic study of developing mesonephric and metanephric renal glomeruli. *Micron* 10:210, 1979.

55. Gersh I: The correlation of structure and function in the developing mesonephros and metanephros. *Contrib Embryol Carnegie Inst Wash* 26:35, 1937.

56. Goormaghtigh N: Existence of an endocrine gland in the media of the renal arterioles. *Proc Soc Exp Biol Med* 42:688, 1939.

57. Granger P, Rojo-Ortega JM, Casado Perez S, et al: The renin-angiotensin system in newborn dogs. *Can J Physiol Pharmacol* 49:134, 1971.

58. Gruskin AB, Edelmann CM Jr, Yuan S: Maturational changes in renal blood flow in piglets. *Pediat Res* 4:7, 1970.

59. Guignard JP, Torredo A, Da Cunha O, et al: Glomerular filtration role in the first three weeks of life. *J Pediatr* 87:268, 1975.

60. Guignard JP: Renal function in the newborn infant. *Pediatr Clin North Am* 29:777, 1982.

61. Hall BV: Further studies of normal structure of renal glomerulus. *In* Metcoff J (ed): *Proceedings of Sixth Annual Conference on Nephrotic Syndrome.* National Nephrosis Foundation, 1955.

62. Hall BV, Roth LE: Preliminary studies on development and differentiation of cells and structures of renal corpuscles. *In Proceedings of Stockholm Conference on Electron Microscopy.* Almqvist and Wiksells International Booksellers, 1956.

63. Hanberg-Sorensen F: Quantitative studies of the renal corpuscle. I. Intraglomerular, interglomerular and interfocal variation in the normal kidney. *Acta Pathol Microbiol Immunol Scand* 80:115, 1972.

64. Hanberg-Sorensen F, Ledel T: Quantitive studies of the renal corpuscles. II. A methodological study. *Acta Pathol Microbiol Immunol Scand* 80:721, 1972.

65. Hay DA, Evan AP: Observations on the development of glomerular capillaries of the puppy kidney. *Scanning Electron Microsc* 1:455, 1984.

66. Hay DA, Evan AP: Maturation of the glomerular visceral epithelium and capillary endothelium in the puppy kidney. *Anat Rec* 193:1, 1979.

67. Hay DA, Evan AP: Maturation of the proximal tubule in the puppy kidney: A comparison to the adult. *Anat Rec* 195:273, 1979.

68. Hodari AA, Hodgkinson CP: Fetal kidney as a source of renin in the pregnant dog. *Am J Obstet Gynecol* 102:691, 1968.

69. Hornych H, Beaufils M, Richet G: The effects of exoge-

nous angiotensin on superficial and deep glomeruli in the rat kidney. *Kidney Int* 2:336, 1972.

70. Horster M: Development of nephron function. *Proc 5th Internat Congr Nephrol* 1:14, 1972.

71. Horster M: Principles of nephron differentiation. *Am J Physiol* 235:F387, 1978.

72. Horster M, Larsson L: Mechanisms of fluid absorption during proximal tubule development. *Kidney Int* 10:348, 1976.

73. Horster M, Lewy JE: Filtration fraction and extraction of PAH during neonatal period in the rat. *Am J Physiol* 219:1061, 1970.

74. Horster M, Valtin H: Postnatal development of renal function: Micropuncture and clearance studies in the dog. *J Clin Invest* 50:779, 1971.

75. Horster M, Kemler BJ, Valtin H: Intracortical distribution of number and volume of glomeruli during postnatal maturation in the dog. *J Clin Invest* 50:796, 1971.

76. Huber CG: On the development and shape of uriniferous tubules of certain higher mammals. *Am J Anat* 4:(S1)1, 1905.

77. Humbert F, Montesano R, Perrelet A, et al: Junctions in developing human and rat kidney: A freeze-fracture study. *J Ultrastruct Res* 56:202, 1976.

78. Ichikawa I: Maturational changes in the dynamics of glomerular ultrafiltration in the rat. *In* Spitzer A (ed): *The kidney during Development, Morphology and Function.* New York, Masson Publ. Co., USA Inc., 1982, p 199.

79. Ichikawa K, Brenner BM: Glomerular actions of angiotensin II. *Am J Med* 76:43, 1984.

80. Ichikawa I, Maddox DA, Brenner BM: Maturational development of glomerular ultrafiltration in the rat. *Am J Physiol* 236:F465, 1979.

81. Imbert MJ, Berjal G, Moss N, et al: Number of nephrons in hypertrophic kidneys after unilateral nephrectomy in young and adult rats: A functional study. *Pflugers Arch* 346:279, 1974.

82. John E, Goldsmith DI, Spitzer A: Quantitative changes in canine glomerular vasculature during development: Physiologic implications. *Kidney Int* 20:223, 1981.

83. Jokelainen P: An electron microscope study of the early development of the rat metanephric nephron. *Acta Anat* (suppl) 52:47, 1963.

84. Jørgensen F, Bentzon MW: The ultrastructure of the normal human glomerulus. Thickness of glomerular basement membrane. *Lab Invest* 18:42, 1968.

85. Jose PA, Logan AG, Slotkoff LM, et al: Intrarenal blood flow distribution in canine puppies. *Pediatr Res* 5:335, 1971.

86. Jose PA, Pelago JC, Felder RE, et al: Maturation of single nephron filtration rate in the canine puppy. Effect of saline loading. *In* Spitzer A (ed): *The Kidney during Development, Morphology and Function.* New York, Masson Publ. Co., USA Inc., 1982, p 139.

87. Kanwar YS: Biology of disease. Biophysiology of glomerular filtration and proteinuria. *Lab Invest* 51:7, 1984.

88. Kanwar YS, Farquhar MG: Presence of heparan sulphate in the glomerular basement membrane. *Proc Natl Acad Sci USA* 76:1303, 1979.

89. Kanwar YS, Farquhar MG: Anionic sites in the glomerular basement membrane. In vivo and in vitro localization to the laminae rarae by cationic probes. *J Cell Biol* 81:137, 1979.

90. Kaylot CT, Carter JM: The early appearance of juxtaglomerular granules in the mouse embryo. *Anat Rec* 151:459, 1965.

91. Kaylor CT, Carter JM: The juxtaglomerular apparatus in fetal and newborn mice. *Anat Rec* 159:171, 1967.

92. Kazimierczak J: Development of the renal corpuscle and the juxtamedullary apparatus. A light and electron microscopic study. *Acta Pathol Microbiol Immunol Scand [A]* (suppl) 218:1, 1971.

93. Kazimierczak J: A study by scanning (SEM) and transmission (TEM) electron microscopy of the glomerular capillaries in developing rat kidney. *Cell Tissue Res* 212:241, 1980.

94. Kazimierczak J: New three-dimensional approach to the morphogenesis of the renal structure. *Acta Med Ped* 21:359, 1980.

95. Kefalides NA: Biochemical properties of human glomerular basement membrane in normal and diabetic kidneys. *J Clin Invest* 53:403, 1974.

96. Kittelson JA: The postnatal growth of the kidney of the albino rat with observations on adult human kidney. *Anat Rec* 13:385, 1971.

97. Kleinman LI, Renter JH: Maturation of glomerular blood flow distribution in the newborn dog. *J Physiol* 228:91, 1973.

98. Knutson BW, Chien F, Bennett CM, et al: Estimation of relative glomerular capillary surface area in normal and hypertrophic rat kidneys. *Kidney Int* 14:437, 1978.

99. Kotchen TA, Strickland AL, Rice TW, et al: A study of the renin-angiotensin system in newborn infants. *J Pediatr* 80:938, 1972.

100. Kunkel PA Jr: The number and size of the glomeruli in the kidney of several mammals. *Bull Johns Hopkins Hosp* 47:285, 1930.

101. Kurtz SM: Electron microscopy of developing human renal glomerulus. *Exp Cell Res* 14:355, 1958.

102. Kurtz SM, McManns JFH: A reconsideration of development, structure and disease of the human renal glomerulus. *Am Heart J* 58:357, 1959.

103. Langeveld JPM, Veerkamp JH, Duyt CMP, et al: Chemical characterization of glomerular and tubular basement membranes of men of different ages. *Kidney Int* 20:104, 1981.

104. Larsson L: The ultrastructure of the developing proximal tubule in the rat kidney. *J Ultrastruct Res* 51:119, 1975.

105. Larsson L: Effects of different fixatives on the ultrastructure of the developing proximal tubule in the rat kidney. *J Ultrastruct Res* 51:140, 1975.

106. Larsson L: Ultrastructure and permeability of intercellular contacts of developing proximal tubule in the rat kidney. *J Ultrastruct Res* 52:100, 1975.

107. Larrson L: The ultrastructure of the developing superficial distal convoluted tubule in the rat kidney. *In* Spitzer A (ed): *The Kidney during Development, Morphology and Function.* New York, Masson Publ. Co., USA Inc., 1982, p 15.

108. Larsson L, Maunsbach AB: The ultrastructural development of the vacuolar apparatus in cells of the developing proximal tubule in the rat kidney. *J Ultrastruct Res* 53:254, 1975.

109. Larsson L, Maunsbach AB: The ultrastructural development of the glomerular filtration barrier in the rat kidney: A morphometric analysis. *J Ultrastruct Res* 72:392, 1980.

110. Larsson L, Aperia A, Wilton P: Effect of normal development on compensatory renal growth. *Kidney Int* 18:29, 1980.

111. Larsson L, Maunsbach AB: The ultrastructural differentiation of the glomerular capillary wall as related to function in the developing kidney. *In* Ritzen A, Aperia A, Hall A, et al (eds): *The Biology of Normal Human Growth.* New York, Raven Press, 1981, p 105.

112. Larsson L, Maunsbach AB: Quantitative ultrastructural changes of the glomerular capillary wall in the developing

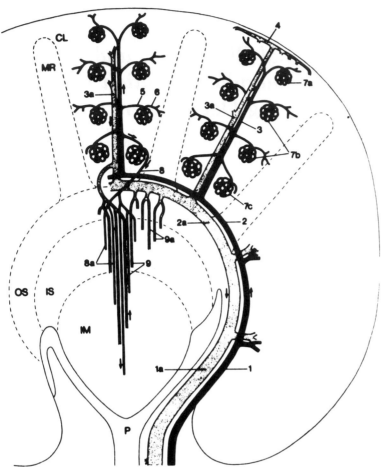

FIG. 3-1. *Schematic representation of the intrarenal blood vessels; peritubular capillaries are not shown. Not drawn to scale. Within the cortex the medullary rays of the cortex (MR) are delineated from the cortical labyrinth (CL) by a dashed line. OS, outer stripe; IS, inner stripe; IM, inner medulla; P, renal pelvis. 1,1a, interlobular artery and vein; 2,2a, arcuate artery and vein; 3,3a, cortical radial artery and vein; 4, stellate vein; 5, afferent arteriole; 6, efferent arteriole; 7a,7b,7c, superficial, midcortical, and juxtamedullary glomeruli; 8,8a, juxtamedullary efferent arteriole, descending vasa recta; 9,9a, ascending vasa recta (those ascending within a vascular bundle and those independent from a bundle). (From Am J Physiol 254:F8, 1988, with permission.)*

stimulated by an angiogenesis factor that is produced by the developing kidney [341].

The maturation of the renal vasculature is not completed by the time of birth, particularly in animal species in which nephrogenesis is continuing. Studies in canine puppies performed by Evan et al. [119,121] revealed substantial differences, both quantitative and qualitative, between the renal vasculature of the newborn and that of the adult animal. These differences were particularly marked in vessels that were located beyond the intralobular arteries. The afferent arterioles were found to vary in origin, length, and number. Most of them originated from the interlobular vessels, but some emerged from the arcuate arteries. The majority of the afferent arterioles were short, but some were extremely long. There was a large variability in the complexity of the glomerular capillary network, noticeable

particularly during the first four weeks after birth. Some of the glomeruli located in the nephrogenic zone had only one glomerular capillary loop. Even the glomeruli located in the inner cortex had a smaller number of capillaries than their counterparts in the adult kidney.

The efferent arterioles of the newborn kidney also showed evidence of immaturity. Those of the outer cortex were short and had a very small, uniform diameter up to a point where they enlarged abruptly to enter venous channels (sinusoids), which were three or four times their size. Just below the nephrogenic zone the efferent arterioles usually extended above their parent glomerulus. Those located deeper within the midcortex extended in various directions. Occasionally two or more of them joined and opened into a common venous channel. A few descended into the medulla to form vasa rectae. Most of the vasa

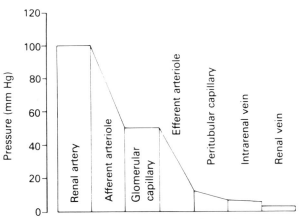

FIG. 3-2. *Hydrostatic pressure profile in the renal vascular tree of the rat. (From Valtin H: Renal Function: Mechanisms Preserving Fluid and Solute Balance in Health. Boston, Little, Brown, 1983, p 101, with permission.)*

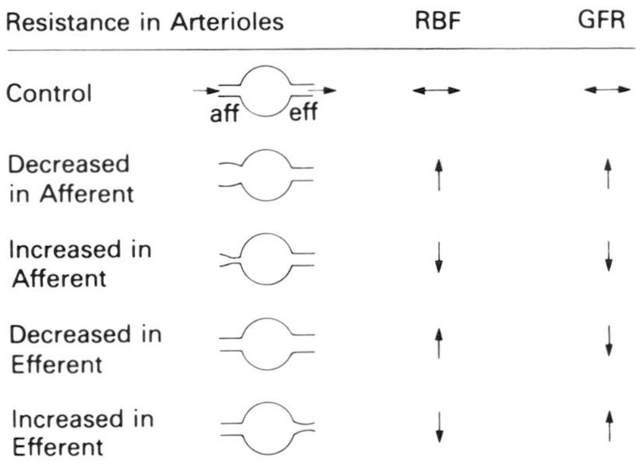

Resistance in Arterioles		RBF	GFR
Control	aff ⤳ eff	↔	↔
Decreased in Afferent		↑	↑
Increased in Afferent		↓	↓
Decreased in Efferent		↑	↓
Increased in Efferent		↓	↑

FIG. 3-3. *The effect of changes in renal arteriolar resistance on renal blood flow (RBF) and glomerular filtration rate (GFR). (From Valtin H: Renal Function: Mechanisms Preserving Fluid and Solute Balance in Health. Boston, Little, Brown, 1983, p 105, with permission.)*

rectae originated from the large diameter efferent arterioles of the inner cortex. The smaller-diameter efferent arterioles branched to form the peritubular capillaries.

The most striking difference between the intrarenal vascular system of the puppy and that of the adult dog was observed at the level of the peritubular capillaries [119,121]. During the first two weeks of extrauterine life the outer cortex contained only sinusoidal vessels that had lake-like dilatations along their course. Even the capillaries of the midcortex and innercortex were large and few in number. Transmission electron microscopy showed these capillaries to have irregular lumens and few areas of fenestrae. The basement membrane was poorly represented. The thick walls and the few fenestrae of the immature capillaries suggest limited permeability, as compared to capillaries of adult animals. The peritubular capillaries did not reach a mature appearance in the puppy until the twentieth week of age. Thus, morphologic changes of the renal vessels cannot explain the rapid and large increase in RBF that occurs almost immediately after birth [191,193,388,389]. Instead, this must be due to a decrease in renovascular resistance.

The Rate of Renal Blood Flow

There is no simple, accurate, reproducible, and noninvasive method to quantify RBF [22,30,220,432,434]. The clearance of para-aminohippurate (PAH) is the standard method for measuring RBF in animals and humans [4,33,72,426]. PAH is a weak acid that is both filtered by the glomerulus and secreted by the organic anion antiporter located in the straight segment of the proximal tubule [70,167,295,403]. The clearance of PAH (C_{PAH}) underestimates the true RBF because the extraction of PAH (E_{PAH}) by the kidney is incomplete, particularly in infants [94,99,137,184,187,384], increasing from 54.8 ± 24.6

(SD) at 8 to 90 days of life to 90.0 ± 4.5 by 5 months of life and to 93.5% in the adult [72]. One reason for the low extraction ratio of PAH by the immature kidney is the preponderance of the juxtamedullary circulation. Blood that is shunted through the vasa rectae fails to perfuse the proximal tubules where PAH secretion occurs [409]. Another reason is the limited ability of the immature proximal tubule to transport weak acids [56,72,216], due to a small number of functional transport sites [121,216,400]. Because the determination of E_{PAH} requires the cannulation of the renal vein, it is virtually never attempted in clinical practice.

Radiolabelled carbonized plastic microspheres are often used to measure RBF and its intrarenal distribution in experimental animals [74,205,215,220,345,350,355,434]. The radiolabelled microspheres must be injected rapidly into the left ventricle or the aorta in order to ensure adequate mixing with the blood [220,432], they should be of sufficient size (10 to 15μ) so that they do not pass through the glomerular capillary, and not so numerous as to impede glomerular blood flow [432]. The RBF is proportional to the number of radioactive counts found in the kidney (or a zone of the kidney). Blood flow to several organs can be determined simultaneously, and sequential measurements can be made in the same animal by using microspheres tagged with different radiolabels [74,215,253,355].

The two kidneys of an average adult male weigh approximately 290 g, constituting only 0.5% of the total body mass. Because of their low relative vascular resistance, they receive 20% to 25% percent of the total cardiac output, which amounts to approximately 1 L/min/1.73 m² body surface area (BSA) [320]. This corresponds to a blood flow of 4 ml/min/g kidney weight (KW) [6], a value similar to that observed in the rat [91,185,434] and in the dog [6,205]. This exceeds the blood flow to other organs of the body by as much as 70-fold [251], supplying more oxygen

tant role in the adjustment of the kidney to postnatal life. The young of several species, such as the dog, the pig, and the guinea pig, are more sensitive to the vasoconstrictor effects of epinephrine and norepinephrine than are their adult counterparts [68,69,141,207,349]. Likewise, transection of the renal nerves increases RBF in piglets but not in mature euvolemic pigs [69]. This has led some investigators to propose that the high renovascular resistance observed early in life is due to a high α-adrenergic receptor density or affinity [126,163,260,359,391].

Other observations speak against this hypothesis. Richer et al. [340] and Robillard et al. [346,349] have reported that in fetal sheep α-adrenergic stimulation decreased RBF to a similar or to a lesser extent than in the grown animal. Segments of renal arteries isolated from fetal, newborn, and adult sheep did not differ significantly in their sensitivity (the concentration required for half-maximal response) to α-adrenergic stimulation [255,256]. The discrepancy between the studies described herein may result from differences in neural-induced intrarenal angiotensin production, in the level of circulating vasoactive compounds, or in the species under investigation.

Despite the immaturity of the nervous system, the circulating levels of norepinephrine are high in the fetus and newborn compared to the adult [346,349]. This, rather than an increased sensitivity of the vessels to α-adrenergic stimuli or an intrinsically greater vascular wall tension, may explain the high vascular resistance present in the newborn. Robillard et al. [347] reported that in sheep hypoxia significantly decreased blood flow to the fetal but not to the neonatal kidney. This effect was associated with an increase in circulating epinephrine, the predominant fetal catecholamine. Other studies from this laboratory have revealed that the resting tension of the renal vasculature in the fetus is not intrinsically higher than in the adult [255]. Studies on segments of renal arteries isolated from the dog, however, revealed an increase in maximal tension to phenylephrine with maturation [376]. This latter report is consistent with in vivo studies that indicated that the extent of renal vasoconstrictive response to α-adrenergic stimulation either did not change or increased with age [141,256]. Thus, while the sensitivity of the renal vasculature to α-adrenergic stimulation is independent of age, and the stiffness of the renal vasculature increases during development, the maximal response to α-adrenergic stimulation appears to differ both with species and stage of maturity. The high levels of circulating epinephrine present in the immature animal [228,312] result in constriction of the renal vascular bed that must account in part for the relatively high renal vascular resistance observed at this age.

Several lines of evidence suggest that the β-adrenergic system contributes to the age-related decrease in renovascular resistance. Administration to dogs or sheep of α-adrenergic antagonists, either alone or in combination with catecholamines or the stimulation of renal nerves, increased RBF to a greater extent in young than in mature animals [207,349]. In the newborn sheep, the vasodilation that is induced by renal nerve stimulation during α-adrenergic blockade was abolished by the intrarenal infusion of the β-adrenergic antagonist ICI 118,551 [282]. Further-

more, the density of β_2-adrenergic receptors in the renal cortex of the sheep has been found to decrease with age [124a]. These findings suggest that the early activation of the renal β-adrenergic system, together with the decline in the circulating level of catecholamines, contribute to the decrease in renovascular resistance that is seen with growth.

Felder et al. [125] have described two different low affinity receptors for dopamine in renal cortical membranes of fetal, newborn, and adult sheep. The density of the D-1 receptor did not change with age, while the density of the D-2 receptor decreased. Although dopamine may alter renal hemodynamics by binding to these receptors [203, 204], the significance of age-related changes in binding density is unclear.

THE PROSTANOIDS

Arachidonic acid, a 20-carbon polyunsaturated fatty acid that is produced by the action of phospholipase A_2 on membrane-bound phospholipids, is the precursor for both the PGs by way of cyclo-oxygenase, and the leukotrienes (through lipoxygenase) [97,111]. The ubiquitous prostanoids are not stored in tissues but are produced in response to specific stimuli, act locally for a brief period of time, and are then inactivated [239].

In the kidney, the unstable but biologically active PGG_1 and PGH_2 yield mostly the end-products PGE_2 and PGI_2 and, to a lesser extent, PGD_2, thromboxane A_2, or the less active $PGF_{2\alpha}$. PGI_2 is in turn rapidly degraded to 6-keto-$PGF_{1\alpha}$ [239]. Synthesis of most of the prostanoids occurs in the renal inner medulla, while their catabolism occurs mostly in the cortex. An exception is PGI_2, which is produced mainly by the arterial vasculature of the cortex. PGE_2 is synthesized mostly in the medulla but is also produced by glomerular mesangial cells [239].

Both PGE_2 and PGI_2 dilate the renal vasculature in a variety of species [143,239,240] and decrease the tone of mesangial cells in culture, resulting in an increase in RBF that is more profound in the inner than in the outer cortex [146]. As can be inferred from their intrarenal distribution, PGE_2 dilates the medullary vasculature, while PGI_2 dilates the vasculature of the renal cortex [433]. $PGF_{2\alpha}$ and thromboxane A_2 are vasoconstrictors [269] but are usually present only in small quantities in the kidney, making their physiologic role obscure.

PGs may exert their influences either directly by binding to specific receptors or indirectly through the action of histamine [45]. They stimulate the release of renin, although they antagonize the pressor effects of AII and norepinephrine [367]. Their role in modulating autoregulation and tubuloglomerular feedback is unclear [190].

In the euvolemic unanesthetized animal, in which the levels of circulating vasoconstrictor hormones are low and the renal nerves are unstimulated, PGs are synthesized at low rates. Under these circumstances, PG-inhibiting drugs do not alter blood flow to the kidney [106,402]. Under different conditions, such as anesthesia, volume depletion, heart failure, or hemorrhage, the renin-angiotensin system, the renal nerves, and vasopressin are all activated to maintain mean arterial blood pressure, albeit at the expense of

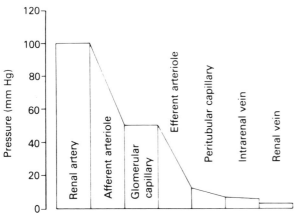

FIG. 3-2. *Hydrostatic pressure profile in the renal vascular tree of the rat. (From Valtin H: Renal Function: Mechanisms Preserving Fluid and Solute Balance in Health. Boston, Little, Brown, 1983, p 101, with permission.)*

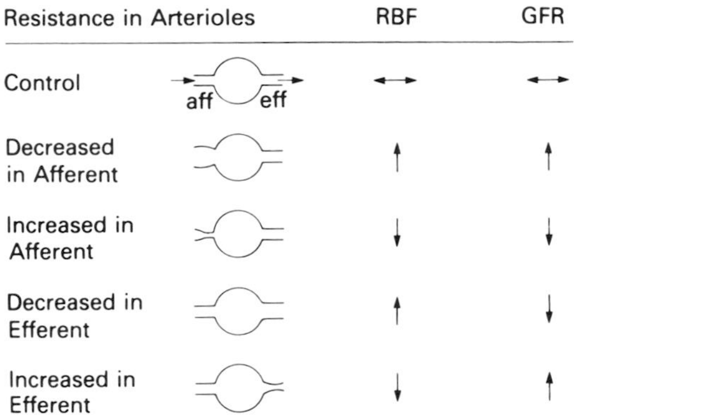

Resistance in Arterioles		RBF	GFR
Control	aff / eff	↔	↔
Decreased in Afferent		↑	↑
Increased in Afferent		↓	↓
Decreased in Efferent		↑	↓
Increased in Efferent		↓	↑

FIG. 3-3. *The effect of changes in renal arteriolar resistance on renal blood flow (RBF) and glomerular filtration rate (GFR). (From Valtin H: Renal Function: Mechanisms Preserving Fluid and Solute Balance in Health. Boston, Little, Brown, 1983, p 105, with permission.)*

rectae originated from the large diameter efferent arterioles of the inner cortex. The smaller-diameter efferent arterioles branched to form the peritubular capillaries.

The most striking difference between the intrarenal vascular system of the puppy and that of the adult dog was observed at the level of the peritubular capillaries [119,121]. During the first two weeks of extrauterine life the outer cortex contained only sinusoidal vessels that had lake-like dilatations along their course. Even the capillaries of the midcortex and innercortex were large and few in number. Transmission electron microscopy showed these capillaries to have irregular lumens and few areas of fenestrae. The basement membrane was poorly represented. The thick walls and the few fenestrae of the immature capillaries suggest limited permeability, as compared to capillaries of adult animals. The peritubular capillaries did not reach a mature appearance in the puppy until the twentieth week of age. Thus, morphologic changes of the renal vessels cannot explain the rapid and large increase in RBF that occurs almost immediately after birth [191,193,388,389]. Instead, this must be due to a decrease in renovascular resistance.

The Rate of Renal Blood Flow

There is no simple, accurate, reproducible, and noninvasive method to quantify RBF [22,30,220,432,434]. The clearance of para-aminohippurate (PAH) is the standard method for measuring RBF in animals and humans [4,33,72,426]. PAH is a weak acid that is both filtered by the glomerulus and secreted by the organic anion antiporter located in the straight segment of the proximal tubule [70,167,295,403]. The clearance of PAH (C_{PAH}) underestimates the true RBF because the extraction of PAH (E_{PAH}) by the kidney is incomplete, particularly in infants [94,99,137,184,187,384], increasing from 54.8 ± 24.6

(SD) at 8 to 90 days of life to 90.0 ± 4.5 by 5 months of life and to 93.5% in the adult [72]. One reason for the low extraction ratio of PAH by the immature kidney is the preponderance of the juxtamedullary circulation. Blood that is shunted through the vasa rectae fails to perfuse the proximal tubules where PAH secretion occurs [409]. Another reason is the limited ability of the immature proximal tubule to transport weak acids [56,72,216], due to a small number of functional transport sites [121,216,400]. Because the determination of E_{PAH} requires the cannulation of the renal vein, it is virtually never attempted in clinical practice.

Radiolabelled carbonized plastic microspheres are often used to measure RBF and its intrarenal distribution in experimental animals [74,205,215,220,345,350,355,434]. The radiolabelled microspheres must be injected rapidly into the left ventricle or the aorta in order to ensure adequate mixing with the blood [220,432], they should be of sufficient size (10 to 15μ) so that they do not pass through the glomerular capillary, and not so numerous as to impede glomerular blood flow [432]. The RBF is proportional to the number of radioactive counts found in the kidney (or a zone of the kidney). Blood flow to several organs can be determined simultaneously, and sequential measurements can be made in the same animal by using microspheres tagged with different radiolabels [74,215, 253,355].

The two kidneys of an average adult male weigh approximately 290 g, constituting only 0.5% of the total body mass. Because of their low relative vascular resistance, they receive 20% to 25% percent of the total cardiac output, which amounts to approximately 1 L/min/1.73 m^2 body surface area (BSA) [320]. This corresponds to a blood flow of 4 ml/min/g kidney weight (KW) [6], a value similar to that observed in the rat [91,185,434] and in the dog [6,205]. This exceeds the blood flow to other organs of the body by as much as 70-fold [251], supplying more oxygen to the kidneys than can be accounted for by their metabolic needs [413]. About one-fifth of this enormous volume of blood is filtered by the kidney to form urine, the major route of excretion of metabolic waste from the body.

CHANGES IN RENAL BLOOD FLOW DURING DEVELOPMENT

The kidneys of the fetus receive approximately 3% of the cardiac output. This corresponds to a blood flow of 1 to 2 ml/min/g KW [39,74,145,157,181], similar to the fetal brain, but only one quarter to one half the rate of blood flow in the adult [315,345,350,353,355]. Renovascular resistance in chronically instrumented fetal sheep was reported to be fourfold greater than in the adult, corresponding to the proportionately lower RBF.

During the first 24 hours after delivery by cesarean section, both RBF and renal vascular resistance remain unchanged [9,181,244,283,284,347]. Thereafter, the vascular resistance decreases precipitously to a proportionately larger extent in the kidneys than in other organs, allowing for a large increase in RBF [196,242,401]. In pigs, RBF was found to increase from 43 to 760 ml/min/m² BSA (17-fold) between 6 hours and 45 days of age [170]. This could not be accounted for by the observed increases in mean arterial blood pressure or cardiac output but coud be explained by the 12-fold fall in renovascular resistance (Fig. 3-4). Studies in the dog [188,205], rat [9,187,410], sheep [347], and human [14,218,355] rendered similar results (Table 3-1). The decrease in renal vascular resistance might be due to decreases in the circulating levels of vasoconstrictor catecholamines, vasopressin, and angiotensin, or to increases in the levels of vasodilator prostaglandins [146,153,279–281,283,285]. Cortisol, which increases abruptly in the plasma of the sheep the day before delivery [182], and growth hormone may also modulate the postnatal changes in renal hemodynamics [183].

The Intrarenal Distribution of Blood Flow

Differences in the distribution of RBF between the cortex and the medulla play an important role in the concentration of urine and possibly in the maintenance of sodium balance [87,434].

Cortical blood flow can be measured by the washout of inert gases [205], the intrarenal distribution of radiolabelled microspheres [205,401,432], extraction of ¹²⁵I-iodoantipyrine-labelled albumin [185], uptake of ⁸⁶Rb-tagged red blood cell, [91,432], or transit renography [220]. In the adult, the cortical blood flow represents about 90% of the total RBF [413], or approximately 5.5 ml/min/g KW [91,185,205, 432], 100 times the rate of blood flow to resting muscle [413].

The distribution of blood flow within the cortex is difficult to quantify accurately due to limitations inherent in the methods of measurement. For example, by using radiolabelled microspheres one overestimates outer cortical and underestimates inner cortical blood flow because of "axial streaming" [220,432], whereas by using ⁸⁶Rb one overestimates the inner cortical blood flow. The best available data indicate that 40% of blood flow to the cortex

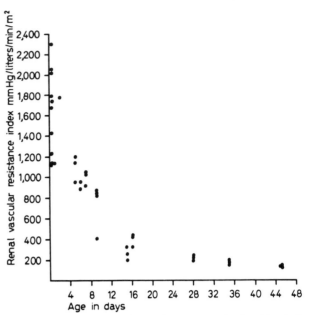

FIG. 3-4. *Changes in renal vascular resistance in the piglet during maturation. (From Gruskin AB, Edelmann CM Jr, Yuan S: Maturational changes in renal blood flow in piglets. Pediatr Res 4:7, 1970, with permission.)*

perfuses the outermost section, and 10% the innermost section, while the remaining 50% is distributed throughout the midcortex.

Blood flow to the medulla accounts for 10% to 15% of the total RBF, corresponding to 1 to 2 ml/min/g KW in the outer medulla, 0.1 to 0.5 ml/min/g KW in the inner medulla, and 0.25 ml/min/g KW in the papilla, as determined by ¹³¹I-albumin extraction [96,432,434]. Measurements of medullary blood flow based on the extraction of ⁸⁶Rb yield, in general, higher values [91,185,432,434]. The rate of blood flow to the medulla is thus similar to that of the brain. Were the blood flow to the medulla similar to that of the renal cortex, the medullary gradient of osmotically active solutes necessary for the counter-current mechanism could not be established [162].

THE INTRARENAL DISTRIBUTION OF BLOOD FLOW DURING DEVELOPMENT

During gestation the rate of RBF per gram kidney remains essentially unchanged; blood flow is distributed evenly throughout the cortex [350]. Following birth, RBF increases more in the outer than the inner cortex [185,205,350]. This was first suggested by the observation that the extraction of PAH increases with age [72,187], which was interpreted to be due mainly to a decrease in the proportion of blood flowing through the vasa rectae [258]. Direct measurements performed by Robillard et al. [350] in sheep and in the dog by Aschinberg et al. [19],

TABLE 3-1. *Postnatal changes in renal blood flow in the human*

Time period after birth	Renal blood flow (ml/min/1.73 m² BSA)
First 12 h	
Early cord clamping	142
Late cord clamping	259
1–2 days	84–92
1–2 weeks	150–200
5–12 months	280–400
1–3 yr	400–650

(*Adapted from* Calcagno PL, Rubin MI: Renal excretion of para-amino-hippurate in infants and children. *J Clin Invest* 42:1632, 1963; Oh W, Oh MA, Lind J: Renal function and blood volume in newborn infant related to placental transfusion. *Acta Pediatr Scand* 55:197, 1966, with permission.)

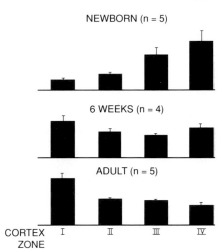

FIG. 3-5. *Relative blood flow per glomerulus in four zones (I = most superficial zone, IV = deepest zone) of the renal cortex in canine. The figure is designed so that the total height of the bars in each age group is equal. (From Olbing H, Blaufox DM, Aschinberg LC, et al: Postnatal changes in renal glomerular blood flow distribution in puppies.* J Clin Invest *52:2885, 1973, with permission.)*

Jose et al. [205], and Olbing et al. [304] confirmed this assumption.

Robillard et al. [350] reported that the glomerular perfusion rate (GPR) was threefold higher in the outer cortex of the 3- to 19-day-old lamb than in chronically instrumented fetal sheep. In contrast, the perfusion rate of glomeruli located in the innermost cortex was similar at both ages. Olbing et al. [304] determined the intrarenal distribution of radionuclide microspheres injected into the thoracic aorta of unanesthetized puppies, ranging in age from 5 hours to 42 days, and in adult dogs (Fig. 3-5). The cortex was divided into four equally thick zones, designated zone I (subcapsular) to zone IV (juxtamedullary). During the first 36 hours of life, the highest blood flow was found in zone II (35.5% ± 2% of injected microspheres per gram of kidney) and the lowest in zone IV (13.4% ± 4% of injected microspheres per gram of kidney). At six weeks of age, zone I had the highest rate of perfusion (48.6% ± 2.1% of injected microspheres per gram of kidney), while flow to zone IV decreased (6.8% ± 0.6% of injected microspheres per gram of kidney). Determination of the number of glomeruli in each zone allowed the investigators to calculate that at birth the perfusion per glomerulus in zone I was only one fifth that in zone IV. By six weeks of age, the pattern had reversed, with perfusion of the outer cortical glomeruli approximately fivefold greater than that of deep glomeruli (zone IV). As a result, the 20-fold increase in RBF with maturation was associated with a 25-fold increase in blood flow to superficial nephrons and a fourfold increase in blood flow to deep glomeruli. The decrease in renovascular resistance that is observed after birth, therefore, must be greater in superficial than in deep renal vascular beds [8,10].

In summary, blood flow to the fetal kidney is similar in magnitude to that of other organs. However, within 48 hours of delivery, blood flow increases by an amount disproportionate to the rest of the body, primarily due to decreased vascular resistance. This increase in RBF is critical to the emergence of the kidney as the organ responsible for the maintenance of body fluid homeostasis. Most of the increase in blood flow occurs in the outermost zones of the cortex. The increase in the rate of blood flow per gram of kidney tissue in a centrifugal distribution is due to proportional decreases in regional vascular resistances.

Glomerular Filtration

Morphology of the Glomerulus

The glomerulus consists of a spherically shaped knot of capillaries enveloped by a basement membrane (GBM) and surrounded by visceral and parietal epithelium that together constitute Bowman's capsule. The glomerular tuft is composed of visceral (podocytic) epithelial cells that lie outside the GBM, endothelial cells that line the capillaries, and mesangial cells that lie between the capillaries, in continuity with the extra-glomerular (lacis) region of the juxtaglomerular apparatus (Fig. 3-6).

The cell bodies of the podocytes lie in Bowman's space and extend tentacle-like major processes that partially encircle the outside of the GBM. The area of basement membrane located between the major processes is covered by narrow cytoplasmic extensions called *foot processes*, which are rich in negatively charged sialoglycoproteins such as podocalyxin [201,235]. Between these foot processes are filtration slits whose 20- to 30-nm wide bases near the GBM are bridged by 4- to 6-nm thick filtration slit diaphragms. The filtration slit diaphragms are composed of arrays of 4×14-nm rectangular pores, about the size of an albumin molecule, surrounding central filaments [351]. Thus, the glomerular epithelium may serve as both a size and charge barrier that excludes negatively charged macromolecules from the urine.

Whereas podocytic and mesangial cells probably have

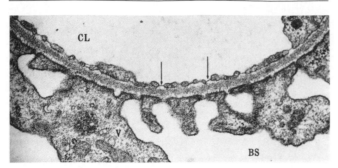

FIG. 3-6. *Transmission electron micrograph illustrating a segment of glomerular capillary wall from a normal rat. The endothelial fenestrations are covered by a thin diaphragm (arrows). CL, capillary lumen; BS, Bowman's space; V, visceral epithelial cell (×60,000). (From Brenner BM, and Rector FC Jr (eds): The Kidney. Philadelphia, W.B. Saunders, 1986, p 13, with permission.)*

common embryologic ancestors, the glomerular vascular endothelium likely derives from cells originating outside the metanephros [117]. Antibodies to the intermediate filament proteins vimentin and desmin bind to epithelial cell podocytes as well as to mesangial cells [392], suggesting they share a common primordial cell. This is not the case with the endothelial cells [392], which orginate outside of the kidney [117]. When developed, the glomerular capillaries contain round fenestrae measuring 40 to 100 nm in diameter, through which the lamina rara externa of the GBM is exposed to the capillary lumen [119].

The GBM is about 150 nm thick in the rat [331] and about 300-nm thick in the human [306]; it lies between the podocyte epithelium and the capillary endothelium. In the adult, it is composed of a central lamina densa, surrounded by the lamina rara externa beneath the epithelium and the lamina rara interna beneath the endothelium. The GBM is composed of collagen types IV and V; laminin, entactin, and various proteoglycans [209]; heparan sulfate, which conveys most of its negative charge [209–211], is located mainly in the lamina rara externa. Heparan sulfate forms a matrix that is both size-selective and charge-selective, preventing the penetration of large, negatively charged molecules, such as albumin, into the urinary space [76,122,209,211–214,354].

THE DEVELOPMENT OF THE GLOMERULAR TUFT

With few notable exceptions (guinea pig and primates), the kidney of mammals is immature at birth, allowing all stages of glomerular development to be seen [120,158,326, 327,334,425]. The most mature glomeruli are found near the medulla, while the least mature are found near the kidney surface. Four stages of glomerular development have been described: the vesicle, the S-body, the capillary loop, and the mature stage [233,334].

In the earliest, or vesicle stage, the glomerulus consists of undifferentiated cells in a cluster. During the so-called S-shaped stage, these undifferentiated cells form a columnar epithelium with a rudimentary 70 to 80 nm base-

ment membrane. These epithelial cells are separated by extracellular matrix from a continuous mesenchymal cell layer, which later differentiates into mesangial and endothelial cells. This mesenchymal cell layer also has a crude basement membrane. The definitive GBM is formed early in the capillary loop stage by fusion of these two primitive basement membranes, with the elimination of the intervening mesenchymal matrix [1,2]. Later in the capillary loop stage, the three layers that constitute the mature GBM become visible. Parallel changes occur in the primitive glomerular endothelium and epithelium. The endothelial fenestrae are initially closed by thin diaphragms that disappear during the capillary loop stage. At the same time, epithelial slits appear.

Experiments in which cationized ferritin was injected into immature rats revealed that, prior to the maturation of the GBM, the primitive unfenestrated endothelium acts as the major glomerular barrier to charged molecules [334]. After the development of endothelial fenestrae, cationic ferritin is trapped either by anionic sites within the GBM or in the intercellular spaces between the early foot processes. With the appearance of the lamina densa, injected cationic ferritin binds to anionic sites in the lamina rara, as in the mature GBM. As the GBM develops into a more effective barrier to charged molecules, it also becomes less permeant to injected anionic (native) ferritin [122,333–335]. Concomitantly, there is a decrease in the number of epithelial slits. This synchronous development of the various components constituting the glomerulus precludes entry of macromolecules into the urinary space during maturation.

THE PERMEABILITY OF THE GLOMERULAR CAPILLARY IN THE ADULT

The glomerular capillary of the adult prevents molecules from passing into the urinary space because of their size, electrical charge, shape, or deformability [55,80,81]. Electron microscopic studies have revealed the existence of a double barrier to the passage of macromolecules through the glomerular capillary. Ferritin enters the endothelial fenestrae but does not penetrate the GBM beyond the lamina rara interna [122]. Catalase and small monomeric forms of ferritin penetrate the lamina densa but are prevented from entering the urinary space by the epithelial slit diaphragms. This suggests that the lamina densa serves as a coarse sieve, while the slit diaphragms serve as an additional fine filter for macromolecules [35]. The classical pore theory has accounted for this phenomemon by postulating the existence of a rigid GBM permeated by circular cylinders, either uniporous or heteroporous, which limit the passage of macromolecules [44,100,101,103,230,231, 314,320]. While the GBM may more nearly resemble a gel than a rigid structure [428], the classical pore theory explains reasonably the permeability of the GBM to neutral dextrans. From clearances of dextrans of various radii, Chang et al. [80] have concluded that the glomerular capillary of the rat contains a single population of pores with a radius of about 48 nm. This is quite similar to earlier estimates of pore size [18,320], which ranged between 24 and 60 nm, or about the size of a molecule of albumin.

Based on a pore radius of 48 nm, one can estimate that 10% of the total glomerular capillary surface area (about 0.002 cm^2) in the adult rat [234] is occupied by pores [80]. This density of pores is substantially higher than in capillaries of skeletal muscle, consistent with the observation that the glomerular capillary is a fenestrated endothelium [320]. Inulin, which has an Einstein-Stokes radius of 14.8 nm, has a fractional clearance of one [320], indicating that there is essentially no restriction to its passage through the glomerular capillary. Albumin, on the other hand, with an Einstein-Stokes radius of 35.5 nm, has a fractional clearance of close to zero, indicating essentially no passage through the glomerulus [320]. This is also true for other large molecules, such as myeloperoxidase (44 nm), catalase (52 nm), and ferritin (61 nm) [122,320].

The glomerulus also restricts passage of molecules based on their shape and flexibility. For example, flexible neutral dextrans pass through the GBM by "reptation." The fractional clearance of neutral dextrans with an effective molecular radius of 28 nm is greater than that of more rigid molecules of similar size, such as albumin, or molecules of both similar size and charge, such as horseradish peroxidase. Sulfation of dextrans results in a decrease in their fractional clearance, in part due to a decrease in their deformability [80].

The fractional clearance of dextrans with radii of 18 to 44 nm is greater for cationic than anionic molecules and intermediate for neutral dextrans [80]. Similarly, the fractional clearances of cationic horseradish peroxidase, albumin, and myoglobin are greater than those of similar sized neutral or negatively charged molecules [57,329]. Thus, the GBM selectively restricts the passage of negatively charged molecules of various shapes and sizes [52]. This is most likely due to the presence of negatively charged heparan sulfate in the lamina rarae, especially in the laminae rara interna [168,212,213]. If heparan sulfate is removed from rat GBM by enzyme digestion, then negatively charged ferritin or ^{125}I-albumin injected into the renal artery appears in the urine [212–214].

Volume expansion of the rat results in an increase in the fractional clearance of 18 to 42 nm neutral dextrans [80,356], while infusion of angiotensin, a potent vasoconstrictor, causes a decrease in molecular clearance [355]. This suggests that changes in RBF result in parallel changes in the permeability of the GBM [109]. If the blood supply to the kidney is interrupted, then previously injected macromolecules, such as albumin or gammaglobulin (IgG), can be found in the urine, whereas the fractional clearance of 30 nm anionic, cationic, or native horseradish peroxidase is unaffected [356,422]. Apparently the GBM serves as an effective barrier to large molecules only in the presence of undisturbed RBF. One hypothesis is that adequate RBF is required for the maintenance of a "concentration-polarization" layer formed by large plasma proteins beneath the endothelial fenestrae [356]. It is assumed that in the absence of blood flow, this barrier disperses, resulting in a more permeable GBM. Support for this theory was provided by experiments performed on isolated perfused kidneys [254]. When albumin was added to the perfusing solution, albuminuria ensued. This was eliminated by the addition of globulin and erythrocytes to the perfusate, sug-

gesting that the larger proteins formed a polarization layer that prevented the passage of smaller proteins. Morphological identification of such a layer, however, has not yet been achieved [254].

An alternative hypothesis to explain the dependence of glomerular permeability on RBF is provided by the pore theory. Under conditions of normal glomerular blood flow, high rates of water flux through the pores or their compaction by the force of blood might limit the passage of albumin. Under conditions of decreased blood flow, there is a decrease in water flux through the pores and less compaction of the pore space, thus allowing for an increase in the passage of albumin [80,231,314]. An increase in RBF should decrease the fractional clearance of all but the smallest and largest molecules, whose passage is least affected by pore size.

The Glomerular Filtration Rate

In 1899, Starling [393,394] proposed that the formation of urine is due to an imbalance between intraglomerular hydrostatic and oncotic pressures that results in ultrafiltration of plasma. Twenty-five years later, Wearn and Richards [421], using micropuncture techniques to sample tubular fluid and microchemical techniques to analyze it, confirmed this assumption. Measurements of the rates at which the glomerular filtrate is formed, however, were not possible until 1926, when Rehberg [337] introduced the concept of clearance. Clearance was later defined by Smith [384] as the virtual volume of plasma that is completely cleared of a test substance "X" by the kidney per unit time. Alternatively, clearance can be defined as the volume of plasma that is required to supply the quantity "Y" of test substance excreted into the urine per unit time. To be a marker of GFR, the test substance should be freely filterable through the glomerular capillary, should be biologically inert, and should be neither reabsorbed nor secreted by the renal tubule. Inulin, a starch-like polymer of fructose with a molecular radius of approximately 15 nm and a molecular weight of approximately 5000 daltons, has alone been shown to fulfill all of these requirements and so has become the gold standard against which all test markers for GFR are compared [384].

Clearance of substance X is described by the equation

$$C = UV/P \tag{1}$$

where U is the concentration of X in the urine, V is the rate of urine flow, and P is the concentration of X in the blood plasma. As UV is equal to the amount of X excreted into the urine per unit time, UV/P is simply the volume of plasma cleared of substance X per unit time.

If substance Y is extracted from the blood exclusively by the kidney, clearance can also be defined as the product

$$C = E \times RPF \tag{2}$$

where E is the fractional extraction of substance Y from the blood by the kidney (A − V/A), and RPF is the renal plasma flow rate.

The Measurement of Glomerular Filtration Rate

The determination of the clearance of inulin is laborious and time-consuming. For this reason, radiolabelled compounds, such as ^{99m}Tc-DTPA, ^{125}I-iothalamate, and ^{51}Cr-EDTA, have been used as alternatives [371]. The claim that clearances of these substances yield measurements similar to those obtained with inulin has been disputed [277,298]. In addition, clinicians are often reluctant to administer radiopharmaceuticals, particularly to children, when alternative methods are available. For these reasons, the clearance of creatinine (C_{CR}), a small molecular weight substance that exists naturally in the blood and urine and can be measured easily in the laboratory, has become the most widely used method to estimate GFR in clinical practice [265]. However, C_{CR} may deviate significantly from C_{IN} [277]. Changes in the rate of production of endogenous creatinine, due, for example, to changes in dietary protein intake or metabolic state [368], may cause the plasma creatinine concentration (P_{CR}) to vary from a true steady-state value. Antibiotics, such as the cephalosporins [386], may interfere with the chromatographic determination of P_{CR}. Even small errors in the measurement of P_{CR} may lead to significant errors in the estimation of GFR. Such mistakes are especially common in children, because the accuracy of the chemical measurement of creatinine diminishes considerably at concentrations below 1 mg/dl [371]. In addition, creatinine is not only filtered through the glomerulus but is also secreted by the renal tubule. The relative amount of urinary creatinine contributed by tubular secretion increases as renal function decreases [36]. As a consequence, C_{CR} overestimates GFR, especially in renal failure. Finally, a marked increase in the rate of urine flow may result in the washout of creatinine present in the tubular lumen or the urinary tract. This will also result in a C_{CR} that overestimates true GFR [250]. Despite these limitations, C_{CR} remains the most practically useful method for estimating GFR.

Developmental Changes in Glomerular Filtration Rate

Soon after it became technically possible to measure GFR in humans, Barnett [33] found that the clearance of inulin was significantly less in infants than in adults, even when corrected for the difference in BSA [259]. This observation revealed that the kidney has its own pattern of maturation, different from that of the body as a whole, and stimulated the investigation into the causes and consequences of the low GFR [113].

Production of urine by the kidney of the fetus is important in the formation of amniotic fluid, which is essential for normal development of the lung [302]. In chronically instrumented fetal sheep, the GFR increased from about 2 ml/min at <120 days of gestation to 3.5 ml/min at >130 days of gestation (term 145 days) [181,348,350]. When expressed per gram KW, however, GFR remained constant at approximately 0.1 ml/min throughout gestation, indicating that the GFR in utero merely increased in parallel with the increase in kidney mass. By 24 hours after delivery by cesarean section, the GFR tripled from 3.5 ml/min to about 10 ml/min, far exceeding any possible increase in kidney mass. The increase in GFR was due apparently to the recruitment of poorly functioning nephrons situated in the outer cortex [9].

An increase in GFR of similar magnitude following birth was noted in the guinea pig, monkey, and human [7,15,218,301]. For example, the C_{CR} of infants born at 25 to 28 weeks' gestation was 11.0 ± 5.4 ml/min/1.73 m^2 BSA, compared to 40.6 ± 14.8 ml/min/1.73 m^2 BSA in infants born at term [371] (Table 3-2). A good correlation between C_{CR} and C_{IN} was noted in 2- to 28-day-old, very-low-birth-weight premature infants (28 to 32 weeks' gestation) [371], possibly due to the immaturity of the creatinine secretory mechanism. This indicates that the difference in C_{CR} between premature and term newborns represents a true difference in GFR.

Following the immediate postnatal period, the GFR con-

TABLE 3-2. *The renal clearance of creatinine in infants*

Gestational age (weeks)	Postnatal age		
	1 week	2–8 weeks	>8 weeks
25 to 28	C 11.0±5.4 (10)*	15.5±6.2 (26)*	47.4±21.5 (9)*+
	A 0.64±0.33*	0.88±0.42*	5.90±5.92*+
29 to 37	C 15.3±5.6 (27)*	28.7±13.8 (27)*+	51.4 (1)
	A 1.22±0.45*	2.43±1.27*+	10.8
38 to 42	C 40.6±14.8 (26)+	65.8±24.8 (20)+	95.7±21.7 (28)+
	A 5.32±1.99	11.15±5.21+	21.0+6.4+

Mean±SD (n) > corrected age up to 15 months.
* Significantly less (p ≤ .05) than corresponding values for full-term infants.
+ Significantly increased (p ≤ .05) compared to previous age group.
C, corrected (ml/min/1.73 m^2 BSA). A = absolute (ml/min).
( ) = number of observations
(*Adapted from* Schwartz GJ, Brion LP, Spitzer A: The use of plasma concentration for estimating glomerular filtration rate in infants, children, and adolescents. *Ped Clin North Am* 34:571, 1987, with permission.)

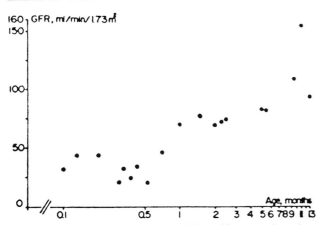

FIG. 3-7. *Glomerular filtration rate (GFR) of human infants during the first year of life, related to the logarithm of age. (From Aperia A, Broberger D, Thodenius K, et al: Development of renal control of salt and fluid homeostasis during the first week of life. Acta Paediatr Scand 64:393, 1975, with permission.)*

tinues to increase in all mammals [188,193,258,338,383, 388], including humans [4,7,15,118,352,371] (Table 3-2). In the rat, between 1 to 3 and 40 days of age, GFR increases by 22-fold, from 0.045 to 1 ml/min/g KW [116]. In the human, GFR, corrected for differences in BSA, doubles from birth to two weeks of age, rises to more than half the adult level by the age of two months, and reaches maturity by about two years of age [33,34,352,426] (Fig. 3-7). Morphogenesis of new nephrons and recruitment of already formed but inadequately perfused superficial glomeruli have been implicated in this process [9]. Morphogenesis continues postnatally in some animal species, such as the rat and the dog [120,158,326,327,425], as well as in infants born before 36 weeks of gestation [327]. In addition, the redistribution of blood flow to the outer cortex results in an increase in the perfusion of poorly functioning nephrons [9]. An increase in the ratio of outer to inner cortical nephron GFR during development was observed in a variety of species [7,10,206]. Neither nephrogenesis nor redistribution of blood flow toward the outer cortex, however, can account for the approximately 25-fold increase in GFR that occurs during maturation. Other variables must be invoked.

The Determinants of Single Nephron Glomerular Filtration Rate (SNGFR)

The rate at which glomerular filtrate is formed is the sum of the filtration rates of various populations of nephrons throughout the kidney. The relationship between those factors favoring and those opposing filtration across each glomerulus is summarized by the Starling equation:

$$SNGFR = P_{uf} \times k \times S \tag{1}$$

where P_{uf} is the average pressure for ultrafiltration across the glomerular capillary, k is the hydraulic conductivity of

the glomerular capillary per unit area, and S is the effective area used for filtration. P_{uf} can be expressed

$$P_{uf} = [(P_{gc} - P_{bs}) - (\pi_{gc} - \pi_t)] \tag{2}$$

where P_{gc} is the mean glomerular capillary hydrostatic pressure, P_{bs} is the hydrostatic pressure in Bowman's space, π_{gc} is the average oncotic pressure in the glomerular capillary, and π_t is the oncotic pressure of the tubular filtrate. As protein concentration in the glomerular filtrate is less than 0.01 mg/dl [60] and P_{bs} is approximately equal to P_t [60], equation 2 simplifies to:

$$P_{uf} = \Delta P - \pi_{gc} \tag{3}$$

where ΔP, the net hydrostatic pressure, is defined as $P_{gc} - P_t$.

If we let $K_f = k \times S$, then equation 1 becomes

$$SNGFR = K_f \times (\Delta P - \pi_{gc}) \tag{4}$$

where K_f is the ultrafiltration coefficient. SNGFR can be measured from the clearance of inulin according to the equation

$$SNGFR = TF/P_{IN} \times V \tag{5}$$

where TF is the concentration of inulin in the renal tubule, P_{IN} is the concentration of inulin in plasma, and V is the rate of tubular fluid flow.

Since the pioneering efforts of Richards in the 1920s [384], measurements of SNGFR and P_{uf} have been obtained by micropuncture. Using sharpened glass micropipettes to collect tubular fluid from superficial nephrons, SNGFR can be calculated from equation 5. When the micropipettes are attached to pressure transducers, P_{uf} can be determined from measurements of P_{gc}, P_t, and π_{gc} (equation 3). P_{gc} can be measured directly in the Munich-Wistar rat, an inbred strain in which some of the glomeruli are subcapsular and thus accessible to micropuncture. Because it cannot be ascertained whether the pressure pipette is introduced closer to the efferent or afferent end of the glomerular capillary, only an average value for P_{gc} can be obtained.

Glomerular pressures have also been measured indirectly in species that lack surface glomeruli [290,309,390]. The flow of tubular fluid is stopped by the introduction of an oil or wax block into the early proximal tubule. As glomerular filtration continues and fluid accumulates in the obstructed tubule segment, the pressure rises until it reaches a stable value, the "stop flow pressure" (P_{sf}). At this point, P_{uf} equals zero, and P_{sf} should be equal to P_{bs}. Substituting into equation 2

$$P_{gc} = P_{sf} + \pi_a, \tag{6}$$

where π_a is the oncotic pressure in the afferent arteriole. It should be noted that the P_{gc} obtained in the absence of filtration should overestimate P_{gc} obtained by direct measurement. Due to the conservation of mass, glomerular blood volume must increase as ultrafiltration decreases, thereby increasing the hydrostatic pressure in the glomerular capillary.

Blantz [49] compared P_{gc} obtained in the hydropenic Munich-Wistar rat by direct measurement to those calculated from P_{sf}. Directly measured P_{gc} rose following the introduction of the oil block, but then it rapidly returned to control values. This biphasic change in P_{gc} might have been due to cessation of glomerular filtration, resulting in a compensatory decrease in afferent arteriole resistance. As a consequence, direct and indirect measurements of P_{gc} coincided. In euvolemic Munich-Wistar rats, however, P_{gc} obtained by indirect measurements overestimated P_{gc} obtained by direct measurements. Ichikawa [191] reported a P_{gc} in the Munich-Wistar rat of approximately 54 mm Hg after the placement of an oil block into the proximal tubule, compared to 47 mm Hg before blockade.

Because surface glomeruli are present in very few species, there is little reliable micropuncture data on animals other than the Munich-Wistar rat [60,250]. Aside from having surface glomeruli, this strain achieves filtration pressure equilibrium so that P_{uf} becomes zero somewhere along the glomerular capillary. This probably does not occur in other mammals, such as the dog [188,309]. These two unique features make it difficult to extrapolate data obtained from this animal species to others, including humans.

Despite these limitations, P_{gc} can be determined and P_t can be measured directly in superficial proximal tubules. In addition, blood can be collected from superficial efferent arterioles, allowing afferent (systemic) and efferent plasma protein concentrations to be estimated. Because the oncotic pressure cannot be determined at each point along the glomerular capillary, only the averge π_{gc} can then be calculated from the formula of Landis [231]:

$$\pi = 2.1C + 0.16C^2 + 0.0009C^3 \qquad (7)$$

where C is the concentration of plasma protein. As oncotic pressure rises along the glomerular capillary, only a maximal value for P_{uf} can be obtained from micropuncture measurements of P_{gc}, P_t, and average π_{gc}. As a consequence, only a minimum value for K_f can be derived from equation 4.

In order to ascertain and to predict changes in intraglomerular hemodynamics, Deen [102] developed a mathematical model in which the glomerular capillary tuft was reduced to a single, straight hollow tube. The radius and hydraulic permeability of this tube were assumed to be constant, the reflection coefficient to protein to be equal to one, and the axial pressure drop along the capillary to be small relative to ΔP. The most convenient model of glomerular filtration would assume a linear profile of ΔP along the glomerular capillary, such that $\pi_{gc} = (\pi_{ea} + \pi_{aa})/2$ (where π_{ea} and π_{aa} are the oncotic pressures in the efferent and afferent arterioles, respectively), as represented by the solid line in Fig. 3-8. $\Delta\pi$, on the other hand, must increase as ultrafiltration proceeds across the glomerular capillary. As oncotic pressure rises within the capillary, the net pressure for ultrafiltration diminishes. This will tend to retard the rate at which plasma oncotic pressure increases along the remainder of the glomerular capillary. As a consequence, π must follow a curvilinear profile along

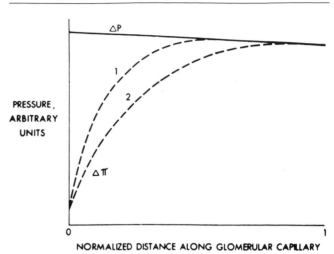

FIG. 3-8. *Hydraulic and colloid-osmotic transcapillary pressure profiles along an idealized glomerular capillary. (From Deen WM, Troy JL, Robertson CR, et al: Dynamics of glomerular ultrafiltration in the rat. IV. Determinants of the ultrafiltration coefficient. J Clin Invest 52:1500, 1973, with permission.)*

the capillary pathway. Because P_{uf} is the difference between ΔP and π, it too must vary along the capillary. This curve cannot be determined from micropuncture measurements. Deen's model, however, predicts that an increase in the plasma flow rate would retard the rate of increase in plasma oncotic pressure along the capillary. Eventually, ΔP would exceed π, such that filtration pressure disequilibrium ensues. Under these circumstances, a unique oncotic pressure curve satisfies the measured values of afferent and efferent arteriolar oncotic pressures, and a unique value of P_{uf} can be derived. Measurements of P_{uf} and SNGFR permit the calculation K_f from equation 4. Alternatively, K_f can be directly measured by independent determinations of glomerular capillary hydraulic conductivity and surface area. These approaches have permitted quantitation of each of the variables that affect the rate of glomerular filtration.

CHANGES IN THE DETERMINANTS OF SNGFR DURING DEVELOPMENT

Changes in SNGFR during development have been measured in the rat [8,191,193,410], dog [188], and guinea pig [388]. In the euvolemic Munich-Wistar rat, SNGFR increased from 16.0 ± 1.2 nl/min at 30 to 45 days of age to 42.8 ± 2.6 nl/min at adulthood [193]. In the dog, in which nephrogenesis is completed by about 14 days of life, SNGFR increased from 3 nl/min at 21 days to 23 nl/min at 77 days of life [188]. In the guinea pig, which is born with a full complement of nephrons, whole kidney GFR increased almost linearly over the first six weeks after birth. SNGFR of superficial nephrons, however, increased little between 1 and 14 days of life and then surged by 20-fold (from 0.9 to 19.3 nl/min) during the ensuing two weeks [388–390] (Fig. 3-9). The filtration rate of the juxtamedullary glomeruli was estimated to increase from 17.2 to

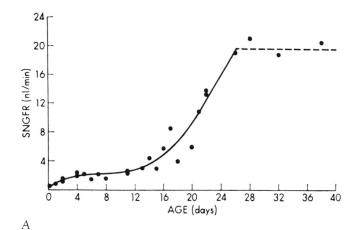

A

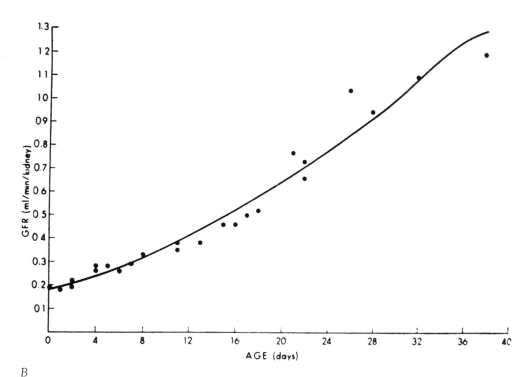

B

FIG. 3-9. *Changes in superficial single-nephron glomerular filtration rate (SNGFR) (A) and in total kidney GFR (B) during the development of the guinea pig. (From Spitzer A, Brandis M: Functional and morphologic maturation of the superficial nephrons. J Clin Invest 53:279, 1974, with permission.)*

42.1 nl/min, or only 2.4 times, during the first two weeks of life, and little, if at all, during the subsequent two weeks of observation. Thus, during the initial period of postnatal development the increase in total kidney GFR was due to an increase in SNGFR of the deep nephrons, whereas during the following period of development it was due entirely to the increase in superficial SNGFR. As discussed in the following sections, measurements performed in the rat and the guinea pig have allowed us to estimate the contribution made by each determinant of glomerular filtration to the overall changes in SNGFR.

The Net Ultrafiltration Pressure

P_{uf} was determined by micropuncture in several animal species. In the guinea pig, the average P_{gc}, calculated from the P_{sf}, was found to increase from 19 to 38 mm Hg between 1 and 49 days of age [388–390]. Concomitantly, P_t increased from 3.6 to 9.9 mm Hg, while π_a increased from 10 to 15.6 mm Hg. As a consequence, P_{uf} increased from 5.4 to 12.5 mm Hg, or 2.5-fold. Most of this increase occurred before the age of 14 days. It is, therefore, not surprising that in the Munich-Wistar rat no increase in P_{uf} was found between 30 days of age and maturity [193,410], and only a slight increase (from 21.7 to 25.6 mm Hg) was noted in the Wistar rat between 21 days of age and adulthood [5]. In the guinea pig, the magnitude of the increase in P_{uf} could explain only about 10% of the increase in GFR observed with maturation. An increase in the surface area or in the permeability of the glomerular capillary, therefore, had to be largely responsible for this process.

The Hydraulic Conductivity of the Glomerular Capillary

There are no direct measurements of hydraulic conductivity (k) during development. Measurements based on the clearance of dextrans of various molecular sizes, however, indicate tht the glomerular capillary is only slightly more restrictive in the newborn than in the mature dog (Fig. 3-10). The estimated increase in k of 1.3-fold observed in dog can account for no more than 5% of the observed increase in SNGFR [152]. There was no difference between one-week and six-week-old puppies in pore size. In contrast, the effective pore area in young puppies was less than one tenth that observed in older animals. As a consequence, the value of K_f was significantly lower in one-week-old puppies (0.010 ± 0.002 ml/sec/mm Hg) than in six-week-old animals (0.093 ± 0.012 ml/sec/mm Hg).

These results are different from those reported previously by Arturson et al. [18] in humans. These authors found a significantly greater restriction to the passage of macromolecules in early infancy than in childhood. Their data were compatible with a two-pore size model of glomerular filtration. Between 6 and 90 days of age, the smaller pores were found to increase from 19.6 ± 0.2 to 25 ± 1.2 nm and the larger pores from 59 ± 3 to 62 ± 3 nm, suggesting a significant increase in permeability with age. Other investigators [191,388], however, citing clinical and theoretical studies, claim that these findings exaggerate the contribution of glomerular permeability to the development of GFR. For example, the permeability of anionic ferritin has been found to decrease with age [122]. In addition, fractional clearance of transferrin (89,000 daltons) was reported to decrease from 2.6 μl/min/1.73 m² BSA in 1- to two-week-old neonates to 1 μl/min/1.73 m² BSA in 10- to 16-year-old children [266]. A similar decrease was noted in the fractional clearance of albumin (69,000 daltons) [266] (Table 3-3). In addition, the model of Deen et al. [102] predicts that the barrier properties of the GBM should improve due to the age-related increase in RBF. The discrepancy in these data can be explained by differences in techniques and by the very small number of infants examined. Taken together, these studies indicate that the changes in the hydraulic conductivity observed during development are very small. Therefore, the development of GFR must be due mainly to increases in capillary surface area (S) used for filtration.

Changes in the Glomerular Capillary Surface Area

In the rat, the length of the glomerular capillary per unit volume of glomerulus (L_v) increases gradually from 4.53 ± 0.28 m/mm³ to 9.68 ± 0.63 m/mm³ between 20 days' gestation and the third postnatal day [302a]. The rate at which L_v increases, however, accelerates between 22 days of gestation and birth. This increase in glomerular capillary surface results in a large increase in GFR after birth.

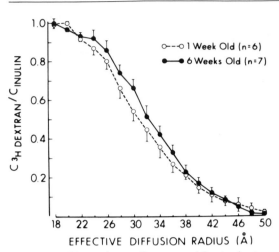

FIG. 3-10. *Glomerular capillary permeability in the 1- and 6-week-old canine measured by the clearance of dextrans. (From Goldsmith DI, Jodorkovsky RA, Sherwinter J, et al: Glomerular capillary permeability in developing canines. Am J Physiol 251:F528, 1986, with permission.)*

Using morphometric measurements of glutaraldehyde-fixed glomeruli of rats, Larsson and Maunsbach [234] found that between 3 and 40 days of age the diameter of superficial glomeruli increased from 50.6 μm to 139.9 μm, whereas the surface density of the glomerular capillaries rose from 0.062 to 0.163 μm²/μm³. They calculated that the surface area of the GBM, epithelial slits, and endothelial fenestrae increased during the same period 28-fold, 30-fold, and 70-fold, respectively. As the surface area of the GBM increased only 1.7-fold when normalized by KW, these investigators concluded that the increase in the surface area of the glomerular capillaries was insufficient to explain the 22-fold increase in GFR observed during the development of the rat. Because most of the increase in KW is due to an increase in the mass of the renal tubules and not of the glomeruli [12], however, it is inappropriate to "correct" the increased glomerular capillary surface for KW. Moreover, these authors ignored their own data regarding the increase in the density of the epithelial slits and endothelial fenestrae. Studies using antiglomerular basement membrane antibodies as a marker of glomerular capillary surface area revealed a threefold to fourfold difference in the amount of antibody bound between rats weighing 50 g and rats weighing 200 g, with no further rise thereafter up to a weight of 400 g [221].

Savin and Terreros [365] harvested isolated glomeruli from cortical tissue by passing it through mesh screens of various sizes. Using a video camera, the glomerular diameter was determined in the presence and absence of a protein-free isotonic bathing solution, The change in glomerular capillary diameter over time was then used to calculate K_f. The K_f increased from 3.77 ± 0.23 nl/min/mm Hg in the immature to 5.52 ± 0.47 nl/min/mm Hg in the mature rabbit, or about twofold. These investigators subsequently determined that, in the human, glomerular

Table 3-3. *Developmental changes in the renal clearance of proteins ($\mu l/min/1.73 \ m^2$ BSA)*

	Neonates (1–2 weeks)	Infants (3–5 months)	Children (10–16 yr)
$C_{Creatinine}$	0.04	0.1	0.1
$C_{Total \ urine \ protein}$	4.1	2.2	1.2
$C_{Globulins}$ (mol wt > 100,000)	0.2	0.4	0.7
$C_{Transferrin}$ (mol wt 89,000)	2.6	2.5	1.0
$C_{Albumin}$ (mol wt 69,000)	2.0	1.2	0.9
$C_{Tubular \ microproteins}$ (mol wt 52,000–12,000)	0.003	0.002	0.0004

(*From* Miltenyi M: Developmental aspects of the glomerular filtration of plasma proteins. *In* Spitzer A (ed): *The Kidney During Development: Morphology and Function.* New York, Masson, 1982, with permission.)

volume increased eightfold, total GBM area increased sevenfold, and K_f increased 2.8-fold (from 6 to 17 nl/min/mm Hg) during development [364]. This is similar to the threefold increase observed in the rat between 40 and 140 days of age [191,193,410] but is less than the tenfold increase in K_f calculated from micropuncture data in the guinea pig between 1 and 30 days of age (from 0.17 to 1.78 nl/min/mm Hg) [388–390]. If one assumes that little of these increase is due to changes in hydraulic conductivity, then glomerular capillary surface area must increase substantially with age.

John et al. [198] measured glomerular capillary surface area directly by quantifying the radioactivation of chromium contained in a silicone rubber compound that was injected into the renal vasculature of one-week-old and adult dogs following fixation of the kidneys with glutaraldehyde. These investigators found an increase in capillary surface area with age of tenfold in superficial and fourfold in deep glomeruli, corresponding to an increase in glomerular capillary surface area of about eightfold for the whole kidney (Fig. 3-11). This is in excellent agreement with micropuncture data obtained in the guinea pig [388–390] and the dextran sieving data obtained in the canine pup [152]. In the latter, the 25-fold increase in SNGFR between 1 and 30 days of age (0.9–19.3 nl/min) can be accounted for by a 2.5-fold increase in P_{uf}, a 1.3-fold increase in k, and an eightfold increase in S [388–390]. Thus, most of the data indicate that the increase in the surface area available for filtration accounts for much of the increase in SNGFR observed during development. It should be pointed out, however, that morphometric analysis does not permit us to assess the glomerular capillary surface area that is actually used for filtration [127].

The Autoregulation of RBF and GFR

Autoregulation is the process by which the kidney maintains RBF and GFR relatively constant despite changes in renal perfusion pressure. Autoregulation occurs in innervated, denervated, and isolated kidneys, indicating that this process is intrinsic to the organ [406,407]. Both GFR

and postglomerular capillary pressure remain stable when renal perfusion pressure changes [129,377,379,407]. Therefore, autoregulation must involve changes in the vascular tone of afferent arterioles.

Although the process affects all renal capillary beds, including those of the cortex [166,288] and medulla [434], the range of perfusion pressures at which autoregulation occurs differs between capillary beds [93]. In the medulla, blood flow is autoregulated between 80 and 120 mm Hg, whereas in the cortex it is autoregulated over a broader range, from 80 to 180 mm Hg [276,434]. As a result, the medulla is more vulnerable to ischemic injury than the cortex.

The myogenic theory of autoregulation, proposed by Bayliss [38] in 1902, asserts that arterial smooth muscle contracts or relaxes to keep wall tension constant over a range of transmural pressures. The observation that an increase in renal perfusion pressure results in a proportional increase in afferent arteriolar resistance [114,278,342] supports this assumption.

The link between the wall tension that develops in response to renal perfusion pressure and the increase in vascular resistance may be an increase in intracellular Ca^{2+} [243]. Fray et al. [130,131] has pointed out that the vascular smooth muscle of juxtaglomerular cells and afferent arterioles has Ca^{2+} channels that are sensitive to voltage, hormones, and stretch. When vascular smooth muscle is stretched, Ca^{2+} permeability, and thus the influx of Ca^{2+} into cells, increases. This augments the tension of the vasculature and thus increases afferent resistance. Using in vivo perfused kidneys of anesthetized dogs, Ogawa and Ono [300] have demonstrated that calcium channel blockers, Ca^{2+} chelators, and calmodulin inhibitors interfered with autoregulation. Autoregulation of RBF could be restored by either the addition of $CaCl_2$ to the perfusate or by the administration of the Ca^{2+} channel activator BAY K 8644. Thus, there appears to be a stretch-sensitive Ca^{2+} channel located within the vascular smooth muscle of the afferent arteriole that mediates the auto-regulatory response of the kidney to changes in renal perfusion pressure [291]. Other proposed modulators of autoregulation, such as the renin-

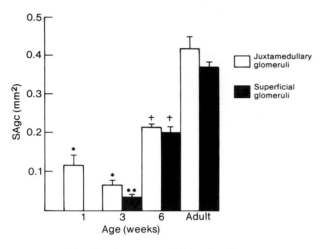

Glomerular Capillary Surface Area (SAgc) in Canine Puppies and Adult Dogs

☐ Juxtamedullary glomeruli

■ Superficial glomeruli

* p<0.01 vs. 6 weeks   ** p<0.001 vs. 6 weeks
+ p<0.001 vs. adult

Values are the means ±S.E.M.

FIG. 3-11. *Glomerular capillary surface area in canine puppies and adult dogs measured by a method based on the radioactivation of chromium contained in a silicone rubber compound injected into the renal vasculature. (From John E, Goldsmith DI, Spitzer A: Quantitative changes in the canine glomerular vasculature during development: Physiologic implications. Kidney Int 20:223, 1981, with permission.)*

angiotensin system [238,293], may ultimately act by affecting the level of intracellular Ca^{2+} [90,159,291].

Tubuloglomerular feedback is another homeostatic process regulating afferent arteriolar resistance wherein changes in delivery of salt or fluid to the distal tubule result in parallel changes in afferent arteriolar tone [40,41, 51,190]. Whether tubuloglomerular feedback is mediated by the renin-angiotensin system [41,160,174,321], adenosine [41,249,316], prostaglandins [41], or other factors is not clear. Changes in either the magnitude or the pulsatile frequency of renal perfusion pressure [252,358] might result in changes in renal tubule interstitial pressure, such that the stimulus for both the autoregulatory and tubuloglomerular feedback response may actually be the same [289, 292]. When the tubuloglomerular response is inhibited by the intratubular administration of furosemide, the autoregulatory response to increased perfusion pressure is attenuated [270]. The vasomotor response to tubuloglomerular feedback signals from the distal nephron is probably mediated by mesangial cell contraction [190,368].

AUTOREGULATION OF RBF AND GFR IN IMMATURE ANIMALS

There are only a few studies of autoregulation of RBF in developing animals [78,208,219,431]. The effect of aortic constriction on RBF and GFR was studied in two groups of lambs, one group 2 to 9 days of age, the other 31 to 48

days of age [11]. Arterial pressure decreased in the first group by 34% and in the second by 39%, while GFR decreased by 50% and 49%, respectively. These results suggest that the renal vasculature of the newborn is as sensitive as that of the older animal to large decreases in renal blood pressure. Unfortunately, because the decrease in blood pressure was not graded, no conclusion can be drawn from this study regarding changes in blood pressure within the autoregulatory range.

In the adult rat, aortic constriction resulting in a decrease in renal perfusion pressure of 30% affected RBF and GFR only slightly [431]. Conversely, a similar reduction in renal perfusion pressure in four- to five-week-old animals resulted in a modest reduction in RBF but a marked decrease in GFR. This suggests that autoregulation changes with age.

Chevalier and Kaiser et al. [85] have shown that autoregulation of RBF in the young rat occurs at renal perfusion pressures between 70 and 100 mm Hg, compared to pressures of 100 to 130 mm Hg in the adult. An increase with age in the set point at which autoregulation occurs has also been found in the dog [208]. To determine the underlying mechanism, Chevalier et al. [83–86] examined the relationship between changes in renal perfusion pressure and the rate of RBF in young and adult rats. All of the animals had one kidney removed prior to study, thus maximizing blood flow to the remnant kidney. In the adult, autoregulation was well maintained in the remaining kidney so that RBF increased proportionately to perfusion pressures of 40 to 100 mm Hg, but RBF did not increase further as perfusion pressure was raised to 130 mm Hg. In contrast, autoregulation of blood flow to the remaining kidney of the young rat was impaired (Fig. 3-12). The administration of prostaglandin (PG) inhibitors to the young, uninephrectomized rats partially restored autoregulation, whereas the administration of angiotensin converting enzyme inhibitors did not. Converting enzyme (ACE) inhibitors did, however, increase RBF at any renal perfusion pressure. The authors speculated that enhanced PG formation after uninephrectomy may have caused an increase in the release of renin and angiotensin, with a resulting vasoconstriction greater in the young than in the old rats [287]. This would suggest that PGs may mediate autoregulation through their effect on renin release, and that their role diminishes with age. Alternatively, the shift in the autoregulatory range may be explained by a change in tubuloglomerular feedback [292]. In rats, the "set point" at which the rate of tubular fluid flow results in autoregulatory changes in glomerular hemodynamics increases with age [61]. Whatever the mechanism may be, autoregulation of RBF occurs in the young and maintains blood flow to the kidney constant over a range of renal perfusion pressures that are physiologic for the age in question.

Factors That Affect RBF and GFR

A variety of factors are known to influence the RBF and GFR [25,37,75,104,112,370,406]. Among the best studied are angiotensin, PGs, and the renal nerves [58,222,251]. These factors act by affecting three different but related variables: (1) mesangial cell contraction, (2) contraction

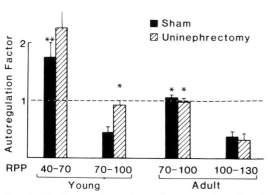

Fig. 3-12. *Autoregulation factor for range of renal perfusion pressure (RPP) of 40–70 mm Hg or 70–100 mm Hg (young rats) and RPP of 70–100 or 100–130 mm Hg (adult rats). A factor equal to or greater than unity denotes lack of autoregulation while a factor of zero indicates perfect autoregulation. Bars show mean ± SE for each group. *, P < 0.05 vs. young sham group and adult groups for RPP of 100–130 mm Hg. **, P < 0.05 vs. young groups for RPP of 70–100 mm Hg and adult groups. (From Chevalier RL, Kaiser DL: Autoregulation of renal blood flow in the rat: Effects of growth and uninephrectomy. Am J Physiol 244:F483, 1983, with permission.)*

TABLE 3-4. *Effect of vasoactive substances on the renal vasculature of the rabbit*

	Interlobular	Afferent	Efferent
Norepinephrine	↑	↑	↑
AII	→	→	↑
Acetylcholine	↓	↓	↓
Dopamine	→↓	↓	↓
Bradykinin	→	→	↓

↑, vasoconstriction; →, no effect; ↓, vasodilation. (*From Edward RM: Segmental effects of norepinephrine and angiotensin II on isolated renal microvessels. Am J Physiol 244:F526, 1983, with permission.*)

or relaxation of vascular smooth muscles, and (3) intrinsic homeostatic mechanisms. The effect of some of these substances on specific segments of the renovasculature is summarized in Table 3-4. Their influence is exerted apparently only under conditions of stress. For example, neither denervation nor PG or converting enzyme inhibition, altered RBF in euvolemic, anesthetized adult animals [406].

The mesangial cell is a modified vascular smooth muscle cell that contracts or relaxes in response to a number of vasoactive agents. Richards and Schmidt [339] noted in 1924 that the number of perfused glomeruli in the superficial cortex of the frog changed with renal nerve stimulation, volume expansion, or the administration of caffeine, epinephrine, or pitressin. The number of open capillary loops, and thus the glomerular capillary area, varied analogously. There is evidence that the glomerular capillary surface available for filtration is also regulated in mammals [368], probably by mesangial cell contraction. Mesangial cells in culture have been found to contract in response to application of angiotensin II (AII), vasopressin, and norepinephrine, a process that is mediated by increases in cytosolic Ca^{2+} [17,23,48,88,303,305]. Atriopeptides, by attaching to specific receptors, activate a guanylate cyclase, resulting in a decrease in cell Ca^{2+} and mesangial cell relaxation [368]. Addition of dopamine or PGE_2 to mesangial cells in culture stimulates cAMP production by activating adenyl cyclase and results in a decrease in basal cell tone [368]. cAMP probably acts by decreasing myosin light chain activity and its phosphorylation and, thus, by dissociating actin from myosin fibers [368].

Endothelial cells react to mechanical force and to neurohumoral mediators by releasing vasoconstrictor or vasodilator substances that control underlying smooth muscle tone and thereby vascular diameter (Fig. 3-13). Furchgott [139,140] called the vasodilators *endothelium-derived relaxing factors* (EDRF), one of which has been identified as nitric oxide [313] and another of which may be ammonia [13,414]. For example, the increase in RBF that follows the infusion of acetylcholine into the rat is abolished by the administration of L-NG-monomethylarginine, an inhibitor of nitric oxide production from arginine [229]. This suggests that acetylcholine-induced vasodilation of the renal vasculature is mediated by nitric oxide. EDRF stimulate the guanylate cyclase of vascular smooth muscle, thereby increasing cGMP with resulting smooth muscle relaxation [322].

Recently, a potent vasoconstrictor peptide, endothelin, has been isolated from the supernatant of porcine aortic endothelial cell culture [380,430]. Administration of small doses of endothelin to isolated strips of renal artery produced significant vasoconstriction [151,430]. Infusion of endothelin into the rat caused a significant decrease in RBF [217]. Conversely, the administration of antibodies to endothelin abolished the decrease in SNGFR observed after stimulation of the renal nerves [224], suggesting that endothelin mediates renal nerve-induced vasoconstriction. Micropuncture studies have revealed that the administration of endothelin results in a decrease in SNGFR due to increased resistance of both the afferent and efferent arterioles [24,225]. Specific binding sites for endothelin have been found in human renal vasculature, with preliminary observations indicating a maximal binding capacity that is greater in fetal than in adult kidney tissue [200,236]. Using Northern blot analysis, MacCumber et al. have detected mRNA for endothelin in the vasa rectae of the renal medulla of the adult rat [248]. The discovery of this peptide has led to the hypothesis that tone in local vascular beds is modulated by the balance between endothelium-derived relaxing and constricting substances [161]. Furthermore, the observation that the number of binding sites for endothelin in the renal vasculature decreases with age might, in part, account for the high renovascular resistance characteristic of immature animals.

THE RENIN-ANGIOTENSIN SYSTEM

Renin is an acid protease whose active form (as distinguished from inactive or prorenin) is secreted from granules

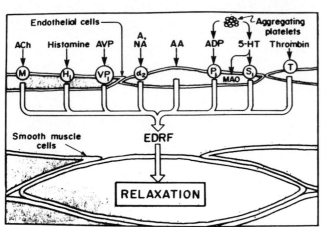

FIG. 3-13. *Generation of a vasoactive substance(s) by the vascular endothelium: various substances activate specific endothelial receptors (circles) and induce the formation of endothelial drived relaxing factors (EDRF) which in turn cause relaxation of arterial vessels. A, adrenaline; Ach, acetylcholine; α_2, alpha-receptor; AA, arachidonic acid; AVP, arginine vasopressin; H_1, histamine receptors; 5-HE, 5-hydroxytryptamine (serotonin); MAO, monoamine oxidase; M, muscarinic receptors; NA, noradrenalin; VP_1, vasopressinergic receptors; P_1, purinergic receptors; S_1, serotonergic receptors; T, thrombin receptors. (From Vanhoutte PM: Vascular physiology: The end of the quest? Nature 327:459, 1987, with permission.)*

located within juxtaglomerular cells, modified vascular smooth muscle cells located predominantly within afferent arterioles [63,67,164,173,272,372]. The release of renin from these granules is promoted by cAMP and inhibited by increases in intracellular Ca^{2+} [88,131]. After renin is released, it may either enter the general circulation by way of the renal veins or enter the lymphatic interstitium surrounding the afferent arterioles [28]. Renin that is secreted into this interstitium may be distributed throughout the juxtaglomerular apparatus, taken up by surrounding capillaries, or circulated within the lymphatic periarterial sheath toward the hilus of the kidney [28].

Whether formed in the general circulation or in the periarterial lymphatics, renin cleaves the N-terminal decapeptide angiotensin I (AI) from the large glycoprotein angiotensinogen, which is produced both by the liver [133] and locally by the proximal convoluted tubule of the kidney [273]. Angiotensin converting enzyme (ACE), synthesized by vascular endothelial cells [299,357], cleaves the carboxy-terminal dipeptide from AI to produce bioactive AII. AII is formed both systemically and within the renal interstitium and may act on the general circulation as well as locally within the kidney [28,63,66,77,98,271,286, 308,314,336,382].

The observation that AI, when infused into the renal artery of the isolated perfused kidney, is rapidly converted to AII demonstrates the presence of biologically active ACE within the kidney [98,328]. To clarify the physiologic significance of intrarenally formed AII, Navar and Rosivall [293] infused AI into one renal artery of a dog that hap-

pened to have two arteries perfusing the same kidney and measured the RBF going to both. RBF decreased only in the area of the kidney perfused by the artery that was infused, indicating that AII was produced and acted only on a well-defined segment of the renal vasculature. Other studies [62,195] have revealed that locally produced AII increased vascular resistance and decreased inner cortical blood flow more than infused AII. These findings suggest that AII formed by the kidney has an important physiologic role in regulating renal hemodynamics [238,242,286, 293,332].

Although its major role is in the conservation of sodium in states of salt or volume depletion [65,175,317,399], AII plays a role in the control of peripheral vascular resistance [3,171,172,385], cardiac contractility [416,429], renal hemodynamics [59,123,124,160,186,189,192], mineralocorticoid secretion [417], adrenal and peripheral nerve catecholamine release [147], thirst [128], neuro-transmission [381], hepatocyte metabolic function [95], salt and water reabsorption from the gut [338], and blood pressure maintenance in volume or sodium depletion [304]. Most studies have revealed that AII administration results in preferential vasoconstriction of the efferent arterioles and to a lesser extent the afferent arterioles [49,50,58,59,90,114,134, 395–398].

The Renin-Angiotensin System During Development

Plasma renin activity (PRA) is elevated in third trimester gravida humans [63,142] and is higher in blood from the umbilical artery than from the umbilical vein [142,148]. Since maternal renin does not cross the placenta [297,307], the elevated renin levels found in the fetus presumably derives from the fetal kidney [155,178,226,323,324,369].

As in the adult [28,63,66,77,173,272,286], all components of the renin-angiotensin system have been identified in the fetal kidney [43,115,155,245,324,408]. Droplets of angiotensinogen and ACE were found in proximal tubules by antisera staining during early stages of differentiation [274,427]. The intensity of antisera staining increased with tubular development. ACE was also found along the afferent and efferent arterioles of the human fetus, whereas in the adult it was characteristically localized to the peritubular capillaries [274]. The physiologic significance of this finding is unclear. Granulated juxtaglomerular cells have been observed in the human kidney by 17 weeks' gestation [115,369], and renin has been detected in kidney vessels and juxtaglomerular apparati during early fetal life [274]. Recently, Gomez and his associates have observed that in the fetus, renin and its mRNA extended to the arcuate and interlobular arteries, whereas in the newborn they were present only in the juxtaglomerular region [154,156] (Fig. 3-14). Finally, receptors for AII have been demonstrated in the renal cortex of the fetal rat [66,262,263,412].

Angiotensinogen levels are low in fetal blood [274], due possibly to excessive consumption by renin [197]. They then increase rapidly to adult levels or greater, perhaps due to estrogen effect on the liver [226]. ACE activity measured from peripheral blood in the first 24 hours of life is higher in premature than in term infants but is similar to the adult [43]. The pattern of ACE distribution in the vasculature of the newborn is intermediate between that of the fetus

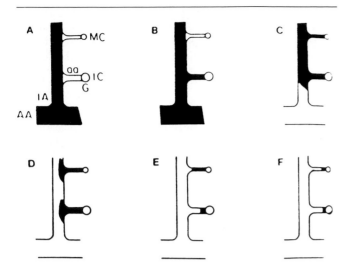

FIG. 3-14. *Schematic representation of the changes in intrarenal distribution of renin during maturation. AA, arcuate artery; IA, interlobular artery; aa, afferent arteriole; G, glomerulus; IC, inner (juxtamedullar) cortex; MC, middle cortex; Shaded areas represent areas containing renin (a) 19-day-old fetus; (b) 20-day-old fetus; (c) newborn 5 days old; (d) newborn 10 days old; (e) postnatal age 20 days; (f) adult 90 days old. (From Gomez RA, Chevalier RL, Sturgill BC, et al: Maturation of the intrarenal renin distribution in Wistar-Kyoto rats. J Hypertens (suppl 5)4:S31, 1986, with permission.)*

and the adult. In many species, the circulating PRA is even greater in the newborn than in the fetus [26,64, 115,164,165,178,323]. After delivery, there is an increase in the content of renin per gram KW [26,66,115,387]. Gomez et al. [154–156] have detected high levels of mRNA for both renin and angiotensin in the kidneys of newborn rats, which decreased with maturation. While birth by cesarean section by itself does not cause the high PRA to increase further [283], vaginal delivery is a powerful stimulus for secretion of renin [197]; the concentration of renin-containing granules in animals delivered vaginally is significantly greater than in those delivered by cesarean section, and much higher than found in the adult [115].

In the human, PRA was reported to be 10 to 12 ng/ml/hr in the term newborn, 5 ng/ml/hr in the one-year-old child, and 1 ng/ml/hr in the six-year-old child [228]. In the sheep, AII levels are high in fetal life, do not change with surgical delivery, but increase further following vaginal delivery [26,283,346]. They then decrease to the levels found in the adult by six to eight weeks of age [64]. It is unclear whether this postnatal activation of the renin-angiotensin system relates to hypoxia [64,424], increased mean arterial blood pressure [169,324], a negative sodium balance [107], or the high levels of circulating catecholamines [280,283,346].

Since the pressor response of the systemic vasculature to AII is present in the fetus [343,344], it is possible that the renin-angiotensin system affects renal hemodynamics starting at very early stages of development. However, the vasopressor and renal vasoconstrictive effects of AII are less in the fetus than in the adult, possibly due to a higher receptor occupancy by endogenous AII [343,344]. Administration of converting enzyme inhibitors did not result in changes in renal hemodynamics in fetal lambs of less than 120 days' gestation (term 145 days) but it did decrease renovascular resistance in older fetuses (>130 days) [343]. The possible role of the renin-angiotensin system in modulating the changes in intrarenal distribution of blood flow that occur with development remains controversial. Some investigators have suggested that the renin-angiotensin system plays a role in this phenomenon [27], whereas others claim that activation of the renin-angiotensin system during development relates more to the need to maintain a positive sodium balance [107].

THE RENAL NERVES

The renal plexus is formed by sympathetic, cholinergic, and dopaminergic nerves from the celiac plexus, the thoracic and lumbar splanchnic nerves, the intermesenteric nerves, and the superior hypogastric plexus, all of which in turn derive from the T-5 to L-3 segments of the spinal cord. The nerves emerging from the renal plexus travel alongside the intrarenal arteries within the periarterial loose connective tissue to innervate the afferent and efferent arterioles, the vasa rectae, and the juxtamedullary apparatuses [31,32,105]. High frequency stimulation of the renal nerves of the rat results in a decrease in RBF, which is attenuated by the administration of Ca^{2+} channel or ACE blockers [318].

Micropuncture studies in the rat have revealed that the decrease in single nephron blood flow and glomerular filtration induced by high frequency renal nerve stimulation is due primarily to an increase in afferent arteriolar resistance [180,223,319]. Norepinephrine and epinephrine have been found to constrict isolated segments of rabbit afferent and efferent arterioles [114], as well as mesangial cells in culture [368]. Under normal physiologic conditions, removal of the renal nerves appears to have little effect on renal circulation [42]. In water-deprived rats, however, denervation of the kidneys resulted in an increase in RBF, more so after the administration of saralasin [224,411]. These studies suggest that renal nerve-mediated vasoconstriction is due not only to the direct effect of catecholamines on the renal vasculature but also to enhanced secretion of renin from the juxtaglomerular apparatus [47,318]. Furthermore, renal nerves contribute little to the basal vasomotor tone of the kidney, exerting their greatest influence under conditions of stress [222].

The Renal Nerves During Development

The innervation of the kidney is underdeveloped in the young [349]. In the sheep fetus, the renal vasculature responds to exogenous norepinephrine but not to tyramine, a catecholamine precursor, indicating metabolic immaturity of the nerve fibers [435]. In the rat and dog, the vasculature of the renal cortex is innervated at birth, while nerve fibers to the vasa rectae cannot be detected until about three weeks of age [141,261]. Despite this, there is convincing evidence that the renal nerves play an important role in the adjustment of the kidney to postnatal life. The young of several species, such as the dog, the pig, and the guinea pig, are more sensitive to the vasoconstrictor effects of epinephrine and norepinephrine than are their adult counterparts [68,69,141,207,349]. Likewise, transection of the renal nerves increases RBF in piglets but not in mature euvolemic pigs [69]. This has led some investigators to propose that the high renovascular resistance observed early in life is due to a high α-adrenergic receptor density or affinity [126,163,260,359,391].

Other observations speak against this hypothesis. Richer et al. [340] and Robillard et al. [346,349] have reported that in fetal sheep α-adrenergic stimulation decreased RBF to a similar or to a lesser extent than in the grown animal. Segments of renal arteries isolated from fetal, newborn, and adult sheep did not differ significantly in their sensitivity (the concentration required for half-maximal response) to α-adrenergic stimulation [255,256]. The discrepancy between the studies described herein may result from differences in neural-induced intrarenal angiotensin production, in the level of circulating vasoactive compounds, or in the species under investigation.

Despite the immaturity of the nervous system, the circulating levels of norepinephrine are high in the fetus and newborn compared to the adult [346,349]. This, rather than an increased sensitivity of the vessels to α-adrenergic stimuli or an intrinsically greater vascular wall tension, may explain the high vascular resistance present in the newborn. Robillard et al. [347] reported that in sheep hypoxia significantly decreased blood flow to the fetal but not to the neonatal kidney. This effect was associated with an increase in circulating epinephrine, the predominant fetal catecholamine. Other studies from this laboratory have revealed that the resting tension of the renal vasculature in the fetus is not intrinsically higher than in the adult [255]. Studies on segments of renal arteries isolated from the dog, however, revealed an increase in maximal tension to phenylephrine with maturation [376]. This latter report is consistent with in vivo studies that indicated that the extent of renal vasoconstrictive response to α-adrenergic stimulation either did not change or increased with age [141,256]. Thus, while the sensitivity of the renal vasculature to α-adrenergic stimulation is independent of age, and the stiffness of the renal vasculature increases during development, the maximal response to α-adrenergic stimulation appears to differ both with species and stage of maturity. The high levels of circulating epinephrine present in the immature animal [228,312] result in constriction of the renal vascular bed that must account in part for the relatively high renal vascular resistance observed at this age.

Several lines of evidence suggest that the β-adrenergic system contributes to the age-related decrease in renovascular resistance. Administration to dogs or sheep of α-adrenergic antagonists, either alone or in combination with catecholamines or the stimulation of renal nerves, increased RBF to a greater extent in young than in mature animals [207,349]. In the newborn sheep, the vasodilation that is induced by renal nerve stimulation during α-adrenergic blockade was abolished by the intrarenal infusion of the β-adrenergic antagonist ICI 118,551 [282]. Further-

more, the density of β2-adrenergic receptors in the renal cortex of the sheep has been found to decrease with age [124a]. These findings suggest that the early activation of the renal β-adrenergic system, together with the decline in the circulating level of catecholamines, contribute to the decrease in renovascular resistance that is seen with growth.

Felder et al. [125] have described two different low affinity receptors for dopamine in renal cortical membranes of fetal, newborn, and adult sheep. The density of the D-1 receptor did not change with age, while the density of the D-2 receptor decreased. Although dopamine may alter renal hemodynamics by binding to these receptors [203, 204], the significance of age-related changes in binding density is unclear.

THE PROSTANOIDS

Arachidonic acid, a 20-carbon polyunsaturated fatty acid that is produced by the action of phospholipase A_2 on membrane-bound phospholipids, is the precursor for both the PGs by way of cyclo-oxygenase, and the leukotrienes (through lipoxygenase) [97,111]. The ubiquitous prostanoids are not stored in tissues but are produced in response to specific stimuli, act locally for a brief period of time, and are then inactivated [239].

In the kidney, the unstable but biologically active PGG_1 and PGH_2 yield mostly the end-products PGE_2 and PGI_2 and, to a lesser extent, PGD_2, thromboxane A_2, or the less active $PGF_{2\alpha}$. PGI_2 is in turn rapidly degraded to 6-keto-$PGF_{1\alpha}$ [239]. Synthesis of most of the prostanoids occurs in the renal inner medulla, while their catabolism occurs mostly in the cortex. An exception is PGI_2, which is produced mainly by the arterial vasculature of the cortex. PGE_2 is synthesized mostly in the medulla but is also produced by glomerular mesangial cells [239].

Both PGE_2 and PGI_2 dilate the renal vasculature in a variety of species [143,239,240] and decrease the tone of mesangial cells in culture, resulting in an increase in RBF that is more profound in the inner than in the outer cortex [146]. As can be inferred from their intrarenal distribution, PGE_2 dilates the medullary vasculature, while PGI_2 dilates the vasculature of the renal cortex [433]. $PGF_{2\alpha}$ and thromboxane A_2 are vasoconstrictors [269] but are usually present only in small quantities in the kidney, making their physiologic role obscure.

PGs may exert their influences either directly by binding to specific receptors or indirectly through the action of histamine [45]. They stimulate the release of renin, although they antagonize the pressor effects of AII and norepinephrine [367]. Their role in modulating autoregulation and tubuloglomerular feedback is unclear [190].

In the euvolemic unanesthetized animal, in which the levels of circulating vasoconstrictor hormones are low and the renal nerves are unstimulated, PGs are synthesized at low rates. Under these circumstances, PG-inhibiting drugs do not alter blood flow to the kidney [106,402]. Under different conditions, such as anesthesia, volume depletion, heart failure, or hemorrhage, the renin-angiotensin system, the renal nerves, and vasopressin are all activated to maintain mean arterial blood pressure, albeit at the expense of renal vasoconstriction [58,239,251]. The resulting increase in the production of vasodilatory PGs usually maintains a normal rate of RBF. The administration of nonsteroidal anti-inflammatory drugs under these circumstances may result in marked renal ischemia, especially to the medulla [110,239].

The Prostaglandins during Development

The excretion of PGE_2 and 6-keto-$PGF_{2\alpha}$ has been found to be fivefold higher in the preterm than in the term newborn and 20-fold greater than in children [16,419,420]. Friedman and Demers examined the renal PG synthetase system in ten preterm newborns ranging from 22 to 40 weeks of gestation who succumbed within 40 hours of birth [135]. Biosynthesis of PGE and PGF occurred mainly in the renal medulla as early as 22 weeks of gestation and increased with gestational age. Their role in the modulation of RBF during development remains controversial.

Some investigators have reported that RBF remained unchanged when either PGs or their inhibitors were infused into fetal lambs [354]. Others claimed that administration of PG inhibitors decreased RBF [257,264] in the fetus. The latter reports are supported by the observation that the decrease in blood flow to the kidney of the fetus due to hypoxia is exacerbated by pretreatment with indomethacin [264] and that long-term use of indomethacin as a tocolytic has resulted in antenatal renal failure and consequent oligohydramnios [89,136].

The infusion of PGI_2 into the renal artery of mature animals increases blood flow to the inner cortex [79], simulating the intrarenal distribution of blood flow observed in the fetus. When PG inhibitors are administered to the fetus, blood flow to the inner cortex decreases substantially [257]. These findings indicate that PGI_2, the major prostanoid produced by the kidney of the fetus at this stage of development [310,311,404,405], might contribute to the relatively high perfusion of the inner cortex. Because the catabolism of PGs increases with postnatal age, while the rate of their synthesis remains unchanged [310], there is a decrease in renal PG concentration with growth. This is accompanied by a shift in production away from PGI_2 and toward PGE_2, the major prostanoid of the mature kidney [146]. The emergence of PGE_2 as the predominant prostanoid might explain the postnatal increase in RBF and its redistribution toward the outer cortex [16].

How these changes in PGs contribute to the development of GFR is unclear [353]. The GFR of 31-day-old rats treated with aspirin for 11 days was similar to that of control animals, even though PGE_2 synthesis was effectively inhibited [267]. In the premature infant, indomethacin used to close patent ductus arteriosus has resulted in transient renal failure that could be attenuated by the administration of furosemide, a diuretic that also stimulates PG production [135]. PGs may thus be more important in moderating the effects of stress-induced vasoconstrictors, such as catecholamines or AII, than in modulating glomerular filtration [257,275,364].

THE ATRIAL NATRIURETIC FACTORS

Atrial natriuretic factors (ANF) are a group of peptides that are released from the atria of the heart in states of fluid accumulation [46,71,179,330]. These peptides act as general circulatory depressants [294,296,325] and exert their greatest effect in conditions of physiologic vasoconstriction [150]. ANF decrease mean arterial blood pressure in the rat, the dog, and the human when infused either intravenously or intra-arterially [53,92,194,296,325,418]. They have been found to be specific dilators of the renal vasculature in the anesthetized rat [54], the isolated perfused rat kidney [378], the conscious rat [294], and the anesthetized dog [109]. Micropuncture studies performed in Munich-Wistar rats have revealed that infusion of ANF increased SNGFR, P_{gc}, and filtration fraction, suggesting afferent arteriole vasodilation and efferent arteriole vasoconstriction [179]. ANF accomplish this by stimulating guanyl cyclase to produce cGMP, which mediates its vasodilatory and mesangial cell relaxant activity [92,138].

In addition, these peptides may reverse the action of AII and epinephrine by decreasing renovascular resistance in states characterized by renovascular constriction [21,246]. There is ample evidence that ANF blunt the production and release of aldosterone from the adrenal gland [20,73,149,202] and reverse the isoproterenol-mediated or diltazepam-mediated increase in renin secretion [227,232,247]. ANF applied to rat mesangial cells in culture decreased basal cell Ca^{2+} and antagonized the AII-mediated rapid rise in intracellular Ca^{2+} content [176,177]. ANF also abolished the AII-induced contraction of isolated glomeruli and mesangial cells in culture [13]. Thus, ANF antagonize the effects of AII at the cellular level.

Atrial Natriuretic Factors during Development

ANF-containing granules have been found in both the atria and ventricles of the heart of the fetus [373,374]. The granules from the ventricles diminish postnatally [423]. Atrial mRNA for ANF increases with postnatal age, while ventricular mRNA decreases rapidly after birth [423].

Using in vitro autoradiography, Scott and Jennes have identified specific receptors for ANF in the kidney and adrenal gland of the fetal rat [375]. Plasma levels of ANF have been reported to be at least twofold higher in fetal sheep, and rat and human membranes than in their mothers [82,84,383a]. In the human the levels increase further from 22 ± 2.5 to 45 ± 5.4 fmol/ml during the first week of life and then decrease to 14 ± 2.1 fmol/ml by ten days of age.

Robillard and his associates [348] have demonstrated that intrarenal infusion of ANF produced renal vasodilatation and increased RBF in a dose-dependent fashion to a similar extent in both fetal and newborn sheep. This contradicts earlier studies in which intravenous infusion of ANF in the sheep fetus resulted in an increase in renovascular resistance [415] and no change in the clearance of PAH in the five- to six-week-old euvolemic puppy [199]. The discrepancy between these reports is likely due to the different routes of ANF administration. When infused intravenously into the anesthetized dog, ANF was tenfold less effective in inducing a decrease in renovascular resistance than when administered intra-arterially [294]. Thus, ANF appear to be potent dilators of the renal vasculature throughout development. Their role in the maturation of renal function remains unclear, however.

References

1. Abrahamson DR: Origin of the glomerular basement membrane visualized after in vivo labeling of laminin in newborn rat kidneys. *J Cell Biol* 100:1988, 1985.
2. Abrahamson DR: Structure and development of the glomerular capillary wall and basement membrane. *Am J Physiol* (Renal Fluid Electrolyte Physiology 22) 253:F783, 1987.
3. Abrams JS: Blood pressure response to the portal infusion of angiotensin II. *Surg Forum* 17:133, 1966.
4. Alexander DP, Nixon DA: Plasma clearance of p-aminohippuric acid by the kidneys of foetal, neonatal, and adult sheep. *Nature* 194:483, 1962.
5. Allison MEM, Lipham EM, Gottschalk CW: Hydrostatic pressure in the rat kidney. *Am J Physiol* 223:975, 1972.
6. Altman PL, Dittmer DS: *Respiration and Circulation.* Committee on Biological Handbooks, Bethesda, Federation of American Societies of Experimental Biology, 1971, p 426.
7. Aperia A, Broberger O, Elinder G, et al: Postnatal changes in glomerular filtration rate in preterm and full-term infants. *In* Spitzer A (ed): *The Kidney during Development: Morphology and Function.* New York, Masson Publishing, 1982, p 133.
8. Aperia A, Broberger O, Herin P: Maturational changes in glomerular perfusion rate and glomerular filtration rate in lambs. *Pediatr Res* 8:758, 1974.
9. Aperia A, Broberger O, Herin P, et al: Renal hemodynamics in the perinatal period. *Acta Physiol Scand* 99:261, 1977.
10. Aperia A, Herin P: Development of glomerular perfusion rate and nephron filtration rate in rats 17–60 days old. *Am J Physiol* 228:1319, 1975.
11. Aperia A, Herin P: Effect of arterial blood pressure reduction on renal hemodynamics in the developing lamb. *Acta Physiol Scand* 98:387, 1976.
12. Aperia A, Larsson L: Correlation between fluid reabsorption and proximal tubule ultrastructure during development of the rat kidney. *Acta Physiol Scand* 105:11, 1979.
13. Appel RG, Wang J, Simonson MS, et al: A mechanism by which atrial natriuretic factor mediates its glomerular actions. *Am J Physiol* 251:F1036, 1986.
14. Arant BS Jr: Developmental patterns of renal functional maturation compared in the human neonate. *Pediatrics* 92:705, 1973.
15. Arant BS Jr: Postnatal development of renal function during the first year of life. *Pediatr Nephrol* 1:308, 1987.
16. Arant BS, Stapleton FB, Eagle WD, et al: Urinary prostaglandin excretion rates and renal function in human infants at birth. *Pediatr Res* 16:317A, 1982.
17. Ardaillou R, Sraer J, Chansel D, et al: The effects of angiotensin II in isolated glomeruli and cultured glomerular cells. *Kidney Int* (suppl 20)31:S74, 1987.
18. Arturson G, Groth T, Grotte G: Human glomerular membrane porosity and filtration pressure: Dextran clearance data analyzed by theoretical models. *Clin Sci* 40:137, 1971.
19. Aschinberg LC, Goldsmith DI, Olbing H, et al: Neonatal changes in renal blood flow distribution in puppies. *Am J Physiol* 228:1453, 1975.
20. Atarashi K, Mulrow PJ, Franco-Saenz R, et al: Inhibition of aldosterone production by an atrial extract. *Science* 224:992, 1984.
21. Atlas SA, Kleinert HD, Camarjo MJF, et al: Purification, sequencing and synthesis of natriuretic and vasoactive rat atrial peptide. *Nature* (Lond) 309:717, 1984.
22. Aukland, K.: Methods for measuring renal blood flow: Total flow and regional distribution. *Ann Rev Physiol* 42:543, 1980.
23. Ausiello DA, Kreisberg JI, Roy C, et al: Contraction of cultured rat glomerular cells of apparent mesangial origin after stimulation with angiotensin II and arginine vasopressin. *J Clin Invest* 65:754, 1980.
24. Badr KF, Murray JJ, Breyer MD, et al: Mesangial cell, glomerular and renal vascular responses to endothelin in the rat kidney. Elucidation of signal transduction pathways. *J Clin Invest* 83:336, 1989.
25. Baer PG, McGiff JC: Hormonal systems and renal hemodynamics. *Annu Rev Physiol* 42:589, 1980.
26. Bailie MD, Derkx FHM, Schalakamp MADH: Release of active and inactive renin by the pig kidney during development. *Dev Pharmacol Ther* 1:47, 1980.
27. Baile MD, Osborn JL, Hook JB: Effect of inhibition of prostaglandin synthetase and angiotensin II on renal function in the newborn piglet. *In* Spitzer A (ed): *The Kidney during Development: Morphology and Function.* New York, Masson Publishing USA, 1982, p 173.
28. Bailie MD, Rector FC Jr, Seldin DM: Angiotensin II in arterial and venous plasma and renal lymph in the dog. *J Clin Invest* 50:119, 1971.
29. Bankir L, Bouby N, Trinh-Trang-Tan MM: Heterogeneity of nephron anatomy. *Kidney Int* (suppl 20)31:S25, 1987.
30. Bankir L, Trinh-Trang-Tan MM, Grunfeld JP: Measurement of glomerular blood flow in rabbit and rats: Erroneous findings with 15μm microspheres. *Kidney Int* 15:126, 1979.
31. Barajas L: Innervation of the renal cortex. *Federation Proc* 37:1192, 1978.
32. Barajas L, Powers K, Wang P: Innervation of the renal cortical tubules: A quantitative study. *Am J Physiol* 247:F50, 1984.
33. Barnett HL: Renal physiology in infants and children. I. Method for estimation of glomerular filtration rate. *Proc Soc Exp Biol Med* 44:654, 1940.
34. Barnett HL, Hare K, McNamara H, et al: Measurement of glomerular filtration rate in premature infants. *J Clin Invest* 27:691, 1948.
35. Batsford SR, Rohrbach R, Vogt A: Size restriction in the glomerular capillary wall: Importance of lamina densa. *Kidney Int* 31:710, 1987.
36. Bauer JH, Brooks CS, Burch RN: Renal function studies in man with advanced renal insufficiency. *Am J Kidney Dis* 2:30, 1982.
37. Baylis C, Brenner BM: The physiologic determinants of glomerular ultrafiltration. *Rev Physiol Biochem Pharmacol* 80:1, 1978.
38. Bayliss WM: On the local reactions of the arterial wall to changes of internal pressures. *J Physiol* (Lond) 28:220, 1902.
39. Behrman RE, Lees MH, Peterson EN, et al: Distribution of the circulation in the normal and asphyxiated fetal primate. *Am J Obstet Gynecol* 108:956, 1970.
40. Bell PD: Luminal and cellular mechanisms for the mediation of tubuloglomerular feedback responses. *Kidney Int* (suppl 12)22:S97, 1982.
41. Bell PD, Navar LG: Intrarenal feedback control of glomerular filtration rate. *Semin Nephrol* 2:289, 1982.
42. Bello-Reuss E, Colindres RE, Pastoriza-Munoz E, et al: Effects of acute unilateral denervation in the rat. *J Clin Invest* 56:208, 1975.
43. Bender JW, Davitt MK, Jose P: Angiotensin-I-converting enzyme activity in term and premature infants. *Biol Neonate* 34:19, 1978.
44. Bertolatus JA, Abuyousef M, Hunsicker LG: Glomerular sieving of high molecular weight proteins in proteinuric rats. *Kidney Int* 31:1257, 1987.
45. Blackshear JL, Orlandi C, Hollenberg NK: Serotonin and

the renal blood supply: Role of prostaglandins and the SHT-2 receptor. *Kidney Int* 30(3):304, 1986.

46. Blaine EH: Atrial natriuretic factor plays a significant role in body fluid homeostasis. *Hypertension* 15:2, 1990.

47. Blair ML, Chen YH, Hisa H: Elevation of plasma renin activity by alpha-adrenoceptor agonists in conscious dogs. *Am J Physiol* 251:E695, 1986.

48. Blanc EB, Sraer J, Sraer JD, et al: Ca^{2+} and Mg^{2+} dependence of angiotensin II binding to isolated rat renal glomeruli. *Biochem Pharmacol* 27:517, 1978.

49. Blantz RC: The glomerular and tubular actions of angiotensin II. *Am J Kidney Dis* 10(suppl 1):2, 1987.

50. Blantz RC, Konnen KS, Tucker BJ: Angiotensin II effects upon the glomerular microcirculation and ultrafiltration coefficient of the rat. *J Clin Invest* 57:419, 1976.

51. Boberg U, Persson AEG: Tubuloglomerular feedback during elevated venous pressure. *Am J Physiol* 249:F524, 1985.

52. Bohrer MP, Baylis C, Humes HD, et al: Permselectivity of the glomerular capillary wall to macromolecules. I. Facilitated filtration of circulating polycations. *J Clin Invest* 61:72, 1978.

53. Bolli P, Muller FB, Linder L, et al: The vasodilation potency of atrial natriuretic peptide in man. *Circulation* 75:221, 1987.

54. Borenstein WB, Cupples WA, Sonnenberg H, et al: The effect of natriuretic atrial extract on renal hemodynamics and urinary excretion in anesthetized rats. *J Physiol* (Lond) 334:133, 1983.

55. Boylan JW: Introduction. *Kidney Int* 16:247, 1979.

56. Braumich H: Hormonal control of postnatal development of renal tubular transport of weak organic acids. *Pediatr Nephrol* 2:151, 1988.

57. Bray J, Robinson GB: Influence of change on filtration across renal basement membrane films in vitro. *Kidney Int* 25:527, 1984.

58. Brenner BM, Badr KF, Schor N, et al: Hormonal influences on glomerular filtration. *Mineral Electrolyte Metab* 4:49, 1980.

59. Brenner BM, Schor N, Ichikawa I: Role of angiotensin II in the physiologic regulation of glomerular filtration. *Am J Cardiol* 49:1430, 1982.

60. Brenner BM, Troy JL, Daugharty TM: The dynamics of glomerular ultrafiltration in the rat. *J Clin Invest* 50:1776, 1971.

61. Briggs JP, Schubert G, Schnermann J: Changes in the operation of the tubuloglomerular feedback mechanism with maturation. *Kidney Int* 21:242, 1982.

62. Britton SL: Intrarenal vascular effects of angiotensin I and angiotensin II. *Am J Physiol* 240:H914, 1981.

63. Brooks UL, Brownfield MS, Reid IA: Measurement and localization of angiotensin like immunoreactivity in juxtaglomerular cells of the rat. *Regulatory Peptides* 4:317, 1982.

64. Broughton PF, Kirkpatrick SML, Lumbers ER, et al: Renin and angiotensin-like levels of foetal, newborn and adult sheep. *J Physiol* (Lond) 315:575, 1974.

65. Brown G, Douglas J: Angiotensin II binding sites in rat and primate isolated renal tubular basolateral membranes. *Endocrinology* 112:2007, 1983.

66. Brown GP, Douglas JG, Krontiris-Litowitz J: Properties of angiotensin II receptors of isolated rat glomeruli: Factors influencing binding affinity and comparative binding of angiotension analogs. *Endocrinology* 106:1923, 1980.

67. Brown JJ, Davies DL, Lever AF, et al: The assay of renin in single glomeruli in the normal rabbit and the appearance of the juxtaglomerular apparatus. *J Physiol* (Lond) 176:418, 1967.

68. Buckley NM, Brazeau P, Gootman PM, et al: Renal circulatory effects of adrenergic stimuli in anaesthetized piglets and mature swine. *Am J Physiol* 237(Heart and Circulatory Physiology 6):H690, 1979.

69. Buckley NM, Charney AN, Brazeau P, et al: Changes in cardiovascular and renal function during catecholamine infusions in developing swine. *Am J Physiol* (Renal Fluid Electrolyte Physiol 9) 240:F276, 1981.

70. Burg M, Orloff J: p-Aminohippurate uptake and exchange in separated renal tubules. *Am J Physiol* 217:1064, 1969.

71. Burnett JC Jr, Kao PC, Hu DC, et al: Atrial natriuretic peptide elevation in congestive heart failure in the human. *Science* 231:1145, 1986.

72. Calcagno PL, Rubin MI: Renal excretion of para-aminohippurate in infants and children. *J Clin Invest* 42:1632, 1963.

73. Cambell WB, Needleman P: Inhibition of aldosterone biosynthesis by atriopeptins in rat adrenal cells. *Clin Res* 57:113, 1985.

74. Carter AM: The blood supply to the abdominal organs of the fetal guinea pig. *J Dev Physiol* 6:407, 1984.

75. Castellino P, Hunt W, DeFronzo RA: Regulation of renal hemodynamics by plasma amino acid and hormone concentrations. *Kidney Int* (suppl 22)32:S15, 1987.

76. Caufield JP: Alterations in the distribution of Alcian blue-staining fibrillar anionic sites in the glomerular basement membrane in aminonucleoside nephrosis. *Lab Invest* 40:503, 1977.

77. Celio MR, Ingagami T: Angiotensin II immunoreactivity coexists with renin in the juxtaglomerular granular epitheloid cells of the rat kidney. *Proc Natl Acad Sci USA* 78:3897, 1981.

78. Celsi G, Larsson L, Aperia A: Proximal tubular reabsorption and Na-K-ATPase activity in remnant kidney of young rats. *Am J Physiol* 251:F588, 1986.

79. Chang LCT, Splawinski JA, Oates JA: Enhanced renal prostaglandin production in the dog. II. Effects on intrarenal hemodynamics. *Circ Res* 36:204, 1975.

80. Chang RLS, Dean WM, Robertson CR, et al: Permselectivity of the glomerular capillary wall to macromolecules. III. Restricted transport of polyanions. *Kidney Int* 8:212, 1975.

81. Chang RLS, Ueki IF, Troy JL, et al: Permselectivity of the glomerular capillary wall to macromolecules. II. Experimental studies in the rat using dextran. *Biophys J* 15:887, 1975.

82. Cheung CY, Gibbs DM, Brace RA: Atrial natriuretic factor in maternal and fetal sheep. *Am J Physiol* 252(2 Pt 1):E279, 1987.

83. Chevalier RL, Carey RM, Kaiser DL: Endogenous prostaglandins modulate autoregulation of renal blood flow in young rats. *Am J Physiol* 253:F66, 1987.

84. Chevalier RL, Gomez A, Carey RM, et al: Renal effects of atrial natriuretic peptide infusion in young and adult rats. *Pediatr Res* 24:333, 1988.

85. Chevalier RL, Kaiser DL: Autoregulation of renal blood flow in the rat: Effects of growth and uninephrectomy. *Am J Physiol* 244:F483, 1983.

86. Chevalier RL, Kaiser DL: Effects of acute uninephrectomy and age on renal blood flow autoregulation in the rat. *Am J Physiol* 249:F672, 1985.

87. Chou SY, Porush JG, Faubert PF: Renal medullary circulation: Hormonal control. *Kidney Int* 37:1, 1990.

88. Churchill PC: Second messengers in renin secretion. *Am J Physiol* 24(9):F175, 1985.

89. Cifuentes RF, Olley PM, Balfe JW, et al: Indomethacin

and renal function in premature infants with persistent ductus arteriosus. *J Pediatr* 95:583, 1979.

90. Click RL, Joyner WL, Gillmore JP: Reactivity of glomerular afferent and efferent arterioles in renal hypertension. *Kidney Int* 15:109, 1979.

91. Coelho JB: Heterogeneity of intracortical peritubular plasma flow in the rat kidney. *Am J Physiol* 233(4):F333, 1977.

92. Cogan MG: Atrial natriuretic factor can increase renal solute excretion primarily by raising glomerular filtration. *Am J Physiol* 250:F710, 1986.

93. Cohen HJ, Marsh DJ, Kayser B: Autoregulation in vasa recta of the rat kidney. *Am J Physiol* 245:F32, 1983.

94. Cole BR, Brocklenbank JT, Capps RG, et al: Maturation of p-aminohippuric acid transport in the developing rabbit kidney: Interrelationships of the individual components. *Pediatr Res* 12:992, 1978.

95. Crane JK, Campanile CP, Garrison JC: The hepatic angiotensin II receptor. *J Biol Chem* 257:4959, 1982.

96. Cupples WA: Renal medullary blood flow: Its measurement and physiology. *Can J Physiol Pharmacol* 64:873, 1986.

97. Currie MG, Needleman P: Renal arachidonic acid metabolism. *Annual Reviews of Physiology* 40:327, 1984.

98. Davalos M, Frega NS, Saker B, et al: Effect of exogenous and endogenous angiotensin II in the isolated perfused rat kidney. *Am J Physiol* 235:F805, 1978.

99. Dean RFA, McCance RA: Inulin, diodone, creatinine, and urea clearances in newborn infants. *J Physiol* (Lond) 106:431, 1947.

100. Deen WM, Bohrer MP, Brenner BM: Macromolecule transport across glomerular capillaries: Application of pore theory. *Kidney Int* 16:353, 1979.

101. Deen WM, Bridges CR, Brenner BM, et al: Heteroporous model of glomerular size selectivity: Application to normal and nephrotic humans. *Am J Physiol* 249:F374, 1985.

102. Deen WM, Robertson CR, Brenner BM: A model of glomerular ultrafiltration in the rat. *Am J Physiol* 223:1178, 1972.

103. Deen WM, Satvat B, Jamieson JM: Theoretical model for glomerular filtration of charged solutes. *Am J Physiol* 238:F126, 1980.

104. Dhaene M, Sabot JP, Philippart Y, et al: Affects of acute protein loads of different sources on glomerular filtration rate. *Kidney Int* (suppl 22)32:S25, 1987.

105. Dieterich HG: Electron microscopic studies of the innervation of the rat kidney. *Z Anat Entwickl* 145:169, 1974.

106. Donker AJ, Arisz L, Brentjens JR, et al: The effect of indomethacin on kidney function and plasma renin activity in man. *Nephron* 17:288, 1976.

107. Drukker A, Goldsmith DI, Spitzer A, et al: The renin angiotensin system in newborn dogs: Developmental patterns and response to acute saline loading. *Pediatr Res* 14:304, 1980.

108. Dunn BR, Ichikawa I, Pfeffer JM, et al: Renal and systemic hemodynamic effects of synthetic atrial natriuretic peptide in the anaesthetized rat. *Circ Res* 59:237, 1986.

109. Duncan KA, Seaton RD, Savin VJ: Filtration by rat glomeruli after expansion of extracellular fluid volume. *J Lab Clin Med* 108:307, 1986.

110. Dunn MG, Zambraski EJ: Renal effects of drugs that inhibit prostaglandin synthesis. *Kidney Int* 18:609, 1980.

111. Dunn MJ: *Renal Prostaglandins* Baltimore, Williams & Wilkins, 1983.

112. Dworkin LD, Ichikawa I, Brenner BM: Hormonal modulation of glomerular function. *Am J Physiol* 244:F95, 1983.

113. Edelmann CM Jr: Introductory remarks. *In* Spitzer A (ed): *The Kidney During Development: Morphology and Function.* New York, Masson Publishing USA, 1982, p xv.

114. Edwards RM: Segmental effects of norepinephrine and angiotensin II on isolated renal microvessels. *Am J Physiol* 244:F526, 1983.

115. Eguchi Y, Yamakawa M, Morikawa Y, et al: Granular cells in the juxtaglomerular apparatus in perinatal rats. *Anat Rec* 181:627, 1974.

116. Ekblom P: Formation of basement membranes in the embryonic kidney. An immuno-histological study. *J Cell Biol* 91:1, 1981.

117. Ekblom P, Sariola H, Karkinen-Jaaskelainen M, et al: The origin of the glomerular endothelium, *Cell Differentiation* 11:35, 1982.

118. Elinder G, Aperia A, Herin P, et al: Effect of isotonic volume expansion on glomerular filtration rate and renal hemodynamics in the developing rat kidney. *Acta Physiol Scand* 108:411, 1980.

119. Evan AP: Maturation of the vascular system of the puppy kidney. *In* Spitzer A (ed): *The Kidney During Development: Morphology and Function.* New York, Masson Publishing USA, 1982, p 3.

120. Evan AP, Gattone VH III, Schwartz GJ: Development of solute transport in rabbit proximal tubule. II. Morphologic segmentation. *Am J Physiol* (Renal Fluid Electrolyte Physiol 14) 245:F391, 1983.

121. Evan AP, Hay DA: Ultrastructure of the developing vascular system in the puppy kidney. *Anat Rec* 199:481, 1981.

122. Farquhar MG, Wissig SL, Palade GE: Glomerular permeability. 1. Ferritin transfer across the normal glomerular capillary wall. *J Exp Med* 113:42, 1961.

123. Faubert PF, Chou SY, Porush JG: Regulation of papillary plasma flow by angiotensin II. *Kidney Int* 32:472, 1987.

124. Faxon DP, Creager MA, Halperin JL, et al: Redistribution of regional blood flow following angiotensin-converting enzyme inhibition. *Am J Med* 76:104, 1984.

124a. Felder CC, Piccio MM, McKelvey AM, et al: Ontogeny of renal beta adrenoceptors in the sheep. *Pediatr Nephrol* 4:635, 1990.

125. Felder RA, Nakamura KT, Robillard JE, et al: Dopamine receptors in the developing sheep kidney. *Pediatr Nephrol* 2:156, 1988.

126. Felder RA, Pelayo JC, Calcagno PL, et al: Alpha-adrenoceptors in the developing kidney. *Pediatr Res* 17:177, 1983.

127. Fetterman GH, Sheeplock NA, Philipp FJ, et al: The growth and maturation of human glomeruli and proximal convolutions from term to adulthood. *Pediatrics* 35:601, 1965.

128. Findlay ALR, Epstein AN: Increased sodium intake is somehow induced in rats by intravenous angiotensin II. *Hormones and Behavior* 14:86, 1980.

129. Foster RP, Maes JP: Effect of experimental neurogenic hypertension on renal blood flow and glomerular filtration rates in intact denervated kidneys of unaesthetized rabbits with adrenal glands demedullated. *Am J Physiol* 150:534, 1947.

130. Fray JC, Lush DJ, Park CS: Interrelationship of blood flow, juxtaglomerular cells, and hypertension: Role of physical equilibrium and Ca. *Am J Physiol* 251:R643, 1986.

131. Fray JCS, Lush DJ, Valentine AND: Cellular mechanisms of renin secretion. *Fed Proc* 42:3150, 1983.

132. Fray JC, Park CS: Forskolin and calcium: Interactions in the control of renin secretion and perfusate flow in the isolated rat kidney. *J Physiol* (Lond) 375:361, 1986.

133. Freeman RH, Rostorfer HH: Hepatic changes in renin

substrate biosynthesis and alkaline phosphatase activity in the rat. *Am J Physiol* 223:364, 1972.

134. Frega, N.S., Davalos, M., Leaf, A.: Effect of endogenous angiotensin on the efferent glomerular arteriole of rat kidney. *Kidney Int* 18:323, 1980.

135. Friedman Z, Demers LM: Prostaglandin synthetase in the human neonatal kidney. *Pediatr Res* 14:190, 1979.

136. Friedman Z, Demers LM, Marks KH, et al: Urinary excretion of prostaglandin E following the administration of furosemide and indomethacin to sick low-birth-rate infants. *J Pediatr* 93:512, 1978.

137. Friis C: Postnatal development of renal function in piglets: Glomerular filtration rate, clearance of PAH and PAH extraction. *Biol Neonate* 35:180, 1979.

138. Fujii K, Ishimatsu T, Kuriyama H: Mechanism of vasodilation induced by alpha-human atrial natriuretic polypeptide in rabbit and guinea-pig renal arteries. *J Physiol* (Lond) 377:315, 1986.

139. Furchgott RF: Role of endothelium in responses of vascular smooth muscle. *Circ Res* 53:557, 1983.

140. Furchgott RF, Zawadzki JV: The obligatory role of endothelial cells in the relaxation of arterial smooth muscle by acetylcholine. *Nature* (Lond) 288:373, 1980.

141. Gallen DD, Cowen T, Griffith SG, et al: Functional and nonfunctional nerve—smooth muscle transmission in the renal arteries of the newborn and adult rabbit and guinea pig. *Blood Vessels* 19:237, 1982.

142. Geelhoed GW, Wander AJ: Plasma renin activities during pregnancy and parturition. *J Clin Endocrinol Metab* 28:412, 1968.

143. Gerber JG, Nies AS: The hemodynamic effects of prostaglandins in the rat. Evidence for important species variation in renovascular responses. *Circ Res* 44:406, 1979.

144. Gersh I: The correlation of structure and function in the developing mesonephros and metanephros. *Contrib Embryol* 153:35, 1937.

145. Gilbert RD: Control of fetal cardiac output during changes in blood volume. *Am J Physiol* (Heart Circ Physiol 6) 620:H80, 1980.

146. Gleason CA: Prostaglandins and the developing kidney. *Semin Perinatol* 11:12, 1987.

147. Glossmann H, Baukal AJ, Catt KJ: Properties of angiotensin II receptors in the bovine and rat adrenal cortex. *J Biol Chem* 249:825, 1974.

148. Godard C, Gaillard R, Yalloton MB: The renin-angiotensin-aldosterone system in mother and fetus at term. *Nephron* 17:353, 1976.

149. Goetz KL: Physiology and pathophysiology of atrial peptides. *Am J Physiol* 254:E1, 1988.

150. Goetz KL: Evidence that atriopeptin is not a physiologic regulator of sodium excretion. *Hypertension* 15:9, 1990.

151. Goetz KL, Wang BC, Madwed JB, et al: Cardiovascular, renal, and endocrine responses to intravenous endothelin in conscious dogs. *Am J Physiol* 255R:1064, 1988.

152. Goldsmith DI, Jodorkovsky RA, Sherwinter J, et al: Glomerular capillary permeability in developing canines. *Am J Physiol* 251:F528, 1986.

153. Goldsmith SR: Vasopressin as vasopressor. *Am J Med* 82:1213, 1987.

154. Gomez AR, Lynch KR, Chevalier RL, et al: Ontogeny of intrarenal renin and angiotensin gene transcriptions in Wistar-Kyoto and spontaneous hypertensive rats. *Pediatr Res* 21:476A, 1987.

155. Gomez RA, Cassis L, Lynch KR, et al: Fetal expression of the angiotensinogen gene. *Endocrinology* 123:2298, 1988.

156. Gomez RA, Chevalier RL, Sturgill BC, et al: Maturation

157. Gomez RA, Meernik JG, Kuehl WD, et al: Developmental aspects of the renal response to hemorrhage during fetal life. *Pediatr Res* 18:40, 1984.

158. Gonchar R, Kaya OA, Dlouha H: The development of various generations of nephrons during postnatal ontogenesis in the rat. *Anat Rec* 182:367, 1975.

159. Goransson A, Isaksson B, Sjoquist M: Whole kidney response to reduced arterial pressure during converting enzyme inhibition in the rat. *Renal Physiol* 9:287, 1986.

160. Goransson A, Sjoquist M, Ulfendahl HR: Superficial and juxtamedullary nephron function during converting enzyme inhibition. *Am J Physiol* 251(1 Pt 2):F25, 1986.

161. Gordon J: Vascular biology: Put out to contract. *Nature* 332:395, 1988.

162. Gottschalk CW: Osmotic concentration and dilution of the urine. *Am J Med* 36:670, 1964.

163. Graham RM, Pettinger WA, Sagalowsky A, et al: Renal alpha-adrenergic receptor abnormality in the spontaneously hypertensive rat. *Hypertension* 4:881, 1982.

164. Granger P, Dalheim H, Tharau K: Enzyme activities of the single juxtaglomerular apparatus in the rat kidney. *Kidney Int* 1:78, 1972.

165. Granger P, Rojo-Ortega JM, Perez SC, et al: The renin-angiotensin system in newborn dogs. *Can J Physiol Pharmacol* 49:135, 1971.

166. Grangjo G, Wolgast M: The pressure-flow relationship in the renal cortical and medullary circulation. *Acta Physiol Scand* 85:228, 1972.

167. Grantham JJ, Chonko AM, Brenner BM, et al (eds): *Contemporary Issues in Nephrology*. Vol 1. New York, Churchill-Livingstone, 1978, p 178.

168. Groggel GC, Stevenson J, Hovingh P, et al: Changes in heparan sulfate correlate with increased glomerular permeability. *Kidney Int* 33:517, 1988.

169. Gross F, Brunner H, Ziegler M: Renin-angiotensin system, aldosterone and sodium balance. *Recent Progr Horm Res* 21:119, 1965.

170. Gruskin AB, Edelmann CM Jr, Yuan S: Maturational changes in renal blood flow in piglets. *Pediatr Res* 4:7, 1970.

171. Gunther S, Alexander RW, Atkinson WJ, et al: Functional angiotensin II receptors in cultured vascular smooth muscle cells. *J Cell Biol* 92:289, 1982.

172. Gunther S, Gimbrone MA Jr, Alexander RW: Identification and characterization of the high affinity vascular angiotensin II receptor in rat mesenteric artery. *Circ Res* 47:278, 1980.

173. Hackenthal E, Metz R, Buhrle CP, et al: Intrarenal and intracellular distribution of renin and angiotensin. *Kidney Int* (suppl 20)31:S4, 1987.

174. Hall JE, Granger JP: Renal hemodynamics actions of angiotensin II: Interactions with tubuloglomerular feedback. *Am J Physiol* 245:R166, 1983.

175. Harris PJ, Young JA: Dose-dependent stimulation and inhibition of proximal tubular sodium reabsorption by angiotensin II in the rat kidney. *Pflugers Arch* 367:295, 1977.

176. Hassid A: Atriopeptins decrease the resting and hormone-elevated cytosolic Ca in cultured mesangial cells. *Am J Physiol* 253:F1077, 1987.

177. Hassid A, Pidikiti N, Gamero D: Effects of vasoactive peptides on cytosolic calcium in cultured mesangial cells. *Am J Physiol* 251:F1018, 1986.

178. Hayduk K, Drause DK, Huenges R, et al: Plasma renin concentration in delivery and during the newborn period in humans. *Experientia* 28:1489, 1972.

of the intrarenal renin distribution in Wistar-Kyoto rats. *J Hypertens* (suppl 5)4:S31, 1986.

266. Miltenyi M: Developmental aspects of the glomerular filtration of plasma proteins. In Spitzer A (ed): The Kidney During Development: Morphology and Function. New York, Masson Publishing USA, 1982, p 147.

267. Moel DI, Cohn RA, Penning J: Renal prostaglandin E_2 synthesis and degradation in the developing rat. Biol Neonate 48:292, 1985.

268. Molitch ME, Rodman E, Hirsch CA: Spurious serum creatinine elevations in ketoacidosis. Ann Int Med 93:280, 1980.

269. Moncada S, Vane JP: Pharmacology and endogenous roles of prostaglandin endoperoxides, thromboxane A_2 and prostacyclin. Pharmacol Rev 30:293, 1979.

270. Moore LC, Casellas D: Autoregulation and tubuloglomerular feedback (TGF) in juxtamedullary afferent arterioles (AA). Kidney Int 37:554, 1989.

271. Moore TJ, Williams GH: Angiotensin II receptors on human platelets. Circ Res 51:314A, 1982.

272. Morgin T, Davis JM: Renin secretion at the individual nephron level. Pflugers Arch 359:23, 1975.

273. Morris BJ, Johnson CI: Renin substrate in granules from rat kidney cortex. Biochem J 154:625, 1976.

274. Mounier F, Hinglais N, Sich M, et al: Ontogenesis of angiotensin I converting enzyme in human kidney. Kidney Int 32:684, 1987.

275. Moutquin JM, Liggins GC: Effects of furosemide on plasma concentrations of renin and prostaglandins E and A in fetal sheep. Prostglandins and Medicine 4:31, 1980.

276. Muller-Suur R, Persson EG, Ulfendahl HR: Tubuloglomerular feedback in juxtamedullary nephrons. Kidney Int (suppl 12)22:S104, 1982.

277. Muther RS: Drug interference with renal function tests. Am J Kidney Dis 111:118, 1983.

278. Myers BD, Deen WM, Brenner BM: Effects of norepinephrine and angiotensin II on the determinants of glomerular ultrafiltration and proximal tubule fluid reabsorption in the rat. Circ Res 37:101, 1975.

279. Nakamura KT, Alden BM, Jose PA, et al: Ontogeny of renal β_2-adrenoceptor vasodilation in fetal (F) and adult (A) sheep using a specific β_2 agonist and antagonist. Pediatr Res 20:455A, 1986.

280. Nakamura KT, Alden BM, Jose PA, et al: Renal β_2-adrenoceptor vasodilation in fetal (F) and adult (A) sheep: Comparison between endogenous catecholamines. Pediatr Res 20:455A, 1986.

281. Nakamura KT, Matherne GP, Jose PA, et al: Effects of epinephrine on the renal vascular bed of fetal, newborn and adult sheep. Pediatr Res 23:181, 1988.

282. Nakamura KT, Matherne GP, Jose PA, et al: Ontogeny of renal beta-adrenoceptor mediated vasodilation in sheep: Comparison between endogenous catecholamines. Pediatr Res 22:465, 1987.

283. Nakamura KT, Matherne GP, McWeeny OS, et al: Renal hemodynamics and functional changes during the transition from fetal to newborn life in sheep. Pediatr Res 21(3):229, 1987.

284. Nakamura KT, McWeeny O, Smith B, et al: Renal hemodynamics and functional changes during the transition from fetal to postnatal life in conscious sheep. Pediatr Res 20:455A, 1986.

285. Nakazawa M, Miyagawa S, Ohno T, et al: Developmental hemodynamic changes in rat embryos at 11 to 45 days of gestation: Normal data of blood pressure and the effect of caffeine compared to data from chick embryo. Pediatr Res 23:200, 1988.

286. Naruse M, Inagami T, Celio MR, et al: Immunohistochemical evidence that angiotensins I and II are forced by intracellular mechanisms in juxtaglomerular cells. Hypertension (suppl 2)4:S70, 1982.

287. Nath KA, Chmielewski DH, Hostetter TH: Regulatory role of prostanoids in glomerular microcirculation of remnant nephrons. Am J Physiol 252:F829, 1987.

288. Navar LG: Renal autoregulation: Perspectives from whole kidney and single nephron studies. Am J Physiol 234(5):F357, 1978.

289. Navar LG, Bell PD, Burke TJ: Role of a macula densa feedback mechanism as a mediator of renal autoregulation. Kidney Int (suppl 12)22:S157, 1982.

290. Navar LG, Bell PD, White RW, et al: Evaluation of the single nephron glomerular coefficient in the dog. Kidney Int 12:137, 1977.

291. Navar LG, Champion WJ, Thomas CE: Effects of calcium channel blockade on renal vascular resistance responses to changes in perfusion pressure and angiotensin-converting enzyme inhibition in dogs. Circ Res 58:874, 1986.

292. Navar LG, Ploth DW, Bell PD: Distal tubular feedback control of renal hemodynamics and autoregulation. Annu Rev Physiol 42:557, 1980.

293. Navar LG, Rosivall L: Contribution of the renin-angiotensin system to the control of intrarenal hemodynamics. Kidney Int 25:857, 1984.

294. Needleman P, Adams SP, Cole BR, et al: Atriopeptins as cardiac hormones. Hypertension 7:469, 1985.

295. New M, McNamara H, Kretchmer N: Accumulation of para-aminohippurate by slices of kidney from rabbits of various ages. Proc Soc Exp Biol Med 102:558, 1959.

296. Nushiro N, Abe K, Seino M, et al: The effects of intravenous injections of alpha-human atrial natriuretic polypeptide on the blood pressure, renal hemodynamics and urinary kinin excretion in anaesthetized rabbits. Tohoku J Exp Med 151:221, 1987.

297. Oakes GK, Fleischman AR, Catt KJ, et al: Plasma renin activity in sheep pregnancy after fetal or maternal nephrectomy. Biol Neonate 31:208, 1977.

298. Odlind B, Hallgren R, Sohtell M, et al: Is ^{125}I-iothalamate an ideal marker for glomerular filtration? Kidney Int 27:9, 1985.

299. Ody C, Junod AF: Converting enzyme activity in endothelial cells isolated from pig pulmonary artery and aorta. Am J Physiol 232(Call Physiology 1):C95, 1977.

300. Ogawa N, Ono H: Different effects of noradrenaline, angiotensin II and BAY K8644 on the abolition of autoregulation of renal blood flow by verapamil. Naunyn Schmiedebergs Arch Pharmacol 333:445, 1986.

301. Oh W, Oh MA, Lind J: Renal function and blood volume in newborn infant related to placental transfusion. Acta Pediatr Scand 55:197, 1966.

302. Oh W, Stern L: Diseases of the respiratory system. In Behrman RE (ed): Neonatal-Perinatal Medicine. Diseases of the Fetus and Infant. Saint Louis, CV Mosby, 1977, p 538.

302a. Okada T, Morikawa Y: Morphometrical studies on perinatal development of glomerular components in rat. Biol Neonate 57:243, 1990.

303. Okuda T, Yamashita N, Kurokawa K: Angiotensin II and vasopressin stimulate calcium—activated chloride conductance in rat mesangial cells. J Clin Invest 78(6):1443, 1986.

304. Olbing H, Blaufox DM, Aschinberg LC, et al: Postnatal changes in renal glomerular blood flow distribution in puppies. J Clin Invest 52:2885, 1973.

substrate biosynthesis and alkaline phosphatase activity in the rat. *Am J Physiol* 223:364, 1972.

134. Frega, N.S., Davalos, M., Leaf, A.: Effect of endogenous angiotensin on the efferent glomerular arteriole of rat kidney. *Kidney Int* 18:323, 1980.

135. Friedman Z, Demers LM: Prostaglandin synthetase in the human neonatal kidney. *Pediatr Res* 14:190, 1979.

136. Friedman Z, Demers LM, Marks KH, et al: Urinary excretion of prostaglandin E following the administration of furosemide and indomethacin to sick low-birth-rate infants. *J Pediatr* 93:512, 1978.

137. Friis C: Postnatal development of renal function in piglets: Glomerular filtration rate, clearance of PAH and PAH extraction. *Biol Neonate* 35:180, 1979.

138. Fujii K, Ishimatsu T, Kuriyama H: Mechanism of vasodilation induced by alpha-human atrial natriuretic polypeptide in rabbit and guinea-pig renal arteries. *J Physiol* (Lond) 377:315, 1986.

139. Furchgott RF: Role of endothelium in responses of vascular smooth muscle. *Circ Res* 53:557, 1983.

140. Furchgott RF, Zawadzki JV: The obligatory role of endothelial cells in the relaxation of arterial smooth muscle by acetylcholine. *Nature* (Lond) 288:373, 1980.

141. Gallen DD, Cowen T, Griffith SG, et al: Functional and nonfunctional nerve—smooth muscle transmission in the renal arteries of the newborn and adult rabbit and guinea pig. *Blood Vessels* 19:237, 1982.

142. Geelhoed GW, Wander AJ: Plasma renin activities during pregnancy and parturition. *J Clin Endocrinol Metab* 28:412, 1968.

143. Gerber JG, Nies AS: The hemodynamic effects of prostaglandins in the rat. Evidence for important species variation in renovascular responses. *Circ Res* 44:406, 1979.

144. Gersh I: The correlation of structure and function in the developing mesonephros and metanephros. *Contrib Embryol* 153:35, 1937.

145. Gilbert RD: Control of fetal cardiac output during changes in blood volume. *Am J Physiol* (Heart Circ Physiol 6) 620:H80, 1980.

146. Gleason CA: Prostaglandins and the developing kidney. *Semin Perinatol* 11:12, 1987.

147. Glossmann H, Baukal AJ, Catt KJ: Properties of angiotensin II receptors in the bovine and rat adrenal cortex. *J Biol Chem* 249:825, 1974.

148. Godard C, Gaillard R, Yalloton MB: The renin-angiotensin-aldosterone system in mother and fetus at term. *Nephron* 17:353, 1976.

149. Goetz KL: Physiology and pathophysiology of atrial peptides. *Am J Physiol* 254:E1, 1988.

150. Goetz KL: Evidence that atriopeptin is not a physiologic regulator of sodium excretion. *Hypertension* 15:9, 1990.

151. Goetz KL, Wang BC, Madwed JB, et al: Cardiovascular, renal, and endocrine responses to intravenous endothelin in conscious dogs. *Am J Physiol* 255R:1064, 1988.

152. Goldsmith DI, Jodorkovsky RA, Sherwinter J, et al: Glomerular capillary permeability in developing canines. *Am J Physiol* 251:F528, 1986.

153. Goldsmith SR: Vasopressin as vasopressor. *Am J Med* 82:1213, 1987.

154. Gomez AR, Lynch KR, Chevalier RL, et al: Ontogeny of intrarenal renin and angiotensin gene transcriptions in Wistar-Kyoto and spontaneous hypertensive rats. *Pediatr Res* 21:476A, 1987.

155. Gomez RA, Cassis L, Lynch KR, et al: Fetal expression of the angiotensinogen gene. *Endocrinology* 123:2298, 1988.

156. Gomez RA, Chevalier RL, Sturgill BC, et al: Maturation

157. of the intrarenal renin distribution in Wistar-Kyoto rats. *J Hypertens* (suppl 5)4:S31, 1986.

157. Gomez RA, Meernik JG, Kuehl WD, et al: Developmental aspects of the renal response to hemorrhage during fetal life. *Pediatr Res* 18:40, 1984.

158. Gonchar R, Kaya OA, Dlouha H: The development of various generations of nephrons during postnatal ontogenesis in the rat. *Anat Rec* 182:367, 1975.

159. Goransson A, Isaksson B, Sjoquist M: Whole kidney response to reduced arterial pressure during converting enzyme inhibition in the rat. *Renal Physiol* 9:287, 1986.

160. Goransson A, Sjoquist M, Ulfendahl HR: Superficial and juxtamedullary nephron function during converting enzyme inhibition. *Am J Physiol* 251(1 Pt 2):F25, 1986.

161. Gordon J: Vascular biology: Put out to contract. *Nature* 332:395, 1988.

162. Gottschalk CW: Osmotic concentration and dilution of the urine. *Am J Med* 36:670, 1964.

163. Graham RM, Pettinger WA, Sagalowsky A, et al: Renal alpha-adrenergic receptor abnormality in the spontaneously hypertensive rat. *Hypertension* 4:881, 1982.

164. Granger P, Dalheim H, Tharau K: Enzyme activities of the single juxtaglomerular apparatus in the rat kidney. *Kidney Int* 1:78, 1972.

165. Granger P, Rojo-Ortega JM, Perez SC, et al: The renin-angiotensin system in newborn dogs. *Can J Physiol Pharmacol* 49:135, 1971.

166. Grangjo G, Wolgast M: The pressure-flow relationship in the renal cortical and medullary circulation. *Acta Physiol Scand* 85:228, 1972.

167. Grantham JJ, Chonko AM, Brenner BM, et al (eds): *Contemporary Issues in Nephrology*. Vol 1. New York, Churchill-Livingstone, 1978, p 178.

168. Groggel GC, Stevenson J, Hovingh P, et al: Changes in heparan sulfate correlate with increased glomerular permeability. *Kidney Int* 33:517, 1988.

169. Gross F, Brunner H, Ziegler M: Renin-angiotensin system, aldosterone and sodium balance. *Recent Progr Horm Res* 21:119, 1965.

170. Gruskin AB, Edelmann CM Jr, Yuan S: Maturational changes in renal blood flow in piglets. *Pediatr Res* 4:7, 1970.

171. Gunther S, Alexander RW, Atkinson WJ, et al: Functional angiotensin II receptors in cultured vascular smooth muscle cells. *J Cell Biol* 92:289, 1982.

172. Gunther S, Gimbrone MA Jr, Alexander RW: Identification and characterization of the high affinity vascular angiotensin II receptor in rat mesenteric artery. *Circ Res* 47:278, 1980.

173. Hackenthal E, Metz R, Buhrle CP, et al: Intrarenal and intracellular distribution of renin and angiotensin. *Kidney Int* (suppl 20)31:S4, 1987.

174. Hall JE, Granger JP: Renal hemodynamics actions of angiotensin II: Interactions with tubuloglomerular feedback. *Am J Physiol* 245:R166, 1983.

175. Harris PJ, Young JA: Dose-dependent stimulation and inhibition of proximal tubular sodium reabsorption by angiotensin II in the rat kidney. *Pflugers Arch* 367:295, 1977.

176. Hassid A: Atriopeptins decrease the resting and hormone-elevated cytosolic Ca in cultured mesangial cells. *Am J Physiol* 253:F1077, 1987.

177. Hassid A, Pidikiti N, Gamero D: Effects of vasoactive peptides on cytosolic calcium in cultured mesangial cells. *Am J Physiol* 251:F1018, 1986.

178. Hayduk K, Drause DK, Huenges R, et al: Plasma renin concentration in delivery and during the newborn period in humans. *Experientia* 28:1489, 1972.

179. Henrich WL: Southwestern internal medicine conference: Renal sodium excretion and atrial natriuretc factor. *Am J Med Sci* 291:199, 1986.
180. Hermansson K, Ojteg G, Wolgast M: The reno-renal reflex: Evaluation from renal blood flow measurements. *Acta Physiol Scand* 120:207, 1984.
181. Hill KJ, Lumbars ER: Renal function in adult and fetal sheep. *J Dev Physiol* 10:149, 1988.
182. Hill KJ, Lumbers ER, Elbourne I: The actions of cortisol on fetal renal function. *J Devel Physiol* 10:85, 1988.
183. Hirschberg R, Kopple JD: Effects of growth hormone on GFR and renal plasma flow in man. *Kidney Int* (suppl 22)32:S21, 1987.
184. Hook JB, Williamson HE, Hirsch GH: Functional maturation of renal PAH transport in the dog. *Can J Physiol Pharmacol* 48:169, 1970.
185. Hope A, Clausen G, Aukland K: Intrarenal distribution of blood flow in rats determined by ^{125}I-iodoantipyrine uptake. *Circ Res* 39:362, 1976.
186. Hornych H, Beaufils M, Richet G: The effect of exogenous angiotensin on superficial and deep glomeruli in the rat kidney. *Kidney Int* 2:336, 1972.
187. Horster M, Lewy JE: Filtration fraction and extraction of PAH during neonatal period in the rat. *Am J Physiol* 219:1061, 1970.
188. Horster M, Valtin H: Postnatal development of renal function: Micropuncture and clearance studies in the dog. *J Clin Invest* 50:779, 1971.
189. Hsu CH, Kurtz TW, Slavicek JM: Effect of exogenous angiotensin II on renal hemodynamics in the awake rat. Measurement of afferent arteriolar diameter by the microsphere method. *Circ Res* 46:646, 1980.
190. Ochikawa I: Hemodynamic influence of altered distal salt delivery on glomerular microcirculation. *Kidney Int* (suppl 12)22:S109, 1982.
191. Ichikawa I: Maturational changes in the dynamics of glomerular ultrafiltration in the rat. *In* Spitzer A (ed): *The Kidney During Development: Morphology and Function.* New York, Masson Publishing USA, 1982, p 119.
192. Ichikawa I, Brenner BM: Glomerular actions of angiotensin II. *Am J Med* 76:43, 1984.
193. Ichikawa I, Maddox D, Brenner BM: Maturational development of glomerular ultrafiltration in the rat. *Am J Physiol* 236(5):F465, 1979.
194. Ishil M, Soyimoto T, Matsooka H, et al: Blood pressure, renal and endocrine responses to alpha-human atrial natriuretic polypeptide in normal volunteers. *Jpn Heart J* 27(6):777, 1988.
195. Itskovitz HD, McGiff JC: Hormonal regulation of the renal circulation. *Circ Res* (suppl 1)34:65, 1974.
196. Iwamoto HS, Oh W, Rudolph AM: Renal metabolism in fetal and newborn sheep. *In* Jones CT, Nathanielsz PW (eds): *The Physiological Development of the Fetus and Newborn.* London, Academic, 1985, p 37.
197. Jelinek J, Hackenfal R, Hilgenfeldt U, et al: The renin angiotensin system in the perinatal period in rats. *J Dev Physiol* 8:33, 1986.
198. John E, Goldsmith DI, Spitzer A: Quantitative changes in the canine glomerular vasculature during development: Physiologic implications. *Kidney Int* 20:223, 1981.
199. John EG, Fornell L: Effect of atrial natriuretic factor (ANF) on developmental renal functions. *Pediatr Res* 21:477A, 1987.
200. Jones CR, Hiley CR, Pelton JT, et al: Autoradiographic localization of endothelin binding sites in kidney. *Eur J Pharmacol* 163:379, 1989.
201. Jones DB: Mucosubstances of the glomerulus. *Lab Invest* 21:119, 1969.
202. Joppich R, Scherer B, Weber PC: Renal prostaglandins: Relationship to the development of blood pressure and concentrating capacity in pre-term and full-term healthy infants. *Eur J Pediatr* 132:253, 1979.
203. Jose PA, Felder RA, Robillard JE, et al: Dopamine-2 receptor in the canine kidney (abstr). *Kidney Int* 29:385, 1986.
204. Jose PA, Eisner GM, Robillard JE: Renal hemodynamics and natriuresis induced by the dopamine-1 agonist, SKF 82526. *Am J Med Sci* 294:181, 1987.
205. Jose PA, Logam AG, Slotkoff LM, et al: Intrarenal blood flow distribution in canine puppies. *Pediatr Res* 5:335, 1971.
206. Jose PA, Pelayo JC, Felder RE, et al: Maturation of single-nephron filtration rate in the canine puppy-effect of saline loading. Spitzer A (ed): *The Kidney During Development: Morphology and function.* New York, Masson Publishing USA, 1982, p 139.
207. Jose PA, Slotkoff LM, Lilienfield LS, et al: Sensitivity of neonatal renal vasculature to epinephrine. *Am J Physiol* 226:796, 1974.
208. Jose PA, Slotkoff LM, Montgomery S, et al: Autoregulation of renal blood flow in the puppy. *Am J Physiol* 229:983, 1975.
209. Kanwar YS: Biophysiology of glomerular filtration proteinuria. *Lab Invest* 51:7, 1984.
210. Kanwar YS, Farquhar MG: Isolation of glycosaminoglycans (heparan sulfate) from glomerular basement membranes. *Proc Natl Acad Sci USA* 76:4493, 1979.
211. Kanwar YS, Farquhar MG: Presence of heparan sulfate in the glomerular basement membrane. *Proc Natl Acad Sci USA* 76:1303, 1979.
212. Kanwar YS, Jakubowski ML: Unaltered anionic sites of glomerular basement membrane in amminonucleoside nephrosis. *Kidney Int* 25:613, 1984.
213. Kanwar YS, Linker YS, Farquhar MG: Increased permeability of the glomerular basement membranes to ferritin after removal of glycosaminoglycans (heparan sulfate). *J Cell Biol* 86:688, 1980.
214. Kanwar YS, Rosenzweig LJ: Clogging of glomerular basement membrane. *J Cell Biol* 93:489, 1982.
215. Kawamura T, Gilbert RD, Power GG: Effect of cooling and heating on the regional distribution of blood flow in fetal sheep. *J Dev Physiol* 8:11, 1986.
216. Kim JK, Hirsch GH, Hook JB: In vitro analysis of organic ion transport in renal cortex of the newborn rat. *Pediatr Res* 6:600, 1972.
217. King AJ, Brenner BM, Anderson S: Endothelin: A potent renal and systemic vasoconstrictor peptide. *Am J Physiol* 256:F1051, 1989.
218. Kleinman LI: Physiology of the perinatal kidney. *In* Stave U (ed): *Physiology of the Perinatal Period.* Vol 2. New York, Appleton-Century-Crofts, 1970, p 679.
219. Kleinman LI, Lubbe, RJ: Factors affecting the maturation of renal PAH extraction in the newborn dog. *J Physiol* (Lond) 223:411, 1972.
220. Knox FG, Ritman EL: The intrarenal distribution of blood flow: Evolution of a new approach to measurement. *Kidney Int* 25:473, 1984.
221. Knutson DW, Chieu FG, Bennet CM, et al: Estimation of relative glomerular capillary surface area in normal and hypertrophic rat kidneys. *Kidney Int* 14:437, 1978.
222. Kon V: Neural control of renal circulation. *Miner Electrolyte Metab* 15:33, 1989.

223. Kon V, Ichikawa I: Effector loci for renal nerve control of cortical microcirculation. *Am J Physiol* 245:F545, 1983.

224. Kon V, Yared A, Ichikawa I: Role of sympathetic nerves in mediating experimental congestive heart failure and acute extracellular fluid volume depletion. *J Clin Invest* 76:1913, 1985.

225. Kon V, Yoshioka T, Fogo A, et al: Glomerular actions of endothelin in vivo. *J Clin Invest* 83:1762, 1989.

226. Kotchen TA, Strickland AL, Rice TW, et al: A study of the renin-angiotensin system in newborn infants. *J Pediatr* 80:938, 1972.

227. Kurtz A, Bruna RD, Pfeilshifter J, et al: Atrial natriuretic peptide inhibits renin release from juxtaglomerular cells by a cGMP-mediated process. *Proc Natl Acad Sci. USA* 83:4769, 1986.

228. Lagercrantz H, Bistoletti P: Catecholamine release in the newborn infant at birth. *Pediatr Res* 11:889, 1977.

229. Lahera V, Salom MG, Fiksen-Olsen MJ, et al: N^G-monomethyl-L-arginine (LNMMA) blocks the renal vasodilatory and natriuretic action of acetylcholine in dogs. *Kidney Int* 37:552A, 1990.

230. Lambert PP, Gassee JP, Verniory A, et al: Measurement of the glomerular filtration pressure from sieving data for macromolecules. *Pflugers Arch* 329:34, 1971.

231. Landis EM, Papenheimer JR: Exchange of substances through the capillary walls. *In* Hamilton DP (ed): *Handbook of Physiology.* Washington, D.C., American Physiology Society, 1963, p 961.

232. Laragh JH: Atrial natriuretic hormone, the renin-aldosterone axis, and blood pressure–electrolyte homeostasis. *N Engl J Med* 313:1330, 1985.

233. Larsson, L.: The ultrastructure of the developing proximal tubule in the rat kidney. *J. Ultrastruct. Res.* 51:119, 1975.

234. Larsson L, Maunsbach AB: Quantitative ultrastructural changes of the glomerular capillary wall in the developing rat kidney. *In* Spitzer A (ed): *The Kidney During Development: Morphology and Function.* New York, Masson Publishing USA, 1982, p 115.

235. Latta H, Johnston WH, Stanley TM: Sialoglycoprotein and filtration barriers in the glomerular capillary wall. *J Ultrastruct Res* 51:354, 1975.

236. Laue A, Grone HJ, Fuchs E: Localization and quantification of endothelin (ET) binding sites in human fetal and adult kidneys. *Kidney Int* 37:372A, 1989.

237. Levens NR, Peach MJ, Carey RM, et al: Changes in an electroneutral transport process mediated by angiotensin II in the rat distal colon in vivo. *Endocrinology* 108:1497, 1981.

238. Levens NR, Peach MJ, Carey RM: Role of the intrarenal renin-angiotensin system in the control of renal function. *Circ Res* 48:157, 1981.

239. Levenson DJ, Simmons CE Jr, Brenner BM: Arachidonic acid metabolism, prostaglandins, and the kidney. *Am J Med* 72:354, 1982.

240. Lifschitz MD: Prostaglandins and renal blood flow: In vivo studies. *Kidney Int* 19:781, 1981.

241. Ljungvist A, Wagermark J: Renal juxtaglomerular granulation in the human foetus and infant. *Acta Pathol Microbiol Scand* 67:257, 1966.

242. Lohmeier TE, Cowley AW, Trippodo NC, et al: Effects of endogenous angiotensin II on renal sodium excretion and renal hemodynamics. *Am J Physiol* 233:F388, 1977.

243. Loutzenhiser R, Epstein M: Effects of calcium antagonists on renal hemodynamics. *Am J Physiol* 249:F619, 1985.

244. Lumbers ER: A brief review of fetal renal function. *J Dev Physiol* 6:1, 1984.

245. Lumbers ER, Lewes JL: The actions of vasoactive drugs on fetal and maternal plasma renin activity. *Biol Neonate* 35:23, 1979.

246. Maack T, Camargo MJF, Kleinert HD, et al: Atrial Natriuretic factor: Structure and functional properties. *Kidney Int* 27:607, 1985.

247. Maack T, Marion DN, Camargo JF, et al: Effects of auriculin (atrial natriuretic factor) on blood pressure, renal function, and the renin-aldosterone system in dogs. *Am J Med* 77:1069, 1984.

248. MacCumber MW, Ross CA, Glazer BM, et al: Endothelin: Visualization of mRNA's by in situ hybridization provides evidence for local action. *Proc Natl Acad Sci USA* 86:7285, 1989.

249. Macias-Nunez JF, Garcia-Iglesias C, Santos JC, et al: Influence of plasma renin content, intrarenal angiotensin II, captopril, and calcium channel blockers on the vasoconstriction and renin release promoted by adenosine in the kidney. *J Lab Clin Med* 106(5):562, 1985.

250. Maddox DA, Deen WM, Brenner BM: Dynamics of glomerular ultrafiltration. VI. Studies in the primate. *Kidney Int* 5:271, 1974.

251. Maher JF: Pathophysiology of renal hemodynamics. *Nephron* 27:215, 1981.

252. Marsh DJ: Frequency response of autoregulation. *Kidney Int* (suppl 12)22:S165, 1982.

253. Masey SA, Koehler RC, Buck JR, et al: Effect of abdominal distension on central and regional hemodynamics in neonatal lambs. *Pediatr Res* 19:1244, 1985.

254. Masri MA, Boyd ND, Mandin H: Role of fibrinogen in the glomerular permeability of the perfused, isolated dog kidney. *Kidney Int* 27:807, 1985.

255. Matherne GP, Nakamura KT, Alden BM, et al: Regional variation of postjunctional alpha-adrenoceptor responses in the developing renal vascular bed of sheep. *Pediatr Res* 25:461, 1989.

256. Matherne GP, Nakamura KT, Robillard JE: Ontogeny of alpha-adrenoceptor responses in renal vascular bed of sheep. *Am J Physiol* 254:R277, 1988.

257. Matson JR, Stokes JB, Robillard JE: Effects of inhibition of prostaglandin synthesis on fetal renal function. *Kidney Int* 20:621, 1981.

258. McCance RA, Widdowson EM: Metabolism, growth and renal function of piglets in the first few days of life. *J Physiol* (Lond) 133:373, 1958.

259. McCance RA, Young WF: The secretion of urine by newborn infants. *J Physiol* (Lond) 99:265, 1941.

260. McGaughran JA Jr, Juno CJ, O'Malley E, et al: The ontogeny of renal alpha-1- and alpha-2-adrenoceptors in the Dahl rat model of experimental hypertension. *J Auton Nerv Syst* 17:1, 1986.

261. McKenna OC, Angelakos ET: Development of adrenergic innervation in the puppy kidney. *Anat Rec* 167:115, 1970.

262. Mendelsohn FAO: Evidence for the local occurrence of angiotensin II in rat kidney and its modulation by dietary sodium intake and converting enzyme blockade. *Clin Sci Mol Med* 57:173, 1979.

263. Mendelsohn FAO, Millan M, Quirion R, et al: Localization of angiotensin II receptors in rat and monkey kidney by in vitro autoradiography. *Kidney Int.* (suppl 20)31:S40, 1987.

264. Millard RW, Baig H, Vatner SF: Prostaglandin control of the renal circulation in response to hypoxemia in the fetal lamb in utero. *Circ Res* 45:172, 1979.

265. Miller BF, Winkler AW: The renal excretion of endogenous creatinine in man. *J Clin Invest* 17:31, 1938.

266. Miltenyi M: Developmental aspects of the glomerular filtration of plasma proteins. *In* Spitzer A (ed): *The Kidney During Development: Morphology and Function.* New York, Masson Publishing USA, 1982, p 147.

267. Moel DI, Cohn RA, Penning J: Renal prostaglandin E_2 synthesis and degradation in the developing rat. *Biol Neonate* 48:292, 1985.

268. Molitch ME, Rodman E, Hirsch CA: Spurious serum creatinine elevations in ketoacidosis. *Ann Int Med* 93:280, 1980.

269. Moncada S, Vane JP: Pharmacology and endogenous roles of prostaglandin endoperoxides, thromboxane A_2 and prostacyclin. *Pharmacol Rev* 30:293, 1979.

270. Moore LC, Casellas D: Autoregulation and tubuloglomerular feedback (TGF) in juxtamedullary afferent arterioles (AA). *Kidney Int* 37:554, 1989.

271. Moore TJ, Williams GH: Angiotensin II receptors on human platelets. *Circ Res* 51:314A, 1982.

272. Morgin T, Davis JM: Renin secretion at the individual nephron level. *Pflugers Arch* 359:23, 1975.

273. Morris BJ, Johnson CI: Renin substrate in granules from rat kidney cortex. *Biochem J* 154:625, 1976.

274. Mounier F, Hinglais N, Sich M, et al: Ontogenesis of angiotensin I converting enzyme in human kidney. *Kidney Int* 32:684, 1987.

275. Moutquin JM, Liggins GC: Effects of furosemide on plasma concentrations of renin and prostaglandins E and A in fetal sheep. *Prostglandins and Medicine* 4:31, 1980.

276. Muller-Suur R, Persson EG, Ulfendahl HR: Tubuloglomerular feedback in juxtamedullary nephrons. *Kidney Int* (suppl 12)22:S104, 1982.

277. Muther RS: Drug interference with renal function tests. *Am J Kidney Dis* 111:118, 1983.

278. Myers BD, Deen WM, Brenner BM: Effects of norepinephrine and angiotensin II on the determinants of glomerular ultrafiltration and proximal tubule fluid reabsorption in the rat. *Circ Res* 37:101, 1975.

279. Nakamura KT, Alden BM, Jose PA, et al: Ontogeny of renal β_2-adrenoceptor vasodilation in fetal (F) and adult (A) sheep using a specific β_2 agonist and antagonist. *Pediatr Res* 20:455A, 1986.

280. Nakamura KT, Alden BM, Jose PA, et al: Renal β_2-adrenoceptor vasodilation in fetal (F) and adult (A) sheep: Comparison between endogenous catecholamines. *Pediatr Res* 20:455A, 1986.

281. Nakamura KT, Matherne GP, Jose PA, et al: Effects of epinephrine on the renal vascular bed of fetal, newborn and adult sheep. *Pediatr Res* 23:181, 1988.

282. Nakamura KT, Matherne GP, Jose PA, et al: Ontogeny of renal beta-adrenoceptor mediated vasodilation in sheep: Comparison between endogenous catecholamines. *Pediatr Res* 22:465, 1987.

283. Nakamura KT, Matherne GP, McWeeny OS, et al: Renal hemodynamics and functional changes during the transition from fetal to newborn life in sheep. *Pediatr Res* 21(3):229, 1987.

284. Nakamura KT, McWeeny O, Smith B, et al: Renal hemodynamics and functional changes during the transition from fetal to postnatal life in conscious sheep. *Pediatr Res* 20:455A, 1986.

285. Nakazawa M, Miyagawa S, Ohno T, et al: Developmental hemodynamic changes in rat embryos at 11 to 45 days of gestation: Normal data of blood pressure and the effect of caffeine compared to data from chick embryo. *Pediatr Res* 23:200, 1988.

286. Naruse M, Inagami T, Celio MR, et al: Immunohistochemical evidence that angiotensins I and II are forced by intracellular mechanisms in juxtaglomerular cells. *Hypertension* (suppl 2)4:S70, 1982.

287. Nath KA, Chmielewski DH, Hostetter TH: Regulatory role of prostanoids in glomerular microcirculation of remnant nephrons. *Am J Physiol* 252:F829, 1987.

288. Navar LG: Renal autoregulation: Perspectives from whole kidney and single nephron studies. *Am J Physiol* 234(5):F357, 1978.

289. Navar LG, Bell PD, Burke TJ: Role of a macula densa feedback mechanism as a mediator of renal autoregulation. *Kidney Int* (suppl 12)22:S157, 1982.

290. Navar LG, Bell PD, White RW, et al: Evaluation of the single nephron glomerular coefficient in the dog. *Kidney Int* 12:137, 1977.

291. Navar LG, Champion WJ, Thomas CE: Effects of calcium channel blockade on renal vascular resistance responses to changes in perfusion pressure and angiotensin-converting enzyme inhibition in dogs. *Circ Res* 58:874, 1986.

292. Navar LG, Ploth DW, Bell PD: Distal tubular feedback control of renal hemodynamics and autoregulation. *Annu Rev Physiol* 42:557, 1980.

293. Navar LG, Rosivall L: Contribution of the renin-angiotensin system to the control of intrarenal hemodynamics. *Kidney Int* 25:857, 1984.

294. Needleman P, Adams SP, Cole BR, et al: Atriopeptins as cardiac hormones. *Hypertension* 7:469, 1985.

295. New M, McNamara H, Kretchmer N: Accumulation of para-aminohippurate by slices of kidney from rabbits of various ages. *Proc Soc Exp Biol Med* 102:558, 1959.

296. Nushiro N, Abe K, Seino M, et al: The effects of intravenous injections of alpha-human atrial natriuretic polypeptide on the blood pressure, renal hemodynamics and urinary kinin excretion in anaesthetized rabbits. *Tohoku J Exp Med* 151:221, 1987.

297. Oakes GK, Fleischman AR, Catt KJ, et al: Plasma renin activity in sheep pregnancy after fetal or maternal nephrectomy. *Biol Neonate* 31:208, 1977.

298. Odlind B, Hallgren R, Sohtell M, et al: Is ^{125}I-iothalamate an ideal marker for glomerular filtration? *Kidney Int* 27:9, 1985.

299. Ody C, Junod AF: Converting enzyme activity in endothelial cells isolated from pig pulmonary artery and aorta. *Am J Physiol* 232(Call Physiology 1):C95, 1977.

300. Ogawa N, Ono H: Different effects of noradrenaline, angiotensin II and BAY K8644 on the abolition of autoregulation of renal blood flow by verapamil. *Naunyn Schmiedebergs Arch Pharmacol* 333:445, 1986.

301. Oh W, Oh MA, Lind J: Renal function and blood volume in newborn infant related to placental transfusion. *Acta Pediatr Scand* 55:197, 1966.

302. Oh W, Stern L: Diseases of the respiratory system. *In* Behrman RE (ed): *Neonatal-Perinatal Medicine. Diseases of the Fetus and Infant.* Saint Louis, CV Mosby, 1977, p 538.

302a. Okada T, Morikawa Y: Morphometrical studies on perinatal development of glomerular components in rat. *Biol Neonate* 57:243, 1990.

303. Okuda T, Yamashita N, Kurokawa K: Angiotensin II and vasopressin stimulate calcium—activated chloride conductance in rat mesangial cells. *J Clin Invest* 78(6):1443, 1986.

304. Olbing H, Blaufox DM, Aschinberg LC, et al: Postnatal changes in renal glomerular blood flow distribution in puppies. *J Clin Invest* 52:2885, 1973.

305. Olsen ME, Hall JE, Montani JP, et al: Mechanisms of angiotensin II natriuresis and antinatriuresis. Am J Physiol 249:F299, 1985.

306. Osawa G, Kimmelstiel P, Seiling V: Thickness of glomerular basement membrane. Am J Clin Path 45:7, 1966.

307. Osborn JL, Hook JB, Baile MD: Effect of saralasin and indomethacin on renal function in developing piglets. Am J Physiol 238:R438, 1980.

308. Osborne MJ, Droz B, Meyer P, et al: Angiotensin II: Renal localization in glomerular mesangial cells by autoradiography. Kidney Int 8:245, 1975.

309. Ott CE, Marchand GR, Diaz-Buxo JA, et al: Determinants of glomerular filtration rate in the dog. Am J Physiol 231:235, 1976.

310. Pace-Asciak CR: Prostaglandin biosynthesis and catabolism in several organs of developing fetal and neonatal animals. Adv Prostaglandin Thromboxane Leukotriene Research 4:45, 1970.

311. Pace-Asciak CR: Prostaglandins biosynthesis and catabolism in the developing fetal sheep kidney. Prostaglandins 13:661, 1977.

312. Padbury JF, Diakomanolts ES, Hobel CJ, et al: Neonatal adaptation: Sympatho-adrenal response to umbilical cord cutting. Pediatr Res 15:1483, 1981.

313. Palmer RMJ, Ferrige AG, Moncada S: Nitric oxide release accounts for the biological activity of endothelium-derived relaxing factor. Nature 327:524, 1987.

314. Pappenheimer JR: Passage of molecules through capillary walls. Physiol Rev 33:387, 1953.

315. Paton JB, Fisher DE, Peterson EN, et al: Cardiac output and organ blood flows in the baboon fetus. Biol Neonate 22:50, 1973.

316. Pawlowska D, Granger JP, Knox FG: Effects of adenosine infusion into renal interstitium on renal hemodynamics. Am J Physiol 252:F678, 1987.

317. Peach MJ: Molecular actions of angiotensin. Biochem Pharmacol 30:2745, 1981.

318. Pelayo JC: Modulation of renal adrenergic effector mechanisms by calcium entry blockers. Am J Physiol 252:F613, 1987.

319. Pelayo JC, Ziegler MG, Blantz RC: Angiotensin II in adrenergic-induced alterations in glomerular hemodynamics. Am J Physiol 247:F799, 1984.

320. Pitts RF: Physiology of the Kidney and Body Fluids Chicago, Year Book Medical Publishers, 1968.

321. Ploth DW, Roy RN: Renin-angiotensin influences on tubuloglomerular feedback activity in the rat. Kidney Int (suppl 22)12:S114, 1982.

322. Pohl U, Busse R: Endothelium-derived relaxant factor inhibits effects of nitrocompounds in isolated arteries. Am J Physiol 252:H307, 1987.

323. Pohlova I, Janovsky M, Jelinek J: Plasma renin activity in the newly born and in young infants. Physiol Bohemoslov 22:233, 1973.

324. Pohlova I, Jelinek J: Components of the renin angiotensin system in the rat during development. Pflugers Arch 351:259, 1974.

325. Pollock DM, Adrenschorst WJ: Effect of atrial natriuretic factor on renal hemodynamics in the rat. Am J Physiol 251:F795, 1986.

326. Potter EL: Normal and Abnormal Development of the Kidney. Chicago, Year Book Medical Publishers, 1972, p 3.

327. Potter EL, Thierstein ST: Glomerular development in the kidney as an index of foetal maturity. J Pediatr 22:695, 1943.

328. Pullman TN, Oparil S, Carone FA: Fate of labeled angiotensin II microinfused into individual nephrons in the rat. Am J Physiol 228:747, 1975.

329. Purtell JN, Pesce AJ, Clyne DH, et al: Isoelectric point of albumin: Effect on renal handling of albumin. Kidney Int 16:366, 1979.

330. Raine ARG, Erne P, Burgisser E, et al: Atrial natriuretic peptide and atrial pressure in patients with congestive heart failure. N Engl J Med 315:533, 1986.

331. Rasch R: Prevention of diabetic glomerulopathy in streptozotocin diabetic rats by insulin treatment. Glomerular basement membrane thickness. Diabetologia 16:319, 1979.

332. Rassier ME, Li T, Zimmerman BG: Analysis of influence of extra- and intrarenally formed angiotensin II on renal blood flow. J Cardiovasc Pharmacol (suppl 10)8:S106, 1986.

333. Reeves W, Caulfield JP, Farquhar MG: Differentiation of epithelial foot processes and filtration slits. Sequential appearance of occluding junctions, epithelial polyanion and slit membranes in developing glomeruli. Lab Invest 39:80, 1979.

334. Reeves WH, Farquhar MG: Maturation and assembly of the glomerular filtration surface in the newborn rat kidney. Studies using electron-dense tracers, cationic probes, and cytochemistry. In Spitzer A (ed): The Kidney During Development: Morphology and Function. New York, Masson Publishing USA, 1982, p 97.

335. Reeves WH, Kanwar YS, Farquhar MG: Assembly of the glomerular filtration surface. Differentiation of anionic sites in glomerular capillaries of newborn rat kidney. J Cell Biol 85:735, 1980.

336. Regoli D, Gunther R: Site of action of angiotensin and other vasoconstrictors of the kidney. Am J Physiol Pharmacol 49:608, 1971.

337. Rehberg PB: Studies on kidney function. II. The excretion of urea and chlorine analysed according to a modified filtration-reabsorption theory. Biochem J 20:461, 1926.

338. Renkin EM, Gilmore JP: Glomerular filtration. In Orloff J, Berliner RW (eds): Handbook of Physiology. Section 8. Renal Physiology. Washington, D.C., American Physiology Society, 1973, p 185.

339. Richard AN, Schmidt CF: A description of the glomerular circulation in the frog's kidney and observations concerning the action of adrenalin and various other substances upon it. Am J Physiol 71:178, 1924.

340. Richer C, Lefevre-Borg F, Lechaire J, et al: Systemic and regional hemodynamic characterization of alpha-1 and alpha-2 adrenoceptor agonists in pithed rats. J Pharmacol Exp Ther 240(3):944, 1987.

341. Risau W, Ekblom P: Production of a heparin-binding angiogenesis factor by the embryonic kidney. J Cell Biol 103:1101, 1986.

342. Robertson CR, Deen WM, Troy JL, et al: Dynamics of glomerular ultrafiltration in the rat. III. Hemodynamics and autoregulation. Am J Physiol 223:191, 1972.

343. Robillard JE: Changes in renal vascular reactivity to angiotensin-II during development in fetal, newborn and adult sheep: Role of A-II vascular receptors occupancy. Pediatr Res 17:355A, 1983.

344. Robillard JE, Gomez RA, VanOrden D, et al: Comparison of the adrenal and renal responses to angiotensin II in fetal lambs and adult sheep. Circ Res 50:140, 1982.

345. Robillard JE, Kisker CT: Effect of metabolic acidosis on fetal hemodynamics. J Dev Physiol 9:105, 1987.

346. Robillard JE, Nakamura KT: Neurohormonal regulation of

renal function during development. *Am J Physiol* 254:F771, 1988.

347. Robillard JE, Nakamura KT, Matherne GP, et al: Renal hemodynamics and functional adjustments to postnatal life. *Semin Perinatol* 12:143, 1988.

348. Robillard JE, Nakamura KT, Varille VA, et al: Plasma and urinary clearance rates of atrial natriuretic factor during ontogeny in sheep. *J Dev Physiol* 10(4):335, 1988.

349. Robillard JE, Nakamura KT, Wilkin MK, et al: Ontogeny of renal hemodynamic response to renal nerve stimulation in sheep. *Am J Physiol* 252:F605, 1987.

350. Robillard JE, Weismann DN, Herin P: Ontogeny of single glomerular perfusion rate in fetal and newborn lambs. *Pediatr Res* 15:1248, 1981.

351. Rodewald R, Karnovsky MJ: Porous structure of the glomerular slit diaphragm in the rat and mouse. *J Cell Biol* 60:423, 1974.

352. Rubin MI, Bruck E, Rapoport M: Maturation of renal function in childhood: Clearance studies. *J Clin Invest* 28:1144, 1949.

353. Rudolph AM, Heymann MA: Circulatory changes during growth in the fetal lamb. *Circ Res* 26:289, 1970.

354. Rudolph AM, Heymann MA: Hemodynamic changes induced by blockers of prostaglandin synthesis in the fetal lamb in utero. *In* Coceani F, Olley PM (eds): *Advances in Prostaglandin Synthesis and Thromboxane Research.* New York, Raven Press, 1978, p 231.

355. Rudolph AM, Heymann MA, Teramo KAW, et al: Studies on the circulation of the previable human fetus. *Pediatr Res* 5:452, 1971.

356. Ryan GB, Karnovsky MJ: Distribution of endogenous albumin in the rat glomerulus: Role of hemodynamic factors in glomerular barrier function. *Kidney Int* 9:36, 1976.

357. Ryan US, Ryan JW, Whitaker C, et al: Localization of angiotensin coverting enzyme (kininase II). II. Immunocytochemistry and immunofluorescence. *Tissue Cell* 8:125, 1976.

358. Sakai T, Craig DA, Wexler AS, et al: Fluid waves in renal tubules. *Biophys J* 50:805, 1986.

359. Sanches A, Vidal MJ, Martines-Sierra R, et al: Ontogeny of alpha-1- and alpha-2-adrenoceptors in spontoneously hypertensive rat. *J Pharmac Exp Ther* 237:972, 1986.

360. Sariola H: Interspecies chemeras: An experimental approach for studies on the embryonic angiogenesis. *Med Biol* 63:43, 1985.

361. Sariola H, Ekblom P, Lehtonen E, et al: Differentiation and vascularization of the metanephric kidney grafted onto the chorioallantoic membrane. *Dev Biol* 96:427, 1983.

362. Sariola H, Peault B, Le Douarin N, et al: Extracellular matrix and capillary ingrowth in interspecies chimeric kidneys. *Cell Differ* 15:43, 1984.

363. Sariola H, Timpl R, von der Mark K, et al: Dual origin of glomerular basement membrane. *Dev Biol* 101:86, 1984.

364. Savin VJ: Ultrafiltration in single isolated human glomeruli. *Kidney Int* 24:748, 1983.

365. Savin VJ, Terreros DA: Filtration in single isolated mammalian glomeruli. *Kidney Int* 20:188, 1981.

366. Saxen L, Lehtonen T: Embryonic kidney in organ culture. *Differentiation* 36:2, 1987.

367. Scharschmidt L, Simonson M, Dunn MJ: Glomerular prostaglandins, angiotensin II, and nonsterodial anti-inflammatory drugs. *Am J Med* (suppl 2B)81:30, 1986.

368. Schlondorff D: The glomerular mesangial cell: An expanding role for a specialized pericyte. *FASEB J* 1:272, 1987.

369. Schmidt D, Forssmann WG, Taugner R: Juxtaglomerular granules of the newborn rat kidney. *Pflugers Arch* 331:226, 1972.

370. Schor N, Ichikawa I, Brenner BM: Mechanism of action of various hormones and vasoactive substances on glomerular ultrafiltration in the rat. *Kidney Int* 20:442, 1981.

371. Schwartz GJ, Brion LP, Spitzer A: The use of plasma concentration for estimating glomerular filtration rate in infants, children, and adolescents. *Pediatr Clin N Am* 34:571, 1987.

372. Schwertschlag U, Hackenthal E: Forskolin stimulates renin release from the isolated perfused rat kidney. *Eur J Pharmacol* 84:111, 1982.

373. Scott JN, Jennes L: Distribution of atrial natriuretic factor in fetal rat atria and ventricles. *Cell Tissue Res* 248:479, 1987.

374. Scott JN, Jennes L: Development of immunoreactive atrial natriuretic peptide in fetal hearts of spontaneously hypertensive Wistar-Kyoto rats. *Anat Embryol* 178:359, 1988.

375. Scott JN, Jennes LH: Ontogeny of atrial natriuretic peptide receptors in fetal rat kidney and adrenal gland. *Histochemistry* 91:395, 1989.

376. Seidel CL, Ross B, Freedman MJ, et al: Maturational changes in the pharmacological characteristics and actomyosin content of canine arterial and venous tissue. *Pediatr Res* 21:152, 1987.

377. Selkurt EE, Hall DW, Spencer MP: Influence of graded arterial pressure decrement on renal clearance of creatinine, p-aminohippurate and sodium. *Am J Physiol* 159:369, 1949.

378. Shimizu T, Nakamura M: Renal effect of atrial natriuretic polypeptide: Comparison with standard saluretics. *Eur J Pharmacol* 127:249, 1986.

379. Shipley RE, Study RS: Changes in renal blood flow, extraction of inulin, glomerular filtration rate, tissue pressure and urine flow with acute alterations of renal artery pressure. *Am J Physiol* 167:676, 1951.

380. Simonson MS, Dunn MJ: Endothelin pathways of transmembrane signalling. *Hypertension* 15:I5, 1990.

381. Sirett NJ, McLean AB, Bray JJ, et al: Distribution of angiotensin II receptors in rat brain. *Brain Res* 122:299, 1977.

382. Skorecki KL, Ballermann BJ, Rennke GH, et al: Angiotensin II receptor regulation in isolated renal glomeruli. *Fed Proc* 42:3064, 1983.

383. Smith FG, Lumbers ER: Changes in renal function following delivery of the lamb by cesarean section. *J Dev Physiol* 10:145, 1988.

383a. Smith FG, Sato T, Varille VA, et al: Atrial natriuretic factor during fetal and postnatal life: A review. *J Dev Physiol* 12:55, 1989.

384. Smith HW: *The Kidney. Structure and Function in Health and Disease.* New York, Oxford University Press, 1964, p 20.

385. Smith JB, Brock TA: Analysis of angiotensin-stimulated sodium transport in cultured smooth muscle cells from rat aorta. *J Cell Physiol* 114:284, 1983.

386. Smith RR, Briggs SL: Positive interference with the Jaffe reaction by cephalosporin antibiotics. *Clin Chem* 23:1340, 1977.

387. Solomon S, Iain A, Eliahau H, et al: Postnatal changes in piglet and renal renin of the rat. *Biol Neonate* 32:237, 1977.

388. Spitzer A: Factors underlying the increase in glomerular filtration rate during postnatal development. Spitzer A (ed): *The Kidney During Development: Morphology and Function.* New York, Masson Publishing USA., 1982, p 127.

389. Spitzer A, Brandis M: Functional and morphologic maturation of the superficial nephrons. *J Clin Invest* 53:279, 1974.

390. Spitzer A, Edelmann CM Jr: Maturational changes in pressure gradients for glomerular filtration. *Am J Physiol* 221:1431, 1971.

391. Sripanidkulchai B, Wyss JM: The development of alpha 2-adrenoceptors in the rat kidney: Correlation with noradrenergic innervation. *Brain Res* 400:91, 1987.

392. Stamenkovic I, Skalli O, Gabbiani G: Distribution of intermediate filament proteins in normal and diseased human glomeruli. *Am J Pathol* 125:465, 1986.

393. Starling EH: On the absorption of fluids from the connective tissue spaces. *J Physiol* (Lond) 19:312, 1896.

394. Starling EH: The glomerular functions of the kidney. *J Physiol* (Lond) 24:317, 1899.

395. Steiner RW, Blantz RC: Acute reversal of saralasin of multiple intrarenal effects of angiotensin II. *Am J Physiol* 237:F386, 1979.

396. Steiner RW, Tucker BJ, Blantz RC: Glomerular hemodynamics in rats with chronic sodium depletion. Effect of saralasin. *J Clin Invest* 64:503, 1979.

397. Steinhausen M, Kucherer H, Parekh N, et al: Angiotensin II control of the renal microcirculation: Effect of blockade by saralasin. *Kidney Int* 30:56, 1986.

398. Steinhausen M, Sterzel RB, Fleming JT, et al: Acute and chronic effects of angiotensin II on the vessels of the split hydronephrotic kidney. *Kidney Int* (suppl 20)31:S64, 1987.

399. Steven K: Effect of peritubular infusion of angiotensin II on rat proximal nephron function. *Kidney Int* 6:73, 1974.

400. Stopp M, Braunlich H: In vitro analysis of postnatal maturation of tubular p-aminohippurate transport in rat kidney. *Acta Biol Med Germ* 39:825, 1980.

401. Stulcova B: Postnatal development of cardiac output distribution measured by radioactive microspheres in rats. *Biol Neonate* 32:119, 1977.

402. Swaim JA, Hyndrickx GR, Boettcher DH, et al: Prostaglandin control of renal circulation in unanaesthetized dog and baboon. *Am J Physiol* 229:826, 1975.

403. Tanner GA, Isenberg MT: Secretion of p-aminohippurate by rat kidney proximal tubules. *Am J Physiol* 219:577, 1970.

404. Terragno NA, McGiff JC, Terragno A: Prostaglandin PGI_2 production by renal blood vessels: Relationship to and endogenous prostaglandin synthesis inhibitor (EPSI). *Clin Res* 26:545, 1978.

405. Terragno NA, Terragno A: Prostaglandin metabolism in fetal and maternal vasculature. *Fed Proc* 38:75, 1979.

406. Thurau K: Renal hemodynamics. *Am J Med* 36:698, 1964.

407. Thurau K, Wober E: Zur Localisation der autoregulativen widerstandsanderungen der Niere. *Pflugers Arch* 274:553, 1962.

408. Trimper CE, Lumbers ER: The renin-angiotensin system in fetal lambs. *Pflugers Arch* 336:1, 1972.

409. Trueta J, Barclay AE, Daniel PM, et al: *Studies of the Renal Circulation*. Oxford, Blackwell Scientific Publications, 1948, p 60.

410. Tucker BJ, Blantz RC: Factors determining superficial nephron filtration in the mature, growing rat. *Am J Physiol* 232(2):F97, 1977.

411. Tucker BJ, Mundy CA, Blantz RC: Adrenergic and angiotensin II influence on renal vascular tone in chronic sodium depletion. *Am J Physiol* 252:F811, 1985.

412. Uva B, Vallarino G, Ghiani P: Heterogeneity of angiotensin II receptors in mechanisms of developing rat metanephros. *Cell Biochem Function* 3:273, 1985.

413. Valtin H: *Renal Function: Mechanisms Preserving Fluid and Solute Balance in Health*. Boston, Little, Brown, 1983.

414. Vanhoutte PM: Vascular physiology: The end of the quest? *Nature* 327:459, 1987.

415. Varille VA, Nakamura KT, McWeeny OJ, et al: Renal hemodynamics response to atrial natriuretic factor in fetal and newborn sheep. *Pediatr Res* 25:291, 1989.

416. Vesely DL: Angiotensin II stimulates guanylate cyclase activity in aorta, heart, and kidney. *Am J Physiol* 240:E391, 1981.

417. Vierhapper H: Effect of human atrial natriuretic peptide on angiotensin II induces secretion of aldosterone in man. *Klin Wochenschr* (suppl 6)64:50, 1986.

418. Wakitani K, Cole BR, Geller DM, et al: Atriopeptins: Correlation between renal vasodilation and natriuresis. *Am J Physiol* 249:F49, 1985.

419. Walker DW, Mitchell MD: Prostaglandins in urine of foetal lambs. *Nature* 271:161, 1978.

420. Walker DW, Mitchell MD: Presence of thromboxane B_2 and 6-keto-prostaglandin F1-alpha in the urine of fetal sheep. *Postgraduate Med* 3:249, 1979.

421. Wearn JT, Richards AN: Observations on the composition of glomerular urine with particular reference to the problem of reabsorption in the renal tubule. *Am J Physiol* 71:209, 1924.

422. Weening JJ, Van-Der-Wall A: Effect of decreased perfusion pressure on glomerular permeability in the rat. *Lab Invest* 57:144, 1987.

423. Wei Y, Rodi CP, Day ML, et al: Developmental changes in the rat atriopeptin hormonal system. *J Clin Invest* 79:1325, 1987.

424. Weisman DN, Robillard JE: Renal hemodynamic responses to hypoxemia during development: Relationships to circulating vasoactive substances. *Pediatr Res* 23:155, 1988.

425. Welling L, Linshaw MA: Structural and functional development of outer versus inner cortical proximal tubules. *Pediatr Nephrol* 2:108, 1988.

426. West JR, Smith HW, Chasis H: Glomerular filtration rate, effective renal blood flow, and maximal tubular excretory capacity in infancy. *J Pediatr* 32:10, 1948.

427. Wigger HJ, Stalcup SA: Distribution and development of angiotensin converting enzyme in the fetal and newborn rabbit. *Lab Invest* 38:581, 1978.

428. Wolgast M, Ojteg G: Electrophysiology of renal capillary membranes: Gel concept applied and Starling model challenged. *Am J Physiol* 254:F364, 1988.

429. Wright GB, Alexander RW, Ekstein LS, et al: Characterization of the rabbit ventricular myocardial receptor for angiotensin II. *Mol Pharmacol* 24:213, 1983.

430. Yanagisawa M, Kurihara H, Kimura S, et al: A novel potent vasoconstrictor peptide produced by vascular endothelial cells. *Nature* 332:411, 1988.

431. Yared A, Yoskioka T: Autoregulation of glomerular filtration in the young. *Semin Nephrol* 9:94, 1989.

432. Yarger WE, Boyd MA, Schrader NW: Evaluation of methods measuring glomerular and nutrient blood flow in rat kidneys. *Am J Physiol* 235(5):H592, 1978.

433. Yoshida M, Ueda S, Soejima H, et al: Effects of prostaglandin E_2 and I_2 on renal cortical and medullary blood flow in rabbits. *Arch Int Pharmacodyn Ther* 282:108, 1986.

434. Zimmerhackl B, Robertson CR, Jamison RL: The microcirculation of the renal medulla. *Circ Res* 57:657, 1985.

435. Zink J, VanPetten GR: Noradrenergic control of blood vessels in the premature lamb fetus. *Biol Neonate* 39:61, 1981.

ently is a dimer of two 85,000-dalton polypeptides. Initial radiation inactivation studies indicated that the molecular weight of the phlorizin-binding moiety of the brush border membrane D-glucose transport protein was 110,000 daltons [158]. Further radiation inactivation studies yielded a molecular weight of 230,000 daltons for the Na^+-dependent phlorizin-binding unit and 345,000 daltons for the Na^+-dependent glucose transporter [89]. These findings suggested that the Na^+-glucose cotransport system is a multimeric structure in which distinct complexes are responsible for phlorizin binding and glucose transport. It is apparent that the precise assignment of molecular weight and structure of the Na^+-glucose cotransport protein is yet to be determined.

The TmG is low in puppies [4] and in human infants [23,59,145,154]. The ratio of TmG to GFR, however, was found to be either higher [4] or similar [23] to that determined later in life. Arant found that glomerulotubular balance was present even in premature babies [3]. These observations invalidate the theory that the larger glomerular-over-tubular mass necessarily translates into functional glomerulotubular imbalance with glomerular predominance [47]. In vitro studies, however, have revealed slower influx and efflux rates in tubular segments isolated from the cortex of newborn compared to those obtained from adult dogs, indicating the existence of intrinsic functional differences in sugar handling [49]. Kinetic analysis revealed a lower (V_{max}), but a similar Km of the transport system for glucose in the newborn compared to the adult. In BBMV from newborn dogs, there appear to be two kinetically distinct transport systems for glucose, as was observed in the adult dog [163]. Two sugar transport systems were also observed in the newborn rat tubule, but only the low affinity system was observed in the adult [118].

Amino Acid Transport

The human kidney of the adult is quite efficient at reabsorbing amino acids. Less than 2% of the filtered load of most amino acids appears in the final urine [178]. Exceptions to this rule are glycine, which is 95% reabsorbed, and histidine, which is 92% reabsorbed. During early infancy, amino acid reabsorption is less complete, especially for threonine, serine, proline, hydroxyproline, glycine, and alanine [24] (Fig. 4-5). Attainment of adult rates of reabsorption occurs at different ages for individual amino acids, consistent with the presence of multiple systems for amino acid transport [22].

The reabsorption of amino acids is an active, energy-requiring process. This was noted by a number of early investigators who, using either thin slices of renal cortex [51,52,114,115,128,136] or separated tubular fragments [66–68,74,117], demonstrated that renal tubule cells could develop intracellular concentrations of amino acids that are significantly higher than in the surrounding media. Anoxia or inhibitors of mitochondrial function decreased or abolished these gradients [66,68,114]. Amino acid uptake was stereospecific, with only the L configuration showing active transport. Studies with these preparations also indicated the presence of multiple amino acid carriers, each

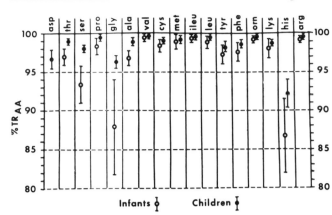

FIG. 4-5. *Tubular reabsorption of free amino acids in infancy and childhood: comparison of percentage of tubular reabsorption (% Taa). Differences between the two groups are statistically significant (p <0.02) with the exception of methionine, isoleucine, leucine, and tyrosine. (From Brodehl J: Renal hyperaminoaciduria. In Edelmann CM Jr (ed): Pediatric Kidney Disease, 1st ed. Boston, Little, Brown, 1978, with permission.)*

subserving the transport of a specific amino acid or a group of structurally similar amino acids. Christensen [32] originally proposed five transport systems for amino acids, but it now appears that this was an oversimplification. For example, cystine [48,130] has two distinct pathways, as do the dibasic amino acids [115,134], glycine [66,96,108], and the iminoamino acids [68,96].

Micropuncture experiments have revealed that amino acid transport is confined principally to the proximal tubule [16,41], with the bulk of the reabsorption occurring in the first one third of this segment. The active step of amino acid transport resides at the luminal membrane, as shown by experiments with BBMV [44,50,93,173] and isolated perfused proximal tubules [122].

Amino acid transport across the brush border membrane is generally coupled to and driven by sodium movement, similar to sugar transport [44,80,93,139] (see Fig. 4-1). Other ion gradients in addition to sodium play a role in driving amino acid transport systems. The efflux of K^+ from BBMV enhanced glutamate uptake, especially in the presence of an inwardly directed Na^+ gradient [25]. Fukuhara and Turner [56] have proposed that Na^+ facilitates the translocation of the glutamate-carrier complex across the brush border membrane and K^+ facilitates the return of the empty carrier to the luminal side of the membrane. An inwardly directed H^+ gradient led to an overshoot of proline uptake in BBMV, indicating a H^+-proline cotransport system [112]. Chloride appears to play a role in taurine transport, because replacement of Cl^- with other anions, both more or less permeable than Cl^-, led to a reduction in BBMV taurine uptake [29].

Movement of amino acids across the basolateral membrane appears to be mainly through facilitated diffusion. Because of the high intracellular amino acid concentration [19], the principal direction of this movement is from the cell to the blood. Thus, the model for amino acid transport

389. Spitzer A, Brandis M: Functional and morphologic maturation of the superficial nephrons. *J Clin Invest* 53:279, 1974.

390. Spitzer A, Edelmann CM Jr: Maturational changes in pressure gradients for glomerular filtration. *Am J Physiol* 221:1431, 1971.

391. Sripanidkulchai B, Wyss JM: The development of alpha 2-adrenoceptors in the rat kidney: Correlation with noradrenergic innervation. *Brain Res* 400:91, 1987.

392. Stamenkovic I, Skalli O, Gabbiani G: Distribution of intermediate filament proteins in normal and diseased human glomeruli. *Am J Pathol* 125:465, 1986.

393. Starling EH: On the absorption of fluids from the connective tissue spaces. *J Physiol* (Lond) 19:312, 1896.

394. Starling EH: The glomerular functions of the kidney. *J Physiol* (Lond) 24:317, 1899.

395. Steiner RW, Blantz RC: Acute reversal of saralasin of multiple intrarenal effects of angiotensin II. *Am J Physiol* 237:F386, 1979.

396. Steiner RW, Tucker BJ, Blantz RC: Glomerular hemodynamics in rats with chronic sodium depletion. Effect of saralasin. *J Clin Invest* 64:503, 1979.

397. Steinhausen M, Kucherer H, Parekh N, et al: Angiotensin II control of the renal microcirculation: Effect of blockade by saralasin. *Kidney Int* 30:56, 1986.

398. Steinhausen M, Sterzel RB, Fleming JT, et al: Acute and chronic effects of angiotensin II on the vessels of the split hydronephrotic kidney. *Kidney Int* (suppl 20)31:S64, 1987.

399. Steven K: Effect of peritubular infusion of angiotensin II on rat proximal nephron function. *Kidney Int* 6:73, 1974.

400. Stopp M, Braunlich H: In vitro analysis of postnatal maturation of tubular p-aminohippurate transport in rat kidney. *Acta Biol Med Germ* 39:825, 1980.

401. Stulcova B: Postnatal development of cardiac output distribution measured by radioactive microspheres in rats. *Biol Neonate* 32:119, 1977.

402. Swaim JA, Hyndrickx GR, Boettcher DH, et al: Prostaglandin control of renal circulation in unanaesthetized dog and baboon. *Am J Physiol* 229:826, 1975.

403. Tanner GA, Isenberg MT: Secretion of p-aminohippurate by rat kidney proximal tubules. *Am J Physiol* 219:577, 1970.

404. Terragno NA, McGiff JC, Terragno A: Prostaglandin PGI$_2$ production by renal blood vessels: Relationship to and endogenous prostaglandin synthesis inhibitor (EPSI). *Clin Res* 26:545, 1978.

405. Terragno NA, Terragno A: Prostaglandin metabolism in fetal and maternal vasculature. *Fed Proc* 38:75, 1979.

406. Thurau K: Renal hemodynamics. *Am J Med* 36:698, 1964.

407. Thurau K, Wober E: Zur Localisation der autoregulativen widerstandsanderungen der Niere. *Pflugers Arch* 274:553, 1962.

408. Trimper CE, Lumbers ER: The renin-angiotensin system in fetal lambs. *Pflugers Arch* 336:1, 1972.

409. Trueta J, Barclay AE, Daniel PM, et al: *Studies of the Renal Circulation.* Oxford, Blackwell Scientific Publications, 1948, p 60.

410. Tucker BJ, Blantz RC: Factors determining superficial nephron filtration in the mature, growing rat. *Am J Physiol* 232(2):F97, 1977.

411. Tucker BJ, Mundy CA, Blantz RC: Adrenergic and angiotensin II influence on renal vascular tone in chronic sodium depletion. *Am J Physiol* 252:F811, 1985.

412. Uva B, Vallarino G, Ghiani P: Heterogeneity of angiotensin II receptors in mechanisms of developing rat metanephros. *Cell Biochem Function* 3:273, 1985.

413. Valtin H: *Renal Function: Mechanisms Preserving Fluid and Solute Balance in Health.* Boston, Little, Brown, 1983.

414. Vanhoutte PM: Vascular physiology: The end of the quest? *Nature* 327:459, 1987.

415. Varille VA, Nakamura KT, McWeeny OJ, et al: Renal hemodynamics response to atrial natriuretic factor in fetal and newborn sheep. *Pediatr Res* 25:291, 1989.

416. Vesely DL: Angiotensin II stimulates guanylate cyclase activity in aorta, heart, and kidney. *Am J Physiol* 240:E391, 1981.

417. Vierhapper H: Effect of human atrial natriuretic peptide on angiotensin II induces secretion of aldosterone in man. *Klin Wochenschr* (suppl 6)64:50, 1986.

418. Wakitani K, Cole BR, Geller DM, et al: Atriopeptins: Correlation between renal vasodilation and natriuresis. *Am J Physiol* 249:F49, 1985.

419. Walker DW, Mitchell MD: Prostaglandins in urine of foetal lambs. *Nature* 271:161, 1978.

420. Walker DW, Mitchell MD: Presence of thromboxane B$_2$ and 6-keto-prostaglandin F1-alpha in the urine of fetal sheep. *Postgraduate Med* 3:249, 1979.

421. Wearn JT, Richards AN: Observations on the composition of glomerular urine with particular reference to the problem of reabsorption in the renal tubule. *Am J Physiol* 71:209, 1924.

422. Weening JJ, Van-Der-Wall A: Effect of decreased perfusion pressure on glomerular permeability in the rat. *Lab Invest* 57:144, 1987.

423. Wei Y, Rodi CP, Day ML, et al: Developmental changes in the rat atriopeptin hormonal system. *J Clin Invest* 79:1325, 1987.

424. Weisman DN, Robillard JE: Renal hemodynamic responses to hypoxemia during development: Relationships to circulating vasoactive substances. *Pediatr Res* 23:155, 1988.

425. Welling L, Linshaw MA: Structural and functional development of outer versus inner cortical proximal tubules. *Pediatr Nephrol* 2:108, 1988.

426. West JR, Smith HW, Chasis H: Glomerular filtration rate, effective renal blood flow, and maximal tubular excretory capacity in infancy. *J Pediatr* 32:10, 1948.

427. Wigger HJ, Stalcup SA: Distribution and development of angiotensin converting enzyme in the fetal and newborn rabbit. *Lab Invest* 38:581, 1978.

428. Wolgast M, Ojteg G: Electrophysiology of renal capillary membranes: Gel concept applied and Starling model challenged. *Am J Physiol* 254:F364, 1988.

429. Wright GB, Alexander RW, Ekstein LS, et al: Characterization of the rabbit ventricular myocardial receptor for angiotensin II. *Mol Pharmacol* 24:213, 1983.

430. Yanagisawa M, Kurihara H, Kimura S, et al: A novel potent vasoconstrictor peptide produced by vascular endothelial cells. *Nature* 332:411, 1988.

431. Yared A, Yoskioka T: Autoregulation of glomerular filtration in the young. *Semin Nephrol* 9:94, 1989.

432. Yarger WE, Boyd MA, Schrader NW: Evaluation of methods measuring glomerular and nutrient blood flow in rat kidneys. *Am J Physiol* 235(5):H592, 1978.

433. Yoshida M, Ueda S, Soejima H, et al: Effects of prostaglandin E$_2$ and I$_2$ on renal cortical and medullary blood flow in rabbits. *Arch Int Pharmacodyn Ther* 282:108, 1986.

434. Zimmerhackl B, Robertson CR, Jamison RL: The microcirculation of the renal medulla. *Circ Res* 57:657, 1985.

435. Zink J, VanPetten GR: Noradrenergic control of blood vessels in the premature lamb fetus. *Biol Neonate* 39:61, 1981.

John W. Foreman
Stanton Segal

4
Tubular Transport of Organic Substances

Our understanding of the nature of organic substrate transport has undergone considerable refinement over the years due to the development of newer, more sophisticated techniques for studying this process, such as measurement of fluxes across each cell membrane. Evaluation of these fluxes has led to a general model for nonelectrolyte transport across the proximal tubule (Fig. 4-1). According to this model, the movement of organic substances that undergo net reabsorption, such as sugars and amino acids, is coupled to the movement of sodium [80,139]. Because the inside of the proximal tubule cell is electrically negative relative to the lumen and the intracellular Na^+ concentration is quite low, there is an electrochemical gradient favoring Na^+ entry into the cell. This, in turn provides the driving force for organic solute uptake. The electrochemical gradient across the luminal membrane is maintained by the active extrusion of Na^+ through the basolateral cell membrane by the enzyme Na^+-K^+-ATPase. Because the entry of organic substrates into the cell is only indirectly linked to the hydrolysis of ATP, organic substrate uptake is termed *secondary active transport*.

The basolateral membrane is composed of the plasma membrane abutting the basement membrane and that defining the lateral spaces between the cells. Movement of organic solutes across this cell boundary is probably carrier mediated because the lipid bilayer is relatively impermeable to most of these substances. Passage from the lateral intercellular spaces across the basement membrane into the interstitium appears to encounter little resistance [174, 123]. Paracellular solute movement can also occur through the tight junctions between proximal tubule cells because they are relatively "leaky" when compared to those between distal tubule cells [18]. This pathway appears to account for a relatively small fraction of the total flux of organic solutes, however.

The sequence of events is reversed for organic compounds that are secreted, such as para-aminohippurate (PAH). The active step of the transport process resides at the basolateral membrane, whereas the exit from the cell, through the luminal membrane, is passive. Some compounds, such as uric acid, can be transported bidirectionally, with active steps being present on both sides of the proximal tubule cell.

Transport of Sugar

Clearance studies in man [144] and animals [137] have shown that the renal reabsorption of sugars, especially of glucose, is extraordinarily efficient. Virtually all of the filtered glucose is reabsorbed within the normal range of blood glucose concentrations. As the plasma glucose concentration is raised, a point is reached at which glucose spills into the urine [137,144]. This plasma level is referred to as the renal threshold for glucose and is approximately 180 mg/dl in normal adults [143]. The rate of sugar reabsorption by the kidney, however, continues to increase as the plasma concentration is further raised, until a maximum (TmG) is achieved, usually 300 to 350 mg/min [42,87,144]. The graphic representation of this relationship, called a *titration curve*, is shown in Figure 4-2. The plot is curvilinear or splayed rather than sharply broken. The splay can be the result of regional differences in renal perfusion leading to saturation of some sites before others or to differences in size and length of the various nephrons [143,144]. Another explanation is that the titration curve is similar to the Michaelis-Menton formulation for enzyme kinetics, and the splay is a measure of the affinity of a substrate for its transport carrier. The threshold and the TmG were initially thought to be constant [137], but it is now clear that they can be altered by changes in either glomerular filtration rate (GFR) or in extracellular fluid volume [37,59,64,79,164,165].

Other physiologically important sugars besides glucose, such as D-galactose [38,57], D-fructose [57] and *myo*-inositol [34,53,102], also undergo net reabsorption. Further, these sugars appear to share the brush border membrane glucose transport system, because glucose loading and the administration of phlorizin, a specific inhibitor of the Na^+-glucose cotransporter, reduced their reabsorption [138, 140,141]. A common transport system was also suggested by the increase in glucose and inositol excretion after infusing glucose in patients with renal glucosuria [53]. This study also suggested the presence of a separate inositol transport system, because the increase in glucose excretion was proportionately greater than that of inositol [53]. D-Mannose loading inhibited fructose reabsorption but had no effect on glucose, galactose, or *myo*-inositol [138,140],

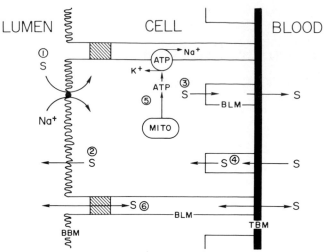

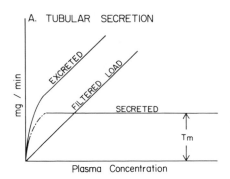

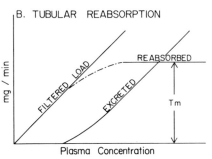

FIG. 4-1. *Model of organic solute (S) transport by the renal proximal tubule cell. Solute uptake by the brush border membrane from the lumen is carrier-mediated coupled to Na^+ influx (1). A favorable electrochemical driving force for luminal Na^+ entry is maintained by the Na^+-K^+-ATPase pump (5). Transported solute is then either used by the cell or returned to the blood across the basolateral membrane through a carrier (3), effecting net transepithelial reabsorption. For transepithelial secretion, the active step may reside on the basolateral membrane (4), with passive movement cross the brush border membrane (2). Paracellular (6) movement of organic solutes can occur in either direction. TBM indicates tubular basement membrane, BBM indicates brush border membrane, and BLM indicates basolateral membrane. (From Foreman JW, Segal S: Fanconi syndrome. In Holliday M, Barratt TM, Venier R (eds): Pediatric Nephrology, 2nd ed. Baltimore, Williams & Wilkins, 1987, with permission.)*

FIG. 4-2. *Tubular titration curves. Tubular secretion (A) and tubular reabsorption (B) of a substrate as a function of the plasma concentration. Tm is the maximal transport rate by the tubule of the substrate. The broken line indicates the splay of the titration curve. (From Foreman JW, Renal handling of urate and organic acids. In Bovee KC (ed): Canine Nephrology. Media, PA: Harwal, 1984, with permission.)*

while fructose loading inhibited mannose reabsorption. These results suggested that a third sugar carrier exists for fructose and mannose transport [138,140]. From these clearance studies, Silverman [139] has proposed a model for luminal sugar transport with a G-transporter primarily for glucose and galactose uptake with some affinity for fructose and *myo*-inositol, an M-transporter for mannose and fructose uptake, and finally a *myo*-inositol transporter for inositol uptake (Fig. 4-3).

Glucose transport is an active, energy-requiring process, as shown by experiment using renal cortical slices from animals [84,133] and humans [129]. Incubation of these cortical slices with α-methylglucoside, a nonmetabolizable glucose analogue, led to intracellular concentrations of this sugar that exceeded those of the media. The higher intracellular concentrations were abolished by anoxia and metabolic inhibitors, indicating an active, energy-requiring transport process. Raising the concentration of α-methylglucoside in the medium led to a nonlinear increase in the transport rate that approached a maximum. Glucose, galactose, and phlorizin inhibited the uptake of α-methylglucoside [132,133]. Taken together, these findings indicate that the transport of glucose is carrier-mediated.

Almost all filtered glucose is reabsorbed in the proximal

tubule, most of it within the first 20% of the tubule length [55,111,167,169]. Tune and Burg [155], using isolated perfused proximal convoluted and proximal straight tubules, have demonstrated that the rate of glucose transport was much greater in the convoluted portion of the proximal tubule than in the straight portion. The concentration of glucose in proximal convoluted cells was higher than that in the perfusing fluid, again indicating active transport across the luminal cell membrane. Movement of glucose from the cells into the peritubular capillaries was found to be facilitated by the higher permeability of the antiluminal cell membrane compared to the luminal cell membrane. The maximal active transport rate (V_{max}) for glucose and the affinity (Km) for glucose decreased along the proximal tubule [11]. The passive movement of glucose from the peritubular blood into the lumen was also lower in the proximal straight tubule compared to the proximal convoluted tubule. These findings suggested the presence of a high capacity, low affinity transport system with a moderate passive leak in the proximal convoluted tubule, followed by a low capacity, high affinity system with a small passive leak in the proximal straight tubule.

Kinne and co-workers, using isolated brush border membrane vesicles (BBMV), confirmed that glucose uptake across the luminal membrane was carrier-mediated and inhibitable by phlorizin [81]. This uptake was stereospecific in that the D but not the L configuration of glucose was

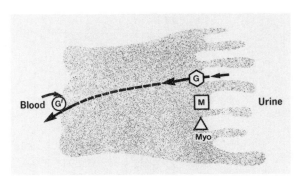

FIG. 4-3. Schematic representation of a proximal tubular cell indicating three sugar transport systems at the brush border membrane; G for the glucose transporter, M for the mannose transporter, and Myo for the myo-inositol transporter. At the antiluminal (basolateral) membrane, a different glucose transporter (G') exists, which is shared with mannose, galatcose, fructose, and myo-inositol. Glucose is reabsorbed from the lumen, diffuses across the cytoplasm, and exits through the G' transporter embedded in the antiluminal membrane. Glucose can also enter the cell from the blood through the antiluminal membrane. (From Silverman M: Glucose Transport in the Kidney. Biochim Biophys Acta 457:334, 1976, with permission.)

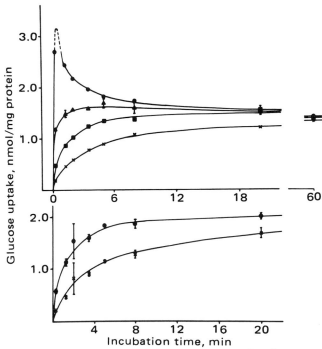

FIG. 4-4. The timed uptake of glucose into BBMV from human kidney. In the upper panel, the uptake of 1 mM D-glucose is shown in the presence of 100 mM NaCl initially only outside the vesicles (●), with 100 mM NaCl both inside and outside the vesicles (▲), and in the presence of 100 μM phlorizin (■). The uptake of 1 mM L-glucose in the presence of 100 mM NaCl outside the vesicles is also plotted (X). In the lower panel, are drawn the uptakes of 1 mM D-glucose (●) and L-glucose (X) in the presence of a 100 mM KCl inwardly directed gradient. (From Turner RJ, Silverman M: Sugar uptake into brush border vesicles from normal human kidney. Proc Natl Acad Sci USA 74:2826, 1977, with permission.)

actively transported. D-Glucose uptake was stimulated by an inwardly directed Na^+ gradient, resulting in a transient accumulation of glucose that exceeded equilibrium levels, termed an *overshoot* (Fig. 4-4). This overshoot was not observed when the Na^+ gradient was replaced by a K^+ gradient, indicating Na^+ dependence of the glucose transport [6,13,14]. Glucose uptake was also found to be driven by the electrical potential present across the BBMV. The glucose overshoot was still observed when the chemical potential energy was obliterated by equilibrating Na^+ across the BBMV, and an electrical potential was created by loading the BBMV with K^+, and then exposing the BBMV to valinomycin [14]. Valinomycin is an ionophore that facilitates K^+ exit from the BBMV and thus induces an electrical potential across the BBMV by rendering the inside of the vesicles negative. As in the other experimental preparations, this transport system was shared with D-galactose [162].

In the dog [162,163] and human [161], glucose uptake by the BBMV occurs through two kinetically distinct transport systems: a high capacity, low affinity system present in BBMV from the outer cortex, and a low capacity, high affinity system in BBMV obtained from the outer medulla [160]. This arrangement is similar to that observed by Barfuss and Schafer in isolated perfused proximal tubules [11]. The outer cortical transport system was reported to be more sensitive to phlorizin inhibition, whereas that of the outer medulla was more sensitive to galactose inhibition [159].

A number of investigators have examined the structural properties of the glucose transporter present in the brush border membrane. Turner and George [157], using reducing agents, identified two disulfide bonds that are important

for the functioning of the glucose transporter, and Lin et al. [90], using reagents that bind to tyrosine, found that tyrosine residues were important for the binding of Na^+ to the transport protein.

The molecular weight of the glucose transporter has been reported to be as low as 30,000 and as high as 345,000 daltons. Studies using labeled N-ethyl-maleimide, which binds to sulfhydryl groups, gave a molecular weight of 60,000 daltons [104]. Photoaffinity-labelling with photosensitive phlorizin analogues suggested that the molecular weight is 72,000 daltons [71]. Affinity chromatography using a phlorizin polymer yielded a protein with a molecular weight between 60,000 and 70,000 daltons that expressed Na^+-dependent D-glucose transport activity when incorporated in artificial liposomes [88]. Koepsell et al. [85] used partial purification and reconstitution procedures to isolate a brush border membrane protein fraction with a molecular weight of 52,000 daltons that had Na^+-dependent D-glucose transport properties. Using similar techniques, Malathi and Preiser [92] found Na^+-dependent D-glucose activity to reside in a fraction containing a single protein band with a molecular weight of 165,000 daltons, which apparently is a dimer of two 85,000-dalton polypeptides. Initial radiation inactivation studies indicated that the molecular weight of the phlorizin-binding moiety of the brush border membrane D-glucose transport protein was 110,000 daltons [158]. Further radiation inactivation studies yielded a molecular weight of 230,000 daltons for the Na$^+$-dependent phlorizin-binding unit and 345,000 daltons for the Na$^+$-dependent glucose transporter [89]. These findings suggested that the Na$^+$-glucose cotransport system is a multimeric structure in which distinct complexes are responsible for phlorizin binding and glucose transport. It is apparent that the precise assignment of molecular weight and structure of the Na$^+$-glucose cotransport protein is yet to be determined.

The TmG is low in puppies [4] and in human infants [23,59,145,154]. The ratio of TmG to GFR, however, was found to be either higher [4] or similar [23] to that determined later in life. Arant found that glomerulotubular balance was present even in premature babies [3]. These observations invalidate the theory that the larger glomerular-over-tubular mass necessarily translates into functional glomerulotubular imbalance with glomerular predominance [47]. In vitro studies, however, have revealed slower influx and efflux rates in tubular segments isolated from the cortex of newborn compared to those obtained from adult dogs, indicating the existence of intrinsic functional differences in sugar handling [49]. Kinetic analysis revealed a lower (V_{max}), but a similar Km of the transport system for glucose in the newborn compared to the adult. In BBMV from newborn dogs, there appear to be two kinetically distinct transport systems for glucose, as was observed in the adult dog [163]. Two sugar transport systems were also observed in the newborn rat tubule, but only the low affinity system was observed in the adult [118].

Amino Acid Transport

The human kidney of the adult is quite efficient at reabsorbing amino acids. Less than 2% of the filtered load of most amino acids appears in the final urine [178]. Exceptions to this rule are glycine, which is 95% reabsorbed, and histidine, which is 92% reabsorbed. During early infancy, amino acid reabsorption is less complete, especially for threonine, serine, proline, hydroxyproline, glycine, and alanine [24] (Fig. 4-5). Attainment of adult rates of reabsorption occurs at different ages for individual amino acids, consistent with the presence of multiple systems for amino acid transport [22].

The reabsorption of amino acids is an active, energy-requiring process. This was noted by a number of early investigators who, using either thin slices of renal cortex [51,52,114,115,128,136] or separated tubular fragments [66–68,74,117], demonstrated that renal tubule cells could develop intracellular concentrations of amino acids that are significantly higher than in the surrounding media. Anoxia or inhibitors of mitochondrial function decreased or abolished these gradients [66,68,114]. Amino acid uptake was stereospecific, with only the L configuration showing active transport. Studies with these preparations also indicated the presence of multiple amino acid carriers, each

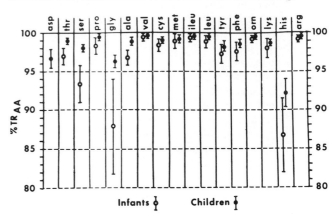

FIG. 4-5. *Tubular reabsorption of free amino acids in infancy and childhood: comparison of percentage of tubular reabsorption (% Taa). Differences between the two groups are statistically significant ($p < 0.02$) with the exception of methionine, isoleucine, leucine, and tyrosine. (From Brodehl J: Renal hyperaminoaciduria. In Edelmann CM Jr (ed): Pediatric Kidney Disease, 1st ed. Boston, Little, Brown, 1978, with permission.)*

subserving the transport of a specific amino acid or a group of structurally similar amino acids. Christensen [32] originally proposed five transport systems for amino acids, but it now appears that this was an oversimplification. For example, cystine [48,130] has two distinct pathways, as do the dibasic amino acids [115,134], glycine [66,96,108], and the iminoamino acids [68,96].

Micropuncture experiments have revealed that amino acid transport is confined principally to the proximal tubule [16,41], with the bulk of the reabsorption occurring in the first one third of this segment. The active step of amino acid transport resides at the luminal membrane, as shown by experiments with BBMV [44,50,93,173] and isolated perfused proximal tubules [122].

Amino acid transport across the brush border membrane is generally coupled to and driven by sodium movement, similar to sugar transport [44,80,93,139] (see Fig. 4-1). Other ion gradients in addition to sodium play a role in driving amino acid transport systems. The efflux of K$^+$ from BBMV enhanced glutamate uptake, especially in the presence of an inwardly directed Na$^+$ gradient [25]. Fukuhara and Turner [56] have proposed that Na$^+$ facilitates the translocation of the glutamate-carrier complex across the brush border membrane and K$^+$ facilitates the return of the empty carrier to the luminal side of the membrane. An inwardly directed H$^+$ gradient led to an overshoot of proline uptake in BBMV, indicating a H$^+$-proline cotransport system [112]. Chloride appears to play a role in taurine transport, because replacement of Cl$^-$ with other anions, both more or less permeable than Cl$^-$, led to a reduction in BBMV taurine uptake [29].

Movement of amino acids across the basolateral membrane appears to be mainly through facilitated diffusion. Because of the high intracellular amino acid concentration [19], the principal direction of this movement is from the cell to the blood. Thus, the model for amino acid transport proposes that the active transport step resides on the luminal membrane, with passive, carrier-mediated movement out of the cell through the basolateral membrane driven by the high intracellular to plasma concentration gradient [9,11,19,52,67,114,115,124]. Not all amino acid transport across the basolateral membrane is by facilitated diffusion, however. A Na$^+$ gradient mechanism has been demonstrated for basolateral membrane transport of the acidic amino acids, glutamate and aspartate [120]. Concentrative glycine uptake across the basolateral membrane has also been documented in isolated proximal tubule segments [10]; however, this transport system is probably not important for transepithelial transport but rather for cell nutrition.

Barfuss and Shafer [10], using isolated segments of the proximal tubule, found the maximal reabsorption rate for glycine in the convoluted portion to be 28.5 pmol/min/mm and in the straight portion to be 2.5 pmol/min/mm, whereas the Km was 11.8 mM in the convoluted portion and 0.7 mM in the straight portion. These investigators found a similar arrangement of cystine transporters [124]. These data led them to suggest that high capacity, low affinity systems for amino acid transport reside in the brush border membrane of the proximal convoluted tubule, while low capacity, high affinity systems are located in the brush border membrane of the proximal straight tubule [122]. This arrangement would allow for the bulk of amino acids to be reabsorbed early in the nephron, with the final clearing of the ultrafiltrate in more distal parts of the proximal tubule. There may be exceptions to this rule, however. Microperfusion studies of histidine transport indicated that the Km for histidine increased along the tubule [91], while similar studies of proline reabsorption suggested the existence of multiple transport systems along the proximal tubule segment [166]. Backflux of amino acids, or movement from the basolateral spaces into the lumen, has also been shown to occur [9,11,124]. For glycine, this movement was not saturable, suggesting a paracellular pathway.

Studies of amino acid handling by the kidney in vivo have revealed a generalized aminoaciduria both in animal [170] and human neonate [24]. The aminoaciduria of the newborn is not due to a lack of specific transport systems; all amino acid transport systems were found to be present in the kidney of the newborn, e.g., proline [73], glycine [108], cystine [72], and taurine [30]. Moreover, most in vitro studies have failed to document differences in amino acid uptake between renal tissue of newborn and adult animals. Exceptions to this are glycine uptake by the dog [94] and taurine uptake by the rat [54], which were lower in the newborn than in the adult. However, renal tissue from immature animals develops much higher intracellular levels of amino acids than adult tissue, especially after long periods of incubation [7,30,72,74,108,116,131,135]. The intracellular amino acid concentrations of proline, serine, threonine, glycine, alanine, and aspartate were higher, while only phenylalanine and histidine were lower in the kidney of newborn compared to adult rats [19]. Thus, the aminoaciduria of the newborn is not due to differences in influx of amino acids. The major reason for decreased amino acid reabsorption by the neonate appears to be

impaired movement of amino acids out of the proximal tubule cell across the basolateral membrane [7,31,54, 94,135], which in turn impedes luminal reabsorption. A small basolateral surface area of the tubule cell [65] and the lack of peritubular capillaries [43] may play a role in this phenomenon.

Organic Acid and Cation Transport

The renal tubule transports a vast array of organic cations and anions, including anions such as bile salts, prostaglandins, and urate, and numerous drugs, such as penicillin and diuretics (Table 4-1). Cations transported include choline, dopamine, and drugs, such as atropine and morphine (Table 4-2). Many of these compounds undergo bidirectional active transport in that both active reabsorption and active secretion occur within the nephron. Significant passive movement of these compounds also occurs, depending on the degree of ionization, which is determined by the extent to which the pK$_a$ or pK$_b$ of the compounds differs from that of physiologic fluids. The pK$_a$ is the pH at which 50% of a weak acid is ionized and the pK$_b$ is the pH at which 50% of a weak base is ionized. The un-ionized acid or base diffuses more easily than the ionized portion into or out of the cell, depending on its lipid solubility. Phenobarbital, a weak acid with a high pK$_a$, is relatively lipid soluble. Alkalinizing the urine and thereby reducing the lipid soluble, nonionized fraction increases the excretion of phenobarbital [168]. This has little or no effect on PAH excretion since the nonionized form is relatively lipid insoluble. Urine flow rates also influence passive movement because lower urine flow rates allow longer contact time of the substrate with the luminal membrane.

PAH, although not normally found in urine, has been used by many investigators as the prototype for organic anion transport. This compound is so avidly secreted by the renal tubule of many animals, including man, that the blood is almost completely cleared of it in a single pass

TABLE 4-1. *Compounds transported by the organic anion pathway*

Endogenous	Exogenous
Bile salts	Amphotericin B
Citrate	Chlorothiazide
Creatinine*	Cimetidine*
cAMP	Cephalosporins
α-Ketoglutarate	Ethacrynic acid
Ketone bodies	Furosemide
Lactate	Nitrofurantoin
Oxalate	PAH
Prostaglandins	Penicillin
Urate	Probenecid
	Pyrazinoate
	Salicylate
	Sulfonamides

* Transported also by the organic cation pathway.

TABLE 4-2. *Compounds transported by the organic cation pathway*

Endogenous	Exogenous
Acetylcholine	Amiloride
Catecholamines	Atropine
Choline	Cimetidine*
Creatinine*	Cisplatin
Histamine	Mecamylamine
Serotonin	Morphine
	Procainamide
	Quinidine
	Tetraethylammonium

* Transported also by the organic anion pathway.

through the kidney when the plasma concentration does not exceed 1 mM. (This property has also prompted investigators to use it for estimating renal blood flow [143].)

PAH secretion occurs principally in the S2 segment of the proximal straight tubule [156]. The active step in its secretion appears to be localized to the basolateral membrane [21,156,171]. This basolateral transport step is stimulated by sodium and inhibited by probenecid [77]. Extrusion across the brush border membrane occurs in exchange for anions, such as bicarbonate, chloride, urate, succinate, lactate, and hydroxyl ions. Cations do not affect this transporter [20,61,75,76]. Karniski and Aronson have found two other anion exchangers in BBMV that appear separate from the broad specificity anion exchanger mediating PAH uptake: one mediates the exchange of Cl^- for formate and the other the exchange of either Cl^- or formate for oxalate [78]. These two anion exchangers appear to play an important role in electroneutral NaCl reabsorption in the proximal tubule [125]. In addition to these anion exchangers in the brush border membrane, there are Na^+-gradient stimulated systems for the reabsorption of monocarboxylic acids [8,58,100], e.g., lactate, acetoacetate, and 3-hydroxybutyrate, and for dicarboxylic and tricarboxylic acids [82,177], e.g., citrate, succinate, malate, and α-ketoglutarate.

Studies in humans [12,35,45,119,175] and a variety of animal species [142–144] have revealed a low clearance of PAH in the young that rises with age. Barnett et al. [12] found the mean PAH clearance of eight premature 3- to 13-day-old infants to be 148 ml/min/1.73m^2 and to rise to 200 ml/min/1.73m^2 by 49 to 107 days of age. Similar results were reported by others [45,175]. Fawer et al. [45] found a progressive rise in PAH clearance between 28 and 35 weeks of gestational age and no further change between 35 weeks and term. Adult values for PAH clearance and TmPAH, when corrected for surface area, were reached by 1 to 2 years of age [27,119].

A number of factors could contribute to the low clearance of PAH in immature animals, including (1) the rate of glomerular filtration; (2) access of PAH to transport sites; (3) surface area available for secretion; and (4) number of PAH carriers and their affinity for PAH. The access of PAH to the transporting sites may be limited in young animals because a large fraction of the total renal blood

flow goes to the vasa recta, bypassing the PAH transport sites present in the proximal tubule [40]. The peritubular capillary network in the immature animal is not as dense as that of the adult, reducing the contact between the blood and basolateral membranes [65]. In addition, the proximal tubule increases in both length and volume with maturation; more importantly, the surface area of the basolateral membrane increases markedly, due to increased infoldings [65]. The increase in basolateral membrane surface area accounts, in part, for the increase in the number of carriers [126]. From studies of PAH transport by isolated perfused proximal straight tubules of developing rabbits, Schwartz et al. [126] estimated that one third of the increase in tubular transport of PAH was due to an increase in surface area and two thirds was due to an increase in the intrinsic capacity of the tubule to transport PAH. The maturation of the transport capacity could be stimulated by the administration of penicillin or PAH to animals [69,70,126] and human neonates [127].

Uric Acid

The importance of uric acid stems from its role in the formation of renal stones and in gout. Uric acid, predominantly ionized to urate at physiologic pH, undergoes net reabsorption in the human kidney. Less than 10% of the filtered load appears in the urine of normal adults [17,63,148,153]. Gutman and Yu [63] infused mannitol and urate in subjects treated with sulfinpyrazone to inhibit the reabsorptive flux and found ratios of urate clearance to inulin clearance that exceeded one. This indicated that there is secretion of urate as well. These experimental data for urate secretion are confirmed by reports describing individuals with a genetic defect in urate reabsorption who have endogenous urate clearance rates that exceed the GFR by as much as 50% [2,106].

The complexity of renal urate transport can be inferred from the conflicting observations published in the literature. Initial investigators of urate transport, primarily using clearance techniques, described either secretion or reabsorption, depending on the animal examined, leading to the assumption that urate was transported in only one direction in any given animal species. With the finding that low doses of salicylate decreased urate excretion and high doses increased excretion in man, bidirectional transport was first proposed [180]. Since then, many studies employing stop-flow, microperfusion, microinjection, isolated tubule perfusion, and clearance techniques have demonstrated bidirectional transport, i.e., both reabsorption and secretion occurring at the same time in the same or different nephron segments.

The vast majority of studies indicate that the proximal tubule is the major site of tubular transport of urate [1,15,86,98,109,121,172]. There is evidence both for [109] and against [86] reabsorption in the pars recta and the loop of Henle. Using stop-flow techniques, bidirectional urate flux was localized to the proximal tubule of the rabbit [15] and the guinea pig [98]. Bidirectional active transport was also detected by micropuncture of the rat, with net reabsorption occurring in the early proximal tubule and net secretion in the late portion of the proximal tubule [1,86].

Weinmann and coworkers, using in vivo microperfusion of the rat proximal tubule, demonstrated saturable transport for both urate reabsorption and secretion with a Km of 0.17 and 0.41 mM, respectively [121,172]. In the dog, the bidirectional transport of urate was documented by stop-flow, clearance, double indicator dilution, and micropuncture techniques [97,110,113,182].

The in vitro studies of urate handling by the kidney have revealed marked species variations. Renal cortical slices from rabbits [103], guinea pigs [103], chickens [33,103], and snakes [33] displayed concentrative uptake of urate that was inhibited by anoxia, 2,4-dinitrophenol, and probenecid. In contrast, concentrative uptake of urate could not be demonstrated in animals that normally exhibit net reabsorption of urate: rat, mongrel dog, monkey, and man [103]. Maximal uptake of urate occurred in the presence of high K^+ concentrations, up to 40 mM in some studies [103]. Media Na^+ concentration also affected uptake, but only when it was lowered to less than 50 mM [83,103]. Reducing the media pH to 6 decreased uptake, but raising it from 7.4 to 7.9 caused little or no change [83,103].

Studies using BBMV indicate that transport of urate across the luminal membrane occurs in exchange for a broad range of anions, including OH^-, Cl^-, HCO_3^-, lactate, and succinate [20,61,75,76]. This anion exchanger also mediates PAH movement into the lumen and is sensitive to inhibition by probenecid and pyrazinoate [75]. Sodium and other cations do not affect BBMV uptake of urate. Basolateral transport of urate occurs also through an anion exchanger [77]. In contrast to the brush border exchanger, the basolateral anion exchanger does not mediate PAH uptake, which occurs through a separate sodium cotransport system [77].

Guggino et al. [61] have postulated that several mechanisms may account for the active urate reabsorption that occurs in rats, dogs, monkeys, and humans (Fig. 4-6). One is through the outwardly directed OH^- gradient created by the exchange of intracellular H^+ for luminal Na^+. Other anions, such as lactate or ketone bodies, which are extruded from the cell through a Na^+-coupled pathway, could also serve as exchange partners for urate. This mechanism may explain the hyperuricemia observed during lactic acidosis and ketosis, although an alternative explanation would be the inhibition of urate secretion. Yet another possibility is that anions actively taken up by the tubular cells across the basolateral membrane are secreted across the brush border membrane in exchange for urate.

The foregoing information constitutes the basis of the model for uric acid transport in man proposed by Chonko and Grantham (Fig. 4-7). There is active reabsorption and secretion throughout the proximal tubule, although the relative magnitudes vary in each segment. In addition, there is a passive flux of urate through the paracellular pathways. In the S1 segment reabsorption predominates, whereas in the S2 segment secretion is dominant. In the S3 segment the active reabsorptive and secretory fluxes are about equal, but because the concentration of urate is much higher in the lumen than in the blood, there is a significant passive reabsorptive flux. This may well be the "postsecretory" reabsorptive site suggested from clearance studies.

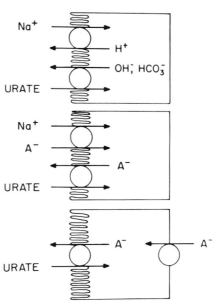

FIG. 4-6. Models for uphill urate absorption through anion exchange across the luminal membrane of the proximal tubular cell. Urate could be exchanged for intracellular OH^- or HCO_3^-. This exchange could be driven by the favorable electrochemical gradient for the movement of OH^- and HCO_3^- out of the cell generated by Na^+–H^+ exchange. Another driving force could be the Na^+-driven uptake of another luminal anion A^-, which could then exchange for luminal urate. Finally, anion A^- transported across the basolateral membrane could exchange for luminal urate. (From Guggino SE, Martin GJ, Aronson PS: Specificity and modes of the anion exchanges in dog renal microvillus membranes. Am J Physiol 244:F612, 1983, with permission.)

Pyrazinamide, an inhibitor of urate secretion, has been used to estimate the magnitude of various renal fluxes in man [150]. The decrement in urate excretion produced by this drug is taken as a measure of the secretion of urate. The rate of urate reabsorption during pyrazinamide administration is thought to reflect the maximal reabsorptive rate. Based on such studies, the fractional reabsorption of urate in man was estimated to be 98%. Urate loading does not affect the reabsorption of urate under these experimental conditions. On the other hand, urate loading of human subjects not receiving pyrazinamide led to increased excretion, suggesting that the secretory flux is sensitive to plasma urate concentrations while the reabsorptive flux is not.

A number of other drugs, in addition to pyrazinamide, affect renal urate transport. Probenecid [142,181], sulfinpyrazone [26], salicylates in high doses (serum levels > 15 mg/dl) [62,181], and phenylbutazone [179] are among agents that are uricosuric. Low doses of salicylates inhibit urate excretion [62,180]. Most diuretics lead to hyperuricemia through volume contraction, although initially they are uricosuric [36,39].

The state of the extracellular fluid volume plays an important role in urate excretion. Expansion of the extracellular volume increases urate excretion [28,149], and contraction decreases excretion [151,152]. This effect appears

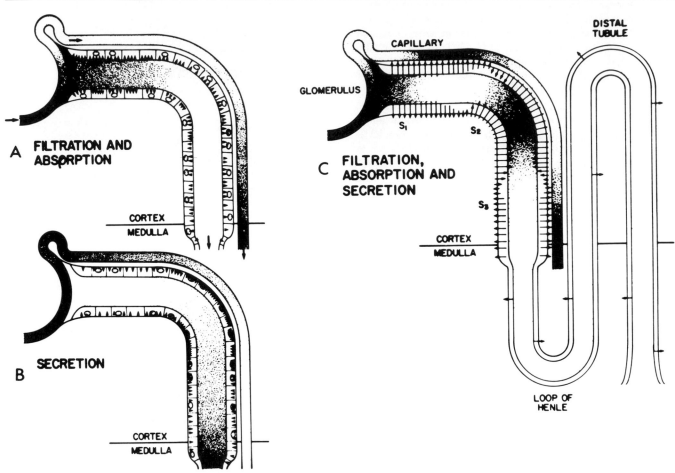

FIG. 4-7. *Model of renal urate handling in man. A. Only filtration and reabsorption are portrayed; secretion is omitted. B. Only secretion is shown; filtration and reabsorption are omitted. C. All components are included. The density of shading in tubule and the capillary indicates the relative amounts of urate, not concentration, in the lumina. (From Chonko AM, Grantham JJ: Disorders of urate metabolism and excretion. In Brenner BM, Rector FC Jr (eds): The Kidney, 2nd ed. Philadelphia, WB Saunders, 1981, with permission.)*

to be independent of urine flow, because urate clearance is enhanced during the syndrome of inappropriate antidiuretic hormone when urine flow is usually reduced but extracellular volume increased [95]. Diabetes insipidus is associated with decreased urate clearance but increased urine flow [60]. Extracellular volume is often diminished in this disease, however.

Finally, certain hormones can influence urate clearance. Angiotensin and norepinephrine markedly reduce the excretion of urate, and this change parallels the reduction in renal blood flow [46]. Estrogens appear to increase urate excretion because women during the childbearing years have lower serum urate levels than age-matched men [176], and men treated with estrogens develop uricosuria [99].

Newborn infants have higher serum urate levels than older infants (mean serum urate 5.2 vs 3.2 mg/dl) in spite of a higher fractional excretion of urate (39% vs 13%–26%) [101,105,107,146,147] and a higher uric acid excretion per unit body weight (20 mg/kg), all apparently due to a higher production rate [101,107,146]. This is especially true for premature infants; the highest serum urate levels are from newborns with the lowest gestational age [146]. Fractional urate excretion is also inversely related to gestational age, with premature infants between 29 and 33 weeks having fractional excretions greater than 50%. Similar observations were made in canine puppies [147].

In children aged 2 to 15 years, the excretion of uric acid increases with advancing age, whereas the excretion of uric acid per kilogram of body weight is inversely related to age [148]. The clearance of uric acid per 1.73 m^2 surface area decreases throughout childhood, as does the fractional excretion of uric acid [148]. Associated with these decreases is an increase in the concentration of uric acid in the serum with increasing age.

References

1. Abramson RG, Levitt M: Micropuncture study of uric acid transport in rat kidney. *Am J Physiol* 214:875, 1975.
2. Akaoka I, Nishizawa T, Yano E, et al: Renal urate excretion in five cases of hypouricemia with an isolated renal defect of urate transport. *J Rheumatol* 4:1, 1977.
3. Arant BS: Developmental patterns of renal functional maturation compared in the human neonate. *J Pediatr* 92:705, 1978.
4. Arant BS Jr, Edelmann CM Jr, Nash MA: The renal reabsorption of glucose in the developing canine kidney. A study of glomerulotubular balance. *Pediatr Res* 3:638, 1974.
5. Arataki M: On the postnatal growth of the kidney with special reference to the number and size of the glomeruli (Albino Rats). *Am J Anat* 36:399, 1926.
6. Aronson PS, Sacktor B: The Na$^+$-gradient dependent transport of D-glucose in renal brush border membranes. *J Biol Chem* 250:6032, 1975.
7. Baerlocher KE, Scriver CR, Mohyuddin F: Ontogeny of iminoglycine transport in mammalian kidney. *Proc Natl Acad Sci USA* 65:1009, 1970.
8. Barac-Nieto M, Murer H, Kinne R: Lactate-sodium cotransport in rat renal brush border membranes. *Am J Physiol* 239:F496, 1980.
9. Barfuss DW, Schafer JA: Active amino acid absorption by proximal convoluted and proximal straight tubules. *Am J Physiol* 236:F149, 1979.
10. Barfuss DW, Schafer JA: Peritubular uptake and transepithelial transport of glycine in isolated proximal tubules. *Am J Physiol* 238:F244, 1980.
11. Barfuss DW, Schafer JA: Differences in active and passive glucose transport along the proximal nephron. *Am J Physiol* 240:F322, 1981.
12. Barnett HL, Hare WK, et al: Influence of postnatal age on kidney function of premature infants. *Proc Soc Exp Biol Med* 69:55, 1948.
13. Beck JC, Sacktor B: Energetics of the Na$^+$-dependent transport of D-glucose in renal brush border membrane vesicles. *J Biol Chem* 250:8674, 1975.
14. Beck JC, Sacktor B: The sodium electrochemical potential-mediated uphill transport of D-glucose in renal brush border membrane vesicles. *J Biol Chem* 253:5531, 1978.
15. Beechwood EC, Berndt WO, Mudge GH: Stop-flow analysis of tubular transport of uric acid in rabbits. *Am J Physiol* 207:1265, 1964.
16. Bergeron M, Morel F: Amino acid transport in rat renal tubules. *Am J Physiol* 216:1139, 1969.
17. Berliner RW, Hilton JG, Yu TF, et al: The renal mechanism for urate excretion in man. *J Clin Invest* 29:396, 1950.
18. Berry CA, Boulpaep EL: Non-electrolyte permeability of the paracellular pathways in the Necturus proximal tubule. *Am J Physiol* 228:581, 1975.
19. Blazer-Yost B, Reynolds R, Segal S: Amino acid content of rat renal cortex and the response to in vitro incubation. *Am J Physiol* 236:F398, 1979.
20. Blomstedt JW, Aronson PS: pH gradient-stimulated transport of urate and p-aminohippurate in dog renal microvillus membrane vesicles. *J Clin Invest* 65:931, 1980.
21. Bordier B, Ornstein L, Weeden RP: The intrarenal distribution of tritiated para-aminohippuric acid determined by a modified technique of section freeze-dry radioautography. *J Cell Biol* 46:518, 1970.
22. Brodehl J: Postnatal development of tubular amino acid reabsorption. *In* Silbernagl S, Lang F, Greger R (eds): *Amino Acid Transport and Uric Acid Transport.* Stuttgart, Georg Thieme Verlag, K.G., 1976, p 128.
23. Brodehl J, Franken A, Gellissen K: Maximal tubular reabsorption of glucose in infants and children. *Acta Paediatr Scand* 61:413, 1972.
24. Brodehl J, Gellissen K: Endogenous renal transport of free amino acids in infancy and childhood. *Pediatrics* 42:395, 1968.
25. Buckhardt G, Kinne R, Stange G, et al: The effects of potassium and membrane potential on sodium-dependent glutamic acid uptake. *Biochim Biophys Acta* 599:191, 1980.
26. Burns JJ, Yu TF, et al: A potent new uricosuric agent, the sulfoxide metabolite of the phenylbutazone analogue, G-25671. *J Pharmacol Exp Ther* 119:418, 1957.
27. Calcagno PL, Rubin MI: Renal extraction of para-aminohippurate in infants and children. *J Clin Invest* 42:1632, 1963.
28. Cannon PJ, Svahn DS, Demartini EF: The influence of hypertonic saline infusions upon the fractional reabsorption of urate and other ions in normal and hypertensive man. *Circulation* 41:97, 1970.
29. Chesney RW, Gusowski N, Dabbagh S, et al: Factors affecting the transport of β amino acids in rat renal brush border membrane vesicles. The role of external chloride. *Biochim Biophys Acta* 812:702, 1985.
30. Chesney RW, Jax DK: Developmental aspects of renal β-amino acid transport. I. Ontogeny of taurine reabsorption of accumulation in rat renal cortex. *Pediatr Res* 13:854, 1979.
31. Chesney RW, Jax DK: Developmental aspects of renal β-amino acid transport. II. Ontogeny of uptake and efflux processes and effects of anoxia. *Pediatr Res* 13:861, 1979.
32. Christensen HN: Recognition sites for material transport and information transfer. *Curr Top Membr Transp* 6:227, 1975.
33. Dantzler WH: Effects of Na, K and oubain on urate and PAH uptake by snake and chicken kidney slices. *Am J Physiol* 217:1510, 1969.
34. Daughaday WH, Larner J: The renal excretion of inositol in normal and diabetic human beings. *J Clin Invest* 33:326, 1954.
35. Dean RFA, McCance RA: Inulin, diodone, creatinine and urea clearances in newborn infants. *J Physiol (Lond)* 106:431, 1947.
36. Demartini FE, Wheaton EA, Healey LA, et al: Effect of chlorothiazide on the renal excretion of uric acid. *Am J Med* 32:572, 1962.
37. Dempster WJ, Eggleton MG, Shuster S: The effect of hypertonic infusions on glomerular filtration rate and glucose reabsorption in the kidney of the dog. *J Physiol (Lond)* 132:213, 1956.
38. Diedrich D: The comparative effects of some phlorizin analogs on the renal reabsorption of glucose. *Biochim Biophys Acta* 71:688, 1963.
39. Duarte CG, Bland JH: Calcium, phosphorus, and uric acid clearances after intravenous administration of chlorothiazide. *Metabolism* 14:211, 1965.
40. Edelmann CM Jr: Maturation of the neonatal kidney. *In* Becker RL (ed): *Proc Third Int Congr Nephrol.* Washington, 1966. Vol 3. Basel, Karger, 1967.
41. Eisenbach GM, Weise M, Stolte H: Amino acid reabsorption in the rat nephron. Free flow micropuncture study. *Pflugers Arch* 357:63, 1975.
42. Elsas LJ, Rosenberg LE: Familial renal glucosuria: A genetic

reappraisal of hexose transport by kidney and intestine. *J Clin Invest* 48:1845, 1969.

43. Evan A: Maturation of the vascular system of the puppy kidney. *In* Spitzer A (ed): *The Kidney During Development: Morphology and Function.* New York, Masson Publishing USA, 1980, p 3.

44. Evers J, Murer H, Kinne R: Phenylalanine uptake in isolated renal brush border membrane vesicles. *Biochim Biophys Acta* 426:598, 1976.

45. Fawer CL, Torrado A, Guigard JP: Maturation of renal function in full-term and premature infants. *Helv Paediatr Acta* 34:11, 1979.

46. Ferris TF, Gorden P: Effect of angiotensin and norepinephrine upon urate clearance in man. *Am J Med* 44:359, 1968.

47. Fetterman GH, Shiplock NA, Phillip FJ, et al: The growth and maturation of human glomeruli and proximal convolutions. *Pediatrics* 35:601, 1965.

48. Foreman JW, Hwang SM, Segal S: Transport interactions of cystine and dibasic amino acids in isolated rat renal tubules. *Metbolism* 29:53, 1980.

49. Foreman JW, Medow MS, Wald H, et al: Developmental aspects of sugar transport by isolated dog renal cortical tubules. *Pediatr Res* 18:719, 1984.

50. Foreman JW, Reynolds RA, Ginkinger K, et al: Effect of acidosis on glutamine transport by isolated rat renal brush border and basolateral membrane vesicles. *Biochem J* 212:713, 1983.

51. Foulkes EC: Effects of heavy metals on renal aspartate transport and the nature of solute movement in kidney cortex slices. *Biochim Biophys Acta* 241:815, 1971.

52. Fox M, Thier S, Rosenberg L, et al: Ionic requirements for amino acid transport in the rat kidney cortex slice. 1. Influence of extracellular ions. *Biochim Biophys Acta* 79:167, 1964.

53. Freinkel N, Goodner CI, Dawson RMC: The relationship between renal glucose and inositol transport. *Clin Res* 8:240, 1960.

54. Friedman AL, Jax DK, Chesney RW: Developmental aspects of renal β-amino acid transport. III. Ontogeny of transport in isolated renal tubule segments. *Pediatr Res* 15:10, 1981.

55. Frohnert P, Hohmann B, Zwiebel R, et al: Free flow micropuncture studies of glucose transport in the rat nephron. *Pflugers Arch Ges Physiol* 315:66, 1970.

56. Fukuhara Y, Turner RJ: Cation dependence of renal outer cortical brush border membrane L-glumate transport. *Am J Physiol* 248:F869, 1985.

57. Gammeltoft A, Kjerulf-Jensen K: The mechanism of renal excretion of fructose and galactose in rabbit, cat, dog and man (with special reference to the phosphorylation theory). *Acta Physiol Scand* 6:368, 1943.

58. Garcia ML, Benavides J, Valdivieso F: Ketone body transport in renal brush border membrane vesicles. *Biochim Biophys Acta* 600:922, 1980.

59. Gekle D, Janovsky M, Slechtova R, et al: Einfluss der glomerularen Filtrationsrate auf die tubulare Glucose reabsorption bei Kindern. *Klin Wochenschr* 45:416, 1967.

60. Gorden P, Robertson GL, Seegmiller JE: Hyperuricemia, a concomitant of congenital vasopressin-resistant diabetes insipidus in the adult. *N Engl J Med* 284:1057, 1971.

61. Guggino SE, Martin GJ, Aronson PS: Specificity and modes of the anion exchanges in dog renal microvillus membranes. *Am J Physiol* 244:F612, 1983.

62. Gutman AB, Yu TF: A three component system for regulation of renal excretion of uric acid in man. *Trans Assoc Am Physicians* 74:353, 1961.

63. Gutman AB, Yu TF, Berger L: Tubular secretion of urate in man. *J Clin Invest* 38:1778, 1959.

64. Handley CA, Sigafoos RB, LaForge M: Proportional changes in renal tubular reabsorption of dextrose and excretion of p-aminohippurate with changes in glomerular filtration. *Am J Physiol* 159:175, 1949.

65. Hay DA, Evans AP: Maturation of the proximal tubule in the puppy kidney: A comparison to the adult. *Anat Rec* 195:273, 1979.

66. Hillman RE, Albrecht I, Rosenberg LE: Identification and analysis of multiple glycine transport systems in isolated mammalian renal tubules. *J Biol Chem* 243:5566, 1968.

67. Hillman RE, Albrecht I, Rosenberg LE: Transport of amino acids by isolated rabbit renal tubules. *Biochim Biophys Acta* 150:528, 1968.

68. Hillman RE, Rosenbergh LE: Amino acid transport by isolated mammalian renal tubules. II. Transport systems for L-proline. *J Biol Chem* 244:4494, 1969.

69. Hirsch GH, Hook JB: Maturation of renal organic acid transport: Substrate stimulation by penicillin. *Science* 165:909, 1969.

70. Hirsch GH, Hook JB: Additional studies on penicillin-induced stimulation of renal PAH transport. *Can J Physiol Pharmacol* 48:550, 1970.

71. Hosang M, Michael-Gibbs E, Diedrich DF, et al: Photoaffinity labeling and identification of (a component of) the small-intestinal Na$^+$,D-glucose transporter using 4-azidophlorizin. *FEBS Letters* 130:244, 1981.

72. Hwang SM, Foreman JW, Segal S: Developmental patterns of cystine transport in isolated rat renal tubules. *Biochim Biophys Acta* 690:145, 1982.

73. Hwang SM, Serabian MA, Roth KS, et al: L-proline transport by isolated renal tubules from newborn and adult rats. *Pediatr Res* 17:42, 1983.

74. Johnston CC, Bartlett P, Podsiadly CJ: Transport of α-aminoisobutyric acid by separated rabbit renal tubules. *Biochim Biophys Acta* 163:418, 1968.

75. Kahn AM, Aronson PS: Urate transport via anion exchange in dog renal microvillus membrane vesicles. *Am J Physiol* 244:F56, 1983.

76. Kahn AM, Branham S, Weinman EJ: Mechanism of urate and p-aminohippurate transport in rat renal microvillus membrane vesicles. *Am J Physiol* 245:F151, 1983.

77. Kahn AM, Shelat H, Weinman EJ: Urate and p-aminohippurate in rat renal basolateral vesicles. *Am J Physiol* 249:F654, 1985.

78. Karniski LP, Aronson PS: Anion exchange pathways for Cl$^-$ transport in rabbit renal microvillus membranes. *Am J Physiol* 253:F513, 1987.

79. Keyes JL, Swanson RE: Dependence of glucose Tm on GFR and tubular volume in the dog kidney. *Am J Physiol* 221:1, 1971.

80. Kinne R: Membrane molecular aspects of tubular transport. *In* Thurau K (ed): *Kidney and Urinary Tract Physiology.* Vol 11. Baltimore, University Park Press, 1976, p 169.

81. Kinne R, Murer H, Kinne-Saffran E, et al: Sugar transport by renal plasma membrane vesicles. Characterization of the systems in the brush border microvilli and basal-lateral plasma membranes. *J Membr Biol* 21:375, 1975.

82. Kippen I, Hirayama B, Klinenberg JR, et al: Transport of tricarboxylic acid cycle intermediates by membrane vesicles fromrenal brush borders. *Proc Natl Acad Sci USA* 76:3397, 1979.

83. Kippen I, Nakata N, Klinenberg JR: Uptake of uric acid by separated renal tubules of the rabbit. I. Characteristics of transport. *J Pharmacol Exp Ther* 201:218, 1977.

84. Kleinzeller A, Kolinska J, Beves I: Transport of glucose and galactose in kidney cortex cells. *Biochem J* 104:843, 1967.

85. Koepsell H, Menuhr H, Ducis I, et al: Partial purification and reconstitution of the Na$^+$-D-glucose cotransport protein from pig renal proximal tubules. *J Biol Chem* 258:1888, 1983.

86. Kramp R, Lassiter WE, Gottschalk CW: Urate-2-14C transport in the rat nephron. *J Clin Invest* 50:35, 1971.

87. Letteri JM, Wesson LG: Glucose titration curves as an estimate of intrarenal distribution of glomerular filtrate in patients with congestive heart failure. *J Clin Lab Med* 65:387, 1965.

88. Lin JT, DaCruz MEM, Reidel S, et al: Partial purification of hog kidney sodium-D-glucose cotransport system by affinity chromatography on a phlorizin polymer. *Biochim Biophys Acta* 640:43, 1981.

89. Lin JT, Kornelia S, Kinne R, et al: Structural state of the Na$^+$/D-glucose cotransporter in calf kidney brush border membranes: Target size analysis of Na$^+$-dependent phlorizin binding and Na$^+$-dependent D-glucose transport. *Biochim Biophys Acta* 777:201, 1984.

90. Lin JT, Stroh A, Kinne R: Renal sodium D-glucose cotransport system: Involvement of tyrosine residues in sodium-transporter interaction. *Biochim Biophys Acta* 692:210, 1982.

91. Lingard J, Rumrich G, Young A: Kinetics of L-histidine transport in the proximal convolution of the rat nephron studied using the stationary microperfusion technique. *Pflugers Arch* 342:13, 1973.

92. Malathi P, Preiser H: Isolation of the sodium-dependent D-glucose transport protein from brush border membranes. *Biochim Biophys Acta* 735:314, 1983.

93. McNamara PD, Ozegovic B, Pepe LM, et al: Proline and glycine uptake by renal brush border membrane vesicles. *Proc Natl Acad Sci USA* 73:4521, 1976.

94. Medow MS, Foreman JW, Bovee KC, et al: Developmental changes of glycine transport in the dog. *Biochim Biophys Acta* 693:85, 1982.

95. Mees EJD, Blom van Assendelft P, Nieuwenhuis MG: Elevation of uric acid clearance caused by inappropriate antidiuretic hormone secretion. *Acta Med Scand* 189:69, 1971.

96. Mohyuddin F, Scriver CR: Amino acid transport in mammalian kidney: Multiple systems for imino acids and glycine in rat kidney. *Am J Physiol* 219:1, 1970.

97. Mudge GH, Cucchi J, et al: Renal excretion of uric acid in the dog. *Am J Physiol* 215:404, 1968.

98. Mudge GH, McAlary B, Berndt WO: Renal transport of uric acid in the guinea pig. *Am J Physiol* 214:875, 1968.

99. Nicholls A, Smith ML, Scott JT: Effect of oestrogen therapy on plasma and urinary levels of uric acid. *Br Med J* 1:449, 1973.

100. Nord EP, Wright SH, Kippen I, et al: Specificity of the Na$^+$-dependent monocarboxylic acid transport pathway in rabbit renal brush border membranes. *J Membr Biol* 72:213, 1983.

101. Passwell JH, Modan M, Brush M, et al: Fractional excretion of uric acid in infancy and childhood. Index of tubular maturation. *Arch Dis Child* 49:878, 1979.

102. Perles R, Colas MC, Blayo MC: Mechanism of renal excretion of inositol in the dog. *Rev Fr Etud Clin Biol* 5:31, 1960.

103. Platts MM, Mudge GH: Accumulation of uric acid by slices of kidney cortex. *Am J Physiol* 200:387, 1961.

104. Poiree JC, Mengual R, Sudaka P: Identification of a protein component of horse kidney brush border D-glucose transport system. *Biochem Biophys Res Commun* 90:1387, 1979.

105. Poulsen H: Uric acid in blood and urine of infants. *Acta Physiol Scand* 33:372, 1955.

106. Praetorius E, Kirk JE: Hypouricemia: With evidence for tubular secretion of urate in man. *J Lab Clin Med* 35:865, 1950.

107. Ravio KO: Neonatal hyperuricemia. *J Pediatr* 88:625, 1976.

108. Reynolds RA, Roth KS, Hwang SM, et al: On the development of glycine transport by rat renal cortex. *Biochim Biophys Acta* 511:274, 1978.

109. Roch-Ramel F, Diezi-Chomety F, De Rougemont D, et al: Renal excretion of uric acid in the rat: A micropuncture and microperfusion study. *Am J Physiol* 230:768, 1976.

110. Roch-Ramel F, Wong NLM, Dirks JH: Renal excretion of urate in mongrel and Dalmatian dogs: A micropuncture study. *Am J Physiol* 231:326, 1976.

111. Rohde R, Deetjen P: Glucose resorption in der Rattenniere: Micropunktionsanalysen der tubularen Glucosekonzent ration bei freiem. *Pflugers Arch Ges Physiol* 302:219, 1968.

112. Roigaard-Peterson H, Jacobsen C, Sheikh MI: H$^+$-L-proline cotransport by vesicles from pars convoluta of rabbit proximal tubule. *Am J Physiol* 253:F15, 1987.

113. Rolan RP, Foulkes EC: Studies on renal urate secretion in the dog. *J Pharmacol Exp Therap* 179:429, 1971.

114. Rosenberg LE, Blair A, Segal S: The transport of amino acids by rat kidney cortex slices. *Biochim Biophys Acta* 54:479, 1961.

115. Rosenberg LE, Downing SJ, Segal S: Competitive inhibition of dibasic amino acid transport in rat kidney. *J Biol Chem* 237:2265, 1962.

116. Roth KS, Hwang SM, London JW, et al: Ontogeny of glycine transport in isolated rat renal tubules. *Am. J. Physiol.* F241, 1977.

117. Roth KS, Hwang SM, Yudkoff M, et al: On the transport of sugars and amino acids by newborn kidney: Use of isolated proximal tubule. *Life Science* 18:1125, 1976.

118. Roth KS, Hwang SM, Yudkoff M, et al: The ontogeny of sugar transport in kidney. *Pediatr Res* 12:1127, 1978.

119. Rubin MI, Bruch E, Rapoport M: Maturation of renal function in childhood clearance studies. *J Clin Invest* 28:1144, 1949.

120. Sacktor B, Rosenbloom IL, Liang CT, et al: Sodium gradient and sodium plus potassium gradient-dependent L-glutamate uptake in renal basolateral membrane vesicles. *J Membr Biol* 60:63, 1981.

121. Samson SC, Senekjian HO, et al: Determination of the apparent transport constants for urate absorption in the rat proximal tubule. *Am J Physiol* 240:F406, 1981.

122. Schafer JA, Barfuss DW: Membrane mechanisms for transepithelial amino acid absorption and secretion. *Am J Physiol* 238:F335, 1980.

123. Schafer JA, Patlak CS, Andreoli TE: A component of fluid absorption linked to passive ion flows in the superficial pars recta. *J Gen Physiol* 66:445, 1975.

124. Schafer JA, Watkins ML: Transport of L-cystine in isolated perfused proximal straight tubules. *Pflugers Arch* 401:143, 1984.

125. Schild L, Giebisch G, Karniski LP, et al: Effect of formate on volume reabsorption in the rabbit proximal tubule. *J Clin Invest* 79:32, 1987.

126. Schwartz GJ, Goldsmith DI, Fine LG: p-Aminohippurate transport in the proximal straight tubule: Development and substrate stimulation. *Pediatr Res* 12:793, 1978.

127. Schwartz GJ, Hegyi TH, Spitzer A: Subtherapeutic dicloxacillin levels in a neonate: Possible mechanisms. *J Pediatr* 89:310, 1976.

128. Scriver CR, Mohyuddin F: Amino acid transport in kidney: Heterogeneity of α-aminoisobutyric uptake. *J Biol Chem* 243:3207, 1968.

129. Segal S, Genel M, Holtzapple P, et al: Transport of alpha-methyl-D-glucoside by human kidney cortex. *Metabolism* 22:67, 1973.

130. Segal S, McNamara PD, Pepe LM: Transport interactions of cystine and dibasic amino acids in renal brush border vesicles. *Science* 197:169, 1977.

131. Segal, S., Rea, C., Smith, I.: Separate transport system for sugar and amino acids in developing rat kidney cortex. *Proc Natl Acad Sci USA* 68:372, 1971.

132. Segal S, Rosenhagen M: The effect of extracellular sodium concentration on α-methyl-D-glucoside transport by rat kidney cortex slices. *Biochim Biophys Acta* 332:278, 1974.

133. Segal S, Rosenhagen M, Rea C: Developmental and other characteristics of alpha-methylglucoside by rat kidney cortex slices. *Biochim Biophys Acta* 291:519, 1973.

134. Segal S, Schwartzman L, Blair A, et al: Dibasic amino acid transport in rat kidney cortex slices. *Biochim Biophys Acta* 135:127, 1967.

135. Segal S, Smith I: Delineation of separate transport systems in rat kidney cortex for L-lysine and L-cystine by developmental patterns. *Biochem Biophys Res Commun* 35:771, 1969.

136. Segal S, Thier SO: Renal handling of amino acids. *In* Orloff J, Berliner RW (eds): *Handbook of Physiology. Renal Physiology.* Washington, DC, Amer Phys Soc, 1973, p 653.

137. Shannon JA, Fisher S: The renal reabsorption of glucose in the normal dog. *Am J Physiol* 122:765, 1938.

138. Silverman M: The chemical and steric determinants governing sugar interactions with renal tubular membranes. *Biochim Biophys Acta* 332:248, 1974.

139. Silverman M: Glucose transport in the kidney. *Biochim Biophys Acta* 457:303, 1976.

140. Silverman M, Aganon MA, Chinard FP: D-Glucose interactions with renal tubule cell surfaces. *Am J Physiol* 218:743, 1970.

141. Silverman M, Black J: High affinity phlorizin receptor sites and their relation to the glucose transport mechanism in the proximal tubule of dog kidney. *Biochim Biophys Acta* 394:10, 1975.

142. Sirota JH, Yu TF, Gutman AB: Effect of benemid (p-di-n-propylsulfamyl-benzoic acid) on urate clearance and other discrete renal functions in gouty subjects. *J Clin Invest* 31:692, 1952.

143. Smith HW: *The Kidney.* London, Oxford University Press, 1958.

144. Smith HW, Goldring W, Chasis H, et al: The application of saturation methods to the study of glomerular and tubular function in the human kidney. *J Mt Sinai Hosp* 10:59, 1943.

145. Stalder G: Funktionen des Tubulesepithels. *Mod Probl Paediatr* 6:22, 1960.

146. Stapleton FB: Renal uric acid clearances in human neonates. *J Pediatr* 103:290, 1983.

147. Stapleton FB, Arant BS Jr: Ontogeny of uric acid excretion in the mongrel puppy. *Pediatr Res* 15:1513, 1981.

148. Stapleton FB, Linshaw MA, Hassanein K, et al: Uric acid excretion in normal children. *J Pediatr* 92:911, 1978.

149. Steele TH: Evidence for altered renal urate reabsorption during changes in volume of the extracellular fluid. *J Lab Clin Med* 74:228, 1969.

150. Steele TH: Urate secretion in man: The pyrazinamide suppression test. *Ann Intern Med* 79:734, 1973.

151. Steele TH, Manuel MA, Boner G: Diuretics, urate excretion and sodium reabsorption: Effects of acetazolamide and urinary alkalinization. *Nephron* 14:48, 1975.

152. Steele TH, Oppenheimer S: Factors affecting urate excretion following diuretic administration in man. *Am J Med* 47:564, 1969.

153. Steele TH, Rieselbach RE: The renal mechanism for urate homostasis in normal man. *Am J Med* 43:868, 1976.

154. Tudvad F: Sugar reabsorption in premature and full term babies. *Scand J Clin Lab Invest* 1:281, 1949.

155. Tune BM, Burg MB: Glucose transport by proximal renal tubules. *Am J Physiol* 221:580, 1971.

156. Tune BM, Burg MB, Patlak CS: Characteristics of p-aminohippurate transport in proximal renal tubules. *Am J Physiol* 217:953, 1969.

157. Turner RJ, George JN: Evidence for two disulfide bonds important to the functioning of the renal outer cortical brush border membrane D-glucose transporter. *J Biol Chem* 258:3565, 1983.

158. Turner RJ, Kempner ES: Radiation inactivation studies of the renal brush border membrane phlorizin-binding protein. *J Biol Chem* 257:10794, 1982.

159. Turner RJ, Moran A: Further studies of proximal tubular brush border membrane D-glucose transport heterogeneity. *J Membr Biol* 70:37, 1982.

160. Turner RJ, Moran A: Heterogeneity of sodium-dependent D-glucose transport sites along the proximal tubule: Evidence from vesicle studies. *Am J Physiol* 242:F406, 1982.

161. Turner RJ, Silverman M: Sugar uptake into brush border vesicles from normal human kidney. *Proc Natl Acad Sci USA* 74:2825, 1977.

162. Turner RJ, Silverman M: Sugar uptake into brush border vesicles from dog kidney. I. Specificity. *Biochem Biophys Acta* 507:305, 1978.

163. Turner RJ, Silverman M: Sugar uptake into brush border vesicles from dog kidney. II. Kinetics. *Biochem Biophys Acta* 511:470, 1978.

164. Van Liew JB, Deetjen P, Boylan JW: Glucose reabsorption in the rat kidney: Dependence on glomerular filtration. *Pflugers Arch* 295:232, 1967.

165. Vitelli A, Cattaneo C, Martini PC: Maximum tubular reabsorption capacity of glucose in diabetes mellitus. *Acta Endocrinol (Copenh)* 50:79, 1965.

166. Voelk H, Silvernagl S, Deetjen P: Kinetics of L-proline reabsorption in the rat kidney by continuous microperfusion. *Pflugers Arch* 382:115, 1979.

167. Von Baeyer H, von Conta C, Haeberle D, et al: Determination of transport constants for glucose in proximal tubules of rat kidney. *Pflugers Arch* 343:273, 1973.

168. Waddel WJ, Bruther TC: The distribution and excretion of phenobarbital. *J Clin Invest* 36:1217, 1957.

169. Walker A, Bott P, Oliver J, et al: The collection and analysis of fluid from single nephrons of the mammalian kidney. *Am J Physiol* 134:580, 1941.

170. Webber WA, Cairns JA: Amino acid excretion patterns in developing rats. *Can J Physiol Pharmacol* 46:165, 1968.

171. Weeden RP: The distribution of p-aminohippuric acid in rat kidney slices. I. Tubular localization. *Kidney Int* 3:205, 1973.

172. Weinmann EJ, Samson SC, et al: Secretion of urate in the proximal convoluted tubule of the rat. *Am J Physiol* 239:F383, 1980.

173. Weiss SD, McNamara PD, Pepe LM, et al: Glutamine and glutamic acid uptake by rat renal brush border membrane vesicles. *J Membr Biol* 43:91, 1978.

174. Welling LW, Grantham JJ: Physical properties of isolated perfused renal tubules and tubular basement membranes. *J Clin Invest* 51:1063, 1972.

175. West JR, Smith HW, Chasis H: Glomerular filtration rate,

effective renal blood flow, and maximal tubular excretory capacity in infancy. *J Pediatr* 32:10, 1948.

176. Wolfson WQ, Hunt HD, Levine R, et al: The transport and excretion of uric acid in man. V. A sex difference in urate metabolism. *J Clin Endocrinol Metab* 9:749, 1949.

177. Wright SH, Kippen I, Klinenberg JR, et al: Specificity of the transport system for tricarboxylic acid cycle intermediates in renal brush borders. *J Membr Biol* 57:73, 1980.

178. Young JA, Freedman BS: Renal tubular transport of amino acids. *Clin Chem NY* 17:245, 1971.

179. Yu TF, Gutman AB: Paradoxical retention of uric acid by uricosuric drugs in low dosage. *Proc Soc Exp Biol Med* 90:542, 1955.

180. Yu TF, Gutman AB: Study of the paradoxical effects of salicylate in low, intermediate and high dosage on the renal mechanisms for excretion of urate in man. *J Clin Invest* 38:1298, 1959.

181. Yu TF, Perel J, Berger L, et al: The effect of the interaction of pyrazinamide and probenecid on urinary acid excretion in man. *Am J Med* 63:723, 1977.

182. Zins GR, Weiner IM: Bidirectional urate transport limited to the proximal tubule in dogs. *Am J Physiol* 215:411, 1968.

ADRIAN SPITZER
ANITA APERIA

5

The Renal Transport of Sodium and Chloride

The renal handling of no other substance has attracted as much interest as that of sodium chloride. This is due mainly to the inextricable relationship between sodium chloride balance and the volume of the extracellular fluid compartment. Sodium salts account, in molar terms, for 95% of the plasma solutes, and, because they are almost completely dissociated, they account for 90% of the osmotic activity of the plasma. Seventy-five percent of this activity is due to sodium chloride.

Sodium and chloride pass freely through the glomerular membrane. The kidney of an adult human filters approximately 14 mmoles of sodium chloride/min, which represents nearly 1.2 kg of salt in a 24-hour period. More than 99% of this amount is reabsorbed during its passage through the renal tubules.

By definition, adults are in zero salt balance, whereas infants and children are in a positive salt balance. Breast-fed puppies excrete in the urine only about 30% of the sodium provided by milk [304], while healthy premature infants, fed a variety of formulas, retain about one-third of the salt present in their diet [154]. Interestingly, the magnitude of this positive balance remains relatively constant within a wide range of sodium intakes [154,303,304,450] and despite the fact that salt intake per unit of body surface area is about twice as high in an adult as in a breast-fed baby. Thus, the immature kidney is able to conserve sodium efficiently, a condition essential for growth, particularly for the accretion of bone.

The situation is different in prematurely born infants who, left to their own devices, tend to go into negative sodium balance, resulting in hyponatremia [1,359]. Fractional sodium excretion correlates inversely with gestational age, being as high as 6% at 20 weeks gestation [10,12,16,395]. Balance studies have demonstrated that infants less than 33 weeks gestation require a minimum of 4 to 5 mEq/kg/day of sodium to offset their renal losses [1,424]. These differences in sodium homeostasis between immature and mature subjects reflect differences in the handling of sodium in various segments of the nephron and in the response of the kidney to factors known to modulate the reabsorption of sodium. Most of the information regarding these issues was obtained from micropuncture and microperfusion experiments. Figure 5-1 describes the rates of sodium reabsorption in different segments of the rabbit nephron. It is apparent that the values are quite variable, reflecting the contribution that each of these segments makes to salt homeostasis.

Sodium Transport Along the Renal Tubule
Proximal Tubule

In the rat, some 50% of the glomerular filtrate is reabsorbed by the end of the convoluted proximal tubule [142]. Since the sodium concentration of the fluid remains relatively constant [155,262], reabsorption in this tubular segment is called isotonic. The capacity for sodium and water transport is believed to diminish gradually along the proximal tubule, being the highest in the S1 segment and the lowest in the S3 segment [233]. It should be emphasized that the reabsorption of other solutes proceeds at different rates from those of sodium. As a consequence, the concentration of these substances changes at different rates as the filtrate proceeds along the proximal tubule. For example, the concentrations of amino acids and glucose decrease rapidly, reaching less than 10% at 25% of proximal tubular length, whereas that of chloride rises due to nearly total lack of reabsorption in the initial segment of the proximal tubule. As a result of these changes, the transepithelial potential difference changes from slightly negative to slightly positive.

The movement of salt and water across the proximal tubular epithelium occurs both through transcellular and paracellular pathways (Fig. 5-2). The proximal tubule is a leaky epithelium [49,331]. The electrical resistance of the mammalian proximal tubular epithelium (S1 segment) is below 50 ohm/cm^2 and the transepithelial electric potential difference is smaller than 5 mV. Since the electrical resistances of the luminal (600 ohm/cm^2) and antiluminal (250 ohm/cm^2) cellular membranes of the proximal tubule are appreciably higher than the transepithelial resistance, a low resistance pathway (paracellular) must exist in parallel with the transcellular pathway [47]. Because the hydraulic conductivity of the proximal convoluted tubule (i.e., the water flow per unit area per unit hydraulic or effective

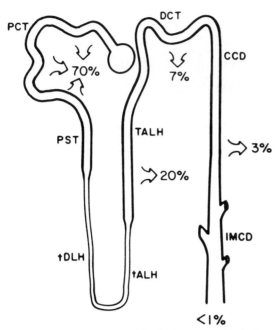

FIG. 5-1. *Percent of filtered load of NaCl reabsorbed in various segments of the nephron under euvolemic conditions. PCT, proximal convoluted tubule; PST, proximal straight tubule; tDLH, thin descending limb of Henle's loop; tALH, thin ascending limb of Henle's loop; TALH, thick ascending limb of Henle's loop; DCT, distal convoluted tubule; CCD, cortical collecting duct; IMCD, inner medullary collecting duct. (From Koeppen BM: Mechanism of segmental sodium and chloride reabsorption. In Seldin DW, Giebisch G (eds): The Regulation of Sodium and Chloride Balance. New York: Raven Press, 1990, p 69, with permission.)*

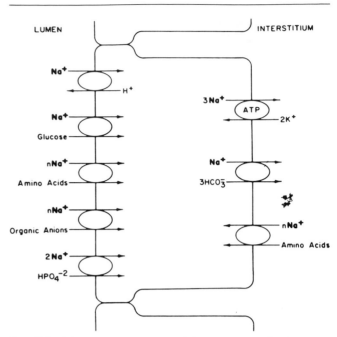

FIG. 5-2. *Schematic representation of the transport mechanisms present in the early portion of the proximal tubule. (From Koeppen BM: Mechanism of segmental sodium and chloride reabsorption. In Seldin DW, Giebisch G (eds): The Regulation of Sodium and Chloride Balance. New York: Raven Press, 1990, p 78, with permission.)*

osmotic pressure difference) is extremely high (240 nl/cm^2/min/mosmol), small effective osmotic pressure gradients (less than 5 mosmol) can induce large transepithelial solvent flows [364]. On the other hand, high hydraulic conductance favors osmotic equilibration [364], making the osmolarity of the reabsorbed fluid similar to those of the luminal and peritubular fluids. It has been estimated that as much as two-thirds of the sodium reabsorption along the S1 segment of the rat proximal convoluted tubule occurs through the paracellular pathway, by diffusion or solvent drag or both, and that only one-third of the sodium reabsorbed in this segment occurs transcellularly [134].

Entry of Na$^+$ into the cell across the luminal membrane occurs in countertransport with H$^+$ [317] or in cotransport with glucose [250], amino acids [121], organic acids [21], and inorganic anions [199]. The extrusion of Na$^+$ across the basolateral membrane is an active process and thus requires energy. The transport at this site occurs via a Na$^+$ pump, which is now recognized to be represented by the Na$^+$ and K$^+$ activated adenosine triphosphatase (Na$^+$-K$^+$-ATPase) [146,230]. Transport of sodium by Na$^+$-K$^+$-ATPase is the most prominent primary active transport process in the kidney (Fig. 5-3). The Na$^+$-K$^+$-ATPase links the transport of sodium to energy metabolism in renal

tubules. The concentration gradient created by the active transport of sodium across cell membranes generates the energy that drives the passive transport of numerous other solids coupled to sodium (secondary active transport). The rate at which sodium and chloride are transported and the factors that affect this transport vary from one segment of the nephron to the other.

Definitive proof that Na$^+$-K$^+$-ATPase is indeed the Na$^+$ pump is based on experiments in which this enzyme was reincorporated into artificial lipid bilayer membranes and shown to transport Na$^+$ and K$^+$ "uphill" in opposite directions, at the expense of ATP hydrolysis [151]. Availability of specific and high affinity labels for the pump has made it possible to estimate that the turnover of the pump is constant (about 100 pump cycles/sec at body temperature) and that differences in rates of transport among various tubular segments are a function of pump density [391]. There is convincing evidence that the Na$^+$ pump extrudes more Na$^+$/cycle than it absorbs K$^+$, i.e., it is electrogenic. The generally accepted value for Na:K transport ratio is 3:2 [138].

It should be pointed out that fluxes across the paracellular pathway, although passive in nature, are dependent in part on the establishment of osmotic and chemical gradients across the epithelium, which are generated by the transcellular transport of solute. It is a combination of these passive fluxes with the active transcellular flux that accounts for the high efficiency of proximal sodium reabsorption. Addition of poorly reabsorbable solute to the

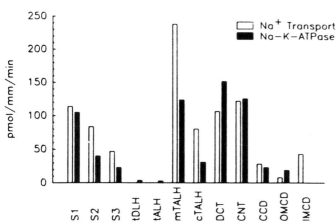

FIG. 5-3. *Net reabsorption of Na+ and Na+,K+-ATPase activity in various segments of rabbit tubules isolated and perfused in vitro. S1, S2, proximal convoluted tubule; S3, proximal straight tubule; tDLH, thin descending limb of Henle's loop; tALH, thin ascending limb of Henle's loop; mTALH, medullary thick ascending limb of Henle's loop; cTALH, cortical thick ascending limb of Henle's loop; DCT, distal convoluted tubule; CNT, connecting tubule; CCD, cortical collecting duct; OMCD, outermedullary collecting duct; IMCD, innermedullary collecting duct. (From Koeppen BM: Mechanism of segmental sodium and chloride reabsorption. In Seldin DW, Giebisch G (eds): The Regulation of Sodium and Chloride Balance. New York: Raven Press, 1990, p 70, with permission.)*

tubular fluid, such as mannitol, substantially reduces proximal reabsorption of salt and water by decreasing the effective transepithelial osmotic gradient. However, renal oxygen consumption remains constant, indicating that the efficiency of the sodium transport is reduced as a consequence of a decrease in passive, paracellular reabsorption of sodium without a change in the active sodium flux [253].

In addition to cell-generated gradients, paracellular fluxes of water and ions are driven by "physical factors," i.e., net hydrostatic and oncotic pressure differences between the tubular lumen and the peritubular capillaries [178]. The concentration of proteins in the peritubular capillaries depends on the plasma protein concentration and the filtration fraction: the hgher the filtration fraction, the higher the peritubular blood protein concentration and, thus, the higher the net oncotic pressure difference between peritubular capillaries and the protein-free proximal luminal fluid. The peritubular capillary hydrostatic pressure is dependent on the efferent arteriolar resistance, the renal venous resistance, and the renal blood flow. Changes in these "physical factors," such as decreases in oncotic pressure or increases in hydrostatic pressure in the peritubular capillaries, as occur during volume expansion, reduce the magnitude of paracellular but not the transcellular fluxes of sodium [37,46]. This results in a decrease in the efficiency of the proximal sodium reaborptive process and contributes to the maintenance of the glomerulotubular balance (Fig. 5-4).

DEVELOPMENTAL CHANGES IN PROXIMAL SODIUM REABSORPTION

During development, the absolute magnitude of the proximal reabsorption of sodium and water changes dramatically. In the guinea pig, the single nephron glomerular filtration rate (SNGFR) and the rate of proximal fluid reabsorption increase by about 20-fold from one day to 40 days of age, while the fractional reabsorption of sodium and water by the proximal convoluted tubule remains relatively constant [404]. Over the same period, the length of the proximal convoluted tubule increases sixfold. Thus, the reabsorptive rate per unit tubule length increases on the average by about threefold during postnatal development [404]. In the rabbit, the reabsorptive flow per unit tubule length in isolated perfused early proximal tubular segments of the juxtamedullary nephrons increases by a factor of three from the first to the sixth week of age [383], most of the change occurring after the fourth week of life (Fig.5-5). In the rat, sixfold increases in kidney weight, GFR, total sodium reabsorption, SNGFR, and proximal tubular sodium reabsorption were observed between the 20th day and the 60th day of extra-uterine life, while the fractional sodium reabsorption along the proximal convoluted tubule remained unchanged (58%) [75]. Since in this species proximal convoluted length increased over the same period of time by about 1.5-fold, sodium reabsorption per unit tubule length must have increased an average of fourfold.

The contributions of the active and passive components to the changes in proximal reabsorptive flow during development have not been completely defined. However, a series of studies indicates that in young animals some of the passive components have a greater influence on the rate of reabsorption than in adult animals.

Fluxes Driven By Hydrostatic Forces
In isolated perfused proximal convoluted tubules from rabbits, reabsorptive flow per unit of hydrostatic pressure difference was as much as seven times higher in young animals than in adults [202] (Fig. 5-6). This indictes that in young rabbits the proximal convoluted tubule has a large hydraulic conductance (LΔP). Whether this high conductance translates into larger reabsorptive flow rates in the proximal convoluted tubule of young than of adult rabbits in vivo is not known.

In the guinea pig, the net hydrostatic pressure difference (ΔP) between proximal tubular lumen and peritubular capillary increases from 1.3 cm H_2O to 2.6 cm H_2O from the first to the third week of age and then stabilizes [241] (Fig. 5-7). In the dog, the net hydrostatic pressure difference between the tubular lumen and peritubular capillaries is 9 cm H_2O in three-week-old puppies and only 2 cm H_2O in the adult animals [204]. Thus, mostly because of high conductance, and in the puppies because of a high driving force, hydrostatic pressure-driven reabsorptive flow (JΔP) is larger in the proximal tubule of newborn than in that of the adult animal.

If the net transtubular hydrostatic pressure difference and the hydraulic conductances are similar in rabbits and guinea pigs, it can be estimated that hydrostatic pressure-

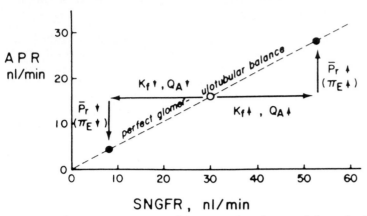

FIG. 5-4. *Schematic representation of the proposed mechanism of glomerulotubular balance. APR, volume of fluid reabsorbed per unit time; Kr, reabsorption coefficient (the product of effective hydraulic permeability and the surface area available for reabsorption); πc and P_c, the mean capillary oncotic and hydrostatic pressures; Kf, glomerular capillary ultrafiltration coefficient (the product of effective hydraulic permeability and the surface area available for filtration); Q_A, initial glomerular plasma flow rate; P_r, net reabsorptive pressure; π_E, oncotic pressure of the blood in the efferent arteriole. (From Mendez RE, Brenner BM: Glomerulotubular balance and the regulation of sodium excretion by intrarenal hemodynamics. In Seldin DW, Giebisch G (eds): The Regulation of Sodium and Chloride Balance. New York: Raven Press, 1990, p 122, with permission.)*

driven flow (~0.005 ml/min/mm) contributes negligibly (<1%) to the total reabsorptive flow of the mature proximal convoluted tubule (~1.2 ml/min/mm). By contrast, in young animals, hydrostatic pressure-driven flow (~0.023 ml/min.mm) accounts for about seven percent of the proximal convoluted tubule reabsorptive flow (~0.33 ml/min/mm). Everything else being equal, the contribution of hydrostatically driven flow to overall fluid reabsorption would be even larger in puppies due to a larger hydrostatic pressure gradient across the proximal convoluted tubule.

Fluxes Driven By Oncotic Forces

Hydraulic conductance to oncotic pressure-driven flow (LΔP) is not necessarily equal to that for hydrostatic pressure-driven flow (JΔP), because distension of the tubules consequent to hydrostatic pressure differences may alter the conductance of the epithelium. In the rabbit, increases in peritubular oncotic pressure, produced by increases in albumin concentration from 6 g/dl to 12 g/dl, induced similar absolute increases in the reabsorptive flow/mm length of proximal convoluted tubule in newborn and adult animals, indicating similar hydraulic conductances for oncotic pressure-driven flows [202]. However, because the plasma protein concentration is lower in the young than in the adult animal, the oncotic pressure difference and thus the associated reabsorptive flow (J$\Delta\pi$) in the proximal convoluted tubule of the newborn was estimated to be about half that in the adult rabbit. In the guinea pig, direct measurements of peritubular oncotic pressure revealed threefold lower values in one-week-old than in 40-day-old animals [241].

If hydraulic conductances and peritubular oncotic pressures are assumed to be similar in rabbits and guinea pigs,

oncotic pressure-driven flow (0.38 ml/min/mm) can account for 31% of the total reabsorptive flow observed in the proximal convoluted tubule of the adult animal. Because of the lower total reabsorptive flow (0.33 ml/min/mm) in the young animals, the oncotic pressure-driven flow (0.14 ml/min/mm) represents a larger proportion of the total in the proximal convoluted tubule of the newborn (42%) than of the adult (31%) animal.

Thus, maturation of proximal tubular function involves a decrease in hydrostatic pressure-driven flow due to a decrease in epithelial hydraulic conductance and, in puppies, a decrease in net transtubular hydrostatic pressure difference. This decrease is more than compensated by twofold to threefold increases in onotic pressure-driven flow, mostly as a result of increased plasma protein concentration, although an increase in filtration fraction may also contribute [241]. The estimated sum of oncotic and hydrostatic pressure-driven flow is of lower absolute magnitude in the proximal convoluted tubule of the young (0.16 nl/min/mm) than of the adult (0.39 nl/min/mm) guinea-pig. However, because the total reabsorptive flow is three to four times lower in the young, this passively driven flow represents a larger proportion of the total (49% vs. 32%) than in the adult. In the dog, the estimated contribution of hydrostatic and oncotic pressure-driven flows to total proximal convoluted tubular reabsorption is even higher in the young animal (85%) than in the adult (32%) as a consequence of the larger hydrostatic pressure difference reported to exist across the proximal convoluted tubule of the canine puppy [204]. The large contribution of these passive fluxes to net sodium reabsorption in the young animal lowers the energy cost for net sodium transport in the proximal convoluted tubule.

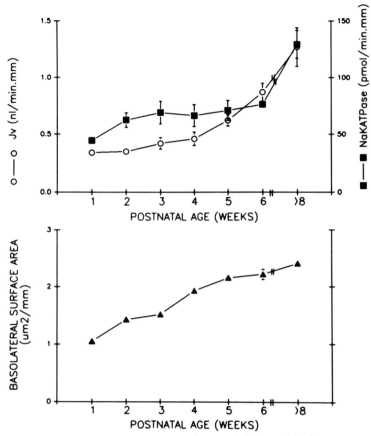

FIG. 5-5. *Relationship between postnatal age and the rate of fluid transport (Jv) (circles), Na$^+$,K$^+$-ATPase activity (squares) and basolateral membrane surface area (triangles) in juxtamedullary proximal tubules of rabbits (From Schwartz GJ, Evan AP: Development of solute transport in rabbit proximal tubule. III. Na-K-ATPase activity. Am J Physiol (Renal Fluid Electrolyte Physiology 15)246:F845, 1984 and Schwartz GJ, Evans AP: Development of solute transport in rabbit proximal tubule. I. HCO$_3$ and glucose absorption. Am J Physiology (Renal Fluid Electrolyte Physiology 14)245:F382, 1983, with permission.)*

Passive Fluxes Associated with Transepithelial Effective Osmotic and Ionic Gradients

In the proximal convoluted tubule of adult rats, the total passive sodium reabsorptive flux (which includes the flow driven by oncotic and hydrostatic pressure-driven differences) had been estimated to be 66% of the total [134]. Thus, passive sodium reabsorption dependent on cell-generated effective osmotic pressure differences and ionic gradients can be estimated to be about 34% of the total in the adult (66% reabsorbed passively less 32% reabsorbed secondary to oncotic and hydrostatic forces). Active transcellular sodium reabsorption represents the other one-third of proximal convoluted tubular reabsorption. It should be pointed out that this analysis is based on the assumption that the coupling of sodium and other ionic fluxes is negligible, an assumption that may result in an underestimation of the active sodium transport [452].

Similar estimates are not available for the proximal convoluted tubule of young animals. There is higher permea-

bility and, thus, lower osmotic reflection coefficients to solids such as mannitol [241] and microperoxidase [202] in the proximal convoluted tubule epithelium of young than of adult animals. The low transtubular HCO$_3$$^-$ gradient that can be generated at low tubular perfusion rates in juxtamedullary proximal convoluted tubules of rabbits before the fourth week of age [382] is consistent with HCO$_3$$^-$ backleak into the lumen due to higher passive permeability. The effective osmotic pressure that could result from transtubular HCO$_3$$^-$, glucose, amino acid, and organic and inorganic anion gradients in the proximal convoluted tubule of young animals may be lower than in adult animals as a consequence of lower reflection coefficients for these solutes, which are preferentially reabsorbed in the late proximal convoluted tubule (S2), resulting in lower associated paracellular fluxes of water and ions. Assuming that paracellular fluxes driven by cell-generated osmotic and ionic gradients are indeed minimal in the proximal convoluted tubule of newborn animals, about half the sodium

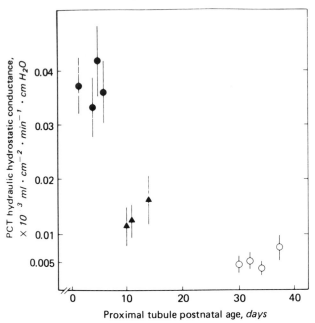

FIG. 5-6. *Hydrostatic hydraulic conductance of the rabbit proximal convoluted tubule (PCT) at three stages of ontogenic differentiation,* (From Horster M, Larson L: *Mechanisms of third absorption during proximal tubule development.* Kidney Int 10:348, 1976, with permission.)

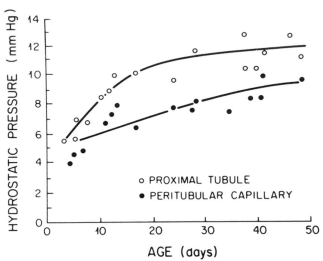

FIG. 5-7. *Hydrostatic pressures (mm Hg) in proximal tubules and adjacent peritubular capillaries of 1- to 50-day-old guinea pigs. The difference represents the net hydrostatic pressure across the proximal tubules* (From Kaskel FJ, Kumar AM, Lockhard EA, et al: *Factors affecting proximal tubular reabsorption during development.* Am J Physiol (*Renal Fluid Electrolyte Physiology 19*)*252:F188, 1987, with permission.*)

reabsorptive flux would be due to active transcellular sodium flux, and the other half would be accounted for by oncotic and hydrostatic pressure-driven paracellular fluxes.

Not considered so far is the fact that development of effective osmotic pressure gradients and the associated volume reabsorption depends not on the absolute values of the reflection coefficients for the preferentialy reabsorbed solutes, but on their relative value with respect to that of chloride. In straight proximal tubules (S3) of adult rabbits the reflection coefficient for HCO_3^- is close to unity, while that for chloride is about 0.8 [370]. This difference is sufficient to generate appreciable effective osmotic pressure gradients and flows across the epithelium when the tubule is bathed with a bicarbonate-rich solution and perfused with an iso-osmolar NaC1 solution [370]. It has been recently reported that tubular fluid obtained from the distal end of the accessible portion of the proximal convoluted tubule of newborn guinea pigs is hyperosmotic relative to plasma (osmolarity ratio = 1.005) and that this hyperosmolarity decreases with age to reach adult values (iso-osmolarity) by 40 days [241] (Fig. 5-8). This finding is consistent with the view tht effective osmotic gradients do exist across the proximal convoluted tubule of the newborn as a consequence of differences in reflection coefficients for preferentially reabsorbed solutes, such as HCO_3^- and glucose, with respect to that of $C1^-$. Such differences in reflection coefficients and the resulting effective osmotic gradient, in the presence of high osmotic water permeability and low perfusion rates that prevail at an early age,

could induce the reabsorption of relatively large volumes of fluid and explain the concurrence of effective osmotic equilibrium and hyperosmolarity of the tubular fluid by the end of the proximal convoluted tubule [370]. To the extent that such passive fluxes participate in net sodium reabsorption, the contribution of the active transcellular component would be decreased from the maximum 50% estimated above.

Development of Transcellular Fluxes in the Proximal Tubule

The developmental changes in transcellular transport of solutes in water are even more difficult to characterize than those through the paracellular pathway. Assuming that no sodium reabsorption is driven by cell-generated osmotic ionic gradients in the proximal convoluted tubule of young animals, all sodium reabsorption not driven by oncotic or hydrostatic pressure differences should be due to transcellular active sodium transport and should represent about 50% of the total (about 25 peq/min/mm). This estimate is to be compared with 60 peq/min/mm of actively reabsorbed Na^+, representing 33% of the total, in proximal convoluted tubules of adult animals [134]. Thus, maturation of proximal convoluted tubular function involves a minimum 2.4-fold increase in active Na^+ reabsorption, similar in magnitude to the threefold increase observed in total reabsorptive flow [383].

During the postnatal development of the rabbit [375,382] and rat [75] there is also a threefold increase in Na^+-K^+-ATPase activity/mm of tubule length (see Fig. 5-5). The apparent proportionality between the increase in enzyme activity and that in reabsorptive flow rate precludes

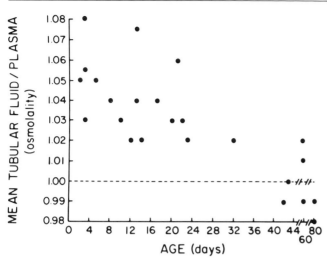

FIG. 5-8. *Mean tubule fluid-to-plasma osmolality ratios measured at the end of proximal tubule of developing guinea pig. Note that iso-osmolality is reached around 44 days of postnatal life (From Kaskel FJ, Kumar AM, Lockhard EA, et al: Factors affecting proximal tubular reabsorption during development. Am J Physiol (Renal Fluid Electrolyte Physiology 19)252:F188, 1987, with permission.)*

us from discerning whether the enzyme develops as a consequence of the increased filtered load or whether the increase in transport is the result of an increase in the abundance of the enzyme. In the juxtamedullary proximal convoluted tubule of the rabbit, a rapid increase in net fluid and solute reabsorption was found to precede the changes in ATPase activity, suggesting that the developmental increase in the enzyme is a consequence rather than a cause of the increase in tubular transport [120,382,383]. Biogenesis of the antiluminal membrane preceded the increase in Na^+-K^+-ATPase activity, as evidenced by the low Na^+-K^+-ATPase activity per unit surface area of basolateral membrane. It appears therefore, that in the newborn, as in the adult, net reabsorption of sodium and water in the proximal convoluted tubule is not limited by the activity of the sodium pump but rather by the influx of Na^+ across the luminal membrane. The developmental characteristics of the various cotransport and exchange mechanisms located in the brush border membrane of the proximal tubule are described in the respective chapters.

Sodium Reabsorption in the Distal Segments of the Nephron

The distal tubular system includes all nephron segments located beyond the pars recta of the proximal tubule, namely, the loop of Henle, the distal tubule, and the collecting duct. In addition to being the segments in which the final regulation of sodium balance is achieved, these parts of the nephron participate in the concentration and dilution of urine, contribute to the regulation of glomerular filtration rate, are the main target sites for hormones that affect the transport of sodium and water, and are the main sites of action of many diuretic drugs.

The Loop of Henle

The loop of Henle can be divided into a thin descending limb (thin DLH), a thin ascending limb (thin ALH), which is better developed in the deep nephrons, and a thick ascending limb (thick ALH). The thin DLH of the superficial nephrons descends to the inner stripe of the outer medulla; that of the juxtamedullary nephrons descends to the inner medulla and even to the papilla. The thick ALH can be subdivided further into medullary and cortical portions, the macula densa, and the first part of the true distal convoluted tubule (DCT), which extends from the macula densa to the kidney surface.

In the nondiuretic state, the loops of Henle reabsorb proprotionately more sodium than water. Consequently, the emerging fluid is hypotonic [156]. When the delivery of filtrate into the loop of Henle is increased, the reabsorption changes proportionately over a wide range [6,274,315]. However, as sodium delivery increases, more sodium escapes reabsorption, both in absolute and relative terms [315]. Moreover, at perfusion rates that exceed 20 nl/min the emerging fluid approaches sodium concentrations similar to those observed at the end of the proximal convoluted tubule, indicating that under these circumstances the difference between the relative sodium and water absorption tends to disappear. A similar phenomenon occurs when the flow rate is decreased below 10 nl/min. The hypotonicity of the fluid leaving the loop of Henle at normal and moderately elevated flow rates is probably due to the abstraction of sodium in the thick ALH, which has a very low permeability to water [180,188,314,351,362]. The disappearance of the difference in the relative sodium and water reabsorption observed at very high perfusion rates is probably due to the short contact time, which blunts the reabsorption of sodium, whereas the increase in NaCl concentration at very slow flow rates is apparently due mainly to net influx of salt in the initial portion of the DCT [377].

The characteristics of transport in the thin DLH have been difficult to investigate in vivo. Studies are limited to juxtamedullary nephrons that can be approached only after surgical exposure of the papilla. Initial experiments performed in desert rodents [96,97,313] appeared to indicate net addition of NaCl along the descending limb. Subsequent experiments in hamsters suggested that the increase in osmolality was due to a large extent to water abstraction [297]. Evidence obtained in rats suggests that secretion of urea contributes to the increase in fluid osmolality along the thin DLH [225,226,337]. In vitro experiments performed in thin DLH isolated from rabbits indicate that the osmotic equilibration occurring in this segment is due to transepithelial water flow along osmotic gradients imposed by various solutes present in the papillary environment, such as NaCl and urea [259–261].

The thin ALH has been as difficult to study by micropuncture techniques as the thin DLH. The observation that osmolality of the fluid passing through this segment was lower than that flowing through the descending segment has been used to justify the assumption that hypertonic fluid is reabsorbed at this level [224,225,297,298]. In vitro microperfusion experiments disclosed that this segment is practically impermeable to water [207,212] and that the passive permeability coefficients for sodium, potassium, and chloride were one to two orders of magnitude higher than in the thin DLH [207,212,214]. Active transport of sodium out of the thin ALH could not be documented [207,212,220]. Thus, as in the thin DLH, outward movement of sodium must occur by diffusion [261].

The thick ALH on the other hand, is endowed with the ability to transport sodium actively [67,351]. This contributes to the build-up of the interstitial osmolality and thus to the efficiency of the concentrating mechanism. In vitro experiments performed in thick ALH isolated from rabbits have consistently shown that NaCl reabsorption in this segment is dependent on the rate of perfusion [67,163,351]. Similar results have been obtained in rats [208,362] and mice [131,180,188,362]. The sodium fluxes appear to be larger in the medullary than in the cortical segments [67,351]. Both the medullary and the cortical portions have high sodium and chloride permeabilities, the former exceeding the latter by a factor of approximately two [351]. According to currently accepted models (Fig. 5-9)), the reabsorption of NaCl at this level is active, mediated by a Na^+ pump located at the basolateral membrane [168]. The entry of Cl^- through the luminal membrane is believed to be passive, coupled to the movement of Na^+ and K^+ [165,166]. The process appears to be electroneutral, with a stoichiometry of 2Cl:1Na:1K [167,316]. There is also evidence for paracellular transport of sodium [207,212, 214]. In summary, the thick ALH is a site of K^+-dependent secondary active NaCl reabsorption through essentially water impermeable membranes. The result is the generation of a hypertonic papillary interstitium and of a hypotonic tubular fluid that is delivered to the distal tubule.

The Distal Convoluted Tubule

The distal tubule (DCT) is generally defined as the segment located between the macula densa and the first confluence of the cortical collecting tubule. Histologic studies have identified at least two distinctive segments: one, the true DCT, is characterized by the presence of a single cell type of light appearance. This portion is very short in the rabbit (<8 mm) [210,312] and somewhat longer in the rat [85,234]. The next portion is the so-called connecting tubule, which is granular in appearance and contains at least two cell types, the connecting tubular cells and the intercalated dark cells, each with specific transport properties [85,232,271]. This is presumably the portion of the nephron where the epithelium of the nephrogenic blastema merges with that of the ureteral bud [329]. Both portions of the distal tubule contain Na^+-K^+-ATPase, the activity being higher in the DCT proper [136,137,242,373].

Micropuncture studies performed in the rat have revealed that in the antidiuretic state some 10% of the

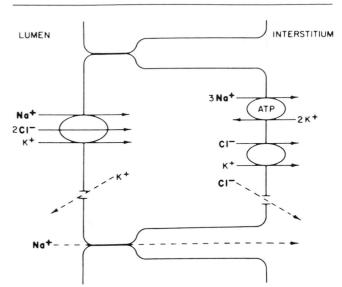

FIG. 5-9. *Schematic representation of Na^+ and Cl^- transport in cells of the thick ascending limb of Henle's loop. (From Koeppen BM: Mechanism of segmental sodium and chloride reabsorption. In Seldin DW, Giebisch G (eds): The Regulation of Sodium and Chloride Balance. New York: Raven Press, 1990, p 87, with permission.)*

filtered load of sodium is reabsorbed in the distal tubule [144,194]. During passage through the DCT, the tubular fluid becomes isotonic to plasma [156,462] due to reabsorption of water in excess of sodium. Net reabsorption of sodium is active, proceeding against an electrochemical gradient [460]. The rate of sodium transport, which overall is approximately one-third that observed in the PCT, decreases along the DCT [246]. Under normal circumstances, fractional reabsorption of sodium in the DCT represents about 80% of the amount delivered to this segment and remains nearly constant over a tenfold range of sodium delivery [144,246]. This proportionality between delivery and reabsorption is maintained even under conditions of extracellular volume expansion [460], indicating that physical forces are inoperative. In vivo microperfusion studies performed in the rat have provided evidence for the existence of a carrier-mediated NaCl cotransport system located in the luminal membrane of the distal tubule.

The DCT is impermeable to urea [71,352]. This contributes to the establishment of high sodium concentration gradients across this nephron segment. In the rat, but not in the dog or monkey, the late portion of the DCT is sensitive to the action of ADH [215].

The presence of Na^+-K^+-ATPase in the peritubular membrane [136,373] and the sensitivity of the transtubular PD to oubain [170] indicate the existence of a Na^+-K^+ exchange mechanism at the contralateral membrane (Fig. 5-10). Sodium is also extruded from the cells of this segment through a Na^+-Ca^{2+} countertransport system [428,460], which accounts, in part, for the relationship that exists between sodium and calcium reabsorption.

The DCTs are relatively leaky epithelia, which explains

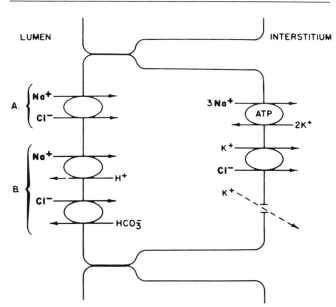

LUMEN

INTERSTITIUM

FIG. 5-10. *Schematic representation of the Na$^+$ and Cl$^-$ transport mechanisms present in cells of the early distal tubule. (From Koeppen BM: Mechanism of segmental sodium and chloride reabsorption. In Seldin DW, Giebisch G (eds): The Regulation of Sodium and Chloride Balance. New York: Raven Press, 1990, p 93, with permission.)*

the effect of changes in transtubular oncotic pressure gradients on transepithelial conductance [34].

The Collecting Tubule

The collecting tubule can be further divided into three portions: the cortical collecting tubule (CCT), which results from fusion of the connecting segments of several nephrons; the outer medullary collecting tubule (OMCT), which extends through the outer and the inner stripes of the outer medulla; and the papillary collecting duct (PCD), which extends from the inner stripe of the outer medulla to the tip of the papilla. The collecting tubule (CT) is made up of two types of cells, the principal cells that apparently are involved in the transport of sodium and potassium, and the intercalated cells that are mainly involved in the transport of protons. Although only some 2% of the filtered sodium and water reach the CT, this segment is crucial to the final adjustments in urine composition. This is particulary true for states of sodium deprivation and osmotic diuresis [293,461]. In the nondiuretic rat, about one-third of the sodium load presented to this segment is reabsorbed [100,410,461].

The reabsorption of sodium occurs against an electrochemical gradient in the CT and is, therefore, active [414]. The reported values for the transepithelial PD cover a wide range [48]. In the absence of transtubular ionic gradients, and when the lumen was perfused with a solution that mimicked the glomerular filtrate, the voltage was generally lumen-negative [48]. Omission of sodium from the perfus-

ate [159,413], inhibition of Na$^+$-K$^+$-ATPase with oubain [68,159,415], and blockade of sodium reabsorption with amiloride [324,325,419] reduce the transtubular electrical PD to zero or even reverse the voltage to lumen-positive values. In addition, the CCT is capable of generating steep transtubular sodium concentration gradients [159,419].

Studies performed in isolated perfused CCT segments obtained from rabbits have revealed the existence of a conductive Na$^+$ pathway in the apical membrane [257] (Fig. 5-11). A second pathway, sensitive to luminal addition of barium and insensitive to amiloride, permits the exit of K$^+$ from the cell. Transport in this segment is particularly sensitive to the action of mineralocorticoids, which affect the activity of the Na$^+$-K$^+$-ATPase [102,103,300,301,309,310,374]. Receptors of high affinity and high specificity for mineralocorticoids have been identified in this segment of the nephron [101,123,124]. A parallelism between sodium reabsorption and Na$^+$-K$^+$-ATPase response to aldosterone has been noted [311] (Fig.5-12). Aldosterone appears to affect both the basolateral and the luminal membranes [257]. The hormone increases the K$^+$ selectivity of the basolateral membrane and the conductance of the apical membrane. Chronic pretreatment of rabbits with DOCA leads to increases in sodium reabsorption and potassium secretion by the isolated CCT [326]. Schwartz and Burg [381] have found that sodium and potassium transport in the CCT in vitro correlated with the plasma aldosterone concentration, which was manipulated by changes in the electrolyte content of the diet.

In the OMCT, the electrical PD is lumen-negative in the outer stripe and lumen-positive in the inner stripe [417]. This difference correlates with the relative proportion of intercalated and dark cells; the PD was found to be negative when the dark cell population exceeded 20% and positive when the dark cell population was less than 10% [414]. The net sodium reabsorption in segments of the outer stripe is about one-third or even less than that in the CCT. No transport of sodium appears to occur in the inner stripe [414]. It would appear, therefore, that composition of the tubular fluid does not change during its passage through this segment.

Active transport of sodium does occur in the PCD. Microcatheterization experiments have revealed that the sodium concentration decreases from about 200 mM at the base of the papilla to about 50 mM at the tip at the papilla [192,228].

The transepithelial PD is lumen-negative but variable [48,342,343]. The PCD has a low permeability for Na$^+$ and Cl$^-$ [353], which may be modulated by mineralocorticoids [438,439].

REABSORPTION OF SODIUM IN THE DISTAL NEPHRON SEGMENTS DURING DEVELOPMENT

Because the fractional reabsorption of sodium in the proximal tubule is either similar to [404] or lower [354] than that of the adult, the retention of sodium observed in growing individuals must be caused by enhanced reabsorption at more distal sites of the nephron. That this might be the case was suggested by clearance experiments per-

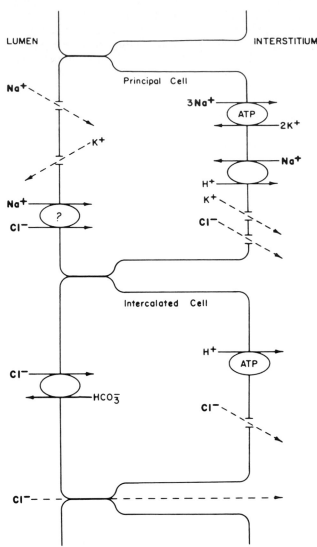

FIG. 5-11. Schematic representation of the Na^+ and Cl^- transport mechanisms present in the principal and HCO_3^- secreting intercalated cells of the cortical collecting duct. (From Koeppen BM: Mechanism of segmental sodium and chloride reabsorption. In Seldin DW, Giebisch G (eds): The Regulation of Sodium and Chloride Balance. New York: Raven Press, 1990, p 97, with permission.)

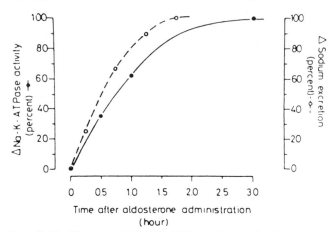

FIG. 5-12. Changes in Na^+,K^+-ATPase (dots) and sodium excretion (circles) as a function of time, in adrenalectomized rats treated with 5 mg/kg/day of aldosterone. (From Mernissi GL, Doucet A: Short-term effect of aldosterone on renal sodium transport and tubular Na-K-ATPase in the rat. Pflugers Arch 399:139, 1983, with permission.)

formed by Kleinman in one-day-old to 23-day-old puppies [252] (Table 5-1). When blockers of distal tubular reabsorption (chlorothiazide and ethacrynic acid) were administered to hydropenic animals, a decrease in fractional Na^+ reabsorption of about 30% ensued, with a further drop of a similar magnitude occurring when a load of isotonic saline, corresponding to about 3% of body weight, was superimposed on the diuretics. Because of the distal blockade, the further decrease in fractional reabsorption, from about 70% to 50%, had to result in large part from proximal inhibition of sodium rebsorption, induced by saline loading. When distal tubule sodium reabsorption was not blocked, saline expansion produced only an insignificant decrease in fractional sodium reabsorption, suggesting that the effect of proximal inhibition was mitigated by increased reabsorption at more distal sites of the nephron. Because newborn dogs excreted less of their filtered sodium than did adult animals during saline expansion, and because the change in proximal fractional reabsorption appeared to be similar in animals of all ages, the distal segments of the newborn nephron must have absorbed a greater fraction of the filtered load than those of the adult dog.

Aperia et al. [13] arrived at a similar conclusion from a study of 23 infants three weeks to 13 months of age who were found to have a higher capacity to form free water than children between 7 and 12 years of age, at comparable rates of distal sodium delivery (approximated by adding the clearance of sodium to the clearance of water). Similar conclusions were reached by Rodriguez-Soriano et al. [354]. These investigators subjected 22 infants varying in age between one-week and 15 months and 17 children between two years and 12 years of age to measurements of water and sodium excretion obtained under conditions of maximal water diuresis induced by the administration of an oral water load of 2 ml/kg, followed by the intravenous infusion of 0.45% saline solution at the rate of 1,000 ml/hr/1.73 m^2 of body surface, over of a period of two hours. Under these circumstances of relative extracellular volume expansion, distal sodium delivery, estimated from the clearance of free water (C_{H_2O}) plus the clearance of sodium (C_{Na}) was found to be 22.4 ± 2.9 ml/dl of glomerular filtrate in the infants and 15.3 ± 2.6 ml/dl in the older children, indicating a lower fractional reabsorption of sodium and water in the proximal tubule of the infants (Fig. 5-13). There was an inverse correlation between the distal sodium delivery and the age of the subjects: the younger the infant, the higher the fractional distal delivery, that is the lower the proportion of filtered load reabsorbed proximally. A

TABLE 5-1. *The effect of distal blockade on sodium reabsorption in canine puppies*

	Control		Saline		Saline + Diuretics
GFR, ml/min per g	0.28 ± 0.02		0.32 ± 0.02		0.45 ± 0.03
P		<0.05		<0.01	
Filtered Na reabsorbed %	99.7 ± 0.1		98.5 ± 0.6		51.2 ± 2.6
P		NS		<0.01	

	Control		Diuretics		Saline + Diuretics
GFR, ml/min/g	0.20 ± 0.01		0.28 ± 0.03		0.40 ± 0.03
P		<0.05		<0.01	
Filtered Na reabsorbed, %	99.8 ± 0.1		70.1 ± 2.8		49.3 ± 2.5
P		<0.01		<0.01	

(*From* Kleinman LI: Renal sodium reabsorption during saline loading and distal blockade in newborn dogs. *Am J Physiol* 228:1403, 1975.)

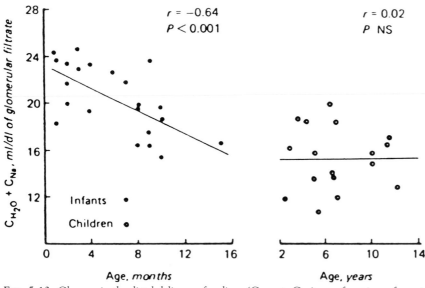

FIG. 5-13. *Changes in the distal delivery of sodium* ($C_{H_2O} + C_{Na}$) *as a function of age in infants and children (From Rodriguez-Soriano J, Vallo A, Castillo G, et al: Renal handling of water in sodium in infancy and childhood: A study using clearance methods during hypotonic saline diuresis. Kidney Int 20:700, 1981, with permission.)*

negative correlation was also observed between free water clearance and the age of the subject. On the other hand, NaCl reabsorption at the diluting segments of the nephron, estimated by the value of C_{H_2O}, was significantly higher in infants than it was in children. This indicates that a proportionately higher amount of the filtrate escaping proximal reabsorption was reabsorbed in the distal nephron segments of the infants than of the older children. As a consequence, the proportion of the sodium load reabsorbed distally (estimated by the ratio $C_{H_2O}/C_{H_2O} + C_{Na} \times 100$) was identical in both groups (90.8 ± 4.5 vs. 90.9 ± 3.3, respectively). Thus, both under hydropenic conditions and under conditions of sodium loading, the infant reabsorbed more sodium than the older child in the distal segments of the nephron. A negative correlation between fractional delivery of sodium to the distal tubule and conceptional age was found by the same investigators in prematurely born babies [355]. However, unlike full-term infants, the distal tubule was unable to compensate, resulting in a high fractional excretion of sodium [355].

Micropuncture studies performed in the rat suggest that this process is not a function of enhanced reabsorption at the level of the thick ascending limb of Henle's loop. The experiments of Zink and Horster [468] demonstrate that the ability of the loop of Henle to generate a hypotonic fluid is low in the newborn and increases only gradually during ontogeny (Fig. 5-14). Aperia and Elinder [14] measured sodium delivery into and sodium reabsorption by the distal convoluted tubules in 24-day-old and 40-day-old hydropenic and volume expanded rats. Under both of these experimental conditions the delivery of fluid into the distal convoluted tubule was larger in the younger than in the older animals, suggesting lower rates of reabsorption in the loop of Henle in the younger rats (Fig. 5-15). However, the fractional reabsorption of sodium along the distal tubule was substantially larger in younger than in the older animals. In hydropenia, the $TF/P_{Na/In}$ ratio fell between the early and late distal tubule by 12-fold in 24-day-old rats and by only threefold in the 40-day-old rats. During volume expansion, the decrease was about sevenfold in the younger animals and only twofold in the older group. Thus, the enhanced reabsorptive capacity of the distal convoluted tubule appears to contribute to the retention of sodium and to the blunted response to saline loading observed during early life. Whether the reabsorption of sodium is also enhanced in the collecting duct cannot be determined from these experiments.

Similar conclusions can be drawn from a micropuncture study performed in guinea pigs [378]. The recollection technique was used to obtain proximal tubular fluid under hydropenic conditions and following expansion with an isoncotic albumin solution corresponding to 5% of body weight. The amount of sodium reabsorbed in the proximal tubule was estimated from changes in TF/P_{In} and the renal fractional reabsorption of sodium was calculated from the urinary to plasma ratio of sodium to inulin. In all age groups there was a marked decrease in proximal reabsorption of fluid following infusion of albumin solution, but the magnitude of the changes did not vary from one age group to another. However, the excretion of sodium was significantly less in the younger animals, suggesting differences in reabsorption in nephron segments located beyond the proximal tubule. Unfortunately, information regarding the transport capacity of various nephron segments obtained by microperfusion of isolated tubular segments are not available in the young.

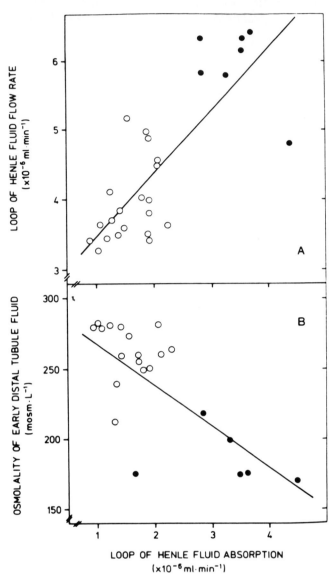

FIG. 5-14. *The reabsorption of fluid in Henle's loops of 12–15 (circles) and 27–35 (dots) day-old rats as a function of flow rate (A) or distal fluid osmolality (B). Inflow was taken as the flow rate in the late proximal tubule and outflow as the rate of flow in the early distal tubule. (From Zink H, Horster M: Maturation of diluting capacity in loop of Henle of rat superficial nephrons Am J Physiol (Renal Fluid Electrolyte Physiology 2)233:F519, 1977, with permission.)*

Reabsorption of Chloride Along the Renal Tubule

Chloride is the most abundant anion in the extracellular fluid. Consequently, variations in total body chloride, like those in sodium, affect the size of the extracellular volume compartment. The mechanism that governs chloride transport varies from one segment of the nephron to the other. In addition, substantial differences exist in this regard between the superficial and the juxtamedullary nephrons.

Proximal Tubule

As soon as micropuncture techniques were applied to the study of proximal tubular transport, it was recognized that the reabsorption of sodium and that of chloride do not proceed pari passu. Unlike the concentration of sodium, the concentration of chloride in the tubular fluid was found to exceed by about 1.5-fold the concentration of this anion in the blood [447]. It was readily recognized that the cre-

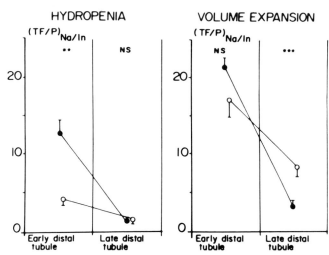

FIG. 5-15. *Changes in the fraction of sodium remaining in distal tubules of hydropenic and volume expanded rats between 24 days (circles) and 40 days (dots) of age. NS = not significant;* ** = *P<0.001;* *** = *P<0.0001. (From Aperia A, Elinder G: Distal tubular sodium reabsorption in the developing rat kidney. Am J Physiol (Renal Fluid Electrolyte Physiology 9)240:F487, 1981, with permission.)*

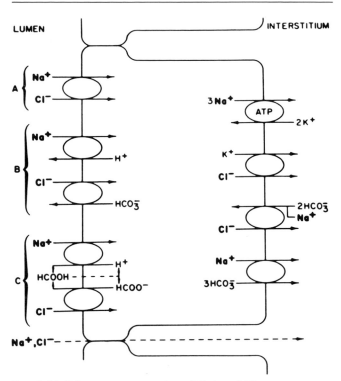

FIG. 5-16. *Schematic representation of Na+ and Cl− transport mechanism present in the late portion of the proximal tubule. (From Koeppen BM: Mechanism of segmental sodium and chloride reabsorption. In Seldin DW, Giebisch G (eds): The Regulation of Sodium and Chloride Balance. New York: Raven Press, 1990, p 79, with permission.)*

ation of this concentration gradient required the preferential reabsorption of a substance such as bicarbonate in the very early portion of the proximal convoluted tubule.

For technical reasons, subsequent information regarding the reabsorption of chloride in the proximal tubule was obtained from studies done in Necturus. Although, in this species the concentration of chloride in the tubular fluid does not rise above that of the plasma, the electrical gradient, which is 5 mV to 10 mV negative compared to the blood, was considered to be sufficient to account for the passive reabsorption of chloride in this segment [143,175,247,454]. Subsequently, the intracellular chloride activity was found to be higher than that prevailing in the tubular fluid [175,406,407], suggesting the existence of an active transport process at the level of the luminal membrane (Fig. 5-16). It appears that the entry of Cl− into the cell occurs via an electrically neutral process, whereby the entry of one Na+ is coupled to the entry of one Cl− [5,248]. The exit of Cl− from the cell may also be coupled to an anion. The existence of a Cl−/HCO3− exchange has been invoked recently [3].

As already indicated, there are considerable differences between the amphibian and the mammalian proximal tubule. Some of these differences, such as the perfusion and the reabsorptive rates, are quantitative. Others, such as the lack of change in chloride concentration and in the electrical negativity of the tubular lumen along the entire length of the proximal tubule, are qualitative. In the mammalian proximal tubule, the concentration of chloride was consistently found to be higher than that prevailing in the plasma [76,240,273,277,294,443,461]. There is general agreement that this concentration gradient is generated by

the more rapid reabsorption of NaHCO3 than that of NaCl. Furthermore, electrical measurements performed in the rat have provided evidence that the majority of chloride transported in the early portion of the proximal tubule is passive [134]. Microperfusion experiments in rabbit proximal tubules indicate, however, that net chloride reabsorption is greater in this initial segment than can be accounted for by electrochemical forces [219]. This has prompted speculation regarding some type of interactive process with the membrane that facilittes the transport of chloride [219]. Beyond the very early portion of the proximal tubule, the concentration gradient is sufficient to account for the passive reabsorption of chloride, despite the fact that the slightly lumen positive PD that prevails along most of the proximal tubule should retard the transport of chloride. There is convincing evidence that in this portion of the proximal tubule the reabsorption of chloride contributes to the reabsorption of sodium and water. Micropuncture experiments performed in the rat [160,288,320] and microperfusion experiments performed in proximal tubular segments from rabbits [218] have made it possible to estimate that this process accounts for 30% to 50% of the fluid reabsorbed at this level. A similar proportion of the fluid is reabsorbed passively in the proximal tubules of the juxtamedullary nephrons, but this is driven both by concentration and electrical gradients [218]. On the other hand, the permeability of the latter segments of the juxtamedullary nephrons for chloride is lower than that of the superficial proximal convoluted tubules [38,221]. Some 10% to 20% of the chloride may also be reabsorbed by solvent drag. There is indeed evidence that the reflection coefficient for NaCl is significantly less than unity. Hierholzer et al. [193] found reflection coefficients for Na^+ of 0.90 and for Cl^- of 0.86. On the other hand, an in vitro micropuncture study has failed to detect significant net transport of chloride under conditions of osmotically induced water flow [222]. Thus, the role of convective forces in the transport of chloride out of the proximal tubule remains uncertain.

As in the proximal convoluted tubule, the reabsorption of sodium in the pars recta is mostly an active process. Isolated pars recta segments perfused with a solution comparable to an ultrafiltrate of plasma have a slightly negative (-2 mV lumen negative) transepithelial PD [8,22,243, 365,368,369]. In pars rectae of superficial tubules the PD becomes slightly lumen-positive when the perfusion fluid has a high chloride concentration, similar to that prevailing in this segment in vivo [8,366,367,451], whereas the PD remains lumen negative when the pars rectae of juxtamedullary nephrons are perfused with a fluid of the same composition [243]. Measurements performed by Andreoli et al. [8] have revealed that the reabsorption of chloride in this segment is equally dependent on diffusion along the favorable transepithelial electrochemical gradient and on solvent drag.

The Loop of Henle

There is no evidence of active NaCl transport either in the thin descending or thin ascending limbs of Henle's loop. In the thin descending limb, the chloride concentration increases as a result of water abstraction [140,197, 200]. The thin ascending limb is highly permeable to chloride [207]. In addition to passive diffusion, there is evidence for a specific carrier-mediated process that is competitively inhibited by bromide [213].

Transport of chloride out of the thick ascending limb occurs against both a chemical and an electrical gradient. Moreover, the lumen-positive potential was found to be dependent on the presence of chloride in the perfusate [67,351]. The existence of a lumen-positive PD has been confirmed by many investigators [50,162,180,188,209, 412,420]. However, whereas the initial studies suggested that the lumen-positive PD is the result of primary active Cl^- transport [67,351], more recent studies indicate that Cl^- transport is dependent on Na^+ [162,164,188,189]. Indeed, when special care was taken to avoid contamination of the tubular fluid with Na^+, the PD decreased, reaching values close to zero [162].

The precise mechanism by which the lumen-positive PD is generated is still a matter of controversy. Among the possibilities that have been entertained and discarded are the backleak of sodium through the paracellular channels [46,164] and a coupling ratio of Cl^- to Na^+ transport

across the luminal membrane of the thick ascending limb greater than unity [164]. It is more likely, however, that two Cl^- ions are coupled to one Na^+ and one K^+ ion and that the lumen-positive PD is the result of K^+ diffusion into the tubule across the luminal membrane (see Fig. 5-9). Support for this model was provided by Greger [164,169] and Hebert et al. [189], who have shown that luminal barium, a presumed inhibitor of K^+ channels, inhibits Cl^- transport. In addition, the apical membrane of the thick ascending limb was found to contain a high K^+ conductance channel, and deletion of K^+ from the perfusing solution resulted in a decrease in the lumen-positive potential [167]. It appears, therefore, that the transport of Cl^- by the thick ascending limb of Henle's loop is secondary active.

Distal Convoluted Tubule

Based on work done in amphibia [45,183,205,327,328, 418,448], Oberleithner et al. [328] have arrived at the conclusion that the cellular mechanism of chloride transport in this segment is similar to that proposed for the thick ascending loop, i.e., the entry of chloride into the cell occurs via a neutral cotransport system that couples two Cl^- to one Na^+ and one K^+. Efflux of Cl^- from the cell occurs along the electrochemical gradient. The system is energized by the active extrusion of Na^+ at the basolateral membrane.

Micropuncture experiments have documented that the transport of chloride in the distal convoluted tubule occurs against a concentration gradient [106,239,245,292,344, 461]. The transport capacity for chloride appears to be about half that of the proximal tubule [444].

There is still some controversy regarding the mechanism of chloride transport in the distal tubule. Initial measurements suggested that the electrical gradient is insufficient to account for the rate of transport observed [344]. This conclusion was challenged by some investigators [87, 239,291] and accepted by others [292]. On balance, the evidence appears to support the contention that at least some of the Cl^- transport is active. This conclusion is based mainly on measurements of intracellular Cl^- activity, which was found to be significantly higher than that predicted by the Nernst equation [327]. The fact that K^+ and particularly Na^+ reabsorption was found to be dependent on the presence of Cl^- in the lumen favors the existence of a coupling between the reabsorption of these three ions [328] (see Fig. 5-10).

Collecting Duct

Electrophysiological and radioisotope studies suggest that the cortical collecting duct has a low permeability to Cl^- [258,419], although the ionic conductance to Cl^- was found to be appreciably higher than that to Na^+ or K^+ [325].

The nature of the chloride transport in the cortical collecting tubule is unsettled, due to a large degree to the high variability observed in transepithelial PD values [182,326,381]. Under most circumstances, the luminal PD is negative, which should favor Cl$^-$ efflux. When cortical collecting tubules from rabbits treated with DOCA were examined, Cl$^-$ was found to be transported against the electrochemical gradient and therefore qualified as being active. This, however, was not the case in non-DOCA treated animals [182]. It would appear, therefore, that depending on the prevailing circumstances, both passive and active transport of chloride may occur in the cortical collecting tubule (see Fig. 5-11).

There is very little information regarding the transport of chloride in the medullary collecting tubule. The information available suggests that only minimal if any chloride reabsorption occurs under control conditions [32,416,459].

The reabsorption of chloride in the papillary collecting duct appears to be load-dependent [196]. This segment is relatively impermeable to Cl$^-$ [342,353]. Consequently, active reabsorption of chloride appears to occur at this site [100,353].

THE RENAL REABSORPTION OF CHLORIDE IN GROWING SUBJECTS

There is very little knowledge regarding the renal handling of chloride in immature animals and humans. The microperfusion study performed by Zink and Horster in loops of Henle of rat superficial nephrons [468] revealed a low capacity for sodium chloride reabsorption at three weeks of age as compared to adult animals. Newborn piglets [305] and newborn infants [9] had a higher excretion of sodium when given sodium bicarbonate than sodium chloride. No such difference was observed between adult dogs and newborn puppies [286], although the newborn animals reabsorbed a higher fraction of the distal tubular load of sodium than the adult dogs, under both experimental conditions (Table 5-2). In addition, in the sodium chloride-expanded puppies, the greater fractional reabsorption of sodium was associated with a greater fractional reabsorption of chloride. There was no difference between the newborn and adult dogs in the fractional reabsorption of the distal potassium load. These findings were interpreted to indicate that the enhanced reabsorption of sodium observed in the newborn occurs together with chloride in a region of the distal nephron that is proximal to the K$^+$/H$^+$ secretory region, probably the thick ascending limb of Henle's loop.

Control of Sodium and Chloride Balance

The control of sodium chloride excretion is intricately related to the maintenance of extracellular homeostasis. It probably is its essential role in the economy of the organism that explains the complexity of the system that controls body fluid homeostasis. The difficulties encountered in distinguishing between the various factors involved in this process explain some of the conflicting results encountered in the vast literature written on this subject. In the normal adult subject, the external balance for sodium is zero. This is due almost exclusively to the fact that the urinary excretion of sodium matches the intake. An increase in sodium intake results in a slight accumulation of fluid, which usually does not exceed 2% to 3% of body weight. At that point, an increase in the excretion of sodium occurs, commensurate with the increase in intake, and a new steady-state is achieved (Fig. 5-17). A return to the basal sodium intake is followed by a short period of increased urinary output, which subsides when the initial weight is reached [19].

The situation is somewhat different in infants. Janovsky et al. [227] fed human milk with a sodium content of about 7 mEq/L to six infants 14 days old to 40 days old, followed by a formula to which salt was added to raise its concentration to 136 mEq/L. As sodium intake increased 20-fold, from 5 mEq/day to 100 mEq/day, the clearance of sodium rose tenfold, from 0.08 to 0.8 ml/min/1.73 m^2. However, the fraction of retained sodium remained at about 60% of intake, resulting in a marked increase in the positive balance. All infants gained an inappropriate amount of weight on the salt-supplemented formula and two-thirds became edematous. A similar response was observed in 5-month-old to 7-month-old infants who were fed diets containing either 50 mEq or 80 mEq of sodium/kg of food [455]. This tendency to retain sodium is also evident under conditions of acute salt loading. Goldsmith et al. [152] subjected puppies and adult dogs to an isotonic load of sodium equal to 10% of body weight. The limited diuretic response of one-week-old puppies in comparison to that of the mature animals was striking; at three hours after administration of saline, the youngest animal had excreted only 5% of the administered load as compared with about 50% in the adult

TABLE 5-2. *Renal function during volume expansion in the dog*

	Newborn NaCl	Adult NaCl	Newborn NaHCO$_3$	Adult NaHCO$_3$	p^a
Glomerular filtration rate (ml/min per g)	0.23 ± 0.02^b	0.88 ± 0.06^b	0.19 ± 0.02^c	0.85 ± 0.061^c	<0.001
Fractional reabsorption Na (%)	99.0 ± 0.3^b	96.6 ± 0.6^{b,e}	98.1 ± 0.7^c	93.2 ± 0.7^{c,e}	<0.001
Fractional reabsorption Cl (%)	97.8 ± 0.5^d	96.9 ± 0.5^e	99.5 ± 0.1^d	99.1 ± 0.3^c	<0.001
Fractional reabsorption K (%)	68.1 ± 5.4^d	79.4 ± 2.6^e	21.7 ± 13.0^{c,d}	54.7 ± 3.6^{c,e}	<0.001

These clearance measurements were made 60 mins after the initiation of a continuous infusion of isotonic NaCl or NaHCO$_3$. Values are means ± SEM. ^{a}one-way analysis of variance. ^{b}P<0.05, newborn NaCl vs. adult NaCl by LSD method. ^{c}P<0.05, newborn NaHCO$_3$ vs. adult NaHCO$_3$ by LSD method. ^{d}P<0.05, newborn NaCl vs. newborn NaHCO$_3$ by LSD method. ^{e}P<0.05, adult NaCl vs. adult NaHCO$_3$ by LSD method.
(*From* Lorenz JM, Kleinman LI, Disney TA: Lack of anion effect on volume expansion natriuresis in developing canine kidney. *J Dev Physiol* 8:395, 1986.)

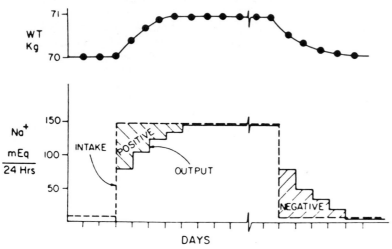

FIG. 5-17. *The effect of acute changes in sodium intake on weight (Wt) and sodium excretion (mEq/ 24 hr) in human. Note that following a few days of sodium retention, a new steady state is achieved (From August JT, Nelson DH, Thorn GW: Response of normal subjects to large amounts of aldosterone. J Clin Invest 37:1549, 1958, with permission.)*

dog (Fig. 5-18). An almost identical response was observed in humans, many years ago by Dean and McCance [95] and more recently by Aperia et al. [11].

The reason for this difference in response between growing and non-growing subjects has to reside with various sensor and effector mechanisms known to be involved in the regulation of extracellular fluid volume. There is substantial evidence that some receptor mechanism must exist within the extracellular fluid compartment. Sonnenberg and Pearce [401] expanded the blood volume of normal, salt-depleted, and salt-loaded dogs by infusing red cells suspended in a saline solution. The degree of natriuresis was directly related to the state of the sodium balance (i.e., the size of the extracellular compartment). Likewise, a higher degree of natriuresis was observed in dogs infused with saline, which distributes within the entire extracellular fluid compartment, than with an equivalent amount of blood, which expands only the intravascular space [463].

There is also evidence that changes in intravascular volume may affect sodium excretion. When human volunteers were emerged to the neck in a water bath, a brisk natriuresis and diuresis ensued, associated with increases in central blood volume, central venous pressure, and right atrial and pulmonary arterial transmural pressure gradients, and a decrease in systemic vascular resistance [18,117]. Natriuresis associated with expansion of the central blood volume was also observed in astronauts on entry into the zero-gravity environment [139].

The Location of Volume Sensors

A number of neural receptors that respond to mechanical stretch or transmural pressure have been identified within the heart and great vessels of the thorax. There are apparently two populations of mechanical receptors in the atria: type A receptors present mainly at the entrance of the

great veins into the atria that respond to changes in the cardiac cycle [333] and type B receptors that discharge in response to atrial stretching [334]. Maneuvers that impede the ability of the atria to expand resulted in a decrease in the renal excretion of sodium [149], whereas increases in left atrial pressure were followed by increases in the urinary excretion of sodium [346]. These effects occurred in the absence of changes in cardiac output or mean arterial pressure and were independent of the state of sodium balance or the presence of mineralocorticoid hormones. There is also some evidence that volume receptors exist in the right ventricle [453] and in the pulmonary interstitium [334].

The signals generated by these receptors travel along the ninth and tenth cranial nerves to the hypothalamic and medullary centers, which integrate the physiological response to these impulses [98,307,363,392].

The existence of baroreceptors in the carotid sinus was first inferred by Guyton and co-workers [176] and confirmed by others [116,244]. Baroreceptors appear also to exist in the juxtaglomerular apparatus, which responds to changes in renal perfusion pressure by changing renin release [90,321,437]. Alterations in the sodium concentration of the blood perfusing the carotid artery and of the cerebral spinal fluid have been reported to affect the excretion of sodium in experimental animals [7], suggesting the presence of sensors in the central nervous system. Finally, an increase in sodium excretion was observed when a solution containing sodium, but not equimolar sucrose, was infused into the portal circulation [335]. Vagotomy abolished this response.

Effectors of Fluid Homeostasis

The excretion of sodium can be modulated either by changes in glomerular filtration rate or by changes in tubular reabsorption. Separating one from the other has not

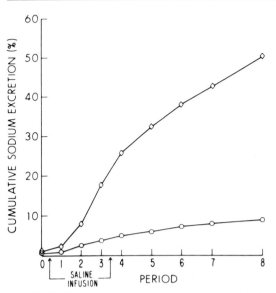

FIG. 5-18. *The natriuretic response of newborns (circles) and adult dogs (squares) to the acute infusion of a normal solution of NaCl in an amount equal to 10% of body weight. (From Goldsmith DI, Drukker A, Blaufox MD, et al: Response of the neonatal canine kidney to acute saline expansion. In ZumWinkel K, Blaufox MD, Funck-Brentano JL (eds): Radionuclides in Nephrology. Stuttgart, Thieme, 1975, p 45, with permission.)*

been easy, due to the fact that these two variables tend to change in parallel. In addition, small changes in filtration rate that may pass undetected may result in very large changes in the filtered load of sodium. deWardener was the first to demonstrate that acute volume expansion results in a marked natriuretic response even in the presence of a decrease in glomerular filtration rate [94]. Ten years later, Brenner et al. [58] discovered and developed the animal model required to access directly the vascular components of superficial glomeruli. This has permitted several investigators to study the effects of alterations in sodium intake on the determinants of glomerular filtration. Sodium deprivation resulted in a decrease in SNGFR, associated with a decrease in renal plasma flow (Q_A) and in glomerular capillary filtration coefficient (K_f) [411,435]. Administration of a competitive antagonist of angiotensin II [411] or of a converting enzyme inhibitor [435] resulted in a return to a normal Q_A but not K_f. Chronic sodium depletion was also found to alter Q_A and K_f, but not SNGFR [379]. The lack of changes in SNGFR was apparently due to the modulating effect of vasodilator prostaglandins, because administration of inhibitors of prostaglandin synthesis produced a marked fall in GFR.

Tubular Control of Sodium Reabsorption
Physical Factors

Decreasing the protein concentration either by addition of isotonic saline to the blood perfusing an isolated heart-lung kidney preparation [408] or by plasmapheresis [445]

was found to result in an increase in sodium excretion. That renal perfusion pressure affects reabsorption of sodium was first suggested by Cushney [86] and supported by the whole animal studies of Shipley and Study [394], and Selkurt [388]. McDonald and deWardener [306] perfused an isolated kidney joined to the circulation of a dog before, during, and after the dog had received a standard intravenous infusion of saline. They found that the increase in sodium excretion by the perfused kidney was directly related to the renal arterial pressure. Earley and Fridler and their co-workers [88,108–113,299] produced unilateral renal vasodilation by infusing acetylcholine into the renal artery. This maneuver produced the expected increase in renal blood flow and in sodium excretion. They then infused either angiotensin or norepinephrine intravenously to raise the systemic arterial pressure to both kidneys. The increase in arterial pressure was accompanied by a further rise in sodium excretion from the vasodilated kidney, although the renal blood flow fell and the glomerular filtration rate did not change significantly. The contralateral kidney had a reduction in blood flow, no significant change in glomerular filtration rate, and no change in urinary sodium excretion. The authors concluded that the natriuretic effect was due to the increase in arterial perfusion pressure, which was probably associated with an increase in the interstitial volume of the kidney. Hypertension induced by bilateral carotid artery ligation and cervical vagotomy [256] and increase in renal venous pressure produced by renal vein occlusion [278] were found to decrease proximal sodium reabsorption. This latter set of experiments also revealed a relationship between the reabsorption of sodium from the proximal tubule and the filtration fraction and, thus, the peritubular plasma oncotic pressure.

Exploration of the relationship between oncotic pressure in the peritubular capillaries and proximal reabsorption of sodium was done by Spitzer and Windhager [405] and by Brenner and associates [54–57,59,89,122]. Perfusion of the peritubular capillaries with a saline solution resulted in a decrease in proximal reabsorptive rate, whereas perfusion with a solution containing 8% dextran increased oncotic pressure and resulted in an increase in reabsorption (Fig. 5-19). A direct relationship between the reabsorptive capacity of the proximal tubule and the oncotic pressure of the fluid perfusing the peritubular capillaries was found to exist [405]. Likewise, perfusion of the efferent arterioles with colloid-free Ringer's solution decreased absolute proximal reabsorption by 45% and fractional fluid reabsorption by 35%, while perfusion with hyperoncotic albumin increased the absolute reabsorption by 41% and the fractional reabsorption by 35%. Similar results have been reported in doubly perfused Necturus proximal tubules [157], perfused salamander proximal tubules [360], and in isolated perfused rabbit proximal tubules [211]. Green et al. [161] measured proximal tubular volume reabsorption when both the tubular lumen and the peritubular capillaries were perfused with Ringer's solution to which variable amounts of albumin had been added. The effects were asymmetrical (luminal vs. peritubular addition of albumin) and nonlinear. Addition of cyanide blunted the effect of oncotic pressure on sodium reabsorption. These results indicate that the effect of the colloid is not due simply to its oncotic force but also to a change in the ability of the proximal tubular

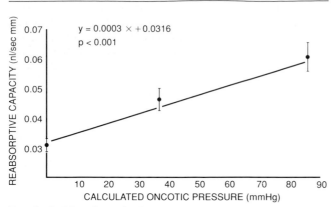

$y = 0.0003 \times + 0.0316$
$p < 0.001$

FIG. 5-19. *The relationship between the rate of fluid reabsorption and the oncotic pressure of the fluid perfusing the peritubular capillaries of rats. (From Spitzer A, Windhager EE: Effect of peritubular oncotic pressure changes on proximal fluid reabsorption. Am J Physiol 218:1188, 1970, with permission.)*

epithelium to transport sodium. It is assumed that the effect of peritubular protein concentration is mediated by changes in renal interstitial pressure, which, in turn, affects the pressure within the lateral intercellular spaces [283]. The mechanism by which this increase in intercellular space pressure results in the backflux of sodium across the tight junction is unknown.

Another hemodynamic mechanism whereby renal perfusion pressure inhibits tubular sodium reabsorption is through an increase in medullary blood flow. Enhanced medullary blood flow decreases sodium reabsorption by a washout mechanism [254]. This effect may be mediated by various hormones, such as prostaglandin E_2 and bradykinin. Carmines et al. [73] have reported that an increase in renal perfusion pressure correlates with an increase in the excretion of prostaglandin E_2 and sodium. Blockade of prostaglandin E_2 production has attenuated the effect of renal perfusion pressure on sodium excretion. These results point toward a relationship between physical and hormonal factors in the control of tubular sodium reabsorption.

Role of Intratubular Factors

There is evidence that the composition of the ultrafiltrate affects the rate of proximal tubular reabsorption. Bartoli and Earley [24] noted a 34% decrease in the reabsorptive rate when the renal tubules were perfused in vivo with a solution of glucose and bicarbonate. Likewise, Haberle et al. [177] noted a higher rate of reabsorption when the tubules were perfused with previously recollected tubular fluid than with Ringer's solution or with an ultrafiltrate of plasma. These authors also noted a correlation between perfusion and reabsorptive rates.

The flow dependence of proximal reabsorption was confirmed by several investigators [457]. It appears to be due to an increase in the transepithelial osmotic gradient, which is associated with an increase in perfusion rate [160].

The role of the intratubular factors in the control of sodium reabsorption under conditions of volume expansion or volume contraction is unknown.

Neural Control of Sodium Excretion

Claude Bernard was the first to report that transection of the great splanchnic nerve resulted in ipsilateral diuresis and that electrical stimulation of the sectioned end of the nerve reversed the diuretic effect [35]. This observation was amply confirmed by both surgical [26,28,30,31,36,39, 40,43,61,99,153,238,322,356,376,426,458] and pharmacologic denervation [206,371]. It was subsequently established that, to a large degree, the natriuretic effect of renal denervation is enhanced by anesthesia [356].

When the renal nerve was stimulated with low level electrical current (less than 1 Hz), there was a decrease in sodium excretion in the absence of changes in renal perfusion pressure, blood flow, glomerular filtration rate, or distribution of glomerular filtration [29,330,398,466]. At high frequencies of renal nerve stimulation (greater than 3 Hz) absolute proximal reabsorption decreased because of a fall in glomerular filtration rate [41]. There is controversy regarding the site of the nephron where this effect occurs. Bello-Reuss et al. [29] and Hermansson et al. [191] reported that renal nerve stimulation affects mainly the proximal reabsorption of sodium and water, a result that could not be confirmed by Kon and Ichikawa [263].

We have already described the effects of atrial distension, which are apparently due to a decrease in efferent renal nerve activity [341]. Stimulation of the stellate ganglion [341] and perfusion of the carotid sinus [466] are also associated with a decrease in nerve traffic and in sodium reabsorption. A recent contender in the modulation of tubular transport of sodium is dopamine, which apparently exerts an inhibitory effect on sodium reabsorption at the level of the pars recta [27].

Renal denervation does not affect urinary flow or sodium excretion in fetal lambs [349], whereas renal nerve stimulation (1 to 2 Hz) decreases sodium excretion to a similar extent in both fetal and adult sheep [348]. Chemical sympathectomy produced a natriuresis in 5-day-old but not in 20-day-old rats [15].

Alpha-adrenergic activity was found to predominate in the kidney of newborn animals [126]. Yet, alpha-adrenergic blockade resulted in greater natriuresis in adult than in young dogs [127]. This may be due either to enhanced reabsorption of sodium at sites distal to the proximal tubule or to the minimal dopaminergic activity present at this age [319], which may be responsible in part for the natriuresis of renal denervation.

A detailed discussion of the role of renal nerves in the modulation of sodium reabsorption can be found in Chapter 12.

Hormonal Control of Sodium Reabsorption

THE RENIN-ANGIOTENSIN-ALDOSTERONE SYSTEM

The role of mineralocorticoids in the maintenance of sodium balance was recognized more than 60 years ago by

Marine and Baumann [296]. It took another quarter of a century until aldosterone was discovered [396], and even longer until the role played by this hormone in edematous states was established [289]. Shortly thereafter, Barger et al. [23] and Ganong and Mulrow [135] described the essential features of the effect of aldosterone on the composition of urine. When aldosterone was injected into the renal artery of dogs, a latent period of some 20 minutes to 60 minutes elapsed before any effects were seen. After that latent period, sodium excretion was reduced, whereas the excretion of potassium and hydrogen ion increased. Despite this compelling evidence that aldosterone affects sodium reabsorption, many investigators have challenged the role of this hormone in the day-to-day regulation of sodium homeostasis. They argued that Addisonian patients are able to tolerate wide variations in sodium intake when maintained on a fixed dose of mineralocorticoids and that normal individuals given daily injections of mineralocorticoids have only a transient period of sodium retention, after which sodium balance is re-established [357]. Finally, dogs treated with aldosterone were found to respond appropriately to volume expansion [94].

It has been pointed out, however, that the evidence quoted herein simply indicates that factors other than mineralocorticoids are involved in the maintenance of sodium balance [387]. Yet, adrenalectomized animals maintained on a high sodium diet and a constant dose of mineralocorticoids, experienced substantially greater increments in extracellular fluid volume than did non-adrenalectomized animals, and became hypertensive. Conversely, adrenalectomized animals receiving a fixed dose of mineralocorticoid but ingesting a low sodium diet had a significant decrease in extracellular fluid volume [361,465]. In addition, adrenalectomized animals receiving low levels of aldosterone replacement were found to be volume-depleted when compared with non-adrenalectomized animals [464]. It is apparent, therefore, that aldosterone contributes to the maintenance of sodium and fluid homeostasis. Micropuncture studies [2,170,171,195] and microperfusion of isolated tubular segments [326,381,416] have localized the action of the hormone to the cortical collecting tubule, and this segment has been shown to contain aldosterone receptors [101,301,440].

There is as yet no consensus regarding the mechanism of action of aldosterone on the renal tubule. Some investigators have proposed that aldosterone stimulates the synthesis of an intracellular protein that increases the intracellular level of ATP [114,249,276]. Others maintain that the hormone increases the permeability of the luminal membrane [83,84,390], whereas a third group places the effect of aldosterone at the basolateral membrane, where it is supposed to stimulate Na^+-K^+-ATPase [203,255,375]. It is possible that the increase in luminal permeability results in enhanced entry of sodium into the cell, which stimulates Na^+-K^+-ATPase activity [338].

In the past, the role of angiotensin II in sodium homeostasis was considered to be limited to its effect on aldosterone synthesis and renal hemodynamics. It is now obvious, however, that angiotensin II affects tubular reabsorption of sodium directly, either through interactions with the sympathetic nervous system or through changes in peritubular capillary Starling forces [184,229,287]. Angiotensin II receptors have been identified in proximal tubular cell membranes [64], and the hormone has been reported to effect water and salt reabsorption in isolated perfused proximal tubular segments [380].

The Renin-Angiotensin-Aldosterone System During Development

All components of the renin-angiotensin-aldosterone system are elevated in the newborn. Kotchen et al. [265] documented high levels of renin in the plasma of infants. Similar findings have been reported by Drukker et al. [105] in puppies. The high plasma renin activity observed during infancy might be due to the presence of stimuli that enhance the synthetic rate of this enzyme, or it might be the result of a poorly developed feedback mechanism. Among the stimulatory factors that have been proposed are a low blood pressure [265], enhanced activity of the sympathetic nervous system [264], and increased sensitivity of the neonatal vasculature to the pressure effect of catecholamines [231]. The lack of appropriate modulation of the renin-angiotensin-aldosterone feedback system is suggested by the measurements of plasma renin activity [105] performed in puppies investigated for their response to infusion of isotonic saline [152] (Fig. 5-20). In all three age groups studied, a significant fall in plasma renin activity was noticed following volume expansion. The decrease was 60% in one-week-old puppies, 70% in two-week-old animals, and 80% in the oldest group. Similar changes were observed following administration of furosemide [158] and after peritoneal dialysis [433]. Thus, in the newborn, plasma renin activity changes in the appropriate direction in response to various stimuli. The degree of suppression following volume expansion, however, increases with age. The incomplete suppression, if attended by parallel changes in plasma aldosterone, might explain the less efficient excretion of a sodium load by the newborn as compared to the adult. Kowarski et al. [266] demonstrated that aldosterone secretion in the newborn is elevated when considered relative to body surface area. This elevation was associated with high plasma concentrations of aldosterone, presumably due to a combination of high secretion rates and low metabolic clearance rates relative to body size [25].

A link between the renin-angiotensin-aldosterone system and the positive sodium balance characteristic of the growing infant was suggested by the close relationship between the drop in plasma renin activity and the amount of sodium excreted in the urine observed in the experiments of Goldsmith et al. [152]. Two-week-old puppies excreted more sodium than three-week-old animals, showed the highest level of renin prior to loading, and underwent the largest absolute drop in plasma renin activity following the administration of the saline load. An inverse relationship between age and plasma aldosterone, on one hand, and between plasma aldosterone concentration and sodium excretion, on the other, was observed both in hydropenic and volume-expanded dogs [216] (Fig. 5-21).

The status of the renin-angiotensin-aldosterone system can also account for the sodium wasting and hyponatremia observed in premature, breast-fed infants during the first

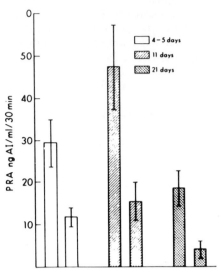

Fig. 5-20. *Plasma renin activity (PRA) before (left column) and after (right column) administration of isotonic sodium to canine puppies of various ages. Note the higher PRA and the larger fall in PRA in younger than in older animals. (From Drukker A, Lee HB, Edelmann CM Jr, et al: Radioimmunoassay of plasma renin activity in small and neonatal animals. Normal values, developmental patterns and response to acute intravenous saline load. In ZumWinkel K, Blaufox MD, Funck-Brentano JL (eds): Radionuclides in Nephrology. Stuttgart, Thieme, 1975, p 108, and Goldsmith DI, Drukker A, Blaufox MD, et al: Response of the neonatal canine kidney to acute saline expansion. In ZumWinkel K, Blaufox MD, Funck-Brentano JL (eds): Radionuclides in Nephrology. Stuttgart, Thieme, 1975, p 45, with permission.)*

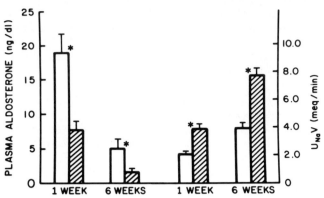

Fig. 5-21. *The effect of an infusion of NaCl solution equal to 10% of body weight on plasma aldosterone concentration and sodium excretion ($U_{Na}V$) of 1- and 6-week-old dogs. Note the inverse relationship between age and plasma aldosterone concentration and between plasma aldosterone concentration and sodium excretion. (From Ito Y, Goldsmith DI, Spitzer A: The role of aldosterone in renal electrolyte transport during development. Pediatr Res 18:370A, 1984, with permission.)*

few weeks of life [1,11,115,201,358,421]. These infants have been found to have high fractional excretion of sodium at any given filtered load [12,358,427] and higher stool losses of sodium than term infants [1]. Sulyok et al. [422–425,442] measured plasma renin activity, plasma aldosterone concentration, and urinary aldosterone excretion, along with sodium and potassium balances, in healthy neonates with gestational ages of 30 weeks to 41 weeks and weights of 1160 g to 4670 g (Fig. 5-22). The highest urinary sodium excretion rates during the first postnatal week were observed in infants of 30 weeks to 32 weeks gestational age (3.1±0.5 mEq/kg/day compared to 1.2±0.4 mEq/kg/day at 36 weeks to 38 weeks gestational age). These infants were in negative sodium balance (about 1 mEq/kg/day) and had the highest plasma renin activity (36.3±6.3 mg.ml^{-1}/h^{-1}) compared with 10.2±2.1 mg.ml^{-1}/h^{-1} in infants born after 39 weeks to 41 weeks gestation. Plasma aldosterone concentration, on the other hand, did not vary with gestational age and the urinary aldosterone excretion was lower in 30-week-old to 32-week-old infants (3.3±0.8 μg/day) than in 39-week-old to 41-week-old infants (7.8±1.4 μg/day). Thus, in response to sodium wasting and the subsequent negative sodium balance, premature infants augment their plasma renal activity to levels exceeding those found in term in-

fants, but their adrenal glands fail to synthesize aldosterone adequately in response to this stimulation.

A partial unresponsiveness of the distal nephron to aldosterone may also contribute to the sodium loss in the hyponatremia of prematurity. During the first three weeks of life, aldosterone excretion is at least as high in premature infants (range 18 to 105 μmol/1.73 m^2 BSA/day) as in term infants. Yet, the premature babies excrete much more sodium than their full-term counterparts, providing further evidence for the partial unresponsiveness of the distal nephron to aldosterone [354,355]. Under these circumstances, free water clearance approximates the reabsorption of NaCl at the distal diluting segment of the nephron. These studies revealed a lower fractional distal tubular reabsorption of sodium (81.9±8.2% SD), resulting in a higher clearance of sodium (2.3 ± 1.8 ml/dl GFR) in babies of 28 weeks to 34 weeks gestation than in neonates 35 weeks to 41 weeks gestational age (88.2±4.5% and 0.9±0.5 ml/dl GFR, respectively). Sulyok et al. [424] found lower values of fractional sodium reabsorption in the distal nephron during the first (69.5±2.4% SE) than during the second (83.7±1.9%) week of life in neonates 27 weeks to 35 weeks gestational age. However, maximal water diuresis was not achieved in these infants, resulting probably in an underestimation of distal sodium reabsorption. This increase occurred concomitantly with a rise in plasma aldosterone concentration and urinary aldosterone excretion from the already high values of 1.7±0.5 mg/ml and 2.6±0.4 ug/day, respectively, to the exceedingly elevated levels of 6.8±3.7 mg/ml and 26.4±2.9 μg/day [424]. Of note is the fact that even this degree of stimulation was insufficient to maintain external sodium balance, and the babies became hyponatremic.

These observations led us to postulate [403] that in growing infants the deposition of sodium, particularly in

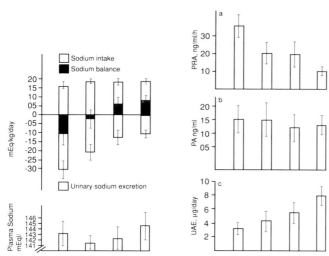

FIG. 5-22. *Sodium balance, plasma sodium concentration (left panel), plasma renin activity (PRA), plasma aldosterone concentration (PA), and urinary adosterone excretion (UAE) in infants of various gestational ages. (From Sulyok E, Nemeth M, Tenyi I, et al: Postnatal development of renin-angiotensin-aldosterone system. RAAS, in relation to electrolyte balance in premature infants. Pediatr Res 13:817, 1979, with permission.)*

bones, creates a state of continuous stimulation for renin release. This in turn increases the amount of circulating angiotensin, which stimulates the production of aldosterone, thereby enhancing the tubular reabsorption of sodium. It is reasonable to assume that during a later period of extrauterine development the rapid rise in GFR observed in the superficial nephrons [404] creates a tendency toward urinary sodium loss. This could lead to the further stimulation of the renin-angiotensin-aldosterone system observed to occur around two or three weeks of age [104,424]. When the rise in aldosterone is insufficient or the distal tubule is unable to respond adequately to this stimulus, as is the case in prematurely born infants, renal loss of sodium and hyponatremia ensue. During a subsequent period of postnatal development, the absolute reabsorption of sodium in the proximal tubule and the intrinsic capacity for reabsorption of the distal tubule rise, resulting in a progressive diminution of the stimuli for renin release and, consequently, a decrease in aldosterone production. Acceptance of this hypothesis should not be construed to imply that other adaptive mechanisms, whether hormonal, neural, or physical in nature, do not play a role in the maintenance of sodium homeostasis during development.

PROSTAGLANDINS

There is little doubt that the prostaglandins play an important role in modulating the response of the renal vasculature to changes in sodium balance. Many of the prostaglandins are either synthesized or metabolized in the kidney. PGE_2 is synthesized by interstitial collecting duct cells located in the renal medulla, and its synthesis is stimulated by angiotensin II [470]. PGI_2 is synthesized by

vascular endothelial cells, largely within the renal cortex, and it apparently mediates baroreceptor but not beta-adrenergic stimulation of renin release [33,133,456]. Both PGE_2 and PGI_2 have a vasodilating effect and antagonize the vasoconstrictor effects of thromboxane A_2 and angiotensin II on the renal vasculature [470], although the latter effect is apparently manifest only under conditions of sodium depletion [190,318].

There is much less certainty regarding the tubular effects of prostaglandins. Studies in whole animals are always open to criticism because of the possible effect of prostaglandins on renal hemodynamics. In addition, whereas some investigators have found that prostaglandin inhibition results in an increase in urinary sodium excretion [145,251,441], others have reported that prostaglandins either have no effect on sodium excretion or are natriuretic [4,118, 197,467].

The in vitro studies are also inconclusive. Some investigators found that PGE_2 increased sodium reabsorption in the toad bladder [285], whereas others reported that PGE_2 inhibits sodium reabsorption in the cortical collecting tubule and the outer medullary collecting duct [469]. Other investigators were unable to detect any effect of PGE, PGA, or PGF on sodium transport [107,128,129]. Therefore, it is fair to conclude that the established role of prostaglandins appears to be confined to their effects on vascular tone.

There is a considerable literature on the status of the prostaglandin system during infancy. Synthesis and metabolism of prostaglandins have been identified as early as fetal life [91,132,332,340,402]. The urinary excretion of PGF_2 $PGF_{2\alpha}$ is high during fetal life and decreases following birth [347,350]. Likewise, the excretion PGE_2 and $PGF_{1\alpha}$ is greater in preterm than in term infants and greater in term infants than in older children [17]. The plasma levels of PGE_2 and $PGF_{2\alpha}$ are high in preterm infants and decrease thereafter, the decrease being accelerated by supplementation of the diet with sodium [119]. It appears, therefore, that, as in adults, the levels of vasodilator prostaglandins are elevated in sodium depletion.

It has been speculated that the high levels of prostaglandins prevailing in infants may account for their limited capacity to concentrate the urine [449]. However, the synthesis of PGE was found to be similar in cortical and medullary collecting tubules of young and adult rabbits [372], and inhibition of prostaglandin synthesis failed to increase the concentrating ability of fetal lambs [302].

Thus, the high levels of prostaglandins in the newborn and infant appear mainly related to the high level of angiotensin II prevailing during this period of life and may contribute to the maintenance of adequate rates of renal blood flow. As in the adult, there is no evidence or a role of prostaglandins in sodium homeostasis.

KININS AND KALLIKREIN

Kinins are generated by the proteolysis of kininogen by kallikrein [150]. The kinins are inactivated by two kinases, kininase I, which is a carboxypeptidase, and kininase II, which is a peptidyl dipeptide hydrolase (angiotensin converting enzyme). Inhibition of kininase II prevents the breakdown of kinins while decreasing angiotensin II production, resulting in a fall in systemic blood pressure [384].

Renal kallikrein release can be stimulated by the administration of mineralocorticoids, angiotensin II, and PGE₂ [74]. High levels of urinary kallikrein have been found in primary hyperaldosteronism and Bartter's syndrome [181]. The potent vasodilatory effect of bradykinin appears to be at least partially mediated by PGE₂ [179]. Their effect, if any, on the transport of sodium is exerted at sites other than the proximal tubule of the superficial nephrons [409].

The excretion rates of kinins and kallikreins are low in newborns and increase with age [147,347,432]. Kinins are considered as possible mediators of neonatal circulatory changes [308] and of the increase in blood pressure and glomerular filtration rate observed with age [397,469]. No relationship has been found between urinary kallikrein and sodium excretion in infants or children [147].

NATRIURETIC HORMONES

The search for a natriuretic substance was spearheaded by the experiments of deWardener and co-workers [94], who found that saline expansion produced a brisk natriuresis in the absence of increased glomerular filtration and in the presence of fixed amounts of mineralocorticoids. This observation was followed by a flurry of activity that continues to this day. Until recently, most of the evidence provided by these studies has been conjectural. On balance, the evidence favored the existence of at least two groups of substances with natriuretic properties: one originating in the hypothalamus and the other in the cardiac atria. During the last few years, the characteristics of the atrial natriuretic hormones have been precisely defined from a chemical and genetic point of view, whereas those of the hypothalamic hormone are still being sought.

The initial search for the existence of a circulating natriuretic substance was based on cross-circulation experiments and experiments in which either transplanted kidneys or isolated perfused kidneys were used in an attempt to control the composition of the perfusate. These experiments established that an increase in sodium excretion occurs in volume expansion in the absence of nervous system activity or detectable changes in GFR or RBF [20,235,279,431]. Efforts were then made to determine whether plasma [79,323] or ultrafiltrates of plasma [63,66,172,345] were able to duplicate the effects of volume expansion. The results favoring the existence of a circulating inhibitor of sodium reabsorption have been more successful when whole plasma, rather than its ultrafiltrate, was used.

Attempts to extract the natriuretic substance from plasma, urine, and brain have been conflicting. Some investigators isolated a substance with a molecular weight greater than 30,000 daltons [148,272,336,385,446], whereas others isolated a substance with a molecular weight of only 1,000 [60,65,77,80,125,172,267,280,386,446]. The chemical properties of either of these substances were not consistent [51,78,82,173,174,268]. More recently, attention has focused on a low molecular weight substance found to be present in human uremic urine and plasma,

which inhibits active sodium transport in the urinary bladder of the toad [53,237]. The origin of this substance appears to be the central nervous system [81], specifically in the hypothalamus [72]. This substance was found to affect ion transport in toad urinary bladder, and to have a high affinity for Na^+-K^+-ATPase in vitro [186]. The hypothalamic factor was also found specifically and reversibly to inhibit Na^+-K^+-ATPase [72,186]. There is still controversy as to whether the hypothalamic factor is a peptide [52,172,185,198,269] or a non-peptide molecule [78,187, 281,282].

A great deal of attention has been placed on the second group of natriuretic substances that originate in the cardiac atria. The search for these substances was generated by the observation that a number of specific granules, which share the electron microscopic characteristics of secretory granules found in endocrine cells [42,70,223], increase in number under conditions of sodium depletion and diminish when sodium chloride or DOCA is administered [92,295]. Homogenates of atria were found to have a natriuretic action [93,434] that was not associated with changes in total or single nephron GFR [62,400]. The mode of action of so-called atrial natriuretic hormone is unclear. It does not inhibit Na^+-K^+-ATPase [284,339,429], but appears to have a vasodilatory effect, particularly in the medullary and papillary areas [44].

Several atrial peptides containing between 23 and 38 amino acids have been identified that possess marked natriuretic activity [130,236,430]. The gene for the antinatriuretic factor has been localized and sequenced, and the protein precursors of the polypeptide and the polypeptide species itself have been identified [290]. The physiological relevance of this atrial peptide is yet to be determined. It would appear that circulating levels of atrial natriuretic peptides increase in response to extracellular fluid volume expansion and that removal of the atrial appendices, the primary source of production, blunts the natriuresis induced by acute volume expansion [141].

Solomon [399] was among the first to postulate that the limited capacity of the newborn animal and human to excrete a sodium load is related to the absence of a circulating natriuretic substance. This investigator volume-expanded young rats by infusing blood obtained either from rats of the same age or from adult rats. A brisk natriuresis was observed after the infusion of blood from either age group, but the rise in urinary sodium excretion was substantially greater after the infusion of the blood from the adult animals. These findings were later confirmed by Krecek et al. [270].

The levels of plasma immunoreactive atrial natriuretic peptide is higher in newborn than in the cord blood [217] (Fig. 5-23) and higher in premature, low-birth-weight than in term infants [389,436]. No correlation, however, was found between the plasma concentration of atrial natriuretic factor and urinary sodium excretion, although the immature kidney was shown to be responsive to the effect of the peptide [393].

Summarizing the evidence to date, Laragh [275] identified four sites at which the atrial natriuretic factor may affect the renin-angiotensin-aldosterone system: (1) the

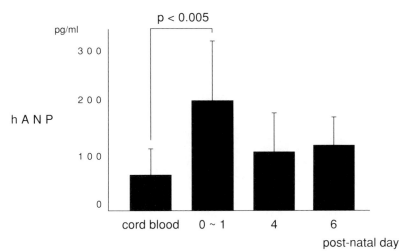

FIG. 5-23. *Concentration (mean ± SD) of natriuretic peptide in the cord blood and plasma of newborns. (From Ito Y, Matsumoto T, Ohbu K, et al: Concentrations of human atrial natriuretic peptide in the cord blood in the plasma of the newborn. Acta Pediatr Scand 77:76, 1988, with permission.)*

conversion of renin substrate to angiotensin I; (2) the stimulation of aldosterone release by angiotensin II; (3) the promotion of renal sodium retention by aldosterone; and (4) the vasoconstrictor effect of angiotensin II. If this applies to the infant, then it is conceivable that the high levels of natriuretic factors found in the newborn may override the effect of the high aldosterone level prevailing at this age and induce a natriuresis [217].

References

1. Al-Dahhan J, Haycock GB, Nichol B, et al: Sodium homeostasis in term and preterm infants. III. The effects of salt supplementation. *Arch Dis Child* 59:945, 1984.
2. Allen GG, Barratt LJ: Effect of aldosterone on the transepithelial potential difference of the rat distal tubule. *Kidney Int* 19:678, 1981.
3. Alpern RJ, Chambers M: Basolateral membrane Cl/HCO₃ exchange in rat proximal convoluted tubule. Na-dependent and independent modes. *J Gen Physiol* 89:581, 1987.
4. Altscheler P, Klahr S, Rosenbaum R, et al: Effects of inhibitors of prostaglandin synthesis on renal sodium excretion in normal dogs and dogs with decreased renal mass. *Am J Physiol (Renal Fluid Electrolyte Physiology 4)*235:F338, 1978.
5. Anagnostopoulos T, Planelles G: Organic anion permeation at the proximal tubule of Necturus. *Pflugers Arch* 381:231, 1979.
6. Anagnostopoulos T, Kinney M, Windhager EE: Salt and water reabsorption by loops of Henle during renal vein constriction. *Am J Physiol* 220:1060, 1971.
7. Andersson B: Central control of body fluid homeostasis. *Proc Aust Physiol Pharmacol Soc* 5:139, 1974.
8. Andreoli TE, Schafer JA, Troutman SL, et al: Solvent drag component of Cl⁻ flux in superficial proximal straight tu-

bules: Evidence for a paracellular component of isotonic fluid absorption. *Am J Physiol (Renal Fluid Electrolyte Physiology 6)*237:F455, 1979.
9. Aperia A, Broberger O, Herin P, et al: A comparative study of the response to an oral NaCl and NaHCO₃ load in newborn preterm and full term infants. *Pediatr Res* 11:1109, 1977.
10. Aperia A, Broberger O, Herin P, et al: Sodium excretion in relation to sodium intake and aldosterone in newborn pre-term and full-term infants. *Acta Paediatr Scand* 68:813, 1979.
11. Aperia A, Broberger O, Thodenius K, et al: Renal response to an oral sodium load in newborn full-term infants. *Acta Paediatr Scand* 61:670, 1972.
12. Aperia A, Broberger O, Thodenius K, et al: Developmental study of the renal response to an oral salt load in preterm infants. *Acta Paediatr Scand* 63:517, 1974.
13. Aperia A, Broberger O, Thodenius K, et al: Development of renal control of salt and fluid homeostasis during the first year of life. *Acta Paediatr Scand* 64:393, 1975.
14. Aperia A, Elinder G: Distal tubular sodium reabsorption in the developing rat kidney. *Am J Physiol (Renal Fluid Electrolyte Physiology 9)*240:F487, 1981.
15. Appenroth D, Braunlich H: Effect of sympathectomy with 6-hydroxy dopamine on the renal excretion of water and electrolytes in developing rats. *Acta Biol Med Ger* 40:1715, 1981.
16. Arant BS: Developmental patterns of renal functional maturation compared in the human neonate. *J Pediatr* 92:705, 1978.
17. Arant BS Jr: Renal disorders of the newborn infant. *Pediatr Nephrol* 12:111, 1984.
18. Arborelius M, Balldin UI, Lilja B, et al: Hemodynamic changes in man during immersion with the head above water. *Aerosp Med* 43:592, 1972.
19. August JT, Nelson DH, Thorn, GW: Response of normal subjects to large amounts of aldosterone. *J Clin Invest* 37:1549, 1958.

20. Bahlman NJ, McDonald SJ, Ventom MG, et al: The effect on urinary sodium excretion of blood volume expansion without changing the composition of blood in the dog. *Clin Sci* 32:403, 1967.

21. Barac-Nieto M, Murer H, Kinne R: Lactate-sodium cotransport in rat renal brush border membranes. *Am J Physiol* (Renal Fluid Electrolyte Physiology 8)239:F496, 1980.

22. Barfuss DW, Schafer JA: Active amino acid absorption by proximal convoluted and proximal straight tubules. *Am J Physiol* (Renal Fluid Electrolyte Physiology 5)236:F149, 1979.

23. Barger AC, Berlin RD, Tulenko JF: Infusion of aldosterone, 9-alpha fluorohydrocortisone and antidiuretic hormone into the renal artery of normal and adrenalectomized unanesthetized dogs: Effect on electrolyte and water excretion. *Endocrinology* 62:804, 1958.

24. Bartoli E, Earley LE: Importance of ultrafilterable plasma factors in maintaining tubular reabsorption. *Kidney Int* 3:142, 1973.

25. Beitins IZ, Bayard F, Levitsky L, et al: Plasma aldosterone concentration at delivery and during the newborn period. *J Clin Invest* 51:386, 1972.

26. Bello-Reuss E, Colindres RE, Pastoriza-Munoz E, et al: Effects of acute unilateral denervation in the rat. *J Clin Invest* 56:208, 1975.

27. Bello-Reuss E, Higashi Y, Kaneda Y: Dopamine decreases fluid reabsorption in straight portions of rabbit proximal tubule. *Am J Physiol* (Renal Fluid Electrolyte Physiology 11)242:F634, 1982.

28. Bello-Reuss E, Pastoriza-Munoz E, Colindres RE: Acute unilateral renal denervation in rats with extracellular volume expansion. *Am J Physiol* (Renal Fluid Electrolyte Physiology 1)232:F26, 1977.

29. Bello-Reuss E, Trevino DL, Gottschalk CW: Effect of renal sympathetic nerve stimulation on proximal water and sodium reabsorption. *J Clin Invest* 57:1104, 1976.

30. Bencsath P, Asztalos B, Szalay L, et al: Renal handling of sodium after chronic renal sympathectomy in the anesthetized rat. *Am J Physiol* (Renal Fluid Electrolyte Physiology 5)236:F513, 1979.

31. Bencsath P, Szalay L, Demeczky L, et al: Effects of chlorothiazide and furosemide on sodium and water excretion after unilateral splanchnicotomy in the dog. *Nephron* 8:329, 1971.

32. Bengele HH, Lechene C, Alexander EA: Sodium and chloride transport along the inner medullary collecting duct: Effect of saline expansion. *Am J Physiol* (Renal Fluid Electrolyte Physiology 7)238:F504, 1980.

33. Berl T, Henrich WL, Erickson AL, et al: Prostaglandins in the beta adrenergic and baroreceptor-mediated secretion of renin. *Am J Physiol* (Renal Fluid Electrolyte Physiology 5)236:F472, 1979.

34. Bermudez DE, Windhager EE: Osmotically induced changes in electrical resistance of distal tubules of rat kidney. *Am J Physiol* 229:1536, 1975.

35. Bernard C: *Lecons sur les proprietes physiologiques des dechets de l'organisme.* Paris, Balliere, 1859.

36. Berne RM: Hemodynamics and sodium excretion of denervated kidney in anesthetized and unanesthetized dogs. *Am J Physiol* 171:148, 1952.

37. Berry CA, Cogan MG: Influence of peritubular protein on solute absorption in the rabbit proximal tubule. *J Clin Invest* 68:506, 1981.

38. Berry CA, Warnock DG, Rector FC, Jr: Ion selectivity and proximal salt reabsorption. *Am J Physiol* (Renal Fluid Electrolyte Physiology 4)235:F234, 1978.

39. Blake WD: Relative roles of glomerular filtration and tubular reabsorption in denervation diuresis. *Am J Physiol* 202:777, 1962.

40. Blake WD, Jurf AN: Renal sodium reabsorption after acute renal denervation in the rabbit. *J Physiol* (Lond) 196:65, 1968.

41. Blantz RC, Pelayo JC: In vivo actions of angiotensin II on glomerular function. *Fed Proc* 42:3071, 1983.

42. Bompiani GD, Rouiller C, Hatt PY: Le tissue de conduction de coeur chez le rat. Etude en microscope electronique. *Arch Mal Coeur* 52:1257, 1959.

43. Bonjour JP, Churchill PC, Malvin RL: Change of tubular reabsorption of sodium and water after renal denervation in the dog. *J Physiol* (Lond) 204:571, 1969.

44. Borenstein HB, Cupples WA, Sonnenberg H, et al: The effect of a natriuretic atrial extract on renal haemodynamics and urinary excretion in anaesthetized rats. *J Physiol* (Lond) 334:133, 1983.

45. Bott PA: Micropuncture study of renal excretion of water K, Na, and Cl in Necturus. *Am J Physiol* 203:662, 1962.

46. Boulpaep EL: Permeability changes of the proximal tubule of Necturus during saline loading. *Am J Physiol* 222:517, 1972.

47. Boulpaep EL: Electrical phenomena in the nephron. *Kidney Int* 9:88, 1976.

48. Boulpaep EL: Electrophysiology of the kidney. *In* Giebisch G, Tosteson DC, Ussing HH (eds): *Membrane Transport in Biology. Vol IVA. Transport Organs.* New York, Springer-Verlag, 1979, p 97.

49. Boulpaep EL, Seely JF: Electrophysiology of proximal and distal tubules in the autoperfused dog kidney. *Am J Physiol* 221:1084, 1971.

50. Bourdeau JE, Burg MB: Voltage dependence on calcium transport in the thick ascending limb of Henle's loop. *Am J Physiol* (Renal Fluid Electrolyte Physiology 5)236:F357, 1979.

51. Bourgoignie J, Kaplan M, Eun C, et al: On the characterization of natriuretic factors. *Clin Res* 23:429A, 1975.

52. Bourgoignie JJ, Favre H, Kaplan MA, et al: On the natriuretic factor of serum and urine from patients with chronic uraemia. *In* Kaufman W, Krause DK (eds): *International Workshop at Cologne on Central Nervous Control of Na⁺ Balance: Relation to the Renin-Angiotensin System.* Stuttgart, Thieme, 1976, p 133.

53. Bourgoignie JJ, Klahr S, Bricker NS: Inhibition of transepithelial sodium transport in the frog skin by a low molecular weight fraction of uremic serum. *J Clin Invest* 50:303, 1971.

54. Brenner BM, Falchuk KH, Keimowitz IR, et al: The relationship between peritubular capillary protein concentration and fluid reabsorption by the renal proximal tubule. *J Clin Invest* 48:1519, 1969.

55. Brenner BM, Galla JH: Influence of postglomerular hematocrit and protein concentration on rat nephron fluid transfer. *Am J Physiol* 220:148, 1971.

56. Brenner BM, Troy JL: Postglomerular vascular protein concentration: Evidence for causal role in governing fluid reabsorption and glomerular tubular balance by the renal proximal tubule. *J Clin Invest* 50:336, 1971.

57. Brenner BM, Troy JL, Daugharty TM: On the mechanism of inhibition of fluid reabsorption by the renal proximal tubule of the volume expanded rat. *J Clin Invest* 50:1596, 1971.

58. Brenner BM, Troy JL, Daugharty TM: The dynamics of glomerular ultrafiltration in the rat. *J Clin Invest* 50:1776, 1971.

59. Brenner BM, Troy JL, Daugharty TM: Quantitative importance of changes in postglomerular colloid osmotic pressure

in mediating glomerular tubular balance in the rat. *J Clin Invest* 52:190, 1973.

60. Bricker NS, Licht A: Natriuretic hormone: Biologic effects and progress in identification and isolation. *In* Lichardus B, Schrier RW, Ponec J (eds): *Hormonal Regulation of Sodium Excretion.* Amsterdam, Elsevier/North Holland Biomedical Press, 1980, p 399.

61. Bricker NS, Staffon RA, Mahoney EP, et al: The functional capacity of the kidney denervated by autotransplantation in the dog. *J Clin Invest* 37:185, 1958.

62. Briggs JP, Steipe B, Schubert G, et al: Micropuncture studies of the renal effects of atrial natriuretic substance. *Pflugers Arch* 395:271, 1982.

63. Brown DC, DuBois M, Knock CA, et al: Absence of antinatriferic and natriuretic activity in plasma ultrafiltrates (mol. wt. less than 50,000) and dialysates from volume expanded dogs. *Kidney Int* 6:388, 1974.

64. Brown GP, Douglas JG: Angiotensin II-binding sites in rat and primate isolated renal tubular basolateral membranes. *Endocrinology* 112:2007, 1983.

65. Buckalew VM Jr, Lancaster CD Jr: Studies of a humoral sodium transport inhibitor in normal dogs and dogs with ligation of the inferior vena cava. *Circ Res* (suppl II)28–29:II-44, 1971.

66. Buckalew VM Jr, Martinez J, Green WE: The effect of dialysates and ultrfiltrates of plasma of saline-loaded dogs on toad bladder sodium transport. *J Clin Invest* 49:926, 1970.

67. Burg MB, Green N: Function of the thick ascending limb of Henle's loop. *Am J Physiol* 224:659, 1973.

68. Burg MB, Isaacson L, Grantham Y, et al: Electrical properties of isolated perfused rabbit tubules. *Am J Physiol* 215:788, 1968.

69. Cameron G, Chambers R: Direct evidence of function in kidney of an early human fetus. *Am J Physiol* 123:482, 1938.

70. Cantin M, Huet M: Chemical nature of atrial specific granules. *In* Fleckenstein A, Rona G (eds): *Recent Advances in Studies on Cardiac Structure and Metabolism. Pathophysiology and Morphology of Myocardial Cell Alterations.* Baltimore, University Park Press, 1975, p 313.

71. Capek K, Rumrich G, Ullrich KJ: Harnstoff-Permeabilitat der cortikalen Tubulusabschnitte von Ratten in Antidiurese und Wasserdiurese. *Pflugers Arch* 290:237, 1966.

72. Carilli CT, Berne M, Cantley LC, et al: Hypothalamic factor inhibits the (Na,K) ATPase from the extracellular surface: Mechanism of inhibition. *J Biol Chem* 260:1027, 1985.

73. Carmines PK, Bell PD, Roman RJ, et al: Prostaglandins in the excretory response to altered renal arterial pressure in dogs. *Am J Physiol* 242:F8, 1985.

74. Carretero OA, Scicli AG: The renal kallikrein-kinin system. *Am J Physiol* (Renal Fluid Electrolyte Physiology 7)238:F247, 1980.

75. Celsi G, Larsson L, Aperia A: Proximal tubular reabsorption and Na-K-ATPase activity in remnant kidney of young rats. *Am J Physiol* (Renal Fluid Electrolyte Physiology 20)251:F588, 1986.

76. Clapp JR, Watson JF, Berliner RW: Osmolality, bicarbonate concentration and water reabsorption in proximal tubule of dog nephron. *Am J Physiol* 205:273, 1963.

77. Clarkson EM, Raw SM, deWardener, HE: Two natriuretic substances in extracts of urine from normal man when salt-depleted and salt-loaded. *Kidney Int* 10:381, 1976.

78. Clarkson EM, Raw SM, deWardener HE: Further observations on a low-molecular weight natriuretic substance in the urine of normal man. *Kidney Int* 16:710, 1979.

79. Clarkson EM, Young DR, Raw SM, et al: The effect of plasma from blood volume expanded dogs on sodium, po-

tassium and PAH transport of renal tubule fragments. *Clin Sci* 38:617, 1970.

80. Clarkson EM, Young DR, Raw SM, et al: Chemical properties, physiological action and further separation of a low molecular weight natriuretic substance in the urine of normal man. *In* Lichardus B, Schrier RW, Ponec J (eds): *Hormonal Regulation of Sodium Excretion.* Amsterdam, Elsevier/North Holland Biomedical Press, 1980, p 333.

81. Cort JH, Rudinger J, Lichardus B, et al: Effects of oxytocin antagonists on the saliuresis accompanying carotid occlusion. *Am J Physiol* 210:162, 1966.

82. Cort MG, Pliska V, Dousa T: The chemical nature and tissue source of the natriuretic hormone. *Lancet* 1:230, 1968.

83. Crabbe J: Site of action of aldosterone on the bladder of the toad. *Nature* 20:787, 1963.

84. Crabbe J: Decreased sensitivity to amiloride of amphibian epithelia treated with aldosterone. Further evidence for an apical hormonal effect. *Pflugers Arch* 383:151, 1980.

85. Crayen M, Thoenes W: Architektur und cytologische Characterisierung des distalen Tubulus der Ratteniere. *Fortschr Zool* 23:270, 1975.

86. Cushny AR: *The Secretion of Urine.* London, Longmans, 1917.

87. Danielson BG, Persson E, Ulfendahl HR: The transport of halide ions across the membrane of distal rat tubules. *Acta Physiol Scand* 78:347, 1970.

88. Daugharty TM, Belleau LJ, Martino JA, et al: Interrelationship of physical factors affecting sodium reabsorption in the dog. *Am J Physiol* 215:1442, 1968.

89. Daugharty TM, Ueki IF, Nicholas DP: Comparative renal effects of isotonic and colloid-free volume expansion in the rat. *Am J Physiol* 222:225, 1972.

90. Davis JO: The control of renin release. *Am J Med* 55:333, 1973.

91. Day NA, Atallah AA, Lee, JB: Presence of prostaglandin A and F in fetal kidney. *Prostaglandins* 5:491, 1974.

92. De Bold AJ: Heart atria granularity. Effects of changes in water-electrolyte balance. *Proc Soc Exp Biol Med* 161:508, 1979.

93. De Bold AJ, Salerno TA: Natriuretic activity of extracts obtained from hearts of different species and from various rat tissues. *Can J Physiol Pharmacol* 61:127, 1983.

94. deWardener HE, Mills IH, Clapham WF, et al: Studies on the efferent mechanism of sodium diuresis which follows the intravenous administration of saline in the dog. *Clin Sci* 21:249, 1961.

95. Dean RFA, McCance RA: The renal response of infants and adults to the administration of hypertonic solutions of sodium chloride and urea. *J Physiol* (Lond) 109:81, 1949.

96. deRouffignac C: Physiological role of the loop of Henle in urinary concentration. *Kidney Int* 2:297, 1972.

97. deRouffignac C, Morel F: Micropuncture study of water, electrolyte and urea movements along to loops of Henle in Psammomys. *J Clin Invest* 48:474, 1969.

98. DeTorrente A, Robertson G, McDonald KM, et al: Mechanism of diuretic response to increased left atrial pressure in the anesthetized dog. *Kidney Int* 8:355, 1975.

99. DiBona GF: The function of the renal nerves. *Rev Physiol Biochem Pharmacol* 94:76, 1982.

100. Diezi J, Michoud P, Aceves J, et al: Micropuncture study of electrolyte transport across papillary collecting duct of the rat. *Am J Physiol* 224:623, 1973.

101. Doucet A, Katz AI: Mineralocorticoid receptors along the nephron: 30H-aldosterone binding in rabbit tubules. *Am J Physiol* (Renal Fluid Electrolyte Physiology 10)241:F605, 1981.

102. Doucet A, Katz AI: Short-term effect of aldosterone on Na-

K-ATPase in single nephron segments. *Am J Physiol* (Renal Fluid Electrolyte Physiology 10)241:F273, 1981.

103. Doucet A, Katz AI, Morel F: Determination of Na-K-ATPase activity in single segments of the mammalian nephron. *Am J Physiol* (Renal Fluid Electrolyte Physiology 6)237:F105, 1979.

104. Drukker A, Goldsmith DI, Spitzer A, et al: The renin angiotensin system in newborn dogs: Developmental patterns and response to acute saline loading. *Pediatr Res* 14:304, 1980.

105. Drukker A, Lee HB, Edelmann CM Jr, et al: Radioimmunoassay of plasma renin activity in small and neonatal animals. Normal values, developmental patterns and response to acute intravenous saline load. In ZumWinkel K, Blaufox MD, Funck-Brentano JL (eds): *Radionuclides in Nephrology.* Stuttgart, Thieme, 1975, p 108.

106. DuBose TD Jr, Seldin DW, Kokko JP: Segmental chloride reabsorption in the rat nephron as a function of load. *Am J Physiol* (Renal Fluid Electrolyte Physiology 3)234:F97, 1978.

107. Dunn MJ, Howe D: Prostaglandins lack a direct inhibitory action on electrolyte and water transport in the kidney and the erythrocyte. *Prostaglandins* 13:417, 1977.

108. Earley LE: Influence of hemodynamic factors on sodium reabsorption. *Ann NY Acad Sci* 139:312, 1966.

109. Earley LE, Daugharty TM: Sodium metabolism. *N Engl J Med* 281:72, 1969.

110. Earley LE, Friedler RM: Observations on the mechanism of decreased tubular reabsorption of sodium and water during saline loading. *J Clin Invest* 43:1928, 1964.

111. Earley LE, Friedler RM: Changes in renal blood flow and possibly the intrarenal distribution of blood during the natriuresis accompanying saline loading in the dog. *J Clin Invest* 44:929, 1965.

112. Earley LE, Friedler RM: The effects of combined renal vasodilation and pressor agents on renal hemodynamics and the tubular reabsorption of sodium. *J Clin Invest* 45:542, 1966.

113. Earley LE, Martino JA, Friedler RM: Factors affecting sodium reabsorption by the proximal tubule as determined during blockade of distal sodium reabsorption. *J Clin Invest* 45:1668, 1966.

114. Edelmann IS, Bororoch R, Porter GA: On the mechanism of action of aldosterone on sodium transport: The role of protein synthesis. *Pflugers Arch* 300:244, 1968.

115. Engelke SC, Shah BL, Vasan U, et al: Sodium balance in very low-birth-weight infants. *J Pediatr* 93:837, 1978.

116. Epstein FH, Post RS, McDowell M: Effects of an arteriovenous fistula on renal hemodynamics and electrolyte excretion. *J Clin Invest* 32:233, 1953.

117. Epstein M, Duncan DC, Fishman LM: Characterization of the natriuresis caused in normal man by immersion in water. *Clin Sci* 43:275, 1972.

118. Epstein M, Lifschitz MD, Hoffman DS, et al: Relationship between renal prostaglandin E and renal sodium handling during water immersion in normal man. *Circ Res* 45:71, 1979.

119. Ertl T, Sulyok E, Nemeth M, et al: The effect of sodium chloride supplementation on the postnatal development of plasma prostaglandin E and $F_{2\alpha}$ values in premature infants. *J Pediatr* 101:761, 1982.

120. Evan AP, Gattone VH II, Schwartz GJ: Development of solute transport in rabbit proximal tubule. II. Morphologic segmentation. *Am J Physiol* (Renal Fluid Electrolyte Physiology 14)245:F391, 1983.

121. Evers J, Murer H, Kinne R: Phenylalanine uptake by isolated renal brush border vesicles. *Biochim Biophys Acta* 426:598, 1976.

122. Falchuk KH, Brenner BM, Tadokoro M: Oncotic and hydrostatic pressure in peritubular capillaries and fluid reabsorption by proximal tubule. *Am J Physiol* 220:1427, 1971.

123. Farman N, Vandewalle A, Bonvalet JP: Aldosterone binding in isolated tubules. II. An autoradiography study of concentration dependency in the rabbit nephron. *Am J physiol* (Renal Fluid Electrolyte Physiology 11)242:F69, 1982.

124. Farman N, Vandewalle A, Bonvalet JP: Binding sites of mineralo- and glucocorticoids along the mammalian nephron (rat and rabbit). In Morel F (ed): *Biochemistry of Kidney Functions, INSERM Symposium No. 21.* Amsterdam, Elsevier, 1982, p 285.

125. Favre H, Hwang KH, Schmidt RW, et al: An inhibitor of sodium transport in the urine of dogs with normal renal function. *J Clin Invest* 56:1302, 1975.

126. Felder RA, Pelayo JC, Calcagno PL, et al: Alpha-adrenoceptors in the developing kidney. *Pediatr Res* 17:177, 1983.

127. Fildes RD, Eisner GM, Calcagno PL, et al: Renal alpha-adrenoceptors and sodium excretion in the dog. *Am J Physiol* (Renal Fluid Electrolyte Physiology 17)248:F128, 1985.

128. Fine LG, Kirschenbaum MA: Absence of direct effects of prostaglandins on sodium chloride transport in the mammalian nephron. *Kidney Int* 19:797, 1981.

129. Fine LG, Trizna W: Influence of prostaglandins on sodium transport of isolated medullary nephron segments. *Am J Physiol* (Renal Fluid Electrolyte Physiology 1)232:F383, 1977.

130. Flynn TG, De Bold ML, De Bold AJ: The amino acid sequence of an atrial peptide with potent diuretic and natriuretic properties. *Biochem Biophys Res Commun* 117:859, 1983.

131. Friedman PA, Andreoli TE: Bicarbonate-stimulated transepithelial voltage and NaCl transport in the mouse renal cortical thick ascending limb (abstr). *Clin Res* 29:462, 1981.

132. Friedman, Z, Demers LM: Prostaglandin synthetase in the human neonatal kidney. *Pediatr Res* 14:190, 1979.

133. Frolich JC, Wilson TW, Sweetman BJ, et al: Urinary prostaglandins: Identification and origin. *J Clin Invest* 55:763, 1975.

134. Fromter E, Rumrich G, Ullrich KJ: Phenomenologic description of Na^+, Cl^-, and HCO_3^- absorption from the proximal tubules of rat kidneys. *Pflugers Arch* 343:189, 1973.

135. Ganong WF, Mulrow PJ: Rate of change in sodium and potassium excretion after injection of aldosterone in the aorta and renal artery of the dog. *Am J Physiol* 195:337, 1958.

136. Garg LC: Chronic effects of mineralocorticoids on Na-K-ATPase in rabbit nephron segments. In Morel F (ed): *Biochemistry of Kidney Functions INSERM Symposium No. 21.* Amsterdam, Elsevier/North Holland Biomedical Press, 1982, p 259.

137. Garg LC, Knepper MA, Burg MB: Mineralocorticoid effects on Na-K-ATPase in individual nephron segments. *Am J Physiol* (Renal Fluid Electrolyte Physiology 9)240:F536, 1981.

138. Garrahan PJ, Glynn IM: Stoichiometry of the sodium pump. *J Physiol* (Lond) 192:217, 1967.

139. Gauer OH, Henry JP: Neurohormonal control of pleuritic volume. *Int Rev Physiol* 9:145, 1976.

140. Gelbart DR, Battilana CA, Bhattacharya J, et al: Transepithelial gradient and fractional delivery of chloride in thin loop of Henle. *Am J Physiol* (Renal Fluid Electrolyte Physiology 4)235:F192, 1978.

141. Genest J, Cantin M: Regulation of body fluid volume. The atrial natriuretic factor. *News Physiol Sci* 1:3, 1986.

142. Gertz KH, Boylan JW: Glomerular-tubular balance. In Or-

loff J, Berliner RW (eds): *Handbook of Physiology. Section 8: Renal Physiology.* Washington, DC, American Physiological Society, 1973, p 173.

143. Giebisch G, Windhager EE: Measurement of chloride movement across single proximal tubules of Necturus kidney. *Am J Physiol* 204:387, 1963.

144. Giebisch G, Windhager EE: Electrolyte transport across renal tubular membranes. In Orloff J, Berliner RW (eds): *Handbook of Physiology. Section 8: Renal Physiology.* Washington, DC, American Physiological Society, 1973, p 315.

145. Gill JR Jr, Alexander RW, Halushka PV, et al: Indomethacin inhibits distal sodium reabsorption in the dog. *Clin Res* 23:431A, 1975.

146. Glynn IM, Karlish SJD: The sodium pump. *Annu Rev Physiol* 37:13, 1975.

147. Godard C, Vallotton MB, Favre L: Urinary prostaglandins, vasopressin and kallikrein excretion in healthy children from birth to adolescence. *J Pediatr* 100:898, 1982.

148. Godon JP: Sodium and water retention in experimental glomerulonephritis. The urinary natriuretic material. *Nephron* 9:109, 1974.

149. Goetz KL, Hermreck AS, Slick GL, et al: Atrial receptors and renal function in conscious dogs. *Am J Physiol* 219:1417, 1970.

150. Golbus MS, Harrison MR, Filly RA: Prenatal diagnosis and treatment of fetal hydronephrosis. *Semin Perinatol* 7:102, 1983.

151. Goldin SM: Active transport of sodium and potassium ions by the sodium and potassium ion-activated adenosine triphosphatase from renal medulla: Reconstitution of the purified enzyme into a well defined in vitro transport system. *J Biol Chem* 252:5630, 1977.

152. Goldsmith DI, Drukker A, Blaufox MD, et al: Response of the neonatal canine kidney to acute saline expansion. In ZumWinkel K, Blaufox MD, Funck-Brentano JL (eds): *Radionuclides in Nephrology.* Stuttgart, Thieme, 1975, p 45.

153. Gordon D, Peart WS, Wilcox CS: Requirement of the adrenergic nervous system for conservation of sodium by the rabbit kidney. *J Physiol* (Lond) 293:24. 1979.

154. Gordon HH, Levine SZ, Marples E, et al: Water exchange of premature infants. Comparison of metabolic (organic) and electrolyte (inorganic) methods of measurement. *J Clin Invest* 18:1878, 1939.

155. Gottschalk CW: Renal tubular function: Lessons from micropuncture. *Harvey Lect* 58:99, 1963.

156. Gottschalk CW, Mylle M: Micropuncture study of the mammalian urinary concentrating mechanism: Evidence for the counter current hypothesis. *Am J Physiol* 196:927, 1959.

157. Grandchamp A, Boulpaep EL: Pressure control of sodium reabsorption and intercellular backflux across proximal kidney tubule. *J Clin Invest* 54:69, 1974.

158. Granger P, Rojo-Ortega JM, Casado Perez S, et al: The renin angiotensin system in newborn dogs. *J Physiol Pharmacol* 49:134, 1971.

159. Granthan JJ, Burg MB, Orloff J: The nature of transtubular Na and K transport in isolated rabbit renal collecting tubules. *J Clin Invest* 49:1815, 1970.

160. Green R, Bishop JHV, Giebisch G: Ionic requirements of proximal tubular sodium transport. III. Selective luminal anion substitution. *Am J Physiol* (Renal Fluid Electrolyte Physiology 5)236:F268, 1979.

161. Green R, Windhager EE, Giebisch G: Protein oncotic pressure effects on proximal tubular fluid movement in the rat. *Am J Physiol* 226:265, 1974.

162. Greger R: Cation selectivity of the isolated perfused cortical thick ascending limb of Henle's loop of rabbit kidney. *Pflugers Arch* 390:30, 1981.

163. Greger R: Chloride reabsorption in the rabbit cortical thick ascending limb of the loop of Henle. *Pflugers Arch* 390:38, 1981.

164. Greger R: Coupled transport of Na and Cl in the thick ascending limb of Henle's loop of rabbit nephron. *Scand Audiol* (suppl)14:1, 1981.

165. Greger R, Schlater E: Properties of the lumen membrane of the cortical thick ascending limb of Henle's loop of rabbit kidney. *Pflugers Arch* 396:315, 1983.

166. Greger R, Schlatter E, Lang F: Evidence for electroneutral sodium chloride cotransport in the cortical thick ascending limb of Henle's loop of rabbit kidney. *Pflugers Arch* 396:308, 1983.

167. Greger R, Schlatter E: Presence of luminal K^+, a prerequisite for active NaCl transport in cortical thick ascending limb of Henle's loop of rabbit kidney. *Pflugers Arch* 392:92, 1981.

168. Greger R, Schlatter E: Properties of the basolateral membrane of the cortical thick ascending limb of Henle's loop of rabbit kidney. A model for secondary active chloride transport. *Pflugers Arch* 396:325, 1983.

169. Greger RF: Coupled transport of 2Cl, 1Na, and 1K at the luminal membrane of the rabbit cortical thick ascending limb of Henle's loop (cTAL) (abstr). *Am Soc Nephrol* 14:147A, 1981.

170. Gross JB, Imai M, Kokko JP: A functional comparison of the cortical collecting tubule and the distal convoluted tubule. *J Clin Invest* 55:1284, 1975.

171. Gross JB, Kokko JP: Effects of aldosterone and potassium sparing diuretics on electrical potential differences across the distal nephron. *J Clin Invest* 59:82, 1977.

172. Gruber KA, Buckalew VM Jr: Further characterization and evidence for a precursor in the formation of antinatriferic factor. *Proc Soc Exp Biol Med* 159:463, 1978.

173. Gruber KA, Buckalew VM Jr: Evidence that natriuretic factor is a cascading peptide hormone system. In Lichardus B, Schrier RW, Ponec J (eds): *Hormonal Regulation of Sodium Excretion.* Amsterdam, Elsevier/North Holland Biomedical Press, 1980, p 349.

174. Gruber KA, Whitaker JM, Buckalew VM Jr: Endogenous digitalis-like substance in plasma of volume-expanded dogs. *Nature* 287:743, 1980.

175. Guggino WB, Boulpaep EL, Giebisch G: Electrical properties of chloride transport across the Necturus proximal tubule. *J Membr Biol* 65:185, 1982.

176. Guyton AC, Scanlon CJ, Armstrong GG: Effects of pressoreceptor reflex and Cushing's reflex on urinary output. *Fed Proc* 11:61, 1952.

177. Haberle DA, Shiigai TT, Maier G, et al: Dependency of proximal tubular transport on the load of glomerular filtrate. *Kidney Int* 20:18, 1981.

178. Haberle DA, VonBaeyer H: Characteristics of glomerulotubular balance. *Am J Physiol* (Renal Fluid Electrolyte Physiology 13)244:F355, 1983.

179. Haddy FJ, Pamnani MB, Clough DL: The sodium-potassium pump in volume expanded hypertension. *Clin Exp Hypertension* 1:295, 1978.

180. Hall DA, Varney DM: Effect of vasopressin on electrical potential difference and chloride transport in mouse medullary thick ascending limb of Henle. *J Clin Invest* 66:792, 1980.

181. Halushka PV, Wohltmann H, Privitera PV, et al: Bartter's Syndrome: Urinary prostaglandin E-like material and kallikrein; indomethacin effects. *Ann Intern Med* 87:281, 1977.

182. Hanley MJ, Kokko JP, Gross JB, et al: An electrophysiologic study of the cortical collecting tubule of the rabbit. *Kidney Int* 17:74, 1980.

183. Hansen L, Teuscher U, Giebisch G, et al: Influence of luminally administered amiloride, ouabain, and amphotericin B on peritubular membrane potential and net volume reabsorption in the distal tubule. *Pflugers Arch* (suppl 12)359:123, 1975.

184. Harris PI, Young JA: Dose-dependent stimulation and inhibition of proximal tubular sodium reabsorption by angiotensin II in the rat kidney. *Pflugers Arch* 367:295, 1977.

185. Haupert GT: Endogenous glycoside-like substances. *In* Hoffman JF, Forbush B (eds): *Current Topics in Membranes and Transport.* Vol 19. New York, Academic, 1983, p. 843.

186. Haupert GT Jr, Carilli CT, Cantley LC: Hypothalamic sodium transport inhibitor is a high affinity reversible inhibitor of (Na,K)ATPase. *Am J Physiol* (Renal Fluid Electrolyte Physiology 16)247:F919, 1984.

187. Haupert GT Jr, Sancho JM: Sodium transport inhibitor from bovine hypothalamus. *Proc Natl Acad Sci USA* 76:4658, 1979.

188. Herbert SC, Culpepper RM, Andreoli TE: NaCl transport in mouse medullary thick ascending limbs. I. Functional nephron heterogeneity and ADH-stimulated NaCl cotransport. *Am J Physiol* (Renal Fluid Electrolyte Physiology 10)241:F412, 1981.

189. Herbert SC, Friedman PA, Andreoli, TE: Cellular conductive properties of mouse medullary thick ascending limbs (mTALH). *Clin Res* 30:449A, 1982.

190. Henrich WL, Berl T, McDonald KM, et al: Angiotensin, renal nerves and prostaglandins in renal hemodynamics during hemorrhage. *Am J Physiol* (Renal Fluid Electrolyte Physiology 4)235:F46, 1978.

191. Hermansson K, Larson M, Kallskog O: Influence of renal nerve activity on arteriolar resistance, ultrafiltration dynamics and fluid reabsorption. *Pflugers Arch* 389:85, 1981.

192. Hierholzer K: Secretion of potassium and acidification in collecting ducts of mammalian kidney. *Am J Physiol* 201:318, 1961.

193. Hierholzer K, Kawamura S, Seldin DW, et al: Reflection coefficients of various substrates across superficial and juxtamedullary proximal convoluted segments of rabbit nephrons. *Miner Electrolyte Metab* 3:172, 1980.

194. Hierholzer K, Wiederholt M: Some aspects of distal tubular solute and water transport. *Kidney Int* 9:198, 1976.

195. Hierholzer K, Wiederholt M, Hozgreve H, et al: Micropuncture study of renal transtubular concentration gradient of sodium and potassium. *Pflugers Arch* 285:193, 1965.

196. Higashihara E, DuBose TD Jr, Kokko JP: Direct examination of chloride transport across papillary collecting duct of the rat. *Am J Physiol* (Renal Fluid Electrolyte Physiology 4)235:F219, 1978.

197. Higashihara E, Stokes JB, Kokko JP, et al: Cortical and papillary micropuncture examination of chloride transport in segments of the rat kidney during inhibition of prostaglandin production. *J Clin Invest* 64:1277, 1979.

198. Hillyard SD, Gonick HD: Further characterization of the natriuretic factor derived from kidney tissue of volume expanded rats. Effects on short-circuit current and sodium-potassium-adenosine triphosphatase activity. *Circ Res* 38:250, 1976.

199. Hoffman N, Thees M, Kinne R: Phosphate transport by isolated renal brush border vesicles. *Pflugers Arch* 362:147, 1976.

200. Hogg RL, Kokko JP: Comparison between the electrical potential profile and the chloride gradients in the thin limbs of Henle's loop in rats. *Kidney Int* 14:428, 1978.

201. Honour JW, Valman HB, Shackletow CHL: Aldosterone and sodium homeostasis in preterm infants. *Acta Paediatr Scand* 66:103, 1977.

202. Horster M, Larsson L: Mechanism of fluid absorption during proximal tubule development. *Kidney Int* 10:348, 1976.

203. Horster M, Schmid H, Schmidt U: Aldosterone in vitro restores nephron Na-K-ATPase of distal segments from adrenalectomized rabbits. *Pflugers Arch* 384:203, 1980.

204. Horster M, Valtin H: Postnatal development of renal function. Micropuncture and clearance studies in the dogs. *J Clin Invest* 50:779, 1971.

205. Hoshi T, Suzuki Y, Ito K: Electrical properties and fluid transport characteristics of the distal tubule of Triturus kidney. *Proc 31st Japanese Congr Nephrol* 1980, p 889.

206. Iino Y, Imai M: Effects of prostaglandins on sodium transport in isolated collecting tubules. *Pflugers Arch* 373:125, 1978.

207. Imai M: Function of the thin ascending limb of Henle of rats and hamsters perfused in vitro. *Am J Physiol* 232:F201, 1977.

208. Imai M: Effect of bumetanide and furosemide on the thick ascending limb of Henle's loop of rabbits and rats perfused in vitro. *Eur J Pharmacol* 41:409, 1977.

209. Imai M: Calcium transport across the rabbit thick ascending limb of Henle's loop perfused in vitro. *Pflugers Arch* 374:255, 1978.

210. Imai M: The connecting tubule: A functional subdivision of the rabbit distal nephron segments. *Kidney Int* 15:346, 1979.

211. Imai M, Kokko JP: Effect of peritubular protein concentration on reabsorption of sodium and water in isolated perfused proximal tubules. *J Clin Invest* 51:314, 1972.

212. Imai M, Kokko JP: Sodium chloride, urea and water transport in the thin ascending limb of Henle. *J Clin Invest* 53:393, 1974.

213. Imai M, Kokko JP: Mechanism of sodium and chloride transport in the thin ascending limb of Henle. *J Clin Invest* 58:1054, 1976.

214. Imai M, Kusano E: Effects of arginine vasopressin on the thin ascending limb of Henle's loop of hamsters. *Am J Physiol* (Renal Fluid Electrolyte Physiology 13)243:F167, 1982.

215. Imbert M, Chabardes D, Montegut M, et al: Vasopressin dependent adenylate cyclase in single segments of rabbit kidney tubule. *Pflugers Arch* 357:173, 1975.

216. Ito Y, Goldsmith DI, Spitzer A: The role of aldosterone in renal electrolyte transport during development. *Pediatr Res* 18:370A, 1984.

217. Ito Y, Matsumoto T, Ohbu K, et al: Concentrations of human atrial natriuretic peptide in the cord blood in the plasma of the newborn. *Acta Pediatr Scand* 77:76, 1988.

218. Jacobson HR: Characteristics of volume reabsorption in rabbit superficial and juxtamedullary proximal convoluted tubules. *J Clin Invest* 63:410, 1979.

219. Jacobson HR: Effects of CO_2 and acetazolamide on bicarbonate and fluid transport in rabbit proximal tubules. *Am J Physiol* (Renal Fluid Electrolyte Physiology 9)240:F54, 1981.

220. Jacobson HR, Gross JB, Kawamura S, et al: Electrophysiologic study of isolated perfused human collecting ducts; ion dependency of the transepithelial potential difference. *J Clin Invest* 58:1233, 1976.

221. Jacobson HR, Kokko JP: Intrinsic differences in various segments of the proximal convoluted tubule. *J Clin Invest* 57:818, 1976.

222. Jacobson HR, Kokko JP, Seldin DW, et al: Lack of solvent drag of NaCl and $NaHCO_3^-$ in rabbit proximal tubules. *Am J Physiol* (Renal Fluid Electrolyte Physiology 12)243:F342, 1982.

223. Jamieson JD, Palade GE: Specific granules in atrial muscle cells. *J Cell Biol* 23:151, 1964.

224. Jamison RL: Micropuncture study of segments of thin loops of Henle in the rat. *Am J Physiol* 215:236, 1968.

225. Jamison RL: The composition and flow of fluid at the bend of Henle's thin loop in water diuresis and antidiuresis. *In* Villarreal H (ed): *Proceedings of the Fifth International Congress of Nephrology.* Vol 2. Basel, Karger, 1972, p 97.

226. Jamison RL, Buerkert J, Lacy F: A micropuncture study of Henle's thin loop in Brattleboro rats. *Am J Physiol* 224:180, 1973.

227. Janovsky M, Martinek J, Stanicova V: The distribution of sodium, chloride and fluid in the body of young infants with increased intake of NaCl. *Biol Neonate* 11:261, 1967.

228. Jarausch KH, Ullrich KJ: Zur Technik der Entnahme von Harnproben aus einzelnen Sammelrohren der Saugetierniere mittels Polyathylen-Capillaren. *Pflugers Archiv* 264:88, 1957.

229. Johnson MD, Malvin RL: Stimulation of renal sodium reabsorption by angiotensin II. *Am J Physiol* (Renal Fluid Electrolyte Physiology 1)232:F298, 1977.

230. Jorgensen PL: Sodium and potassium ion pump in kidney tubule. *Physiol Rev* 60:864, 1980.

231. Jose PA, Slotkoff LM, Lillienfield L, et al: Sensitivity of neonatal renal vasculature to epinephrine. *Am J Physiol* 226:796, 1974.

232. Kaissling B: Ultrastructural characterization of the connecting tubule and the different segment of the collecting duct system in the rabbit kidney. *In* Guder WG, Schmidt U (eds): *Biochemical Nephrology.* Bern, Hans Huber, 1978, p 435.

233. Kaissling B, Kriz W: *Ulrastructural Analysis of the Rabbit Kidney.* Berlin, Springer-Verlag, 1979, p 1.

234. Kaissling B, Peter S, Kriz W: The transition of the thick ascending limb of Henle's loop into the distal convoluted tubule in the nephron of the rat kidney. *Cell Tissue Res* 182:111, 1977.

235. Kaloyanides GJ, Azer M: Evidence for a humoral mechanism in volume expansion natriuresis. *J Clin Invest* 50:1603, 1971.

236. Kangawa K, Matsuo H: Purification and complete amino acid sequence of a-human atrial natriuretic polypeptide(a-hANP). *Biochem Biophys Res Commun* 118:131, 1984.

237. Kaplan MA, Bourgoignie JJ, Rosecan J, Bricker NS: The effects of the natriuretic factor from uremic urine on sodium transport, water and electrolyte content, and pyruvate oxidation by the isolated toad bladder. *J Clin Invest* 53:1568, 1974.

238. Kaplan SA, Rapaport S: Urinary excretion of sodium and chloride after splanchnicotomy. Effect on the proximal tubule. *Am J Physiol* 164:175, 1951.

239. Kashgarian M, Stockle H, Gottschalk CW, et al: Transtubular electrochemical potentials of sodium and chloride in proximal and distal renal tubules of rats during antidiuresis and water diuresis (diabetes insipidus). *Pflugers Archiv* 277:89, 1963.

240. Kashgarian M, Warren Y, Levitin, H: Micropuncture study of proximal renal tubular chloride transport during hypercapnea in the rat. *Am J Physiol* 209:655, 1965.

241. Kaskel FJ, Kumar AM, Lockhard EA: et al: Factors affecting proximal tubular reabsorption during development. *Am J Physiol* (Renal Fluid Electrolyte Physiology 19)252:F188, 1987.

242. Katz AI, Doucet A, Morel F: Na-K-ATPase activity along the rabbit, rat and mouse nephron. *Am J Physiol* (Renal Fluid Electrolyte Physiology 6)237:F114, 1979.

243. Kawamura S, Imai M, Seldin DW, et al: Characteristics of salt and water transport in superficial and juxtamedullary straight segments of proximal tubules. *J Clin Invest* 55:1269, 1975.

244. Keeler R: Natriuresis after unilateral stimulation of carotid receptors in unanesthetized rats. *Am J Physiol* 226:507, 1974.

245. Khuri RN, Agulian SK, Bogharian K: Electrochemical potentials of chloride in distal renal tubule of the rat. *Am J Physiol* 227:1352, 1974.

246. Khuri RN, Wiederholt M, Strieder N, et al: The effect of graded solute diuresis on renal tubular sodium transport in the rat. *Am J Physiol* 228:1262, 1975.

247. Kimura G, Spring KR: Transcellular and paracellular tracer chloride fluxes in Necturus proximal tubule. *Am J Physiol* (Renal Fluid Electrolyte Physiology 4)235:F617, 1978.

248. Kimura G, Spring KR: Luminal Na entry into Necturus proximal tubule cells. *Am J Physiol* (Renal Fluid Electrolyte Physiology 5)236:F295, 1979.

249. Kinne R, Kirsten R: Der Einfluss von Aldosteron aus die Aktivitat mitochondrialer und cytoplasmatischer Enzyme in der Rattenniere. *Pflugers Arch* 300:244, 1968.

250. Kinne R, Murer H, Kinne-Saffran, E, et al: Sugar transport by renal plasma membrane vesicles: Characteristics of the systems in brush-border microvilli and basolateral plasma membranes. *J Membr Biol* 21:275, 1975.

251. Kirschenbaum MA, Stein JH: The effect of inhibition of prostaglandin synthesis on urinary sodium excretion in the conscious dog. *J Clin Invest* 57:517, 1976.

252. Kleinman LI: Renal sodium reabsorption during saline loading and distal blockade in newborn dogs. *Am J Physiol* 228:1403, 1975.

253. Knox FG, Fleming JS, Rennie DW: Effect of osmotic diuresis on sodium reabsorption and oxygen consumption of kidney. *Am J Physiol* 210:751, 1966.

254. Knox FG, Granger GP: Control of sodium excretion: The kidney produces under pressure. *News Physiol Sci* 2:26, 1987.

255. Knox WH, Sen AD: Mechanism of action of aldosterone with particular reference to (Na^+, K^+)-ATPase. *Ann NY Acad Sci USA* 242:471, 1974.

256. Koch KM, Aynedjian HS, Bank N: Effect of acute hypertension on sodium reabsorption by the proximal tubule. *J Clin Invest* 47:1969, 1968.

257. Koeppen BM, Biagi, BA, Giebisch G: Intracellular microelectrode characterization of the rabbit cortical duct. *Am J Physiol* (Renal Fluid Electrolyte Physiology 13)244:F35, 1983.

258. Koeppen BM, Helman, SI: Acidification of luminal fluid by the rabbit cortical collecting tubule perfused in vitro. *Am J Physiol* (Renal Fluid Electrolyte Physiology 11)242:F521, 1982.

259. Kokko JP: Sodium, chloride and water transport in the descending limb of Henle. *J Clin Invest* 49:1838, 1970.

260. Kokko JP: Urea transport in the proximal tubule and the descending limb of Henle. *J Clin Invest* 51:1999, 1972.

261. Kokko JP: Transport characteristics of the thin limbs of Henle. *Kidney Int* 22:449, 1982.

262. Kokko JP, Burg MB, Orloff, J: Characteristics of NaCl and water transport in the renal proximal tubule. *J Clin Invest* 50:69, 1971.

263. Kon V, Ichikawa I: Effector loci for renal nerve control of cortical microcirculation. *Am J Physiol* (Renal Fluid Electrolyte Physiology 14)245:F545, 1983.

264. Kotchen TA, Hartley LH, Rice TW, et al: Renin, norepinephrine and epinephrine responses to graded exercise. *J Appl Physiol* 31:178, 1971.

265. Kotchen TA, Strickland AL, Rice TW, et al: A study of the renin-angiotensin system in the newborn infant. *J Pediatr* 80:938, 1972.

266. Kowarski A, Katz H, Migeon CJ: Plasma aldosterone concentration in normal subjects from infancy to adulthood. *J Clin Endocrinol Metab* 39:159, 1977.

267. Kramer HJ, Backer A, Kruck F: Antinatriferic activity in

human plasma following acute and chronic salt-loading. *Kidney Int* 12:214, 1977.

268. Kramer HJ, Kruck F: Plasma natriuretic activity in oedematous states. *In* Moorhead JF (ed): *Dialysis, Transplantation, Nephrology. Proceedings of the European Dialysis and Transplant Association.* Vol 12. Kent, Pitman Medical, 1976, p S321.

269. Kramer HJ, Rietzel C, Klingmuller D, et al: Further studies on isolation and purification of a small molecular weight natriuretic hormone. *In* Lichardus B, Schrier RW, Ponec J (eds): *Hormonal Regulation of Sodium Excretion.* Amsterdam, Elsevier/North Holland Biomedical Press, 1980, p 313.

270. Krecek J, Dlouha H, Lavrova JA, et al: Sensitivity of prepubertal rats to the hypertensinogenic effect of salt—a lack of natriuretic factor. *In* Lichardus B, Schrier RW, Ponec J (eds): *Hormonal Regulation of Sodium Excretion.* Amsterdam, Elsevier/North Holland Biomedical Press, 1980, p 289.

271. Kriz W, Kaissling B, Pszalla, M: Morphological characterization of the cells in Henle's loop and the distal tubule. *In* Vogel HG, Ullrich KJ (eds): *New Aspects of Renal Function.* Amsterdam, Excerpta Medica, 1978, p 67.

272. Kruck F: Influence of humoral factors on renal tubular sodium handling. *Nephron* 6:205, 1969.

273. Kunau RT Jr: The influence of the carbonic anhydrase inhibitor, benzolamide (CL-11,366), on the reabsorption of chloride, sodium, and bicarbonate in the proximal tubule of the rat. *J Clin Invest* 51:294, 1972.

274. Landwehr DM, Klose RM, Giebisch G: Renal tubular sodium and water reabsorption in the isotonic sodium chloride loaded rat. *Am J Physiol* 212:1327, 1967.

275. Laragh JH: Atrial natriuretic hormone, the renin aldosterone axis and blood pressure-electrolyte homeostasis. *N Engl J Med* 313:1330, 1985.

276. Law PY, Edelman IS: Induction of citrate synthase by aldosterone in the rat kidney. *J Membr Biol* 41:41, 1978.

277. Le Grimellec C: Micropuncture study along the proximal convoluted tubule: Electrolyte reabsorption in first convolutions. *Pflugers Arch* 354:133, 1975.

278. Lewy JE, Windhager EE: Peritubular control of proximal tubular fluid reabsorption in the rat kidney. *Am J Physiol* 214:943, 1968.

279. Lichardus B, Nizet A: Water and sodium excretion after blood volume expansion under conditions of constant arterial venous and plasma oncotic pressure and constant hematocrit. *Clin Sci* 42:701, 1972.

280. Lichardus B, Pliska V, Uhrin, V, et al: The cow as a model for investigating natriuretic activity. *Lancet* 1:127, 1968.

281. Licht A, Stein S, McGregor CW, et al: Progress in isolation and purification of an inhibitor of sodium transport obtained from dog urine. *Kidney Int* 21:339, 1982.

282. Lichtstein D, Samuelov S: Endogenous ouabain-like activity in rat brain. *Biochem Biophys Res Commun* 96:1518, 1980.

283. Liedtke CM, Hopfer U: Mechanism of Cl⁻ translocation across small intestinal brush-border membrane. I. Absence of Na⁺-Cl⁺ cotransport. *Am J Physiol (Gastrointest Liver Physiology 5)*242:G263, 1982.

284. Link WT, Pamani MB, Huot SJ, et al: Effect of atrial extract on vascular Na⁺-K⁺ pump activity. *Physiologist* 24:59, 1981.

285. Lipson LC, Sharp GWG: Effect of prostaglandin E1 on sodium transport and osmotic water flow in the toad bladder. *Am J Physiol* 220:1046, 1971.

286. Lorenz JM, Kleinman LI, Disney TA: Lack of anion effect on volume expansion natriuresis in developing canine kidney. *J Dev Physiol* 8:395, 1986.

287. Lowitz HD, Stumpe KO, Ochwadt B: Micropuncture study of the action of angiotensin II on tubular sodium and water reabsorption in the rat. *Nephron* 6:173, 1969.

288. Lucci MS, Warnock DG: Effects of anion-transport inhibitors on NaCl reabsorption in the rat superficial proximal convoluted tubule. *J Clin Invest* 64:570, 1979.

289. Luetscher JA Jr, Johnson BB: Observations on the sodium retaining corticoid (aldosterone) in the urine of children and adults in relation to sodium balance and edema. *J Clin Invest* 23:1441, 1954.

290. Mack T, Camargo MJF, Kleinert HD, et al: Atrial natriuretic factor: Structure and functional properties. *Kidney Int* 27:607, 1985.

291. Malnic G, De Mello Aires M, Vieira F: Chloride excretion in nephrons of rat kidney during alterations of acid-base equilibrium. *Am J Physiol* 218:20, 1970.

292. Malnic G, Giebisch G: Some electrical properties of distal tubular epithelium in the rat. *Am J Physiol* 223:797, 1972.

293. Malnic G, Klose RM, Giebisch, G: Micropuncture study of distal tubular potassium and sodium transport in rat nephron. *Am J Physiol* 211:529, 1966.

294. Marchand GR, Ott CE, Cuche JL, et al: Comparison of proximal tubule fluid-to-plasma ultrafiltrate chloride ratio in rats and dogs. *J Appl Physiol* 4:1009, 1976.

295. Marie JP, Guillemot H, Hatt PY: Le degre de granulation des cardiocytes auriculaires. *Pathol Biol (Paris)* 24:549, 1976.

296. Marine D, Baumann J: Duration of life after suprarenalectomy in cats and attempts to prolong it by injections of solutions containing sodium salts, glucose and glycerol. *Am J Physiol* 81:86, 1927.

297. Marsh DJ: Solute and water flows in thin limbs of Henle's loop in the hamster kidney. *Am J Physiol* 218:824, 1970.

298. Marsh DJ, Azen SP: Mechanism of NaCl reabsorption by hamster thin ascending limbs of Henle's loops. *Am J Physiol* 228:71, 1975.

299. Martino JA, Earley LE: Demonstration of a role of physical factors as determinants of the natriuretic response to volume expansion. *J Clin Invest* 46:1963, 1967.

300. Marver D: Aldosterone receptors in rabbit renal cortex and red medulla. *Endocrinology* 106:611, 1980.

301. Marver D, Schwartz MJ: Identification of mineralocorticoid target sites in the isolated rabbit cortical nephron. *Proc Natl Acad Sci USA* 77:3672, 1980.

302. Matson JR, Stokes JB, Robillard JE: Effects of inhibition of prostaglandin synthesis on fetal renal function. *Kidney Int* 20:621, 1981.

303. McCance RA, Widdowson EM: Metabolism, growth and renal function of piglets in the first days of life. *J Physiol (Lond)* 133:373, 1956.

304. McCance RA, Widdowson EM: The response of the newborn puppy to water, salt and food. *J Physiol (Lond)* 141:81, 1958.

305. McCance RA, Widdowson EM: The effect of administering sodium chloride, sodium bicarbonate and potassium bicarbonate to newly born piglets. *J Physiol (Lond)* 165:569, 1963.

306. McDonald SJ, deWardener HE: The relationship between the renal arterial perfusion pressure and the increase in sodium excretion which occurs during an infusion of saline. *Nephron* 2:1, 1965.

307. Mellander S, Oberg B: Transcapillary fluid absorption and other vascular reactions in the human forearm during reduction of the circulating blood volume. *Acta Physiol Scand* 71:37, 1967.

308. Melmon KL, Cline MJ, Hughes T: Kinins: Possible mediators of neonatal circulatory changes in man. *J Clin Invest* 47:1295, 1968.

309. Mernissi GL, Doucet A: Sites and mechanism of mineralocorticoids action along the rabbit nephron. *In* Morel F (ed): *Biochemistry of Kidney Functions, INSERM Symposium*

No. 21. Amsterdam, Elsevier/North Holland Biomedical Press, 1982, p 269.

310. Mernissi GL, Doucet A: Short-term effects of aldosterone and dexamethasone on Na-K-ATPase along the rabbit nephron. Pflugers Arch 399:147, 1983.

311. Mernissi GL, Doucet A: Short-term effect of aldosterone on renal sodium transport and tubular Na-K-ATPase in the rat. Pflugers Arch 399:139, 1983.

312. Morel F, Chabardes D, Imbert M: Functional segmentation of the rabbit distal tubule by microdetermination of hormone-dependent adenylate cyclase activity. Kidney Int 9:264, 1976.

313. Morel F, deRouffignac C: Micropuncture study of urea medullary recycling in desert rodents. In Schmidt-Nielsen B (ed): Urea and the Kidney. Amsterdam, Excerpta Medica, 1970, p 401.

314. Morgan T, Berliner RW: Permeability of the loop of Henle, vasa recta, and collecting duct to water, urea, and sodium. Am J Physiol 215:108, 1968.

315. Morgan T, Berliner RW: A study by continuous microperfusion of water and electrolyte movements in the loop of Henle and distal tubule of the rat. Nephron 6:388, 1969.

316. Murer H, Greger R: Membrane transport in the proximal tubule and thick ascending limb of Henle's loop: Mechanisms and their alterations. Klin Wochenschr 60:1103, 1982.

317. Murer H, Hopfer U, Kinne R: Sodium/proton antiport in brush border membrane vesicles isolated from small intestine and kidney. Biochem J 154:597, 1985.

318. Muther RS, Potter DM, Bennett WM: Aspirin-induced depression of glomerular filtration rate in normal humans: Role of sodium balance. Ann Intern Med 94:317, 1981.

319. Nakamura KT, Felder RA, Jose PA, et al: Effects of dopamine in the renal vascular bed of fetal, newborn and adult sheep. Am J Physiol (Regulatory Integrative Comp Physiology 21)252:R490, 1987.

320. Neumann KH, Rector FC: Mechanism of NaCl and water absorption in the proximal convoluted tubule of rat kidney. J Clin Invest 58:1110, 1976.

321. Niijima A: Observation on the localization of mechanoreceptors in the kidney and afferent nerve fibers in the renal nerves in the rabbit. J Physiol (Lond) 245:81, 1975.

322. Nomura G, Takabatake T, Arai S, et al: Effect of acute unilateral renal denervation on tubular sodium reabsorption in the dog. Am J Physiol (Renal Fluid Electrolyte Physiology 1)232:F16, 1977.

323. Nutbourne DM, Howse JD, Schrier RW, et al: The effects of expanding the blood volume of a dog on the short-circuit current across an isolated frog skin incorporated in the dog's circulation. Clin Sci 38:629, 1970.

324. O'Neil RG: Potassium secretion by the cortical collecting tubule. Fed Proc 40:2403, 1981.

325. O'Neil RG, Boulpaep EL: Ionic conductive properties and electrophysiology of the rabbit cortical collecting tubule. Am J Physiol (Renal Fluid Electrolyte Physiology 12)243:F81, 1982.

326. O'Neil RG, Helman SI: Transport characteristics of renal collecting tubules: Influences of DOCA and diet. Am J Physiol (Renal Fluid Electrolyte Physiology 2)233:F544, 1977.

327. Oberleithner H, Guggino W, Giebisch G: Mechanism of distal tubular chloride transport in Amphiuma kidney. Am J Physiol (Renal Fluid Electrolyte Physiology 11)242:F331, 1982.

328. Oberleithner H, Lang F, Wang W, et al: Effects of inhibition of chloride transport on intracellular sodium activity in distal amphibian nephron. Pflugers Arch 394:55, 1982.

329. Osathandonh V, Potter EL: Development of human kidney by microdissection. III. Formation and interrelationship of collecting tubules and nephrons. Arch Pathol Lab Med 756:290, 1963.

330. Osborn JL, Holdaas H, Thames MD, et al: Renal adrenoceptor mediation of antinatriuretic and renin secretion response to low frequency renal nerve stimulation in the dog. Circ Res 53:298, 1983.

331. Oschman JL: Morphological correlates of transport. In Giebish G, Tosteson DC, Ussing HH (eds): Membrane Transport in Biology. Vol III. New York, Springer-Verlag, 1987, p 55.

332. Pace-Asciak CR: Prostaglandin biosynthesis in the developing fetal sheep kidney. Prostaglandins 13:661, 1977.

333. Paintal AS: A study of right and left atrial receptors. J Physiol (Lond) 120:596, 1953.

334. Paintal AS: Vagal sensory receptors and their reflex effects. Physiol Rev 53:159, 1973.

335. Passo SS, Thornborough JR, Rothballer, AB: Hepatic receptors in control of sodium excretion in anesthetized cats. Am J Physiol 224:373, 1972.

336. Pearce JW, Veress AT: Concentration and bioassay of a natriuretic factor in plasma of volume expanded rats. Can J Physiol Pharmacol 53:742, 1975.

337. Pennell JP, Lacy FB, Jamison RL: An in vivo study of the concentrating process in the descending limb of Henle's loop. Kidney Int 5:337, 1974.

338. Petty KJ, Kokko JP, Marver D: Secondary effect of aldosterone on Na-K ATPase activity in the rabbit cortical collecting tubule. J Clin Invest 68:1514, 1981.

339. Pollock DM, Mullins MM, Banks RO: Failure of atrial myocardial extract to inhibit renal Na-K-ATPase. Renal Physiol 6:295, 1983.

340. Prezyna AP: The renomedullary body—an organ of prostaglandin production. Summary of recent observations (abstr). In Samuelsson B, Paoletti R (eds): Advances in Prostaglandin and Thromboxane Research. Vol 2. New York, Raven Press, 1976, p 956.

341. Prosnitz EH, DiBona GF: Effect of decreased renal sympathetic nerve activity on renal tubular sodium reabsorption. Am J Physiol (Renal Fluid Electrolyte Physiology 4)235:F557, 1978.

342. Rau WS, Fromter E: Electrical properties of the medullary collecting ducts of the golden hamster kidney. I. The transepithelial potential difference. Pflugers Arch 351:99, 1974.

343. Rau WS, Fromter E: Electrical properties of the medullary collecting ducts of the golden hamster kidney. II. The transepithelial resistance. Pflugers Arch 351:113, 1974.

344. Rector FC, Clapp JR: Evidence for active chloride reabsorption in the distal renal tubule of the rat. J Clin Invest 41:101, 1962.

345. Rector FC, Martinez-Maldonado M, Kurtzman NA, et al: Demonstration of a hormonal inhibitor of proximal tubular reabsorption during expansion of extracellular volume with isotonic saline. J Clin Invest 47:761, 1968.

346. Reinhardt HW, Eisele R, Kaczmarczyk G, et al: The control of sodium excretion by reflexes from the low pressure system independent of adrenal activity. Pflugers Arch 384:171, 1980.

347. Robillard JE, Lawton WJ, Weismann DN, et al: Developmental aspects of the renal kallikrein-like activity in fetal and newborn lambs. Kidney Int 22:594, 1982.

348. Robillard JE, McWeeny OJ, Smith B, et al: Ontogeny of neurogenic regulation of renal tubular reabsorption in sheep (abstr). Pediatr Res 23:545A, 1988.

349. Robillard JE, Nakamura KT, DiBona GF: Effects of renal denervation on renal responses to hypoxemia in fetal lambs. Am J Physiol (Renal Fluid Electrolyte Physiology 19)250:F294, 1986.

350. Robillard JE, Weismann DN, Gomez RA, et al: Renal and adrenal responses to converting enzyme inhibition in fetal and newborn life. *Am J Physiol* (Regulatory Integrative Comp Physiology 13)244:R249, 1983.

351. Rocha AS, Kokko JP: Sodium chloride and water transport in the medullary thick ascending limb of Henle. Evidence for active chloride transport. *J Clin Invest* 52:612, 1973.

352. Rocha AS, Kokko JP: Permeability of the medullary nephron segments to urea and water: Effects of vasopressin. *Kidney Int* 6:146, 1974.

353. Rocha AS, Kudo LH: Water, urea, sodium chloride, and potassium transport in the in vitro isolated perfused papillary collecting duct. *Kidney Int* 22:485, 1982.

354. Rodriguez-Soriano J, Vallo A, Castillo G, et al: Renal handling of water and sodium in infancy and childhood: A study using clearance methods during hypotonic saline diuresis. *Kidney Int* 20:700, 1981.

355. Rodriguez-Soriano J, Vallo A, Oliveros R, et al: Renal handling of sodium in premature and full-term neonates: A study using clearance methods during water diuresis. *Pediatr Res* 17:1013, 1983.

356. Rogenes PR, Gottschalk CW: Renal function in conscious rats with chronic unilateral denervation. *Am J Physiol* (Renal Fluid Electrolyte Physiology 11)242:F140, 1982.

357. Rosenbaum JD, Papper S, Aschley MM: Variations in renal excretion of sodium independent of changes in adrenal cortical hormone dosage in patients with Addison's disease. *J Clin Endocrinol Metab* 15:1459, 1958.

358. Ross B, Cowett RM, Oh W: Renal functions of low birth weight infants during the first two months of life. *Pediatr Res* 11:1162, 1977.

359. Roy RN, Chance GW, Radde IC, et al: Late hyponatremia in very low birth weight infants (<1.3 kilograms). *Pediatr Res* 10:526, 1978.

360. Sackin H, Boulpaep EL: Isolated perfused salamander proximal tubule: Methods, electrophysiology, and transport. *Am J Physiol* (Renal Fluid Electrolyte Physiology 10)241:F39, 1981.

361. Samuals AI, Miller ED, Fray JCS, et al: Renin-antagonists and the regulation of blood pressure. *Fed Proc* 35:2512, 1976.

362. Sasaki S, Imai M: Effects of vasopressin on water and NaCl transport across the thick ascending limb of Henle's loop of mouse, rat, and rabbit kidneys. *Pflugers Arch* 383:215, 1980.

363. Schad H, Seller H: Reduction of renal nerve activity by volume expansion in conscious cats. *Pflugers Arch* 363:155, 1976.

364. Schafer JA: Mechanisms coupling the absorption of solutes, and water in the proximal nephron. *Kidney Int* 25:708, 1984.

365. Schafer JA, Andreoli TE: Anion transport processes in the mammalian superficial proximal straight tubule. *J Clin Invest* 58:500, 1976.

366. Schafer JA, Patlak CS, Andreoli TE: A component of fluid absorption linked to passive ion flows in the superficial pars recta. *J Gen Physiol* 66:445, 1975.

367. Shafer JA, Patlak CS, Andreoli TE: Fluid absorption and active and passive ion flows in the rabbit superficial pars recta. *Am J Physiol* (Renal Fluid Electrolyte Physiology 2)233:F154, 1977.

368. Schafer JA, Troutman SL, Andreoli TE: Volume reabsorption, transepithelial differences, and ionic permeability properties in mammalian superficial proximal straight tubules. *J Gen Physiol* 64:582, 1974.

369. Schafer JA, Toutman SL, Watkins MD, et al: Volume absorption in the pars recta. I. "Simple" active Na transport. *Am J Physiol* (Renal Fluid Electrolyte Physiology 3)234:F332, 1978.

370. Schafer JA, Troutman SL, Watkins ML, et al: Flow dependence of fluid transport in the isolated superficial pars recta: Evidence that osmotic disequilibrium between external solutions drives isotonic fluid transport. *Kidney Int* 20:588, 1981.

371. Schambelan M, Sebastian A, Biglieri EG: Control of aldosterone secretion in hyporeninemic hypoaldosteronism. *Clin Res* 25:466A, 1977.

372. Schlondorff D, Satriano JA, Schwartz GH: Synthesis of prostaglandin E2 in different segments of isolated collecting tubules from adult and neonatal rabbits. *Am J Physiol* (Renal Fluid Electrolyte Physiology 17)248:F134, 1985.

373. Schmidt U, Dubach A, Morel F: Action of (Na^+-K^+)-stimulated adenosine triphosphatase in the rat nephron. *Pflugers Arch* 306:219, 1969.

374. Schmidt U, Dubach UC: Sensitivity of Na-K-adenosine triphosphatase activity in various structures of the rat nephron: Studies with adrenalectomy. *Eur J Clin Invest* 1:307, 1971.

375. Schmidt U, Horster M: Na-K-activated ATPase activity: Maturation in rabbit nephron segments dissected in vitro. *Am J Physiol* (Renal Fluid Electrolyte Physiology 2)233:F55, 1977.

376. Schneider E, Mclane-Vega L, Hanson R, et al: Effect of chronic bilateral renal denervation on daily sodium excretion in the conscious dog. *Fed Proc* 37:645, 1978.

377. Schnermann J, Schubert G, Briggs J: Rise in NaCl concentration along the early post-macula densa distal tubule due to net NaCl influx. *Pflugers Arch* 391:R20, 1981.

378. Schoeneman MJ, Spitzer A: The effect of intravascular volume expansion on proximal tubular reabsorption during development. *Proc Soc Exp Biol Med* 165:319, 1980.

379. Schor N, Ichikawa I, Brenner BM: Glomerular adaptations to chronic dietary salt restriction or excess. *Am J Physiol* (Renal Fluid Electrolyte Physiology 7)238:F428, 1980.

380. Schuster VL, Kokko JP, Jacobson HR: Angiotensin II directly stimulates sodium transport in rabbit proximal convoluted tubules. *J Clin Invest* 73:507, 1984.

381. Schwartz GJ, Burg MB: Mineralocorticoid effects on cation transport by cortical collecting tubules in vitro. *Am J Physiol* (Renal Fluid Electrolyte Physiology 4)235:F576, 1978.

382. Schwartz GJ, Evans AP: Development of solute transport in rabbit proximal tubule. I. HCO_3^- and glucose absorption. *Am J Physiol* (Renal Fluid Electrolyte Physiology 14)245:F382, 1983.

383. Schwartz GJ, Evan AP: Development of solute transport in rabbit proximal tubule. III. Na-K-ATPase activity. *Am J Physiol* (Renal Fluid Electrolyte Physiology 15)246:F845, 1984.

384. Schwartz SL, Williams GH, Hollenberg NK, et al: Captopril-induced changes in prostaglandin production. *J Clin Invest* 65:1257, 1980.

385. Sealey JE, Kirshman JD, Laragh JH: Natriuretic activity in plasma and urine of salt-loaded men and sheep. *J Clin Invest* 48:2210, 1969.

386. Sedlakova E, Lichardus B, Cort JH: Plasma saluretic activity: Its nature and relation to oxytocin analogues. *Science* 164:580, 1969.

387. Seely JF, Levy M: Control of extracellular fluid volume. *In* Brenner BM, Rector FC (eds): *The Kidney.* Philadelphia, WB Saunders, 1981, p 371.

388. Selkurt EE: Effect of pulse pressure and mean arterial pressure modification on renal hemodynamics and electrolyte and water excretion. *Circulation* 4:541, 1951.

389. Shaffer SG, Greer PG, Goetz KL: Elevated atrial natriuretic factor in neonates with respiratory distress syndrome. *J Pediatr* 109:1028, 1986.

390. Sharp GWG, Coggins CH, Lichtenstein NS, et al: Evidence for a mucosal effect of aldosterone on sodium transport in the toad bladder. *J Clin Invest* 45:1640, 1966.

391. Shaver JL, Stirling C: Ouabain binding to renal tubules of the rabbit. *J Cell Biol* 76:278, 1978.

392. Shepherd JT: Intrathoracic baroreflexes. *Mayo Clin Proc* 48:426, 1973.

393. Shine P, McDougall JG, Towstoless MK, et al: Action of atrial natriuretic peptide in the immature ovine kidney. *Pediatr Res* 22:11, 1987.

394. Shipley RE, Study RS: Factors regulating renal blood flow and urine flow following acute changes in renal artery perfusion pressure. *Am J Physiol* 163:650, 1950.

395. Siegel S.R, Oh W: Renal function as a marker of human fetal maturation. *Acta Pediatr Scand* 65:481, 1976.

396. Simpson SA, Tait JR, Wettstin A, et al: Konstitution des Aldosterons des neuen Mineral Corticoids. *Experientia* 10:132, 1954.

397. Sinaiko AR, Glasser RJ, Gillum RF, et al: Urinary kallikrein excretion in grade school children with high and low blood pressure. *J Pediatr* 100:938, 1982.

398. Slick L, Aguilera AJ, Zambraski EJ, et al: Renal neuroadrenergic transmission. *Am J Physiol* 299:60, 1975.

399. Solomon S: Evidence that the renal response of volume expansion involves a blood borne factor. *Biol Neonate* 35:113, 1979.

400. Sonnenberg H, Cupples WA, De Bold AJ, et al: Intrarenal localization of the natriuretic effect of cardiac atrial extract. *Can J Physiol Pharmacol* 60:1149, 1982.

401. Sonnenberg HN, Pearce JW: Renal response to measured blood volume expansion in differently hydrated dogs. *Am J Physiol* 203:344, 1962.

402. Speziale N, Speziale E, Terragno A, et al: Mobilization and metabolism of arachidonic acid in developing rat kidney. *In* Spitzer A (ed): *The Kidney During Development: Morphology and Function.* New York, Masson Publishing USA, 1982, p 187.

403. Spitzer A: The role of the kidney in sodium homeostasis during maturation. *Kidney Int* 21:539, 1982.

404. Spitzer A, Brandis M: Functional and morphologic maturation of the superficial nephrons. Relationship to total kidney functions. *J Clin Invest* 53:279, 1974.

405. Spitzer A, Windhager EE: Effect of peritubular oncotic pressure changes on proximal fluid reabsorption. *Am J Physiol* 218:1188, 1970.

406. Spring KR, Kimura G: Chloride reabsorption by renal proximal tubules of Necturus. *J Membr Biol* 38:233, 1978.

407. Spring KR, Kimura G: Intercellular ion activities in Necturus proximal tubule. *Fed Proc* 38:2729, 1979.

408. Starling EH, Verney EB: The secretion of urine as studied on the isolated kidney. *Proc R Soc Lond (Biol)* 97:321, 1925.

409. Stein JH, Congbalay RC, Karsh DL, et al: The effect of bradykinin on proximal tubular sodium reabsorption in the dog: Evidence for functional nephron heterogeneity. *J Clin Invest* 51:1709, 1972.

410. Stein JH, Osgood RW, Kunau RT: Direct measurement of papillary collecting duct of sodium transport in the rat. *J Clin Invest* 58:767, 1976.

411. Steiner RW, Tucker BJ, Blantz RC: Glomerular hemodynamics in rats with chronic sodium depletion: Effect of saralasin. *J Clin Invest* 64:503, 1979.

412. Stokes JB: Effect of prostaglandin E2 on chloride transport across the rabbit thick ascending limb of Henle. Selective inhibition of the medullary portion. *J Clin Invest* 64:495, 1979.

413. Stokes JB: Potassium secretion by cortical collecting tubule: Relation to sodium absorption, luminal sodium concentration, and transepithelial voltage. *Am J Physiol* (Renal Fluid Electrolyte Physiology 10)241:F395, 1981.

414. Stokes JB: Ion transport by the cortical and outer medullary collecting tubule. *Kidney Int* 22:473, 1982.

415. Stokes JB: Sodium and potassium transport across the cortical and outer medullary tubule of the rabbit: Evidence for diffusion across the outer medullary portion. *Am J Physiol* (Renal Fluid Electrolyte Physiology 11):242:F514, 1982.

416. Stokes JB, Ingram MJ, Williams AD, et al: Heterogeneity of the rabbit collecting tubule: Localization of mineralocorticoid hormone action to the cortical portion. *Kidney Int* 20:340, 1981.

417. Stokes JB, Tisher CC, Kokko P: Structural functional heterogeneity along the rabbit collecting tubule. *Kidney Int* 14:585, 1978.

418. Stoner LC: Isolated, perfused amphibian renal tubules: The diluting segment. *Am J Physiol* 233:F438, 1977.

419. Stoner LC, Burg MB, Orloff J: Ion transport in cortical collecting tubule: Effect of amiloride. *Am J Physiol* 227:453, 1974.

420. Suki WN, Rouse D, Ng RCK, et al: Calcium transport in the thick ascending limb of Henle. Heterogeneity of function in the medullary and cortical segments. *J Clin Invest* 66:1004, 1980.

421. Sulyok E: The relationship between electrolyte and acid-base balance in the premature infant during early postnatal life. *Biol Neonate* 66:103, 1971.

422. Sulyok E, Heim T, Soltesz G, et al: The influence of maturity on renal control of acidosis in newborn infants. *Biol Neonate* 21:418, 1972.

423. Sulyok E, Nemeth M, Tenyi I, et al: Postnatal development of renin-angiotensin-aldosterone system, RAAS, in relation to electrolyte balance in premature infants. *Pediatr Res* 13:817, 1979.

424. Sulyok E, Varga F, Gyory E, et al: Postnatal development of renal sodium handling in premature infants. *J Pediatr* 95:787, 1979.

425. Sulyok E, Varga F, Gyory E, et al: On the mechanisms of renal sodium handling in newborn infants. *Biol Neonate* 37:75, 1980.

426. Takas L, Bencsath P, Szalay L: Decreased proximal tubular transport capacity after renal sympathectomy. *Proc Int Cong Nephrol* 8:553, 1978.

427. Tarnow-Mordi WO, Shaw JCL, Liv D, et al: Iatrogenic hyponatremia of the newborn due to maternal fluid overload: A prospective study. *Br Med J* 283:639, 1981.

428. Taylor A: Role of microtubules and microfilaments in the action of vasopressin. *In* Andreoli TE, Grantham J, Rector R (eds): *Disturbances in Body Fluid Osmolality.* Washington, DC: *American Physiological Society,* 1977, p 97.

429. Thibault G, Garcia R, Cantin M, et al: Atrial natriuretic factor. Characterisation and partial purification. *Hypertension* (suppl 1)5:I-75, 1983.

430. Thibault G, Garcia R, Siedah NG, et al: Purification of three rat atrial natriuretic factors and their amino acid composition. *FEBS Letters* 164:286, 1983.

431. Tobian L, Coffee K, McCrea P: Evidence for a humoral factor of non-renal and non-adrenal origin which influences renal sodium excretion. *Trans Assoc Am Physicians* 80:200, 1967.

432. Tortorolo G, Porcelli G, Cuatalo P: Urinary kallikreins in premature, small at term and normal newborns and in children. *In* Pisano JJ, Austen KF (eds): *Chemistry and Biolgy of Kallikrein: Kinin System in Health and Disease.* Washington, DC, DHEW (NIH), 1974, p 76.

433. Trimper CE, Lambers ER: The renin-angiotensin system in foetal lambs. *Pflugers Arch* 336:1, 1972.

434. Trippodo NC, MacPhee AA, Cole FF: Partially purified human and rat atrial natriuretic factor. *Hypertension* (suppl 1)5:I-81, 1983.

435. Tucker BJ, Blantz RC: Mechanism of altered glomerular hemodynamics during chronic sodium depletion. *Am J Physiol* (Renal Fluid Electrolyte Physiology 13)244:F11, 1983.

436. Tulassay T, Rascher W, Ceyberth HW, et al: Role of atrial natriuretic peptide in sodium homeostasis in premature infants. *J Pediatr* 109:1023, 1986.

437. Uchida J, Kamishaha K, Heda H: Two types of renal mechanoreceptors. *Jpn Heart J* 12:233, 1971.

438. Uhlich E, Baldamus CA, Ullrich KJ: Einfluss von Aldosteron auf den Natriumtransport in den Sammelrohren der Saugetierniere. *Pflugers Arch* 308:111, 1969.

439. Uhlich E, Halback R, Ullrich KJ: Influence of aldosterone on ^{24}Na efflux in collecting ducts of rats. *Pflugers Arch* 320:261, 1970.

440. Vandewalle A, Farman N, Bencsath P, et al: Aldosterone binding along the rabbit nephron: An autoradiographic study on isolated tubules. *Am J Physiol* (Renal Fluid Electrolyte Physiology 9)240:F172, 1981.

441. Vanherwegman JL, Duchobu J, D'Hollander A: Effect of indomethacin on renal hemodynamics and on water and sodium excretion by the isolated dog kidney. *Pflugers Arch* 357:232, 1975.

442. Varga F, Sulyok E, Nemeth M, et al: Activity of the renin-angiotensin-aldosterone system in full-term newborn infants during the first week of life. *Acta Paediatr Hung* 22:120, 1981.

443. Vari RC, Ott CE: In vivo proximal tubular fluid-to-plasma chloride concentration gradient in the rabbit. *Am J Physiol* (Renal Fluid Electrolyte Physiology 11)242:F575, 1982.

444. Velazquez H, Wright FS, Good DW: Luminal influences on potassium secretion: Chloride replacement with sulfate. *Am J Physiol* (Renal Fluid Electrolyte Physiology 11)242:F46, 1982.

445. Verderstraeten P, Toussaint C: Effects of plasmapheresis on renal hemodynamics and sodium excretion in dogs. *Pflugers Arch* 306:92, 1969.

446. Veress AT, Miloyevic S, Sonnenberg H: Characterization of the natriuretic activity in the plasma of hypervolaemic rats. *Clin Sci* 59:183, 1980.

447. Walker AM, Bott PA, Oliver J, et al: The collection and analysis of fluid from single nephrons of the mammalian kidney. *Am J Physiol* 134:580, 1941.

448. Walker AM, Hudson CL, Findley T Jr, et al: The total molecular concentration and the chloride concentration of fluid from different segments of the renal tubule of amphibia: The site of chloride reabsorption. *Am J Physiol* 118:121, 1937.

449. Walker DW, Mitchell MD: Prostaglandins in urine of foetal lambs. *Nature* (Lond) 271:161, 1978.

450. Wallace WM, West WB, Taylor A: *Water and Electrolyte Metabolism in Relation to Age and Sex.* Boston, Little, Brown, 1958.

451. Warnock DG, Burg MB: Urinary acidification: CO_2 transport by the rabbit proximal straight tubule. *Am J Physiol* (Renal Fluid Electrolyte Physiology 1)232:F20, 1977.

452. Weinstein AM, Windhager EE: Sodium transport along the proximal tubule. *In* Seldin DW, Giebisch G (eds): *The*

453. Wennergren G, Henriksson BA, Weiss LB, et al: Effects of stimulation of nonmedullated cardiac afferents on renal water and sodium excretion. *Acta Physiol Scand* 97:261, 1976.

454. Whittembury G, Diezi F, Diezi J, et al: Some aspects of proximal tubular sodium chloride reabsorption in Necturus kidney. *Kidney Int* 7:293, 1975.

455. Whitten CF: Metablic data on the handling of NaCl by infants. *J Pediatr* 74:819, 1969.

456. Whorten AR, Smigel M, Oates JA, et al: Regional differences in prostacyclin formation by the kidney: Prostacyclin is a major prostaglandin of renal cortex. *Biochim Biophys Acta* 529:176, 1978.

457. Wiederholt M, Hierholzer K, Windhager EE, et al: Microperfusion study of fluid reabsorption in proximal tubules of rat kidneys. *Am J Physiol* 213:809, 1967.

458. Wilson DR, Honath U, Sole M: Effect of acute and chronic denervation on renal function after release of unilateral ureteral obstruction in the rat. *Can J Physiol Pharmacol* 57:731, 1979.

459. Wilson DR, Honrath U, Sonnenberg H: Prostaglandin synthesis inhibition during volume expansion: Collecting duct function. *Kidney Int* 22:1, 1982.

460. Windhager EE: Sodium chloride transport. *In* Giebisch G, Tosteson DC, Ussing HH (eds): *Membrane Transport in Biology.* Vol 4A. Berlin, Springer-Verlag, 1979, p 145.

461. Windhager EE, Giebisch G: Micropuncture study of renal tubular transfer of sodium chloride in the rat. *Am J Physiol* 200:581, 1961.

462. Wirz H, Dirix R: Urinary concentration and dilution. *In* Orloff J, Berliner RW (eds): *Handbook of Physiology. Section 8: Renal Physiology.* Washington, DC, Am Physiol Soc, 1973, p 415.

463. Wright FS, Davis JO, Johnston CI, et al: Renal sodium excretion after volume expansion with saline and blood. *Proc Soc Exp Biol Med* 128:1044, 1968.

464. Young DB, Guyton AC: Steady state aldosterone dose-response relationships. *Circ Res* 40:138, 1977.

465. Young DB, McCaa RE, Pan YJ, et al: Effectiveness of the aldosterone sodium and potassium feedback control system. *Am J Physiol* 231:945, 1976.

466. Zambraski EJ, DiBona GF, Kaloyanides GJ: Effect of sympathetic blocking agents on the antinatriuresis of reflex renal nerve stimulation. *J Pharmacol Exp Ther* 198:464, 1976.

467. Zambraski EJ, Dunn MJ: Renal prostaglandin E2 secretion and excretion in conscious dogs. *Am J Physiol* (Renal Fluid Electrolyte Physiology 5)236:F552, 1979.

468. Zink H, Horster M: Maturation of diluting capacity in loop of Henle of rat superficial nephrons. *Am J Physiol* (Renal Fluid Electrolyte Physiology 2)233:F519, 1977.

469. Zinner SH, Margolius HS, Rosner B: Stability of blood pressure rank and urinary kallikrein concentration in childhood: An eight-year follow-up. *Circulation* 58:908, 1978.

470. Zusman RM, Keiser HR: Prostaglandin biosynthesis by rabbit renomedullary interstitial cells in tissue culture: Mechanism of stimulation by angiotensin II, bradykinin and arginine vasopressin. *J Biol Chem* 252:2069, 1977.

LISA M. SATLIN
GEORGE J. SCHWARTZ

6

Renal Regulation of Potassium Homeostasis

General Features of Potassium Balance

Potassium is the most abundant cation in the intracellular fluid. Maintenance of a high cellular concentration of potassium is essential for several vital cellular processes, including growth [57,101,190], synthesis of protein and nucleic acids, [103,104,174], enzyme activation [18,29,69], control of cell volume [186,193], and regulation of intracellular pH [1]. The steep potassium concentration gradient that normally exists across the cell membrane is a requisite for the transmission of electrical impulses by excitable tissue, such as muscle and nerve, and net potassium secretion by transporting epithelia of the kidney and colon.

Body Potassium Content

The total body potassium in the adult male has been estimated to be approximately 50 mEq/kg body weight [41,130]. Approximately 98% of this potassium is located within cells, primarily in muscle. Although the concentration of potassium in the intracellular fluid ranges between 100 mEq/L and 150 mEq/L, the activity, or effective concentration that is ionically active, may be 50% lower [25,88,99]. Only about 2% of the total body potassium is found in the extracellular fluid, where it is present in the adult within a narrow concentration range of 3.5 mEq/L to 5.0 mEq/L. The high ratio of intracellular to extracellular potassium is generated and maintained by the action of Na-K-adenosine triphosphatase (Na-K-ATPase), an enzyme pump located in the cell membranes of all animal cells. Na-K-ATPase catalyzes the hydrolysis of ATP, thereby providing energy for the active transport of two potassium ions into the cell at the expense of three sodium ions extruded [84]. The unequal exchange ratio creates a negative voltage within the cell.

Total body potassium (gm) increases at a predictable rate when plotted against either height or weight (Fig. 6-1) [2,47,48,101], without sex-related differences below 135 cm and 30 kg, respectively [47,48]. Thereafter, girls accrue less potassium/kg body weight and potassium/cm height than do boys, presumably reflecting those physio-logic and endocrinologic changes of puberty unique to that sex [47,48].

In infancy, the accretion of body potassium/cm length is more rapid than it is later in childhood [47,48] (Fig. 6-2), probably reflecting both actual cellular growth and a maturation in intracellular chemical composition. Potassium concentration in human muscle water has been estimated to be approximately 72 mEq/L at birth, reaching adult levels (134 mEq/L) after seven months of age [33].

Potassium is readily absorbed from the gastrointestinal tract and enters the extracellular fluid. Constancy of the concentration of potassium in the plasma during entry of potassium into the extracellular fluid is maintained by hormonally mediated temporary shifts of this cation into cells [14]. Although the average dietary intake of potassium in the adult ranges between 80 mEq/day and 120 mEq/day [193], minimal potassium needs could be provided by a daily intake of as little as 20 mEq to 30 mEq [173a]. Assuming that an average adult ingests 2000 calories/day to 2500 calories/day, the latter value would translate to a minimal daily potassium requirement of approximately 1 mEq/100 kcal. Zero external potassium balance in the adult requires that intake equal excretion. Growing infants and children, in a state of positive potassium balance, must conserve potassium to incorporate into newly formed cells. The minimal daily potassium requirement during childhood has been estimated to be higher than in the adult, averaging 2 mEq/100 kcal of energy expended [121].

The kidney is the primary route for elimination of potassium, responsible for excreting about 90% of the daily intake [57]. The colon is also capable of potassium secretion, a route that assumes greater importance in conditions of reduced renal function [11]. In general, urinary potassium excretion parallels dietary intake. The speed of the renal adaptation to variations in intake depends on the preceding potassium intake, the magnitude of the change in dietary potassium, and the species studied (see Potassium Adaptation, following). Adaptation to step changes in potassium intake is more rapid in some animals (e.g., sheep) than in humans, occurring within 1 day to 2 days of altered dietary intake [132].

In man, extreme adjustments in the rate of renal potas-

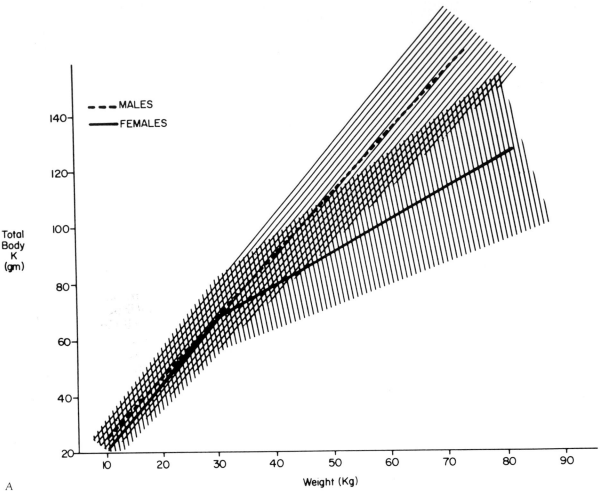

A

FIG. 6-1. *Total body potassium as a function of weight (panel A) and height (panel B) in males and females 3 to 18 years of age. The shaded area represents the mean ± 1 standard deviation. (Reproduced from Flynn MA, Woodruff C, Clark J, et al: Total body potassium in normal children. Pediatr Res 6:239, 1972, with permission.)*

sium conservation cannot be achieved as rapidly as for sodium, nor are the adjustments as complete. Specifically, urinary sodium can be virtually eliminated within three days to four days of sodium restriction, yet a minimal urinary potassium loss of about 10 mEq/day persists in the adult, even after several weeks of severe potassium restriction [150]. This minimal daily renal loss of potassium coupled to obligatory extrarenal losses necessitates a daily basal potassium intake in the adult of at least 20 mEq.

Sites of Potassium Transport
Renal Handling of Potassium

Samples of tubular fluid can be obtained by micropuncture only from those nephron sites exposed to the cortical surface (proximal and distal convolutions of superficial neph-

rons) or papillary tip (thin loops of Henle of juxtamedullary nephrons and terminal collecting ducts). The relative contributions to overall renal potassium handling of the nephron segments inaccessible to micropuncture have been assessed by in vitro microperfusion of nephron segments isolated from rabbit and rat kidney. Thus, our limited understanding of potassium handling by successive segments of the kidney reflects a synthesis of data obtained from both superficial and juxtamedullary nephrons, by microperfusion and by micropuncture, in two different species.

In vivo free-flow micropuncture studies in the hydropenic rat provided much of the original description of potassium transport characteristics of various segments of superficial nephrons. These studies demonstrated that the renal handling of potassium involves the processes of filtration, reabsorption, and secretion. As a general rule,

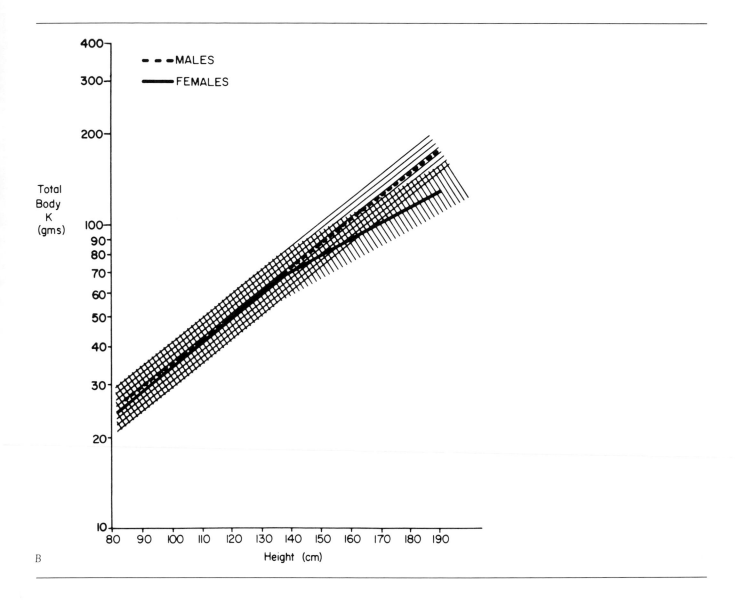

filtered potassium is almost completely reabsorbed in proximal parts of the nephron, whereas the potassium excreted in urine derives largely from distal secretion.

CORTICAL NEPHRON

Potassium is freely filtered at the glomerulus. Approximately 50% of the filtered load of potassium is reabsorbed along the initial two-thirds of the proximal tubule that is accessible to micropuncture (Fig. 6-3), a fraction similar to that of water and sodium reabsorption along this segment [105]. Thus, the concentration of potassium at any given site along the proximal convoluted tubule remains near or slightly below that of plasma [105, 106].

Approximately 5% to 15% of the filtered load of potassium reaches the superficial early distal tubule (see Fig. 6-3) [105,106], indicating further net potassium reabsorption in the interposed nephron segments. Potassium secretion by the distal tubule is responsible for net urinary

potassium secretion, which can approach 20% to 50% of the filtered load (see Fig. 6-3) [105]. The rate of potassium secretion along the distal tubule is highly variable and depends on the metabolic state of potassium balance.

JUXTAMEDULLARY NEPHRON

Samples of tubular fluid collected by micropuncture at the tip of the rodent renal papilla have indicated that the rate of delivery of potassium to the end of the descending limb of deep juxtamedullary nephrons can exceed the filtered load (see Fig. 6-3) [12,77]. This observation suggests that potassium must be secreted at some proximal site in the juxtamedullary nephron. Evidence from microperfusion studies indicates that potassium can be secreted into the end-proximal tubule and the descending limb of the loop of Henle [76]. Both active and passive transport may contribute to the net secretion of a small amount of potassium that has been demonstrated to occur in both the isolated

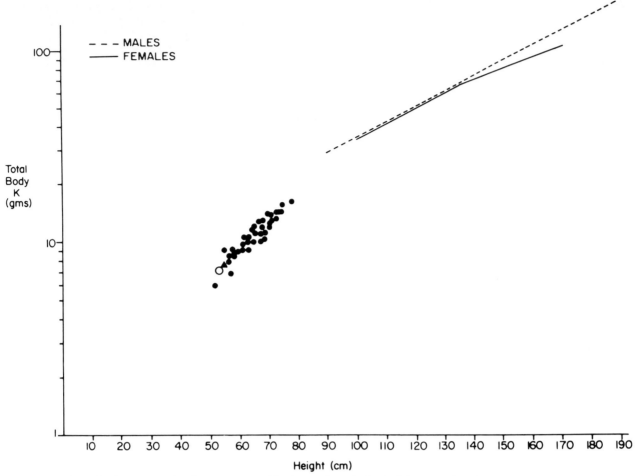

FIG. 6-2. *Relationship between total body potassium and height in infants (individual data points) and children 3 to 18 years of age (linear regression line and data same as in Figure 6-1). (Reproduced from Flynn MA, Woodruff C, Clark J, et al: Total body potassium in normal children. Pediatr Res 6:239, 1972, with permission.)*

perfused superficial and juxtamedullary proximal straight tubule, or pars recta [62,183,192].

The juxtamedullary pars recta [192] and descending limb of the loop of Henle [137] possess a relatively high potassium permeability, suggesting that an elevated potassium concentration in the medullary interstitium could facilitate significant diffusional potassium entry into the fluid perfusing these segments. The existence of a transepithelial potassium gradient appears likely in view of studies that have demonstrated a high potassium concentration in the vasa recta plasma and inner medullary interstitium of the rat during antidiuresis [12,20,34].

If delivery of potassium to the distal convoluted tubule of deep nephrons is substantially reduced to only 5% to 15% of the filtered load, as it is in the superficial nephron, the bulk of the potassium delivered to the loop of Henle must be reabsorbed by the thin and thick ascending limbs of both populations of nephrons. Thick ascending limbs of

juxtamedullary nephrons perfused in vitro reabsorb potassium [169]. Little net flux is measured across cortical thick ascending limbs [21,151]; however, it is likely that the rate of transport is enhanced by increasing the luminal potassium concentration [151], a situation that presumably occurs in vivo as potassium is secreted between the proximal convoluted tubule and the tip of the loop of Henle. As for juxtamedullary nephrons in vivo, a progressive fall in interstitial potassium concentration between the papillary tip and outer medulla may further favor net reabsorption [21,169].

DISTAL NEPHRON

The portion of the nephron that has traditionally been referred to as the "distal tubule" in micropuncture studies comprises at least four morphologically and functionally heterogeneous subdivisions [82,83,85,117,118,127]. Spe-

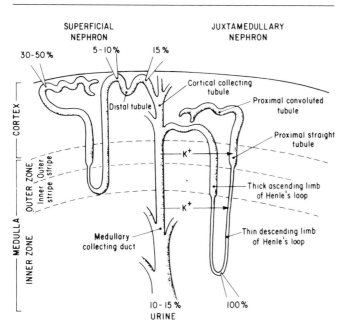

FIG. 6-3. *Fractional delivery of potassium to various sites in superficial and juxtamedullary nephrons as a percentage of the filtered load. Arrows indicate direction of net potassium transport (reabsorption vs. secretion). (Reproduced from Giebisch G, Malnic G, Berliner RW: Renal transport and control of potassium excretion. In Brenner BM, Rector FC Jr (eds): The Kidney, Philadelphia, WB Saunders, 1986, with permission.)*

cifically, the anatomic segment originating at the macula densa and terminating at the first confluence with another distal tubule consists of a short segment of thick ascending limb, followed by the distal convoluted tubule, connecting segment, and initial collecting tubule, sequentially [82,83]. These segments can be distinguished not only by morphology, but also with respect to Na-K-ATPase activity [85], hormonal sensitivity [117,118], and embryologic development [127].

Direct examination of the transport characteristics of the individual segments comprising the distal nephron in the rabbit indicates that the connecting tubule [75,152] and cortical collecting duct [61] are major regulatory sites of potassium secretion; in fact, the isolated perfused cortical collecting duct can generate potassium concentrations in excess of 100 mM if allowed sufficient contact time with the luminal fluid [61]. The earliest convolutions of the distal tubule, examined directly by in vivo microperfusion, contribute at most a constant small amount to total potassium secretion [144,163]. The rate of potassium secretion in the late distal tubule and cortical collecting duct can be enhanced dramatically by administration of mineralocorticoids or by potassium loading of the animal [147,160,161] and is associated with marked morphologic changes in the connecting and collecting ducts (see below) [163,182].

In contrast to the potassium secretion characteristic of the cortical collecting duct, the outer medullary collecting duct exhibits passive potassium efflux down its electro-chemical gradient [167,168]. As a result of earlier potassium secretion and water abstraction, the potassium concentration of the tubular fluid delivered to the medullary collecting duct is high. The combination of the lumen-positive voltage therein [168] and high mass flow of potassium entering this segment create a driving force favoring passive reabsorption of potassium.

The final collecting duct segment, the papillary collecting duct, when perfused in vitro, has the capacity to absorb small amounts of potassium actively, i.e., in the absence of electrical and chemical gradients [138]. In addition, this segment possesses a relatively high potassium permeability that may allow passive potassium secretion in vivo if, as is likely, there exists a potassium concentration gradient between the papillary interstitium and tubular lumen [138]. However, papillary micropuncture and microcatheterization studies have not shown significant net potassium transport in this segment in vivo [155a].

POTASSIUM RECYCLING

The concentrations of potassium in the inner medullary interstitium [20] and blood from the vasa recta [12,34] are high, exceeding that of peripheral plasma. The accumulation of potassium at these sites is believed to arise not only from reabsorption from the medullary collecting duct [168], but also from net potassium reabsorption by the thick ascending limb of Henle's loops [169]. This potassium may then diffuse from the interstitium into the pars recta and thin descending limb to produce the high mass flow rate of potassium, exceeding the filtered load, measured near the bends of the long loops of Henle [77].

Thus, potassium is essentially trapped in the medullary interstitium by a countercurrent exchange mechanism between the ascending and descending limbs of the loop of Henle. It has been suggested that this recycling of potassium involving the loops of Henle in the renal medulla may be responsible in some way for regulating net urinary potassium secretion [76,169]. Specifically, it now appears that conditions requiring increased potassium excretion (e.g., high potassium diet) are associated with enhanced potassium recycling. Conversely, recycling can be depressed by potassium deprivation [5,37].

Potassium Handling by the Gastrointestinal Tract

The overall pattern of potassium handling by the nephron, i.e., proximal reabsorption and distal secretion, is repeated in the gastrointestinal tract. Most dietary potassium is passively reabsorbed from the small intestine. Net potassium excretion of 10% to 15% (7 mEq to 15 mEq in the adult) of the daily potassium intake is provided by colonic secretion [129,177]. The rate of potassium secretion is determined in large part by the electrical gradient arising from sodium reabsorption [42]. Additional factors that influence stool potassium excretion are mineralocorticoid activity [10,46] and stool volume [129]. Aldosterone increases colonic reabsorption of sodium and potassium secretion [10,46,135]. Unlike the kidney, however, "escape" from the sodium retention (see below) is not observed [50]. Although ileal fluid is relatively low in potassium content, averaging approximately 10 mEq/L [41], losses of this cation can become substantial with severe or chronic diarrhea [49,183a].

Cellular Mechanisms of Renal Potassium Transport

Proximal Tubule

The mechanisms responsible for potassium reabsorption across the proximal tubular epithelium are incompletely understood. Both active and passive transport mechanisms appear to be important. In the early proximal convoluted tubule, the transepithelial potential is oriented lumen-negative [51] and the concentration of potassium in the tubular fluid may fall below that of the plasma [56]. Under these circumstances, potassium reabsorption would require active transport processes. The transepithelial potential changes to lumen-positive in the late proximal convoluted tubule [51] and may provide a favorable driving force for passive diffusion of potassium along the extensive paracellular shunt pathway (Fig. 6-4a) [56,193]. Such intercellular transport would presumably be coupled to and be driven by sodium-dependent fluid reabsorption [57]. Evidence to support this process arises from studies showing a close correlation between inhibition of proximal tubular fluid reabsorption, either by volume expansion or induction of an osmotic diuresis, and reduction in proximal reabsorption of potassium [16,86].

Thick Ascending Limb

Potassium transport across the thick ascending limb of the loop of Henle occurs primarily through a secondary active transport mechanism. This process involves the cotransport of one sodium and one potassium with two chloride ions (Fig. 6-4b) [21,64,92]. The driving force is ultimately provided by Na-K-ATPase activity at the basolateral membrane, which creates a low intracellular sodium concentration and provides a concentration gradient for sodium entry into the cell. In addition, the lumen-positive transepithelial voltage may provide a route for passive potassium reabsorption through paracellular channels [193]. There are also passive conductance pathways for potassium movement across both luminal and basolateral membranes (Fig. 6-4b) [64,65]. Potassium back-leak into the lumen provides a continuous supply of potassium for cotransport with sodium and chloride [65].

Collecting Duct

The potassium-secreting epithelium of the collecting duct comprises several different cell types. Principal cells, the most numerous cells in the cortical collecting duct, absorb sodium and secrete potassium (Fig. 6-4c). The model for potassium secretion in this cell considers potassium to be actively transported into the cell against a large concen-

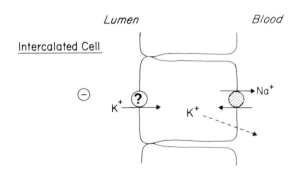

FIG. 6-4. *Possible pathways of transepithelial potassium transport in (A) the proximal tubule, (B) thick ascending limb, (C) principal cells of the cortical collecting duct, and (D) intercalated cells of the cortical collecting duct. Broken arrows indicate passive pathways whereas solid arrows depict active or facilitated transport mechanisms. (Adapted from and reproduced from Giebisch G, Malnic G, Berliner RW: Renal transport and control of potassium excretion. In Brenner BM, Rector FC Jr (eds): The Kidney, Philadelphia, WB Saunders, 1986, with permission.)*

tration gradient in exchange for sodium at the basolateral membrane (see Fig. 6-4c). This 3-Na for 2-K electrogenic exchange, driven by the enzyme Na-K-ATPase [84], results in a high intracellular potassium concentration and negative voltage within the cell.

Chemical measurements of the intracellular potassium concentration in single segments of collecting duct range from 100 mM to 150 mM [122,133,142,171]. However, it is the activity and not the chemical concentration that determines the electrochemical driving force for potassium movement across the epithelium. Microelectrode measurements of the potassium activity in single cells of distal tubules (45 mM to 75 mM) [88,123] are much lower than chemical concentrations and may reflect the consequence of substantial amounts of binding to intracellular protein and substrates or the compartmentalization of potassium within the cell [25].

The electrical potential gradient generated by sodium reabsorption in the cortical collecting duct is oriented with lumen-negative and provides the favorable electrical driving force for potassium secretion [17,61,147,167]. Potassium passively moves from cell to lumen primarily across the apical membrane, which has a significant potassium conductance [93,125,168] (see Fig. 6-4c). Thus, the electrical gradient in the cortical collecting duct and high cellular concentration of potassium favor the exit of cellular potassium into the tubular fluid. Similar cellular transport pathways are probably found in the connecting tubule cell [160,163].

Morphologic studies have shown that maneuvers that alter potassium transport result in ultrastructural changes of these specific tubular cells (Fig. 6-5a-c). Stimulation of net potassium secretion, either by chronic potassium loading, mineralocorticoid administration, or reduction in renal mass, augments the basolateral surface area of cortical principal cells as well as connecting duct cells [81,134, 158,163,182,199]. The microplicated surface of intercalated cells (mitochondria-rich cells; dark cells), scattered among the principal cells of the collecting duct, may be markedly reduced by this maneuver (see Fig. 6-5c) [42a,134], thereby highlighting the unique responsibility of principal and connecting duct cells for regulation of potassium secretion. Conversely, elimination of dietary potassium in the rat is associated with an increase in apical surface area of medullary intercalated cells (see Fig. 6-5b) [42a], suggesting that this specific cell, also involved in transepithelial acid-base transport [141,149], may be responsible for potassium reabsorption [134,163,165]. In contrast to the extensive information available concerning the cellular mechanisms underlying potassium secretion, little is known about how cells reabsorb potassium (Fig. 6-4d). Potassium may be reabsorbed by an apical ATP-coupled H^+-K^+ pump that secretes hydrogen ions in exchange for potassium reabsorption [191a].

Factors Regulating Potassium Transport

The net urinary excretion of potassium depends on the interaction of the various luminal and circulatory factors capable of influencing renal potassium transport. The magnitude of potassium secretion is determined by the movement of this cation from cell to luminal fluid along an electrochemical gradient and by the permeability of the luminal membrane to potassium. Factors that enhance the electrochemical driving force or permeability favor potassium secretion.

Plasma Potassium Concentration

An increase in potassium intake (dietary or by infusion) tends to increase plasma potassium transiently [97], which stimulates renal potassium excretion [132,161,196] and aldosterone secretion by the adrenal gland [13]. The temporary increase in plasma potassium reduces the concentration gradient across the basolateral membrane against which the Na-K-ATPase pump must function and thereby favors an increase in cellular uptake of potassium. Indeed, a 20% rise in plasma potassium can increase the intracellular potassium activity by 30% [89]. This consequent increase in intracellular potassium activity in the renal tubular epithelium [89,123] enhances secretion into the luminal fluid by promoting potassium diffusion down its electrochemical gradient. Hyperkalemia may further augment the chemical driving force favoring potassium secretion in the distal nephron due to its inhibitory effect on proximal tubular sodium and bicarbonate reabsorption, with resulting increase in urinary flow rate [19,45,80]. This suppression of proximal reabsorption presumably follows a decrease in intracellular proton concentration [1], an increase in cell pH, and finally, inhibition of proximal reabsorption of bicarbonate [19,52,136]. The increased cellular potassium activity and distal flow rate, as well as aldosterone effects (see below) that follow an acute elevation of potassium, together increase the rate of potassium excretion, serving to maintain plasma potassium within a constant range.

Rates of excretion of potassium correlate to some extent with plasma potassium concentration, independent of aldosterone effects [161,197]. Elevation of plasma potassium had a direct stimulatory effect on potassium secretion by the microperfused initial collecting duct of the rat, reaching an apparent maximal secretory rate at a plasma potassium concentration of about 6 mEq/L at constant tubular flow rate [161]; the attainment of a maximal secretory rate may reflect the inability of tubular cells to increase intracellular potassium concentration above a certain limiting value [161].

Effect of Potassium Intake

Micropuncture experiments performed in control, potassium-deprived, and potassium-loaded rats demonstrate similar patterns of potassium transport in the superficial proximal tubule and loop of Henle, resulting in similar potassium concentration ratios at the early distal tubular puncture site (probably the distal convoluted tubule) (see Fig. 6-6) [105]. The nearly 200-fold difference in rate of urinary potassium excretion between the two extreme states of potassium balance derives almost entirely from variations

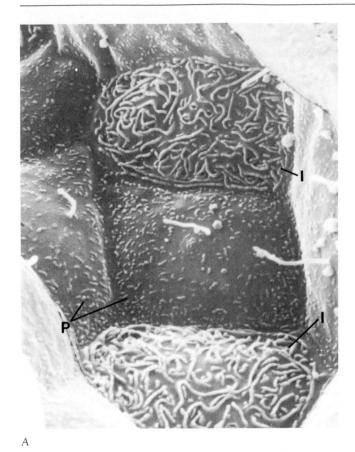

A

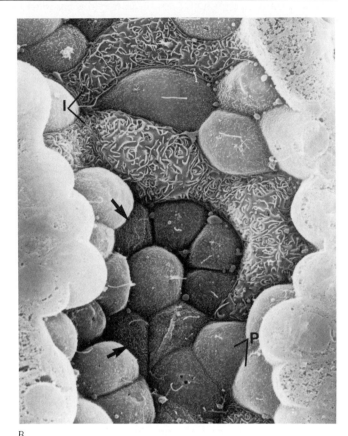

B

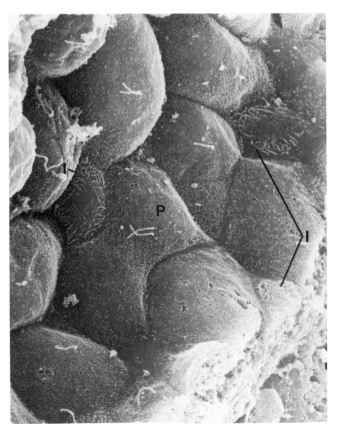

C

FIG. 6-5. Scanning electron micrographs of cortical collecting ducts from the rat. (A) Control animal. Two distinct cell types are noted: principal cells (P) and intercalated cells (I). The apical surface of the intercalated cell possesses an elaborate system of microplicae, while the principal cell has a few short microvilli and a cilium. The apical cell outline of both cell types is approximately hexagonal. ×8,000. (B) Animal fed a low-potassium diet. The apical surfaces of many of the intercalated cells (I) are enlarged and irregular compared to the control state. These cells possess a complex arrangement of microplicae. However, there are some intercalated-like cells (arrows) that possess microplicae, but in a reduced amount compared to the other intercalated cells of the same collecting tubule. The principal cells (P) appear to be normal, except for some showing an irregular apical cell shape. ×3,800. (C) Animal maintained on a high potassium diet. The apical surface of the intercalated cells (I) are characteristically small, possessing a less elaborate array of microplicae than in the control and potassium-depleted animals. No changes are noted in the principal cells (P). ×4,500 before 33% reduction. (Micrographs kindly provided by Dr. A. Evan.)

in the rate of potassium secretion in distal parts of the nephron. Animals provided with a low potassium diet (Fig. 6-6c) demonstrate only a slight rise in potassium concentration along the distal tubule, compared to the steep increase in concentration observed along the distal tubule in the potassium-loaded animals (Fig. 6-6b). In the latter case, net potassium secretion increases the tubular concentration such that by the time the fluid reaches the mid-distal tubule, the delivery of potassium greatly exceeds the filtered load. In the absence of dietary potassium, supression of potassium secretion is observed with conversion to a state of net reabsorption in superficial distal tubules [105,106].

Tubular Flow Rate

Potassium secretion by distal segments of the nephron is strongly influenced by the rate of flow through the tubule and the concentration of potassium in the tubular lumen [59]. At low rates of flow, distal potassium secretion results in a gradual increase in the tubular fluid concentration of potassium [59,89]. With increases in flow rate, within the physiological range, the tubular fluid potassium concentration remains constant or falls [40,59], thereby preserving or enhancing the favorable chemical gradient against which potassium secretion must occur. Thus, a rise in urinary flow rate, as occurs with extracellular volume expansion or diuretic therapy, creates a more favorable concentration gradient for potassium secretion and thereby stimulates potassium entry into the tubular fluid.

Effects of Diuretic Agents

In general, diuretics increase distal delivery of fluid and sodium, thereby enhancing net potassium secretion. Mannitol, the most widely used osmotic diuretic, is freely filtered and poorly absorbed by the proximal tubule. Its presence in high concentration in the luminal fluid reduces water and sodium reabsorption, increasing distal rates of flow [172].

Micropuncture and microperfusion studies have shown that carbonic anhydrase inhibitors, such as acetazolamide, reduce sodium bicarbonate reabsorption in the proximal tubule by 40% to 80% [23,27,111]. This results in increased distal delivery of sodium and water as well as increased negativity of the distal transepithelial voltage due to the presence of the nonreabsorbable anion bicarbonate [27,58,172]. The fractional excretion of potassium to levels approaching 70% has been observed following administration of acetazolamide [58].

Thiazide diuretics inhibit sodium chloride reabsorption in the distal convoluted tubule; the kaliuresis, which may exceed the filtered load, results predominantly from the increased distal tubular delivery of sodium and fluid [58,96].

Some diuretics have a specific effect on renal potassium transport in addition to increasing distal delivery of tubular fluid. The powerful loop diuretics, furosemide and ethacrynic acid, specifically inhibit the Na-Cl-Cl-K cotransport mechanism in the thick ascending limb of Henle's loop [22,24,92]. The kaliuresis following administration of these potent agents may reach two times to five times the baseline levels, or 80% to 100% of the filtered load [40,58]. Amiloride, a potassium sparing diuretic, reduces the sodium conductance of the apical membrane of distal cells [126]. As a result of diminished cell sodium entry, the cell becomes hyperpolarized and the lumen-negative transepithelial voltage is decreased [9], thereby reducing the driving force favoring diffusion of potassium from cell to lumen. Spironolactone, another potassium-sparing diuretic acting at the level of the cortical collecting duct, competitively antagonizes the action of aldosterone [100].

Luminal Sodium Concentration

It has long been recognized that changes in urinary sodium excretion are accompanied by parallel changes in the rate of urinary potassium excretion. Expansion of the extracellular fluid volume [36,105,185], administration of diuretics [40], or contralateral nephrectomy [35] are followed by increases in the excretion of both sodium and potassium. The kaliuresis is due in large part to the increased tubular fluid flow rate reaching distal potassium secretory sites, a consequence of reduced reabsorption of sodium and water within each nephron.

The specific contribution of luminal sodium concentration in mediating potassium secretion has been examined using in vivo and in vitro continuous microperfusion at constant tubular fluid flow rates. Luminal sodium concentrations exceeding 35 mM do not affect net potassium secretion; however, potassium secretion is markedly inhibited when tubular fluid sodium concentration is reduced to less than 10 mM [60,166]. Since in vivo measurements of tubular fluid sodium concentration in the rat distal tubule range between 35 mM to 70 mM [60], it is unlikely that luminal sodium concentration plays a significant role in regulating distal potassium secretion under physiological conditions. However, under conditions of maximal sodium retention when the urinary sodium concentration may be as low as 1 mM [57], this phenomenon may be responsible for the concomitant fall in urinary potassium excretion.

Transepithelial Voltage

Micropuncture studies of the distal tubule and microperfusion of isolated cortical collecting ducts have indicated that the transepithelial potential difference, generated in large part by active reabsorption of sodium and oriented lumen-negative, is a major determinant of the rate of potassium secretion [53,166]. Maneuvers that reduce the active transport of sodium in vitro (and thereby decrease the transepithelial voltage), such as replacement of luminal sodium with choline or addition of ouabain to the peritubular surface, diminish potassium secretion [61,107]. Modification of the transepithelial voltage by perfusion with solutions containing impermeant ions (e.g., sulfate) markedly increases potassium secretion [105,181]. High concentrations of impermeant anions in the tubular lumen would cause the lumen-negative voltage to increase, thereby en-

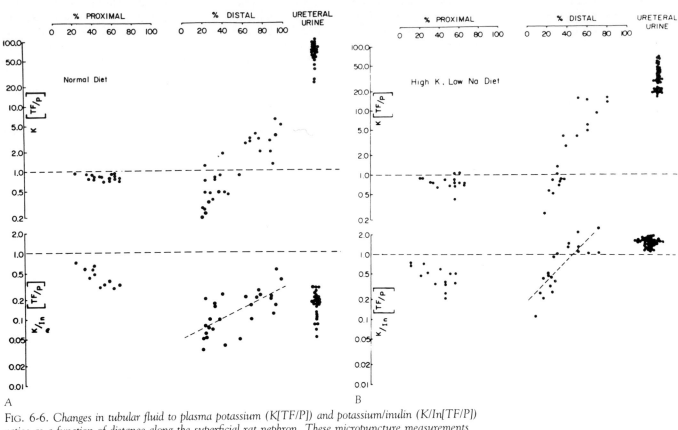

FIG. 6-6. *Changes in tubular fluid to plasma potassium (K[TF/P]) and potassium/inulin (K/In[TF/P]) ratios as a function of distance along the superficial rat nephron. These micropuncture measurements were obtained from rats on a (A) control diet, (B) high potassium diet, and (C) low potassium diet. (Reproduced from Malnic G, Klose RM, Giebisch G: Micropuncture study of renal potassium excretion in the rat. Am J Physiol 206:674, 1964, with permission.)*

hancing the electrical gradient favoring potassium movement into the luminal fluid, i.e., enhancing potassium secretion.

Hormonal Effects

MINERALOCORTICOIDS

Aldosterone is the most important circulating hormone that influences potassium excretion. High circulating levels of hormone result in an enhancement of net urinary potassium excretion and, initially, sodium retention [6,43,72,114].

Examination of single nephron segments has established that the primary targets of mineralocorticoid action are the late distal tubule (connecting tubule) [159,160] and cortical collecting duct [147,160,170,191]. Chronic pretreatment of animals with mineralocorticoids increases net sodium absorption, net potassium secretion, and lumen-negative voltage in the isolated perfused cortical collecting duct [67,124,147,191]. Rates of potassium transport in isolated perfused cortical collecting ducts in vitro correlate well with in vivo plasma aldosterone concentrations (Fig.

6-7), varied by altering the electrolyte content in the diet [147]. At the cellular level, aldosterone enhances the permeability of the apical membrane to potassium and sodium [93,124,140,170], the degree of basolateral membrane infolding [81,182], the level of Na-K-ATPase activity [55,120,128], and the rate of basolateral active uptake of potassium, resulting in an increase in intracellular potassium activity [188,189].

Although aldosterone appears to play an important role in regulating potassium excretion on a long-term basis [197,198], its short-term influence on potassium metabolism has yet to be fully evaluated. The effects of an acute infusion of aldosterone on tubular transport in the distal nephron of adrenalectomized rats, assessed by in vivo and in vitro microperfusion (constant luminal fluid composition and flow rate), include increases in both sodium reabsorption and potassium secretion [45,159], evident after a lag period of one hour to two hours [43,45,191]. However, an effect on net urinary potassium excretion in clearance collections is not consistently observed during this time period [43,191]. The failure to observe a kaliuresis in intact animals may result from the reduction in urinary flow rate often seen following an acute aldosterone infusion

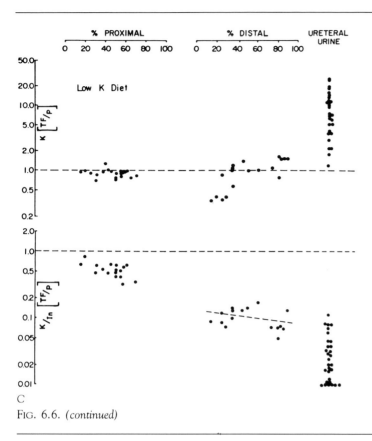

C

FIG. 6.6. (continued)

[43,191]. A decrease in luminal flow rate through the distal nephron would be expected to reduce potassium secretion, thereby opposing the direct stimulatory effect of aldosterone on the distal tubule.

Prolonged administration of mineralocorticoid (over several days) results in increased potassium secretion but only transient renal sodium retention [6,72,114,194]. This phenomenon, termed mineralocorticoid escape, is specific for sodium and does not occur for potassium [68a,114].

GLUCOCORTICOIDS

Clearance studies have demonstrated that exogenous glucocorticoid administration increases net excretion of potassium [15,45,179]. This response is generally thought to represent an indirect effect of the enhanced glomerular filtration, distal delivery of sodium, and rate of urinary flow routinely observed with glucocorticoid infusion [179]. Indeed, dexamethasone was shown not to alter the rate of potassium secretion in isolated cortical collecting ducts perfused in vitro [147] and in distal tubules microperfused at constant rate [45], although clearance studies revealed an increase in urinary flow and a kaliuresis [45].

CORTISOL

The rates of urinary excretion of potassium and water follow a diurnal cycle, with a nadir in the early morning and peak in the late afternoon [115,131,184], in synchrony with the circadian rhythm of cortisol release. Although this pattern is not observed in adrenalectomized animals provided with continuous infusions of cortisol, it can be re-established by administering the hormone as a single morning dose, suggesting that the normal circadian rhythm of plasma cortisol concentration may modulate potassium excretion [116].

ADH

Administration of vasopressin to intact animals frequently causes an increase in urinary excretion of potassium despite a reduction in urinary flow rate [8,79,156]. Direct examination of collecting ducts perfused at constant luminal flow rate has shown that antidiuretic hormone and its nonpressor analogue dDAVP directly enhance potassium secretion [44,175] and sodium reabsorption [30,175]. This effect appears to be mediated by an increase in potassium permeability of the luminal membrane, induced by hormone binding at the basolateral cell membrane [43,68,71].

CATECHOLAMINES

High levels of circulating catecholamines are associated with a reduction in the renal excretion of potassium and sodium [32,78]. However, because of the multiple hormonal, metabolic, and hemodynamic effects of catecholamines, it has been difficult to determine whether inhibition of transport represents a direct tubular effect or a

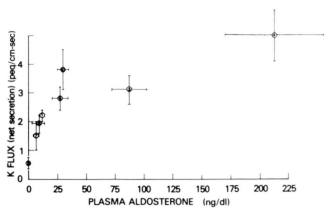

FIG. 6-7. *Potassium secretion (peq/cm-sec), measured across isolated perfused rabbit cortical collecting ducts, plotted as a function of plasma aldosterone concentration (ng/dl). Means are represented by circles and 2SE by the lengths of the lines. The numbers within the circles refer to different diets. (Adapted from and reproduced from Schwartz GJ, and Burg MB: Mineralocorticoid effects on cation transport by cortical collecting tubules in vitro. Am J Physiol 235:F576, 1978, with permission.)*

secondary effect. Adrenergic receptors are present in all nephron segments, including the potassium secretory epithelium of the distal tubule and collecting duct [7], suggesting that catecholamines are capable of directly affecting this epithelium.

Micropuncture studies have demonstrated that pharmacologic stimulation of alpha-adrenoreceptors increases the urinary excretion of sodium, potassium, and water by inhibiting reabsorption of these substances at a nephron site beyond the distal tubule, most likely the collecting duct [162]; the saliuresis and diuresis may result from an inhibition of vasopressin action, with increased distal tubular flow enhancing potassium secretion [162]. Beta-adrenergic agents have been shown to directly inhibit potassium secretion in the isolated perfused cortical collecting duct [43,90]. This inhibition may be mediated by a depolarization of the transepithelial potential difference [90] or a decrease in the apical membrane potassium permeability of this nephron segment [26,43].

Acid-base Balance

Changes in systemic acid-base balance can induce alterations in the rate of excretion of potassium in the urine [108,176]. At any level of plasma potassium, acute metabolic acidosis decreases and acute metabolic alkalosis increases urinary pH and the rate of urinary potassium excretion [176]. Tracer flux experiments [112] and microelectrode measurements [88] in the mammalian distal tubule have demonstrated an increase in intracellular potassium in response to alkalosis and a decrease in acidosis. It is likely that the observed changes in potassium excretion derive in part from changes in the cellular concentration

of potassium, possibly mediated by changes in cytoplasmic pH in the potassium-secreting epithelium of the distal nephron.

Moreover, acidification of the tubular fluid reaching the cortical collecting duct in itself inhibits potassium secretion [17], possibly by closing pH-sensitive potassium channels in the luminal membrane. Under these conditions, the negative transepithelial voltage normally present in the cortical collecting duct is increased [17], presumably due to a reduction in movement of positive electrical charge, carried by potassium, into the lumen [17].

The effects of chronic disturbances in acid-base homeostasis on net potassium excretion are complex and may be influenced by modifications in the rate of tubular flow, composition of glomerular filtrate, and circulating aldosterone levels [57]. The reduction in net potassium excretion by acute acidosis may be offset by an increase in distal flow rate with prolonged acidosis. Indeed, a kaliuresis may be seen under conditions of chronic acidemia, associated with a reduced extracellular concentration of bicarbonate, reflecting the inhibition of proximal reabsorption of sodium and water [63,180]. In chronic metabolic alkalosis, potassium depletion may result from an initial stimulation of potassium excretion, such that cellular potassium decreases and inhibits its own secretion [112].

Potassium Adaptation

Chronic potassium loading leads to "potassium adaptation," characterized by the ability of the animal to tolerate otherwise lethal acute potassium loads [57]. A similar tolerance is seen in chronic renal insufficiency, an adaptive response that serves to maintain potassium balance during the course of many forms of progressive renal disease [95,145,146]. This adaptation is mediated by an increased ability of the potassium secretory epithelium of the distal nephron [70,195] and colon [14,46,70] to excrete potassium.

The cellular mechanisms that may be responsible for this response include stimulation of Na-K-ATPase activity [38,54,70,119,154], amplification of basolateral cell surface area [163], increase in intracellular potassium activity [88], and enhanced transepithelial potential difference [70]. The sum effect of these changes in potassium secreting epithelia is to create a more favorable electrochemical gradient for potassium diffusion from the cell to the luminal fluid.

Gastrointestinal potassium adaptation is observed in response to potassium loading [46] and renal insufficiency [11]. Indeed, fecal potassium excretion can triple in patients with severe renal insufficiency and thereby serve to better maintain potassium balance [70,145].

Maturation of Renal Potassium Transport
Renal Potassium Handling in Infancy and Childhood

Clearance studies in the newborn consistently demonstrate low rates of potassium excretion [173] (Table 6-1), an

TABLE 6-1. *Plasma levels and renal clearances of potassium in infants and children on regular diets without significant renal disease*

Age (yr)	n	P_K (mEq/L)	C_{cr} (ml/min/1.73m²)	C_K (ml/min/1.73m²)	FEK (%)	$U_{Na/K}$
0–0.3	13	5.2 ± 0.8* +	62 ± 26* + @	5 ± 3* + @	8.5 ± 3.8* +	1.1 ± 1.1
0.4–1	10	4.9 ± 0.5* +	99 ± 38* +	14 ± 6*	14.6 ± 5.0	0.8 ± 0.9
3–10	19	4.2 ± 0.5	141 ± 30	20 ± 11	14.5 ± 8.9	1.5 ± 1.1
11–20	17	4.3 ± 0.3	137 ± 21	21 ± 8	16.2 ± 8.2	1.4 ± 0.8

Mean ± standard deviation
Ccr and C_K were each calculated as: rate of renal excretion/plasma level
FEK: fractional excretion of potassium, or the percentage of filtered potassium appearing in the final urine:
$$FEK = \frac{urinary\ potassium\ (mEq/L)}{plasma\ potassium\ (mEq/L)} \times \frac{plasma\ creatinine\ (mg/dl)}{urinary\ creatinine\ (mg/dl)} \times 100\%$$
(Satlin, L.M. and Schwartz, G.J. unpublished observations)
* $p < 0.05$ vs (11–20) yr
+ $p < 0.05$ vs. (3–10) yr
@ $p < 0.05$ (0–.3) yr vs. (.4–1) yr

observation that may reflect the neonatal requirement of potassium for cellular growth [190] or immature renal potassium secretory mechanisms or both. The renal potassium clearance (C_K), even when corrected for the low glomerular filtration rate (C_{Cr}) in infancy, is reduced compared to that measured in the older child (see Table 6-1). Children and adults ingesting a regular diet containing sodium in excess of potassium excrete a urine with a sodium-to-potassium ratio greater than one [139,173] (see Table 6-1). Although the sodium-to-potassium ratio of breast milk and infant formulas is in the range of 0.5 to 0.6, the newborn (0 to 0.3 years) demonstrates significant renal potassium retention with an average urinary sodium-to-potassium ratio also exceeding one (see Table 6-1).

The relative conservation of potassium in the newborn and immature animal is generally associated with a higher plasma potassium concentration than in the adult [98,139,173,187]. Indeed, an inverse relationship has been demonstrated between plasma potassium and gestational age in premature infants [173]. Low-birth-weight infants may excrete urine with a sodium-to-potassium ratio in excess of two, suggesting significant salt wasting in addition to enhanced potassium retention and a relative hyporesponsiveness of the immature kidney to mineralocorticoid stimulation [173].

Infants, like adults administered a potassium load, can excrete potassium at a rate that exceeds its filtration, indicating net renal tubular secretion [178]. However, the newborn is unable to excrete such a potassium load as efficiently or as rapidly as the adult [87,102,110]. Balance studies performed in potassium-loaded newborn piglets showed an increase in net urinary potassium excretion within the first 40 hours of life; however, progressive retention of potassium in these animals led to dramatic hyperkalemia and death [110]. Rats subjected to potassium-loading demonstrated a low rate of excretion per unit body weight during the first two weeks of life, with a rapid increase in the response thereafter [87].

As described above, net potassium excretion in the adult derives almost entirely from potassium secretion in the late distal tubule and cortical collecting duct. Micropuncture experiments performed in suckling rats have shown that approximately 50% of the filtered load of potassium is reabsorbed along the proximal tubule, similar to the fractional reabsorption observed in the adult [98,155]. However, up to 40% of the filtered load of potassium reaches the superficial distal tubule of the newborn, far exceeding the distal delivery measured in the adult [98]; thus, functional maturation of the intervening segment, i.e., the loop of Henle, occurs postnatally [98,200]. Comparison of early distal fluid and final urine in the newborn would suggest that the distal tubule and cortical collecting duct secrete less potassium during the newborn period than in the adult animal [98]. Clearance experiments in saline-expanded puppies have also provided indirect evidence for a diminished capacity of the immature distal nephron to secrete potassium [91].

Renal potassium secretion is influenced by a number of factors, as outlined earlier in the chapter. In the presence of adequate urine flow, the higher plasma potassium concentration generally observed in the newborn would be expected to stimulate the basolateral uptake of potassium, enhance intracellular potassium activity, and augment net secretion. The reduced serum bicarbonate concentration characteristic of the infant might be expected to increase distal sodium and water delivery and thereby result in a kaliuresis [63,180]; on the other hand, acidemia might decrease the intracellular potassium activity in the potassium secretory epithelium and thereby mitigate against the flow effect. In fact, as discussed above, evidence suggests that the distal nephron secretes less potassium in the newborn than in the adult. Possible explanations for a diminished potassium secretory rate in the newborn include immaturity of the potassium secretory epithelium, low tubular flow rates, low Na-K-ATPase activity, insensitivity to mineralocorticoids, and increased backleak of potassium through paracellular routes. It is possible that reduced transepithelial voltage and diminished permeability of the luminal membrane to potassium also limit potassium secretion in the newborn.

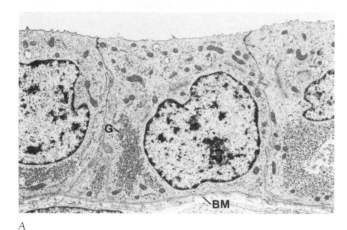

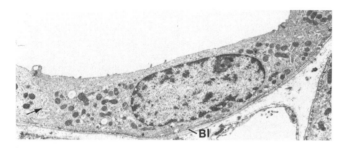

FIG. 6-8. (A) Transmission electron micrograph of a mid-cortical collecting duct from a newborn rabbit showing several principal cells resting on a thin basement membrane (BM). Note the few organelles, simple apical and basal cell surfaces, and glycogen deposits (G) ×10,000. (B) Transmission electron micrograph of a mid-cortical collecting duct from an adult rabbit. The single principal cell shown has varying amounts of basal infolding (BI), fingerlike processes (arrow) at the lateral cell surface, and many short mitochondria. ×4,500 before 51% reduction. (Reproduced from Satlin LM, Evan AP, Gattone VH, et al: Postnatal maturation of the rabbit cortical collecting duct. Pediatr Nephrol 2:135, 1988, with permission.)

Maturity of the Cortical Collecting Duct

Studies of the rabbit cortical collecting duct indicate that this nephron segment, responsible for the final regulation of potassium secretion in the adult, is morphologically and functionally immature at birth [142]. The principal cell of the newborn rabbit possesses few organelles, simple apical and basal cell surfaces, and occasional areas of glycogen deposition (Fig. 6-8a) [142]. The basal cell surface of the adult principal cell appears to possess many more infoldings than that of the newborn, more organelles and mitochondria, and no glycogen (compare Figures 6-8a and b) [142].

Measurements of tubular volume, dry weight, and cell number per unit of tubular length, as well as cell volume, are all significantly lower in the neonatal collecting duct than in the adult segment (Fig. 6-9) [142]. Indeed, significant growth does not begin until after the fourth week of

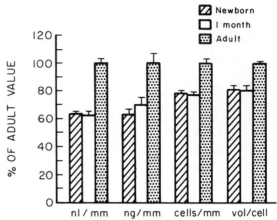

FIG. 6-9. Maturational profile of the cortical collecting duct of the rabbit. Columns represent, left to right, tubular volume, tubular weight, cell number, and cell volume. Values are expressed as a percentage of the adult value, with mean ± SE. All values in the newborn and 1-month-old rabbits are significantly less than the corresponding values from mature animals. (Reproduced from Satlin LM, Evan AP, Gattone VH, et al: Postnatal maturation of the rabbit cortical collecting duct. Pediatr Nephrol 2:135, 1988, with permission.)

life, around the time of weaning, at which point cellular hyperplasia and hypertrophy occur (see Fig. 6-9).

Estimates of the cellular potassium concentration (mEq/L intracellular water) in individual cortical collecting ducts are remarkably constant after birth (Fig. 6-10) [142]. In contrast, potassium concentration (mEq/L tissue water) in thigh skeletal muscle, a non-secreting tissue taken from the same rabbits, significantly increases with age, in large part due to loss of muscle water content [142]. Thus, despite the mature concentration of potassium in the cell water of the neonatal collecting duct, this segment appears morphologically immature.

Tubular Flow Rate

An important mediator of potassium secretion is the rate of delivery of sodium and water into the distal nephron. Increased delivery reduces the luminal potassium concentration, thereby favoring potassium secretion. Flow rates in the cortical collecting duct cannot be measured in animals in vivo. However, it is well known that in newborn mammals, glomerular filtration rates [98,157] and distal flow rates [3,98] are low, even when appropriate correction is made for the small body size. Low flow rates of the collecting tubular fluid would lead to higher concentrations of potassium in the tubular fluid, creating a less favorable cell-to-lumen concentration gradient and thereby limiting potassium secretion. A postnatal increase in single nephron glomerular filtration rate, as demonstrated in vivo in the maturing guinea pig during the second two weeks of extrauterine life [157], may lead to the opening up of previously nonfiltering superficial nephrons that drain into the

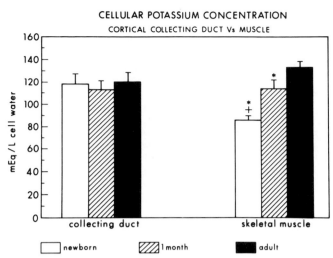

FIG. 6-10. *Comparison of cellular potassium concentration in the cortical collecting duct and skeletal muscle of newborn, 1-month-old, and adult rabbits. Mean values ±SE are given at each age group. Asterisk (*) denotes a statistical difference (p < 0.05) compared to the adult value. The plus (+) denotes a statistical difference (p < 0.05) compared to the 1-month value.*

cortical collecting duct and increase rates of distal tubular flow and delivery of sodium, resulting in the enhancement of potassium secretion with maturation.

Although potassium secretion per kg body weight or potassium per g kidney weight was less in the newborn than in the adult dog during potassium loading, potassium secretion per ml glomerular filtrate was not different between the two age groups, suggesting that the limited secretory capacity in the newborn dog is due to a lower glomerular filtration rate or distal flow [102]. A low tubular flow rate would contribute to the reduced capacity for potassium secretion in the neonatal kidney.

Na-K-ATPase

As stated above, the potassium concentration in the neonatal collecting duct is at mature levels, in contrast to muscle, a nonsecreting tissue [142]. The high intracellular potassium is generated and maintained by the enzyme Na-K-ATPase. Measurement of Na-K-ATPase activity (expressed per unit dry weight) in the neonatal rabbit cortical collecting duct has been reported to be only 50% of that measured in the mature nephron [143], suggesting that potassium secretory ability, unlike the steady state cellular levels [142], is limited in the neonate.

Mineralocorticoid Activity

Although plasma aldosterone levels are elevated in the newborn and immature animal when compared to the adult [39,94,153,173] and would be expected to stimulate po-

tassium secretion, the immature kidney appears to be relatively insensitive to this hormone [73,164,173]. The currently accepted model for aldosterone action requires initial hormone-receptor binding, followed by translocation of this complex to the nucleus where specific genes are stimulated to code for physiologically active proteins, such as Na-K-ATPase [109]. Studies have shown an equivalent number of aldosterone binding sites and similar nuclear binding of hormone-receptor complexes in rats ages seven to 30 days, suggesting that the hyposensitivity to aldosterone observed in the first two weeks of life in this model represents a postreceptor phenomenon [164].

Paracellular Conductance

There is evidence to suggest that immature proximal tubules and cortical collecting ducts have an increased hydraulic (paracellular) conductance when compared with tubules isolated from adult animals [73,74]. If this is true, then greater potassium backleak from lumen to interstitium in the cortical collecting duct could potentially limit potassium secretion. At any given tubular flow rate, net potassium secretion by the "leakier" immature cortical collecting duct would be expected to be less than that by its mature "tight" counterpart. Thus, at the low tubular flow rates found in the immature kidney, which result in increased tubular fluid potassium concentrations, enhanced paracellular backleak of potassium may severely limit net potassium secretion.

Transepithelial Voltage

A reduced capacity for potassium secretion in the newborn distal nephron may be due to differences in the electrochemical gradient across the epithelium or the relative rates of potassium exit across the apical membrane versus basolateral membrane [167]. Since the mean transepithelial voltage across the newborn cortical collecting duct has not been determined, the role of the electrical gradient in mediating potassium secretion is unknown. Nevertheless, we can speculate that the potential difference across this membrane is diminished in the newborn, when compared to the adult, since a reduced transepithelial voltage has been demonstrated in the neonatal outer medullary collecting duct [73].

Permeability of Cell Membranes

Measurements of the apical and basolateral permeability of the newborn potassium secretory epithelium have not been performed. In the case of potassium permeability in the collecting duct, the driving force is predominantly due to the difference between the high intracellular potassium concentration and the low potassium concentration in the tubular fluid. Since the intracellular potassium concentration in the collecting duct may be similar in the newborn and adult [142], a diminished potassium secretory rate in this immature segment could possibly be due to a decreased number of potassium channels in the apical membrane.

References

1. Adler S, Fraley DS: Potassium and intracellular pH. *Kidney Int* 11:433, 1977.
2. Anderson EC, Langham WH: Average potassium concentration of the human body as a function of age. *Science* 130:713, 1959.
3. Aperia A, Elinder G: Distal tubular sodium reabsorption in the developing rat kidney. *Am J Physiol* 240:F487, 1981.
5. Arrascue JF, Dobyan DC, Jamison RL: Potassium recycling in the renal medulla: Effects of acute potassium chloride administration to rats fed a potassium-free diet. *Kidney Int* 20:348, 1981.
6. August JT, Nelson DH, Thorn GW: Response of normal subjects to large amounts of aldosterone. *J Clin Invest* 37:1549, 1958.
7. Barajas L, Powers K, Wang P: Innervation of the renal cortical tubules: A quantitative study. *Am J Physiol* 247:F50, 1984.
8. Barraclough MA, Jones NF: The effect of vasopressin on the reabsorption of sodium, potassium and urea by the renal tubules in man. *Clin Sci* 39:517, 1970.
9. Barratt LJ: The effect of amiloride on the transepithelial potential difference of the distal tubule of the rat kidney. *Pflugers Arch* 361:251, 1976.
10. Bastl CP, Binder HJ, Hayslett JP: Role of glucocorticoids and aldosterone in maintenance of colonic cation transport. *Am J Physiol* 238:F181, 1980.
11. Bastl CP, Hayslett JP, Binder HJ: Increased large intestinal secretion of potassium in renal insufficiency. *Kidney Int* 12:9, 1977.
12. Battilana CA, Dobyan DC, Lacy FB, et al: Effect of chronic potassium loading on potassium secretion by the pars recta or descending limb of the juxtamedullary nephron in the rat. *J Clin Invest* 62:1093, 1978.
13. Bauer JH, Gautner WC: Effect of potassium chloride on plasma renin activity and plasma aldosterone during sodium restriction in normal man. *Kidney Int* 15:286, 1979.
14. Bia MJ, DeFronzo RA: Extrarenal potassium homeostasis. *Am J Physiol* 240:F257, 1981.
15. Bia MJ, Tyler K, DeFronzo RA: The effect of dexamethasone on renal electrolyte excretion in the adrenalectomized rat. *Endocrinology* 111:882, 1982.
16. Bomsztyk K, Wright FS: Effects of transepithelial fluid flux on transepithelial voltage and transport of calcium, sodium, chloride, and potassium by renal proximal tubule. *Kidney Int* 21:269, 1981.
17. Boudry JF, Stoner LC, Burg MB: Effect of acid lumen pH on potassium transport in renal cortical collecting tubules. *Am J Physiol* 230:239, 1976.
18. Boyer PD, Lardy HA, Phillips PH: Further studies on the role of potassium and other ions in phosphorylation of adenylic system. *J Biol Chem* 149:529, 1943.
19. Brandis M, Keyes J, Windhager EE: Potassium induced inhibition of proximal tubular reabsorption in rats. *Am J Physiol* 222:421, 1972.
20. Bulger RE, Beeuwkes R III, Saubermann AJ: Application of scanning electron microscopy to x-ray analysis of frozen-hydrated sections. III. Elemental content of cells in the rat renal papillary tip. *J Cell Biol* 88:274, 1981.
21. Burg MB: Thick ascending limb of Henle's loop. *Kidney Int* 22:454, 1982.
22. Burg M, Green N: Effect of ethacrynic acid on the thick ascending limb of Henle's loop. *Kidney Int* 4:301, 1973.
23. Burg M, Green N: Bicarbonate transport by isolated perfused rabbit proximal convoluted tubules. *Am J Physiol* 233:F307, 1977.
24. Burg M, Stoner LV, Cardinal J, et al: Furosemide effect on isolated perfused tubules. *Am J Physiol* 255:119, 1973.
25. Civan MM: Intracellular activities of sodium and potassium. *Am J Physiol* 234:F261, 1978.
26. Clausen T, Flatman JA: The effect of catecholamines on Na-K transport and membrane potential in rat soleus muscle. *J Physiol* 270:383, 1977.
27. Cogan MG, Maddox DA, Warnock DG, et al: Effect of acetazolamide on bicarbonate reabsorption in the proximal tubule of the rat. *Am J Physiol* 237:F447, 1979.
28. Cole BR, Brocklebank JT, Murray BN, et al: Maturation of the developing rabbit kidneys: Variations in cellular size and contents. *Pediatr Res* 15:916, 1981.
29. Conn JW: Hypertension, the potassium ion and impaired carbohydrate tolerance. *N Engl J Med* 273:1135, 1965.
30. Costanzo LS, Windhager EE: Effects of PTH, ADH and cyclic AMP on distal tubular Ca and Na reabsorption. *Am J Physiol* 239:F478, 1980.
32. DeFronzo RA, Bia M, Birkhead G: Epinephrine and potassium homeostasis. *Kidney Int* 20:83, 1981.
33. Dickerson JWT, Widdowson EM: Chemical changes in skeletal muscle during development. *Biochem J* 74:247, 1960.
34. Diezi J, Michoud P, Aceves J, et al: Micropuncture study of electrolyte transport across papillary collecting duct of the rat. *Am J Physiol* 224:623, 1973.
35. Diezi J, Michoud P, Grandchamp A, et al: Effects of nephrectomy on renal salt and water transport in the remaining kidney. *Kidney Int* 10:450, 1976.
36. Dirks JH, Seely JF: Effect of saline infusions and furosemide on the dog distal nephron. *Am J Physiol* 219:114, 1970.
37. Dobyan DC, Lacy FB, Jamison RL: Potassium recycling in the renal medulla by short term potassium deprivation. *Kidney Int* 16:704, 1979.
38. Doucet A, Katz AI: Renal potassium adaptation: Na-K-ATPase activity along the nephron after chronic potassium loading. *Am J Physiol* 238:F380, 1980.
39. Drukker A, Goldsmith D, Spitzer A, et al: The renin-angiotensin system in newborn dogs: Developmental patterns and response to acute saline loading. *Pediatr Res* 14:304, 1980.
40. Duarte CG, Chomety F, Giebisch G: Effect of amiloride, ouabain, and furosemide on distal tubule function in the rat. *Am J Physiol* 221:632, 1971.
41. Edelman IS, Liebman J: Anatomy of body water and electrolytes. *Am J Med* 27:256, 1959.
42. Edmonds CJ: Transport of sodium and secretion of potassium and bicarbonate by the colon of normal and sodium-depleted rats. *J Physiol* (Lond) 193:589, 1967.
42a. Evan A, Huser J, Bengele HH, et al: The effect of alterations in dietary potassium on collecting system morphology in the rat. *Lab Invest* 42:668, 1980.
43. Field MJ, Giebisch GH: Hormonal control of renal potassium excretion. *Kidney Int* 27:379, 1985.
44. Field MJ, Stanton BA, Giebisch G: Influence of ADH on renal potassium handling: A micropuncture and microperfusion study. *Kidney Int* 25:502, 1984.
45. Field MJ, Stanton BA, Giebisch G: Differential acute effects of aldosterone, dexamethasone, and hyperkalemia on distal tubular potassium secretion in the rat kidney. *J Clin Invest* 74:1792, 1984.
46. Fisher KA, Binder HJ, Hayslett JP: Potassium secretion by colonic mucosal cells after potassium adaptation. *Am J Physiol* 231:987, 1976.
47. Flynn MA, Woodruff C, Clark J, et al: Total body potassium in normal children. *Pediatr Res* 6:239, 1972.
48. Flynn MA, Clark J, Reid JC, et al: A longitudinal study

of total body potassium in normal children. *Pediatr Res* 9:834, 1975.

49. Fordtran JS, Dietschy JM: Water and electrolyte movement in the intestine. *Gastroenterology* 50:263, 1966.

50. Fourman BH, Mulrow PJ: Effect of corticosteroids on water and electrolyte metabolism. *In* Greep RO, Astwood EB (eds): *Handbook of Physiology. Endocrinology.* Washington, DC, American Physiological Society, 1973, p 179.

51. Fromter E, Gessner K: Free flow potential profile along rat kidney proximal tubule. *Pflugers Arch* 351:69, 1974.

52. Fuller GR, MacLeod MB, Pitts RF: Influence of administration of potassium salts on the renal tubular reabsorption of bicarbonate. *Am J Physiol* 182:111, 1955.

53. Garcia-Filho E, Malnic G, Giebisch G: Effects of changes in electrical potential difference on tubular potassium transport. *Am J Physiol* 238:F235, 1980.

54. Garg LC, Narang N: Renal adaptation to potassium in the adrenalectomized rabbit. Role of distal tubular sodium-potassium adenosine triphosphatase. *J Clin Invest* 76:1065, 1985.

55. Garg LC, Knepper MA, Burg MB: Mineralocorticoid effects on Na-K-ATPase in individual nephron segments. *Am J Physiol* 240:F536, 1981.

56. Giebisch G: Renal potassium transport. *In* Giebisch G, Tosteson DC, Ussing HH (eds): *Membrane Transport in Biology.* Vol IVA. Berlin, Springer-Verlag, 1978, p 215.

57. Giebisch G, Malnic G, Berliner RW: Renal transport and control of potassium excretion. *In* Brenner BM, Rector FC Jr (eds): *The Kidney.* Philadelphia, WB Saunders, 1986, p 177.

58. Goldberg M: The renal physiology of diuretics. *In* Orloff JJ, Berliner RW (eds): *Handbook of Physiology. Renal Physiology.* Washington, DC, American Physiological Society, 1973, p 1003.

59. Good DW, Wright FS: Luminal influences of potassium secretion: Sodium concentration and fluid flow rate. *Am J Physiol* 236:F192, 1979.

60. Good DW, Velasquez H, Wright FS: Luminal influences on potassium secretion: Low sodium concentration. *Am J Physiol* 246:F609, 1984.

61. Grantham JJ, Burg MB, Orloff J: The nature of transtubular Na and K transport in rabbit collecting tubules. *J Clin Invest* 49:1815, 1970.

62. Grantham JJ, Qualizza PB, Irwin RL: Net fluid secretion in proximal straight renal tubules in vitro: role of PAH. *Am J Physiol* 226:191, 1974.

63. Green R, Giebisch G: Some ionic requirements of proximal tubular sodium transport. I. The role of bicarbonate and chloride. *Am J Physiol* 229:1205, 1975.

64. Greger R, Schlatter E: Presence of luminal K$^+$, a prerequisite for active NaCl transport in the cortical thick ascending limb of Henle's loop of rabbit kidney. *Pflugers Arch* 392:92, 1981.

65. Greger R, Schlatter E: Properties of the lumen membrane of the cortical thick ascending limb of Henle's loop of rabbit kidney. *Pflugers Arch* 396:315, 1983.

66. Greger R, Schlatter E: Properties of the basolateral membrane of the cortical thick ascending limb of Henle's loop of rabbit kidney. A model for secondary active chloride transport. *Pflugers Arch* 396:325, 1983.

67. Gross JB, Kokko JP: Effects of aldosterone and potassium sparing diuretics on electrical potential differences across the distal nephron. *J Clin Invest* 59:82, 1977.

68. Guggino SE, Suarez-Isla BA, Guggino WB, et al: Forskolin and antidiuretic hormone stimulate a Ca^{+2} activated K$^+$ channel in cultured kidney cells. *Am J Physiol* 249:F448, 1985.

68a. Haas JA, Berndt TJ, Youngberg SP, et al: Collecting duct sodium reabsorption in deoxycorticosterone-treated rats. *J Clin Invest* 63:211, 1979.

69. Hastings AB, Buchanan JM: The role of intracellular cations on liver glycogen formation in vitro. *Proc Natl Acad Sci USA* 28:478, 1942.

70. Hayslett JP, Binder HJ: Mechanism of potassium adaptation. *Am J Physiol* 243:F103, 1982.

71. Hebert SC, Friedman PA, Andreoli TE: Effect of antidiuretic hormone on cellular conductive pathways in mouse medullary thick ascending limbs of Henle. I. ADH increases transcellular conductance pathways. *J Membr Biol* 80:201, 1984.

72. Hierholzer K, Lange S: The effects of adrenal steroids on renal function. *In* Thurau K (ed): *MTP International Review Science. Kidney and Urinary Tract Physiology.* London, Butterworth, 1975, p 273.

73. Horster M: Expression of ontogeny in individual nephron segments. *Kidney Int* 22:550, 1982.

74. Horster M, Larsson L: Mechanisms of fluid absorption during proximal tubule development. *Kidney Int* 10:348, 1976.

75. Imai M, Nakamura R: Function of distal convoluted and connecting tubules studied by isolated nephron segments. *Kidney Int* 22:465, 1982.

76. Jamison RL, Work J, Schafer JA: New pathways for potassium transport in the kidney. *Am J Physiol* 242:F297, 1982.

77. Jamison RL, Lacy FB, Pennell JP, et al: Potassium secretion by the descending limb of pars recta of juxtamedullary nephron in vivo. *Kidney Int* 9:323, 1976.

78. Johnson MD, Barger CA: Circulating catecholamines in control of renal electrolyte and water excretion. *Am J Physiol* 240:F192, 1981.

79. Johnson MD, Kinter LB, Beeuwkes R: Effect of AVP and DDAVP on plasma renin activity and electrolyte excretion in conscious dogs. *Am J Physiol* 236:F66, 1979.

80. Kahn M, Bohrer NK: Effect of potassium-induced diuresis on renal concentration and dilution. *Am J Physiol* 211:1365, 1967.

81. Kaissling B: Structural aspects of adaptive changes in renal electrolyte excretion. *Am J Physiol* 243:F211, 1982.

82. Kaissling B, Kriz W: *Structural Analysis of the Rabbit Kidney.* Berlin, Springer-Verlag, 1979, p 13.

83. Kaissling B, Peter S, Kriz W: The transition of the thick ascending limb of Henle's loop into the distal convoluted tubule in the nephron of the rat kidney. *Cell Tissue Res* 182:111, 1977.

84. Katz AI: Renal Na-K-ATPase: Its role in tubular sodium and potassium transport. *Am J Physiol* 242:F207, 1982.

85. Katz AI, Doucet A, Morel F: Na-K-ATPase activity along the rabbit, rat and mouse nephron. *Am J Physiol* 237:F114, 1979.

86. Kaufman JS, Hamburger RJ: Passive potassium transport in the proximal convoluted tubule. *Am J Physiol* 248:F228, 1985.

87. Kerstein L, Mohr C, Braunich H: Der Mechanismus der renalen ausscheidung von Natrion und Kalium und seine altersabhangigi Entwicklung ber Ratten Vom 5 bis 240 Levenstag. *Acta Biol Med Ger* 27:327, 1971.

88. Khuri RN, Agulian SK, Kalloghlian A: Intracellular potassium in cells of the distal tubule. *Pflugers Arch* 335:297, 1972.

89. Khuri RN, Wiederholt M, Strieder N, et al: Effects of flow rate and potassium intake on distal tubular potassium transfer. *Am J Physiol* 228:1249, 1975.

90. Kimmel PL, Goldfarb S: Effects of isoproterenol on potas-

sium secretion by the cortical collecting tubule. *Am J Physiol* 246:F804, 1984.

91. Kleinman LI, Banks RO: Segmental nephron sodium and potassium reabsorption in newborn and adult dogs during saline expansion. *Proc Soc Exp Biol Med* 173:231, 1983.

92. Koenig B, Ricapito S, Kinne R: Chloride transport in the thick ascending limb of Henle's loop: Potassium dependence and stoichiometry of the NaCl cotransport system in plasma membrane vesicles. *Pflugers Arch* 399:173, 1983.

93. Koeppen BM, Biagi BA, Giebisch GH: Intracellular microelectrode characterization of the rabbit cortical collecting duct. *Am J Physiol* 244:F35, 1983.

94. Kowarski A, Katz H, Migeon CJ: Plasma aldosterone concentration in normal subjects from infancy to adulthood. *J Clin Endocrinol Metab* 38:489, 1974.

95. Kunau RT, Whinnery MA: Potassium transfer in distal tubule of normal and remnant kidneys. *Am J Physiol* 235:F186, 1978.

96. Kunau RT Jr, Weller DR, Webb HL: Clarification of the site of action of chlorothiazide in the rat nephron. *J Clin Invest* 56:401, 1975.

97. Laragh JH, Capeci NE: Effect of administration of potassium chloride on serum sodium and potassium concentration. *Am J Physiol* 180:539, 1955.

98. Lelievre-Pegorier M, Merlet-Benichou C, Roinel N, et al: Developmental pattern of water and electrolyte transport in rat superficial nephrons. *Am J Physiol* 245:F15, 1983.

99. Lev AA: Determination of activity and activity coefficients of potassium and sodium ions in frog muscle fibers. *Nature* 201:1132, 1964.

100. Liddle GW: Specific and non-specific inhibition of mineralocorticoid activity. *Metabolism* 10:1021, 1961.

101. Linshaw MA: Potassium homeostasis and hypokalemia. *In* Gruskin AB (ed): *Pediatric Nephrology. Pediatric Clinics of North America* 34(3). Philadelphia, WB Saunders, 1987, p 649.

102. Lorenz JM, Kleinman LI, Disney TA: Renal response of newborn dog to potassium loading. *Am J Physiol* 251:F513, 1986.

103. Lubin M: Intracellular potassium and control of protein synthesis. *Fed Proc* 23:994, 1964.

104. Lubin M: Intracellular potassium and macromolecular synthesis in mammalian cells. *Nature* 213:451, 1967.

105. Malnic G, Klose RM, Giebisch G: Micropuncture study of renal potassium excretion in the rat. *Am J Physiol* 206:674, 1964.

106. Malnic G, Klose RM, Giebisch G: Micropuncture study of distal tubular potassium and sodium transport in rat nephron. *Am J Physiol* 211:529, 1966.

107. Malnic G, Klose RM, Giebisch G: Microperfusion study of distal tubular potassium and sodium transfer in rat kidney. *Am J Physiol* 211:548, 1966.

108. Malnic G, de Mello-Aires M, Giebisch G: Potassium transport across renal distal tubules during acid-base disturbances. *Am J Physiol* 221:1192, 1971.

109. Marver D, Kokko JP: Renal target sites and the mechanism of action of aldosterone. *Miner Electrolyte Metab* 9:1, 1983.

110. McCance RA, Widdowson EM: The response of the newborn piglet to an excess of potassium. *J Physiol* 141:88, 1958.

111. McKinney TD, Burg MB: Bicarbonate and fluid absorption by renal proximal straight tubules. *Kidney Int* 12:1, 1977.

112. de Mello-Aires M, Malnic G: Renal handling of sodium and potassium during hypochloremic alkalosis in the rat. *Pfluegers Arch* 331:215, 1972.

113. de Mello-Aires M, Giebisch G, Malnic G: Kinetics of potassium transport across single distal tubules of rat kidney. *J Physiol* 1232:47, 1973.

114. Mohring HJ, Mohring B: Reevaluation of DOCA escape phenomenon. *Am J Physiol* 223:1237, 1972.

115. Moore-Ede MC, Herd JA: Renal electrolyte circadian rhythms: Independence from feeding and activity patterns. *Am J Physiol* 232:F128, 1977.

116. Moore-Ede MC, Schmelzer WS, Kass DA, et al: Cortisol mediated synchronization of circadian rhythm in urinary potassium excretion. *Am J Physiol* 233:R230, 1977.

117. Morel F: Sites of hormone action in the mammalian nephron. *Am J Physiol* 240:F159, 1981.

118. Morel F, Chabardes D, Imbert M: Functional segmentation of the rabbit distal tubule by microdetermination of hormone-dependent adenylate cyclase activity. *Kidney Int* 9:264, 1976.

119. Mujais SK, Chekal MA, Hayslett JP, et al: Regulation of renal Na$^+$-K$^+$-ATPase in the rat: Role of increased potassium transport. *Am J Physiol* 251:F199, 1986.

120. Mujais SK, Chekal MA, Jones WJ, et al: Modulation of renal Na-K-ATPase by aldosterone. Effect of high physiologic levels on enzyme activity in isolated rat and rabbit tubules. *J Clin Invest* 76:170, 1985.

121. National Research Council, National Academy of Sciences. *Recommended Dietary Allowances*, 9th rev ed. Washington, DC, 1980, p 169.

122. Natke E Jr, Stoner LC: Na$^+$ transport properties of the peritubular membrane of cortical collecting tubule. *Am J Physiol* 242:F664, 1982.

123. Oberleithner H, Kubota T, Giebisch G: Potassium transport and intracellular potassium activity in distal tubules of Amphiuma. *Fed Proc* 39:1079, 1980.

124. O'Neil RG, Helman SI: Transport characteristics of renal collecting tubules: Influence of DOCA and diet. *Am J Physiol* 233:F544, 1977.

125. O'Neil RG, Boulpaep EL: Ionic conductance properties and electrophysiology of the rabbit cortical collecting tubule. *Am J Physiol* 243:F81, 1982.

126. O'Neil RG, Sansom SC: Characterization of apical cell membrane Na$^+$ and K$^+$ conductances of cortical collecting duct using microelectrode techniques. *Am J Physiol* 247:F14, 1984.

127. Osathandonh V, Potter EL: Development of human kidney as shown by microdissection. III. Formation and interrelationship of collecting tubules and nephrons. *Arch Pathol Lab Med* 756:290, 1963.

128. Petty KJ, Kokko JP, Marver D: Secondary effect of aldosterone on Na-K-ATPase activity in the rabbit cortical collecting tubule. *J Clin Invest* 68:1514, 1981.

129. Phillips SF: Absorption and secretion by the colon. *Gastroenterology* 56:966, 1969.

130. Pierson RN Jr, Lin DHY, Phillips RA: Total body potassium in health: Effects of age, sex, height and fat. *Am J Physiol* 226:206, 1974.

131. Rabinowitz L, Wynder CJ, Smith KM, et al: Diurnal potassium excretory cycles in the rat. *Am J Physiol* 250:F930, 1986.

132. Rabinowitz L, Sarason RL, Yamauchi H, et al: Time course of adaptation to altered potassium intake in rats and sheep. *Am J Physiol* 247:F607, 1984.

133. Rajerison RM, Faure M, Morel F: Effects of temperature, ouabain and diuretics on the cell sodium and potassium contents of isolated rat kidney tubules. *Pflugers Arch* 406:285, 1986.

134. Rastegar A, Biemesderfer D, Kashgarian M, et al: Changes in membrane surfaces of collecting duct cells in potassium adaptation. *Kidney Int* 18:293, 1980.

135. Richards P: Clinical investigation of the effects of adrenal corticosteroid excess on the colon. *Lancet* 1:437, 1969.

136. Roberts HE, Magida MG, Pitts RF: Relationship between potassium and bicarbonate in blood and urine. *Am J Physiol* 172:47, 1952.

137. Rocha AS, Kokko JP: Membrane characteristics regulating potassium transport out of the isolated perfused descending limb of Henle. *Kidney Int* 4:326, 1973.

138. Rocha AS, Kudo LH: Water, urea, sodium, chloride, and potassium transport in the in vitro isolated perfused papillary collecting duct. *Kidney Int* 22:485, 1982.

139. Rodriguez-Soriano J, Vallo A, Castillo G, et al: Renal handling of water and sodium in infancy and childhood: A study using clearance methods during hypotonic saline diuresis. *Kidney Int* 20:700, 1981.

140. Sansom SC, O'Neil RG: Mineralocorticoid regulation of apical cell membrane Na$^+$ and K$^+$ transport of the cortical collecting duct. *Am J Physiol* 248:F858, 1985.

141. Satlin LM, Schwartz GJ: Postnatal maturation of rabbit renal collecting duct: intercalated cell function. *Am J Physiol* 253:F622, 1987.

142. Satlin LM, Evan AP, Gattone VH, et al: Postnatal maturation of the rabbit cortical collecting duct. *Pediatr Nephrol* 2:135, 1988.

143. Schmidt U, Horster M: Na-K-activated ATPase: Activity maturation in rabbit nephron segments dissected in vitro. *Am J Physiol* 233:F55, 1977.

144. Schnermann J, Steipe B, Briggs JP: In situ studies of distal convoluted tubule in rat. II. K secretion. *Am J Physiol* 252:F970, 1987.

145. Schon DA, Silva P, Hayslett JP: Mechanism of potassium excretion in renal insufficiency. *Am J Physiol* 227:1323, 1974.

146. Schultze RG, Taggart DD, Shapiro H, et al: On the adaptation in potassium excretion associated with nephron reduction in the dog. *J Clin Invest* 50:1061, 1971.

147. Schwartz GJ, Burg MB: Mineralocorticoid effects on cation transport by cortical collecting tubules in vitro. *Am J Physiol* 235:F576, 1978.

149. Schwartz GJ, Barasch J, Al-Awqati Q: Plasticity of functional epithelial polarity. *Nature* 318:368, 1985.

150. Schwartz WB: Potassium and the kidney. *N Engl J Med* 253:601, 1955.

151. Shareghi GR, Agus ZS: Magnesium transport in the cortical thick ascending limb of Henle's loop of the rabbit. *J Clin Invest* 69:759, 1982.

152. Shareghi GR, Stoner LC: Calcium transport across segments of the rabbit distal nephron in vitro. *Am J Physiol* 235:F367, 1978.

153. Siegel SR, Fischer DA: Ontogeny of the renin-angiotensin-aldosterone system in the fetal and newborn lamb. *Pediatr Res* 14:99, 1980.

154. Silva P, Brown RS, Epstein F: Adaptation to potassium. *Kidney Int* 11:466, 1977.

155. Solomon S: Absolute rates of sodium and potassium reabsorption by proximal tubules of immature rats. *Biol Neonate* 25:340, 1974.

155a. Sonnenberg H, Ching C: Comparison of micropuncture and microcatheterization in papillary collecting duct. *Am J Physiol* 239:F92, 1980.

156. Sonnenberg H, Honrath U, Wilson DR: Effect of vasopressin analogue (dDAVP) on potassium transport in medullary collecting duct. *Am J Physiol* 252:F986, 1987.

157. Spitzer A, Brandis M: Functional and morphologic maturation of the superficial nephrons. Relationship to total kidney function. *J Clin Invest* 53:279, 1974.

158. Stanton BA: Role of adrenal hormones in regulating distal

159. Stanton BA: Regulation by adrenal corticosteroids of sodium and potassium transport in loop of Henle and distal tubule of rat. *J Clin Invest* 78:1612, 1986.

160. Stanton BA: Regulation of Na$^+$ and K$^+$ transport by mineralocorticoids. *Sem Nephrol* 7:82, 1987.

161. Stanton BA, Giebisch GH: Potassium transport by the renal distal tubule: Effects of potassium loading. *Am J Physiol* 243:F487, 1982.

162. Stanton B, Puglisi E, Gellai M: Localization of alpha$_2$-adrenoceptor-mediated increase in renal Na$^+$, K$^+$, and water excretion. *Am J Physiol* 252:F1016, 1987.

163. Stanton BA, Biemesderfer D, Wade JB, et al: Structural and functional study of the rat distal nephron: Effects of potassium adaptation and depletion. *Kidney Int* 19:36, 1981.

164. Stephenson G, Hammet M, Hadaway G, et al: Ontogeny of renal mineralocorticoid receptors and urinary electrolyte responses in the rat. *Am J Physiol* 247:F665, 1984.

165. Stetson DL, Wade JB, Giebisch G: Morphologic alterations in the rat medullary collecting tubule following potassium depletion. *Kidney Int* 17:45, 1980.

166. Stokes JB: Potassium secretion by cortical collecting tubule: Relation to sodium absorption, luminal sodium concentration, and transepithelial voltage. *Am J Physiol* 241:F395, 1981.

167. Stokes JB: Ion transport by the cortical and outer medullary collecting tubule. *Kidney Int* 22:473, 1982.

168. Stokes JB: Na and K transport across the cortical and outer medullary collecting tubule of the rabbit: evidence for diffusion across the outer medullary portion. *Am J Physiol* 242:F514, 1982.

169. Stokes JB: Consequences of potassium recycling in the renal medulla. Effects on ion transport by the medullary thick ascending limb of Henle's loop. *J Clin Invest* 70:219, 1982.

170. Stokes JB: Mineralocorticoid effect on K$^+$ permeability of the rabbit cortical collecting tubule. *Kidney Int* 28:640, 1985.

171. Sudo J, Morel F: Na$^+$ and K$^+$ cell concentrations in collagenase-treated rat kidney tubules incubated at various temperatures. *Am J Physiol* 246:C407, 1984.

172. Suki W, Stinebaugh BJ, Frommer JP, et al: Physiology of diuretic agents. *In* Seldin DW, Giebisch G (eds): *The Kidney. Physiology and Pathophysiology*. New York, Raven Press, 1985, p 2127.

173. Sulyok E, Nemeth M, Tenyi I, et al: Relationship between maturity, electrolyte balance and the function of the renin-angiotensin-aldosterone system in newborn infants. *Biol Neonate* 35:60, 1979.

173a. Tannen RL: Potassium disorders. *In* Kokko JP, Tannen RL (eds): *Fluids and Electrolytes*. Philadelphia, WB Saunders, 1986, p 150.

174. Toback FG, Ekelman KB, Ord'onez NG: Stimulation of DNA synthesis in kidney epithelial cells in culture by potassium. *Am J Physiol* 247:C14, 1984.

175. Tomita K, Pisano JJ, Knepper MA: Control of sodium and potassium transport in the cortical collecting duct of the rat. Effects of bradykinin, vasopressin, and deoxycorticosterone. *J Clin Invest* 76:132, 1985.

176. Toussaint C, Vereerstraeten P: Effects of blood pH changes on potassium excretion in the dog. *Am J Physiol* 202:768, 1962.

177. Turnberg LA: Electrolyte absorption from the colon. *Gut* 11:1049, 1970.

178. Tuvdad F, McNamara H, Barnett HL: Renal response of

159. [nephron structure and ion transport. *Fed Proc* 44:2717, 1985.]

premature infants to administration of bicarbonate and potassium. *Pediatrics* 13:4, 1964.

179. Uete T, Venning EH: Interplay between various adrenal cortical steroids with respect to electrolyte excretion. *Endocrinology* 71:768, 1967.

180. Ullrich KJ, Radtke HW, Rumrich G: The role of bicarbonate and other buffers on isotonic fluid reabsorption in the proximal convolution of the rat kidney. *Pflugers Arch* 330:149, 1971.

181. Velasquez H, Wright FS, Good DW: Luminal influences on potassium secretion: chloride replacement with sulfate. *Am J Physiol* 242:F46, 1982.

182. Wade JB, O'Neil RG, Pryor JL, et al: Modulation of cell membrane area in renal collecting tubules by corticosteroid hormones. *J Cell Biol* 81:439, 1979.

183. Wasserstein AG, Agus ZS: Potassium secretion in the rabbit proximal straight tubule. *Am J Physiol* 245:F167, 1983.

183a. Watten RH, Morgan FM, Songkhla YN: Water and electrolyte studies in cholera. *J Clin Invest* 38:1879, 1959.

184. Wesson LG Jr: Electrolyte excretion in relation to diurnal cycles of renal function. *Medicine* 43:547, 1964.

185. West CD, Rapoport S: Urine flow and solute excretion of hydrogenic dog under "resting" conditions and during osmotic diuresis. *Am J Physiol* 163:159, 1950.

186. Whittembury G, Grantham JJ: Cellular aspects of renal sodium transport and cell volume regulation. *Kidney Int* 9:103, 1976.

187. Widdowson EM, McCance RA: The effect of development on the composition of the serum and extracellular fluid. *Clin Sci* 15:361, 1956.

188. Wiederholt M, Schoormans W, Fischer F, et al: Mechanisms of action of aldosterone on potassium transfer in the rat kidney. *Pflugers Arch* 345:159, 1973.

189. Wiederholt M, Agulian SK, Khuri RN: Intracellular potassium in the distal tubule of the adrenalectomized and aldosterone treated rat. *Pflugers Arch* 347:117, 1974.

190. Wilde W: Potassium. *In* Comar CL, Bronner F (eds): *Mineral Metabolism.* Vol IIB. New York, Academic, 1962, p 73.

191. Wingo CS: Effect of ouabain on K secretion in cortical collecting tubules from adrenalectomized rabbits. *Am J Physiol* 247:F588, 1984.

191a. Wingo CS: Active proton secretion and potassium absorption in the rabbit outer medullary collecting duct: functional evidence for H-K activated adenosine triphosphatase. *J Clin Invest* 84:361, 1989.

192. Work J, Troutman SL, Schafer JA: Transport of potassium in the rabbit pars recta. *Am J Physiol* 242:F226, 1982.

193. Wright FS, Giebisch G: Regulation of potassium excretion. *In* Seldin DW, Giebisch G (eds): *The Kidney. Physiology and Pathophysiology.* New York, Raven Press, 1985, p 1223.

194. Wright FS, Knox FG, Howards SS, et al: Reduced sodium reabsorption by the proximal tubule of DOCA-escaped dogs. *Am J Physiol* 216:869, 1969.

195. Wright FS, Strieder N, Fowler NB, et al: Potassium secretion by distal tubule after potassium adaptation. *Am J Physiol* 221:437, 1971.

196. Young DB: Relationship between plasma potassium concentration and renal potassium excretion. *Am J Physiol* 242:F599, 1982.

197. Young DB, Paulsen AW: Interrelated effects of aldosterone and plasma potassium on potassium excretion. *Am J Physiol* 244:F28, 1983.

198. Young DB, Smith MJ Jr, Jackson TE, et al: Multiplicative interaction between angiotensin II and K concentration in stimulation of aldosterone. *Am J Physiol* 247:E328, 1984.

199. Zalups RK, Stanton BA, Wade JB: Structural adaptation in initial collecting tubule following reduction in renal mass. *Kidney Int* 27:636, 1985.

200. Zink H, Horster M: Maturation of diluting capacity in loop of Henle of rat superficial nephrons. *Am J Physiol* 233:F519, 1977.

ADRIAN SPITZER
RUSSELL W. CHESNEY

7

Role of the Kidney in Mineral Metabolism

Calcium, phosphate, and magnesium are of paramount importance to body function, particularly during periods of growth, owing both to their quantity as main constituents of the skeleton and to their participation in a variety of cellular processes. Despite recent progress, however, our knowledge regarding the role played by the kidney in the homeostasis of these minerals remains incomplete. Reasons accounting for this include the tendency of calcium, phosphate, and magnesium to bind to plasma proteins and to form complexes with other ions and the difficulty of separating the role of the gastrointestinal tract from that of the kidney in the maintenance of external balance.

Calcium

The concentration of calcium in the extracellular fluid averages 10 mg/dl (2.5 mmol/liter) in the adult. The plasma concentration is somewhat higher in the fetus than in the mother, reflecting active transport of Ca^{2+} by the placenta [57,61,88] and probably contributing to the low parathyroid hormone (PTH) levels found in the newborn [35]. When the placental input is interrupted at birth, the serum calcium concentration falls, reaching its nadir at 24 to 48 months of age. Concomitant with the low levels of calcium in serum, phosphate is elevated, as compared with the adult [54,113], a situation that is unique to the growing child and is as yet unexplained in physiologic terms. Subsequently, the serum concentration of calcium rises [63,113], reaching a maximal concentration in early childhood, and then decreases slowly until the age of 16 years [8]. There is a negative correlation between Ca^{2+} and serum immunoreactive PTH levels, indicating the existence of a feedback mechanism.

Calcium is present in biologic fluids in free form as divalent calcium ions (Ca^{2+}), and bound to a variety of intracellular and extracellular constituents. In the plasma, calcium is reversibly bound to serum proteins (~40%) and also forms complexes with citrate, phosphate, bicarbonate, and sulfate (~10%). The remaining approximately 50% of plasma calcium is in free form. In the cell cytosol, the concentration of free Ca^{2+} is believed to be very low

($10^{-6} - 10^{-7}$M) [34,81]. Most of the intracellular calcium is either sequestered in intracellular organelles or complexed with macromolecules. Whether the intracellular concentration of Ca^{2+} in the kidney and elsewhere varies as a function of age is unknown.

Although extracellular proteins, in general, exhibit relatively low affinity for Ca^{2+} ($K_d \sim 10^{-3}$M), certain intracellular proteins have a very high and specific affinity for Ca^{2+} [73]. The ability of Ca^{2+} to mediate cellular signals is dependent on the fact that these Ca^{2+}-binding proteins are able to respond swiftly to fluctuations in cytosolic Ca^{2+} activity. Among the Ca^{2+}-binding proteins are the calcium-controlled protein of the muscle, troponin C [25]; the vitamin D–induced, calcium-binding protein, which exists both in the intestinal and in the renal epithelial cells [128]; and the calcium-dependent regulator protein, calmodulin [22]. Calmodulin, which is likely one of the most important Ca^{2+}-binding proteins in transporting epithelia, has been identified in intestinal epithelial cells [62], extracts of rat renal medulla [33], and toad urinary bladder [55,78]. This protein is believed to mediate the control of a large number of target enzymes by Ca^{2+}, including adenylate cyclase, cyclic nucleotide phosphodiesterase, Ca^{2+}-adenosinetriphosphatase (ATPase), myosin light-chain kinase, and acylhydrolase [22,70,89] as well as a class of Ca^{2+}-dependent protein kinases [106].

Because calcium, either bound to protein or complexed with other ions, is physiologically inactive, considerable efforts have been invested in the measurement of the ionized fraction. According to Walser [125], the concentration of free ionic calcium in the plasma of adult men is 1.34 ± 0.03 mM and that of the complexed fraction is 0.17 ± 0.02 mM. Both fractions pass through the glomerular capillary membrane [59,75], but the tubule can reabsorb calcium only in its free form. These facts must be taken into consideration when interpreting data concerning the renal handling of this mineral.

The amount of calcium excreted in the urine during a 24-hour period ranges between 5 and 10 mEq/day (100 to 200 mg/day) in the adult, which represents 1% to 2% of the filtered load. Reabsorption of most filtered calcium permits the maintenance of an appropriate external balance and contributes to the regulation of the plasma concentration of ionized calcium. However, unlike the plasma concentration of Pi and Mg, which are primarily controlled by the kidney, the plasma concentration of calcium is primarily affected by alterations in the blood-bone equilibrium.

Clearance studies have failed to reveal the existence of a Tm-limited mechanism for calcium reabsorption [21,98–100]. This may be due to the fact that the concentration of calcium in plasma cannot be increased to the same degree as that of glucose, Pi, or Mg without producing serious side effects [84]. Alternatively, a whole kidney Tm may not exist, owing to the fact that the reabsorption of Ca^{2+}, at least in the proximal tubule, is proportional to that of Na^+ and H_2O, and thus an upper limit for reabsorption may not exist in this nephron segment.

Peacock et al. [99] have suggested that Ca^{2+} reabsorption may be limited by a concentration gradient, rather than by Tm [98]. Studies performed in normal subjects and in patients with hypoparathyroidism and hyperparathyroidism have allowed these investigators to construct a curve that describes the relationship between calcium excretion and serum calcium concentration. The extrapolated regression line intercepts the abscissa at about 9.5 mg/dl of total calcium, or 5.5 mg/dl ultrafiltrable calcium (UF_{Ca}), which Mioni et al. [91] termed the "theoretical" renal calcium threshold. These authors suggested that the calcium titration curve may be interpreted to be the result of two reabsorptive processes: one that is gradient-time-limited (a constant fraction of delivered solute is reabsorbed), and another that is Tm-limited. At plasma concentrations of ultrafiltrable calcium [UF_{Ca}] below the theoretical renal threshold, most filtered calcium is reabsorbed and excretion is low, whereas above the threshold an increasing fraction of filtered calcium is excreted. As a consequence, the plasma UF_{Ca} is maintained at a value near the renal calcium threshold.

Dietary deprivation of calcium has little or no effect on the plasma concentration of calcium, as a result of enhanced tubular reabsorption brought about by PTH secretion [83]. This is unlike Pi and Mg, for which an increase in tubular reabsorption is secondary to a fall in their plasma concentration and a decrease in the filtered load [96].

Very little is known concerning the relationship between changes in serum calcium and its handling by the kidney during development. Arant [7] performed measurements of urinary calcium-creatinine ratios ($U_{Ca/Cr}$) in 99 healthy newborn infants of 26 to 43 weeks gestational age. During the first week of life, the $U_{Ca/Cr}$ was found to be greater in infants of less than 30 weeks gestation (0.11 ± 0.06) than in full-term infants (0.03 ± 0.01). Ghazali and Barratt [50] have calculated that the $U_{Ca/Cr}$ was 0.25 in children, a value slightly higher than that observed in the adult [93], suggesting that the fractional reabsorption of Ca^{2+} might be lower during childhood than later on in life. Between one and 15 years of age, the excretion of calcium appeared to vary directly as a function of body weight [50], amounting to 2.4 ± 0.7 (SD) mg/kg/24 hours for a sample of children studied in Great Britain and to 3.6 ± 2.4 mg/kg/24 hours for a sample of Swiss children. Possible explanations for these differences are variations in intake of calcium,

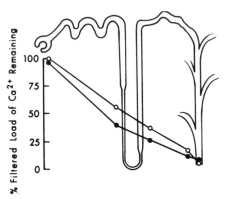

FIG. 7-1. *Fraction of the filtered load of calcium remaining in the renal tubule of normal and thyroparathyroidectomized rats. (Data from Agus ZS, Gardner LB, Beck LH, et al: Effects of parathyroid hormone on renal tubular reabsorption of calcium, sodium and phosphate. Am J Physiol 224:1143, 1973; and Agus ZS, Chiu PJ, Goldberg M: Regulation of urinary calcium excretion in the rat. Am J Physiol 232:F545, 1977, with permission.)*

sodium, and vitamin D, which render such values of little physiologic significance.

Calcium Transport Along the Renal Tubule

Application of micropuncture and microperfusion techniques have provided information concerning the characteristics of Ca^{2+} transport in each nephron segment (Fig. 7-1). It is generally agreed that Ca^{2+} is reabsorbed along the entire nephron proportional to Na^+, that is, some 50% to 60% in the proximal tubule, 10% in pars recta, 20% to 25% in the loop of Henle, 5% to 10% in the distal tubule, and the remainder in the collecting duct.

The ratio of tubular fluid (TF_{Ca}) to UF_{Ca} concentration is consistently greater than unity along the entire proximal tubule [115] and remains remarkably constant, even after experimental maneuvers that increase or decrease the renal reabsorption of Ca^{2+} [85]. This has led to the view that the reabsorption of Ca^{2+} in the renal proximal tubule is a passive process, coupled to active transport of Na^+. That this is indeed the case was confirmed by the experiments of Ullrich et al. [124], who found that only about 20% of the Ca^{2+} reabsorbed in this segment can be due to active transport. In addition, these experiments showed that in the proximal tubule the efflux of Ca^{2+} across the contraluminal membrane occurs at least in part via Na^+-Ca^{2+} exchange. These findings were later confirmed by Lee et al. [76].

In the straight portion of the proximal tubule (pars recta) as much as 70% of the Ca^{2+} reabsorbed appears to be active [104], since only approximately 30% of the Ca^{2+} reabsorbed can be attributed to Na^+ and H_2O transport [5,104]. Because ouabain did not affect the active transport of Ca^{2+} in this segment, while cooling of the tubules did [104], a role for Ca^{2+}-ATPase in the active transport of Ca^{2+} was claimed. However, the activity of the enzyme is not sufficient to account for the entire amount of Ca^{2+} actively transported at this site [38].

There is very little if any reabsorption of calcium in the thin descending and thin ascending limbs of Henle's loop. In the thick ascending limb, the reabsorption of Ca^{2+} can be dissociated from that of Na^+, making this segment important in the regulation of Ca^{2+} absorption. Bourdeau and Burg [14] found Ca^{2+} reabsorption in this segment to be voltage-dependent, a finding that is generally compatible with passive movement. However, the slope of the relationship between calcium fluxes and transepithelial voltage was greater than that predicted for strictly passive calcium movement. The investigators interpreted this to represent single-file pore diffusion, whereby the interaction of the ion with the transport pathway allows for greater transport per unit driving force than would be predicted. Further evidence for passive, paracellular transport of calcium in this segment is provided by studies that demonstrated that the reabsorption of calcium was dependent on the magnitude of its concentration gradient [14].

In the distal tubule, calcium transport occurs against an electrochemical gradient and, therefore, must be active. A vitamin D–dependent Ca^{2+}-binding protein identified in this segment has generated speculation about its involvement in this process [121]. The fact that vitamin D_3 has been found to increase the transport of Ca^{2+} in this segment provides support for this assumption [17].

In the cortical collecting duct, most of the calcium is reabsorbed in the early portion, which contains granular cells similar to those of the late distal tubule [108]. Some calcium movement was also detected in the late portion of this segment, which contains "light" cells. Yet, the Ca^{2+}-ATPase activity and the amount of vitamin D–dependent, Ca^{2+}-binding protein are very high in this segment [38], suggesting that they may be involved in the maintenance of intracellular Ca^{2+} concentration rather than in transepithelial Ca^{2+} transport.

Mechanisms of Transepithelial Ca^{2+} Transport

The transport of Ca^{2+} across the renal epithelium occurs both through transcellular and through paracellular pathways [48] (Fig. 7-2). Passage between the cells is regulated by physical forces and applies mainly to leaky epithelia, such as the proximal tubule, whereas in tight epithelia, such as the distal tubule and the collecting duct, the transcellular pathway is the only route taken by Ca^{2+} [31]. Because the Ca^{2+} activity in proximal tubule cells is maintained within a very low range, several-fold below that prevailing in the tubular lumen, and the intracellular voltage is negative, the entry of Ca^{2+} into the cell can occur along a favorable electrical gradient [124]. For the same reasons, however, extrusion of Ca^{2+} across the contraluminal membrane must be an active, energy-dependent process.

In tissues other than the kidney there is evidence that Ca^{2+} entry into the cell is facilitated by Ca^{2+} channels and Ca^{2+}-binding proteins that act as carriers [123]. The

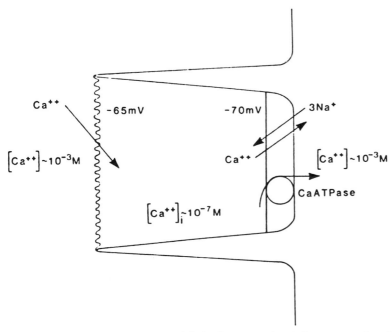

Fig. 7-2. Cellular model of transepithelial calcium transfer. Calcium enters the cell through the luminal membrane along an electrochemical gradient and exits the cell across the basolateral membrane via primary and secondary active transport mechanisms. Paracellular transport of calcium may also occur in the mammalian proximal tubule.

entry may involve phosphorylation of membrane proteins or depolarization of the cell membrane, processes that open Ca^{2+} channels and thereby increase permeability [90]. There is preliminary evidence that phosphorylation of membrane phospholipids in renal microvilli may increase Ca^{2+} binding and uptake by these membranes [64,65,111].

The efflux of Ca^{2+} from the cell is driven in part by a Na^+-Ca^{2+} exchange. The process is energized by the Na^+ gradient and is therefore secondarily active. The exchanger is present in many tissues [124], including the kidney, where it appears to play important roles, both in transcellular Ca^{2+} transport and in the regulation of intracellular Ca^{2+} concentration [51,124]. The in vitro studies suggest that the exchange process is electrogenic and, at least in toad bladder, has a stoichiometry of three Na^+ to one Ca^{2+} [20].

The role of Ca^{2+}-ATPase in the transepithelial transport of Ca^{2+} remains unsettled [38]. As already indicated, the enzyme does not appear to possess sufficient activity to account for a significant portion of Ca^{2+} transport in those segments of the renal tubule where the transport appears to be active, such as the late portion of the distal tubule and early portion of the cortical collecting duct. Its role in the segments in which Ca^{2+} transport is predominantly (proximal tubule and medullary ascending limb) or exclusively (cortical collecting tubule) passive remains unknown.

Factors Affecting Calcium Reabsorption

SODIUM

The parallelism between Ca^{2+} and Na^+ reabsorption in the proximal tubule is maintained under a variety of experimental circumstances designed to decrease reabsorption of Na^+, such as the infusion of saline or mannitol [21,41] or acute administration of diuretics [36,39,43,105]. The proportionally greater urinary excretion of Ca^{2+} observed by some investigators under such circumstances appears to be the consequence of differential inhibition of tubular reabsorption at sites beyond the loop of Henle [2]. This dissociation has been used as evidence in favor of an independent Ca^{2+} transport mechanism located in the distal nephron, probably in the collecting duct [6,43].

Thiazide diuretics, while variably affecting Ca^{2+} excretion when administered acutely [6,16,29,40,94,95,127], consistently result in a decrease in Ca^{2+} excretion when given chronically [132]. The latter effect, which benefits patients with hypercalciuria and a propensity for the formation of renal stones, is believed to be the consequence of enhanced reabsorption of Ca^{2+} in both the proximal and the distal nephron segments. Proximal reabsorption apparently is increased nonspecifically as a result of the extracellular volume contraction induced by the diuretic [16,116,132]. Enhanced distal reabsorption might be explained by the potentiating effect of thiazides on PTH [16], intact parathyroid glands apparently being necessary for the effect to be manifested fully [16,95]. Amiloride has also been shown to decrease Ca^{2+} excretion [30] and increase its distal tubular reabsorption in the rat [27]. This effect is presumably due to a decrease in the distal nephron potential that would ordinarily oppose Ca^{2+} transport.

HYPERCALCEMIA

Hypercalcemia has multiple effects on renal function. Infusion of calcium in the Munich-Wistar rat produced a fall both in kidney and in single nephron glomerular filtration rate (GFR), associated with a decrease in ultrafiltration coefficient (K_f), possibly secondary to contraction of the mesangial cells, which may diminish the glomerular capillary surface area [66]. Hyercalcemia also produced a fall in proximal tubule fluid reabsorption [44,126], which was accompanied by a degree of calciuresis that exceeded the natriuresis. This discrepancy suggests a distal inhibition of calcium reabsorption that may be due to the suppression of PTH secretion by the increase in plasma Ca^{2+} concentration.

INORGANIC PHOSPHATE

Phosphate loading enhances the renal reabsorption of calcium, independently of PTH, plasma calcium, and renal Na^+ handling, at sites within and possibly beyond the distal convoluted tubule of the superficial nephrons [23,74]. The mechanism by which acute infusion of phosphate results in a decrease in calcium excretion is not well understood, although it apparently is related to the elevation of plasma phosphate concentration [24].

Phosphate depletion causes hypercalciuria [24,82], which is blunted by administration of PTH [24,52,53,131]. The impairment in Ca^{2+} reabsorption appears to occur in Henle's loop [131].

MAGNESIUM

The infusion of magnesium salts causes an increase in the urinary excretion of calcium that is more rapid and larger than that induced by saline infusion [37,86,103]. The effect does not appear to be mediated by the decrease in PTH [86]. Magnesium appears to affect Ca^{2+} reabsorption both at the level of proximal tubule and at the loop of Henle [37,103].

DISTURBANCES IN ACID–BASE BALANCE

There are numerous reports showing that both chronic and acute metabolic acidosis are associated with increases in calcium excretion [13,46,49,77,92,112,118]. Conversely, metabolic alkalosis induced by infusion of bicarbonate has been found to enhance Ca^{2+} reabsorption [45,97,122]. The effect appears to be exerted mainly at the level of the distal nephron [118].

PARATHYROID HORMONE

Administration of PTH results in a fall in urinary calcium excretion [3,42,130], whereas parathyroidectomy has the opposite effect [11,71,119,120]. The predominant role of the distal nephron segments in the renal regulation of calcium excretion is highlighted by the fact that the hypocalciuric effect of PTH occurs in spite of a concomitant decrease in fractional and absolute reabsorption of calcium in the proximal tubule [3]. Direct evidence has been obtained for a PTH effect in the distal convoluted tubule and the granular portion of the collecting duct [32,108]. These

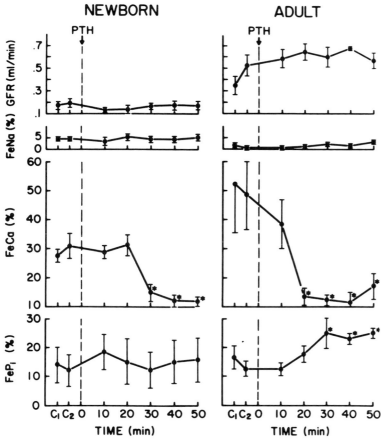

FIG. 7-3. *Glomerular filtration rates and fractional excretions of sodium* (FE_{Na}), *calcium* (FE_{Ca}), *and phosphate* (FE_{Pi}) *during control periods and following additions of PTH to perfused isolated kidneys of newborn and mature animals. Values are means + SE. * Significantly different from control values* ($P > 0.001$) *by analysis of variance (From Johnson V, Spitzer A: Renal reabsorption of phosphate during development: Whole kidney events. Am J Physiol (Renal Fluid Electrolyte Physiology 20)251:F251, 1986, with permission.)*

sites of action correlate closely with the presence of PTH-sensitive adenylate cyclase activity in the rabbit renal tubule [19].

Serum PTH levels are low in the newborn [35], possibly owing to the high plasma concentration of calcium prevailing at this age. That this may indeed be the case is indicated by the fact that ethylenediaminetetraacetate (EDTA)-induced hypocalcemia resulted in increased levels of serum PTH in sheep fetuses [110]. Administration of parathyroid extract to fetal sheep did not affect the excretion of calcium, although, apparently, it did increase the excretion of phosphate [4]. On the other hand, addition of PTH to the fluid perfusing the isolated kidney of newborn guinea pigs was reported to increase calcium reabsorption while failing to influence phosphate excretion [68] (Fig. 7-3). This relative resistance of the immature renal tubule to the effect of PTH does not appear to be related to the adenylate cyclase system, because activation of adenyl cyclase has been found to result in an increase in aden-

osine 3':5'-cyclic phosphate (cAMP) in renal parenchyma of fetal and neonatal rabbits [79]. Likewise, addition of PTH to the perfusate of newborn guinea pig kidney resulted in an increase in cAMP excretion similar in magnitude to that observed in adult animals [68].

VITAMIN D AND OTHER HORMONES

The effect of vitamin D and its metabolites on Ca^{2+} reabsorption in the kidney is unclear. It was known for a long time that administration of vitamin D results in increased calcium excretion [15,80]. This effect has been found to be secondary to a decrease in PTH and an increase in the filtered load of Ca^{2+}, rather than to a direct effect of vitamin D on the renal tubule. In animal experiments, when both PTH and serum calcium concentration were maintained constant [28], an increase in Ca^{2+} reabsorption in response to vitamin D, probably localized to the proximal tubule, was clearly demonstrated. Similar results were obtained with $25(OH)D_3$ and $1,25(OH)_2D_3$ [101,102]. The physiologic relevance of these observations remains unclear.

The developmental aspects of vitamin D metabolism and the effect of vitamin D on kidney function are discussed in detail in the last section of this chapter.

Calcitonin [12,18,56,109], thyroid hormone [1,9,26, 72], growth hormone [10,47,58,60,67,69], and mineralocorticoids [87,126], have a predominant hypercalciuric effect, although not necessarily resulting from direct action on the renal tubule. For instance, expansion of the extracellular space was shown to account for this effect in acromegaly [60,114]; mineralocorticoid administration [87,117,126] and increased bone resorption might explain the hypercalciuria of patients with Cushing's syndrome.

Phosphate

The plasma contains about 14 mg/dl phosphorus, of which 8 to 9 mg is complexed to lipids; the remainder is mostly inorganic phosphate (Pi). The Pi exists in the blood in two ionic forms, divalent (HPO_4^{2-}) and monovalent ($H_2PO_4^{-}$). The pK of this buffer pair is 6.8, so that at the normal blood pH of 7.4 the ratio of divalent to monovalent Pi is 4:1.

The concentration of Pi in the plasma varies with age. The concentration is as high as 15 mg/dl (4.8 mmol/liter) in the fetus [73], 7 to 10.9 mg/dl (2.3 to 3.5 mmol/liter) in prematurely born infants [38], and 5.8 to 9.3 mg/dl (1.9 to 3.0 mmol/liter) in full-term newborns [109]. The plasma concentration of Pi decreases slowly thereafter to reach the normal adult values of 3 to 4.5 mg/dl by the second decade of life (Table 7-1) [165].

Close to 90% of plasma Pi is ultrafiltrable. The fraction of the filtered Pi that is reabsorbed by the kidney varies with age and with the need of the organism, being 99% in the newborn [109], 95% in the infant, and 80% in the adult [64].

The relationship between the filtered load of Pi (GFR $\times$ U_{Pi}) and the total urinary excretion of Pi ($U_{Pi}V$) has been studied in the adult and immature of several species. In most of these studies the filtered load of Pi was altered by increasing either the rate of Pi infusion or its concentration in the infusate. Although the concentration of Pi in the plasma may in itself affect the reabsorption of Pi, studies of this kind have contributed substantially to our understanding of the renal handling of Pi. They revealed that the renal Pi transport system is a saturable process

with no appreciable first order component. As a consequence, the excretion of Pi can approach zero when the plasma concentration of Pi decreases below the threshold (Fig. 7-4). As plasma Pi is raised, Pi reabsorption at first increases but rapidly reaches a maximum (Tm_{Pi}), above which increments in plasma Pi are associated with proportional increases in $U_{Pi}V$. The point at which the straight line drawn through the dot (see Fig. 7-4) intercepts the line describing the plasma Pi concentration has been called the theoretical threshold. In the absence of splay, Tm_{Pi} will be equal at this point with the filtered load of Pi or GFR $\times$ Pi threshold. Thus, Tm_{Pi} = GFR $\times$ Pi threshold and hence Pi threshold = Tm_{Pi}/GFR. The kidney tends to maintain the plasma Pi concentration close to the value of the Pi threshold. At any plasma level above Tm, the fractional excretion of Pi will vary with the filtered load of Pi. This has led Parfitt and Frame [166] to question the use of fractional excretion of Pi as an indicator of the capacity of the renal tubule to transport Pi; Bijvoet [28,29] proposed that Tm_{Pi}/GFR is a more appropriate index of renal Pi transport capacity. In the normal adult, Tm_{Pi}/GFR varies between 2.5 and 4.2 mg/dl. It should be pointed out, however, that this ratio should not be used for comparing changes in the renal reabsorption of Pi during development. This is due to the fact that the numerator and the denominator of this ratio change independently and at different rates during growth. For this reason the maximal reabsorptive capacity (Tm) remains the best standard of comparison between subjects of different ages.

There are very few studies in which Tm_{Pi} was determined properly in growing subjects. McCrory et al. [151] induced acute elevations in serum Pi by administering a single dose of Pi (0.5 to 1.5 g NaH_2PO_4/kg) to six normal newborn infants. Despite increases in serum Pi to at least 12 mg/dl, these authors did not observe any measurable increase in the rate of tubular reabsorption of Pi. They concluded that these infants were reabsorbing Pi at a maximal rate, even before the oral administration of phosphate. Brodehl et al. [37] determined the renal handling of Pi by short-term clearance studies in 51 infants (6 to 12 months of age) and 143 children (1 to 15 years of age). They confirmed that fractional Pi reabsorption was significantly higher in infancy than in childhood and that the tubular Pi reabsorption in fasting infants and children was already very near or equal to its maximum value [36]. These investigators further noted that at each level of fractional Pi reabsorption, infants had higher plasma Pi concentrations than children or, conversely, that at a given plasma Pi level, fractional Pi reabsorption was lower in infants than in older

TABLE 7-1. *Normal ranges of serum calcium, phosphorus, and magnesium levels at various ages*

	Calcium		Phosphorus		Magnesium	
	mg/dl	mmol/l	mg/dl	mmol/l	mg/dl	mmol/l
Premature	6.1–11.0	1.5–2.8	7.0–10.9	2.3–3.5	1.1–2.4	0.6–1.0
Newborn	7.0–12.0	1.8–3.0	5.8–9.3	1.9–3.0	1.6–2.6	0.7–1.1
Child	8.8–10.8	2.2–2.7	4.5–6.5	1.5–2.1	1.4–1.9	0.6–0.8
Adult	8.4–10.2	2.1–2.6	3.0–4.5	0.9–1.5	1.4–2.0	0.6–8.0

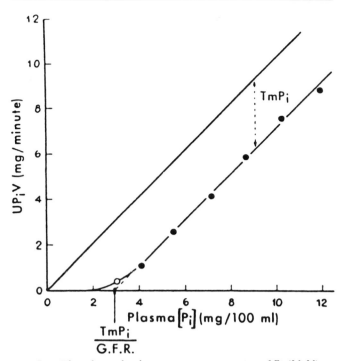

FIG. 7-4. *The relationship between urinary excretion of Pi ($U_{Pi}V$) and plasma Pi in a healthy individual, during fasting (circles) and during an infusion of phosphate (dots). The upper line depicts the filtered Pi. The vertical distance between the curves is proportional to the tubular reabsorption of Pi.*

lowering the Pi content of the diet from 0.8 to 0.2 g/100 g BW, resulted in an attenuated and delayed enhancement in maxTRP/ml GFR in adult animals as compared with the response observed in the young rats.

Thus, rapidly growing animals adjust renal reabsorption of Pi to maintain the concentration of Pi in plasma higher than in adult animals. The renal alterations in Pi handling in response to variations in dietary Pi occur independently of plasma Pi concentration, GFR, or filtered load of Pi.

That the enhanced renal reabsorption of Pi observed during growth is due to factors intrinsic to the renal tubule was conclusively demonstrated by the studies of Johnson and Spitzer [116]. Kidneys obtained from guinea pigs less than 7 or greater than 30 days of age were perfused in vitro with a Krebs-Hensleit bicarbonate buffer solution containing fraction V serum albumin in concentrations appropriate to the age of the animal, and Na^+ or KH_2PO_4 in concentrations varying between 3 and 15 mg/dl. The absolute rate of Pi reabsorption per unit of kidney weight was 2.5-fold higher in the newborn than in the more mature animal over the entire range of filtered loads (Fig. 7-5). The filtered load at which the maximal tubular reabsorption of Pi was reached in the newborn was 24.3 ± 2.8 mg/min, a value that exceeded by 2.5-fold the filtered load of Pi encountered under physiologic conditions. Thus, an increase in the filtered load of Pi could be easily accommodated by the renal tubule of the newborn guinea pig, allowing for the conservation of Pi required by the growing organism. In the adult, the Tm_{Pi} was 53.9 ± 2.6 mg/minute, a value only slightly higher than the average normal

children. Further analysis of the data led them to surmise that age-dependent low GFR leads to the greater retention of Pi observed in infants. This conclusion, which is similar to that arrived at by McCrory et al. [151], was challenged by Russo and Nash [188]. These investigators performed experiments in puppies that were Pi depleted by being given aluminum hydroxide, a Pi binder, or were phosphate loaded with sodium phosphate. Puppies in both groups were found to have a higher Pi plasma concentration than adult dogs. Plasma Pi concentration and the rate of excretion of Pi were independent of GFR. At any filtered load of Pi, the excretion of Pi was greater and the rate of reabsorption lower in Na^+-loaded than in Na^+-restricted animals. The maximal rate of reabsorption was higher in the Pi-loaded than in the Pi-restricted animals.

Further light was shed on this issue by studies performed by Caverzasio et al. [46] on young growing and adult rats. Maximal net Pi reabsorption per unit volume of glomerular filtrate (maxTRP/ml GFR) was determined during acute Pi infusion in intact, young (2-month-old) and adult (8- to 9-month-old) rats maintained on similar intakes of Pi (0.8 g/100 g body weight). MaxTRP/ml GFR was significantly lower in adult (1.44 ± 0.06 mmol/ml) as compared with young animals (2.22 ± 0.12 mmol/ml). This difference was observed even after thyroparathyroidectomy and was not associated with differences in urinary excretion of cAMP, GFR, renal handling of Na^+, plasma calcium concentration, or acid–base status. Phosphate depletion, induced by

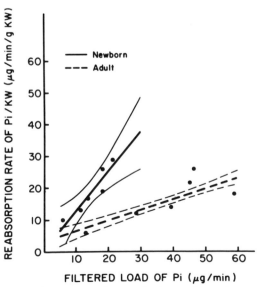

FIG. 7-5. *Regression lines and 95% confidence limits of the relationship between reabsorption of Pi per gram of kidney weight (gKW) and filtered load of Pi by isolated perfused kidneys of newborn (y = 1.25x + 0.09, r = 0.92) guinea pigs. Slopes of regression lines are significantly different (P < 0.01). (From Johnson V, Spitzer A: Renal reabsorption of phosphate during development: Whole kidney events. Am J Physiol (Renal Fluid Electrolyte Physiology 20)251:F251, 1986, with permission.)*

filtered load of Pi encountered at this age. The Tm_{Pi}-GFR ratio was significantly higher in the newborn (117.4 ± 10.8 g/min/ml) as compared with the adult animals (82.6 ± 3.6 g/min/ml). It should be noted, furthermore, that the difference in the reabsorption of Pi between the newborn and the adult guinea pig would be considerably greater than 2.5-fold if expressed per unit of proximal tubule length or luminal membrane surface area [215].

Localization of Pi Transport Along the Renal Tubule

PROXIMAL CONVOLUTED TUBULE

There is general agreement that the proximal convoluted tubule is the major site of Pi reabsorption in the kidney (Fig. 7-6). This was suggested by initial observations made with clearance techniques [150] and confirmed by micropuncture studies [5]. Under normal circumstances, the earliest convolutions display greater capacity to reabsorb Pi than the later ones [204,216]. In vitro microperfusion studies, carried out in rabbit isolated nephron segments, also indicate that the intrinsic transport capacity for Pi is greater in the early than in the late portions of the proximal convoluted tubule [153]. There is now convincing evidence that Pi reabsorption also occurs in the pars recta of the proximal tubule [89,140,141,204]. The rate of reabsorption, measured in isolated perfused segments of rabbit nephrons, was one-third of that observed in the proximal convoluted tubule [23].

LOOP OF HENLE

Most of the evidence is against significant reabsorption of Pi at this site [90,140,173,204].

DISTAL CONVOLUTED TUBULE AND COLLECTING DUCT

The observation of Amiel et al. [4] that the Pi delivery at the end of the accessible superficial distal tubule was significantly greater than in the final urine has been generally confirmed [90,133,173]. There is controversy, however, whether this difference is due to reabsorption of Pi in the terminal parts of the renal tubule or to functional heterogeneity between cortical and juxtamedullary nephrons [40,89,94,197].

The only micropuncture study done in developing animals leaves the same uncertainty, although it did disclose a difference between newborn and adult animals. The experiments were performed on euvolemic, non-fasted guinea pigs, 5 to 14 and 42 to 49 days of age, maintained on a standard guinea pig diet (0.76% Pi) [118]. By the end of the proximal convoluted tubule, the fraction of the filtered load of Pi reabsorbed was significantly higher in immature ($76.7\% \pm 2.8\%$) than in mature ($67.2\% \pm 2.7\%$) guinea pigs. Measurements of urinary excretion of Pi indicated the further reabsorption of $15.6\% \pm 2.1\%$ in the newborn and $10.5\% \pm 1.8\%$ of the filtered load of Pi in the adult. This may represent reabsorption of Pi in tubular segments located beyond the proximal tubule, or it may reflect a higher

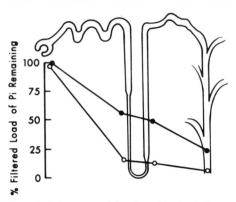

Fig. 7-6. *Fraction of the filtered load of phosphate remaining in the renal tubule of normal and thyroparathyroidectomized rats. (Data from Greger R, Lang F, Marchand G, et al: Site of renal phosphate reabsorption. Micropuncture and microinfusion study. Pflugers Arch 359:111, 1977, with permission.)*

fractional reabsorption of Pi by the deep than by the superficial nephrons of the newborn animals. This issue could not be resolved by micropuncture performed in guinea pigs because in this animal species the distal convoluted tubules do not reach the surface of kidney.

Thus, Pi reabsorption in the proximal tubule involves events in two populations of nephrons, each consisting of at least three different tubule segments (early convoluted, late convoluted, and pars recta) that appear to have different Pi transport capacities and may react differently to regulatory factors.

Cellular Mechanism of Pi Transport in the Proximal Tubule

Transport of Pi across a proximal tubule epithelium involves three steps: (1) uptake from the lumen across the brush border membrane (BBM); (2) transport through the cell cytosol; and (3) efflux from the cell into the peritubular fluid through the basolateral membrane (Fig. 7-7). Because of the small but significant binding of Pi in the serum, the concentration of Pi in the glomerular filtrate is considerably lower than that predicted by Donnan equilibrium, being on the average 0.87 of the plasma Pi concentration [69]. In the rat, at plasma Pi of 2.5 mM, the concentration of Pi in the fluid that enters the proximal tubule is approximately 2.2 mM, a value that is similar to that in the peritubular interstitium. Phosphate concentration in the fluid leaving the proximal tubule is usually only slightly lower than in the glomerular filtrate, although substantially lower concentrations have been observed in the absence of PTH or in Pi-depleted animals [19,93]. Data regarding the concentration of Pi in the cytosol are more difficult to obtain. Phosphate content in frozen clamped kidney tissue is 4 to 5 mmol/g wet weight or about 5 mmol/kg tissue water [106,110]. However, measurements of intracellular Pi concentration by nuclear magnetic resonance (NMR) spectroscopy in isolated perfused kidneys revealed that only about 27% of the total intracellular Pi was visible and

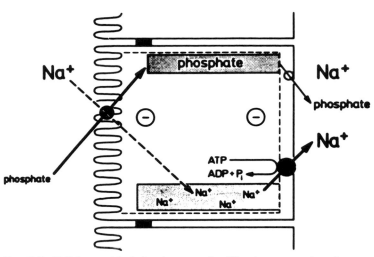

Fig. 7-7. Cellular model of phosphate transfer. Phosphate enters the cell across the brush border membrane in symport with sodium and exits the cell across the basolateral membrane along an electrochemical gradient.

therefore free in solution [77]. In rat kidneys perfused with Pi-free solution, the cytoplasmic concentration of NMR visible Pi was only 0.6 to 0.7 mM [77]. These data suggest that a large pool of intracellular Pi is bound or otherwise immobilized and therefore does not contribute to transport and possibly metabolism.

Because the renal proximal tubule cells are 60 to 65 mV negative with respect both to tubular lumen and to peritubular fluid, the free cellular Pi concentration at equilibrium should be in the range of 0.20 to 0.25 mmol. The actual free Pi concentration in the cells seems to be almost three-fold higher than this equilibrium value, which suggests that Pi has to enter the cell across the luminal membrane against an electrochemical potential gradient and to leave the cell at the contraluminal side down an electrochemical potential gradient. These calculations also indicate that the distribution of Pi among various compartments is not determined by thermodynamic driving forces but rather by the kinetics of specific transport systems located in the brush border and the basolateral membranes.

The overall picture is similar in the newborn, although the various electrochemical gradients affecting Pi transport across the proximal tubule epithelium may be quantitatively different from those observed in the adult. As already indicated, the concentration of Pi in plasma is higher in the newborn than in the adult, while the concentration of protein is lower, at least during the first few months of postnatal life. As a consequence, the concentration of Pi in the glomerular filtrate approaches 3.0 mM. A similar concentration is expected to prevail in the peritubular interstitium. There is no direct information regarding the concentration of Pi in the fluid leaving the proximal tubule. However, in view of the fact that the fractional reabsorption of Pi is known to be higher in the newborn than it is in the adult animal, whereas the reabsorption of water seems to be similar at both ages, the concentration

of Pi in the fluid leaving the proximal tubule is expected to be lower than that observed in the adult, probably similar to that found in parathyroidectomized or in Pi-depleted animals. Information is available regarding the intracellular concentration of Pi in proximal tubule cells. Measurements performed in perfused kidneys of the guinea pig have revealed values that are substantially lower in the newborn (0.91 ± 0.14 mM) than in the adult (1.85 ± 0.23 mM) [15]. Unfortunately, there is no information regarding the electrical potential difference across various cell boundaries in the proximal tubule of the newborn. This makes it impossible to calculate equilibrium values for phosphate across the membranes of this tubular segment. There is, however, evidence that, like in the adult, the entry of Pi into the cell requires energy.

TRANSPORT OF PI ACROSS THE BRUSH BORDER MEMBRANE

The existence of a relationship between tubular reabsorption of Na^+ and Pi was inferred on the basis of clearance and micropuncture studies that revealed a parallelism between the reabsorption of Na^+ and that of Pi [19,78, 79,148]. Hoffmann and associates [108], showed that in vesicles of brush border membranes (BBM), like in proximal tubule segments, the uptake of Pi is saturable and inhibited by arsenate. When a Na^+ gradient was present, Pi uptake exceeded transiently the equilibrium value, indicating the presence of an active transport process. Replacement of Na^+ in the medium by K^+ reduced uptake to minimal values, indicating that the transport of Pi across the BBM requires the presence of Na^+. Subsequent studies have indicated that each Pi was cotransported with two Na^+ and that divalent phosphate was transported in preference to monovalent phosphate [108].

At pH 7.4, the Na^+-Pi cotransport is not sensitive to

membrane potential. However, at more acid extravesicular or tubular pH values, an electrogenic component of Pi transport becomes apparent [41,189]. It appears that in BBM prepared from superficial kidney cortex of the rat there are two symporters that have different K_m but similar V_{max} values [39]. Only one system was identified in vesicles prepared from deep kidney cortex. Gmaj and Murer [85] have calculated that in order to be in equilibrium with the Na^+ gradient and the 2.0 mM Pi present in the tubular fluid, the intracellular concentration of Pi should be about 160 mM, whereas, as already indicated, this value is < 1 mM. Thus, the Na^+-Pi cotransport system in the BBM is far from the equilibrium point, being limited by the turnover rate of the transport system rather than by the electrochemical driving forces.

The Na^+-Pi symporter has not yet been isolated, owing mainly to the lack of a specific label that binds tightly to the transporter.

PI TRANSPORT ACROSS THE BASOLATERAL MEMBRANE

There is relatively little and conflicting information regarding the efflux of Pi from the proximal tubule cells. Unlike the BBM, which can be easily isolated and form a nearly homogeneous population of tightly sealed, rightside-out oriented vesicles, the basolateral membrane preparations are composed of a mixture of inside-out and rightside-out vesicles, only a small fraction of which are tightly sealed and therefore suitable for transport studies [84]. In addition, contamination by BBM is almost impossible to avoid. It would appear that a Na^+-independent transport pathway, possibly an anion exchanger, provides the main route for the exit of Pi from the cell [33,108]. In addition, a Na^+-dependent mechanism was described that may account for the entry of Pi into the cells when the luminal Pi uptake is restricted [190,191].

There is no information available regarding the exit of Pi from proximal tubule cells of immature animals. The fact that the intracellular concentration of Pi is low in the newborn diminishes the possibility that the exit of Pi at the contraluminal membrane proceeds along the electrochemical gradient and makes it more likely that a carrier-mediated mechanism is in place.

COUPLING BETWEEN THE LUMINAL ENTRY AND BASOLATERAL EXIT OF PI

Experiments performed by Freeman et al. [77] and by Barac-Nieto et al. [15] on isolated perfused kidneys of rat and guinea pig demonstrate that the intracellular concentration of Pi remains nearly constant for several hours in the absence of Pi in the perfusion media. This finding indicates the existence of a tight coupling between the entry of Pi across the BBM and the exit of Pi across the basolateral membrane. In isolated perfused tubules of rabbits, omission of Pi from the luminal perfusate blunts the reabsorption of fluids, whereas omission of Pi from the peritubular bath has no effect on transport [34]. When Pi is absent from both the luminal and the contraluminal sides of the cell, there is a considerable reduction in the transport of fluid associated with the decrease in O_2 con-

sumption. This effect does not occur when glucose is omitted or replaced by 2-deoxy glucose, a nonmetabolizable sugar [34]. This effect was ascribed to the incorporation of Pi into glycolytic intermediates, which makes it unavailable for oxidative phosphorylation and glycolysis (the Crabtree effect) [130]. These observations indicate that the uptake of Pi at the contraluminal side of the cell is insufficient to maintain the intracellular concentration of Pi within normal range. In addition, it suggests that the Pi entering the cell comes into equilibrium with the cytosolic Pi pool, rather than being transported across the cell via a discrete pathway, such as vesicular transport.

Regulation of Na^+-Pi Cotransport

Gmaj and Murer [85] have provided a lucid description of the subject by placing it within the framework of classic enzymology. Their assumptions were: (1) that the Na^+-Pi cotransport system catalyzes the transfer of Pi from compartment A to compartment B, not unlike an enzyme that catalyzes the conversion of substance A to substance B; and (2) that the events that produce changes in Pi transport or activity fall into two categories, short-term and long-term regulation. Two types of short-term regulation seem to be especially important: allosteric regulation, which occurs when a regulating substance changes the enzyme activity by binding to the enzyme molecule at a regulatory site different from the substrate binding site, and activation-inactivation, which usually involves reversible covalent modification of the enzyme molecule (e.g., phosphorylation, ribosylation, methylation) and is catalyzed by an additional set of regulatory enzymes, such as protein kinases and protein phosphatases. The regulatory enzymes may themselves be subject to regulation. Long-term regulation or adaptation usually involves the de novo synthesis of the enzyme (transporter) molecules and allows for sustained cellular response when the intensity of the original stimulus has subsided. Transport and insertion of protein into target membranes may be involved. These processes may have different time courses and kinetics than the protein synthesis and may be subject to regulation.

Integration of the information available in such a model is hampered by the lack of information regarding the molecular properties of the transporting system and the effects that changes in the intracellular concentration of Pi, Na^+, and H^+ may have on the transporters.

ALLOSTERIC REGULATION BY NA^+ AND H^+

With the exception of the rabbit [23,95], the rate of Pi reabsorption in the proximal tubule increases with increasing pH [7,41,54]. In one of these studies [7], the Pi uptake increased several-fold on increasing the pH of the medium from 6.0 to 8.0. The effect of pH was greatest at low Na^+ concentration. Phosphate had no effect on the apparent affinity for Na^+, whereas Na^+ increased affinity of the transport system for Pi, at both high and low pH. The stoichiometry of the Na^+-Pi cotransport was apparently not affected by changes in pH. These findings suggest that Na^+ and H^+ are powerful allosteric modulators of brush border Pi transport that interact with the transporter at

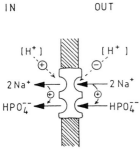

FIG. 7-8. *Schematic representation of interactions of Pi, Na+, and H+ with the Na+-Pi cotransport system of renal BBM (allosteric regulation). Broken lines and minus and plus signs denote inhibition and stimulation, respectively, of reactions indicated by solid arrows. (From Gmaj, P, Murer H: Cellular mechanisms of inorganic phosphate transport in kidney. Physiol Rev 66:36, 1986, with permission.)*

sites different from the Pi binding site and, by mutual interaction, control the affinity of the symporter for Pi (Fig. 7-8).

In summary, the evidence suggests that H^+ acts on both sides of the BBM to decrease the affinity of the Na^+-Pi cotransport system for Na^+. As a consequence, H^+ inhibits Pi transport from the luminal side but stimulates it from the cytosolic side. Because the sensitivity of the Na^+-Pi cotransport system to pH is higher at low Na^+ concentrations, it is expected that changes in cytosolic pH would affect Pi transport to a larger extent than changes in luminal pH. Finally, owing to the fact that changes in pH affect the affinity of the cotransporter, they can be effective only at nonsaturating Pi concentrations.

COVALENT MODIFICATIONS
Cyclic AMP-dependent Phosphorylation
It is well recognized that the phosphaturic effect of PTH is associated with an increased excretion of cAMP [50] and that the effect of PTH can be mimicked by administration of dibutyryl cAMP [75]. Moreover, PTH-stimulated adenylate cyclase activity has been described in proximal tubule basolateral membranes from rat [193] and dog [21, 191]. Cyclic AMP is thought to exert its effect in mammalian cells by activating a group of enzymes designated as cAMP-dependent protein kinases. Kinne et al. [124] found that these enzymes are localized preferentially in the BBM. It has been postulated, therefore, that the asymmetric cAMP-dependent phosphorylation of the proximal tubular cell membrane might underlie the effect of PTH on renal transport processes [124–127]. According to the model proposed by Hammerman [96a], PTH binds to its receptor located in the basolateral membrane of the proximal tubular cell and activates adenylate cyclase located at that site. Increased levels of intracellular cAMP resulting from such activation stimulate the activity of cAMP-dependent protein kinase in the BBM, and solute transport across the BBM is decreased consequent to phosphorylation of specific BBM proteins. Dephosphorylation of phospho-

proteins mediated by phosphoprotein phosphatase and perhaps by reduction in levels of cAMP affects the activity of phosphodiesterase in BBM and thus reverses the action of PTH. Hammerman and Hruska [101] identified by gel electrophoresis and autoradiography two bands that appear to be phosphorylated: one with an M_r of 62,000 and another with an M_r of 96,000. Addition of cAMP to the media of transiently lysed vesicles was found to affect both phosphorylation and inhibition of Pi transport in a concentration related manner [101]. Both cAMP-dependent phosphorylation and inhibition of Na^+-stimulated Pi transport were greater in vesicles from kidneys of parathyroidectomized dogs as compared with control animals. Similar findings were reported in the mouse [97].

Biber et al. [24] were unable to duplicate these results. They found no relationship between cAMP-dependent phosphorylation of BBM from kidneys of rats and inhibition of Na^+-dependent Pi transport in the membranes. No effect of cAMP on either K_m or V_{max} of the Na^+-Pi cotransport system could be demonstrated, although specific phosphorylation of several protein bands was evident. None of these proteins, however, was in the 62,000 M_r band.

Interpretation of these discrepant results is made difficult by potential effects of nucleotides on Pi transport in isolated BBM [158]. When added to membrane suspensions, nucleotides are rapidly hydrolyzed by a variety of enzymes [70,142,206]. In addition, in order to allow them exposure to the cytosolic side of the membranes, the vesicles have to be lysed and then resealed, a maneuver that may affect the regulatory system. Finally, it is possible that the protein phosphorylation is measured in leaky vesicles, which are permeable to the nucleotides but do not transport Pi, whereas the Na^+-Pi cotransport is measured in sealed vesicles that had not been phosphorylated. There is also question as to the specificity of the proteins that were found to be phosphorylated. The possibility exists that these proteins are not intrinsic to the membrane but that they belong to the cytoskeleton or to other contaminants of BBM preparation. Hence, the role played by protein phosphorylation in the regulation of Na^+-Pi cotransport remains unsettled.

Adenosine Diphosphate Ribosylation
Another type of covalent modification that may affect the transport of Pi may be induced by changes in intracellular levels of nicotinamide-adenine dinucleotide (NAD). Kempson et al. [121] were the first to propose this hypothesis. These investigators noted that a number of stimuli known to modulate the reabsorption of Pi in the renal proximal tubule also affect the NAD-NADH ratio. Injection of nicotinamide in Pi-depleted rats increased the levels of intracellular NAD and the NAD-NADH ratio in renal cortex and decreased renal reabsorption of Pi and the Na^+-Pi cotransport in BBM vesicles prepared from rat kidneys [121]. Administration of PTH to thyroparathyroidectomized rats increased the NAD-NADH ratio [22], while injection of nicotinamide in phosphate-depleted rats partially restored the phosphaturic action of PTH or of dibutyryl cAMP in these animals. Because PTH-induced cAMP generation in phosphate-depleted rats was not affected by nic-

otinamide, it was concluded that nicotinamide acts at a step beyond the generation of cAMP. This conclusion was supported by the finding that administration of nicotinamide restored phosphaturia induced by administration of dibutyryl cAMP.

Experiments on BBM vesicles appeared to confirm that NAD inhibits Na^+-dependent Pi transport [99,100]. It became apparent, however, that breakdown of NAD resulted in release of free Pi and dilution of the radioisotope used to measure Na^+-dependent Pi transport [98,206]. Subsequent experiments, performed by Hammerman et al. [98] and by Kempson et al. [123], revealed NAD-induced inhibition of Na^+-dependent Pi transport that could not be explained by hydrolysis of the nucleotide. On the other hand, Tenenhouse and Chu [206] and Gmaj et al. [83] were unable to detect any inhibition of Na^+-dependent Pi transport when NAD hydrolysis was prevented. When NAD was introduced into the intravesicular space and removed from the extravesicular space, stimulation rather than inhibition of Na^+-Pi cotransport was observed [83]. Moreover, in isolated perfused kidneys [13] and in isolated perfused proximal tubules [220,221], the oxidation and reduction of intracellular NAD with pyruvate and lactate, respectively, resulted in no appreciable change in Pi reabsorption.

Proponents of the theory maintain that NAD modifies covalently the membrane proteins by transferring the ADP-ribose moiety of NAD to an amino acid acceptor molecule in the protein [105]. This process can be catalyzed by ADP-ribosyl-transferase or can occur nonenzymatically through the formation of ADP-ribose and subsequent covalent attachment to amine groups in protein through formation of a Schiff base [222]. The latter process can result from the action of the enzyme NAD-glycohydrolase to hydrolase NAD [131]. Kempson and co-workers [122] have been indeed able to identify the presence of both ADP-ribosyl-transferase and NAD-glycohydrolase [120] in rat kidney. Thus, the membrane itself can serve as a substrate for ADP ribosylation in vitro.

In spite of this body of evidence, the role of NAD ribosylation in modulating the Na^+-dependent Pi transport across the luminal cell membrane of proximal tubules remains in question. One can only surmise that although both cAMP-dependent protein phosphorylation and ADP ribosylation have been demonstrated in isolated BBM preparations, the evidence supporting a role for these reactions in the regulation of Pi transport remains speculative.

Adaptation of Pi Transport to Supply and Demand

Renal adaptation of Pi transport to changes in supply or demand has been demonstrated consistently [20,51,53, 71,102,202]. Characteristically, the adaptive response is reflected in changes in the V_{max} of the Na^+-Pi cotransport, whereas the K_m remains unaltered [39,53,75,111,119, 145,159,209]. The increase of Na^+-Pi cotransport activity in Pi depletion is prevented by inhibitors of protein synthesis [192], whereas the increase of Na^+-Pi cotransport activity in response to thyroxin is inhibited by cytoskeletal

inhibitors [223]. It appears, therefore, that both protein synthesis and membrane recycling are involved in adaptive responses.

Experiments performed in LLC-PK$_2$ cells in culture revealed two phases in the adaptation to low Pi concentration in the media: a rapid increase in Pi transport by about 30% that occurred within 10 minutes, and a slow increase thereafter resulting in a doubling of Pi transport rate by 15 hours [25,47]. Both the rapid and the long-term adaptations were characterized by increases in V_{max}, but only the long-term adaptation was inhibited by cycloheximide and actinomycin D, suggesting that protein synthesis is involved only in the long-term adaptation to Pi deprivation. The magnitude of the up and down regulation was small in cells grown in a medium with high Pi concentration but large in cells adapted to low Pi concentration [47]. These results are consistent with the hypothesis that protein synthesis and membrane recycling are involved in the adaptation of the brush border Na-Pi$^+$ cotransport system to changes in Pi supply.

Factors That Affect Renal Handling of Pi

GLOMERULAR FILTRATION RATE

The plasma concentration of Pi is tightly controlled by the kidney. As already indicated, there is, in general, a constant relationship between the filtered load and the tubular reabsorption of Pi. This is likely due to the fact that Pi reabsorption is tightly linked to Na^+ reabsorption. Consequently, the glomerular tubular balance that exists for Na extends to Pi. The plasma concentration of Pi, and thus Pi body homeostasis, is affected only when either the filtered load of Pi or the tubular reabsorption of Pi is altered drastically [88]. Bijvoet [26] has shown that under conditions of fasting the plasma concentration of Pi is maintained owing to an increase in Tm_{Pi}/GFR, whereas increases in GFR as large as 50% are associated with slight decreases in plasma Pi. However, reductions in GFR below 30 ml/min lead to hyperphosphatemia [105]. Bricker [35] proposed that sequential, albeit small, elevations in plasma Pi cause an increase in parathyroid hormone secretion, accounting for the hyperparathyroidism observed in chronic renal failure [184,185]. Reduction in Pi intake, proportional to the decrease in GFR, prevented the development of hyperparathyroidism [194–196]. Yet, Pi homeostasis was preserved as well in dogs subjected to parathyroidectomy as in parathyroid-intact uremic animals [205]. Thus, although the retention of Pi that occurs in renal failure is probably responsible for the development of hyperparathyroidism, the parathyroid glands are not essential to the maintenance of Pi balance.

ROLE OF EXTRACELLULAR FLUID VOLUME

Expansion of the extracellular fluid compartment by the infusion of saline decreases tubular reabsorption of Pi [216]. Infusion of hyperoncotic albumin has no effect on Pi reabsorption, provided that the plasma level of ionized calcium is maintained constant [129]. Hence, it would appear that it is not the expansion of the extracellular fluid volume but the increased delivery of Na^+ that affects the reabsorption of Pi. Interestingly, saline loading does not affect urinary excretion of Pi in thyroparathyroidectomized animals [19,79,129], presumably because the increased amount of Pi escaping reabsorption in the proximal tubule is reclaimed at more distal sites of the nephron.

EFFECT OF PI INTAKE

It has been recognized for a long time that changes in the dietary intake of Pi cause adaptive changes in the renal reabsorption of Pi, even in hypoparathyroid human subjects [166]. Troehler at al. [208] were among the first to report that the tubular reabsorption of Pi was consistently higher in rats fed a low Pi diet than in rats fed a high Pi diet, even when the parathyroid glands were removed. Similar effects have been observed in dogs [87,178,217]. Micropuncture experiments have revealed that Pi reabsorption is threefold higher in rats subjected to a low Pi diet than in those fed a high Pi diet. Administration of PTH to the animals on a low Pi diet reduced Pi reabsorption in the late proximal convolution but failed to affect the reabsorption of Pi in the early convolutions of the proximal tubule [211]. In rabbit, Pi depletion resulted in an enhancement in Pi reabsorption in the S2 but not in the S1 segment [152].

The adaptation to low Pi diet develops relatively quickly. Enhanced Pi reabsorption is already detectable by two to four hours of Pi deprivation [45,145] and is fully expressed by 3 days [208]. The response to Pi overload produced by infusion of Pi appears to be even faster, a decrease in Pi reabsorption being detectable by 1 hr [51]. These changes in the renal reabsorption of Pi are expressed at the level of the BBM, being characterized by an increase in V_{max} [51,53,71,122,192,202,203]. In Pi-deprived rats, Pi excretion is augmented by metabolic acidosis and is further increased by administration of PTH [92,119,214]. The increase in Na^+-Pi cotransport activity observed in Pi-deprived animals is inhibited by actinomycin D, suggesting that de novo protein synthesis is involved in this process [192]. Thus, Pi reabsorption in animals adapted to low Pi diet does not seem to be resistant to the acute inhibitory effects of acidosis and PTH that are primarily mediated by allosteric regulation of the Na^+-Pi cotransport systems in the BBM.

Adaptive changes to manipulations in Pi intake have also been observed in developing animals, but, at least quantitatively, they differ from those occurring in adult subjects. Mulroney and Haramati [156] measured the maximal reabsorption of Pi per unit of GFR (maxRPi/GFR) in rats of various ages who were fed a low (0.007%), normal (0.7%), or high (1.8%) Pi diet for four days and were acutely parathyroidectomized prior to the experiments. On all dietary regimens, the maxRPi/GFR was highest in immature rats (three to four weeks of age) and decreased with age. Immature rats fed a low Pi diet had, on the average, a 68% percent increase in maxRPi/GFR, as compared with 38% in adult (12- to 13-week-old) rats. Conversely, in response to a diet high in Pi, the decrease in maxRPi/GFR was smaller in immature (42%) than in the mature (61%) rats.

Neiberger et al. [161] compared the kinetics of Pi trans-

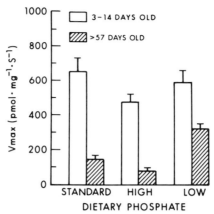

FIG. 7-9. Effect of variations in Pi intake on the V_{max} of Na^+-Pi cotransport in BBM vesicles of newborn (3- to 14-day-old) and adult (>57-day-old) guinea pigs. Within each dietary group the differences in V_{max} between newborn and adult animals were all statistically significant (P < 0.01). Within each age group, effects of changes in dietary Pi on V_{max} were significant in adult (P < 0.01) and Pi-supplemented newborn guinea pigs (P < 0.05). (From Neiberger RE, Barac-Nieto M, Spitzer A: Renal reabsorption of phosphate during development: Transport kinetics in BBMV. Am J Physiol (Renal Fluid Electrolyte Physiology 26)257:F268, 1989, with permission.)

port in BBM vesicles prepared from kidneys of 3- to 14-day-old guinea pigs with animals greater than 57 days of age. For the preceding five days, the animals were fed a standard diet, nominally free of Pi, or a diet high in Pi (Fig. 7-9). On the standard diet, the V_{max} of the Na^+-Pi cotransport system was substantially higher in BBM vesicles from the newborn (650 ± 77 pmol/mg/s) than from adult (144 ± 17 pmol/mg/s) guinea pigs. A low dietary Pi did not affect significantly the V_{max} of the Na^+-Pi cotransport in BBM of newborn animals, but it did up-regulate the system in the adult (from 144 ± 17 to 318 ± 32 pmol/mg/s). Thus, the increase in maxRPi/GFR observed by Mulroney and Haramati [156] in Pi deprived animals was probably due to increases in Pi reabsorption in distal segments of the nephron. An increase in Pi intake resulted in a smaller relative decrease in V_{max} in the newborn than in the adult (27 vs 44%). There were no significant differences in the apparent K_m of the Na^+-Pi cotransport system between newborn and adult guinea pigs on either diet. The serum Pi concentration was similar in newborn and adult animals on a standard diet (1.8 ± 0.1 vs 2.1 ± 0.2 mM). In the newborn, the serum Pi decreased substantially on a low Pi diet (from 1.8 ± 0.1 to 0.8 ± 0.1) and rose by twofold on the high Pi diet (from 1.8 ± 0.1 to 3.5 ± 0.2 mM). In the adult, there were no significant changes in serum Pi with changes in Pi intake.

Somewhat different results have been reported in older rats by Caverzasio et al. [47]. These authors observed a higher Na^+-dependent Pi uptake by BBM vesicles of young growing (two-month-old) than adult (eight- to nine-month-old) rats only under conditions of a low Pi diet.

The results demonstrate that in the newborn the Na^+-Pi cotransport system is characterized by a high transport capacity but a low adaptability to changes in dietary Pi. The tendency to retain Pi and the inability to adapt to changes in Pi intake may explain the hyperphosphatemia observed in newborns fed a cow's milk diet, which is rich in Pi [55,81]. The mechanisms that account for these adaptive responses of the kidney to Pi loading and Pi depletion remain unknown.

EFFECT OF CALCIUM

An acute increase in plasma concentration of calcium generally has been associated with a decrease in the urinary excretion of Pi [4,143]. Likewise, an increase in Pi excretion was observed during acute hypocalcemia induced by the administration of Ca^{2+} complexing agents such as EGTA or EDTA [181]. Consistent with this type of response, Ullrich and co-workers [212] observed that a decrease in the calcium concentration in the fluid perfusing peritubular capillaries resulted in a diminution of the Pi reabsorptive flux in proximal convoluted tubule, whereas Amiel and colleagues [4] found that an elevation in plasma calcium from low to normal levels increased the Pi reabsorptive capacity of the proximal tubule, loop of Henle, and terminal nephron segments. Other investigators, however, have reported that calcium infusion produced inhibition of Pi transport [216] or had no affect on Pi excretion in the absence of PTH [60]. The calcium ionophore A23187 when given intravenously was reported to enhance Pi reabsorption in the presence of PTH at nephron sites other than the early or the late proximal tubule [210]. Furthermore, a decrease in fractional Pi reabsorption of superficial proximal tubule was observed in thyroparathyroidectomized dogs in response to calcium chloride infusion [86]. However, this response was not accompanied by an increase in fractional Pi excretion, indicating enhanced reabsorption at other sites along the nephron.

The decrease in the fractional reabsorption of Pi associated with acute elevation in the plasma concentration of calcium may be due, at least in part, to the increase in the concentration of total and ultrafilterable Pi that occurs in this experimental condition. Thus, the effect of calcium on Pi transport may differ with the basal level of plasma calcium concentration, and it may affect differently various segments of the nephron and various populations of nephrons.

Changes in Pi reabsorption consequent to chronic changes in plasma calcium concentrations are more consistent and predictable than those due to acute changes in plasma calcium. As already mentioned, chronic elevation of plasma calcium in hypoparathyroid human subjects is associated with a decrease in the tubular reabsorption of Pi [30,62,74]. In thyroparathyroidectomized rats the tubular reabsorptive capacity for Pi was found to be inversely related to the level of plasma calcium [31]. This change could not be ascribed to variations in the dietary intake or intestinal absorption of Pi or to any change in PTH, calcitonin, or endogenous production of $1,25(OH)_2D_3$. As is the case for acute changes in plasma concentration, the

mechanism by which chronic changes in plasma calcium affect the renal transport of Pi is unknown.

EFFECTS OF CHANGES IN ACID–BASE STATUS

Clearance studies performed in dogs [149] and humans [80] revealed that infusion of bicarbonate caused phosphaturia, even in the absence of PTH. This was thought to be due either to competition for the transporting sites or to an increase in the divalent to monovalent phosphate ratio due to tubular fluid alkalinization [14]. Microperfusion experiments performed in rat proximal tubule appeared to support this assumption. Reabsorption of 2.0 mM Pi from otherwise unbuffered perfusion solution was found to be faster at acid than at alkaline pH [14]. It was only later shown that the pH of poorly buffered perfusion solutions changes rapidly in the tubule and may achieve steady state values long before the tubular fluid sample is recollected [139]. Similar results were observed when rat proximal tubules were perfused with 100 [43] or 10 [95] mM Pi. The presence of HCO_3^- in the perfusion fluid did not affect the pH dependence of Pi reabsorption. On the other hand, when the concentration of phosphate in the tubular perfusate was only 2 mM, reabsorption was twice as high at a luminal pH of 7.4 than at 6.8. Reabsorption of Pi was considerably reduced in chronically alkalotic rats, whether the luminal pH was alkaline or acid [17]. Micropuncture experiments in which the tubule and the peritubular capillaries were independently perfused yielded concordant results. Reabsorption of Pi from stationary droplets was stimulated by alkaline luminal pH but inhibited by intracellular alkaline pH [213].

The apparent discrepancy between these results was resolved in part by the experiments of Lang et al. [139], who found that Pi reabsorption in the rat proximal tubule was stimulated by increases in luminal pH when the concentration of Pi in the luminal fluid was low but was inhibited by pH increases when luminal Pi concentration was high. Quamme and Wong [180] found Pi reabsorption to be twice as high at a luminal pH of 7.65 than at a pH of 6.50. Systemic infusion of Pi inhibited Pi reabsorption to a larger extent at alkaline than at acid pH in the lumen. A similar reduction in pH dependence of Pi reabsorption was observed in animals fed a high Pi diet [179]. Clearance experiments performed in rats rendered results that were consistent with those generated by in vitro experiments. Alkalosis was found to stimulate and acidosis to inhibit Pi reabsorption, but only at nonsaturating plasma Pi concentrations [103]. It would appear therefore that Pi reabsorption is stimulated by increases in pH in the lumen only when the concentration of Pi in the tubule or in the cell is low; at high Pi concentrations, the pH dependence of Pi reabsorption is diminished or lost [17,139,179,180,213]. These findings are in good agreement with those obtained in BBM vesicles. Na^+-Pi cotransport was found to be stimulated at alkaline pH of the media but inhibited when the interior of the vesicles (i.e., the cytosolic surface of the membrane) was alkaline [7].

These results may be interpreted to indicate that at nonsaturating Pi concentrations of Pi at the luminal side of the membrane the pH affects the affinity of the cotransporter for Na^+-Pi; at Pi concentrations in the lumen above saturation, the luminal pH no longer has an effect on the Pi carrier interaction. However, the cytosolic pH may still affect the rate of Pi transport by changing the rate of Pi dissociation from the carrier at the cytosolic surface of the membrane.

It should be also pointed out that disturbances in acid–base balance may affect Pi transport indirectly, through alterations in cell metabolism. For instance, alkalosis, by stimulating glycolysis [63,106,135,136,160], results in an increased incorporation of Pi into glycolytic intermediates. The ensuing hypophosphatemia may, in turn, stimulate renal reabsorption of Pi [110]. Acidosis, on the other hand, is associated with stimulation of renal glycogenesis and thus with release of Pi from glycolytic intermediates and with increased conversion of anionic substrate to either glucose or CO_2. The ensuing increase in cell pH and in Pi availability may inhibit the dissociation of Pi on the cytosolic surface of the BBM and thus contribute to the inhibition of Pi transport observed in metabolic acidosis [92,138,199].

In chronic metabolic acidosis a large decrease in the V_{max} of the Na^+-Pi cotransport is observed in the absence of changes in K_m [119,146]. This is consistent with changes either in the number or the activity of the symporters, an adaptive effect that must be distinguished from the direct allosteric effects of H^+ on Pi transport described by Gmaj and Murer [85].

In summary, alkalinity of the tubular lumen enhances, and acidity inhibits, reabsorption of Pi in the proximal tubule. The effects of luminal pH are predominant at nonsaturable Pi concentrations in lumen, whereas the effects of cell pH become apparent at high Pi concentrations in the tubular fluid. Changes in Pi reabsorption observed in chronic acid–base disturbances are due to changes in the number or the activity of the cotransporters.

EFFECTS OF HORMONES
Parathyroid Hormone
PTH has multiple effects on tubular function, including inhibition of Pi, HCO_3^-, Na^+, and fluid reabsorption [68,112,117,154] and stimulation of gluconeogenesis [91,134,135,160,182]. Chase and Auerbach [50] were the first to suggest that the effect of PTH on Pi transport was mediated by an increase in intracellular cAMP. Agus and co-workers [2] were able to show that infusion of dibutyryl cAMP mimicked the phosphaturic action of PTH.

Both the proximal and the distal collecting tubules appear to respond to acute changes in the plasma level of PTH [6,168,176,211]. The proximal tubule effect was shown in one study to be localized at the level of the early convoluted tubule [96], whereas in another study [66] the effect was ascribed to the late proximal convolutions and pars recta. Dennis and co-workers [65,66] reported subsequently that, in the proximal convoluted tubule of the rabbit, PTH produced inhibition of fluid reabsorption, which was dependent on the presence of bicarbonate, but did not affect the reabsorption of Pi. By contrast, in the pars recta, both fluid reabsorption and Pi reabsorption were significantly inhibited by PTH, but only inhibition of fluid

was dependent on the presence of bicarbonate. The lack of PTH effect on the reabsorption of Pi in the early segments of the proximal tubule is at odds with observations made by other investigators [1,16,211] who found comparable degrees of inhibition of Pi transport in the early and late segments of the proximal tubule.

Baumann and co-workers [16] have reported that PTH has a preferential effect on fluid reabsorption when applied on the contraluminal side of the epithelium, whereas cAMP inhibits fluid reabsorption preferentially when applied on the luminal side. The effects were not additive. These observations are consistent with the view that PTH binds to receptors located on the basolateral membrane of the proximal tubule cells [132] to activate adenyl cyclase and generate cAMP; cAMP acts then at the luminal membrane, perhaps by activating a protein kinase, to bring about its effects on fluid and Pi reabsorption. The effects are terminated by dephosphorylation, and cAMP is inactivated by tubule cell phosphodiesterase [76]. The cAMP moiety that escapes the effects of this enzyme is excreted in the urine. The fact that cAMP, which is generated in the cell, has effects similar to those of PTH on tubule transport is due to its binding to BBM receptors, which makes it resistant to hydrolysis by phosphodiesterase [115]. It is possible, but not proved, that the same receptors may be accessible from the cytosolic side.

In vitro studies were carried out in BBM vesicles of rats and dogs [75,111,203] or on renal cortical slices from mice [52] exposed to PTH added to the incubation medium. In all these experiments, a decrease in Na^+-dependent Pi uptake was observed, but the effect was relatively small, compared with that observed in vivo. This finding strengthens the argument of those who believe that PTH may also act at sites of the nephron located beyond the proximal tubule.

The effects of chronic changes in PTH availability on Pi transport appear to be due not only to changes in cAMP [163] but also to changes in calcium and vitamin D levels [3,32,59,62,74,162,187]. Indeed, it should not be forgotten that PTH is primarily a calcium regulating hormone and that the production of PTH is not regulated by the concentration of Pi in the extracellular compartment. Moreover, the kidney is able to adjust its rate of Pi reabsorption in the presence of PTH [30].

The role played by PTH in the control of Pi reabsorption during development is unclear. The serum levels of PTH are known to be low during the first few days after birth [61], which may explain the very high fractional reabsorption of Pi observed during this period of life [55]. Shortly thereafter, the PTH levels appear to increase dramatically, becoming higher during infancy than during middle childhood [11]. Infusion of exogenous PTH during the early newborn period resulted in a minimal depression of renal Pi reabsorption [147]. By 7 days of age, however, full-term infants manifest an adequate phosphaturic response to the acute administration of the hormone. This is associated with an increase in the urinary excretion of cAMP. In contrast, other authors have found a low adenylate cyclase response to PTH stimulation in the renal cortex of neonatal rats [82], suggesting a degree of end-organ unresponsiveness to PTH. Addition of PTH to the fluid perfusing the isolated kidney preparation of guinea-pig resulted in a phosphaturic effect in adult animals but not in the newborn [116]. The effect on Ca^{2+} reabsorption was present at both ages. No difference in cAMP excretion was detected. These results support the contention that the immature kidney is less sensitive to the phosphaturic effect of PTH than the adult kidney. This difference may be due to the low intracellular Pi concentration, as has been shown to be the case in phosphate-depleted adult animals [200]. Alternatively, the lack of a phosphaturic response to PTH in the newborn may be a consequence of age-related differences in the distribution of Pi reabsorption along the renal tubule. It is possible that the reabsorption of Pi in the newborn is completed by the time that the tubular fluid reaches the pars recta, the segment of the nephron at which, according to Dennis and co-workers [67], PTH acts on Pi transport.

The simultaneous inhibition of Pi and HCO_3^- reabsorption and stimulation of gluconeogenesis by PTH and/or cAMP has suggested to Gmaj and Murer [85] that these responses may be triggered by some common cellular mechanism. According to these investigators, binding of PTH to the receptors results in stimulation of adenylate cyclase, increased synthesis of cAMP, and increased influx of Ca^{2+} into the cells [182]. Calcium and cAMP stimulate gluconeogenesis [135,137,160]. Increased incorporation of anionic precursors into glucose results in increased proton consumption and alkaline shift of cell pH. Increased cell pH inhibits both Na^+-Pi cotransport and Na^+-H exchange via direct allosteric effects on these transport systems. In addition, Na^+-Pi cotransport may be inhibited directly by Pi release from phosphorylated glycolytic intermediates (product inhibition), and Na^+-H exchange may be inhibited directly by Ca^{2+} [49,219]. This hypothesis is compatible with the fact that resistance to the phosphaturic affect of PTH or cAMP occurs in starvation [19,128], in Pi depletion [19,30,198,200], in respiratory alkalosis [110], after lithium administration [9,12], and in type 2 pseudohypoparathyroidism [72]. In all these conditions, sensitivity to PTH and cAMP can be restored by manipulations that affect systemic or cellular pH. Alternatively, the effect of PTH on Pi transport by proximal tubule cells may be mediated by phosphorylation of BBM proteins, as proposed by Hammerman [97,99–101]. It should be pointed out, however, that neither of these hypotheses is sufficiently backed by experimental evidence. The former suffers particularly from the lack of information regarding the interactions between changes in the intracellular milieu and the cytosolic side of the Na^+-Pi cotransporter. The latter suffers from the lack of evidence that phosphorylation of BBM proteins causes specific changes in the microenvironment of the Na^+-Pi cotransporters that result in changes in their activity.

Effect of Vitamin D Metabolites
Not unlike PTH, $1,25(OH)_2D_3$ is a hormone, the primary function of which is to increase the reabsorption of Ca^{2+} by the intestine and the renal tubule and to promote its deposition into bone. Its effect on Pi transport may be only incidental. When given in pharmacologic amounts, vitamin D metabolites were found to stimulate the tubular

reabsorption of Pi in animals deprived of parathyroid glands [58,104]. The effect was rather small and apparently dependent on the concomitant administration of other hormones such as ADH, PTH, calcitonin, or glucagon [164,169,171,175–177). At least some of these factors may affect the renal adenylate cyclase system [169,170,172]. The vitamin D metabolites themselves could interfere with the renal generation of cAMP [170,172], at least when present in pharmacologic amounts. Finally, as in the case of PTH, rats deficient in vitamin D adapt well to Pi deprivation [201].

Contrary to its acute phosphaturic effect, vitamin D_3 was found to increase the urinary excretion of Pi when given in large amounts for a prolonged period of time. This observation, made initially in humans by Albright and Reifenstein [3], was largely confirmed. Thyroparathyroidectomized animals have been found to have a similar response to the administration of vitamin D [59,162] or vitamin D metabolites [32,62,187]. Administration of $1,25(OH)_2D_3$ to thyroparathyroidectomized rats was found to restore completely their ability to adjust to changes in Pi intake [32]. It is possible, therefore, that vitamin D plays a role in the maintenance of a high tubular Pi reabsorptive capacity in chronic hypoparathyroidism. The effect of $1,25(OH)_2D_3$ on the renal handling of Pi may be mediated, at least in part, by its calcemic effect. Indeed, an increase in serum calcium induced by a rise in the calcium content of the diet was found to decrease the tubular reabsorption of Pi in thyroparathyroidectomized rats [31] and in hypoparathyroid patients [62,74]. Micropuncture studies have revealed that $1,25(OH)_2D_3$ affects the tubular reabsorption of Pi in the same segments as those involved in the response to dietary manipulations of Pi [155] and is expressed at the level of the BBM [203]. Moreover, the phosphaturic effect of $1,25(OH)_2D_3$ observed in hypoparathyroid animals and humans does not occur in euparathyroid subjects [32,144]. Taken together, these observations indicate that $1,25(OH)_2D_3$ does not have a direct effect on the renal transport of Pi.

Growth Hormone
Phosphate reabsorption is increased in acromegaly [42] and decreased in pituitary dwarfism [107]. Administration of growth hormone increases Pi reabsorption in men [18,57,107,113] and in animals [44,56]. The effect is associated with an increase in V_{max} of the Na^+-Pi transport in BBM [102].

The high levels of growth hormone present in infants and children may explain, in part, the high rates of Pi reabsorption observed during these periods of life. That this may indeed be the case is demonstrated by the fact that administration of growth hormone release inhibitory factor (GHRIF) to newborn rats resulted in a decrease in the renal reabsorptive capacity for Pi [157]. On the other hand, dietary Pi deprivation did not alter the pattern of secretion or the average plasma concentration of growth hormone [207], but it did result in up-regulation of Pi-cotransport both in control [48] and in hypophysectomized rats [207]. Thus, the up-regulatory response in renal Pi cotransport to decrease Pi supply does not appear to be mediated by growth hormone. It is more likely that hypophysectomy and administration of GHRIF lead to increases in the demand for Pi, associated with a decrease in growth rate. The mechanism by which this change affects the transport of Pi by the renal tubule remains to be established. Potential mediators are changes in the intracellular concentration of Pi or in the level of $1,25(OH)_2D_3$. The lack of an acute effect of growth hormone on renal Pi reabsorption in the adult dog [218] may be due to the fact that the action of the hormone is indirect, being mediated by somatomedin (insulin-like growth factor 1, IGF_1).

Steroid Hormones

Mineralocorticoids have not been found to affect the reabsorption of Pi [183], but glucocorticoids have a marked inhibitory effect on Na^+-Pi cotransport [8,114,186]. The action appears to be mediated by a nuclear mechanism, suggesting hormone-dependent synthesis of an inhibitory protein.

Thyroid Hormones

Acute administration of triiodothyronine in humans produces a decrease in Pi reabsorption [21]. Yet, in thyrotoxicosis, serum Pi is elevated in association with an increase in the fractional reabsorption of Pi [167]. This apparent paradox may be the result of parathyroid gland suppression by the increase in serum calcium observed in this condition [27].

Magnesium

Magnesium is predominantly an intracellular ion, only about 1% of the total body magnesium (approximatly 2000 mEq in the adult subject) being present in the extracellular fluid compartment. The plasma concentration of Mg varies between 1.1 and 2.6 mg/dl (0.6 and 1.1 mmol/liter) [36], approximately half being bound to proteins and ions. About 80% of the Mg present in the plasma is ultrafilterable (UF_{Mg}) [37]. No age-related differences in serum concentation appear to exist (see Table 7-1) [1,2], although the levels may be lower in low-birth-weight infants [35]. The kidneys play an important role in regulating the extracellular concentration of Mg. Hypermagnesemia results in a substantial reduction in Mg reabsorption, whereas hypomagnesemia is associated with an increase in the reabsorption of Mg. Titration studies performed in dogs [21] revealed a maximum reabsortion rate of 140 μg/min/kg BW, which was achieved at a filtered load of Mg of 280 μg/min. The Tm-like mechanism appears to reflect the behavior of two nephron segments involved in the reabsorption of Mg, namely the proximal tubule, which reabsorbs a constant fraction of the filtered load, and the thick ascending limb of Henle's loop, which responds to hypermagnesemia with a decrease in the reabsorption of Mg [39]. Secretion of Mg has been postulated by some [15,38] and contested by others [6,7].

Reabsorption of Mg Along the Renal Tubule

Most of the filtered load of Mg is reabsorbed in the ascending limb of Henle's loop (50% to 70%) (Fig. 7-10)

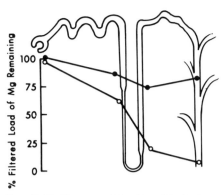

FIG. 7-10. *Fraction of the filtered load of magnesium remaining in the renal tubule of dogs under control conditions (dots) and following infusion of magnesium sulfate (circles). (Data from Wen SF, Eranson Rl, Dirks JH: Am J Physiol 219:570, 1970, with permission.)*

[13,24]. The proximal tubule reabsorbs 25% to 50% (depending on the animal species) [5,13,16,23,25], and the distal nephron reabsorbs about 5% of the filtered load [16,38]. About 10% of the filtered Mg is excreted in the urine.

PROXIMAL TUBULE

Several micropuncture studies [8,23,33,38] have revealed that the TF/UF_{Mg} is about 1.5 by the end of the proximal convoluted tubule, whereas the TF/P_{In} is more than 2.0. This indicates that the reabsorption of Mg in the proximal tubule is not isotonic, suggesting a lower permeance of Mg than that of the other ions transported in this nephron segment. The TF/UF_{Mg} concentration was found to remain relatively constant in experimental conditions such as volume expansion, metabolic changes in the acid–base status, and changes in the plasma levels of calcium and Pi. Microperfusion experiments performed in the rat [4] and dog [31] revealed very little back-flux of Mg into the proximal tubule, indicating that Mg transport is mainly a uni-directional process, probably transcellular. The rate of transport in this nephron segment is proportional to the load and is not saturable even at luminal Mg concentrations that exceed by tenfold that of the plasma UF_{Mg} [31].

LOOP OF HENLE

Several micropuncture studies have provided evidence that the loop of Henle is the segment of the nephron where most of the filtered Mg is reabsorbed and where the factors that modulate the excretion of Mg exert their effect. There is no apparent transport of Mg in the descending limb of Henle's loop [5,13]. It is likely, therefore, that reabsorption of Mg is accomplished by the thick ascending limb of the loop. Like the proximal tubule, the loop of Henle is largely impermeable to the backflux of Mg into the tubular fluid and able to increase its reabsorptive capacity as luminal Mg concentration increases. In the dog [31], the fractional reabsorption remained at about 80% of the delivered load into the loop of Henle at any level of luminal Mg concentration up to 10 mEq/liter. On the other hand, hypermagnesemia blunted the reabsorption of Mg, together with that of Ca^{2+}, but did not affect the reabsorption of Na^+. The cellular mechanism that accounts for this behavior remains unknown. It is assumed that transport of Mg across the luminal membrane of this segment is largely passive along an electrical but against a concentration gradient [34]. If this is indeed the case, the system would be driven by the secondary-active reabsorption of Cl^- and would be inhibited by loop diuretics such as furosemide and ethacrynic acid. Experimental evidence, to be described subsequently, supports this assumption [14,28].

DISTAL CONVOLUTED TUBULE AND COLLECTING DUCT

Mg transport in the early distal tubule is negligible, and the underlying mechanism has not been studied [5]. Microperfusion studies of the distal tubule indicate an increase in Mg reabsorption with increased load [31]. The reabsorption has to be active since the transtubular potential difference is markedly negative. The late distal tubule and the collecting duct do not appear to reabsorb Mg [6]. It is of interest that both the U/P_{In} and the U/UF_{Mg} were lower in these animals than in those used for measurements of proximal tubule reabsorption. These animals excreted a urine that was about 40% less concentrated and contained about 50% less Mg than that of the animals used for studies of proximal function. Because measurements in papillary collecting ducts can be done only in very young animals (weighing 50 to 100 g), it is reasonable to speculate that the differences were at least in part age-related.

Factors Affecting Renal Reabsorption of Mg

GLOMERULAR FILTRATION RATE

Variations in the rate of glomerular filtration have little effect on Mg excretion [22]. An increase in Mg excretion is observed in chronic renal disease when the GFR decreases below 30 ml/min [26,27].

Infusion of saline results in proportionate increases in the excretion of Na^+, Mg, and Ca^{2+} [19]. Volume expansion decreases the reabsorption of Mg at the level of proximal tubule, which, at least in the dog [12], is not compensated by increases in the reabsorption of Mg in the loop of Henle. The reason for this lack of compensatory response is not known.

HYPERMAGNESEMIA AND HYPOMAGNESEMIA

As already described, acute infusion of Mg results in an increase in the excretion of Mg. This is the combined result of an increase in the filtered load of Mg and a decrease in the fractional but not absolute reabsorption in the proximal tubule and a decrease both in fractional and absolute reabsorption in the thick ascending loop of Henle [31]. Hypomagnesemia results in a decrease in the excretion of Mg owing almost exclusively to increased reabsorption in the thick ascending limb of Henle's loop.

HYPERCALCEMIA AND HYPOCALCEMIA

As already described, infusion of calcium results in a decrease in Mg reabsorption, while infusion of Mg decreases the reabsorption of calcium [21]. Hypercalcemia appears to diminish the reabsorption of Mg in the proximal tubule and even more so in the loop of Henle [17,30]. The reabsorption of Mg at this latter site was greater than that of calcium, whereas the reabsorption of Na^+ was not affected. Taken together, these studies suggest competition between Ca^{2+} and Mg transport in this nephron segment.

PHOSPHATE DEPLETION

Phosphate depletion was described by some [11] but not by others [32] to produce an increase in Mg excretion.

PARATHYROID HORMONE

Acute administration of PTH has been found to enhance the renal reabsorption of Mg [3,21]. This effect, however, can be obscured by the hypercalcemia ensuing PTH administration. As already indicated, hypercalcemia inhibits Mg reabsorption in the loop of Henle. The effect of PTH on Mg transport appears to be mediated by cAMP [9].

CALCITONIN

Calcitonin [29] and glucocorticoids and mineralocorticoids [18,20] do not appear to have direct effects on the renal transport of Mg.

LOOP DIURETICS

Loop diuretics such as furosemide cause decreases in Mg reabsorption that exceed the inhibition of Na^+ reabsorption [14]. The reason for this difference is not known. Thiazide diuretics [40] have little effect on the renal handling of Mg. The same applies to disturbances in acid–base balance.

No studies have been done on the renal control of Mg excretion during maturation.

The Vitamin D–Endocrine System

Substantial progress has been made in elucidating the vitamin D–endocrine system and the description of the sequential metabolic steps required for vitamin D to become active. However, only a limited number of studies have focused on the developmental aspects of vitamin D metabolism and on the role played by this secosteroid in the maintenance of calcium homeostasis in the rapidly growing subject. Neither the factors regulating the absorption of calcium from the intestine nor those controlling its accretion into bone have been delineated. Most of the information that is available comes from animal studies. Attempts to extrapolate it to the human lead often to what appear, on the surface, to be conflicting conclusions.

To appreciate the role of vitamin D and PTH in the regulation of body calcium and phosphate homeostasis, a review of the vitamin D–endocrine system is required (Fig. 7-11). Vitamin D_3 (cholecalciferol) is produced by the

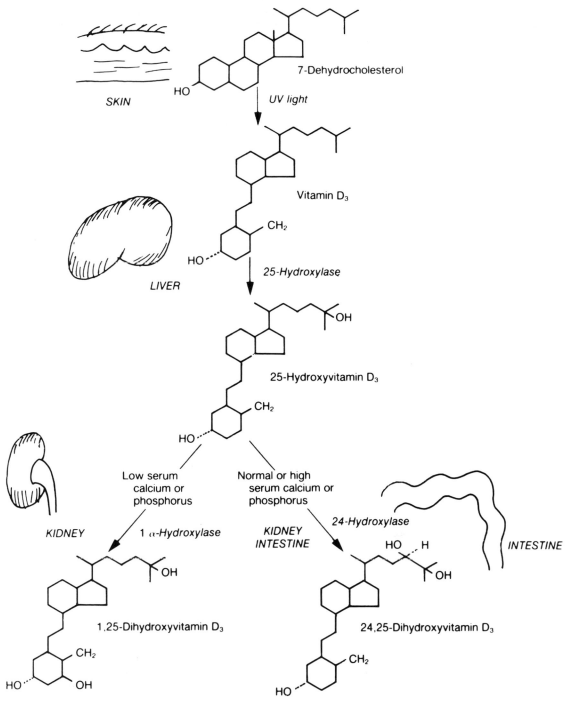

Fig. 7-11. *The metabolism of vitamin D in man and factors influencing the production of various metabolites. (From Chesney RW: Metabolic bone diseases. Pediatr Rev 5:227, 1984, with permission.)*

thermal conversion of pre-vitamin D_3, which, in turn, results from photolysis of 7-dehydrocholesterol in the skin by ultraviolet B irradiation at 288 nm [20,58]. A specific vitamin D–binding protein (DBP) (molecular weight 52,000 daltons) transports vitamin D to the liver, where a microsomal enzyme within the hepatocyte adds an hydroxyl group at carbon-25 by incorporating the oxygen molecule. This step is not strongly feedback-regulated, as indicated by the fact that animals or humans develop very high serum values of 25-hydroxyvitamin D [25(OH)D] when given large doses of vitamin D [12]. After sunshine exposure or an oral dose of vitamin D, the parent vitamin D compound is either stored in fat or converted to 25(OH)D. This latter compound is the main form of vitamin D found in serum, circulating at concentrations of 20 to 80 ng/ml in humans [26]. The serum values of vitamin D are lower, approximating 1 to 2 ng/ml [70]. However, since DBP binds avidly to 25(OH)D and other vitamin D metabolites, the free levels of these compounds are considerably less than the total levels measured in plasma or serum.

The 25(OH)D is transported to the kidney via DBP. Within the proximal tubule of the kidney reside two enzymes with hydroxylase activity: 25(OH)D-1α-hydroxylase and 25(OH)D-24-hydroxylase [25,59]. The major activity of 1α-hydroxylase is confined to the mitochondria, and it is mixed with a monooxygenase that incorporates oxygen at the 18-position of the secosteroid molecule [20,25,58]. Enzyme activity was also detected in the placenta of mammalian species. This is considered to account for the high concentrations of 1,25(OH)$_2$D in the serum of pregnant women [47]. The main regulators of the 1α-hydroxylase activity are a low serum calcium, low serum phosphate, and elevated PTH concentration, although other factors, including estrogens, androgens, growth hormone, and insulin, may play secondary, indirect roles in promoting synthesis of 1,25-dihydroxyvitamin D [1,25(OH)$_2$D or calcitriol] [20,58,70].

The other major vitamin D metabolite produced in the kidney is 24,25-dihydroxyvitamin D [24,25(OH)$_2$D]. The enzyme producing this metabolite operates in counterpoint to 1α-hydroxylase. Consequently, 24,25(OH)$_2$D values are higher whenever: (1) serum Ca and PO$_4$ are normal; (2) PTH is normal; and (3) vitamins D$_2$, D$_3$, or 25(OH)D are provided in large quantities in vivo to patients or in vitro to renal cortex homogenates or isolated tubule preparations [12,20,58,59]. Although this metabolite can also be made in the intestine or bone, serum values of 24,25(OH)$_2$D are low in children with chronic renal failure and in pregnant women [11].

The vitamin D endocrine system regulates serum calcium level by a typical closed feedback loop system [20]. Hypocalcemia with resultant decreased ionized serum calcium causes PTH secretion, which in turn stimulates 1α-hydroxylase activity. The newly synthesized 1,25(OH)$_2$D combines with receptors in the intestine and stimulates the active transport of calcium and phosphate from the lumen of the gut into the bloodstream. With regard to intestinal effects, its potency is not matched by any other vitamin D compound. The precise mechanism of 1,25(OH)$_2$D action on the enterocyte and the final gene product is not yet established, although a role for 1,25(OH)$_2$D-dependent, DNA-directed protein synthesis appears important to active calcium transport. The 1,25(OH)$_2$D can also act in concert with PTH to promote active bone resorption with subsequent release of calcium and phosphate into the circulation from mineralized osteoid. However, the higher iPTH levels also cause an increase in urinary phosphate excretion. On balance, serum calcium concentration increases while that of phosphate remains the same. The now higher level of calcium suppresses PTH secretion, and 1,25(OH)$_2$D synthesis declines.

The synthesis of 1,25(OH)$_2$D is tightly feedback-regulated, and because it is made at one site (the renal cortex) and has its biological actions at other sites (intestine or bone) that are reached via the bloodstream, the active form of vitamin D should be considered a hormone. When PTH secretion is impaired, as in hypoparathyroidism, or when the biological activity of PTH is blunted, as in pseudohypoparathyroidism, serum calcium values are low and serum phosphate values are high. The synthesis of 1,25(OH)$_2$D likewise is attenuated so that calcium transport from the gut is limited and bone resorption is blunted [12,20,58].

The other limb of the vitamin D endocrine system is stimulated by hypophosphatemia. Hypophosphatemia cannot cause PTH secretion, but it probably stimulates 1,25(OH)$_2$D synthesis at the level of the renal tubule, which results in augmented intestinal calcium and phosphate absorption. The kidney, in turn, excretes calcium and retains phosphate because iPTH values are normal or low. As a result, serum phosphate concentrations become normal, slowing down 1,25(OH)$_2$D synthesis. Higher 1,25(OH)$_2$D values occur when hypophosphatemia is not associated with increased PTH secretion, and in thyroparathyroidectomized animals.

Fetoplacental Unit

During the last five months of pregnancy the calcium content of the human fetus increases from 0.1 to 30 g [29]. Calcium translocation rate via the placenta ranges from 24 to 203 mg/kg/24 hours in the rat and sheep, respectively, and averages 150 to 170 mg/kg/24 hours in humans [29,31].

There are at least five reports supporting the assumption that 1,25(OH)$_2$D is an important regulator of placental calcium translocation (Table 7-2). First, activity of the enzyme 25(OH)D-1α-hydroxylase can be detected in the placenta of humans and several other mammalian species [29,30,89,94]. The enzyme activity is greatest in the maternal side of the placenta, where 24,25(OH)$_2$D synthesis is also evident [30,48]. Second, 25(OH)D, a necessary substrate for the 1α-hydroxylase enzyme, is able to pass from the maternal to the fetal circulation [8,29,31]. This transfer is essential to the synthesis of 1,25(OH)$_2$D by both the placenta and the fetal kidney: maternal vitamin D deficiency prevents both fetal and placental production of 1,25(OH)$_2$D or 24,25(OH)$_2$D [33,34]. Binding to DBP also appears to be an important factor in the transfer rates of 25(OH)$_2$D across the human placenta [69]. Third, fetal nephrectomy in the lamb results in reversal of the vectorial or net transfer of calcium from mother to fetus, and, thus, in the absence of fetal 1,25(OH)$_2$D synthesis, calcium transfer is impaired [29]. Fourth, the high calcium concentration in the fetus, as reflected by elevated cord blood calcium values [31] in comparison to those of the mother, indicates active, uphill Ca^{2+} transfer, a process that, at least in the gut, is vitamin D–dependent [20,58]. Fifth, calcium-binding protein (CaBP), a vitamin D–dependent cytosolic protein found in the gut and brain [91], is also present in the placenta of vitamin D–replete animals but not vitamin D–deficient animals [29]. Since this protein is

TABLE 7-2. Feto-maternal vitamin D kinetics

	Metabolites synthesized			
	Vitamin D	25(OH)D	1,25(OH)$_2$D	24,25(OH)$_2$D
Mother	X	X	X	X
Placenta			X	
Fetus		X	X	
	Direction of transfer			
	Vitamin D	25(OH)D	1,25(OH)$_2$D	24,25(OH)$_2$D
Predominant direction Mother→fetus	X	X	X	X
Minor direction Fetus→mother		X	X	

TABLE 7-3. Relative calcium, phosphorus, vitamin D, and calciotropic hormone status in the newborn infant at birth and at 24 hours of age

	Cord blood vs. maternal blood	Infant blood at 24 hr. vs. cord blood
Calcium	↑	↓
Ionized calcium	↑	↓
Phosphate	↑	↑
Parathyroid hormone	↓	↓ →?
Calcitonin	↑	↑
1,25(OH)$_2$-vitamin D*	↓	↑ →?
25-hydroxyvitamin D*	↓	→?
24,25(OH)$_2$-vitamin D*	↓	?
Vitamin D binding protein*	↓	→

* Assumes no vitamin D supplements in first 24 hr. of life.
(From Greer FR, Chesney RW: Disorders of calcium metabolism in the neonate. *Semin Nephrol* 3:100, 1983, with permission.)

a reasonable candidate for a gene product or vitamin D–dependent, DNA-directed protein synthesis [91], it is plausible to speculate that calcium transfer may be related to vitamin D action.

The placenta permits the passage of several lipophilic vitamin D metabolites in either direction, including vitamin D, 25(OH)D, and 1,25(OH)$_2$D, and evidence for maternal to fetal 24,25(OH)$_2$D transfer has been found [8,29,31]. The bi-directional transfer of vitamin D and the fetal and placental production of various vitamin D metabolites (Table 7-3) make it difficult to ascertain where a given molecule of 1,25(OH)$_2$D or 24,25(OH)$_2$D is synthesized in the pregnant woman.

Maternal vs. Cord Blood Levels

In general, the concentrations of vitamin D metabolites are lower in cord than in maternal blood [8,29,31,95] (Table 7-3). This is opposite to total calcium, ionized

calcium, and phosphate values [31]. In human cord blood, 25(OH)D values are lower than maternal values, although they do correlate [27,95]. Other investigators have found similar values of 25(OH)D in maternal and cord blood [31,84]. Because vitamin D–binding protein levels are 50% higher in maternal than in cord serum, the free 25(OH)D values actually may be higher in cord blood [6]. Calculations indicate that the maternal-fetal gradient for free 25(OH)D is in the opposite direction of that for total 25(OH)D. Yet, 25(OH)D synthesis by the human fetal liver may be minimal if, like in the fetal rat and lamb, the P-450 oxidase system needed for 25(OH)D production develops after birth [29,31]. The origin of the high free 25(OH)$_2$D remains unknown.

All studies to date have demonstrated a much higher 1,25(OH)$_2$D concentration in the maternal than the cord blood [6,8,27,29,31,84,95]. However, when examined in light of the differences in DBP, the calculated concentration of free 1,25(OH)$_2$D may be similar or slightly higher in the fetus [5] than in the mother. Even though total

1,25(OH)₂D concentration is higher in maternal than in cord blood, a correlation exists between these two values [6,27].

The value for 24,25(OH)₂D may be higher in the fetuses of certain mammalian species, such as lamb and rat, but in the human the concentration of this metabolite in the mother may be higher or not different from that of the fetus [41]. A good correlation appears to obtain between maternal and fetal values [5,95].

Changes in Vitamin D–Binding Protein

Low serum DBP values are found in the cord blood of premature infants and remain low for the first nine weeks of life [38]. At 12 weeks of age (42 weeks post-conception), the levels of DBP are 490 ± 130 μg/ml, similar to those found in adults. Only after 12 weeks of age is a correlation between serum 25(OH)D and DBP evident. This may indicate that the maturation of the protein synthetic capacity of the liver occurs concomitantly with that in the absorption and/or hepatic 25-hydroxylation of vitamin D. Thus, although DBP is lower in cord and preterm infant blood, it is difficult to infer that the reduced values of 25(OH)D found in the serum of some, but not all, infants can be fully accounted for by the age-related difference in DBP.

Vitamin D Metabolism and Function in Premature Infants

The ability of the premature infant to convert vitamin D to 25(OH)D and further to 1,25(OH)₂D is probably similar to that of the adult [8,31,36,90], although not all investigators have confirmed this observation [37,52].

All studies to date indicate that the conversion of 25(OH)D to 1,25(OH)₂D proceeds in an unimpaired fashion in the preterm infant (Fig. 7-12) [8,28,31,54,85]. Although the values of 1,25(OH)₂D are lower in cord blood than in maternal blood, within 24 hours of birth neonatal 1,25(OH)₂D is found to equal adult values [84]. In premature infants, the plasma concentration of 1,25(OH)₂D appears to rise above the levels encountered in the adult, so that by five to 10 weeks of post-natal age, the mean serum concentration is 100 pg/ml, compared with 30 pg/ml in the adult [28,54,85] (Fig. 7-13). The studies of Glorieux et al. [28] revealed no impairment of 1,25(OH)₂D synthesis, despite the relatively high plasma concentration of phosphate prevailing in the preterm infant. Further studies by Steichen et al. [83] indicated that low dietary phosphate intake, in the form of soy protein formulas and human breast milk, results in even higher circulating values for 1,25(OH)₂D, indicating that hypophosphatemia may serve as a further stimulus for the synthesis of this vitamin D compound.

The metabolism of 25(OH)D to 24,25(OH)₂D also appears to proceed at similar rates in the preterm neonate and in adults; a correlation was found between the serum concentrations of 25(OH)D and 24,25(OH)₂D [54,96].

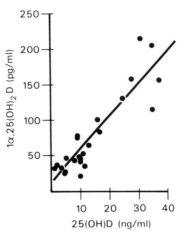

FIG. 7-12. *Relationship between circulating 1,25(OH)₂D and 25(OH)D in preterm infants (r = 0.90, P < 0.0005). (From Glorieux FH, Salle BL, Delvin EE, et al: Vitamin D metabolism in preterm infants: Serum calcitriol values during the first five days of life. J Pediatr 99:640, 1981, with permission.)*

Nonetheless, the value found in neonates (0.3 to 0.6 ng/ml) is significantly lower than that usually present in children (1.7 ± 0.5 ng/ml) [70] or in adults (3.5 ± 10 ng/ml) [54]. It has been speculated that this low level of 24,25(OH)₂D in the presence of a high value of 1,25(OH)₂D is appropriate to the need for increased intestinal calcium (and phosphate) absorption required to effect rapid bone mineral accretion.

Hypocalcemia during the first 72 to 96 hours of life is quite common in neonates [31]. Attempts at either preventing or treating this condition with vitamin D metabolites have met with variable success [4,10,24,40,53, 61,77,78,92].

Rickets develops with some frequency in preterm infants, particularly in those developing bronchopulmonary dysplasia or receiving low-phosphate-containing milk [3,13–16,46,53,72]. The rickets can occur despite seemingly adequate supplementation with 400 to 800 IU (10 to 20 μg) of vitamin D. Although a variety of etiologic factors have been suggested, including increased need for minerals and vitamin D owing to rapid growth postnatally, mineral deficiencies, abnormal vitamin D metabolism, and inappropriate hormonal response, little evidence exists that vitamin D metabolism is impaired [3,13,53]. In several cases of rickets of very-low-birth-weight premature infants, the circulating values of 25(OH)D, 24,25(OH)₂D, and 1,25(OH)₂D were appropriate to the intake of calcium and phosphate and to the serum values for these minerals [13,53,83,85]. Commonly, 25(OH)D and 24,25(OH)₂D levels are normal and those for 1,25(OH)₂D are elevated, as would be anticipated with hypophosphatemia [72]. These data suggest that dietary mineral deficiency, rather than impaired vitamin D metabolism, causes the rickets [3,13,53,72].

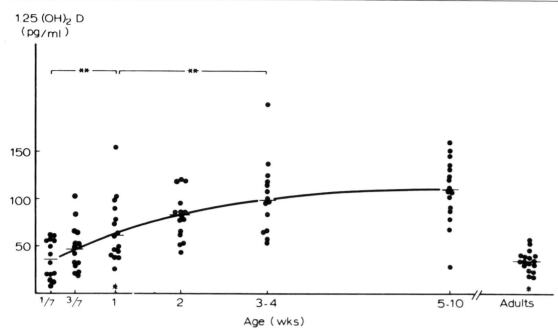

Fig. 7-13. *Plasma concentration of 1,25(OH)₂D with increasing age in preterm infants and adults. (From Markestad T, Aksnes L, Finne PH, et al: Plasma concentrations of vitamin D metabolites in premature infants. Pediatr Res 18:269, 1984, with permission.)*

Vitamin D Metabolism and Function in Term Infants

Hypocalcemia, rickets, and abnormalities of the vitamin D–PTH endocrine axis are quite rare among term neonates. In contrast to preterm infants, the placenta has transferred from the mother the 30 g or so of calcium necessary to the development of the fetus by the moment of delivery. Although there is a decline in both serum and ionized calcium during the first 24 hours of life [73], the level of calcium usually exceeds 8.0 mg/dl. The metabolism of vitamin D in term infants appears to proceed in a normal fashion [39,55], and the ultimate stabilization of serum calcium concentration is largely determined by the intake of calcium and phosphate, the secretion of PTH and calcitonin, the presence or absence of hypomagnesemia, and the presence of a medical condition (e.g., infant of a diabetic mother) that can impair calcium homeostasis [31,39,74].

A hypocalcemic stimulus, such as an exchange transfusion, was found to stimulate the production of 1,25(OH)₂D synthesis in that the concentration of this metabolite in the plasma of term infants rebounded rapidly after transfusion with blood products whose 1,25(OH)₂D concentration was lower than that found in the neonates [55]. This study indicates that a decline in ionized calcium leads to rapid production of 1,25(OH)₂D, since the response was evident in the final aliquot of blood taken during exchange. In contrast, the values of 25(OH)D and 24,25(OH)₂D remained precisely the same as those in the donor blood.

Mechanism of Intestinal Phosphate Absorption

It has long been known that intestinal phosphate absorption is regulated by vitamin D [12,20,58]. However, the role of vitamin D at a cellular and membrane level is not established and is poorly studied [70]. Since the regulation of phosphate reabsorption largely occurs within the kidney [20,47], the gut does not appear to be a major regulatory site of whole body phosphate homeostasis. Recent balance studies in preterm infants do not indicate any great change in intestinal phosphate absorption brought about by different levels of vitamin D intake [77,78] or by differences in fat content of the formula, which can influence vitamin D absorption [44]. Indeed, the efficiency of phosphate absorption remained in the range of 80% to 94% of intake.

Parathyroid Hormone
Maternal vs. Fetal

PTH secretion is governed by the prevailing concentration of ionized calcium reaching the parathyroid gland [70]. Factors that can acutely alter ionized calcium concentrations, such as alkalosis or the infusion of EDTA, enhance glandular secretion rates, and intravenous calcium infusion reduces these rates [80]. The status of PTH secretion and action during pregnancy is as confusing as that found for vitamin D. In thyroparathyroidectomized pregnant sheep, acutely induced maternal hypocalcemia fails to alter serum calcium values in the fetus, implying that placental calcium transport is independent of PTH [9]. In animals, PTH cannot cross the placenta because there is no placental mechanisms for transfer of this 84 amino-acid peptide hormone [60,80]. Moreover, in thyroparathyroidectomized pregnant ewes with chronic hypocalcemia, fetal plasma calcium levels are maintained [71].

Despite the finding of a normal serum calcium in fetal sheep whose mothers have no circulating PTH, human pregnancy is a period of extensive changes in PTH secretion. Menstrual cyclicity of calcium-regulating hormones has been reported [29,65,70], and the most logical hypothesis is that estrogen inhibits PTH-induced bone resorption, thereby lowering serum ionized calcium and causing a rise in iPTH values [65]. Indeed, PTH levels rise progressively through the follicular phase of the cycle and fall through the luteal phase. Then, with the reduction of estrogen levels, calcium levels rise and iPTH values fall [65]. Appropriate changes in serum $1,25(OH)_2D$ values have been reported [70]. In pregnancy, both total and ionic calcium values fall progressively with each trimester [63]. In response, iPTH values rise progressively during pregnancy so that at term they are 50% above early pregnancy levels and 33% above puerperal levels [56]. Pitkin [64] has introduced the concept that pregnancy is associated with maternal hyperparathyroidism. Since the GFR increases during pregnancy, these changes cannot be blamed on an inability of the maternal kidney to degrade the PTH molecule [80].

PTH has been detected in the human fetal blood as early as the 12th or 13th week of gestation [75]. Data on PTH measurements in cord blood measured at term are confusing in that both low [74,76] and normal [62,84] concentrations have been found. The response of the parathyroid gland and the human fetus to mild hypercalcemia has been examined indirectly by making simultaneous measurements in samples of amniotic fluid and maternal serum [18]. Amniotic fluid calcium falls from 7.6 ± 0.7 mg/dl at weeks 14 to 15 of gestation to 6.4 ± 0.5 mg/dl at term, with a comparable fall in the ionized calcium component. In contrast to the rise in PTH values in maternal serum, the fetal amniotic fluid PTH level falls, and no correlation was found between amniotic fluid PTH and amniotic fluid total and ionized calcium values, amniotic fluid phosphate level, or maternal serum PTH. The authors attributed the fall in amniotic fluid PTH level to the relative hypercalcemia of the fetus during the latter stages of the third trimester.

Perhaps the best indication of the independence of fetal from maternal PTH is the finding that amniotic PTH values were found to be reduced below maternal values in a woman with primary hyperparathyroidism [21]. After removal of the adenoma, maternal PTH levels fell, and fetal amniotic fluid values rose in response to hypocalcemia. Finally, the known association of transient neonatal hypocalcemia with maternal hyperparathyroidism indicates that the fetal gland is responding to higher fetal serum calcium concentrations brought about by transfer of calcium from the hypercalcemic mother to her fetus [11,31].

The response of the fetal sheep to PTH is dose-dependent [1,45,81], in as much as low doses of PTH fail to raise fetal serum calcium. The phosphaturic effect of PTH

can also be demonstrated in the chronically catheterized fetal sheep; in addition, urinary cyclic AMP excretion is increased. However, the magnitude of the phosphaturia and that of cyclic AMP excretion is less than that in adult sheep or human at comparable doses of PTH [1].

Mechanism of Action of Parathyroid Hormone

Although whole body calcium homeostasis is regulated through the action of $1,25(OH)_2D$, which facilitates active calcium absorption from the gut, total body phosphate homeostasis is regulated by the kidney [11,20,70]. Renal reabsorption of phosphate is markedly inhibited by PTH [22,47].

Our understanding of the mechanism by which PTH blocks phosphate reabsorption and causes urinary phosphate excretion has been greatly facilitated by understanding the molecular structure of PTH, by use of highly purified fragments of PTH, by use of isolated renal plasma membranes, by knowledge of the complex adenylate cyclase system derived from studies in other tissues, and, finally, from cleverly designed clinical studies of patients with pseudohypoparathyroidism and hyperparathyroidism [2,7,22,23,49,66]. An extensive description of the sequence of events leading to an elucidation of the mechanism of PTH action is beyond the scope of this chapter and, thus, only a summary emphasizing major points is given.

PTH is a 1-84 amino acid product of the parathyroid glands derived from a 115-amino acid precursor called prepro-parathyroid hormone [22]. Prepro-PTH is cleaved within the gland to a 1-84 peptide and to amino (N) and carboxyterminal (C) fragments. In the circulation, 1-84 PTH is then cleaved in the liver and kidney into further N and C fragments, accounting for the heterogeneity of PTH species detected by early radioimmune assays [2]. The C-terminal fragments have a half-life of 20 to 40 minutes, whereas the N-terminal fragments have a half-life of less than 10 minutes. Because the C-terminal fragments are cleared by the kidney, renal insufficiency results in a substantial increase in their half-life. The component of PTH with renal action is the 1-34 amino acid N-terminal fragment [2,22,66]. This 1-34 fragment binds to specific receptors found in the plasma membrane of renal cells (Fig. 7-14), presumably in the basolateral membrane [2,22]. A complex sequence of events ensues, resulting in the activation of adenylate cyclase [2,22,23,49,66]. The PTH receptor combines with a regulatory protein called the guanine nucleotide regulatory protein (the G or the N protein) [32]. This G-protein consists of at least three polypeptide units and has both stimulatory and inhibitory properties on adenylate cyclase activation [32,87]. The 1-34 PTH becomes a stimulator of the G protein after combining with its receptor and with the stimulatory component of G protein. The 3-34 PTH is an agonist, at least in vitro, and combines with the inhibitory component of G protein. Because the G protein can combine with the adenylate cyclase complex, binding the guanosine triphosphate (GTP) to G protein must occur; this dissociates the PTH and permits adenylate cyclase to become active. Adenylate

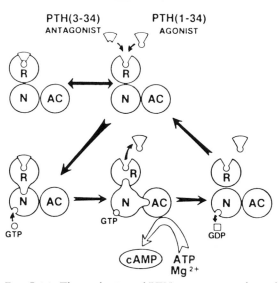

FIG. 7-14. *The mechanism of PTH action on membrane-bound adenylate cyclase. The biologically active PTH agonist (1-34) and the biologically inactive PTH antagonist (3-34) are capable of binding to the PTH receptor (R). However, only PTH (3-34) is capable of converting the receptor to a high-affinity state, so that guanyl nucleotide regulatory protein (N) can be stimulated to bind guanosine triphosphate (GTP). The binding of GTP to N converts R to a low-affinity state, inducing dissociation of PTH (1-34) and the formation of an N-adenylate cyclase complex (AC), leading to the activation of this enzyme and the increased production of intracellular cAMP. In contrast, the binding of PTH (3-34) to R does not induce an affinity change in R, so that it is not possible for R to interact with N and, as in the case of the binding of PTH (1-34), to induce activation of adenylate cyclase. (From Arnaud CD, Kolb FO: The calciotropic hormones and metabolic bone disease. In Greenspan FS, Forsham PH: Basic and Clinical Endocrinology. Los Altos, CA, Lange, 1984, p 187, with permission.)*

cyclase converts Mg^{2+}-ATP to cAMP [32,87]. Certain bacterial toxins can block G protein from combining with adenylate cyclase by inducing ADP-ribosylation of the G protein. Cholera toxin inactivates the stimulatory unit, and pertussis toxin activates the inhibitory segment [87]. In summary, the hormone binds to the receptor, inducing changes in G protein that activate adenylate cyclase. This is why, after a patient is injected with PTH, the urinary content of cAMP [2,7,22] and the intracellular cAMP concentration rise.

High renal cell levels of cAMP induce phosphorylation and dephosphorylation of intracellular and membrane proteins, which appear to block the uptake of phosphate by the luminal membrane [35]. The mechanism by which protein phosphorylation blocks Na^+-dependent phosphate transport is uncertain. Distal nephron phosphate reabsorption does not appear to be regulated by this process; cAMP does not alter distal phosphate and calcium handling [22]. Enhancement of distal calcium reabsorption relates to the influence of PTH in its role as a calcium ionophore [43]. The process involves enhanced calcium binding to renal membranes, greater calcium translocation, and the poten-

tial for mitochondrial sequestration of calcium [43]. Voltage-independent transport of calcium also is enhanced by PTH in the thick ascending limb of Henle [79,88]. Active calcium transport by BBM vesicles has been reported, but these reports have not accounted for the extensive calcium binding that occurs in association with PTH administration [43]. PTH administration also may be associated with changes in membrane phospholipid content, particularly relating to phosphoinositol turnover, which enhances calcium binding [68]. No current data indicate that PTH affects the Ca^{2+}-activated ATPase, and virtually all studies indicate that cAMP does not enhance Ca^{2+} reabsorption or cellular uptake [43,79].

Influence of Parathyroid Hormone on the Immature Nephron

As noted previously, infusion of PTH into the sheep fetus during the third trimester has been shown to increase serum calcium levels [45], but smaller doses of PTH did not alter serum calcium [122,123]. This calcium-raising property of PTH in the fetus could be the result of hormone-induced bone resorption and release of calcium into the extracellular fluid. A dose-dependent response of calcium release to PTH was observed by Raisz [67] and Stern et al. [86] in the fetal rat limb bone assay system. This PTH-induced bone resorption resulted in higher calcium values in the bathing media, even in vitamin D–deficient animals [86].

Kooh et al. [45] have also demonstrated that PTH infusion in fetal sheep reduces the tubular reabsorption of phosphate and increases, albeit little, the urinary excretion of cAMP. This demonstrates responsivity of the fetal kidney to relatively high-dose PTH.

The few studies done in newborn animals suggest a blunted response of the renal tubule of PTH, particularly in relation to the high serum concentration of phosphate. The response of neonatal guinea pig kidney to PTH has been discussed previously in this chapter. The phosphaturic response to a high dose (30 U/kg) of PTH infused into immature thyroparathyroidectomized rats was significantly lower at three to six weeks than at 20 weeks of age [93]. The fractional excretion of phosphate after a similar dose of PTH was 8.0% at age three weeks and 21.3% at 20 weeks. Despite these changes in phosphate excretion, the urinary excretion of cAMP was not different, suggesting that the blunting of the PTH effect observed at early age is at a step beyond cAMP generation. Further, a right-shifted dose response curve to PTH was found in young rats. This relative tubular insensitivity of the tubule to PTH may help the young animal to maintain the positive phosphate balance required for growth [82].

Studies on the human newborn indicate a similar state of affairs. Urinary cAMP excretion is low on the first day of life and rises over the first three days [50]. Term newborns demonstrate a reduced phosphaturic response to PTE on day one as compared with day three [17]. Fewer studies are available in preterm infants. One study detected a positive correlation between body weight and PTH-stimulated cAMP excretion in three-day-old preterm infants, which implies a correlation between renal PTH response and gestational age [51].

No direct measurements are available regarding the effect of PTH on $1,25(OH)_2D$ production in the newborn. If we can infer that the enhanced 1α-hydroxylase activity observed in neonatal hypocalcemia is at least indirectly related to PTH secretion, the immature renal tubule appears to respond to PTH.

References
Calcium

1. Adams PH, Jowsey J, Kelly PJ, et al: Effects of hyperthyroidism on bone and mineral metabolism in man. *Q J Med* 36:1, 1967.
2. Agus ZS, Chiu PJ, Goldberg M: Regulation of urinary calcium excretion in the rat. *Am J Physiol* 232(Renal Fluid Electrolyte Physiol 1):F545, 1977.
3. Agus ZS, Gardner LB, Beck LH, et al: Effects of parathyroid hormone on renal tubular reabsorption of calcium, sodium and phosphate. *Am J Physiol* 224:1143, 1973.
4. Alexander DP, Nixon DA: Effect of parathyroid extract in foetal sheep. *Biol Neonate* 14:117, 1969.
5. Almeida ALJ, Kudo LH, Rochia AS: Calcium transport in isolated perfused pars recta of proximal tubule. Abstracts and Proceedings of the VII International Congress of Nephrology, Montreal. Munich, S Karger, 1978, p E16.
6. Antoniou LD, Eisner GM, Slotkoff LM, et al: Relationship between sodium and calcium transport in the kidney. *J Lab Clin Med* 74:410, 1969.
7. Arant BS Jr: Renal handling of calcium and phosphorus in normal human neonates. *Semin Nephrol* 3:94, 1983.
8. Arnaud SB, Goldsmith RS, Stickler GB, et al: Serum parathyroid hormone and blood minerals: Interrelationships in normal children. *Pediatr Res* 7:485, 1973.
9. Aub JC, Bauer W, Heath C, et al: Studies of calcium and phosphorus metabolism. III. The effects of the thyroid hormone and thyroid disease. *J Clin Invest* 7:97, 1929.
10. Bauer W, Aub JC: Studies of calcium and phosphorus metabolism. XVI. The influence of the pituitary gland. *J Clin Invest* 20:295, 1941.
11. Biddulph DM, Hirsch PF, Cooper CW, et al: Effect of thyroparathyroidectomy and parathyroid hormone on urinary excretion of calcium and phosphate in the golden hamster. *Endocrinology* 87:1346, 1970.
12. Bijvoet OLM, van der Stuys Veer J, de Vries HR, et al: Natriuretic effect of calcitonin in man. *N Engl J Med* 284:681, 1971.
13. Bogert LJ, Kirkpatrick EE: Studies in inorganic metabolism. II. The effects of acid-forming and base-forming diets upon calcium metabolism. *J Biol Chem* 54:375, 1922.
14. Bourdeau JE, Burg M: Voltage dependence of calcium transport in the thick ascending limb of Henle's loop. *Am J Physiol* 236(Renal Fluid Electrolyte Physiol 5):F357, 1979.
15. Brickman AS, Coburn JW, Norman AW, et al: Short-term effects of 1,25-dihydroxycholecalciferol on disordered calcium metabolism of renal failure. *Am J Med* 57:28, 1974.
16. Brickman AS, Massry SG, Coburn JW: Changes in serum and urinary calcium during treatment with hydrochlorothiazide: Studies on mechanisms. *J Clin Invest* 51:945, 1972.
17. Bronner F: Calcium homeostasis. *In* Bronner F, Coburn JW (eds): *Disorders of Mineral Metabolism. Calcium Physiology,* Vol II. New York, Academic, 1982, p 43.
18. Cannigia A, Gennari C: Azione della tirocalcitonina nell'uomo. *Minerva Med* 59:279, 1968.
19. Chabardes D, Imbert M, Clique A, et al: PTH-sensitive adenyl cyclase activity in different segments of the rabbit nephron. *Pflugers Arch* 354:229, 1975.
20. Chase HS, Al-Awqati W: Regulation of the sodium permeability of the luminal border of toad bladder by intracellular sodium and calcium. *J Gen Physiol* 79:693, 1981.
21. Chen PS Jr, Neuman WF: Renal excretion of calcium by the dog. *Am J Physiol* 180:623, 1955.
22. Cheung WY: Calmodulin plays a pivotal role in cellular regulation. *Science* 207:19, 1980.
23. Coburn JW, Hartenbower DL, Massry SG: Modification of calciuretic effect of extracellular volume expansion by phosphate infusion. *Am J Physiol* 220:337, 1971.
24. Coburn JW, Massry SG: Changes in serum and urinary calcium during phosphate depletion: Studies in mechanisms. *J Clin Invest* 49:1073, 1970.
25. Collins JH: Structure and evolution of troponin C and related proteins. *In* Ducan CJ (ed): *Calcium in Biological Systems.* Cambridge, MA, Cambridge University Press, 1976, p 303.
26. Cook PB, Nassim JR, Collins J: The effects of thyrotoxicosis upon the metabolism of calcium, phosphorus and nitrogen. *Q J Med* 28:505, 1959.
27. Costanzo LS, Conrad MP, Beahm LS: Effect of amiloride on calcium transport by the distal convoluted tubule: In vivo microperfusion study. *Abst Am Soc Nephrol* 15:4A, 1982.
28. Costanzo LS, Sheehe PR, Weiner IM: Renal actions of vitamin D in D-deficient rats. *Am J. Physiol* 226:1490, 1974.
29. Costanzo LS, Weiner IM: On the hypocalciuric action of chlorothiazide. *J Clin Invest* 54:628, 1974.
30. Costanzo LS, Weiner IM: Relationship between clearances of Ca and Na: Effect of distal diuretics and PTH. *Am J Physiol* 230:67, 1976.
31. Costanzo LS, Windhager EE: Calcium and sodium transport by the distal convoluted tubule of the rat. *Am J Physiol* 235(Renal Fluid Electrolyte Physiol 4):F492, 1978.
32. Costanzo LS, Windhager EE: Effect of parathyroid hormone and cyclic AMP on calcium and sodium transport in the distal tubule (abstr). *Kidney Int* 14:638, 1978.
33. Craven PA, DeRubertis FR: Effects of vasopressin and urea on Ca^+-calmodulin-dependent regulation of renal prostaglandin E. *Am J Physiol* 241(Renal Fluid Electrolyte Physiol 10):F649, 1981.
34. Crutch B, Taylor A: Measurement of cytosolic free Ca^{2+} concentration in epithelial cells of toad urinary bladder. *J Physiol* (Lond) 345:109, 1983.
35. David L, Anast CS: Calcium metabolism in newborn infants. *J Clin Invest* 54:287, 1974.
36. Demartini FE, Briscoe AM, Ragan C: Effect of ethacrynic acid on calcium and magnesium excretion. *Proc Soc Exp Biol Med* 124:320, 1967.
37. DiBona GF: Effect of hypermagnesemia on renal tubular sodium handling in the rat. *Am J Physiol* 221:53, 1971.
38. Doucet A, Katz AI: High-affinity Ca-Mg-ATPase along the rabbit nephron. *Am J Physiol* 242(Renal Fluid Electrolyte Physiol 11):F346, 1982.
39. Duarte CG: Effects of ethacrynic acid and furosemide on urinary calcium, phosphate and magnesium. *Metabolism* 17:867, 1968.
40. Duarte CG: Effects of chlorothiazide and amipramizide (MK 870) on the renal excretion of calcium, magnesium and phosphate. *Metabolism* 17:420, 1968.

41. Duarte CG, Watson JF: Calcium reabsorption in proximal tubule of the dog nephron. *Am J Physiol* 212:1355, 1967.

42. Edwards BR, Baer PG, Sutton RAL, et al: Effects of parathyroid hormone (PTH) on renal tubular calcium reabsorption in the dog. *Clin Res* 20:956, 1972.

43. Edwards BR, Baer PG, Sutton RAL, et al: Micropuncture study of diuretic effects on sodium and calcium reabsorption in the dog nephron. *J Clin Invest* 52:2418, 1973.

44. Edwards BR, Sutton, RAL, Dirks JH: Effect of calcium infusion on renal tubular reabsorption in the dog. *Am J Physiol* 227:13, 1974.

45. Edwards NA, Hodgkinson A: Metabolic studies in patients with idiopathic hypercalciuria. *Clin Sci* 29:143, 1965.

46. Farquharson RF, Salter WT, Tibbeitts DM, et al: Studies of calcium and phosphorus metabolism. XII. The effect of the ingestion of acid-producing substances. *J Clin Invest* 10:221, 1931.

47. Fraser R, Harrison MT: Effect of growth hormone on urinary calcium excretion. *Ciba Found Colloq Endocrinol* 13:135, 1960.

48. Friedman AP: Renal calcium transport: Sites and insights. *News Physiol Sci* 3:17, 1988.

49. Gerhardt D, Schlesinger W: Uber die Kalk und Magnesiaausscheidung beim diabetes mellitus und ihre Beziehung zur Ausscheidung abnormer Sauren (Acidose). *Naunyn Schmeidebergs Archiv für Pharmakologie* 43:83, 1899.

50. Ghazali S, Barratt TM: Urinary excretion of calcium and magnesium in children. *Arch Dis Child* 49:97, 1974.

51. Gmaj P, Murer H, Kinne R: Calcium ion transport across plasma membranes isolated from the rat kidney cortex. *Biochem J* 178:549, 1979.

52. Goldfarb S, Westby GR, Goldberg M, et al: Renal tubular effects of chronic phosphate depletion. *J Clin Invest* 59:770, 1977.

53. Grabie M, Lau K, Agus ZS, et al: Role of parathyroid hormone in the hypercalciuria of chronic phosphate depletion. *Miner Electrolyte Metab* 1:279, 1978.

54. Greenberg BG, Winters RW, Graham JB: The normal range of serum inorganic phosphorus and its utility as a discriminant in the diagnosis of congenital hypophosphatemia. *J Clin Endocrinol Metab* 20:364, 1960.

55. Grosso A, Cox JA, Malnoe A, et al: Evidence for a role of calmodulin in the hydrosmotic action of vasopressin in toad bladder. *J Physiol* (Paris) 78:270, 1982.

56. Haas HG, Dambacher MA, Guncaga J, et al: Renal effects of calcitonin and parathyroid extract in man: Studies in hypoparathyroidism. *J Clin Invest* 50:2689, 1971.

57. Hallman N, Salmi I: On plasma calcium in cord blood and in the newborn. *Acta Paediatr* 42:126, 1953.

58. Hanna S, Harrison MT, MacIntyre I, et al: Effects of growth hormone in calcium and magnesium metabolism. *Br Med J* 2:12, 1961.

59. Harris CA, Baer PG, Chirito E, et al: Composition of mammalian glomerular filtrate. *Am J Physiol* 227:972, 1974.

60. Henneman PH, Forbes AP, Moldawer M, et al: Effects of human growth hormone in man. *J Clin Invest* 39:1223, 1960.

61. Hohenauer L, Rosenberg TF, Oh W: Calcium and phosphorus homeostasis on the first day of life. *Biol Neonate* 15:49, 1970.

62. Howe CL, Mooseker MS, Graves TA: Brush-border calmodulin. A major component of the isolated microvillus core. *J Cell Biol* 85:916, 1980.

63. Howland J, Kramer B: Calcium and phosphorus in the serum in relation to rickets. *Am J Dis Child* 22:105, 1921.

64. Hruska K, Khalifa S, Hammerman M: Parathyroid hormone administration mimics the effects of phosphorylation of brush border membrane vesicles on phospholipid composition and calcium translocation. *Clin Res* 30:451A, 1982.

65. Hruska KA, Mills S, Hammerman M: Calcium translocation in brush border membrane vesicles is stimulated by membrane phosphorylation (abstr). *Kidney Int* 21:134, 1982.

66. Humes HD, Ichikawa I, Troy JL, et al: Evidence for a parathyroid hormone-dependent influence of calcium on the glomerular ultrafiltration coefficient. *J Clin Invest* 61:32, 1978.

67. Ikkos D, Lufft R, Geinzell CA: The effect of human growth hormone in man. *Acta Endocrinol* (Copenh) 32:341, 1959.

68. Johnson V, Spitzer A: Renal reabsorption of phosphate during development: Whole kidney events. *Am J Physiol* 251(Renal Fluid Electrolyte Physiol 20):F251, 1986.

69. Karam J, Harrison MT, Hartog M, et al: Renal citrate and urinary calcium excretion: The effects of growth hormone contrasted with those of sodium fluoroacetate. *Clin Sci* 21:265, 1961.

70. Klee CB, Crouch TH, Richman PG: Calmodulin. *Annu Rev Biochem* 49:489, 1980.

71. Kleeman CR, Bernstein D, Rockney R, et al: Studies on the renal clearance of diffusible calcium and the role of the parathyroid glands in its regulation. *Yale J Biol Med* 34:1, 1961.

72. Krane SM, Brownell GL, Stanbury JB, et al: The effect of thyroid disease on calcium metabolism in man. *J Clin Invest* 35:874, 1956.

73. Kretsinger RH: Structure and evolution of calcium-modulated proteins. *CRC Crit Rev Biochem* 8:119, 1980.

74. Law K, Goldfarb S, Goldber M, et al: Effects of phosphate administration on tubular calcium transport. *J Lab Clin Med* 99:317, 1982.

75. LeGrimellec C, Poujeol P, de Rouffignac C: ³H inulin and electrolyte concentrations in Bowman's capsule in rat kidney. *Pflugers Arch* 354:117, 1975.

76. Lee CO, Taylor A, Winghager EE: Cytosolic calcium ion activity in epithelial cells of Necturus kidney. *Nature* (Lond) 287:859, 1980.

77. Lemann J Jr, Litzow JR, Lennon EJ: Studies of the mechanism by which chronic metabolic acidosis augments urinary calcium excretion in man. *J Clin Invest* 46:1318, 1967.

78. Levine SD, Kachadorian WA, Levin DN, et al: Effects of trifluoperazine on function and structure of toad urinary bladder. *J Clin Invest* 67:662, 1981.

79. Linarelli LG, Bobik G, Bobik C: The effect of parathyroid hormone on rabbit renal cortex adenyl cyclase during development. *Pediat Res* 7:878, 1973.

80. Litvak J, Moldawer MP, Forbes AP, et al: Hypocalcemic hypercalciuria during vitamin D and dihydrotachysterol therapy of hypoparathyroidism. *J Clin Endocrinol Metab* 18:246, 1958.

81. Lorenzen M, Lee CO, Windhager EE: Effect of quinidine and ouabain on intracellular calcium (iCa) and sodium (iNa) ion activities in isolated perfused proximal tubules of Necturus kidney. *Kidney Int* 21:281, 1982.

82. Lotz M, Zisman E, Bartter FC: Evidence for a phosphorus-depletion syndrome in man. *N Engl J Med* 278:409, 1968.

83. MacFadyen IJ, Nordin BEC, Smith DA, et al: Effect of variation in dietary calcium on plasma concentration and urinary excretion of calcium. *Br Med J* 1:161, 1965.

84. Marshall DH: Calcium and phosphate kinetics. *In* Nordin BEC (ed): *Calcium, Phosphate, and Magnesium Metabolism: Clinical Physiology and Diagnostic Procedures.* New York, Churchill-Livingstone, 1976, p 257.

velopment: Whole kidney events. *Am J Physiol* 251(Renal Fluid Electrolyte Physiol 20):F251, 1986.

117. Karlinsky ML, Sanger DS, Kurtzman NA, et al: Effect of parathormone and cyclic adenosine monophosphate on renal bicarbonate reabsorption. *Am J Physiol* 227:1226, 1974.

118. Kaskel FJ, Kumar AM, Feld LG, et al: Renal reabsorption of phosphate during development: Tubular events. *Pediatr Nephrol* 2:129, 1988.

119. Kempson SA: Effect of metabolic acidosis on renal brush border membrane adaptation to low phosphorus diet. *Kidney Int* 22:225, 1982.

120. Kempson SA: NAD-glychoydrolase in renal brush border membranes. *Am J Physiol* 249(Renal Fluid Electrolyte Physiol 18):F366, 1985.

121. Kempson SA, Colon-Otero G, Lise Ou SY, et al: Possible role of nicotinamide-adenine dinucleotide as an intracellular regulator of renal transport of phosphate in the rat. *J Clin Invest* 67:1347, 1981.

122. Kempson SA, Curthoys NP: NAD$^+$-dependent ADP-ribosyltransferase in renal brush-border membranes. *Am J Physiol* 245(Cell Physiol 14):C449, 1983.

123. Kempson SA, Turner ST, Yusufi ANK, et al: Actions of NAD$^+$ on renal brush border transport of phosphate in vivo and in vitro. *Am J Physiol* 249(Renal Fluid Electrolyte Physiol 18):F948, 1985.

124. Kinne R, Schlatz LJ, Kinne-Saffran E, et al: Distribution of membrane-bound cyclic AMP-dependent protein kinase in plasma membranes of cells of the kidney cortex. *J Membr Biol* 24:145, 1975.

125. Kinne R, Schwartz IL: Asymmetric distribution of renal epithelial cell membrane function in the action of antidiuretic hormone and parathyroid hormone. *In* Andreoli TE, Grantham JJ, Rector FC (eds): *Disturbances in Body Fluid Osmolality*. Bethesda, American Physiological Society, 1977, p 37.

126. Klahr S, Hammerman MR, Martin K, et al: Renal effects of parathyroid hormone and calcitonin. *In* Dunn MJ (ed): *Renal Endocrinology*. Baltimore, Williams & Wilkins, 1983, p 269.

127. Klahr S, Peck WA: Cyclic nucleotides in bone and mineral metabolism. II. Cyclic nucleotides and the renal regulation of mineral metabolism. *Adv Cyclic Nucleotide Protein Phosphorylation Res* 13:133, 1980.

128. Knox FG, Preiss J, Kim JK, et al: Mechanisms of resistance to the phosphaturic effect of the parathyroid hormone in the hamster. *J Clin Invest* 59:657, 1977.

129. Knox FG, Schneider EG, Willis LR, et al: Proximal tubule reabsorption after hyperoncotic albumin infusion. *J Clin Invest* 53:501, 1974.

130. Koobs DH: Phosphate mediation of the Crabtree and Pasteur effects. *Science* 178:127, 1972.

131. Kun E, Chang ACY, Sharma ML, et al: Covalent modification of proteins by metabolites of NAD$^+$. *Proc Natl Acad Sci USA* 73:3131, 1976.

132. Kuntziger H, Amiel C: Recent progress in renal handling of phosphate. *Adv Exp Med Biol* 103:3, 1978.

133. Kuntziger H, Amiel C, Gaudebout C: Phosphate handling by the rat nephron during saline diuresis. *Kidney Int* 2:318, 1972.

134. Kurokawa K: Mechanism of renal action of parathyroid hormone. *Adv Exp Med Biol* 81:291, 1977.

135. Kurokawa K, Ohno T, Rasmussen H: Ionic control of renal gluconeogenesis. II. The effects of Ca^{2+} and H$^+$ upon the response to parathyroid hormone and cyclic AMP. *Biochim Biophys Acta* 313:32, 1973.

136. Kurokawa K, Rasmussen H: Ionic control of renal gluco-

neogenesis. I. The interrelated effects of calcium and hydrogen ions. *Biochim Biophys Acta* 313:17, 1973.

137. Kurokawa K, Rasmussen H: Ionic control of renal gluconeogenesis. III. The effects of changes in pH, pCO$_2$, and bicarbonate concentration. *Biochim Biophys Acta* 313:42, 1973.

138. Landberg H, Hartmann A, Kill F: Glomerular filtration rate and plasma pH as determinants of phosphate reabsorption. *Kidney Int* 26:128, 1984.

139. Lang F, Greger R, Knox FG, et al: Factors modulating renal handling of phosphate. *Renal Physiol* 4:1, 1981.

140. Lang F, Greger R, Marchand GR, et al: Stationary microperfusion study of phosphate reabsorption in proximal and distal nephron segments. *Pflugers Arch* 368:45, 1977.

141. Lang F, Greger R, Marchand GR, et al: Saturation kinetics of phosphate reabsorption in rats. *Adv Exp Med Biol* 81:153, 1977.

142. Lang RP, Yanagawa N, Nord EP, et al: Nucleotide inhibition of phosphate transport in the renal proximal tubule. *Am J Physiol* 245(Renal Fluid Electrolyte Physiol 14):F263, 1983.

143. Lavender AR, Pullman TN: Changes in inorganic phosphate excretion induced by renal arterial infusion of calcium. *Am J Physiol* 205:1025, 1963.

144. Lemann J, Maierhofer WJ, Adams ND, et al: Increased serum 1,25-(OH)$_2$-vitamin D concentrations fail to affect serum or urine phosphate in humans. *Adv Exp Med Biol* 151:375, 1982.

145. Levine BS, Ho K, Hodsman A, et al: Early renal brush border membrane adaptation to dietary phosphorus. *Miner Electrolyte Metab* 10:222, 1984.

146. Levine BS, Ho K, Kraut JA, et al: Effect of metabolic acidosis on phosphate transport by the renal brush border membrane. *Biochim Biophys Acta* 727:7, 1983.

147. Linarelli LG, Bobik J, Bobik C: Newborn urinary cyclic AMP and developmental renal responsiveness to parathyroid hormone. *Pediatrics* 50:14, 1972.

148. Maesaka JK, Levitt MF, Abramson RG: Effects of saline infusion on phosphate transport in intact and thyroparathyroidectomized rats. *Am J Physiol* 225:1421, 1973.

149. Malvin RL, Lotspeick WD: Relationship between tubular transport of inorganic phosphate and bicarbonate in the dog. *Am J Physiol* 187:51, 1956.

150. Malvin RL, Wilde WS, Sullivan LP: Localization of nephron transport by stop-flow analysis. *Am J Physiol* 194:135, 1958.

151. McCrory WW, Forman CW, McNamara H, et al: Renal excretion of inorganic phosphate in newborn infants. *J Clin Invest* 4:357, 1952.

152. McKeown JW, Brazy PG, Dennis VW: Axial heterogeneity of phosphate transport along proximal convoluted tubules: Influence of phosphate restriction. *American Society of Nephrology* 11th Ann. Meeting, New Orleans, 1972.

153. McKeown JV, Brazy PC, Dennis VW: Intrarenal heterogeneity for fluid, phosphate and glucose absorption in the rabbit. *Am J Physiol* 237(Renal Fluid Electrolyte Physiol 6):F312, 1979.

154. McKinney TD, Myers P: PTH inhibition of bicarbonate transport by proximal convoluted tubules. *Am J Physiol* 239(Renal Fluid Electrolyte Physiol 8):F127, 1980.

155. Muhlbauer RC, Bonjour JP, Fleisch H: Tubular handling of phosphate along the nephron of thyroparathyroidectomized rats injected with ethane-1-hydroxy-1, 1-diphosphonate. *Clin Sci* 60:171, 1981.

156. Mulroney SE, Haramati A: Renal adaptation to changes in dietary phosphate intake during development. *Fed Proc* 46:1288, 1987.

157. Mulroney SE, Lumpkin MD, Haramati A: Antagonist to GH-releasing factor inhibits growth and renal Pi reabsorption in immature rats. *Am J Physiol* 257(Renal Fluid Electrolyte Physiol 26):F29, 1989.

158. Murer H, Biber J, Gmaj P, et al: Cellular mechanisms in epithelial transport: Advantages and disadvantages of studies with vesicles. *Mol Physiol* 6:55, 1984.

159. Murer H, Stern H, Burckhardt G, et al: Sodium-dependent transport of inorganic phosphate across the renal brush border membrane. *Adv Exp Med Biol* 128:11, 1980.

160. Nagata N, Rasmussen H: Parathyroid hormone. 3′,5′-AMP, Ca^{++} and gluconeogenesis. *Proc Natl Acad Sci* USA 64:368, 1970.

161. Neiberger RE, Barac-Nieto M, Spitzer A: Renal reabsorption of phosphate during development: Transport kinetics in BBMV. *Am J Physiol* 257(Renal Fluid Electrolyte Physiol 26):F268, 1989.

162. Ney RL, Kelley C, Bartter FC: Actions of vitamin D independent of the parathyroid glands. *Endocrinology* 82:760, 1968.

163. Nickols GA, Carnes DL, Anast GS, et al: Parathyroid mediated refractoriness of the rat kidney cyclic AMP system. *Am J Physiol* 236(Endocrinol Metab Gastrointest Physiol 5):E401, 1979.

164. Nseir NI, Szramowski J, Puschett JB: Mechanism of the renal tubular effects of 25-hydroxy and 1,25-dihydroxy vitamin D_3 in the absence of parathyroid hormone. *Miner Electrolyte Metab* 1:48, 1978.

165. Owen GM, Garry P, Fomon SJ: Concentrations of calcium and inorganic phosphorus in serum of normal infants receiving various feedings. *Pediatrics* 31:495, 1963.

166. Parfitt AM, Frame B: Phosphate loading and depletion in vitamin D treated hypoparathyroidism. *In* Avioli L, Bortier P, Fleish H, et al (eds): Homeostasis of Phosphate and other Minterals. The Second International Workshop. Paris, Armour Montagu Cis, 1975, p 251.

167. Parsons V, Anderson J: The maximum renal tubular reabsorptive rate for inorganic phosphate in thyrotoxicosis. *Clin Sci* 27:313, 1964.

168. Pastoriza-Munoz E, Colindres RE, Lassiter WE, et al: Effect of parathyroid hormone on phosphate reabsorption in rat distal convolution. *Am J Physiol* 235(Renal Fluid Electrolyte Metab 4):F321, 1978.

169. Popovtzer MM, Blum MS, Flus RS: Evidence for interference of 25(OH)vitamin D_3 with phosphaturic action of calcitonin. *Am J Physiol* 232(Endocrinol Metab Gastrointest Physiol 3):E515, 1977.

170. Popovtzer MM, Robinette JB: Effect of 25(OH)vitamin D_3 on urinary excretion of cyclic adenosine monophosphate. *Am J Physiol* 229:907, 1975.

171. Popovtzer MM, Robinette JB, DeLuca HF, et al: The acute effect of 25-hydroxycholecalciferol on renal handling of phosphorus. Evidence for a parathyroid hormone-dependent mechanism. *J Clin Invest* 53:913, 1974.

172. Popovtzer MM, Wald H: Evidence for interference of 25(OH)vitamin D_3 with phosphaturic action of glucagon. *Am J Physiol* 240(Renal Fluid Electrolyte Physiol 9):F269, 1981.

173. Poujeol P, Charbardes D, Roinel N, et al: Influence of extracellular fluid volume expansion on magnesium, calcium, and phosphate handling along the rat nephron. *Pflugers Arch* 365:203, 1976.

174. Puschett JB: Renal tubular effects of parathyroid hormone: An update. *Clin Orthop* 135:249, 1978.

175. Puschett JB, Fernandez PC, Boyle IT, et al: The acute renal tubular effects of 1,25-dihydroxycholecalciferol. *Proc Soc Exp Biol Med* 141:379, 1972.

176. Puschett JB, Kuhrman MS: Renal tubular effects of 1,25-dihydroxyvitamin D_3: Interactions with vasopressin and parathyroid hormone in the vitamin D-depleted rat. *J Lab Clin Med* 92:895, 1978.

177. Puschett JB, Moranz J, Kurnick WS: Evidence for a direct action of cholecalciferol and 25 hydroxycholecalciferol on the renal transport of phosphate, sodium and calcium. *J Clin Invest* 51:373, 1972.

178. Quamme GA, O'Callaghan T, Wong NLM, et al: Hypercalciuria in the phosphate-depleted dog: A micropuncture study. *Kidney Int* 10:492, 1976.

179. Quamme GA, Whiting SJ, Wong NLM: Influence of luminal pH on the adaptation of proximal phosphate transport to changes in dietary phosphate (abstr). *Kidney Int* 23:109, 1983.

180. Quamme GA, Wong NLM: Phosphate transport in the proximal convoluted tubule: Effect of intraluminal pH. *Am J Physiol* 246(Renal Fluid Electrolyte Physiol 15):F323, 1984.

181. Rasmussen H, Anast C, Arnaud C: Thyrocalcitonin, EGTA, and urinary electrolyte excretion. *J Clin Invest* 46:746, 1967.

182. Rasmussen H, Goodman DBP, Friedmann N, et al: Ionic control of metabolism. *In* Greep RO, Astwood EB (eds): *Handbook of Physiology. Section 7: Endocrinology.* Vol VII. Washington, DC, 1976, American Physiological Society, p 255.

183. Rastegar A, Agus Z, Connor TB, et al: Renal handling of calcium and phosphate during mineralocorticoid "escape" in man. *Kidney Int* 2:279, 1972.

184. Reiss E, Canterbury JM: Genesis of hyperparathyroidism. *Am J Med* 50:679, 1971.

185. Reiss E, Canterbury JM, Kanter A: Circulating parathyroid hormone concentration in chronic renal insufficiency. *Arch Intern Med* 124:417, 1969.

186. Roberts LE, Pitts RF: The effects of cortisone and desoxycorticosterone on the renal tubular reabsorption of phosphate and the excretion of titratable acid and potassium in dogs. *Endocrinology* 52:224, 1953.

187. Rosen JF, Fleischmann AR, Finberg L, et al: 1,25-dihydroxycholecalciferol: Its use in the long term management of idiopathic hypoparathyroidism in children. *J Clin Endocrinol Metab* 45:457, 1977.

188. Russo JC, Nash MA: Renal response to alterations in dietary phosphate in the young beagle. *Biol Neonate* 38:1, 1980.

189. Samarazija I, Molnar V, Froemter E: pH dependence of phosphate absorption in rat renal proximal tubule. Vol 19. *Proc Eur Dialysis Transplant Assoc* 1983, p 779.

190. Schwab SJ, Klahr S, Hammerman MR: Uptake of Pi in basolateral vesicles after release of unilateral obstruction. *Am J Physiol* 247(Renal Fluid Electrolyte Metab 16):F543, 1984.

191. Schwab SJ, Klahr S, Hammerman MR: Na^+ gradient-dependent P_i uptake in basolateral membrane vesicles from dog kidney. *Am J Physiol* 246(Renal Fluid Electrolyte Physiol 15):F663, 1984.

192. Shah SV, Kempson SA, Northrup TE, et al: Renal adaptation to low phosphate diet in rats. Blockade by actinomycin D. *J Clin Invest* 64:955, 1979.

193. Shlatz LJ, Schwartz IL, Kinne-Saffran E, et al: Distribution of parathyroid hormone-stimulated adenylate cyclase in plasma membranes of cells of the kidney cortex. *J Membr Biol* 24:131, 1975.

194. Slatopolsky E, Bricker NS: The role of phosphorus restriction in the prevention of secondary hyperparathyroidism in chronic renal disease. *Kidney Int* 4:141, 1973.

195. Slatopolsky E, Caglar E, Gradowska L, et al: On the pre-

vention of secondary hyperparathyroidism in experimental chronic renal disease using "proportional reduction" of dietary phosphorus intake. *Kidney Int* 2:147, 1972.

196. Slatopolsky E, Caglar S, Pennell JP, et al: On the pathogenesis of hyperparathyroidism in chronic experimental renal insufficiency in the dog. *J Clin Invest* 50:492, 1971.

197. Staum BB, Hamburger RJ, Goldberg M: Tracer microinjection study of renal tubular phosphate reabsorption in the rat. *J Clin Invest* 51:2271, 1972.

198. Steele TH: Renal resistance to parathyroid hormone during phosphate deprivation. *J Clin Invest* 58:1461, 1976.

199. Steele TH, Challoner-Hue L, Gottstein JH, et al: Acid-base maneuvers and phosphate transport in the isolated rat kidney. *Pflugers Arch* 392:178, 1981.

200. Steele TH, DeLuca HF: Influence of dietary phosphorus on renal phosphate reabsorption in the parathyroidectomized rat. *J Clin Invest* 57:867, 1976.

201. Steele TH, Engle JE, Tanaka Y, et al: Phosphatemic action of 1,25-dihydroxyvitamin D_3. *Am J Physiol* 229:489, 1975.

202. Stoll R, Kinne R, Murer H: Effect of dietary phosphate transport by isolated rat renal brush-border vesicles. *Biochem J* 180:465, 1979.

203. Stoll R, Kinne R, Murer H, et al: Phosphate transport by rat renal brush border membrane vesicles: Influence of dietary phosphate, thyroparathyroidectomy, and 1,25-dihydroxyvitamin D_3. *Pflugers Arch* 380:47, 1979.

204. Strickler JC, Thompson DD, Klose RM, et al: Micropuncture study of inorganic phosphate excretion in the rat. *J Clin Invest* 43:1596, 1964.

205. Swenson RS, Weisinger JR, Ruggeri JL, et al: Evidence that parathyroid hormone is not required for phosphate homeostasis in renal failure. *Metabolism* 24:199, 1975.

206. Tenenhouse HS, Chu YL: Hydrolysis of nicotinamide-adenine dinucleotide by purified renal brush border membranes. *Biochem J* 204:635, 1982.

207. Tenenhouse HS, Klugerman AH, Gurd W, et al: Pituitary involvement in renal adaptation to phosphate deprivation. *Am J Physiol* 255(Regulatory Integrative Comp Physiol 24):R373, 1988.

208. Troehler U, Bonjour JP, Fleisch H: Inorganic phosphate homeostasis. Renal adaptation to the dietary intake in intact and thyroparathyroidectomized rats. *J Clin Invest* 57:264, 1976.

209. Turner ST, Kiebzak GM, Dousa TP: Mechanism of glucocorticoid effect on renal transport of phosphate. *Am J Physiol* 243(Cell Physiol 12):C227, 1982.

210. Ullrich KJ: Mechanisms of cellular phosphate transport in rat kidney proximal tubule. *Adv Exp Med Biol* 103:21, 1978.

211. Ullrich KJ, Rumrich G, Kloss S: Phosphate transport in the proximal convolution of the rat kidney. I. Tubular heterogeneity, effect of parathyroid hormone in acute and chronic parathyroidectomized animals, and effect of phosphate diet. *Pflugers Arch* 372:269, 1977.

212. Ullrich KJ, Rumrich J, Kloss S: Phosphate transport in the proximal convolution of rat kidneys. II. Effect of extracellular Ca^{2+} and application of Ca^{2+} ionophore A 23187 in chronic PTX animals. *Pflugers Arch* 375:97, 1978.

213. Ullrich K, Rumrich J, Kloss S: Phosphate transport in the proximal convolution of the rat kidney. III. Effect of extracellular and intracellular pH. *Pflugers Arch* 337:33, 1978.

214. Webb RK, Woodhall PB, Tisher CC, et al: Relationship between phosphaturia and acute hypercapnia in the rat. *J Clin Invest* 60:829, 1977.

215. Welling LW, Evan AP, Gattone VH II, et al: Correlation of structure and function in developing proximal tubule of guinea pig. *Am J Physiol* 256(Renal Fluid Electrolyte Metab 25):F13, 1989.

216. Wen SF: Micropuncture studies of phosphate transport in the proximal tubule of the dog. The relationship to sodium reabsorption. *J Clin Invest* 53:143, 1974.

217. Wen SF: Phosphate transport in the phosphate-depleted dog (abstr). *Kidney Int* 8:405, 1975.

218. Westby GR, Goldfarb S, Goldberg M, et al: Acute effects of bovine growth hormone on renal calcium and phosphate excretion. *Metabolism* 26:525, 1977.

219. Windhager EE, Taylor A: Regulatory role of intracellular calcium ions in epithelial Na^+ transport. *Annu Rev Physiol* 45:519, 1983.

220. Yanagawa N, Nagami G, Joe OK, et al: Dissociation of gluconeogenesis from fluid and phosphate reabsorption in isolated rabbit proximal tubules. *Kidney Int* 25:869, 1984.

221. Yanagawa N, Nagami GT, Kurokawa K: Cytosolic redox potential and phosphate transport in the proximal tubule of the rabbit. A study in the isolated perfused tubules. *Mineral Electrolyte Metab* 11:57, 1985.

222. Yayaishi O, Ueda K: Poly(ADP-ribose) and ADP-ribosylation of proteins. *Annu Rev Biochem* 46:95, 1977.

223. Yusufi ANK, Holets RJ, Dousa TP: Stimulation of renal brush border membrane (BBM) transport of phosphate (P_i) by thryoid hormones: Mechanism of action (abstr). *Fed Proc* 43:663, 1984.

Magnesium

1. Anast CS: Serum magnesium levels in the newborn. *Pediatrics* 33:969, 1964.

2. Bajpai PC, Sugden D, Ramos A, et al: Serum magnesium levels in the newborn and older child. *Arch Dis Child* 41:424, 1966.

3. Bethune JE, Turpin RA, Inque H: Effect of parathyroid extract on divalent ion excretion in man. *J Clin Endocrinol Metab* 28:673, 1968.

4. Brunette MG, Aras M: A microinjection study of nephron permeability to calcium and magnesium. *Am J Physiol* 221:114, 1971.

5. Brunette MG, Vigneault N, Carriere S: Micropuncture study of magnesium transport along the nephron in the young rat. *Am J Physiol* 227:891, 1974.

6. Brunette MG, Vigneault N, Carriere S: Micropuncture study of renal magnesium transport in magnesium-loaded rats. *Am J Physiol* 229:1695, 1975.

7. Brunette MG, Vigneault N, Carriere S: Magnesium handling by the papilla of the young rat. *Pflugers Arch* 373:229, 1979.

8. Brunette MG, Wen SF, Evanson RL, et al: Micropuncture study of magnesium reabsorption in the proximal tubule of the dog. *Am J Physiol* 216:1510, 1969.

9. Burnatowska MA, Harris CA, Sutton RAL, et al: Effects of PTH and cAMP on renal handling of calcium, magnesium, and phosphate in the hamster. *Am J Physiol* 233(Renal Fluid Electrolyte Physiol 2):F514, 1977.

10. Carney SL, Wong NLM, Quamme GA, et al: Effect of magnesium deficiency on renal magnesium and calcium transport in the rat. *J Clin Invest* 65:180, 1980.

11. Coburn JW, Massry SG: Changes in serum and urinary calcium during phosphate depletion: Studies on mechanisms. *J Clin Invest* 49:1073, 1970.

12. Dematini FE, Briscoe AM, Ragan C: Effect of ethacrynic acid on calcium and magnesium excretion. *Proc Soc Exp Biol Med* 124:320, 1967.

13. de Rouffignac C, Morel F, Moss N, et al: Micropuncture study of water and electrolyte movements along the loop of Henle in Psammomys, with special reference to magnesium, calcium and phosphorus. *Pflugers Arch* 344:309, 1973.

14. Eknoyan G, Suki WN, Martinez-Maldonado M: Effect of diuretics on urinary excretion of phosphate, calcium, and magnesium in thyroparathyroidectomized dogs. *J Lab Clin Med* 76:257, 1970.

15. LeGrimellec CL, Roinel N, Morel F: Simultaneous Mg, Ca, P, K, Na, and Cl analysis in rat tubular fluid. II. During acute Mg plasma loading. *Pflugers Arch* 340:197, 1973.

16. LeGrimellec CL, Roinel N, Morel F: Simultaneous Mg, Ca, P, K, Na and Cl analysis in rat tubular fluid perfusion of either inulin or ferrocyanide. *Pflugers Arch* 340:181, 1973.

17. LeGrimellec CL, Roinel N, Morel F: Simultaneous Mg, Ca, P, K, Na, and Cl analysis in rat tubular fluid. III. During acute Ca plasma loading. *Pflugers Arch* 346:171, 1974.

18. Lemann J Jr, Piering WF, Lennon EJ: Studies on the acute effects of aldosterone and cortisol on the interrelationship between renal sodium, calcium, and magnesium excretion in normal man. *Nephron* 7:117, 1970.

19. Massry SG, Coburn JW, Chapman LW, et al: Effect of NaCl infusion on urinary Ca^{++} and Mg^{++} during reduction in their filtered loads. *Am J Physiol* 213:1218, 1967.

20. Massry SG, Coburn JW, Chapman LW, et al: The acute effect of adrenal steroids on the interrelationship between the renal excretion of sodium, calcium, and magnesium. *J Lab Clin Med* 70:563, 1967.

21. Massry SG, Coburn JW, Kleeman CR: Renal handling of magnesium in the dog. *Am J Physiol* 216:1460, 1969.

22. Massry SG, Kleeman CR: Calcium and magnesium excretion during acute rise in glomerular filtration rate. *J Lab Clin Med* 80:645, 1972.

23. Morel F, Roinel N, LeGrimellec C: Electron probe analysis of tubular fluid composition. *Nephron* 6:350, 1969.

24. Mudge GH, Taggart JV: Effects of acetate on the renal excretion of p-aminohippurate in the dog. *Am J Physiol* 161:191, 1950.

25. Murayama Y, Morel F, LeGrimellec C: Phosphate, calcium and magnesium transfers in proximal tubules and loops of Henle, as measured by single nephron microperfusion experiments in the rat. *Pflugers Arch* 333:1, 1972.

26. Popovtzer MM, Massry SG, Coburn JW, et al: The interrelationship between sodium, calcium, and magnesium excretion in advanced renal failure. *J Lab Clin Med* 73:763, 1969.

27. Popovtzer MM, Schainuck LI, Massry SG, et al: Divalent ion excretion in chronic kidney disease: Relation to degree of renal insufficiency. *Clin Sci* 38:297, 1970.

28. Quamme GA: Effect of intraluminal furosemide on calcium and magnesium transport in the loop of Henle and the role of PTH. *Kidney Int* 14:642, 1978.

29. Quamme GA: Effect of calcitonin on calcium and magnesium transport in the rat nephron. *Am J Physiol* 238(Endocrinol Metab 1):573, 1980.

30. Quamme GA, Dirks JH: Effect of magnesium (Mg) on calcium (Ca) and Mg transport in the rat: A microperfusion study. Abstracts of 7th Annual Meeting of the International Society of Nephrology, Montreal, Munich: S Karger, 1978, p E12.

31. Quamme GA, Dirks JH: Intraluminal and contraluminal magnesium on magnesium and calcium transfer in the rat nephron. *Am J Physiol* 238(Renal Fluid Electrolyte Physiol 7):F187, 1980.

32. Quamme GA, O'Callaghan T, Wong NLM, et al: Hypercalciuria in the phosphate-depleted dog: A micropuncture study. *Kidney Int* 10:492, 1976.

33. Quamme GA, Wong NLM, Dirks JH, et al: Magnesium handling in the dog kidney: A micropuncture study. *Pflugers Arch* 377:95, 1987.

34. Sharegi GR, Agus ZS: Magnesium transport in the cortical

thick ascending limb of Henle's loop of rabbit. *J Clin Invest* 69:759, 1982.

35. Tsang RC, Oh W: Serum magnesium levels in low birth weight infants. *Am J Dis Child* 120:44, 1970.

36. Walser M: Magnesium metabolism. *Ergeb Physiol* 59:185, 1967.

37. Walser M: Divalent cations: Physicochemical state in glomerular filtrate and urine and renal excretion. In Orloff J, Berliner RW (eds): *Handbook of Physiology*, Section 8: *Renal Physiology*. Washington, DC, American Physiological Society, 1973, p 555.

38. Wen SF, Evanson RL, Dirks JH: Micropuncture study of renal magnesium transport in proximal and distal tubule of the dog. *Am J Physiol* 219:570, 1970.

39. Wong NLM, Quamme GA, Dirks JH: Tubular maximum reabsorptive capacity for magnesium in the dog. (abstr). *Kidney Int* 16:658, 1979.

40. Yendt ER, Cohanim M: Prevention of calcium stones with thiazides. *Kidney Int* 13:397, 1978.

The Vitamin D–Endocrine System
Parathyroid Hormone

1. Alexander DP, Nixon DA: Effect of parathyroid extract in fetal sheep. *Biol Neonate* 14:117, 1969.

2. Arnaud CD, Kolb FO: The calciotropic hormones and metabolic bone disease. In Greenspan FS, Forsham PH (eds): *Basic and Clinical Endocrinology*. Los Altos, CA, Lange, 1984, p 187.

3. Atkinson SA: Calcium and phosphorus requirements of low-birthweight infant: A nutritional and endocrinological perspective. *Nutr Rev* 41:69, 1983.

4. Barak Y, Milbauer B, Weisman Y, et al: Response of neonatal hypocalcemia to 1,25-hydroxyvitamin D. *Arch Dis Child* 54:642, 1979.

5. Bouillon R: Vitamin D metabolites in human pregnancy. In Holick MF, Gray TK, Anast CS (eds): *Perinatal Calcium and Phosphorus Metabolism*. New York, Elsevier, 1983, p 291.

6. Bouillon R, Van Assche FA, Van Baelen H, et al: Influence of the vitamin D-binding protein on the serum concentration of 1,25-dihydroxyvitamin D: Significance of the free 1,25-dihydroxyvitamin D concentration. *J Clin Invest* 67:589, 1981.

7. Broadus AE, Mahaffey JE, Bartter FC, et al: Nephrogenous cyclic adenosine monophosphate as a parathyroid function test. *J Clin Invest* 60:771, 1977.

8. Bruns ME, Bruns DE: Vitamin D metabolism and function during pregnancy and the neonatal period. *Ann Clin Lab Sci* 13:521, 1983.

9. Care AD: Calcium homeostasis in the fetus. *J Devel Physiol* 2:85, 1980.

10. Chan GM, Tsang RC, Chen IW, et al: The effects of $1,25(OH)_2D$ supplementation in premature infants. *J Pediatr* 93:91, 1978.

11. Chesney RW: Metabolic bone diseases. *Pediatr Rev* 5:227, 1984.

12. Chesney RW: Current clinical applications of vitamin D metabolite research. In Urist MR (ed): *Clinical Orthopaedics and Related Research*. Philadelphia, Lippincott, 1989, p 285.

13. Chesney RW, Hamstra AJ, DeLuca HF: Rickets of prematurity: Supranormal levels of serum 1,25-dihydroxyvitamin D. *Am J Dis Child* 135:34, 1981.

14. Chudley AE, Brown DR, Holzman IR, et al: Nutritional rickets in two very-low-birthweight infants with chronic lung disease. *Arch Dis Child* 55:687, 1980.

15. Cifuentes RF, Kooh SW, Radde IC: Vitamin D deficiency in

a calcium-supplemented very low-birthweight infant. 96:252, 1980.

16. Comment: Vitamin D metabolism in the rickets of very-low-birthweight, premature infants. Nutr Rev 39:234, 1981.

17. Connelly JP, Crawford JD, Watson J: Studies of neonatal hyperphosphatemia. Pediatrics 30:425, 1962.

18. Cruikshank DP, Pitkin RM, Reynolds WA, et al: Calcium-regulating hormones and ions in amniotic fluid. Am J Obstet Gynecol 136:621, 1980.

19. Davies M, Klimiuk PS, Adams PH, et al: Familial hypocalciuric hypercalcemia and acute pancreatitis. Br Med J 282:1023, 1981.

20. DeLuca HF: The vitamin D system in the regulation of calcium and phosphorus metabolism. Nutrit Rev 37:161, 1979.

21. Dorey LG, Gell JW: Primary hyperparathyroidism during the third trimester of pregnancy. Obstet Gynecol 45:469, 1975.

22. Drezner MK, Neelon FA: Pseudohypoparathyroidism. In Stanbury JB, Wyngaarden JB, Fredrickson DS, et al (eds): The Metabolic Basis of Inherited Disease. New York, McGraw-Hill, 1983, p 1508.

23. Farfel Z, Bourne HR: Deficient activity of receptor-cyclase coupling protein in platelets of patients with pseudohypoparathyroidism. J Clin Endocrinol Metab 51:1202, 1980.

24. Fraser DR: Regulation of the metabolism of vitamin D. Physiol Rev 60:551, 1980.

26. Fraser DR: The physiological economy of vitamin D. Lancet 1:969, 1983.

27. Gertner JM, Glassman MS, Coustan DR, et al: Fetomaternal vitamin D relationships at term. J Pediatr 97:637, 1980.

28. Glorieux FH, Salle BL, Delvin EE, et al: Vitamin D metabolism in preterm infants: Serum calcitriol values during the first five days of life. J Pediatr 99:640, 1981.

29. Gray TK: Vitamin D metabolism during pregnancy. In Kumar R (ed): Vitamin D. The Hague, Martinus Nijoff, 1984, p 217.

30. Gray TK, Lester GE: Vitamin D metabolism in the pregnant rat. In Cohn DV, Talmage RV, Matthews JL (eds): Hormonal Control of Calcium Metabolism. Proceedings of the Seventh International Conference of Calcium-Regulating Hormones. New York, Elsvier, 1981, p 236.

31. Greer FR, Chesney RW: Disorders of calcium metabolism in the neonate. Semin Nephrol 3:100, 1983.

32. Habener JF, Potts JT: Biosynthesis of parathyroid hormone. N Engl J Med 29:580, 1978.

33. Halloran BP, Barthell EN, DeLuca HF: Vitamin D metabolism during pregnancy and lactation in the rat. Proc Natl Acad Sci USA 76:5549, 1979.

34. Halloran BP, DeLuca HF: Calcium regulation during the mammalian reproductive cycle: The role of vitamin D. In Cohn DV, Talmage RV, Matthews JL (eds): Hormonal Control of Calcium Metabolism, Proceeding of the Seventh International Conference on Calcium-Regulating Hormones. New York, Elsevier, 1981, p 230.

35. Hammerman MR, Hansen VA, Morrissey JJ: Cyclic-AMP-dependent protein phosphorylation and dephosphorylation alter phosphate transport in canine renal brush border vesicles. Biochim Biophys Acta 755:10, 1983.

36. Hillman LS, Haddad JG: Human perinatal vitamin D metabolism. I. 25-Hydroxyvitamin D in maternal and cord blood. J Pediatr 84:742, 1974.

37. Hillman LS, Haddad JG: Perinatal vitamin D metabolism. II. Serial 25-hydroxy-vitamin D concentrations in sera of term and premature infants. J Pediatr 86:928, 1975.

38. Hillman LS, Haddad JG: Serial analyses of serum vitamin D-binding protein in preterm infants from birth to postconceptual maturity. J Clin Endocrinol Metab 56:189, 1983.

39. Hillman LS, Rojanasathit S, Slatopolsky E, et al: Serial measurments of serum calcium, magnesium, parathyroid hormone, calcitonin, and 25-hydroxy-vitamin D in premature and term infants during the first week of life. Pediatr Res 11:739, 1977.

40. Hillman LS, Salmons SJ, Haussler MR, et al: Serial 1,25-dihydroxyvitamin D serum concentrations in premature infants on varying feeding regimens (abstr). Pediatr Res 17:290A, 1983.

41. Hillman LS, Slatopolsky E, Haddad JG: Perinatal vitamin D metabolism. IV. Maternal and cord serum 24,25-dihydroxyvitamin D concentrations. J Clin Endocrinol Metab 47:1073, 1978.

42. Holloran BP, DeLuca HF: Calcium regulation during the mammalian reproductive cycle: The role of vitamin D. In Cohn DV, Talmage RV, Matthews JL (eds): Hormonal Control of Calcium Metabolism. Proceedings of the Seventh International Conference on Calcium-Regulating Hormones. New York, Elsevier, 1981, p 230.

43. Hruska KA, Khalifa S, Meltzer V, et al: Calcium as a mediator of the physiologic and pathophysiologic effects of parathyroid hormone. Semin Nephrol 4:159, 1984.

44. Huston RK, Reynolds JW, Jensen C, et al: Nutrient and mineral retention and vitamin D absorption in low-birthweight infants: Effect of medium-chain triglycerides. Pediatrics 72:44, 1983.

45. Kooh SW: Parathyroid hormone responsiveness in the sheep fetus and newborn lamb. Can J Physiol Pharmacol 58:934, 1980.

46. Kulkarni PB, Hall RT, Rhodes PG, et al: Rickets in very low-birthweight infants. J Pediatr 96:249, 1980.

47. Lester GE: Vitamin D metabolism in small animals. In Anast C, Gray T, Holick M (eds): Perinatal Mineral Metabolism. New York, Elsevier, 1983, p 25.

48. Lester GE, Gray TK, Lorenc RS: Evidence for maternal and fetal differences in vitamin D metabolism. Proc Soc Exp Biol Med 159:303, 1978.

49. Levine MD, Downs RW Jr, Singer M, et al: Deficient activity of guanine nucleotide regulatory protein in erythocytes from patients with pseudohypoparathyroidism. Biochem Biophys Res Commun 94:1319, 1980.

50. Linarelli LG, Bobik J, Bobik C: Newborn urinary cyclic AMP and developmental renal responsiveness to parathyroid hormone. Pediatrics 50:14, 1972.

51. Mallet E, Basuyau JP, Brunelle P, et al: Neonatal parathyroid secretion and renal receptor maturation in premature infants. Biol Neonate 33:304, 1978.

52. Markestad T, Aksnes L, Finne PH, et al: Vitamin D nutritional status of premature infants supplemented with 500IU vitamin D2 per day. Acta Paediatr Scand 72:517, 1983.

53. Markestad T, Aksnes L, Finne PH, et al: Plasma concentrations of vitamin D metabolites in a case of rickets of prematurity. Acta Paediatr Scand 72:759, 1983.

54. Markestad T, Aksnes L, Finne PH, et al: Plasma concentrations of vitamin D metabolites in premature infants. Pediatr Res 18:269, 1984.

55. Markestad T, Asknes L, Finne PH, et al: Effect of exchange transfusions with citrated blood on plasma concentrations of vitamin D metabolites in neonates. Pediatr Res 18:429, 1984.

56. Marx SJ, Spiegel AM, Brown EM, et al: Familial hypercalciuric hypercalcemia. In DeLuca HF, Anast CS (eds): Pediatric Diseases Related to Calcium. New York, Elsevier, 1980, p 413.

57. Marx SJ, Spiegel AM, Levine MA, et al: Familial hypocalciuric hypercalcemia: The relation to primary parathyroid hyperplasia. N Engl J Med 307:416, 1982.

58. Norman AW, Henry HL, Malluche HH: 24R,25-Dihydroxyvitamin D3 are both indispensable for calcium and phosphorus homeostasis. Life Sci 27:229, 1980.

59. Norman AW, Schaefer K, von Herrath D, et al: *Vitamin D: Chemical, Biochemical and Clinical Endocrinology of Calcium Metabolism.* New York, Walter de Gruyter, 1982, p 157.

60. Northrop G, Misenhimer HR, Becker FO: Failure of parathyroid hormone to cross the nonhuman primate placenta. *Am J Obstet Gynecol* 129:449, 1977.

61. Peterson S, Christensen NC, Fogh-Anderson N: Effect of serum calcium on 1,25(OH)$_2$D supplementation in infants of low birthweight, infants with perinatal asphyxia and infants of dibaetic mothers. *Acta Paediatr Scand* 70:897, 1981.

62. Pitkin RM, Cruikshank DP, Schauberger CW, et al: Fetal calciotropic hormones and neonatal calcium homeostasis. *Pediatrics* 66:77, 1980.

63. Pitkin RM, Gebhardt MP: Serum calcium concentrations in human pregnancy. *Am J Obstet Gynecol* 127:775, 1977.

64. Pitkin RM, Reynolds WA, Williams GA, et al: Calcium metabolism in normal pregnancy: A longitudinal sudy. *Am J Obstet Gynecol* 133:781, 1979.

65. Pitkin RM, Reynolds WA, Williams GA, et al: Calcium-regulating hormones during the menstrual cycle. *J Clin Endocrinol Metab* 47:626, 1978.

66. Potts JT: Pseudohypoparathyroidism. *In* Stanbury JB, Wyngaarden JB, Fredrickson DS (eds): *The Metabolic Basis of Inherited Disease.* New York, McGraw-Hill, 1983, p 1350.

67. Raisz LG: Bone resorption in tissue culture: Factors influencing the response to parathyroid hormone. *J Clin Invest* 44:103, 1965.

68. Rappaport MS, Stern PH: Parathyroid hormone enhances inositol incorporation into phospholipids in bone organ culture (abstr). Sixth Annual Meeting of the American Society for Bone and Mineral Research, 1984, p A58.

69. Ron M, Levitz M, Chuba J, et al: Transfer of 25 hydroxy-vitamin D$_3$ and 1,25-dihydroxyvitamin D$_3$ across the perfused human plancenta. *Am J Obstet Gynecol* 148:370, 1984.

70. Rosen JF, Chesney RW: Circulating calcitriol concentrations in health and disease. *J Pediatr* 103:1, 1983.

71. Ross R, Care AD, Robinson JS, et al: Perinatal 1,25-dihydroxycholecalciferol in the sheep and its role in the maintenance of the transplacental calcium gradient. *J Endocrinol* 87:17, 1980.

72. Rowe JC, Wood DH, Rowe DW, et al: Nutritional hypophosphatemic rickets in a premature infant fed breast milk. *N Engl J Med* 300:293, 1979.

73. Schauberger CW, Pitkin RM: Maternal-perinatal calcium relationships. *Obstet Gynecol* 53:74, 1979.

74. Schedewie HK, Odell WD, Fisher DA, et al: Parathormone and perinatal calcium homeostasis. *Pediatr Res* 13:1, 1979.

75. Scothorne RJ: Functional capacity of fetal parathyroid glands with reference to their clinical use as homografts. *Ann NY Acad Sci* 120:669, 1964.

76. Seino Y, Ishida M, Yamaoka K, et al: Serum calcium-regulating hormones in the perinatal period. *Calcif Tissue Int* 34:331, 1982.

77. Senterre J, David L, Salle B: Effects of 1,25-dihydroxy-cholecalciferol on calcium, phosphorus and magnesium balance and on circulating parathyroid hormone and calcitonin in preterm infants. *In* Stern L, Salle B (eds): *Intensive Care in the Newborn.* Vol II. New York, Masson, 1980, p 115.

78. Senterre J, Salle B: Calcium and phosphorus economy of the preterm infant and its interaction with vitamin D and its metabolites. *Acta Paediatr Scand* (suppl) 296:85, 1982.

79. Shareghi GR, Agus ZS: Magnesium transport in the cortical thick ascending limb of Henle's loop of the rabbit. *J Clin Invest* 69:759, 1982.

80. Slatopolsky E, Martin K, Morrissey J, et al: Current concepts of the metabolism and radioimmunoassay of parathyroid hormone. *J Lab Clin Med* 99:309, 1982.

81. Smith FG, Tinglof BO, Meuli J, et al: Fetal response to parathyroid hormone in sheep. *J Appl Physiol* 27:276, 1969.

82. Spitzer A, Kaskel F, Feld L, et al: Renal regulation of phosphate homeostasis during growth. *Semin Nephrol* 3:87, 1983.

83. Steichen JJ, Schell D, Tsnag R: Effect of soy-based or cow-milk-based formula feeding on bone mineral content, mineral, vitamin D and iron metabolism in term infants (abstr). *Pediatr Res* 17:202A, 1983.

84. Steichen JJ, Tsang RC, Gratton TL, et al: Vitamin D homeostasis in the perinatal period: 1,25-dihydroxyvitamin D in maternal cord and neonatal blood. *N Engl J Med* 302:315, 1980.

85. Steichen JJ, Tsang RC, Greer FR, et al: Elevated serum 1,25-dihyroxyvitamin D concentrations in rickets of very low-birthweight infants. *J Pediatr* 99:293, 1981.

86. Stern PH, Halloran BP, DeLuca HF, et al: Responsiveness of vitamin D-deficient fetal rat limb bones to parathyroid hormonc in culture. *Am J Physiol* 244(Endocrinol Metab 7):E421, 1983.

87. Stiles GL, Caron MG, Lefkowitz RJ: β-adrenergic receptors: Biochemical mechanisms of physiologic regulation. *Physiol Rev* 64:661, 1984.

88. Suki WN, Rouse D, Ng RCK, et al: Calcium transport in the thick ascending limb of Henle: Heterogeneity of function in the medullary and cortical segments. *J Clin Invest* 66:1004, 1980.

89. Tanaka Y, Halloran B, Schnoes HD, et al: In vitro production of 1,25(OH)$_2$D$_3$ by rat placental tissue. *Proc Natl Acad Sci USA* 76:5033, 1979.

90. Tsang RC, Greer FR, Steichen JJ: Perinatal metabolism of vitamin D: Transition from fetal to neonatal life. *Clin Perinatal* 8:287, 1981.

91. Taylor AN: Intestinal vitamin D-induced calcium-binding protein: Time-course of immunocytological localization following 1,25-dihydroxyvitamin D$_3$. *J Histochem Cytochem* 31:426, 1983.

92. Venkataraman P, Buckley D, Neumann V, et al: Profound neonatal hypocalcemia in very low birthweight infants with unresponsive parathyroid glands, refractory to 1,25-dihydroxyvitamin D$_3$ (abstr). *Pediatr Res* 17:340A, 1983.

93. Webster SK, Haramati D: Developmental changes in the phosphaturic response to parathyroid hormone in the rat. *Am J Physiol* 249(Renal Fluid Electrolyte Physiol 18):F251, 1985.

94. Weisman Y, Harrell A, Edelstein S, et al: 1,25(OH)$_2$D$_3$ and 24,25(OH)$_2$D$_3$ in vitro synthesis in human decidua and placenta. *Nature* 281:317, 1979.

95. Weisman Y, Occhipinti M, Knox G, et al: Concentrations of 24,25-dihydroxyvitamin D and 25-hydroxyvitamin D in paired in maternal-cord sera. *Am J Obstet Gynecol* 103:704, 1978.

96. Weisman Y, Reiter E, Root A: Measurement of 24,25-dihydroxyvitamin D in sera of neonates and children. *J Pediatr* 91:904, 1977.

SHERMAN D. LEVINE

8
Concentrating and Diluting Mechanisms

Overview and Perspective

In the healthy adult or child, maintenance of a normal plasma osmolality is achieved through two mechanisms acting in concert: (1) States of water excess are met by a decrease in plasma levels of antidiuretic hormone, resulting in the excretion of a dilute urine, and (2) states of water depletion are corrected by a combination of increased water intake and increased antidiuretic hormone release, the latter leading in turn to increased renal water reabsorption and the excretion of a highly concentrated urine. Newborn and young infants, on the other hand, lack the ability to vary their intake of solute-free water independently and thus must depend on their caretakers and their renal concentrating system as defenses against water depletion.

Both glomerular filtrate and the subsequent proximal reabsorbate are isosmotic to plasma, so that the fluid that enters the more distal nephron segments is perforce isosmotic as well. Events within the distal nephron, however, can effect the formation of a urine whose osmolality can range from as low as 30 mOsm/kg to as high as 1200 mOsm/Kg in human adults, and considerably higher in many smaller mammals. This chapter focuses on the physiology and ontogeny of the mechanisms by which the kidney can elaborate this dilute or concentrated urine.

Renal Concentrating and Diluting Ability in Humans

Infants can dilute their urine very well [2,11]. The water-loaded newborn can achieve a urine osmolality of 30–50 mOsm, comparable to levels achieved in the adult [118]. Studies using clearance techniques during hypotonic saline loading have demonstrated free water clearances averaging 19% of the glomerular filtration rate (GFR) in infants (1 week to 15 months of age) and 14% of the GFR in older children (2 to 12 years old). Approximately 90% of the salt delivered to the distal nephron was absorbed in the process of urinary dilution [118]. Once again, these values are quite comparable to those obtainable in adults and suggest that excretion of ingested water is limited by the child's relatively low GFR (as discussed in Chapter 3)

rather than by the distal nephron's ability to remove salt from the filtered fluid. The diluting ability of the premature's kidney is diminished, however, at least in part as a consequence of a limitation in the ability to reabsorb sodium, and premature infants can develop a diminished plasma sodium concentration when sodium depleted [5].

In contrast, the human infant's kidney does not concentrate urine to the same extent as the adult kidney. That is, although the adult human can excrete a urine having an osmolality as high as 1200 mOsm in the face of water deprivation, the maximum level achievable in the 30- to 35-week preterm newborn is 360 mOsm [143], and that in the full-term newborn is 380–800 mOsm [38,143]. The capacity to raise the urine osmolality to adult levels is not achieved until an age of about 1½ years [154].

The diminished ability to excrete a concentrated urine is the consequence of two factors. The first is that the infant ingests a diet relatively low in protein, most of which is used for tissue growth. Thus only a small fraction of the ingested dietary nitrogen is converted to urea and excreted in the urine. Under these circumstances, the urinary osmolality is low because the urine contains little urea (compared with the nonanabolic adult ingesting a high protein diet), not because it contains too much water. The urinary electrolyte concentration of a newborn with a urinary osmolality of 600 mOsm is much higher than the comparable concentration in an adult with the same measured osmolality, because the adult's urine contains a great deal more urea.

The second factor, quantitatively less important, represents a true diminution in the kidney's ability to reabsorb water and is a consequence of immaturity of both tubular structure and function.

General Principles of Renal Concentration and Dilution

It is relatively simple for an epithelium to create a dilute fluid from a more concentrated one, requiring only a tissue that can reabsorb salt while remaining impermeable to water. In the mammalian kidney, these characteristics are

Table 8-1. *Properties of nephron segments involved in concentration and dilution*

Segment	Active NaCl Transport	Passive Permeabilities (Vasopressin Absent)			Effect of Vasopressin
		NaCl	Water	Urea	
Henle's loop					
Descending limb	0	+	+ +	+	None
Thin ascending limb	0	+ +	0	+	None
Thick ascending limb	+ +	+	0	+	Increased active NaCl reabsorption
Distal tubule	+	+	0	0	None
Collecting duct	+	+	0	0	Increased water permeability
Cortex					and NaCl reabsorption
Outer medulla	+	+	0	0	Increased water permeability and NaCl reabsorption
Inner medulla/ papilla	+	+	0	+	Increased water and urea permeabilities

Permeability: 0 = very low; + = low; + + = high.

shared by the cortical and medullary thick ascending limbs of Henle's loop, the distal tubule, and, in the absence of vasopressin, the cortical and medullary collecting tubules (Table 8-1).

The production of a concentrated fluid, in comparison, is far more complex. The salt-excreting organs of certain animals that ingest sea water (e.g., the dogfish rectal gland) possess epithelial cells that can directly secrete a salt-rich fluid containing very little water, thereby maintaining external balance despite an extremely hypertonic intake. Mammalian tissues lack this ability to secrete hypertonic fluids directly and thus must create a concentrated tubular fluid in a far more complex manner.

In brief, the mammalian kidney generates a hypertonic interstitial environment within the renal medulla, largely the responsibility of the ascending and descending limbs of Henle's loop, and then permits a relatively small fraction of the tubular fluid to traverse a water-permeant epithelium (the vasopressin-stimulated medullary collecting tubule) within this hypertonic environment and to equilibrate with it by extraction of water, thereby making the tubular fluid hypertonic as well.

We might then ask, how can the medullary interstitium be made hypertonic to plasma? This is in no sense a trivial question; the continued appearance in the literature of very sophisticated mathematical models of the renal medulla and their inability to duplicate precisely measured medullary solute concentration patterns suggests that there is much yet to be learned about the details of the concentrating mechanism. Nonetheless we will begin by presenting a very simple model, whose relevance to the renal medullary concentrating system was first noted by Schmidt-Nielsen [133], in the hope that it will yield some intuitive insight.

A Simple "Countercurrent Multiplier"

Off the coast of Peru lies one of the world's richest fishing grounds, a consequence of a large-scale countercurrent sys-

tem. As shown in Figure 8-1, a deep Pacific Ocean current flows east toward the coast, rises, and returns to the west (white arrows). Particulate organic matter, rich in nutrients, is carried in the deep current toward the coast, then to the surface, and finally away. Since the nutrient particles are heavier than water, they are driven by gravity back down into the shore-directed flow of water (black arrows), thereby becoming trapped at the tip of the water flow loop, in the water adjacent to the shore.

Several characteristics of the model deserve particular comment. First, as a consequence of gravity-driven particulate movement, the concentration in the shoregoing limb of the loop at any given distance from shore (i.e., along any black arrow) exceeds the concentration in the seagoing limb. Second, although the concentration difference between seagoing and shoregoing limbs at any given distance from shore can be quite small, the concentration achieved at the tip of the loop can be extremely large. Finally, abolition of the local gradients (removal of "gravity") or disturbing the pattern of water flow will eliminate the overall concentration gradient; indeed such disturbances in the ocean currents are known to diminish the local fishing harvest significantly.

This model demonstrates the importance of the two factors critical to establishment of a countercurrent system: (1) a hairpin structure with countercurrent flow of fluid and (2) a mechanism for establishing a local gradient between the two paths' fluid movement. The flow toward and away from shore corresponds to flow through the descending and ascending limbs of Henle's loop, respectively, whereas "gravity" corresponds to salt transport by the ascending limb.

Extrapolation to the Renal Medulla: The Renal Countercurrent Multiplier

The aforementioned model is an oversimplification in a number of important ways. (1) Instead of direct solute transfer from ascending to descending limbs of the loop,

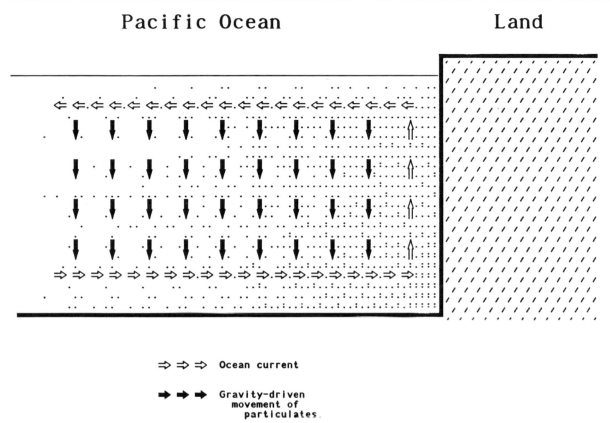

FIG. 8-1. *A simple countercurrent system found in nature.* (Adapted from *Schmidt-Nielsen K: Countercurrent systems in animals.* Sci Am 244:118, 1981.)

solute (primarily sodium chloride) is transported from the ascending limb to the interstitium, thereby creating an osmotic gradient that pulls water from the water-permeant descending limb into the interstitium. This fluid eventually leaves via the medullary capillary network, the vasa recta. (2) Active sodium pumping by Na-K-ATPase occurs only in the thick portion of the ascending limb and not in the thin ascending limb. Nonetheless, there is new salt movement from the thin ascending limb into the interstitium. Urea plays a critical role in mediating this salt efflux.

MECHANISM OF SALT EFFLUX FROM THE THIN ASCENDING LIMB

Although the mathematical analysis is extremely complex, the following explanation may provide some intuitive insight.

1. Active NaCl reabsorption from the thick ascending limb yields a hypo-osmolar tubular fluid (Fig. 8-2).
2. In the vasopressin-stimulated cortical collecting tubule, water moves from tubule to interstitium, thereby achieving isotonicity with plasma and concentrating urea in that urea-impermeant segment. (It is worth considering that ⅚ of the fluid must be removed to bring its osmo-

lality from 50 to 300, assuming no solute transport by the collecting tubule.)
3. In the vasopressin-stimulated medullary collecting tubule, water is further reabsorbed and urea concentration further increased (Fig. 8-3).
4. At the tip of the papilla, urea permeability is high in the presence of vasopressin, so that urea moves from tubular fluid into the papillary interstitium.

The above-mentioned steps accomplish the generation of an extremely high urea concentration at the tip of the papilla. We turn now to the events in the thin limb:

5. The descending limb is permeable to water, but not to NaCl. Permeability to urea is low. As a consequence, water leaves the descending limb as fluid moves into a region of increasing urea concentration. The concentration of NaCl in the tubular fluid thereby progressively increases to levels exceeding those of the interstitium (Figs. 8-2, 8-4).
6. The ascending limb is permeable to NaCl, but not to water. NaCl therefore leaves the tubule by moving down its concentration gradient into the interstitium (Fig. 8-4).

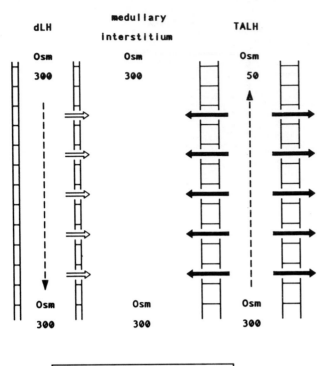

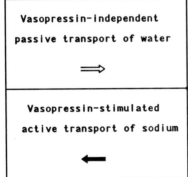

FIG. 8-2. *Transport of water and solutes in descending limb of Henle's loop (dLH) and thick ascending limb of Henle's loop (TALH).*

tip in the medulla, and water and permeant solutes (including dissolved oxygen to a significant extent) move out of the descending limb, through the interstitium, and into the ascending limb along the entire loop. Erythrocytes remain within the loop, although they shrink as they approach the tip and re-expand as they approach the cortex. Capillary plasma protein concentration increases and then decreases as blood flows around the loop. In this manner, the medullary osmotic gradient is preserved by a "counter-current exchanger" while nutrients are still delivered and wastes removed.

Renal Medullary Osmolytes

Renal medullary cells, like all others, must maintain osmotic equilibrium with the local interstitial milieu. It is well known that inorganic ions such as sodium, potassium, and chloride tend to denature macromolecules, so that the maintenance of cell function within the medulla has been a matter of scientific interest.

Studies have shown that the medullary cells maintain their osmolality in significant part by the accumulation of betaine, glycerophosphorylcholine, and the polyols sorbitol and inositol [8,10]. These solutes tend to maintain molecules in their native form [138,156] and thus counteract the effects of the high salt concentrations.

Sorbitol has been a solute of particular interest to investigators, since certain cell lines believed to be derived from renal papillary pelvic epithelium possess high levels of aldose reductase, the enzyme that catalyzes the conversion of glucose to sorbitol. Furthermore, these cells respond to incubation in high NaCl medium by increasing aldose reductase activity, thereby accumulating sorbitol to concentrations sufficient to maintain cell volume without increasing cell electrolyte content [9,21]. They respond also to replacement in normal medium by rapidly increasing sorbitol efflux [21]. A role for increased sorbitol levels in the pathogenesis of diabetic nephropathy has also been proposed [14].

Sorbitol concentration patterns during development have not been examined.

This outline, albeit incomplete, emphasizes the role of urea as a mediator of thin ascending limb salt transport and thereby provides an explanation for the reduced ability of newborn and young infants to concentrate their urine.

Medullary Blood Flow and the Vasa Recta

The medullary vasculature, like that of all other tissues, must deliver nutrients and oxygen and remove waste products and carbon dioxide. In addition, it has the task of removing the salt and water that move from the various tubular segments into the interstitium. If the capillary bed were to run directly from cortex to medullary tip, the medullary osmotic gradient would rapidly dissipate. Instead, the network is arranged in a hairpin loop with its

Vasopressin Stimulation of Water Permeability in the Distal Nephron

The control of urine osmolality, from maximally dilute to maximally concentrated, is primarily the consequence of a single effect of a single hormone—the enhancement of the water permeability of the luminal membrane of cortical and medullary collecting tubule cells by vasopressin. This is clearly a fundamental process in vertebrate physiology; indeed, much of the data describing the mechanisms that underlie vasopressin stimulation of water flow have come from studies of amphibian urinary bladder. Although there remain some important "missing links," many of the details of vasopressin-stimulated transport have been clarified over the past several years.

The cell responsible for vasopressin-stimulated water

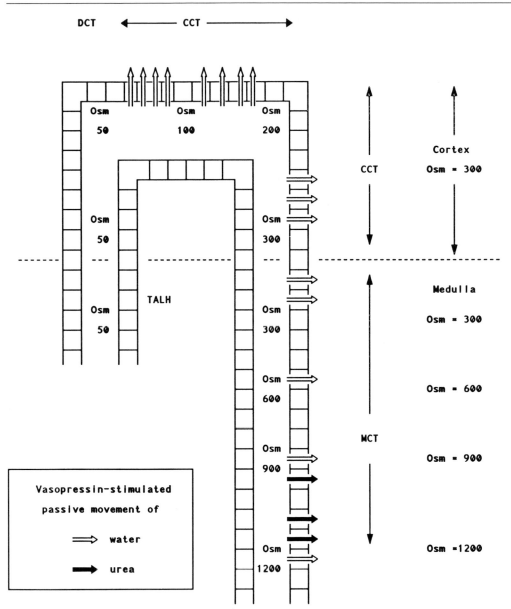

FIG. 8-3. *Water and urea transport pathways in cortical collecting tubule (CCT) and medullary collecting tubule (MCT).*

transport is the "principal" cell of the collecting tubule and the "granular" cell of the amphibian urinary bladder. These cells make up the majority of their respective epithelia, and, except where noted, they are the subject of the subsequent discussion.

Vasopressin Stimulation of Adenylate Cyclase

The vasopressin-stimulated toad urinary bladder was among the very first tissues in which both a hormone-responsive increase in cyclic adenosine monophosphate (AMP) levels

and cyclic AMP-responsive tissue function could be demonstrated [53]. Vasopressin's antidiuretic action is mediated by binding of the hormone to receptors on the tubular cell's serosal (blood-side) surface, followed by the receptor-mediated stimulation of adenylate cyclase, the enzyme that converts adenosine triphosphate (ATP) to cyclic AMP. Vasopressin binding to cortical collecting tubule is limited to principal cells [86], consistent with localization of the water permeability response to those cells [86] (Fig. 8-5).

Adenylate cyclase, like many other hormone-stimulated enzymes, consists of at least three subunits: (1) a "V2" receptor (R); (2) one of several guanosine triphosphate

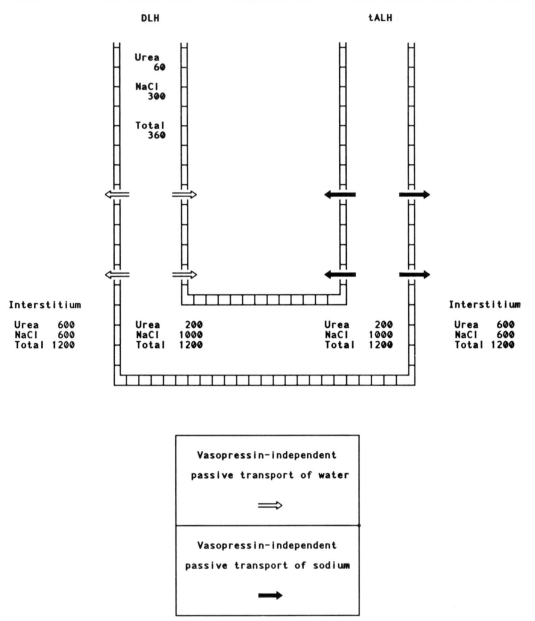

FIG. 8-4. *Development of gradient for passive efflux of sodium from thin ascending limb of Henle's loop (tALH) consequent to water efflux from descending limb (dLH).*

(GTP)-dependent guanine nucleotide regulatory proteins (G), which may have either stimulatory (Gs) or inhibitory (Gi) actions; and (3) a catalytic subunit (C) that performs the conversion of ATP to cyclic AMP. (Vasopressin may also activate a "V1" receptor, with consequences to be discussed in the subsequent section of this chapter.) Evidence for the G-protein mediation of vasopressin stimulation of adenylate cyclase has come from studies of the effect of cholera toxin, which selectively ADP-ribosylates and activates Gs and also stimulates water permeability in rabbit cortical collecting tubule [103] and toad urinary bladder

[69]. Computer models of vasopressin-stimulated adenylate cyclase in LLC-PK1 cells, a cultured pig kidney epithelial cell line, have characterized the very complex interactions among the subunits in detail [7,119,120,136]. These studies suggest that vasopressin directly stimulates only Gs, but that Gi activity is modulated by availability of GTP and receptor.

Of potential relevance to the attenuation of the concentrating mechanism in the developing kidney is the observation that the responsiveness of LLC-PK1 cell adenylate cyclase to vasopressin is increased when the cells are

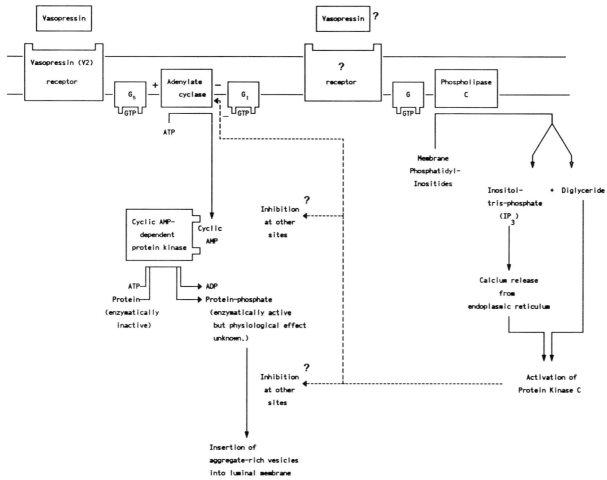

FIG. 8-5. *Intracellular mediation and modulation of vasopressin-stimulated water permeability in collecting tubule.*

incubated in hypertonic sodium chloride [135]; this finding may explain the inability of rats with chronic diabetes insipidus (in which medullary osmolality is chronically low) to concentrate their urine acutely after vasopressin [57]. It perhaps also accounts at least in part for the attenuated responsiveness of the developing kidney in which medullary osmolality is chronically diminished.

Cyclic AMP-Dependent Kinase

Cyclic AMP-dependent protein kinase (kinase A) is the primary intracellular receptor for cyclic AMP. Vasopressin stimulation of kinase A activity has been described in renal medullary tubular cells [35,36] and in cells from toad urinary bladder [124]. Although the substrate phosphorylated by kinase A has not yet been defined, studies have suggested that the kinase can influence cytoskeletal structure in other tissues [1,88], thereby suggesting a possible mode of action for the enzyme.

Interactions Among Vasopressin, Calcium, and Phospholipid Derivatives

In the kidney and amphibian bladder, as in many other tissues, hormone-stimulated events involve interactions between calcium and cyclic AMP as cellular messengers. These interactions can occur both via interregulation of the concentrations of the messengers themselves and at more distal steps modulating the responses to the individual messages. Furthermore, agents and experimental maneuvers that greatly increase or decrease cell calcium can influence (typically diminish) vasopressin-stimulated water flow [95].

These interactions are not limited to the kidney. In smooth muscle and liver, for example, vasopressin-stimulated responses are mediated not by the V2 receptor–stimulated adenylate cyclase, but by a vasopressin-stimulated phospholipase C, consequent to vasopressin-binding to a V1 receptor. Studies have suggested that products of phospholipase C activation may play an important role in modulating vasopressin-stimulated water flow and that vasopressin may activate phospholipase C in tubular cells.

The products of phospholipase C hydrolysis of the membrane lipid phosphatidylinositol bis phosphate include 1,4,5 inositol triphosphate and diglyceride. The inositol trisphosphate can release calcium from intracellular stores [104,147], whereas the diglyceride activates a phospholipid-dependent kinase, now known as protein kinase, C and increases its sensitivity to calcium [45,104]. Protein kinase C in turn is able to phosphorylate several proteins, among them several that are also phosphorylated by cyclic AMP–dependent kinase [45].

PROTEIN KINASE C

Evidence supporting a role for protein kinase C as a modulator of vasopressin action has been facilitated by studies examining the effects of phorbol esters, which mimic the stimulatory effect of diglycerides on both protein kinase C activation and on the physiologic response to hormones in other tissues [23,104,116], and membrane permeant diglycerides such as dioctanoyl glycerol [116]. In the toad urinary bladder, both phorbol myristate acetate (PMA—an active phorbol ester) and dioctanoyl glycerol inhibit water flow stimulated by vasopressin, but not flow stimulated by forskolin (when prostaglandin synthesis was inhibited) or exogenous cyclic AMP [125]. Stimulation by 8-bromo cyclic AMP, a nonhydrolyzable analog, was inhibited by PMA, consistent with an additional "post–cyclic AMP" site of action. The pattern of action suggests that PMA inhibits primarily at the level of the receptor or GTP-regulatory protein of adenylate cyclase, rather than at the catalytic portion of the enzyme.

Similar effects of PMA on both vasopressin-stimulated water flow and 8-bromo-cyclic AMP–stimulated water flow have been reported in rabbit cortical collecting tubule [4]. Consistent with a site of action at adenylate cyclase, PMA decreases both cell cyclic AMP content and the in-situ level of cyclic AMP–dependent protein kinase in toad bladder [125]. The toad bladder data are consistent with other reports demonstrating that phorbol esters elicit downregulation of adenylate cyclase [34,136].

In contrast to the toad bladder data, which demonstrate calcium modulation of submaximally stimulated water permeability, studies in rabbit cortical collecting tubule suggest that kinase C inhibits flow only when the tissue is exposed to very high (nonphysiologic) concentrations of vasopressin and not to concentrations of vasopressin attainable in vivo [3].

Calcium and Calmodulin

At least some of the effects of calcium on cell metabolism may be mediated via its modulation of calmodulin, a virtually ubiquitous calcium-binding protein. Calmodulin is known to regulate the activities of many enzymes that are potentially relevant to mediation or modulation of vasopressin-stimulated water permeability, including adenylate cyclase, phosphodiesterase, calcium ATPase, myosin light chain kinase, and phospholipase [25]. In particular, calmodulin can regulate vasopressin-sensitive adenylate cyclase in LLC-PK1 cells (see previously) [6]. Other investigations into the role of calmodulin have focused on the effects of trifluoperazine and W-7, two agents that bind to calmodulin in a calcium-dependent manner, thereby blocking its ability to activate calmodulin-regulated enzymes. In the toad urinary bladder, both trifluoperazine and W-7 inhibit vasopressin-stimulated water permeability with a pattern suggesting a "post–cyclic AMP" site of action [13,50,93,157].

The response to these agents in the kidney is somewhat different. Both trifluoperazine and W-7 inhibit stimulation of cyclic AMP production by vasopressin in cultured rat papillary collecting tubule cells [76]. Blockade of calmodulin-dependent enzymes may also mediate the clinically relevant inhibition of renal concentrating ability by tetracycline antibiotics [126]. Taken together, these data suggest that calcium may enhance vasopressin-stimulated water permeability via activation of calmodulin-dependent enzymes.

These observations support the view that calcium can have both stimulatory and inhibitory effects on vasopressin-stimulated water transport across responsive epithelial cells. However, they do not deal with the important question of whether the normal response to vasopressin requires some steady-state level of cytosolic free calcium in order to take place or whether indeed vasopressin-elicited changes in calcium play a regulatory role in the response to hormone. Defining the answers to these questions is complicated by the need to evaluate the very low concentration of free cytoplasmic calcium as compared with the high calcium concentrations in the extracellular fluid and cell organelles.

One laboratory has demonstrated that both vasopressin and the phosphodiesterase inhibitor theophylline decrease fluorescence of quin-2, an indicator of free calcium concentration, with a time course paralleling the enhancement of water transport in toad urinary bladder, suggesting that these stimuli of water permeability also diminish intracellular calcium [20]. However, another laboratory [144] demonstrated no such effect.

In the rabbit renal cortical collecting tubule, vasopressin has been shown to elicit a small calcium transient in the water transporting principal cells, which could not be reproduced by the selective V_2 agonist desmopressin, 1-(3-mercaptopropionic acid)-8-D-arginine vaso-pressin (dDAVP) [22], suggesting thereby that the cells contained V_2 responsive phospholipase C.

PROSTAGLANDINS

Measurement of phospholipid turnover and prostaglandin synthesis has offered another approach to the question of whether vasopressin alters calcium and phospholipid metabolism via V2 receptors. Exposure to vasopressin increases the synthesis of phosphatidic acid and phosphatidylinositol in toad bladder epithelial cells, presumably by activation of phospholipase C, whereas incubation with phosphodiesterase inhibitor did not increase synthesis, suggesting a direct effect of vasopressin, rather than cyclic AMP [127]. Furthermore, vasopressin, but not cyclic AMP, stimulates the production of prostaglandins by toad bladder epithelial cells [15,19,158], suspensions of cortical and medullary collecting tubules [128], and cultured cells of cortical tubular origin [44]. Since prostaglandins are metabolites of phospholipid-bound arachidonic acid, these data would support the view that there is indeed increased turnover of membrane phospholipid after exposure to vasopressin, presumably mediated by V2 receptors. The prostaglandins in turn have been shown to inhibit water permeability by actions at several sites within the stimulatory cascade [48,105,123], including G proteins and post–cyclic AMP sites.

Events at the Luminal Membrane

Although the binding of vasopressin to its receptors occurs at the basolateral surface of the epithelial cell, the eventual increase in epithelial cell permeability to water occurs via alterations in the cell's luminal membrane [47]. In the absence of vasopressin, the permeability of the luminal membrane (best measured in the rabbit cortical collecting tubule) is extremely low compared with that of most other cell membranes. After exposure to vasopressin, luminal membrane permeability increases many-fold, but remains only about one-seventh that of the basolateral membrane [141], at least in part because the latter has a far greater area. Thus, in the collecting tubule, the luminal membrane provides virtually all the resistance to flow in the absence of hormone and when it is present.

Data obtained using freeze-fracture electron microscopy, first in amphibian urinary bladders and subsequently in renal tubules, have linked this response to the appearance within the luminal membrane of clusters (called "aggregates") of 80 Å diameter particles [26,56,85] (Fig. 8-6).

Numerous studies have specifically related the aggregates to water permeability and not to the ability to transport either urea or sodium [84,94]. Membrane vesicles rich in aggregates have been shown to have an extremely high water permeability [151], consistent with this formulation. There is a close correlation between aggregate turnover and urine osmolality (and presumably with collecting tubule water permeability as well) in rats with diabetes insipidus before and after the infusion of vasopressin [90].

The transport characteristics of the vasopressin-elicited water pathway (and presumably, although not definitively, those of the aggregate particles) support the view that the pathway is a channel, sufficiently narrow to exclude molecules even as small as urea [41,92] and equal to 6 to 12 water molecule diameters in length [61,91,92,107]. The water permeability of the pathway may not be constant, but may vary with changes in the cell pH [27,108] and perhaps other factors as well. The structure of the transport system has not yet been characterized, although significant progress toward isolation has been made in this regard [52,58].

The relationship between the vasopressin-induced water channel and the channel believed to be constitutively present in erythrocyte membranes [137] has been a provocative one [109]. Mercurial reagents such as p-chloromercuribenzene sulfonic acid (pCMBS) and HgCl2 are known to inhibit flow across erythrocyte water channels

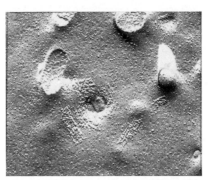

Fig. 8-6. *Freeze-fracture replica of vasopressin-elicited particle aggregates from granular cell luminal membrane of toad urinary bladder, a tissue whose permeability to water increases after vasopressin. Note proximity of aggregates to fused aggrephores.*

[99], and studies [68] have demonstrated similar effects of these agents in toad urinary bladder, suggesting that the structures may have features in common.

Cellular Events Mediating Aggregate Appearance and Recovery

How do these important structures reach their place in the luminal membrane? Using toad urinary bladder, Wade [152] and Humbert et al. [74] have demonstrated that the aggregates exist preformed within the walls of intracellular tubular structures. These structures, referred to as "aggrephores," then fuse with the luminal membrane on exposure to vasopressin [102]. Thus, the vasopressin-elicited increase in water permeability does not require acute synthesis of new transport pathways, but only the insertion of preformed ones (Fig. 8-7).

The onset of water flow begins rapidly upon vasopressin stimulation, with a delay in collecting tubule of only 20 to 30 seconds for onset of flow, and 3.5 minutes for half-maximal flow [87]. In toad urinary bladder, flow response times are similar, and increases in membrane capacitance, consistent with the addition of aggrephore membrane to the luminal surface, also occur very rapidly [106,140].

The mode of aggregate delivery to the surface varies from species to species. In toad bladder, the primary delivery pattern involves fusion of intact aggrephores with the luminal surface [60,102]. The aggrephore heads are often coated with clathrin, suggesting a mechanism for their movement to the surface. In frog urinary bladder and rat renal collecting tubule, on the other hand, fused aggrephores are unusual [32,33], and the aggregates may well be delivered predominantly via small clathrin-coated vesicles [17,43], which may have budded either from the aggrephores or from the Golgi complex, where the aggregate particles are presumed to be synthesized.

Cytoskeletal elements appear to mediate the movement of aggregates from the cell interior to its surface. Vasopressin induces polymerization of monomeric actin into

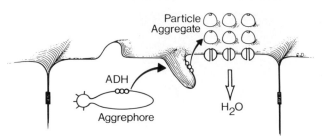

FIG. 8-7. *Model of particle delivery to luminal membrane (courtesy of Dr. Richard M. Hays).*

filamentous actin in toad bladder cells [30]. An intact cytoskeleton is required for the vasopressin response; exposure of tissues to the microtubule-disrupting agent colchicine or to the microfilament inhibitor cytochalasin B leads to inhibition of subsequent vasopressin-stimulated water flow [83,145,146]. These studies are complicated, however, by a lack of specificity. Colchicine has been shown to stimulate prostaglandin E_2 formation [12,18], and cytochalasin B can disrupt tissue architecture during water flow [55].

When vasopressin is removed from responsive tissues, water permeability falls rapidly, and luminal membrane aggregate frequency diminishes. Transcellular water flow (i.e., the presence of an osmotic gradient between tubular fluid and cell) accelerates this process [59]. In toad urinary bladder, fused aggrephores, still containing a large number of aggregates, detach from the luminal membrane after vasopressin removal [28], and endocytosis of luminal membrane via coated pits has been demonstrated in cortical collecting tubule [142].

Vasopressin Stimulation of Other Renal Tissues

Vasopressin Stimulation of NaCl Reabsorption by Thick Ascending Limb

In contrast to many other discoveries of renal physiology, the first evidence that vasopressin might enhance salt reabsorption by thick ascending limb was derived from a systematic segmental analysis of hormone-stimulated adenylate cyclase and not from transport experiments [75,101]. Shortly afterwards, workers from several laboratories demonstrated that vasopressin enhances cyclic AMP–dependent protein kinase activity in rat medullary thick ascending limb tubules [40] and increases sodium chloride reabsorption by medullary, but not cortical, thick ascending limb tubules isolated from rat and mouse, but not from rabbit [51,63,122]. Exogenous vasopressin also increases NaCl reabsorption by medullary tubules of Brattleboro rats, as assessed by micropuncture and microperfusion [31,155]. Vasopressin does not appear to increase cyclic AMP production in medullary thick ascending limbs isolated from pump-perfused human kidneys [24]. However, the sugges-

tion has been made that this unresponsiveness may derive from epithelial damage during pump perfusion [65].

Two potential sites of vasopressin's action are currently under active investigation. One group of studies localizes the primary site of vasopressin's action to the basolateral chloride conductance pathway [49]. Increases in basolateral chloride conductance increase chloride movement from cell to blood down its electrochemical gradient and diminishes cell chloride, thereby increasing the gradient for transport from lumen to cell.

A second line of evidence supports the view that vasopressin increases the rate of salt reabsorption by medullary thick ascending limb by increasing the number of functional Na-K-2Cl cotransport units in the epithelium's apical membrane [62,64]. In the absence of furosemide, vasopressin increases total transcellular conductance, with the majority of that increase attributable to the basolateral membrane. However, when luminal furosemide (which specifically blocks Na-K-2Cl entry into the cell) is present, vasopressin alters neither total transcellular conductance nor the individual membrane conductances. Thus, the increase in the basolateral conductance, although large, is considered in this formulation to be a secondary phenomenon, attributable to a primary increase in salt (in particular chloride) [65,100] entry across the apical membrane.

The stimulation of NaCl reabsorption by vasopressin could enhance renal concentrating capacity in several ways. First, any increase in interstitial osmolality adjacent to the thick ascending limb cells would enhance water reabsorption from the adjacent outer medullary collecting tubules, thereby increasing fluid osmolality and decreasing downstream flow. Second, this water removal would increase the concentration of urea in the collecting duct fluid as it passes toward the inner medulla. All else being the same, this increased urea concentration would cause more urea to be delivered to the inner medullary interstitium, where it would lead to increased reabsorption of water from the descending thin limbs of long-looped nephrons, and eventually thereby to increased passive salt reabsorption by the thin ascending limbs, a step necessary for function of the countercurrent multiplier in regions that lack active salt reabsorption.

Vasopressin Stimulation of Urea Permeability in Terminal Collecting Tubule

As discussed earlier, the recycling of urea and its delivery to the medullary interstitium are critical components of the passive model of the countercurrent multiplier. In contrast to amphibian urinary bladder, the urea permeability of collecting tubule segments is low and is not increased by exposure to vasopressin.

The sole exception to this is the terminal two-thirds of the inner medullary collecting duct, where basal urea permeability is high (1.7 μ/second) and increases to the extremely high level of 6.9 μ/second after vasopressin [121]. One would anticipate that the combination of vasopressin-stimulated water reabsorption in the cortical and medullary collecting tubules (which would greatly increase the concentration of urea within the tubular lumen), together with the above-mentioned increase in urea permeability at the very end of the medullary collecting tubule, would maximize efflux of urea from the terminal medullary collecting tubule and its appearance in the interstitium of the medullary tip. At that site, it would effect maximum enhancement of water removal from the thin descending limb and the eventual passive reabsorption of sodium from the thin ascending limb.

Effects of Vasopressin on Renal Vasculature

Vasopressin selectively decreases inner medullary flow [148], and this can be inhibited by V_1 antagonists [78], suggesting V_1 mediation of the vasoconstriction. Some laboratories [29,150], but not others [77], have demonstrated that vasopressin increases GFR of juxtamedullary nephrons. The mechanism of this effect is currently unknown.

Ontogeny of Renal Concentrating Ability

Maximum urinary osmolality in newborns is approximately one-half that observed in older members of the same species in humans [39,54,112,154], rats [66,149], and rabbits [42]. The modest increase in minimum urine flow rate, and therefore in requisite water intake, is of little consequence so long as the newborn is otherwise healthy and has adequate access to water but may become life-threatening in clinical settings characterized by extrarenal fluid losses in the face of inadequate intake.

The newborn's limitation in urinary concentrating ability has been attributed to combinations of several factors, among them the availability of medullary solute (particularly urea), medullary anatomy, salt reabsorption by distal nephron segments, and the responsiveness of tubular water permeability to vasopressin.

Availability of Medullary Solute

Under usual circumstances, in both children and adults, about half the papillary solute is salt and the remainder urea. Infants typically ingest a diet that is limited in protein and are in an anabolic state. As a result, the production and eventual excretion rates for urea are low compared with those of older children. Furthermore, the concentration of urea in the papilla is also low—only about one-fourth of the total solute.

If full-term infants are administered a high protein diet or fed urea, urinary osmolality increases almost to adult levels, with the additional urinary solute consisting entirely of urea. The proportion of urea to salt in the urine increases as well [37,39]. Urea feeding does not diminish urine volume, nor does it alter salt excretion. These data suggest that the low rate of urea production and consequent diminished medullary accumulation, rather than any abnormality of tubular function or anatomy, are responsible for much of the newborn human's limited urine osmolality. That is, the urine osmolality is low primarily because the urine contains relatively little urea and not because it contains too much water.

In this regard, one could make the case that the human full-term newborn, although not the preterm infant, does not have a meaningful concentrating defect because he or she can concentrate salt (the only solutes relevant to cell and extracellular fluid volumes) to the same extent as the adult can. Nonetheless, significant differences have been observed in medullary structure and function, and are considered in the following sections.

Circulating Vasopressin Levels

Early studies [67,79] suggested that the newborn had diminished pituitary stores and plasma levels of vasopressin, although vasopressin could be demonstrated in the urine of newborns. More recent studies using immunoassay methods, however, have demonstrated that plasma vasopressin levels in the fetus [117,153] and the newborn [89,134] respond appropriately to volume and osmolar stimuli. Furthermore, very high levels of vasopressin have been demonstrated in cord blood [111]. Thus, low vasopressin levels are not the cause of diminished concentrating ability.

Vasopressin-Stimulated Cyclic AMP Production

Immaturity of vasopressin-stimulated adenylate cyclase has been suggested as a contributor to the diminished concentrating ability of the developing kidney. Vasopressin causes smaller increases in cyclic AMP levels in medullary slices obtained from 1- to 14-day-old puppies than in slices obtained from adult animals [98]. In addition, tissues from neonatal rats demonstrate decreased vasopressin stimulation of adenylate cyclase both in kidney homogenates [46] and in renal medullary membranes [113]. This diminished responsiveness correlated with a decrease in the number of vasopressin binding sites in the developing rat renal medulla, suggesting that a deficiency of receptor sites accounted at least in part for the decrease in cyclase activation [113]. Direct comparison of vasopressin-stimulated adenylate cyclase activity in isolated cortical collecting tubules by Schlondorff and co-workers [131] showed that the activity in tubules obtained from 10-day-old rabbits was less than one-tenth that of tubules from adults. Sodium fluoride–stimulated enzyme activity was diminished as well, to about one-fifth of adult levels, suggesting a decrease beyond the receptor level in the isolated tubules. Finally, the activity of cAMP phosphodiesterase appears to be increased in developing rats [46], whereas the activity of both cyclic AMP and cyclic AMP–dependent kinase is diminished [129,130].

In one-day-old piglets, exogenous administration of dDAVP, a nonmetabolizable but biologically active vasopressin analog, neither decreased urine volume nor increased renal medullary cyclic AMP content. In contrast, simultaneous infusion of dDAVP with dibutyryl cyclic AMP, a permeant analog of cyclic AMP that resists degradation by phosphodiesterase, caused a marked decrease in urine flow rate, an increase in urine osmolality, and an

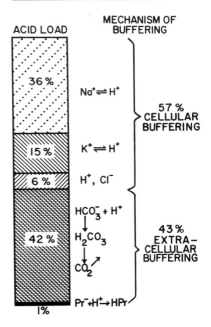

FIG. 9-1. *Mechanisms of buffering of nonvolatile acid in acute metabolic acidosis.* (From *Swan RC, Pitts RF: Neutralization of infused acid by nephrectomized dogs.* J Clin Invest 34:205, 1955, with permission.)

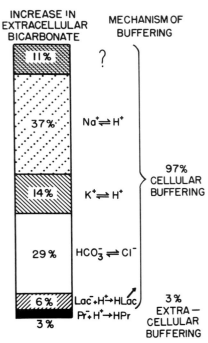

FIG. 9-2. *Mechanisms of buffering of CO_2 in respiratory acidosis.* (From *Giebisch G, Berger L, Pitts RF: The extra renal response to acute acid–base disturbances of respiratory origin.* J Clin Invest 34:231, 1955, with permission.)

cellular buffering [194,257]. Primary changes in pCO_2, causing respiratory acidosis (Fig. 9-2) or alkalosis, are not well buffered extracellularly because HCO_3^- does not serve as a good buffer for H_2CO_3 in the absence of respiratory control [86a,194]. Rather, these disturbances are buffered by cellular Na^+/H^+, K^+/H^+, and Cl^-/HCO_3^- exchange [86a,194].

Acid–base disorders are observed when the renal or respiratory functions are abnormal or when a load of acid or base overwhelms the defense mechanisms. A disturbance that tends to cause the extracellular pH to fall ([H^+] rises) is called acidosis; a disturbance causing it to rise ([H^+] falls) is called alkalosis. If the disturbance is associated primarily with a change in HCO_3^- concentration, it is called metabolic. An abnormally low level of blood pH is designated acidemia; the converse is referred to as alkalemia. If the rate of alveolar ventilation is abnormal, causing a change in pCO_2, the disturbance is called respiratory. Thus, there are four primary acid–base disorders: metabolic acidosis, metabolic alkalosis, respiratory acidosis, and respiratory alkalosis.

Generally, there is a compensatory response by the unaffected system to restore the extracellular pH toward normal. For example, metabolic acidosis, which is associated primarily with acidemia due to a reduced concentration of extracellular HCO_3^-, is partially compensated for by a decrease in pCO_2, resulting from an increased rate of alveolar ventilation. The loss of CO_2 through the lungs in

response to addition of strong acid results in temporary and incomplete correction of the blood pH (Eqn 3) at the expense of further lowering of plasma HCO_3^- concentration. Respiratory alkalosis, which is associated with alkalemia due to a primarily increased rate of alveolar ventilation, is partially compensated for by a reduced concentration of HCO_3^-, brought about by increased renal excretion of base.

Note that the renal compensation for a primary respiratory disturbance is relatively slow, requiring at least a few days to reach a new steady state [197]. During the early adaptive period, little change in plasma HCO_3^- concentration is noted, despite even a large change in pCO_2 and thereby in extracellular pH. As the renal response develops, the plasma HCO_3^- concentration rises and extracellular pH is shifted toward normal.

Confidence bands for plasma pH and HCO_3^- concentration as functions of pCO_2 have been established for adults with acute and chronic acid–base disorders [16,233] but not for children (Fig. 9-3).

Acute cellular buffering results in an increase of 1 mM HCO_3^- for each 10-mm increase in pCO_2 [16,33]. Thus, acute respiratory acidosis, with a pCO_2 of 80 mm Hg will result in a 4-mM increase in plasma HCO_3^- and a fall in pH to 7.17. The renal response occurs much more slowly than cellular buffering, but when complete will minimize the change in blood pH by compensating with a 3.5-mM rise in plasma HCO_3^- for each 10-mm increase in pCO_2.

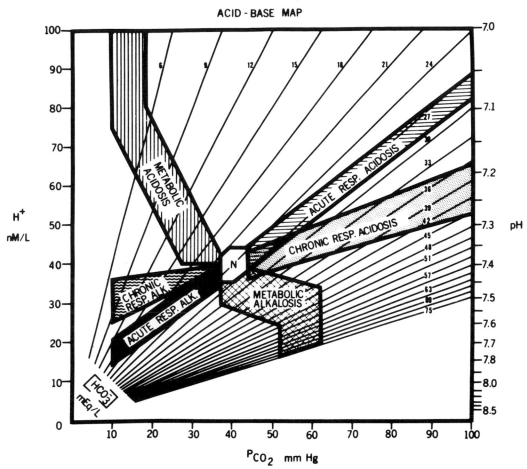

FIG. 9-3. *Acid–base map constructed from the arterial blood gas values from patients with various acid–base disorders. Normal adult values are in the area labeled N. (From Goldberg M, Green SB, et al: Computer-based instruction and diagnosis of acid–base disorders. JAMA 223:269, 1973, with permission.)*

Because of renal compensation, chronic respiratory acidosis and a pCO_2 of 80 mm will result in a rise in plasma HCO_3^- concentration of 14 mm and thus a fall in pH only to 7.30 [233,268].

Mixed acid–base disturbances are observed commonly. In the nursery the severely acidemic infant with sepsis and respiratory distress syndrome may be noted to have both a reduced plasma HCO_3^- concentration (metabolic acidosis) and an elevated pCO_2 (respiratory acidosis). In other situations the extracellular pH may be close to normal, but associated with large reductions in both plasma HCO_3^- concentration and pCO_2, reflecting a mixed metabolic acidosis and respiratory alkalosis, as may be seen in the septic baby with respiratory distress syndrome who is mechanically overventilated. Care must be taken not to interpret this as metabolic acidosis with respiratory compensation, since compensation is almost never complete. Rather, the normal pH suggests a mixed disorder.

Metabolic Aspects

The study of acid–base balance requires knowledge of net protons added to the body fluids by metabolism and growth. A simplified approach to this system [104] relies on the electric charge of the reactants and products to determine whether a process generates or consumes protons. For instance, if a neutral substance A^0 is metabolized to a product B^0, no net protons are generated:

$$A^0 \rightarrow B^0,$$

where superscripts are used to denote net charge on the reactants.

On the other hand, if A^0 is metabolized to the anion C^- in the cell water, this reaction generates a proton to preserve electrical neutrality:

$$A^0 \rightarrow C^- + H^+$$

or

$$A^0 + OH^- \rightarrow C^-$$

Similarly, if A^0 is metabolized to the cation D^+, a proton must have been consumed (or a hydroxyl ion generated).

$$A^0 \rightarrow D^+ + OH^-$$

or

$$A^0 + H^+ \rightarrow D^+$$

In general, the oxidation of most carbohydrates and triglycerides to CO_2 and water generates no net protons [104]. For instance, complete oxidation of glucose to CO_2 and water generates no net protons:

$$Glucose^0 \rightarrow CO_2^0 + H_2O^0$$

But the partial oxidation of glucose leads to the production of lactic acid and possibly to lactic acidosis:

$$Glucose^0 \rightarrow Lactate^- + H^+$$

The metabolism of neutral amino acids fails to generate net acid. But when sulfur-containing neutral amino acids are converted into sulfate anions, sulfuric acid is produced:

$$Met^0 \text{ or } Cys^0 \rightarrow Glucose^0 + Urea^0 + SO_4^{-2} + 2H^+$$

The conversion of cationic amino acids into neutral products will also generate protons:

$$Arg^+ \rightarrow Glucose^0 + Urea^0 + H^+$$

In contrast, metabolism of dietary and organic anions (acetate, citrate, gluconate) to neutral end products will consume protons:

$$Lactate^- + H^+ \rightarrow Glucose^0 + CO_2^0 + H_2O^0$$

Renal Excretion of NH_4^+

Although sulfuric and hydrochloric acid cannot be destroyed directly by metabolic processes, they can be removed by H^+-consuming processes and the renal excretion of NH_4^+. The conversion of glutamine in the kidney to glucose results in the consumption of two protons:

$$Glutamine^0 \rightarrow 2NH_4^+ + \text{Carboxylate anion}^{-2}$$
$$\text{Carboxylate anion}^{-2} + 2H^+ \rightarrow Glucose^0 + CO_2$$

If the carboxylate anion is consumed with an equivalent

amount of protons and ammonium ions are excreted into the urine, net acid is eliminated from the body. Note that the excretion of ammonium generated from glutamine metabolism per se does not eliminate net acid from the body. The consumption of carboxylate anions occurs during gluconeogenesis from glutamine in the kidney. However, if the ammonium is converted to urea, and not excreted as NH_4^+, net proton consumption is prevented:

$$2NH_4^+ + CO_2 \rightarrow Urea^0 + 2H^+$$

Although ammonium excretion per se does not eliminate net acid from the body, because the pK of ammonia and amino groups is so alkaline that these nitrogen groups have already combined with protons at physiologic pH, ammonium excretion does preserve other cations and does prevent urea synthesis (and H^+ production) from the glutamine-derived ammonium [104]. Thus, the measurement of urinary ammonium serves as a useful marker of the extent of proton removal by the kidney.

Renal Excretion of H_2PO_4

An analysis of phosphate intake and its contribution to titratable acid excretion requires knowledge of the ratio $H_2PO_4^- - HPO_4^{-2}$ in both diet and urine.

The major constituent of titratable acid in the urine is $H_2PO_4^-$. For its excretion HPO_4^{-2} must be filtered at the glomerulus, escape reabsorption by the tubules, and then be converted to $H_2PO_4^-$ by H^+ ions secreted by tubular cells. To analyze whether this excretion of $H_2PO_4^-$ participates in the elimination of protons generated from the oxidation of protein, one must know the nature of the dietary phosphate. If dietary phosphate is HPO_4^{-2} and is excreted as $H_2PO_4^-$, this would lead to the elimination of part of the acid load derived from protein. On the other hand, if dietary phosphate is in the form of $H_2PO_4^-$, the excretion of urinary $H_2PO_4^-$ cannot assist in getting rid of the protons generated from the oxidation of protein [104]. But 80% of dietary $H_2PO_4^-$ is converted to extracellular HPO_4^{-2} (at pH 7.40). Therefore, the excretion of $H_2PO_4^-$ is usually important in maintaining the systemic pH during the metabolism of protein.

Ratios of $H_2PO_4^- - HPO_4^{-2}$ in meat muscle, cow's milk, and fruits and vegetables are 14:14, 2:4, and 4:1, respectively [104]. These data suggest that the urinary phosphate excretion of the infant on a major milk diet or a child on a high quality meat diet represents a substantial vehicle for the net elimination of protons produced from protein oxidation and thereby contributes to acid–base balance. Nevertheless, since the excretion of phosphate is regulated to control phosphate balance rather than acid–base balance, phosphate excretion is not increased in response to acidosis, and titratable acid excretion becomes progressively less important with increasing degrees of metabolic acidosis.

From elaborate acid balance studies performed in healthy premature infants, Kildeberg et al. [134] have shown that the deposition of base in bone (hydroxyapatite) during active skeletal growth contributes substantially to the metabolic proton load. During the process of skeletal mineralization, hydroxyapatite synthesis is associated with a release of protons:

$$10 \, Ca^{+2} + 4.8 \, HPO_4^- + 1.2 \, H_2PO_4^- + 2 \, H_2O \rightarrow$$
$$[Ca_3 \, (PO_4)_2]_3 \cdot Ca \, (OH)_2 + 9.2 \, H^+$$

The incorporation of one g of calcium into the growing skeleton causes the release of 20 mEq of protons [134,135]. Thus, in the healthy premature infant, a gain of 50–60 mg of calcium from skeletal hydroxyapatite deposition results in the generation of approximately one mEq of proton that must be excreted by the kidney or be neutralized by the gastrointestinal absorption of base [134,135]. This burden is superimposed on the acid load generated from endogenous acid production, from urinary organic anion excretion, and from sulfuric acid production, which total approximately 2 mEq/kg/day [134,135].

These studies have been extended to full-term infants and growing children by Chan [46], who found that endogenous acid production consistently exceeded that of adults (1 mEq/kg/day) by 0.5–1 mEq/kg/day [46]. No wonder that the growing infant, with relatively immature mechanisms for renal excretion [129,251] and rapid mineralization of the skeleton, is generally hypobasemic compared with the adult [75,76,228] and at risk of developing metabolic acidosis during periods of stress or increased catabolism.

Segmental Analysis of Renal H$^+$ Transport

The reabsorption of filtered HCO$_3^-$ and the excretion of net acid are accomplished by H$^+$ secretion from the renal tubular cell into the lumen. The segments that are responsible for H$^+$ secretion include the proximal tubule, the collecting duct, and, to a lesser extent, the distal tubule, connecting tubule, and thick ascending limb of the loop of Henle (Fig. 9-4) [14,141,155]. The three ultrastructurally distinct segments of the proximal tubule contribute to the reabsorption of as much as 90% of the filtered HCO$_3^-$ (Fig. 9-5) [14,141]. Studies of isolated perfused proximal tubular segments have shown that the straight portion reabsorbs HCO$_3^-$ at a rate substantially below that of the convoluted portion (Fig. 9-6) [29,123], perhaps in keeping with the smaller amounts of filtered HCO$_3^-$ escaping the early proximal tubule.

The thick limb of the loop of Henle has been thought to play little role in urinary acidification [14,29,141]. Studies of isolated perfused thick ascending limbs from rabbit or mouse have not shown significant HCO$_3^-$ absorption [83,121]. However, experiments in cortical and medullary thick ascending limbs taken from rats have shown HCO$_3^-$ absorptive rates of 5–10 pmol/min/mm [98], which are lower than that of the rabbit proximal straight tubule [179] and less than 5% of that measured in the in vivo perfused rat proximal convoluted tubule [11]. Nevertheless, such transport rates would be capable of reclaiming a substantial

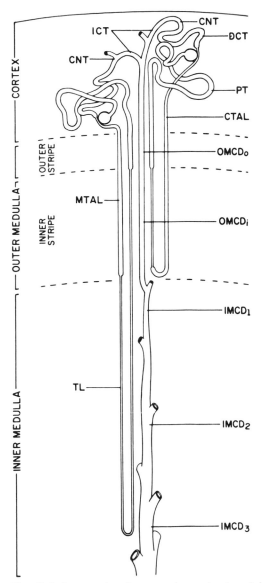

Fig. 9-4. *Structural and segmental organization of the mammalian kidney. Diagram of a superficial and juxtamedullary nephron. CNT, connecting tubule; ICT, initial collecting tubule; PT, proximal tubule; CTAL, cortical thick ascending limb; OMCD$_o$, outer medullary collecting duct from outer stripe; MTAL, medullary thick ascending limb; OMCD$_i$, outer medullary collecting duct from inner stripe; OMCD$_1$, outer third of inner medullary collecting duct; IMCD$_2$, middle third of inner medullary collecting duct; IMCD$_3$, inner third of inner medullary collecting duct; TL, thin limb of Henle's loop. (From Madsen KM, Tisher CC: Structural-functional relationships along the distal nephron. Am J Physiol 250:F1, 1986, with permission.)*

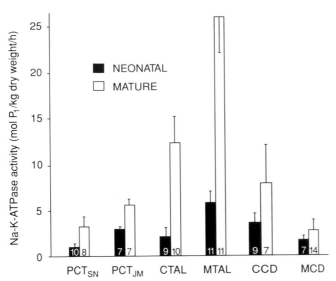

FIG. 10-3. *Distribution of ATPase activity in neonatal and mature rabbit nephron. Values are means ± SD. Numbers in bars indicate the number of analyzed tubular segments. Abbreviations: PCT$_{SN}$, proximal convoluted tubules (early segment) of subcapsular nephron; PCT$_{JM}$, proximal convoluted tubule (early segment) from juxtamedullary nephron. CTAL, cortical thick ascending loop of Henle. MTALH, medullary thick ascending loop of Henle. CCD, cortical collecting duct. MCD, medullary collecting duct. (From Schmidt U, Horster M: Na-K-activated ATPase: Activity maturation in rabbit nephron segments dissected in vitro. Am J Physiol 233:F55, 1977, with permission.)*

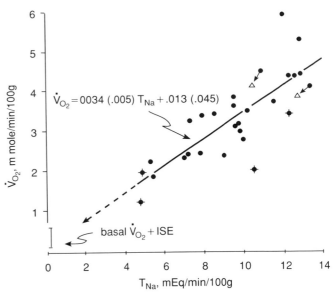

FIG. 10-4. *Relationship between O_2 consumption (VO_2) and net Na^+ reabsorption (T_{Na}) during water diuresis (●), water diuresis plus elevated ureteral pressure (+), or following Pitressin infusion (Δ) sufficient to inhibit water diuresis without affecting blood flow. Symbols are means of two or more consecutive clearance periods. (From Knox FG, Fleming JS, Rennie DW: Effect of osmotic diuresis on sodium reabsorption and oxygen consumption of kidney. Am J Physiol 210:751, 1966, with permission.)*

the paracellular pathway, by diffusion or solvent drag or both, and that only one-third of the Na^+ reabsorbed in these segments occurs through active transcellular transport [99]. Na^+ crosses the luminal membranes of proximal cells in countertransport with H^+ [194] or in cotransport (Fig. 10-7) with glucose [159], amino acids [84], organic acids (e.g., lactate) [21], and inorganic anions (e.g., phosphate) [131], and most of it is actively extruded from the cells at the basolateral side by the ouabain inhibitable Na^+-K^+-ATPase (Fig. 10-8). One-third of the Na^+ that enters the cell in exchange for H^+ exits across the basolateral membrane in cotransport with HCO_3^- rather than through the Na^+-K^+-ATPase [4]. This basolateral HCO_3^- coupled Na^+ extrusion represents net Na^+ reabsorption not coupled directly to ATP utilization and hence contributes to the high efficiency of Na^+ transport in the proximal tubule.

The preferential reabsorption of $NaHCO_3$ and of cotransported organic solutes in the early segments of the proximal tubules establishes transepithelial Cl^- and HCO_3^- gradients [196] and small electrical potential and effective osmotic pressure differences across the PCT epithelium [7]. These driving forces, in turn, induce osmotic and ionic flows across the paracellular pathway (see Fig. 10-7). These fluxes, although passive in nature, are dependent on the establishment of osmotic and electrochemical potential gradients for Cl^-, HCO_3^-, and preferentially reabsorbed solutes across the epithelium generated by the

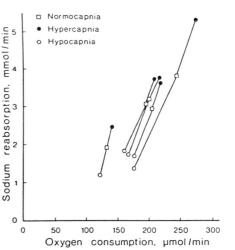

FIG. 10-5. *Changes in sodium reabsorption and oxygen consumption induced by raising (open circles) or reducing (closed circles) plasma PCO_2, at constant plasma bicarbonate concentration ($32 ± 1$ mM) in five dogs, during continuous infusion of ethacrynic acid. Average change in Na^+ reabsorption per μmol change in oxygen consumption, at constant GFR, was $48 ± 2$ μEq. (From Mathisen O, Montclair T, Kiil F: Oxygen requirement of bicarbonate dependent sodium reabsorption in the dog kidney. Am J Physiol 238:F175, 1980, with permission.)*

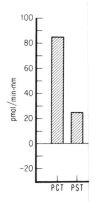

100

80

60

40

20

0

−20

pmol/min·mm

PCT PST

FIG. 9-6. Rates c
rabbit nephron. N
bules at 37°C wii
both luminal and
bule; PST, proxin
Henle's loop; CC
bits; CCD/ACID
rabbits; CCD/AL
rabbits; CCD/DC
ticosterone acetate
outer medullary c
medullary collecti
121,123,124,16

I and II [277,2
II, but unlike t
with an enzyme
than cytosolic,

Functional I

From a histori
quilibrium pH c
in situ and th
equilibrated wi
showing that a
occurred by H
HCO_3^- reabso
disequilibrium
have confirmed
and distal tubu
medullary colle

Carbonic an
several mechan
that carbonic a
to H_2CO_3 intr
luminal pump.
OH^- to HCO
alkalinization c
ary to proton pi

active skeletal growth contributes substantially to the metabolic proton load. During the process of skeletal mineralization, hydroxyapatite synthesis is associated with a release of protons:

$$10\ Ca^{+2} + 4.8\ HPO_4^- + 1.2\ H_2PO_4^- + 2\ H_2O \rightarrow$$
$$[Ca_3\ (PO_4)_2]_3 \cdot Ca\ (OH)_2 + 9.2\ H^+$$

The incorporation of one g of calcium into the growing skeleton causes the release of 20 mEq of protons [134,135]. Thus, in the healthy premature infant, a gain of 50–60 mg of calcium from skeletal hydroxyapatite deposition results in the generation of approximately one mEq of proton that must be excreted by the kidney or be neutralized by the gastrointestinal absorption of base [134,135]. This burden is superimposed on the acid load generated from endogenous acid production, from urinary organic anion excretion, and from sulfuric acid production, which total approximately 2 mEq/kg/day [134,135].

These studies have been extended to full-term infants and growing children by Chan [46], who found that endogenous acid production consistently exceeded that of adults (1 mEq/kg/day) by 0.5–1 mEq/kg/day [46]. No wonder that the growing infant, with relatively immature mechanisms for renal excretion [129,251] and rapid mineralization of the skeleton, is generally hypobasemic compared with the adult [75,76,228] and at risk of developing metabolic acidosis during periods of stress or increased catabolism.

Segmental Analysis of Renal H$^+$ Transport

The reabsorption of filtered HCO_3^- and the excretion of net acid are accomplished by H^+ secretion from the renal tubular cell into the lumen. The segments that are responsible for H^+ secretion include the proximal tubule, the collecting duct, and, to a lesser extent, the distal tubule, connecting tubule, and thick ascending limb of the loop of Henle (Fig. 9-4) [14,141,155]. The three ultrastructurally distinct segments of the proximal tubule contribute to the reabsorption of as much as 90% of the filtered HCO_3^- (Fig. 9-5) [14,141]. Studies of isolated perfused proximal tubular segments have shown that the straight portion reabsorbs HCO_3^- at a rate substantially below that of the convoluted portion (Fig. 9-6) [29,123], perhaps in keeping with the smaller amounts of filtered HCO_3^- escaping the early proximal tubule.

The thick limb of the loop of Henle has been thought to play little role in urinary acidification [14,29,141]. Studies of isolated perfused thick ascending limbs from rabbit or mouse have not shown significant HCO_3^- absorption [83,121]. However, experiments in cortical and medullary thick ascending limbs taken from rats have shown HCO_3^- absorptive rates of 5–10 pmol/min/mm [98], which are lower than that of the rabbit proximal straight tubule [179] and less than 5% of that measured in the in vivo perfused rat proximal convoluted tubule [11]. Nevertheless, such transport rates would be capable of reclaiming a substantial

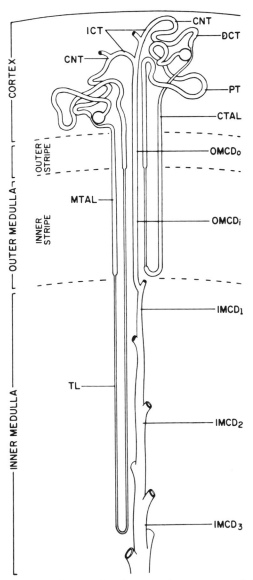

FIG. 9-4. *Structural and segmental organization of the mammalian kidney. Diagram of a superficial and juxtamedullary nephron. CNT, connecting tubule; ICT, initial collecting tubule; PT, proximal tubule; CTAL, cortical thick ascending limb; OMCD$_o$, outer medullary collecting duct from outer stripe; MTAL, medullary thick ascending limb; OMCD$_i$, outer medullary collecting duct from inner stripe; OMCD$_1$, outer third of inner medullary collecting duct; IMCD$_2$, middle third of inner medullary collecting duct; IMCD$_3$, inner third of inner medullary collecting duct; TL, thin limb of Henle's loop. (From Madsen KM, Tisher CC: Structural-functional relationships along the distal nephron. Am J Physiol 250:F1, 1986, with permission.)*

pH = 7.4
Pco_2 = 40
$[HCO_3]$ = 24

FIG. 9-5.
of Henle's
Basic mec

portion
the prox

The d
in resorb
ever, se\
stimulate

The c
is a hete
ism [127
the inter
acid–bas
the colle
or net F
are prelo
The tran
of maxir
than 5%
convolut
accomm
delivered
tions, h
served at

The o
within t
approach
9-6) [29]
medullar
[161] or
[161].

the proximal tubule where these gradients become important. Against the net flux of 12 pmol/minute/mm is a paracellular backleak of HCO_3^- from peritubular to luminal fluids of 26 pmol/minute/mm and a proton leak from lumen to blood of 2 pmol/minute/mm, to yield a net transcellular H^+ secretory rate of 40 pmol/minute/mm. Because the luminal fluid is more acidic than is the cell [215], and the interior of the cell is 60 mV negative with respect to the luminal fluid [30], there will be a passive lumen to cell proton flux of 12 pmol/minute/mm [122]. This leads to an overall calculated rate of luminal membrane H^+ secretion of 52 pmol/minute/mm at the end of the proximal tubule [14].

In the proximal convoluted tubule of the rat, H^+ secretion is a saturable function of luminal HCO_3^- concentration with an apparent Km of 16 mM and a V_{max} of 200 pmol/minute/mm [11]. In the early proximal tubule, where gradients for HCO_3^- and H^+ have not been developed, the rate of active H^+ secretion closely approximates the rate of net H^+ secretion. As gradients develop along the tubule, leak of HCO_3^- from blood to luminal fluid may approach 30% and a partially offsetting H^+ leak may reach 5% of the active rate of H^+ secretion [11,14,29,213]. By the end of the accessible proximal tubule, the active H^+ secretory rate may be twice the net rate because HCO_3^- backleak, enhanced by the reduced concentration of HCO_3^- in the tubular fluid (see Fig. 9-5), substantially offsets the H^+ secretory rate [11,14,141]. The HCO_3^- permeability is an important determinant of HCO_3^- delivery out of the proximal tubule, and thus of the substrate available for transport by the thick ascending limb and collecting duct of the kidney.

Loop of Henle

The loop of Henle may reabsorb up to 15% to 20% of filtered HCO_3^- [71,141] (some of this should be attributed to the proximal straight tubule, which is not accessible to micropuncture) (see Fig. 9-5). The cortical proximal straight tubule may absorb HCO_3^- at rates approaching 25% of the proximal convoluted tubule (see Fig. 9-6) [29,71,179]. Some HCO_3^- may also be reabsorbed in the descending limb, as water is abstracted in the medulla and luminal HCO_3^- concentration rises. Because the pCO_2 of the medullary interstitium is less than that of the cortex [71], loss of CO_2 alkalinizes the luminal fluid so that HCO_3^- is lost by the reaction:

$$HCO_3^- + HB \overset{C.A.}{\rightleftharpoons} B^- + H_2CO_3 \rightleftharpoons CO_2 + H_2O + B^-,$$

as well as by diffusion from a higher luminal to a lower interstitial HCO_3^- concentration. Thus, in the descending limb HCO_3^- reabsorption is catalyzed by carbonic anhydrase [67] in the absence of active H^+ secretion [14].

The thick ascending limb of the rat has been shown in in vitro microperfusion experiments to absorb HCO_3^- [98]. The measured rate is calculated to be of sufficient magnitude to account for much of the 10% to 15% of filtered HCO_3^- that is absorbed from loops of Henle of rats in vivo [98]. The mechanism of HCO_3^- absorption is dependent on carbonic anhydrase and Na-K-ATPase, can be inhibited by 1 mM amiloride, and is stimulated by furosemide [96]. The results suggest that HCO_3^- is absorbed primarily by apical Na^+-H^+ exchange, the driving force for luminal entry of Na^+ being maintained by Na-K-ATPase on the basolateral membrane [96]. Stimulation of HCO_3^- absorption by furosemide can be explained by competition for apical Na^+ entry between Na^+-H^+ exchange and Na^+-K^+-$2Cl^-$ co-transport [96]. The thick ascending limb of the rabbit or mouse does not absorb HCO_3^- in vitro (see Fig. 9-6) [83,121].

Distal Convoluted Tubule

Luminal fluid in the distal convoluted tubule is usually low in HCO_3^- (5–7 mEq/liter) and pH (6.5–6.7) (see Fig. 9-5) [39,73]. Segments of the distal nephron usually reabsorb the remaining HCO_3^- and further acidify the luminal fluid to titrate filtered buffers and trap ammonium. The surface distal tubule of the rat demonstrates little HCO_3^- absorption under normal circumstances [155]. Severe metabolic acidosis [154,164], starvation [157a], and protein loading [144a] stimulate distal tubular HCO_3^- reabsorption.

It is not clear whether any of the unique cell types of the distal convoluted tubule amenable to micropuncture are capable of H^+ secretion. Several experts have attributed absorption of HCO_3^- to the intercalated cells of the contiguous connecting segment and initial collecting duct [14,155,189]; however, rigorous studies of individually identified cells in the distal tubule or connecting segment have not yet been performed. It is possible, based on the numbers of intercalated cells in the connecting segment [127,155], that this later segment is normally involved in acid–base transport.

Collecting Duct

There are two types of cells in the collecting duct: principal cells and intercalated cells. Principal cells, the majority cell type, are active in absorbing Na^+ and secreting K^+ in the cortical collecting duct. The intercalated cell of the collecting duct is responsible for acid–base transport. It comprises approximately one-third of all cells in the cortical collecting duct, one-fifth in the outer medullary collecting duct, and fewer than one-tenth in the inner medullary collecting duct [52,127,151]. The pH of intercalated cells exceeds that of principal cells by approximately 0.4 units [216,223], and most likely exceeds 7.2 [216,223].

Studies have shown that there may be at least two types of intercalated cells, judged originally from the ultrastructural appearance of the cytoplasm and matrix, as "black" ("dark") and "gray" ("light") [127]. The most prominent distinguishing features are the spherical and flat-shaped apical vesicles of the "light" or "gray" form, of which some open into the lumen [127]. Others [170,270] find this cell to resemble the microplicated carbonic anhydrase-rich "alpha" type (mitochondria-rich) cell of the turtle bladder [146].

The "dark" form resembles the "beta" type (mitochon-

active skeletal growth contributes substantially to the metabolic proton load. During the process of skeletal mineralization, hydroxyapatite synthesis is associated with a release of protons:

$$10\ Ca^{+2}\ +\ 4.8\ HPO_4^-\ +\ 1.2\ H_2PO_4^-\ +\ 2\ H_2O \rightarrow$$
$$[Ca_3\ (PO_4)_2]_3 \cdot Ca\ (OH)_2\ +\ 9.2\ H^+$$

The incorporation of one g of calcium into the growing skeleton causes the release of 20 mEq of protons [134,135]. Thus, in the healthy premature infant, a gain of 50–60 mg of calcium from skeletal hydroxyapatite deposition results in the generation of approximately one mEq of proton that must be excreted by the kidney or be neutralized by the gastrointestinal absorption of base [134,135]. This burden is superimposed on the acid load generated from endogenous acid production, from urinary organic anion excretion, and from sulfuric acid production, which total approximately 2 mEq/kg/day [134,135].

These studies have been extended to full-term infants and growing children by Chan [46], who found that endogenous acid production consistently exceeded that of adults (1 mEq/kg/day) by 0.5–1 mEq/kg/day [46]. No wonder that the growing infant, with relatively immature mechanisms for renal excretion [129,251] and rapid mineralization of the skeleton, is generally hypobasemic compared with the adult [75,76,228] and at risk of developing metabolic acidosis during periods of stress or increased catabolism.

Segmental Analysis of Renal H$^+$ Transport

The reabsorption of filtered HCO_3^- and the excretion of net acid are accomplished by H^+ secretion from the renal tubular cell into the lumen. The segments that are responsible for H^+ secretion include the proximal tubule, the collecting duct, and, to a lesser extent, the distal tubule, connecting tubule, and thick ascending limb of the loop of Henle (Fig. 9-4) [14,141,155]. The three ultrastructurally distinct segments of the proximal tubule contribute to the reabsorption of as much as 90% of the filtered HCO_3^- (Fig. 9-5) [14,141]. Studies of isolated perfused proximal tubular segments have shown that the straight portion reabsorbs HCO_3^- at a rate substantially below that of the convoluted portion (Fig. 9-6) [29,123], perhaps in keeping with the smaller amounts of filtered HCO_3^- escaping the early proximal tubule.

The thick limb of the loop of Henle has been thought to play little role in urinary acidification [14,29,141]. Studies of isolated perfused thick ascending limbs from rabbit or mouse have not shown significant HCO_3^- absorption [83,121]. However, experiments in cortical and medullary thick ascending limbs taken from rats have shown HCO_3^- absorptive rates of 5–10 pmol/min/mm [98], which are lower than that of the rabbit proximal straight tubule [179] and less than 5% of that measured in the in vivo perfused rat proximal convoluted tubule [11]. Nevertheless, such transport rates would be capable of reclaiming a substantial

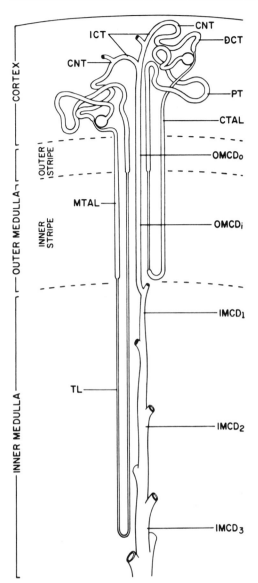

FIG. 9-4. *Structural and segmental organization of the mammalian kidney. Diagram of a superficial and juxtamedullary nephron. CNT, connecting tubule; ICT, initial collecting tubule; PT, proximal tubule; CTAL, cortical thick ascending limb; OMCD_o, outer medullary collecting duct from outer stripe; MTAL, medullary thick ascending limb; OMCD_i, outer medullary collecting duct from inner stripe; OMCD_1, outer third of inner medullary collecting duct; IMCD_2, middle third of inner medullary collecting duct; IMCD_3, inner third of inner medullary collecting duct; TL, thin limb of Henle's loop. (From Madsen KM, Tisher CC: Structural-functional relationships along the distal nephron. Am J Physiol 250:F1, 1986, with permission.)*

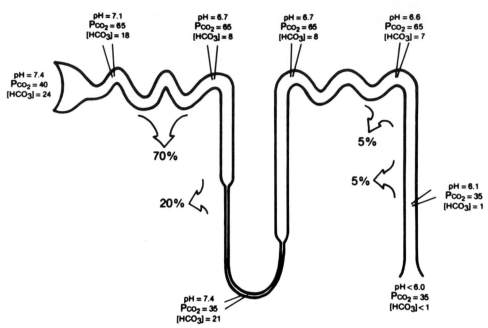

FIG. 9-5. *Profile of acid–base parameters along the superficial nephron of the rat; the data from the tip of Henle's loop represent the function of juxtamedullary nephrons. (From Koeppen BM, Steinmetz PR: Basic mechanisms of urinary acidification. Med Clin North Am 67:753, 1983, with permission.)*

portion of the HCO_3^- that had escaped reabsorption in the proximal convoluted and straight tubules [98].

The distal convoluted tubule may not play a major role in resorbing HCO_3^- under normal conditions [164]. However, severe chronic acidosis, protein loading, and fasting stimulate distal tubular HCO_3^- reabsorption [45,154,164].

The collecting duct from the cortex and outer medulla is a heterogeneous segment that exhibits cellular dimorphism [127,151]. Approximately one-third of the cells are the intercalated cells that are known to participate in net acid–base transport [168,222,223]. The cortical portion of the collecting duct is capable of net HCO_3^- reabsorption or net HCO_3^- secretion, depending on whether animals are preloaded with acid or base, respectively [21,180,223]. The transport rates in this segment, even under conditions of maximal stimulation, are rather small, attaining less than 5% of the HCO_3^- reabsorptive rate in the proximal convoluted tubule (see Fig. 9-6) [29], but sufficient to accommodate the remaining volume of glomerular filtrate delivered to this segment in vivo. Under normal conditions, however, very little net HCO_3^- transport is observed at this level of the nephron [161,180].

The outer medullary collecting duct, especially that from within the inner stripe, absorbs HCO_3^- at a rate that approaches that of the proximal straight tubule (see Fig. 9-6) [29]. But unlike the cortical collecting duct, the outer medullary segment has not been found to secrete HCO_3^- [161] or to respond dramatically to acid or alkali loading [161].

The papillary (inner medullary) collecting duct, which has a paucity of intercalated cells [52,127], is capable of significant net HCO_3^- reabsorption in vivo. The rate of H^+ secretion can be stimulated by metabolic acidosis [101]; data are not available to compare these rates with those of other segments.

Carbonic Anhydrase
General Characteristics

Carbonic anhydrase is an important zinc-containing metalloenzyme of 30,000 molecular weight [59] and several isomeric forms [159,239,262] that is present in cells in which there is rapid exchange between CO_2 and HCO_3^- or acid–base secretion [173]. In the kidney carbonic anhydrase facilitates H^+ secretion, whether by Na^+/H^+ exchange or H^+ATPase [72,203,271]. Most renal carbonic anhydrase exists free in the cytosol and is identical to the high activity isozyme type II that is found in red cells [35,67,159,239,262]. It has a very high turnover number ($10^6 \, sec^{-1}$ at pH 9) [159].

A small fraction of carbonic anhydrase (3% to 5%) exists in a different isomeric form (type IV) [277,278] and is membrane bound, especially to brush border and basolateral membranes of the proximal tubule [67,141,162, 277,278]. This isoenzyme has a molecular weight of 68,000 and is antigenically different from carbonic anhydrase types

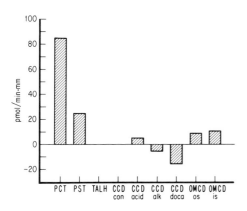

FIG. 9-6. *Rates of bicarbonate absorption in various segments of the rabbit nephron. Measurements were made in isolated perfused tubules at 37°C with 25 mEq/liter HCO_3^- and 40 mm Hg pCO_2 in both luminal and bathing solutions. PCT, proximal convoluted tubule; PST, proximal straight tubule; TALH, thick ascending limb of Henle's loop; CCD/CON, cortical collecting duct from control rabbits; CCD/ACID, cortical collecting duct taken from acid loaded rabbits; CCD/ALK, cortical collecting duct taken from alkali loaded rabbits; CCD/DOCA, cortical collecting duct taken from deoxycorticosterone acetate (mineralocorticoid) loaded rabbits; OMCD/OS, outer medullary collecting duct from outer stripe; OMCD/IS, outer medullary collecting duct from inner stripe. (Data from 41,85,120, 121,123,124,161,180,183,184,213,218,223,241,248.)*

I and II [277,278]. Its turnover number is lower than type II, but unlike the latter, is sensitive to halides, in keeping with an enzyme that is in contact with extracellular, rather than cytosolic, fluid [277].

Functional Roles

From a historic series of experiments in which the disequilibrium pH or difference between the pH of tubular fluid in situ and the pH obtained after the tubular fluid has equilibrated with the in situ pCO_2, evidence was obtained showing that acidification of the proximal tubular fluid occurred by H^+ secretion, rather than by direct ionic HCO_3^- reabsorption [203,271]. Further studies estimating disequilibrium pH in various segments along the nephron have confirmed this mechanism of acidification in proximal and distal tubules [72,145,203,271] and outer and inner medullary collecting ducts [70,102,241].

Carbonic anhydrase may facilitate HCO_3^- transport by several mechanisms [67,141]. Traditionally it is believed that carbonic anhydrase accelerates the hydration of CO_2 to H_2CO_3 intracellularly, thereby generating H^+ for the luminal pump. It may also catalyze the neutralization of OH^- to HCO_3^-, thereby buffering the resulting cellular alkalinization caused by the accumulation of OH^- secondary to proton pumping. Either of these mechanisms permits

ongoing luminal H^+ secretion by preventing the local depletion of substrate (H^+). This is true for proximal tubule and collecting duct intercalated cells.

The brush border of early proximal tubule cells also contains carbonic anhydrase [278] that is in contact with the luminal fluid. At this location, the enzyme permits the buffering of secreted protons by luminal HCO_3^- by catalyzing the dehydration of carbonic acid (H_2CO_3) to the reabsorbable products, CO_2 and water [277,278].

There may also be functional evidence for carbonic anhydrase at the basolateral membrane. Since membrane-bound carbonic anhydrase (type IV) has been shown to form cation-selective channels in lipid bilayers [66], it is possible that the basolateral carbonic anhydrase may facilitate base exit by allowing protons to enter the cell and titrate the OH^- generated from the dehydration of HCO_3^- [14]. Whether this is a major mechanism for accelerating transepithelial H^+ secretion is not yet clear.

Membrane-bound carbonic anhydrase has also been demonstrated functionally in the luminal membrane of the inner stripe of the outer medullary collecting duct [241], but not in that of the outer stripe [241] nor in the distal convoluted tubule [72], medullary proximal straight tubule [145], or papillary collecting duct [70,102]. These findings indicate that the luminal fluid is not in contact with carbonic anhydrase, presumably along most of the length of the distal nephron.

Carbonic anhydrase has been localized along the nephron by histochemical and immunocytochemical techniques. Despite some differences in results between these methods as well as some species differences, an overall schema has evolved (Fig. 9-7) [67,68,162]. In general, acid–base transporting segments are rich in carbonic anhydrase. Glomeruli are universally negative. Enzyme activity is very high in cytoplasm and both apical (brush border) and basolateral membranes of the proximal convoluted tubule. Less activity is found in the proximal straight tubule. For reasons that are not yet clear, outer medullary portions of the thin descending limbs of Henle's loop of most species (excluding rabbit) are strongly positive in the cytoplasm and both apical and basolateral membranes [67,68,162].

Distal tubule, connecting tubule, and cortical principal cells of the distal nephron show little or no carbonic anhydrase activity; when present it is located in the basal regions of the cytoplasm or plasmalemma. Strong carbonic anhydrase activity is located in the intercalated cells of the distal nephron (see Fig. 9-7). Intense cytoplasmic staining as well as luminal and basolateral membrane staining [68] of intercalated cells of all of these segments indicates that the cytosolic location of carbonic anhydrase does not determine the polarity of H^+ flux across the cell [67]. Rather, the generation of protons for export across the apical or basolateral membrane is determined by the locations of H^+ pumps and HCO_3^- exit paths on the respective membranes. The inner medullary collecting duct shows fewer intercalated cells and the principal cells show staining that becomes progressively less as the duct descends from the inner zone of the outer medulla into the papillary tip [67,162,239] (see Fig. 9-7).

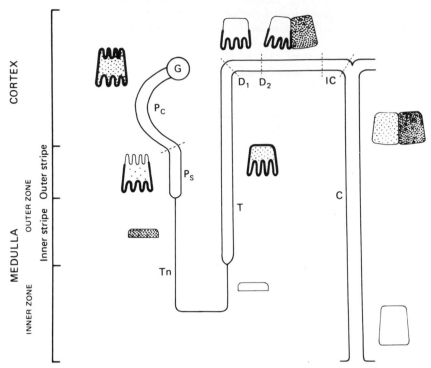

FIG. 9-7. *Distribution of carbonic anhydrase histochemical activity in segments of rat kidney. Individual tubular cells are oriented with the luminal side at the top of the figure. Heavy lines indicate membrane bound activity, dotted areas indicate intracellular enzyme. G, glomerulus; Pc, proximal convoluted tubule; Ps, proximal straight tubule; Tn, thin limb of Henle's loop; T, thick ascending limb; D_1, early distal convoluted tubule; D_2, late distal convoluted tubule; IC, initial collecting tubule or connecting segment; C, collecting duct. The two kinds of enzyme carrying cells in C are also in IC; the intercalated cell contains much more activity than the other cell type in IC or C. (From Lonnerholm G, Ridderstrale Y: Intracellular distribution of carbonic anhydrase in the rat kidney. Kidney Int 17:162, 1980, with permission.)*

Tubular Acidification Mechanisms
Proximal Tubule

The proximal convoluted tubule reabsorbs approximately 75% of filtered HCO_3^-, decreases luminal HCO_3^- concentration to about 8 mEq/liter, and in the presence of a pCO_2 of 60 mm Hg [73] results in acidification of the tubular fluid to pH 6.70 [57,73] (see Fig. 9-5). Further HCO_3^- reabsorption occurs in the proximal straight tubule, albeit at lower transport rates (see Fig. 9-6) [41,179], such that about 90% of filtered HCO_3^- is reabsorbed by the end of the proximal tubule [71,141].

The major mechanism of H^+ secretion is via a reversible Na^+-H^+ exchanger in the luminal membrane (Fig. 9-8) [17,136a,190,220]. This process is electrically neutral and uses the energy derived from the cellular entry of Na^+ down its chemical gradient across the luminal membrane to secrete H^+ into the luminal fluid [17]. Indeed, the direction of transport (Na^+ absorption, H^+ secretion) is determined by the balance of the concentration gradients for Na^+ and H^+ across the brush border membrane. The

cell pH is nearly the same as that of the initial luminal filtrate (approximately 7.20) [215,281]; however, the cell Na^+ is approximately 10% of that in the luminal fluid. Thus, the Na^+-H^+ exchanger normally allows Na^+ to enter the cell and H^+ to be extruded. This apical Na^+ gradient is maintained by the Na-K-ATPase–dependent extrusion of Na^+ across the basolateral membrane in exchange for K^+.

As protons are secreted, HCO_3^- builds up in the cell and exits conductively, most likely in the symport form, $Na(HCO_3)_3^{-2}$ across the basolateral membrane [9,10]. The Na^+-H^+ exchanger therefore effects the translocation of Na^+ and HCO_3^- across the proximal tubular epithelium, but the energy input is indirect (secondary active) and is used only to extrude Na^+ by Na-K-ATPase [17].

There is another mechanism in the proximal tubule for secreting protons whose quantitative contribution is not yet known. Studies in membrane vesicles [136] as well as in isolated perfused proximal tubules [220] have consistently shown Na^+-independent acidification (see Fig. 9-8). The luminal membrane of the proximal tubule contains an electrogenic proton-translocating ATPase that

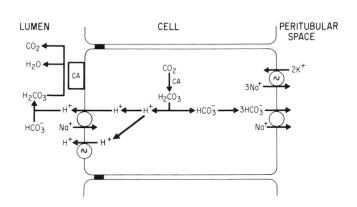

FIG. 9-8. *Model of luminal acidification by proximal convoluted tubule cell. The circles enclosing "~" indicate primary active transport; those without "~" represent exchangers. CA is carbonic anhydrase.*

pumps protons at the direct expense of ATP. Inhibition of H^+ATPase by dicyclohexylcarbodiimide (DCCD) reduces proximal tubule HCO_3^- absorption by 21% without affecting glucose or fluid (Na^+) absorption [23]. There is also some evidence that proton-translocating ATPases may shuttle back and forth from the brush border to cytoplasmic vesicles to regulate the rate of proton secretion [4,81,206, 209,222,250].

Efforts to quantify the relative contribution of these two processes to proximal tubular HCO_3^- reabsorption are fraught with difficulty. The effects of Na^+ removal and ouabain inhibition of Na-K-ATPase are not only to reduce HCO_3^- absorption markedly, but also to inhibit cell metabolism and reduce the generation of CO_2 that is required for buffering the cellular base resulting from H^+ secretion [41,179,231,232]. Microperfusion studies of proximal tubules in vivo show that inhibition of Na^+-H^+ exchange by 1 mM amiloride reduces HCO_3^- absorption by only 21% to 36%, much less than expected from this dose when used in isolated brush border vesicles [23,114]. On the other hand, even in the absence of Na^+, some net H^+ secretion goes on [50,51,220], but the maintenance of the cellular pCO_2 under these conditions cannot be rigorously ensured. Calculations put this rate at 10% to 20% of that observed in proximal tubules exposed to Na^+ [14,50].

Finally, it appears that the exit of some HCO_3^- or base across the basolateral membrane requires the presence of ambient and cellular Na^+ [9,10]. If the HCO_3^- exit step requires Na^+, net HCO_3^- absorption may be Na^+-dependent even in the absence of a significant amount of luminal Na^+-H^+ exchange (other Na^+-dependent entry processes would still be ongoing). Obviously, further and more creative studies are needed to quantify the roles of Na^+-H^+ exchange and H^+-translocating ATPase in mediating proximal HCO_3^- transport.

When protons are secreted from the cell into the lumen, a base equivalent (OH^-) accumulates in the cytosol. Cy-

toplasmic carbonic anhydrase mediates the buffering reaction ($OH^- + CO_2 = HCO_3^-$) that mitigates in part the cellular alkalinity (see Carbonic Anhydrase). Ultimately, for H^+ secretion to continue, this moiety must be excreted across the basolateral membrane at a rate equivalent to the acidification process. The exit of HCO_3^- is most likely to be conductive and passive, driven by the electrochemical gradient [40,281]. There is some evidence that the HCO_3^- conductance is coupled to the co-transport of Na^+ [9,10], in the approximate ratio Na^+-HCO_3^- = 1:3. This would allow HCO_3^- exit to be regulated by small changes in cell pH because the driving forces would be closer to electrochemical equilibrium than a simple HCO_3^- conductance [9,10] (see Fig. 9-8). The conductive movement of HCO_3^- across the basolateral membrane, especially in its coupling to Na^+ ($Na[HCO_3]_3^{-2}$), could be an important system for regulating cell pH and thereby the rate of H^+ secretion by Na^+-H^+ exchange [9,10,141].

The role of simple anion exchange mechanisms in mediating HCO_3^- transport across the plasmalemma may be of only minor importance across the basolateral [41,212] or luminal [14,43, 221,236] membrane of proximal tubular cells.

Leak pathways also affect the rate of transepithelial acidification, because pH and HCO_3^- gradients will be developed from this process, especially beyond the early proximal tubule. At the end of the proximal tubule, under free flow conditions, the HCO_3^- concentration is 8 mEq/liter and pH is 6.70 (see Fig. 9-5) [57,73]. Given a peritubular HCO_3^- concentration of 24 mEq/liter and pH of 7.30, the rate of net H^+ secretion will be reduced by the adverse gradient for H^+ and by the passive leak of protons out of and HCO_3^- into the luminal fluid [11,14]. Note that CO_2 rapidly permeates the proximal tubular epithelium, so that it is unlikely that a significant pCO_2 gradient would develop between tubular fluid and peritubular blood and limit active H^+ secretion [73,229].

The leak components may be mediated through transcellular or paracellular (trans-junctional) routes. Proximal tubular H^+/OH^- permeability has been estimated from changes in H^+ fluxes in response to pH gradients. Such measurements are complicated by the various contributions to H^+ movement, such as H^+ diffusion, Na^+-H^+ exchange, and non-ionic diffusion of organic buffers. Transepithelial H^+ permeability in rabbit proximal tubule ranges from 0.3 to 5 cm/sec; removal of Na^+ alone reduces H^+ permeability by 40% to 50% [106,220,221]. In the late proximal tubule, where organic buffer concentration is low, the approximate backleak of protons (from lumen to blood) would be only 2 pEq/minute/mm [14,106,221].

Bicarbonate permeability, on the other hand, appears to be quite small, about $1–3 \times 10^{-5}$ cm/sec [11,112,213,272]. However, in view of the high concentrations and large transepithelial HCO_3^- difference (luminal HCO_3^- 8 mEq/liter, peritubular 24 mEq/liter), this could amount to a leak of HCO_3^- of 6–30 pmol/minute/ mm from the blood back into the luminal fluid [14].

The data from these calculations can be summarized to show the difference between net transepithelial H^+ secretion (12 pmol/minute/mm) [11,14] and luminal membrane active H^+ secretion (52 pmol/minute/mm) at the end of the proximal tubule where these gradients become important. Against the net flux of 12 pmol/minute/mm is a paracellular backleak of HCO_3^- from peritubular to luminal fluids of 26 pmol/minute/mm and a proton leak from lumen to blood of 2 pmol/minute/mm, to yield a net transcellular H^+ secretory rate of 40 pmol/minute/mm. Because the luminal fluid is more acidic than is the cell [215], and the interior of the cell is 60 mV negative with respect to the luminal fluid [30], there will be a passive lumen to cell proton flux of 12 pmol/minute/mm [122]. This leads to an overall calculated rate of luminal membrane H^+ secretion of 52 pmol/minute/mm at the end of the proximal tubule [14].

In the proximal convoluted tubule of the rat, H^+ secretion is a saturable function of luminal HCO_3^- concentration with an apparent Km of 16 mM and a V_{max} of 200 pmol/minute/mm [11]. In the early proximal tubule, where gradients for HCO_3^- and H^+ have not been developed, the rate of active H^+ secretion closely approximates the rate of net H^+ secretion. As gradients develop along the tubule, leak of HCO_3^- from blood to luminal fluid may approach 30% and a partially offsetting H^+ leak may reach 5% of the active rate of H^+ secretion [11,14,29,213]. By the end of the accessible proximal tubule, the active H^+ secretory rate may be twice the net rate because HCO_3^- backleak, enhanced by the reduced concentration of HCO_3^- in the tubular fluid (see Fig. 9-5), substantially offsets the H^+ secretory rate [11,14,141]. The HCO_3^- permeability is an important determinant of HCO_3^- delivery out of the proximal tubule, and thus of the substrate available for transport by the thick ascending limb and collecting duct of the kidney.

Loop of Henle

The loop of Henle may reabsorb up to 15% to 20% of filtered HCO_3^- [71,141] (some of this should be attributed to the proximal straight tubule, which is not accessible to micropuncture) (see Fig. 9-5). The cortical proximal straight tubule may absorb HCO_3^- at rates approaching 25% of the proximal convoluted tubule (see Fig. 9-6) [29,71,179]. Some HCO_3^- may also be reabsorbed in the descending limb, as water is abstracted in the medulla and luminal HCO_3^- concentration rises. Because the pCO_2 of the medullary interstitium is less than that of the cortex [71], loss of CO_2 alkalinizes the luminal fluid so that HCO_3^- is lost by the reaction:

$$HCO_3^- + HB \overset{C.A.}{\rightleftharpoons} B^- + H_2CO_3 \rightleftharpoons CO_2 + H_2O + B^-,$$

as well as by diffusion from a higher luminal to a lower interstitial HCO_3^- concentration. Thus, in the descending limb HCO_3^- reabsorption is catalyzed by carbonic anhydrase [67] in the absence of active H^+ secretion [14].

The thick ascending limb of the rat has been shown in in vitro microperfusion experiments to absorb HCO_3^- [98]. The measured rate is calculated to be of sufficient magnitude to account for much of the 10% to 15% of filtered HCO_3^- that is absorbed from loops of Henle of rats in vivo [98]. The mechanism of HCO_3^- absorption is dependent on carbonic anhydrase and Na-K-ATPase, can be inhibited by 1 mM amiloride, and is stimulated by furosemide [96]. The results suggest that HCO_3^- is absorbed primarily by apical Na^+-H^+ exchange, the driving force for luminal entry of Na^+ being maintained by Na-K-ATPase on the basolateral membrane [96]. Stimulation of HCO_3^- absorption by furosemide can be explained by competition for apical Na^+ entry between Na^+-H^+ exchange and Na^+-K^+-$2Cl^-$ co-transport [96]. The thick ascending limb of the rabbit or mouse does not absorb HCO_3^- in vitro (see Fig. 9-6) [83,121].

Distal Convoluted Tubule

Luminal fluid in the distal convoluted tubule is usually low in HCO_3^- (5–7 mEq/liter) and pH (6.5–6.7) (see Fig. 9-5) [39,73]. Segments of the distal nephron usually reabsorb the remaining HCO_3^- and further acidify the luminal fluid to titrate filtered buffers and trap ammonium. The surface distal tubule of the rat demonstrates little HCO_3^- absorption under normal circumstances [155]. Severe metabolic acidosis [154,164], starvation [157a], and protein loading [144a] stimulate distal tubular HCO_3^- reabsorption.

It is not clear whether any of the unique cell types of the distal convoluted tubule amenable to micropuncture are capable of H^+ secretion. Several experts have attributed absorption of HCO_3^- to the intercalated cells of the contiguous connecting segment and initial collecting duct [14,155,189]; however, rigorous studies of individually identified cells in the distal tubule or connecting segment have not yet been performed. It is possible, based on the numbers of intercalated cells in the connecting segment [127,155], that this later segment is normally involved in acid–base transport.

Collecting Duct

There are two types of cells in the collecting duct: principal cells and intercalated cells. Principal cells, the majority cell type, are active in absorbing Na^+ and secreting K^+ in the cortical collecting duct. The intercalated cell of the collecting duct is responsible for acid–base transport. It comprises approximately one-third of all cells in the cortical collecting duct, one-fifth in the outer medullary collecting duct, and fewer than one-tenth in the inner medullary collecting duct [52,127,151]. The pH of intercalated cells exceeds that of principal cells by approximately 0.4 units [216,223], and most likely exceeds 7.2 [216,223].

Studies have shown that there may be at least two types of intercalated cells, judged originally from the ultrastructural appearance of the cytoplasm and matrix, as "black" ("dark") and "gray" ("light") [127]. The most prominent distinguishing features are the spherical and flat-shaped apical vesicles of the "light" or "gray" form, of which some open into the lumen [127]. Others [170,270] find this cell to resemble the microplicated carbonic anhydrase-rich "alpha" type (mitochondria-rich) cell of the turtle bladder [146].

The "dark" form resembles the "beta" type (mitochondria-rich) cell of the turtle bladder [246] and has vesicular membrane structures throughout the cytoplasm, few microprojections on the luminal surface, and an extensive basolateral plasma membrane [170,270]. Both types in the collecting duct are rich in mitochondria [127,216,219], carbonic anhydrase [34,162], and H^+ pumps [89,222,223].

Because the light type predominates in the outer medullary collecting duct, whereas the dark type is more prevalent in the cortical collecting duct [127,170,270], it is possible that the light cells are involved in H^+ secretion and the dark cells in HCO_3^- secretion. This is supported by fluorescent studies showing at the functional level that most intercalated cells in the cortical collecting duct of the rabbit show a luminal Cl^-/HCO_3^- exchanger, while most in the outer medulla show a basolateral Cl^-/HCO_3^- exchanger [223,224]. Some of the H^+ secreting cells appear to regulate by exocytosis the number of H^+ pumps on the luminal membrane in response to CO_2 [222]. When CO_2 is acutely lowered they remove H^+ pumps from the membrane by endocytosis and store them in the apical cytoplasm [222,224]. For this group of H^+-secreting intercalated cells the control of acidification is accomplished by regulating the number of pumps on the membrane, in addition to the rates of these pumps [4,222,223].

The major intercalated cell type in the rabbit cortical collecting duct binds peanut agglutinin to the apical membrane [152,219,223]. It is likely that these are HCO_3^--secreting intercalated cells [219,223].

Antibodies to the membrane domain of the red blood cell anion exchanger, band 3, have been found to cross-react with the basolateral Cl^-/HCO_3^- exchanger of the H^+-secreting intercalated cell [69,219]. The antibodies do not distinguish functional subtypes of H^+-secreting cells in the outer medulla but, as do the fluorescent dyes, indicate that a majority of the intercalated cells in the rabbit outer medullary collecting duct are involved in H^+ secretion, whereas only a minority secrete H^+ in the cortical collecting duct [219,223].

Urinary acidification is mediated by H^+ secretion in the distal convoluted tubule, cortical, and inner medullary collecting ducts (see discussion in Carbonic Anhydrase) [70,72,102,241]. The H^+ secretion has been shown in isolated perfused cortical and medullary collecting ducts to be electrogenic and unaffected by Na^+ removal or Na-K-ATPase inhibition [142,181,249]. Since the cortical (but not the medullary) segment absorbs Na^+, changes in Na^+ transport, by altering the transepithelial voltage, will affect secondarily the rate of H^+ secretion [14,142,149].

The H^+ pump is a proton translocating ATPase [87,90], located on the luminal membrane [89], with characteristics different from those of the H^+-ATPase of mitochondria and lysosomes [4].

In H^+-secreting cells HCO_3^- exits via a Cl^-/HCO_3^- exchanger located in the peritubular membrane [248] (Fig. 9-9). There is controversy regarding the fate of the cellular chloride, which may exit the cell via a chloride conductance channel through the luminal membrane [248] or, more likely, may exit across the basolateral membrane and enter the lumen paracellularly via the tight junction, driven by the lumen positive voltage of H^+ secretion [14,140,141].

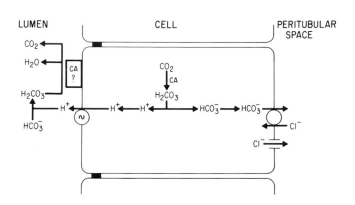

FIG. 9-9. *Model of luminal acidification by rabbit outer medullary collecting duct cell. The circles enclosing "~" indicate primary active transport; those without "~" indicate exchangers. CA is carbonic anhydrase, which is in contact with the luminal fluid only in the inner stripe segment.*

Cortical collecting ducts isolated from acid loaded rabbits secrete H^+ (reabsorb HCO_3^-) (see Fig. 9-6) [161,180,181,223]. The characteristics of H^+ secretion are similar to those of the medullary segment, but the net fluxes are smaller (see Fig. 9-6). Whether this reflects the fewer numbers of H^+-secreting cells or lower H^+ secretion rates of cortical versus medullary intercalated cells, in addition to the partially offsetting HCO_3^- secretion in the cortical segment, is not yet clear (see following).

HCO_3^- secretion has been occasionally observed in perfused collecting ducts isolated from normal rabbits [223] and more consistently from rabbits and rats that received alkali [21,180,182] or mineralocorticoids [85,139,240]. The secretory process is sensitive to acetazolamide but not to ouabain or Na^+ removal [182,240,244] and requires chloride in the lumen [150,240]. The model for HCO_3^- secretion by intercalated cells of the cortical collecting duct that fits best the experimental data requires a luminal Cl^-/HCO_3^- exchanger and a basolateral chloride conductance (Fig. 9-10) [141,223,240,244].

To summarize, there are two major subtypes of intercalated cells: those that secrete H^+ and those that secrete HCO_3^-. HCO_3^--secreting cells predominate in the rabbit cortical collecting duct, bind peanut agglutinin to their apical surfaces, and have an apical Cl^-/HCO_3^- exchanger, which does not cross react with band 3 antibodies [69,219]. H^+-secreting intercalated cells can be further divided into endocytic and nonendocytic subtypes, both of which are common in the outer medullary collecting duct, less common in the inner cortical collecting duct, and uncommon in the mid-cortical collecting duct [219,223, 224]. H^+-secreting cells have an apical H^+ pump and basolateral Cl^-/HCO_3^- exchanger that cross reacts with band 3 antibodies [69,219]. The physiologic role of endocytosis in distinguishing one functional subtype of intercalated cell has not been fully evaluated. The distribution

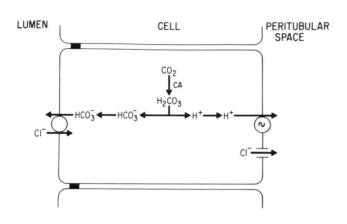

FIG. 9-10. *Model of luminal HCO_3^- secretion by rabbit cortical collecting duct cell. The legend is described in Figure 9-9.*

of intercalated cell subtypes has not yet been established in the rat collecting duct [270].

Leak pathways are rather small in the cortical collecting tubule, consistent with its being a tight epithelium [105,109,211]. The inner medullary (papillary) collecting duct absorbs HCO_3^- [102,205,266], in part by H^+ secretion, that is independent of Na^+ [70,102,198]. There is evidence for substantial carbonic anhydrase–dependent as well as some carbonic anhydrase–independent HCO_3^- absorption in this segment [205,275], although there is little carbonic anhydrase in these cells [35,67,162] and few intercalated cells [52].

Following HCO_3^- loading the elevated CO_2 tension in the alkaline urine is due in part to H^+ secretion in the collecting duct with delayed dehydration (in the absence of luminal carbonic anhydrase) of generated H_2CO_3 to CO_2. Also, counter-current trapping of CO_2 adds to the CO_2 tension in the medullary collecting duct [70,100]. These factors explain the high pCO_2 gradient between urine and blood that is observed during HCO_3^- diuresis.

Regulation of Acidification
Proximal Tubule

The regulation of renal acidification has been studied at the level of the single nephron by free flow micropuncture and by microperfusion of isolated segments in vitro and in vivo. The paracellular diffusion of HCO_3^- critically affects net HCO_3^- reabsorption (H^+ secretion) in the proximal tubule. Consequently, the factors influencing the rate of acidification are discussed in the context of either active transcellular proton secretion or passive HCO_3^- diffusion.

HCO_3^- CONCENTRATION

The proximal tubule is extremely sensitive to concentration gradients. Reabsorption of HCO_3^- is directly propor-

tional to mean luminal HCO_3^- concentration [11,171, 213] up to a concentration of approximately 45 mEq/liter. Within the physiologic range of HCO_3^- concentrations, the major effect of luminal HCO_3^- is to stimulate active H^+ secretion by reducing the chemical gradient for protons across the luminal membrane [14]. Peritubular HCO_3^- concentration also substantially influences active H^+ secretion. Increased peritubular HCO_3^- concentration (at constant pCO_2 and therefore at higher pH) inhibits HCO_3^- absorption and vice versa [10,49,64,213].

The effect of reduced peritubular HCO_3^- concentration on stimulating active proton secretion into the lumen is mediated in part by decreasing cell pH via the $Na(HCO_3)_3^{-2}$ symporter [9,10,14]. The increase in cell proton concentration makes more substrate available for luminal Na^+-H^+ exchange (H^+ secretion), increases the chemical driving force for luminal H^+ secretion, and activates the Na^+-H^+ exchanger allosterically [17,18] (see following). In brush border membrane vesicles taken from acidotic animals, there is an increased V_{max} for Na^+-H^+ exchange, which may be due to either an increased number of transporters or an increased turnover rate per exchanger [58,137,264]. Conversely, chronic metabolic alkalosis induces a decrease in the V_{max} of the Na^+-H^+ exchange, possibly by reducing the number of exchange sites [32].

pCO_2

The ambient pCO_2 also plays a major role in regulating proximal tubular acidification via changes in cell and peritubular pH. Acute increases in pCO_2 stimulate and acute decreases in pCO_2 reduce HCO_3^- absorption in proximal segments [49,64,123,213].

The reduction in cell pH with hypercapnia causes an increased conversion of intracellular OH^- to HCO_3^- [123,141,143], provides more substrate for H^+ secretion across the luminal membrane, and, most importantly, allosterically stimulates the activity of the Na^+/H^+ exchanger [18]. Such allosteric stimulation is not observed when the external site of the antiporter is exposed to an acid medium [19].

Another possible consequence of acute hypercapnia, by acidifying the cytosol, is to cause an increase in cell calcium that mediates exocytic insertion of proton pumps from cytoplasmic vesicles into the luminal membrane [4,44,222,223]. The action of these newly inserted pumps helps to restore cell pH to normal and to increase the rate of transepithelial H^+ secretion [4,44,88,222].

FILTERED HCO_3^- LOAD

The foregoing data would suggest that metabolic alkalosis and respiratory alkalosis depress, while metabolic acidosis and respiratory acidosis stimulate, proximal tubular HCO_3^- reabsorption. However, free flow micropuncture studies do not consistently show an effect of acute hypercapnia on HCO_3^- transport [54,153]. The stimulatory effect may be counterbalanced by changes in luminal HCO_3^- concentration and the limited filtered load (see following). Associated with acute hypercapnia is vasodilatation and a concomitant reduction in glomerular filtration rate and proximal HCO_3^- delivery [146]. Likewise, hyperchloremic metabolic acidosis, which would be expected to stimulate proximal HCO_3^- transport, in fact is associated with a reduction in HCO_3^- reabsorption, as the rate of HCO_3^- delivery to the proximal tubule falls [57,156].

When glomerular filtration rate rises, the rate of HCO_3^- absorption increases [166a,196]. With increasing luminal flow rate, there is less of a fall in luminal HCO_3^- concentration and less of a gradient opposing H^+ secretion [11,12,14,49,166a]. Increased luminal flow rate can also dissipate the luminal diffusion barrier for HCO_3^- (and an opposing local pH gradient) in the vicinity of the proximal tubular Na^+/H^+ antiporters, which results in enhanced HCO_3^- absorption [12]. This flow dependence of HCO_3^- reabsorption occurs only when HCO_3^- concentrations are not so high as to saturate the reabsorptive mechanisms; at higher HCO_3^- concentrations, flow dependence, and thus glomerulo-tubular balance, is blunted [12].

EXTRACELLULAR FLUID VOLUME

The relationship between change in extracellular volume and rates of proximal tubular HCO_3^- reabsorption is not entirely clear. Clearance studies indicate that volume expansion results in reduced HCO_3^- reabsorption [147,199]. Studies done by micropuncture or microperfusion of isolated tubule segments have generally documented that volume expansion results in a major inhibition of NaCl transport and little or no inhibition of HCO_3^- absorption [13,28,53,57,157]. Even though extracellular volume expansion can increase proximal tubular HCO_3^- permeability by approximately 50% [13], the baseline permeability is so low that the increase has little effect on HCO_3^- absorption until large gradients develop. This rarely occurs with the isohydric solutions commonly used in microperfusion of proximal segments in vitro and in vivo. But when large gradients are present, as in the late proximal tubule under free-flow conditions, it is probable that back-leak of HCO_3^- contributes to the reduction in the net HCO_3^- transport observed in the whole kidney.

Another factor that is relevant to the volume-induced reduction in HCO_3^- reabsorption is the generation of a diffusion barrier to HCO_3^- in the cell or on the peritubular side of the cell [8]. As the local concentration of HCO_3^- builds up, the pH increases and secondarily inhibits H^+ secretion. Volume absorption, by carrying away the HCO_3^- and reducing the local pH, secondarily stimulates H^+ secretion [8]. According to these studies, inhibition of fluid and NaCl absorption by extracellular volume expansion could lead to a small reduction in net HCO_3^- absorption [8,14].

POTASSIUM DEPLETION

Potassium deficiency may sometimes lead to alkalosis and increased proximal reabsorption of HCO_3^- [144,148]. However, potassium deficiency does not always influence proximal HCO_3^- reabsorption in free flow micropuncture studies [56,158,166], perhaps because of the limiting filtered load of HCO_3^-. Acute reductions in peritubular or bath potassium do not stimulate HCO_3^- absorption [49,183,214]. Glomerular filtration rate often decreases in metabolic alkalosis associated with potassium depletion

[56]. When proximal tubules are microperfused in vivo, so that delivery of HCO_3^- is maintained at an optimal rate, potassium depletion does result in a substantial increase in HCO_3^- absorption [49]. Thus, chronic potassium depletion may lead to alkalosis and increased proximal HCO_3^- reabsorption if the delivery of HCO_3^- can be maintained.

PARATHYROID HORMONE

Parathyroid hormone (PTH) inhibits HCO_3^- absorption in proximal tubules [22,77,120,184] through inhibition of active H^+ secretion [184,185]. In the absence of HCO_3^-, PTH has no effect on proximal fluid absorption [65]. In view of the major effect of PTH on active H^+ secretion in brush membrane vesicles [58], it is surprising to see that in vivo administration of PTH inhibits proximal HCO_3^- reabsorption only modestly. PTH has no effect on whole kidney HCO_3^- reabsorption [22], since the distal nephron segments reabsorb the excess HCO_3^- rejected from the proximal tubule [14,22]. The differences between the in vivo and in vitro findings are not easy to reconcile; the in vivo response may be modulated by the multiple interactions among PTH, calcium, phosphate, and vitamin D.

OTHER FACTORS

Acute changes in calcium and phosphate appear to have little effect on HCO_3^- absorption by proximal tubules [186,204].

Adrenergic nerve stimulation causes increased proximal water and HCO_3^- reabsorption [48,55].

Distal Nephron

ELECTROCHEMICAL PH GRADIENT

The effect of luminal pH on distal H^+ transport has been best studied in the turtle bladder, a model for the mammalian collecting duct. Because the passive permeability to protons is very small [243], the inhibition of acidification with decreasing mucosal pH can be attributed only to a decreased rate of active H^+ secretion [5,242,243]. Further studies show that not only the pH gradient but the transepithelial electrical gradient determines the rate of H^+ secretion [5]. That is, either a decrease in mucosal pH or an applied positive transepithelial voltage will inhibit acidification; an opposing electrochemical gradient of 3 pH units or 180 mV will stop H^+ transport [5]. It is likely that qualitatively similar results will be obtained in the collecting duct.

pCO2

The effect of pCO_2 on distal (and proximal) acidification has already been noted. H^+ secretion is acutely stimulated by an increase in pCO_2 [5,88,124,222,230,231,232]. Studies with fluorescent probes have revealed that CO_2 causes vesicles containing H^+ pumps to fuse with the luminal membrane (exocytosis) and thus provide additional H^+ pumps for transepithelial H^+ secretion [88,222]. Ultrastructural studies have confirmed the importance of exocytosis in the regulation of distal acidification [168,245]. Whether a more chronic exposure to high pCO_2 would result not only in exocytosis of preformed H$^+$ pumps but also in the synthesis of additional H$^+$ pumps is not yet determined.

ANION DELIVERY

The distal delivery of Na$^+$ and its accompanying anion substantially affects distal acidification. Avidity for Na$^+$ (volume contraction or mineralocorticoid loading) markedly stimulates urine acidification [234]. Impermeant anions, such as sulfate, phosphate, and ferrocyanide, stimulate acidification to a much greater extent than more permeant ions, such as Cl$^-$ and thiocyanate, probably by affecting transepithelial voltage in the collecting duct [24]. Inasmuch as H$^+$ secretion in the collecting duct is electrogenic and dependent on the transepithelial electrochemical gradient [5], voltage changes due to alterations in the rate of Na$^+$ transport will affect the rate of acidification [142,149]. Changes in transepithelial voltage due to different anion gradients should also affect the rate of acidification in the cortical and medullary collecting ducts.

In the medullary collecting duct in vitro replacement of luminal Cl$^-$ by gluconate stimulates HCO$_3^-$ absorption independently of voltage [248]. Thus, the distal delivery of a fluid that is low in Cl$^-$ will inhibit HCO$_3^-$ secretion by the cortical collecting duct [85] and stimulate H$^+$ secretion by the medullary collecting duct [248]. These effects should contribute to the maintenance of hypochloremic metabolic alkalosis and explain the efficacy of Cl$^-$ administration for its correction [128].

MINERALOCORTICOIDS

Mineralocorticoids stimulate acidification independently of changes in extracellular volume, serum potassium, or ammonia synthesis [166,177,235]. The effects of distal Na$^+$ and anion delivery on acidification are evident only when mineralocorticoid levels are not suppressed [234]. Mineralocorticoids increase luminal electronegativity by enhancing Na$^+$ absorption [192,225], thereby facilitating electrogenic H$^+$ secretion by the cortical collecting duct. A reduction in lumen negative voltage by partial replacement of Na$^+$ or inhibition of Na-K-ATPase markedly reduces HCO$_3^-$ absorption in cortical collecting ducts taken from acidotic rabbits [149]. Moreover, mineralocorticoids directly stimulate H$^+$ secretion by turtle bladders and medullary collecting ducts in the absence of Na$^+$ transport [6,249]. It is likely that they act in the same way on responsive cells in the cortical collecting duct [142]. If this is indeed the case, mineralocorticoids will stimulate both cortical and medullary segments to secrete protons, until the resulting metabolic alkalosis somehow acts to change the direction of transport in the cortical collecting duct (see following) [85,180].

Accordingly, acid loading of mineralocorticoid-stimulated rabbits inhibits HCO$_3^-$ secretion by the cortical collecting ducts taken from these animals [85]. Unidirectional flux studies have shown that acid loading markedly reduces the HCO$_3^-$ secretory flux without affecting the HCO$_3^-$ absorptive flux [85]. It is not clear what happens to the numbers of H$^+$- and HCO$_3^-$-secreting cells or the density of their pumps under either mineralocorticoid loading or mineralocorticoid plus acid loading.

POTASSIUM DEPLETION

Potassium depletion may cause changes in systemic acid-base status. By suppressing aldosterone secretion, K$^+$ depletion may lead to reduced collecting duct acidification [142,249]. Metabolic acidosis develops in dogs [42,86,118] and rabbits [183]; however, metabolic alkalosis is frequently observed with severe K$^+$ depletion in humans [125,258] and rats [86,158,165,172,279]. It is not clear why different species respond differently to K$^+$ depletion; chronic or acute reductions in potassium do not stimulate collecting duct acidification, at least in the rabbit [124,183].

There is, however, morphologic evidence of stimulation in rat medullary collecting duct intercalated cells [107,247]. K$^+$ depletion causes a reduction in the volume of apical vesicles along with an increase in luminal membrane area [247] (see Chapter 6), similar to the exocytic membrane insertion seen after acute hypercapnia and chronic metabolic acidosis [168,169]; this morphologic response would be consistent with enhanced H$^+$ secretion by the rat collecting duct.

A more important effect of K$^+$ depletion is to stimulate ammonia synthesis [3,259,260,261]. By consuming protons (see previously) and providing additional buffer to the distal nephron, increased ammonia production facilitates net H$^+$ secretion because the luminal pH is maintained higher. All things being equal, for the same H$^+$ secretion rates, additional buffer allows more net acid excretion. This effect may balance or overshadow the hypoaldosteronism observed with K$^+$ depletion and may result, in some species, in metabolic alkalosis.

PARATHYROID HORMONE

PTH inhibits proximal acidification but stimulates acidification at more distal renal sites [22]. Indeed, the isolated toad bladder shows this directly [82], and thyroparathyroidectomy inhibits acidification in the papillary collecting duct [26]. On the other hand, calcium inhibits acidification by the isolated turtle bladder [20].

ADAPTATION TO ACID-BASE STATUS

The cortical collecting tubule can secrete H$^+$ or HCO$_3^-$ in vitro depending on the acid-base status of the animal from which the segment is obtained (see Fig. 9-6) [21,161,180,181,182]. These effects persist for hours after the tubule has been removed from the animal and immersed in artificial solutions at pH 7.4, indicating that adaptive changes, probably including structural alterations at the cellular level, have occurred [107,168,169,170].

Ultrastructural examination of the turtle bladder has revealed that mitochondria-rich (carbonic anhydrase-rich) cells exist in two forms: microvillated and microplicated [119,242]. The luminal surface area is greater in the microplicated state. Maneuvers that raise cell pH inhibit H$^+$ secretion by the bladder and cause microplicated cells to become microvillated, thereby reducing mucosal surface area [119]. On the other hand, the addition of CO$_2$ to turtle bladders increases the number of microplicated cells and thus of apical surface area without changing the total number of carbonic anhydrase–rich cells [245]. The increase in apical surface is due to exocytic insertion of apical cytoplasmic vesicles containing H^+ pumps into the luminal membrane [44,88,245].

Respiratory acidosis and chronic metabolic acidosis lead to an increase in density of the luminal membrane associated with a decrease in volume of tubulovesicular structures in the apical cytoplasm of the intercalated (carbonic anhydrase–rich) cell of the rat medullary collecting duct (168,169).

Acidosis may also result in major changes that convert the cortical collecting tubule from HCO_3^- secretion to H^+ secretion; these may be so extensive as to require cellular remodeling of cytoskeletal and transport proteins [223]. Under control conditions cortical collecting ducts from rabbits secrete HCO_3^-, have a lumen negative transepithelial voltage, few H^+-secreting cells, and many HCO_3^--secreting cells per millimeter of tubule [223]. After the animals are acid loaded, the tubules appear different under the same in vitro conditions. They now absorb HCO_3^- (see Fig. 9-6), have a less negative voltage, 10-fold more H^+-secreting cells, and half as many HCO_3^--secreting cells [223]. It is probable that the increase in number of H^+-secreting cells is caused in part by a reversal of the functional polarity of some intercalated cells; this reversal may mediate the conversion of the tubule from net HCO_3^- secretion to H^+ secretion [223].

In contrast to the in vivo acid–base induced changes in HCO_3^- transport in cortical collecting ducts perfused in vitro, no such effects are seen in outer medullary collecting ducts [161]. However, there is some correlation of in vitro acidification rates in outer medullary collecting ducts to in vivo urine pH in rabbits subjected to starvation [149]. Moreover, acute reduction of peritubular pH by reducing HCO_3^- concentration stimulates HCO_3^- absorption in this segment; alkalinization, by raising peritubular HCO_3^-, has the opposite effect [124].

In the inner medullary collecting duct, metabolic acidosis increases markedly the rate of acidification [101,266]. Microperfusion of distal tubules in vivo has demonstrated that severe metabolic acidosis stimulates HCO_3^- absorption, independent of the HCO_3^- load delivered or of rates of Na^+ and K^+ transport [154,164].

HCO$_3^-$ SECRETION

Secretion of HCO_3^- by isolated cortical collecting ducts requires luminal Cl^- and is stimulated by removal of basolateral Cl^-, in keeping with an apical Cl^-/HCO_3^- exchanger and basolateral Cl^- conductance (see Fig. 9-10) [223,240]. The rate of HCO_3^- secretion in vitro is stimulated by in vivo alkali or mineralocorticoid loading [21,85,139,180,218,240]. Moreover, HCO_3^- secretion in the rabbit collecting duct is stimulated by isoproterenol [218], suggesting that it may be under beta-adrenergic control. In contrast, HCO_3^- secretion in the rat, but not the rabbit [218], collecting duct is inhibited by vasopressin, either directly or by stimulation of concomitant H^+ secretion [263].

Net Acid Excretion

Net acid excretion is calculated by subtracting urinary HCO_3^- from the sum of titratable acid and ammonium; it is usually expressed as mEq/minute/1.73m^2 body surface area (BSA). Nearly 90% of the filtered HCO_3^- is reabsorbed in the proximal tubule; additional HCO_3^- may be absorbed in the loop of Henle and possibly distal tubule (see Fig. 9-5). When acid urine is being formed, the remaining HCO_3^- is reabsorbed distally and net acid excretion results. The collecting ducts secrete protons to acidify the tubular fluid from a value of 6.6 to below 6.0 (see Fig. 9-5). The titration of urinary buffers, especially dibasic phosphate and ammonia, results in the excretion of net acid. Under special conditions, the cortical collecting duct may secrete HCO_3^-, and the urinary pH may exceed 6.5.

Titratable Acid

The main urinary buffer is phosphate (pK = 6.8). Other urinary buffers such as creatinine (pK 5.0) and uric acid (pK 5.7) are quantitatively less important, whereas beta-hydroxybutyrate (pK 4.8) plays a role only during diabetic ketoacidosis. Because urinary acidification is limited to a gradient of 3 pH units (pH 4.5), the excretion of strong acid is accomplished primarily by excretion of the anion with ammonium. By titrating the urinary pH back up to that of blood, one can determine the number of equivalents of protons secreted by the kidney.

In the proximal tubule the fluid is acidified to a pH of about 6.7 and is thus quantitatively the major site of generation of titratable acid (see Fig. 9-5) [39]. Further addition of titratable acid occurs in the collecting duct (see Fig. 9-5) [39]. At a plasma pH of 7.4, approximately 80% of the filtered phosphate is in the form of HPO_2^{-2} ($HPO_4^{-2} + H^+ \rightleftharpoons H_2PO_4^-$; pK = 6.8). In the end proximal or distal tubular fluid, wherein the pH is about 6.7 [39], slightly less than half (44%) of the phosphate remains untitrated as HPO_4^{-2}. As the pH falls in the collecting duct to below pH 6.0, nearly all the remaining alkaline phosphate has been titrated to $H_2PO_4^-$. Metabolic acidosis causes a 35% increase in titratable acid excretion, with the proximal tubule contributing to most of the increment, followed by the medullary collecting duct [39]. Therefore, the doubling or tripling of net acid excretion during acidosis results primarily from the increase in ammonium production and titration [39] (see following).

Ammonium Transport

Ammoniagenesis and its regulation as well as renal ammonia handling are discussed elsewhere (see Chap. 10). A brief summary of the nephron segments that produce and transport ammonia follows. Proximal tubule cells, especially those of the S1 and S2 segments, are the major sites of ammonia production, although all nephron segments can produce ammonia from glutamine [97]. Metabolic acidosis increases production by 60% in the S1 and 150% in S2, without affecting any other segment [97].

Under normal acid–base conditions, ammonia entry into

the proximal tubule can totally account for that amount excreted in the urine [38]. However, the majority of ammonia present at the end of the proximal tubule is not found in the superficial distal convoluted tubule [38,210]. Thus, ammonium is absorbed in the loop of Henle. Finally, ammonia enters the tubular fluid along the distal nephron and prior to the inner medullary collecting duct [38].

Transport of ammonia in the loop of Henle occurs by several mechanisms. First, water abstraction in the descending limb raises the concentration of ammonium and alkalinizes the tubular fluid, thereby back-titrating the ammonium and enabling ammonia to diffuse into the medullary interstitium. The more acidic fluid of the medullary collecting duct then traps this ammonia in the lumen for excretion as ammonium. In addition, there is direct ammonium absorption by cortical and medullary thick ascending limbs [96], and the rates are sufficient to account for the difference between proximal and distal ammonia deliveries [38,96]. Ammonium is absorbed passively or is co-transported with Na^+ and Cl^- [96,98]. Non-ionic diffusion of ammonia is much less likely because the limbs also absorb HCO_3^- and acidify, rather than alkalinize, the tubular fluid [96,98].

In the collecting duct ammonia is added to the final urine by nonionic diffusion and trapped as ammonium in the acidic medullary collecting duct fluid [38,139,241]. Cortical collecting ducts may also trap ammonia by generating an acid disequilibrium pH in the luminal fluid near the cell surfaces [139]. This acid disequilibrium occurs even in cortical collecting ducts that are secreting HCO_3^- and are thereby alkalinizing the tubular fluid [139]. The acid disequilibrium pH may also add to the tubular trapping of ammonia in the outer medullary collecting duct of the outer stripe, which acidifies the tubular fluid [241]. Thus, the generation of an acid disequilibrium pH in the area of H^+-secreting cells in cortical as well as in medullary collecting ducts facilitates net urinary acidification, especially when the delivery of other urinary buffers is limited.

Maturation of Renal Acid–Base Transport
Blood pH, HCO_3^-, and pCO_2

It is well established that infants maintain lower values of pH and concentrations of HCO_3^- and buffer base in the blood than older children or adults [34,237,273,274] (Table 9-1). Moreover, the infant is prone to the development of acidosis during periods of sickness and poor dietary intake. This limited ability to regulate acid–base balance under stress, as well as the "physiologic acidosis" of the newborn, have led investigators to determine the blood parameters of acid–base status (tCO_2, pH, pCO_2, HCO_3^-) and assess renal responses to endogenous and exogenous acid loads. These studies have revealed that the immature kidney is able to maintain acid–base balance in the healthy infant and that the "physiologic acidosis" is not attributable solely to immature kidney function but also to the byproducts of growth and metabolism. Yet, the response to exogenous acid loads is limited in the neonate and most probably contributes to the frequency of metabolic acidosis seen during illness and stress.

Fetal Acid-Base Status

The fetus is exposed to an environment quite different from that prevailing in the mother [280]. Studies done on chronically catheterized fetal sheep have shown that fetal arterial blood pH is less than maternal pH by 0.1–0.2 units and pCO_2 is 10–15 mm Hg higher, whereas no differences are apparent in HCO_3^- concentrations [1,2,61,130,269]. Similar differences have been noted between human fetuses and their mothers [280]. Although the fetus is able to acidify its urine [178], the contribution of the kidney to fetal acid–base homeostasis is probably small [130,177, 269]. The renal acidifying capacity, estimated from the response to acid loading, is much less than that of the adult. The dose of mineral acid per kg body weight required to bring the urinary pH of the sheep down to approximately 5.8 is threefold higher in the fetus than in the adult [269]. The placenta probably excretes most of the acid load [61,238,269].

RESPONSE OF FETUS TO ACID–BASE DISTURBANCES IN MOTHER

Respiratory acid–base disorders in the mother result in changes in pH of the fetus because of the rapid diffusion of CO_2 between maternal and fetal circulatory systems. For instance, maternal hyperventilation associated with mild respiratory alkalosis will result in the diffusion of CO_2 from fetus to mother and an increased blood pH in the fetus. Such an increase may mask the presence of fetal distress (acidosis).

Adjustment of the fetus to maternal metabolic acid–base disturbances takes longer and may not be identical to that of the mother [273]. This reflects not only immature fetal kidney function but also the rapidity of transplacental equilibration of CO_2 versus that of HCO_3^- and protons [31,61]. In maternal metabolic acidosis, there is immediate hyperventilation with partial correction of the acidosis in the mother, but there is "respiratory" alkalosis in the fetus. Such fetal alkalosis in the presence of maternal acidosis could also mask true acidosis in the fetus.

The normal adult respiratory volume of 5 liters/minute generally doubles during pregnancy, reflecting the progesterone-stimulated chronic hyperventilation leading to reduced arterial pCO_2 (26–37 mm Hg) [115,273]. During labor the ventilatory rate increases to as much as 35 liters/minute, resulting in a further decrease in maternal pCO_2 [115]. Yet, during early labor, fetal blood pH is approximately 7.35 (7.25 to 7.45), decreases to 7.30 (7.25 to 7.35) in the second stage, and to 7.25 (7.11 to 7.36) at the time of birth [115,200,273,276a]. Fetal pCO_2 is about 46 mmHg (44 to 48) during early labor and increases to 51 (37 to 79) at birth [160,273,276a]. Although these values are associated with fetal pO_2 levels of 22 mm Hg (16–24 mm Hg) during early labor and only 8–24 mm Hg during delivery [115,160,273,276a], there is no evidence that the fetus is sick from this hypoxemia. Compensatory mechanisms, including high hematocrit, high cardiac output, and shift to the left of the oxyhemoglobin dissociation curve, allow for adequate availability of oxygen. However,

Table 9-1. *Acid-base data in the blood of normal infants, children, and adults*

Group	pH	pCO$_2$ (mm Hg)	tCO$_2$ (mM)	n
Preterm Infants[a]	7.35 ± 0.04	32 ± 3*	17.9 ± 2.2*	6
Term Infants[b]	7.34 ± 0.03*	37 ± 1*	20.0 ± 0.8*	10
Children[b]	7.41 ± 0.04	39 ± 3*	25.2 ± 1.6	10
Male Adults[c]	7.39 ± 0.01	41 ± 2	25.2 ± 1.0	25

Values are given as Mean ± SD.
Postnatal ages were approximately 1 month for preterm, 1–12 months for term infants, 7–12 years for children, and 22–34 years for adults.
Data from [a]Sulyok E, Heim T: Assessment of maximal urinary acidification in premature infants. *Biol Neonate* 19:200, 1971; [b]Edelmann CM Jr, Rodriguez Soriano J, Boichis H, et al: Renal biocarbonate reabsorption and hydrogen ion excretion in normal infants. *J Clin Invest* 46:1309, 1967; and [c]Madias NE, Androgue HJ, Horotwitz GL, et al: A redefinition of normal acid-base equilibrium in man: Carbon dioxide tension as a key determinant of normal plasma bicarbonate concentrations. *Kidney Int* 16:612, 1979.
* Significantly different from adult (P<0.05) by multiple range test.

the stress of labor and delivery most probably affects the acid–base status of the neonate (see following).

Changes in Blood pH, HCO$_3^-$, and pCO$_2$ After Birth

Immediately after birth the neonatal acid–base state resembles that of the fetus, until the lungs and kidneys assume their functions [126,187,237,276,276a]. One hour after birth the normal neonate is in a state of metabolic acidosis with an averge blood pH of 7.30 (range 7.20–7.48), pCO$_2$ of 39 mm Hg, total CO$_2$ of 20–21 mEq/liter, and buffer base of 41 mEq/liter [103,237,273,274]. By 24 hours of age some of these values tend to approach median adult levels: pH reaches 7.39 (adult 7.40), pCO$_2$ 34 mm Hg (adult 41), total CO$_2$ 21 mEq/liter (adult 24 mm Hg), and buffer base 45 mEq/liter (adult 49 mm Hg) [237]. Note that a similar blood pH value is achieved at lower pCO$_2$ and total CO$_2$ values in the newborn compared with the adult. These findings may reflect the varying postnatal rates of brain stem, pulmonary, and renal maturation. That is, to achieve the blood pH of 7.4 set by chemoceptors and brain stem in the presence of renal immaturity, the infant compensates with a centrally driven hyperventilation. In clinical terms, and compared with the adult, the infant has a mixed acid–base disturbance of metabolic acidosis and respiratory alkalosis. As the kidney matures the respiratory drive diminishes.

The low serum bicarbonate concentration observed at birth is associated with about twice the concentration of lactic acid in cord blood as in maternal blood [25]. Lactic acid is also found in higher concentration in umbilical artery than in vein [25]. This difference is considerably larger after an asphyxic birth [73a,110,237]. These findings indicate that lactic acid is produced by the fetus and removed by the placenta until birth.

Response to Acid Loading

Compared with the adult, the term newborn exhibits a larger fall in blood pH and total CO$_2$, a smaller and less rapid fall in urinary pH, and much smaller increases in

urinary titratable acid and ammonium excretion per unit of surface area in response to a comparable acid load per kg body weight [60,80,92,99,108,129,176]. Larger doses of acid per kg body weight are needed in the newborn to promote increased urinary acid excretion [92,108,138, 176,269] as compared with the adult.

The immaturity of the renal response mechanisms of the infant combined with the lower serum buffer base account for the relatively large decreases in pH resulting from minor changes in diet. For example, high protein feeding may result in metabolic acidosis during the first two to three weeks after birth, whereas it has no effect on the acid–base status of infants over two months of age [47,62, 111,175,255]. Although phosphate preloading of one-week-old infants can increase acid excretion by 150% [108,176], the rate of titratable acid excretion only approaches half that of the adult [138].

These limitations in acid excretion disappear during the first month of life [187a,256]. Acid loading studies performed in infants older than one month have shown that the infant acidifies the urine to the same degree as do older children (Table 9-2); that is, with regard to minimum urinary pH and net acid excretion per 1.73 m^2 BSA, there is no limitation in the ability of a healthy infant to excrete metabolically produced protons, yet infants can be rendered acidotic more easily than adults [76]. (Note that in the studies included in Table 9-2 the adults received less NH$_4$Cl per kg and therefore may not have responded as completely as the infants and children.) This is due to the fact that during acidosis older subjects can double or triple their baseline rates of net acid excretion, whereas the infant is limited in this response [75,76,108,176].

The renal response to an acid load appears to increase with both gestational and postnatal ages. Net acid excretion, including rates of excretion of both titratable acid and ammonium, increases by approximately 50% during the first three weeks of life [129,251,256]. Premature infants of 34 to 36 weeks gestational age and 1 to 3 weeks postnatal age exhibit only half the rates of net acid, titratable acid, and ammonium excretion as do term babies of comparable postnatal age [256]. After NH$_4$Cl loading, urinary pH in preterm infants does not consistently decrease below 5.9 until the second postnatal month, whereas in one- to three-week-old term infants it decreases to below

Table 9-2. *Renal response to acute acid load*

Group	Glomerular Filtration Rate (ml/min/1.73m²)	Urinary pH (minimum)	TA	NH⁴ (µEq/min/1.73m²)	NAE	n
Preterm Infants[a]	61 ± 3*	5.2 ± 0.2*	54 ± 20*	37 ± 10*	90 ± 24	8
Term Infants[b]	84 ± 30	4.9 ± 0.1	62 ± 16*	57 ± 14	119 ± 30*	11
Children[b]	123 ± 38	4.9 ± 0.2	50 ± 10	80 ± 12*	130 ± 14*	10
Adults[c]	109 ± 32	4.8 ± 0.2	39 ± 10	52 ± 12	91 ± 21	9

Values are given as Mean ± SD; TA = titratable acid; NAE = net acid excretion.
NH_4Cl was given orally at 4–5 mEq/kg in infants and children, 1.9 mEq/kg for adults.
Urine was collected 3–5 hours after acid load, at which time plasma tCO_2 had fallen 4–6 mEq/L.
Postnatal ages were 3–4 months for preterm infants, 1–12 months for term infants, 7–12 years for children, and 29–64 years for adults.
Data from [a]Schwartz GJ, Haycock GB, Edelmann CM Jr, et al: Late metabolic acidosis: A reassessment of the definition. *J Pediatr* 95:102, 1979; [b]Edelmann CM Jr, Rodriguez Soriano J, Boichis H, et al: Renal bicarbonate reabsorption and hydrogen ion excretion in normal infants. *J Clin Invest* 46:1309, 1967; and [c]Wrong O, Davies HEF: The excretion of acid in renal disease. *Q J Med* 28:259, 1959.
* Significantly different from adult (P<0.05) by multiple range test.

pH 5 [251–254,256] (see Table 9-2). Thus, during the neonatal period premature infants are limited in their ability to excrete an acid load and do not quite achieve the performance exhibited by term infants, even by four to six weeks of age [47,251,256] (see Table 9-2).

The increment in renal net acid excretion in the neonatal premature infant following acid loading is half that observed during the second month, indicating that early in life acid excretion is normally at close to the maximal rate [256]. The blunted response to acid loading of premature infants compared with term infants may be related to immaturity of acid secretory mechanisms or to the relative unresponsiveness of the distal tubule and collecting duct to aldosterone. Protein loading can enhance net renal acid excretion, primarily by increasing the availability of phosphate and thus stimulating titratable acid excretion (rather than ammonium excretion) [47,256]. The increase in plasma base deficit and decrease in plasma tCO_2 associated with protein loading may reflect in part the increased catabolism of excess dietary protein to nonvolatile acids and the immaturity of renal acid excretory mechanisms.

TITRATABLE ACID

The limited ability of the immature kidney to respond to acid loading is due in part to insufficient excretion of urinary buffers. This is due not only to the low glomerular filtration rate but also to the low dietary supply of phosphate and the retention of this anion for the process of growth. Before feeding begins, only 10% to 25% of renal acid is excreted as titratable acid [177]. In one-week-old babies fed cow's milk formulas, which are rich in phosphate, net acid excretion per kg per day is high, and 60% of the urinary acid is titratable acid [177]. On the other hand, one-week-old breast-fed infants (ingesting low phosphate milk) excreted 60% less net acid than infants fed cow's milk, and only 20% of this was as titratable acid [177]. In some cases breast-fed babies excrete 10-fold less titratable acid than do infants fed cow's milk [47,80]. However, net acid excretion is appropriately lower with breast milk feeding, because human milk contains less protein than does cow's milk, which reduces the metabolic production of acid [138].

AMMONIUM

Limitations in ammonia production and excretion may also contribute to the inability of the immature kidney to excrete acid loads or regulate acid–base balance during stress. At similar urinary values of pH, there is a lower rate of synthesis of ammonia in the newborn than in the adult [60,92]. Other factors accounting for the low rates of urinary excretion of ammonia include lower concentration of renal glutamine and lower activities of renal glutaminase and glutamine synthetase (approximately one-third of adult levels in one- to two-week-old rats) [93]. Renal gluconeogenic capacity, measured as the rate of conversion of glutamate to glucose by cortical slices, is low in newborn rats [94]. In addition, the lowering of renal glutamate concentration (an inhibitor of glutaminase) following acid loading is not observed in the young rat, consistent with a lack of stimulation of ammonia synthesis and secretion in response to acidosis [93]. All of these factors approach those of the adult rat by two to three weeks postnatally, but may take as long as one to two years in the human [75,76,138]. The relevance of these in vitro findings to in vivo renal ammonia production by the human infant is, at best, tenuous.

Bicarbonate Reabsorption

In addition to limitations in proton secretion, infants are faced with a lower plasma HCO_3^- concentration, which is attributable to a lower renal threshold for HCO_3^- reabsorption [75] (Table 9-1); (Fig. 9-11). During the first year of life infants have a HCO_3^- threshold of 21.5–22.5 mM, significantly lower than that of adults (24–28 mM) (Fig. 9-11) [7,75,103,167,202]. Consequently, infants have 20% less HCO_3^- buffer per unit of plasma volume than do adults.

In a state of acid–base balance, the level of the HCO_3^- threshold, rather than the maximal rate of reabsorption of HCO_3^-, determines HCO_3^- concentration in plasma. The renal HCO_3^- threshold is primarily a property of the proximal tubule, from which nearly 85% of the filtered HCO_3^- is reabsorbed [14,141]. Several studies have confirmed the lower HCO_3^- threshold of the infant, despite

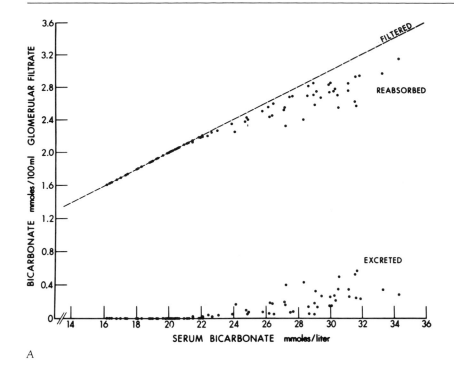

A

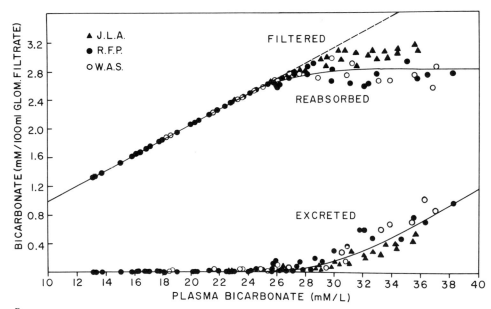

B

FIG. 9-11. *Reabsorption and excretion of filtered* HCO_3^- *in infants (A) and adults (B). Although the maximum rates of* HCO_3^- *reabsorption are similar, infants show a lower threshold. (From Edelmann CM Jr, Rodriguez Soriano J, Boichis H, et al: Renal bicarbonate reabsorption and hydrogen ion excretion in normal infants. J Clin Invest 46:1309, 1967; and Pitts RF, Ayer JL, Schiess WA: The renal regulation of acid–base balance in man. J Clin Invest 28:35, 1949, with permission.)*

the fact that the maximal rates of HCO_3^- reabsorption (Tm HCO_3^-) are in the range of those reported for adults [195] (2.5 to 2.6 mEq/dl of glomerular filtration rate) (Fig. 9-11) [75,254,265]. This same situation also applies to the lower plasma concentration of HCO_3^- in premature in-

fants in whom the reabsorption of HCO_3^- is also nearly complete (see Table 9-1) [228,254,265].

Studies performed in puppies have confirmed that there is good agreement between resting levels of plasma HCO_3^- concentration and the renal threshold for HCO_3^-, both of which at 18 mEq/liter are substantially less than mature levels of 23–26 mEq/liter [188]. Gastric aspiration combined with the infusion of sodium and potassium bicarbonate progressively increased plasma HCO_3^- concentrations in the absence of volume expansion, while raising the renal threshold for HCO_3^- to 25 mEq/liter (the adult level); there was no transport maximum for HCO_3^- reabsorption [188]. Thus, the low threshold for HCO_3^- in the infant appears not to be due to a limitation in the maximal transport capacity for HCO_3^-. It may reflect greater nephron heterogeneity, a response to the large extracellular volume prevailing at this age [84], or it may be a consequence of a low fractional reabsorption of sodium in the proximal tubule [76].

Metabolic Acidosis of Prematurity

As noted previously, full-term infants beyond the first day or two of postnatal life are able to maintain plasma pH values that are comparable to those of adults [7,237,274]; this is accomplished at low total CO_2 and pCO_2 values (see Table 9-1) [7,75,274]. Although there is no satisfactory explanation for the low pCO_2, it is likely that respiration is adjusted to the reduced renal threshold for HCO_3^- to generate a "normal" plasma pH.

The situation in the low-birth-weight (LBW) or premature infant is complicated by a relative metabolic acidosis (pH approximately 7.3), which tends to persist beyond the first day of postnatal life [34,37,103,174, 202,254]. The condition is generally that of simple metabolic acidosis [103,129,193,202,237,251]. Depending on a variety of factors, including the gestational age, birth weight, and feeding history of the LBW infant, acid–base variables tend to reach values comparable to those in a full-term infant by three to six weeks of postnatal life (Fig. 9-12; Table 9-1) [129,228,251]. By this time blood pH nears 7.4 and plasma total CO_2 20–22 mEq/liter, indicating that pCO_2 must still be low (approximately 35 mm Hg) [129,228]. Therefore, healthy premature infants attain a normal blood pH only by hyperventilating, much like term infants (see Table 9-1). The stimulus of the respiratory center is unknown, but it is not hypoxia [237].

The chronic state of hypobasemia and hyperpnea in premature infants suggests a continuing source of acid that may be due to the persistence of fetal metabolic processes. An overproduction of lactic and pyruvic acid would result in a reduction of buffer base and contribute to metabolic acidosis. Indeed, the plasma content of organic acids of premature infants is two to three times as great as that of full-term infants or adults [34,237]. Normal premature infants 3 to 58 days of age (1.1–2.2 kg) excrete two to five times more organic acid per body weight per day than does the normal adult [34]. Ketone bodies are not responsible for this excess of organic acids, and lactic acid constitutes less than 20% of the total excretion of organic acids [34,131]. The difference is made up in large part by pyruvic acid [95,237]. The presence of excess lactic and pyruvic acids suggests incomplete carbohydrate metabolism, as observed in the fetus [73a,95,110], but this may not be the only explanation [237]. This temporarily persistent fetal

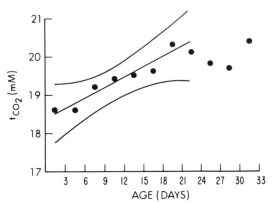

FIG. 9-12. *Regression and confidence limits of plasma tCO_2 values as a function of postnatal age in low-birth-weight infants. Each point represents the mean for a three-day interval; 385 separate determinations from 114 infants are included. (From Schwartz, et al: J Pediatr 95:102, 1979, with permission).*

metabolic pattern cannot result from prolonged asphyxia, since oxygen tension is greater in the neonate than in the fetus; however, as a consequence of hypoxia during labor and delivery, combustible organic acids, including lactate, may accumulate and contribute to metabolic acidosis [131].

Studies of acid–base balance in LBW infants (1–2 kg body weight) have shown that total CO_2 concentrations range between 16.7 and 18.8 mEq/liter during the first four weeks of postnatal life, while base deficit exceeds 6 mEq/liter (Table 9-1) [252]. By the sixth week of postnatal life, total CO_2 goes up to 21 mEq/liter, and the base deficit decreases to less than 4 mEq/liter [252]. A similar study performed in the United States revealed that total CO_2 values of 20 mEq/liter or greater are generally achieved by three postnatal weeks (see Fig. 9-12) [228].

Late Metabolic Acidosis

Late metabolic acidosis was originally described by Kildeberg [132] in a group of apparently healthy two- to three-week-old prematurely born infants, fed cow's milk formulas, with delayed weight gain. The net acid excretion was generally increased in these patients, but not sufficiently to offset the high endogenous rate of acid production, presumably caused by excessive catabolism of dietary constituents in the context of a delayed growth response [132,133]. Supporting this interpretation is the observation that the spontaneous correction of the acid–base imbalance was usually associated with a rapid gain in body weight.

Subsequently late metabolic acidosis was defined more broadly to include acidotic infants with appropriate rates of growth and those with "feeding acidosis" due to excessive protein intake [201,217]. We studied 114 healthy premature infants who were fed 2.5 to 3 g/kg of protein per day (to maximize growth but prevent feeding acidosis) and monitored their acid–base status (plasma tCO_2) during the first three weeks of life. Plasma tCO_2 values as low as

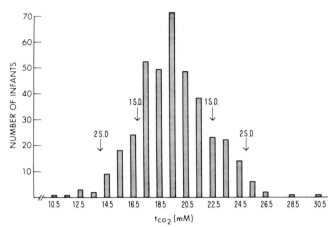

FIG. 9-13. *Frequency distribution of plasma tCO$_2$ values from 385 determinations in 114 healthy low birth weight infants. (From Schwartz GJ, Haycock GB, Edelmann CM Jr, et al: Late metabolic acidosis: A reassessment of the definition. J Pediatr 95:102, 1979, with permission.)*

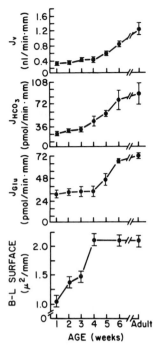

FIG. 9-14. *Maturational increases in water, HCO$_3^-$, and glucose absorption by isolated perfused juxtamedullary proximal convoluted tubules of rabbits and compared with changes in basolateral surface area. Jv, fluid absorption; J$_{HCO_3}$, HCO$_3^-$ absorption; Jglu, glucose absorption; BL-SURFACE, basolateral surface area. (From Schwartz GJ, Evan AP: Development of solute transport in rabbit proximal tubule. I. HCO$_3^-$ and glucose absorption. Am J Physiol 245:F382, 1983, with permission.)*

14.5 mM were found to fall within 2 SD of the mean tCO$_2$ value (19.5 mM) [228]. A histogram showed no deviations from normality (Fig. 9-13). There was no difference in the rate of weight gain between infants with tCO$_2$ values above or below 18 mM. Moreover, therapy with HCO$_3^-$, sufficient to bring the tCO$_2$ to 21 mM, did not affect the rate of weight gain [228].

These studies confirm that healthy premature infants have plasma tCO$_2$ values below those of full-term newborns. Average values are 18.6 mM at birth and increase to 20 mM by the first month (see Fig. 9-12) [228]. True hypobasemia at this age means a plasma tCO$_2$ value below 14.5 mM (see Fig. 9-13), a much more stringent criterion for metabolic acidosis than previously employed [228]. Late metabolic acidosis thus should be a diagnosis confined only to the premature infant who is hypobasemic and failing to grow [132,133,228].

Experimental Data Concerning Maturation of Acid–Base Mechanisms

HCO$_3^-$ REABSORPTION

The foregoing data suggest that the mechanism for reabsorption of HCO$_3^-$, primarily a property of the proximal tubule, is fully developed at birth. Although fractional reabsorption of HCO$_3^-$ approaches 100%, the threshold for HCO$_3^-$ reabsorption is set lower in term and preterm infants than in older children and adults [75,228,254]. Studies in proximal tubule segments isolated from maturing rabbits and perfused in vitro have provided some pertinent information. First, in the early proximal tubule taken from rabbits of various ages, HCO$_3^-$ absorption is directly proportional to net Na$^+$ transport (Jv), indicating that this is primarily a Na$^+$-dependent process [226]. Second, there is tremendous heterogeneity in the postnatal maturation of

proximal tubular structure and function, such that marked variability in the rate of HCO$_3^-$ absorption would be expected between superficial and deep nephron segments during this period [78,226]. Third, HCO$_3^-$ absorption is at one-third of the adult level in the juxtamedullary proximal tubule during the first three weeks of life (26–30 pmol/minute/mm) and rises acutely (160%) during the next three weeks before reaching the adult range by 8–12 weeks (89 ± 18 pmol/minute/mm) (Fig. 9-14) [226].

A similar maturational change has been observed in the near-steady-state gradient for tCO$_2$ that can be achieved by the segment at very slow flow rates. This variable provides information about the rates of HCO$_3^-$ absorption balanced against its leak back into the lumen (pump versus leak) and gives an approximate value for the steady state end-proximal pH. The gradient was 8–9 mM during the first two weeks of life (pH 7.2) and thereafter doubled (to approximately 18 mM) in four- to five-week-old animals to equal that of adult rabbits (pH 6.8) [226] (see Fig. 9-5). Ouabain caused the gradient to decline to 1–4 mM at all ages. Thus, the maturational increase in HCO$_3^-$ gradient generated by the juxtamedullary proximal tubule parallels the surge in net HCO$_3^-$ transport and is mediated in large part by increased Na$^+$/H$^+$ exchange. Whether the increased Na$^+$/H$^+$ exchange is due to increased number of exchangers or increased driving forces for H^+ secretion via the same exchangers is considered in the following morphologic and functional studies.

Morphologic studies in rabbit kidney showed inner cortical proximal tubules to be mature by four weeks of postnatal life (see Fig. 9-14), midcortical by five to six weeks, and outer cortical by seven weeks [78]. It is probable that transport capacity parallels the morphologic maturation [15]. Therefore, major differences in transport capabilities would be expected in proximal segments taken from different locations in the cortex during postnatal maturation, and major imbalances between nephron HCO_3^- filtration and reabsorption could be manifested by a greater splay and reduced threshold for HCO_3^- reabsorption [75,76]. This conclusion becomes more powerful if it can be established that the superficial nephrons are filtering but are not capable of reabsorbing solutes. In this regard, micropuncture studies have shown that fluid reabsorptive capacity in young rats is approximately 40% of that of mature rats, while single nephron glomerular filtration rates are less than 20% of mature values [15]. These studies indicate that proximal tubular HCO_3^- reabsorptive capacity is more than adequate for the rate of nephron glomerular filtration and should rule out an insufficient rate of Na^+ or HCO_3^- transport as a cause of the low renal HCO_3^- threshold.

The maturational surge in HCO_3^- absorption may be caused by at least two factors: an increase in the number of luminal Na^+-H^+ exchangers and an increase in the driving forces for luminal Na^+ entry (and thereby H^+ secretion). The latter would be consequent to an increase

in basolateral Na-K-ATPase activity and thus in the extrusion of Na^+ across the basolateral membrane. These possibilities were investigated by measuring the maturation of glucose absorption, which is co-transported with Na^+ and thus, like HCO_3^-, is dependent on the lumen to cell gradient for Na^+ [226]. The results proved that the maturation of glucose absorption parallels that of HCO_3^- (see Fig. 9-14), indicating that the luminal transporters mature synchronously or that the availability of Na-K-ATPase determines the maturation of both transport pathways. The finding that the surface area of the luminal membrane reaches mature levels before the increases in transport [78] suggests that the structure of the luminal membrane does not limit solute transport in the maturing proximal tubule. Moreover, the increase in basolateral membrane surface area, taken to be proportional to Na-K-ATPase activity [227], precedes the maturational surges in solute transport (see Fig. 9-14).

The relationship between Na-K-ATPase and the maturation of HCO_3^- transport was investigated by measuring Na-K-ATPase activity (Vmax) in individual juxtamedullary proximal tubules [227]. The maturation of HCO_3^- transport was found to precede that of maximal Na-K-ATPase activity (Fig. 9-15), indicating that the change in Na-K-ATPase activity is secondary to the maturation of HCO_3^- transport [227]. Therefore, the rise in HCO_3^- absorption must be a function of the number of Na^+-H^+ exchangers present in the luminal membrane. It is likely that their numbers increase according to a determined postnatal maturational pattern, as suggested by the increase in Na^+-glucose transporters. The resulting increase in intracellular Na^+ concentration then stimulates Na-K-

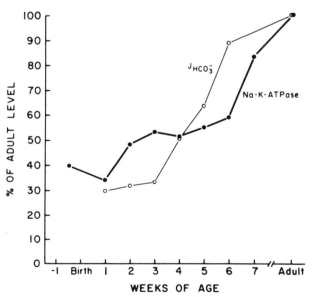

FIG. 9-15. Maturational increases in HCO_3^- absorption and maximal Na-K-ATPase activity as percentage of adult level in isolated juxtamedullary proximal convoluted tubules of the rabbit. (From Schwartz GJ, Evan AP: Development of solute transport in rabbit proximal tubule. III. Na-K-ATPase activity. Am J Physiol 246:F845, 1984, with permission.)

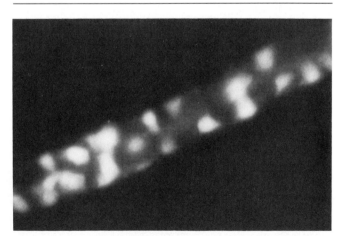

FIG. 9-16. Cortical collecting duct isolated from mature rabbit kidney and stained with the pH sensitive dye 6-carboxyfluorescein. Bright staining cells are rich in carbonic anhydrase and have an alkaline cell pH; they are intercalated cells. The darker areas represent principal cells, which do not take up this dye in high concentration. Real magnification was ×100 before 26% reduction. (From Satlin LM, Schwartz GJ: Postnatal maturation of rabbit renal collecting duct: Intercalated cell function. Am J Physiol 253:F622, 1987, with permission.)

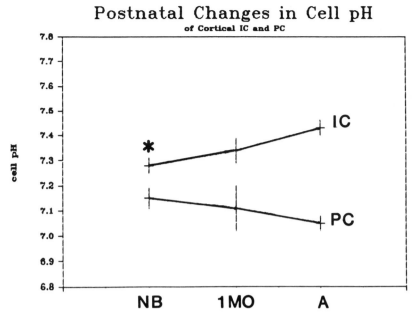

FIG. 9-17. *Maturational changes in pH of intercalated (IC) and principal (PC) cells of isolated cortical collecting ducts of the newborn (NB), one-month-old (1 MO), and adult (A) rabbits. (From Satlin LM, Schwartz GJ: Postnatal maturation of rabbit renal collecting duct: Intercalated cell function. Am J Physiol 253:F622, 1987, with permission.)*

ATPase activity, which in turn restores intracellular Na^+ concentration toward the initial values [227].

CARBONIC ANHYDRASE

No differences in carbonic anhydrase activity were found in renal homogenates from prematures, term infants, and adults [27,63,163], although the concentration increases during maturation in the kidneys of several laboratory animals [79,173]. However, histochemical studies in the 26-week human fetus have revealed that in the inner cortex proximal tubular staining was of similar intensity to that seen in the adult cortex, while in the fetal outer cortex (newly formed nephrons) little evidence for carbonic anhydrase was found [163]. Also, there was significant carbonic anhydrase activity in some fetal collecting duct cells in cortex and outer medulla but less staining than in mature cells [163]. A postnatal study showed marked immuno-histochemical heterogeneity in nephronal carbonic anhydrase activity, the intensity of staining increasing with maturation in all zones of the kidney [35]. Despite these changes, it is not clear whether lack of carbonic anhydrase is the factor limiting H^+ secretion in premature infants. The catalytic activity or turnover number for carbonic anhydrase is so high that only small amounts are required to sustain H^+ secretion [173].

INTERCALATED CELLS

To investigate the final renal regulation of net H^+ secretion at the cellular level, we isolated cortical and medullary collecting ducts from maturing rabbits and measured cell pH using the fluorescent pH sensitive dye 6-carboxyfluorescein [216]. This dye permits not only the measurement of cell pH, but also an estimate of cytosolic carbonic anhydrase activity [44,113,216,223]. Indeed, the green fluorescence of 6-carboxyfluorescein was concentrated selectively in mature intercalated cells, the intensity being three- to tenfold higher than in neighboring principal cells (Fig. 9-16) [216].

We also found that the mature intercalated cell was 0.4 ± 0.1 pH units more alkaline (pH 7.43 ± 0.03) than the principal cell (Fig. 9-17). With these techniques the neonatal intercalated cell was not identifiable in the outer cortical collecting duct but was found in the mid-cortex (Fig. 9-18). Its intracellular pH was significantly less alkaline (7.28 ± 0.03) than that of the mature animal but still more alkaline than that of the adjacent principal cell (Fig. 9-17). The lower pH in the immature intercalated cell is attributable to a paucity of proton pumps and reduced mitochondrial potential [216].

As maturation progresses, the number of 6-carboxyfluorescein-identified intercalated cells/millimeter of tubule doubled in the mid-cortex, while less differentiated intercalated cells appeared in the outer cortex. During the second postnatal month, the intercalated cells from the mid-cortex appeared more differentiated, as assessed by the more alkaline pH (see Fig. 9-17), larger mitochondrial potential, and a greater density of H^+ pumps [216]. Intercalated cells from the neonatal outer medullary collecting duct had a cell pH similar to that measured in

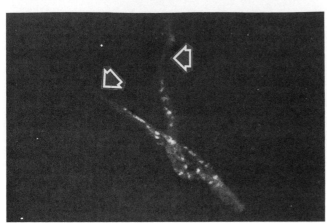

FIG. 9-18. *Fluorescence micrograph of isolated newborn branched collecting duct stained with 6-carboxyfluorescein. Bright staining cells are rich in carbonic anhydrase and have an alkaline cell pH; they are localized to the inner cortex and outer medulla. Note the relative absence of dye uptake in the most superficial cortex (arrowheads), consistent with the absence of intercalated cells in the immature outer cortex. Real magnification was ×25 before 26% reduction. (From Satlin LM, Schwartz GJ: Postnatal maturation of rabbit renal collecting duct: Intercalated cell function. Am J Physiol 253:F622, 1987, with permission.)*

mature ducts (7.27 ± 0.04 versus 7.28 ± 0.04; p = NS), as well as numerous acidic cytoplasmic vesicles and significant mitochondrial potentials. There was no increase in number of intercalated cells/millimeter in this segment with maturation [216].

These data show that in the rabbit the intercalated cells of the outer medullary segment are nearly mature, whereas those of the cortical collecting duct proliferate and differentiate during postnatal life (see Fig. 9-18). The centrifugal pattern of postnatal renal maturation is recapitulated in the collecting duct, but the nature of the signals directing cell proliferation and cytodifferentiation are presently unknown [216]. The immature state of the neonatal cortical collecting duct, in particular of the intercalated cells, suggests that this segment may not be capable of responding significantly to changes in acid–base state. This may explain in part the severity of acidosis seen in the neonate during periods of stress and disease, especially if the outer medullary (more mature) intercalated cells are already secreting protons at near maximal rates to support normal metabolism and growth.

References

1. Adams FH, Fujiwara T, Rowshan S: The nature and origin of the fluid in the fetal lamb lung. *J Pediatr* 63:881, 1963.
2. Adams FH, Moss AJ, Fagan L: The tracheal fluid in the fetal lamb. *Biol Neonate* 5:151, 1963.
3. Adam WR, Simpson DP: Renal mitochondrial glutamine metabolism and dietary potassium and protein content. *Kidney Int* 7:325, 1975.
4. Al-Awqati Q: Proton-translocating ATPases. *Ann Rev Cell Biol* 2:179, 1986.
5. Al-Awqati Q, Mueller A, Steinmetz PR: Transport of H+ against electrochemical gradients in turtle urinary bladder. *Am J Physiol* 233:F502, 1977.
6. Al-Awqati Q, Norby LH, Mueller A, et al: Characteristics of stimulation of H+ transport by aldosterone in turtle urinary bladder. *J Clin Invest* 58:351, 1976.
7. Albert MS, Winters RW: Acid-base equilibrium of blood in normal infants. *Pediatrics* 37:728, 1966.
8. Alpern RJ: Bicarbonate-water interactions in the rat proximal convoluted tubule: An effect of volume flux on active proton secretion. *J Gen Physiol* 84:753, 1984.
9. Alpern RJ: Mechanism of basolateral H+/OH−/HCO3− transport in the rat proximal tubule: A sodium-coupled electrogenic process. *J Gen Physiol* 86:613, 1985.
10. Alpern RJ, Chambers M: Cell pH in the rat proximal convoluted tubule: Regulation by luminal and peritubular pH and sodium concentration. *J Clin Invest* 78:502, 1986.
11. Alpern RJ, Cogan MG, Rector FC Jr: Effect of luminal bicarbonate concentration on proximal acidification in the rat. *Am J Physiol* 243:F53, 1982.
12. Alpern RJ, Cogan MG, Rector FC Jr: Flow dependence of proximal tubular bicarbonate absorption. *Am J Physiol* 245:F478, 1983.
13. Alpern RJ, Cogan MG, Rector FC Jr: Effects of extracellular fluid volume and plasma bicarbonate concentration on proximal acidification in the rat. *J Clin Invest* 71:736, 1983.
14. Alpern RJ, Warnock DG, Rector FC Jr: Renal acidification mechanisms. *In* Brenner BM, Rector FC Jr (eds): *The Kidney*, 3rd ed. Philadelphia, Saunders, 1986, p 206.
15. Aperia A, Larsson L: Correlation between fluid reabsorption and proximal tubule ultrastructure during development of the rat kidney. *Acta Physiol Scand* 105:11, 1979.
16. Arbus GS, Herbert LA, Levesque PR, et al: Characterization and clinical application of the "significance band" for acute respiratory alkalosis. *N Engl J Med* 280:117, 1969.
17. Aronson PS: Mechanism of active H+ secretion in the proximal tubule. *Am J Physiol* 245:F647, 1983.
18. Aronson PS, Nee J, Suhm MA: Modifier role of internal H+ in activating the Na+-H+ exchanger in renal microvillus membrane vesicles. *Nature* 299:161, 1982.
19. Aronson PS, Suhm MA, Nee J: Interaction of external H+ with the Na+-H+ exchanger in renal microvillus membrane vesicles. *J Biol Chem* 258:6767, 1983.
20. Arruda JAL: Calcium inhibits urinary acidification: Effect of the ionophore A23187 on the turtle bladder. *Pflugers Arch* 183:107, 1979.
21. Atkins JL, Burg MB: Bicarbonate transport by isolated perfused rat collecting ducts. *Am J Physiol* 249:F485, 1985.
22. Bank N, Aynedjian HS: A micropuncture study of the effect of parathyroid hormone on renal bicarbonate reabsorption. *J Clin Invest* 58:336, 1976.
23. Bank N, Aynedjian HS, Mutz BF: Evidence for a DCCD-sensitive component of proximal bicarbonate reabsorption. *Am J Physiol* 249:F636, 1985.
24. Bank N, Schwartz WB: The influence of anion penetrating ability on urinary acidification and the excretion of titratable acid. *J Clin Invest* 39:1516, 1960.
25. Bell B: The metabolism and acidity of the foetal tissues and fluids. *Br Med J* 1:126, 1928.
26. Bengele HH, McNamara ER, Alexander EA: Effect of acute thyroparathyroidectomy on nephron acidification. *Am J Physiol* 246:F569, 1984.
27. Berfenstam R: Carbonic anhydrase activity in fetal organs. *Acta Paediatr [Uppsala]* 41:310, 1952.

28. Berry CA, Cogan MG: Influence of peritubular protein on solute absorption in the rabbit proximal tubule: A specific effect on NaCl transport. *J Clin Invest* 68:506, 1981.

29. Berry CA, Warnock DG: Acidification in the in vitro perfused tubule. *Kidney Int* 22:507, 1982.

30. Biagi B, Kubota T, Sohtell M, et al: Intracellular potentials in rabbit proximal tubules perfused in vitro. *Am J Physiol* 240:F200, 1981.

31. Blechner JN, Meschia G, Barron GH: A study of the acid-base balance of fetal sheep and goats. *Q J Exp Physiol* 45:60, 1960.

32. Blumenthal SS, Ware RA, Kleinman JG: Proximal tubule hydrogen ion transport processes in diuretic-induced metabolic alkalosis. *J Lab Clin Med* 106:17, 1985.

33. Brackett NC, Cohen JJ, Schwartz WB: Carbon dioxide titration curve of normal man. Effect of increasing degrees of acute hypercapnia on acid-base equilibrium. *N Engl J Med* 272:6, 1965.

34. Branning WS: The acid-base balance of premature infants. *J Clin Invest* 21:101, 1942.

35. Brown D, Kumpulainen T, Roth J, et al: Immunohistochemical localization of carbonic anhydrase in postnatal and adult rat kidney. *Am J Physiol* 245:F110, 1983.

36. Brown D, Orci L: The "coat" of kidney intercalated cell tubulovesicles does not contain clathrin. *Am J Physiol* 250:C605, 1986.

37. Bucci G, Scalamandre A, Savignoni PG, et al: Acid-base status of "normal" premature infants in the first week of life. *Biol Neonate* 8:81, 1965.

38. Buerkert J, Martin D, Trigg D: Ammonium handling by superficial and juxtamedullary nephrons in the rat: Evidence for an ammonia shunt between the loop of Henle and the collecting duct. *J Clin Invest* 70:1, 1978.

39. Buerkert J, Martin D, Trigg D: Segmental analysis of the renal tubule in buffer production and net acid formation. *Am J Physiol* 244:F442, 1983.

40. Burckhardt B Ch, Cassola AC, Fromter E: Electrophysiological analysis of bicarbonate permeation across the peritubular cell membrane of rat kidney proximal tubule. II. Exclusion of HCO_3^-- effects on other ion permeabilities and of coupled electroneutral HCO_3^--transport. *Pflugers Arch* 401:43, 1984.

41. Burg M, Green N: Bicarbonate transport by isolated perfused rabbit proximal tubules. *Am J Physiol* 233:F307, 1977.

42. Burnell JM, Teubner EM, Simpson DP: Metabolic acidosis accompanying potassium deprivation. *Am J Physiol* 227:329, 1974.

43. Burnham C, Munzesheimer C, Rabon E, et al: Ion pathways in renal brush border membranes. *Biochim Biophys Acta* 685:260, 1982.

44. Cannon C, van Adelsberg J, Kelly S, et al: Carbon-dioxide-induced exocytotic insertion of H^+ pumps in turtle bladder luminal membrane: Role of cell pH and calcium. *Nature* 314:443, 1985.

45. Capasso G, Kinne R, Malnic G, et al: Renal bicarbonate reabsorption in the rat. I. Effects of hypokalemia and carbonic anhydrase. *J Clin Invest* 78:1558, 1986.

46. Chan JCM: Acid-base and mineral disorders in children: A review. *Int J Pediatr Nephrol* 1:54, 1980.

47. Chan LL, Balfe JW, Exeni R, et al: Net acid excretion during first week of life. *Int J Pediatr Nephrol* 2:37, 1981.

48. Chan YL: Adrenergic control of bicarbonate absorption in the proximal convoluted tubule of the rat kidney. *Pflugers Arch* 388:159, 1980.

49. Chan YL, Biagi B, Giebisch G: Control mechanisms of bicarbonate transport across the rat proximal convoluted tubule. *Am J Physiol* 242:F532, 1982.

50. Chan YL, Giebisch G: Relationship between sodium and bicarbonate transport in the rat proximal convoluted tubule. *Am J Physiol* 240:F222, 1981.

51. Chantrelle B, Cogan MG, Rector FC Jr: Evidence for coupled sodium/hydrogen exchange in the rat superficial proximal tubule. *Pflugers Arch* 395:186, 1982.

52. Clapp WL, Madsen KM, Verlander JW, et al: Intercalated cells of the rat inner medullary collecting duct. *Kidney Int* 31:1080, 1987.

53. Cogan MG: Volume expansion predominately inhibits proximal reabsorption of NaCl rather than $NaHCO_3$. *Am J Physiol* 245:F272, 1983.

54. Cogan MG: Effect of acute alterations in Pco_2 on proximal HCO_3^-, Cl^-, and H_2O reabsorption. *Am J Physiol* 246:F21, 1984.

55. Cogan MG: Neurogenic regulation of proximal bicarbonate and chloride reabsorption. *Am J Physiol* 250:F22, 1986.

56. Cogan MG, Liu FY: Metabolic alkalosis in the rat: Evidence that reduced glomerular filtration rather than enhanced tubular bicarbonate reabsorption is responsible for maintaining the alkalotic state. *J Clin Invest* 71:1141, 1983.

57. Cogan MG, Maddox DA, Lucci MS, et al: Control of proximal bicarbonate reabsorption in normal and acidotic rats. *J Clin Invest* 64:1168, 1979.

58. Cohn DE, Klahr S, Hammerman MR: Metabolic acidosis and parathyroidectomy increase Na^+/H^+ exchange in brush border vesicles. *Am J Physiol* 245:F217, 1983.

59. Coleman JE: Carbonic anhydrase: Zinc and the mechanism of catalysis. *Ann NY Acad Sci* 429:26, 1984.

60. Cort JH, McCance RA: The renal response of puppies to an acidosis. *J Physiol (Lond)* 124:358, 1954.

61. Daniel SS, Baratz RA, Bowe ET, et al: Elimination of hydrogen ion by the lamb fetus and newborn. *Pediatr Res* 6:584, 1972.

62. Darrow DC, daSilva MM, Stevenson SS: Production of acidosis in premature infants by protein milk. *J Pediatr* 27:43, 1945.

63. Day R, Franklin J: Renal carbonic anhydrase in premature and mature infants. *Pediatrics* 7:182, 1951.

64. deMello-Aires M, Malnic G: Peritubular pH and Pco_2 in renal tubular acidification. *Am J Physiol* 288:1766, 1975.

65. Dennis VW: Influence of bicarbonate on parathyroid hormone-induced changes in fluid absorption by the proximal tubule. *Kidney Int* 10:373, 1976.

66. Diaz E, Sandblem JP, Wistrand PJ: Selectivity properties of channels induced by a reconstituted membrane-bound carbonic anhydrase. *Acta Physiol Scand* 116:461, 1982.

67. Dobyan DC, Bulger RE: Renal carbonic anhydrase. *Am J Physiol* 243:F311, 1982.

68. Dobyan DC, Magill LS, Friedman PA, et al: Carbonic anhydrase histochemistry in rabbit and mouse kidneys. *Anat Rec* 204:185, 1982.

69. Drenckhahn D, Schluter K, Allen DP, et al: Colocalization of band 3 with ankyrin and spectrin at the basal membrane of intercalated cells in the rat kidney. *Science* 230:1287, 1985.

70. DuBose TD Jr: Hydrogen ion secretion by the collecting duct as a determinant of the urine to blood Pco_2 gradient in alkaline urine. *J Clin Invest* 69:145, 1982.

71. DuBose TD Jr, Lucci MSD, Hogg RJ, et al: Comparison of acidification parameters in superficial and deep nephrons of the rat. *Am J Physiol* 244:F497, 1983.

72. DuBose TD Jr, Pucacco LR, Carter NW: Determination of disequilibrium pH in the rat kidney in vivo: Evidence for hydrogen ion secretion. *Am J Physiol* 240:F138, 1981.

73. DuBose TD Jr, Pucacco LR, Lucci MS, et al: Micropuncture determination of pH, Pco_2, and total CO_2 concentra-

tion in accessible structures of the rat renal cortex. *J Clin Invest* 64:476, 1979.

73a. Eastman NJ, McLane CM: The lactic acid content of umbilical cord blood under various conditions. *Bull Johns Hopkins Hosp* 48:261, 1931.

74. Edelmann CM Jr, Boichis H, Rodriguez Soriano J, et al: The renal response of children to acute ammonium chloride acidosis. *Pediatr Res* 1:452, 1967.

75. Edelmann CM Jr, Rodriguez Soriano J, Boichis H, et al: Renal bicarbonate reabsorption and hydrogen ion excretion in normal infants. *J Clin Invest* 46:1309, 1967.

76. Edelmann CM Jr, Spitzer A: The maturing kidney. A modern view of well-balanced infants with imbalanced nephrons. *J Pediatr* 75:509, 1969.

77. Emmett M, Goldfarb S, Agus ZS, et al: The pathophysiology of acid-base changes in chronically phosphate-depleted rats. Bone-kidney interactions. *J Clin Invest* 59:291, 1977.

78. Evan AP, Gattone VH, Schwartz GJ: Development of solute transport in rabbit proximal tubule. II. Morphologic segmentation. *Am J Physiol* 245:F391, 1983.

79. Fisher DA: Carbonic anhydrase activity in fetal and young rhesus monkeys. *Proc Soc Exp Biol Med* 107:359, 1961.

80. Fomon SJ, Harris DM, Jensen RL: Acidification of the urine by infants fed humen milk or whole cow's milk. *Pediatrics* 23:113, 1958.

81. Forgac M, Cantley L, Wiedemann B, et al: Clathrin-coated vesicles contain an ATP-dependent proton pump. *Proc Natl Acad Sci USA* 80:1300, 1983.

82. Frazier LW: Effects of parathyroid hormone on H^+ and NH_4^+ excretion in toad urinary bladder. *J Membr Biol* 30:187, 1976.

83. Friedman PA, Andreoli TE: CO_2-stimulated NaCl absorption in the mouse renal cortical thick ascending limb of Henle. Evidence for synchronous Na/H and Cl/HCO_3 exchange in apical plasma membranes. *J Gen Physiol* 80:683, 1982.

84. Friis-Hansen B: Body water compartments in children: Changes during growth and related changes in body composition. *Pediatrics* 28:169, 1961.

85. Garcia-Austt J, Good DW, Burg MB, et al: Deoxycorticosterone-stimulated bicarbonate secretion in rabbit cortical collecting ducts: Effects of luminal chloride removal and in vivo acid loading. *Am J Physiol* 249:F205, 1985.

86. Garella S, Chang B, Kahn SI: Alterations of hydrogen ion homeostasis in pure potassium depletion: Studies in rats and dogs during the recovery phase. *J Lab Clin Med* 93:321, 1979.

86a. Giebisch G, Berger L, Pitts RF: The extra renal response to acute acid-base disturbances of respiratory origin. *J Clin Invest* 34:231, 1955.

87. Gluck S, Al-Awqati Q: An electrogenic proton-translocating adenosine triphosphatase from bovine kidney medulla. *J Clin Invest* 73:1704, 1984.

88. Gluck S, Cannon C, Al-Awqati Q: Exocytosis regulates urinary acidification in turtle bladder by rapid insertion of H^+ pumps into the luminal membrane. *Proc Natl Acad Sci USA* 79:4327, 1982.

89. Gluck S, Hirsch S, Brown D: Immunocytochemical localization of H^+ATPase in rat kidney (abstr). *Kidney Int* 31:167, 1986.

90. Gluck S, Kelly S, Al-Awqati Q: The proton translocating ATPase responsible for urinary acidification. *J Biol Chem* 275:9230, 1982.

91. Goldberg M, Green SB, Moss, ML, et al: Computer-based instruction and diagnosis of acid-base disorders. *JAMA* 223:269, 1973.

92. Goldstein L: Renal ammonia and acid excretion in infant rats. *Am J Physiol* 218:1394, 1970.

93. Goldstein L: Ammonia metabolism in kidneys of suckling rats. *Am J Physiol* 220:213, 1971.

94. Goldstein L, Harley-de Witt S: Renal gluconeogenesis and mitochondrial NAD^+/NADH ratios in nursing and adult rats. *Am J Physiol* 224:752, 1973.

95. Gonzalez RF, Gardner LI: Concentration of pyruvic acid in the blood of the newborn infant. *Pediatrics* 19:844, 1957.

96. Good DW: Sodium-dependent bicarbonate absorption by cortical thick ascending limb of rat kidney. *Am J Physiol* 248:F821, 1985.

97. Good DW, Burg MB: Ammonia production by individual segments of the rat nephron. *J Clin Invest* 73:602, 1984.

98. Good DW, Knepper MA, Burg MB: Ammonia and bicarbonate transport by thick ascending limb of rat kidney. *Am J Physiol* 247:F35, 1984.

99. Gordon HH, McNamara H, Benjamin HR: The response of young infants to ingestion of ammonium chloride. *Pediatrics* 2:290, 1948.

100. Graber ML, Bengele HH, Alexander EA: Elevated urinary Pco_2 in the rat: An intrarenal event. *Kidney Int* 21:795, 1982.

101. Graber ML, Bengele HH, Mroz E, et al: Acute metabolic acidosis augments collecting duct acidification rate in the rat. *Am J Physiol* 241:F669, 1981.

102. Graber ML, Bengele HH, Schwartz JH, et al: pH and pCO_2 profiles of the rat inner medullary collecting duct. *Am J Physiol* 241:F659, 1981.

103. Graham BD, Wilson JL, Tsao MU, et al: Development of neonatal electrolyte homeostasis. *Pediatrics* 8:68, 1951.

104. Halperin ML, Jungas RL: Metabolic production and renal disposal of hydrogen ions. *Kidney Int* 24:709, 1983.

105. Hamm LL, Pucacco LR, Kokko JP, et al: Hydrogen ion (H^+) permeability of isolated perfused tubules (abstr). *Kidney Int* 21:234, 1981.

106. Hamm LL, Pucacco LR, Kokko JP, et al: Hydrogen ion permeability of the rabbit proximal convoluted tubule. *Am J Physiol* 246:F3, 1984.

107. Hansen GP, Tisher CC, Robinson RR: Response of the collecting duct to disturbances of acid-base and potassium balance. *Kidney Int* 17:326, 1980.

108. Hatemi N, McCance RA: Renal aspects of acid-base control in the newly born. III. Response to acidifying drugs. *Acta Paediatr [Uppsala]* 50:603, 1961.

109. Helman SI, Grantham JJ, Burg MB: Effect of vasopressin on electrical resistance of renal cortical collecting tubules. *Am J Physiol* 220:1825, 1971.

110. Hendricks CH: Studies on lactic acid metabolism in pregnancy and labor. *Am J Obstet Gynecol* 73:492, 1957.

111. Hoffman WS, Parmalee AH, Grossman A: Mechanism of production of acidosis in premature infants by protein milk. *Am J Dis Child* 75:637, 1948.

112. Holmberg C, Kokko JP, Jacobson HR: Determination of chloride and bicarbonate permeabilities in proximal convoluted tubules. *Am J Physiol* 241:F386, 1981.

113. Hopkinson DA, Coppock JS, Muhlemann MF, et al: The detection and differentiation of the products of the human carbonic anhydrase loci, CA I and CA II, using fluorogenic substrates. *Ann Hum Genet* 38:155, 1974.

114. Howlin KJ, Alpern RJ, Rector FC Jr: Amiloride inhibition of proximal tubular acidification. *Am J Physiol* 248:F773, 1985.

115. Huch R, Huch A: Fetal and maternal $Ptco_2$ monitoring. *Crit Care Med* 9:694, 1981.

116. Hulter HN, Ilnicki LP, Harbottle JA, et al: Impaired renal H^+ secretion and NH_3 production in mineralocorticoid-

deficient glucocorticoid-replete dogs. *Am J Physiol* 232:F136, 1977.

117. Hulter HN, Licht JH, Glynn RE, et al: Renal acidosis in mineralocorticoid deficiency is not dependent on NaCl

depletion or hyperkalemia. *Am J Physiol* 236:F283, 1979.

118. Hulter HN, Sebastian A, Sigala JF, et al: Pathogenesis of renal hyperchloremic acidosis resulting from dietary potassium restriction in the dog: Role of aldosterone. *Am J Physiol* 238:F79, 1980.

119. Husted RF, Mueller AL, Kessel RG, et al: Surface characteristics of carbonic anhydrase-rich cells in turtle urinary bladder. *Kidney Int* 19:491, 1981.

120. Iino Y, Burg MB: Effect of parathyroid hormone on bicarbonate absorption by proximal tubules in vitro. *Am J Physiol* 236:F387, 1979.

121. Iino Y, Burg MB: Effect of acid-base status in vivo on bicarbonate transport by rabbit renal tubules in vitro. *Jap J Physiol* 31:99, 1981.

122. Ives HE: Proton/hydroxyl permeability of proximal tubule brush border vesicles. *Am J Physiol* 248:F78, 1985.

123. Jacobson HR: Effects of CO_2 and acetazolamide on bicarbonate and fluid transport in rabbit proximal tubules. *Am J Physiol* 240:F54, 1981.

124. Jacobson HR: Medullary collecting duct acidification. Effects of potassium, HCO_3 concentration, and pCO_2. *J Clin Invest* 74:2107, 1984.

125. Jones JW, Sebastian A, Hulter HN, et al: Systemic and renal acid-base effects of chronic dietary potassium depletion in humans. *Kidney Int* 21:402, 1982.

126. Kaiser IH: Hydrogen ion concentration of human fetal blood in utero at term. *Science* 118:29, 1953.

127. Kaissling B, Kriz W: Structural analysis of the rabbit kidney. *Adv Anat Embryol Cell Biol* 56:1, 1979.

128. Kassirer JP, Berkman PM, Lawrenz DR, et al: The critical role of chloride in the correction of hypokalemic alkalosis in man. *Am J Med* 38:172, 1965.

129. Kerpel-Fronius E, Heim T, Sulyok E: The development of the renal acidifying processes and their relation to acidosis in low-birth-weight infants. *Biol Neonate* 15:156, 1970.

130. Kesby GJ, Lambers ER: Factors affecting renal handling of sodium, hydrogen ions, and bicarbonate by the fetus. *Am J Physiol* 251:F226, 1986.

131. Kildeberg P: Disturbances of hydrogen ion balance occurring in premature infants. I. Early types of acidosis. *Acta Paediatr [Uppsala]* 53:505, 1964.

132. Kildeberg P: Disturbances of hydrogen ion balance occurring in premature infants. II. Late metabolic acidosis. *Acta Paediatr [Uppsala]* 53:517, 1964.

133. Kildeberg P: Late metabolic acidosis of premature infants. *In* Winters RW (ed): *The Body Fluids in Pediatrics.* Boston, Little, Brown, 1973, p 338.

134. Kildeberg P, Engel K, Winters RW: Balance of net acid in growing infants. Endogenous and trans-intestinal aspects. *Acta Paediatr Scand* 58:321, 1969.

135. Kildeberg P, Winters RW: Balance of net acid: Concept, measurement and applications. *Adv Pediatr* 25:349, 1978.

136. Kinne-Saffran E, Beauwens R, Kinne R: An ATP-driven proton pump in brush-border membranes from rat renal cortex. *J Membr Biol* 64:67, 1982.

136a. Kinsella JL, Aronson PS: Properties of the Na^+-H^+ exchanger in renal microvillus membrane vesicles. *Am J Physiol* 238:F461, 1980.

137. Kinsella JL, Cujkid T, Sacktor B: Na^+-H^+ exchange activity in renal brush-border membrane vesicles in response to metabolic acidosis: The role of glucocorticoids. *Proc Natl Acad Sci USA* 81:630, 1984, p 589.

138. Kleinman LI: The kidney. *In* Stave U (ed): *Perinatal Physiology.* New York, Plenum, 1978.

139. Knepper MA, Good DW, Burg MB: Mechanism of ammonia secretion by cortical collecting ducts of rabbits. *Am J Physiol* 247:F729, 1984.

140. Koeppen BM: Conductive properties of the rabbit outer medullary collecting duct: Inner stripe. *Am J Physiol* 248:F500, 1985.

141. Koeppen B, Giebisch G, Melnic G: Mechanism and regulation of renal tubular acidification. *In* Seldin DW, Giebisch G (eds): *The Kidney. Physiology and Pathophysiology.* New York, Raven, 1985, p 1491.

142. Koeppen BM, Helman SI: Acidification of luminal fluid by the rabbit cortical collecting tubule perfused in vitro. *Am J Physiol* 242:F521, 1982.

143. Koeppen BM, Steinmetz PR: Basic mechanisms of urinary acidification. *Med Clin North Am* 67:753, 1983.

144. Kunau RT, Frick A, Rector FC, et al: Micropuncture study of the proximal tubular factors responsible for the maintenance of alkalosis during potassium deficiency in the rat. *Clin Sci* 34:223, 1968.

144a. Kunau RT, Walker KA: Effect of oral acid ingestion and amiloride on total CO_2 absorption in the rat superficial distal tubule (abstr). *Kidney Int* 27:284, 1985.

145. Kurtz I, Star R, Balaban RS, et al: Spontaneous luminal disequilibrium pH in S_3 proximal tubules. Role in ammonia and bicarbonate transport. *J Clin Invest* 78:989, 1986.

146. Kurtzman NA: Relationship of extracellular volume and CO_2 tension to renal bicarbonate reabsorption. *Am J Physiol* 219:1299, 1970.

147. Kurtzman NA: Regulation of renal bicarbonate reabsorption by extracellular volume. *J Clin Invest* 49:586, 1970.

148. Kurtzman NA, White MG, Rogers PW: The effect of potassium and extracellular volume on renal bicarbonate reabsorption. *Metabolism* 22:481, 1973.

149. Laski ME, Kurtzman NA: Characterization of acidification in the cortical and medullary collecting tubule of the rabbit. *J Clin Invest* 72:2050, 1983.

150. Laski ME, Warnock DG, Rector FC Jr: Effects of chloride gradients on total CO_2 flux in the rabbit cortical collecting tubule. *Am J Physiol* 244:F112, 1983.

151. LeFurgey A, Tisher CC: Morphology of rabbit collecting duct. *Am J Anat* 155:111, 1979.

152. LeHir M, Kaissling B, Koeppen BM, et al: Binding of peanut lectin to specific epithelial cell types in the kidney. *Am J Physiol* 242:C117, 1982.

153. Levine DZ: Effect of acute hypercapnia on proximal tubular water and bicarbonate absorption. *Am J Physiol* 221:1164, 1971.

154. Levine DZ: An in vivo microperfusion study of distal tubule bicarbonate reabsorption in normal and ammonium chloride rats. *J Clin Invest* 75:588, 1985.

155. Levine DZ, Jacobson HR: The regulation of renal acid secretion: New observations from studies of distal nephron segments. *Kidney Int* 29:1099, 1986.

156. Levine DZ, Nash LA: Effect of chronic NH_4Cl acidosis on proximal tubular H_2O and HCO_3 reabsorption. *Am J Physiol* 225:380, 1973.

157. Levine DZ, Nash LA, Chan T, et al: Proximal bicarbonate reabsorption during Ringer and albumin infusions in rat. *J Clin Invest* 57:1490, 1976.

157a. Levine DZ, Nash LA, Iacovitti M: Distal tubule bicarbonate reabsorption ($JtCO_2$) in vivo: Modulation by overnight fasting (abstr). *Clin Res* 35:551A, 1987.

158. Levine DZ, Walker T, Nash LA: Effects of KCl infusions on proximal tubular function in normal and potassium-depleted rats. *Kidney Int* 4:318, 1973.

159. Lindskog S, Engberg P, Forsman C, et al: Kinetics and mechanism of carbonic anhydrase isoenzymens. *Ann NY Acad Sci* 429:61, 1984.

160. Litschgi M, Tschumi A: Diagnostische Kriterien der neonatalen Azidose in den ersten 60 Minuten post partum. *Schweiz Med Weshr* 110:85, 1980.

161. Lombard WE, Kokko JP, Jacobson HR: Bicarbonate transport in cortical and outer medullary collecting tubules. *Am J Physiol* 244:F289, 1983.

162. Lonnerholm G, Ridderstrale Y: Intracellular distribution of carbonic anhydrase in the rat kidney. *Kidney Int* 17:162, 1980.

163. Lonnerholm G, Wistrand PJ: Carbonic anhydrase in the human fetal kidney. *Pediatr Res* 17:390, 1983.

164. Lucci MS, Puccaco LR, Carter NW, et al: Evaluation of bicarbonate transport in the rat distal tubule: Effects of acid-base status. *Am J Physiol* 243:F335, 1982.

165. Luke RB, Levitin H: Impaired renal conservation of chloride and the acid-base changes associated with potassium depletion in the rat. *Clin Sci* 32:511, 1967.

166. Maddox DA, Gennari FJ: Proximal tubular bicarbonate reabsorption and Pco_2 in chronic metabolic alkalosis in the rat. *J Clin Invest* 72:1385, 1983.

166a. Maddox DA, Gennari FJ: Load dependence of HCO_3 and H_2O reabsorption in the early proximal tubule of the Munich-Wistar rat. *Am J Physiol* 248:F113, 1985.

167. Madias NE, Androgue HJ, Horotwitz GL, et al: A redefinition of normal acid-base equilibrium in man: Carbon dioxide tension as a key determinant of normal plasma bcarbonate concentration. *Kidney Int* 16:612, 1979.

168. Madsen KM, Tisher CC: Cellular response to acute respiratory acidosis in rat medullary collecting duct. *Am J Physiol* 245:F670, 1983.

169. Madsen KM, Tisher CC: Response of intercalated cells of rat outer medulary collecting duct to chronic metabolic acidosis. *Lab Invest* 51:268, 1984.

170. Madsen KM, Tisher CC: Structural-functional relationships along the distal nephron. *Am J Physiol* 250:F1, 1986.

171. Malnic G, de Mello-Aires M: Kinetic study of bicarbonate reabsorption in proximal tubule of the rat. *Am J Physiol* 220:1759, 1971.

172. Manitius A, Levitin H, Beck D, et al: On the mechanism of impairment of renal concentrating ability in potassium deficiency. *J Clin Invest* 39:684, 1960.

173. Maren TH: Carbonic anhydrase: Chemistry, physiology, and inhibition. *Physiol Rev* 47:595, 1967.

174. Marples E, Lippard VW: Acid-base balance of new-born infants. II. Consideration of low alkaline reserve of normal newborn infants. *Am J Dis Child* 44:31, 1932.

175. Marples E, Lippard VW: Acid-base balance of newborn infants. III. Influence of cow's milk on acid-base balance of blood of newborn infants. *Am J Dis Child* 45:294, 1933.

176. McCance RA, Hatemi N: Control of acid-base stability in the newly born. *Lancet* 1:293, 1961.

177. McCance RA, Widdowson EM: Renal aspects of acid-base control in the newly born. I. Natural development. *Acta Paediatr [Uppsala]* 49:409, 1960.

178. McCance RA, Widdowson EM: The acid-base relationships of the foetal fluids of the pig. *J Physiol* 151:484, 1960.

179. McKinney TD, Burg MB: Bicarbonate and fluid absorption by renal proximal straight tubules. *Kidney Int* 12:1, 1977.

180. McKinney TD, Burg MB: Bicarbonate transport by rabbit cortical collecting tubules. *J Clin Invest* 60:766, 1977.

181. McKinney TD, Burg MB: Bicarbonate absorption by rabbit cortical collecting tubules in vitro. *Am J Physiol* 234:F141, 1978.

182. McKinney TD, Burg MB: Bicarbonate secretion by rabbit cortical collecting tubules in vitro. *J Clin Invest* 61:1421, 1978.

183. McKinney TD, Davidson KK: Effect of potassium depletion and protein intake in vivo on renal tubular bicarbonate transport in vitro. *Am J Physiol* 252:F509, 1987.

184. McKinney TD, Myers P: Bicarbonate transport by proximal tubules: Effect of parathyroid hormone and dibutyryl cyclic AMP. *Am J Physiol* 238:F166, 1980.

185. McKinney TD, Myers P: PTH inhibition of bicarbonate transport by proximal convoluted tubules. *Am J Physiol* 239:F127, 1980.

186. McKinney TD, Myers P: Effect of calcium and phosphate on bicarbonate and fluid transport by proximal tubules in vitro. *Kidney Int* 21:433, 1982.

187. Meschia G, Cotter JR, Breathnach CS, et al: The hemoglobin, oxygen, carbon dioxide and hydrogen ion concentrations in the umbilical bloods of sheep and goats as sampled via in dwelling plastic catheters. *Q J Exp Physiol* 50:185, 1965.

187a. Monnens L, Schretlen E, van Munster P: The renal excretion of hydrogen ions in infants and children. *Nephron* 12:29, 1973.

188. Moore ES, Fine BP, Satrasook SS, et al: Renal reabsorption of bicarbonate in puppies: Effect of extracellular volume contraction on the renal threshold for bicarbonate. *Pediatr Res* 6:859, 1972.

189. Morel F, Chabardes D, Imbert M: Functional segmentation of the rabbit distal tubule by microdetermination of hormone-dependent adenylate cyclase activity. *Kidney Int* 9:264, 1976.

190. Murer H, Hopfer U, Kinne R: Sodium-proton antiport in brush-border membrane vesicles isolated from rat small intestine and kidney. *Biochem J* 154:597, 1976.

191. Nagami GT, Kurokawa K: Regulation of ammonia production by mouse proximal tubules perfused in vitro. Effect of luminal perfusion. *J Clin Invest* 75:844, 1985.

192. O'Neil RG, Helman SI: Transport characteristics of renal collecting tubules: Influences of DOCA and diet. *Am J Physiol* 233:F544, 1977.

193. Pincus JB, Gittleman IF, Saito M, et al: A study of plasma values of sodium, potassium, chloride, carbon dioxide, carbon dioxide tension, sugar, urea and the protein base-binding power, pH, and hematocrit in prematures on the first day of life. *Pediatrics* 18:39, 1956.

194. Pitts RF: *Physiology of the Kidney and Body Fluids*, 3rd ed. Chicago, Year Book, 1974, p 179.

195. Pitts RF, Ayer JL, Schiess WA: The renal regulation of acid-base balance in man. III. The reabsorption and excretion of bicarbonate. *J Cin Invest* 28:35, 1949.

196. Pitts RF, Lotspeich WD: Bicarbonate and the renal regulation of acid-base balance. *Am J Physiol* 147:138, 1946.

197. Polack A, Haynie GD, Hays RM, et al: Effects of chronic hypercapnia on electrolyte and acid-base equilibrium. I. Adaptation. *J Clin Invest* 40:1223, 1961.

198. Prigent A, Bichara M, Paillard M: Hydrogen transport in papillary collecting duct of rabbit kidney. *Am J Physiol* 248:C241, 1985.

199. Purkerson ML, Lubovitz H, White RW, et al: On the influence of extracellular fluid volume expansion on bicarbonate reabsorption in the rat. *J Clin Invest* 48:1754, 1969.

200. Raiha NCR, Kauraniemi TV: Carbon dioxide tension and acid-base balance of humen amniotic fluid at the end of gestation. *Biol Neonate* 4:25, 1962.

201. Ranlov P, Siggaard-Andersen O: Late metabolic acidosis in premature infants. Prevalence and significance. *Acta Paediatr Scand* 54:531, 1965.

202. Reardon HS, Graham BD, Wilson JL, et al: Studies of

acid-base equilibrium in premature infants. *Pediatrics* 6:753, 1950.

203. Rector FC Jr, Carter NW, Seldin DW: The mechanism of bicarbonate reabsorption in the proximal and distal tubules of the kidney. *J Clin Invest* 44:278, 1965.

204. Richardson RMA: Effect of acute hypercalcemia (HC) on renal HCO_3 handling in the rat (abstr). *Kidney Int* 23:238, 1983.

205. Richardson RMA, Kunau RT Jr: Bicarbonate reabsorption in the papillary collecting duct: Effect of acetazolamide. *Am J Physiol* 243:F74, 1982.

206. Rodman JS, Kerjaschki D, Merisko E, et al: Presence of an extensive clathrin coat on the apical plasmalemma of the rat kidney proximal tubular cell. *J Cell Biol* 98:1630, 1984.

207. Rose BD: *Clinical Physiology of Acid-Base and Electrolyte Disorders*. New York: McGraw-Hill, 1977, p 165.

208. Rubin MI, Calcagno PL, Ruben DL: Renal excretion of hydrogen ions: A defense against acidosis in premature infants. *J Pediatr* 59:848, 1961.

209. Sabolic I, Haase W, Burckhardt G: ATP dependent H^+ pump in membrane vesicles from rat kidney cortex. *Am J Physiol* 248:F835, 1985.

210. Sajo IM, Goldstein MB, Sonnenberg H, et al: Sites of ammonia addition to tubular fluid in rats with chronic metabolic acidosis. *Kidney Int* 20:353, 1981.

211. Sansom SC, Weinman EJ, O'Neil RG: Microelectrode assessment of chloride-conductive properties of cortical collecting duct. *Am J Physiol* 247:F291, 1984.

212. Sasaki S, Berry CA: Mechanism of bicarbonate exit across basolateral membrane of the rabbit proximal convoluted tubule. *Am J Physiol* 246:F889, 1984.

213. Sasaki S, Berry CA, Rector FC Jr: Effect of luminal and peritubular HCO_3^- concentrations and Pco_2 on HCO_3^- reabsorption in rabbit proximal convoluted tubules perfused in vitro. *J Clin Invest* 70:639, 1982.

214. Sasaki S, Berry CA, Rector FC Jr: Effect of potassium concentration on bicarbonate reabsorption in the rabbit proximal convoluted tubule. *Am J Physiol* 244:F122, 1983.

215. Sasaki S, Shiigai T, Takeuchi J: Intracellular pH in the isolated perfused rabbit proximal straight tubule. *Am J Physiol* 249:F417, 1985.

216. Satlin LM, Schwartz GJ: Postnatal maturation of rabbit renal collecting duct: Intercalated cell function. *Am J Physiol* 253:F622, 1987.

217. Schan RJ, O'Brien K: Longitudinal studies of acid-base status in infants with low birth weights. *J Pediatr* 70:885, 1967.

218. Schuster VL: Cyclic adenosine monophosphate-stimulated bicarbonate secretion in rabbit cortical collecting tubules. *J Clin Invest* 75:2056, 1985.

219. Schuster VL, Bonsib SM, Jennings ML: Two types of collecting duct mitochondria-rich (intercalated) cells: Lectin and band 3 cytochemistry. *Am J Physiol* 251:C347, 1986.

220. Schwartz GJ: Na^+-dependent H^+ efflux from proximal tubule: Evidence for reversible Na^+-H^+ exchange. *Am J Physiol* 241:F380, 1981.

221. Schwartz GJ: Absence of Cl^--OH^- or Cl^--HCO_3^- exchange in the rabbit renal proximal tubule. *Am J Physiol* 245:F462, 1983.

222. Schwartz GJ, Al-Awqati Q: Carbon dioxide causes exocytosis of vesicles containing H^+ pumps in isolated perfused proximal and collecting tubules. *J Clin Invest* 75:1638, 1985.

223. Schwartz GJ, Barasch J, Al-Awqati Q: Plasticity of epithelial polarity. *Nature* 318:368, 1985.

224. Schwartz GJ, Bergmann JE: Cellular heterogeneity of the rabbit collecting duct (CD) (abstr). *Kidney Int* 31:415, 1987.

225. Schwartz GJ, Burg MB: Mineralocorticoid effects on cation transport by cortical collecting tubules in vitro. *Am J Physiol* 235:F576, 1978.

226. Schwartz GJ, Evan AP: Development of solute transport in rabbit proximal tubule. I. HCO_3^- and glucose absorption. *Am J Physiol* 245:F382, 1983.

227. Schwartz GJ, Evan AP: Development of solute transport in rabbit proximal tubule. III. Na-K-ATPase activity. *Am J Physiol* 246:F845, 1984.

228. Schwartz GJ, Haycock GB, Edelman CM Jr, et al: Late metabolic acidosis: A reassessment of the definition. *J Pediatr* 95:102, 1979.

229. Schwartz GJ, Weinstein AM, Steele RE, et al: Carbon dioxide permeability of rabbit proximal convoluted tubules. *Am J Physiol* 240:F231, 1981.

230. Schwartz JH, Finn JH, Vaughn G, et al: Distribution of metabolic CO_2 and the transported ion species in acidification by turtle bladder. *Am J Physiol* 226:283, 1974.

231. Schwartz JH, Steinmetz PR: CO_2 requirements for H^+ secretion by the isolated turtle bladder. *Am J Physiol* 220:2051, 1971.

232. Schwartz JH, Steinmetz PR: Metabolic energy and pCO_2 as determinants of H^+ secretion by turtle urinary bladder. *Am J Physiol* 233:F145, 1977.

233. Schwartz WB, Brackett NC, Cohen JJ: The response of extracellular hydrogen ion concentration to graded degrees of chronic hypercapnia: The physiologic limits of the defense of pH. *J Clin Invest* 44:291, 1965.

234. Schwartz WB, Jenson RL, Relman AS: Acidification of the urine and increased ammonium excretion without change in acid-base equilibrium: Sodium reabsorption as a stimulus to the acidifying process. *J Clin Invest* 34:673, 1955.

235. Sebastian A, Schambelan M, Lindenfeld S, et al: Amelioration of metabolic acidosis with fludrocortisone therapy in hyporeninemic hypoaldosteronism. *N Engl J Med* 297:576, 1977.

236. Seifter JL, Knickelbein R, Aronson PS: Chloride transport in rabbit renal microvillus membrane vesicles: Evidence against Cl^-/OH^- exchange and NaCl cotransport. *Am J Physiol* 247:F753, 1984.

237. Smith CA: *The Physiology of the Newborn Infant*, 3rd ed. Springfield, Ill., Charles C Thomas, 1959, p 320.

238. Smith FG, Schwartz A: Response of the intact lamb fetus to acidosis. *Am J Obstet Gynecol* 106:52, 1970.

239. Spicer SS, Sens MA, Hennigar RA, et al: Implications of the immunohistochemical localization of the carbonic anhydrase isozymes for their function in normal and pathologic cells. *Ann NY Acad Sci* 429:382, 1984.

240. Star RA, Burg MB, Knepper MA: Bicarbonate secretion and chloride absorption by rabbit cortical collecting ducts. Role of chloride/bicarbonate exchange. *J Clin Invest* 76:1123, 1985.

241. Star RA, Burg MB, Knepper MA: Luminal disequilibrium pH and ammonia transport in outer medullary collecting duct. *Am J Physiol* 252:F1148, 1987.

242. Steinmetz PR: Cellular mechanisms of urinary acidification. *Physiol Rev* 54:890, 1974.

243. Steinmetz PR, Lawson LR: Effect of luminal pH on ion permeability and flows of Na^+ and H^+ in turtle bladder. *Am J Physiol* 220:1573, 1971.

244. Stetson DL, Beauwens R, Palmisano J, et al: A double-membrane model for urinary bicarbonate secretion. *Am J Physiol* 249:F546, 1985.

245. Stetson DL, Steinmetz PR: Role of membrane fusion in CO_2 stimulation of proton secretion by turtle bladder. *Am J Physiol* 245:C113, 1983.

246. Stetson DL, Steinmetz PR: "A" and "B" types of carbonic

anhydrase-rich cells in turtle bladder. *Am J Physiol* 249:F553, 1985.

247. Stetson DL, Wade JB, Giebisch G: Morphological alterations in the rat medullary collecting duct following potassium depletion. *Kidney Int* 17:45, 1980.

248. Stone DK, Seldin DW, Kokko JP, et al: Anion dependence of rabbit medullary collecting duct acidification. *J Clin Invest* 71:1505, 1983.

249. Stone DK, Seldin DW, Kokko JP, et al: Mineralocorticoid modulation of rabbit medullary collecting duct acidification. A sodium-independent effect. *J Clin Invest* 72:77, 1983.

250. Stone DK, Xie XS, Racker E: An ATP driven proton pump in clathrin-coated vesicles. *J Biol Chem* 258:4059, 1983.

251. Sulyok E, Heim T: Assessment of maximal urinary acidification in premature infants. *Biol Neonate* 19:200, 1971.

252. Sulyok E: The relationship between electrolyte and acid-base balance in the premature infant during early postnatal life. *Biol Neonate* 17:227, 1971.

253. Sulyok E, Heim T, Soltesz G, et al: The influence of maturity on renal control of acidosis in newborn infants. *Biol Neonate* 21:418, 1972.

254. Svenningsen NW: Renal acid-base titration studies in infants with and without metabolic acidosis in the postneonatal period. *Pediatr Res* 8:659, 1974.

255. Svenningsen NW, Lindquist B: Incidence of metabolic acidosis in term, preterm and small-for-gestational age infants in relation to dietary protein intake. *Acta Paediatr Scand* 62:1, 1973.

256. Svenningsen NW, Lindquist B: Postnatal development of renal hydrogen ion excretion capacity in relation to age and protein intake. *Acta Paediatr Scand* 63:721, 1974.

257. Swan RC, Pitts RF: Neutralization of infused acid by nephrectomized dogs. *J Clin Invest* 34:205, 1955.

258. Tannen RL: The effect of uncomplicated potassium depletion on urine acidification. *J Clin Invest* 49:813, 1970.

259. Tannen RL: Relationship of renal ammonia production and potassium homeostasis. *Kidney Int* 11:453, 1977.

260. Tannen RL, Kunin AS: Effect of potassium on ammoniagenesis by renal mitochondria. *Am J Physiol* 231:44, 1976.

261. Tannen RL, McGill J: Influences of potassium on renal ammonia production. *Am J Physiol* 231:1178, 1976.

262. Tashian RE, Hewett-Emmett D, Dodgson SJ, et al: The value of inherited deficiencies of human carbonic anhydrase isoenzymes in understanding their cellular roles. *Ann NY Acad Sci* 429:262, 1984.

263. Tomita K, Pisano JJ, Burg MB, et al: Effects of vasopressin and bradykinin on anion transport by the rat cortical collecting duct. Evidence for an electroneutral sodium chloride pathway. *J Clin Invest* 77:136, 1986.

264. Tsai CJ, Ives HE, Alpern RJ, et al: Increased Vmax for Na^+/H^+ antiporter activity in proximal tubule bursh-border vesicles from rabbits with metabolic acidosis. *Am J Physiol* 247:F339, 1984.

265. Tudvad F, McNamara H, Barnett HL: Renal response of premature infants to administration of bicarbonate and potassium. *Pediatrics* 13:4, 1954.

266. Ullrich KJ, Papavassiliou F: Bicarbonate reabsorption in the papillary collecting duct of rats. *Pflugers Arch* 389:271, 1981.

267. Van Slyke DD, Sendroy J Jr, Hastings AB, et al: Studies of gas and electrolyte equilibria in blood. X. The solubility of carbon dioxide at 38° in water, salt solution, serum, and blood cells. *J Biol Chem* 78:765, 1928.

268. Van Ypersele de Strihou C, Brasseur L, de Coninck J: "Carbon Dioxide Response Curve" for chronic hypercapnia in man. *N Engl J Med* 275:117, 1966.

269. Vaughn D, Kirschbaum H, Bersentes T, et al: Fetal and neonatal response to acid loading in the sheep. *J Appl Physiol* 24:135, 1968.

270. Verlander JW, Madsen KM, Tisher CC: Two populations of intercalated cells exist in the cortical collecting duct of the rat (abstr). *Clin Res* 33:501A, 1985.

271. Vieira FL, Malnic G: Hydrogen ion secretion by rat renal cortical tubules as studied by an antimony microelectrode. *Am J Physiol* 214:710, 1968.

272. Warnock DG, Yee VJ: Anion permeabilities of the isolated perfused rabbit proximal tubule. *Am J Physiol* 242:F395, 1982.

273. Weisberg HF: Acid-base pathophysiology in the neonate and infant. *Ann Clin Lab Sci* 12:245, 1982.

274. Weisbrot IM, James LS, Prince CE, et al: Acid-base homeostasis of the newborn infant during the first 24 hours of life. *J Pediatr* 52:395, 1958.

275. Wesson DE, Frommer JP: Carbonic-anhydrase-independent HCO_3 reabsorption in the rat: Effect of ethoxzolamide (abstr). *Kidney Int* 27:290, 1985.

276. Weston P, Brinkman CR III, Ladner C, et al: Fetal and neonatal response to base loading. *Biol Neonate* 16:261, 1970.

276a. Wible JL, Petrie RH, Koons A, et al: The clinical use of umbilical cord acid-base determinations in perinatal surveillance and management. *Clin Perinatol* 9:387, 1982.

277. Wistrand PJ: Properties of membrane-bound carbonic anhydrase. *Ann NY Acad Sci* 429:195, 1984.

278. Wistrand PJ, Kinne R: Carbonic anhydrase activity of isolated brush-border and basal-lateral membranes of renal tubular cells. *Pflugers Arch* 370:121, 1977.

279. Wright FS, Strieder N, Fowler NB, et al: Potassium secretion by distal tubule after potassium adaptation. *Am J Physiol* 221:437, 1971.

280. Yamada N: Respiratory environment and acid-base balance in the developing fetus. *Biol Neonate* 16:222, 1970.

281. Yoshitomi K, Fromter E: Cell pH of rat renal proximal tubule in vivo and the conductive nature of peritubular HCO_3^- (OH^-) exit. *Pflugers Arch* 402:300, 1984.

282. Zeidel ML, Silva P, Seifter JL: Intracellular pH regulation and proton transport by rabbit renal medullary collecting duct cells: Role of plasma membrane H^+ATPase. *J Clin Invest* 77:113, 1986.

283. Zweymuller E: Renal aspects of acid-base control in the newly-born. II. The organic acids. *Acta Paediatr [Uppsala]* 49:591, 1960.

Mario Barac-Nieto
Aaron Friedman
David P. Simpson

10
Renal Metabolism

Renal Energy Metabolism

The kidneys perform a variety of energy requiring transport functions, such as the reabsorption of Na^+ and Ca^{2+} from the glomerular filtrate and the secretion of H^+ into the tubular fluid. In addition, energy-requiring biosynthesis of glucose, serine, proteins, and lipids also occurs in the kidney. These functions are sustained through generation of ATP by mitochondrial aerobic oxidation of various substrates and, to a lesser extent, through glycolytic oxidation of glucose to lactate and substrate level phosphorylations involving anaerobic dismutations. Different cells along the nephron effect specific transport and metabolic functions. Final differentiation of these cells involves drastic changes in these characteristics. In this section we review information pertinent to the major renal energy requiring (endergonic) functions, their relationship to renal exergonic (energy generating) metabolic processes, and their changes during postnatal development.

Renal O₂ Delivery

The rate of renal O_2 consumption per unit of tissue weight exceeds that in other organs such as brain and liver and is second only to that of the heart (Table 10-1). Although the renal mass represents less than 1% of body weight, the kidneys are responsible for about 10% of the body's resting energy turnover. Yet, because the kidneys receive a large percentage of the resting cardiac output (about 20%), the renal arteriovenous difference for O_2 is only about 1 μmole O_2 per ml blood, the renal O_2 extraction approximately 10%, and the renal venous O_2 content (18 vol O_2 per dl blood) and O_2 tension (about 70 mm Hg) are higher than in the venous effluent of most organs. Thus, the energy metabolism of the mature kidney is not thought to be limited by the O_2 supply. However, not all regions of the kidney are exposed to these relatively high O_2 tensions. Because of the peculiar arrangement of the vasae rectae in the renal medulla and the countercurrent exchange of O_2 between descending and ascending limbs of the vasae rectae, the tissue O_2 tension decreases progressively from the cortex to the tip of the papilla (Fig. 10-1). However, even

at the tip of the papilla, the tissue O_2 tension of 10 to 20 mm Hg exceeds by far the level at which it becomes limiting for mitochondrial function [52].

Measurements of the tissue concentration of reduced cytochrome a, a_3 have indicated that in the renal medulla there is considerable reduction of the electron transport chain, suggesting a limited O_2 supply to this area. This state of reduction can be alleviated by furosemide, an inhibitor of Na^+-K^+-Cl^- cotransport in the thick ascending limbs of Henle's loops [82]. Similarly, the urinary PO_2, which reflects the medullary O_2 tension, rises when the transport of Na^+ in the thick ascending limbs is reduced by ethacrynic acid or when medullary blood flow is increased by water diuresis [285]. Thus, in the medullary nephron segments the balance between O_2 supply and demand is thought to determine the oxidoreduction state of the mitochondria. The medullary thick ascending limbs were found to be particularly vulnerable to hypoxic damage during perfusion of the isolated kidney, and this vulnerability may be of relevance to the pathophysiology of ischemic acute renal failure [36].

The cells of the renal thick ascending limbs and proximal tubules have abundant mitochondria (Fig. 10-2), suggesting high rates of aerobic metabolism at these nephron sites [265]. These cells, particularly those of the thick ascending limbs, have also high Na^+-K^+-ATPase activity (Fig. 10-3) indicative of high rates of Na^+ transport [232].

Thus, although the rate of O_2 delivery to most areas of the kidney is ample, the O_2 supply to specific regions, such as the medullary thick ascending limbs, may be limiting under certain conditions, particularly when the rates of active transport of Na^+ are high. In such case, the glycolytic capacity of the cells becomes important to the sustenance of an adequate level of function.

The Major Renal Endergonic Function: Na⁺ Reabsorption

The relationship between energy supply and demand in the kidney is expressed in the large decreases in renal O_2 consumption associated with reductions in the filtered loads and thus in the reabsorption of solutes. A direct correlation

TABLE 10-1. *Comparison of blood flow and O_2 utilization rates of several organs in man*

Region or Organ	Mass gm	Blood flow rate ml/100 g · min	ml/min	A-V diff. O_2 μmol/100 ml	O_2 consumption μmol/ min	μmol/100 g · min
Heart	300	84	252	508	1295	431
Kidney	300	420	1260	63	804	267
Brain	1400	54	750	276	2053	147
Hepato-portal	2600	58	1500	151	2277	87.5
Skin	3600	13	460	111	535	15
Skeletal muscle	31000	2.7	840	267	2232	7.2
Residual	24000				1964	8.2
Total	63200		5400		11160	

Adapted from Lambertson CJ, *in* P Bard (ed): *Medical Physiology.* St. Louis, CV Mosby, 1961, p 594.

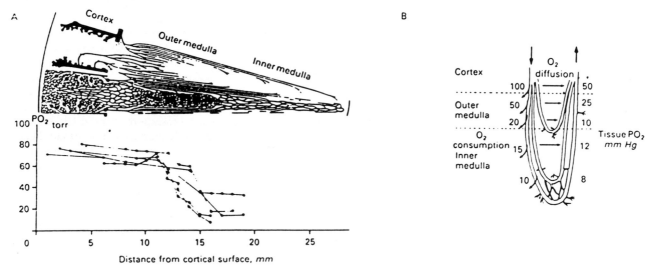

FIG. 10-1. *Heterogeneity of renal oxygenation. A. Renal tissue oxygen tension in different parts of the kidney. The upper part illustrates schematically the renal vascular pattern. B. Countercurrent exchange of oxygen in the vasa recta: diffusion of oxygen between arterial and venous limbs minimizes the dissipation of the corticomedullary gradient of tissue oxygen tension. (From Brezis M, Rosen S, Silva P, et al: Renal ischemia: A new perspective. Kidney Int 26:375, 1984, with permission.)*

exists between renal O_2 uptake and Na^+ reabsorption (Fig. 10-4), indicating that a major fraction of the O_2 consumed by the kidney supports the tubular reabsorption of Na^+. From the slope of this relationship, it is estimated that approximately 30 equivalents of Na^+ are reabsorbed per mole of O_2 consumed by the adult dog kidney [164]. The renal Na^+/O_2 ratio is higher than in other ion-transporting tissues, such as the frog skin [300] or the toad bladder [172], in which 18 equivalents of Na^+ are transported per mole of O_2 consumed. The high efficiency of renal Na^+ transport is due to the characteristics of the proximal convoluted tubule (PCT) epithelium across which most (65% to 70%) of the filtered Na^+ and H_2O are reabsorbed [156]. Studies of proximal Na^+ reabsorption in the kidney of dogs

treated with ethacrynic acid to prevent changes in distal Na^+ transport have shown that the molar ratio of proximal Na^+ reabsorbed to O_2 uptake is 48 ± 2 (Fig. 10-5), higher than that measured in the absence of ethacrynic acid (30:1) [188]. These observations are consistent with the view that the efficiency of proximal Na^+ reabsorption is higher than that of more distal nephron segments [156,164]. By contrast, in suspensions of K^+-depleted rabbit proximal tubules, the simultaneous changes in ouabain-sensitive K^+ and O_2 uptakes that occur immediately following increases in the extracellular K^+ from 0 to 5 mM (Fig. 10-6), yielded a ratio of 11.7 equivalents of K^+ reaccumulated in the cells per mole O_2 consumed [127]. This K^+/O_2 is almost identical to that predicted from the known stoichiometry

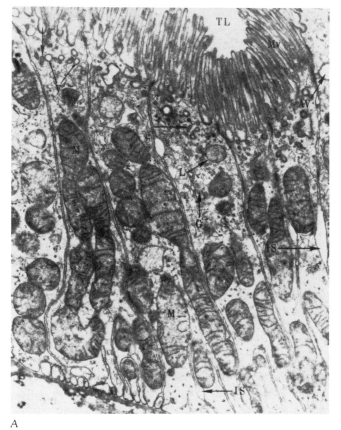

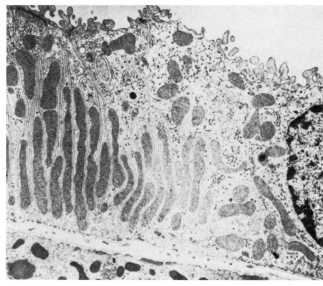

A B

FIG. 10-2. A. *Electron micrograph of the pars convoluta of the proximal tubule from a normal human kidney. The mitochondria (M) are elongated and tortuous, occasionally doubling back on themselves. The endocytic apparatus composed of apical vacuoles (AV), apical vesicles (V), and apical dense tubules (arrows) is well developed. (G = Golgi appartus. IS = intercellular space. Mv = microvilli forming the brush border. TL = tubule lumen. L = lysosome.) Magnification ×15.000 B. Electron micrograph of the pars recta segment of the distal tubule of the rat. Note especially the deep, complex invaginations of the basal plasmalemma, which encloses elongated mitochondrial profiles and extends into the apical region of the cell. Magnification ×10,000 before a 3% enlargement. From Tisher CC: Anatomy of the kidney. In Brenner BM, Rector FC (eds): The Kidney. 2nd ed. Vol. 1, Philadelphia, WB Saunders, 1981, p 25, with permission.)*

[145] of the purified Na^+-K^+-ATPase in vitro (3 equivalents of Na^+ and 2 equivalents of K^+ transported per mole of ATP hydrolyzed), and a mitochondrial P/O = 3 (moles of ATP synthesized per gram atom of O_2 used) [127]. Based on these stoichiometries one would predict that, in the steady state, for 6 moles of ATP used by the Na^+-K^+-ATPase (and hence for each mole of O_2 consumed in their synthesis), there would be 18 Eq of Na^+ extruded by the cells and 12 Eq of K^+ accumulated in the cells; this is what is observed in epithelia such as the frog skin and in suspensions of kidney tubules. Thus, active K^+ accumulation and Na^+ extrusion by isolated proximal tubule cells in vitro appear to have the same energy requirement as that of the Na^+-K^+-ATPase in vitro. Yet, the efficiency of net transepithelial Na^+ transport in intact proximal tubules in vivo is much higher.

COUPLING OF ACTIVE AND PASSIVE NA^+ REABSORPTION IN THE PROXIMAL TUBULES: ITS INFLUENCE ON THE EFFICIENCY OF NA^+ TRANSPORT

The proximal tubule is a "leaky" epithelium [33,202]. The electrical resistance of the mammalian proximal epithelium (S_1 segment) is low (<50 ohms/cm^2), and the transepithelial electrical potential difference is small (<5 mV). Because the electrical resistances of the luminal (600 ohms/cm^2) and antiluminal (250 ohms/cm^2) membranes of renal proximal tubule cells are appreciably higher than the transepithelial resistance, a low resistance pathway (paracellular) must exist in parallel with the transcellular pathway [32]. It has been estimated that about two thirds of the Na^+ reabsorption along the PCT of the rat occurs through

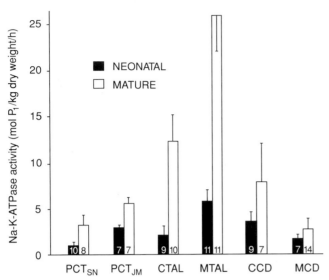

FIG. 10-3. *Distribution of ATPase activity in neonatal and mature rabbit nephron. Values are means ± SD. Numbers in bars indicate the number of analyzed tubular segments. Abbreviations: PCT$_{SN}$, proximal convoluted tubules (early segment) of subcapsular nephron; PCT$_{JM}$, proximal convoluted tubule (early segment) from juxtamedullary nephron. CTAL, cortical thick ascending loop of Henle. MTALH, medullary thick ascending loop of Henle. CCD, cortical collecting duct. MCD, medullary collecting duct. (From Schmidt U, Horster M: Na-K-activated ATPase: Activity maturation in rabbit nephron segments dissected in vitro. Am J Physiol 233:F55, 1977, with permission.)*

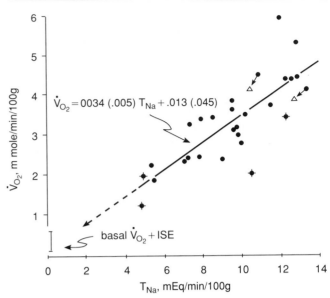

FIG. 10-4. *Relationship between O_2 consumption (VO_2) and net Na^+ reabsorption (T_{Na}) during water diuresis (●), water diuresis plus elevated ureteral pressure (+), or following Pitressin infusion (Δ) sufficient to inhibit water diuresis without affecting blood flow. Symbols are means of two or more consecutive clearance periods. (From Knox FG, Fleming JS, Rennie DW: Effect of osmotic diuresis on sodium reabsorption and oxygen consumption of kidney. Am J Physiol 210:751, 1966, with permission.)*

the paracellular pathway, by diffusion or solvent drag or both, and that only one-third of the Na^+ reabsorbed in these segments occurs through active transcellular transport [99]. Na^+ crosses the luminal membranes of proximal cells in countertransport with H^+ [194] or in cotransport (Fig. 10-7) with glucose [159], amino acids [84], organic acids (e.g., lactate) [21], and inorganic anions (e.g., phosphate) [131], and most of it is actively extruded from the cells at the basolateral side by the ouabain inhibitable Na^+-K^+-ATPase (Fig. 10-8). One-third of the Na^+ that enters the cell in exchange for H^+ exits across the basolateral membrane in cotransport with HCO_3^- rather than through the Na^+-K^+-ATPase [4]. This basolateral HCO_3^- coupled Na^+ extrusion represents net Na^+ reabsorption not coupled directly to ATP utilization and hence contributes to the high efficiency of Na^+ transport in the proximal tubule.

The preferential reabsorption of $NaHCO_3$ and of cotransported organic solutes in the early segments of the proximal tubules establishes transepithelial Cl^- and HCO_3^- gradients [196] and small electrical potential and effective osmotic pressure differences across the PCT epithelium [7]. These driving forces, in turn, induce osmotic and ionic flows across the paracellular pathway (see Fig. 10-7). These fluxes, although passive in nature, are dependent on the establishment of osmotic and electrochemical potential gradients for Cl^-, HCO_3^-, and preferentially reabsorbed solutes across the epithelium generated by the

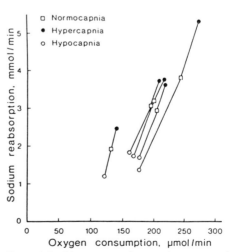

FIG. 10-5. *Changes in sodium reabsorption and oxygen consumption induced by raising (open circles) or reducing (closed circles) plasma PCO_2, at constant plasma bicarbonate concentration (32 ± 1 mM) in five dogs, during continuous infusion of ethacrynic acid. Average change in Na^+ reabsorption per μmol change in oxygen consumption, at constant GFR, was 48 ± 2 μEq. (From Mathisen O, Montclair T, Kiil F: Oxygen requirement of bicarbonate dependent sodium reabsorption in the dog kidney. Am J Physiol 238:F175, 1980, with permission.)*

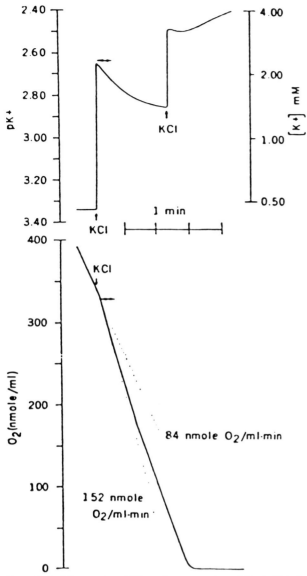

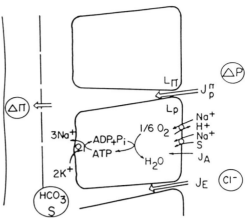

FIG. 10-7. *Schematic representation of pathways and reabsorptive driving forces in proximal tubule (S_1) cells. L_π = hydraulic conductance (oncotic) of paracellular pathway; L_P = hydraulic conductance (hydrostatic) of paracellular pathway; ($\triangle P$) = net transtubular hydrostatic pressure difference; ($\triangle \pi$) = lumen to capillary net oncotic pressure difference. J_P^π = hydrostatic and oncotic pressures driven flow; S = Na^+ dependent cotransported solutes. J_A = trancellular active flux; $3Na^+:2K^+$: (ATP $\rightarrow$ ADP + P_i) is the molar stoichiometry of the transport ATPase; 1/6 ($O_2 \rightarrow H_2O$) : 1(ADP + Pi $\rightarrow$ ATP) is the molar stoichiometry of oxidative phosphorylation coupled to NADH-linked respiration; HCO_3^- and S = transtubular gradients of bicarbonate and preferentially reabsorbed cotransported solutes; Cl^- transtubular gradient of chloride; J_E = paracellular flux driven by cell-generated transtubular effective osmotic and ionic gradients. (From Barac-Nieto M, Spitzer A: The relationship between renal metabolism and proximal tubule transport during ontogeny. Pediatr Nephrol 2:356, 1988, with permission.)*

FIG. 10-6. *The uptake of K^+ and consumption of O_2 in K^+-depleted isolated renal tubules. Double-headed arrows indicate the initial rate period. During this 18-second interval the K^+ uptake was 230 nmol per ml of suspension and the incremental oxygen consumption was 20.4 nmol per ml of suspension, yielding a K^+/O_2 ratio of 11.7. The experimental apparatus contained 5.5 ml of tubule suspension (9 mg protein/ml) and KCl additions were in the form of 10 μl portions of a stock solution. (From Harris SI, Balaban RS, Mandel LJ: Oxygen consumption and cellular ion transport: Evidence for adenosine triphosphate to O_2 ratio near 6 in intact cell. Science 208:1146, 1980, with permission.)*

transcellular transport of solutes (Fig. 10-9). The combination of passive paracellular fluxes with active transcellular fluxes accounts for the high efficiency of net proximal Na^+ reabsorption. When poorly reabsorbable solutes (e.g., mannitol) are present in the tubular fluid, there is substantial reduction in proximal reabsorption of Na^+ and H_2O. Yet, in mannitol diuresis the renal O_2 consumption does not change, indicating that the reduction in Na^+ transport is a consequence of a decrease in passive reabsorption of Na^+ [164].

ENERGY COST OF NA$^+$ TRANSPORT BEYOND THE PROXIMAL TUBULE NEPHRON SEGMENTS

Na^+ reabsorption across nephron segments other than the proximal tubule is also due to a combination of passive and energy-requiring processes. Thus, in the thin segments of Henle's loop (Table 10-2), Na^+ reabsorption occurs along chemical concentration gradients [140,166,167]. The influx of Na^+ from the tubule lumen into the thick ascending limb cells is mediated by a furosemide-sensitive Na^+-K^+-$2Cl^-$ cotransport pathway. An equivalent amount of Na^+ is reabsorbed in the thick ascending limbs passively through the paracellular pathway (Fig. 10-10). By contrast, most of the Na^+ reabsorbed by tight epithelia, such as the distal tubules and the collecting ducts, occurs through the transcellular pathway, mediated by entry of Na^+ from the lumen into the cells through amiloride-sensitive, aldosterone-responsive Na^+ channels. In these segments, active efflux of Na^+ from the cells into the interstitial fluid is driven by the Na^+-K^+-ATPase at the basolateral cell membranes [42,43]. Accordingly, the efficiency of Na^+ transport in

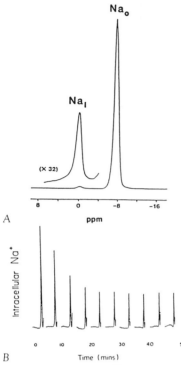

A.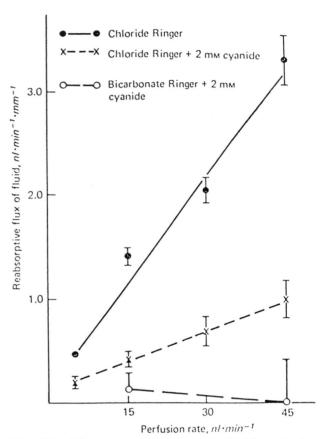

FIG. 10-8. A. *Typical $^{23}Na^+$-NMR spectrum of a suspension of renal cortical tubules. Na_i and Na_o represent intracellular and extracellular Na^+ peaks, respectively. Lower trace: N_i is displayed relative to Na_o. Upper trace: Na_i is enlarged 32-fold over lower trace. Suspension contained 4.1 mg protein/ml. B. Experiment showing efflux of intracellular Na^+ as tubules are warmed to 37°C. Tubules suspensions were kept cold (4°C) during their preparation, resulting in an accumulation of intracellular Na^+. When placed in the NMR, suspensions reached 37°C within 10 min. Each spectrum is a 5 min accumulation of intracellular Na^+ only. Extracellular Na^+ peaks have been omitted. Ouabain (10^{-3} M) inhibited completely the decrease in Na_i. (From Gullans SR, Avison M, Takshi O, et al: NMR measurements of intracellular sodium in the rabbit proximal tubule. Am J Physiol 249:F160, 1985, with permission.)*

FIG. 10-9. *Relationship between reabsorptive fluid flux and tubule perfusion rate in proximal tubule in the presence of transtubular Cl^- and HCO_3 gradients (Chloride Ringer), in the absence or presence of 2 mM cyanide; and in cyanide-poisoned tubules perfused in the absence of transtubular Cl^- and HCO_3 gradients (Bicarbonate Ringer ± 2 mM cyanide). (From Green R, Moriarty RJ, Giebisch G: Ionic requirements of proximal tubular fluid reabsorption: Flow dependency of fluid transport. Kidney Int 20:580, 1981, with permission.)*

distal tubules and collecting ducts is that of the transcellular transport process and hence heavily reflects the metabolic coupling stoichiometry of the Na^+-K^+-ATPase (18 equivalents of Na^+ per mole O_2). In the thick ascending limbs, where approximately equal amounts of Na^+ are transported through the transcellular and the paracellular pathways, the Na^+/O_2 is expected to be about 36 equivalents per mole.

Renal Active Transport Processes Other Than That of Na^+

There are other primary active transport processes besides that of Na^+. Such is the case of some of the Ca^{2+}, which enters passively into the cells and is, in part, actively

extruded across the basolateral membranes by a Ca^{2+}-ATPase [73,149]. However, the Ca^{2+}-ATPase represents only a minor fraction (5% to 10%) of the Na^+-K^+-ATPase activity (Fig. 10-11) and thus probably consumes little of the ATP generated in the renal cells. Increases in cytosolic Ca^{2+} are rapidly counteracted by reaccumulation of Ca^{2+} in the endoplasmic reticulum through the activity of a Ca^{2+}-ATPase, so that its concentration is maintained at the nanomolar level. Rapid changes in cytosolic Ca^{2+} concentration serve as regulatory signals in the modulation of many intracellular processes. The rate of energy expenditure associated with the regulation of cytosolic Ca^{2+} by the Ca^{2+}-ATPase in the endoplasmic reticulum is not known.

The H^+-secreting, mitochondria-rich cells of the cortical and medullary collecting ducts effect Na^+-independent, substrate-requiring net secretion of H^+ into the tubule lumen (Fig. 10-12) through an H^+-ATPase [235]. This

TABLE 10-2. *Determinants of transport across thin limbs of Henle as determined by in vitro perfusion techniques*

Parameter	Descending	Ascending
Transepithelial PD	0	0
Net solute flux	0	0
Na^+ flux	bidirect. equal	bidirect. equal
Osmotic permeability, $L_p \times 10^{-4}$ ml/cm^2/sec/atm	1.6–1.7	0
Passive permeability $\times 10^{-5}$ cm/sec		
P_{Na}	0.16–1.9	22–80
P_{Cl}	—	93–196
Purea	1.0–1.5	7–22
P_K	2.5	22–80
P_{Ca}	0.8	1.4
P_{PO_4}	0.5	0.6
Reflection coefficient		
NaCl	0.95	—
Urea	0.96	—

Transepithelial PD, net solute, and Na^+ fluxes were determined with identical lumen and bath solutions. *From Kokko JP: Transport characteristics of the thin limbs of Henle. Kidney Int 22:449, 1982, with permission.*

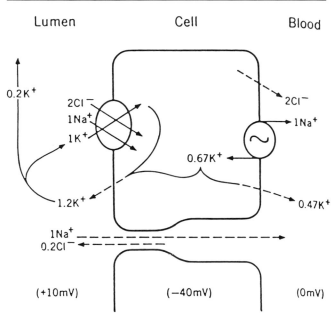

FIG. 10-10. *Model for NaCl absorption in mouse medullary thick ascending limb of Henle (mTALH). conductive pathways are denoted by dashed arrows. All flux values are normalized to an electroneutral Na^+-K^+-Cl^- cotransport mechanism in apical plasma membrane with a stoichiometry of 1:1:2. Stoichiometry of Na^+-K^+-ATPase is assumed to be $3Na^+$-$2K^+$. Depicted in the lower cell is ADH-dependent voltage profile across mouse mTALH. (From Herbert SC, Andreoli TE: Control of NaCl transport in the thick ascending limb. Am J Physiol 246:F745, 1984, with permission.)*

transporting enzyme was recently identified in luminal membranes of proximal tubule cells (D. Brown, personal communication), possibly accounting for the observation that not all proximal H^+ secretion is mediated through Na^+-coupled pathways [271]. It appears, therefore, that a fraction of the H^+ secreted into the proximal tubule lumen

and most of that secreted into the collecting ducts require expenditure of ATP. Assuming that 20% of the renal reabsorption of HCO_3^- is mediated by the H^+-ATPase and that the molar ratio of H^+ secretion to ATP utilization is 3:1, as in the toad bladder [72], active bicarbonate reabsorption would require the expenditure of ~1.7 μmole ATP per minute and per gram kidney. If the total rate of renal ATP turnover is 36 μmole/min/g kidney (O_2 uptake = 6 μmole/min/g and P/O = 3), the energy expenditure for bicarbonate reabsorption through primary active H^+ secretion would represent about 5% of the renal O_2 consumption.

There is controversy as to whether the secretion of certain organic anions (p-aminohippurate) and cations (tetraethylammonium) by the proximal tubules is mediated by primary active (ATP energized) or secondary active (ion gradient coupled) processes [132,190,230,273]. By contrast, it is recognized that the reabsorption of glucose, amino acids, organic and inorganic anions such as phosphate and sulfate [270], as well as a major fraction of the luminal entry of protons in this nephron segment [217] is mediated by secondary active Na^+-coupled transport systems. In the thick ascending limb, another secondary active process, the coupled cotransport of Na^+-K^+ and Cl^-, mediates the transfer of these ions from tubular lumen into the cells [165]. Tertiary coupling between Na^+-H^+ exchange, formate-Cl^- exchange, and nonionic diffusion of formic acid may mediate the electroneutral transfer of NaCl across the luminal membrane of proximal cells [231]. This Cl^- influx pathway together with Cl^- conductive channels at the basolateral membrane participates in the transcellular reabsorption of NaCl across the epithelium of the late proximal tubules. These secondary and tertiary active transport process are driven by the electrochemical potential gradient for Na^+ across the cell membranes and do not by themselves effect consumption of metabolic energy. However, to the extent that they constitute pathways for Na^+ influx into the cells, they ultimately require the low intracellular Na^+ concentration maintained through the

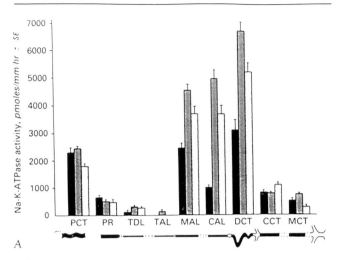

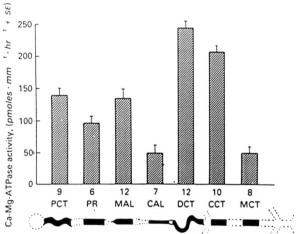

Fig. 10-11. *Distribution of ATPases along the nephron. A. Na⁺-K⁺-ATPase activity along rabbit, rat, and mouse nephron. Abbreviations: JM, juxtamedullary; PCT, proximal convolute tubule; PR, pars recta; TDL, thin descending limb; TAL, thin ascending limb; MAL, medullary, and CAL, cortical thick ascending limb; DCT, distal convolute tubule; CCT, cortical collecting tubule; MCT, medullary collecting tubule. Rabbit, dark bars; rat, cross-hatched bars; mouse, open bars. B. Ca²⁺-Mg²⁺-ATPase along the rabbit nephron. (From Katz AI: Distribution and function of classes of ATPases along the nephron. Kidney Int 29:21, 1986, with permission.)*

ATP-dependent activity of the Na⁺ pump. Nevertheless, this energy expenditure is not additional to that required for Na⁺ transport. Through these Na⁺ coupled transport processes, the renal epithelial cells achieve active reabsorption of many solutes without additional energy expenditure.

Renal Endergonic Synthetic Processes

The kidneys support a variety of synthetic processes. Thus, renal production of glucose from lactate, prominent in starved obese humans [205], is energy requiring. Generation of 1 mmole of glucose from pyruvate requires con-

sumption of 12 mmoles of ATP and 2 mmoles of O_2 (Fig. 10-13). The rate of renal gluconeogenesis (0.1 mmole glucose per minute) from lactate, pyruvate, and glycerol, observed in starved humans in vivo, could account for a considerable fraction (20%) of the renal O_2 consumption [205]. By contrast, gluconeogenesis from glutamine involves the prior partial oxidation of the glutamine carbon skeleton to pyruvate and is a net exergonic (energy producing) process, generating 14 mmoles of ATP for each mmole of glucose produced from 2 mmoles of glutamine (Fig. 10-13).

The nitrogens derived from renal glutamine metabolism can be excreted in the urine as NH_4^+ or can be transferred to the liver in nontoxic form as alanine. In metabolic acidosis, there is an increase in the net synthesis of alanine by the kidney [280]. The alanine derives from partial oxidation of glutamine to pyruvate, coupled with transamination of glutamate (derived from glutamine) and pyruvate. Stimulation of renal alanine synthesis by lactate results from increased transamination of the pyruvate derived from lactate metabolism with glutamate derived from glutamine utilization (Fig. 10-14). These incomplete oxidation processes result in net generation rather than expenditure of ATP, as they involve the partial oxidation of glutamine or lactate or both and thus do not contribute to the renal energy demand but rather to renal energy production.

Infusion of glycine results in significant increases in the heat production (and O_2 consumption) by the kidneys [143]. Glycine serves as substrate for various metabolic processes (Fig. 10-15). The proximal tubule is the major site in the body for synthesis of serine from glycine [182]. Serine is then used by the liver to synthesize glucose and is an important constituent of phospholipids and proteins. A renal glycine-arginine transamidinase mediates the synthesis of guanidoacetic acid from glycine and arginine. Guanidoacetic acid produced in the kidney is methylated, in kidney or liver, to produce methyl-guanidoacetate, i.e., creatine, which is stored mainly in muscle. Increases in the dietary supply of arginine, threonine, or aspartate induce the activity of the renal transamidinase. Increases in dietary or plasma creatine levels inhibit the renal synthesis of guanidoacetic acid, which normally accounts for about one-third of the daily production of creatine in the body. In chronic renal failure, extrarenal synthesis of guanidoacetate and creatine compensates for the decreased renal production of these substances [55].

Conjugation of endogenous and exogenous substrates with glycine (e.g., benzoyl, acyl), glucuronides (e.g., methyl, phenyl, resorcinyl, salicyl, 17-keto and hydroxysteroids), acetate (e.g., benzylhomocysteine, p-amino-hippurate), or sulfate (e.g., phenol, menthol, resorcinol) plays an important role in the renal elimination of these conjugates from the body and is energy requiring. The quantitative contribution of these conjugations to the renal O_2 consumption is not known.

Carnitine is essential in the transfer of long chain fatty acids across the mitochondrial membrane and thus promotes their uptake and oxidation in kidney cortex [16]. The kidney contributes to conservation of filtered carnitine through an Na⁺-dependent reabsorptive transport [138]

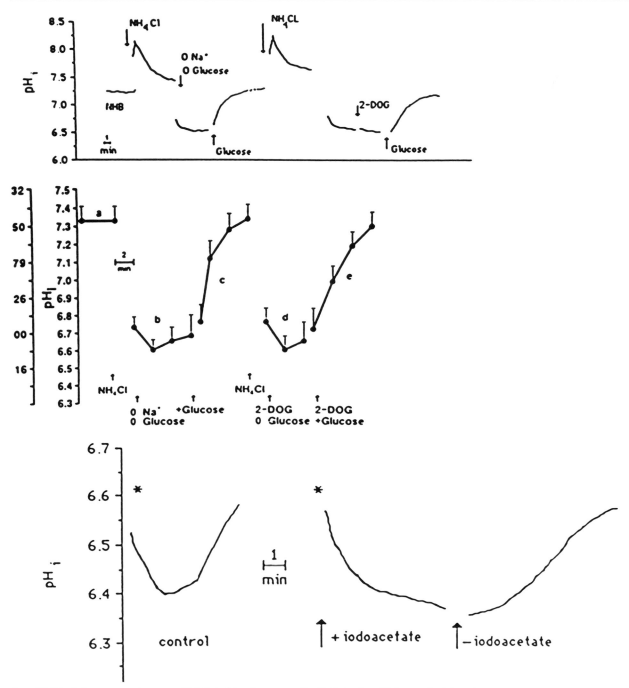

FIG. 10-12. *Substrate requirement of Na⁺-independent cytosolic alkalinization (H⁺ secretion) in cultured inner medullary collecting duct cells, following an NH₄Cl load.* **Middle panel:** *Changes in pH_i when monolayers are bathed in media of the following composition and pH_o held constant at 7.2–110 mM NaCl (a); after a 20 mM NH₄Cl pulse in Na⁺ and glucose-free choline-Cl (b); addition of 5 mM glucose (c); after 20 mM pulse in Na⁺ and glucose-free choline Cl and addition of 5 mM 2-deoxyglucose at arrow (d) and addition of glucose (e). Values are means ± SE, n = 6.* **Top panel:** *Representative example of the above experiments. pH_i value during period that monolayers were exposed to NH₄Cl may not be accurate because they are above the calibration values.* **Bottom panel:** *Effect of iodoacetate on Na⁺-independent cytosolic alkalinization. Changes in pH_i were continuously monitored after a brief exposure to NH₄Cl (*), which was replaced by Na⁺-free, 5 mM glucose choline buffer (pH_o 7.2) (control), then by a similar solution containing 1 mM iodoacetate (+ iodoacetate), and finally in iodoacetate-free buffer (− iodoacetate). (From Selvaggio AM, Schwartz JM, Bengele HH, et al: Mechanisms of H⁺ secretion by inner medullary collecting duct cells. Am J Physiol 254:F391, 1988, with permission.)*

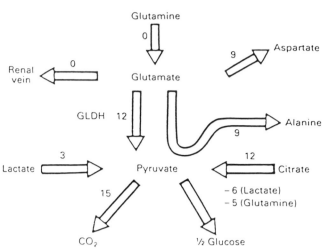

FIG. 10-13. *ATP metabolism associated with renal glutamine, lactate, and citrate utilization. The quantity of ATP produced in each segment of the metabolic pathway is as follows: Each turnover of NADH is equivalent to the turnover of 3 ATP. The number of ATP generated when glutamine, lactate, and citrate are metabolized to oxaloacetate or pyruvate are indicated by the numbers close to each arrow. The two arrows linking glutamate and pyruvate represent flux through glutamic dehydrogenase (12 ATP) and alanine aminotransferase (9 ATP). One less NADH, and therefore 3 less ATP, are generated via the transaminase pathway than through the dehydrogenase pathway. When pyruvate is converted to glucose 6 ATP are consumed (−6 ATP). However, for gluconeogenesis from glutamine, the synthesis of oxaloacetate by pyruvate carboxylase enzyme is not required, and only 5 ATP are consumed. In both cases, 0.5 mole of glucose is formed per mole of glutamine or lactate utilized. (From Vinay P, Lemieux G, Gougoux A, et al: Regulation of glutamine metabolism in the dog kidney in vivo. Kidney Int 29:68, 1986, with permission.)*

and participates in carnitine biosynthesis. Methylation of lysine results in formation of trimethyl-lysine, which in the kidney serves as precursor of butyrobetaine. In rats, butyrobetaine produced in the kidney is converted to carnitine mostly in the liver. In humans, the kidneys synthesize carnitine from butyrobetaine. Renal metabolism of circulating trimethyl-lysine appears to be critical to the endogenous synthesis of carnitine. The extent to which trimethyl-lysine produced from proteolysis is liberated into the circulation is not well defined, and extrarenal synthesis of butyrobetaine and carnitine from locally produced trimethyl-lysine can also occur [224]. Carnitine deficiency, due to genetic defects in its renal reabsorption [81], to dietary deficiencies, and also frequently during hemodialysis [28], is associated with accumulation of lipids in several tissues and generalized muscular weakness [80]. It is not known if developmental changes in tissue carnitine levels, in synthesis of carnitine or of its precursors, or in the activity of acylcarnitine transferases or translocase, occur in the kidney, particularly in association with high lipid intake, such as during breast feeding.

In vitro, renal proximal tubules can synthesize triglycerides from fatty acids, lactate, and glutamine [17,293]. In vivo, fatty acids injected into the renal arterial inflow are rapidly incorporated into neutral lipids and phospholipids in renal tissue and in the renal venous effluent [19]. The contribution of energy-requiring lipid synthesis to the renal O_2 consumption in vivo is unknown.

Synthesis of renal hormones such as renin, erythropoietin, and 1,25 hydroxy-vitamin D require consumption of ATP. Finally, the turnover of cell constituents such as nucleoproteins, proteins, lipids, and carbohydrates, the production of autocrine and paracrine growth factors, and the synthesis of extracellular matrix constituents are all energy-requiring processes. Many intracellular regulatory processes involve phosphorylation-dephosphorylation sequences that imply consumption of high-energy phosphates and thus impinge on renal O_2 consumption. The contributions of these endergonic processes to the energy metabolism of the kidneys remains to be quantified.

Relationship Between Renal Na^+ Reabsorption and Other Synthetic or Transport Endergonic Processes

DEPENDENCE OF RENAL ENDERGONIC PROCESSES ON GFR

Some of the metabolic functions of the kidney, as well as the net reabsorption of Na^+, vary in proportion to the filtered load of substrates and thus contribute to the proportionality observed between renal O_2 uptake and glomerular filtration rate (GFR) [56]. To the extent that the rates of energy-requiring processes other than Na^+ reabsorption vary in proportion to the GFR, the slope of the regression line correlating changes in renal Na^+ reabsorption and in O_2 consumption (30 Eq/mole) will result in an underestimate of the efficiency of Na^+ transport in the kidney, as some of the change in O_2 uptake associated with changes in GFR relates not to the change in Na^+ transport activity but to those of other energy-requiring processes [53]. For example, the selective absorption of small molecular weight proteins and peptides through receptor-mediated endocytosis involves the continuous internalization of membrane vesicles from the cell surface into the cytosol and the recycling of the receptors from the endosomal membrane vesicles back to the cell surface; this process is energy dependent [284], and its rate may vary in proportion to changes in the filtered loads of small molecular weight proteins and peptides. The synthesis of serine from glycine in proximal tubule cells depends on the supply of substrate to these cells [212], which is in part a function of the filtered glycine load. Similarly, the rate of primary active H^+ secretion along the nephron may be dependent on the HCO_3^- load [272], and thus, its energy requirement may also vary in proportion to changes in GFR.

COUPLING BETWEEN RENAL METABOLIC AND TRANSPORT FUNCTIONS

The proportional changes in reabsorption of Na^+ and solutes such as bicarbonate, phosphate, glucose, amino acids, and lactate may play a role in the maintenance of the balance between glomerular and tubular functions [42].

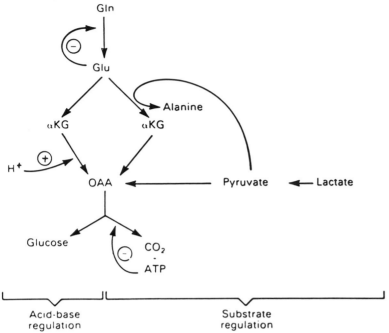

FIG. 10-14. *Metabolism of glutamine in dog proximal tubule cells. Regulation by pH and by substrate availability. The diagram illustrates that glutamate, Glu (and secondarily, glutamine, Gln), utilization can be promoted through faster deamination (because of faster alpha-ketoglutarate, KG, removal as during stimulation by decreases in pH, H⁺[+]) or by faster transamination (because of elevated pyruvate concentration as during regulation by increases in availability of lactate). The oxaloacetate OAA, generated from KG, is converted to pyruvate, which then is mostly oxidized to CO_2 and water or converted to glucose or alanine. In dog kidney both pathways coexist and are responsible for the bulk of ammonia production in physiologic situations. In both cases the rate of alpha-ketoglutarate metabolism is limited by the cell ATP turnover, which may therefore limit the overall rate of renal glutamine utilization. (From Vinay P, Lemieux G, Gougoux A, et al: Regulation of glutamine metabolism in the dog kidney in vivo. Kidney Int 29:68, 1986, with permission.)*

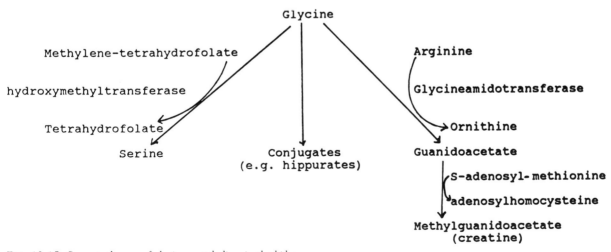

FIG. 10-15. *Some pathways of glycine metabolism in the kidney.*

Increases in filtration rate result in increased delivery of organic solutes as well as of water and salts to the proximal tubules. The filtered organic solutes are virtually completely reabsorbed by the end of the early proximal tubule segment (S_1). On increases in GFR, the concentrations of organic solutes, phosphate, and HCO_3^- in the tubular fluid of late proximal segments rise, increasing the rates of cotransport with Na^+ into the cells and the rate of Na^+-H^+ exchange. The higher cellular Na^+ influx can in turn stimulate the activity of the basolateral Na^+-K^+-ATPase, the generation of adenosine diphosphate (ADP), and the rate of aerobic oxidation of the cotransported organic solutes. Whether such increases in solute delivery also stimulate other metabolic pathways is not yet known, but if it does, it may have a bearing on the hypertrophic growth of the tubules that occurs as a consequence of hyperfiltration [90]. A similar adjustment of tubular transport and metabolic functions may be operative during postnatal development of proximal tubules when increases in tubular reabsorption occur "pari passu" with increases in GFR.

COMPETITION BETWEEN RENAL METABOLIC AND TRANSPORT FUNCTIONS

In the perfused rat kidney, an inverse relationship was observed between the rates of glucose production from pyruvate and the rates of Na^+ reabsorption [241]. In isolated proximal tubules, inhibition of Na^+ transport by ouabain stimulated glucose production [98]. These observations led to the hypothesis that there is competition for ATP between two endergonic processes, gluconeogenesis from pyruvate and Na^+ transport. However, competition was observed neither in the perfused kidney supplied with adequate substrates and O_2 [56], nor in proximal tubule suspensions [121]. In isolated perfused proximal straight tubules, changes in gluconeogenesis induced by addition of metabolic precursors or by mercaptopicolinate, an inhibitor of phosphoenolpyruvate carboxykinase, a rate-limiting gluconeogenic enzyme, failed to alter the rates of fluid and Na^+ reabsorption [297]. In the dog in vivo, renal gluconeogenesis is increased by infusion of lactate without a decrease in net renal Na^+ reabsorption [70]. Thus, competition for energy between renal gluconeogenesis and Na^+ transport only occurs under special circumstances.

An interrelationship has been proposed to exist between tubular Na^+ reabsorption and renal ammoniagenesis. In the acidotic dog, a decrease in Na^+ reabsorption due to administration of ouabain or secondary to renal artery constriction results in proportional decreases in glutamine use, ammoniagenesis, and O_2 consumption [123]. Because use of glutamine for generation of ATP cannot exceed the rate of ATP consumption, it was proposed that the rate of ATP use sets a limit to the rate of renal use of glutamine and thus to ammoniagenesis. In the developing kidney, the low absolute rate of ATP use linked to Na^+ reabsorption may limit the rates of renal glutamine use and ammoniagenesis.

In summary, a tight coupling exists between renal transport and metabolic functions. Changes in renal O_2 consumption can reflect changes in Na^+ transport as well as changes in synthetic functions of the kidney. Renal metabolic processes such as the aerobic oxidation of substrates can vary in proportion to changes in Na^+ transport, thus coupling energy-requiring and energy-producing processes. In turn, under certain circumstances, the rates of renal Na^+ transport can set a limit on the rates of renal metabolic functions such as ammoniagenesis and gluconeogenesis.

Developmental Changes in the Major Energy-requiring Processes: Proximal Na⁺ Reabsorption

The absolute magnitude of the renal blood flow, the GFR, and the proximal reabsorption of Na^+ and water change dramatically during postnatal development. In the guinea pig, single nephron glomerular filtration rate (SNGFR) and the rate of proximal fluid reabsorption increase by ~ 20-fold from 1 to 40 days of age, whereas fractional reabsorption of Na^+ and H_2O remain relatively constant. Over the same period, the length of the PCT increases by ~ sixfold. Thus, in the guinea pig the reabsorptive rate per unit PCT length increases by an average of about threefold during development [256].

The reabsorptive flow per unit tubule length in isolated perfused early proximal juxtamedullary segments of rabbit also increases by a factor of 3 from the 1st to the 6th week of age [236] (Fig. 10-16). However, in S1 and S2 segments of superficial nephrons, which in the rabbit are very immature at birth, the postnatal increases in Na^+ and fluid reabsorption are much more pronounced. In the rat, sixfold increases in kidney weight, GFR, total Na^+ reabsorption, SNGFR, and proximal tubular Na^+ reabsorption occurred from the 20th to the 60th day of extrauterine life [48]; the fractional Na^+ reabsorption along the accessible PCT remained constant (58%). Because, in rat, PCT length increased over the same period by ~1.5-fold [48], Na^+ reabsorption per unit tubule length must have increased by an average of ~fourfold. In view of the fact that both proximal tubular and whole kidney fractional Na^+ reabsorption were found to be constant and independent of age, there appears to be no change in the proportion of filtered Na^+ and water reabsorbed by the PCT and that reabsorbed by more distal nephron segments during postnatal development.

A centrifugal pattern of nephron development and maturation occurs postnatally in several species (rat, rabbit, guinea pig, dog); juxtamedullary nephrons reach maturity at an earlier age than superficial nephrons [288]. Hence, with development a progressively larger fraction of the filtered Na^+ is reabsorbed by the superficial nephrons. It is not presently known if the ratio of Na^+ transport to O_2 use differs in superficial and juxtamedullary nephrons. If such difference exists, the kidney of the neonate would tend to reflect more heavily than that of the adult the Na^+/O_2 ratio of juxtamedullary nephrons.

Role of the Na⁺-K⁺-ATPase in the Development of Transcellular Fluxes in the Renal Tubules

During postnatal development of PCT in rabbits [234,236] and rats [48], there is a threefold increase in Na^+-K^+-

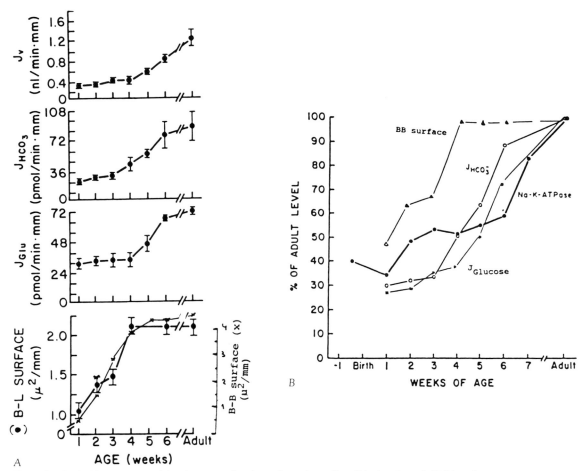

Fig. 10-16. A. Time course of development of reabsorptive volume flux (J_v), basolateral (B-L) and brush border (B-B) membrane areas, net HCO^3 and glucose reabsorption in juxtamedullary proximal convoluted tubule of rabbits. (From Schwartz GJ, Evan AP: Development of solute transport in rabbit proximal tubule. I. HCO₃⁻ and glucose absorption. Am J Physiol 245:F382, 1983, with permission.) B. Time course of development of basolateral membrane surface area (triangles), reabsorptive volume flow (x), net bicarbonate (J_{HCO3}–) reabsorption and Na⁺-K⁺-adenosine-triphosphatase activity (Na⁺-K⁺-ATPase), in juxtamedullary proximal convoluted tubule of rabbits. Data are expressed as percent of values at maturity. (Adapted from [83,236,237], with permission.)

ATPase activity per millimeter of tubule length. The apparent proportionality between the increase in enzyme activity and that in net reabsorptive flow rate [48,234] makes it impossible to determine whether the enzyme develops as a consequence of increased load or whether the rise in transport occurs as a consequence of increased availability of the enzyme. In growing and unilaterally nephrectomized rats, a good correlation has been found between the total Na⁺-K⁺-ATPase activity along the PCT and the rate of net proximal Na⁺ reabsorption, leading to the suggestion that increases in Na⁺-K⁺-ATPase activity are necessary to support increases in proximal Na⁺ reabsorption [48]. Adaptation to nephrectomy is achieved in the growing rat, transiently, through increases in the density of the enzyme at the basolateral membrane and then through increases in tubular length, without changes in the density of transport

enzyme or in the surface of basolateral membrane per unit tubule length [48].

In the juxtamedullary PCT of the rabbit, postnatal increases in basolateral and luminal cell membrane surface per millimeter of tubule length were complete by about 4 weeks of age [83]. Biogenesis of the cell membrane surface areas preceded the increase in Na⁺-K⁺-ATPase activity, as evidenced by the fact that the basolateral cell membrane synthesized from the 2nd to the 4th week of age was low in Na⁺-K⁺-ATPase activity. Administration of glucocorticoids to developing rats results in accelerated maturation of Na⁺-K⁺-ATPase activity without increases in the basolateral membrane area [139]. Thus, membrane biosynthesis and increases in Na⁺-K⁺-ATPase activity during postnatal development occur independently.

In developing rabbit juxtamedullary PCT, the surge in

the net reabsorption of HCO_3^-, glucose, and water [236] preceded the increase in Na^+-K^+-ATPase activity (Fig. 10-16). This sequence of events suggests that the developmental rise in the activity of the Na^+-K^+-ATPase is a consequence rather than a cause of the increase in tubular transport. Thus, the developmental surge in net reabsorption of Na^+ and H_2O in PCT is not limited by the activity of the Na^+-K^+-ATPase. Rather, luminal influx of Na^+ determines the overall rate of transcellular Na^+ transport. If cellular influx, rather than efflux, limits Na^+ transport by the immature PCT, one would expect the intracellular Na^+ concentration to be lower in cells from immature than from mature animals. Consistent with this presumption is the observation that both the intracellular Na^+ concentration and Na^+-K^+-ATPase were found to be lower in primary cultures of proximal tubular cells derived from 10-day-old rats than in those from adults, suggesting that influx of Na^+ is more limited in the cells from the immature animals [176]. The fact that the rate of net gain of Na^+ that occurs in these cells on inhibition of the Na^+-K^+-ATPase with ouabain increases with maturation [175] provides further support for this hypothesis.

The major pathways for luminal Na^+ influx that set the pace of active Na^+ transport in PCT cells are the Na^+-H^+ exchange and the Na^+-dependent cotransport systems. Development of net reabsorption of HCO_3^- (a Na^+-H^+ exchange-dependent process) and of glucose (a Na^+-coupled cotransport process) in rabbit juxtamedullary PCT occurred between the 4th and the 6th week of age, almost simultaneously with that of fluid transport [236], but subsequent to the completion of the biogenesis of luminal cell membrane surface area [83], suggesting that maturation of the area of luminal cell membrane precedes its functional development. Whether the luminal (brush border) membrane synthesized up to the 4th week had its full complement of glucose and H^+ transporters, or these appear concomitantly with the surge in net HCO_3^- and glucose reabsorption, cannot be determined from these data. However, high- and low-capacity Na^+-dependent cotransport systems for glucose have been found in renal brush border membranes derived from dog kidney superficial cortex and outer medulla, respectively [269]. In the guinea pig, the V_{max} of the high-capacity glucose cotransport system increases less than twofold with development [238]. Developmental changes in Na^+-dependent cotransport of alpha-methylglucoside of similar magnitude have been observed in suspensions of rat PCT [227]. These data suggest that the luminal membranes of PCT in newborn guinea pigs and rats, as those in the fetal rat [26], do not have a full complement of glucose cotransporters, and that these develop postnatally.

The capacity for Na^+-H^+ exchange also increases during postnatal development, as evidenced by a significantly higher amiloride-sensitive Na^+ influx in primary cultures of renal proximal cells obtained from 15-day-old rats compared with that of cells from 10-day-old rats [8].

The fractional reabsorption of various amino acids that are transported out of the tubular lumen through Na^+-cotransport systems is low during the early postnatal period. Increases in Na^+-dependent proline cotransport have been observed during the first month of age in brush border membrane vesicles derived from maturing rats [192]. Similarly, taurine-Na^+ cotransport is lower in brush border membrane vesicles from 7-day-old rats than in those from adult animals [51]. It is likely that these lower rates of uptake are due to a low number of cotransporters. Alternatively, the low rates of cotransport of these amino acids in membrane vesicles from neonates may be due to a more rapid dissipation of the Na^+ gradient than in vesicles from adult animals [192]. Thus, although the net uptake of amino acids may be reduced, the influx of Na^+ across the luminal membrane actually may be larger in newborn than in adult rats.

In proximal cells in primary culture, the amiloride-insensitive Na^+ influx was found to be higher in cells from immature than from mature rats [8]. In addition, Na^+ influx into renal brush border membranes vesicles derived from immature rats has been reported to be higher than into those from adult animals [192,299]. Na^+-dependent phosphate influx into brush border membranes of newborn guinea pigs [197] and young rats [154] was also higher than in those of the adult animals. Furthermore, in rapidly growing tumor or normal cells, the intracellular Na^+ concentration is higher than in nondividing cells [47]. In immature erythroid cells, Na^+-coupled amino acid influx was found to be higher than in the fully differentiated cells and was related to the high rates of protein synthesis present in the growing cells [173]. Thus, although certain pathways for Na^+ influx may be higher in immature than in mature proximal cells, others are not, and it is not yet established if in differentiating proximal cells in vivo the net influx of Na^+, the intracellular Na^+ concentration, and the fractional saturation of the Na^+ pump are higher than in the mature cells.

These data provide a controversial picture of the development of luminal and antiluminal transport processes in the proximal tubular cells. Some data suggest that postnatal development of the energy-requiring transcellular Na^+ flux is limited, at least in the juxtamedullary proximal convoluted tubule of rabbits and in rat proximal cells in culture, by development of luminal Na^+ influx through Na^+-H^+ exchange and glucose-Na^+ cotransport, which together account for a major fraction of the Na^+ influx into mature PCT cells [125]. Whether these same or other pathways account for most of the Na^+ influx into the developing PCT cells remains to be established, as other data suggest that certain pathways for Na^+ influx (amiloride-insensitive, phosphate cotransport) are higher in immature than in mature PCT.

Development of Ouabain-Sensitive O_2 Consumption in Proximal Tubule

Measurements of the O_2 consumption in isolated proximal tubular suspensions provide insight into the factors limiting the development of the active component of Na^+ reabsorption in PCT. The ouabain-sensitive O_2 consumption of PCT suspensions of adult rats was 13 ± 1 pmoles O_2 per minute per microgram protein (Fig. 10-17). Assuming P/O = 3, Na^+/ATP = 3, and that all ouabain-sensitive O_2 uptake is only associated with the activity of Na^+-K^+-

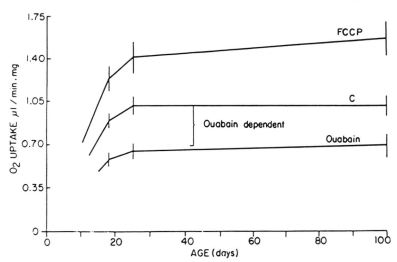

FIG. 10-17. *Time course of development of O_2 consumption ($\mu l/min/mg$ protein) in suspensions of proximal tubules of rats. Tubules were incubated at 37°C, for 5–10 min, in Krebs Ringer's bicarbonate solution, equilibrated with 95 percent O_2 −5 percent CO_2, supplemented with 5 mM glucose, 5 mM lactate, and 1 mM glutamine (C) and exposed to 1 mM ouabain (Ouabain), or to 5 μM carbonyl-cyanide trifluorophenylhydrazone (FCCP). Incubations were carried out in a closed 2 ml chamber of a polarographic O_2 electrode (YSI). Ouabain-dependent O_2 uptake was calculated as the differences between (C) and (Ouabain). Data are means and standard deviations of triplicate determinations at each age. (From Barac-Nieto M, Spitzer A: The relationship between renal metabolism and proximal tubule transport during ontogeny. Pediatr Nephrol 2:356, 1988, with permission.)*

ATPase, we can estimate the active Na^+ flux to be 234 pEq/min/μg protein. Using a dry tissue weight/tubule length ratio of 0.37 μg/mm [234] and a protein/dry weight ratio of 0.66 [39,256], an active Na^+ flux of 57 pEq/mm/min is calculated. This is similar to the transcellular active Na^+ flux estimated to occur in rat PCT in vivo [99]. Comparison of this Na^+ transport rate with the maximal rate of transport (390 pEq/mm/min) calculated from the optimal activity of the Na^+-K^+-ATPase measured in vitro [237] and an Na^+/ATP = 3 indicates that the enzyme operates at 15% saturation, which, at nonlimiting concentrations of ATP, K^+, and Mg^{2+}, would correspond to an intracellular Na^+ concentration of about 20 mEq/L, similar to that directly measured in rat PCT cells in vivo [298].

Ouabain-sensitive O_2 uptake in PCT suspensions obtained from 2- to 3-week-old rats was 11 ± 1 pmoles/min/μg protein, somewhat lower but not significantly different from that in PCT of adult rats. Using the same P/O and Na^+/ATP ratios as above, the active Na^+ flux is estimated to be 198 pEq/min/μg protein. When corrected for a dry weight/tubule length ratio of 0.29 μg/mm [234] and a protein/dry weight ratio of 0.56 in tubules of young animals [39,256], a value of 32 pEq/min/mm tubule length is arrived at for the active Na^+ efflux from PCT cells of young rats. This represents two-thirds of the total Na^+ reabsorption observed in PCT of young rats in vivo [48], as compared with one third in mature PCT, and would indicate that active Na^+ flux is relatively higher in PCT of newborn than adult rats. This estimate is based on the assumption that the ouabain-sensitive O_2 consumption measured in isolated PCT suspensions in vitro reflects quantitatively

the rate of active Na^+ extrusion by the Na^+-K^+-ATPase in the intact PCT in vivo. Although the magnitude of the net transepithelial Na^+ reabsorptive flux in PCT of newborn rats is known [48], the magnitude of the active component of Na^+ reabsorption in developing PCT in vivo is not. Consequently the active Na^+ flux, estimated from the ouabain-sensitive O_2 consumption in vitro, cannot be compared with its value in vivo. The estimated active flux represents 25% of the maximal flux calculated from the optimal activity of the ouabain-sensitive ATPase activity of immature PCT, assessed in vitro [237]. This indicates that the enzyme operates at a higher level of saturation and that the intracellular Na^+ concentration should be higher in immature than in mature PCT. This conclusion is at variance with the observation of lower intracellular Na^+ concentration in 2-day primary cultures of PCT cells from young than in those from mature rats [176]. Primary culture conditions differ markedly from those used for incubation of proximal tubules suspensions. Thus, the rates of Na^+ transport in primary cultures of immature proximal cells may be limited by the Na^+ influx, whereas in suspensions of PCT tubules in vitro, Na^+ influx may be higher in young than in adult rats. Which of these preparations reflects the conditions prevailing in vivo cannot be decided at present.

The relatively high rates of ouabain-sensitive O_2 consumption in PCT suspensions derived from immature rats may be associated with high rates of biosynthesis of proteins, lipids, and carbohydrates. Inhibition of the Na^+-K^+-ATPase with ouabain may reduce not only transcellular Na^+ transport, but also the cellular influx of metab-

TABLE 10-3. *Renal blood flow, glomerular filtration rate, fractional sodium excretion, O_2 consumption, and Na/O_2 ratio during hydropenia (HP) and volume expansion (VE) in 24- and 40-day-old rats*

Group	RBF ml/min/100 g	GFR ml/min/100 g	FENa$^+$ %	VO$_2$ μM/min/100 g	Na/O$_2$ μM/μM
24-day HP	1.33 ± 0.94[bcd]	0.27 ± 0.10[bcd]	0.9 ± 0.4[d]	3.21 ± 0.94[bcd]	14.5 ± 1.7[b]
24-day VE	2.65 ± 0.69[a]	0.52 ± 0.15[a]	1.1 ± 0.5[d]	4.31 ± 0.84[a]	19.6 ± 3.1[acd]
40-day HP	2.50 ± 0.60[a]	0.47 ± 0.11[a]	1.2 + 0.8[d]	4.90 ± 0.90[a]	15.3 ± 2.3[b]
40-day VE	2.80 ± 0.71[a]	0.54 ± 0.17[a]	2.7 ± 1.2[a]	5.11 ± 0.81[a]	16.7 ± 1.5[b]

Values are means ± SD; g refer to body weight.
[a] P < 0.05 vs. 24-day HP.
[b] P < 0.05 vs. 24-day VE.
[c] P < 0.05 vs. 40-day HP.
[d] P < 0.05 vs. 40-day VE. *From* Elinder C, Aperia A: Renal oxygen consumption and sodium reabsorption during isotonic volume expansion in the developing rat. *Pediatr Res* 16:351, 1982, with permission.

olites necessary for such biosynthesis, as amino acids, whose entry into the cells depends on the electrochemical Na$^+$ gradient. Because biosynthetic processes are prominent in the immature PCT, they can account for a relatively large part of the ouabain-sensitive component of the O$_2$ consumption in PCT of young rats. Consequently, the O$_2$ cost of net Na$^+$ transport would appear to be higher in immature than in mature PCT, as endergonic processes other than Na$^+$ transport may be inhibited by ouabain.

The Na$^+$/O$_2$ ratio in the kidney of 24-day-old rats in vivo (Table 10-3) has been reported to be 15 Eq/mole, a value similar to that reported for 40-day-old animals [78], but lower than those observed in the kidney of the adult rat [206,287]. Quantification of the effect of changes in the rates of biosynthetic processes on the O$_2$ consumption of immature proximal cells should help us to define the contribution of biosynthesis to the renal energy turnover during development and their influence on the apparently high O$_2$ cost of Na$^+$ transport in the kidney of the neonate.

It is possible that a larger backflux of Na$^+$ into the lumen in the immature than in the mature PCT, due to a higher permeability of the paracellular pathway, contributes to the low metabolic efficiency of net Na$^+$ reabsorption [78]. Measurements of the unidirectional fluxes of Na$^+$ across the proximal tubule of developing animals are not yet available to support or deny this assumption.

Development of Renal Cortical Metabolic Pathways

AEROBIC METABOLISM

Studies of the changes in kidney metabolism that occur during postnatal development are scarce. The kidney of the fetal sheep consumes O$_2$ at a rate 7.5 times lower than that of the newborn sheep [141], whose rate, in turn, does not differ from that of the adult animal (Table 10-4). In the hydropenic rat, the renal O$_2$ uptake was similar at 24 and at 40 days of age [78]. Comparisons of the rates of O$_2$ consumption per unit wet tissue weight in renal cortical slices [44,69] and proximal tubule suspensions [22] have revealed only small (10%–20%) age-related differences (Figs. 10-17, 10-18). These findings indicate that, even at

birth, the kidney has a high potential for aerobic metabolism.

The renal blood flow is much lower in the neonate (<1 ml/min/g kidney) than in the adult animal (~6 ml/min/g). Because the rates of O$_2$ uptake per unit kidney weight are similar in newborn and adult animals, the arterio-venous O$_2$ difference and the fractional O$_2$ extraction must be higher in the kidney of the neonate than in the adult. This is, indeed, the case in the newborn sheep [141], where renal O$_2$ extraction was found to be 35%, as compared with 10% in adult sheep. In young rats the renal arteriovenous difference for O$_2$ was 2.4 vs 1.98 μmol/ml in adult animals, while the blood hemoglobin concentration, the renal blood flow, and thus the renal O$_2$ delivery, were lower than in the adult [78], indicating a higher renal O$_2$ extraction in the younger than in the older rats (~34% versus 22%). These observations imply that the renal venous O$_2$ tension, and thus the O$_2$ tension in some regions of the kidney of newborn animals, are lower than in the adult and may limit energy turnover.

TABLE 10-4. *Renal blood flow, oxygen delivery, and oxygen consumption in fetal and newborn sheep*

	Fetus	Newborn
Oxygen content, mM		
Aorta	2.71 ± 0.18	5.48 ± 0.14
Renal vein	2.04 ± 0.17	3.61 ± 0.19
Renal blood flow (ml/min/100 g)	154 ± 9	406 ± 32
Oxygen delivery (μmol/min/100 g)	418 ± 38	2231 ± 127
Oxygen consumption (μmol/min/100 g)	104 ± 10	785 ± 79
Oxygen extraction, %	25 ± 2	35 ± 3

Values are means ± SEM; g refer to kidney weight. *From* Iwamoto HS, Oh W, Rudolph AM: Renal metabolism in fetal and newborn sheep. *In* Jones CT, Nathanielsz PW (eds): *The Physiological Development of the Fetus and Newborn.* New York, Academic, 1985, p 37, with permission.

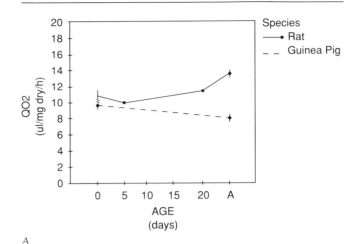

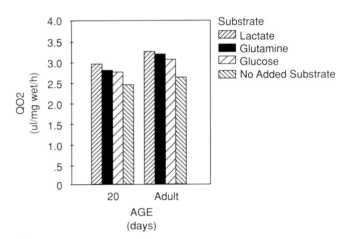

FIG. 10-18. *Oxygen consumption in kidney cortex slices of developing and adult animals. A. O₂ consumption in μg per mg dry tissue weight per h. (From Dicker SE, Shirley DG: Rates of oxygen consumption and anaerobic glycolysis in renal cortex and medulla of adult and newborn rats and guinea pigs. J Physiol (Lond) 212:235, 1971, with permission.) B. In rat kidney slices measurements were made in the absence or in the presence of 18.75 mM lactate, glutamine, or glucose and expressed in μl O₂ per mg wet tissue weight per h. (From Caldwell T, Solomon S: Changes in oxygen consumption of kidney during maturation. Biol Neonate 25:1, 1975, with permission.)*

When incubated at 37°C in Krebs-Ringer bicarbonate solution supplemented with 5 mM lactate, 5 mM glucose, and 1 mM glutamine, PCT suspensions from 2-week-old and adult rats used O_2 at rates of 40 ± 1 and 45 ± 0.9 pmoles/μg protein/min, respectively (Fig. 10-17, data expressed in pmoles using 22.4 μl O_2 per μmole). The small magnitude of this difference is, however, misleading because of the changes in tissue protein/dry weight ratio [39] and in the ratio of dry weight/tubule length that occur during development [234]. When corrected for these var-

iables, the O_2 consumptions per millimeter of tubule length in PCT suspensions of young and adult rats were calculated to be 6.5 and 11 pmoles/mm/min, respectively, a 70% increase in O_2 uptake with age.

The respiratory capacity of a tissue is an index of the aerobic oxidation potential. Respiratory capacity is measured as the rate of uncoupled respiration and reflects the maximal rate of mitochondrial oxidation, in the absence of limitations imposed by coupled oxidative phosphorylation. In PCT suspensions, the rates of uncoupled O_2 consumption were 1.3 and 1.58 μl O_2 per milligram protein per minute in immature and mature rats, respectively (see Fig. 10-17). When expressed in pmoles O_2 per millimeter tubule length, these values are 9.4 and 17.2 pmoles/min/mm tubule length in 2-week-old and adult rats, respectively, representing an 83% increase in aerobic potential with age. That the aerobic metabolic capacity of the renal proximal tubules increases with postnatal development is also indicated by the 50% increase in mitochondrial membrane surface area per unit cell volume (Table 10-5) observed to occur over the first 4 weeks of postnatal development in rabbit juxtamedullary PCT [83]. This change was much more pronounced (threefold increase) in superficial PCT, which reach maturity at a later age. The total activity per unit tissue weight of isocitrate dehydrogenase [39], a Krebs cycle enzyme, increases by 4.5-fold from birth to the 3rd week of age in rat kidneys. Similar increases have been reported for other Krebs cycle enzymes, such as fumarase [301], malate dehydrogenase [282], and citrate synthetase [199] (Table 10-6) in renal cortex and outer medulla of developing rat and mice. These studies indicate that in rats, mice, and rabbits, renal aerobic metabolism reaches near mature levels at a relatively early age (3 to 4 weeks of postnatal life). By contrast, the major developmental surge in net transport rates across the PCT epithelium of the early maturing juxtamedullary nephrons in the rabbit occurs between 4 and 6 weeks of age and that in PCT of rats starts during the 3rd week and continues up to the 8th week of age.

In conclusion, postnatal developmental changes in transcellular Na^+ reabsorption in PCT in vitro do not appear to be limited by the cellular concentrations of enzymes of the pathways of aerobic metabolism. However, whether the O_2 supply might be limiting PCT function in the neonate in vivo remains to be established.

PCT of young and adult rats were found to respire in vitro at about 65% of capacity (Fig. 10-17), similar to findings in PCT of adult rabbits [127]. In PCT of young and adult rats, ouabain-sensitive respiration represented 18.9% and 18.4% of the respiratory capacity, respectively (Fig. 10-17). At low intracellular Na^+ concentration (20 mEq/L), the Na^+-K^+-ATPase operates at about one-sixth of its capacity and is not limited by the supply of ATP but by the Na^+ influx rates. Indeed, the O_2 consumption by PCT of both young and adult rats and of adult rabbits can be increased by increasing cellular Na^+ influx with cationophores [127]. The aerobic reserve (respiratory capacity minus rate of basal respiration) of immature and mature PCT can accomodate a twofold increase in active Na^+ transport. In sum, there exists already at birth a large

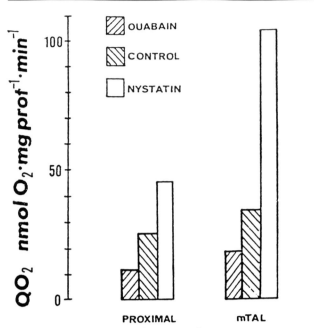

FIG. 10-20. *A comparison of the rates of oxygen consumption (QO$_2$) of the proximal tubules and the medullary thick ascending limbs of Henle's loop (mTAL) measured using suspensions of rabbit renal tubules. The control QO$_2$ of tubules respiring in normal physiological media is compared with the respiration observed when the Na,K,ATPase is maximally inhibited by the addition of ouabain or stimulated by addition a cationophore (nystatin). (From Sotloff SP: Coupling renal metabolism to ion transport in renal epithelia. Semin Nephrol 7:20, 1987, with permission.)*

In renal cortex of 5-day-old rats, the rates of O$_2$ uptake and glycolysis were found to be 7.5 and 3.8 nmoles/mg dry weight per minute, corresponding to 45 and 3.8 nmoles/mg dry weight per minute of ATP synthesized, respectively [69]. Thus, in young rats the glycolytic potential for ATP production was 8.4% of the aerobic rate of ATP synthesis, higher than in adult animals but still only a minor fraction of the total energy turnover of the kidney under aerobic conditions. The glycolytic potential of renal cortical tissue (Fig. 10-21) decreases with maturation [69]. This change is associated with a progressive fall during the first weeks of extrauterine life in the activity of rate-limiting glycolytic enzymes such as hexokinase [199,283], phosphofructokinase [134], and pyruvate kinase [40] in the kidney cortex (Fig. 10-22). Similar changes in glycolytic enzyme activity also have been observed in microdissected isolated proximal convoluted tubules [134].

The absence of significant reserves of high-energy phosphates, particularly phosphocreatine, in the kidneys (see Fig. 10-19) makes this organ very susceptible to ischemic damage. The high glycolytic potential of the renal cortical structures of newborn animals, becomes important during periods of renal ischemia (Fig. 10-23). Although in the kidney of adult rabbits the ATP content of the tissue drops from 10 to 1 μmol/g dry weight within 5 minutes of ischemia, a similar ischemic period in the kidney of newborn

rabbits reduces the ATP content from 12 to 9 μmoles/g dry [91]. Thus, the level of high-energy phosphate is better preserved after short periods of ischemia in the kidney of newborn than in that of adult rabbits. Glycolysis as well as other anaerobic ATP-generating reactions [117] can contribute to the maintenance of the ATP content in kidneys of young animals after short periods of ischemia.

The activities of two glycolytic enzymes, phosphofructokinase and pyruvate kinase, in the thick ascending limbs and the collecting ducts of rabbits are low at birth and increase with age [134], indicating that the glycolytic potential (aerobic, anaerobic, or both) in these segments continues to develop postnatally. Increased Na$^+$ transport by the thick ascending limbs during osmotic diuresis is associated with increases in the concentration of lactate in the medulla, as lactate produced from glycolysis by the medullary structures is trapped by the countercurrent exchange system [66]. Increased glycolytic lactate production suggests limitation in the rates of medullary mitochondrial energy metabolism in response to increases in energy demand. Maturation of the glycolytic capacity of the thick ascending limb may contribute to the ability of this nephron segment to accommodate increases in Na$^+$ load due to changes in GFR. Similarly, maturation of the H$^+$ secretory capacity at the medullary collecting ducts may be associated with the maturational increase in their capacity for glycolysis.

OXIDATION-REDUCTION POTENTIAL

The addition of short chain fatty acids or succinate to proximal tubules from adult rabbits, incubated in vitro, induces proportionate increases in O$_2$ uptake, mitochondrial NADH/NAD, and ouabain-sensitive O$_2$ consumption [12]. This suggests that increases in the rate of aerobic oxidation of these substrates enhance the mitochondrial reductive potential and, presumably, the phosphorylation potential and thus the activity of the Na$^+$ pump. Whether the increased ouabain-sensitive O$_2$ consumption is due only to the increase in Na$^+$ transport activity or also to stimulation of biosynthetic processes by the addition of the substrates is not clear, because such biosynthesis may be affected by ouabain-induced changes in intracellular ionic composition.

A higher reductive potential (higher mitochondrial NADH/NAD ratio) is observed in kidney cortex (Fig. 10-24) of young than of adult rats [108]. This indicates, if one assumes no specific limitation in O$_2$ delivery, that development of the potential for the oxidation of substrates (and thus for generation of NADH) precedes the development of the potential for oxidation of NADH to NAD through coupled respiration. The high mitochondrial NADH/NAD may result from a relatively slow development of respiratory pace-setting ATP utilization processes such as active ion transport, which in juxtamedullary PCT of rabbits reaches mature levels by 7 weeks of age [236]. By contrast, substrate oxidation processes such as the β-oxidation of fatty acids, the aerobic oxidation of lactate, and the turnover of substrates in the Krebs cycle, may reach mature levels earlier. In agreement with this view is the absence during postnatal development of changes in

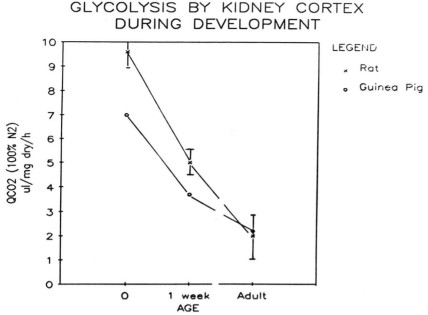

FIG. 10-21. *Glycolysis in kidney cortex slices of newborn and adult animals. The rate of production of* CO_2 *from $NaHCO_3$ titrated by lactic acid generated by the tissue during incubation under anaerobic conditions (100% N_2), in the presence of 5 mM glucose, expressed in $\mu l/mg$ dry tissue weight per h. (From Dicker SE, Shirley DG: Rates of oxygen consumption and anaerobic glycolysis in renal cortex and medulla of adult and newborn rats and guinea pigs. J Physiol (Lond) 212:235, 1971, with permission.)*

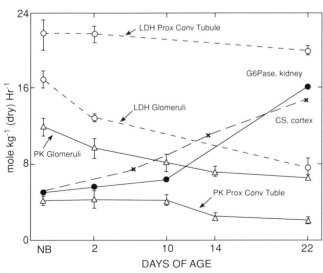

FIG. 10-22. *Maturational changes in the activity of glycolytic (pyruvate kinase, PK, lactate dehydrogenase LDH), gluconeogenic (glucose-6-phosphatase, filled circles) and Krebs cycle (citrate synthetase CS) enzymes in whole kidney, renal cortex, glomeruli (G), or proximal convoluted tubule (PCT). Adapted from [39,40,199].*

the activity of renal cortical enzymes in the major pathways for substrate utilization, such as hydroxyacyl dehydrogenase, an enzyme in the fatty acid β-oxidation pathway [199] and lactic dehydrogenase (H-type isoenzyme), which mediates the first step of lactate utilization [40]. The activities of these enzymes are high already at birth and are not rate limiting for the oxidation of these substrates in the PCT of young animals.

As noted before, the aerobic respiratory capacity in PCT of rat kidney and the activity of various Krebs cycle enzymes of rat kidney cortex reach mature levels by 3 to 4 weeks of age. By contrast, the activity of the Na^+-K^+-ATPase in the PCT starts to increse during the 3rd week and continues to rise until the 8th week of age [134]. The high mitochondrial redox potential in kidney cortex of young animals may poise the differentiating PCT cells for high rates of synthesis of lipids, complex carbohydrates, nucleic acids, and proteins associated with biosynthesis of membranes and transport proteins during final differentiation.

GLUCONEOGENESIS

Twofold to threefold increases in gluconeogenesis from glutamate [108] and from lactate [302] occur during the first 2 weeks of postnatal life in the rat (Fig. 10-25). This

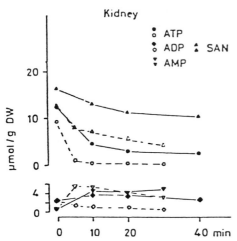

FIG. 10-23. Adenine nucleotides in kidney of newborn rabbits (solid symbols) before and after ischemia for 10, 20, or 40 min. Reference values (open symbols) are for kidneys of adult animals. Triangles, sum of adenine nucleotides; circles, ATP; diamonds, ADP; inverted triangles, AMP. (From Fisher JH, Isselhard A: Metabolic patterns in several tissues of newborn rabbits during ischemia. Biol Neonate 27:235, 1975, with permission.)

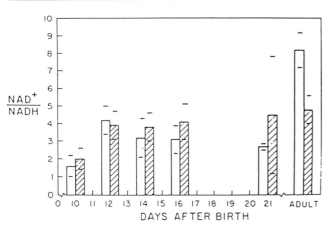

FIG. 10-24. Mitochondrial $NAD^+/NADH$ ratios in kidneys from nursing and adult rats. Open bars show mean values ± SE for control (H_2O) rats, and shaded bars show values for acidotic (5 mmoles NH_4Cl/Kg) rats. Values for control nursing rats are all significantly different from control adults (P < 0.05 or less). Values from acidotic nursing rats are not significantly different from acidotic adults (P > 0.05). (From Goldstein L, Harley-DeWitt S: Renal gluconeogenesis and mitochondrial NAD/NADH ratios in nursing and adult rats. Am J Physiol 224:752, 1973, with permission.)

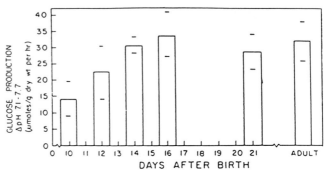

FIG. 10-25. Response of gluconeogenesis in renal cortical slices of nursing and adult rats to medium acidification. Slices were incubated for 90 min in Krebs-Ringer bicarbonate solution (pH 7.1 and 7.7) containing 10 mM glutamate. Values are mean differences ± SEM (between values at pH 7.1 and at pH 7.7). Value for 10-day-old rats is significantly different from adult value (P < 0.05); values for nursing rats 12 days old and older are not significantly different from adult (P > 0.05). (From Goldstein L, Harley-DeWitt S: Renal gluconeogenesis and mitochondrial NAD/NADH ratios in nursing and adult rats. Am J Physiol 224:752, 1973, with permission.)

increase is associated with similar rises in the activity of rate-limiting gluconeogenetic enzymes (Fig. 10-26) such as glucose-6-phosphatase [39,65,302], phosphoenolpyruvate carboxykinase [301,302], and fructose diphosphatase [90] in kidney cortex of rat [302] and mice [301] and in isolated PCT of rabbits [134]. Consequently, by 2 weeks of age the generation of ADP during renal gluconeogenesis from lac-

tate or pyruvate can contribute significantly to the renal energy turnover, and the rate of gluconeogenesis does not appear to be limiting for the partial oxidation of glutamine and ammonia production by the kidney of the young rat [108].

HEXOSE-MONOPHOSPHATE PATHWAY

The activities of renal enzymes in the hexosemonophosphate (HMP) shunt pathway, such as glucose-6-phosphate and 6-phosphogluconate dehydrogenase (Fig. 10-26), are maximal near birth and decrease ~1.5-fold by 3 weeks of age [39]. The activity of the HMP pathway has been associated with the generation of pentoses for nucleic acids and complex carbohydrate synthesis, and with the generation of cytosolic-reducing potential (NADPH) for synthesis of lipids. Increases in the activity of HMP pathway enzymes have been found associated with compensatory renal growth [86] and with the renal hypertrophy of diabetes mellitus [6] and chronic metabolic acidosis [71]. Thus, the activity of this pathway appears to be increased during normal and abnormal kidney growth.

Renal Substrate Metabolism

In the adult organism the kidney can use a variety of substrates for generation of ATP. These include lactate, glucose, fatty acids, citrate, glutamine, ketoacids [55], and, when infused into the circulation, a variety of metabolic intermediates such as pyruvate, ketoglutarate, succinate, alanine, and glutamate [55]. The contribution of each substrate to the generation of ATP varies according to the plasma concentration of the substrates and the metabolic state of the animal [55]. For example, during acidosis, renal utilization of glutamine increases without increases in its concentration in plasma [204]. However, the contribution

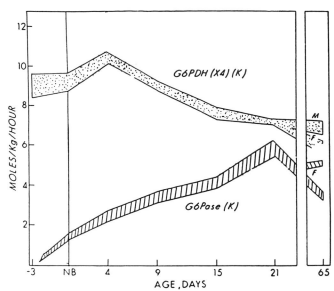

FIG. 10-26. *Developmental changes in the activity of a hexose-mono-phosphate pathway enzyme (glucose-6-phosphate dehydrogenase) and a gluconeogenic (glucose 6-phosphatase) enzyme in the rat kidney. (From Burch HB, Kuhlman AM, Skerjance J, et al: Changes in patterns of enzymes of carbohydrate metabolism in the developing rat kidney. Pediatrics 47:199, 1971, with permission.)*

of each substrate to the renal production of ATP has not been defined quantitatively.

LACTATE AND GLUTAMINE

Estimates of renal decarboxylation rates of lactate and glutamine obtained by administering labeled substrates to the dog indicate that they could account for most (60%) of the renal O_2 uptake. Lactate decarboxylation can account for 40% of the renal O_2 consumption in alkalosis [177], whereas glutamine decarboxylation can account for 40% of the renal O_2 uptake in acidosis [215]. The rates of decarboxylation of lactate and glutamine may, however, overestimate the rates of oxidation of these substrates in part because of recirculation of the labeled metabolites generated by extrarenal metabolism of the labeled substrates. When corrected for recirculation of label, the oxidation of lactate by the dog kidney was found to contribute only about 20% to the renal O_2 uptake [34]. In addition, intrarenal randomization of label in pools of intermediates common to metabolic pathways, such as the Krebs cycle and gluconeogenesis, results in further overestimate of the rates of lactate and glutamine oxidation from measurements of decarboxylation rates [286]. Labeling of CO_2 with ^{14}C from labeled lactate [70] or glutamine [281] used for glucose production can occur, because of the incorporation of ^{14}C into pools of metabolites common to the gluconeogenic and the oxidative pathways (e.g., oxaloacetate, malate). Thus, decarboxylation rates overestimate the rates of substrate oxidation to CO_2 and H_2O.

In rat [118], dog [25], and rabbit [121] proximal tubule

suspensions, glucose production from lactate and glutamine is stimulated by fatty acids, such as oleate, suggesting that the major fate of lactate and glutamine is their conversion to glucose. However, recent in vivo and in vitro metabolic balance studies of renal lactate and glutamine metabolism in the acidotic dog indicate that there is little conversion of glutamine and lactate to glucose and that, instead, they are mostly oxidized to CO_2 and H_2O [123,186]. Studies that allow quantitation of the relative fluxes of substrates through the oxidative and the gluconeogenic pathways [152] are needed to determine if these apparent differences in renal metabolism of glutamine and lactate are the result of differences in methodology or of differences between species.

Lactate is produced mainly in the medullary structures [178] and used in the renal cortex [207], particularly in the cortical thick ascending limbs, but not in the proximal tubules [162]. Although synthesis of glutamine occurs in the renal cortex of rat, it does not occur in dog renal cortex, which lacks glutamine synthetase. Most of the renal utilization of glutamine occurs in the proximal tubules [279].

In summary, under conditions of normal acid base balance, when little glutamine is used by the kidney, lactate oxidation accounts for less than 20% of the renal O_2 uptake. Thus, other substrates must be used for aerobic oxidation, particularly by the proximal tubules, where lactate oxidation is apparently minimal.

LIPIDS

Endogenous tissue lipids [289], as well as extracellular long-chain [119] and short-chain fatty acids [255] can be used by proximal tubules [294] and thick ascending limbs [49]; their relative magnitude is not yet well defined. Renal uptake of non-esterified fatty acids (FFA) depends on their concentration in plasma [18], more specifically on the fatty acid to albumin molar ratio, as most of the plasma fatty acids exist bound to albumin and are in equilibrium, with a minor fraction occurring in the free form. The free form is also in equilibrium with membrane or intracellular fatty acid binding sites or both [200], so that their rate of cellular uptake is saturable, and agents that interact with those binding sites can inhibit their uptake [16]. Only a small fraction (10%) of the FFA taken up by the kidney is directly decarboxylated; most is incorporated into triglycerides and phospholipids [19]. This may represent an intermediate step in their intrarenal oxidation.

Endogenous tissue lipids may be a major source of fatty acids for oxidation and generation of ATP by the kidney [289]. In the kidney perfused in the absence of exogenous substrates [93], inhibition of the oxidation of fatty acids results in a decrease in renal Na^+ reabsorption. However, because of the dilution in specific activity of infused labeled fatty acids by the endogenous renal fatty acid pools, the contribution of fatty acid oxidation to the generation of ATP by the kidney has not been quantified.

Metabolism of long-chain fatty acids by the kidney also involves their esterification in triacylglycerols and phospholipids. Incorporation and net synthesis of triacylglycerols from FFA have been demonstrated in renal cortical

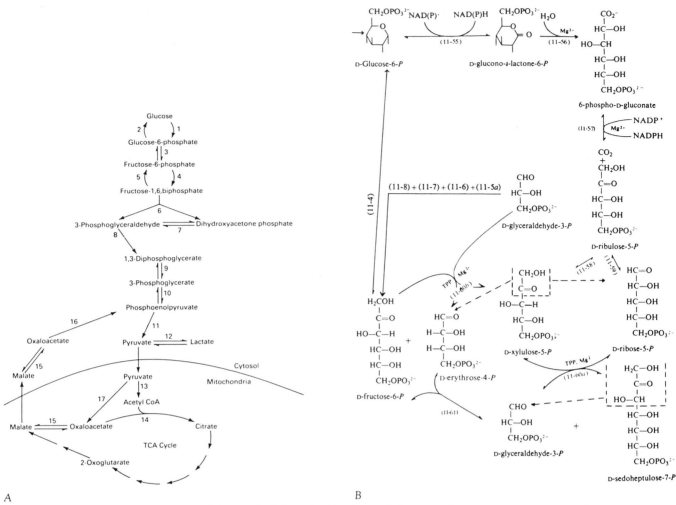

A   B

FIG. 10-27. *Some pathways of glucose metabolism in the kidney. A. Glycolytic and gluconeogenic pathways. B. Hexose monophosphate pathway. C. Glucuronate pathway. Adapted from [55,226].*

tubules in vitro [17,293]. Infused labeled fatty acids are rapidly incorporated into renal tissue lipids and into lipids that leave the kidney in the renal venous blood [19]. The extent to which net synthesis of triacylglycerols, phospholipids, and cholesterol esters occurs in the developing and the mature kidneys in vivo is not defined.

The esterified fatty acids turn over at a much higher rate than the phosphate, glycerol, or inositol moieties of phosphatidylcholine and phosphatidylinositols [264]. These phospholipids are particularly abundant in cell membranes, and their relatively high turnover reflects the activity of phospholipase-mediated second messenger systems that participate in the transduction and amplification of receptor—agonist interactions [27].

Increased synthesis of phosphatidylcholine is one of the earliest metabolic events during compensatory renal growth [267]. Renal synthesis of lipids may also be high during postnatal development, particularly during the breast-feeding period when lipid intake is relatively high [290].

Glycerophosphorylcholine, a methylamine, is prominent in the renal medulla, where it plays a role in the volume regulation of the cells exposed to the hyperosmotic medullary environment [11]. Its synthesis or degradation thus may vary with the state of hydration of the organism and, during the postnatal period, with the development of renal concentrating ability.

GLUCOSE

Measurements of a positive arteriovenous difference and of a decrease in the specific activity of labeled glucose across the kidney indicate that glucose is both used and produced by the kidney [60]. Significant decarboxylation of labeled glucose occurs in the dog kidney in vivo, suggesting its oxidation to CO_2 and H_2O [102]. In the isolated perfused kidney, addition of glucose to an otherwise substrate-free perfusate increases GFR and fractional reabsorption of Na^+. Insulin stimulates glucose decarboxylation and in-

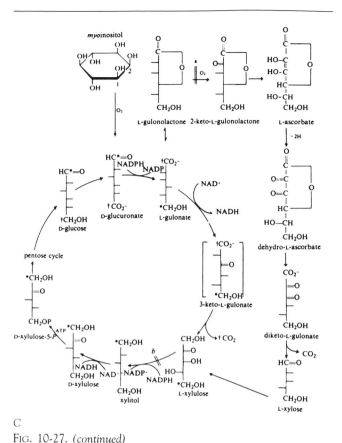

C

FIG. 10-27. (continued)

creases fractional reabsorption of Na^+. Thus, glucose oxidation can support a fraction of the net renal Na^+ transport [115].

The ability to metabolize glucose varies from one nephron segment to another (Fig. 10-27). The capacity for glucose utilization is high in the thick ascending limb and in the collecting duct [118] and low in the proximal nephron, which is mostly gluconeogenic. Using ^{14}C-labeled glucose, the contribution of glucose oxidation to renal CO_2 production in vivo has been estimated at about 13% [102]. In the medulla, glucose may be partially oxidized to lactate or completely oxidized to CO_2 and H_2O, depending on the balance between energy supply and demand. In addition, glucose is a precursor of sorbitol, an intracellular solute important in the volume regulation of cells exposed to the hyperosmotic medullary environment [11]. In the renal cortex, synthesis of myoinositol from glucose occurs at daily rates several times larger than that of dietary myoinositol absorption [268]. Myoinositol is a precursor of membrane phosphatidylinositols, which participate in the intracellular transduction of receptor–agonist interactions at the cell membranes [27]. The kidney reabsorbs filtered myoinositol through a Na^+-dependent cotransport process inhibited by high glucose concentrations [124]. The kidney is also the major site for myoinositol catabolism to CO_2 [136] and to glucose [171], for which it must first undergo conversion to glucuronate. Formation of glucuronides is important for

the urinary excretion of xenobiotics and bile salts [76]. Furthermore, glucuronate is an important substrate for the synthesis of mucopolysaccharides, which are present in abundant quantities in the extracellular matrix of the renal medulla [85] and are also important constituents of the glomerular mesangial matrix and of the glomerular and tubular basement membranes [193]. It is very likely that the glucuronate pathway of glucose metabolism plays an important role in the synthesis of these structures during development.

Renal Substrate Metabolism During Maturation

Utilization of fatty acids by renal cortex slices of fetal and newborn rats is very low compared with that of 10-day-old or adult animals [97]. Oxidation of fatty acids to CO_2 increases continuously from fetal life, to birth, to 30 days of age [97]. Because the concentration of fatty acids in blood is low during fetal life and they cannot be readily used by the fetal cortex, it is reasonable to assume that fatty acids are not a major metabolic substrate for the kidney at this age. Fetal rat kidney cortex can oxidize lactate to CO_2 quite rapidly [96]. After birth, breast milk provides fatty acids and ketoacids for renal metabolism at a time when the capacity to use these substrates for oxidation and lipid synthesis matures [97,290]. Availability of these substrates is probably important for the postnatal growth of the kidney, as suggested by the fact that synthesis of certain phospholipids such as phosphatidylcholine occurs promptly on stimulation of renal growth [267].

In summary, at birth renal cortical structures have the metabolic characteristics of tissues engaged in biosynthetic processes, namely high levels of hexosemonophosphate shunt dehydrogenase and a high reducing potential. Enzymes involved in the oxidation of substrates, such as hydroxyacyl and lactate dehydrogenases, are already at mature levels of activity at birth, whereas in various species enzymes of the Krebs cycle develop later, simultaneously with early increases in mitochondrial membrane surface density and aerobic respiratory capacity. Maturation of renal gluconeogenic function follows a similar time course, perhaps because certain enzymatic steps are common to the Krebs cycle and to gluconeogenesis.

The glycolytic capacity of the proximal tubules decreases after birth, whereas that of the thick ascending limbs and collecting ducts increases. Although the fetal kidney tissue uses lactate and glucose as the major energy fuels, 2 or 3 weeks after birth the kidney may use keto acids and fatty acids as the major metabolic substrates. This change in metabolism may be important for final differentiation of the renal cells, which involves active biosynthesis of cellular membranes. Later during postnatal development, maturation of specific transepithelial transport processes for glucose, bicarbonate, and the associated net fluid reabsorption occurs. Cell-generated transepithelial solute gradients can only be effectively coupled to net solute and fluid reabsorption on maturation of the permeability properties of the paracellular pathway, resulting in the high rates of

Na^+ transport per mole of O_2 consumed, charcteristic of the mature kidney.

Renal Ammoniagenesis

Hydrogen Ion Homeostasis and NH_4^+ Excretion

As part of its homeostatic function, the kidney varies the rate of urinary excretion of titratable acid and NH_4^+ to meet changes in the pools of bicarbonate in the body fluids. Significant quantities of bicarbonate are generated in the kidney through the excretion of titratable acid, such as acidic phosphate salts. For each mole of dibasic phosphate converted to monobasic phosphate, through H^+ secretion into the luminal fluid, and excreted in the urine, 1 mole of $NaHCO_3$ is generated in the renal cells and conserved in the body fluids after transport across the basolateral cell membrane. Of the total renal bicarbonate generation in the adult of 1 mEq/kg/day, approximately 40% stems from the renal excretion of titratable acid. The rest derives from renal NH_4^+ excretion.

The catabolism of ingested or endogenously derived amino acids generates approximately equimolar amounts of NH_4^+ and HCO_3^-, which, in the most part, are used for urea synthesis in the liver. In the kidney, glutamine catabolism results in production of NH_4^+ and HCO_3^-. The NH_4^+ produced is, in part, transported from the cells into the tubule lumen and excreted as NH_4Cl in the urine, whereas equimolar amounts of $NaHCO_3$ are conserved in the body fluids, resulting in a net gain of $NaHCO_3$. The net renal generation of $NaHCO_3$ is, thus, stoichiometrically related to the rate of urinary NH_4^+ excretion. The renal excretion of titratable acid and NH_4^+ generates HCO_3^- in amounts that balance its continuous loss (as CO_2 and H_2O) due to metabolic generation of strong acid, such as results from the catabolism of sulfur-containing and cationic amino acids.

The pools of HCO_3^- in the body fluids can decrease under several circumstances. Balance studies performed during ammonium chloride [179,244] or methionine ingestion [181] have shown that an increase in NH_4^+ excretion ensues that, when a new steady state is reached, is almost equal to the decrease in HCO_3^- stores (the difference is accounted for by bone and intracellular buffering) [180].

Most of the NH_4^+ in the urine is derived from synthesis in the kidney. Glutamine delivered to the kidney by the renal arterial blood is the major substrate. Persistent decreases in HCO_3^- stores result in corresponding increases in ammonia formation from glutamine. It is this ability to vary NH_4^+ synthesis and excretion in response to changes in demand for HCO_3^- generation that makes ammoniagenesis of unique importance to acid–base homeostasis.

THE RENAL AMMONIUM POOL

NH_4^+ is a weak acid that releases a hydrogen ion in the reaction:

$$NH_4^+ \rightarrow NH_3 + H^+$$

The weakness of NH_4^+ as an acid is reflected in the very low dissociation constant (10^{-9}), or high pK (9.1) for this reaction. This means that at any physiologic pH nearly all of the ammonium is in the NH_4^+ form and only a small amount is present as NH_3 (the term *ammonium* will be used to designate the total amount of NH_4^+ plus NH_3 present; NH_3 and NH_4^+ will be used to indicate the individual specific components of the reaction). For example, in blood at pH 7.4, nearly 99% of the ammonium is in the NH_4^+ form and only 1% is NH_3. At pH levels below 7.4, such as in tubular fluid and urine, even greater proportions of the total are present as NH_4^+.

Despite the very small concentrations of NH_3 present in biologic fluids, this moiety plays an important role in the transfer of ammonium into the tubular fluid. Because of its positive charge, NH_4^+ penetrates cell membranes poorly. In contrast, NH_3, which is uncharged and lipid soluble, diffuses rapidly across cell membranes. An increase in ammonium inside a cell increases the concentration of NH_3 in the intracellular fluid. If the concentration of NH_3 on the other side of the cell membrane is less than that inside, NH_3 will diffuse across the membrane, forming NH_4^+ in the extracellular fluid. The amount of NH_4^+ formed depends on the pH of the extracellular fluid; the lower the pH, the more NH_4^+ formed. Thus, NH_3 serves as the transfer form of ammonium and causes rapid equilibration of ammonium across cell membranes and transfer of ammonium from one region of the kidney to another. A cortico-medullary gradient of ammonium exists in the kidney, generated by the reabsorptive transport of NH_4^+ in the thick ascending limbs of Henle's loop [111,157,158] and diffusion trapping of NH_3 by the countercurrent exchangers [110]. The concentration of NH_4^+ varies within different compartments of the kidney, depending on the pH of each compartment.

For discussion of the dynamics of renal ammonium metabolism, the kidney can be considered to have one large ammonium pool. Any change in the amount of ammonium entering this pool is rapidly reflected by changes in the amount of ammonium throughout the organ. An impressive demonstration of the rapid distribution of ammonium throughout the kidney is provided by an experiment performed by Fulgraff and Pitts [100], in which creatinine and ^{15}N-ammonium were injected simultaneously into the renal artery of a dog. The creatinine passed across the glomerular membranes and followed the tortuous course of the nephron before reaching the final urine. The transit time from renal artery to urine for creatinine was over 100 seconds. The labeled ammonium, however, moved across cell membranes. As a result, it diffused rapidly from the arterial blood into the terminal segments of the nephron. Excretion of ^{15}N-ammonium was detectable in less than half the time it took for creatinine to appear in the urine.

Two sources contribute to the renal ammonium pool. Under normal conditions in man, ammonium present in the renal arterial blood contributes about 40% of the total ammonium and ammonium synthesized in the kidney makes up the remainder [214,257]. Figure 10-28 shows schematically the dynamic properties of the renal ammonium pool.

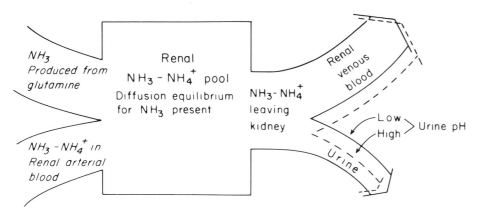

FIG. 10-28. *Routes of entry into and exit from renal ammonium pool. The influence of changes in urine pH on the distribution of NH_4^+ between urine and renal venous blood is shown diagrammatically. (From Simpson DP: Control of hydrogen ion homeostasis and renal acidosis. Medicine 50:503, 1971, with permission.)*

NONIONIC DIFFUSION

The mechanism generally considered responsible for shifts in ammonium excretion with changes in urine pH is nonionic diffusion, which depends on two properties of ammonium mentioned earlier [201]. First, NH_3 penetrates cell membranes much more readily than NH_4^+. Second, the lower the pH of a solution, the greater the amount of NH_3 that diffuses into that solution, forming NH_4^+. The pH of the blood remains relatively constant, whereas the pH of the tubular fluid, especially in more distal parts of the nephron, can vary over a range of 3 pH units or more (representing a thousandfold change in H^+ concentration). When increased H^+ secretion causes tubular fluid to become more acidic, more NH_4^+ will be formed from NH_3 diffusing into that fluid and less NH_4^+ will be present in renal venous blood. If tubular fluid pH rises, the direction of NH_3 diffusion will be reversed, causing urine NH_4^+ excretion to fall and venous NH_4^+ concentration to rise. Although the mechanism of non-ionic diffusion provides an adequate explanation for most of the acute shifts in NH_4^+ distribution within the kidney, it is possible that other mechanisms also play a role; active secretion or reabsorption of NH_4^+ could contribute to some of the phenomena presently attributed to nonionic diffusion [111,157,158].

TUBULAR TRANSPORT OF NH_4^+

Along the proximal tubules, the major site of NH_4^+ production in the nephron [109], NH_4^+ is preferentially secreted into the tubular lumen, probably by an amiloride sensitive exchange for Na^+ [160,195]. Along the thick ascending limbs, most NH_4^+ is reabsorbed as a result of a secondary active process in which NH_4^+ instead of K^+ is transported through the Na^+- and $2Cl^-$- dependent symporter present in the luminal cell membrane [111,157,158]. The medullary nephron segments and vasa recta operate as a countercurrent multiplier for NH_4^+, and similar to Na^+, an ammonium corticomedullary gradient is generated [110]. The NH_4^+ in the medullary interstitium is then secreted across the collecting duct epithelium into the tubular lumen by a combination of active H^+ secretion, which acidifies the urine, and passive NH_3 movement along the established pH gradient, resulting in a high concentration of NH_4^+ in the final urine [163]. Whether regulation of ammonium transport across the renal cell membranes participates in the regulation of the renal excretion of NH_4^+ during acid–base imbalances remains to be explored.

Other conditions can also cause a change in NH_4^+ excretion without alteration in renal ammonia formation. An increase (or decrease) in delivery of ammonium to the kidney will increase (or decrease) the ammonium pool, resulting in a corresponding change in NH_4^+ excretion [67, 203]. Such changes in NH_4^+ delivery occur if the concentration of ammonium in the blood rises or falls or if marked alteration in renal blood flow occurs. Changes in urine flow rate also may affect NH_4^+ excretion [185,201]. These effects are usually minor or transient and may play little role in acid–base homeostasis.

RESPONSE OF NH_4^+ EXCRETION TO METABOLIC ACIDOSIS

When the HCO_3^- stores decrease abruptly, the rate of renal HCO_3^- generation initially is less than that required to compensate for the decrease, and a metabolic acidosis ensues. This acid–base disturbance serves as a strong stimulus to renal ammoniagenesis. With time, ammonium production increases, resulting in an increase in the renal ammonium pool and a rise in NH_4^+ excretion. When a new steady state is achieved, NH_4^+ excretion will have increased sufficiently to almost balance the decrease in HCO_3^- stores.

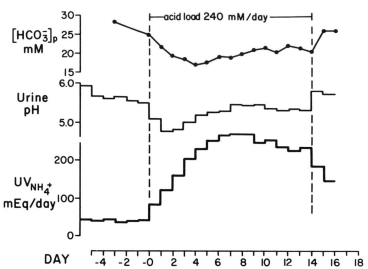

FIG. 10-29. *Response of normal adult to a large increase in hydrogen ion load. Daily changes in plasma HCO₃⁻, urine pH, and NH₄⁺ excretion are shown. During the first six days, NH₄⁺ excretion steadily rises until a new steady state of acid–base balance is achieved. (From Simpson DP: Control of hydrogen ion homeostasis and renal acidosis. Medicine 50:503, 1971, with permission.)*

The pattern of change in ammoniagenesis in response to metabolic acidosis reveals important features of this homeostatic adaptation [229,244]. Figure 10-29 shows the response of an adult man to a large acid load given orally in the form of ammonium chloride. Ammonium chloride is absorbed in the intestine and carried through the portal circulation to the liver where the NH_3 is removed, leaving HCl behind [75]. During the first day of acidosis, urine pH falls and a modest increase in NH_4^+ excretion occurs; this initial increase is due in large part to increased nonionic diffusion of NH_3 into the acidic urine and only to a small degree to an increase in renal synthesis of ammonium. Subsequently, urine pH stabilizes and then rises slightly. NH_4^+ excretion, however, increases steadily, reaching its maximum in about 6 days. Measurements of arterial-venous differences for ammonium across the kidney have confirmed that the change in NH_4^+ excretion in chronic metabolic acidosis is associated with increased ammonium production [204,240]. In man [204], administration of a modest amount of ammonium chloride for 6 to 9 days resulted in a doubling of ammonium production by the kidney; the rate of delivery of ammonium to the kidney in the arterial blood did not change, whereas the renal ammonium pool increased by 50%. Excretion of NH_4^+ in the urine almost doubled, and the ammonium leaving the kidney through the renal vein increased by a third. Similar but more extensive studies have been carried out in dog [240].

OTHER CONDITIONS ASSOCIATED WITH INCREASED RENAL AMMONIAGENESIS

In contrast to metabolic acidosis, data on the influence of *respiratory acidosis* on renal ammoniagenesis are sparse. In man, NH_4^+ excretion during hypercapnea may be slightly increased, but the dramatic rise seen with metabolic acidosis is lacking. In dog, NH_4^+ excretion increases in acute respiratory acidosis. Gougoux et al. [113] found that when pCO_2 was raised sufficiently to lower blood pH to 7.0 or below, renal glutamine extraction and ammonium production doubled within a couple of hours.

Potassium depletion is accompanied by an increase in renal ammoniagenesis [10,101] and in NH_4^+ excretion [260]. Because potassium depletion is also believed to cause an intracellular acidosis in the kidney, it is likely that the basic mechanism is the same as in metabolic acidosis, that is, decreases in intracellular pH and bicarbonate trigger a rise in renal ammonium formation.

SOURCES FOR RENAL AMMONIUM SYNTHESIS

Glutamine is the most abundant amino acid in the blood, being present in a concentration of around 0.5 mM. Because of the high rate of renal blood flow, it is delivered to the kidney in large amounts. Moreover, each molecule of glutamine can provide two molecules of ammonium, one derived from the amide nitrogen and one from the amine group.

Van Slyke et al. [276] first suggested that glutamine may serve as a substrate for ammoniagenesis when they noted that glutamine was extracted from the kidney in sufficient amount to account for most of the ammonium excreted in the urine and was added to the renal venous blood. Subsequently, Shaloub et al. [240] investigated in detail amino acid metabolism by the intact dog kidney. When renal arteriovenous differences for a large number of amino acids were measured in chronically acidotic dogs, only glutamine and glycine were extracted in significant amounts by the kidney. The small quantity of glycine removed could contribute little to total renal ammonium synthesis. If both the amide and amine nitrogens were quantitatively converted to ammonium, the amount of glutamine extracted was sufficient to account for all of the ammonium produced by the kidney. Expanding these studies, the same group used ^{15}N-labeled amino acids to define more precisely the role of glutamine in ammoniagenesis [214]. When glutamine labeled with ^{15}N in the amide position was infused into one renal artery of an acidotic dog, about 40% of the NH_4^+ in the urine could be accounted for by this source. When ^{15}N was present instead in the amine nitrogen of glutamine, it contributed about 20% of the NH_4^+ in the urine. By combining these findings with those of other studies, Pitts estimated that the amide N of glutamine accounted for about 60% of the ammonium synthesized in the kidney, the amine N for about 30%, and that the remaining 10% derived from other amino acids.

Thus, in both man and dog, glutamine metabolism is responsible for 90% or more of the ammonium formed in the kidney in chronically acidotic states. It should be noted that experiments with labeled glutamine were carried out in dogs with chronic metabolic acidosis; the extent to which the results apply to nonacidotic animals has not been established. Owen and Robinson [204] found that in normal man the amount of ammonium formed in the kidney was less than the total nitrogen in glutamine removed from the blood. The amide group of glutamine appears to make a considerably larger contribution to ammonium production than the amine group, some of which may be removed from the kidney as serine or other amino acids, particularly in humans in the acidotic state.

One would expect that there would be a steady increase in glutamine use as ammonium synthesis increases during development of acidosis. However, this does not appear to be the case. Tizzianello and colleagues [266] studied amino acid extraction in man in control subjects and after 1 day of ammonium chloride loading. As expected, in the control subjects glutamine extraction exceeded renal ammonium production. However, after 24 hours of ammonium chloride acidosis, ammonium synthesis had increased by over 50%, whereas glutamine extraction was unchanged. The extraction of glycine and ornithine by the kidney, although small in amount, rose during the first 24 hours of acidosis, and their sum was sufficient to account for the increment in ammonium formation. Whether a change in the pathways of glutamine metabolism occurs in the first 24 hours of acidosis, and more of the glutamine nitrogens are converted to ammonia rather than transferred to other amino acids, remains to be demonstrated. Further studies are needed to define the changes in amino acid extraction and metabolism during the entire 6-day course of adaptation to acidosis.

LOCALIZATION WITHIN NEPHRON

The sites at which ammonium is added to the tubular fluid and the sites at which it is produced in the kidney are not identical. Ammonium is produced primarily in the proximal convoluted segments of the nephron, but it is added to the tubular fluid mainly in the collecting ducts [228,253]. The major factors determining the entry of ammonium to the tubular fluid are the pH of that fluid and the concentration of NH_3 in adjacent tissue. Within the nephron, tubular fluid pH is lowest in the collecting duct. Hence this segment is the site at which most of the ammonium present in the final urine is added.

The site of greatest ammonium production corresponds to the location of enzymes involved in ammoniagenesis and intermediary metabolism. Glutaminase [63], glutamate dehydrogenase, and the enzymes of the citric acid cycle [233] are located in greatest concentration in the proximal convoluted tubule, corresponding to the large number of mitochondria in cells of this region. The predominance of the convoluted tubules as well as the concentration of enzymes makes these segments the chief source of ammonium synthesized in the kidney. The enzymes of gluconeogenesis, which may play a role in disposing of the carbon skeleton of glutamine under some conditions, are also located in greatest quantity in the cells of the proximal convoluted tubules [41,275].

Renal Glutamine Metabolism and Ammoniagenesis

PATHWAYS OF GLUTAMINE METABOLISM AND COMPARTMENTALIZATION

Glutamine filtered by the glomerulus is efficiently reabsorbed by the tubule so that less than 1% of the filtered load reaches the urine. Even when the filtered load is greatly increased by infusion of glutamine, insignificant quantities are present in urine [213]. Under normal acid–base conditions, the amount of glutamine reabsorbed by the tubule exceeds the total amount of glutamine extracted by the kidney. Thus, some of the reabsorbed glutamine must be released into the blood on the peritubular side of the cell and escapes metabolism [242]. However, after chronic acidosis develops, net glutamine extraction exceeds the filtered load, demonstrating that glutamine is taken up on the peritubular side of the tubule as well [242]. Some peritubular uptake as well as efflux of glutamine probably occur also in nonacidotic states.

The removal of glutamine from tubular fluid against a concentration gradient implies the existence of a glutamine transporter in the renal tubule. Studies in isolated membrane vesicles have demonstrated Na^+-dependent glutamine transport in brush border preparations [2,288,291]. Similarly, renal cortical basolateral membrane vesicles exhibit transport of glutamine [94,291]. Although glutamine levels in renal cortex approximate those in plasma, carriers for glutamine on the two sides of the cell may be necessary for the efficient uptake of glutamine from the tubular and peritubular fluid for subsequent metabolism in the cell.

MITOCHONDRIAL TRANSPORT AND METABOLISM

After transport into the cell from tubular or peritubular fluid glutamine is metabolized predominantly by glutaminase located inside mitochondria [189]. The outer mitochondrial membrane is freely permeable to small molecules and ions; in contrast, the inner membrane is practically impermeable to passive movement of small, charged molecules. Specific substrate carriers are present in this membrane [174,245]. Among these carriers there is one for glutamine. When this carrier is blocked, by low temperature or sulfhydryl inhibitors, entry of glutamine into renal mitochondria is reduced and metabolism of glutamine almost ceases [1,169,248]. Unfortunately, detailed study of the properties of the glutamine transporter have been greatly hampered by the close link between it and glutaminase; thus far it has been difficult to study the separate properties of these two units within the framework of intact mitochondria [251].

After glutamine enters mitochondria, it is converted to glutamate by the hydrolytic action of glutaminase (phosphate-dependent glutaminase; glutaminase I; glutamine amidohydrolase), which releases the amide nitrogen as NH_4^+. Glutaminase has many peculiar characteristics [103]: dependence on high concentrations of phosphate and glutamine for maximum activity, a high pH optimum of around 8.0, and existence of monomer and dimer subunits. These characteristics are at variance with conditions likely to be encountered in vivo, and it is unclear to what extent these unusual properties are artifacts produced by the extraction procedure.

Once glutamate has been formed from glutamine, three routes are available for its subsequent metabolism. Glutamate can be transported on its own specific inner membrane carrier, out of the mitochondria into the cytoplasm; it can be converted within mitochondria to other amino acids; or it can be converted to α-ketoglutarate by glutamate dehydrogenase, forming NH_4^+ in the process. The latter is the major route of metabolism of glutamate derived from glutamine in the kidney. This reaction serves to link glutamine metabolism to the citric acid cycle and to the various metabolic pathways available to the substrates of this cycle. Sites of regulation within the citric acid cycle may thus influence glutamine metabolism and ammoniagenesis.

α-Ketoglutarate entering the citric acid cycle can be disposed of by three main routes: formation of CO_2, transamination, and synthesis of glucose. In the Krebs cycle conversion of α-ketoglutarate to malate releases a molecule of CO_2 when succinate is formed. The oxaloacetate, which results from the conversion of malate by malate dehydrogenase in the mitochondrial matrix, combines with acetyl Co-A to form citrate. Subsequent revolutions of the citric acid cycle result in net decarboxylation of the acetyl group. Further net catabolism of the malate carbons can only occur after its transport into the cytosol and conversion by cytosolic malate dehydrogenase to oxaloacetate, the substrate for phosphoenolpyruvate carboxykinase, generating phosphoenol-pyruvate (PEP), a branch point in determining the subsequent fate of its carbons. PEP can be converted to pyruvate, then to acetyl C0-A, to CO_2 and H_2O through the Krebs cycle, or to alanine through transamination. Alternatively, PEP can be converted to 2-phosphoglycerate and then to glucose through the gluconeogenic pathway.

These multiple pathways for the disposal of the carbon skeleton of glutamine provide a large number of sites at which regulation of glutamine metabolism can occur. It is

this multiplicity of possibilities that has made the study of the regulation of ammoniagenesis a subject of such interest and controversy over the years.

NONMITOCHONDRIAL PATHWAYS OF GLUTAMINE METABOLISM

Glutamine can be metabolized by two enzyme systems that reside outside mitochondria. Glutamine ketoacid amino transferase (glutaminase II) forms ammonium from the amine nitrogen of glutamine, releasing an unstable intermediate, α-ketoglutaramate; this is converted to α-ketoglutarate by γ-amidase, forming ammonium from the amide nitrogen of glutamine [58]. Glutamine also can be metabolized by γ-glutamyl transpeptidase located in the brush border membrane [62,263]. This enzyme, at one time referred to as phosphate independent glutaminase, can react with glutamine, especially when maleate is present. However, it is doubtful that glutamine is an important substrate for this enzyme in vivo, where its role is probably predominantly that of a transpeptidase.

Glutamate can form aspartate through the action of aspartate aminotransferase, which is located both in the cytoplasm and in mitochondria. Aspartate (Asp) can serve as a source of NH_4^+ through a series of reactions in the cytoplasm, which are referred to as the purine nucleotide cycle; a molecule of fumarate is the other product of this cycle [31]:

$$AMP + H_2O \rightarrow IMP + NH_3 \tag{1}$$

$$IMP + GTP + Asp \rightarrow Adenylosuccinate + GDP + Pi \tag{2}$$

$$Adenylosuccinate \rightarrow AMP + Fumarate \tag{3}$$

$$Asp + GTP + H_2O \rightarrow Fumarate + GDP + Pi + NH_3 \tag{Net}$$

With aspartate as a substrate, ammonia production was high in S1 segments, with a value exceeding that from glutamine. Segments derived from chronically acidotic rats produced more ammonia from aspartate than those from control rats. An inhibitor of adenylosuccinase, 6-mercaptopurine, significantly inhibited ammonia production from aspartate and from glutamine [259]. These findings suggests that the purine nucleotide cycle also participates in renal ammoniagenesis by S1 segments of the nephron.

REGULATION OF AMMONIAGENESIS

Hems [130] perfused kidneys from control and chronically acidotic animals with medium at pH 7.4 and glutamine as the sole substrate. The kidney from animals with acidosis of 7 to 10 days duration used twice as much glutamine and produced twice as much ammonium as the controls. No change in ammoniagenesis by control kidneys occurred when the perfusate pH was lowered from 7.4 to 7.1.

With identical medium pH, kidney slices from acidotic animals used more glutamine and produced more ammonium and CO_2 than slices from alkalotic dogs [246]. Similar results have been obtained with slices of rat kidney cortex [112]. Ammonium production and glutamine utilization are significantly greater in mitochondria from chronically acidotic animals than controls [38,106,261]. Thus, one site of metabolic alteration that leads to enhanced ammoniagenesis in acidosis resides in the mitochondrion. Additional adaptive sites, elsewhere in the cell, have not been excluded.

When mitochondria are incubated with the metabolic inhibitor rotenone, glutamine metabolism is blocked at the glutamate dehydrogenase step. Under such conditions, ammonium is formed from the amide nitrogen of glutamine and glutamate is produced intramitochondrially. The steps present in glutamine metabolism in such preparations are reduced to two: glutamine transport by its inner membrane carrier and the action of glutaminase. When mitochondria from chronically acidotic dog or rat kidney are studied in the presence of rotenone, enhanced glutamate and ammonium formation compared with controls is found [1,248]. These studies indicate that adaptation of glutamine metabolism has occurred either at the mitochondrial transport step or at glutaminase. Although an increase in glutaminase activity in the rat kidney has long been known to occur in acidosis, no change in the concentration of this enzyme has been found in dog [216,225]; even in rat, evidence exists indicating that the change in glutaminase activity is not essential for enhanced ammoniagenesis in acidosis [104] and that the time course of the adaptation to acidosis of glutaminase activity does not follow that seen for ammoniagenesis in the intact animal [1,261]. By contrast, adaptation in rotenone-inhibited mitochondria of rats can be seen very early in the course of acidosis [1]. Based on these considerations, a strong case can be made for an adaptation in the glutamine carrier located in the inner membrane as a site of major importance in regulating ammoniagenesis [1]. In chronic acidosis, an increase in the number of active carrier units should cause increased delivery of glutamine into mitochondria and thus more substrate for formation of ammonium.

Glutaminase would seem a likely site for regulation of ammonium production, but, as noted in the preceding paragraph, demonstration of enhanced activity of the extracted enzyme in acidosis has been shown not to be involved in the adaptation of ammoniagenesis in dogs. More subtle changes in in situ glutaminase activity, not demonstrable in extracts, are, however, possible. For example, a lower, rather than a higher concentration of glutamine in the matrix, has been found to occur in purified mitochondria derived from chronically acidotic rats than in those from control rats [64]. This indicates that in the adaptation to acidosis an increased conversion of intramitochondrial glutamine to glutamate predominates, rather than an increased entry of glutamine into the mitochondria. Increased conversion of glutamine to glutamate could be due to activation of glutaminase I, without an increase in the abundance of this enzyme.

Phosphoenolpyruvate carboxykinase was proposed as a regulator of glutamine metabolism [3]. This enzyme plays an important role in controlling the metabolism of the carbon skeleton of glutamine, but is remote from the initial steps of glutamine metabolism in mitochondria; recent finding indicate that it is not a regulatory factor in ammoniagenesis from glutamine [278]. Another suggested site of regulation is the purine nucleotide cycle. Some evidence

for enhanced activity of this cycle in acidosis has been obtained in rat kidney [31]. Information on the activity of this pathway in the dog and on the time course of this adaptation in the rat are not available.

Recently, the total rate of ATP synthesis has been suggested as a limiting factor in ammoniagenesis [122]. It seems reasonable that conservation of cellular energy would impose some upper limit on the rate of metabolism of any substrate. How such a limit could serve to adjust glutamine metbolism between control and chronically acidotic conditions remains to be described, particularly because renal oxygen consumption does not change in acidosis.

Additional potential sites for the regulation of glutamine metabolism, before its transport into mitochondria, are the brush border and basolateral membranes of the proximal tubule cells where carriers for this amino acid have recently been identified. Because nearly all of the filtered glutamine is reabsorbed, it is unlikely that enhancement of glutamine transport at the brush border side of the cell could play a significant role in the adaptation to acidosis; increased transport of glutamine by brush border vesicles from acidotic rat kidney has, however, been demonstrated [2,94], but the metabolic significance of this observation is uncertain. Adaptation in acidosis of glutamine transport in the basolateral side of the cell could be a means of providing more glutamine intracellularly for subsequent metabolism. The evidence for such an adaptation is conflicting. In dog, one group has found increased uptake of glutamine by vesicles of basolateral membranes prepared from kidneys of animals with chronic metabolic or acute respiratory acidosis [105,292]. No such change in glutamine transport was detected in basolateral preparations from the rat [94]. Because both in dog and rat there is increased glutamine utilization in acidosis, it would seem likely that the underlying mechanism responsible for this increase is similar in the two species. Clarification of these conflicting results in different species is necessary before the role of basolateral membrane transport in the regulation of ammoniagenesis can be assessed.

DEVELOPMENTAL ASPECTS OF AMMONIUM EXCRETION AND FORMATION

Fetal pigs have been found to have a more acidic allantoic fluid (pH 6.0), containing larger amounts of ammonium [191] at 46 days than at 22 days of gestation. Ammonium production from glutamine has also been demonstrated in renal tissue slices from pigs of 46 days gestation [222]. Thus, the enzymatic machinery for ammonium production is present during fetal life, but the extent to which ammonium is actually produced by the fetal kidney (as opposed to formation elsewhere and passive entry into the allantoic fluid by diffusion) has not been established.

After birth the protein content of the diet has an important influence on the amount of NH_4^+ in the urine. In premature infants, studied up to 3 weeks after birth, Svenningsen and Lindqvist [258] have found that NH_4^+ excretion was significantly greater on a high-protein than on a low-protein diet; diet did not influence NH_4^+ excretion in premature infants studied 4 to 6 weeks after birth. Others have found a large effect of diet in full-term infants several months after birth. Fomon et al. [92] compared NH_4^+ excretion of infants fed cow's milk with that of infants on human milk. The infants on cow's milk excreted several times as much NH_4^+ as those receiving the lower protein- and phosphate-containing diet of human milk.

Factors implicated in mediating the influence of diet on NH_4^+ excretion in the newborn are the dietary acid load, the amount of substrate delivery to the kidney, and changes in urine pH and thus in nonionic diffusion of ammonia. Edelmann and Wolfish [77] found that in premature infants a high-protein diet led to increases in both inulin and PAH clearances. The increase in PAH clearance, presumably reflecting a rise in renal blood flow, was almost equal to the twofold increase in NH_4^+ excretion. The increased delivery rate of NH_4^+ and of glutamine in the high-protein group may have contributed to the renal NH_4^+ pool and thus may account for the increase in NH_4^+ excretion. Although in this study no difference in urine pH was observed between the two groups, others have reported that a high protein intake is accompanied by a reduction in urine pH in both premature and full-term infants [77,92]; the change in urine pH by promoting nonionic diffusion of ammonia could be responsible for the increase in NH_4^+ excretion. In these latter studies, no measurements of renal blood flow were made, so the role of substrate delivery cannot be assessed.

When an ammonium chloride load is given to a full-term infant so that an acute metabolic acidosis is produced, urine pH falls promptly and NH_4^+ excretion rises [92]. In premature infants of 1 to 3 weeks of age, ammonium chloride administration is accompanied by a smaller decrease in urine pH and a lower rate of NH_4^+ excretion than in full-term infants [258]. This difference is still present, although considerably reduced, at 4 to 6 weeks of age.

Striking impairment of NH_4^+ excretion in response to an acute metabolic acidosis was demonstrated in newborn puppies by Cort and McCance [59]. Basal NH_4^+ excretion in puppies was only about half that in adults. During 6 hours of observation after an NH_4Cl load, adult dogs increased NH_4^+ excretion over 10-fold, but almost no change occurred in puppies. Changes in urine pH were similar in the two groups, so that the lack of response of the puppies to an acid challenge cannot be explained by a difference in ability to acidify the urine. The findings suggest a marked limitation in ammoniagenesis in puppies, but the limiting factor in this response has not been identified. In a similar study in piglets, Hatemi and McCance [128] found lower basal NH_4^+ excretion in 1- to 2-day-old than in 10- to 12-week-old animals; the diet of the piglets was not controlled. A modest increase in NH_4^+ excretion occurred in both groups of animals during the 8 hours that followed NH_4Cl administration, but no comparison with the response in adult pigs was made.

Goldstein [107] studied ammonium excretion in rats of different ages. Basal NH_4^+ excretion and urine pH were slightly lower in rats less than 16 days old than in older animals. NH_4^+ excretion rose about threefold within 4 hours after NH_4Cl administration in 20-day-old or adult rats, but the increase in 9-day-old animals was half that observed in adult rats. Urine pH was similar in the different age groups, suggesting that factors other than the effect of pH gradients on nonionic diffusion of ammonia were involved in the diminished response of the younger animals. This study also provided information on the effects of more prolonged acidosis on NH_4^+ excretion in young rats. When given NH_4Cl for up to 2 days, the increase in NH_4^+ excretion in 10-day-old rats was similar to that seen in adults; however, because basal NH_4^+ excretion was lower in the younger animals, in absolute terms, NH_4^+ excretion remained less than in adults. Concordant with these observations are the findings that both glutamine and glutaminase in the renal cortex of young rats were found to be 50% and 30%, respectively, of those of the adult [105,107].

In summary, decreases in nonionic diffusion of ammonia can account for some of the reduced NH_4^+ excretion observed in the newborn. The increase in NH_4^+ excretion in response to increases in protein intake in the newborn may involve other factors, such as increases in dietary acid load and in substrate delivery to the kidneys. The ability to increase NH_4^+ excretion is greatly impaired in various animals (dogs, rats) in the first few days of life, but confirmatory data on humans is only available for premature infants. Substrate availability, glutamine transport by cellular or mitochondrial membranes, or enzymatic formation of ammonium could each play a role in diminished ammonium formation at birth.

Acid–Base State and Citric Acid Cycle Metabolites

Metabolic alkalosis induces a profound increase in the urinary excretion of citrate and, to a lesser extent, of α-ketoglutarate [61,243]. Plasma concentrations of these substances change only slightly in alkalosis, so the effect is intrarenal in origin. By contrast, in metabolic acidosis, urinary excretion of organic anions, such as citrate, decreases. Loss of endogenously generated metabolizable organic anions in the urine represents net loss of bicarbonate from the body fluids. Had the organic anion been retained and metabolized to neutral products such as glucose, CO_2, and H_2O, the bicarbonate titrated to CO_2 and H_2O by the organic acid produced would have been regenerated. The loss of bicarbonate on urinary excretion of endogenously produced organic anions is in contrast to urinary loss of ingested nonmetabolized organic anions, which do not contribute to changes in acid–base balance. It is also in contrast to the net alkalinizing effect of ingestion and metabolism of the salts of metabolizable organic anions. For example, addition of sodium citrate to the diet results in a rise in HCO_3^- concentration in the body fluids as the citrate is metabolized to CO_2 and H_2O, glucose, or lipid, and the Na^+ is conserved as $NaHCO_3$.

Transport of Citrate and α-Ketoglutarate in Renal Tubules

Under normal acid–base conditions there is net utilization of citrate and α-ketoglutarate in the kidney [13,14,57,243].

The uptake exceeds the amounts of citrate or α-ketoglutarate filtered, indicating that these solutes are taken up from both the tubular and peritubular sides of the cells. Both citrate and α-ketoglutarate reabsorption by the nephron exhibit a tubular maximum [5,13,57], which are not affected by acute metabolic acidosis.

Most of the filtered citrate and α-ketoglutarate are removed from the proximal tubule fluid against concentration gradients, the levels of citrate and α-ketoglutarate in renal cortex being severalfold greater than in plasma. This suggests the existence of tubular transport mechanisms for citrate and α-ketoglutarate. Studies in vesicles prepared from brush border and basolateral proximal cell membranes have demonstrated the presence of Na^+-dependent polycarboxylate carrier systems in kidney cortex [144,147,161, 295]. The brush border citrate carrier is sodium gradient driven, pH dependent, and electrogenic [15,161]. It transports not only the monoprotonated form of citrate, but also succinate, α-ketoglutarate, and other dicarboxylate anions as well [15,161,295]. The transporters for these organic acids in the brush border and basolateral membranes may play an important role in establishing and maintaining intracellular levels of substrates at concentrations exceeding those in the plasma.

Net renal secretion of α-ketoglutarate has been shown during metabolic alkalosis [14,57]. Micropuncture studies have localized this secretion to the proximal convoluted tubule and to a more distal site in the nephron. Secretion of citrate by the nephron has been more difficult to demonstrate conclusively, although clearances slightly exceeding the filtered load have been found when citrate reabsorption is inhibited by malate infusion [23]. Citrate secretion has also been observed in certain pathologic states in which its excretion exceeds the filtered load manyfold [68].

Excretion of Citrate and α-Ketoglutarate in Acid–Base Disturbances

When metabolic alkalosis is produced, there is an increase in early proximal tubular fluid pH [228], which inhibits the Na^+-coupled cotransport of citrate [15,296]. The pH dependence of the luminal citrate transporter is indirect [15,296]. Decreases in the luminal transport of citrate when pH increases are due to pH-dependent decreases in the concentration of the substrate, monoprotonated citrate, and, to a lesser extent, to increases in the concentration of the nontransported but inhibitory nonprotonated form of citrate [15] rather than to effects of pH on the carrier system. α-Ketoglutarate or succinate cotransport with Na^+ is not affected by pH changes [296]. The pH dependency of citrate cotransport is important in the regulation of citrate reabsorption by the proximal tubules during acute acidosis and alkalosis [35]. In addition, chronic metabolic alkalosis did not alter, but chronic metabolic acidosis increased the capacity (V_{max}) for Na^+-citrate cotransport in renal brush border membrane vesicles [142]. The adaptive increase in V_{max} can contribute to the decrease in citrate excretion observed in chronic acidosis.

Other factors besides luminal pH may be involved in the regulation of renal citrate transport. In K^+-depleted rats, urinary citrate excretion decreases. When K^+-depleted rats are given excess oral bicarbonate, citrate excretion increases little in spite of elevations in extracellular and intratubular pH [151]. The presence of intracellular acidosis in K^+-depleted animals may play a role in promoting citrate reabsorption in K^+-depleted animals. Similar to systemic acidosis, K^+-depletion may result in upregulation of the Na^+-citrate cotransport system.

Changes in intracellular pH also promote (acidosis) or inhibit (alkalosis) mitochondrial metabolism of citrate in the kidney, altering the tissue citrate levels and perhaps contributing to the corresponding changes in renal citrate reabsorption [243].

In addition to its effects on acid–base balance, the increase in citrate clearance that accompanies metabolic alkalosis has an important pathophysiologic role. In renal distal tubular acidosis, for example, relatively alkaline urine is excreted. The systemic acidosis, and presumably the decreases in proximal tubular fluid pH and in intracellular pH, lead to diminished citrate excretion in the urine [37,198]. In distal renal tubular acidosis, citrate excretion, may be so low as to be unmeasurable. The lack of chelation of calcium by citrate is a major factor in the stone formation and nephrocalcinosis that are characteristic of this condition. Generally, treatment of distal renal tubular acidosis with alkali decreases the reabsorption and the metabolism of citrate in the kidney, increases its urinary excretion, which, by chelating more calcium, diminishes the risk of stone formation.

Changes in Substrate Levels in Kidney

The changes in citrate and α-ketoglutarate metabolism caused by changes in systemic acid–base balance are accompanied by alterations in intracellular concentrations of these and related compounds. Metabolic alkalosis increases the concentration of all citric acid cycle intermediates, and decreases in these occur with metabolic acidosis [245]. These alterations occur very rapidly. In the rat, sharp decreases or increases in renal tissue concentrations of citrate, α-ketoglutarate, malate, and pyruvate occur within 5 minutes of administration of an acid or alkali load, respectively. The acute changes in the cellular concentration of metabolic intermediates have been used to develop several possible explanations for the increase in renal ammonium production in acidosis [128]. However, except perhaps in the rat, there is little evidence to suggest that acute changes in ammonium production from glutamine play a significant role in altering NH_4^+ excretion. In humans, the modest increase in ammonium production on the first day of acidosis does not appear to stem from increased metabolism of glutamine [266], but rather from increases in nonionic diffusion of NH_3. In dog, increased ammonium production with acute metabolic acidosis has generally not been demonstrable [87,88,277]. Thus, although the changes in tissue levels of Krebs cycle intermediates in acute acidosis and alkalosis reflect important metabolic events, they may have relatively little bearing on the regulation of renal ammoniagenesis.

In tissue slices, citrate utilization and oxidation to CO_2 diminish with an increase in the alkalinity of the medium. Tissue concentration of citrate is greater after incubation of slices in high rather than low bicarbonate-containing media. A similar pattern is observed with α-ketoglutarate as substrate [243]. Mitochondrial oxidation and utilization of citrate have also been shown to be inhibited at high bicarbonate concentrations in the medium, supporting the view that the effects of acid–base changes on renal citrate metabolism are exerted at this subcellular level. These in vitro results resemble closely the changes observed in the intact kidney.

Mechanism of Regulation of Citric Acid Cycle Metabolism by Acid–Base Changes

Passage of substrates of the citric acid cycle (and of many other compounds as well) across the inner mitochondrial membrane is accomplished by transport on specific carriers. The rate of transport by each of these carriers depends, among other things, on the magnitude of the pH gradient across the inner mitochondrial membrane (ΔpH) [249, 250]; the greater ΔpH, the more rapidly a substrate will be transported into mitochondria and the more slowly it will be shifted out. The interior of mitochondria is relatively alkaline compared with the outside. In the presence of bicarbonate and phosphate, the mitochondrial pH gradient (ΔpH) at medium pH 7.1 may be four times higher than that at pH 7.7. Consequently, concomitant changes in cytosolic pH and $[HCO_3^-]$ by altering ΔpH [250] can influence the rates of transport of substrates across the mitochondrial membrane and the size of the pools of metabolites of the Krebs cycle.

Based on these observations, one can construct an overall description of the changes that occur in renal tissue substrate levels in response to acid–base changes (Fig. 10-30) [243]. Normally, the pool of citric acid cycle intermediates in the renal cortex consists of a large cytoplasmic component and a smaller intramitochondrial one. The distribution of a substrate between the cytoplasmic and mitochondrial compartments is determined by the equilibrium conditions established across the inner mitochondrial membrane. Addition or removal of substrate by metabolic events in one compartment will result, through rapid readjustment of equilibrium across the inner mitochondrial membrane, in changes in pool size in both compartments. If ΔpH increases, as occurs when cytoplasmic pH and bicarbonate diminish, substrate will be removed from the cytoplasmic pool and added to the mitochondrial compartment, increasing substrate availability to the enzymes of the citric acid cycle. The action of these enzymes will remove some of the additional substrate that entered the mitochondria, tending to restore the pool size of this compartment to its previous level. The net effect of these changes is a reduction in the cytoplasmic pool with little or no change in the mitochondrial pool; total metabolite

concentration in the tissue diminishes. Opposite changes occur in metabolic alkalosis, in which increases in pH and bicarbonate reduce ΔpH.

This scheme also accounts for changes in renal citrate and α-ketoglutarate utilization in response to acid–base changes. Citrate transported into the cytoplasmic pool by its plasma membrane carriers enters mitochondria at a rate governed by the citrate carrier in the inner mitochondrial membrane. When ΔpH is diminished in metabolic alkalosis, for example, the rates of mitochondrial citrate uptake and utilization decrease, and the concentration of citrate in the cell rises. Alternatively, high HCO_3^- or pH may have direct inhibitory effects on the mitochondrial substrate carriers [247].

Other attempts to explain the acute affects of acid–base disturbances on renal metabolism have generally been based on the assumption that changes in pH affect a single enzyme of intermediary metabolism, such as α-ketoglutarate dehydrogenase, as the tissue level of α-ketoglutarate falls sharply in acidosis and rises in alkalosis [183,263]. Effects of acidosis and alkalosis on levels of substrates preceding α-ketoglutarate, such as glutamate and citrate, presumably arise from a mass action effect of the intramitochondrial α-ketoglutarate pool. How such changes in a single enzyme could account for effects on substrates more remote from α-ketoglutarate, such as malate or pyruvate, is unclear.

Perfusion of isolated kidney of the rat with a bicarbonate-rich, alkaline perfusate, using citrate as the only exogenous substrate, failed to produce an increase in tissue citrate but inhibited citrate reabsorption. This indicates that accumulation of citrate in the kidney during alkalosis may be related to the availability of other substrates and their conversion to citrate [5]. The activity of citrate synthetase is optimal at an alkaline pH [168], and activation of this enzyme in alkalosis, could result in an expansion of the pools of intermediates in the Krebs cycle. The net decrease in renal utilization of citrate in alkalosis may thus be the result of a combination of increased synthesis and decreased utilization of citrate.

The Metabolic Roles of Citrate in the Kidney

Utilization of organic anions, such as citrate and succinate, occurs in proximal tubular segments [12] but not in the thick ascending limbs [49], perhaps due to the absence of polycarboxylate cotransport systems in the latter. Renal oxidation of citrate in vivo may account for a minor fraction ($\frac{1}{10}$) of the renal oxygen consumption [24]. Citrate plays an important role in the regulation of the glycolytic rate through its allosteric inhibition of phosphofructokinase (PFK) [30,50]. In the absence of acid–base changes, increases in the intracellular citrate concentration association, with increased rate of aerobic oxidation, inhibit glycolysis, contributing to the so-called Pasteur effect (inhibition of glycolysis by aerobic metabolism). Citrate stimulates fructose diphosphatase, a gluconeogenic enzyme. Thus, increases in tissue citrate, at normal or acidic pH,

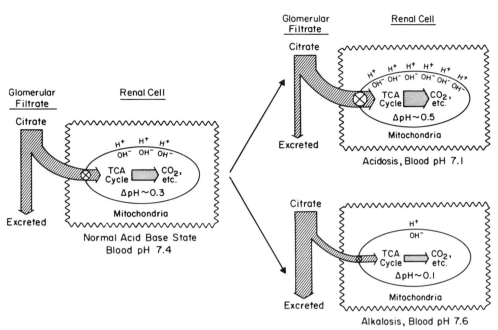

FIG. 10-30. *Proposed role of changes in mitochondrial pH gradient (ΔpH) in regulating citrate excretion, reabsorption, and metabolism. On left are shown conditions during normal acid–base state. When metabolic acidosis develops (upper right), ΔpH increases, stimulating transport of citrate into the mitochondria by the citrate carrier, cytoplasmic citrate levels fall, enabling enhanced transport of citrate out of the tubular fluid. In metabolic alkalosis (lower right), a reduction in ΔpH causes opposite changes from those in acidosis. (From Simpson DP: Citrate excretion: A window on renal metabolism. Am J Physiol 244:F223, 1983, with permission.)*

inhibit glycolysis and promote gluconeogenesis [207]. At an alkaline pH, as in metabolic alkalosis, the inhibitory effect of citrate on PFK is minimized, and the renal glycolytic rate increases in spite of increased tissue citrate concentration. Citrate also plays an important role in the regulation of "de novo" synthesis of lipids from carbohydrates or amino acids. Citrate activates acetyl CoA carboxylase [274], a rate-limiting enzyme in fatty acid synthesis. It also participates in the transfer of intramitochondrial acetyl groups and reducing equivalents to the cytosol for fatty acid synthesis [29].

Renal Citrate Metabolism During Development

The capacity for "de novo" synthesis of fatty acids in the adult kidney is believed to be limited [9]. By contrast, in the newborn rat, significant incorporation of labeled ketoacids into renal tissue fatty acids has been observed [290], suggesting active fatty acid synthesis in the kidney at this age. We are not aware of studies of the developmental changes in renal lipogenic capacity and of their role in the structural and functional maturation of the kidney. The ability of the developing kidney to respond to changes in acid–base balance with changes in citrate metabolism and transport has not, to our knowledge, been explored.

Renal Metabolism of Polypeptides

The liver and kidney account for most of the metabolism of peptide hormones [184]. Glomerular filtration is the major route of renal peptide removal from plasma. Therefore the GFR affects the circulating hormone levels [219]. Other factors that affect the rate of renal filtration of peptides are the size, shape, and charge of the molecule and glomerular permeability. Large peptides such as insulin do not pass through the glomerular membrane easily, whereas small molecules such as vasopressin or angiotensin are freely permeant.

Small polypeptides are absorbed nearly completely by the proximal tubule. Larger molecular weight peptides, such as insulin, enter the proximal tubule by endocytosis [155]. Although there is charge binding (nonspecific) of peptides to the luminal membrane, specific receptor binding is quantitatively more important [146,220]. Subsequently endosomal vesicles form, migrate to the cytosol, fuse with lysosomes, and the peptides contained within are degraded into their constituent amino acids or smaller polypeptides. These degradation products then leave the cell across the basolateral membrane or are metabolized. Smaller polypeptides may be degraded by peptidases at the luminal membrane brush border and are absorbed from the proximal tubule lumen fluid as amino acids and oligopeptides [46,209]. This is not an all or none phenomenon.

TABLE 10-7. *Renal metabolism of peptide hormones*

Polypeptide	Circulating hormone removed by kidney %	Membrane site of removal	% Urinary excretion
Insulin	50	60% luminal 40% basolateral	<1
Glucagon	30	Mostly luminal	<1
Parathyroid hormone	30	Mostly luminal Some basolateral	<1
Calcitonin	65	Mostly luminal	<1
Growth hormone	70	Mostly luminal	2
Vasopressin	50	Mostly luminal	25–70
Prolactin	70	Mostly luminal	~1

Luminal membrane removal involves filtration at the glomerulus and then transport into the renal epithelium with or without prior intraluminal hydrolysis by peptidases. Basolateral removal involves receptor-mediated binding or transport from the circulation. Derived from [46,47,137,155,208,209,210,211].

For example, angiotensin and bradykinin are nearly completely hydrolyzed at the brush border and transported into the proximal tubule cell as the individual constituent amino acids [47]. Pullman and co-workers showed that the addition of unlabeled free amino acids inhibits the uptake of labeled angiotensin across renal luminal membrane [218]. Brush border membrane vesicles were found to degrade this peptide hormone [210]. However, where a more complex structure is present, such as oxytocin, which is a cyclic peptide, absorption is slow and the luminal membrane is incapable of hydrolyzing it [210]. In a study comparing glucagon and insulin handling, Peterson et al. showed that glucagon is hydrolyzed by the proximal tubule brush border enzymes and the products reabsorbed [208]. This does not occur at the distal tubule. Degradation by brush border enzymes also occurs in the case of insulin, but is incomplete and less efficient than the degradation observed for glucagon. Most insulin is absorbed through endocytosis at the proximal tubule. Peterson et al. concluded that these uptake systems are not mutually exclusive and both endocytosis and luminal hydrolysis in varying degrees may be used as transport and degradation pathways.

Some polypeptides are taken up by the proximal tubule through the basolateral membrane as well. Sixty percent of insulin uptake is across the brush border membrane, with the remaining 40% occurring across the basolateral membrane [208,150]. The precise mechanism of movement of insulin across the basolateral membrane is unclear, but may also be receptor-mediated endocytosis [211]. Parathormone is also removed from the circulation, in part through the basolateral membrane, but most is cleared through filtration, followed by luminal endocytosis and degradation [137,187]. Data regarding the renal handling of polypeptide hormones are summarized in Table 10-7.

In renal failure, the circulating levels of polypeptide hormones are usually elevated [79]. This increase is due to decreased metabolism, but may be further altered by changes in extrarenal metabolism and, theoretically, by increased hormone secretion. Because of the low glomerular filtration rate, little hormone is delivered for degra-

dation by the proximal tubules. In addition, proximal tubular damage present in progressive renal disease impairs the tubular transport and metabolism of polypeptides and results in an increase in fractional urinary hormone clearance [221,252].

The finding of high circulatory levels of polypeptide hormones had led to the suggestion that they may represent uremic toxins. Parathormone, in particular, has been considered as a potential toxin in patients with chronic renal failure [252]. Rabkin and Kitaji [219] point out that, although the circulating levels of hormones may be high, the biologic effects may be minimal. In some instances the "hormone" measured may actually represent various degradation products. This has been demonstrated to be true for calcitonin, glucagon, insulin, and parathormone. End-organ unresponsiveness has been reported to occur in uremia, which would minimize the effects of elevated circulating peptide hormone levels. Further, the accumulation of hormones with opposing physiologic functions would diminish the effects of an elevated plasma hormone level and can result, through feedback, in inhibition of the hormone release.

We are unaware of studies regarding the relationship between the clearance of peptide hormones and their blood levels during postnatal development. However, changes in GFR during chronic renal disease may have a profound impact on the humoral regulation of growth and maturation.

References

1. Adam W, Simpson DP: Glutamine transport in rat kidney mitochondria in metabolic acidosis. *J Clin Invest* 54:165, 1974.
2. Alleyne GAO, McFarlane-Anderson N, Scott B: Glutamine uptake by cortical slices and luminal brush border vesicles of rat kidney. *Biochem J* 12:99, 1980.
3. Alleyne GAO, Scullard GH: Renal metabolic response to acid-base changes. I. Enzymatic control of ammoniagenesis in the rat. *J Clin Invest* 48:364, 1969.

4. Alpern RJ: Mechanism of basolateral $H^+/OH^-/HCO_3^-$ transport in the rat proximal convoluted tubule: A sodium coupled electrogenic process. *J Gen Physiol* 86:613, 1985.

5. Anaizi NH, Cohen JJ, Black AJ, et al: Renal tissue citrate: Independence from citrate utilization, reabsorption and pH. *Am J Physiol* 251:F547, 1986.

6. Anderson JW, Stowring L: Gycolytic and gluconeogenic enzyme activities in renal cortex of diabetic rats. *Am J Physiol* 224:930, 1973.

7. Andreoli TE, Schafer JA, Troutman SL, et al: Solvent drag component of Cl^- flux in superficial straight tubules: Evidence for a paracellular component of isotonic fluid reabsorption. *Am J Physiol* 237:F455, 1979.

8. Aperia A, Fukuda Y, Lechene C: Ontogenic increase in Na^+-H^+ exchange induces increase Na^+-K^+ ATPase activity in rat proximal convoluted tubule. *Kidney Int* 33:415, 1988.

9. Arbex R, Rous S, Pavarger P: Incorporation du [1,5-^{1}a4C] citrate dans les differents acides gras de la souris vivante. *Biochim Biophys Acta* 218:11, 1970.

10. Baertl JM, Sancetta SM, Gabuzda GJ: Relation of acute potassium depletion to renal ammonium metabolism in patients with cirrhosis. *J Clin Invest* 42:696, 1963.

11. Bagnasco S, Balaban R, Fales HM, et al: Predominant osmotically active organic solutes in rat and rabbit renal medullas. *J Biol Chem* 261:5872, 1986.

12. Balaban RS, Mandel LJ: Metabolic substrate utilization by rabbit proximal tubule. An NADH fluorescence study. *Am J Physiol* 254:F407, 1988.

13. Balagura S, Pitts RF: Renal handling of α-ketoglutarate by the dog. *Am J Physiol* 207:483, 1964.

14. Balagura S, Stone WJ: Renal tubular secretion of α-ketoglutarate in dog. *Am J Physiol* 212:1319, 1967.

15. Barac-Nieto M: Effects of pH, calcium and succinate on sodium citrate cotransport in renal microvilli. *Am J Physiol* 247:F282, 1984.

16. Barac-Nieto M: Renal uptake of p-aminophippuric acid in vitro. Effects of palmitate and 1-carnitine. *Biochim Biophys Acta* 233:446, 1971.

17. Barac-Nieto M: Effects of lactate and glutamine on palmitate metabolism in rat kidney cortex. *Am J Physiol* 231:14, 1976.

18. Barac-Nieto M, Cohen JJ: Non-esterified fatty acid uptake by dog kidney: Effects of probenecid and chlorothiazide. *Am J Physiol* 215:98, 1968.

19. Barac-Nieto M, Cohen JJ: The metabolic fates of palmitate in the dog kidney in vivo. Evidence for incomplete oxidation. *Nephron* 8:488, 1971.

20. Barac-Nieto M, Gupta RK, Spitzer A: NMR studies of phosphate metabolism in the isolated perfused kidney of developing rats. *Pediatric Nephrology* 4:329, 1990.

21. Barac-Nieto M, Murer H, Kinne R: Lactate sodium cotransport in rat renal brush border membranes. *Am J Physiol* 239:F496, 1980.

22. Barac-Nieto M, Spitzer A: The relationship between renal metabolism and proximal tubule transport during ontogeny. *Pediatr Nephrol* 2:356, 1988.

23. Baruch SB, Burich RL, Eun CE, et al: Renal metabolism of citrate. *Med Clin North Am* 59:569, 1975.

24. Baruch S, Burich RL, King VF: Effects of alkalosis on renal citrate metabolism in dogs infused with citrate. *Am J Physiol* 225:385, 1973.

25. Bavarel G, Bonnard M, deCastanet EDA, et al: Lactate and pyruvate metabolism in isolated renal tubules of normal dogs. *Kidney Int* 14:567, 1978.

26. Beck JC, Lipkowitz MS, Abramson RG: Characterization of the fetal glucose transporter in rabbit kidney. Comparison with the adult brush border electrogenic Na^+-glucose symporter. *J Clin Invest* 82:379, 1988.

27. Berridge MJ: Cell signaling through phospholipid metabolism. *J Cell Sci* (suppl) 4:137, 1986.

28. Bertoli M, Battistella PD, Vergani L, et al: Carnitine deficiency induced during hemodialysis and hyperlipidemia. Effect of replacement therapy. *Am J Clin Nutr* 34:1496, 1981.

29. Bhaduri A, Srere PA: The incorporation of citrate carbon into fatty acids. *Biochim Biophys Acta* 70:221, 1963.

30. Bock PE, Frieden C: Phosphofructokinase. I. Mechanism of the pH-dependent inactivation and reactivation of the rabbit muscle enzyme. *J Biol Chem* 254:5630, 1976.

31. Bogusky RT, Lowenstein LM, Lowenstein JM: The purine necleotide cycle. A pathway for ammonia production in the rat kidney. *J Clin Invest* 58:326, 1976.

32. Boulpaep EL: Electrical phenomena in the nephron. *Kidney Int* 9:88, 1976.

33. Boulpaep EL, Seely JF: Electrophysiology of proximal and distal tubules in the autoperfused dog kidney. *Am J Physiol* 221:1084, 1971.

34. Brand P, Cohen JJ, Bignall MC: Independence of lactate oxidation from net Na^+ reabsorption in dog kidney in vivo. *Am J Physiol* 227:1255, 1974.

35. Brennan S, Hering-Smith K, Hamm LL: Effect of pH on citrate reabsorption in the proximal convoluted tubule. *Am J Physiol* 255:F301, 1988.

36. Brezis M, Rosen S, Silva P, et al: Renal ischemia: A new perspective. *Kidney Int* 26:375, 1984.

37. Brodwall EK, Westlie L, Myhre E: The renal excretion and tubular reabsorption of citric acid in renal tubular acidosis. *Acta Med Scand* 192:137, 1972.

38. Brosnan JT, Hall B: The transport and metabolism of glutamine by kidney cortex mitochondria from normal and acidotic rats. *Biochem J* 164:331, 1977.

39. Burch HB, Kuhlman AM, Skerjance J, et al: Changes in patterns of enzymes of carbohydrate metabolism in the developing rat kidney. *Pediatrics* 47:199, 1971.

40. Burch HB, Lowry OH, Perry SG, et al: Effect of age on pyruvate kinase and lactate dehydrogenase distribution in rat kidney. *Am J Physiol* 226:1227, 1974.

41. Burch HB, Narins R, Chu C, et al: Distribution along the rat nephron of three enzymes of gluconeogenesis in acidosis and starvation. *Am J Physiol* (Renal Fluid Elect Physiol) 235:F246, 1978.

42. Burg MB: Renal handling of sodium chloride, water, aminoacids and glucose. *In* Brenner BM, Rector FC (eds): *The Kidney*. Vol 1, 2nd ed. Philadelphia, WB Saunders, 1981, p 238.

43. Burg M, Green N: Function of the thick ascending limb of Henle's loop. *Am J Physiol* 224:659, 1973.

44. Caldwell T, Solomon S: Changes in oxygen consumption of kidney during maturation. *Biol Neonate* 25:1, 1975.

45. Cameron IL, Smith NRK, Pool TB, et al: Intracellular concentration of sodium and other elements as related to mitogenesis and oncogenesis in vivo. *Cancer Res* 40:1493, 1980.

46. Carone FA, Peterson DR: Hydrolysis and transport of small peptides by the proximal tubules. *Am J Physiol* 238:F151, 1980.

47. Carone FA, Pullman TN, Oparil S, et al: Micropuncture evidence of rapid hydrolysis of bradykinin by rat proximal tubule. *Am J Physiol* 230:1420, 1976.

48. Celsi G, Larsson L, Aperia A: Proximal tubular reabsorption and Na-K-ATPase activity in remnant kidney of young rats. *Am J Physiol* 20:F588, 1986.

49. Chamberlin ME, Mandel LJ: Substrate support of medullary

thick ascending limb oxygen consumption. *Am J Physiol* 251:F758, 1986.

50. Cheema-Dhadli S, Robinson BH, Halperin ML: Properties of the citrate transporter in rat heart: Implications for regulation of glycolysis by cytosolic citrate. *Can J Biochem* 54:561, 1976.

51. Chesney RW, Gusowski N, Zeilkovic I, et al: Developmental aspects of renal B-amino acid transport. V. Brush border membrane transport in nursing animals—effect of age and diet. *Pediatr Res* 20:890, 1986.

52. Cohen JJ: Is the function of the renal papilla coupled exclusively to an anaerobic pattern of metabolism? *Am J Physiol* 236:F426, 1979.

53. Cohen JJ: Relationship between energy requirements for Na⁺ reabsorption and other renal functions. *Kidney Int* 29:32, 1986.

54. Cohen JJ, Barac-Nieto M: Renal metabolism of substrates in relation to renal function. *In* Berliner RW, Orloff J (eds): *Handbook of Physiology. Section 8: Renal Physiology.* Washington, DC, American Physiological Society, 1973, p 909.

55. Cohen JJ, Kamm DE: Renal Metabolism: Relation to renal function. *In* Brenner BM, Rector FC (eds): *The Kidney.* Vol 1, 2nd ed. Philadelphia, WB Saunders, 1981, p 144.

56. Cohen JJ, Merkens LS, Peterson OW: Relationship of Na⁺ reabsorption to utilization of O_2 and lactate in the perfused rat kidney. *Am J Physiol* 238:F415, 1980.

57. Cohen JJ, Wittmann E: Renal utilization and excretion of α-ketoglutarate in dog: Effect of alkalosis. *Am J Physiol* 204:795, 1963.

58. Cooper AJL, Meister A: Isolation and properties of a new glutamine transaminase from rat kidney. *J Biol Chem* 249:2554, 1974.

59. Cort JH, McCance RA: The renal response of puppies to an acidosis. *J Physiol (Lond)* 124:358, 1954.

60. Costello J, Scott JM, Wilson P, et al: Glucose utilization and production by the dog kidney in vivo in metabolic acidosis and alkalosis. *J Clin Invest* 52:608, 1973.

61. Crawford MA, Milne MD, Scribner BH: The effects of changes in acid-base balance on urinary citrate in the rat. *J Physiol* 149:413, 1959.

62. Curthoys NP, Kuhlenschmidt T: Phosphate independent glutaminase from rat kidney. Partial purification and identity with γ-glutamyltranspeptidase. *J Biol Chem* 250:2099, 1975.

63. Curthoys NP, Lowry OH: The distribution of glutaminase isoenzymes in the various structures of the cytoplasm in normal, acidotic, and alkalotic rat kidney. *J Biol Chem* 248:162, 1973.

64. Curthoys NP, Shapiro RA: Effect of metabolic acidosis and of phosphate on the presence of glutamine within the matrix pace of rat renal mitochondria during glutamine transport. *J Biol Chem* 253:63, 1978.

65. Dawkins MJ: Changes in glucose 6 P'tase activity in kidney and liver after birth. *Nature* 191:72, 1968.

66. Dell RB, Winters RW: Lactate gradients in the kidney of the dog. *Am J Physiol* 213:301, 1967.

67. Denis G, Preuss H, Pitts R: The P_{NH_3} of renal tubular cells. *J Clin Invest* 43:571, 1964.

68. DeToni E, Nordio S: The relationship between calcium phosphorus metabolism, the "Krebs cycle" and steroid metabolism. *Arch Dis Child* 34:371, 1959.

69. Dicker SE, Shirley DG: Rates of oxygen consumption and anaerobic glycolysis in renal cortex and medulla of adult and new born rats and guinea pigs. *J Physiol (Lond)* 212:235, 1971.

70. Dies F, Herrera J, Matos M, et al: Substrate uptake by dog kidney in vivo. *Am J Physiol* 218:405, 1970.

71. Dies F, Lotspeich WD: Hexosemonophosphate shunt in the kidney during acid base and electrolyte imbalance. *Am J Physiol* 212:61, 1967.

72. Dixon TE, Al-Awgati Q: H⁺/ATP stoichiometry of proton pump of turtle urinary bladder. *J Biol Chem* 255:3237, 1980.

73. Doucet A, Katz AI: High affinity Ca-Mg-ATPase along the rabbit nephron. *Am J Physiol* 242:F346, 1982.

74. Dowd TL, Barac-Nieto M, Gupta RK, et al: ³¹P NMR and saturation transfer studies in the isolated perfused rat kidney. *Renal Physiol Biochem* 12:161, 1989.

75. Duda GD, Handler P: Kinetics of ammonia metabolism in vivo. *J Biol Chem* 232:303, 1958.

76. Dutton GJ, Stevenson IH: Synthesis of glucuronides and uridine diphosphate glucuronic acid in kidney cortex and gastric mucosa. *Biochim Biophys Acta* 31:568, 1959.

77. Edelmann CM, Wolfish NM: Dietary influence on renal maturation in premature infants. *Pediatr Res* 2:421, 1968.

78. Elinder C, Aperia A: Renal oxygen consumption and sodium reabsorption during isotonic volume expansion in the developing rat. *Pediatr Res* 16:351, 1982.

79. Emmanouel DA, Linheimer MD, Katz AI: Pathogenesis of endocrine abnormalities in uremia. *Endocr Rev* 1:28, 1980.

80. Engel AG, Angelini L: Carnitine deficiency of human skeletal muscle with associated lipid storage myopathy. *Science* 179:899, 1973.

81. Engel AG, Rebouche CJ, Wilson DM, et al: Primary systemic carnitine deficiency. II. Renal handling of carnitine. *Neurology* 31:819, 1981.

82. Epstein FH, Balaban RS, Ross BD: Redox state of cytochrome aa₃ in isolated perfused rat kidney. *Am J Physiol* 43:F356, 1982.

83. Evan AP, Gattone VH II, Schwartz GJ: Development of solute transport in rabbit proximal tubule. II. Morphologic segmentation. *Am J Physiol* 245:F391, 1983.

84. Evers J, Murer H, Kinne R: Phenylalanine uptake by isolated renal brush border vesicles. *Biochim Biophys Acta* 426:598, 1976.

85. Farber SJ, Von Praag D: Composition of glycosaminoglycans (mucopolysaccharides) in rabbit renal papilla. *Biochim Biophys Acta* 208:219, 1970.

86. Farquhar JK, Scott WN, Coe FL: Hexosemonophosphate shunt activity in compensatory renal hypertrophy. *Proc Soc Exp Biol Med* 129:809, 1968.

87. Fine A: Effects of acute metabolic acidosis on renal, gut, liver and muscle metabolism of glutamine and ammonia in the dog. *Kidney Int* 21:439, 1982.

88. Fine A, Bennett FI, Alleyne GAO: Effects of acute acid-base alterations in glutamine metabolism and renal ammoniagenesis in the dog. *Clin Sci Mol Med* 54:503, 1978.

89. Fine L: The biology of renal hypertrophy. *Kidney Int* 29:619, 1986.

90. Fine LH, Kaplan NO, Kuftinee D: Developmental changes in mammalian lactic dehydrogenase. *Biochemistry* 2:116, 1963.

91. Fisher JH, Isselhard A: Metabolic patterns in several tissues of newborn rabbits during ischemia. *Biol Neonate* 27:235, 1975.

92. Fomon SJ, Harris DM, Jensen RL: Acidification of the urine by infants fed human milk and whole cow's milk. *Pediatrics* 23:113, 1959.

93. Fonteles MC, Cohen JJ, Black AJ, et al: Support of kidney function by long chain fatty acids derived from renal tissue. *Am J Physiol* 244:F235, 1983.

94. Foreman JW, Reynolds RA, Pepe LM, et al: Glutamine transport into isolated renal membrane vesicles from normal and acidotic rats. *Contrib Nephrol* 31:101, 1982.

95. Freeman D, Bartlett S, Radda G, et al: Energetics of sodium transport in the kidney. Saturation transfer ^{31}P-NMR. *Biochim Biophys Acta* 762:235, 1983.

96. Freund N, Sedraoui M, Geloso JP: Oxidative metabolism in fetal rat kidney during late gestation. *J Dev Physiol* 4:215, 1982.

97. Freund N, Sedraoui M, Geloso JP: Fatty acid oxidation by developing kidney. *Biol Neonate* 45:183, 1984.

98. Friedrichs D, Schoner W: Stimulation of gluconeogenesis by inhibition of the sodium pump. *Biochim Biophys Acta* 304:142, 1973.

99. Fromter E, Rumrich G, Ullrich KJ: Phenomenologic description of Na^+, Cl^-, and HCO_3^- absorption from the proximal tubules of rat kidneys. *Pflugers Arch* 343:189, 1973.

100. Fulgraff G, Pitts RF: Kinetics of ammonia production and excretion in the acidotic dog. *Am J Physiol* 209:1206, 1965.

101. Gabuzda GJ, Hall PW: Relation of potassium depletion to renal ammonium metabolism and hepatic coma. *Medicine* 45:481, 1966.

102. Garza-Quintero R, Cohen JJ, Brand PH, et al: Steady state glucose oxidation by the dog kidney in vivo: Relation to Na^+ reabsorption. *Am J Physiol* 228:549, 1975.

103. Godfrey S, Kuhlenschmidt T, Gurthoys NP: Correlation between activation and dimer formation of rat renal phosphate-dependent glutaminase. *J Biol Chem* 252:1927, 1977.

104. Goldstein L: Actinomycin D inhibition of the adaptation of renal glutaminedeaminating enzymes in the rat. *Nature* 205:1330, 1965.

105. Goldstein L: Ammonia metabolism in kidneys of suckling rats. *Am J Physiol* 220:213, 1971.

106. Goldstein L: Glutamine transport by mitochondria isolated from normal and acidotic rats. *Am J Physiol* 229:1027, 1975.

107. Goldstein L: Renal ammonia and acid excretion in infant rats. *Am J Physiol* 218:1394, 1970.

108. Goldstein L, Harley-DeWitt S: Renal gluconeogenesis and mitochondrial NAD/NADH ratios in nursing and adult rats. *Am J Physiol* 224:752, 1973.

109. Good DW, Burg MB: Ammonia production by individual segments of the rat nephron. *J Clin Invest* 73:602, 1984.

110. Good DW, Knepper MA: Ammonia transport in the mammalian kidney. *Am J Physiol* 248:F459, 1985.

111. Good DW, Knepper MA, Burg MB: Ammonia absorption by the thick ascending limb of Henle's loop. *Am J Physiol* 247:F35, 1984.

112. Goorno W, Rector FC, Seldin DW: Relation of renal gluconeogenesis to ammonia production in the dog and rat. *Am J Physiol* 213:969, 1967.

113. Gougoux A, Vinay P, Cardoso M, et al: Immediate adaptation of the dog kidney to acute hypercapnia. *Am J Physiol* (Renal Fluid Elect Physiol) 243:F227, 1982.

114. Green R, Moriarty RJ, Giebisch G: Ionic requirements of proximal tubular fluid reabsorption: Flow dependency of fluid transport. *Kidney Int* 20:580, 1981.

115. Gregg CM, Cohen JJ, Black AJ, et al: Effects of glucose and insulin on metabolism and function of perfused rat kidney. *Am J Physiol* 235:F52, 1978.

116. Grollman AP, Harrison HC, Harrison HE: The renal excretion of citrate. *J Clin Invest* 40:1290, 1961.

117. Grownow GHJ, Cohen JJ: Substrate support for renal functions during hypoxia in the perfused rat kidney. *Am J Physiol* 247:F618, 1984.

118. Guder WG, Ross BD: Enzyme distribution along the nephron. *Kidney Int* 26:101, 1984.

119. Guder WG, Wirthensohn G: Metabolism of isolated kidney tubules: Interactions between lactate, glutamine and oleate metabolism. *Eur J Biochem* 99:577, 1979.

120. Gullans SR, Avison M, Takshi O, et al: NMR measurements of intracellular sodium in the rabbit proximal tubule. *Am J Physiol* 249:F160, 1985.

121. Gullans SR, Brazy PC, Dennis V, et al: Interactions between gluconeogenesis and sodium transport in rabbit proximal tubules. *Am J Physiol* 246:F859, 1984.

122. Halperin ML, Jungas RL, Pichette C, et al: A quantitative analysis of renal ammoniagenesis and energy balance: A theoretical approach. *Can J Physiol Pharmacol* 60:1431, 1982.

123. Halperin ML, Vinay P, Gougoux A, et al: Regulation of the maximum rate of renal ammoniagenesis in the acidotic dog. *Am J Physiol* 248:F607, 1985.

124. Hammerman MR, Sacktor B, Doughaday WH: Myoinositol transport in renal brushborder vesicles and its inhibition by glucose. *Am J Physiol* 239:F113, 1980.

125. Harris RC, Seifter JL, Lechene C: Coupling of Na-H exchange and Na-K pump activity in cultured rat proximal tubule cells. *Am J Physiol* 251:C815, 1986.

126. Harris SI, Balaban RS, Barret L, et al: Mitochondria respiratory capacity and Na^+ and K^+ dependent adenosinetriphosphatase mediated ion transport in the intact renal cell. *J Biol Chem* 256:10319, 1981.

127. Harris SI, Balaban RS, Mandel LJ: Oxygen consumption and cellular ion transport: Evidence for adenosine triphosphate to O_2 ratio near 6 in intact cell. *Science* 208:1146, 1980.

128. Hatemi N, McCance RA: The response of piglets to ammonium chloride. *J Physiol (Lond)* 157:603, 1961.

129. Herbert SC, Andreoli TE: Control of NaCl transport in the thick ascending limb. *Am J Physiol* 246:F745, 1984.

130. Hems DA: Metabolism of glutamine and glutamic acid by isolated perfused kidneys of normal and acidotic rats. *Biochem J* 130:671, 1972.

131. Hoffman N, Thees M, Kinne R: Phosphate transport by isolated renal brush border vesicles. *Pflugers Arch* 362:147, 1976.

132. Holohan PD, Ross CR: Mechanisms of organic cation transport in kidney plasma membrane vesicles. 2. Delta pH studies. *J Pharmacol Exp Ther* 216:294, 1981.

133. Horster M: Loop of Henle functional differentiation. In vitro perfusion of the isolated thick ascending limb segment. *Pflugers Arch* 378:15, 1978.

134. Horster M, Schmidt U: In vitro electrolyte transport and enzyme activity of single dissected and perfused nephron segments during differentiation. *In* Guder W, Schmidt U (eds): *Current Problems in Clinical Biochemistry.* Vol 8: *Biochemical Nephrology.* Bern, Stuttgart, Vienna, Hans Huber Publishers, 1978, p 98.

135. Horster M, Valtin H: Postnatal development of renal function. Micropuncture and clearance studies in the dog. *J Clin Invest* 50:779, 1971.

136. Howard CF, Anderson L: Metabolism of myoinositol in animals. II. Complete catabolism of ^{14}C myoinositol by rat kidney slices. *Arch Biochem Biophys* 118:332, 1967.

137. Hruska KA, Martin K, Mennes P, et al: Degradation of parathyroid hormone and fragment production by the isolated perfused dog kidney. *J Clin Invest* 60:501, 1977.

138. Huth PJ, Shug AL: Properties of carnitine transport in rat kidney cortex slices. *Biochim Biophys Acta* 602:621, 1980.

139. Igarashi Y, Aperia A, Larsson L, et al: Effect of betamethasone on Na^+-K^+-ATPase activity and basal and lateral cell membranes in proximal tubules during early development. *Am J Physiol* 245:F232, 1983.

140. Imai M, Kokko JP: Mechanisms of sodium and chloride

transport in the thin ascending limb of Henle. *J Clin Invest* 58:1054, 1976.

141. Iwamoto HS, Oh W, Rudolph AM: Renal metabolism in fetal and newborn sheep. *In* Jones CT, Nathanielsz PW (eds): *The Physiological Development of the Fetus and Newborn.* New York, Academic, 1985, p 37.

142. Jenkins AD, Dousa TP, Smith LH: Transport of citrate across renal brush border membrane: Effects of dietary acid and alkali loads. *Am J Physiol* 249:F590, 1985.

143. Johannes J, Lie M, Kiil F: Effect of glycine and glucagon on glomerular filtration and renal metabolic rates. *Am J Physiol* 233:F61, 1977.

144. Jorgenson KE, Kragh-Hansen U, Rigaard-Petersen H, et al: Citrate uptake by basolateral and luminal membrane vesicles from rabbit kidney cortex. *Am J Physiol* (Renal Fluid Elect Physiol) 244:F686, 1983.

145. Jorgensen PL: Structure, function and regulation of Na,K-ATPase in the kidney. *Kidney Int* 29:10, 1986.

146. Just M, Habermann E: Interactions of a protease inhibitor and other peptides with isolated brush border membranes from rat renal cortex. *Archiv Pharmazie* 280:161, 1973.

147. Kahn AM, Branham S, Weinman EJ: Mechanisms of L-malate transport in rat renal basolateral membrane vesicles. *Am J Physiol* (Renal Fluid Elect Physiol) 246:F779, 1984.

148. Kaskel FJ, Kumar A, Lockhart EA, et al: Factors affecting proximal tubular reabsorption during development. *Am J Physiol* 252:F188, 1987.

149. Katz AI: Distribution and function of classes of ATPases along the nephron. *Kidney Int* 29:21, 1986.

150. Katz AI, Rubenstein AH: Metabolism of proinsulin, insulin and C-peptide in the rat. *J Clin Invest* 52:1113, 1973.

151. Kaufman AM, Kahn T: Complementary role of citrate and bicarbonate excretion in acid base balance in the rat. *Am J Physiol* 255:F182, 1988.

152. Kelleher JK: Gluconeogenesis from labeled carbon. Estimating isotope dilution. *Am J Physiol* 250:E296, 1986.

153. Kelly S, Dixon TE, Al-Awqati Q: Metabolic pathways coupled to H^+ transport in turtle urinary bladder. *J Membr Biol* 54:237, 1980.

154. Kiebzak GM, Sacktor B: Effect of age on renal conservation of phosphate in the rat. *Am J Physiol* 251:F399, 1986.

155. King AC, Cuatrecasas P: Peptide hormone-induced receptor and mobility, aggregation, and internalization. *N Engl J Med* 305:77, 1981.

156. Kinne R: Metabolic correlates of tubular transport. *In* Giebisch G, Tosteson DC, Ussing HH(eds): *Membrane Transport in Biology, 4B.* Berlin, Springer, 1979, p 529.

157. Kinne R, Kinne-Saffran E, Schuetz H, et al: Ammonium transport in medullary thick ascending limb of rabbit kidney: Involvement of the $Na^+-K^+-2Cl^-$ cotransporter. *J Membr Biol* 94:279, 1986.

158. Kinne R, Koening J, Hannafin J, et al: The use of membrane vesicles to study the NaCl/KCl cotransporter involved in active transepithelial chloride transport. *Pflugers Arch* (suppl 1) 405:S101, 1985.

159. Kinne R, Murer H, Kinne-Saffran E, et al: Sugar transport by renal plasma membrane vesicles: Characteristics of the systems in brush-border microvilli and basolateral plasma membranes. *J Membr Biol* 21:275, 1975.

160. Kinsella JL, Aronson PS: Interaction of NH_4^+ and Li^+ with the renal microvillus membrane Na^+-H^+ exchanger. *Am J Physiol* 241:C220, 1981.

161. Kippen I, Hirayama B, Klinenberg JR, et al: Transport of tricarboxylic acid cycle intermediates by membrane vesicles from renal brush border. *Proc Natl Acad Sci USA* 76:3397, 1979.

162. Klein KL, Wang MS, Torikai S, et al: Substrate oxidation by isolated single nephron segments of the rat. *Kidney Int* 20:20, 1981.

163. Knepper MA, Packet R, Good DW: Ammonia transport in the kidney. *Physiol Rev* 69:179, 1989.

164. Knox FG, Fleming JS, Rennie DW: Effect of osmotic diuresis on sodium reabsorption and oxygen consumption of kidney. *Am J Physiol* 210:751, 1966.

165. Koenig BS, Ricapito S, Kinne R: Chloride transport in the thick ascending limb of Henle's loop: Potassium dependency and stoichiometry of the NaCl cotransport system in plasma membrane vesicles. *Pflugers Arch* 399:173, 1983.

166. Kokko JP: Sodium chloride and water transport in the descending limb of Henle. *J Clin Invest* 49:1838, 1970.

167. Kokko JP: Transport characteristics of the thin limbs of Henle. *Kidney Int* 22:449, 1982.

168. Kosicki GW, Srere PA: Kinetic studies on the citrate condensing enzyme. *J Biol Chem* 236:2560, 1961.

169. Kovacevic Z, McGivan JD: Mitochondrial metabolism of glutamine and its physiological significance. *Physiol Rev* 63:547, 1983.

170. Krebs HA, Hems R, Weidemann MJ, et al: The fate of isotopic carbon in kidney cortex synthesizing glucose from lactate. *Biochem J* 101:242, 1966.

171. Krebs HA, Lund P: Formation of glucose from hexoses, pentoses, polyols and related substances in kidney cortex. *Biochem J* 98:210, 1963.

172. Labarca P, Canessa M, Leaf A: Metabolic cost of sodium transport in the toad bladder. *J Membr Biol* 32:383, 1977.

173. Lannigan DA, Knauf PA, Macara IG: Relationship of the decrease in protein synthesis and intracellular Na^+ during Friend Murine Erytrolukemic Cell Differentiation. *J Biol Chem* 31:14430, 1986.

174. Lanou KF, Schoolwerth AC: Metabolite transport in mitochondria. *Annu Rev Biochem* 48:871, 1979.

175. Larsson S, Aperia A, Lechene C: Studies on final differentiation of rat renal proximal cells in culture. *Am J Physiol* 251:C455, 1986.

176. Larsson SH, Aperia A, Lechene C: Studies on terminal differentiation of rat renal proximal tubular cells in culture: Ouabain-sensitive transport. *Acta Physiol Scand* 132(2):129, 1988.

177. Leal-Pinto E, Park HC, King F, et al: Metabolism of lactate by the intact functioning kidney of the dog. *Am J Physiol* 224:1463, 1973.

178. Lee JB, Peter HM: Effect of oxygen tension on glucose metabolism in rabbit kidney cortex and medulla. *Am J Physiol* 217:1464, 1969.

179. Lemann J, Lennon EJ, Goodman AD, et al: The net balance of acid in subjects given large loads of acid or alkali. *J Clin Invest* 44:507, 1965.

180. Lemann J, Litzow JR, Lennon EJ: The effects of chronic acid loads in normal man: Further evidence for participation of bone mineral in the defense against chronic metabolic acidosis. *J Clin Invest* 45:1608, 1966.

181. Lemann J, Relman AS: The relation of sulfur metabolism to acid-base balance and electrolyte excretion. The effects of DL-methionine in normal man. *J Clin Invest* 38:2215, 1959.

182. Lowry M, Hall DE, Brosnan JT: Serine synthesis in rat kidney: Studies with perfused kidney and cortical tubules. *Am J Physiol* 250:F649, 1986.

183. Lowry M, Ross BD: Activation of oxoglutarate dehydrogenase in the kidney in response to acute acidosis. *Biochem J* 190:711, 1980.

184. Mack T, Johnson V, Kau ST, et al: Renal filtration transport and metabolism of low molecular weight proteins: A review. *Kidney Int* 16:251, 1979.

185. MacKnight ADC, MacKnight JM, Robinson JR: The effect of urinary output upon the excretion of ammonia in man. *J Physiol (Lond)* 163:314, 1962.

186. Manillier C, Vinay P, Lalonde L, et al: ATP turnover and renal response of dog tubules to pH changes in vitro. *Am J Physiol* 251:F919, 1986.

187. Martin KJ, Hruska KA, Lewis J, et al: The renal handling of parathyroid hormone: Role of peritubular uptake and glomerular filtration. *J Clin Invest* 60:808, 1977.

188. Mathisen O, Montclair T, Kiil F: Oxygen requirement of bicarbonate dependent sodium reabsorption in the dog kidney. *Am J Physiol* 238:F175, 1980.

189. Maunsbach AB: Ultrastructure of the proximal tubule. *In* Orloff J, Berliner RW (eds): *Renal Physiology.* Washington, DC, American Physiological Society, 1973, p 31.

190. Maxild J, Moller JV, Sheikh MI: Involvement of the Na^+-K^+-ATPase in p-aminohippurate transport by rabbit kidney tissue. *J Physiol (Lond)* 315:189, 1981.

191. McCance RA, Widdowson EM: The acid-base relationships of the foetal fluids of the pig. *J Physiol (Lond)* 151:484, 1960.

192. Medow MS, Roth KS, Goldmann DR, et al: Developmental aspects of proline transport in rat renal brush border membranes. *Proc Natl Acad Sci USA* 83:7561, 1986.

193. Michael AF, Blau E, Vernier RL: Glomerular polyanion. Alteration in aminonucleoside nephrosis. *Lab Invest* 23:649, 1970.

194. Murer H, Hopfer U, Kinne R: Sodium/proton antiport in brush border membrane vesicles isolated from small intestine and kidney. *Biochem J* 154:597, 1985.

195. Nagami GT: Luminal secretion of ammonia in the mouse proximal tubule perfused in vitro. *J Clin Invest* 81:159, 1988.

196. Neumann KH, Rector FC: Mechanism of NaCl and water reabsorption in the proximal convoluted tubule of rat kidney: Role of chloride concentration gradients. *J Clin Invest* 58:1110, 1976.

197. Neiberger R, Barac-Nieto M, Spitzer A: Renal reabsorption of phosphate during development: transport kinetics in BBMV. *Am J Physiol* 257:F268, 1989.

198. Norman ME, Feldman NI, Cohn RM, et al: Urinary citrate excretion in the diagnosis of distal renal tubular acidosis. *J Pediatr* 92:394, 1978.

199. Novakova J, Capek K, Bass A, et al: Postnatal changes of some enzymatic activities of energy supplying metabolism in the cortex, inner and outer medulla of rat kidney. *Physiol Bohemoslov* 29:289, 1980.

200. Ockner RK, Manning JA, Popenhausen RB, et al: A binding protein for fatty acids in cytosol of intestinal mucosa, liver, myocardium and other tissues. *Science* 177:56, 1972.

201. Orloff J, Berliner RW: The mechanism of the excretion of ammonia in the dog. *J Clin Invest* 35:223, 1956.

202. Oschman JL: Morphological correlates of transport. *In* Giebish G III, Tosteson DC, Ussing HH (eds): *Membrane Transport in Biology.* Berlin, Springer, 1978, p 55.

203. Owen EE, Johnson JH, Taylor MP: The effect of induced hyperammonemia on renal ammonia metabolism. *J Clin Invest* 40:215, 1961.

204. Owen EE, Robinson RR: Aminoacid extraction and aminoacid metabolism by the human kidney during prolonged administration of ammonium chloride. *J Clin Invest* 42:263, 1963.

205. Owen OE, Felig P, Morgan AP, et al: Liver and kidney metabolism during prolonged starvation. *J Clin Invest* 48:574, 1969.

206. Parekh N, Veith U: Renal hemodynamics and oxygen consumption during post-ischemic acute renal failure in the rat. *Kidney Int* 19:306, 1981.

207. Pashley DH, Cohen JJ: Substrate interconversion in dog kidney cortex slices. Regulation by ECF pH. *Am J Physiol* 225:1519, 1973.

208. Peterson DR, Carone FA, Oparil S, et al: Differences between renal tubular processing of glucagon and insulin. *Am J Physiol* 242:112, 1982.

209. Peterson DR, Chrabaszez G, Peterson WR, et al: Mechanism for renal tubular handling of angiotensin. *Am J Physiol* 236:F365, 1979.

210. Peterson DR, Oparil S, Flourel G, et al: Handling of angiotensin II and oxytocin by renal tubular segments perfused in vitro. *Am J Physiol* 232:F319, 1977.

211. Peterson J, Kitaji J, Duckworth WC, et al: Fate of 125 I-insulin removed from the peritubular circulation of isolated perfused rat kidney. *Am J Physiol* 243:F126, 1982.

212. Pitts RF, Damian A, MacLeod M: Synthesis of serine by rat kidney in vivo and in vitro. *Am J Physiol* 219:584, 1970.

213. Pitts RF, Pilkington LA: The relation between plasma concentrations of glutamine and glycine and utilization of their nitrogens as sources of urinary ammonia. *J Clin Invest* 45:86, 1960.

214. Pitts RF, Pilkington LA, de Haas JCM: N^{15} tracer studies on the origin of urinary ammonia in the acidotic dog, with notes on the enzymmatic synthesis of labeled glutamic acid and glutamines. *J Clin Invest* 44:731, 1965.

215. Pitts RF, Pilkington LA, MacLeod MB, et al: Metabolism of glutamine in the intact functioning kidney of the dog. Studies in metabolic acidosis. *J Clin Invest* 51:557, 1972.

216. Pollak VE, Mattenheimer H, DeBruin H, et al: Experimental metabolic acidosis: The enzymatic basis of ammonia production by the dog kidney. *J Clin Invest* 44:169, 1965.

217. Preisig PA, Ives HE, Cragoe EJ, et al: Role of Na^+/H^+ antiporter in rat proximal tubule bicarbonate absorption. *J Clin Invest* 80:970, 1987.

218. Pullman TN, Carone FA, Oparil S, et al: Effects of constituent amino acids on tubular handling of microinfused angiotensin II. *Am J Physiol* 234:F325, 1978.

219. Rabkin R, Kitaji J: Renal metabolism of peptide hormones. *Miner Electrolyte Metab* 9:212, 1983.

220. Rabkin R, Peterson J, Mamelok R: Binding and degradation of insulin by isolated renal brush border membranes. *Diabetes* 31:618, 1982.

221. Rabkin R, Simon NM, Steiner S, et al: Effect of renal disease on renal uptake and excretion of insulin in man. *N Engl J Med* 282:182, 1970.

222. Radde IC, McCance RA: Glutaminase activity of the foetal membranes and kidneys of pigs. *Nature* 183:115, 1959.

223. Rane S, Aperia A: Ontogeny of Na-K-ATPase activity in thick ascending limb and of concentrating capacity. *Am J Physiol* 249:F723, 1985.

224. Rebouche CJ: Sites and regulation of carnitine biosynthesis in mammals. *Fed Proc* 41:2848, 1982.

225. Rector FC Jr, Orloff J: The effect of the administration of sodium bicarbonate and ammonium chloride on the excretion and production of ammonia. The absence of alteractions in the activity of renal ammonia-producing enzymes in the dog. *J Clin Invest* 38:366, 1959.

226. Ross B, Espinal J, Silva P: Glucose metabolism in renal tubular function. *Kidney Int* 29:54, 1986.

227. Roth KS, Hwang SM, Yudkoff M, et al: The ontogeny of sugar transport in kidney. *Pediatr Res* 12:1127, 1978.

228. Sajo DM, Goldstein MB, Sonnenberg H, et al: Sites of ammonia addition to tubular fluid in rats with chronic metabolic acidosis. *Kidney Int* 20:353, 1981.

229. Sartorius OW, Roemmelt JC, Pitts RF: The renal regulation of acid-base balance in man. IV. The nature of the renal

compensations in ammonium chloride acidosis. *J Clin Invest* 28:423, 1949.

230. Schali C, Schild L, Overney J, et al: Secretion of tetramethylammonium by proximal tubules of rabbit kidneys. *Am J Physiol* 245:F238, 1983.

231. Schild L, Giebish G, Karniski LP, et al: Effect of formate on volume absorption in the rabbit proximal tubule. *J Clin Invest* 79:32, 1987.

232. Schmidt U, Dubach UC: Activity of the $Na^+ + K^+$ stimulated adenosine triphosphatase in the rat nephron. *Pflugers Arch* 306:219, 1969.

233. Schmidt U, Guder WG: Sites of enzyme activity along the nephron. *Kidney Int* 9:233, 1976.

234. Schmidt U, Horster M: Na-K-activated ATPase: Activity maturation in rabbit nephron segments dissected in vitro. *Am J Physiol* 233:F55, 1977.

235. Schwartz GJ, Barash J, Al-Awgati Q: Plasticity of functional epithelial polarity. *Nature* 318:368, 1985.

236. Schwartz GJ, Evans AP: Development of solute transport in rabbit proximal tubule. I. HCO_3^- and glucose absorption. *Am J Physiol* 245:F382, 1983.

237. Schwartz GJ, Evan AP: Development of solute transport in rabbit proximal tubule. III. Na-K-ATPase activity. *Am J Physiol* 246:F845, 1984.

238. Seigle R, Kinne R, Spitzer A: Glucose transport in newborn guinea pig brush border membrane fragments. *Kidney Int* 21:287, 1982.

239. Selvaggio AM, Schwartz JM, Bengele HH, et al: Mechanisms of H^+ secretion by inner medullary collecting duct cells. *Am J Physiol* 254:F391, 1988.

240. Shaloub R, Webber W, Glabman S, et al: Extraction of amino acids from and their addition to renal blood plasma. *Am J Physiol* 204:181, 1963.

241. Silva P, Hallac R, Spokes K: The relationship among gluconeogenesis, QO_2 and Na^+ transport in the perfused rat kidney. *Am J Physiol* 242:F506, 1982.

242. Silverman M, Vinay P, Shinola L, et al: Luminal and antiluminal transport of glutamine in dog kidney: Effect of metabolic acidosis. *Kidney Int* 20:359, 1981.

243. Simpson DP: Citrate excretion: A window on renal metabolism. *Am J Physiol* 244:F223, 1983.

244. Simpson DP: Control of hydrogen ion homeostasis and renal acidosis. *Medicine* 50:503, 1971.

245. Simpson DP: Mitochondrial transport functions and renal metabolism. *Kidney Int* 23:785, 1983.

246. Simpson DP: Pathways of glutamine and organic acid metabolism in renal cortex in chronic metabolic acidosis. *J Clin Invest* 51:1969, 1972.

247. Simpson DP: Dissociation of acid base effects on substrate accumulation and pH in dog mitochondria. *Am J Physiol* 254:F863, 1988.

248. Simpson DP, Adam W: Glutamine transport and metabolism by mitochondria from dog renal cortex. General properties and response to acidosis and alkalosis. *J Biol Chem* 250:8148, 1975.

249. Simpson DP, Hager SR: pH and bicarbonate effects on mitochondrial anion accumulation. Proposed mechanism for changes in renal metabolite levels in acute acid-base disturbances. *J Clin Invest* 63:704, 1979.

250. Simpson DP, Hager SR: Bicarbonate-carbon dioxide buffer system: A determinant of the mitochondrial pH gradient. *Am J Physiol* 247:F44, 1984.

251. Simpson DP, Hecker J: Glutamine distribution in mitochondria from normal and acidotic rat kidneys. *Kidney Int* 21:774, 1982.

252. Slatopolsky E, Martin K, Hruska K: Parathyroid hormone

253. Sonnenberg H, Cheema-Dhadli S, Goldstein MB, et al: Ammonia addition into the medullary collecting duct of the rat. *Kidney Int* 19:281, 1981.

254. Sotloff SP: Coupling renal metabolism to ion transport in renal epithelia. *Semin in Nephrol* 7:20, 1987

255. Sotloff SP, Mandel LJ: Active ion transport in the renal proximal tubule. III. The ATP dependence of the Na pump. *J Gen Physiol* 84:643, 1984.

256. Spitzer A, Brandis M: Functional and morphologic maturation of the superficial nephrons. Relationship to total kidney functions. *J Clin Invest* 53:279, 1974.

257. Stone WJ, Balagura S, Pitts RF: Diffusion equilibrium for ammonia in the kidney of the acidotic dog. *J Clin Invest* 46:1603, 1967.

258. Svenningsen NW, Lindquist B: Postnatal development of renal hydrogen ion excretion capacity in relation to age and protein intake. *Acta Paediatr Scand* 63:721, 1974.

259. Tamura K, Endou H: Contribution of purine nucleotide cycle to intranephron ammoniagenesis in rats. *Am J Physiol* 255:F1122, 1988.

260. Tannen RL: The effect of uncomplicated potassium depletion on urine acidification. *J Clin Invest* 49:813, 1970.

261. Tannen RL, Kunin AS: Effect of pH on ammonia production by renal mitochondria. *Am J Physiol* 231:1631, 1976.

262. Tannen RL, Sastrasinh S: Response of ammonia metabolism to acute acidosis. *Kidney Int* 25:1, 1984.

263. Tate SS, Meister A: Stimulation of the hydrolytic activity and decrease of the transpeptidase activity of γ-glutamyl transpeptidase by maleate: Identity of a rat kidney maleate-stimulated glutaminase and γ-glutamyl transpeptidase. *Proc Natl Acad Sci USA* 71:3329, 1974.

264. Tinker DO, Hanahan DJ: Phospholipid metabolism in the kidney biosynthesis of phospholipids from radioactive precursors in rabbit renal cortex slices. *Biochemistry* 5:423, 1966.

265. Tisher CC: Anatomy of the kidney. *In* Brenner BM, Rector FC (eds): *The Kidney.* Vol. I, 2nd ed. Philadelphia, WB Saunders, 1981, p 25.

266. Tizzianello A, Deferrari G, Garibotto G, et al: Renal ammoniagenesis in an early stage of metabolic acidosis in man. *J Clin Invest* 69:240, 1982.

267. Toback FG, Smith PD, Lowenstein LM: Phospholipid metabolism in the initiation of renal compensatory growth after acute reduction in renal mass. *J Clin Invest* 53:91, 1974.

268. Toyer DA, Schwertz DW, Kreisberg JI, et al: Inositol phospholipid metabolism in the kidney. *Ann Rev Physiol* 48:51, 1986.

269. Turner RJ, Silverman M: Sugar uptake into brush border vesicles from dog kidney. II. Kinetics. *Biochim Biophys Acta* 511:470, 1978.

270. Ullrich KJ: Sugar, aminoacid and Na^+ cotransport in the proximal tubule. *Ann Rev Physiol* 41:181, 1979.

271. Ullrich KJ, Capasso G, Rumrich G, et al: Coupling between proximal tubular transport processes: Studies with ouabain, SITS and HCO_3^- free solutions. *Pflugers Arch* 368:245, 1977.

272. Ullrich KJ, Papavassiliou F: Bicarbonate reabsorption in the papillary collecting duct of rats. *Pflugers Arch* 389:271, 1981.

273. Ullrich KJ, Rumrich G, Fritzsch G, et al: Contraluminal p-aminohippurate transport in the proximal tubule of the rat kidney. I. Kinetics, influence of anions, cations and capillary preperfusion. *Pflugers Arch* 409:229, 1987.

274. Vagelos PR: Regulation of fatty acid biosynthesis. *Curr Top Cell Regul* 4:119, 1971.

metabolism and its potential as a uremic toxin. *Am J Physiol* 239:F1, 1980.

275. Vandervalle A, Wirthensohn G, Heidrich HG, et al: Distribution of hexokinase and phosphoenolpyruvate carboxykinase along the rabbit nephron. *Am J Physiol* (Renal Fluid Elect Physiol) 240:F492, 1981.

276. VanSlyke DD, Phillips RA, Hamilton PB, et al: Glutamine as source material of urinary ammonia. *J Biol Chem* 150:481, 1943.

277. Vinay P, Allignet E, Pichette C, et al: Changes in renal metabolite profile and ammoniagenesis during acute and chronic metabolic acidosis in dog and rat. *Kidney Int* 17:312, 1980.

278. Vinay P, Coutlee F, Martel P, et al: Effect of phosphoenolpyruvate carboxykinase inhibition on renal metabolism of glumamine: In vivo studies in the dog and rat. *Can J Biochem* 58:103, 1980.

279. Vinay P, Gougoux A, Lemieux G: Isolation of a pure suspension of rat proximal tubules. *Am J Physiol* 241:F403, 1981.

280. Vinay P, Lemieux G, Gougoux A, et al: Regulation of glutamine metabolism in the dog kidney in vivo. *Kidney Int* 29:68, 1986.

281. Vinay P, Mapes JP, Krebs HA: Fate of glutamine carbon in renal metabolism. *Am J Physiol* 234:F123, 1978.

282. Wacker G, Kissane JM: Quantitative histochemistry of the developing rat kidney. *Lab Invest* 11:690, 1962.

283. Waldman RH, Burch HB: Rapid method of study of enzyme distribution in rat kidney. *Am J Physiol* 204:749, 1963.

284. Wall DA, Maack T: Endocytic uptake, transport and catabolism of proteins by epithelial cells. *Am J Physiol* 248:C12, 1985.

285. Washington JA, Holland JH: Urine oxygen tension: Effect of osmotic and saline diuresis and of ethacrynic acid. *Am J Physiol* 210:243, 1966.

286. Weinman EO, Strisover EH, Chaikoff IL: Conversion of fatty acids to carbohydrates: Application of isotopes to this problem and role of the Krebs cycle as a synthetic pathway. *Physiol Rev* 37:252, 1957.

287. Weinstein SW: Micropuncture study on renal tubular effects of 2,4 dinitrophenol in the rat. *Am J Physiol* 223:583, 1972.

288. Welling L, Linshaw MA: Structural and functional development of outer versus inner cortical proximal tubules. *Pediatr Nephrol* 2:108, 1988.

289. Wiedeman MJ, Krebs HA: The fuel of respiration of rat kidney cortex. *Biochem J* 112:149, 1969.

290. Williamson DH: Ketone body metabolism during development. *Fed Proc* 44:2342, 1985.

291. Windus DW, Cohn DE, Klahr S, et al: Glutamine transport in renal basolateral vesicles from dogs with metabolic acidosis. *Am J Physiol* (Renal Fluid Elect Physiol) 246:F78, 1984.

292. Windus DW, Klahr S, Hammerman MR: Glutamine transport in basolateral vesicles from dogs with acute respiratory acidosis. *Am J Physiol* 247:F403, 1984.

293. Wirthenson G, Guder W: Triacylglycerol metabolism in isolated rat kidney cortex tubules. *Biochem J* 186:317, 1980.

294. Wirthenson G, Guder WG: Renal lipid metabolism. *Miner Electrolyte Metab* 9:203, 1983.

295. Wright SH, Kippen I, Wright EM: Stoichiometry of Na^+-succinate co-transport in renal brush border membranes. *J Biol Chem* 257:1773, 1982.

296. Wright SH, Kippen I, Wright EM: Effect of pH on the transport of Krebs cycle intermediates in renal brush border membranes. *Biochim Biophys Acta* 684:287, 1982.

297. Yaganawa N, Nagami G, Jo O, et al: Dissociation of gluconeogenesis from fluid and phosphate reabsorption in isolated rabbit proximal tubules. *Kidney Int* 25:869, 1984.

298. Yoshitomi K, Fromter E: How big is the electrochemical potential differences for Na^+ across rat renal proximal tubular cell membranes in vivo? *Pflugers Arch* 405:S121, 1985.

299. Zelikovic I, Stejskal E, Lohstroh P, et al: Na^+/H^+ exchange is increased in renal brushborder vesicles from neonatal rat. *Kidney Int* 33:430, 1988.

300. Zerhan K: Oxygen consumption and active sodium transport in the isolated short-circuited frog skin. *Acta Physiol Scand* 36:300, 1956.

301. Zorzoli A: Gluconeogenesis in the mouse kidney cortex. II. Glucose production and enzyme activities in newborn and early postnatal animals. *Dev Biol* 17:400, 1968.

302. Zorzoli A, Turkenkopf IJ, Mueller VL: Gluconeogenesis in developing rat kidney cortex. *Biochem J* 111:181, 1969.

MICHAEL D. BAILIE
THOMAS L. KENNEDY, III

11
Development of the Endocrine Function of the Kidney

The kidney produces several hormones and autocoids* (Table 11-1). Some of the hormones, such as angiotensin II and vitamin D, act not only as modulators of kidney function but also as physiologic regulators of other systems. Hormones produced outside the kidney, such as aldosterone, antidiuretic hormone, atrial natriuretic peptide, parathyroid hormone, calcitonin, and catecholamines and, to a lesser extent, insulin, thyroid hormone, progesterone, and estrogens also affect renal function under a variety of circumstances. Recently, studies have demonstrated that the vascular endothelium produces peptide hormone(s), endothelin(s), which can also modify renal function [251,261]. Finally, the kidney is an important site for the metabolism of several protein and peptide hormones [40,41]. For a detailed discussion of the role of the kidney as an endocrine organ, see the review by Dunn [62].

Renin-Angiotensin System

In 1898, two Danish workers discovered a pressor substance in extracts of renal cortex, which they named renin [282]. Renin is an acid protease that hydrolyzes a protein substrate, angiotensinogen, to form a decapeptide, angiotensin I (AI) (Fig. 11-1). Angiotensinogen is an alpha 2-globulin produced in the liver. AI has no intrinsic activity but is converted to an octapeptide, angiotensin II (AII) by angiotensin I converting enzyme (ACE), a carboxy-terminal dipeptidyl peptidase [108,191]. While ACE is found in a number of organs and tissues, the majority of AII in the systemic circulation is produced when AI is hydrolyzed during passage of blood through the lung [108,192]. Angiotensin II and renin are metabolized primarily in the liver and kidney. It should be noted that ACE is also the enzyme responsible for the degradation of bradykinin.

While renin is produced in a number of organs, the enzyme present in the circulation comes mainly from the kidney [108,192]. Renin is produced at the vascular pole of the glomerulus where the juxtaglomerular (JG) cells of

the afferent arteriole and the macula densa cells of the distal tubule make contact (Fig. 11-1). This region has been referred to as the juxtaglomerular apparatus (JGA). The JG cells are modified smooth muscle cells that contain storage granules of renin [108,147]. Immunoreactive renin is found in the myoepithelioid cells of the JGA as well as in proximal afferent arterioles and interlobular arteries [147]. Renin appears to be synthesized in the rough endoplasmic reticulum and stored in the golgi apparatus. The secretion of renin is primarily by exocytosis of the renin granules, although there may be other ways that renin leaves the cell [147].

The secretion of renin is complex and is regulated by multiple factors (Table 11-2) [54,55,93,121,130]. The kidney acts as a baroreceptor via the granulated JG cells in the afferent arteriole (Fig. 11-2). Increases in renal perfusion pressure inhibit and decreases stimulate renin secretion. In addition, the macula densa of the distal tubule acts as part of a feedback loop that responds to changes in the concentration or rate of delivery of solutes to the distal tubule. Recent studies utilizing the isolated perfused JGA of the rabbit have demonstrated that renin secretion rate increases with decreases in the concentration of sodium chloride at the macula densa and decreases with increasing concentrations [149]. While the rate of delivery of sodium chloride to the macula densa (changes in the flow rate of the tubular fluid) can also affect renin secretion, changes

TABLE 11-1. *Hormones and autocoids produced by the kidney*

1. Renin and angiotensin
2. Prostaglandins and thromboxanes
3. Kallikrein-kinin
4. Vitamin D metabolites
5. Erythropoietin
6. Histamine
7. Serotonin
8. Vasodepressor lipids
9. Dopamine

*A substance produced locally that has its action at or near the site of production—a "local hormone" [59].

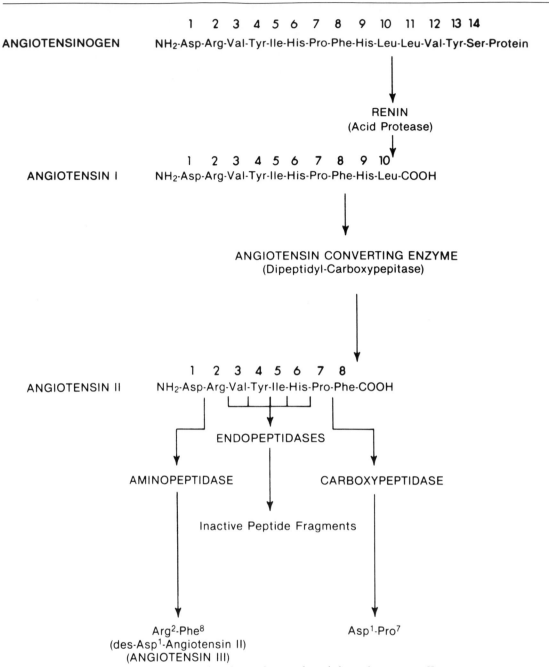

FIG. 11-1. *The enzymatic sequence involved in the synthesis and catabolism of angiotensin II.*

associated with varying the rate of delivery are considerably less than those produced by varying the concentration.

The JG cells are innervated by both cholinergic and dopaminergic nerves. Stimulation of β-adrenergic receptors and dopaminergic nerves results in an increase in the release of renin. Beta-adrenergic blockade inhibits renin secretion. Alpha-adrenergic stimulation probably is inhibitory to renin secretion [130]. Finally, several humoral agents modify the release of renin from the kidney (Table 11-2). One of the more important is the feedback regulation produced by AII. AII has a direct inhibitory effect on the JG cells. Also, by increasing systemic blood pressure, AII causes the baroreceptor suppression of renin release.

The renin-angiotensin system plays a role in a variety of pathologic and physiologic conditions [16,107,142,193]. The renin-angiotensin system has been implicated in several forms of hypertension, including renovascular hypertension, essential hypertension, hypertension of chronic

TABLE 11-2. *Factors regulating the secretion of renin*

1. Renal afferent arteriolar baroreceptors
2. Macula densa feedback
3. Sympathetic nervous system
4. Humoral factors
   Angiotensin II
   Catecholamines
   Dopamine
   Prostaglandins
   Antidiuretic hormone
   Atrial natriuretic factor(s)
5. Sodium, potassium, calcium

renal disease and malignant hypertension [193]. Angiotensin II may also be important in the pathogenesis of numerous non-hypertensive disturbances, including congestive heart failure, nephrotic syndrome, liver failure, hypotension, and shock [107,142]. AII also has been implicated in the regulation of intrarenal blood flow, glomerular filtration rate, and renal water and electrolyte homeostasis [142,184,193].

Utilizing the techniques of molecular biology, it has been possible to greatly expand our knowledge of the control of renin synthesis and secretion [65,67,100,101,120]. The renin gene has been studied and the regulation of gene expression, synthesis-secretion coupling, and tissue expression studied [65]. These techniques allow the study of not only the local production of renin but also of angiotensinogen [65,120]. Ingelfinger et al. found angiotensinogen mRNA expression in the rat was localized to the proximal tubule although there was some expression in the distal tubule and glomerulus [120]. Angiotensinogen gene expression was enhanced by low-salt diet. They postulated that angiotensin II could be formed in the proximal tubule and act as a local hormone. Gomez and co-workers have demonstrated that inhibition of ACE enhances the intrarenal production of renin by the induction of expression of the renin gene in cells that were not previously involved in the secretion of renin [100].

This use of molecular biology in conjunction with physiological studies has greatly aided the investigtion of the effects of the renin-angiotensin system on proximal tubular function. A variety of studies has now demonstrated that AII has a significant effect on sodium transport in the S1 segment of the proximal tubule [50,23]. AII augments primarily sodium bicarbonate transport in the SI segment and acts at both the luminal and basolateral membranes [50]. AII has been shown to stimulate the Na^+-H^+ exchanger. It is proposed that this effect of AII is an important regulator of sodium chloride transport by the proximal tubule and can account for an amount of sodium reabsorption greater than that regulated by aldosterone.

The relationships between the renin-angiotensin system and the renal prostaglandins and between the sympathetic nervous system and the regulation of glomerular function have been reviewed extensively [7,24,118,136,232,254]. Numerous studies have demonstrated the existence of a

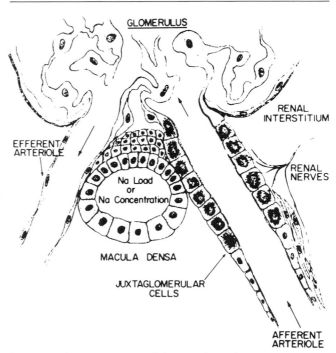

FIG. 11-2. *Diagramatic view of the juxtaglomerular apparatus. From Davis JO, Freeman RH: Mechanisms regulating renin release. Physiol Rev 56:1, 1976, with permission of the American Heart Association, Inc.*

complex interaction between AII and other vasoactive hormones. AII receptors have been found to be present not only in the renal arterioles but also in the glomerulus and renal tubules [23,24,50,118,254]. AII clearly has effects on factors that modify glomerular hemodynamics, including increasing glomerular hydrostatic pressure and reducing the glomerular ultrafiltration coefficient. In addition to being a potent vasopressor, AII is also a stimulator of aldosterone secretion by the adrenal gland [192], which enhances distal tubular sodium reabsorption and potassium excretion. Finally, it is now becoming clear that production of renin and angiotensinogen in several tissues in addition to kidney (brain, heart, adrenal gland, vascular endothelium) can lead to local production of AII [64]. This local generation of AII may be important in the regulation of blood pressure and organ function.

The measurement of renin in plasma depends on the determination of the concentration of AI formed after a timed incubation of the sample. Conversion of AI to AII is blocked by adding inhibitors of ACE. Plasma renin activity (PRA) is determined by the amount of AI formed from the angiotensinogen present in the sample. Plasma renin concentration (PRC) is determined after the addition of an excess amount of angiotensinogen to the sample [108]. PRA and PRC are usually expressed as nanograms of AI formed per milliliter of plasma per hour (ng/ml/hr). However, some laboratories do use other units of concentration and time. With the isolation of the renin gene, the direct assay of renin is now possible but not in clinical use.

Development of the Renin-Angiotensin System

The concentration of AII in the systemic circulation or at local receptor sites depends on the concentration of all of the intermediate constituents of the system, i.e., angiotensinogen, renin, AI, ACE, and angiotensinases. During growth and development, a quantitative change may occur in any of these components, either because of changes in their rate of production or in their rate of catabolism. In addition, the number or affinity of the AII receptors may change with age.

Because of the complex nature of the control of renin release, the study of the regulation of PRA is difficult at best. This is especially true in the newborn and developing animal where many of the regulatory factors may change rapidly because of normal growth and development. Granular JG cells have been identified in the kidneys of fetal and newborn animals and humans [56,148,233,253, 277,278]. The presence of these cells suggests that the kidney can produce renin in utero. Gomez et al. have studied the expression and distribution of the renin and angiotensinogen genes in the developing rat kidney [101,102]. They found that renal renin concentration was higher in newborn than in adult rats. The distribution of renin in the newborn kidney was seen throughout the length of the afferent and interlobular vessels. As the animals matured, the distribution pattern changed to that of the adult with primary localization in the JGA. Angiotensinogen mRNA was found in both the newborn and adult kidneys. Renin mRNA levels were eightfold higher in the newborn than in the adult. Renin mRNA was found in kidney of fetal rats at 20 days of gestation. El-Dahr et al. have utilized these techniques to study the changes in renal renin in rats with unilateral ureteral obstruction carried out in the first month of life [67]. They found increased distribution of immunoreactive renin in both kidneys in animals with unilateral ureteral obstruction. These studies support previous physiologic observations that ureteral obstruction leads to an increase of renin content of both kidneys, and that the ACE inhibitor, enalapril, modifies the changes in renal hemodynamics associated with ureteral obstruction [46,47].

Studies have directly demonstrated the ability of the kidney of the fetus and newborn of several species to secrete renin [13,60,61,245,255,272]. Changes in PRA and in the factors that regulate renin secretion have been studied in a number of animal models and in the human both during prenatal and postnatal development [13,22,29,45,58,60, 61,95,96,115,128,133,195,209,210,211,214,218,219, 223,243–245,246,248,255,25., 258,270–274,283,284, 287,293,296,299].

PRA in the human is high at birth and during early childhood [95,96,115,133,211,230,272,284,287] compared to the normal adult. Following birth, there is a gradual fall in PRA, with adult values being reached near puberty [115,272,284,287]. Hiner et al. [115] reported that PRA decreased from a mean value of 2.37 ng/ml/hr in children two to four years of age to 1.08 ng/ml/hr by 16 or 17 years of age. Van Acker and co-workers [284] found that the PRA in three-month-old to 12-month-old infants averaged 6.27 ng/ml/hr and had decreased to 2.07 ng/ml/

hr in teenagers. The highest levels are found in the newborn period, where values as high as 17.2 ng/ml/hr have been reported [95]. Plasma renin is also higher in premature infants as young as 30 weeks gestational age [218,271]. Measurements in rodents, lambs, dogs, pigs, and rabbits have revealed similar high values at birth [13,61,206, 214,244,255].

Renin in the plasma of the fetus and newborn could be maintained at an elevated level by several factors, including (1) a high rate of renin release from the kidney, (2) a relatively small volume of distribution of renin in relation to the rate of release, and (3) a slower rate of degradation of renin by the immature liver and kidney. Most studies demonstrate that the factors that trigger the release of renin in the adult are also effective in the newborn and fetus. For example, the human newborn, the fetal lamb, and newborn piglet release renin in response to furosemide [13,209,246,248,274,283]. Hypoxia and asphyxia also increase PRA in the newborn lamb and piglet [13,299]. Decreased renal perfusion pressure, isoproterenol, hemorrhage, and inhibition of AII or inhibition of ACE activity result in an increase in PRA in the newborn [13,224, 245,255]. Renin is suppressed by volume expansion, AII, and propranolol in the fetus and newborn of several species [13,61,247,248].

Only a few investigators have measured the rate of secretion of renin from the kidney of the newborn [13,299]. The results of studies in the piglet suggest that PRA may not be determined by the rate of renin release [13]. Indeed, while the concentration of renin in the plasma of these animals decreased by fivefold and sixfold during the first 50 days of life, the rate of renin release remained relatively constant. Thus, PRA may be more dependent on the volume of distribution of renin or its rate of degradation than on the rate of renin release.

Osborn et al. [195] and Solomon et al. [258] have studied the catabolism of renin in newborns. In the nephrectomized piglet, the half-life of renin in the circulation decreased from 17 minutes in one-day-old to five-day-old animals to 12 minutes at 50 days of age [195]. The half-life of renin also has been reported to decrease in the developing rat [258]. While the direction of this change may explain a fall in PRA with age, the difference between the half-lives was not statistically significant. Additional work is needed to clarify whether or not the metabolism of renin changes with age.

Finally, in addition to the active form of renin usually measured in plasma, an inactive form of the enzyme has been identified [237,238]. Inactive renin is released by the kidney of the newborn piglet and by the kidney of the fetal lamb in response to a variety of stimuli, including decreased renal perfusion pressure and isoproterenol infusion into the renal artery [13,248]. The secretion of active and inactive renin from renal cortical tissues slices obtained from fetal, newborn, and adult sheep has been measured [180]. Veratridine, which promotes the release of norepinephrine from nerve terminals, stimulated the secretion of active renin but **not inactive** renin in slices from fetal and newborn animals. This response could be blocked with propranolol, indicating that active renin secretion in the fetal and newborn sheep was in part dependent on the β-adrenoceptors. Active and inactive renin have been measured in the plasma of children [25,26,74,304]. In one study, the concentration of active renin was higher in children than in adults but inactive renin was not found in plasma of most children under one year of age [25]. Other studies have demonstrated inactive renin in the plasma of newborns and infants and have found values greater than those seen in adults [74,304]. The physiologic significance of circulating prorenin in children or adults remains unclear.

Circulating angiotensinogen is produced in the liver [108,192], and changes in concentration of the substrate for renin could result in changes in PRA. The concentration of angiotensinogen in the plasma of the pregnant human or animal is elevated [45,96,133], probably secondary to the effect of estrogen on its production by liver [113]. Several studies have revealed that the concentration of substrate in cord plasma is considerably less than that in maternal plasma [96,128,133]. However, whether or not the concentration of angiotensinogen is significantly greater in human infants than in older children or adults is not clear. Two studies have demonstrated that the difference in plasma angiotensinogen concentration between non-pregnant and pregnant women is approximately fourfold, while the difference between the newborn and the non-pregnant adult is less than twofold [96,133]. On the other hand, a low substrate concentration has been demonstrated during childhood, suggesting that substrate concentration may be a limiting factor in the determination of PRA [29]. It is possible that the high concentration of renin in plasma may result in the utilization of substrate at a rate greater than it can be formed.

Carver and Mott found that the substrate concentration was lower in the fetal lamb than in maternal plasma [45]. Nephrectomy of the fetus has resulted in a threefold increase in substrate concentration, consistent with the ability of the kidney to synthesize renin. In one study in rats, the concentration of substrate in the plasma was found to change little during the first 80 days of life [214]. Another study suggests that the concentration of substrate in plasma of rats at birth is not rate-limiting and may increase with age [293]. Yet another study indicates that changes in substrate concentration in rat plasma over the first eight to ten weeks of life may well affect PRA [296]. Lee et al. have demonstrated angiotensinogen mRNA in rat embryos, suggesting a biological function for the renin-angiotensin system in early development [139]. Additional studies are clearly needed to determine if changes in the concentration of substrate in plasma are important in regulating the final concentration of AII in plasma during development.

ACE is a peptidyldipeptide hydrolase that catalyzes the cleavage of the carboxy terminus dipeptide of AI, converting it to the active component, AII. While ACE is present in a number of tissues and in plasma, only that in the lung appears capable of affecting the concentration of AII in plasma [191]. Limitation of the concentration or the activity of pulmonary ACE during early development could result in lower concentrations of AII in plasma.

Studies in rats have demonstrated developmental changes in pulmonary ACE [295,298]. In the fetal rat lung, ACE became detectable at 18 days gestation and increased by approximately sixfold during the remaining three days of pregnancy [295]. Following birth, there is a further increase in the activity of pulmonary ACE [294]. Kinetic analysis suggests that this rise in ACE activity in lung tissue is due to an increase in enzyme content and not to a change in enzyme-substrate affinity.

Immunochemical techniques have been used to determine the presence of ACE in kidneys from human fetuses and children [172]. ACE was detected in fetal kidneys between 11 weeks and 14 weeks of gestation and was located on the basolateral membranes and primary apical microvilli of cells in the early proximal tubule. In addition, ACE was found on glomerular endothelial cells. The same distribution was found in kidneys from infants and children. ACE also has been measured in plasma from developing rat fetuses and was found to be higher than that in the maternal plasma [205]. Neither the source nor the significance of this increased concentration of ACE in fetal plasma is known.

A relationship between the developmental changes in ACE and AII generation is suggested in the rat by the coincidence between the peak in plasma AII concentration and the rapid increase in pulmonary ACE activity that occurs during the fifth postnatal week. No similar information is available for the human neonate.

Angiotensin II is degraded by several different enzymes, including a carboxypeptidase, an aminopeptidase, and an endopeptidase. While angiotensinases are present in plasma, studies suggest that peripheral capillary beds, including those in the kidney, are the most important sites of AII degradation [41,191,192]. In vivo and in vitro studies have revealed that there is an increase in angiotensinase activity in both rats and rabbits during development [30,214,297]. Whether or not these changes affect the plasma concentration of AII remains unknown.

While the factors regulating the release of renin in the newborn and fetus are reasonably well defined, the role played by the renin-angiotensin system during this period of life is less well understood. A number of investigators have attempted to fill this void [22,61,103,195,208,219,223, 224,242,255,272,283,293,299] but have encountered several problems that made the interpretation of their findings precarious. Prominent among these are the difficulties in measuring hemodynamic variables, including cardiac output and the distribution of blood flow, in newborn animals and humans. Furthermore, the suggestion that the sensitivity of the target organs to AII may be different in newborn and adult animals [224,242,305] complicates further the interpretation of data.

Studies in the newborn animal and fetus have revealed an increase in plasma renin in response to adverse conditions such as hypoxia, asphyxia, and hemorrhage [5,103, 255,299]. Hypoxemia causes an increase in PRA in both newborn piglets and lambs [5,299]. In the fetal lamb at 120 days of gestation (term 140 days), Smith et al. [270] found that constriction of the aorta above the renal arteries results in a twofold to 2.5-fold increase in PRA. These investigators also found that a reduction in the blood volume of the fetal-placental unit by 8% to 10% resulted in an increase in PRA from approximately 4 ng/ml/hr to 55 ng/ml/hr. Changes in renal blood flow, mean arterial blood pressure, and renal vascular resistance have been determined in response to hemorrhage in the 120-day and 130-day fetal lamb with and without pretreatment with the ACE inhibitor, captopril [103]. Captopril did not modify the response in the 120-day-old fetus. However, in the older fetus captopril treatment resulted in a decrease in blood pressure during hemorrhage, which was not seen in the untreated animals.

The role of the renin-angiotensin system in the regulation of fetal and neonatal fluid and electrolyte homeostasis has also been studied [61,95,223,272]. Drukker et al. [61] demonstrated that in the newborn dog between one week and three weeks of age, plasma renin concentration (PRC) fell in response to intravascular volume expansion. They were unable to demonstrate any correlation between age-related changes in renal blood flow. Robillard et al. [223] found a positive correlation between PRA and plasma aldosterone concentration in the fetal lamb. Since the slope of the line relating PRA and aldosterone concentration was greater before than after birth, they suggested that the fetal adrenal gland was more sensitive to aldosterone than that of the animal after birth. An inverse correlation between urinary sodium to potassium concentration ratio and plasma aldosterone suggested that aldosterone was in part responsible for the decrease in the ratio seen with increasing fetal age.

In the human newborn, relationships between PRA,

aldosterone, and sodium balance have been determined [95,272]. The results of these studies suggest there is a role for the renin-angiotensin system and aldosterone in the changing sodium balance of the healthy newborn infant.

Prostaglandins

The prostaglandins and thromboxanes are formed from the 20-carbon essential fatty acid, arachidonic acid, in many tissues, including the kidney [63,171]. Our knowledge of the chemistry and the physiologic significance of these autocoids has expanded at a rapid rate since their discovery in 1930, and their biochemistry and physiology have been extensively reviewed [52,63,171]. Arachidonic acid can be oxygenated by two major pathways, one involving lipoxygenase leading to the formation of leukotrienes, and the other via cyclo-oxygenase leading to the formation of the prostaglandins and thromboxane (Fig. 11-3). A third pathway involving a cytochrome P-450 monooxygenase has also been described [52]. At least 24 of the potential cyclo-oxygenase derivatives can be produced by the kidney [63]. The most important renal prostaglandins and their site of synthesis are shown in Table 11-3.

The study of prostaglandin synthesis and physiology has been difficult because these compounds have a very short half-life and their actions are diverse. In addition, the rapid

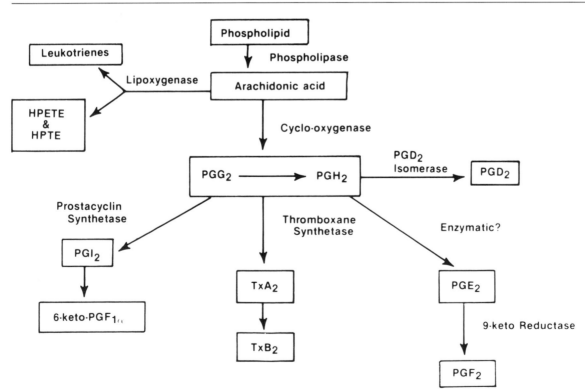

FIG. 11-3. *The prostaglandin cascade. 6-keto-PGF$_1$ and TxB$_2$ are stable degradation products of the parent compounds.*

TABLE 11-3. *Renal prostaglandins and their site of synthesis*

PG	Site
1. PGE_2	Glomeruli, CCT, MCT, MTHAL, MIC
2. PGF_2	Glomeruli, MCT, MTHAL, MIC
3. PGI_2	Glomeruli, Arterioles, MCT
4. TxA_2	Glomeruli, MCT

CCT = cortical collecting tubule, MCT = medullary collecting tubule, MTHAL = medullary thick ascending limb, MIC = medullary interstitial cells, PGI_2 = Prostacycin

TABLE 11-4. *Factors affecting the regulation of renal prostaglandin synthesis*

A. Hormones
 1. Angiotensin
 2. Catecholamines
 3. Vasopressin
 4. Kinins
B. Drugs
 1. Diuretics
 2. Calcium
 3. ATP
C. Pathological Conditions
 1. Renal failure
 2. Hydronephrosis
 3. Hypertension
 4. Renal ischemia
 5. Bartter's syndrome
 6. Glomerulonephritis

catabolism of prostaglandins in the lungs makes the concentrations in the systemic circulation low and not necessarily representative of local tissue levels. The discovery of stable metabolic products, 6-keto-$PGF_{1\alpha}$ for prostacyclin and TxB_2 for thromboxane A_2, has improved the ability to determine their presence in body fluids.

Prostaglandins are produced in both the renal cortex and medulla (Table 11-3). It had been suggested that only one type of prostaglandin was synthesized in any segment of the nephron [9,63,276]. However, studies now indicate that several prostaglandins may be synthesized at the same site [9,111]. Since prostaglandins are not stored, increased release reflects increased synthesis. Prostaglandin synthesis may be affected by a number of factors, including changes in renal hemodynamics, certain drugs, renal and non-renal hormones, and a number of pathologic states (Table 11-4).

TxA_2 is produced in very low amounts by the normal kidney. However, in pathologic conditions such as hydronephrosis and acute renal failure, increased urinary excretion has been observed [63,137,213]. Reingold et al. found that there was increased release of PGE_2, PGI_2, and TxA_2 by the hydronephrotic rabbit kidney [216]. However, the response of the hydronephrotic cat kidney was much less and no TxA_2 was seen. These data suggest species differences in this response. Kühl and coworkers determined prostaglandin excretion in 24 newborns and young children with obstructive uropathy and found increased excretion of PGE_2 and TxB_2, the stable metabolic product of TxA_2. However, it is not clear whether the TxA_2 produced under these conditions is synthesized by renal cells or by inflammatory cells that invade the hydronephrotic kidney or by platelets that become trapped in the damaged kidney [63]. Furthermore, the physiologic significance of these changes in prostaglandin production on glomerular or tubular function is unknown.

The renal prostaglandins have been implicated in a number of regulatory functions, including renal vascular resistance, glomerular filtration, renin release, vasopressin release, and modulation of its end-organ action and in the modulation of the renal kallikrein-kinin system [69,90, 106,114,181,232,234]. These relationships are complex, and some are species specific.

Development of Renal Prostaglandins

Pace-Asciak studied developmental changes in renal prostaglandin metabolism [199]. In the newborn rat kidney at ten and 19 days of age, he found relatively small differences in prostaglandin synthesis compared to adult animals. However, activities of catabolizing enzymes changed as much as 60-fold in relation to adult values. On the other hand, Friedman et al. found that between 22 weeks and 40 weeks of gestational age there is increasing ability of the renal cortex and the medulla of the human to produce prostaglandins E_2 and $F_{2\alpha}$ [88]. Biosynthesis was greater in the medulla than in the cortex and the production of PGE_2 was consistently greater than that of $PGF_{2\alpha}$. Increases in cyclo-oxygenase activity were observed by Stygles et al. to occur between four weeks and 15 weeks of age in kidneys of spontaneously hypertensive rats [267].

Several investigators have demonstrated the presence of prostaglandins in the urine and plasma of fetal animals. PGE_2, $PGF_{2\alpha}$, 6-keto-$PGF_1\alpha$, and TxB_2 have been found in the urine and amniotic fluid of fetal sheep and the pregnant ewe [170,291,292]. Silver et al. also determined PGE_2 and $PGF_{2\alpha}$ in the plasma of fetal horses [250]. Prostaglandin concentration generally increased during gestation.

There are several studies on the concentration of prostaglandins in urine and plasma of premature and full-term newborns, infants, and children [31,69,97,119,126,249, 275]. The plasma concentration and the urinary excretion of PGE_2 excretion are low in the newborn and increase as the individual matures [31,119,249]. In premature infants between 29 weeks and 33 weeks gestational age, Sulyok et al. found a threefold increase in PGE_2 excretion during the first three weeks of postnatal life [275]. Sodium chloride supplementation caused a more rapid decrease in the plasma concentration of PGE_2 and $PGF_{2\alpha}$ than in infants who were not supplemented. The authors speculate that the high concentration of prostaglandins in the plasma of the premature infants may balance the vasoconstriction resulting from an elevated PRA. The relationship between the concentration of the prostaglandins in the plasma and the rate of urinary excretion needs to be clarified further.

As with other hormones, the developmental changes in prostaglandin levels depend mainly on the relative activity of enzymes involved in their synthesis and catabolism. Pace-Asciak has extensively studied the development of the prostaglandin catabolizing enzymes, prostaglandin 15-hydroxydehydrogenase (15-PGDH), prostaglandin 9-hydroxydehydrogenase (9-PGDH), and prostaglandin 13-reductase (13-PGR) in renal tissue as well as other organs of the rat and lamb [197–199]. The results demonstrate that the pattern of development varies from enzyme to enzyme, organ to organ, and species to species. For example, in the rat kidney, 15-PGDH reaches peak activity at 19 days of age, being some 60 times greater than in the adult kidney. In the rat lung, this peak is seen at one day of postnatal age and is only 2.5 times the adult value [198]. In the lamb lung the peak occurs at 115 days gestational age (term, 140 days) and is four times that of the adult, while the peak in the kidney occurs at 120 days and is the same as that seen in the adult animal [198,199]. The physiologic significance of this variability remains to be determined.

While understanding of the role of prostaglandins in the regulation of renal function in the fetus and newborn has remained behind that achieved in the adult, studies have been undertaken to define the response to inhibition of prostaglandin synthesis [11,14,86,87,143,159,196,199, 306]. Winther et al. reported that in the newborn lamb indomethacin caused a reduction in effective renal plasma flow and urine flow rate without altering glomerular filtration rate [306]. Similarly, in the fetal lamb, indomethacin caused a decrease in renal blood flow in the absence of changes in glomerular filtration rate [159]. A fall in PRA was also noticed in these animals. These studies suggest that the renal prostaglandins participate in the regulation of renal hemodynamics and affect renin release in the fetal lamb. In newborn piglets, Osborn and co-workers found no change in renal blood flow or the intrarenal distribution of blood flow following administration of indomethacin [14,196]. There is no explanation for these species differences. Recently, Meléndez et al. measured PGE_2 receptors in the kidney of the developing rat [167]. They reported a higher affinity for PGE_2 in the 5-day-old animal when compared to the adult. They also found that the newborn animal had a greater rate of excretion of PGE_2 than the 21-day-old animal, suggesting greater rate of synthesis. Inhibition of prostaglandin synthesis by indomethacin or acetaminophen blocked the renal response of the 5-day-old rat to water deprivation while enhancing the response in the more mature animal. They speculate that the differences in physiological response may be related to the differences in affinity to PGE_2 at the various ages.

In the human neonate, the effects of inhibition of prostaglandin synthesis on renal function have been studied during treatment for patent ductus arteriosis and lung disease [48,88]. Results of these studies suggest that a transient fall in glomerular filtration rate takes place during treatment. It is apparent that the studies performed so far have not generated a clear picture of the relationship between changes in prostaglandins and changes in renal function or in systemic cardiovascular control with age [86,143].

Kallikrein-Kinin System

The kallikrein-kinin system was first described in 1937 [301]. It consists of a sequence of proteins with distinct physiologic activity that results from enzymatic proteolysis. Several excellent reviews of this system are available [42,143,154,188,213,236]. Because of difficulties in developing reliable assays, because the system exhibits multifactorial regulation, and because the effects of kinins are not easily distinguishable from those of other hormones, progress in understanding this system has been slow.

Furthermore, understanding is complicated because there are two kallikrein-kinin systems, one present in plasma and one present in certain other tissues. The first involves a kallikrein that has a molecular weight of approximately 100,000 daltons. The other, known as glandular kallikrein, is found in exocrine glands and their secretions, lung, pancreas, and kidney and has a molecular weight of 24,000 daltons to 44,000 daltons [42]. In plasma and kidney, kallikrein exists as a zymogen, prekallikrein, which is involved in the activation of factor XI of the intrinsic clotting mechanism [8]. Once activated, kallikreins are serine proteases, are very similar to pancreatic trypsin, and act on substrates, kininogens, to form vasoactive peptides, kinins (Fig. 11-4).

Two forms of kininogen exist. Both are synthesized in the liver [33]: one is of high molecular weight (HMW), while the other is of low molecular weight (LMW). Plasma kallikrein preferentially activates the HMW substrate to form bradykinin, while glandular kallikrein can act on both to form lysbradykinin or kallidin (Fig. 11-4) [42]. Kinins are inactivated by two enzymes, arginine carboxypeptidase, or Kininase I, and peptidyl carboxylase, or Kininase II. This latter enzyme is identical to ACE (Figs. 11-1 and 11-4).

Plasma kallikrein, also known as Fletcher factor, has three recognized functions. First, it is the most potent activator of Hageman factor and, therefore, is involved in both coagulation and fibrinolysis [173]. Second, it is chemotactic for polymorphonuclear leukocytes. Third, it generates the potent vasodilator, bradykinin and, therefore, may be involved in the regulation of blood pressure. Plasma kallikrein also may contribute to the activation of the complement system [260].

The precise role of the renal kallikrein-kinin system is uncertain. It is evident that it is an integral part of a number of intrarenal hormonal systems, including renin-angiotensin [239,286], aldosterone [153,286], prostaglandins [164,182], and vasopressin [154]. As such, the renal kallikrein-kinin system may play an important role in the control and distribution of renal blood flow and the regulation of salt and water excretion. Urinary kallikrein mediates the conversion of inactive to active renin *in vitro* [239] and may stimulate intrarenal renin release [280].

Urinary kallikrein excretion shows a direct correlation with plasma aldosterone concentration in subjects placed on varying sodium intakes [153,286], to the extent that

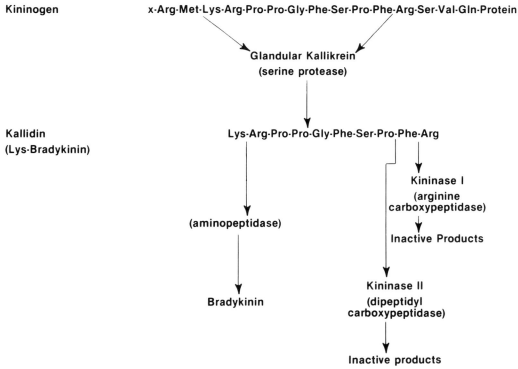

FIG. 11-4. *The enzymes of the kallikrein-kinin system.*

the rate of kallikrein excretion can be used as an index of circulating levels of salt retaining hormone. Further, the kallikrein-kinin system stimulates the production of renal prostaglandins, including PGE_2 and PGI_2 [164], which in turn modulate the reactivity of the renal vessels to pressor hormones [182]. Finally, the renal kallikrein-kinin system may play a role in several pathophysiologic states, including essential hypertension [161,169], chronic renal insufficiency [144], and conditions associated with high aldosterone concentrations such as Bartter's syndrome [163], although a definite connection to any disease remains unproven [151].

The activity of the renal kallikrein-kinin system is usually assessed by measuring urinary kallikrein, since all kallikrein in the urine is believed to originate in the kidney. Several methods are available, all with certain limitations [44]. Some involve the measurement of kinin-releasing activity, and some measure the protein quantitatively [236]. Urinary kinins appear to reflect kinins generated by kallikrein in the kidney rather than those present in the plasma. In several species, renal kallikrein synthesis has been localized to the granular segment of the distal tubule and of the cortical collecting tubule [43,187,189,194]. Recently, renal kallikrein has been identified in the human nephron in the connecting tubule cells [72]. This is of particular interest since kininogen is found in the intermingled principal cells of the cortical collecting tubules while the inactivating kininases are concentrated in the proximal nephron [72]. The release of renal kallikrein is stimulated by mineralocorticoids, sodium restriction, diuretics, and vasodilator agents [144,288]. Among inhibitors of the system are indomethacin [20] and amiloride [152].

Development of the Renal Kallikrein-Kinin System

There are only limited studies dealing with the developmental aspects of the kallikrein-kinin system. The physiological importance of this system in the regulation of renal blood flow, natriuresis, or water excretion in the fetus or newborn remains to be determined [221,222]. Urinary kallikrein activity and total excretion have been measured in small groups of newborns and is lower through the first year of life than in older children, even when corrected for body weight [17,20,98]. There is speculation that the reduced activity may reflect decreased distal nephron mass and/or maturity, including diminished responsiveness to hormones such as aldosterone [289]. The levels correlate directly with levels of urinary prostaglandins and inversely with PRA [98]. Indomethacin administration to preterm infants leads to a decrease in urinary kallikrein, perhaps secondary to suppression of kallikrein synthesis [20].

Prekallikrein levels in the serum of premature infants are low and increase with gestational as well as postnatal age [6]. The normal temporal increase in prekallikrein is delayed in sick infants but occurs when the infant recovers

milk [109,166]. However, there is maternal influence on fetal erythropoiesis in instances when oxygen delivery is markedly impaired, for example, in severe maternal hypoxemia [110], anemia [311], or placental insufficiency [165]. Recognizing that the fetus will respond to chronic intrauterine hypoxia and stress with an elevation of erythropoietin in both serum [185,228] and amniotic fluid [290], recent studies have demonstrated the utility of erythropoietin levels as a marker of fetal distress and central nervous system injury [227]. In maternal diabetes mellitus, the high fetal insulin levels, secondary to hyperglycemia, correlate directly with cord erythropoietin levels [303]. Although these results could suggest a role for insulin in fetal erythropoietin production, a more likely explanation is that erythropoietin increases in response to the effect of insulin to increase tissue oxygen consumption, resulting in fetal hypoxemia [303]. This increase in oxygen demand may exceed the oxygen carrying capacity of the blood causing a relative hypoxic state in the fetus [158]. Recently, however, insulin [266] and perhaps other erythropoietic stimulating factors [229] have been shown to stimulate fetal erythropoiesis independent of erythropoietin. Nevertheless, it appears that erythropoietin is the major erythropoietic growth factor and hypoxia is the primary stimulus for erythropoietin production. This is true antenatally as well as postnatally [307], although the response of the fetus or newborn to a hypoxic insult is blunted when compared to an older infant [264,265]. Erythropoietin levels are variable but are generally above adult normals. The levels fall shortly after birth and remain very low in the first month of life and then increase to adult normal, which persist throughout childhood [112,165]. The fall after birth temporally precedes the decline in erythropoiesis and the "physiologic anemia" of the second and third months of life.

The levels of erythropoietin observed in response to similar degrees of hypoxia are lower in newborns than in adults [37]. While there is some evidence that this may be due to the fact that erythroid progenitor cells of the newborn are more sensitive to erythropoietin [145], it is generally agreed that CFU-E targets are equally responsive in the newborn and adults. According to the "adaptive theory" of Finne and Halvorsen [73], the shift from hemoglobin F to hemoglobin A and the increase in 2,3-diphosphoglycerate in red cells in the newborn, which allow more effective tissue oxygenation, makes the observed fall in erythropoietin levels understandable and even predictable. Additionally, one might speculate that erythropoietin levels may not truly reflect the numbers or sensitivity of erythroid progenitor cells or that low serum erythropoietin levels may be due in part to rapid internalization and degradation in a bone marrow whose volume almost equals that of the adult [135,183].

Erythropoietin levels also may be low during the newborn period because of the presence of erythropoietin inhibitors that have been isolated from the urine of two-day-old infants and persist throughout the first month of life [21,146,253]. The nature and the role of these inhibitors are not known.

The liver, probably the Kupffer cell, is the major source of erythropoietin in the fetus [37,235,308]. Although there is some interspecies variation [150], it is clear that some time after birth, there is a shift from hepatic to renal synthesis of erythropoietin. This switch does not appear to reflect the site of erythropoiesis [4] or the type of hemoglobin being produced [201]. In sheep, the switch begins during the third trimester, is complete by 40 days after birth, and is characterized by a gradual decrease in hepatic synthesis and an increase in renal erythropoietin formation [309]. That certain factors may influence this shift in site of production is demonstrated in the fetal sheep, where the absence of thyroid hormone delays the switch, while excess thyroxin accelerates it [309]. In rat neonates, the switch to renal synthesis is hastened by hypoxia [49]. The timing of the transition in the human is not known. In the premature infant, the fetal pattern persists, supporting the idea that hepatic synthesis is less sensitive to hypoxia than the kidney and defends against the polycythemia that could result from reduced intrauterine PO_2 [53]. Once the transition has occurred, the kidney becomes the major source of erythropoietin, accounting for 90% to 95% of the erythropoietin produced in response to hypoxia [122]. Although intrarenal oxygen sensing appears to be most important in erythropoietin synthesis [15], there is also evidence for a role for extrarenal hypoxia sensors, perhaps involving the hypothalamus [200].

In summary, the "physiologic anemia" of the newborn and the "anemia of prematurity" appear to result from insufficient levels of erythropoietin. The number and responsiveness of erythroid progenitors are normal, and, therefore, a rationale exists for the possible use of recombinant erythropoietin in infants with these anemias. Such use is not without potential problems, and the considerations for clinical trials are well summarized in a recent review [240].

Histamine and Serotonin

The formation of serotonin (5-hydroxytryptamine) (Fig. 11-5) requires two steps: L-tryptophan is hydroxylated by tryptophan-5-hydroxylase to L-5-hydroxytryptophan (L-5-HTP), which is then converted by aromatic L-amino acid decarboxylase to serotonin. Histamine (Fig. 11-5) is formed by the action of L-histidine decarboxylase on histidine. All the enzymes required to produce these vasoactive autocoids have been identified in renal tissue [1].

At least two studies have demonstrated the formation of serotonin by the kidney. Stier et al. [263] infused the amino acid precursor of serotonin, L-5-HTP, into the isolated non-blood perfused rat kidney and found an increase in the concentration of serotonin in the urine and in the venous effluent. Furthermore, carbidopa, a decarboxylase inhibitor, and ketanserin, a serotonin-2 receptor antagonist, blocked the increase in renal vascular resistance associated with the infusion of L-5-HTP. Pirotzky and co-workers [212] not only demonstrated the renal release of serotonin but also demonstrated the release of histamine, slow-reacting substance, and platelet-activating factor following the infusion of a calcium ionophore in the isolated rat kidney. These findings support the concept that several mediators of inflammation are produced by the kidney

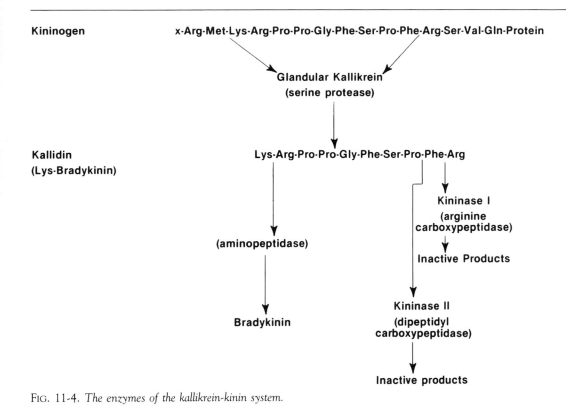

FIG. 11-4. *The enzymes of the kallikrein-kinin system.*

the rate of kallikrein excretion can be used as an index of circulating levels of salt retaining hormone. Further, the kallikrein-kinin system stimulates the production of renal prostaglandins, including PGE_2 and PGI_2 [164], which in turn modulate the reactivity of the renal vessels to pressor hormones [182]. Finally, the renal kallikrein-kinin system may play a role in several pathophysiologic states, including essential hypertension [161,169], chronic renal insufficiency [144], and conditions associated with high aldosterone concentrations such as Bartter's syndrome [163], although a definite connection to any disease remains unproven [151].

The activity of the renal kallikrein-kinin system is usually assessed by measuring urinary kallikrein, since all kallikrein in the urine is believed to originate in the kidney. Several methods are available, all with certain limitations [44]. Some involve the measurement of kinin-releasing activity, and some measure the protein quantitatively [236]. Urinary kinins appear to reflect kinins generated by kallikrein in the kidney rather than those present in the plasma. In several species, renal kallikrein synthesis has been localized to the granular segment of the distal tubule and of the cortical collecting tubule [43,187,189,194]. Recently, renal kallikrein has been identified in the human nephron in the connecting tubule cells [72]. This is of particular interest since kininogen is found in the intermingled principal cells of the cortical collecting tubules while the inactivating kininases are concentrated in the proximal nephron [72]. The release of renal kallikrein is stimulated by mineralocorticoids, sodium restriction, diuretics, and vasodilator agents [144,288]. Among inhibitors of the system are indomethacin [20] and amiloride [152].

Development of the Renal Kallikrein-Kinin System

There are only limited studies dealing with the developmental aspects of the kallikrein-kinin system. The physiological importance of this system in the regulation of renal blood flow, natriuresis, or water excretion in the fetus or newborn remains to be determined [221,222]. Urinary kallikrein activity and total excretion have been measured in small groups of newborns and is lower through the first year of life than in older children, even when corrected for body weight [17,20,98]. There is speculation that the reduced activity may reflect decreased distal nephron mass and/or maturity, including diminished responsiveness to hormones such as aldosterone [289]. The levels correlate directly with levels of urinary prostaglandins and inversely with PRA [98]. Indomethacin administration to preterm infants leads to a decrease in urinary kallikrein, perhaps secondary to suppression of kallikrein synthesis [20].

Prekallikrein levels in the serum of premature infants are low and increase with gestational as well as postnatal age [6]. The normal temporal increase in prekallikrein is delayed in sick infants but occurs when the infant recovers

[6]. Plasma kallikrein and prekallikrein levels are low in infants with respiratory distress syndrome [231] but appear to play no important pathophysiological role. On the other hand, the renal kallikrein-kinin system may be significant in the newborn spontaneously hypertensive rat where depressed kallikrein activity appears to be related to an inherited defect in prekallikrein activation [3].

Cord blood kininogen has been found to be one-third to one-half of adult plasma level and appears to be depressed in infants who suffer birth asphyxia [168,279]. Kinin levels in cord blood vary considerably from infant to infant but, on average, are significantly greater than in plasma of adults [168]. Kininase activity, on the other hand, does not appear to be low at birth [168] or change throughout childhood [75].

The fact that levels of kallikrein-kinin system proteins are low in the newborn should not be construed to mean that the kallikrein-kinin system is unimportant at this age. Bradykinin is capable of constricting smooth muscle from the umbilical artery [68] and producing significant pulmonary vasodilation, dependent in part on PGI_2 [83]. Umbilical smooth muscle constriction appears to be favored by oxygen tensions close to the physiologic range [68] and thus may play a role in the regulation of the transitional circulation [83]. In fetal lambs, exogenously administered bradykinin is capable of significant cardiovascular effects, including profound systemic vasodilation, increased pulmonary blood flow, increased left ventricular output, and constriction of umbilical artery and ductus arteriosus [12].

Using the fetal and newborn lamb, Robillard et al. [220] explored the relationships between kallikrein on the one hand and aldosterone, prostaglandins, and renal hemodynamics on the other. The rate of urinary kallikrein excretion increased in the fetus throughout the third trimester and continued to rise after birth. The increase in urinary kallikrein excretion in the fetal lamb was not entirely dependent on changes in GFR, renal mass, or urine flow rate. In fetal animals older than 120 days, urine kallikrein excretion correlated positively with plasma aldosterone and negatively with sodium excretion, supporting the concept that urinary kallikrein excretion reflects the sodium retaining activity of aldosterone. Paralleling the continuous increase in kallikrein through gestation was an associated increase in cord blood kininogen [220].

The same study also demonstrated no relationship between kallikrein excretion and prostaglandin excretion in the fetus or newborn lamb, despite the fact that kinins have been shown to stimulate renal prostaglandins. The finding could indicate that in sheep, urinary kallikrein levels do not reflect increased renal kinin activity. Finally, the increase in urinary kallikrein excretion correlated with a rise in renal blood flow, suggesting a possible cause and effect relationship [224].

The relation of urinary kallikrein excretion and hypertension is complex [161,169,241]. The exact role of the kallikrein-kinin system in regulation of blood pressure is complicated by interactions with the renin-angiotensin system, prostaglandins, and by effects on renal function. Urinary kallikrein excretion has been studied as a marker of a variety of hypertensive states [151] and has been found to be decreased in some patients with essential as well as other forms of hypertension. The potential of this system to be a marker in children for future hypertension is seen in the study by Berry et al. [18]. These investigators studied 405 normotensive adults and 391 normotensive young individuals. They found evidence for a gene for high urinary kallikrein excretion, which appeared to be protective for the development of hypertension.

Vitamin D

The rapid growth and the large amount of bone mineralization taking place in the fetus require adequate supplies of vitamin D and its metabolites. Since the metabolism and action of vitamin D are reviewed in detail in this volume (see Chap. 7) and elsewhere [27,57,91,105,141, 225], they will be discussed only briefly here.

Vitamin D originating from dietary ingestion of ergocalciferol (vitamin D_2) or cholecalciferol (vitamin D_3) or from the activation of a provitamin in the skin by sunlight is transported to the liver by a vitamin D binding protein [27,141]. In the liver, it is converted to 25-hydroxyvitamin D_3 (25-OH-D_3 or calcidiol), which is then transported to the kidney where it is converted to the most active metabolite, 1,25-dihydroxyvitamin D_3 [1,25-$(OH)_2$-D_3- or calcitriol]. Other metabolites, including 24,25-dihydroxyvitamin D_3, are also produced in the kidney. It is not known whether these latter metabolites are regulators of calcium metabolism or represent degradation products of 1,25-$(OH)_2$-D_3 [57,141]. Although the kidney is the most important site of synthesis of 1,25-$(OH)_2$-D_3, other tissues, including placenta, have been reported to synthesize the hormone [57].

Understanding the regulation of vitamin D in the fetus depends upon knowledge of several factors, including (1) the ability of the various metabolites to cross the placenta; (2) the ability of the liver to hydroxylate vitamin D; (3) the ability of the kidney to convert calcidiol to calcitriol; (4) the presence of various factors that normally control the concentration of vitamin D metabolites (calcium, phosphate, PTH, and other hormones); and (5) production of vitamin D metabolites by the maternal liver and kidney, and by the placenta.

The source of vitamin D and its metabolites made available to the feto-placental unit is not clear. Some studies demonstrate that nephrectomy of the fetus results in altered serum calcium concentration, implying a role for the fetal kidney. In the fetal rat, however, evidence suggests that the site of production of calcitriol may be other than the kidney. Calcitriol synthesized by the maternal kidney appears to cross the placenta in sheep but not in rats or cows [105]. Most of the evidence suggests that calcidiol can cross the placenta in humans. The plasma concentration of calcidiol in the newborn human was found to be directly related to the plasma concentration in the mother [27,28,92,105]. Another study suggests that calcidiol but not calcitriol may cross the human placenta [262], while yet another suggests that calcitrol can cross the placenta [157]. In the fetal calf, the concentration of calcidiol but not calcitriol correlated with that in the maternal serum [99], indicating transplacental passage. Some studies indicate that the fetal kidney and the placenta can convert 25-$(OH)D_3$ to 1,25-$(OH)_2$-D_3 [226]. However, Kooh and Vieth [132] failed to detect calcitriol in plasma or 1-hydroxylase enzyme in renal tissue of the sheep fetus [132].

The ability of the liver and the kidney to hydroxylate vitamin D is present in preterm infants between 28 weeks and 37 weeks gestational age [94,156]. The concentration of calcitriol in cord blood and in serum is greater in infants than in adults [94,155,156]. One study suggests that the concentration of calcitriol in the fetus is affected by the concentrations of calcium, phosphorus, and parathyroid hormone [82]. Thus, the fetus appears to have an adequate supply of vitamin D metabolites. The contribution of placental passage or the production by the liver and kidney to the concentration vitamin D in plasma of the fetus remains to be determined. The role of the fetal kidney in the catabolism of vitamin D also needs further elaboration. The development of the 25-hydroxy vitamin D_3-1-hydroxylase system is a case in point.

Erythropoietin

Erythropoietin is a glycoprotein hormone that is the primary regulator of erythropoiesis. The hormone acts to stimulate the replication and differentiation of committed erythroid progenitors into mature red blood cells. Erythropoietin is produced primarily, although not exclusively, in the kidney (Table 11-5) [84,85,129,217,281]. The site of production of erythropoietin within the kidney has not been definitely identified [78], but the renal cortex appears the most likely site [80,162]. Some studies suggest that this hormone may be produced in the glomerulus [35,36, 78,138]. The specific cell type involved is not known, although there is evidence to support both mesangial cells [138] and peritubular cortical interstitial cells [134].

Although the primary stimulus for erythropoietin synthesis and release is renal cellular hypoxia, a number of other factors have also been reported to be involved (Table 11-6) [32,66,77,79,104,124,125,186,202,203,207]. It is

TABLE 11-5. *Factors that increase erythropoietin production*

1. Hypoxemic hypoxia
2. Anemic hypoxia
3. Ischemic hypoxia
4. Renin-angiotensin
5. Glucocorticoids
6. ACTH
7. Growth hormone
8. Thyroid hormone
9. Prolactin
10. Serotonin
11. Vasopressin
12. Cobalt
13. Proximal tubular function
14. Adenosine
15. Androgens*
16. Prostaglandins*
17. Beta-adrenergic agonists*

* Also thought to enhance erythropoietin effect

TABLE 11-6. *Sites of erythropoietin production*

1. Renal Cortex
2. Liver
3. Macrophages
4. Tumors
   a. Renal carcinoma
   b. Other (including lung, CNS, thymus, liver, adrenal, ovary, uterus)

hypothesized that hypoxia, perhaps through the release of external messengers and their action on cell membranes [81], causes an influx of calcium into cells that activates phospholipase A, which in turn releases arachidonic acid. This fatty acid is the substrate for the cyclo-oxygenase system and triggers the prostaglandin cascade, leading to the production of increased amounts of prostaglandins (Fig. 11-3). Finally, the prostaglandins stimulate adenylate cyclase, leading to the formation of cyclic adenosine monophosphate (cyclic AMP). The cyclic AMP triggers a protein kinase that enhances the production of erythropoietin [78]. Additional pathways via the β-adrenergic nervous system also may be involved in the generation of erythropoietin [78].

Erythropoietin was first recognized in 1906 as a humoral factor that could stimulate the production of red blood cells [38]. However, understanding its mode of the action has developed slowly [259]. Recent advances, including the development of sensitive assays [39], such as the commonly used radioimmunoassay [89], the erythropoietin gene identification sequencing [116], and the isolation of monoclonal anti-erythropoietin antibody [300], made it possible to expand considerably our knowledge in this area. There are several comprehansive reviews [6,76,78] on the control of erythropoietin production and its relationship to other intrarenal hormones, including the prostaglandins [203] and the renin-angiotensin system [104]. The regulation of erythropoiesis in the fetus and newborn has also been reviewed [110,307].

Development of Erythropoietin

Several distinct events take place during the development of the erythropoietin system. First, the site of red blood cell production changes twice, from the yolk sac to the liver and then from the liver to the bone marrow. Second, the type of hemoglobin being produced changes from hemoglobin F to hemoglobin A with the conversion from gamma-chain to beta-chain production. Third, the site of erythropoietin biosynthesis transfers from the liver to the kidney. That the kidney is neither essential nor central to erythropoietin production in the fetus is illustrated by the fact that anephric newborns may have normal erythropoiesis [109,160,310] and normal levels of erythropoietin [302] and that yolk sac red blood cell formation begins before the kidney develops [73].

The regulation of erythropoiesis by the fetus [185,186,311] is independent of maternal erythropoietin, which does not cross the placenta [109] or appear in breast milk [109,166]. However, there is maternal influence on fetal erythropoiesis in instances when oxygen delivery is markedly impaired, for example, in severe maternal hypoxemia [110], anemia [311], or placental insufficiency [165]. Recognizing that the fetus will respond to chronic intrauterine hypoxia and stress with an elevation of erythropoietin in both serum [185,228] and amniotic fluid [290], recent studies have demonstrated the utility of erythropoietin levels as a marker of fetal distress and central nervous system injury [227]. In maternal diabetes mellitus, the high fetal insulin levels, secondary to hyperglycemia, correlate directly with cord erythropoietin levels [303]. Although these results could suggest a role for insulin in fetal erythropoietin production, a more likely explanation is that erythropoietin increases in response to the effect of insulin to increase tissue oxygen consumption, resulting in fetal hypoxemia [303]. This increase in oxygen demand may exceed the oxygen carrying capacity of the blood causing a relative hypoxic state in the fetus [158]. Recently, however, insulin [266] and perhaps other erythropoietic stimulating factors [229] have been shown to stimulate fetal erythropoiesis independent of erythropoietin. Nevertheless, it appears that erythropoietin is the major erythropoietic growth factor and hypoxia is the primary stimulus for erythropoietin production. This is true antenatally as well as postnatally [307], although the response of the fetus or newborn to a hypoxic insult is blunted when compared to an older infant [264,265]. Erythropoietin levels are variable but are generally above adult normals. The levels fall shortly after birth and remain very low in the first month of life and then increase to adult normal, which persist throughout childhood [112,165]. The fall after birth temporally precedes the decline in erythropoiesis and the "physiologic anemia" of the second and third months of life.

The levels of erythropoietin observed in response to similar degrees of hypoxia are lower in newborns than in adults [37]. While there is some evidence that this may be due to the fact that erythroid progenitor cells of the newborn are more sensitive to erythropoietin [145], it is generally agreed that CFU-E targets are equally responsive in the newborn and adults. According to the "adaptive theory" of Finne and Halvorsen [73], the shift from hemoglobin F to hemoglobin A and the increase in 2,3-diphosphoglycerate in red cells in the newborn, which allow more effective tissue oxygenation, makes the observed fall in erythropoietin levels understandable and even predictable. Additionally, one might speculate that erythropoietin levels may not truly reflect the numbers or sensitivity of erythroid progenitor cells or that low serum erythropoietin levels may be due in part to rapid internalization and degradation in a bone marrow whose volume almost equals that of the adult [135,183].

Erythropoietin levels also may be low during the newborn period because of the presence of erythropoietin inhibitors that have been isolated from the urine of two-day-old infants and persist throughout the first month of life [21,146,253]. The nature and the role of these inhibitors are not known.

The liver, probably the Kupffer cell, is the major source of erythropoietin in the fetus [37,235,308]. Although there is some interspecies variation [150], it is clear that some time after birth, there is a shift from hepatic to renal synthesis of erythropoietin. This switch does not appear to reflect the site of erythropoiesis [4] or the type of hemoglobin being produced [201]. In sheep, the switch begins during the third trimester, is complete by 40 days after birth, and is characterized by a gradual decrease in hepatic synthesis and an increase in renal erythropoietin formation [309]. That certain factors may influence this shift in site of production is demonstrated in the fetal sheep, where the absence of thyroid hormone delays the switch, while excess thyroxin accelerates it [309]. In rat neonates, the switch to renal synthesis is hastened by hypoxia [49]. The timing of the transition in the human is not known. In the premature infant, the fetal pattern persists, supporting the idea that hepatic synthesis is less sensitive to hypoxia than the kidney and defends against the polycythemia that could result from reduced intrauterine PO_2 [53]. Once the transition has occurred, the kidney becomes the major source of erythropoietin, accounting for 90% to 95% of the erythropoietin produced in response to hypoxia [122]. Although intrarenal oxygen sensing appears to be most important in erythropoietin synthesis [15], there is also evidence for a role for extrarenal hypoxia sensors, perhaps involving the hypothalamus [200].

In summary, the "physiologic anemia" of the newborn and the "anemia of prematurity" appear to result from insufficient levels of erythropoietin. The number and responsiveness of erythroid progenitors are normal, and, therefore, a rationale exists for the possible use of recombinant erythropoietin in infants with these anemias. Such use is not without potential problems, and the considerations for clinical trials are well summarized in a recent review [240].

Histamine and Serotonin

The formation of serotonin (5-hydroxytryptamine) (Fig. 11-5) requires two steps: L-tryptophan is hydroxylated by tryptophan-5-hydroxylase to L-5-hydroxytryptophan (L-5-HTP), which is then converted by aromatic L-amino acid decarboxylase to serotonin. Histamine (Fig. 11-5) is formed by the action of L-histidine decarboxylase on histidine. All the enzymes required to produce these vasoactive autocoids have been identified in renal tissue [1].

At least two studies have demonstrated the formation of serotonin by the kidney. Stier et al. [263] infused the amino acid precursor of serotonin, L-5-HTP, into the isolated non-blood perfused rat kidney and found an increase in the concentration of serotonin in the urine and in the venous effluent. Furthermore, carbidopa, a decarboxylase inhibitor, and ketanserin, a serotonin-2 receptor antagonist, blocked the increase in renal vascular resistance associated with the infusion of L-5-HTP. Pirotzky and co-workers [212] not only demonstrated the renal release of serotonin but also demonstrated the release of histamine, slow-reacting substance, and platelet-activating factor following the infusion of a calcium ionophore in the isolated rat kidney. These findings support the concept that several mediators of inflammation are produced by the kidney

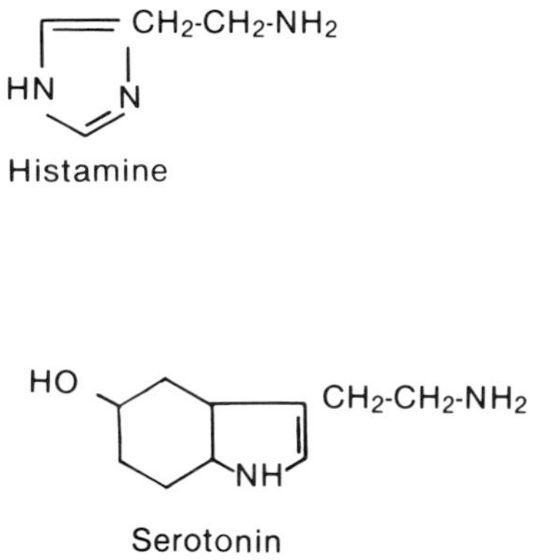

CH₂-CH₂-NH₂

HN N

Histamine

HO

CH₂-CH₂-NH₂

NH

Serotonin

FIG. 11-5. *Chemical structures of histamine and serotonin.*

and that some of them may have effects on renal hemodynamics.

Histochemical and biochemical studies have localized the site of histamine formation in the kidney to the glomerulus [1,2,127]. A dose-related increase in histamine excretion in urine was observed when L-histidine was given to normal individuals [117].

The effects of histamine and serotonin on renal function depend in part on the species studied, on the route of administration, and on the dose of the drug [1]. Histamine has been reported to produce vasodilation in the blood-perfused dog kidney and vasoconstriction when the perfusate is Krebs solution. Serotonin usually produces vasoconstriction of the renal vasculature. Histamine generally produces a diuresis and natriuresis while serotonin produces the opposite result. There is no information available regarding the changes in physiologic effects or the biosynthetic pathways for serotonin or histamine in the kidney during development.

Dopamine

Dopamine has recently been recognized as an important intrarenal hormone, in addition to its role as a metabolic precursor of epinephrine and norepinephrine and as a neurotransmitter [71,140,268]. In the kidney, endogenously produced dopamine can come from two sources. A small amount is derived from dopaminergic nerves and can be evaluated by the determination of dopamine in the renal venous effluent, while the majority appears to be derived from conversion of L-DOPA to dopamine by the enzyme, L-aromatic amino acid decarboxylase, located in the S1 and S2 segments of the proximal tubule [71,140]. Two types of dopamine receptors have been identified outside the central nervous system, DA1 and DA2 corresponding to the D1/D2 receptors in the central nervous system. DA1 receptor stimulation produces increases in RBF and inhibits water and electrolyte transport in the proximal tubule. Aperia, Bertorello, and Seri demonstrated that dopamine caused a reversible inhibition of Na^+-K^+-ATPase in the

proximal tubule and suggested that the intrarenal production of dopamine is an important natriuretic hormone [10]. Bertorello et al. also have shown in the rat that a high sodium diet will result in inhibition of Na^+-K^+-ATPase by endogenous dopamine acting through the DA1 receptor [19]. The nature of the dopamine receptor and renal effects of dopamine have recently been reviewed [71].

Studies on the importance of dopamine and dopamine receptors in the developing kidney have been limited. Buckley and co-workers [34] and Vane et al. [285] infused dopamine into anesthetized piglets. The former demonstrated that dopamine produced an increase in renal vascular resistance in piglets younger than two weeks of age compared to vasodilatation in adult animals. Thus, the vasodilatory response to dopamine in the pig kidney develops over time after birth. The latter authors reported that dopamine interfered with the autoregulatory response in three-week-old to four-week-old piglets but had no effect on renal blood flow at this age. Studies carried out in anesthetized newborn puppies confirm that there is an age-related change in the response of renal vascular resistance to dopamine [204]. Furthermore, while GFR and sodium excretion increased in older and younger animals in response to dopamine, the response was greater in the more mature animals [204]. These data suggest that there is a maturational pattern in either the number of dopamine receptors or their responsiveness. However, a study by Nakamura et al. in unanesthetized fetal, newborn, and adult sheep gave different results [179]. They found that the intrarenal arterial infusion of dopamine produced a vasodilatory response at all three ages when renal α- and β-adrenoceptors were blocked [179]. The difference in various studies may be related to the species used or to the use of anesthesia. Felder et al. [70] and Kinoshita, Jose, and Felder [131] studied dopamine receptors in sheep and rat kidney during development, respectively. They found in the sheep that DA1 receptor density and affinity do not change with age and there was a decrease in DA2 receptor density. In the rat, while DA1 receptor density increased over the first three weeks of life, there was a decrease in efficiency of the coupling between the DA1 receptor and adenylate cyclase. It appears that the maturational increase in the vasodilatory response and natriuretic response to dopamine may be related to an increase in the efficiency of the coupling mechanism [71].

The importance of the renal dopamine system in the regulation of neonatal salt and water handling remains to be fully evaluated. A few studies have been carried out in preterm infants in which the effects of dopamine infusion or the administration of the dopamine receptor antagonist, metoclopramide, have been examined. Sulyok et al. studied the effect of high and low sodium intake on the excretion of dopamine in well preterm infants (28 to 31 weeks gestational age, GA) [269]. They found increased dopamine excretion was associated with the low sodium diet and sodium depletion, while the reverse was true on the high sodium intake. In another study on nine premature infants (28 to 35 weeks, GA) who required ventilatory support, Sulyok and colleagues infused dopamine at a rate of 2 μg/kg-min [273]. They found an increase in urine flow rate and sodium excretion associated with an increase in

PRA and no change in plasma aldosterone concentration. Blood pressure did not change. They suggested that the failure of the rise in aldosterone was due to the inhibitory effect of dopamine. Furthermore, in another study, they found that the dopamine antagonist, metoclopramide, inhibited tubular sodium reabsorption [268]. There is no clear explanation for the discrepancy between these studies as well as the known association between increased excretion of dopamine and sodium and the inhibitory effect of dopamine on Na^+-K^+-ATPase. It is possible that the clinical state of the infants under study may have modified the responses.

Vasodepressor Renal Lipids

A number of investigators have demonstrated that the kidney produces substances that have an anti-hypertensive action. Muirhead [174–178] has proposed that there is an antihypertensive lipid produced by the interstitial cells of the renal medulla. At least three lipids have been found in the renal interstitial cells of the renal medulla, prostaglandins, alkyl ethers of phosphatidylcholine, and a neutral lipid [174]. While the major prostaglandin of the renal medulla, PGE_2, may have local effects, there is little evidence that it affects systemic blood pressure. On the other hand, the other lipids may have significant antihypertensive action [174–177,215,256]. Muirhead and co-workers have isolated a lipid of low polarity, which they called ANRL (antihypertensive neutral renomedullary lipid). They have subsequently suggested that this substance be renamed medullipin I. Additional studies now suggest that medullipin I is released by the kidney and is activated to medullipin II by the liver [176–178]. The latter substance is a vasodilator and suppresses sympathetic activity and can cause a natriuresis and diuresis. The medullipin system appears to be responsible for the amelioration of renoprival hypertension as well as the return of blood pressure toward normal when animals with one-kidney, one clip hypertension, are unclipped [176,177]. Whether or not these vasodepressors are important in the regulation of blood pressure in the premature and term newborn infant is unknown.

References

1. Abboud HE: Histamine and Serotonin. *In* Dunn MJ (ed): *Renal Endocrinology*. Baltimore, Williams & Wilkins, 1983, p 429.
2. Abboud HE, Ou SL, Velosa JA, et al: Dynamics of renal histamine in normal rat kidney and in nephrosis induced by aminonucleoside of puromycin. *J Clin Invest* 69:327, 1982.
3. Ader JL, Tran-Van T, Praddaude F: Renal tissue kallikrein in newborn and young SHR. *Am J Hypertens* 1:S53, 1988.
4. Alter BP, Jackson BT, Lipton JM, et al: Control of the simian fetal hemoglobin switch at the progenitor cell level. *J Clin Invest* 67:458, 1981.
5. Alward CA, Hook JB, Helmrath TA, et al: Effects of respiratory distress on renal function in the newborn piglet. *Pediatr Res* 12:225, 1978.
6. Andrew M, Bhogal M, Karpatkin M: Factors XI & XII &

7. prekallikrein in sick and healthy premature infants. *N Engl J Med* 305:1130, 1981.
7. Andrews PM, Coffey AK: Cytoplasmic contractile elements in glomerular cells. *Federation Proc* 42:3046, 1983.
8. Abdrew M, Paes B, Johnston M: Development of the hemostatic system in the neonate and young infant. *Am J Pediatr Hematol Oncol* 12:95, 1990.
9. Anggard E, Oliw E: Formation and metabolism of prostaglandins in the kidney. *Kidney Int* 19:771, 1981.
10. Aperia A, Bertorello A, Seri I: Dopamine causes inhibition of Na^+-K^+-ATPase activity in rat proximal convoluted tuule segments. *Am J Physiol* 252:F39, 1987.
11. Arant BS: Relationship between blood volume, prostaglandin synthesis, and arterial blood pressure in neonatal puppies. *In* Spitzer A (ed): *The Kidney During Development: Morphology and Function*. New York, Masson Publishing USA, 1982, p 167.
12. Assali NS, Johnson GH, Brinkman CR, et al: Effects of bradykinin on fetal circulation. *Am J Physiol* 221:1375, 1971.
13. Bailie MD, Derkx FHM, Schalekamp MADH: Release of active and inactive renin by the pig kidney during development. *Dev Pharmacol Ther* 1:47, 1980.
14. Bailie MD, Osborn JL, Hook JB: Effect of inhibition of prostaglandin synthetase and angiotensin II on renal function in the newborn piglet. *In* Spitzer A (ed): *The Kidney During Development: Morphology and Function*. New York, Masson Publishing USA, 1982, p 173.
15. Bauer C, Kurtz A: Oxygen sensing in the kidney and its relation to erythropoietin production. *Annu Rev Physiol* 51:845, 1989.
16. Bell PD, Navar LG: Macula densa feedback control of glomerular filtration: Role of cytosolic calcium. *Miner Electrolyte Metab* 8:61, 1982.
17. Bergman I, Binder C, Rana H, et al: Urinary kallikrein excretion in healthy young infants. *Adv Exp Med Biol* 198a:211, 1986.
18. Berry TD, Hasstedt SJ, Hunt SC, et al: A gene for high urinary kallikrein may protect against hypertension in Utah kindreds. *Hypertension* 13:3, 1989.
19. Bertorello A, Hökfelt T, Goldstein M, et al: Proximal tubule Na^+-K^+-ATPase activity is inhibited during high-salt diet: Evidence for DA-mediated effect. *Am J Physiol* 254:F795, 1988.
20. Betkerur MV, Yeh TF, Miller K, et al: Indomethacin and its effect on renal function and urinary kallikrein excretion in premature infants with patent ductus arteriosus. *Pediatrics* 68:99, 1981.
21. Biljanovic-Paunovic L, Pavlovic-Kentera V, Nikoloc R, et al: Erythropoietin in premature infants. *Acta Paediatr Scand* 71:75, 1982.
22. Binder ND, Anderson DF, Potter DM, et al: Normal arterial blood pressure in the nephrectomized fetal lamb. *Biol Neonate* 42:50, 1982.
23. Blantz RC: The glomerular and tubular actions of angiotensin II. *Am J Kidney Dis* (suppl 1)10:2, 1987.
24. Blantz RC, Pelayo JC: In vivo actions of angiotensin II on glomerular function. *Fed Proc* 42:3071, 1983.
25. Blazy I, Dechaux M, Guillot F, et al: Inactive renin in infants and children: Evidence for its physiological response to orthostasis in children. *J Clin Endocrinol Metab* 59:321, 1984.
26. Blazy I, Guillot F, Laborde K, et al: Comparison of plasm renin and prorenin in healthy infants and children as determined with an enzymatic method and a new direct immunoradiometric assay. *Scand J Clin Lab Invest* 49:413, 1989.

27. Bouillon R, Van Assche FA: Perinatal vitamin D metabolism. *Dev Pharmacol Ther* (suppl 1, vol 4)4:38, 1982.

28. Bouillon R, Van Baelen H, De Moor P: 25-hydroxyvitamin D and its binding protein in maternal and cord serum. *J Clin Endocrinol Metab* 45:679, 1977.

29. Brons M, Thayssen P: Plasma renin concentration, activity and substrate in normal children. *Inter J Pediatr Nephrol* 4:43, 1983.

30. Broughton-Pipkin FB: Hepatic inactivation of val⁵-angiotensin II amide (hypertensin), val⁵-angiotensin II free acid and adrenalin in immature and adult rabbits. *J Physiol* (Lond) 225:35, 1972.

31. Brouhard BH, Alpin CE, Cunningham RJ, et al: Immunoreactive urinary prostaglandins A and E in neonates, children and adults. *Prostaglandins* 15:881, 1978.

32. Brown JE, Adamson JW: The influence of beta-adrenergic agonists on erythroid colony formation. *J Clin Invest* 60:70, 1977.

33. Bryan FT, Ryan JW, Neimeyer RS: Bradykininogen synthesis by liver. *In* Back N, Frank F, Sicuteri F (eds): *Vasopeptides: Chemistry, Pharmacology and Pathophysiology.* New York, Plenum Press, 1972, p 43.

34. Buckley NM, Charney AN, Brazeau P, et al: Changes in cardiovascular and renal function during catecholamine infusions in developing swine. *Am J Physiol* 240:f276, 1981.

35. Burlington H, Cronkite EP, Reinecke U, et al: Erythropoietin production in culture of goat renal glomeruli. *Proc Nat Acad Sci USA* 69:3547, 1972.

36. Busuttil RW, Roh BL, Fisher JW: Further evidence for the production of erythropoietin in the dog kidney. *Acta Haematol* (Basel) 47:238, 1972.

37. Carmena AO, Howard D, Stohlman F: Regulation of erythropoiesis: Erythropoietin production in the newborn animal. *Blood* 32:376, 1968.

38. Carnot P, DeFlandre C: Sur l'activite hematopoietique des differents organes aur cours de la regeneration du sang. *CR Acad Sci Paris* 143:384, 1906.

39. Caro J, Ersler AJ: Erythropoietin assays and their use in the study of anemia. *Contrib Nephrol* 66:54, 1988.

40. Carone FA, Peterson DR, Flouret G: Renal tubular processing of small peptide hormones. *J Lab Clin Med* 100:1, 1982.

41. Carone FA, Peterson DR, Oparil S, et al: Renal tubular transport and catabolism of proteins and peptides. *Kidney Int* 16:271, 1979.

42. Carretero OA, Scicli AG: The renal kallikrein-kinin system. *In* Dunn MJ (ed): *Renal Endocrinology.* Baltimore, Williams & Wilkins, 1983, p 96.

43. Carretero OA, Scicli AG: Renal kallikrein: Its localization and possible role in renal function. *Fed Proc* 35:194, 1976.

44. Carretero OA, Scicli AG, Nasjletti A: Glandular kallikrein-kinin system: Methodology for its measurement. *In* Radzialowski FM (ed): *Hypertension Research Methods and Models.* Vol 19. New York, Marcel Dekker, 1981, p 195.

45. Carver JG, Mott JC: Renin substrate in plasma of unanesthetized pregnant ewes and their foetal lambs. *J Physiol* 276:395, 1978.

46. Chevalier RL, Gomez RA: Response of the renin-angiotensin system to relief of neonatal ureteral obstruction. *Am J Physiol* 255:F1070, 1988.

47. Chevalier RL, Peach MJ: Hemodynamic effects of enalapril on neonatal chronic partial ureteral obstruction. *Kidney Int* 28:891, 1985.

48. Cifuentes RF, Olley PM, Balfe JW, et al: Indomethacin and renal function in premature infants with persistent ductus arteriosus. *J Pediatr* 95:583, 1979.

49. Clemons GK, Fitzsimmons SL, DeManincor D: Immuno-reactive erythropoietin concentrations in fetal and neonatal rats and the effects of hypoxia. *Blood* 68:892, 1986.

50. Cogan MG: Angiotensin II: A powerful controller of sodium transport in the early proximal tubule. *Hypertension* 15:451, 1990.

51. Cotes PM, Bangham DR: Bioassay of erythropoietin in mice made polycythaemic by exposure to air at reduced pressure. *Nature* (Lond) 191:1065, 1961.

52. Currie MG, Needleman P: Renal arachidonic acid metabolism. *Annu Rev Physiol* 40:327, 1984.

53. Dallman PR: Erythropoietin and the anemia of prematurity. *J Pediatr* 105:756, 1984.

54. Davis JO: What signals the kidney to release renin? *Circ Res* 28:301, 1971.

55. Davis JO, Freeman RH: Mechanisms regulating renin release. *Physiol Rev* 56:1, 1976.

56. de Martino C, Zamboni LA: Morphologic study of the sonephros of the human embryo. *J Ultrastruct Res* 16:399, 1966.

57. DeLuca HF: Recent advances in the metabolism of vitamin D. *Ann Rev Physiol* 43:199, 1981.

58. Dillon MJ, Gillen MEA, Ryness JM, et al: Plasma renin activity and aldosterone concentration in the human newborn. *Arch Dis Child* 51:537, 1976.

59. Garrison JC, Rall TW: Autacoids: Drug therapy of inflammation. *In* Gilman AG, Rall TW, Nies AS, et al (eds): *The Pharmacological Basis of Therapeutics.* New York, Pergamon Press, 1990, p 574.

60. Drukker A, Donoso VS, Linshaw MA, et al: Intrarenal distribution of renin in the developing rabbit. *Pediatr Res* 17:762, 1983.

61. Drukker A, Goldsmith DI, Spitzer A, et al: The renin angiotensin system in newborn dogs: Developmental patterns and response to acute saline loading. *Pediatr Res* 14:304, 1980.

62. Dunn MJ: *Renal Endocrinology.* Baltimore, Williams & Wilkins, 1983.

63. Dunn MJ: *Renal Prostaglandins. In* Dunn MJ (ed): *Renal Endocrinology.* Baltimore, Williams & Wilkins, 1983, p 1.

64. Dzau VJ: Significance of the vascular renin-angiotensin pathway. *Hypertension* 7:554, 1986.

65. Dzau VJ, Burt DW, Pratt RE: Molecular biology of the renin-angiotensin system. *Am J Physiol* 255:563, 1988.

66. Eckhardt KU, Kurtz A, Bauer C: Regulation of erythropoietin production is related to proximal tubular function. *Am J Physiol* 256:F942, 1989.

67. El-Dahr SS, Gomez RA, Gray MS, et al: In situ localization of renin and its mRNA in neonatal uretal obstruction. *Am J Physiol* 258:F854, 1990.

68. Eltherington LG, Stoff J, Hughes T, et al: Constriction of human umbilical arteries: Interaction between oxygen and bradykinin. *Circ Res* 22:747, 1968.

69. Ertl T, Sulyok E, Nemeth M, et al: The effect of sodium chloride supplementation on the postnatal development of plasma prostaglandin E and F₂alpha in preterm infants. *J Pediatr* 101:761, 1982.

70. Felder RA, Nakamura KT, Robillard JE, et al: Dopamine receptors in the developing sheep kidney. *Pediatr Nephrol* 2:156, 1988.

71. Felder RA, Felder CC, Eisner GM, et al: The dopamine receptor in adult and maturing kidney. *Am J Physiol* 257:F315, 1989.

72. Figueroa CD, MacIver AG, MacKenzie JC, et al: Localisation of immunoreactive kininogen and tissue kallikrein in the human nephron. *Histochemistry* 89:437, 1988.

73. Finne PH, Halvorsen S: Regulation of erythropoiesis in the fetus and newborn. *Arch Dis Child* 47:683, 1972.

74. Fiselier T, Derkx F, Monnens L, et al: The basal levels of active and inactive plasma renin concentration in infancy and childhood. *Clin Sci* 67:383, 1984.

75. Fiselier TJW, Lijnen P, Monnens L, et al: Levels of renin, angiotensin I & II, angiotensin-converting enzyme and aldosterone in infancy and childhood. *Eur J Pediatr* 141:3, 1983.

76. Fisher JW: Control of erythropoietin production. *Proc Soc Exp Biol Med* 173:289, 1983.

77. Fisher JW, Langston JW: The influence of hypoxemia and cobalt on erythropoietin production in the isolated perfused dog kidney. *Blood* 29:115, 1967.

78. Fisher JW, Nelson PK, Beckman B, et al: Kidney control of erythropoietin production. *In* Dunn MJ (ed): *Renal Endocrinology*. Baltimore, Williams & Wilkins, 1983, p 142.

79. Fisher JW, Roh BL, Halvorsen S: Inhibition of erythropoietic effects of hormones by erythropoietin antisera in mildly plethoric mice. *Proc Soc Exp Biol Med* 126:97, 1967.

80. Fisher JW, Taylor G, Porteous DD: Localization of erythropoietin in the glomeruli of sheep kidney using a fluorescent antibody technique. *Nature.* 205:611, 1965.

81. Fisher JW, Ueno M: External messengers and erythropoietin production. *Bull NY Acad Med* 554:9, 1989.

82. Fleischman AR, Rosen JF, Cole J, et al: Maternal and fetal serum 1,25-dihydroxyvitamin D levels at term. *J Pediatr* 97:640, 1980.

83. Frantz E, Soifer S, Clyman RI, et al: Bradykinin produces pulmonary vasodilation in fetal lambs: Role of prostaglandin production. *J Appl Physiol* 76:1512, 1989.

84. Fried W: The liver as a source of extrarenal erythropoietin production. *Blood* 40:671, 1972.

85. Fried W, Anagnostou A: Extrarenal erythropoietin production. *In* Fisher JW (ed): *Kidney Hormones*. London, Academic, 2, 1977, p 231.

86. Friedman WF, Fitzpatrick KM: Effects of prostaglandins, thromboxanes, and inhibitors of their synthesis on renal and gastrointestinal function in the newborn period. *Semin Perinatol* 4:143, 1980.

87. Friedman Z, Demers LM: Prostaglandin synthesis in the human neonatal kidney. *Pediatr Res* 14:190, 1979.

88. Friedman Z, Demers LM, Marks KH, et al: Urinary excretion of prostaglandin E following the administration of furosemide and indomethacin to sick low-birthweight infants. *J Pediatr* 93:512, 1978.

89. Garcia JF, Ebbe SN, Hollander L, et al: Radioimmunoassay of erythropoietin: Circulating levels in normal and polycythemic human beings. *J Lab Clin Med* 99:624, 1982.

90. Gerber JG, Olson RD, Nies AS: Interrelationship between prostaglandins and renin release. *Kidney Int* 19:816, 1981.

91. Gertner JM: Developmental changes in renal vitamin D activation. *Semin Nephrol* 3:139, 1983.

92. Gertner JM, Glassman MS, Coustan DR, et al: Fetomaternal vitamin D relationships at term. *J Pediatr* 97:637, 1980.

93. Gibbons GH, Dzau VJ, Farhi ER, et al: Interaction of signals influencing renin release. *Annu Rev Physiol* 46:291, 1984.

94. Glorieux FH, Salle BL, Delvin EE, et al: Vitamin D metabolism in preterm infants: Serum calcitriol values during the first five days of life. *J Pediatr* 99:640, 1981.

95. Godard C, Geering J-M, Geering K, et al: Plasma renin activity related to sodium balance, renal function and urinary vasopressin in the newborn infant. *Pediatr Res* 13:742, 1979.

96. Godard C, Gaillard R, Vallotton MB: The renin-angiotensin-aldosterone system in mother and fetus at term. *Nephron* 17:353, 1976.

97. Godard C, Vallotton MB, Favre L: Urinary prostaglandins, vasopressin, and kallikrein excretion in healthy children from birth to adolescence. *J Pediatr* 100:898, 1982.

98. Godard CM, Dale HD, Favre H, et al: Urinary prostaglandins and kallikrein in healthy children from birth to adolescence. *Pediatr Res* 15:178, 1981.

99. Goff JP, Horst R, Littledike ET: Effect of the maternal vitamin D status at parturition on the vitamin D status of the neonatal calf. *J Nutr* 112:1387, 1982.

100. Gomez AR, Lynch KR, Chevalier RL, et al: Renin and angiotensinogen gene expression and intrarenal distribution during ACE inhibition. *Am J Physiol* 254:F900, 1988.

101. Gomez AR, Lynch KR, Chevalier DW, et al: Renin and angiotensinogen gene expression in maturing rat kidney. *Am J Physiol* 254:F852, 1988.

102. Gomez AR, Lynch KR, Sturgill BC, et al: Distribution of renin mRNA and its protein in the developing kidney. *Am J Physiol* 257:F850, 1989.

103. Gomez RA, Robillard JE: Developmental aspects of the renal responses to hemorrhage during converting-enzyme inhibition in fetal lambs. *Circ Res* 54:301, 1984.

104. Gould AB, Goodman S, Dewolf R, et al: Interrelationship of the renin system and erythropoietin in rats. *J Lab Clin Med* 96:523, 1980.

105. Greer FR, Chesney RW: Disorders of calcium metabolism in the neonate. *Semin Nephrol* 3:100, 1983.

106. Gross PA, Schrier RW, Anderson RJ: Prostaglandins and water metabolism: A review with emphasis on in vivo studies. *Kidney Int* 19:839, 1981.

107. Haber E: The role of renin in normal and pathological cardiovascular homeostasis. *Circulation* 54:849, 1976.

108. Haber E, Carlson W: The biochemistry of the renin-angiotensin system. *In* Genest J, Kuchel O, Hamet P, et al (eds): *Hypertension: Pathology and Treatment*. New York, McGraw-Hill, 1983, p 171.

109. Haga P, Kristiansen S: Role of the kidney in foetal erythropoiesis: Erythropoiesis and erythropoietin levels in newborn mice with renal agenesis. *J Embryol Exp Morph* 61:165, 1981.

110. Halvorsen K, Haga P, Halvorsen S: Regulation of erythropoiesis in the foetus and neonate. *In* Nakao K, Fisher JW, Takaku F (eds): *Erythropoiesis*. Proceedings of the Fourth International Conference on Erythropoiesis. Baltimore, University Park Press, 1974.

111. Hassid A, Dunn M: Biosynthesis and metabolism of prostaglandins in human kidney in vitro. *In* Dunn MJ, Patrono C, Cinotti GA (eds): *Prostaglandins and the Kidney: Biochemistry, Physiology and Clinical Applications*. New York, Plenum Press, 1983.

112. Hellebostad M, Haga P, Cotes PM: Serum immunoreactive erythropoietin in healthy normal children. *Br J Haematol* 70:247, 1988.

113. Helmer OM, Judson WE: Influence of high renin substrate levels on renin-angiotensin system in pregnancy. *Am J Obstet Gynecol* 99:9, 1967.

114. Henrich WL: Role of prostaglandins in renin secretion. *Kidney Int* 19:822, 1981.

115. Hiner LB, Gruskin AB, Baluarte HJ, et al: Plasma renin activity in normal children. *J Pediatr* 89:258, 1976.

116. Hirth P, Wieczorek L, Scigalla P: Molecular biology of erythropoietin. *Contrib Nephrol* 66:38, 1988.

117. Horakova Z, Keiser HR, Beaven MA: Blood and urine histamine levels in normal and pathological states as measured by a radiochemical assay. *Clin Chim Acta* 79:447, 1977.

118. Ichikawa I, Kon V: Glomerular mesangium as an effector

locus for the tubuloglomerular feedback system and renal sympathetic innervation. *Federation Proc* 42:3075, 1983.

119. Ignatowska-Switalska M, Januezewicz P: Urinary prostaglandins E2 and F2-alpha in healthy newborns, infants, children and adults. *Prostaglandins and Medicine* 5:289, 1980.

120. Ingelfinger JR, Zuo WM, Fon EA, et al: In situ hybridization evidence for angiotensinogen messenger RNA in the rat proximal tubule: An hypothesis for the intrarenal angiotensin system. *J Clin Invest* 85:147, 1990.

121. Jackson EK, Branch RA, Oates JA: Participation of prostaglandins in the control of renin release. In Oates JA (ed): *Prostaglandins and the Cardiovascular system.* New York, Raven Press, 1982.

122. Jacobson LO, Marks EK, Gaslon EO, et al: Studies on erythropoiesis. IX. Reticulocyte response of transfusion-induced polycythemic mice to anemic plasma from nephrectomied mice and to plasma from nephrectomized rats exposed to low oxygen. *Blood* 14:635, 1959.

123. Jelkmann W: Renal erythropoietin: Properties and production. *Rev Physiol Biochem Pharmacol* 104:140, 1986.

124. Jepson JH, Friesen HG: The mechanism of action of human placental lactogen on erythropoiesis. *Acta Haematol* (Basel) 15:465, 1968.

125. Jepson JH, McGarry EE, Lowenstein L: Erythropoietin excretion in a hypopituitary patient. *Arch Intern Med* 122:265, 1968.

126. Joppich R, Scherer B, Weber PC: Renal prostaglandins: Relationships to the development of blood pressure and concentrating capacity in pre-term and full term healthy infants. *Eur J Pediatr* 132:253, 1979.

127. Juhlin L: Determination of histamine in small biopsies and histological sections. *Acta Physiol Scand* 71:30, 1967.

128. Katz FH, Beck P, Makowski EL: The renin-aldosterone system in mother and fetus at term. *Am J Obstet Gynecol* 118:51, 1974.

129. Kazal LA, Erslev AJ: Erythropoietin production in renal tumors. *Ann Clin Lab Sci* 5:98, 1975.

130. Keeton TK, Campbell WB: The pharmacologic alteration of renin release. *Pharmacol Rev* 31:81, 1981.

131. Kinoshita S, Jose PA, Felder RA: Ontogeny of the dopamine (DA₁) receptor in rat renal proximal convoluted tubule (PCT). *Pediatr Res* 25:68A, 1989.

132. Kooh SW, Vieth R: 25-hydroxyvitamin D metabolism in the sheep fetus and lamb. *Pediatr Res* 14:360, 1980.

133. Kotchen TA, Strickland AL, Rice TW, et al: A study of the renin-angiotensin system in newborn infants. *J Pediatr* 80:938, 1972.

134. Koury MJ, Koury ST, Bondurint MC, et al: Correlation of the molecular and anatomical aspects of renal erythropoietin production. *Contrib Nephrol* 76:24, 1989.

135. Krantz SB, Sawyer ST, Sawada K-I: The role of erythropoietin in erythroid cell differentiation. *Contrib Nephrol* 66:25, 1988.

136. Kreisberg JJ: Contractile properties of the glomerular mesangium. *Federation Proc* 42:3053, 1983.

137. Kühl PG, Schönig G, Schweer H, et al: Increased renal biosynthesis of prostaglandin E₂ and thromboxane B₂ in human congentital obstructive uropathy. *Pediatr Res* 27:103, 1990.

138. Kurtz AW, Jelkmann W, Bauer C: Mesangial cells derived from rat glomeruli produce an erythropoiesis stimulating factor in cell culture. *Fed Eur Biomed Sco Letter* 137:129, 1982.

139. Lee HU, Campbell DJ, Habener JF: Developmental expression of angiotensinogen gene in rat embryos. *Endocrinology* 121:1335, 1987.

140. Lee MR: Dopamine and the kidney. *Clin Sci* 62:439, 1982.

141. Lemmann J Jr, Gray RW: Vitamin D metabolism and the kidney. In Dunn MJ (ed): *Renal Endocrinology.* Baltimore, Williams & Wilkins, 1983.

142. Levens NR, Peach MJ, Carey RM: Role of the intrarenal renin-angiotensin system in the control of renal function. *Circ Res* 48:157, 1981.

143. Levin DL: Effects of inhibition of prostaglandin synthesis on fetal development, oxygenation, and the fetal circulation. *Semin Perinatol* 4:35, 1980.

144. Levinsky NG: The renal kallikrein-kinin system. *Circ Res* 44:441, 1979.

145. Linch DC, Knotl LJ, Rodesh CH, et al: Studies of circulating hemopoietic progenitor cells in human fetal blood. *Blood* 59:976, 1982.

146. Lindemann R: Erythropoietin and erythropoiesis inhibitors in the neonatal period. In Nakao K (ed): *Erythropoiesis.* Baltimore, University Park Press, 1974.

147. Lindop GBM: Morphological aspects of renin synthesis, processing, storage and secretion. *Kidney Int* (suppl 20)31:S-18, 1987.

148. Ljungquist A, Wagermark J: Renal juxtaglomerular granulation in the human foetus and infant. *Acta Pathol Microbiol Scand* 67:257, 1966.

149. Lorenz JN, Weihprecht H, Schnermann J, et al: Characterization of the macula densa stimulus for renin secretion. *Am J Physiol* 259:F186, 1990.

150. Lucarelli G, Porcellini A, Carnevali C, et al: Fetal and neonatal erythropoiesis. *Ann NY Acad Sci* 149:544, 1968.

151. Margolius HS: Tissue kallikreins and kinins: Roles in human disease and target for new drug development. *Adv Exp Med Biol* 247A:1, 1989.

152. Margolius HS, Chao J, Perlman B, et al: Identification of amphibian kallikrein and studies of kallikrein inhibition by amiloride. In Gross F, Vogel HG (eds): *Enzymatic Release of Vasoactive Peptides.* New York, Raven Press, 1980, p 313.

153. Margolius HS, Horwitz D, Keller RG, et al: Urinary kallikrein excretion in normal man: Relationship to sodium intake and sodium-retaining steroids. *Circ Res* 35:812, 1974.

154. Marin-Grez M: Multihormonal regulation of renal kallikrein. *Biochem Pharmacol* 31:3941, 1982.

155. Markestad T: Plasma concentration of 1,25-dihydroxyvitamin D, 24,25-dihydroxyvitamin D, and 25,26-dihydroxyvitamin D in the first year of life. *J Clin Endocrinol Metab* 57:755, 1983.

156. Markestad T, Aksnes L, Finne PH, et al: Plasma concentrations of vitamin D metabolites in premature infants. *Pediatr Res* 18:269, 1984.

157. Marx SJ, Swart EG Jr, Hamstra AJ, et al: Neonatal intrauterine development of the fetus of a woman receiving extraordinary high doses of 1,25-dihydroxyvitamin D. *J Clin Endocrinol Metab* 51:1138, 1980.

158. Matoth Y, Zaizov R: Regulation of erythropoiesis in the fetal rat. *Isr J Med Sci* 7:839, 1971.

159. Matson JR, Stokes JB, Robillard JE: Effects of inhibition of prostaglandin synthesis on fetal renal function. *Kidney Int* 20:621, 1981.

160. Mauer SM, Dobrin RS, Vernier RL: Unilateral and bilateral renal agenesis in monoamniotic twins. *J Pediatr* 84:236, 1974.

161. Mayfield RK, Margolius HS: Renal kallikrein-kinin system: Relation to renal function and blood pressure. *Am J Nephrol* 3:145, 1983.

162. McDonald TP, Martin DH, Simmons ML, et al: Preliminary results of erythropoietin production by bovine kidney cells in culture. *Life Sci* 8:949, 1969.

163. McGiff JC: Bartter's syndrome results from an imbalance of vasoactive hormones. *Ann Intern Med* 87:369, 1977.

164. McGiff JC, Itskovitz HD, Terragno A, et al: Modulation and mediation of the action of the renal kallikrein-kinin system by prostaglandins. *Fed Proc* 35:175, 1976.

165. Meberg A: Haemoglobin concentrations and erythropoietin levels in appropriate and small for gestational age infants. *Scand J Haematol* 24:162, 1980.

166. Meberg A, Haga P, Johansen M: Plasma erythropoietin levels in mice during the growth period. *Brit J Haematol* 45:569, 1980.

167. Meléndez E, Reyes JL, Escalante BA, et al: Development of receptors of prostaglandin E2 in the rat kidney and neonatal renal function. *Dev Pharmacol Ther* 14:125, 1990.

168. Melmon KL, Cline MJ, Hughes T, et al: Kinins: Possible mediators of neonatal circulatory changes in man. *J Clin Invest* 47:1295, 1968.

169. Mills IH: Kallikrein, kininogen and kinins in control of blood pressure. *Nephron* 23:61, 1979.

170. Mitchell MD, Robinson JS, Thorburn GD: Prostaglandins in fetal tracheal and amniotic fluid from late pregnant sheep. *Prostaglandins* 14:1005, 1977.

171. Moncada S, Flower RJ, Vane JR: Prostaglandins, prostacyclin and thromboxane. *In* Gilman AG, Goodman LS, Gilman A (eds): *The Pharmacological Basis of Therapeutics*. New York, Macmillan, 1980.

172. Mounier F, Hinglais N, Sich M, et al: Ontogenesis of angiotensin-I converting enzyme in human kidney. *Kidney Int* 32:684, 1987.

173. Movat HZ: The kinin system: Its relation to blood coagulation, fribrinolysis and the formed elements of the blood. *Rev Physiol Biochem Pharmacol* 84:143, 1978.

174. Muirhead EE: Vasodepressor renal medullary lipids. *In* Dunn MJ (ed): *Renal Endocrinology*. Baltimore, Williams & Wilkins, 1983, p 75.

175. Muirhead EE: Antihypertensive functions of the kidney. *Hypertension* 2:444, 1980.

176. Muirhead EE, Byers LW, Brooks B, et al: The liver converts the antihypertensive hormone of the kidney: The renohepatic axis. *Hypertension* (suppl II)8:II-117, 1986.

177. Muirhead EE: The renomedullary system of blood pressure control. *Am J Med Sci* 295:231, 1988.

178. Muirhead EE: Discovery of the renomedullary system of blood pressure control and its hormones. *Hypertension* 15:114, 1990.

179. Nakamura KT, Felder RA, Jose PA, et al: Effects of dopamine in the renal vascular bed of fetal, newborn, and adult sheep. *Am J Physiol* 252:R490, 1987.

180. Nakamura KT, Klingefus JM, Smith FG, et al: Ontogeny of neuronally released norepinephrine on renin secretion in sheep. *Am J Physiol* 257:R765, 1989.

181. Nasjletti A, Malik KU: Renal kinin-prostaglandin relationship: Implications for renal function. *Kidney Int* 19:860, 1981.

182. Nasjletti A, Malik KU: The renal kallikrein-kinin and prostaglandin systems interaction. *Ann Rev Physiol* 43:597, 1981.

183. Nathan DG: The beneficence of neonatal hemopoiesis. *N Engl J Med* 321:190, 1989.

184. Navar LG, Rosivall L: Contribution of the renin-angiotensin system to the control of intrarenal hemodynamics. *Kidney Int* 25:857, 1984.

185. Notti I, Bessler H, Djaldetti M: Increased erythropoiesis in embryonic spleen of polycythemic mice: An indicator for erythropoietin production by the embryo. *Biol Neonate* 40:269, 1981.

186. Noveck RJ, Fisher JW: Erythropoietic effects of 5-hydroxytryptamine. *Proc Soc Exp Biol Med* 138:103, 1971.

187. Nustad K, Vaaje K, Pierce JV: Syntheis of kallikreins by rat kidney slices. *Br J Pharmacol* 53:229, 1975.

188. Obika LFO: Recent developments in urinary kallikrein research. *Life Sci* 23:765, 1978.

189. Omata K, Carretero OA, Scicli AG, et al: Localization of active and inactive kallikrein (kininogenase activity) in the microdissected rabbit nephron. *Kidney Int* 22:602, 1982.

190. Omini C, Vigano T, Marini A, et al: Angiotensin II: A releaser of PGI_2 from fetal and newborn rabbit lungs. *Prostaglandins* 25:901, 1983.

191. Oparil S, Bailie MD: Mechanism of renal handling of angiotensin II in the dog. *Circ Res* 50:119, 1971.

192. Oparil S, Haber E: The renin-angiotensin system (First of two parts). *N Engl J Med* 291:389, 1974.

193. Oparil S, Haber E: The renin-angiotensin system (Second of two parts). *N Engl J Med* 291:446, 1974.

194. Orstavik TB, Nustad K, Brandtzaeg P: Localization of glandular kallikreins in rat and man. *In* Gross F, Vogel HG (eds): *Enzymatic Release of Vasoactive Peptides*. New York, Raven Press, 1980, p 137.

195. Osborn JL, Hook JB, Bailie MD: Regulation of plasma renin in developing piglets. *Dev Pharmacol Ther* 1:217, 1980.

196. Osborn JL, Hook JB, Bailie MD: Effect of saralasin and indomethacin on renal function in developing piglets. *Am J Physiol* 238:R438, 1980.

197. Pace-Asciak C: Activity profiles of prostaglandin 15- and 9-hydroxydehydrogenase and 13-reductase in the developing rat kidney. *J Biol Chem* 250:2795, 1975.

198. Pace-Asciak CR: Developmental aspects of the prostaglandin biosynthetic and catabolic systems. *Semin Perinatol* 4:15, 1980.

199. Pace-Asciak CR: Prostaglandin biosynthesis and catabolism in several organs of developing fetal and neonatal animals. *Adv Prost Thromboxane Research* 4:45, 1978.

200. Pagel H, Jelkmann W, Weiss C: O_2-supply to the kidneys and the production of erythropoietin. *Respir Physiol* 77:111, 1989.

201. Papayannoupoulou TH, Brice M, Stamatoyannopoulos G: Stimulation of fetal hemoglobin synthesis in bone marrow cultures from adult individuals. *Proc Natl Acad Sci USA* 73:2033, 1976.

202. Paul P, Rothmann SA, Meagher RC: Modulation of erythropoietin production by adenosine. *J Lab Clin Med* 112:168, 1988.

203. Paulo LG, Wilkerson RD, Roh BL, et al: The effect of prostaglandin E1 on erythropoietin production. *Proc Soc Exp Biol Med* 142:771, 1973.

204. Pelayo JC, Fildes RD, Jose PA: Age-dependent renal effects of intrarenal dopamine infusion. *Am J Physiol* 247:R212, 1984.

205. Peleg E, Peleg D, Yaron A, et al: Perinatal development of angiotensin converting enzyme in the rats blood. *Gynecol Obstet Invest* 25:12, 1988.

206. Pernollet MG, Devynck MA, Macdonald GJ, et al: Plasma renin activity and adrenal angiotensin II receptors in fetal, newborn, and adult and pregnant rabbits. *Biol Neonate* 36:119, 1979.

207. Peschle C, Sasso GF, Mastroberardino G, et al: The mechanism of endocrine influences on erythropoiesis. *J Lab Clin Med* 78:20, 1971.

208. Pipkin FB, Mott JC, Robertson NRC: Angiotensin II-like activity in circulating arterial blood in immature and adult rabbits. *J Physiol* 218:385, 1971.

209. Pipkin FB, Ousey J, Rosedale PD: The effect of furosemide on the renin-angiotensin-aldosterone system (RAAS) in the conscious newborn foal. *Int J Pediatr Nephrol* 4:288, 1983.

210. Pipkin FB, Symonds EM, Craven DJ: The fetal renin-an-

giotensin system in normal and hypertensive pregnancy. *Isr J Med Sci* 12:225, 1976.

211. Piplin FB, Smales ORC, O'Callaghan MJ: Renin and angiotensin levels in children. *Arch Dis Child* 56:298, 1981.

212. Pirotzky E, Bidault J, Burtin C, et al: Release of platelet-activating factor, slow-reacting substance, and vasoactive amines from isolated rat kidneys. *Kidney Int* 25:404, 1984.

213. Pisano JJ, Marks ES: The renal kallikrein-kinin system: A look at the controversies. *Adv Exp Med Biol* 198A:192, 1986.

214. Pohlova I, Jelinek J: Components of the renin-angiotensin system in the rat during development. *Pflugers Arch* 351:259, 1974.

215. Prewitt RL, Leach BE, Byers LW, et al: Antihypertensive polar renomedullary lipid, a semisynthetic vasodilator. *Hypertension* 1:299, 1979.

216. Reingold DF, Watters K, Holmberg S, et al: Differential biosynthesis of prostaglandins by hydronephrotic rabbit and cat kidneys. *J Pharmacol Exp Ther* 216:510, 1981.

217. Rich IN, Heit W, Kubanek B: Extra-renal erythropoietin production by macrophages. *Blood* 60:1007, 1982.

218. Richer C, Hornych H, Amiel-Tison C, et al: Plasma renin activity and its postnatal developmental in preterm infants. *Biol Neonate* 31:301, 1977.

219. Robillard JE, Gomez RA, Van Orden D, et al: Comparison of the adrenal and renal responses to angiotensin II in fetal lambs and adult sheep. *Circ Res* 50:140, 1982.

220. Robillard JE, Lawton WJ, Weismann DW, et al: Developmental aspects of the renal kallikrein-like activity in fetal and newborn lambs. *Kidney Int* 22:594, 1982.

221. Robillard JE, Nakamura KT: Neurohormonal regulation of renal function during development. *Am J Physiol* 254:F771, 1988.

222. Robillard JE, Nakamura KT: Hormonal regulation of renal function during development. *Biol Neonate* 53:201, 1988.

223. Robillard JE, Ramberg E, Sessions C, et al: Role of aldosterone on renal sodium and potassium excretion during fetal and newborn period. *Dev Pharmacol Ther* 1:201, 1980.

224. Robillard JE, Weismann DN, Gomez RA, et al: Renal and adrenal responses to converting-enzyme inhibition in fetal and newborn life. *Am J Physiol* 244:R249, 1983.

225. Rosen JG, Chesney RW: Circulating calcitriol concentrations in health and disease. *J Pediatr* 103:1, 1983.

226. Ross R, Care AD, Robinson JS, et al: Perinatal 1,25-dihydroxycholecalciferol in the sheep and its role in the maintenance of the transplacental calcium gradient. *J Endocrinol* 87:17P, 1980.

227. Ruth V, Autti-Ramo I, Granstrom M-L, et al: Prediction of perinatal brain damage by cord plasma vasopressin, erythropoietin and hypoxanthine values. *J Pediatr* 113:880, 1988.

228. Ruth V, Fyhrquist F, Clemons G, et al: Cord plasma vasopressin, erythropoietin and hypoxanthine as indices of asphyxia at birth. *Pediatr Res* 24:490, 1988.

229. Sanengen T, Myhre K, Halvorsen S: Erythropoietic factors in plasma from neonatal mice. In vivo studies by the ex-hypoxic polycythaemic mice assay for erythropoietin. *Acta Physiol Scand* 129:381, 1987.

230. Sassard J, Sann L, Vincent M, et al: Plasma renin activity in normal subjects from infancy to puberty. *J Clin Endocrinol Metab* 40:524, 1975.

231. Saugstad OD, Harvie A, Langslet A: Activation of the kallikrein-kinin system in premature infants with respiratory distress syndrome. *Acta Paediatr Scand* 71:965, 1982.

232. Scharschmidt LA, Lianos E, Dunn MJ: Arachidonate metabolites and the control of glomerular function. *Fed Proc* 42:3058, 1983.

233. Schmidt D, Forssmann WG, Taugner R: Juxtaglomerular granules of the newborn rat kidney. *Pflugers Arch* 331:226, 1972.

234. Schnermann J, Briggs JP: Participation of renal cortical prostaglandins in the regulation of glomerular filtration rate. *Kidney Int* 19:802, 1981.

235. Schooley JC, Mahlmann LJ: Extrarenal erythropoietin production by the liver of the weanling rat. *Proc Soc Exp Biol Med* 145:1081, 1974.

236. Scicli AG, Carretero OA: Renal kallikrein-kinin system. *Kidney Int* 29:120, 1986.

237. Sealey JE, Atlas SA, Laragh JH: Plasma prorenin: Physiological and biochemical characteristics. *Clin Sci* 63:113s, 1982.

238. Sealey JE, Atlas SA, Laragh JH: Prorenin in plasma and kidney. *Fed Proc* 42:2681, 1983.

239. Sealey JE, Atlas SA, Laragh JH: Linking the kallikrein and renin systems via activation of inactive renin. *Am J Med* 65:994, 1978.

240. Shannon KM: Anemia of prematurity: Progress and prospects. *Am J Pediatr Hematol Oncol* 12:14, 1990.

241. Sharma JN: Interrelationships between the kallikrein-kinin system and hypertension: A review. *Gen Pharmacol* 19:177, 1988.

242. Siegel S: Decreased vascular and increased adrenal and renal sensitivity to angiotensin II in the newborn lamb. *Circ Res* 48:34, 1981.

243. Siegel SR: Amniotic fluid concentrations of renin and aldosterone during development in the fetal sheep. *Pediatr Res* 15:1419, 1981.

244. Siegel SR, Fisher DA: Ontogeny of the renin-angiotensin-aldosterone system in the fetal and newborn lamb. *Pediatr Res* 14:99, 1980.

245. Siegel SR, Fisher DA: The effects of angiotensin II blockade and nephrectomy on the renin-angiotensin-aldosterone system in the newborn lamb. *Pediatr Res* 13:603, 1979.

246. Siegel SR, Leake RD, Weitzman RE, et al: Effects of furosemide and acute salt loading on vasopressin and renin secretion in the fetal lamb. *Pediatr Res* 14:869, 1980.

247. Siegel SR, Oaks G, Palmer S: Effects of angiotensin II on blood pressure, plasma renin activity, and aldosterone in the fetal lamb. *Dev Pharmacol Ther* 3:144, 1981.

248. Siegel S, Parkhill T: The effects of angiotensin II, saralasin, and furosemide on inactive renin in the fetal lamb. *Pediatr Res* 14:1353, 1980.

249. Siegler RL, Walker MB, Crouch RH, et al: Plasma prostaglandin E concentrations from birth through childhood. *J Pediatr* 91:734, 1977.

250. Silver M, Barnes RJ, Comline RS, et al: Prostaglandins in maternal and fetal plasma and in allantoic fluid during the second half of gestation in the mare. *J Reprod Fertil* (suppl) 27:531, 1979.

251. Simonson MS, Dunn MJ: Endothelin: Pathways of transmembrane signaling. *Hypertension* (suppl I)15:I-5, 1990.

252. Sippell WG, Bidlingmaier F, Knorr D: Development of endogenous glucocorticoids, mineralocorticoids and progestins in the human fetal and perinatal period. *Eur J Clin Pharmacol* 18:95, 1980.

253. Skjaelaaen P, Halvorsen S: Inhibition of erythropoiesis by plasma from newborn infants. *Acta Paediatr Scand* 60:301, 1971.

254. Skorecki KL, Ballermann BJ, Rennke HG, et al: Angiotensin II receptor regulation in isolated renal glomeruli. *Federation Proc* 42:3064, 1983.

255. Smith FG Jr, Lupu AN, Barajas L, et al: The renin-angiotenin system in the fetal lamb. *Pediatr Res* 8:611, 1974.

256. Smith KA, Prewitt RL, Byers LW, et al: Analogues of

phosphatidylcholine: Alpha-adrenergic antagonists from the renal medulla. *Hypertension* 3:460, 1981.

257. Solomon S, Iaina A, Eliahou H, et al: Possible determinants of plasma renin activity in infant rats. *Proc Soc Exp Biol Med* 153:309, 1976.

258. Solomon S, Iaina A, Eliahou H, et al: Postnatal changes in plasma and renal renin of the rat. *Biol Neonate* 32:237, 1977.

259. Spivak JL: The mechanism of action of erythropoietin. *Int J Cell Cloning* 4:136, 1986.

260. Spragg J, Austen KF: Plasma factors: The Hagaman-factor-dependent pathways and the complement sequence. *In* Hadden JW, Coffey RG, Spreafico F (eds): *Immunopharmacology.* New York, Plenum Press, 1977, p 125.

261. Stacy DL, Scott JW, Granger JP: Control of renal function during intrarenal infusion of endothelin. *Am J Physiol* 258:F1232, 1990.

262. Steichen JJ, Tsang RC, Gratton TL, et al: Vitamin D homeostasis in the perinatal period: 1,25-dihydroxyvitamin D in maternal, cord and neonatal blood. *N Engl J Med* 302:315, 1980.

263. Stier CT Jr, McKendall G, Itskovitz HD: Serotonin formation in nonblood-perfused rat kidneys. *J Pharmac Exp Ther* 228:53, 1984.

264. Stockman JA III, Garcia JF, Oski FA: The anemia of prematurity: Factors governing the erythropoietin response. *N Engl J Med* 296:647, 1977.

265. Stockman JA, Graber JE, Clark DA, et al: Anemia of prematurity: Determinants of the erythropoietic response. *J Pediatr* 105:786, 1984.

266. Stonestreet BS, Goldstein M, Oh W, et al: Effect of prolonged hyperinsulinemia on erythropoiesis in fetal sheep. *Am J Physiol* 257:R1199, 1989.

267. Stygles VG, Smith WL, Reinke DA, et al: Prostaglandin-forming cyclooxygenase in renal medulla of spontaneously hypertensive rats during development. *Biol Neonate* 33:309, 1978.

268. Sulyok E, Ertl T, Varga L, et al: The effect of metaclopramide administration on electrolyte status and activity of renin-angiotensin-aldosterone system in premature infants. *Pediatr Res* 19:192, 1985.

269. Sulyok E, Gyódi G, Ertl T, et al: The influence of NaCl supplementation on the postnatal development of urinary excretion of noradrenalin, dopamine, and serotonin in premature infants. *Pediatr Res* 19:5, 1985.

270. Sulyok E, Németh M, Tényi I, et al: The possible role of prostaglandins in the hyperfunction of the renin-angiotensin-aldosterone system in the newborn. *J Obstet Gynecol* 86:205, 1979.

271. Sulyok E, Németh M, Tényi I, et al: Relationship between maturity, electrolyte balance and the function of the renin-angiotensin-aldosterone system in newborn infants. *Biol Neonate* 35:60, 1979.

272. Sulyok E, Németh M, Tényi I, et al: Postnatal development of renin-angiotensin-aldosterone system, RAAS, in relation to electrolyte balance in premature infants. *Pediatr Res* 13:817, 1979.

273. Sulyok E, Seri I, Tulassay T, et al: The effect of dopamine administration on the activity of therenin-angiotensin-aldosterone system in sick preterm infants. *Eur J Pediatr* 143:191, 1985.

274. Sulyok E, Varga F, Nemeth M, et al: Furosemide-induced alterations in the electrolyte status, the function of renin-angiotensin-aldosterone system, and the urinary excretion of prostaglandins in newborn infants. *Pediatr Res* 14:765, 1980.

275. Sulyok E, Ertl T, Csaba IF, et al: Postnatal changes in

urinary prostaglandin E excretion in premature infants. *Biol Neonate* 37:192, 1980.

276. Sun FF, Taylor BM, McGuire JC, et al: Metabolism of prostaglandins in the kidney. *Kidney Int* 19:760, 1981.

277. Sutherland LE, and Hartroft PM: Comparative morphology of juxtaglomerular cells. II. The presence of juxtaglomerular cells in embryos. *Canad J Zool* 46:257, 1968.

278. Sutherland LE, Hartroft PM: Juxtaglomerular cells are present in early metanephroi of the hog embryo. *Anat Rec* 148:342, 1964.

279. Suzuki S: A biochemical study on the kinetics of kininogen in asphyxiated newborns. *Adv Exp Med Biol* 156:1067, 1983.

280. Suzuki S, Franco-Saenz R, Tan SY, et al: Direct action of rat urinary kallakrein on rat kidney to release renin. *J Clin Invest* 66:757, 1980.

281. Tharling EB, Ersbak J: Erythrocytosis and hypernephroma. *Scand J Haematol* 1:38, 1964.

282. Tigersted R, Bergman PG: Niere und Kreislauf. *Scand Arch Physiol* 8:223, 1898.

283. Trimper CE, Lumbers ER: The renin-angiotensin system in foetal lambs. *Pflugers Arch* 336:1, 1972.

284. Van Acker KJ, Scharpe SL, Deprettere AJR, et al: Renin-angiotensin-aldosterone system in the healthy infant and child. *Kidney Int* 16:196, 1979.

285. Vane DW, Weber TR, Careskey J, et al: Systemic and renal effects of dopamine in the infant pig. *J Surg Res* 32:477, 1982.

286. Vinci JM, Zusman RM, Izzo JL, et al: Human urinary and plasma kinins: Relationship to Na-retaining steroids and plasma renin activity. *Circ Res* 44:228, 1979.

287. Vincent M, Dessart Y, Annat G, et al: Plasma renin activity, aldosterone and dopamine b-hydroxylase activity as a function of age in normal children. *Pediatr Res* 14:894, 1980.

288. Vio CP, Figueroa CD: Evidence for a stimutory effect of high potassium diet on renal kallikrein. *Kidney Int* 31:1327, 1987.

289. Vio CP, Olavarrio F, Krause S, et al: Kallikrein excretion: Relationship with maturation and renal function in human neonates at different gestational ages. *Biol Neonate* 52:121, 1987.

290. Voutilainen PEJ, Widness JA, Clemons GK, et al: Amniotic fluid erythropoietin predicts fetal distress in Rh-immunized pregnancies. *Am J Obstet Gynecol* 160:429, 1989.

291. Walker DW, Mitchell MD: Presence of thromboxane B2 and 6-keto-prostaglandin F$_1$alpha in the urine of fetal sheep. *Prost and Med* 3:249, 1979.

292. Walker DW, Mitchell MD: Prostaglandins in urine of foetal lambs. *Nature* 271:161, 1978.

293. Wallace KB, Bailie MD: Age-related differences in the stoichiometry of the renin-angiotensinogen reaction in rat plasma. *Dev Pharmacol Ther* 4:190, 1982.

294. Wallace KB, Bailie MD, Hook JB: Angiotensin-converting enzyme in developing lung and kidney. *Am J Physiol* 234:R141, 1978.

295. Wallace KB, Bailie MD, Hook JB: Development of angiotensin-converting enzyme in fetal rat lungs. *Am J Physiol* 236:R57, 1979.

296. Wallace KB, Hook JB, Bailie MD: Postnatal development of the renin-angiotensin system in rats. *Am J Physiol* 238:R432, 1980.

297. Wallace KB, Oparil S, Bailie MD: Angiotensin II metabolism by tissues from developing rats. *Pediatr Res* 15:1088, 1981.

298. Wallace KB, Roth RA, Hook JB, et al: Age-related differences in angiotensin I metabolism by isolated perfused rat lungs. *Am J Physiol* 238:R395, 1980.

299. Weismann DN, Williamson HE: Hypoxemia increases renin secretion rate in anesthetized newborn lambs. *Life Sci* 29:1887, 1981.

300. Weiss TL, Kavinsky CJ, Goldwasser E: Characterization of monoclonal antibody to human erythropoietin. *Proc Nat Acad Sci USA* 79:5465, 1982.

301. Werle E: Uber die wirkung des Kallikreins auf den isolierten darm und uber eine neue darmkontrahierende substanz. *Biochem Z* 289:217, 1937.

302. Widness JA, Phillipps AF, Clemons GK: Erythropoietin levels and erythropoiesis at birth in infants with Potter syndrome. *J Pediatr* 116:155, 1990.

303. Widness JA, Susa JB, Garcia JF: Increased erythropoiesis and elevated erythropoietin in infants born to diabetic mothers and in hyperinsulinemic rhesus fetuses. *J Clin Invest* 67:637, 1981.

304. Wilson DM, Stevenson DK, Luetscher JA: Plasma prorenin and renin in childhood and adolescence. *Am J Dis Child* 142:1070, 1988.

305. Wilson TA, Kaiser DL, Wright EM Jr, et al: Importance of plasma angiotensin concentrations in a comparative study of responses to angiotensin in the maturing newborn lamb. *Hypertension* (suppl II)3:II-18, 1981.

306. Winther JB, Hoskins E, Printz MP, et al: Influence of indomethacin on renal function in conscious newborn lambs. *Biol Neonate* 38:76, 1980.

307. Zanjani ED, Poster J, Mann LI, et al: *Regulation of erythropoiesis in the fetus. Kidney Hormones. II.* London, Academic, 1977.

308. Zanjani ED, Poster J, Burlington H, et al: Liver as the primary site of erythropoietin production in the fetus. *J Lab Clin Med* 89:641, 1977.

309. Zanjani ED, Ascensao JL, Mcglave PB, et al: Studies on the liver to kidney switch of erythropoietin formation. *J Clin Invest* 67:1183, 1981.

310. Zanjani ED, Banisadre M: Hormonal stimulation of erythropoietin production and erythrpoiesis in anephric sheep fetuses. *J Clin Invest* 64:1181, 1979.

311. Zanjani ED, Peterson EN, Gorden AS, et al: Erythropoietin production in the fetus: Role of the kidney and maternal anemia. *J Lab Clin Med* 83:281, 1974.

312. Zivny J, Kobilkova J, Neuwirt J, et al: Regulation of erythropoiesis in fetus and mother during normal pregnancy. *Obstetrics* 60:77, 1982.

PEDRO A. JOSE
ROBIN A. FELDER

12
Renal Nerves

Renal Innervation

It has been estimated that the kidney, relative to its size, has a richer innervation than any other abdominal viscera, except the adrenal glands [369,400]. In the adult, the renal nerves are composed of fibers from the celiac plexus, thoracic and lumbar splanchnic nerves, intermesenteric nerves, and the superior hypogastric plexus, all of which ultimately arise from spinal cord segments T-6 to L-4 [306,307,412]. These nerve fibers make up the renal plexus and are associated with the aortic renal ganglion, which is located near the junction of the aorta and the renal artery [338,339,369]. Renal nerves contain both afferent and efferent nerves. The main renal nerve plexus divides into secondary plexuses that lie alongside the branches of the renal artery and accompany the vessels into the parenchyma of the kidney [369]; a few fibers first approach the kidney at its hilum.

Nerve fibers are more common in the cortex than in the medulla. The medulla is innervated from offshoots of nerve bundles that lie alongside the arcuate arteries and accompany the arteriole rectae spuriae. The anatomy appears to be similar in the human newborn [306].

The nerve impulses to the kidney (efferent impulses) are carried by sympathetic nerves, which are mainly noradrenergic. The actions of these nerves are mediated by specific neurotransmitters such as norepinephrine (noradrenergic nerves), dopamine (dopaminergic nerves), and several peptides (peptidergic nerves).

The impulses from the kidney (afferent impulses) travel to the central nervous system through the same sympathetic nerves that provide efferent innervation. Some of these afferent nerves contain substance P, a transmitter of sensory impulses.

Neurotransmitters convey messages to the effector cells by occupying specific receptors (Fig. 12-1). These receptors can be located at the nerve terminal proximal to the synapse (presynaptic or prejunctional receptors) or distal to the synapse (postjunctional receptors); the receptors in immediate proximity to the nerve terminal are called postsynaptic receptors and those beyond the limits of the nerve terminal are called extrasynaptic receptors. Each class of

receptor has several subtypes according to function and pharmacologic profile. For example, alpha-adrenoceptors are subclassified as $alpha_1$ or $alpha_2$, beta-adrenoceptors as $beta_1$ or $beta_2$, dopamine receptors as $dopamine_1$ and $dompamine_2$. Based on molecular characteristics each subtype can be subdivided further (e.g., $alpha_{1a}$, $alpha_{1b}$). $Subtype_1$ receptors are always postjunctional whereas $subtype_2$ receptors can be either prejunctional or postjunctional receptors. The prejunctional (presynaptic) receptors function mainly to regulate norepinephrine release by the nerves and thus affect the target cell indirectly. Prejunctional $alpha_2$ and $dopamine_2$ receptors inhibit norepinephrine release, and prejunctional $beta_2$-receptors facilitate norepinephrine release. The postjunctional receptors directly affect the target cell. The functions of the various subtypes of receptors are listed in Tables 12-1 and 12-2.

Efferent Nerves

NORADRENERGIC NERVES

The efferent renal axons originate from cell bodies in the paravertebral sympathetic ganglia (T-6 to L-4) and in the prevertebral solar plexus [412]. The postganglionic sympathetic fibers are derived mainly from the celiac ganglion [172]. The noradrenergic input appears to originate primarily from prevertebral ganglia, whereas the dopaminergic input appears to originate from the paravertebral ganglia [412]. The renal autonomic innervation, which is mainly noradrenergic, reaches the afferent and efferent arterioles, vasa rectae, and juxtaglomerular apparatuses. Using fluorescence and electron microscopic methods and autoradiography, Barajas et al. [27,31] and other investigators [117,128] have demonstrated that adrenergic terminals are also in direct contact with tubular basement membranes. The branches that innervate the renal tubules arise from perivascular bundles and are thinner than the arterial nerve bundles. The proximal tubules have the greatest innervation, followed by the thick ascending limbs of Henle, the distal convoluted tubules, and the collecting ducts [28].

Histochemical studies of the kidney have demonstrated the existence of cholinesterase-containing fibers [30,298] with a distribution similar to that of the noradrenergic

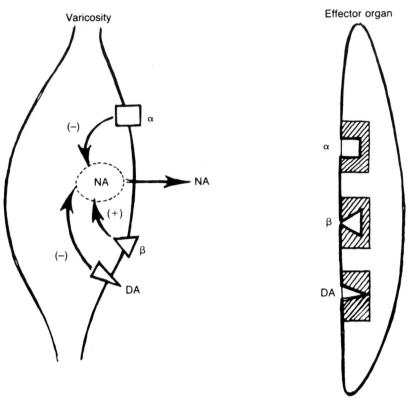

FIG. 12-1. *Diagram of a neuroeffector junction in the peripheral nervous system showing prejunctional and postjunctional adrenergic and dopamine receptors. Adapted from Langer SZ: Presynaptic regulation of catecholamine release.* Biochem Pharmacol 23:1793, 1974.

nerves. Both adrenergic and acetylcholinesterase-containing fibers disappear after the administration of 6-(OH) dopamine (which selectively destroys noradrenergic and dopaminergic nerves), suggesting that the acetylcholinesterase containing fibers may represent adrenergic nerves containing acetylcholine. Indeed, acetylcholinesterase activity and norepinephrine uptake have been shown to coexist in the same axon of a renal nerve [30]. By using horseradish peroxidase-wheat germ agglutinin, which when injected into the kidney is taken up by the nerve fibers and transported retrogradely, neurons were found in the celiac, nodosal, and dorsal root ganglia but not in the brain stem or spinal cord, indicating that the kidney has efferent sympathetic but not parasympathetic innervation [172].

DOPAMINERGIC NERVES

Both norepinephrine and dopamine are present within all noradrenergic neurons [128], but there is evidence that renal neuronal dopamine may be released from a subset of dopaminergic nerves [39,205,313]. This evidence is multifactorial.

The terminal regions of some renal axons contain high levels of dopa decarboxylase (which converts dopa to dopamine), an enzyme absent from terminal noradrenergic axons but characteristic of known dopaminergic axons in the brain [196a]. In addition, some of the catecholamin-

ergic neurons supplying the kidney lack dopamine-beta-hydroxylase, an enzyme necessary to convert dopamine to norepinephrine. Both the cell bodies and terminal regions of some renal sympathetic neurons contain more dopamine than required for the synthesis of norepinephrine.

The dopamine-to-norepinephrine ratio has been used as an index of dopaminergic nerve activity [41,42]. In the dog, the proportion of dopamine to norepinephrine is about fivefold higher in the kidney than in peripheral sympathetic neural tissues, suggesting the presence of a source of dopamine other than the noradrenergic neurons. A higher dopamine-to-norepinephrine ratio (compared with other tissues) has also been described in the renal cortex of cat, dog, and goat, but not in that of guinea pig, ferret, or rat [40,41,125,297]. In the rat, the dopamine-to-norepinephrine ratio in the renal cortex was similar to that in the atrium, spleen, and mesenteric artery, but greater than that found in the vas deferens [40]. Other studies have shown that in the rat the dopamine-to norepinephrine ratio is higher in the inner and outer medulla than in the cortex [160]. In human kidneys, dopamine is mainly found in juxtamedullary and outer medullary areas, whereas norepinephrine is found mainly in the cortex [39].

Release of dopamine from renal nerves may not be solely a consequence of co-release with norepinephrine. Hydralazine administration increases renal venous overflow of dopamine to a greater extent than norepinephrine, whereas

TABLE 12-1a. *Subtypes of alpha-adrenergic receptors.*

	Alpha$_1$	Alpha$_2$
Agonist potency series	E ≥ NE >> PE >> I	E ≥ NE >> PE >> I
Physiologic Responses	Smooth muscle contraction in blood vessels and genitourinary tract	Smooth muscle relaxation in gastroinestinal tract
	Activation of glycogenolysis (rat liver) Inhibition of lipolysis in adipose cells (human, hamster) Platelet aggregation (human, rabbit) Inhibition of insulin release by pancreatic islet cells	
Location	Presynaptic, postsynaptic (e.g., platelets)	Presynaptic, postsynaptic, and nonsynaptic
Mechanism	Stimulation of phospholipase C activity Acterations in cellular calcium-ion fluxes	Inhibition of adenylate cyclase activity

E = epinephrine, NE = norepinephrine, I = isoproterenol, and PE = phenylephrine
(*Adapted from* Leftowitz RJ, Caron MG, Stiles GL: Mechanisms of membrane-receptor regulation. Biochemical, physiological, and clinical insights derived from studies of the adrenergic receptors. *N Engl J Med* 310:1570, 1984.

TABLE 12-1b. *Subtypes of beta-adrenergic receptors.*

	Beta$_1$	Beta$_2$
Agonist potency series*	I > E ≥ NE > PE	I > E >> NE > PE
Physiologic responses	Stimulation of rate and force of cardiac contraction	Smooth muscle relaxation in bronchi, blood vessels, and genitourinary and gastrointestinal tracts
	Stimulation of lipolysis	
		Increase glycogenolysis and gluconeogenesis in liver
	Stimulation of amylase secretion by salivary glands	Increased glucogenolysis in muscle
		Increased insulin and glucagon secretion by pancreatic cells
Location	Postsynaptic	Presynaptic, postsynaptic, and nonsynaptic; neutrophils
Mechanism	Stimulation of adenylate cyclase activity	Stimulation of adenylate cyclase activity

*E = epinephrine, NE = norepinephrine, I = isoproterenol, and PE = phenylephrine
(*Adapted from* Leftowitz RJ, Caron MG, Stiles GL: Mechanisms of membrane-receptor regulation. Biochemical, physiological, and clinical insights derived from studies of the adrenergic receptors. *N Engl J Med* 310:1570, 1984.

isometric handgrip selectively activates noradrenergic nerves [205,206]. Morgunov and Baines have also demonstrated a direct relationship between vagal afferent activity and renal nerve release of dopamine, the opposite of that noted with norepinephrine [313].

The basal dopamine/norepinephrine ratio (0.15) is not influenced by the degree of renal nerve stimulation, but is increased (0.25) by pretreatment with guanethidine [66–69]. Guanethidine decreases renal norepinephrine but does not affect dopamine concentration, again indicating the presence of dopaminergic nerves distinct from noradrenergic nerves [43,68]. Surgical or chemical renal denervation decreases renal tissue norepinephrine content to a greater extent than dopamine content [19,125,199]. Histofluorometric studies have also demonstrated dopaminergic nerves in kidneys of cows, sheep, dogs, and rats [125,126]. In the dog, the arcuate arteries contain mainly norepinephrine, whereas the cortical radial (interlobular) arteries contain both norepinephrine and dopaminergic nerves. At the vascular pole of the glomerulus, at all cortical locations, the innervation is predominantly do-

paminergic. The major renal vessels contain predominantly norepinephrine. As the vessels branch into the renal cortex the percentage of dopaminergic fibers increases and the predominant neurotransmitter becomes dopamine [125,126]. However, the functional role of the dopaminergic nerves remains unclear [23,43,66,210]. Chapman et al. [95,96] reported that renal nerve stimulation after alpha-adrenergic blockade produced vasodilatation, diuresis, and natriuresis that was blocked by sulpiride, a dopamine antagonist. Conversely, renal nerve stimulation in the dog after alpha-adrenergic blockade was not associated with vasodilatation, which should have occurred if there were functional renal dopaminergic nerves [207].

Maturation of the Adrenergic Innervation
In the canine puppy, as in the adult dog, the adrenergic fibers enter the kidney with the renal arteries and follow the arterial route into the inner cortex [299]. At birth, the nephrogenic zone occupies the outer half to two thirds of the cortex, and the nerve fibers are the only structures that can be identified by fluorescence microscopy. By the 14th

Table 12-2. *Physiologic effects of occupation of adrenergic and dopaminergic receptors in renal vasculature and nephron.*

Location	Effect	Receptor Subtype
Renal vascular bed	Relax	DA_1, ?DA_2, $Beta_1$, $Beta_2$
	Constrtict	$Alpha_1$, $Alpha_2$
Afferent arteriole	Relax	DA_1, ?Beta
	Constrict	$Alpha_1$
Efferent arteriole	Relax	DA_1, ?Beta
	Constrict	$Alpha_1$
Glomerulus	GFR (+)	DA_2
	Variable effect	DA_1
	GRF (−)	Alpha
	GFR (0)	Beta
Juxtaglomerular apparatus	Renin (+)	$Beta_1$, $Alpha_1$
	Renin (−)	$Alpha_1$, $Alpha_2$?
PT	Transport (−)	DA_1
	Transport (+)	$Alpha_1$, $Alpha_2$, Beta, ?DA_2
TAL	Transport (+)	$Alpha_1$, Beta
CCD	Antagonize DOCA effect	DA
	Transport (+)	$Beta_1$
	Antagonize ADH effect	$Alpha_2$, ?DA_2

+ = stimulate or increase, − = inhibit or decrease, 0 = no effect, ADH = antidiuretic hormone
DOCA = deoxycorticosterone, PT = proximal tubule, TAL = thick ascending limb, CCD = cortical collecting duct, DA_1 = dopamine₁ receptor, DA_2 = dopamine₂ receptor
The functional effects of receptor subtype occupation are not consistent from species to species or even within species; the predominating renal effects of receptor subtype occupation are summarized in this table. The text should be consulted for detailed discussion of the varying effects of catecholamines on renal function. (*Adapted from* Felder RA, Felder CC, Eisner GM, et al: Renal dopamine receptors. *In* McGrath B, Bell C (eds): *Peripheral Actions of Dopamine.* London, McMillan, 1988, p 124.

day, glomerulogenesis is completed and fluorescence can no longer be detected in this area. In the rest of the cortex, fluorescent fibers are seen in the proximity of the cortical radial artery and afferent arterioles. After the second week of life, the distribution of fluorescent nerves in the cortex remains constant, but the density of the fibers increases. In the medulla, single fluorescent nerve fibers accompanying the vasa rectae appear only after 21 days of age. The nerves emerge in bundles from the arcuate connective tissue sheath before joining the vasa rectae in the outer medulla. The renal tissue levels of norepinephrine correlate with the density of fluorescent nerve fibers. At birth and at 7 days of age, when fluorescent fibers are found only in a narrow region of the inner cortex, the level of norepinephrine is low in the cortex. The subsequent rise in norepinephrine is greater in the inner than in the outer cortical zone [237,299], establishing the pattern encountered in the adult dog.

In the rat kidney, norepinephrine is present in low concentrations at 21 days of fetal life. After birth renal norepinephrine concentration increases steadily until it surpasses adult levels, peaks at 21 days of life, and then decreases to adult levels by 60 days [190,413]. Renal sympathetic innervation parallels the changes in renal norepinephrine during maturation.

Electron microscopic studies of the human fetus have shown that the glomeruli, macula densa, and segments of metanephric distal convoluted tubules are innervated by unmyelinated nerve fibers [468].

PEPTIDERGIC NERVES

Nonadrenergic, noncholinergic neural vasoactive transmitters have been described in the peripheral circulation, including the kidney [58,166]. Some of these fibers are efferent and some are afferent. The substances that mediate the actions of these nerves include substance P (a tachykinin), neurotensin, somatostatin, and vasocative intestinal peptide (VIP) [166,169,170]. Retrograde fluorescent dye labeling and indirect immunofluorescent techniques identified substance-P–containing afferent (see below) neurons in the dorsal root ganglia from L1 to L3 [268]. Substance-P–immunoreactive nerve fibers were also found in renal blood vessels, cortical proximal and distal tubules, and renal pelvis. Occasional fibers were also seen in glomeruli [159]. Neurotensin and VIP have been found in the juxtaglomerular apparatus [166]. Somatostatin, neurotensin, and VIP have also been found in large renal arteries [166].

Afferent Nerves

Electrical activity generated in afferent fibers located within the kidney is conveyed to the central nervous system through the same sympathetic nerves that provide efferent renal innervation [316]. The central projections of renal afferent fibers have been identified by electrical stimulation and antegrade and retrograde transport of horseradish peroxidase by nerve fibers [129,267,399]. In the rat, sensory afferent fibers are derived mainly from the nodosal and dorsal root ganglia [172]. Based on peaks in compound action potential and differences in after-potential, nerve fibers can be classified into three groups, designated as A, B, and C [70]. A fibers have a short, pronounced negative after-potential and minimal positive after-potential. Based on mean conduction velocity and therefore fiber size (diameter), A fibers can be further subdivided into subgroups: A-alpha (12–22 μ), A-beta (5–12 μ), A-delta (2–5 μ), and A-gamma (1–2 μ). B fibers show no negative after-potential, but have a large positive after-potential. A and B fibers are myelinated, and C fibers are unmyelinated and hence have a very slow conduction velocity.

Most of the renal afferent nerves are myelinated [29,124]. A-delta fibers carry information mainly from renal arterial mechanoreceptors [82,100,333], whereas C fibers carry information mainly from renal chemoreceptors [82,100,364]. There are only a few A-beta fibers, and their function has not been determined [10,82]. Afferent fibers from the left kidney enter the spinal cord at the T-8 to L-2 level; afferent fibers from the right kidney enter the spinal cord at the T-7 to L-1 level (the entry points at which the fiber density is the greatest are T-10 to L-1 for the left kidney and T-9 to T-13 for the right kidney) [130]. Most of the afferent renal nerves enter the spinal cord along the medial aspect of the ipsilateral dorsal horn, and a few fibers enter through the contralateral dorsal horn.

Kuo et al. reported that both the peripheral and the central axonal branches are better labeled with horseradish peroxidase in kittens than in adult cats [267]; this may represent the anatomic counterpart of the high renal adrenergic activity noted in the newborn of some species [75,155,163,238].

Monosynapses of afferent nerves with preganglionic sympathetic neurons at the level of Lissauer's tract, lamina VI, and dorsal gray commissure (of the spinal cord) may be responsible for renorenal reflexes. Other somatic and visceral inputs can also be integrated in these areas [339,442]. The information from the afferent fibers is relayed to the nucleus gracilis and subsequently to the nucleus tractus solitarius [396], where cardiovascular afferent interactions are integrated [157]. Afferent renal nerves activate the lateral tegmental field, paramedian reticular nucleus, and the dorsal vagal complex, an important area of cardiovascular regulation in the medulla. Stimulation of renal afferent nerves also activates the lateral preoptic, lateral, and paraventricular nuclei in the hypothalamus [81]. Efferent sympathetic responses to afferent renal nerve stimulation are abolished in the rat by lesions in the region of the anteroventral third ventricle, indicating that this is a site of renal functional regulation. Many of the nuclei activated by afferent renal nerves are also activated by carotid sinus nerves. For example, the paraventricular nucleus, which can influence release of ADH and ACTH, and the lateral hypothalamus, which can affect renin secretion, can be activated by afferent inputs from renal or carotid sinus nerves. Some areas, like the thirst-related preoptic area, are activated by afferent renal nerves, but not by carotid sinus nerves [81].

Renal Neurotransmitters
Catecholamines

Catecholamines leaving the kidney through the urine, lymph, and renal venous blood come from four sources: (1) renal nerves, (2) non-neuronal renal tissue, (3) arterial plasma, and (4) direct adrenal-renal vascular anastomoses [19,20,25,67–69,244,258,312,342,394,422]. Increasing renal nerve activity directly (stimulation of renal nerves) [67,68,258] or indirectly (carotid occlusion, hind limb compression, mental stress, hand grip) [70,205,206,342] results in an increase in renal venous outflow of both dopamine and norepinephrine. Renal nerve stimulation (0.5 to 4 Hz) causes a frequency-dependent increase in renal venous outflow of norepinephrine and dopamine [258]. Renal nerve stimulation at 0.65 Hz results in renal venous catecholamine overflow similar to that noted at basal states; 0.84 Hz is similar to that noted with bilateral carotid occlusion, and about 1.6 Hz with hindquarter compression [67–70].

Urinary norepinephrine reflects mainly arterial rather than renal levels [68], whereas urinary dopamine is derived from renal non-neuronal (i.e., tubular) sources [19,422]. Proximal tubules (S1 and S2 segments) can synthesize dopamine from circulating dihydroxyphenylalanine (DOPA), tyrosine, and conjugated dopamine [108,195, 422,451]. Acute renal denervation increases dopamine excretion but decreases norepinephrine excretion [312]. Chronic renal denervaton reduces the excretion of both norepinephrine and dopamine [312]. However, after chronic renal denervation, the reduction in norepinephrine excretion is greater than that of dopamine, indicating the existence of a pool of dopamine separate from norepinephrine. The natriuresis seen after acute renal denervation may be related to the increase in urinary dopamine, dopamine/norepinephrine ratio, and/or a decrease in urinary norepinephrine [232,312].

The concentration of norepinephrine is similar, whereas the concentration of dopamine is lower in renal lymph than in arterial blood [422]. Because lymph flow is only about 1 μl/min, the amount of catecholamine cleared by this route is small. The low catecholamine levels in renal lymph suggest that catecholamine levels are low within the renal interstitium, except for the synaptic cleft [422].

Approximately 65% to 70% of norepinephrine and dopamine and 80% to 90% of epinephrine present in the renal artery blood are extracted by the kidney [67–70]. The fractional extractions of catecholamines are not influenced by moderate renal activity [68], but may be reduced by high nerve activity (2–4 Hz). Ten percent of the filtered catecholamines are reabsorbed (mainly by the proximal tubule) [20]. Norepinephrine and dopamine released into the peritubular space are methylated, and both amines and their methylated derivatives are secreted into the tubular lumen [20]. The tubular secretion of dopamine (and metabolites) is much greater than that of norepinephrine (and metabolites) [20,185].

Salt depletion increases norepinephrine levels in plasma and renal venous blood [84,274,288,343]. A low-salt diet reduces the release of dopamine from renal nerves but not of norepinephrine [19]. Salt loading or extracellular fluid volume expansion results in an increase in urinary dopamine excretion and a decrease in norepinephrine excretion [6,26,65,88,144]. Both sodium and chloride are important in modulating the increases in dopamine excretion [26].

There are no studies comparing the release of renal catecholamines in the newborn with that in the adult. Very high levels of plasma catecholamines are observed during birth [270,346], the predominant circulating catecholamine being norepinephrine (epinephrine in adults) [223]. The catecholamines may play a role in adaptation to extrauterine life, including cardiovascular regulation and normal maintenance of blood sugar concentration, nonshivering thermogenesis, and free fatty acid metabolism [204]. The circulating catecholamine levels initially decrease with age [309], and then increase after 20 years of age [256].

Urinary catecholamines are low at birth and increase with maturation [110,111,325]. A low-sodium diet increases urinary norepinephrine in low-birth-weight infants [426] and adults [6,26]. Dopamine excretion increases only in infants [426], whereas it decreases in adults [26].

Adrenal medullary activity, when compared with noradrenergic activity, is lower at birth and during the first year of life. Beyond 1 year of age, the development of noradrenergic and adrenomedullary activity proceed at a similar pace, reaching full maturation at about 5 years of age [110,111]. Adrenosympathetic activity is initially less in girls than boys, but similar by 5 years of age.

Neuropeptides and Other Neurotransmitters in the Kidney

A discussion regarding neurotransmitters other than catecholamines is beyond the scope of this chapter.

Renal Receptors
Afferent Receptors

Several afferent receptors have been described in the kidney, including mechanoreceptors, chemoreceptors, and possibly nociceptors.

MECHANORECEPTORS

Mechanoreceptors have been demonstrated in the kidneys of several species [17,316,333–335], including nonhuman primates [178]. These receptors have been localized in the cortex, medulla, pelvis, and the renal arteries and veins. Elevation in subcapsular, ureteral, venous, or interstitial pressure increases discharge in ipsilateral afferent nerves [335,445]. Pressure on the surface of the kidney also activates renal mechanoreceptors [17,178]. The activity of renal arterial mechanoreceptors varies directly with arterial blood pressure [316]; both pulse synchronous and asynchronous receptors have been described [178,316]. Occlusion of the renal artery results in the disappearance of pulse synchronous but not asynchronous afferent nerve activity. Stimulation of renal afferent mechanoreceptors may elicit

excitatory and inhibitory effects on the function of the contralateral kidney [259] and systemic vascular effects [178,259,317]. Renal mechanoreceptors exhibit rapid adaptation to a sustained stimulus [37]. The physiologic role of renal afferent nerves is discussed in a later section.

CHEMORECEPTORS

Renal chemoreceptors have been identified in the rat [259,260,363–365,377], but not in the dog [259]. Two types of chemoreceptors have been described. R-1 are receptors with no resting discharge that are activated by renal ischemia. The discharge consists of a train of impulses that cease abruptly when renal blood flow returns. R-1 receptors are not responsive to changes in renal perfusion, renal venous, or ureteral pressure [316,365]. R-2 chemoreceptors, which are more numerous than R-1 chemoreceptors, exhibit a basal discharge and continue to discharge in the face of a sustained stimulus [364]. The resting discharge is highest in the nondiuretic state and declines under diuretic conditions, e.g., during extracellular fluid volume expansion. Like R-1 chemoreceptors, R-2 chemoreceptors are activated by ischemia [365], renal artery stenosis [142], backflow of urine into the pelvis, or perfusion of the pelvis with mannitol, potassium, or sodium chloride solutions. Adenosine, prostaglandins, and kinins may also stimulate the chemoreceptors [142,243,245,401] and produce an increase in ipsilateral afferent nerve activity [363,365]. As with mechanoreceptors, the effects of chemoreceptor stimulation on efferent fibers may not be homogeneous; some fibers may be excitatory and others inhibitory [259,377]. The functional consequences of chemoreceptor activation are discussed in a later section.

NOCICEPTORS

The existence of nociceptive receptors in the renal pelvis and capsule is suggested by the painful sensation elicited by distention of the kidney [116].

Efferent Receptors
CLASSIFICATION OF ADRENERGIC AND DOPAMINERGIC RECEPTORS

Neurotransmitters convey specific messages by binding to receptors on the cell membrane surface. Receptors are linked to membrane-bound, signal-transducing binding proteins [177], which act as intermediaries in the generation of second messengers that elicit biologic responses [278]. Ahlquist divided the responses to catecholamines (epinephrine, norepinephrine) into those resulting from activation of alpha-adrenergic and beta-adrenergic receptors [3]. Subsequently other investigators have subdivided these receptors into alpha$_1$, alpha$_2$, beta$_1$, beta$_2$, adrenoceptor subtypes [55,271,272]. Additional data suggest that both alpha$_1$ and alpha$_2$ adrenoceptors can be further subdivided into alpha-a and alpha-b sub-subtypes [79,165]. The cloning, sequencing, and expression of the gene coding for the beta$_1$, beta$_2$, and alpha$_2$ adrenoceptors have been reported [253].

Dopamine, the other endogenous catecholamine, was initially thought to function exclusively as a precursor of epinephrine and norepinephrine. Robison et al. first suggested that dopamine may play an important role as a neurotransmitter within the central nervous system [376]. In 1979, Kebabian and Calne provided evidence for the existence of two dopamine receptor subtypes, dopamine$_1$ and dopamine$_2$ [247]. At least five dopamine receptor subtypes have been cloned.

ADRENERGIC AND DOPAMINERGIC RECEPTORS IN THE KIDNEY

Both adrenergic and dopaminergic receptors have been described in the kidney (Tables 12-1 and 12-2). Similar to receptors found elsewhere, the renal adrenergic and dopaminergic receptors are linked to membrane-bound, signal-transducing guanosine triphosphate (G)-binding proteins. The G proteins function as intermediaries in transmembrane signaling pathways that consist of three proteins: receptors, G proteins, and effectors [177]. Beta$_1$ and beta$_2$ adrenoceptors and dopamine$_1$ receptors stimulate adenylate cyclase activity through the stimulatory G protein (G$_s$). Alpha$_2$ adrenoceptors and dopamine$_2$ receptors inhibit adenylate cyclase activity through the inhibitory G protein (G$_i$). Actions on adenylate cyclase lead to an increase (G$_s$) or decrease (G$_i$) of the second messenger cyclic AMP. Alpha$_1$ adrenoceptors stimulate phospholipase C (PL-C) activity, leading to the breakdown of phosphoinositides into two second messengers, inositol phosphate and diacylglycerol [54,361]. Alpha$_1$ adrenoceptors may be linked to a G protein (Gq) other than G$_s$ or G$_i$ [439]. Dopamine$_1$ receptors also may increase PL-C activity in the kidney [145,151]; dopamine$_2$ receptors may decrease PL-C activity in some cells [395]; however, no such effect has been described in renal tissue. Neurotransmitters may also activate phospholipase A$_2$, leading to the formation of biologically active arachidonate metabolites [398].

Receptors can be located in the axon (presynaptic or prejunctional) or in the target cell (postsynaptic or extrasynaptic, depending on proximity to the nerve terminal) (Fig. 12-1). Presynaptic alpha$_2$ adrenoceptors and DA$_2$ receptors inhibit the release of norepinephrine, whereas presynaptic beta$_2$ adrenoceptors increase norepineprhine release [97,240,273,416]. In the rat kidney both alpha$_1$ and alpha$_2$ adrenoceptors may modulate neurotransmitter release [379]; beta$_2$ adrenoceptor facilitation of neurotransmitter release is usually masked by the dominant alpha adrenoceptor system [389]. In the adult kidney, presynaptic modulation of catecholamine release is not physiologically important [287,372,389]. The role of presynaptic receptors in the developing kidney is not known.

Location of Postsynaptic or Extrasynaptic Adrenergic and Dopaminergic Receptors Along the Nephron

The use of radioligands and autoradiograph methods has made it possible to identify and localize various types and subtypes of neurotransmitter receptors in the kidney. These techniques and neurotransmitter-adenylate cyclase linkage have been used to identify receptors in specific nephron segments.

Alpha Adrenoceptors

The renal vasculature contains many more alpha$_1$ than alpha$_2$ adrenoceptors [318,319,420,421,428,430]. The density of alpha$_2$ adrenoceptors varies with species, decreasing in the order: mouse > rat > rabbit > dog > man [98,331]. More alpha$_2$ than alpha$_1$ adrenoceptors are present in renal cortical tubules [112,184,300,386,406,428]. There are fewer alpha adrenoceptors in medulla than cortex, and most are of the alpha$_2$ subtype [318,319,420,421, 428]. Two subtypes of alpha$_2$ adrenoceptors are present in renal tissue [414,437]. Alpha$_1$ adrenoceptors are not present in guinea pig kidney, and the alpha$_2$ adrenoceptor present has a much lower affinity than in other species [226,331]. In the adult dog, most of the alpha adrenoceptors (both alpha$_1$ and alpha$_2$) are in medullary blood vessels [421,430]; neither adrenoceptor could be identified in renal tubules by autoradiography [421,430] or radioligand binding [155]. Except for the guinea pig, glomeruli contain alpha$_2$ but not alpha$_1$ adrenoceptors [302,318,319,430, 448]. Alpha$_1$ and alpha$_2$ adrenoceptors are present in proximal convoluted tubule [269,318,319,420,421,447,465]; alpha$_2$ adrenoceptors have been described in descending thin limb of Henle [449], and cortical [89,447] and medullary collecting duct [447]. No alpha$_{1-2}$ adrenoceptors were detected in proximal straight tubule [269,447] or in medullary or cortical thick ascending limb [269,447]; alpha$_1$ adrenoceptors were not found in cortical collecting duct [269] (Table 12-2).

Beta Adrenoceptors

Beta adrenoceptors are mainly located in the cortex and outer stripe of the medulla [9,197,281,320,427,429]. Few beta adrenoceptors are seen in renal vasculature [429], being localized mainly in the afferent arterioles [197]. Beta$_1$ adrenoceptors predominate in the rat [407,429] and beta$_2$ adrenoceptors predominate in the dog [282] and guinea pig [281], and seem to be equal in distribution in the sheep [236]. Beta$_1$ adrenoceptors are found in glomeruli [219,263, 281,282,303,410,429,430,452], juxtaglomerular apparatus [282,320,429], distal convoluted tubule [217,218,330,429], and cortical [197,217,218,330,429] and medullary collecting ducts [217,218,310,311,330]. Beta$_2$ adrenoceptors are present in glomeruli of the rat [78,164,429]. There are also beta adrenoceptors in mesangial cells and in the thick ascending limb of the rat, but the subtype was not determined [197].

There is controversy regarding the presence of beta receptors in the proximal tubule. In the rabbit, the presence of beta-adrenoceptor–linked adenylate cyclase has been identified by some investigators [148,321], but not by others [310]. In the rat, beta adrenoceptors were detected in vitro by adenylate cyclase linkage and immunohistochemical and radioligand-binding studies [9,225,431], but not by autoradiographic studies [197,320,427,429]. No beta-adrenoceptor–linked adenylate cyclase activation was detected in the isolated proximal convoluted tubule of rat [310,311] or dog [321]. Beta$_2$ adrenoceptors have been detected by autoradiography in the proximal straight tubule of the dog [282] and guinea pig [281]. Beta-adrenoceptor–linked adenylate cyclase activity was also found in the proximal tubule pars recta of the dog [321] and baboon [211], but not of the rat [310,311,321] or man [211]. The reasons for these discrepancies are not clear.

Dopaminergic Receptors

Dopamine₁ [5,7,8,71,167,180,181,285,322] receptors have been identified in renal vasculature from the major renal arteries to the afferent arteriole [438]. Dopamine₂ [305] receptors may also be present in these vessels, but in smaller quantities than dopamine₁ receptors. Dopamine₂ receptors predominate in glomeruli [149,390], whereas dopamine₁ receptors have been identified only in cultured mesangial cells [392]. Dopamine₁ receptors are present mainly in the cortex and have been localized in proximal convoluted and straight tubule [148,151,250] and cortical collecting duct, but not in cortical thick ascending limb [250] and distal convoluted tubule. Dopamine₂ receptors are present in both cortex and medulla [152], but their localization to specific nephron segments is unknown. Like the alpha₂ adrenoceptors [362], dopamine₁ and dopamine₂ receptors are present in basolateral membranes [147]. There is also evidence for the presence of alpha [337], beta [187], and dopamine [145–147] receptors in brush border membranes. The location of adrenergic receptors in specific segments of the nephron, as identified by radioligand binding, autoradiography, or adenylate cyclase linkage, is summarized in Table 12-3 (adrenergic) and Table 12-4 (dopaminergic).

In summary, the renal vasculature contains alpha₁, beta₁, and beta₂ adrenoceptors and dopamine₁ receptors.

There is abundant evidence for the presence of alpha₁ and alpha₂ adrenoceptors and dopamine₁ receptors in the proximal convoluted tubules. Beta₂ adrenoceptors and dopamine₁ receptors are present in proximal tubular pars rectae. Alpha₂ and beta₁ adrenoceptors are present in collecting ducts. Beta adrenoceptors (subtype not determined) are also present in the distal tubules. There is no agreement on the location and subtypes of autonomic receptors.

CONSEQUENCES OF OCCUPATION OF ADRENERGIC AND DOPAMINERGIC RECEPTORS

The physiologic consequences of the occupation of postjunctional (postsynpatic or extrasynaptic) receptors in some nonrenal and renal tissues are listed in Tables 12-1 and 12-2, respectively. Renal vasoconstriction occurs when postjunctional vascular alpha₁ and alpha₂ adrenoceptors are occupied by agonists [133,182,212,423,443,461,462]. Renal vasodilatation is associated with beta₁ [435] and beta₂ adrenoceptors [326,328,329,435], and with dopamine₁ receptors [71,167,180,181,285,385]. Glomerular filtration rate is decreased by alpha₁ and alpha₂ agonists, and variably affected by beta (subtype not determined) and dopamine₁ agonists. Sodium reabsorption is increased by alpha₁ and beta (subtype not determined) adrenergic agonists [21,22,44,117,119,457], whereas sodium excretion is increased by dopamine₁ agonists [23,46,231,232,351]. The effect of alpha₂ and dopamine₂ agonists on sodium transport is discussed more extensively in other sections.

Table 12-3. Current state of knowledge concerning adrenergic receptors in specific nephron segments based on radioligand binding (RB), autoradiography (AR), adenylate cyclase (AC) linkage, or immunohistochemical (IH) techniques.

Nephron Segment	Alpha Adrenoceptor	Ref	Beta Adrenoceptor	Ref
Arterioles	A₂ (AR), A₁ (AR)	318,319	B(RB)	9
Glomerulus	A₂ (RB,AR,ACᵃ)	302,430,448	B₁(RB,AR)	197,303,429
	A₁ absent (AR)	112,318	B₂(AR)	429
Proximal tubule				
PCT	A₂ (AR)	319,428,465	B(AC)	148,310
	A₁ (RB,AR)	269,318,428		
PT	A₂ (RB,AC)	224,337,431	B(RB,IH,AC)	9,225,431
	A₁(RB)	431		
PST	A₂ absent(AC)	447	B₂(AR,AC)	281,282,321
	A₁ absent(RB)	269		
Intermediate tubule				
DTL	A₂ (AC)	449		
Distal tubule				
MTAL	A₂ absent (AC)	448	B(AR)	320,429
			no AC linkage	310
CTAL	A₂ absent (AC)	448	B(AR,AC)	310,320
DCT			B₁(AR,AC,RB)	310,320,330
CCD	A₂ (ACᵇ)	89,269,448	B₁(AR,AC)	310,320,330,427
MCD	A₂ (ACᵇ,AR)	89,448,168a	B(AC,RB,AR)	168a,310,330

ᵃ Inhibits effects of PTH and serotonin [448].
ᵇ Inhibits effect of AVP only [358].
Abbreviations: PCT = proximal convoluted tubule, PT = proximal tubule, PST = proximal straight tubule, DTL = descending limb of Henle, MTAL = medullary thick ascending limb of Henle, CTAL = cortical ascending limb of Henle, DTC = distal convoluted tubule, CCD = cortical collecting duct, MCD = medullary collecting duct.

Table 12-4. *Evidence for dopamine receptors in renal vasculature and renal tubule based on radioligand binding and adenylate cyclase studies.*

Location	Receptor subtype	Species	References
Renal artery	DA_1, DA_2	Rabbit, dog	7, 8, 305, 322
Glomerulus	DA_2	Rat	149
Mesangial cell	DA_1	Rat	392
PCT	DA_1	Rabbit, rat	148, 250
PST	DA_1	Rabbit, rat	148, 250
PT (BBMV, BLMV)	DA_1, DA_2	Dog	147
CCD	DA_1	Rabbit, rat	151, 250
Medulla	DA_2	Rat	151

DA_1 = dopamine-1 receptor
DA_2 = dopamine-2 receptor
PT = proximal tubule
BBMV = brush border membrane vesicles
BLMV = basolateral membrane vesicles

PCT = proximal convoluted tubule
PST = proximal straight tubule
CCD = cortical collecting duct

Potassium excretion is decreased by $beta_1$ adrenoceptors [21,113,114,246] and may be increased by dopamine$_1$ agonists [59]. The hydroosmotic effect of vasopressin is antagonized by alpha$_2$ [89,266] and dopamine (probably through the dopamine$_2$ receptor) agonists [323]. Renin secretion is increased by beta$_1$ [119,257,345], by dopamine$_1$ agonists [59], and decreased by alpha$_2$ agonists [405] and dopamine$_2$ receptors [463]. Alpha$_1$ adrenergic agonists increase renin secretion in vivo [60], but decrease it in vitro [294]. Erythropoietin production may be increased by beta (presumed to be beta$_2$ adrenoceptor) adrenergic agonists [78,164,429].

Alpha Adrenoceptors

Infusion of pharmacologic doses of epinephrine or norepinephrine into the renal artery causes vasoconstriction and decreases in glomerular filtration rate and in the excretion of sodium and potassium [21,22,24,347,386]. Glomerular filtration rate decreases to a lesser extent than renal plasma flow, resulting in an increase in filtration fraction [347]. When low doses of norepinephrine or epinephrine are infused, glomerular filtration remains nearly constant because of an increase in transglomerular capillary hydrostatic pressure gradient and an increase in glomerular ultrafiltration coefficient in the face of a decrease in glomerular plasma flow [62]. Myers et al. concluded from their studies in rats that norepinephrine affects mainly the tone of efferent arterioles [324]. In contrast, in the isolated perfused rabbit kidney, norepinephrine was reported to increase mainly afferent arteriolar resistance [366]. In the hamster pouch—renal transplant preparation, norepinephrine constricted both afferent and efferent arterioles [101]. On isolated renal vessels of rabbits, norepinephrine had a greater vasoconstrictor effect on cortical radial (interlobular) arteries and afferent arterioles than on efferent arterioles [140]. Thus, alpha adrenergic agonists appear to affect mainly the tone of preglomerular vessels; greater effects on postglomerular vessels observed by some are probably due to adjustments to perturbations in systemic blood pressure.

The renal vasoconstrictor effect of norepinephrine is primarily mediated by alpha$_1$ adrenoceptors [119,141, 212,345]. This is in agreement with the radioligand binding studies, suggesting a predominance of alpha$_1$ over alpha$_2$ adrenoceptors [318,319,420] in blood vessels. Alpha$_2$ adrenergic agonists can decrease renal blood flow [133,202,212,461,462] but are much less potent vasoconstrictors than alpha$_1$ adrenergic agonists. Under certain conditions the alpha$_2$ adrenoceptors normally situated extrasynaptically assume a postsynaptic position, which is the normal location of alpha$_1$ adrenoceptors. In this situation, alpha$_2$ adrenoceptors can be activated by norepinephrine released at nerve terminals and by circulating catecholamines [357,358]. This may explain why alpha$_2$-adrenergic agonists were ineffective vasoconstrictors in the rat studied in vivo [462], whereas they were effective vasoconstrictors (albeit to a lesser extent than alpha$_1$ adrenergic agonists) in the isolated rat kidney [21].

Although alpha$_1$ and to a lesser extent alpha$_2$ adrenergic blockers can attenuate the vasoconstrictor effects of norepinephrine and of renal nerve stimulation, the intrarenal infusion of alpha-adrenergic antagonsist into the kidney does not alter renal blood flow [99,119,162,424]. Under physiologic conditions, there appears to be minimal alpha adrenergic influence of circulating catecholamines on renal hemodynamics, at least in the adult.

The infusion of alpha-adrenergic antagonists into the renal artery of anesthetized dogs induces a natriuresis without changing glomerular filtration rate or renal blood flow [99,162,424]. Alpha-adrenergic agonists have an antinatriuretic effect, which has been demonstrated both in vivo and in vitro [21,22,203,347,357]. This is due mainly to an increase in sodium transport in the proximal convoluted tubule [44,90,91,168,457] and is mediated by alpha$_1$ adrenoceptors [21,22,119,201-203]. The renal effects of alpha$_2$ adrenoceptor stimulation have been variable. Studies have shown that this maneuver increases [21,401-405], decreases [173,415,423], or does not alter [119,203] sodium reabsorption. Insel et al. [224] and Nord et al. [337] reported that alpha$_2$ but not alpha$_1$-adrenoceptors affected sodium transport in rabbit proximal tubular cells, and Fildes et al. reported that in dogs alpha$_2$ adrenergic blockade increased sodium excretion [162]. In the isolated perfused rat kidney, stimulation of alpha$_2$ adrenoceptors reverses the diuretic effect of furosemide [402] or arachidonic acid

[358]. However, the intravenous infusion of alpha$_2$ adrenoceptor agonists increased sodium and water excretion [173,415,423].

In an attempt to reconcile these apparently divergent findings, Pettinger et al. [357,358] suggested that the physiologic effects of α_2-adrenoceptor activation depends on the preactivation of adenylate cyclase and the nature of the hormone activating the adenylate cyclase. They further proposed separate roles for alpha adrenoceptor subtypes in the handling of water and electrolytes. According to this scheme, renal nerve stimulation is associated with sodium and water reabsorption, because the alpha$_1$-adrenoceptors are located postsynaptically [403]. Renal alpha$_2$-adrenoceptors, when in their usual extrasynaptic location, are not responsive to renal nerve stimulation, but respond to circulating catecholamines and other hormones [404]. Thus, alpha$_2$-adrenoceptors can cause a natriuresis and diuresis by antagonizing the effects of vasopressin in distal tubular cells [89,266,403]. Under certain circumstances, alpha$_2$-adrenoceptors can increase in number and locate in postsynaptic sites; in this state, they can mediate antinatriuretic effects, possibly by stimulating the Na^+/H^+ antiport in proximal tubular cells [337]. In addition, alpha$_1$ adrenoceptors stimulate renal gluconeogenesis [21,301,450], and their effect on renal sodium reabsorption apparently requires glucose metabolism [22].

Alpha$_1$-adrenoceptors may increase sodium transport by stimulating phospholipase C activity, leading to activation of protein kinase C [332]. Protein kinase C activation stimulates Na^+/H^+ antiport activity at the brush border membrane in some cells, including those of the proximal tubule [304]. Cyclic AMP decreases Na^+/H^+ activity [241], and because alpha$_2$ adrenoceptors decrease adenylate cyclase activity, a decrease in cAMP leads to an increase in Na^+/H^+ activity [284a]. A direct effect of alpha$_2$ adrenergic agonists [93,131,337] is also possible because the alpha$_2$ adrenoceptor may be the same as the Na^+/H^+ antiporter [340]. Alpha adrenoceptors can also increase sodium transport at the basolateral membrane by increasing Na^+/K^+ ATPase activity [38].

In addition to effects on sodium and water transport, alpha-adrenergic agonists increase bicarbonate, chloride, and phosphate reabsorption [21,22,90]. The subtypes of alpha-adrenergic receptors that mediate these effects are not fully characterized; Baines and Ho suggested that the antiphosphaturic effect may be due to alpha$_2$ adrenoceptors [21].

Beta Adrenoceptors

The infusion of the nonselective beta-adrenergic agonist isoproterenol (nM range) into the renal artery of dogs results in an increase in renal blood flow and variable changes in glomerular filtration rate [314,347]. When isoproterenol, in the micromolar range, is infused into the renal artery of dogs, renal vasoconstriction occurs because of stimulation of alpha receptors and the consequent decrease in systemic pressure due to overflow of the agonists into the systemic circulation [292,314]. Both beta$_1$ and beta$_2$ adrenoceptors mediate the renal vasodilatory effect of isoproterenol [435]. Glomerular filtration rate is not usually affected by beta-adrenergic stimulation, apparently because of the counter-balancing effect of decreased glomerular ultrafiltration coefficient and increased glomerular capillary hydrostatic pressure gradient [62].

Under basal conditions, renal beta-adrenergic blockade does not alter renal blood flow [209]. However, when renal function is decreased, renal blood flow and glomerular filtration rate may be further decreased by beta-adrenergic blockade with propranolol [36,132,456]. Thus, in pathologic states, beta adrenoceptors may be important modulators of renal hemodynamics. The effect of beta-adrenergic blockade on sodium excretion is variable [87,209,440,456].

The effects of beta-adrenergic agonists on water and electrolyte excretion depends on the route of administration, dose, and state of fluid and electrolyte balance [391]. Systemic administration of beta-adrenergic agonists results in a decrease in excretion of sodium, chloride, potassium, and water [186–188, 280], due to increased reabsorption in the proximal and distal convoluted tubules [186]; reabsorption in the loop of Henle is decreased [186]. These effects could be mediated in part by a decrease in renal perfusion pressure and an increase in renin-angiotension [367] and vasopressin activity or levels [279,391]. However, isoproterenol increases water and electrolyte reabsorption in rats with congenital diabetes insipidus [280] and in rats treated with the angiotensin II antagonist, saralasin [188]. The antidiuretic, antinatriuretic, and antikaliuretic effects of beta adrenergic stimulation were also demonstrated in the isolated perfused kidney [21,57,277].

Gill and Casper [175] reported that the infusion of isoproterenol (nM range) into the renal artery during alpha-adrenergic blockade in hypophysectomized dogs undergoing a water diuresis increased urine flow and free water clearance in the absence of changes in glomerular filtration rate. Because sodium excretion was not affected, the authors concluded that beta-adrenergic stimulation decreases proximal tubular reabsorption and increases distal sodium reabsorption. Reid et al. [367] also reported that isoproterenol increases free water clearance in the dog undergoing a water diuresis, but this effect was associated with an increase in glomerular filtration rate and a decrease in renal vascular resistance. Cyclic AMP was found to mimic the effects of isoproterenol or proximal sodium transport in the dog [176]. However, other investigators using similar dosages (nM range) could not demonstrate an effect of isoproterenol on sodium transport by either micropuncture studies of the proximal tubule or whole animal clearances [63,418]. Because the latter studies were performed during hydropenia, a proximal tubular effect may have been masked by increased transport at more distal sites along the nephron [186]. The inability to detect an effect of beta-adrenergic agonists by micropuncture was probably due to the fact that in the dog beta adrenoceptors are present only in the straight segment of the proximal tubule [321], which is not amenable to micropuncture. In the rat, where beta adrenoceptors have been detected in the proximal convoluted tubule [9], the perfusion of the peritubular capillaries with epinephrine during alpha-adrenergic blockade (thus a state of beta agonist stimulation) decreased proximal tubular fluid absorption [91]. However, other investigators reported that isoproterenol increases transport in the proximal convoluted tubule [44,168,186,187,457]. This apparent discrepancy may be due to differences in specificity of agents for the beta adrenoceptor. In the latter studies [168,186,187,457] the drugs have been used in concentrations such that other adrenoceptors (e.g., alpha adrenoceptors) also may have been occupied.

In the cortical thick ascending limb of the mouse [359], perfused in vitro beta-adrenergic stimulation increases chloride transport. In the rabbit cortical collecting tubule, beta-adrenergic stimulation increases chloride transport [216–218] and decreases potassium secretion [249]; osmotic water permeability and sodium transport are not affected [216]. The changes in sodium, chloride, and potassium excretion are due to beta$_1$-adrenergic stimulation [246], whereas the decrease in urine flow is related to beta$_2$-adrenergic stimulation [391]. Kimmel and Goldfarb suggest that the decrease in potassium secretion in the cortical collecting tubule is secondary to the increase in chloride transport [249] induced by changes in cAMP [115,249,310, 311,434]; cAMP may inhibit Na$^+$-K$^+$-ATPase in rat and rabbit tubule [56,393]. Another possibility is that the beta-adrenoceptors' effects are due to different G protein-ion linkage [464a]. A beta-adrenoceptor may be associated to G protein linked to chloride and potassium transport in principal cells of the cortical collecting ducts; no such linkage would be present in the proximal tubule.

In summary, renal vasodilatation is due to occupation of both beta$_1$- and beta$_2$-adrenoceptors. Occupation of renal beta$_1$-adrenoceptors results also in a decrease in sodium, chloride, and potassium excretion due to effects on proximal and distal convoluted tubule and cortical collecting duct transport. Under certain circumstances in some species (e.g., during water diuresis and alpha-adrenergic blockade in the dog), sodium and water transport can be decreased in the proximal tubule. This may be due to occupation of beta$_2$-adrenoceptors.

Dopamine Receptors

Dopamine modulates renal hemodynamics and affects electrolyte and water reabsorption [4,71,95,96,151,167,180, 181,196,220,221,276,285]. Low doses of dopamine given directly into the renal artery induce vasodilation that is not inhibited by alpha- and beta-adrenergic antagonists, but is blocked by dopamine antagonists [180]. As with most vasodilators, the increase in renal blood flow [94,196], occurs predominantly in the inner cortex and outer medulla [417]. The effect is mediated by dopamine$_1$ receptors [71,167,180,181,231,285,384,385]; dopamine$_1$ receptors linked to activation of adenylate cyclase have been demonstrated in renal arteries [7,103,305,322]. The presence of other dopamine receptor subtypes in the renal vascular bed is not well established. Presynaptic [35,136] and postsynaptic [305,390] dopamine$_2$ receptors are present in the renal vascular bed, but whether they play a role in dopamine induced vasodilatation is not yet established [151,233,285,286,390]. Dopamine has been shown to vasodilate the main renal arteries, the arcuate and cortical radial arteries, and the efferent and afferent arterioles [12,139,360,419]. Dopamine$_1$ receptors have been so far

identified only in the main renal arteries and the afferent and efferent arterioles [7,138a,322,438]. The role of prostaglandins and kinins in the vasodilatory action of dopamine is controversial [151,231,291].

Intravenous infusion of dopamine blockers does not decrease renal blood flow [167,351], indicating that in the adult animal under basal conditions there is minimal dopaminergic influence on renal circulation, a situation similar to that noted for alpha- and beta-adrenoceptors [163,456].

The effect of dopamine on glomerular filtration rate is less predictable [23,59,107,167,222,231,390]. Imbs et al. reported that dopamine increases glomerular filtration rate in hydropenic but not in water-loaded dogs [222]. We found that the dopamine$_1$ agonist SKF 38393 increases glomerular filtration rate in rats with denervated but not innervated kidneys [156]. The dopamine$_1$ agonist fenoldopam increases single-nephron blood flow without affecting single-nephron filtration rate and glomerular pressure; this suggests that the glomerular ultrafiltration coefficient was decreased [360]. Barnett et al. have reported that dopamine attenuates the contractile response to angiotensin II of isolated rat glomeruli and cultured mesangial cells [34].

The renal vasodilation produced by administration of dopamine and dopamine$_1$ agonists is associated with natriuresis and diuresis [86,167,180,181,220,221,231], due in part to alterations in peritubular physical factors controlling renal sodium transport. Dopamine-induced alterations in water and electrolyte excretion, however, can also occur in the absence of changes in renal blood flow or glomerular filtration rate [231,296], suggesting a direct tubular effect. Dopamine also has a phosphaturic effect [242], which persists after the renal hemodynamic changes have subsided [107].

Dopamine decreases transport of solute in rat renal proximal convoluted tubule [14,56,92] and rabbit proximal straight tubule [46] by inhibiting Na$^+$-K$^+$-ATPase activity [14,56]. The dopamine$_1$ agonist fenoldopam also may decrease Na$^+$/H$^+$ antiport activity in renal cortical brush border membranes [146]. Dopamine may also act through presynaptic dopamine$_2$ receptors to decrease norepinephrine release and thus sodium reabsorption [34a]. The inhibitory effect of dopamine on sodium transport is not mediated by prostaglandins or the kallikrein system [231]. Like alpha$_2$ adrenoceptors [89,266,403], dopamine receptors antagonize the hydro-osmotic effect of vasopressin in cortical collecting ducts [323]. In addition, dopamine antagonizes the effect of deoxycorticosterone acetate (DOCA) on transtubular potential difference [323]. The dopamine receptor subtype mediating these effects is not known. In denervated kidneys, dopamine increases sodium transport [34a,275].

The natriuresis of acute and chronic sodium loading may be in part regulated by dopamine [6,15,234,265,351,408]. High-NaCl diet is associated with increased renal dopamine levels; the opposite is noted with a low-sodium diet [6,19,26,341]. The natriuresis of saline loading and unilateral renal denervation is attenuated by dopamine blockers [234,265,351], through the dopamine$_1$ receptor [232].

There are also reports suggesting that dopamine participates in the natriuresis induced by atrial natriuretic factor [356].

Function of Renal Nerves
Efferent Nerves

Spontaneous renal efferent nerve activity has been recorded in several animal species, including rat, cat, rabbit, and dog. Basal efferent renal nerve activity occurring in polysynchronous rhythmic bursts at about 1 to 2 Hz has been described in both anesthetized and unanesthetized states [2,192,193,251,371,436]. Basal renal nerve activity averaged 1.7 Hz in the chloralose-urethane–anesthetized normotensive rat and 3.8 Hz in the spontaneously hypertensive rat [289]. In cats, discharge frequencies of renal sympathetic nerves may reach 4 Hz during severe hypotension [248].

Efferent sympathetic discharge to the kidneys can be influenced by supraspinal centers [72,81,396], by carotid and cardiopulmonary reflexes [11,191,194,339,355,368, 442,453], and by inputs from somatic nerves [208,227,248] and viscera [453–455], including the kidney (renorenal reflexes) [259–261,363,365]. Stimulation of mechanoreceptors in the atrium and carotid/aortic nerves is inhibitory to afferent nerve activity and is accompanied by an increase in renal blood flow and urine flow and a decrease in renin secretion [227]. In the rabbit, the impulses are carried through barosensory A and C fibers of aortic nerves. The natriuresis of extracellular fluid volume expansion is associated with decreased renal nerve activity [122,315]. The natriuresis that follows closure of a chronic arteriovenous fistula or acute unilateral nephrectomy may also be due to changes in efferent renal nerve activity [18,213,370]. Carotid sinus denervation and bilateral occlusion of the carotid arteries interfere with both the hemodynamic and renal functional changes caused by unilateral nephrectomy, indicating that carotid baroreceptors constitute the major afferent pathway mediating the renal response to acute unilateral nephrectomy [18,370].

Stimulation of nociceptive receptors carried by C fibers is excitatory to renal nerve efferent activity and is associated with a decrease in renal blood flow, an increase in renin secretion, and antidiuresis [189,227,339]. A reflex increase in efferent renal sympathetic nerve activity (induced by hypercapneic acidosis, reduction in carotid sinus pressure, head-up tilt, heart failure, or sodium depletion) is associated with an antinatriuresis [11,33,118,120].

EFFECTS OF RENAL NERVE STIMULATION ON RENAL FUNCTION

Varying frequencies of renal nerve stimulation affect different aspects of renal function in the dog [345,441,467]. Renal nerve stimulation at 0.25 Hz does not affect renal blood flow, sodium excretion, or renin secretion [117]. However, this level of renal nerve stimulation augments renin secretion caused by other stimuli. Renal nerve stimulation at 0.5 Hz increases renin secretion without affecting renal blood flow or urinary sodium excretion. Renal nerve stimulation at 1.0 Hz increases sodium reabsorption and renin secretion; renal blood flow may [127,199,257] or may not be decreased [397,466]. Higher frequencies of renal nerve stimulation decrease renal blood flow and sodium excretion; renin secretion is increased. The renal blood flow response reaches its maximum at 6 Hz [342].

The effect of the frequency of renal nerve stimulation on renal function is less consistent in the rat. Bello-Reuss et al. [48] and DiBona and Sawin [121] reported that renal nerve stimulation in the rat at 1 Hz decreased urine flow and sodium excretion without affecting renal blood flow. Other investigators have noted that renal blood flow and sodium excretion decrease concomitantly [254] at this frequency of renal nerve stimulation. Hermansson et al. found an inverse relationship between renal blood flow and renal nerve stimulation from 2 to 10 Hz [198,200]. The increase in renin secretion observed during nerve stimulation is mediated by beta$_1$ adrenoceptors, whereas the increase in sodium reabsorption is mediated by alpha$_1$ adrenoceptors [119,345].

Renal Nerve Stimulation and Glomerular Hemodynamics

In the rat, renal nerve stimulation at 2 to 5 Hz results in decreases in single-nephron blood flow and glomerular filtration. At this frequency, afferent arteriolar resistance increases to a greater extent than efferent resistance, leading to a decrease in glomerular capillary hydrostatic pressure [62,200,254]. The alterations in preglomerular and postglomerular resistances are due to angiotensin II and adrenergic regulated calcium movement across membranes of vascular smooth muscle [348,353]. Vasodilatory prostaglandins may modulate the vasoconstrictive effects of renal nerves on the renal microcirculation [344,349]. In addition, renal nerve stimulation (through adrenergic nerves and angiotensin II) decreases the glomerular capillary surface area available for filtration and thus decreases the glomerular ultrafiltration coefficient [254]. The response becomes more apparent when prostaglandin synthesis is inhibited [350]. This effect is thought to be due to glomerular mesangial cell contraction [137,138,214,388]. Beta-adrenergic stimulation by catecholamines, by increasing cAMP, also may result in mesangial cell contraction and thus constriction of glomerular capillaries; this effect is inhibited by prostaglandin E$_2$ [264]. Additionally, the renal nerves regulate glomerular ultrafiltration by affecting endothelial cells or contractile elements of the glomerular epithelial cells [13].

Renal Nerve Stimulation and Sodium Reabsorption

Stimulation of renal nerves (less than 1 Hz) can decrease sodium excretion in the absence of changes in renal perfusion pressure, renal blood flow, glomerular filtration rate, or distribution of glomerular filtration [48,345,397,466]. At higher frequencies of renal nerve stimulation (greater than 3 Hz), absolute proximal reabsorption decreases because of a fall in glomerular filtration rate [62]. Bello-Reuss et al. [48] and Hermansson et al. [198] found that the nephron segment mainly responsible for the increase in sodium and water reabsorption associated with renal nerve stimulation is in the superficial proximal convoluted tubule. Kon and Ichikawa were unable to confirm these results [254]. They suggested that the predominant effect occurs in deeper nephrons not accessible to micropunture, or parts of the nephron distal to the proximal convoluted tubule. Supporting this assumption is the fact that low-frequency (less than 1 Hz) renal nerve stimulation increased sodium and chloride transport in Henle's loop of the rat [121]. The effect of renal nerve stimulation on sodium reabsorption is mediated by alpha$_1$ adrenoceptors located at the basolateral membrane [119,345,403].

EFFECTS OF RENAL DENERVATION

Acute renal denervation in volume-expanded or euvolemic rat increases water and electrolyte excretion in the absence of changes in renal blood flow, glomerular filtration rate, and perfusion pressure [45,47,354]. The determinants of glomerular ultrafiltration are also not affected. Different results were obtained in the hydropenic rat, in which renal adrenergic activity is greater than that in the euvolemic or volume-expanded animal [215,290,350]. Under these conditions the glomerular ultrafiltration coefficient was decreased by denervation, but single-nephron filtration rate was not altered, due to an offsetting increase in transglomerular hydrostatic pressure. The latter was due to a decrease in afferent arteriolar resistance and a near constancy of efferent arteriolar resistance. The changes in glomerular dynamics after denervation may be due in part to an increase in intrarenal angiotensin II [350].

Renal Denervation and Sodium Reabsorption

The natriuresis, kaliuresis, and diuresis associated with renal denervation were initially ascribed to an increase in filtered load [53]. Subsequent studies, however, have shown that the natriuresis of renal denervation is primarily due to a decrease in tubular reabsorption rather than to changes in renal blood flow, glomerular filtration rate, or intrarenal distribution of glomerular filtrate [45,61,64, 102,312,336,354]. Micropuncture studies have identified the superficial proximal tubule as one site where sodium, chloride, and bicarbonate reabsorption are decreased [45,47,49,102,354]. In the studies of Pelayo et al. [354], reductions in fractional and absolute proximal tubular reabsorption were not accompanied by changes in factors that affect passive movement of fluid and solute across the proximal tubule epithelium, suggesting that the effect of denervation on proximal tubular reabsorption is a primary epithelial event. Acute renal denervation also resulted in a decrease in sodium reabsorption in the loop of Henle and early distal convoluted tubule [52]. The magnitude of the diuresis and natriuresis depends on the degree of reabsorption in the nephron segments beyond the proximal tubule [45,49]. In sodium-depleted rats, the depression of proximal tubular reabsorption produced by acute renal denervation can be completely compensated by an increase in distal reabsorption so that no change in overall sodium excretion occurs [432].

The decreased reabsorption in the proximal tubule may be due to a decrease in norepinephrine or an increase in dopamine excretion [312]. Blockade of dopamine$_1$ receptors [232] or of prostaglandin synthesis [32] attenuate the natriuresis of renal denervation [232]. Presumably, dopamine exerts its effects at the proximal tubule and cortical collecting duct, where dopamine$_1$ receptors are located [148,250], whereas the effects of prostaglandin blockade are confined to a distal nephron segment [32].

Afferent Nerves

Renal afferent nerves can influence kidney function directly and indirectly, the latter through cardiovascular effects mediated by the sympathetic nervous system [243]. Renal afferent nerves may contribute to the coordination of function between the two kidneys through renorenal reflexes [261,316]. Stimulation of renal afferent nerves results in an increase in ipsilateral afferent nerve activity, whereas the effects on ipsilateral or contralateral efferent nerve activity, kidney function, and systemic arterial pressure are variable. Inhibition of contralateral or ipsilateral efferent nerve activity has been reported in the rabbit, dog, and cat [1,259,262,446] whereas excitatory effects have been reported in the rat and dog [105,200,259]. Afferent nerve stimulation may result in increases [83,334], decreases [1,446], or no change [18] in blood pressure. Contralateral renal function was also variably altered [1,83, 259,333]. The inconsistency could be due to the simultaneous stimulation of a mixed population of afferent nerves, because renal nerves contain a heterogeneous group of mechanoreceptive, chemoreceptive, and possibly nociceptive receptor afferent fibers [116]. Differences in nature or intensity of the stimuli and in the animal species are also important variables to consider [259]. For example, stimulation of chemoreceptors in rats (by retrograde pelvic perfusion with isotonic NaCl) and mechanoreceptors (by increasing ureteral pressure) increased contralateral urine flow and sodium excretion without affecting mean arterial pressure, heart rate, renal blood flow, or glomerular filtration rate [259]. In dogs, stimulation of mechanoreceptors (by increasing ureteral pressure) increased ipsilateral renal blood flow and renin secretion; contralateral blood flow was decreased without any changes in sodium and water excretion or renin secretion. Retrograde perfusion of the pelvis with normal saline did not elicit chemoreceptor responses in dogs. Thus, in dogs renal mechanoreceptor stimulation results in a contralateral excitatory renorenal reflex, whereas in rats renal mechanoreceptor and chemoreceptor stimulation produce a contralateral inhibitory reflex [259]. Ipsilateral or contralateral renal denervation or spinal cord section at the T-6 level abolishes the renorenal reflex [259,363]. Stimulation of renal mechanoreceptors by venous compression yields the same results as those obtained with elevation in ureteral pressure, i.e., an increase in ipsilateral afferent nerve activity and a decrease in ipsilateral and contralateral efferent renal nerve activity, resulting in an increase in ipsilateral urinary sodium excretion and contralateral urine flow rate and sodium excretion [105,259,261]. Increasing renal venous pressure in one kidney results in inhibition of cardiopulmonary sympathetic nerve activity, leading to a fall in systemic blood pressure without increasing heart rate [259,262].

Constriction of the renal artery is associated with an increase in blood pressure dependent on intact renal nerves and independent of the renin-angiotensin system or the sinoaortic baroreflex [143]. This pressor reflex is due to stimulation of renal chemoreceptors; prostaglandins and kinins, but not adenosine, have been implicated in this response [142].

Acute unilateral renal denervation in anesthetized volume-expanded rats is associated with ipsilateral diuresis and natriuresis in the denervated kidney, in the absence of changes in renal blood flow, glomerular filtration rate, or blood pressure [104,232,312]. The innervated, contralateral kidney responds with antidiuresis and antinatriuresis [104,232,312]; renal blood flow and glomerular filtration rate also may decrease. The changes in the ipsilateral kidney (following ipsilateral renal denervation) are due to lack of noradrenergic activity [312] and to increases in dopaminergic [232,312] and prostaglandin activities [32]. The changes in contralateral renal function (after ipsilateral renal denervation) are due to increased nerve traffic and norepinephrine excretion [104,312].

Acute unilateral nephrectomy is also associated with an increase in sodium and potassium excretion by the remaining kidney due in part to disappearance of renal nerve activity. This reflex needs an intact nervous supply to the remaining kidney (and to the kidney to be removed) [370] and a normal pituitary gland. The renal excretory changes of acute unilateral nephrectomy have been found to be associated with a gamma-melanocyte–stimulating hormonelike peptide [284]. Thus, renal nerves affect ipsilateral and contralateral renal function and systemic hemodynamics not only by changing in sympathetic activity but also by influencing other neurohormonal systems. In normotensive rats, renal denervation increases norepinephrine and decreases dopamine content in the hypothalamus, but does not affect blood pressure [80]. In hypertensive rats, renal denervation is associated with a decrease in norepinephrine, but not dopamine content of the hypothalamus [243,459]. Renal denervation delays the development and attenuates the full expression of hypertension in spontaneously hypertensive rats [460]. Alterations in central nervous system catecholamine content [243,459] as well as increases in renal sodium excretion [460] may account for this phenomenon.

Function of Adrenergic Nerves in Conscious Animals

Although it is well established that renal nerves participate in the regulation of tubular reabsorption of salt and water in anesthetized animals, their role in conscious animals is still debated. In conscious dogs there are no detectable differences in sodium handling between innervated and chronically denervated kidneys during control states or after hemorrhage or volume expansion [283]. Mizelle et al. reported that conscious dogs on a low-sodium diet (5 mEq/ day) excreted the same amount of sodium whether or not the kidneys were denervated [308]. Sadowski et al. also reported that renal nerves do not play any role in the maintenance of sodium balance in conscious dogs [380,381]. Fractional lithium clearances were also not different between the denervated and innervated state, indicating that proximal sodium reabsorption was also unaffected [308]. Varying the circulating levels of catecholamines within physiologic range is not associated with changes in urinary sodium excretion [229]. Bencsath et al. reported that rats with prior bilateral renal denervation lowered their daily sodium excretion to the same level as rats with sham denervation when given a diet of boiled rice and water (15 μmol sodium intake/rat/day) [50,51]. Fernandez-Repollet et al. also reported that conscious rats can maintain a positive sodium balance on a low-sodium diet (95 μmol sodium intake/rat/day) in the absence of renal nerves [161]. However, chronic unilateral renal denervation in conscious rats is associated with ipsilateral increases in the excretion of sodium, potassium, and water [378]. Other studies indicate that renal nerve activity may play a role in the renal response to changes in extracellular fluid volume, baroreflex stimulation, and perfusion pressure in conscious animals [122,191,192,315,383,411]. In conscious dogs, bilateral carotid artery occlusion is associated with increased renal nerve activity and decreased renal blood flow [192]. Renal nerve activity varies inversely with sodium intake; volume expansion is associated with a decrease in renal nerve activity, diuresis, and natriuresis [122]. Rats on a low-sodium diet, which had a higher renal nerve activity than rats on a normal or high-sodium diet, also had the greatest reduction in renal nerve activity and the biggest natriuretic response after volume expansion [122].

These studies suggest that renal nerve activity affects sodium and water excretion but not renal hemodynamics [315]. The role played by the renal nerves in the control of sodium excretion appears to be more prominent in sodium depleted subjects. Conscious dogs [387], rabbits [183], and rats [120] with denervated kidneys are unable to maintain a positive sodium balance when subjected to dietary sodium restriction. Gill and Barter [174] reported that humans in whom autonomic insufficiency was produced by guanethidine administration were unable to lower urinary sodium excretion sufficiently to avoid a negative sodium balance. Patients with autonomic failure also have a decreased ability to conserve sodium, which is not corrected by the administration of mineralocorticoids [458].

The reasons for the differences in results from different laboratories are not readily apparent. Mizelle et al. [308] suggested that compensatory changes may obscure conclusions regarding the importance of direct effects of renal nerves on long-term regulation of sodium balance, decreases in blood pressure associated with bilateral denervation [161,308] or development of renal hypersensitivity to catecholamines [432] may mask any inherent defect in renal sodium reabsorption. Differences in basal adrenergic activity may also be involved; in the studies of Bencsath et al., the rats with denervated kidneys that were able to maintain a sodium balance had an increase in sodium excretion when subjected to anesthesia [50]. The state of sodium balance or nutrition may also play a role. Denervation natriuresis was observed in fasted but not in fed conscious rats [433].

Ontogeny of Adrenergic and Dopaminergic Receptors

Studies performed by us and others have indicated that adrenergic and dopaminergic effects on renal hemodynamics and function undergo changes during development [73–77,151,153,230,235–238,293,327–329,352,374,425]. There seem to be species differences in the ontogenetic pattern, and some variation in results may be due to the experimental conditions (e.g., influence of anesthesia).

Alpha Adrenoceptors

The development of alpha adrenoceptors in the kidney has been examined in the rat and dog. In the rat, renal alpha$_1$ and alpha$_2$ adrenoceptor density do not change [382], increase [295,413], or decrease [184] with age. The receptor affinity was reported to remain the same [184,382] or to decrease [295,413]. Sripanidkulchai and Wyss [413] found only high-affinity alpha$_2$ adrenoceptors in the fetal and neonatal rat up to 4 days of age; both high and low affinity were detected thereafter. The density of low-affinity receptors reached adult levels at 2 months and that of high-affinity receptors at 3 to 4 months [413,414]. These studies did not distinguish between vascular, mesangial, and renal tubular receptors. In the dog [155] and sheep [178a], we have found that the density of renal cortical tubular alpha$_1$ and alpha$_2$ adrenoceptors decreased with age.

The effect of renal nerve stimulation on renal hemodynamics during development has been studied in several animal species [76,171,374,375]. In both anesthetized pig and unanesthetized sheep, renal nerve stimulation (less than 3 Hz) resulted in a greater increase in renal vascular resistance in fetal than newborn or adult sheep; 1- to 2-week-old piglets were similarly more reactive than mature swine [76,375]. Piglets less than 4 days old had comparable or lesser response than mature swine [76]. The response to electrical stimulation of the isolated renal artery of the rabbit was also less in adults compared with neonates [171]. Renal nerve stimulation greater than 5 Hz, however, increased the renal vascular resistance to a greater extent in adults than younger animals [76,375]. In the adult rat, spontaneous renal nerve activity in the conscious state is about 1 to 2 Hz in normotensive animals and about 4 Hz in spontaneously hypertensive rats [289]. The significance and mechanism for the increased sensitivity of the immature renal vasculature to low-level renal nerve stimulation remain to be determined.

Surgical renal denervation did not alter baseline renal blood flow in fetal lambs [373,375], but it increased renal blood flow and decreased renal vascular resistance in piglets [77]. These results suggest that the renal circulation of the pig is under tonic neural vasoconstrictor influence [75,76], whereas that of the sheep is not [374].

The effects of alpha-adrenergic agents on renal hemodynamics seem to be dependent not only on the animal species but on the experimental conditions. In the rabbit, norepinephrine vasoconstricted the isolated renal arteries to a greater extent in adults than newborns [171]. In the anesthetized swine, the intravenous infusion of equipressor concentrations of norepinephrine increased renal vascular resistance to the greatest extent in 2-week-old piglets, but 1-week-old piglets had a lesser response than mature swine [77] (at low epinephrine concentrations, 1-week-old piglets had the greatest change in renal vascular resistance). A greater vasoconstrictor response to epinephrine was also noted in anesthetized immature dogs [238] and the isolated renal artery of newborn guinea pig [171] compared with their adult counterparts. Norepinephrine also constricted the isolated renal artery to a greater extent in younger than older animals when the intramural pressure was low [106]. In the unanesthetized sheep, the intrarenal arterial infusion of the alpha$_1$-adrenergic agonist phenylephrine as a bolus ($\geq 1.8 \times 10^{-7}$M) induced the greatest vasoconstriction in adults and least in the newborns (adult > fetus > newborns) [293]. At low concentrations ($\leq 1.8 \times 10^{-7}$M), phenylephrine had a similar vasoconstrictor effect in all groups. The alpha$_2$-adrenergic agonist guanabenz decreased renal blood flow to an extent similar to that observed with higher concentrations ($\geq 1.8 \times 10^{-7}$M) of phenylephrine (i.e., adults > fetus > newborn) [293]. In isolated renal arteries, both alpha$_1$ and alpha$_2$ agonists induced greater vasoconstriction in fetal than in older sheep [292a].

In the anesthetized dog, renal alpha-adrenergic blockade with the nonselective alpha-adrenergic blocker phentolamine [162] resulted in an increase in renal blood flow in puppies but not adult dogs. The increase in renal blood flow with renal alpha-adrenergic blockade was greater in younger than older puppies [162]. In unanesthetized sheep, alpha-adrenergic blockade did not increase renal blood flow in fetal, newborn, or adult sheep [374].

It appears that in the basal state, renal nerves exert a negligible influence on the renal vasculature of sheep, but may increase the tone of these vessels in immature dogs and in pigs of all ages.

Sensitivity of the renal vasculature to exogenous catecholamines seems to be greatest in adult rabbit, neonatal pigs and dogs (1 to 3 weeks), and newborn guinea pigs. A heightened renal vascular response to alpha-adrenergic stimulation correlates with denser renal innervation (guinea pig) [171] and a higher density of alpha-adrenergic receptors (canine puppies) [155]. The renal vasculature of the immature sheep appears to be particularly sensitive to alpha-adrenergic stimulation (in vitro), but this sensitivity may be obscured in vivo by counterregulatory mechanisms (e.g., vasodilator prostaglandins).

Beta Adrenoceptors

Robillard and co-workers reported that renal nerve stimulation during alpha-adrenergic blockade in conscious sheep produced vasodilatation in fetal and newborn but not adult animals [375]. The intrarenal arterial infusion of epinephrine or norepinephrine during alpha-adrenergic blockade increased renal blood flow at all ages [328,329], but the greatest vasodilatation occurred in fetuses. The renal vasodilatory response was blocked by beta$_2$-adrenergic blockers but not by cholinergic or dopaminergic antagonists, indicating involvement of beta$_2$-adrenoceptors [328,329, 375]. Selective beta$_2$-adrenergic activation (by terbutaline) was less prominent than when beta-adrenergic receptors were stimulated by epinephrine and norepinephrine (which stimulate both beta$_1$ and beta$_2$ adrenoceptors) [326]. In sheep, the vasodilatory activity induced by direct activation of adenylate cyclase (by forskolin) did not vary throughout development [326]. The greater vasodilatory effect of beta-adrenoceptor stimulation observed in fetal and newborn sheep may, therefore, be related to greater production of cAMP. Radioligand binding studies have shown that the sheep fetal kidneys have mainly beta$_2$ receptors, whereas adult kidneys have both beta$_1$ and beta$_2$ adrenoceptors; beta-adrenoceptor density is similar in adult and fetal sheep kidneys [236].

There are no studies in the sheep on the ontogeny of the relationship between beta-adrenergic stimulation and adenylate cyclase activity. Judes et al. [239], however, reported that beta-receptor activation with the nonselective beta-adrenergic agonist isoproterenol resulted in greater production of cAMP in glomeruli from younger than older rats. The vasoconstriction induced by renal nerve stimulation alone or alpha-adrenergic stimulation was not enhanced by beta-adrenergic blockade, indicating that beta-adrenergic vasodilation does not counteract alpha-adrenergic vasoconstrictor responses during development [328,329,375]. The physiologic role of beta-adrenergic–mediated vasodilatation in immature sheep remains to be determined.

The effect of beta-adrenergic stimulation in the developing pig is different from that noted in sheep [73,76]. The renal vasodilator effects of intravenous isoproterenol increased with age, peaking at 2 weeks of age (alpha-adrenergic vasoconstriction with norepinephrine seemed to be greatest at 1 week of age) [73,76]. In conscious dogs, the intravenous infusion of isoproterenol [134] did not increase renal blood flow in either puppies or adults. However, any direct renal vasodilatation could have been obscured by the fall in systemic blood pressure. We reported that the intrarenal arterial infusion of isoproterenol increased outer cortical blood flow in 6- to 8-week-old puppies but not in adult dogs [235]. No such effect was noted in 1-week-old puppies (unpublished observations). The density of the beta-adrenergic receptors (subtype not determined) in the renal cortex also increases with age, with the outer cortex maturing earlier than the inner cortex [153].

In the newborn puppy, as in the piglet, there is little beta-adrenergic effect on renal blood flow; responsiveness increases with age, to a level greater than that noted in adults. In the sheep there is high beta-adrenergic responsiveness at a young age.

Dopamine Receptors

Intravenous dopamine (2 μg/kg/min) increases renal blood flow in adults without changing blood pressure; in the young, renal blood flow does not increase or actually decreases [74,158,228]. This is due to the immaturity of the dopamine receptors, which allows dopamine to occupy alpha adrenoceptors [327]. However, when systemic blood pressure and cardiac output are increased by dopamine, renal blood flow may also increase, even in the newborn [135]. In anesthetized dogs, the infusion of dopamine into the renal artery increased renal blood flow in 50-day-old puppies but not in those younger than 1 month [352]. In piglets [75] and puppies [352], dopamine administered during alpha-adrenergic blockade increased renal blood flow in an age-related fashion. This apparently does not occur in the sheep [327]. In dogs and sheep, renal cortical dopamine$_1$ receptor density does not change with age [153,154]; in sheep renal cortical dopamine$_2$ receptor density decreases with age [154].

In summary, dopamine exerts less of a vasodilator effect in newborns than in adults. The vasoconstrictor effect in piglets and dogs seems to be mediated by increased alpha-adrenergic activity. The vasodilatory response induced by dopamine increases with maturation in pigs and dogs. In sheep, the magnitude of the renal vasodilatory response, which is modest compared with other animals, does not change with maturation. This is probably due to a low affinity of dopamine for the vasodilatory dopamine$_1$ receptors.

Adrenergic Regulation of Renal Sodium Transport During Maturation

Renal nerve stimulation (1 to 2 Hz) decreases sodium excretion to a similar extent in fetal and adult sheep [372a]. Renal denervation [373] does not alter urine flow or urinary electrolyte excretion in fetal lambs. However, in 5-day-old rats, chemical sympathectomy with 6-hydroxydopamine (which destroys both noradrenergic and dopaminergic nerves) induces a natriuresis; after the 20th day of life sodium and potassium excretion decreases, probably as a consequence of denervation hypersensitivity [16]. This phenomenon also occurs in adult dogs, in which chronic renal denervation increases the sensitivity of the kidney to the effects of circulating catecholamines [432].

In the unanesthetized uninephrectomized sheep, the intrarenal arterial infusion of the alpha$_1$-adrenergic agonist phenylephrine decreased sodium excretion to a greater extent in neonatal than in older animals [375a]. In the anesthetized dog, the infusion of the nonselective alpha-adrenergic blocker, phentolamine, into the renal artery induced a dose-related increase in sodium excretion in both puppies and adults [162]. The effect was greater in adult dogs than in young puppies. The intrarenal infusion of dopamine tended to decrease sodium excretion in young puppies; alpha- and beta-adrenergic blockade during intrarenal dopamine infusion (to maximize dopaminergic effects) induced a dose-related natriuresis that increased with age [352]. In human infants, dopamine administered intravenously increased creatinine clearance and sodium excretion, effects qualitatively similar to those observed in adults [444]. However, endogenous dopamine may have different effects in newborn infants. Sodium depletion caused enhanced sodium reabsorption in both low-birth-weight infants and adults, but dopamine increased only in the former [426]. When the effect of dopamine was blocked by administering metoclopramide, a predominantly dopamine$_2$ antagonist, sodium excretion increased in low-birth-weight infants [426] and decreased in the adults [400a]. This effect was associated with decreases in plasma aldosterone and arginine vasopressin levels in the low-birth-weight infants and increases in the adults [85,426].

Receptor studies indicate that alpha-adrenergic activity predominates in the kidneys of newborn and ovine newborns [155]. Therefore, alpha-adrenergic blockade should result in greater natriuresis in puppies than in adult dogs. Yet, the opposite was seen [162]. It is possible that increased distal tubular avidity for sodium in the newborn [409] obscures proximal tubular events (where most of the alpha-adrenergic receptors are located) [269,465]. Alternatively, alpha-adrenergic antagonists may induce natriuresis by blocking alpha adrenoceptors and allowing the expression of endogenous beta-adrenergic and dopamine effects. Renal denervation induces a natriuresis in part by increasing dopaminergic activity [232,312]. The effect of dopamine on sodium excretion is minimal in the puppy. Consequently, blockade of alpha adrenoceptors, although eliminating the alpha antinatriuretic effect, is not accompanied by the natriuresis associated with dopamine receptors (and probably beta adrenoceptors). In contrast, in the adult dog, in which alpha-adrenoceptor density is low and beta adrenoceptors and dopamine receptors are many, alpha-adrenergic blockade does not only obliterate the antinatriuretic effects of the alpha adrenoceptors, but it also unmasks the inhibitory effects of dopamine and beta-adrenoceptor stimulation or sodium reabsorption in the proximal tubule.

The high density of the renal alpha adrenoceptors [155,178a] may explain in part the high degree of sodium retention observed in the newborn animals [409]. Conversely, the blunted natriuretic effect of dopamine in the young does not appear to be related to differences in dopamine receptor density, but rather to postreceptor events [150,153,250a].

Although variations in responses to catecholamines may explain the differences in salt handling between the young and adult, other factors may be incriminated. Increased levels of sodium-retaining hormones have been proposed as the cause of the increased avidity for sodium in the young (e.g., aldosterone) [409]. This may also be due to a limited ability of the newborn to elaborate a natriuretic factor(s) (e.g., atrial natriuretic factor, ANF) or failure of this factor(s) to effect a natriuretic response. An interaction among natriuretic and antinatriuretic factors is known to occur. In the adult, dopamine and ANF inhibit aldosterone secretion [85,179], whereas in the young, dopamine may actually increase serum aldosterone levels [426]. The natriuretic effect of ANF is decreased when adrenergic activity is increased [123]. A relationship may exist between the adrenergic system, substance P, and kinins. The ability of the newborn to excrete a salt load is enhanced by substance P, an undecapeptide tachykinin [163]. Increased adrenergic activity decreases substance P production [248a]. The sympathetic nervous system also regulates ANF levels and effects [179]. If the adrenergic nervous system regulates substance P levels in the kidney, it is anticipated that the high alpha-adrenergic activity prevailing in the newborn would result in decreased substance P levels, and therefore in renal kallikreins, limiting the ability of the puppy to excrete a salt load. Increased adrenergic activity would also limit the natriuretic effects of ANF.

References

1. Aars H, Akre S: Reflex changes in sympathetic activity and arterial blood pressure evoked by afferent stimulation of the renal nerve. Acta Physiol Scand 78:184, 1970.
2. Adrian ED, Bronk DW, Phillips G: Discharges in mammalian sympathetic nerves. J Physiol (Lond) 74:115, 1921.
3. Ahlquist RP: A study of adrenotropic receptors. Am J Phsiol 153:586, 1948.
4. Akpaffiong MJ, Redfern PH, Woodward B: An investigation of the importance of the adrenal gland to the action of dopamine in the rat kidney. Br J Pharmacol 79:103, 1983.
5. Alessandrini C, Calvallotti C, De Rossi M, et al: Localization of dopamine receptors in the rabbit renal artery: A histoautoradiographic study. Pharmacology 29:17, 1984.
6. Alexander RW, Gill JR Jr, Yamabe H, et al: Effects of dietary sodium and of acute saline infusion on the interrelationship between dopamine excretion and adrenergic activity in man. J Clin Invest 54:194, 1974.
7. Alkadhi KA, Sabouni MH, Ansari AF, et al: Activation of DA$_1$ receptors by dopamine or fenoldopam increases cyclic AMP levels in the renal artery but not in the superior cervical ganglion of the rat. J Pharmacol Exp Ther 238:547, 1986.
8. Amenta F: Density and distribution of dopamine receptors in the cardiovascular system and in the kidney. J Auton Pharmacol 10(suppl 1)s11, 1990.
9. Amenta F, Cavallotti C, De Rossi M, et al: Beta-adrenoceptors in the rat kidney. Immunohistochemical study. Naunyn Schmiedebergs Arch Pharmacol 324:94, 1983.
10. Ammons WS: Renal afferent input to thoracolumbar spinal neurons of the cat. Am J Physiol (Regulatory Integrative Comp Physiol 19)250:R435, 1986.
11. Anderson RJ, Henrich WL, Gross PA, et al: Role of renal nerves, angiotensin II, and prostaglandins in the antinatriuretic response to acute hypercapnic acidosis in the dog. Circ Res 50:294, 1982.
12. Andreucci VE, Dal Canton A, Corradi A, et al: Role of the efferent arteriole in glomerular hemodynamic of superficial nephrons. Kidney Int 9:475, 1976.
13. Andrews PM, Coffey AK: Cytoplasmic contractile elements in glomerular cells. Fed Proc 42:3046, 1983.
14. Aperia A, Bertorello A, Seri I: Dopamine causes inhibition of Na$^+$-K$^+$-ATPase activity in rat proximal convoluted tubule segments. Am J Physiol (Renal Fluid Electrolyte Physiol 21)252:F39, 1987.
15. Aperia A, Bertorello A, Seri I: Dopamine (DA) is an intrarenal natriuretic hormone (abstr). Kidney Int 32:258, 1987.
16. Appenroth D, Braunlich H: Effect of sympathectomy with 6-hydroxy dopamine on the renal excretion of water and electrolytes in developing rats. Acta Biol Med Ger 40:1715, 1981.
17. Astrom A, Crafoord J: Afferent activity recorded in the kidney nerves of rats. Acta Physiol Scand 70:10, 1967.
18. Ayus JC, Humphreys MH: Hemodynamic and renal functional changes after acute unilateral nephrectomy in the dog: Role of carotid sinus baroreceptors. Am J Physiol (Renal Fluid Electrolyte Physiol 11)242:F181, 1982.

19. Baines AD: Effects of salt intake and renal denervation on catecholamine catabolism and excretion. *Kidney Int* 21:316, 1982.

20. Baines AD, Craan H, Chan W, et al: Tubular secretion and metabolism of dopamine, norepinephrine, methoxytyramine and normetanephrine by the rat kidney. *J Pharmacol Exp Ther* 208:144, 1979.

21. Baines AD, Ho P: Specific α_1-, α_2-, and β-responses to norepinephrine in pyruvate perfused rat kidneys. *Am J Physiol* (Renal Fluid Electrolyte Physiol 21)252:F170, 1987.

22. Baines AD, Drangova R, Ho P: α_1-adrenergic stimulation of renal Na reabsorption requires glucose metabolism. *Am J Physiol* (Renal Fluid Electrolyte Physiol 22)253:F810, 1987.

23. Baines AD, Drangova R: Neural not tubular dopamine increases glomerular filtration rate in perfused rat kidneys. *Am J Physiol* (Renal Fluid Electrolyte Physiol 19)250:F674, 1986.

24. Balint P, Chatel R: Die Wirkung von adrenalin und von noradrenalin auf die Nierenhamodynamik bein Hund. *Naunyn Schmiedebergs Arch Pharmacol* 258:24, 1967.

25. Ball SG, Gunn IG, Douglas IH: Renal handling of dopa, dopamine, norepinephrine, and epinephrine in the dog. *Am J Physiol* (Renal Fluid Electrolyte Physiol 11)242:F56, 1982.

26. Ball SG, Oates NS, Lee MR: Urinary dopamine in man and rat: Effects of inorganic salts on dopamine excretion. *Clin Sci Mol Med* 55:167, 1978.

27. Barajas L: Innervation of the renal cortex. *Fed Proc* 37:1192, 1978.

28. Barajas L, Powers K, Wang P: Innervation of the renal cortical tubules: A quantitative study. *Am J Physiol* (Renal Fluid Electrolyte Physiol 16)247:F50, 1984.

29. Barajas L, Wang P: Myelinated nerves of the rat kidney. A light and electron microscopic autoradiographic study. *J Ultrastruc Res* 65:148, 1978.

30. Barajas L, Wang P: Simultaneous ultrastructural visualization of acetylcholinesterase activity and tritiated norepinephrine uptake in renal nerves. *Anat Rec* 205:185, 1983.

31. Barajas L, Wang P, Powers K, et al: Identification of renal neuroeffector junctions by electron microscopy of reembedded light microscopic autoradiograms of semithin sections. *J Ultrastruct Res* 77:379, 1981.

32. Barber JD, Harrington WW, Moss NG, et al: Prostaglandin blockade impairs denervation diuresis and natriuresis in the rat. *Am J Physiol* (Renal Fluid Electrolyte Physiol 19)250:F895, 1986.

33. Barger AC, Muldowney FP, Liebowitz MR: Role of the kidney in the pathogenesis of congestive heart failure. *Circulation* 20:273, 1959.

34. Barnett R, Singhal PC, Scharschmidt LA, et al: Dopamine attenuates the contractile response to angiotensin II in isolated rat glomeruli and cultured mesangial cells. *Circ Res* 59:529, 1986.

34a. Bass AS: DA$_2$ dopamine receptor mediated renal effects of LY 141865 in rats subjected to acute unilateral denervation (abstr). *Kidney Int* 35:477, 1989.

35. Bass AS, Robie NW: Stereoselectivity of S- and R-sulpride for pre- and postsynaptic dopamine receptors in the canine kidney. *J Pharmacol Exp Ther* 229:67, 1984.

36. Bauer JH, Brooks CS: The long-term effect of propranolol therapy on renal function. *Am J Med* 66:405, 1979.

37. Beacham WS, Kunze DL: Renal receptors evoking spinal vasomotor reflex. *J Physiol (Lond)* 201:73, 1969.

38. Beach RE, Schwab SJ, Brazy PC, et al: Norepinephrine increases Na$^+$-K$^+$-ATPase and solute transport in rabbit proximal tubules. *Am J Physiol* (Renal Fluid Electrolyte Physiol 21)252:F215, 1987.

39. Bell C, Ferguson M, Petrovic T: Neurochemistry of dopaminergic nerves. *In* McGrath B, Bell C (eds): *Peripheral Actions of Dopamine*. London, McMillan 1988, p 41.

40. Bell C, Gillespie JS: Dopamine and noradrenaline levels in peripheral tissues of several mammalian species. *J Neurochem* 36:703, 1981.

41. Bell C, Lang WJ, Laska F: Dopamine-containing vasomotor nerves in the dog kidney. *J Neurochem* 31:77, 1978.

42. Bell C, Lang WJ, Laska F: Dopamine-containing axons supplying the arterio-venous anastomoses of the canine paw pad. *J Neurochem* 31:1329, 1978.

43. Bell C, Lang WJ: Neural dopaminergic vasodilator control in the kidney. *Nature* 246:27, 1973.

44. Bello-Reuss E: Effect of catecholamines on fluid reabsorption by the isolated proximal convoluted tubule. *Am J Physiol* (Renal Fluid Electrolytes Physiol 7)238:F347, 1980.

45. Bello-Reuss E, Colindres RE, Pastoriza-Munoz E, et al: Effects of acute unilateral renal denervation in the rat. *J Clin Invest* 56:208, 1975.

46. Bello-Reuss E, Higashi Y, Kaneda Y: Dopamine decreases fluid reabsorption in straight portions of rabbit proximal tubule. *Am J Physiol* (Renal Fluid Electrolyte Physiol 11)242:F634, 1982.

47. Bello-Reuss E, Pastoriza-Munoz E, Colindres RE: Acute unilateral renal denervation in rats with extracellular volume expansion. *Am J Physiol* (Renal Fluid Electrolyte Physiol 1)232:F26, 1977.

48. Bello-Reuss E, Trevino DL, Gottschalk CW: Effect of renal sympathetic nerve stimulation on proximal water and sodium reabsorption. *J Clin Invest* 57:1104, 1976.

49. Bencsath PL, Asztalos B, Szalay L, et al: Renal handling of sodium after chronic renal sympathectomy in the anesthetized rat. *Am J Physiol* (Renal Fluid Electrolyte Physiol 5)236:F513, 1979.

50. Bencsath P, Fekete MI, Kanyicska, et al: Renal excretion of sodium after bilateral renal sympathectomy in the anaesthetized and conscious rat. *J Physiol (Lond)* 331:443, 1982.

51. Bencsath P, Szenasi G, Tackacs L: Renal nerves and sodium conservation in conscious rats (letter). *Am J Physiol* (Renal Fluid Electrolyte Physiol 17)248:F616, 1985.

52. Bencsath P, Szenasi G, Takacs L: Water and electrolyte transport in Henle's loop and distal tubule after renal sympathectomy in the rat. *Am J Physiol* (Renal Fluid Electrolyte Physiol 18)249:F308, 1985.

53. Berne RM: Hemodynamics and sodium excretion of denervated kidney in anesthetized and unanesthetized dog. *Am J Physiol* 171:148, 1952.

54. Berridge MJ: Inositol trisphosphate and diacylglcerol: Two interacting second messengers. *Annu Rev Biochem* 56:159, 1987.

55. Berthelsen S, Pettinger WA: A functional basis for classification of alpha-adrenergic receptors. *Life Sci* 21:595, 1977.

56. Bertorello A, Aperia A: Both DA$_1$ and DA$_2$ receptor agonists are necessary to inhibit NaK-ATPase activity in proximal tubules from rat kidney. *Acta Physiol Scand* 132:441, 1988.

57. Besarab A, Silva P, Landsberg L, et al: Effect of catecholamines on tubular function in the isolated rat kidney. *Am J Physiol* (Renal Fluid Electrolyte Physiol 2)233:F39, 1977.

58. Bevan JA, Brayden JE: Non adrenergic neural vasodilator mechanisms. *Circ Res* 60:309, 1987.

59. Bhat S, Churchill M, Churchill P, et al: Renal effects of SK&F 82526 in anesthetized rats. *Life Sci* 38:1565, 1986.

60. Blair ML, Chen YH, Izzo JL Jr: Influence of renal perfusion pressure on α- and β-adrenergic stimulation of renin release. *Am J Physiol* (Endocrinol Metab 11)248:E317, 1985.

61. Blake WD, Jurf AN: Renal sodium reasorption after acute renal denervation in the rabbit. *J Physiol (Lond)* 196:65, 1968.

62. Blantz RC, Pelayo JC: In vivo actions of angiotensin II on glomerular function. *Fed Proc* 42:3071, 1983.

63. Blendis LM, Auld RB, Alexander EA, et al: Effect of renal beta- and alpha-adrenergic stimulation on proximal sodium reabsorption in dogs. *Clin Sci* 43:569, 1972.

64. Bonjour JP, Churchill PC, Malvin RL: Change of tubular reabsorption of sodium and water after renal denervation in the dog. *J Physiol (Lond)* 204:571, 1969.

65. Boren DR, Henry DP, Selkurt EE, et al: Renal modulation of urinary catecholamine excretion during volume expansion in the dog. *Hypertension* 2:383, 1980.

66. Bradley T, Frederickson ED, Goldberg LI: Effect of DA_1 receptor blockade with SCH 23390 on the renal response to electrical stimulation of the renal nerves. *Proc Soc Exp Biol Med* 181:492, 1986.

67. Bradley T, Hjemahl P, DiBona GF: Increased release of norepinephrine and dopamine from canine kidney during bilateral carotid occlusion. *Am J Physiol (Renal Fluid Electrolyte Physiol* 21)252:F240, 1987.

68. Bradley T, Hjemdahl P: Further studies on renal nerve stimulation induced release of noradrenaline and dopamine from the canine kidney in situ. *Acta Physiol Scand* 122:369, 1984.

69. Bradley T, Hjemdahl P: Renal overflow of noradrenaline and dopamine to plasma during hindquarter compression and thoracic inferior vena cava obstruction in the dog. *Acta Physiol Scand* 127:205, 1986.

70. Brinley FJ Jr: Excitation and conduction in nerve fibers. *In* Mountcastle VB (ed): *Medical Physiology*. St. Louis, CV Mosby, 1970, p 46.

71. Brodde OE: Vascular dopamine receptors: Demonstration and characterization by in vitro studies. *Life Sci* 31:289, 1982.

72. Brody MJ, Johnson AK: Role of the arterioventral third ventricle region in fluid and electrolyte balance, arterial pressure regulation in hypertension. *In* Martini L, Ganong WF (eds): *Frontiers in Neuroendocrinology*. New York, Raven Press, 1980, p 249.

73. Buckley NM, Brazeau P, Charney AN, et al: Cardiovascular and renal effects of isoproterenol infusions in young swine. *Biol Neonate* 45:69, 1984.

74. Buckley NM, Brazeau P, Frasier ID: Cardiovascular effects of dopamine in the developing swine. *Biol Neonate* 43:50, 1983.

75. Buckley NM, Brazeau P, Frasier ID: Renal blood flow autoregulation in developing swine. *Am J Physiol (Heart Circ Physiol* 14)245:H1, 1983.

76. Buckley NM, Brazeau P, Gootman PM, et al: Renal circulatory effects of adrenergic stimuli in anesthetized piglets and mature swine. *Am J Physiol (Heart Circ Physiol* 6)237:H690, 1979.

77. Buckley NM, Charney AN, Brazeau P, et al: Changes in cardiovascular and renal function during catecholamine infusions in developing swine. *Am J Physiol (Renal Fluid Electrolyte Physiol* 9)240:F276, 1981.

78. Busuttil RW, Roh BL, Fisher JW: The cytological localization of erythropoietin in the human kidney using the fluorescent antibody technique. *Proc Soc Exp Biol Med* 137:327, 1971.

79. Bylund DB: Heterogeneity of alpha-2 adrenergic receptors. *Pharmacol Biochem Behav* 22:835, 1985.

80. Calaresu FR, Ciriello J: Altered concentrations of catecholamines in the hypothalamus of the rat after renal denervation. *Can J Physiol Pharmacol* 59:1274, 1981.

81. Calaresu FR, Ciriello J: Renal afferent nerves affect discharge rates of medullary and hypothalamic single units in the cat. *J Auton Nerv Syst* 3:311, 1981.

82. Calaresu FR, Kim P, Nakamura H, et al: Electrophysiological characteristics of renorenal reflexes in the cat. *J Physiol (Lond)* 283:141, 1978.

83. Calaresu FR, Stella A, Zanchetti A: Hemodynamic responses and renin release during stimulation of afferent renal nerves in the cat. *J Physiol (Lond)* 255:687, 1976.

84. Campese VM, Romoff MS, Levitan D, et al: Abnormal relationship between sodium intake and sympathetic nervous system activity in salt-sensitive patients with essential hypertension. *Kidney Int* 21:371, 1982.

85. Carey RM, Thorner MO, Ortt EM: Dopaminergic inhibition of metoclopramide-induced aldosterone secretion in man. *J Clin Invest* 66:10, 1980.

86. Carey RM, Stote RMK, Duff JW, et al: Selective peripheral dopamine-1 receptor stimulation with fenoldopam in human essential hypertension. *J Clin Invest* 74:2198, 1984.

87. Carrara MC, Baines AD: Propranolol induces acute natriuresis by β blockade and dopaminergic stimulation. *Can J Physiol Pharmacol* 54:683, 1976.

88. Carriere S, Lalumiere G, Gaigneault A, et al: Sequential changes in catecholamine plasma levels during isotonic volume expansion in dogs. *Am J Physiol (Renal Fluid Electrolyte Physiol* 4)235:F119, 1978.

89. Chabardes D, Montegut M, Imbert-Teboul M, et al: Inhibition of α_2-adrenergic agonists on AVP-induced cAMP accumulation in isolated collecting tubule of the rat kidney. *Mol Cell Endocrinol* 37:263, 1984.

90. Chan YL: Adrenergic control of bicarbonate absorption in the proximal convoluted tubule of the rat kidney. *Pflugers Arch* 388:159, 1980.

91. Chan YL: The role of norepinephrine in the regulation of fluid absorption in the rat proximal convoluted tubule. *J Pharmacol Exp Ther* 215:65, 1980.

92. Chan YL, Chatsudthipong V, Su-Tsai SM, et al: The role of calcium in the dopaminergic effect on the proximal convoluted tubule of rat kidney (abstr). *Fed Proc* 45:508, 1986.

93. Chang EB, Field M, Miller RJ: Alpha 2-adrenergic receptor regulation of ion transport in rabbit ileum. *Am J Physiol (Gastrointest Liver Physiol* 5)242:G237, 1982.

94. Chapman BJ, Horn NM, Munday KA, et al: The actions of dopamine and of sulpiride on regional blood flows in the rat kidney. *J Physiol (Lond)* 298:437, 1980.

95. Chapman BJ, Horn NM, Robertson MJ: Renal blood-flow changes during renal nerve stimulation in rats tested with α-adrenergic and dopaminergic blockers. *J Physiol (Lond)* 325:67, 1982.

96. Chapman BJ, Munday KA, Radhi ARAH: The effects of renal nerve stimulation in rats treated with α-adrenergic and dopaminergic blockers. *J Physiol (Lond)* 341:65P, 1983.

97. Chassaing C, Duchene-Marullaz P, Veyrac MJ: Effects of catecholamines on cardiac chronotropic response to vagal stimulation in the dog. *Am J Physiol (Heart Circ Physiol* 14)245:H721, 1983.

98. Cheung YD, Barnett DB, Nahorski SR: Heterogeneous properties of alpha$_2$ adrenoceptors in particulate and soluble preparations of human platelet and rat and rabbit kidney. *Biochem Pharmacol* 35:3767, 1986.

99. Chou SY, Liebman PH, Ferder LF, et al: Effects of α-adrenergic blockade on sodium excretion in normal and chronic salt retaining dogs. *Can J Physiol Pharmacol* 54:209, 1976.

100. Ciriello J, Calaresu FR: Central projections of afferent renal fibers in the rat: An anterograde transport study of horseradish peroxidase. *J Auton Nerv Syst* 8:273, 1983.

101. Click RL, Joyner WL, Gilmore JP: Reactivity of glomerular

the rabbit kidney (proceedings). *J Physiol (Lond)* 293:24P, 1979.

184. Graham RM, Pettinger WA, Sagalowsky A, et al: Renal alpha-adrenergic receptor abnormality in the spontaneously hypertensive rat. *Hypertension* 4:881, 1982.

185. Grantham JJ, Chonko AM: Renal handling of organic anions and cations; metabolism and excretion of uric acid. *In* Brenner BM, Rector FC Jr (eds): *The Kidney*. WB Saunders, Philadelphia, 1986, p 663.

186. Greven J, Heidenreich O: A micropuncture study of the effect of isoprenaline or renal tubular fluid and electrolyte transport in the rat. *Naunyn Schmiedebergs Arch Pharmacol* 287:117, 1975.

187. Greven J, Klein H: Effects of dopamine on whole kidney function and proximal transtubular volume fluxes in the rat. *Naunyn Schmiedebergs Arch Pharmacol* 296:289, 1977.

188. Greven J, Pantel J: Failure of an angiotensin II antagonist to influence isoprenaline-induced antidiuresis in rats. *Naunyn Schmiedebergs Arch Pharmacol* 332:271, 1986.

189. Grignolo A, Koepke JP, Obrist PA: Renal function, heart rate, and blood pressure during exercise and avoidance in dogs. *Am J Physiol* (Regulatory Integrative Comp Physiol 11)242:R482, 1982.

190. Grignolo A, Seidler FJ, Bartolome M, et al: Norepinephrine content of the rat kidney during development: Alterations induced by perinatal methadone. *Life Sci* 31:3009, 1982.

191. Gross R, Hackenberg H, Hackenthal E: Interaction between perfusion pressure and sympathetic nerves in renin release by carotid baroreflex in conscious dogs. *J Physiol (Lond)* 313: 237, 1981.

192. Gross R, Kirchheim H: Effects of bilateral carotid and auditory stimulation on renal blood flow and sympathetic nerve activity in the conscious dog. *Pflugers Arch* 383:233, 1980.

193. Gross R, Kirchheim HR, Ruffman K: Effect of carotid occlusion and of perfusion pressure on renal function in conscious dogs. *Cir Res* 48:774, 1981.

194. Guo GB, Thames MD, Abboud FM: Differential baroreflex control of heart rate and vascular resistance in rabbits. Relative role of carotid, aortic, and cardiopulmonary baroreceptors. *Circ Res* 50:554, 1982.

195. Hagege J, Richet G: Proximal tubule dopamine histofluorescence in renal slices incubated with L-dopa. *Kidney Int* 27:3, 1985.

196. Hardaker WT, Wechsler AS: Redistribution of renal intracortical blood flow during dopamine infusion in dogs. *Circ Res* 33:437, 1973.

196a. Harris T, Muller B, Cotton RGH, et al: Dopaminergic and noradrenergic nerves of the dog have different dopa decarboxylase activities. *Neurosci Lett* 65:155, 1986.

197. Healy DP, Munzel PA, Insel PA: Localization of β_1- and β_2- adrenergic receptors in rat kidney by autoradiography. *Circ Res* 57:278, 1985.

198. Hermansson K, Larson M, Kallskog O, et al: Influence of renal nerve activity in arteriolar resistance, ultrafiltration dynamics and fluid reabsorption. *Pflugers Arch* 389:85, 1981.

199. Hermansson K, Ojteg G, Wolgast M: The cortical and medullary blood flow at different levels of renal nerve activity. *Acta Physiol Scand* 120:161, 1984.

200. Hermansson K, Ojteg G, Wolgast M: The reno-renal reflex: Evaluation from renal blood flow measurements. *Acta Physiol Scand* 120:207, 1984.

201. Hesse IFA, Johns EF: The subtype of α-adrenoceptor involved in the neural control of renal tubular sodium reabsorption in the rabbit. *J Physiol (Lond)* 352:527, 1984.

202. Hesse IFA, Johns EJ: An in vivo study of the alpha-adre-

noceptor subtypes on the renal vasculature of the anesthetized rabbit. *J Auton Pharmacol* 4:145, 1984.

203. Hesse IFA, Johns EJ: The role of α-adrenoceptors in the regulation of renal tubular reasorption and renin secretion in the rabbit. *Br J Pharmacol* 84:715, 1985.

204. Heymann MA, Iwamoto HS, Rudolph AM: Factors affecting changes in the neonatal systemic circulation. *Annu Rev Physiol* 43:371, 1981.

205. Hjemdahl P, Bradley T, Tidgren B: Release of dopamine from the kidney in vivo. *In* McGrath B, Bell C (eds): *Peripheral Actions of Dopamine*. London, McMillan 1988, p 56.

206. Hjemdahl P, Tidgren B: Differential changes of norepinephrine (NE) and dopamine (DA) overflow from the human kidney in response to different stressors (abstr). *Circulation* 76:IV-272, 1987.

207. Holdaas H, DiBona GF: On the existence of renal vasodilator nerves. *Proc Soc Exp Biol Med* 176:426, 1984.

208. Holdaas H, DiBona GF: Stimulatory and inhibitory reflexes from somatic receptors: Effect on renin release. *Am J Physiol* (Regulatory Integrative Comp Physiol 15)246:R1005, 1984.

209. Hollenberg NK, Adams DF, McKinstry DN, et al: Beta adrenoceptor-blocking agents and the kidney: Effect of nadolol and propranolol on the renal circulation. *Br J Clin Pharmacol* (suppl 2)7:219S, 1979.

210. Hom GJ, Jandhyala BS: Effects of cerebroventricular administration of ouabain on renal hemodynamics in anesthetized dogs: Evidence for the participation of renal dopaminergic vasodilator fibers. *J Pharmacol Exp Ther* 230:275, 1984.

211. Homma S, Murayama N, Gapstur S, et al: β-adrenoceptors coupled to adenylate cyclase in human and baboon nephron (abstr). *Clin Res* 36:520A, 1988.

212. Horn PT, Kohli JD, Listinsky JJ, et al: Regional variation in the alpha-adrenergic receptors in the canine resistance vessels. *Naunyn-Schmiedebergs Arch Pharmacol* 318:166, 1982.

213. Humphreys MH, Al-Bander H, Eneas JF, et al: Factors determining electrolyte excretion and renin secretion after closure of an arteriovenous fistula in the dog. *J Lab Clin Med* 918:89, 1981.

214. Ichikawa I, Kon V: Glomerular mesangium as an effector locus for the tubuloglomerular feedback system and renal sympathetic innervation. *Fed Proc* 42:3075, 1983.

215. Ichikawa K, Maddox DA, Cogan MG, et al: Dynamics of glomerular ultrafiltration in euvolemic Munich-Wistar rats. *Renal Physiol* 1:121, 1978.

216. Iino Y, Troy JL, Brenner BM: Effects of catecholamines on electrolyte transport in cortical collecting tubule. *J Membr Biol* 61:67, 1981.

217. Imai M: The connecting tubule: A functional subdivision of the rabbit distal nephron segment. *Kidney Int* 15:346, 1979.

218. Imai M, Nakamura R: Function of distal convoluted and connecting tubules studied by isolated nephron segments. *Kidney Int* 22:465, 1982.

219. Imbert M, Chabardes D, Morel F: Hormone-sensitive adenylate cyclase in isolated rabbit glomeruli. *Mol Cell Endocrinol* 1:295, 1984.

220. Imbs JL, Schmidt M, Ehrhardt JD, et al: The sympathetic nervous system and renal sodium handling: Is dopamine involved? *J Cardiovasc Pharmacol* (suppl 1)6:S171, 1984.

221. Imbs JL, Schmidt M, Schwartz J: Characteristiques pharmacologiques des recepteurs dopaminergiques renaux: Perspectives therapeutiques. *J Pharmacol (Paris)* (suppl III)14:5, 1983.

222. Imbs JL, Schmidt M, Schwartz J: Renal vascular effects of

61. Blake WD, Jurf AN: Renal sodium reasorption after acute renal denervation in the rabbit. *J Physiol (Lond)* 196:65, 1968.

62. Blantz RC, Pelayo JC: In vivo actions of angiotensin II on glomerular function. *Fed Proc* 42:3071, 1983.

63. Blendis LM, Auld RB, Alexander EA, et al: Effect of renal beta- and alpha-adrenergic stimulation on proximal sodium reabsorption in dogs. *Clin Sci* 43:569, 1972.

64. Bonjour JP, Churchill PC, Malvin RL: Change of tubular reabsorption of sodium and water after renal denervation in the dog. *J Physiol (Lond)* 204:571, 1969.

65. Boren DR, Henry DP, Selkurt EE, et al: Renal modulation of urinary catecholamine excretion during volume expansion in the dog. *Hypertension* 2:383, 1980.

66. Bradley T, Frederickson ED, Goldberg LI: Effect of DA_1 receptor blockade with SCH 23390 on the renal response to electrical stimulation of the renal nerves. *Proc Soc Exp Biol Med* 181:492, 1986.

67. Bradley T, Hjemahl P, DiBona GF: Increased release of norepinephrine and dopamine from canine kidney during bilateral carotid occlusion. *Am J Physiol (Renal Fluid Electrolyte Physiol* 21)252:F240, 1987.

68. Bradley T, Hjemdahl P: Further studies on renal nerve stimulation induced release of noradrenaline and dopamine from the canine kidney in situ. *Acta Physiol Scand* 122:369, 1984.

69. Bradley T, Hjemdahl P: Renal overflow of noradrenaline and dopamine to plasma during hindquarter compression and thoracic inferior vena cava obstruction in the dog. *Acta Physiol Scand* 127:205, 1986.

70. Brinley FJ Jr: Excitation and conduction in nerve fibers. *In* Mountcastle VB (ed): *Medical Physiology*. St. Louis, CV Mosby, 1970, p 46.

71. Brodde OE: Vascular dopamine receptors: Demonstration and characterization by in vitro studies. *Life Sci* 31:289, 1982.

72. Brody MJ, Johnson AK: Role of the arterioventral third ventricle region in fluid and electrolyte balance, arterial pressure regulation in hypertension. *In* Martini L, Ganong WF (eds): *Frontiers in Neuroendocrinology*. New York, Raven Press, 1980, p 249.

73. Buckley NM, Brazeau P, Charney AN, et al: Cardiovascular and renal effects of isoproterenol infusions in young swine. *Biol Neonate* 45:69, 1984.

74. Buckley NM, Brazeau P, Frasier ID: Cardiovascular effects of dopamine in the developing swine. *Biol Neonate* 43:50, 1983.

75. Buckley NM, Brazeau P, Frasier ID: Renal blood flow autoregulation in developing swine. *Am J Physiol (Heart Circ Physiol* 14)245:H1, 1983.

76. Buckley NM, Brazeau P, Gootman PM, et al: Renal circulatory effects of adrenergic stimuli in anesthetized piglets and mature swine. *Am J Physiol (Heart Circ Physiol* 6)237:H690, 1979.

77. Buckley NM, Charney AN, Brazeau P, et al: Changes in cardiovascular and renal function during catecholamine infusions in developing swine. *Am J Physiol (Renal Fluid Electrolyte Physiol* 9)240:F276, 1981.

78. Busuttil RW, Roh BL, Fisher JW: The cytological localization of erythropoietin in the human kidney using the fluorescent antibody technique. *Proc Soc Exp Biol Med* 137:327, 1971.

79. Bylund DB: Heterogeneity of alpha-2 adrenergic receptors. *Pharmacol Biochem Behav* 22:835, 1985.

80. Calaresu FR, Ciriello J: Altered concentrations of catecholamines in the hypothalamus of the rat after renal denervation. *Can J Physiol Pharmacol* 59:1274, 1981.

81. Calaresu FR, Ciriello J: Renal afferent nerves affect discharge rates of medullary and hypothalamic single units in the cat. *J Auton Nerv Syst* 3:311, 1981.

82. Calaresu FR, Kim P, Nakamura H, et al: Electrophysiological characteristics of renorenal reflexes in the cat. *J Physiol (Lond)* 283:141, 1978.

83. Calaresu FR, Stella A, Zanchetti A: Hemodynamic responses and renin release during stimulation of afferent renal nerves in the cat. *J Physiol (Lond)* 255:687, 1976.

84. Campese VM, Romoff MS, Levitan D, et al: Abnormal relationship between sodium intake and sympathetic nervous system activity in salt-sensitive patients with essential hypertension. *Kidney Int* 21:371, 1982.

85. Carey RM, Thorner MO, Ortt EM: Dopaminergic inhibition of metoclopramide-induced aldosterone secretion in man. *J Clin Invest* 66:10, 1980.

86. Carey RM, Stote RMK, Duff JW, et al: Selective peripheral dopamine-1 receptor stimulation with fenoldopam in human essential hypertension. *J Clin Invest* 74:2198, 1984.

87. Carrara MC, Baines AD: Propranolol induces acute natriuresis by β blockade and dopaminergic stimulation. *Can J Physiol Pharmacol* 54:683, 1976.

88. Carriere S, Lalumiere G, Gaigneault A, et al: Sequential changes in catecholamine plasma levels during isotonic volume expansion in dogs. *Am J Physiol (Renal Fluid Electrolyte Physiol* 4)235:F119, 1978.

89. Chabardes D, Montegut M, Imbert-Teboul M, et al: Inhibition of α_2-adrenergic agonists on AVP-induced cAMP accumulation in isolated collecting tubule of the rat kidney. *Mol Cell Endocrinol* 37:263, 1984.

90. Chan YL: Adrenergic control of bicarbonate absorption in the proximal convoluted tubule of the rat kidney. *Pflugers Arch* 388:159, 1980.

91. Chan YL: The role of norepinephrine in the regulation of fluid absorption in the rat proximal convoluted tubule. *J Pharmacol Exp Ther* 215:65, 1980.

92. Chan YL, Chatsudthipong V, Su-Tsai SM, et al: The role of calcium in the dopaminergic effect on the proximal convoluted tubule of rat kidney (abstr). *Fed Proc* 45:508, 1986.

93. Chang EB, Field M, Miller RJ: Alpha 2-adrenergic receptor regulation of ion transport in rabbit ileum. *Am J Physiol (Gastrointest Liver Physiol* 5)242:G237, 1982.

94. Chapman BJ, Horn NM, Munday KA, et al: The actions of dopamine and of sulpiride on regional blood flows in the rat kidney. *J Physiol (Lond)* 298:437, 1980.

95. Chapman BJ, Horn NM, Robertson MJ: Renal blood-flow changes during renal nerve stimulation in rats tested with α-adrenergic and dopaminergic blockers. *J Physiol (Lond)* 325:67, 1982.

96. Chapman BJ, Munday KA, Radhi ARAH: The effects of renal nerve stimulation in rats treated with α-adrenergic and dopaminergic blockers. *J Physiol (Lond)* 341:65P, 1983.

97. Chassaing C, Duchene-Marullaz P, Veyrac MJ: Effects of catecholamines on cardiac chronotropic response to vagal stimulation in the dog. *Am J Physiol (Heart Circ Physiol* 14)245:H721, 1983.

98. Cheung YD, Barnett DB, Nahorski SR: Heterogeneous properties of alpha$_2$ adrenoceptors in particulate and soluble preparations of human platelet and rat and rabbit kidney. *Biochem Pharmacol* 35:3767, 1986.

99. Chou SY, Liebman PH, Ferder LF, et al: Effects of α-adrenergic blockade on sodium excretion in normal and chronic salt retaining dogs. *Can J Physiol Pharmacol* 54:209, 1976.

100. Ciriello J, Calaresu FR: Central projections of afferent renal fibers in the rat: An anterograde transport study of horseradish peroxidase. *J Auton Nerv Syst* 8:273, 1983.

101. Click RL, Joyner WL, Gilmore JP: Reactivity of glomerular

afferent and efferent arterioles in renal hypertension. *Kidney Int* 15:109, 1979.

102. Cogan MG: Neurogenic regulation of proximal bicarbonate and chloride reabsorption. *Am J Physiol* (Renal Fluid Electrolyte Physiol 19)250:F22, 1986.

103. Collier WL, Cavallotti C, De Rossi M, et al: Dopamine-sensitive adenylate cyclase in rabbit renal artery. *Neurosci Lett* 43:197, 1983.

104. Colindres RE, Spielman WS, Moss NG, et al: Functional evidence for renorenal reflexes in the rat. *Am J Physiol* (Renal Fluid Electrolyte Physiol 8)239:F265, 1980.

105. Corradi A, Arendhorst WJ: Rat renal hemodynamics during venous compression: Roles of nerves and prostaglandins. *Am J Physiol* (Renal Fluid Electrolyte Physiol 17)248:F810, 1985.

106. Cox RH, Jones AW, Swain ML: Mechanics and electrolyte composition of arterial smooth muscle in developing dogs. *Am J Physiol* 231:77, 1976.

107. Cuche JL, Marchand GR, Greger RF, et al: Phosphaturic effect of dopamine in dogs. Possible role of intrarenally produced dopamine in phosphate regulation. *J Clin Invest* 58:71, 1976.

108. Cuche JL: Sources of circulating dopamine. *In* McGrath B, Bell C (eds): *Peripheral Actions of dopamine.* London, McMillan, 1988, p 1.

109. Dale HH: On some physiological action of ergot. *J Physiol (Lond)* 34:163, 1906.

110. Dalmaz Y, Peyrin L: Sex-differences in catecholamine metabolites in human urine during development and at adulthood. *J Neural Transm* 54:193, 1982.

111. Dalmaz Y, Peyrin L, Sann L, et al: Age-related changes in catecholamine metabolites of human urine from birth to adulthood. *J Neural Transm* 46:153, 1979.

112. Dashwood MR: Autoradiographic localization of prazosin binding sites in rat kidney. *Eur J Pharmacol* 94:163, 1983.

113. DeFronzo RA, Bia M, Birkhead G: Epinephrine and potassium homeostasis. *Kidney Int* 20:83, 1981.

114. DeFronzo RA, Stanton B, Klein-Robbenhaar G, et al: Inhibitory effect of epinephrine on renal potassium secretion: A micropuncture study. *Am J Physiol* (Renal Fluid Electrolyte Physiol 14)245:F303, 1983.

115. De Rouffignac C, Elalouf JM: Hormonal regulation of chloride transport in the proximal and distal nephron. *Annu Rev Physiol* 50:123, 1988.

116. DeWolf WC, Fraley EE: Renal pain. *Urology* 6: 403, 1975.

117. DiBona GF: Neurogenic regulation of renal tubular sodium reabsorption. *Am J Physiol* (Renal Fluid Electrolyte Physiol 2)233:F73, 1977.

118. DiBona GF, Johns EJ: A study of the role of renal nerves in the renal responses to 60° head-up tilt in the anesthetized dog. *J Physiol (Lond)* 299:117, 1980.

119. DiBona GF, Sawin LL: Role of renal α_2-adrenergic receptors in spontaneously hypertensive rats. *Hypertension* 9:41, 1987.

120. DiBona GF, Sawin LL: Renal nerves in renal adaptation to dietary sodium restriction. *Am J Physiol* (Renal Fluid Electrolyte Physiol 14)245:F322, 1983.

121. DiBona GF, Sawin LL: Effect of renal nerve stimulation on NaCl and H_2O transport in Henle's loop of the rat. *Am J Physiol* (Renal Fluid Electrolyte Physiol 12)243:F576, 1982.

122. DiBona GF, Sawin LL: Renal nerve activity in conscious rats during volume expansion and depletion. *Am J Physiol* (Renal Fluid Electrolyte Physiol 17)248:F15, 1985.

123. DiBona GF, Sawin LL: Role of renal nerves in congestive heart failure. *Kidney Int* 33:418, 1988.

124. Dieterich HG: Electron microscopic studies of the inner-

vation of the kidney. *Z Anat Entwickl* 145:169, 1974.

125. Dinerstein RJ, Jones RT, Goldberg LI: Evidence for dopamine-containing renal nerves. *Fed Proc* 42:3005, 1983.

126. Dinerstein RJ, Vannice J, Henderson RC, et al: Histofluorescence techniques provide evidence for dopamine-containing neuronal elements in canine kidney. *Science* 205:497, 1979.

127. DiSalvo J, Fell C: Changes in renal blood flow during renal nerve stimulation. *Proc Soc Exp Biol Med* 136:150, 1971.

128. Dolezel S: Monoaminergic innervation of the kidney. Aorticorenal ganglion—A sympathetic, monoaminergic ganglion supplying the renal vessels. *Experientia* 23:109, 1967.

129. Donovan MK, Winternitz SR, Wyss JM: An analysis of the sensory innervation of the urinary system in the rat. *Brain Res Bull* 11:321, 1983.

130. Donovan MK, Wyss JM, Winternitz SR: Localization of renal sensory neurons using the fluorescent dye technique. *Brain Res* 259:119, 1983.

131. Donowitz M: Ca^{2+} in the control of active intestinal Na and Cl transport: Involvement in neurohormonal action. *Am J Physiol* (Gastrointest Liver Physiol 8)245:G165, 1983.

132. Dreslinski GR, Aristimuno GG, Messerli FH, et al: Effects of beta blockade with acetobutalol on hypertension, hemodynamics, and fluid volume. *Clin Pharmacol Ther* 26:562, 1979.

133. Drew GM, Whiting SB: Evidence for two distinct types of postsynaptic α-adrenoceptor in vascular smooth muscle in vivo. *Br J Pharmacol* 67:207, 1979.

134. Driscoll DJ, Fukushige J, Hartley CJ, et al: The comparative hemodynamic effects of isoproterenol in chronically instrumented puppies and adult dogs. *Dev Pharmacol Ther* 2:91, 1981.

135. Driscoll DJ, Gillete PC, Lewis RM: Comparative hemodynamic effects of isoproterenol, dopamine, and dobutamine in the newborn dog. *Pediatr Res* 13:1006, 1979.

136. Dupont AG, Vanderniepen P, Lefebvre RA, et al: Pharmacological characterization of neuronal dopamine receptors in the rat hindquarters, renal and superior mesenteric vascular beds. *J Auton Pharmacol* 6:305, 1986.

137. Dworkin LD, Ichikawa I, Brenner BM, et al: Hormonal modulation of glomerular function. *Am J Physiol* (Renal Fluid Electrolyte Physiol 13)244:F95, 1983.

138. Dzau VJ, Kresiberg J: Cultured glomerular mesangial cells contain renin: Influence of calcium and isoproterenol. *J Cardiovasc Pharmacol* (suppl 10)8:S6, 1986.

138a. Edwards RM: Comparison of the effects of fenoldopam, SK&F R-87516 and dopamine on renal arterioles in vitro. *Eur J Pharmacol* 126:167, 1986.

139. Edwards RM: Response of isolated arterioles to acetylcholine, dopamine and bradykinin. *Am J Physiol* (Renal Fluid Electrolyte Physiol 17)248:F183, 1985.

140. Edwards RM: Segmental effects of norepinephrine and angiotensin II on isolated renal microvessels. *Am J Physiol* (Renal Fluid Electrolyte Physiol 13)244:F526, 1983.

141. Edwards RM, Trizna W: Characterization of α-adrenoceptors on isolated rabbit renal arterioles. *Am J Physiol* (Renal Fluid Electrolyte Physiol 23)254:F178, 1988.

142. Faber JE: Role of prostaglandins and kinins in the renal pressor reflex. *Hypertension* 10:522, 1987.

143. Faber JE, Brody MJ: Afferent renal nerve-dependent hypertension following acute renal artery stenosis in the conscious rat. *Circ Res* 57:676, 1985.

144. Faucheux B, Buu NT, Kuchel O: Effects of saline and albumin on plsma and urinary catecholamines in dogs. *Am J Physiol* (Renal Fluid Electrolyte Physiol 1)232:F123, 1977.

145. Felder CC, Blecher MM, Jose PA: Dopamine-1 (DA-1) but not dopamine 2 (DA-2) stimulated phospholipase C

(PL-C) activity in renal cortical membranes (abstr). *Kidney Int* 31:166, 1987.

146. Felder CC, Blecher MM, Jose PA: Dopamine-1 regulated sodium transport in rat renal brush border membrane vesicles (abstr). *Kidney Int* 33:263, 1988.

147. Felder CC, McKelvey TC, Blecher M, et al: Dopamine receptors (DA-R) in proximal tubular basolateral (BLM) and brush border membranes (BBM) (abstr). *Pediatr Res* 21:475A, 1987.

148. Felder RA, Blecher M, Calcagno PL, et al: Dopamine receptors in the proximal tubule of the rabbit. *Am J Physiol* (Renal Fluid Electrolyte Physiol 16)247:F499, 1984.

149. Felder RA, Blecher M, Eisner GM, et al: Cortical tubular and glomerular dopamine receptors in the rat kidney. *Am J Physiol* (Renal Fluid Electrolyte Physiol 15)246:F557, 1984.

150. Felder RA, Blecher M, Schoelkopf L, et al: Renal dopamine receptors during maturation (abstr). *Pediatr Res* 17:148A, 1983.

151. Felder RA, Felder CC, Eisner GM, et al: Renal dopamine receptors. *In* McGrath B, Bell C (eds): *Peripheral Actions of Dopamine*. London, McMillan 1988, p 124.

152. Felder R, Garland DS: Renal dopamine receptor in the spontaneously hypertensive rat (SHR) (abstr). *Pediatr Nephrol* 1:C61, 1987.

153. Felder RA, Jose PA: Development of adrenergic and dopamine receptors in the kidney. *In* Strauss J (ed): *Homeostasis, Nephrotoxicity, and Renal Anomalies in the Newborn.* Boston, Martinus Nijhoff, 1986, p 3.

154. Felder RA, Nakamura KT, Robillard JE, et al: Dopamine receptors in the developng kidney. *Pediatr Nephrol* 2: 156, 1988.

155. Felder RA, Pelayo JC, Calcagno PL, et al: Alpha-adrenoceptors in the developing kidney. *Pediatr Res* 17:177, 1983.

156. Felder RA, Seikaly MG, Eisner GM, et al: Renal dopamine-1 defect in the spontaneously hypertensive rat. *Contrib Nephrol* 67:71, 1988.

157. Felder RB: Excitatory and inhibitory interactions among renal and cardiovascular afferent nerves in dorsomedial medulla. *Am J Physiol* (Regulatory Integrative Comp Physiol 19)250:R580, 1986.

158. Feltes TF, Hansen TN, Martin CG, et al: The effects of dopamine infusion on regional blood flow in newborn lambs. *Pediatr Res* 21:131, 1987.

159. Ferguson M, Bell C: Substance P-immunoreactive nerves in the rat kidney. *Neurosci Lett* 60: 183, 1985.

160. Fernandez-Pardal J, Saavedra JM: Catecholamines in discrete kidney regions. Changes in salt-sensitive Dahl hypertensive rats. *Hypertension* 4:821, 1982.

161. Fernandez-Repollet E, Silva-Netto CR, Colindres RE, et al: Role of renal nerves in maintaining sodium balance in unrestrained conscious rats. *Am J Physiol* (Renal Fluid Electrolyte Physiol 18)249:F819, 1985.

162. Fildes RD, Eisner GM, Calcagno PL, et al: Renal alpha adrenoceptors and sodium excretion in the dog. *Am J Physiol* (Renal Fluid Electrolyte Physiol 17)248:F128, 1985.

163. Fildes R, Sohaug M, Eisner GM, et al: Enhancement of sodium excretion by substance P during saline loading in the canine puppy. *Pediatr Res* 17:737, 1983.

164. Fink GD, Fisher JW: Stimulation of erythropoiesis by beta adrenergic agonists. I. Characterization of activity in polycythemic mice. *J Pharmacol Exp Ther* 202:192, 1977.

165. Flavahan NA, Vanhoutte PM: α_1-adrenoceptor subclassification in vascular smooth muscle. *Trends Pharmacol Sci* 7:347, 1986.

166. Forssmann WG, Reinecke M: Organ-specific innervation by autonomic nerve fibers as revealed by electron microscopy and immunohistochemistry. *Front Horm Res* 12:59, 1984.

167. Frederickson ED, Bradley T, Goldberg LI: Blockade of renal effects of dopamine in the dog by DA₁ antagonist SCH 23390. *Am J Physiol* (Renal Fluid Electrolyte Physiol 18)249:F236, 1985.

168. Fulgraff G, Heidenreich O, Heintze K, et al: Wirkung von alpha-und beta-sympathomimetica und sympatholytica auf die renale exkretion und resorption von flussigkeit und electrolyten in ausscheidungs-und mikropunktionsversuchen an ratten. *Naunyn Schmiedebergs Arch Pharmacol* 262:295, 1969.

168a. Fuchs E, Neumann P, Salzbrunn B, et al: α- and β-adrenergic binding sites in human kidney detected by autoradiography. (abstr) *Kidney Int* 35:311, 1989.

169. Furness JB, Costa M, Papka RE, et al: Neuropeptides contained in peripheral cardiovascular nerves. *Clin Exp Hypertens [A]* 6:91, 1984.

170. Furness JB, Papka RE, Della NG, et al: Substance P-like immunoreactivity in nerves associated with the vascular system of guinea-pigs. *Neuroscience* 7:447, 1982.

171. Gallen DD, Cowen T, Griffith SG, et al: Functional and non-functional nerve—smooth muscle transmission in the renal arteries of the newborn and adult rabbit and guinea pig. *Blood Vessels* 19:237, 1982.

172. Gattone VH, Marfurt CF, Dallie S: Extrinsic innervation of the rat kidney: A retrograde tracing study. *Am J Physiol* (Renal Fluid Electrolyte Physiol 19)250:F189, 1986.

173. Gellai M, Ruffolo RR Jr: Renal effects of selective alpha-1 and alpha-2 adrenoceptor agonists in conscious, normotensive rats. *J Pharmacol Exp Ther* 240:723, 1987.

174. Gill JR, Bartter FC: Adrenergic nervous system in sodium metabolism. II. Effects of guanethidine on the renal response to sodium deprivation in normal man. *N Engl J Med* 275:1466, 1966.

175. Gill JR Jr, Casper AG: Depression of proximal tubular sodium reabsorption in the dog in response to renal beta adrenergic stimulation by isoproterenol. *J Clin Invest* 50:112, 1971.

176. Gill JR Jr, Casper AG: Renal effects of adenosine 3′,5′-cyclic monophosphate and dibutyryl adenosine 3′,5′-cyclic monophosphate. Evidence for a role for adenosine 3′,5′-cyclic monophosphate in the regulation of proximal tubular sodium reabsorption. *J Clin Invest* 50:1231, 1971.

177. Gilman AG: G proteins: Transducers of receptor-generated signals. *Annu Rev Biochem* 56:615, 1987.

178. Gilmore JP, Tomomatsu E: Renal mechanoreceptors in nonhuman primates. *Am J Physiol* (Regulatory Integrative Comp Physiol 17)248:R202, 1985.

178a. Gitler MS, Piccio MM, Robillard JE, et al: Ontogeny of renal alpha adrenoceptor subtypes in the sheep (abstr). *Pediatr Res* 25:340A, 1989.

179. Goetz KL: Physiology and pathophysiology of atrial peptides. *Am J Physiol* (Endocrinol Metab 7)254:E1, 1988.

180. Goldberg LI, Glock BB, Kohli JD, et al: Separation of peripheral dopamine receptors by a selective DA₁ antagonist, SCH 23390. *Hypertension* (suppl I)6:I25, 1984.

181. Goldberg LI, Kohli ID: Differentiation of dopamine receptors in the periphery. *In* Kaiser C, Kebabian JW (eds): *The Dopamine Receptors.* Washington, DC, American Chemical Society, 1983, p 101.

182. Goldberg MR, Robertson D: Yohimbine: A pharmacological probe for the study of the a₂-adrenoceptor. *Pharmacol Rev* 35:143, 1983.

183. Gordon D, Pert WS, Wilcox CS: Requirement of the adrenergic nervous system for conservation of sodium by

the rabbit kidney (proceedings). *J Physiol (Lond)* 293:24P, 1979.

184. Graham RM, Pettinger WA, Sagalowsky A, et al: Renal alpha-adrenergic receptor abnormality in the spontaneously hypertensive rat. *Hypertension* 4:881, 1982.

185. Grantham JJ, Chonko AM: Renal handling of organic anions and cations; metabolism and excretion of uric acid. *In* Brenner BM, Rector FC Jr (eds): *The Kidney.* WB Saunders, Philadelphia, 1986, p 663.

186. Greven J, Heidenreich O: A micropuncture study of the effect of isoprenaline or renal tubular fluid and electrolyte transport in the rat. *Naunyn Schmiedebergs Arch Pharmacol* 287:117, 1975.

187. Greven J, Klein H: Effects of dopamine on whole kidney function and proximal transtubular volume fluxes in the rat. *Naunyn Schmiedebergs Arch Pharmacol* 296:289, 1977.

188. Greven J, Pantel J: Failure of an angiotensin II antagonist to influence isoprenaline-induced antidiuresis in rats. *Naunyn Schmiedebergs Arch Pharmacol* 332:271, 1986.

189. Grignolo A, Koepke JP, Obrist PA: Renal function, heart rate, and blood pressure during exercise and avoidance in dogs. *Am J Physiol* (Regulatory Integrative Comp Physiol 11)242:R482, 1982.

190. Grignolo A, Seidler FJ, Bartolome M, et al: Norepinephrine content of the rat kidney during development: Alterations induced by perinatal methadone. *Life Sci* 31:3009, 1982.

191. Gross R, Hackenberg H, Hackenthal E: Interaction between perfusion pressure and sympathetic nerves in renin release by carotid baroreflex in conscious dogs. *J Physiol (Lond)* 313: 237, 1981.

192. Gross R, Kirchheim H: Effects of bilateral carotid and auditory stimulation on renal blood flow and sympathetic nerve activity in the conscious dog. *Pflugers Arch* 383:233, 1980.

193. Gross R, Kirchheim HR, Ruffman K: Effect of carotid occlusion and of perfusion pressure on renal function in conscious dogs. *Cir Res* 48:774, 1981.

194. Guo GB, Thames MD, Abboud FM: Differential baroreflex control of heart rate and vascular resistance in rabbits. Relative role of carotid, aortic, and cardiopulmonary baroreceptors. *Circ Res* 50:554, 1982.

195. Hagege J, Richet G: Proximal tubule dopamine histofluorescence in renal slices incubated with L-dopa. *Kidney Int* 27:3, 1985.

196. Hardaker WT, Wechsler AS: Redistribution of renal intracortical blood flow during dopamine infusion in dogs. *Circ Res* 33:437, 1973.

196a. Harris T, Muller B, Cotton RGH, et al: Dopaminergic and noradrenergic nerves of the dog have different dopa decarboxylase activities. *Neurosci Lett* 65:155, 1986.

197. Healy DP, Munzel PA, Insel PA: Localization of β_1- and β_2- adrenergic receptors in rat kidney by autoradiography. *Circ Res* 57:278, 1985.

198. Hermansson K, Larson M, Kallskog O, et al: Influence of renal nerve activity in arteriolar resistance, ultrafiltration dynamics and fluid reabsorption. *Pflugers Arch* 389:85, 1981.

199. Hermansson K, Ojteg G, Wolgast M: The cortical and medullary blood flow at different levels of renal nerve activity. *Acta Physiol Scand* 120:161, 1984.

200. Hermansson K, Ojteg G, Wolgast M: The reno-renal reflex: Evaluation from renal blood flow measurements. *Acta Physiol Scand* 120:207, 1984.

201. Hesse IFA, Johns EF: The subtype of α-adrenoceptor involved in the neural control of renal tubular sodium reabsorption in the rabbit. *J Physiol (Lond)* 352:527, 1984.

202. Hesse IFA, Johns EJ: An in vivo study of the alpha-adre-

203. Hesse IFA, Johns EJ: The role of α-adrenoceptors in the regulation of renal tubular reasorption and renin secretion in the rabbit. *Br J Pharmacol* 84:715, 1985.

204. Heymann MA, Iwamoto HS, Rudolph AM: Factors affecting changes in the neonatal systemic circulation. *Annu Rev Physiol* 43:371, 1981.

205. Hjemdahl P, Bradley T, Tidgren B: Release of dopamine from the kidney in vivo. *In* McGrath B, Bell C (eds): *Peripheral Actions of Dopamine.* London, McMillan 1988, p 56.

206. Hjemdahl P, Tidgren B: Differential changes of norepinephrine (NE) and dopamine (DA) overflow from the human kidney in response to different stressors (abstr). *Circulation* 76:IV-272, 1987.

207. Holdaas H, DiBona GF: On the existence of renal vasodilator nerves. *Proc Soc Exp Biol Med* 176:426, 1984.

208. Holdaas H, DiBona GF: Stimulatory and inhibitory reflexes from somatic receptors: Effect on renin release. *Am J Physiol* (Regulatory Integrative Comp Physiol 15)246:R1005, 1984.

209. Hollenberg NK, Adams DF, McKinstry DN, et al: Beta adrenoceptor-blocking agents and the kidney: Effect of nadolol and propranolol on the renal circulation. *Br J Clin Pharmacol* (suppl 2)7:219S, 1979.

210. Hom GJ, Jandhyala BS: Effects of cerebroventricular administration of ouabain on renal hemodynamics in anesthetized dogs: Evidence for the participation of renal dopaminergic vasodilator fibers. *J Pharmacol Exp Ther* 230:275, 1984.

211. Homma S, Murayama N, Gapstur S, et al: β-adrenoceptors coupled to adenylate cyclase in human and baboon nephron (abstr). *Clin Res* 36:520A, 1988.

212. Horn PT, Kohli JD, Listinsky JJ, et al: Regional variation in the alpha-adrenergic receptors in the canine resistance vessels. *Naunyn-Schmiedebergs Arch Pharmacol* 318:166, 1982.

213. Humphreys MH, Al-Bander H, Eneas JF, et al: Factors determining electrolyte excretion and renin secretion after closure of an arteriovenous fistula in the dog. *J Lab Clin Med* 918:89, 1981.

214. Ichikawa I, Kon V: Glomerular mesangium as an effector locus for the tubuloglomerular feedback system and renal sympathetic innervation. *Fed Proc* 42:3075, 1983.

215. Ichikawa K, Maddox DA, Cogan MG, et al: Dynamics of glomerular ultrafiltration in euvolemic Munich-Wistar rats. *Renal Physiol* 1:121, 1978.

216. Iino Y, Troy JL, Brenner BM: Effects of catecholamines on electrolyte transport in cortical collecting tubule. *J Membr Biol* 61:67, 1981.

217. Imai M: The connecting tubule: A functional subdivision of the rabbit distal nephron segment. *Kidney Int* 15:346, 1979.

218. Imai M, Nakamura R: Function of distal convoluted and connecting tubules studied by isolated nephron segments. *Kidney Int* 22:465, 1982.

219. Imbert M, Chabardes D, Morel F: Hormone-sensitive adenylate cyclase in isolated rabbit glomeruli. *Mol Cell Endocrinol* 1:295, 1984.

220. Imbs JL, Schmidt M, Ehrhardt JD, et al: The sympathetic nervous system and renal sodium handling: Is dopamine involved? *J Cardiovasc Pharmacol* (suppl 1)6:S171, 1984.

221. Imbs JL, Schmidt M, Schwartz J: Characteristiques pharmacologiques des recepteurs dopaminergiques renaux: Perspectives therapeutiques. *J Pharmacol (Paris)* (suppl III)14:5, 1983.

222. Imbs JL, Schmidt M, Schwartz J: Renal vascular effects of

dopaminomimetics. *In* Gessa GL, Corsini GU (eds): *Apomorphine and Other Dopaminomimetics.* New York, Raven Press, 1981, p 265.

223. Insel PA, Snavely MD: Catecholamines and the kidney: Receptors and renal function. *Annu Rev Physiol* 43:625, 1981.

224. Insel PA, Snavely MD, Healy DP, et al: Radioligand binding and functional assays demonstrate postsynaptic alpha$_2$-receptors on proximal tubules of rat and rabbit kidney. *J Cardiovasc Pharmacol* (suppl 8)7:S9, 1985.

225. Jacobs WR, Chan YL: Evidence for the presence of functional beta-adrenoceptor along the proximal tubule of the rat kidney. *Biochem Biophys Res Commun* 141:334, 1986.

226. Jarrot B, Louis WJ, Summers RN: The characteristics of ^{3}H-clonidine binding to an alpha-adrenoceptor in membranes from guinea pig kidney. *Br J Pharmacol* 65:663, 1979.

227. Johansson B: Circulatory responses to stimulation of somatic afferents with special reference to depressor effects from muscle nerves. *Acta Physiol Scand* (suppl 198)57:1, 1962.

228. John E, Assadi F, Fornell L: Dose related effect of dopamine (D) on renal function (RF) during ontogeny (abstr). *Pediatric Nephrol* 1:C27, 1987.

229. Johnson MD, Barger CA: Circulating catecholamines in control of renal electrolyte and water excretion. *Am J Physiol* (Renal Fluid Electrolyte Physiol 9)240:F192, 1981.

230. Jose PA: *Adrenergic Regulation of Blood Pressure.* NHLBI Workshop on Juvenile Hypertension, Proc Symposium. New York, Biomedical Information Corp, 1984, p 205.

231. Jose PA, Eisner GM, Robillard JR: Renal hemodynamics and natriuresis induced by the dopamine-1 agonist, SKF 82526. *Am J Med Sci* 294:181, 1987.

232. Jose PA, Felder RA, Holloway RR, et al: Dopamine receptors modulate sodium excretion in denervated kidney. *Am J Physiol* (Renal Fluid Electrolyte Physiol 19)250:1033, 1986.

233. Jose PA, Felder RA, Robillard JE, et al: Dopamine-2 receptor in the canine kidney (abstr). *Kidney Int* 28:385, 1986.

234. Jose PA, Holloway RR, Campbell TW, et al: Dopamine blockade attenuates the natriuresis of saline loading in the adrenalectomized rat. *Nephron* 48:54, 1988.

235. Jose P, Logan A, Slotkoff L, et al: Intrarenal blood flow distribution in the maturing kidney. Proceedings of the 1st International Symposium *"Radionuclides in Nephrology,"* New York, Grune and Stratton, 1972, p 9.

236. Jose PA, McKelvey T, Felder CC, et al: Ontogeny of renal beta adrenoceptors in the sheep. *Pediatr Nephrol* (submitted)

237. Jose PA, Pelayo JC, Felder RA, et al: Maturation of single nephron filtration rate in the canine puppy—effect of saline loading. *In* Spitzer A (ed): *The Kidney During Development: Morphology and Function.* New York, Masson Publishing USA, 1982, p 139.

238. Jose PA, Slotkoff LM, Lilienfield LS, et al: Sensitivity of neonatal renal vasculature to epinephrine. *Am J Physiol* 226:796, 1974.

239. Judes C, Helwig JJ, Bollavck C, et al: Isoproterenol-sensitive adenylate cyclase in glomeruli isolated from young and adult rat renal cortex. *Gen Pharmacol* 16:205, 1985.

240. Kahan T, Dahlof C, Hjemdahl P: Facilitation of nerve stimulation evoked noradrenaline overflow by isoprenaline but not by circulating adrenaline in the dog *in vivo.* *Life Sci* 40:1811, 1987.

241. Kahn AM, Dolson GM, Hise MK, et al: Parathyroid hormone and dibutyryl cAMP inhibit Na$^+$/H$^+$ exchange in renal brush border vesicles. *Am J Physiol* (Renal Fluid Electrolyte Physiol 17)248:F212, 1985.

242. Kaneda Y, Bello-Reuss E: Effect of dopamine on phosphate reabsorption in isolated perfused rabbit proximal tubules. *Miner Electrolyte Metab* 9:147, 1983.

243. Katholi RE: Renal nerves in the pathogenesis of hypertension in experimental animals and humans. *Am J Physiol* (Renal Fluid Electrolyte Physiol 14)245:F1, 1983.

244. Katholi RE, Bishop SP, Oparil S, et al: Renal function during reflexly activated catecholamine flow through an adrenorenal rete. *Am J Physiol* (Renal Fluid Electrolyte Physiol)240:F30, 1981.

245. Katholi RE, Hageman GR, Whitlow PL, et al: Hemodynamic and afferent renal nerve response to intrarenal adenosine in the dog. *Hypertension* (suppl I)5:I491, 1983.

246. Katz LD, D'Avella J, DeFronzo RA: Effect of epinephrine on renal potassium excretion in the isolated perfused rat kidney. *Am J Physiol* (Renal Fluid Electrolyte Physiol 16)247:F331, 1984.

247. Kebabian JW, Calne DB: Multiple receptors for dopamine. *Nature* 277:93, 1979.

248. Kendrick E, Oberg B, Wennergren G: Vasoconstrictor fibre discharge to skeletal muscle, kidney, intestine and skin at varying levels of arterial baroreceptor activity in the cat. *Acta Physiol Scand* 85:464, 1972.

248a. Kessler JA, Adler JE, Bohn MC, et al: Substance P in principal sympathetic nerves: Regulation by impulse activity. *Science* 242:1403, 1981.

249. Kimmel PL, Goldfarb S: Effects of isoproterenol on potassium secretion by the cortical collecting tubule. *Am J Physiol* (Renal Fluid Electrolyte Physiol 15)246:F804, 1984.

250. Kinoshita S, Canada M, Felder RA: DA-1 receptors identified in rat renal homogenates, slices, and microdissected nephrons with ^{125}I-SCH23982 (abstr). *Kidney Int* 33:419, 1988.

250a. Kinoshita S, Jose PA, Felder RA: Ontogeny of the dopamine$_1$ (DA$_1$) receptor in rat renal proximal convoluted tubule (PCT) (abstr). *Pediatr Res* 25:68A, 1989.

251. Kirchheim HR, Gross R: Response of renal blood flow and renal sympathetic nerve ativity to baroreceptor and emotional stimuli in the conscious dog. *In* Bauer RD, Bussew R (eds): *The Arterial System.* Berlin, Heidelberg, New York, Springer, 1978, p 203.

252. Knight DS, Bazer GT: Visualization of intrarenal catecholamine containing elements: Flourescence histochemistry and electron microscopy. *J Auton Nerv Syst* 1:173, 1979.

253. Kobilka BK, Matsui H, Kobilka TS, et al: Cloning, sequencing, and expression of the gene coding for the human platelet α_2-adrenergic receptor. *Science* 238:650, 1987.

254. Kon V, Ichikawa I: Effector loci for renal nerve control of cortical microcirculation. *Am J Physiol* (Renal Fluid Electrolyte Physiol 14)245:F545, 1983.

255. Kopin IJ: Catecholamine metabolism (and the biochemical assessment of sympathetic activity) *Clin Endocrinol Metab* 6:525, 1977.

256. Kopin IJ, Goldstein DS, Feurstein GZ: The sympathetic nervous system and hypertension. *In* Laragh JS, Buhler FR, Seldin DW (eds): *Frontiers in Hypertension Research.* New York, Springer-Verlag, 1981, p 283.

257. Kopp U, Aurell M, Nilsson IM, et al: The role of beta-1 adrenoceptors in the renin release response to graded sympathetic stimulation. *Pflugers Arch* 387:107, 1980.

258. Kopp U, Bradley T, Hjemdahl P: Renal venous outflow and urinary excretion of norepinephrine, epinephrine and dopamine during graded renal nerve stimulation. *Am J Physiol* (Endocrinol Metab 7)244:E52, 1983.

259. Kopp UC, Olson LA, DiBona GF: Renorenal reflex re-

sponses to mechano- and chemoreceptor stimulation in the dog and rat. *Am J Physiol* (Renal Fluid Electrolyte Physiol 15)246:F67, 1984.

260. Kopp UC, Smith LA, DiBona GF: Impaired renorenal reflexes in spontaneously hypertensive rats. *Hypertension* 9:69, 1987.

261. Kopp UC, Smith LA, DiBona GF: Renorenal reflexes: Neural components of ipsilateral and contralateral renal responses. *Am J Physiol* (Renal Fluid Electrolyte Physiol 18)249:F507, 1985.

262. Kostreva DR, Seagard JL, Castaner A, et al: Reflex effects of renal afferents on the heart and kidney. *Am J Physiol* (Regulatory Integrative Comp Physiol 10)241:R286, 1981.

263. Kotake C, Hoffman PC, Goldberg LI, et al: Comparison of the effects of dopamine and beta-adrenergic agonists on adenylate cyclase of renal glomeruli and striatum. *Mol Pharmacol* 20:429, 1981.

264. Kreisberg JI, Venkatachalam MA, Patel PY: Cyclic AMP associated shape change in mesangial cells and its reversal by prostaglandin E$_2$. *Kidney Int* 25:874, 1984.

265. Krishna GG, Danovitch GM, Beck FWJ, et al: Dopaminergic mediation of the natriuretic response to volume expansion. *J Lab Clin Med* 105:214, 1985.

266. Krothapalli RK, Suki WN: Functional characterization of the alpha adrenergic receptor modulating the hydroosmotic effect of vasopressin on the rabbit cortical collecting tubule. *J Clin Invest* 73:740, 1984.

267. Kuo DC, Nadelhaft I, Hisamitsu T, et al: Segmental distribution and central projections of renal afferent fibers in the cat studied by transganglionic transport of horseradish peroxidase. *J Comp Neurol* 216:162, 1983.

268. Kuo DC, Oravitz JJ, Eskay R, et al: Substance P in renal afferent perikarya identified by retrograde transport of fluorescent dye. *Brain Res* 323:168, 1984.

269. Kusano E, Nakamura R, Asano Y, et al: Distribution of alpha-adrenergic receptors in the rabbit nephron. *Tohoku J Exp Med* 142:275, 1984.

270. Lagercrantz H, Bistoletti P: Catecholamine release in the newborn infant at birth. *Pediatr Res* 11:889, 1977.

271. Lands AM, Arnold A, McAuliff JP, et al: Differentiation of receptor systems activated by sympathomimetic amines. *Nature* 214:597, 1967.

272. Langer SZ, Cavero I, Massingham R: Recent developments in noradrenergic neurotransmission and its relevance to the mechanism of action of certain antihypertensive agents. *Hypertension* 2:372, 1980.

273. Langer SZ: Presynaptic regulation of catecholamine release. *Biochem Pharmacol* 23:1793, 1974.

274. Lansberg L, Young JB: Sympathetic nervous system in hypertension. *In* Brenner BM, Stein JH (eds): *Contemporary Issues in Nephrology, Hypertension.* London, Churchill-Livingstone, 1981, p 100.

275. Laradi A, Sakhrani LM, Massry SG: Effect of dopamine on sodium uptake by renal proximal tubule cells of rabbit. *Miner Electrolyte Metab* 12:303, 1986.

276. Lee MR: Dopamine and the kidney. *Clin Sci* 62:439, 1982.

277. Lees P, Lockett MF: Some actions of isoprenaline and orciprenaline on perfused cat kidneys. *Br J Pharmacol* 25:152, 1965.

278. Leftowitz RJ, Caron MG, Stiles GL: Mechanisms of membrane-receptor regulation. Biochemical, physiological, and clinical insights derived from studies of the adrenergic receptors. *N Engl J Med* 310:1570, 1984.

279. Levi J, Coburn J, Kleeman CR: Mechanism of the antidiuretic effect of β-adrenergic stimulation in man. *Arch Intern Med* 136:25, 1976.

280. Levi J, Grinblat J, Kleeman CR: Effect of isoproterenol on water diuresis in rats with congenital diabetes insipidus. *Am J Physiol* 221:1728, 1971.

281. Lew R, Summers RJ: Autoradiographic localization of B-adrenoceptor subtypes in the guinea-pig kidney. *Br J Pharmacol* 85:341, 1985.

282. Lew R, Summers RJ: The distribution of beta-adrenoceptors in dog kidney: An autoradiographic analysis. *Eur J Pharmacol* 140:1, 1987.

283. Lifschitz MD: Lack of a role for the renal nerves in renal sodium reabsorption in conscious dogs. *Clin Sci Mol Med* 54:567, 1978.

284. Lin S-Y, Chaves C, Widemann E, et al: A γ-melanocyte stimulating hormone-like peptide causes reflex natriuresis after acute unilateral nephrectomy. *Hypertension* 10:619, 1987.

284a. Liu FY, Cogan MG: Angiotensin II stimulates early proximal bicarbonate absorption in the rat by decreasing cyclic adenosine monophosphate. *J Clin Invest* 84:93, 1989.

285. Lokhandwala MF, Barrett RJ: Cardiovascular dopamine receptors: Physiological, pharmacological and therapeutic implications. *J Auton Pharmacol* 3:189, 1982.

286. Lokhandwala MF, Steenberg ML: Evaluation of effects of SKF 82526 and LY 171555 on presynaptic (DA2) and postsynaptic (DA1) dopamine receptors in rat kidney. *J Auton Pharmacol* 4:273, 1984.

287. Lokhandwala MF, Steenberg ML: Selective activation by LY 141865 and apomorphine of presynaptic dopamine receptors in the rat kidney and influence of stimulation parameters in the action of dopmaine. *J Pharmacol Exp Ther* 288:161, 1984.

288. Luft FC, Rankin LI, Henry BP, et al: Plasma and urinary norepinephrine values of extremes of sodium intake in normal man. *Hypertension* 1:261, 1979.

289. Lundin S, Rickste SE, Thoren P: Renal sympathetic activity in spontaneously hypertensive rats and normotensive controls, as studied by three different methods. *Acta Physiol Scand* 120: 265, 1984.

290. Maddox DA, Price DC, Rector FC Jr: Effects of surgery on plasma volume and salt and water excretion in rats. *Am J Physiol* (Renal Fluid and Electrolyte Physiol 2)233:F600, 1977.

291. Manoogian C, Nadler J, Ehrlich L, et al: The renal vasodilating effect of dopamine is mediated by calcium flux and prostacycline release in man. *J Clin Endocrinol Metab* 67:678, 1988.

292. Mark AL, Eckstein JW, Abboud FM, et al: Renal vascular responses to isoproterenol. *Am J Physiol* 217:764, 1969.

292a. Matherne GP, Nakamura KT, Alden BM, et al: Regional variation of postjunctional alpha-adrenoceptor responses in the developing renal vascular bed of the sheep. *Pediatr Res* 25:461, 1989.

293. Matherne GP, Nakamura KT, Robillard JE: Ontogeny of α-adrenoceptor responses in renal vascular bed of sheep. *Am J Physiol* (Regulatory Integrative Comp Physiol 23)254:R277, 1988.

294. Matsumura Y, Miyawaki N, Sasaki Y, et al: Inhibitory effects of norepinephrine, methoxamine and phenylephrine on renin release from rat kidney cortical slices. *J Pharmacol Exp Ther* 233:782, 1985.

295. McCaughran JA Jr, Juno CJ, O'Malley E, et al: The ontogeny of renal alpha1- and alpha2-adrenoceptors in the Dahl rat model of experimental hypertension. *J Auton Nerv Syst* 17:1, 1986.

296. McGrath B, Bode K, Luxford A, et al: Effects of dopamine on renal function in the rat isolated perfused kidney. *Clin Exp Pharmacol Physiol* 12:343, 1985.

297. McGrath BP, Lim AE, Bode K, et al: Differentiation of noradrenergic and dopaminergic nerves in the rat kidney: Evidence against significant dopaminergic innervation. *Clin Exp Pharmacol Physiol* 10:543, 1983.

298. McKenna OC, Angelakos ET: Acetylcholinesterase containing nerve fibers in the canine kidney. *Circ Res* 23:645, 1968.

299. McKenna OC, Angelakos ET: Development of adrenergic innervation in the puppy kidney. *Anat Rec* 167:115, 1970.

300. McPherson GA, Summers RJ: ^{3}H-prazosin and ^{3}H-clonidine binding to alpha adrenoceptors in membranes prepared from regions of rat kidney. *J Pharm Pharmacol* 33:189, 1981.

301. McPherson GA, Summers RJ: A study of alpha 1-adrenoceptors in rat renal cortex: Comparison of ^{3}H-prazosin binding with the alpha 1-adrenoceptor modulating gluconeogenesis under physiological conditions. *Br J Pharmacol* 77:177, 1982.

302. McPherson GA, Summers RJ: Evidence from binding studies for alpha 2-adrenoceptors directly associated with glomeruli from rat kidney. *Eur J Pharmacol* 90:333, 1983.

303. McPherson GA, Summers RJ: Evidence from binding studies for β_1-adrenoceptors associated with glomeruli isolated from rat kidney. *Life Sci* 33:87, 1983.

304. Mellas J, Hammerman MR: Phorbol ester-induced alkalinization of canine renal proximal tubular cells. *Am J Physiol* (Renal Fluid Electrolyte Physiol 19)250:F451, 1986.

305. Missale C, Pizzi M, Memo M, et al: Postsynaptic D$_1$ and D$_2$ dopamine receptors are present in rabbit renal and mesenteric arteries. *Neurosci Lett* 61:207, 1985.

306. Mitchell GAG: The nerve supply of the kidneys. *Acta Anat* (Basel) 10:1, 1950.

307. Mitchell GAG: Intrinsic renal nerves. *Acta Anat* (Basel) 13:1, 1951.

308. Mizelle HL, Hall JE, Woods LL, et al: Role of renal nerves in compensatory adaptation to chronic reductions in sodium intake. *Am J Physiol* (Renal Fluid Electrolyte Physiol 21)252:F291, 1987.

309. Mongeau JG, de Champlain J, Davignon A: A study of sympathetic activity in adolescents suffering from essential hypertension. Preliminary data on plasma catecholamines. In Giovanelli G, New MI, Gorin SC (eds): *Hypertension in Children and Adolescents.* New York, Raven Press, 1981, p 151.

310. Morel F, Doucet A: Hormonal control of kidney functions at the cell level. *Physiol Rev* 66:377, 1986.

311. Morel F, Imbert-Teboul M, Chabardes D: Distribution of hormone dependent adenylate cyclase in the nephron and its physiological significance. *Annu Rev Physiol* 43:569, 1981.

312. Morgunov N, Baines AD: Renal nerves and catecholamine excretion. *Am J Physiol* (Renal Fluid Electrolyte Physiol 9)240:F75, 1981.

313. Morgunov N, Baines AD: Vagal afferent activity and renal nerve release of dopamine. *Can J Physiol Pharmacol* 63:636, 1985.

314. Morimoto S, Abe Y, Yamamoto K: Diuretic action of isoproterenol in the dog. *Jpn Circ J* 35: 601, 1971.

315. Morita H, Vatner SF: Effects of volume expansion on renal nerve activity, renal blood flow, and sodium and water excretion in conscious dogs. *Am J Physiol* (Renal Fluid Electrolyte Physiol 18)249:F680, 1985.

316. Moss NG: Renal function and renal afferent and efferent nerve activity. *Am J Physiol* (Renal Fluid Electrolyte Physiol 12)243:F425, 1982.

317. Moss NG, Harrington WW: Reinnervation of the kidney following nerve crush (abstr). *Fed Proc* 40:553, 1981.

318. Muntz KH, Garcia C, Hagler HK: α_1-receptor localization in rat heart and kidney using autoradiography. *Am J Physiol* (Heart Circ Physiol 18)249:H512, 1985.

319. Muntz KH, Meyer L, Gadol S, et al: Alpha-2 adrenergic receptor localization in the rat heart and kidney using autoradiography and tritiated rauwolscine. *J Pharmacol Exp Ther* 236:542, 1986.

320. Munzel PA, Healy DP, Insel PA: Autoradiographic localization of β-adrenergic receptors in rat kidney slices using [^{125}I]-iodocyanopindolol. *Am J Physiol* (Renal FLuid Electrolyte Physiol 15)246:F240, 1984.

321. Murayama N, Ruggles BT, Gapstur SM, et al: Evidence for beta adrenoceptors in proximal tubules. Isoproterenol-sensitive adenylate cyclase in pars recta of canine nephron. *J Clin Invest* 76:474, 1985.

322. Murthy VV, Gilbert JC, Goldberg LI, et al: Dopamine sensitive adenylate cyclase in canine renal artery. *J Pharm Pharmacol* 28:567, 1976.

323. Muto S, Tabei K, Asano Y, et al: Dopaminergic inhibition of the action of vasopressin on the cortical collecting tubule. *Eur J Pharmacol* 114:393, 1985.

324. Myers BD, Deen WM, Brenner BM: Effects of norepinephrine and angiotensin II on determinants of glomerular ultrafiltration and proximal tubule fluid reabsorption in the rat. *Circ Res* 37:101, 1975.

325. Nakai T, Yamada R: Urinary catecholamine excretion by various age groups with special reference to clinical value of measuring catecholamines in newborns. *Pediatr Res* 17:456, 1983.

326. Nakamura KT, Alden BM, Matherne GP, et al: Ontogeny of renal hemodynamic response to terbutaline and forskolin in sheep. *J Pharmacol Exp Ther* 247:453, 1988.

327. Nakamura KT, Felder RA, Jose PA, et al: Effects of dopamine in the renal vascular bed of fetal, newborn and adult sheep. *Am J Physiol* (Regulatory Integrative Comp Physiol 21)252:R490, 1987.

328. Nakamura KT, Matherne GP, Jose PA, et al: Effects of epinephrine on the renal vascular bed of fetal, newborn, and adult sheep. *Pediatr Res* 23:181, 1988.

329. Nakamura KT, Matherne GP, Jose PA, et al: Ontogeny of renal β-adrenoceptor mediated vasodilation in sheep: Comparison between endogenous catecholamines. *Pediatr Res* 22:465, 1987.

330. Nakamura R, Imai M: Nephron distritution of [^{3}H]-dihydroalprenolol binding and its physiological significance. *Jpn J Nephrol* 5:70, 1982.

331. Neylon CB, Summers RJ: [^{3}H]-rauwolscine binding to α_2-adrenoceptors in the mammalian kidney: Apparent receptor heterogeneity between species. *Br J Pharmacol* 85:349, 1985.

332. Neylon CB, Summers RJ: Stimulation of alpha$_1$-adrenoceptors in rat kidneys mediates increased inositol phospholipid hydrolysis. *Br J Pharmacol* 91:367, 1987.

333. Niijima A: Afferent discharges from arterial mechanoreceptors in the kidney of the rabbit. *J Physiol* (Lond) 219:477, 1971.

334. Niijima A: The effect of efferent discharges in renal nerves on the activity of arterial mechanoreceptors in the kidney in rabbit. *J Physiol* (Lond) 222:335, 1972.

335. Niijima A: Observation on the localization of mechanoreceptors in the kidney and afferent nerve fibres in the renal nerves in the rabbit. *J Physiol* (Lond) 245:81, 1975.

336. Nomura G, Takabatake T, Arai S, et al: Effect of acute unilateral renal denervation on tubular reabsorption in the dog. *Am J Physiol* (Renal Fluid Electrolyte Physiol 1)232:F16, 1977.

337. Nord EP, Howard MJ, Hafezi A, et al: Alpha2 adrenergic

agonists stimulate Na$^+$-H$^+$ antiport activity in the rabbit renal proximal tubule. *J Clin Invest* 80:1755, 1987.

338. Norvell JE: The aorticorenal ganglion and its role in renal innervation of the kidney. *J Auton Nerv Syst* 8:291, 1983.

339. Numao Y, Saito M, Terui N, et al: Physiological and pharmacological properties of the three subsystems constituting the aortic nerve-renal sympathetic reflex in the rabbit. *J Auton Nerv Syst* 9:361, 1983.

340. Nunnari JM, Repaske MG, Brandon S, et al: Regulation of porcine brain α_2-adrenergic receptors by Na$^+$, H$^+$ and inhibitors of Na$^+$/H$^+$ exchange. *J Biol Chem* 262:12387, 1987.

341. Oates NS, Ball SG, Perkins CM, et al: Plasma and urine dopamine in man given sodium chloride in the diet. *Clin Sci* 56:261, 1979.

342. Oliver JA, Pinto J, Sciacca RR, et al: Basal norepinephrine overflow into the renal vein: Effect of renal nerve stimulation. *Am J Physiol* (Renal Fluid Electrolyte Physiol 8)239:F371, 1980.

343. Oliver JA, Pinto J, Sciacca RR, et al: Increased renal secretion of norepinephrine and prostaglandin E$_2$ during sodium depletion in the dog. *J Clin Invest* 66:748, 1980.

344. Oliver JA, Sciacca RR, Pinto J, et al: Role of the prostaglandin in norepinephrine release during augmented renal sympathetic nerve activity in the dog. *Circ Res* 48:835, 1981.

345. Osborn JL, Holdaas H, Thames MD, et al: Renal adrenoceptor mediation of antinatriuretic and renin secretion response to low frequency renal nerve stimulation in the dog. *Circ Res* 53:298, 1983.

346. Padbury JF, Diakomanolis ES, Hobel CJ, et al: Neonatal adaptation: Sympatho-adrenal response to umbilical cord cutting. *Pediatr Res* 15:1483, 1981.

347. Pearson JE, Williams RL: Analysis of direct renal actions of alpha and beta adrenergic stimulation upon sodium excretion compared to acetylcholine. *Br J Pharmacol* 33:223, 1968.

348. Pelayo JC: Modulation of renal adrenergic effector mechanisms by calcium entry blockers. *Am J Physiol* (Renal Fluid Electrolyte Physiol 21)252:F613, 1987.

349. Pelayo JC: Renal adrenergic effector mechanisms: Glomerular sites for prostaglandin interaction. *Am J Physiol* (Renal Fluid Electrolyte Physiol 23)254:F184, 1988.

350. Pelayo JC, Blantz RC: Analysis of renal denervation in the hydropenic rat: Interactions with angiotensin II. *Am J Physiol* (Renal Fluid Electrolyte Physiol 15)246:F87, 1984.

351. Pelayo JC, Fildes RD, Eisner GM, et al: Effects of dopamine blockade on renal sodium excretion. *Am J Physiol* (Renal Fluid Electrolyte Physiol 14)245:F247, 1983.

352. Pelayo JC, Fildes RD, Jose PA: Age-dependent renal effects of intrarenal dopamine infusion. *Am J Physiol* (Regulatory Integrative Comp Physiol 16)247:R212, 1984.

353. Pelayo JC, Ziegler MG, Blantz RC: Angiotensin II in adrenergic-induced alterations in glomerular hemodynamics. *Am J Physiol* (Renal Fluid Electrolyte Physiol 16)247:F799, 1984.

354. Pelayo JC, Ziegler MG, Jose PA, et al: Renal denervation in the rat: Analysis of glomerular and proximal tubular function. *Am J Physiol* (Renal Fluid Electrolyte Physiol 13)244:F70, 1983.

355. Pelletier CL, Shepherd JT: Relative influence of carotid baroreceptors and muscle receptors in the control of renal and hind-limb circulations. *Can J Physiol Pharmacol* 53:1042, 1975.

356. Pettersson A, Hedner J, Hedner T: The diuretic effect of atrial natriuretic peptide (ANP) is dependent on dopaminergic activation. *Acta Physiol Scand* 126:619, 1986.

357. Pettinger WA, Smyth DD, Umemura S: Renal α_2-adrenoceptors, their locations and effects on sodium excretion. *J Cardiovasc Pharmacol* (suppl 8)7:S24, 1985.

358. Pettinger WA, Umemura S, Smyth DD, et al: Renal a$_2$-adrenoceptors and the adenylate cyclase-cAMP system: Biochemical and physiological interactions. *Am J Physiol* (Renal Fluid Electrolyte Physiol 21)252:F199, 1987.

359. Polhemus RE, Hall DA: Effect of catecholamines on potential difference and chloride efflux in the mouse thick ascending limb of Henle's loop (abstr). *Kidney Int* 19:253, 1981.

360. Pollock DM, Arendshorst WJ: Maintenance of tubuloglomerular feedback activity during DA1-induced renal vasodilation in the rat (abstr). *Federation Proc* 46:636, 1987.

361. Rasmussen H, Kojima I, Apfeldorf W, et al: Cellular mechanism of hormone action in the kidney: Messenger function of calcium and cyclic AMP. *Kidney Int* 29:90, 1986.

362. Raymond JR, Regan JW, Beach RE, et al: Enrichment of alpha-2 adrenergic receptors of rabbit proximal tubule basolateral membranes (BLM) (abstr). *Kidney Int* 31:178, 1987.

363. Recordati G, Genovesi S, Cerati D: Renorenal reflexes in the rat elicited upon stimulation of renal chemoreceptors. *J Auton Nerv Syst* 6:127, 1982.

364. Recordati GM, Moss NG, Genovesi S, et al: Renal receptors in the rat sensitive to chemical alterations of their environment. *Circ Res* 46:395, 1980.

365. Recordati G, Moss NG, Genovesi S, et al: Chemoreceptors. *J Auton Nerv Syst* 3:237, 1981.

366. Regoli D, Gauthier R: Site of action of angiotensin and other vasoconstrictors on the kidney. *Can J Physiol Pharmacol* 49:608, 1971.

367. Reid IA, Schrier RW, Earley LE: An effect of extrarenal beta adrenergic stimulation on the release of renin. *J Clin Invest* 51:1861, 1972.

368. Reison DS, Oliver J, Sciacca RR, et al: Release of norepinephrine from sympathetic nerve efferents by bilateral carotid occlusion. *Am J Physiol* (Heart Circ Physiol 14)245:H635, 1983.

369. Renner O: Die Innervation der Niere. *In Muller's Die Lebensnerven.* Berlin, Springer, 1924.

370. Ribstein J, Humphreys MH: Renal nerves and cation excretion after acute reduction in functioning renal mass in the rat. *Am J Physiol* (Renal Fluid Electrolyte Physiol 15)246:F260, 1984.

371. Ricksten SE, Noresson E, Thoren P: Inhibition of renal sympathetic nerve traffic from cardiac receptors in normotensive and spontaneously hypertensive rats. *Acta Physiol Scand* 106:17, 1979.

372. Robie NW: Evaluation of presynaptic alpha-adrenoceptor function in the canine renal vascular bed. *Am J Physiol* (Heart Circ Physiol 8)239:H422, 1980.

372a. Robillard JE, McWeeny OJ, Smith B, et al: Ontogeny of neurogenic regulation of renal tubular reabsorption in sheep (abstr). *Pediatr Res* 23:545A, 1988.

373. Robillard JE, Nakamura KT, DiBona GF: Effects of renal denervation on renal responses to hypoxemia in fetal lambs. *Am J Physiol* (Renal Fluid Electrolyte Physiol 19)250:F294, 1986.

374. Robillard JE, Nakamura KT: Neurohormonal regulation of renal function during development. *Am J Physiol* (Renal Fluid Electrolyte Physiol 23)254:F771, 1988.

375. Robillard JE, Nakamura KT, Wilkin MK, et al: Ontogeny of renal hemodynamic response to renal nerve stimulation in sheep. *Am J Physiol* (Renal Fluid Electrolyte Physiol 21)252:F605, 1987.

375a. Robillard JE, Smith FG, McWeeney OJ, et al: Ontogeny

of the renal response to alpha$_1$-adrenoceptor stimulation in sheep (abstr). *Pediatr Res* 25:347A, 1989.

376. Robison GA, Butcher RW, Sutherland EW: *Cyclic AMP.* New York, Academic, 1971.

377. Rogenes PR: Single-unit and multiunit analysis of reno-renal reflexes elicited by stimulation of renal chemoreceptors in the rat. *J Auton Nerv Syst* 6:143, 1982.

378. Rogenes PR, Gottschalk CW: Renal function in conscious rats with chronic unilateral renal denervation. *Am J Physiol* (Renal Fluid Electrolyte Physiol 11)242:F140, 1982.

379. Rump LC, Majewski H: Modulation of norepinephrine release thorough α$_1$- and α$_2$-adrenoceptors in the rat isolated kidney. *J Cardiovasc Pharmacol* 9:500, 1987.

380. Sadowski J, Kurkus J, Gellert R: Denervated and intact kidney responses to saline load in awake and anesthetized dogs. *Am J Physiol* (Renal Fluid Electrolyte Physiol 6)237:F262, 1979.

381. Sadowski J, Kurkus J, Gellert R: Reinvestigation of denervation diuresis and natriuresis in conscious dogs. *Arch Int Physiol Biochim* 87:663, 1979.

382. Sanchez A, Vidal MJ, Martinez-Sierra R, et al: Ontogeny of renal alpha-1 and alpha-2 adrenoceptors in the spontaneously hypertensive rat. *J Pharmacol Exp Ther* 237:972, 1986.

383. Schad H, Seller H: Reduction of renal nerve activity by volume expansion in conscious cats. *Pflugers Arch* 363:155, 1976.

384. Schmidt M, Imbs JL, Giesen EM, et al: Blockade of dopamine receptors in the renal vasculature by isomers of flupenthixol and sulpiride. *J Cardiovasc Pharmacol* 5:86, 1983.

385. Schmidt M, Krieger JP, Giesen-Crouse EM, et al: Vascular effects of selective dopamine receptor agonists and antagonists in the rat kidney. *Arch Int Pharmacodyn Ther* 286:195, 1987.

386. Schmitz JM, Graham RM, Sagalowsky A, et al: Renal alpha-1 and alpha-2 adrenergic receptors: Biochemical and pharmacological correlations. *J Pharmacol Exp Ther* 219:400, 1981.

387. Schneider E, McLane Vega L, Hanson R, et al: Effect of chronic bilateral renal denervation on daily sodium excretion in the conscious dog (abstr). *Fed Proc* 37:645, 1978.

388. Schor N, Ichikawa I, Brenner BM: Mechanisms of action of various hormones and vasoactive substances on glomerular ultrafiltration in the rat. *Kidney Int* 20:442, 1981.

389. Schwartz DD, Eikenberg DC: Enhanced endogenous neurotransmitter overflow in the isolated perfused rat kidney after chronic epinephrine administration: Lack of a prejunctional beta adrenoceptor influence. *J Pharmacol Exp Ther* 244:11, 1988.

390. Seri I, Aperia A: Contribution of dopamine$_2$ receptors to dopamine-induced increase in glomerular filtration rate. *Am J Physiol* (Renal Fluid Electrolyte Physiol 23)254:F196, 1988.

391. Shibouta Y, Inada Y, Terashita ZI, et al: Antidiuresis induced by β$_1$- and β$_2$-adrenergic agonists in ethanol anesthetized rats. *Eur J Pharmacol* 47: 149, 1978.

392. Shultz PJ, Sedor JR, Abboud HE: Dopaminergic stimulation of cAMP accumulation in cultured rat mesangial cells. *Am J Physiol* (Heart Circ Physiol 22)253:H358, 1987.

393. Silva P, Koenig B, Lear S, et al: Dibutyryl cyclic AMP inhibits transport dependent QO$_2$ in cells dissected from the rabbit medullary ascending limb. *Pflugers Arch* 409:74, 1987.

394. Silva P, Landsberg L, Besarb A: Excretion and metabolism of catecholamines by the isolated perfused rat kidney. *J Clin Invest* 64:850, 1979.

395. Simmonds SH, Strange PG: Inhibition of inositol phospholipid breakdown by D$_2$ dopamine receptors in dissociated bovine anterior pituitary cells. *Neurosci Lett* 60:267, 1985.

396. Simon OR, Schramm LP: The spinal course and medullary termination of myelinated renal afferents in the rat. *Brain Res* 290:239, 1984.

397. Slick L, Aguilera AJ, Zambraski EJ, et al: Renal neuroadrenergic transmission. *Am J Physiol* 299:60, 1975.

398. Slivka SR, Insel PA: α$_1$-Adrenergic receptor-mediated phosphoinositide hydrolysis and prostaglandin E$_2$ formation in Madin-Darby canine kidney cells. Possible parallel activation of phospholipase C and phospholipase A$_2$. *J Biol Chem* 262:4200, 1987.

399. Slotkin TA, Levant B, Orband-Miller L, et al: Do sympathetic neurons coordinate cellular development in the heart and kidney? Effects of neonatal central and peripheral catecholaminergic lesions on cardiac and renal nucleic acids and proteins. *J Pharmacol Exp Ther* 244:166, 1988.

400. Smith HW: *The Physiology of the Kidney.* London, Oxford University Press, 1937.

400a. Smit AJ, Meijer S, Wesseling H, et al: Effect of metoclopramide on dopamine-induced changes in renal function in healthy controls and in patients with renal disease. *Clin Sci* 75:421, 1988.

401. Smits JFM, Brody MJ: Activation of afferent renal nerves by intrarenal bradykinin in conscious rats. *Am J Physiol* (Regulatory Integrative Comp Physiol 16)247:R1003, 1984.

402. Smyth DD, Umemura S, Pettinger WA: Alpha-2 adrenoceptors and sodium reabsorption in the isolated perfused rat kidney. *Am J Physiol* (Renal Fluid Electrolyte Physiol 16)247:F680, 1984.

403. Smyth DD, Umemura S, Pettinger WA: Renal nerve stimulation causes α$_1$-adrenoceptor-mediated sodium retention but not α$_2$-adrenoceptor antagonism of vasopressin. *Circ Res* 57:304, 1985.

404. Smyth DD, Umemura S, Pettinger WA: Renal α$_2$-adrenergic receptors multiply and mediate sodium retention after prazosin treatment. *Hypertension* 8:323, 1986.

405. Smyth DD, Umemura S, Yang E, et al: Inhibition of renin release by alpha adrenoceptor stimulation in the isolated perfused rat kidney. *Eur J Pharmacol* 140:33, 1987.

406. Snavely MD, Insel PA: Characterization of alpha-adrenergic receptor subtypes in the rat renal cortex. Differential regulation of alpha 1- and alpha 2-adrenergic receptors by guanyl nucleotides and Na. *Mol Pharmacol* 22:532, 1982.

407. Snavely MD, Motulsky HJ, Moustafa E, et al: β-adrenergic receptor subtypes in the rat renal cortex. Selective regulation of β$_1$-adrenergic receptors by pheochromocytoma. *Circ Res* 51:504, 1982.

408. Sowers JR, Crane PD, Beck FW, et al: Relationship between urinary dopamine production and natriuresis after acute intravascular volume expansion with sodium chloride in dogs. *Endocrinology* 115:2085, 1984.

409. Spitzer A: The role of the kidney in sodium homeostasis during maturation. *Kidney Int* 21: 539, 1982.

410. Sraer J, Ardaillou R, Loreau N, et al: Evidence for parathyroid hormone sensitive adenylate cyclase in rat glomeruli. *Mol Cell Endocrinol* 1:285, 1974.

411. Sreeharan N, Kappagoda CT, Linden RJ: The role of renal nerves in the diuresis and natriuresis caused by stimulation of atrial receptors. *Q J Exp Physiol* 66:163, 1981.

412. Sripairojthikoon W, Wyss JM: Cells of origin of the sympathetic renal innervation in rat. *Am J Physiol* (Renal Fluid Electrolyte Physiol 21)252:F957, 1987.

413. Sripanidkulchai B, Wyss JM: The development of α$_2$-ad-

renoceptors in the rat kidney: Correlation with noradrenergic innervation. *Brain Res* 400:91, 1987.

414. Sripanidkulchai B, Dawson R, Oparil S, et al: Two renal
α₂-adrenergic receptor sites revealed by p-aminoclonidine
binding. *Am J Physiol* (Renal Fluid Electrolyte Physiol
21)252:F283, 1987.

415. Stanton B, Puglisi E, Gellai M: Localization of α₂-adre-
noceptor-mediated increase in renal Na⁺, K⁺, and water
excretion. *Am J Physiol* (Renal Fluid Electrolyte Physiol
21)252:F1016, 1987.

416. Steenberg ML, Ekas RD Jr, Lokhandwala MF: Effect of
epinephrine on norepinephrine release rate from rat kidney
during sympathetic nerve stimulation. *Eur J Pharmacol*
93:137, 1983.

417. Stein JH, Ferris TF, Huprich JE, et al: Effect of renal
vasodilatation on the distribution of cortical blood flow in
the kidney of the dog. *J Clin Invest* 50:1429, 1971.

418. Stein JH, Osgood RW, Ferris TF: The effect of beta adrenergic stimulation on proximal tubular sodium reabsorption. *Proc Soc Exp Biol Med* 141:901, 1972.

419. Steinhausen M, Weis S, Fleming J, et al: Responses of in
vivo renal microvessels to dopamine. *Kidney Int* 30:361,
1986.

420. Stephenson JA, Summers RJ: Light microscopic autoradiography of the distribution of [³H] rauwolscine binding
to α₂-adrenoceptors in rat kidney. *Eur J Pharmacol* 116:271,
1985.

421. Stephenson JA, Summers RJ: Autoradiographic evidence
for a heterogeneous distribution of ³H-prazosin in rat, dog,
and human kidney. *J Auton Pharmacol* 6:109, 1986.

422. Stephenson RK, Sole MJ, Baines AD: Neural and extra-
neural catecholamine production by rat kidneys. *Am J
Physiol* (Renal Fluid Electrolyte Physiol 11)242:F261, 1982.

423. Strandhoy JW: Role of alpha-2 receptors in regulation of
renal function. *J Cardiovasc Pharmacol* (suppl 8)7:S28,
1985.

424. Strandhoy JW, Schneider EG, Willis LR, et al: Intrarenal
effects of phenoxybenzamine on sodium reabsorption. *J Lab
Clin Med* 83:263, 1974.

425. Su C, Bevan JA, Assali NS, et al: Regional variation of
lamb blood vessel responsiveness to vasoactive agents during fetal development. *Circ Res* 41:844, 1977.

426. Sulyok E: Dopaminergic control of neonatal salt and water
metabolism. *Pediatr Nephrol* 2:163, 1988.

427. Summers RJ, Kuhar MJ: Autoradiographic localization of
β-adrenoceptors in rat kidney. *Eur J Pharmacol* 91:305,
1983.

428. Summers RJ: Renal α-adrenoceptors. *Fed Proc* 43:2917,
1984.

429. Summers RJ, Stephenson JA, Kuhar MJ: Localization of
beta adrenoceptor subtypes in rat kidney by light microscopic autoradiography. *J Pharmacol Exp Ther* 232:561,
1985.

430. Summers RJ, Stephenson JA, Lipe S, et al: α₂-adrenoceptors in dog kidney: Autoradiographic localization and putative functions. *Clin Sci* (suppl 10)68:105S, 1985.

431. Sundaresan PR, Fortin TL, Kelvine SL: α- and β-adrenergic receptors in proximal tubules of rat kidney. *Am J
Physiol* (Renal Fluid Electrolyte Physiol 22)253:F848, 1987.

432. Szenasi G, Bencsath P, Takacs L: Proximal tubular transport and urinary excretion of sodium after renal denervation in sodium depleted rats. *Pflugers Arch* 403:146, 1985.

433. Szenasi G, Bencsath P, Szalay L, et al: Fasting induces
denervation natriuresis in the conscious rat. *Am J Physiol*
(Renal Fluid Electrolyte Physiol 18)249:F753, 1985.

434. Tago K, Schuster VL, Stokes JB: Regulation of chloride
self exchange by cAMP in cortical collecting tubule. *Am
J Physiol* (Renal Fluid Electrolyte Physiol 20)251:F40, 1986.

435. Taira N, Yabuuchi Y, Yamashita S: Profile of β-adrenoceptors in femoral, superior mesenteric and renal vascular
beds of dogs. *Br J Pharmacol* 59:577, 1977.

436. Takeuchi J, Iino S, Hanada S, et al: Experimental studies
on the nervous control of the renal circulation. *Jpn Heart
J* 6:543, 1965.

437. Tam LT, Pettinger WA, Hjerpe KS, et al: High dietary
NaCl increases high affinity renal α₂-adrenoceptor binding
sites by 600% in Dahl salt sensitive but not in Dahl salt
resistant rats (abstr). *Fed Proc* 46:1238, 1987.

438. Tamaki T, Hura CE, Kunau RT: Dopamine increases
cAMP accumulation in canine afferent arterioles (abstr).
Clin Res 35:637A, 1987.

439. Terman BI, Slivka SR, Hughes RJ, et al: α₁-adrenergic
receptor-linked guanine nucleotide-binding protein in muscle and kidney epithelial cells. *Mol Pharmacol* 31:12, 1987.

440. Textor SC, Fouad FM, Bravo EL, et al: Redistribution of
cardiac output to the kidneys during oral nadolol admin-
stration. *N Engl J Med* 307:601, 1982.

441. Thames MD, DiBona GF: Renal nerves modulate the secretion of renin mediated by nonneural mechanisms. *Circ
Res* 44:645, 1979.

442. Thames MD, Abboud FM: Interaction of somatic and cardiopulmonary receptors in control of renal circulation. *Am
J Physiol* (Heart Circ Physiol 6)237:H560, 1979.

443. Timmermans PB, Van Zweiten PA: The postsynaptic
alpha₂ receptors. *J Auton Pharmacol* 1:171, 1981.

444. Tulassay T, Seri I, Machay T, et al: Effects of dopamine
on renal functions in premature neonates with respiratory
distress syndrome. *Int J Pediatr Nephrol* 4:19, 1983.

445. Uchida Y, Kamisaka K, Ueda H: Two types of renal mechanoreceptors. *Jpn Heart J* 12:233, 1971.

446. Ueda H, Uchida Y, Kamisaka K: Mechanism of reflex
depressor effect by the kidney in dog. *Jpn Heart J* 8:597,
1967.

447. Umemura S, Marver D, Smyth DD, et al: α₂-Adrenoceptors and cellular cAMP levels in single nephron segments
from the rat. *Am J Physiol* (Renal Fluid Electrolyte Physiol
18)249:F28, 1985.

448. Umemura S, Smyth DD, Pettinger WA: α₂-Aadrenoceptor
stimulation and cellular cAMP levels in microdissected rat
glomeruli. *Am J Physiol* (Renal Fluid Electrolyte Physiol
19)250:F103, 1986.

449. Umemura S, Smyth DD, Pettinger WA: Regulation of
renal cellular cAMP levels by prostaglandins and α₂-adrenoceptors: Microdissection studies. *Kidney Int* 29:703,
1986.

450. Veiga JA, Saggerson ED: Gluconeogenesis in guinea pig
renal tubular fragments—effects of noradrenaline, 3':5'
cyclic AMP and angiotensin II. *Comp Biochem Physiol [C]*
74:409, 1983.

451. Wahbe F, Hagege J, Loreau N, et al: Endogenous dopamine
synthesis and dopa-decarboxylase activity in rat renal cortex. *Mol Cell Endocrinol* 27:45, 1982.

452. Wargo AA, Slotkoff LM, Jose PA, et al: Cyclic nucleotide
response to stimulation in isolated glomeruli from dog kidney. *Nephron* 32:165, 1982.

453. Weaver LC: Cardiac sympathetic afferent influences on
renal nerve activity. *J Auton Nerv Syst* 3:253, 1981.

454. Weaver LC, Danos LM, Oehl RS, et al: Contrasting reflex
influences of cardiac afferent nerves during coronary occlusion. *Am J Physiol* (Heart Circ Physiol 9)240:H620, 1981.

455. Weaver LC, Fry HK, Meckler RL: Differential renal and
splenic nerve responses to vagal and spinal afferent inputs.
Am J Physiol (Regulatory Integrative Comp Physiol
15)246:R78, 1984.

456. Weber MA, Drayer JIM: Renal effects of beta-adrenoceptor
blockade. *Kidney Int* 18:686, 1980.

457. Weinman EJ, Sansom SC, Knight TF, et al: Alpha and beta adrenergic agonists stimulate water absorption in the rat proximal tubule. *J Membr Biol* 69:107, 1982.

458. Wilcox CS, Aminoff MJ, Slater JD: Sodium homeostasis in patients with autonomic failure. *Clin Sci Mol Med* 53:321, 1977.

459. Winternitz SR, Katholi RE, Oparil S: Decrease in hypothalamic norepinephrine content following renal denervation in the one-kidney, one clip Goldblatt hypertensive rat. *Hypertension* 4:369, 1982.

460. Winternitz SR, Katholi RE, Oparil S: Role of the renal sympathetic nerves in the development and maintenance of hypertension in the spontaneously hypertensive rat. *J Clin Invest* 66:971, 1980.

461. Wolff DW, Buckalew VM Jr, Strandhoy JW: Renal α_1- and α_2-adrenoceptor mediated vasoconstriction in dogs: Comparison of phenylephrine, clonidine, and guanabenz. *J Cardiovasc Pharmacol* 6:S793, 1984.

462. Wolff DW, Gesek FA, Strandhoy JW: In vivo assessment of rat renal alpha adrenoceptors. *J Pharmacol Exp Ther* 241:472, 1987.

463. Worth DP, Harvey JN, Brown J, et al: Domperidone treatment in man inhibits the fall in plasma renin activity induced by intravenous γ-L-glutamyl-L-dopa. *Br J Clin Pharmacol* 21:497, 1986.

464. Yamaguchi I, Kopin IJ: Differential inhibition of alpha-1 and alpha-2 adrenoceptor-mediated pressor responses in pithed rats. *J Pharmacol Exp Ther* 214: 275, 1980.

464a. Yatani A, Brown AM: Rapid beta-adrenergic modulation of cardiac calcium channel currents by a fast G protein pathway. *Science* 245:71, 1989.

465. Young WS, Kuhar MJ: Alpha-2 adrenergic receptors are associated with renal proximal tubules. *Eur J Pharmacol* 67:493, 1980.

466. Zambraski EJ, DiBona GF, Kaloyanides GJ: Effect of sympathetic blocking agents on the antinatriuresis of reflex renal nerve stimulation. *J Pharmacol Exp Ther* 198:464, 1976.

467. Zimmerman BG, Gisslen J: Pattern of renal vasoconstriction and transmitter release during sympathetic stimulation in presence of angiotensin and cocaine. *J Pharmacol Exp Ther* 163:320, 1968.

468. Zimmermann HD: Elektronenmikroskopische befunde zur innervation des nephron nach untersuchungen an der fetalen nachniere des menschen. *Z Zellforsch Mikrosk Anat* 129:65, 1972.

II
Mechanisms of Renal Injury

ALLISON EDDY
ALFRED F. MICHAEL

13

Immune Mechanisms of Renal Injury

The kidney is frequently the prime target of immunological disease in man. Indeed, most forms of glomerulonephritis are now felt to be the result of an immune process. Although our knowledge of the pathogenesis of tubulo-interstitial disease is just in its naissance, similar processes appear to be important here as well. Until recently it was understood, based largely on immunofluorescence findings, that most glomerular diseases were initiated by humoral mechanisms, usually by the entrapment of immune complexes from the circulation (producing granular deposits of antibody along the glomerular capillary wall) and very occasionally by the interaction of an antibody with intrinsic components of the glomerular basement membrane (associated with linear deposition of antibody) (Fig. 13-1).

Within the last decade the problem has become more complex and has actually posed more questions than have been answered. It now appears that a third and possibly additional primary immunological reactions may initiate glomerulonephritis. Nephritogenic immune complexes may form in situ within the glomerular capillary wall by the interaction either of an autoantibody binding to an autologous (non-basement membrane) glomerular antigen or of an antibody formed in response to a foreign antigen "planted" within the glomerulus. In addition, it has been proposed, although not clearly demonstrated, that cellular immunity might initiate renal disease in a manner analagous to a delayed-type hypersensitivity reaction. Finally, the detection of significant renal deposits of complement usually occurs in the presence of other immune reactants, with the notable exception of mesangiocapillary glomerulonephritis in man. This observation has led some to speculate that the alternative pathway of complement might be activated within the kidney through an antibody-independent mechanism. Such a mechanism has yet to be demonstrated in an experimental model of renal disease.

Studies of the pathogenesis of renal injury in humans are limited for obvious reasons, not the least of which is the fact that the disease process is generally well established by the time patients first seek medical attention. Fortunately, there are several well characterized models of renal disease in animals that share many pathological features in common with human renal disease. It has largely been through the study of these models that our current understanding of the pathogenesis of immunological renal disease has evolved. In this chapter we will attempt to review this area, which has been divided into three parts. The first of these describes the classical models of immunologically initiated glomerulonephritis. The second discusses in greater detail the mediator systems that may be secondarily activated to produce glomerular injury. In the third section, our current understanding of the immunological mechanisms of tubulo-interstitial diseases is reviewed.

Structure of the Glomerular Capillary Wall and Mesangium

Some understanding of structural relationships within the glomerulus is required to appreciate fully the complexities of immunological renal disease. The intraglomerular capillary network is separated from the urinary space by the ultrafiltration unit of the glomerular capillary wall, which in turn is composed of two cell types, the epithelial and endothelial cells, and their interposed extracellular matrices, which fuse to form the unique glomerular basement membrane (GBM) [227,230,326,499] (Fig. 13-2). With heavy metal stains, electron microscopy shows the GBM, which measures between 240 nm and 340 nm in man, to be a trilaminar structure composed of a tightly packed lamina densa sandwiched between the relatively electron lucent lamina rara interna on the subendothelial side and the lamina rara externa in the subepithelial position. The GBM is believed to be made up of a network of microfibrils that are closely packed in the lamina densa and much less so in the laminae rarae [304,392]. Chemical analysis has shown the GBM to consist largely of nonpolar collagen-like glycoproteins (approximately 80% of the extracellular protein) with a lesser amount of relatively polar, noncollagenous glycoproteins. Biochemical, morphologic and immunohistochemical studies have identified a number of these components (Table 13-1). However, controversy remains regarding the precise way in which these components are interlinked. The basement membrane collagens, type

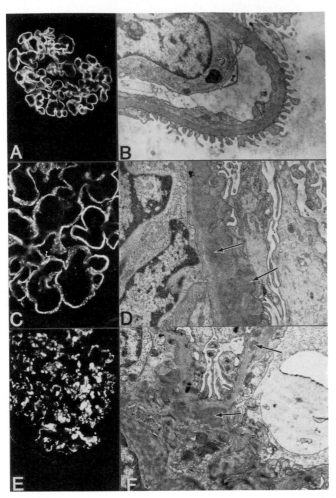

FIG. 13-1. *Immunofluorescence and electron microscopic features of three distinct patterns of immunological renal injury. In anti-glomerular basement membrane (GBM) nephritis, IgG is deposited in a linear pattern along the GBM (A); however, electron dense immune deposits are not detectable with electron microscopy (B). Membranous nephropathy, which can be reproduced experimentally in the rat model of Heymann nephritis, is characterized by the typical granular deposition of IgG and C3 (C) along the subepithelial aspect of the glomerular capillary wall, which corresponds to the subepithelial electron dense deposits (arrows) identified with electron microscopy (D). Immune complex-induced glomerulonephritis is characterized by the deposition of immunoglobulin and complement (E) within the glomerular capillary wall and mesangium. Electron microscopy reveals electron dense deposits (arrows) in similar locations (F).*

IV and probably type V, are the major structural support within the GBM [83,197,419,422,512]. The Goodpasture antigen, namely that part of the GBM reactive with autoantibodies obtained from the serum or eluted from the kidneys of patients with the Goodpasture syndrome, is a component that has still not been fully characterized. It has been shown to reside along the internal aspect of the GBM [446], and recent work by Wieslander et al. [510]

suggests that it resides on the collagenase-resistant globular domain (NC1) of type IV collagen. Laminin, a large glycoprotein composed of several identifiable subunits, which probably functions as a cell attachment protein, is present within the laminae rarae [83,131,303,421,512]. Entactin, a sulphated glycoprotein, is thought also to participate in the adhesion of cells to extracellular material [33,190].

Closely associated with these glycoproteins are glycosaminoglycans, the most abundant of which is heparan sulfate. The presence of heparan sulfate proteoglycan in the GBM was first described by Kanwar and Farquhar in 1979 [223–226]. Small amounts of other glycosaminoglycans, including chondroitin sulphate, hyaluronic acid, and dermatin sulphate, have been reported, but evidence suggests that these minor components may be mesangial contaminants present in preparations of GBM [226,269,359]. These components are extremely interesting because the anionic charge sites of the laminae rarae have been shown to be rich in heparan sulfate and, although constituting only 1% of the dry weight of the GBM, they may contribute significantly to the charge selective properties of the ultrafiltration unit (Fig. 13-3). At the present time it is unknown whether other glycoproteins present in the GBM also contribute to its negative charge. Serum amyloid P has been identified within the GBM [109]. No doubt, future studies will identify additional components within the GBM. Even now monoclonal antibodies are available that are reactive with human GBM, binding to antigenic determinants of unknown identity [328,328] (Fig. 13-4). Another recent study reported the unique binding of anionic plasma proteins, including albumin and IgG_4, to the basement membrane of human kidneys, suggesting the possibility that normal anionic plasma components may bind electrostatically to positive charge sites present within the GBM [323]. In vivo perfusion studies had previously concluded that such sites do not exist since anionic probes failed to bind to the GBM [396]. An alternative explanation could be that cationic charge sites do exist, but are normally abrogated by binding of circulating anionic plasma proteins.

The cellular components of the glomerular capillary wall are also important, not only because of the assumption that the endothelial and epithelial cells synthesize the extracellular matrix (the exact nature of the cellular synthesis remains to be determined), but also since they contribute directly to the permselectivity of the ultrafiltration unit both with respect to size and charge [227,230]. The endothelium is very thin and attenuated; its cytoplasm is traversed by multiple large fenestrae, which lack slit diaphragms or limiting membranes. Through these fenestrae the lamina rara interna is readily accessible to the bloodstream—one of the few mammalian basement membranes in direct contact with the circulation. The epithelial cells form the outer aspect of the ultrafiltration barrier, with the body of each cell extending freely into the urinary space on one side while multiple interdigitating podocytes anchor it to the GBM on the opposite side. Between these foot processes are filtration slits that are bridged by slit diaphragms, forming reticulated pores thought to play an important role in the permselectivity functions of the glo-

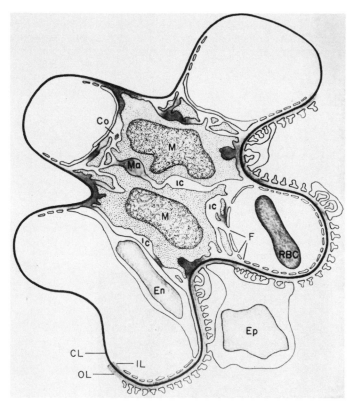

FIG. 13-2. *Diagram illustrating a glomerular mesangial region surrounded by capillaries. The central layer (CL) or lamina densa of the glomerular basement membrane envelops the capillaries like a sheet and also passes over the mesangial region. The thickness of the outer layer (OL) or lamina rara externa and inner layer (IL) or lamina rara interna of the basement membrane have been drawn thicker than they actually are to highlight their relationships to the adjacent cells. Mesangial cells (M) are partially surrounded by mesangial matrix (Ma). The capillary boundary of the mesangium is formed by the axial portions of endothelial cells (En). Fenestrations (F) of the endothelium allow passage of macromolecules and plasma into intercapillary and intercellular channels (IC). Epithelial cell bodies (Ep) extend primary processes, which branch to form the foot processes. The diameter of the capillary lumen is usually slightly larger than the diameter of a red blood cell (RBC). (Reprinted with permission from Latta H, J Ultrastruct Res 4:455, 1960 and American Physiological Society Handbook of Physiology, 1973, pp 1–29.)*

merular capillary wall. Although both cell types are surrounded by a polyanionic extracellular coat, that of the epithelium has been of greater interest due to its prominence—800 A° in greatest thickness versus 120 A° for that of the endothelium. This glycocalyx is rich in sialoproteins that are thought to form the basis of the anionic radicals. This negatively charged cell coat of the epithelial cells is often referred to as the glomerular polyanion and more recently as podocalyxin [240,499]. The glomerular epithelial (visceral) cells in man are also known to have receptors on their surface for C3b (CR1) [149] and to have intracytoplasmic intermediate filaments of vimentin [196].

As plasma perfuses through the glomerulus certain components migrate from the capillary lumen across the semipermeable glomerular capillary wall to form an ultrafiltrate of plasma within the urinary space. In addition, it is known that plasma also traffics through the mesangial regions,

presumably gaining access through the fenestrae of the endothelium [326]. The mesangium, that region occupying a centrolobular position between the capillary loops and extending from the hilum of the glomerulus to the peripheral capillary lobule, is composed of mesangial cells and their matrix. The mesangium is bounded by the endothelium, which separates it from the capillary lumen and the mesangial reflection of the basement membrane (Fig. 13-2). At the vascular pole it merges with the extraglomerular mesangial zone, which forms part of the juxtaglomerular apparatus. The mesangial cells are now thought to be derived from smooth muscle cells and as such have retained contractile functions felt to be important in the regulation of the size of the capillary surface area for filtration [29,260,419,420]. The mesangial cells can phagocytose certain macromolecules as they travel through this region, but this function appears to be restricted. Sub-

Table 13-1. *Biochemical composition of the glomerulus*

Component	M.W.	Glomerular basement membrane	Mesangial matrix
Collagen-Type IV	500,000	+	+
-Type V	300,000	+	+
Entactin	158,000	+	−
Fibronectin	450,000	+	+
Laminin	900,000	+*	+
Heparan Sulfate	130,000	+*	+
Chondroitin Sulfate	130,000	−	+
Goodpasture Antigen[x]	26,000	+	−
Amyloid P	235,000	+	−
Anionic Plasma Proteins		+	−

* Distributed along the LRI and LRE
[x] Reactive epitope on NC1 region of Type IV collagen (Wieslander et al, 1984)

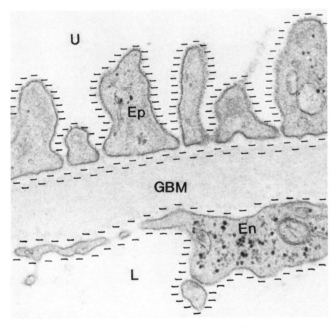

Fig. 13-3. *Electron micrograph of the glomerular filtration barrier of a normal human kidney. L: capillary lumen; En: endothelial cell; GBM: glomerular basement membrane; Ep: visceral epithelial cell foot process; U: urinary space. The fixed anionic charge sites found in the distribution depicted by dashes contribute significantly to the charge selective properties of the ultrafiltration unit. The negative charge sites on the visceral epithelial surface are related to sialic acid in the glomerular polyanion (podocalyxin) whereas those present in the lamina rara interna and externa are derived from heparan sulfate proteoglycan. (Modified from Melvin et al: In* Contemp Issues Nephrol, *12:191, 1983.)*

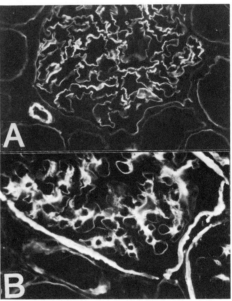

Fig. 13-4. *Biochemical composition of the normal human glomerulus demonstrated by immunofluorescence microscopy employing monoclonal antibodies. Monoclonal antibody MBM15 identifies an antigen present along the GBM, TBM, and the internal aspect of Bowman's capsule (A). Monoclonal antibody MBM4 (anti-type IV collagen) stains the internal aspect of the GBM, the mesangium, the full thickness of Bowman's capsule and TBM (B). (Reprinted from Michael AF et al:* Kidney Int *24:74, 1983, with permission.)*

stances that have been identified within mesangial cells of animals following parenteral administration include thorium dioxide, colloidal gold, colloidal carbon, iron dextran, dextran, polyvinyl alcohol polymers, horse radish peroxidase, myeloperoxidase, catalase, ferritin, and aggregated albumin [326]. Although the localization of aggregated IgG and immune complexes is largely within the matrix, recent evidence suggests limited uptake by mesangial cells [298]. Thus, it seems that one important function of the mesangial cell is its role of scavenger, keeping the glomerular filter free of macromolecules. A bone marrow-derived phagocytic cell identifiable by surface 1a antigens has been shown to make up 1% to 2% of the rat glomerular cells residing in the mesangial zone [431,432]. The presence of such a subpopulation of bone marrow-derived cells has not been demonstrated in the human glomerulus.

The structure of the extracellular matrix of the mesangium is not well defined since the relative inaccessibility of this region precludes exact analysis. It shares many structural components in common with GBM (Types IV and V collagen, laminin, fibronectin) but lacks certain constituents (e.g., Goodpasture antigen) present in the GBM [304,326,328]. Studies on the distribution of fibronectin and cold-soluble globulin have been somewhat inconclusive, but it now appears that fibronectin extends from the mesangial zone along the subendothelial zone of the GBM. Fibronectin is a multifunctional protein with specific binding regions for a number of molecules, including fibrinogen, collagen, heparan, heparan sulfate, hyaluronic acid, actin, and cell surface components. Its functions within the mesangial matrix have not been determined. Anionic charge sites are also known to be present within the mesangial matrix and are probably composed of heparan sulfate, which is the major glycosaminoglycan present in the mesangium, although smaller amounts of chondroitin sulfate may also contribute [226].

Plasma components appear to gain access to the mesangium through the endothelial fenestrae, bypassing the glomerular basement membrane. As they percolate through the mesangial zone toward the vascular pole, macromolecules are primarily detected in extracellular channels. The mechanisms controlling mesangial uptake of macromolecules are still largely unknown, although this is in part determined by certain characteristics and the blood level of the macromolecule itself, hemodynamic factors, and intrinsic characteristics of the glomerular capillary wall [326]. The disposition of such molecules trapped within the mesangium is likewise undetermined, but the possibilities at present seem limited and include backflow, returning to the capillary space, uptake by cells within the mesangium, biochemical degradation in situ, or egress at the glomerular stalk region into the interstitial space or lymphatics. There is no experimental evidence that mesangial traffic gains access to the urinary space, even though this zone is contiguous with cells of the distal tubule at the site of the juxtaglomerular apparatus.

Humoral Mechanisms

Interaction of Antibodies with Intrinsic Components of the Glomerular Basement Membrane (GBM)

Several of the known structural components of the GBM can be identified in the developing human fetus, and they persist through adult life. Even the so-called human Goodpasture antigen(s) can be demonstrated in human fetal kidneys, although at this early time period the antigen is occasionally "hidden," and kidney tissue sections require denaturation in order to expose them before they bind antibodies obtained from the serum of patients with Goodpasture syndrome [528]. Thus, in the normal situation circulating, immunologically responsive cells have acquired a state of tolerance to the autoantigens of the GBM. Indeed, the spontaneous development of anti-GBM antibodies is a rare event in man and perhaps even more unusual

in animals, where the spontaneous development of anti-GBM antibodies has been described only in three horses and certain strains of mice [19,20,519]. Anti-GBM nephritis can be experimentally induced either by the passive administration of heterologous anti-GBM antibodies to normal animals (nephrotoxic serum nephritis or Masugi nephritis) or by active immunization of animals with heterologous GBM in Freund's complete adjuvant, which induces the subsequent development of autoantibodies (experimental autoimmune glomerulonephritis). A review of each of these models provides insight into the pathogenesis of glomerular injury induced by antibodies interacting with intrinsic components of the GBM—the fundamental mechanisms of immune injury in the Goodpasture syndrome in man.

NEPHROTOXIC SERUM NEPHRITIS (ACUTE OR HETEROLOGOUS PHASE)

In 1900 Lindemann [286] reported the development of proteinuria and uremia in rabbits injected with heterologous anti-kidney antisera. The pathology of the renal lesion was extensively studied in the 1930s by Masugi [305], and in 1951 Krakower et al. [256] reported that the major site of reactivity of the antibody was to nephritogenic antigen(s) within the GBM. Since that time, the pathogenesis of the glomerular injury resulting from the interaction of heterologous nephrotoxic serum (NTS) with the GBM has been extensively studied in many animals, including rat, rabbit, sheep, dog, and guinea pig. In this section an attempt will be made to summarize the major observations on the immune mechanisms of renal injury during the heterologous phase of nephrotoxic serum nephritis. Basement membrane antigens obtained from vascular and connective tissue from a variety of organs can induce production of anti-basement membrane antibodies, although the best sources are kidney, lung, and placenta [28,171, 256,257,438].

Following the injection of nephrotoxic serum, the subsequent lesions differ in their character and severity depending upon the type and quantity of antibody used, the animal species chosen for immunization, and the stage of the disease being examined [182,232,233,309,486,519]. Antibody-binding to glomeruli occurs rapidly following intravenous administration and probably accounts for some of the immediate structural and functional changes observed. Within ten minutes of injection, 60% to 80% of this antibody fixes to rat glomerular antigens exposed to the circulation, and maximum fixation, close to 90%, occurs within one hour. This extremely short antibody half-life contrasts with the much longer half-life of heterologous antibodies reactive with antigens not readily available to the circulation [496]. The degree of antibody binding is influenced by the GBM anionic charge sites. In a study of anti-GBM nephritis in rats, the binding of cationic antibody was four times greater than that observed for comparable doses of anionic antibody [292a]. By indirect immunofluorescence, the heterologous antibody is observed in a continuous linear pattern along the GBM (see Fig. 13-1). Immediate hemodynamic changes detected by micropuncture studies during this early phase are associated with a decline in GFR [43,44]. With large doses of antibody, complete anuria has been observed. Evidence for immediate ultrastructural changes of the GBM include the observations of focal foot process widening reported as early as ten minutes after injection [441] and loss of discrete anionic binding sites, which has been demonstrated by colloidal iron staining at 30 minutes [259] and by polyethyleneimine staining at one hour following administration of NTS [380]. The cellular components of the glomerular capillary wall also show evidence of early injury. Several investigators have reported endothelial swelling and displacement, leaving a denuded GBM—observed as early as 10 to 15 minutes following injection [145,305, 441,453]. Pilia et al. [380], in a model of NTS in Munich Wistar rats, described focal changes primarily in the epithelial cells at one hour, consisting of cellular swelling and detachment from the GBM. In an ultrastructural study of NTS in the rat, Kreisberg et al. [259] reported the influx of mononuclear cells resembling lymphocytes in the capillary lumina as early as 15 minutes, with heavy infiltration by 30 minutes after the administration of NTS. A role for these cells in the pathogenesis of proteinuria was supported by the observation that rats pretreated with total lymphoid irradiation or anti-lymphocyte serum were found to have decreased 24-hour protein excretion and no loss of negative charge from the filtration barrier at 15, 30, and 120 minutes, as was demonstrated by colloidal iron staining in the rats that were not pretreated.

Indirect immunofluorescence studies demonstrate that heterologous anti-GBM antibodies react in vitro not only with all renal basement membranes but also with other visceral basement membranes, including lung, liver, spleen, placenta, and choroid plexus. However, following in vivo injection of these antibodies, damage is usually confined to the kidney, an observation that is probably related to their weaker fixation in and more rapid disappearance from other organs. Occasionally, pulmonary edema and hemorrhage have developed following the administration of nephrotoxic antibody [69,138,484,486].

A second phase of injury begins one hour following the administration of NTS, predominates over the next few hours, and generally subsides by 24 hours. This is the period of inflammation caused by the transient infiltration of polymorphonuclear leucocytes (PMN) that are thought to be chemotactically attracted by complement components bound to GBM-anti-GBM immune complexes (Fig. 13-5). Considerable experimental data summarized in Table 13-2 supports a definite role for complement-PMN mediated mechanisms of glomerular injury in the heterologous phase of experimental anti-GBM nephritis, similar to that observed in the classical cutaneous Arthus reaction [75]. However, it is becoming increasingly appreciated that other factors also participate in the pathogenesis of nephritis at this early period, and glomerular damage may ensue under certain specified experimental conditions (Table 13-3) even in the absence of complement and PMN. The mediating factors are not well understood in this latter set of circumstances, although likely candidates may include mononuclear cells, platelets and their vasoactive amines, fibrinogen, and the Hageman factor related kinin-forming system.

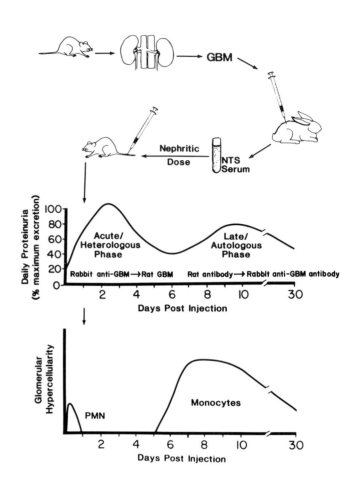

FIG. 13-5. *Summary of the sequence of key events in the classical experimental model of anti-GBM nephritis. Injection of a rat with anti-GBM antibodies prepared by immunization of rabbits produces a biphasic model of glomerulonephritis. In the acute phase the heterologous rabbit anti-rat GBM antibody binds to the rat GBM and produces proteinuria through a sequence of events dependent upon complement fixation and glomerular infiltration of polymorphonuclear leucocytes (PMN). The late phase begins as autologous (rat) antibody binds to the foreign protein (heterologous rabbit antibody) now bound to the GBM and acting as a planted antigen within the glomerulus. Production of proteinuria during the autologous phase is dependent on the glomerular infiltration of monocytes; the participation of complement and PMNs is not required. (Modified from Unanue et al: Textbook of Immunology, 1984.)*

With time, an entirely new period of glomerular injury appears, heralded by the activation of the host's immune responses to the heterologous antibody (a "planted" antigen) bound to its GBM. This phase of nephritis resulting from the interaction of host autologous antibody to a foreign antigen (heterologous antibody) now planted within the GBM is referred to as the autologous phase of NTS nephritis and is discussed in further detail in the following section as an example of "in situ" antigen-antibody interaction.

TABLE 13-2. *Heterologous phase of experimental anti-GBM nephritis—evidence for complement-polymorphonuclear leucocyte mechanisms*

1. Demonstration of complement components by indirect immunofluorescence in numerous studies.
2. Complement depletion prevents accumulation of PMN and proteinuria in rats [483] and rabbits [73,75].
3. Demonstration of PMN infiltration by electron microscopy.
4. PMN depletion by nitrogen mustard or specific antibody prevents heterologous phase in rats and rabbits [73,75].

TABLE 13-3. *Heterologous phase of experimental anti-GBM nephritis—evidence for complement-polymorphonuclear leucocyte independent mechanisms*

1. Non-complement fixing anti-GBM antibodies induced injury in the absence of overt C-PMN participation [182,375,483].
2. Gamma-2 fraction sheep anti-rabbit GBM causes injury in normal and PMN-depleted rabbits [186].
3. Complement-fixing Fc fragment of nephrotoxic antibody not required for glomerular injury [251,444].
4. Induction of renal disease in animals with genetic complement deficiencies: C4 deficient guinea pigs [444], C5 deficient mice [487], C6 deficient rabbits [400].
5. Proteinuria develops in guinea pigs given nephrotoxic serum after C3 depletion by cobra venom factor [86].
6. Absence of PMN and complement deposition in Munich Wistar rats given nephrotoxic serum [380].

ANTIBODIES TO DEFINED STRUCTURAL COMPONENTS OF THE GBM

Recent experiments have attempted to define the nature of the antigenic determinant of the GBM involved in the experimental models of NTS nephritis through the passive administration of antibodies reactive with known antigens of the GBM. Following the injection of mice with rabbit anti-type IV collagen antisera, Yaar et al. [527] observed linear deposition of the rabbit antibody and mouse C3 along the GBM during the first 48 hours of study (heterologous phase) with minimal morphological evidence of injury, including occasional intratubular hemorrhages, glomerular cell degeneration, and rare polymorphonuclear cells. During this period the animals failed to develop proteinuria. Following the passive administration of rabbit anti-laminin antibody, the same group noted linear deposition of rabbit antibody along the GBM and tubular basement membranes (TBM). However, these animals failed to develop proteinuria or morphological evidence of renal disease during the heterologous phase. Abrahamson et al. [1] studied the effects of passive administration of sheep anti-laminin antisera to rats and reported the linear binding of the heterologous antibody to the rat GBM, mesangium, and some TBM. However, during the early phase they failed to detect deposition of complement, morphological changes, or proteinuria. In contrast, Wick et al. [512] reported the development of edema and exudation in the kidneys of mice five hours following the injection of antibodies to type IV collagen or laminin. Several monoclonal

antibodies reactive with other undefined components of the rat basement membrane have now been developed, but to date there are no reports of renal pathology resulting from the in vivo administration and binding of these probes to rat GBM [325]. Thus, the nature of the nephritogenic antigen in experimental models of anti-GBM nephritis is at present unknown, and in the final analysis multiple determinants may be involved.

In humans, the non-collagenous globular domain (NCl) of type IV collagen, having a molecular weight of 26,000 (reduced monomeric form), has recently been isolated from human GBM and shown to be reactive with the circulating antibodies obtained from seven of seven patients with Goodpasture syndrome, suggesting that it is an important antigenic determinant in the pathogenesis of anti-GBM disease in man [510].

An extremely interesting experiment of nature occurring in man has recently provided new insights into the pathogenesis of anti-GBM nephritis. A subset of patients with hereditary nephritis (Alport's syndrome), after receiving a renal transplant, subsequently developed anti-GBM nephritis de novo in the renal allograft [216,218,311,333, 366]. Patients with hereditary nephritis have a structural defect of the glomerular basement membrane easily appreciated by electron microscopy, which reveals the typically thickened GBM with longitudinal splitting, reticulation, and fragmentation, adjacent to extremely thin and attenuated basement membranes. Some of these patients lack the so-called "Goodpasture antigen," which means that antibody obtained from the serum of patients with Goodpasture syndrome fails to bind to the Alport GBM in the linear pattern universally seen with kidneys from normal individuals (Fig. 13-6). Transplantation of a normal renal allograft containing the Goodpasture antigen into such individuals may immunize them, leading to the production of antibodies to this foreign antigen and the development of anti-GBM nephritis. The ensuing glomerular injury may be severe enough to result in allograft failure. Although the biochemical defect of the renal basement membrane in Alport's syndrome is at present unknown, further investigations of this disease may provide insight into the nature of potentially nephritogenic antigens in man.

EXPERIMENTAL AUTOIMMUNE GLOMERULONEPHRITIS

In 1962 Steblay [452] reported that sheep immunized with human GBM in Freund's adjuvant developed a proliferative and crescentic glomerulonephritis characterized by the linear deposition of sheep immunoglobulin G and complement along the glomerular basement membrane. Since several structural components of the GBM are shared in common by most animals, it was suggested that this active immunization resulted in the formation of antibodies against the immunizing human GBM, some of which were autoantibodies cross-reactive with antigenic determinants of the host sheep GBM. Renal injury was similarly observed if sheep were immunized with preparations of heterologous GBM prepared from monkeys, rabbits, dogs, rats, and human lung basement membrane preparations, and occasionally even with preparations of homologous sheep GBM

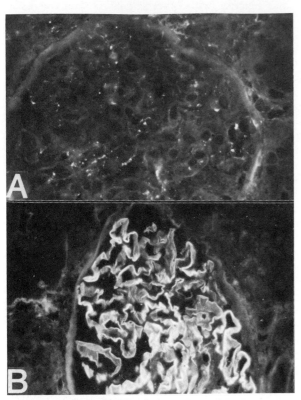

FIG. 13-6. *Illustration of the absence of Goodpasture antigen in a male patient with familial nephritis. Antibody against Goodpasture antigen(s) eluted from the kidney of a patient with this disease fails to react with the glomeruli of a boy with familial nephritis (A). Such a patient is at risk of developing anti-GBM nephritis following the transplantation of a normal renal allograft. This patient's sister demonstrates the normal staining pattern with the Goodpasture antigen distributed in a linear pattern along the GBM (B). (Reprinted from Jeraj et al: Am J Kidney Dis, Vol II, 626, 1983, with permission.)*

creted in the urine [277,313]. In 1968, Lerner et al. [277] noted that 10 of 27 normal rabbits injected with membrane components obtained from their own urine developed anti-GBM nephritis that could be passively transferred by injecting the nephrotoxic antibodies eluded from the kidney into normal rabbits. Such studies suggested the possibility that in these animals the basement membrane antigens themselves were altered in such a way as to no longer be recognized as "self" or that the normal state of tolerance to GBM components was overcome in yet undefined ways, resulting in the formation of antibodies directed against the glomerular basement membrane antigens.

Although basement membranes are the extracellular matrices found in every organ of the body and they share several structural components in common, to date all experimental models of anti-GBM nephritis have failed to show significant extrarenal pathology except for the minimal pulmonary lesions reported in rabbits immunized with choroid plexus [314] and the deposition of host immunoglobulin noted in the alveolar walls of mice chronically immunized with purified laminin [342]. In fact, Steblay et al. [456] reported that sheep injected with preparations of heterologous (human) lung basement membrane in Freund's complete adjuvant developed progressive anti-GBM nephritis but failed to bind autoantibodies in their lungs or to develop Goodpasture-like pulmonary lesions. These observations are particularly perplexing if one wishes to extrapolate the observations made from the study of animal models of anti-GBM nephritis to the disease observed in man, in whom pulmonary involvement (Goodpasture's syndrome) is common. However, studies by Jennings et al. [101,217] have documented that passively-administered antibodies react with alveolar capillary basement membrane of rats, but only after exposure of the alveoli to high concentrations of oxygen, which leads to an increase in capillary permeability. Other important pathogenic factors will no doubt be clarified once the nature of the nephritogenic antigen(s) is identified.

Recent studies have begun to evaluate the nephritogenic potential of the known components of GBM both by active as well as passive immunization. Murphy-Ullrich et al. [341] described pathological changes in the glomerulus and hepatic pulmonary vasculature of mice immunized with autologous or heterologous guinea pig denatured fibronectin. More recently, the same group repeatedly immunized mice over nine months with preparations of laminin purified from the murine Engelbreth-Holm-Swarm (EHS) sarcoma and reported mild mesangial hypercellularity, deposition of mouse IgG without C3 along capillary loops and within the mesangium, and evidence of changes within the GBM by electron microscopy [342]. Circulating anti-laminin antibodies could not be detected. Mouse IgG was also seen along tubules, in the alveolar wall, and in blood vessels.

GLOMERULAR INJURY INDUCED BY MERCURIC CHLORIDE

An interesting pattern of glomerular injury has been observed in rabbits [9,398a] and Brown Norway rats [416] chronically injected with mercuric chloride ($HgCl_2$). In

injected in adjuvant, suggesting that under such circumstances the normal state of tolerance to native GBM antigens was overcome [453–457]. A critical role for the autoantibodies in the pathogenesis of the renal damage is further suggested by the observation that circulating antibodies recovered from nephritic sheep will passively transfer nephritis to uninephrectomized naive sheep [276, 401,457]. The nephritic antibody does not appear to be transmitted transplacentally nor through colostrum, as lambs born of nephritic sheep do not have detectable glomerulonephritis. Preparations of heterologous GBM injected in adjuvant have also induced nephritis in goats [518], monkeys [372,454], rats [518], rabbits [488,489], guinea pigs [84], and chickens [48], although there is considerable variability in the severity of the injury.

It has been observed that urine of normal individuals contains antigens that are cross-reactive with the GBM and that similar antigens are detectable in the circulation following nephrectomy, suggesting that these are breakdown products, resulting from the turnover of basement membranes, which under normal circumstances are ex-this biphasic model of renal injury, the animals first demonstrate linear deposits of IgG along the GBM and TBM. The anti-GBM antibodies are usually detectable by two weeks. A few animals manifest very transient proteinuria at this point. Although the nature of the reactive GBM antigen has not been identified, it appears to be more widely distributed than that involved in nephrotoxic serum nephritis. $HgCl_2$-treated rabbits form antibodies reactive with GBM, TBM, vessel walls in several organs, splenic reticulum, hepatic sinusoids, intestinal lamina propria and basal lamina, and perimysium and endomysium of skeletal and cardiac muscles; the antibody eluted from the kidneys of $HgCl_2$-injected rats cross-reacts with the basement membranes associated with arterioles [9,398a,416].

The pattern of glomerular deposition of the immune reactants in rabbits changes after four to five weeks, appearing as granular sub-epithelial deposits of IgG and C3. By two to three months the rabbits have developed severe membranous glomerulopathy. The nature of these immune complexes is unknown although there is some evidence to suggest that the antibody is similar to that found in the early phase of the disease and that at least some antigens participating in the immune complex formation are derived from soluble polysaccharide components of the collagenous matrix of the GBM.

The glomerular response to the administration of $HgCl_2$ in rats is more variable. Brown Norway rats demonstrate a biphasic pattern of disease similar to that observed in rabbits, while most other rat strains develop monophasic disease, characterized by the immune complex-associated pattern of glomerular injury [103,104]. As yet unidentified, it appears most likely that the antigen-antibody complexes formed in rats differ from those that develop in the rabbit. It has been reported that subepithelial deposits in Brown Norway rats occur only when immune complexes are detectable in the circulation [198]. Antinuclear antibodies detectable in several of the diseased rats but not rabbits suggest that these might be important in the pathogenesis of glomerular disease in the rat [508]. It is conceivable that some of the immune complexes form in situ in both animals models by the interaction of antibody with normal glomerular antigens modified by exposure to mercuric chloride, but as yet this mechanism has not been clearly demonstrated.

Interaction of Antibodies with Glomerular (non-GBM) Antigens

PASSIVE HEYMANN NEPHRITIS

Rats injected with an extract of homologous kidney in Freund's complete adjuvant were first reported to develop nephrotic syndrome by Heymann et al. in 1959 [187]. Since that time this model of experimental nephritis has received much attention, not only because the glomerular lesions have been shown to be immunologically induced, but because the resulting subepithelial immune deposits are indistinguishable from those seen in membranous nephropathy in man [10,22,87,121,470,492]. The greater susceptibility of certain strains of rats (especially Lewis, Sprague-Dawley, and Wistar) to Heymann nephritis is in part controlled by major histocompatibility-linked genes [245, 426,464].

The nature of the immunogen present in the homologous kidney extract has been further identified. The major antigen is a component of the luminal brush border of proximal tubules and is referred to as Fx1A [114,115,165,174, 175,238,295,296,329,347]. Isolation of Fx1A involved ultracentrifugation of the supernatant remaining after rat kidney cortex obtained by passage through graded sieves was centrifuged at low speed to remove glomeruli and intact tubule fragments. Kerjaschki et al. [238] further purified the nephritogenic antigen obtained from the isolated membranes of tubular microvilli and identified it as a glycoprotein of molecular weight 330,000 (gp330). The carbohydrate moiety has been shown by binding with concanavalin A to contain mannose or glucose residues or both. The key observation leading to a better understanding of the immunopathology of Heymann nephritis was the report that an antigen cross-reactive with the tubular brush border antigen was also present along the subepithelial aspect of the glomerular capillary wall of normal rats [239]. With the use of polyclonal and monoclonal antibodies to gp330, it was shown that the glomerular antigen was concentrated within invaginations of the epithelial cell surface membrane, usually in clathrin-coated pits, structures known to be involved in receptor mediated endocytosis (Fig. 13-7). The nephritic antigen was also noted to be associated with intracellular structures such as the rough endoplasmic reticulum and Golgi apparatus, suggesting that the epithelial cells synthesized this antigen.

The model of passive Heymann nephritis induced by injecting rats with anti-Fx1A antibody is now generally felt to be a model of in situ immune complex formation, developing as the injected antibody binds to the glomerular antigen, producing large subepithelial immune deposits composed of anti-Fx1A antibody and complement (heterologous phase) [22,87,89,121,292,349,492] (Fig. 13-8). Within five days the rats develop proteinuria in the absence of evidence of glomerular inflammatory changes. This

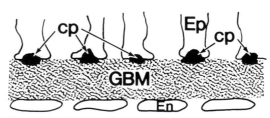

FIG. 13-7. Diagram illustrating the nephritogenic glomerular antigen (glycoprotein of MW 330 kd) participating in the in situ formation of subepithelial immune deposits observed in rats with Heymann nephritis. Small immune deposits (dark deposits) are found in the coated pits (cp) at the base of the foot processes of glomerular epithelial cells (Ep) and extending into the lamina rara externa of the GBM. With the use of a purified antibody to gp330, this coated-pit antigen has been identified within the glomeruli of normal Lewis rats where it is restricted to glomerular epithelial cells and is distinctly absent from endothelial cells (En). (Based on the work of Kerjaschki et al: J Exp Med 157:667, 1983.)

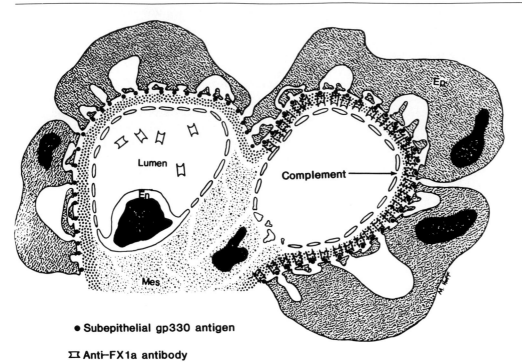

● **Subepithelial gp330 antigen**

⌶ **Anti–FX1a antibody**

FIG. 13-8. *Schematic illustration of the pathogenesis of membranous nephropathy in the model of passive Heymann nephritis in rats. The glomerular antigen gp330 (depicted by black dots) is found in the normal rat glomerulus concentrated within the coated pits of the epithelial cells (Ep) (see Figure 13-7). Following the passive administration of Fx1A antiserum, large subepithelial immune deposits develop. Proteinuria begins following the fixation of complement to these deposits, producing a glomerular lesion that morphologically resembles membranous nephropathy in man.*

mechanism was first suggested in 1978 by the studies of Van Damme et al. [492] showing early fixation of heterologous Fx1A antibody to presumed subepithelial glomerular antigens within one to three hours after infusion of the antibody and by the studies of Couser et al. [87] showing early fixation of heterologous Fx1A in the subepithelial spaces in the isolated perfused rat kidney. Unlike anti-GBM antibodies, which rapidly bind to glomeruli following intravenous injection, glomerular deposition of heterologous anti-Fx1A occurs more gradually, increasing steadily over a five-day period. It has been suggested that this difference in kinetics is due to restricted access of the antibody to antigenic sites, which are not in direct contact with the circulation, and that factors such as the size and charge of the antibody may be rate-limiting. The mechanisms by which intact IgG antibodies cross the relatively impermeable capillary wall to react with the pit antigen have not been determined. It has been observed that rats rendered proteinuric with the aminonucleoside of puromycin prior to active immunization with the Fx1A antigen develop very few subepithelial deposits when compared to non-treated rats, suggesting that alterations in the charge and antigenicity of the epithelium of the glomerular capillary wall hinder the subsequent development of subepithelial immune deposits [88]. However, a similar injury induced by injection of adriamycin had no effect on the subsequent development of passive Heymann nephritis [36].

Induction of renal injury and the development of proteinuria in the model of passive Heymann nephritis is dependent upon complement activation but not on the presence of neutrophils as occurs in the heterologous phase of anti-GBM nephritis and the classical Arthus reaction [87,411,412]. Sequential immunofluorescence studies of kidneys obtained from rats after injection of anti-Fx1A shows early and prominent participation of rat C3 in the subepithelial deposits (Fig. 13-1). Rats depleted of C3 with cobra venom factor prior to antibody administration showed deposition of the antibody in the subepithelial space similar to untreated rats, but they failed to develop proteinuria [411]. Normocomplementemic rats developed proteinuria beginning five days after antibody administration. Similarly, administration of heterologous anti-Fx1A as F(ab')$_2$ fragments or as the IgG$_2$ antibody fractions that are unable to fix complement failed to induce proteinuria after subepithelial immune deposit formation [413]. However, depletion of neutrophils using an anti-neutrophil serum did not alter the pathological changes [411].

It is unknown why chemotaxins generated during complement activation fail to attract neutrophils in this model unless such chemotaxins remain inaccessible to the circulating cells. Thus, the presumed cell-independent mechanism by which complement alters glomerular permeability inducing nephrotic syndrome remains unknown. It has been suggested that these changes may be mediated through membrane lysis similar to that observed for the terminal complement components that lyse red blood cells [41]. Bieseker et al. [42] demonstrated components of the membrane-attack complex of complement (C5b-9) along the glomerular capillary wall in rats with active Heymann nephritis. Adler et al. [6] and deHeer et al. [93] have also confirmed the presence of the terminal complement components within these subepithelial immune deposits. Studies by Noble et al. [361] add further support to a role for complement in the induction of proteinuria in this model. Rats actively immunized with Fx1A antigen who failed to develop proteinuria were distinguished by the absence of deposition of complement in the subepithelial immune deposits, despite similar deposition of immunoglobulins.

The autologous phase of passive Heymann nephritis initiated by the production of rat antibodies to the heterologous anti-Fx1A antibody planted in the subepithelial glomerular deposits has not been well studied. It is known that the early phase of passive Heymann nephritis marked by the onset of proteinuria at five days is not dependent on an autologous phase reaction since minimal rat immunoglobulin is present in the glomeruli at this time and the onset of disease is not modified by depletion of recipient lymphocytes with total lymphoid irradiation or cyclophosphamide therapy [411,412]. However, autologous antibodies probably participate at later time periods since rat immunoglobulin is present in the subepithelial deposits by the seventh day [3,4]. Adler et al. [5] avoided the heterologous phase of passive Heymann nephritis by injecting rats with subnephritic doses of the non-complement fixing γ2 fraction of sheep anti-Fx1A, which produced subepithelial deposits of sheep immunoglobulin without morphological or functional evidence of glomerular injury. Three days later the kidneys were transplanted into bilaterally nephrectomized rats presensitized to sheep immunoglobulin, and within five days post-transplant the subepithelial deposits of sheep γ2 (now acting as a planted glomerular antigen) had bound rat immunoglobulin and complement, and the rats had developed proteinuria. Glomerular injury was shown to require autologous antibody production and the presence of complement, but not the presence of neutrophils.

The immune mechanism of glomerular injury in Heymann nephritis becomes more difficult to unravel when the disease is actively induced by immunization of rats with the isolated Fx1A antigen. Under these experimental conditions, proteinuria usually develops in six to eight weeks. Until the studies of Van Damme and Couser, it was thought that disease under these circumstances resulted from the glomerular deposition of circulating Fx1A-anti-Fx1A immune complexes. Studies by Abrass et al. [4] suggest that manipulation of the mononuclear phagocytic system by splenectomy delays clearance of Fx1A-anti-Fx1A immune complexes, leading to increased accumulation of glomerular deposits and accelerated loss of renal function in the model of active Heymann nephritis. It is probable that the formation of immune complexes both in situ

within the glomerulus and within the circulation play a role in the active model, although the predominant mechanism remains controversial [2,4,89,291]. Immune complex-induced renal disease is discussed in greater detail in the next section.

As previously mentioned, the histological lesions of passive Heymann nephritis in rats are identical to those observed in humans with membranous nephropathy. However, there is no conclusive evidence that autologous tubular antigens participate in the human disease. Naruse et al. [346] detected tubular antigens in the peripheral capillary loop deposits in three of seven patients with idiopathic membranous nephropathy. However, this finding has not been confirmed by others except in one patient reported by Douglas et al. [100], who also had a circulating antibody reactive with the brush border of proximal tubules. Now that the nephritogenic antigen of passive Heymann nephritis has been isolated, characterized, and localized, not only to the brush border of proximal tubules but also to the subepithelial aspect of the normal GBM, it might be more fruitful to approach human membranous nephropathy from this vantage point, seeking to identify similar antigens normally present within the glomerular capillary wall that might react in situ with an autoantibody under the appropriate pathological circumstances.

Interaction of Antibodies with Exogenous Antigens Planted within the Glomerular Capillary Wall

The idea that circulating antibodies might bind to antigenic determinants within the glomerulus that are not structural components of the glomerular capillary wall has been known for some time and is illustrated by the sequence of events that follow the administration of heterologous anti-GBM antibody. Indeed, current evidence suggests that intact circulating immune complexes cannot move across a normal GBM to become lodged in a subepithelial position. Subepithelial immune deposits associated with glomerular disease have not been seen experimentally following the infusion of preformed immune complexes, except in studies that have used low avidity antibodies, that is, complexes that may readily undergo spontaneous intravascular dissociation [160].

The presence of subepithelial electron dense deposits is the hallmark of membranous nephropathy, and large subepithelial "humps" are suggestive of post-streptococcal glomerulonephritis, two very important causes of glomerular disease in man. The principle that immune complexes may form "in situ" in the kidney by two sequential steps, namely, deposition of an exogenous antigen followed by the binding of a circulating antibody, provides an attractive alternative explanation for the formation of subepithelial immune complexes. There is every reason to believe that the same process may account for the formation of immune deposits at other locations within the kidney as well. It was through the careful study of certain experimental models of renal disease in animals that this mechanism of renal injury was first proposed.

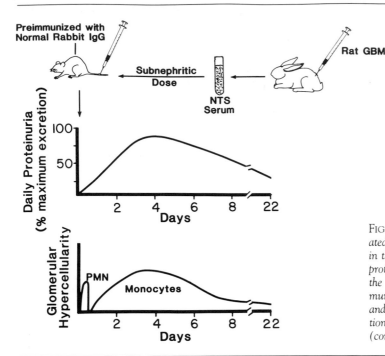

FIG. 13-9. *Schematic summary of the experimental model of accelerated anti-GBM nephritis. The autologous phase of glomerular injury in the model of anti-GBM nephritis (identified by the presence of proteinuria) can be accelerated by pre-immunizing the recipient rat to the heterologous (rabbit) immunoglobulin. This insures a high immune response to the heterologous (planted) antibody and an early and prominent autologous phase of renal injury. Glomerular infiltration of monocytes begins much earlier than in the classical model (compare with Fig. 13-5).*

NEPHROTOXIC SERUM NEPHRITIS (LATE OR AUTOLOGOUS PHASE)

The acute phase of glomerular injury induced by the binding of heterologous anti-GBM antibody (discussed in the previous section) becomes quiescent within a few days following antibody injection. However, a second phase of glomerular injury subsequently develops as the host's immune system begins to produce antibodies to the foreign protein (heterologous anti-GBM antibody) now bound to the GBM and acting as a planted antigen (Fig. 13-5). This second phase develops slowly, usually seven to ten days after administration of the antibody, and may ensue even if the acute phase induced by injection of very small amounts of heterologous anti-GBM antibody fails to induce significant pathological changes. The quantitative studies of Unanue and Dixon [484,485] showed that 75 μg of antibody bound per gram of kidney is necessary for heterologous injury in the rat (15 μg/g kidney in rabbits and 5 μg/g kidney in sheep), whereas just 2 μg/g can induce the autologous phase of injury. This autologous phase of glomerular injury can be accelerated by pre-immunizing the recipient animal to the heterologous immunoglobulin, thus insuring a high immune response to the heterologous anti-GBM antibody and an early and prominent autologous phase of renal injury (accelerated form of nephrotoxic serum nephritis) (Fig. 13-9).

A key role for autologous antibodies in the induction of this secondary phase of renal injury is further supported by the observation that this phase can also be induced by passive administration of antibody directed against the heterologous immunoglobulin [484–486] (Fig. 13-10). Further evidence is suggested by the observation that treatment of rats with total lymphoid irradiation eight days after induction of an accelerated autologous form of NTS is associated with a decrease in proteinuria, improved histology, and decreased levels of circulating antibody to the planted heterologous antibody [290,291].

The production of glomerular damage during the autologous phase does not appear to require the presence of complement or polymorphonuclear leukocytes, although the latter are known to participate [344,445,479,483,487] (Table 13-3). Recent studies support a key role for mononuclear cells in the pathogenesis of this injury. Morphologic studies have attributed some of the glomerular hypercellularity to infiltrating macrophages, and large numbers of macrophages have been detected by glomerular cell culture during the autologous phase of anti-GBM induced antibody injury (summarized in Table 13-4). These macrophages appear to participate in glomerular injury, because prior depletion of macrophages by irradiation in the rat [106,430,433] or by treatment with nitrogen mustard or antimacrophage serum in the rabbit [191–193] has abrogated the glomerular lesion and prevented proteinuria. In addition, abrogation of renal injury in association with nitrogen mustard pretreatment can in part be restored in the rabbit by subsequent repletion of macrophages in the form of peritoneal macrophages obtained from unsensitized rabbits [195]. Furthermore, it was shown that local irradiation of the kidney failed to prevent the development of glomerulonephritis; renal disease resembled that in the nonirradiated contralateral kidney, suggesting that proliferation of intrinsic glomerular cells is not necessary for the induction of proteinuria [66]. However, normal rats exposed to nephrotoxic serum under an accelerated protocol show evidence of proliferation of intrinsic glomerular cells. The work of Sterzl et al. [465] suggests that these cells undergo early mitosis beginning at a time when monocytic infiltration is not yet detectable.

At present, the factors attracting macrophages to the

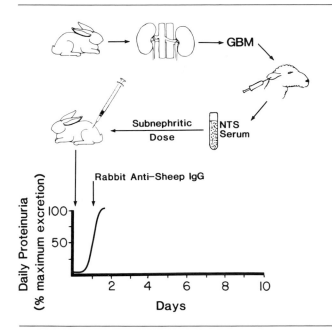

FIG. 13-10. *The autologous phase of anti-GBM nephritis can be induced rapidly and reproducibly by the passive administration of autologous antibody. Rabbits immunized with subnephritic doses of sheep anti-rabbit GBM antibody bind 90% of this antibody to their GBM within one hour. The second (autologous) phase of renal injury usually begins several days later as the rabbit produces antibodies to the heterologous (sheep) antibody, which is now acting as a foreign antigen planted within the glomerulus. However, this phase of injury can be accelerated and initiated abruptly if rabbit anti-sheep IgG is passively injected following immunization with nephrotoxic serum (NTS). Glomerular injury in this model is mediated by the infiltration of macrophages.*

TABLE 13-4. *Participation of monocytes in the autologous phase of anti-GBM nephritis*

Model	Glomerular Preparation		Observation
	Tissue Selection	Culture	
I. Classical Model (rabbit)			
1. Kondo [263]	+		—Mo* observed in crescents
2. Thomson [480]	+	+	—Mo slightly increased in heterologous phase, peaked day 12–14 autologous phase
3. Cattell [66]	+		—irradition of one kidney—developed same hypercellularity as shielded kidney
II. Accelerated Model (rat)			
1. Schreiner [430]	+		—Mo prominent days 2–4 —TBI** decreased cellularity and proteinuria
2. Dubois [106]	+	+	—outgrowth of Mo and possibly endothelial cells; increased mesangial cells —TBI decreased cellularity and proteinuria
3. Sterzel [465]	+		—proliferation of intrinsic cells observed day 1 before significant Mo infiltration
III. Passive Autologous Model (rabbit)			
1. Holdsworth [193]	+	+	—disease abrogated by anti-Mo serum
2. Holdsworth [194]	+	+	—use of F(ab')₂ anti-GBM failed to induce disease seen with intact antibody
3. Holdsworth [195]	+	+	—disease abrogated by nitrogen mustard; partially restored by infusion of peritoneal Mo

* Mo = Macrophage
** TBI = Total body irradiation

glomerulus during the autologous phase are not entirely understood. The binding of macrophages through surface receptors specific for the Fc-fragment of the heterologous antibody (immune adherence) is important since equiva-lent amounts of the F(ab')₂ fragments of the heterologous anti-GBM antibody prevent the glomerular accumulation of macrophages in rabbits, cause no significant histological changes, and induce minimal proteinuria during the autologous phase [194]. Bhan et al. [37] showed that lymphocytes sensitized to the heterologous antibody, which is bound to the GBM, may attract monocytes to the glomerulus in a delayed-type hypersensitivity reaction. However, Lowry et al. [290] failed to show a correlation between antigen-specific delayed-type hypersensitivity and albuminuria in a model of accelerated autologous nephrotoxic serum nephritis in intact rats. A role for other monocyte chemotactic factors and cellular adhesion molecules has not been explored in any detail. It is known that monocytic accumulation occurs in the absence of complement or fibrin [498]. Thus, in contrast to the heterologous phase of nephrotoxic serum nephritis, which shares features with the classical Arthus reaction, dependent on complement and polymorphonuclear leukocytes for production of glomerular injury, the autologous phase proceeds in the absence of these mediators, although renal damage requires glomerular infiltration of macrophages.

OTHER PLANTED GLOMERULAR ANTIGENS

Exogenous antigens may become planted within the glomerulus by a variety of mechanisms and subsequently become the target of an antibody-mediated immune response. Macromolecular antigens may become transiently trapped within the glomerular mesangium as a result of its normal filtration function. Mauer et al. [306] demonstrated that administration of aggregated human IgG to rabbits, followed by infusion of anti-human IgG antisera, resulted in a formation of immune complexes in situ within the mesangium, accompanied by leukocytic infiltration and proteinuria. Trapping of circulating immune complexes was avoided in this model by transplantion of the aggregate-containing kidneys into normal rabbits prior to passive administration of antiserum.

Foreign antigens may become trapped within the kidney due to electrostatic binding to native glomerular charge sites. Batsford et al. [26,362,502,503] demonstrated that cationized proteins (pI > 8.5) of molecular weight in the range of 500 kilodaltons to 900 kilodaltons, such as cationized ferritin and human IgG, are bound to anionic charge sites along the glomerular capillary wall when administered to rats. These positively charged macromolecules then rapidly disappeared unless they were complexed with antibody, which was experimentally achieved by passive administration of specific antibody. Under this set of conditions, electron dense deposits formed in the subepithelial spaces and, following deposition of C3, proteinuria developed. Izui et al. [213] suggested that DNA may bind to the glomerular basement membrane and serve as a planted antigen for reaction with anti-DNA antibodies in the autoimmune disease of NZB/W mice, a disorder that has many similarities to systemic lupus erythematosus of man. Although the basis for this DNA-GBM binding is not known, it may very well be on the basis of electrostatic charge.

Specific chemical interactions may explain the trapping of other exogenous antigens within the glomerulus. For example, lectins (proteins with carbohydrate binding sites) can bind to the GBM and serve as planted antigens, which upon reaction with anti-lectin antibody form immune com-

plexes in situ. Golbus et al. [167,518] injected rats with concanavalin A (a lectin that binds to residues of mannose and glucose) followed by anti-concanavalin A antibodies and observed the formation of subendothelial immune complexes and the subsequent development of proliferative glomerulonephritis. It is noteworthy that many infectious organisms pathogenic to man contain lectin-like materials, raising the possibility that similar mechanisms could induce human post-infectious glomerulonephritis.

This concept of the trapping of foreign molecules within the kidney, thereby setting the scene for in situ formation of immune complexes, raises many exciting possibilities for the induction of renal disease in man, especially when glomerulonephritis develops in association with antecedent or concomitant systemic illness or exposure to drugs or toxins.

Glomerular Deposition of Circulating Immune Complexes

Soluble immune complexes formed in the circulation by the reaction of antibodies with non-renal antigens are currently thought to be involved in the pathogenesis of many forms of glomerulonephritis in man. The kidney is unique among the body's major organ systems in its peculiar susceptibility to injury induced by the deposition of immune complexes. However, it must be emphasized that circulating immune complexes are in a dynamic state of continual formation and elimination as the immune system deals with foreign antigens, and yet glomerular deposition and injury from such complexes is, overall, a relatively uncommon event.

The challenge of unraveling the pathogenetic mechanisms of immune complex-induced glomerular injury has made considerable gains since Von Pirquet, in 1911, [504] first recognized that a relationship existed between the host's response to a foreign serum component and the development of serum sickness. Many important observations were made in the 1950s by the studies of Germuth [162–155] and Dixon [96–98] and their respective coworkers, establishing a role for immune complexes in the induction of glomerulonephritis seen in experimental models of serum sickness in rabbits. Our understanding of the participating mechanisms has become rather complicated during the past 25 years and still continues to draw heavily from the study of animal models. Evaluation of glomerulonephritic human kidneys by immunofluorescence microscopy frequently reveals the presence of immunoglobulins and complement proteins, and the detection of electron dense immune deposits by electron microscopy provides supporting evidence for the participation of immune complexes; yet, identification of the antigen-antibody systems involved has frequently not been possible.

Animal Models of Immune Complex Glomerulonephritis

The factors that participate in the development of immune-complex glomerulonephritis are summarized in this section.

It is important to emphasize at the outset that this network is in a state of constant change; the immune complexes are not fixed within the glomeruli, but rather are in a state of dynamic equilibrium with participating components remaining in the circulation.

ACUTE SERUM SICKNESS

Acute serum sickness in rabbits is the classic model of immune complex-induced tissue injury. In 1943 Rich & Gregory [397] first reported the development of acute diffuse proliferative glomerulonephritis following a one-shot intravenous injection of heterologous serum protein. Subsequent studies have generally involved the use of purified plasma proteins such as serum albumin or ovalbumin. The concept that this injected foreign protein subsequently participated in the formation of immune complexes that were nephrotoxic to some rabbits evolved through careful evaluation of the fate of the antigen after injection and its temporal relationship to the development of glomerular lesions [96,98,152,163,267] (Fig. 13-11). A significant amount of the protein (two-thirds to three-quarters) leaves the vascular compartment during the first 24 to 48 hours following intravenous administration, establishing a state of equilibrium with extravascular spaces. During the next several days the protein is slowly catabolized, disappearing at an exponential rate. The third phase, that of immune elimination, begins at about the fifth day with the appearance of antibodies that initiate the formation of immune

complexes. At first these are small, soluble immune complexes formed in great antigen excess and, as such, are not readily phagocytosed but continue to circulate. As antibody production continues, the complexes increase in size and are readily removed by the mononuclear phagocytic system. Antigen and immune complexes have disappeared from the circulation by approximately day ten, leaving behind only free antibody. The early studies of Germuth [152], later confirmed by Dixon [96] and colleagues, demonstrated that the inflammatory vascular and glomerular lesions developed during the immune phase of antigen elimination, associated with the glomerular deposition of the antigen and rabbit gamma globulin, which were detectable by immunofluorescence.

The clinicopathological features of acute serum sickness in rabbits in many ways resemble those of acute poststreptococcal glomerulonephritis in man. The glomerular injury begins abruptly during the phase of immune elimination of the antigen and is associated with significant morphological changes in the kidney and the onset of proteinuria (Fig. 13-12). Thereafter, the lesions heal rapidly, so that the glomeruli appear normal again within two to three weeks. By light microscopy, the glomerular lesions consist of diffuse hypercellularity due to endothelial cell swelling and proliferation and, perhaps more importantly, the infiltration of mononuclear phagocytes. By immunofluorescence, fine granular deposits of the foreign antigen together with rabbit IgG and C3 are usually found along the glomerular capillary wall. With progression of the disease, the IgG and C3 content increases and the deposits enlarge, supporting the contention that the glomerular bound immune complexes are not static but continue to interact with components from the circulation [129]. Within two weeks of onset of the disease, C3 is often the only remaining protein detectable by immunofluorescence. By electron microscopy, these immunoreactants have been shown to correspond to the presence of electron dense deposits initially found along the subendothelial and subepithelial aspects of the glomerular capillary wall [123]. Numerous large subepithelial humps are observed later in the course of the disease [129].

CHRONIC SERUM SICKNESS

Chronic immune complex glomerulonephritis may be induced in rabbits by prolonged daily administration of a heterologous protein (usually bovine serum albumin, BSA). Under these conditions several variables become important in predicting the development of glomerular injury, as not all animals so treated subsequently develop nephritogenic immune complexes. In addition, a variety of patterns of renal injury may occur, usually beginning five to eight weeks after initiation of immunization and ranging in severity from minimal disease to extensive membranous and proliferative changes, occasionally associated with necrotizing glomerulonephritis and crescent formation [97]. Immunofluorescence studies show impressive coarse granular glomerular deposits of antigen along with rabbit C3 and IgG (Fig. 13-1). The presence of numerous electron dense deposits is confirmed by electron microscopy. Unlike the rabbits with acute serum sickness, animals repeatedly

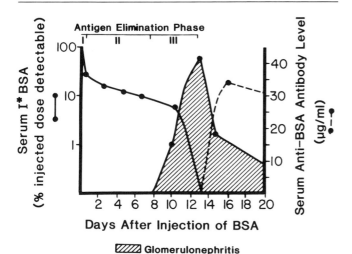

FIG. 13-11. *Diagram summarizing the fate of antigen (BSA) in rabbits with acute serum sickness (solid line). These early studies reported by Dixon et al: (Arch of Pathol 65:18, 1958) provided the key observation that glomerulonephritis did not develop until anti-BSA antibodies were produced (dashed line) associated with the appearance of immune complexes within the circulation. Following the formation of antibodies, the antigen is rapidly eliminated from the circulation (immune elimination phase III). Antigen elimination phase I represents escape of antigen from the circulation, establishing a state of equilibrium with extravascular compartments. The second phase of antigen elimination represents catabolism of the antigen.*

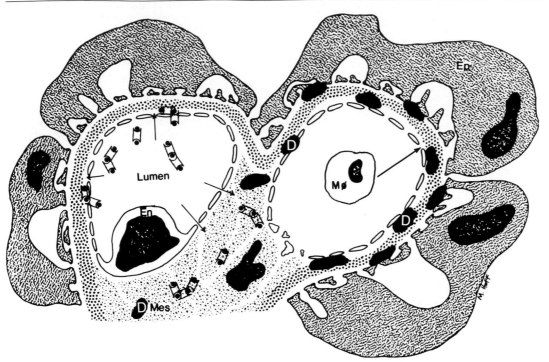

FIG. 13-12. *Schematic illustration of the pathogenesis of immune complex glomerulonephritis. Appropriately sized soluble complexes of antigen (●) and antibody (□) present within the glomerular microcirculation may become trapped within the glomerulus under the appropriate conditions. The pattern of immune complex deposition is influenced by several factors, such as immune complex size, avidity, and charge, leading to deposition of deposits within the mesangium (MES) and/or along the glomerular capillary wall in a subepithelial (Ep) and/or subendothelial (En) distribution. Within the glomerulus these complexes undergo further rearrangement, enlarging to form deposits (D) of a stable lattice structure. Once nephritogenic immune complexes stabilize within the glomerulus, they trigger a sequence of events that induce glomerular injury. Macrophages (Mø) derived from circulating blood monocytes have been shown to play an important role in this active phase of glomerular damage.*

exposed to nephritogenic immune complexes ultimately die from renal failure. Even if antigen administration is discontinued after the onset of proteinuria, only some animals show a gradual improvement, while others continue to progress and ultimately die from irreversible renal disease. As will be discussed in greater detail in the following section, the nephrotoxic potential of immune complexes is determined by several factors that ultimately dictate their size and fate. Thus, rabbits with a poor immune response remain in a state of extreme antigen excess and fail to develop glomerulonephritis [56,57,97,154,156,167,515, 516]. Animals mounting a strong antibody response are at risk of anaphylactic reactions, but those that survive develop acute glomerulonephritis resembling that seen with acute serum sickness, resolving over two to three weeks with minimal evidence of chronic pathology. It has been assumed that a large antibody response results in formation of large immune complexes that are rapidly eliminated by cells of the mononuclear phagocytic system before they can be taken up by glomeruli. Only animals that produce an intermediate amount of antibody develop chronic renal disease, presumably because small soluble immune com-

plexes are slowly cleared from the circulation and thus have prolonged exposure to the glomerular capillary system.

For reasons that are not understood, histologic lesions developing in the course of chronic serum sickness are usually confined to the kidney, whereas acute serum sickness may result in more widespread deposition of immune complexes, producing arteritis, endocarditis, synovitis, and immune deposits in the choroid plexus, in addition to glomerulonephritis [96,152,254]. However, this is not true for rabbits with a vigorous antibody response injected repeatedly to maintain a state of antigen excess. Under these circumstances, deposits of immune complexes can be found in many tissues, including the renal interstitium, lungs, heart, intestine, adrenals, choroid plexus, and spleen [8,56,57,377,379,516]. Although the renal disease of chronic serum sickness has been most extensively studied in the rabbit, glomerulonephritis has been described in rats and mice following repeated injection of a foreign protein. However, modifications in the immunization protocols are frequently necessary to establish reproducible model systems in these animals [14,45,124,235,318–320].

PASSIVE SERUM SICKNESS

Several recent studies have turned to the evaluation of passive serum sickness, usually induced in mice or rats by the administration of immune complexes preformed in vitro [67,143,147,148,208]. The value of this approach has been the ability to study the effects of a uniform population of immune complexes c. predetermined characteristics. To date, however, most work has been focused on morphological studies detailing the pattern of complex deposition, while little emphasis has been placed on whether such entrapment induces the histological and functional changes that would be anticipated in glomerulonephritis. In those few studies in which injury has been examined, the glomerular damage has often been mild and transient. It must also be cautioned that these immune complexes preformed in vitro may undergo considerable change following parenteral administration such that any conclusions made based on the original nature of the complex may be erroneous. Nonetheless, these models of passive serum sickness have expanded our understanding of factors that may be influential in the glomerular deposition of immune complexes.

OTHER EXPERIMENTAL MODELS OF IMMUNE COMPLEX GLOMERULONEPHRITIS

A role for circulating immune complexes in the induction of renal disease has been suggested in several other animal models. Participating exogenous antigens identified to date include several viruses (Table 13-5), of which chronic lymphocytic choriomeningitis infection in mice has been most extensively studied [61,189,222,363–365], and other infectious agents, including bacteria, plasmodia, shistosoma, and toxoplasma [309,339,519]. Endogenous antigens have been implicated in other situations, particularly in the model of active Heymann nephritis in which rats are immunized with the FX1A antigen prepared from the renal tubule brush border and in animals immunized with preparations of thyroglobulin [158,228,229,345,500,509].

MURINE MODELS OF SYSTEMIC LUPUS ERYTHEMATOSUS

The most striking and extensively studied spontaneous model of immune complex disease involving endogenous antigens is that which occurs in certain strains of mice— a disease that shares many features with systemic lupus erythematosus, including a fatal form of immune complex glomerulonephritis. The most thoroughly studied strain is the F1 hybrid of New Zealand Black and New Zealand White mice (NZB/NZW) F1. More recently the BXSB and MRL/1 murine strains have been reported to manifest a similar disease. The natural history and pathogenesis of the immune complex disease developing in these mice have been extensively studied and will not be reviewed in detail here, except to summarize a few salient features (reviewed in detail in references 462,463,475,477).

The renal disease involves a significant proliferative glomerulonephritis, frequently associated with inflammatory changes within the interstitium; it is the major cause of death in all strains, even though each has its own unique

Table 13-5. *Viruses associated with glomerulonephritis in animals*

Cats	Retrovirus
Dogs	Canine Adenovirus
Hamsters	SV40
Hogs	Hog Cholera
Horses	Equine Infectious Anemia
Mastomys (multi-mammate mouse)	Retrovirus
Mice	Coxsackie B, ECHO 9
	Cytomegalovirus
	Encephalomyocarditis Virus
	Lactic Dehydrogenase Virus
	Lymphocytic Choriomeningitis Virus
	Mammary Tumor Virus
	Murine Leukemia Viruses
	Polyoma
Mink	Aleutian Disease Virus

This table was based on material referenced from 339,448,519,525.

features. Morphological studies support the hypothesis that the glomerular injury is induced by immune complexes, detected by immunofluorescence as the deposition of IgG and C3 and as electron dense deposits most prominent in the mesangial zone but also present on both sides of the glomerular capillary wall (being more prominent in the subepithelial region) [11,53,236]. Elution of antibodies from diseased kidneys is fraught with technical limitations, but in most instances antibodies against native DNA have been recovered and constitute the major group of antibodies in the glomerular immune deposits [11]. However, other antibody-antigen systems also participate to a variable extent; the best characterized are those involving a glycoprotein from the envelope of the endogenous murine retrovirus (gp 70)—a virus that is normally present in all mice [214]. Based on the detection of similar immune complexes within the circulation and evidence of polyclonal B cell hyperactivity, it is widely accepted that renal injury follows the deposition of nephritogenic immune complexes. Antibody elution studies reporting that the majority of IgG anti-DNA antibodies isolated from nephritic kidneys have a high isoelectric point (pI 8.0 to 9.0) suggest that the interaction of circulating immune complexes may in part be on the basis of electrostatic binding to anionic sites within the glomerulus [92,113]. However, the report by Izui et al. [213] that isolated DNA will bind to glomerular basement membrane and collagen suggests the possibility that some of these immune deposits are formed in situ after initial trapping of DNA antigens.

The nature of the primary defect of SLE in man and in the murine models is unknown; the bulk of the evidence to date suggests that it is a syndrome rather than a single disease entity [437,462,463,477]. Studies of murine SLE have suggested that the genetic predisposition to this autoimmune disease exists in a variety of genetic backgrounds. The fundamental abnormality appears to reside in the lymphohematopoietic cells, as evidenced by the protection provided by normal bone marrow cells transferred to lethally irradiated NZB mice, whereas irradiated non-autoimmune mice reconstituted with marrows from

NZB donors developed an autoimmune state. The factor responsible for polyclonal B cell activation is still unknown and, although it is associated with a variety of abnormalities in the function of T cells and in the production of and response to certain cytokines, these abnormalities are different in the various strains of mice and may equally result from the disease process rather than be involved in its initiation. At the present time the change induced by a single factor cannot adequately explain all of the data available on the etiopathogenesis of murine SLE.

Factors Influencing Glomerular Deposition and Phlogistic Potential of Immune Complexes

It is becoming increasingly apparent that the formation of immune complexes and their subsequent entrapment within the kidney is a dynamic process undergoing constant change, so that even a minor alteration at one step will ultimately be expressed throughout the entire system. Furthermore, under normal circumstances the kidney is totally oblivious to the process of immune complex formation, even though small quantities may filter through the glomerular mesangium on a regular basis. It is only in very unusual situations that antigen-antibody complexes become trapped within the kidney and induce pathological changes in renal structure and function. Each important variable in this scheme will now be reviewed.

THE ANTIGEN

As the signal triggering the specific immune response, it is interesting that thus far the role of the antigen per se has received very little attention. Obviously, it must be immunogenic and in certain experimental models this is in part determined by the antigen dose and route of administration. The antigen must persist in the circulation in adequate concentration in order to allow antibody binding. It is now generally agreed that the size of the immune complex, as determined predominantly by the antigen to antibody ratio, is a critical factor controlling the rate of immune complex clearance [102]. The size of the antigen and the number of antigenic determinants influences this ratio [74,153,299,467]. Studies by Koyama et al. [255] of passive serum sickness in mice showed a role for antigen valency in determining the pattern of glomerular deposition of immune complexes. Immune complexes containing high valency antigens appeared in the mesangial stalk region, whereas those of low valency deposited in the glomerular capillary wall if the complexes were of low antigen to antibody ratio.

In addition, it has recently been suggested that the biochemical nature of the antigen may affect the rate of elimination of complex. Finbloom et al. [128] demonstrated that mice injected with immune complexes of identical size prepared from the same purified antibody and differing only in the presence or absence of exposed galactose sugars on the terminal side chains of the antigen were handled in very different ways following parenteral administration. It appeared that galactose receptors present on hepatocytes mediated rapid clearance of complexes with exposed galactose sugars on the antigen ($T\frac{1}{2}$-15 min), whereas the immune complexes lacking exposed galactose terminals were eliminated much more slowly by binding to Fc-receptors (i.e., antibody-dependent) on the Kupffer cells ($T\frac{1}{2} > 300$ min), suggesting that some immune complexes may be removed from the circulation through receptors specific for the antigen as well as for the antibody. Since the renal deposition of immune complexes may depend on the interaction of electrostatic charges and given that the isoelectric point of the serum immunoglobulins generally ranges between five and eight, the fate of immune complexes may be directed by the charge on the antigen, which has greater potential for variation.

Persistence of high circulating levels of antigen after the induction of renal injury may actually diminish the severity of disease. Valdes et al. [491] demonstrated that rabbits with chronic serum sickness given a large intravenous boost of antigen rapidly dissolved the glomerular deposits and healed the glomerular lesions. Subendothelial and mesangial deposits induced in mice by the passive administration of immune complexes likewise were removed following the administration of high dose antigen (human serum albumen) [301]. It has been assumed that antigen in extreme excess, as established in the above experimental models, interacts with glomerular-bound immune complexes, promoting conversion of large latticed complexes to small soluble complexes and resulting in dissolution of the antigen-antibody precipitates. Thus, the view that antigen is merely passive, serving to aggregate the biologically active Fc fragments of many antibodies and thereby accelerating interaction with complement components and leucocyte Fc receptors, underestimates the active role that antigens may play in the pathogenesis of immune complex-induced glomerulonephritis.

Unfortunately, in only a few immune complex-mediated diseases is the specific antigen known or even suspected in man. Most commonly implicated are antigens derived from micro-organisms. As reviewed in Chapter 69, this includes several bacteria and viruses, while some parasites, fungi, mycoplasma, and actinomyces are suspected occasionally. Other exogenous antigens such as certain drugs, including gold, penicillamine, sulfa compounds, mercurial salts, and trimethadione [519], toxoids, and foreign serum proteins have been associated with a clinical picture of acute serum sickness [161,212,336]. Endogenous antigens rarely have the opportunity to react with autoantibodies, but, when such a situation develops, glomerulonephritis is occasionally observed. Nuclear antigens, tumor-associated antigens [82,85,281,370,474,511], thyroglobulin [220,368,384], and immunoglobulin G (cryoglobulin for example) [24,80, 105,122,168,315,321,386,398,447) have been implicated.

ANTIBODY PRODUCTION AND IMMUNE COMPLEX FORMATION

It is generally accepted that production of the participating antibody requires an intact cellular immune system, including monocytes, T lymphocytes, and B lymphocytes. Yet, this aspect of serum sickness has been poorly studied. The nature of the antibody response—including its quantity, avidity, and affinity—all play a role in determining the physical characteristics of the immune complexes subsequently formed. Such variables ultimately determine not only the rate of removal of circulating immune complexes by the mononuclear phagocytic system, and thus susceptibility to and severity of glomerulonephritis, but also influence the site of glomerular deposition of complexes as being predominantly mesangial, subendothelial, or subepithelial. Although the class of the antibody dictates the pathway of clearance of immune complexes within the mononuclear phagocytic system, antibody class per se may not significantly influence the pattern of immune complex-induced renal injury. In studies by Border et al. [52], rabbits immunized with DNA denatured by ultraviolet light developed IgG-antiDNA antibodies and mesangial proliferative glomerulonephritis identical to that seen in rabbits immunized with heat denatured DNA that developed only IgG-antiDNA antibodies. In the majority of examples of immune complex-induced renal injury studied to date, both in experimental animals and in man, IgG rather than IgM appears to be the major antibody subclass.

The ability of soluble immune complexes formed in the circulation to become lodged within glomeruli initially depends upon the ability of such complexes to survive in the circulation for long enough periods of time and in sufficient concentrations to receive adequate exposure to the glomerular capillary network. The size of the immune complexes, as determined by the antigen to antibody ratio, predicts their circulating half-life. Large latticed complexes formed near equivalence are very efficiently cleared by the mononuclear phagocytic system and thus do not deposit in glomeruli [74,299,307]. At the other extreme, the smallest complexes containing one or two molecules of antibody are too small to be trapped and retained within glomeruli. It is now generally accepted that intermediate-sized complexes are most likely to produce glomerular deposits. Early studies by Wilson [516] and Dixon [97] of acute serum sickness in rabbits suggested that glomerulonephritis developed only in those rabbits with appreciable levels of immune complexes with sedimentation coefficients greater than 19S in sucrose gradients, that is, BSA-antiBSA complexes larger than Ag2Ab2.

The nature of the antibody response may influence immune complex size in several ways. The quantity of the antibody available is important. In studies of apoferritin-induced serum sickness in inbred mouse strains genetically disparate with respect to quantity of antibody produced, Iskander et al. [209] reported that the high antibody responders developed severe necrotizing glomerulonephritis with immune deposits initially localized to the mesangium when immunized with high doses of antigen; they developed less severe to no disease when immunized with low doses of antigen (i.e., in extreme antibody excess, complexes rapidly removed by the mononuclear phagocytic system). By contrast, the low antibody response group did not develop disease when immunized with high doses of antigen (i.e., extreme antigen excess complexes that lack propensity for tissue deposition), whereas immunization with low doses of antigen produced a glomerulopathy associated with deposits along the glomerular capillary wall. Such studies emphasize the role of the antigen-to-antibody ratio in determining nephritogenic potential.

The strength of the bond between antigen and antibody is very important in determining immune complex stability since this interaction is through reversible noncovalent forces that enable complexes to dissociate again after initial contact. The strength of this union is determined by the affinity constant for each univalent binding site. In biological systems this is often discussed in terms of the antibody avidity, that is, the summation of the strengths of interaction at the multiple potential antigen-antibody binding sites. Antibody avidity affects not only the incidence but also the pattern of the glomerular lesion. Several recent studies of serum sickness in mice have confirmed that the very low affinity antibodies produce immune complexes that deposit within the glomerular capillary wall, whereas complexes composed of high affinity antibodies lodge in the glomerular mesangium [159,160,177,210, 255,279,280] (Fig. 13-13). It must be cautioned that these studies did not control for complex charge, which is now known to influence their site of deposition, as discussed later. The persistence of poorly avid antibodies may partly explain the increased severity of glomerular injury in certain individuals [450]. In the normal situation maturation of the antibody response following exposure to a foreign protein is associated with a transition from the production of low to high affinity antibodies [156]. Induction of serum sickness in a mouse line selectively bred for its production of low affinity antibodies by repeated injection of human serum albumin produced glomerulonephritis associated with deposits in the glomerular capillary wall. Within this line, mice lacking the ability to mount an increasing antibody avidity response with time were more susceptible to severe renal disease [94,466].

It has been suggested that antibody avidity plays a role in the pattern of glomerular injury seen in patients with systemic lupus erythematosus. Patients with the membranous pattern of disease, identified by the restriction of immune complex deposition to the peripheral capillary loops in a subepithelial position, appear to be unique among patients with lupus nephritis in that their circulating antibodies to native DNA are of low avidity (i.e., nonprecipitating) [140,141]. It is interesting that these patients often have a normal serum complement profile as well. In contrast, the avidity of anti-native DNA antibodies eluted from the kidneys of four patients who died with advanced proliferative glomerulonephritis was more than tenfold higher than those obtained from the serum of patients with active glomerulonephritis [522].

Although it is widely accepted that immune complexes induce glomerulonephritis in man, a need for some healthy skepticism still exists; experimentally it has not been possible to reproduce the full spectrum of disease by infusion of preformed immune complexes into animals. This perplexing problem is most apparent for immune complexes in the subepithelial location. To date, only two experimental protocols have convincingly demonstrated subepithelial deposition of deposits. The first protocol involved the infusion of mice with egg albumin complexed with low avidity antibodies [160]. In the second effective protocol, reviewed in greater detail in a later section, preformed cationic immune complexes were identified in a subepithelial location following intravenous infusion. It is equally

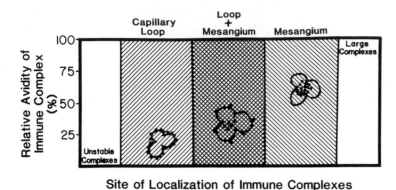

FIG. 13-13. *Schematic illustration of the influence of immune complex avidity on the site of glomerular deposition of immune complexes determined by the injection of mice with preformed soluble immune complexes. Weakly avid complexes were detected along the glomerular capillary wall. With increasing avidity a greater proportion of the immune complexes were deposited within the mesangium. Poorly avid complexes fail to form stable complexes and thus do not appear within the glomerulus. Highly avid complexes form large macromolecules, which are rapidly cleared by mononuclear phagocytes before tissue deposition can occur. (These experiments did not control for immune complex charge, which also influences the site of immune complex localization.) (Modified from Germuth et al: Lab Invest 41:360, 1979.)*

conceivable that these complexes quickly dissociated after infusion and reformed again in situ in the subepithelial space after the initial binding of the antigen in this site. Thus, the actual mechanism by which these complexes attach to the glomeruli is at present unknown and, in the final analysis, may involve both the trapping of preformed complexes and reassembly of complexes in situ [67,143, 147,148,503]. In addition, studies of circulating immune complexes in man have been very confusing since such complexes may co-exist with diseases that are not thought to be related to immune complex pathology, whereas in other situations circulating immune complexes cannot be detected in disease states that are widely accepted as immune complex in origin [89a,309].

IMMUNE COMPLEX ELIMINATION BY THE MONONUCLEAR PHAGOCYTIC SYSTEM

Immune complex induced glomerulonephritis could be considered an immunodeficiency disease that develops due to the host's inability to efficiently eliminate the offending antigen. The role of the mononuclear phagocytic system in the clearance of circulating immune complexes was clearly shown by Benacerraf in 1959 [32]. Wilson and Dixon [176] suggested that this system affords protection from nephritis through the removal of circulating immune complexes until the phagocytes become saturated, after which time glomerular damage develops. It is now clear that additional factors influence the efficiency of the mononuclear phagocytic system in the elimination of immune complexes. Some of these variables depend upon characteristics of the complexes themselves. Soluble immune complexes are removed principally by the liver, and the

rate of removal is directly proportional to the size of the complex [12,13,127,229,230]. Particulate complexes such as autologous erythrocytes sensitized with IgM are also dependent upon hepatic elimination, whereas those sensitized with IgG are removed primarily in the spleen [116,136,427]. The phagocytic uptake of immune complexes is thought to depend largely on binding of the Fc fragment present on immunoglobulin G to specific membrane receptors (FcR) present on macrophages and Kupffer cells. Similar receptors have not been described in man for the Fc portion of the IgM molecules. Immune complexes prepared with reduced and alkylated antibodies show impaired binding to Fc and C3 receptors and, when injected into mice, demonstrate decreased hepatic localization and enhanced and prolonged glomerular deposition, as compared to similar complexes made with intact antibodies [178].

Several recent clinical studies have suggested that patients with systemic lupus erythematosus have defective FcR mediated clearance of particulate immune complexes [21,181,231,493,494]. Frank et al. [137] reported that the clearance of autologous erythrocytes sensitized with the non-complement-fixing IgG anti-RhD was defective in patients with SLE and that the degree of abnormality correlated with clinical disease activity and the level of detectable circulating immune complexes. Parris et al. [374] reported that this defect in FcR-mediated splenic clearance was more marked in patients with renal disease. At the present time the nature of this defect is controversial, although it does not appear to be on the basis of a primary genetic defect. Some studies have suggested that the defect is due to decreased numbers of available Fc receptors, which could be due to either decreased receptor expression or to competitive inhibition by autoantibodies or soluble immune complexes. It has recently been suggested by Fries et al. [142] and Salmon et al. [414], based on studies with peripheral blood monocytes, that the number of FcR is actually increased rather than decreased and that the functional defect appears to be on the basis of an abnormality in the actual mechanisms of phagocytosis once the complexes are receptor-bound. However, it should be restated that these studies have been done with particulate antigens and that a defective clearance of soluble immune clearances, such as those considered pathogenic in SLE, has not been described.

Lymphohemopoietic cells and phagocytes also carry membrane receptors for several of the complement components [399,429]. However, until recently it had been thought that complement and its receptors did not play a role in the clearance of soluble immune complexes; this is probably true for non-primate animals. The clearance of soluble complexes such as aggregated IgG is not altered in rabbits [12,75], rats [390], or mice [330] depleted of complement by cobra venom factor. However, Cornacoff et al. [81] recently studied the clearance of BSA anti-BSA complexes injected into baboons and rhesus monkeys and showed that these complexes rapidly bind to erythrocytes and are subsequently removed by the liver. It has been proposed that such binding is complement-dependent, occurring through the erythrocyte receptor for C3b (CR1), and that, as such, this mechanism represents an adaptation of primates, which are the only animals with large numbers of C3b receptors on erythrocytes. In this situation, baboons depleted of complement show decreased binding of complexes to erythrocytes and increased deposition of immune complexes in sites outside the mononuclear phagocytic system [507]. An increased fractional uptake of immune complexes by the kidney was not detected in that study. Quantitative studies of the erythrocyte CR1 in humans with systemic lupus erythematosus have shown decreased receptor numbers that Wilson et al. [206,334,520,521] conclude to be a primary genetic defect inherited in an autosomal co-dominant manner. It is unclear whether such an abnormality is involved in the pathogenesis of disease or whether it simply represents a disease marker. Such studies deserve further attention and raise the important possibility that the function of the mononuclear phagocytic system may be unique in primates, an observation that cautions against liberal extrapolation from experimental models to man.

Several studies have reported that manipulations of the mononuclear phagocytic system affect the number of immune complexes deposited in glomeruli. Decreased glomerular uptake is observed following stimulation of mice with endotoxin [134] or corynebacterium [23], rats with zymosan [390], and guinea pigs with BCG [17]. In contrast, the depression of the systemic macrophage system induced in mice by the intravenous injection of colloidal carbon has been associated with increased glomerular deposition of immune complexes [134]. Paswell et al. [376] reported that inbred strains of mice with depressed phagocytic activity, as measured by the rate of clearance of carbon, were those strains most susceptible to immune complex disease.

GLOMERULAR HEMODYNAMICS AND PERMEABILITY

The kidney is the organ that suffers most from immune complex pathology; explanations for this have included a possible role of hemodynamic factors, such as the high renal blood flow and transcapillary hydrostatic pressure gradient. The severity of serum sickness in rabbits is increased in the presence of systemic hypertension [130,513]. Progression of glomerular damage is diminished in spontaneously hypertensive rats suffering from ferritin-anti-ferritin immune complex nephritis when compared to Dahl salt-sensitive hypertensive rats with similar nephritis [391]. The difference between these two rat models is that the spontaneously hypertensive rats develop pre-renal vasoconstriction, which thus appears to offer protection from the injurious effects of intrarenal hypertension observed in the Dahl rats. Other evidence that hemodynamic factors play a role include the observation that the vascular lesions of serum sickness are more severe at sites of vascular bifurcations [249,250], decreased glomerular filtration rate decreases glomerular immune complex deposition [155], and renal artery stenosis protects the kidney in immune complex disease [371]. The administration of angiotensin II to rats has been shown to result in an increase in mesangial sequestration of macromolecules, presumably due to the changes in the glomerular microcirculation and permeability induced by this hormone [461].

Factors leading to an increase in the permeability of the glomerular capillary wall might be expected to increase the deposition of immune complexes. Vasoactive amines were first shown to play such a role by Benacerraf in 1959 [31]. Injection of vasoactive amines into mice increased the glomerular deposition of circulating colloidal carbon. The additional observation that the passive administration of immune complexes had a similar effect suggested that the formation of circulating immune complexes in vivo might trigger the release of endogenous amines and thereby promote vascular deposition of immune complexes. Since these early observations, attempts to elucidate the exact role of endogenous vasoactive amines in immune complex nephritis have been very complicated. In rabbits with acute serum sickness, immune reactions simultaneously trigger IgE-mediated release from basophils of histamine and platelet-activating factor, the latter initiating release of additional amines from platelets. Antagonists of histamine and serotonin have no effect in chronic serum sickness in rabbits and passive serum sickness in mice [519].

ROLE OF IMMUNE COMPLEX CHARGE

The role of the glomerular capillary wall as a charge selective filtration barrier repelling anionic and attracting cationic molecules may be important in renal immunopathology as well as renal physiology. The influence of glomerular anionic charges on the binding and persistence of immune complexes has just recently received attention, but certain observations made to date are worthy of review. In studies of passive serum sickness in mice using complexes of predetermined charge, it has been suggested that electrochemical interactions influence the site of glomerular deposition of antigen-antibody complexes (summarized in Table 13-6). Of note is the observation that cationic com-

TABLE 13-6. *Passive serum sickness—influence of antigen charge*

Animal	Immune Complex (IC)	Charge	Predominant Location of Immune Deposits			Reference
			Mesangial	Subendothelial	Subepithelial	
1) Mice	BGG-anti-BGG*	i) cationic IC		+	+	Gallo [143]
		ii) anionic IC	−	−	−	
2) Mice	HSA-anti-HSA**	i) cationic Ab	+ (14 days)	+ (12 hr–72 hr)	+ (14 days)	Gauthier [147]
3) Mice	Dextran-IgA Antidextran	i) small cationic IC	±	+		Isaacs [208]
		ii) large cationic IC	±			
		iii) neutral IC	+			
		iv) anionic IC	+			
4) Mice	Nondissociating BGG-anti-BGG	i) cationic IC	+	+	+	Caulin-Glaser [67]
		ii) cationic Ag	+	+	+	
		iii) native IC	+	−	−	
		iv) anionic IC	±	−	−	
5) Mice	HSA-anti-HSA	i) native IC	+			Gauthier [148]
		ii) anionic Ab	+			
		iii) cationic Ag	+	+ (1–48 hr)	+ (3–14 days)	

* BGG-Bovine gamma globuline
** HSA-Human serum albumen

plexes may form electron dense deposits in the subepithelial space, a situation that more recently has been considered secondary to the formation of immune complexes in situ. Indeed, the sequential studies of Gauthier et al. [148], using preformed complexes of cationic antigens, raise the possibility that complexes initially trapped in the subendothelial region may dissociate and reassociate again in a subepithelial position after electrostatic attraction of the cationic antigen to anionic sites in the lamina rara externa. However, studies by Caulin-Glaser et al. [67] involving the passive administration of non-dissociating complexes have shown that cationic complexes can cross the glomerular capillary wall intact to form subepithelial deposits. The charge and the size of immune complexes work together to influence the site of glomerular localization, as shown by studies of Isaacs et al. [208], in which small cationic complexes accumulated in the mesangium. Despite the presence of anionic sites within the mesangium, anionic immune complexes have been reported to deposit there occasionally. It is noteworthy that the rate of clearance of immune complexes by the mononuclear phagocytic system may be influenced by charge [150]. At this point it is important to caution that conclusions drawn from studies of passive serum sickness must take into consideration that complex charge may become altered and complexes may dissociate following infusion and before glomerular deposition.

Studies of active serum sickness induced by antigens of variable charge are somewhat confusing, as it is difficult to know whether the charge is influencing the antibody response or the net charge of the immune complex formed, or indeed whether it is being trapped within the kidney eliciting in situ immune complex formation. However, studies to date have suggested that cationic antigens induce more nephrotoxic immune responses than neutral or anionic antigens. This was demonstrated by Border et al. [51] in rabbits injected with BSA of predetermined charge and by Gallo et al. [144] who studied the response in mice following the intravenous administration of preparations of bovine gamma globulin of varying charge (Fig. 13-14). Both groups of investigators observed the formation of deposits in the subepithelial region only with cationic antigens.

Immunization of experimental animals with polysaccharides has generally been ineffective in producing glomerulonephritis. However, a study by Isaacs et al. [207] reported that mice injected with dextrans develop glomerulonephritis associated with the deposition of IgA-containing immune complexes. Although the pattern of glomerular injury was influenced by the charge and size of the antigen, subepithelial deposits could not be produced either by passive administration of cationic complexes or by active immunization with cationic dextran antigen.

IN SITU MODIFICATION OF IMMUNE COMPLEXES

Immune complexes lodged within glomeruli remain for relatively short periods of time unless they undergo further rearrangement, enlarging their lattice structure (to the point where they are generally detectable by electron microscopy) and thus stabilizing the complex [7,135,302]. Thereafter, these complexes become considerably more difficult to eliminate. At the present time it is unclear whether small immune complexes transiently deposited in the glomeruli are able to induce inflammatory changes. Alteration of the lattice structure requires the participation of precipitating antigen-antibody systems and the alteration of bonds between the antigens and antibodies. Mannik et

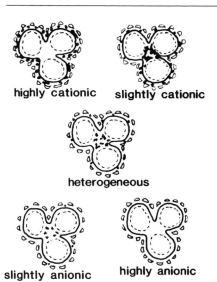

highly cationic   slightly cationic

heterogeneous

slightly anionic   highly anionic

Fig. 13-14. *Schematic illustration of the influence of immunogen (bovine gamma globulin) charge on the pattern of glomerular deposition of immune complexes (represented as closed circles). Highly cationic immunogen (pI 9.5–11.5) deposits along the subepithelial aspect of the GBM (solid black line) possibly attracted to this locale, which is rich in anionic sites, due to electrostatic forces. In contrast, a highly anionic immunogen (pI 2.0–5.0) fails to deposit within the glomerulus. Heterogenous or weakly charged immunogens are detected along the GBM and within the mesangium. (Modified from Gallo et al: Lab Invest 48:353, 1983, with permission.)*

al. [302] have shown that covalently cross-linked immune complexes (i.e., complexes of fixed lattice structure) injected into mice fail to persist in glomeruli as well as non-cross-linked complexes. In the latter situation the electron dense deposits persisting in the mesangium were shown to be larger than the original complexes administered, supporting the theory that lattice enlargement is involved in complex stabilization.

Changes in the immune complex structure may involve the participation of several additional components from the circulation other than the original immunogen and its antibodies. The immune response usually involves polyclonal B cell activation; thus, a heterogeneous group of antibodies participate. The addition of antibodies of increasing affinity may provide further stability to the complex. The fixation of complement components to immune deposits is frequently observed by immunofluorescence studies [129]. The entire immune complex may act as a planted antigen encouraging the participation of other antibody systems. Likely candidates include rheumatoid factors, which are IgG and IgM antibodies reactive with antigenic determinants on the Fc domain of IgG, anti-idiotypic antibodies reactive with antigenic determinants unique to the variable region of the Fab portion of a given antibody [169,533], and immunoconglutinins, IgM antibodies binding to sites on activated fragments of C3 and C4 [309].

In other situations subsequent modifications of the early immune deposits lead to their diminution and elimination.

Under conditions of extreme antigen excess, the complexes may solubilize [179,301,482,491]. Complement fixation may actually accelerate the elimination of glomerular immune complexes. Bartolotti et al. [25] have reported that decomplemented rabbits with acute serum sickness show a significantly decreased rate of clearance of glomerular immune complexes as compared to normocomplementemic controls. These studies may reflect the role of the alternative complement pathway in solubilization of immune complexes, as demonstrated by Nussenzweig et al. [91,331]. It is clear that immune deposits may move from their original site of deposition. Occasionally, such changes are involved in the stabilization of complexes, but at other times it represents passage of complexes through mesangial channels, leading to their egress at the vascular pole. Removal of immune complexes by mesangial phagocytosis is at present a point of controversy [298,326]. Mesangial cells are able to internalize a variety of substances, but their role in the clearance of immune complexes is uncertain, since recent studies of acute serum sickness have suggested that the phagocytic clearance is accomplished primarily by monocytes infiltrating the glomeruli.

SECONDARY MEDIATORS OF IMMUNE COMPLEX-INITIATED GLOMERULAR INJURY

Once nephritogenic immune complexes stabilize within the glomerulus, it is presumed that they trigger a sequence of events that induce glomerular inflammation. There is no direct evidence that immune complexes per se produce renal injury. Polymorphonuclear leucocytes do not appear to contribute to the glomerular hypercellularity of acute serum sickness, and their depletion by nitrogen mustard does not alter the course of disease, supporting the concept that glomerulonephritis in these models is independent of polymorphonuclear leukocytes. Although complement proteins are frequently detected in the glomerular bound immune deposits, there is no evidence that complement participates directly in the glomerular inflammation, since complement depletion with cobra venom factor does not render protection or alter mononuclear cell infiltation or proteinuria [76]. However, both complement and polymorphonuclear leucotyes are required for the production of the extrarenal vasculitis of acute serum sickness [248].

Marrow-derived monocytes are emerging as the critical mediator of immune complex induced renal damage (summarized in Table 13-7). Not only have monocytes been shown to contribute substantially to the glomerular hypercellularity, but their infiltration peaks at the time of immune elimination and onset of proteinuria, and depletion of macrophages with antimacrophage serum largely prevents glomerular hypercellularity and proteinuria. Such observations strengthen the concept that infiltration of monocytes plays a key role in the production of the inflammatory changes of renal disease in serum sickness.

Why monocytes accumulate in the glomerulus is unknown. It is possibly on the basis of immune adherence to Fc fragments of the participating antibodies or binding to activated C3 components, although immune complexes made of reduced and alkylated antibodies that are unable to bind to Fc or C3 receptors appear to be equally effective

TABLE 13-7. *Participation of monocytes in serum sickness*

Animal	Model	Glomerular Preparation		Identification		Comments	Reference
		Tissue section	Cell culture	EM	Histochemical		
1) Rabbit	Acute	+		+			Sano [415]
2) Mice	Passive	+		+		—giant lysosomes of Chediak-Higashi mice identified infiltrating monocytes	Striker [468]
3) Rabbit	Acute	+		+	+	—pulse labelling quantitated role of cell division as small	Hunsicker [203]
4) Rabbit	Acute & Chronic	+	+	+	+		Holdsworth [192]
5) Rabbit	Acute	+	+	+		—disease abrogation by anti-macrophage serum	Holdsworth [193]
6) Rabbit	Acute	+		+		—attenuation of disease with anti-macrophage serum	Lavelle [271]
7) Rabbit	Chronic	+	+	+	+		Becker [30]

in the induction of monocytic infiltration [178]. In addition, complement depletion does not inhibit monocytic infiltration, suggesting that binding to C3 receptors does not play a role in this process. The role of other potentially chemotactic factors, cellular adhesion molecules, or a direct monocytic response to glomerular alterations associated with immune complex deposition has not been well examined. Other work suggests the possibility that monocytic infiltration may be a manifestation of cellular rather than humoral immunity under the direction of sensitized T-lymphocytes in a delayed-type hypersensitivity reaction. Bhan et al. [38] have reported that lymphocytes, presensitized to immune complex components, which were passively transferred to rats 24 hours after they received intravenous immune complexes that had become deposited in the mesangium, resulted in an influx of monocytes 48 hours after the time of cell transfer. The production of acute serum sickness in rabbits treated with cyclosporine resulted in the usual glomerular deposition of immune complexes, but hypercellularity was inhibited and proteinuria profoundly decreased [350]. Cyclosporine has no known direct effects on the function of B cells or monocytes, but is thought to act preferentially on proliferating T cells, suggesting that inhibition of a delayed-type hypersensitivity reaction prevented the glomerular inflammation of acute serum sickness in that study. In the model of experimental glomerulonephritis associated with infection of rabbits with *Trypanosoma rhodesiense*, monocytic infiltration and glomerular injury clearly precedes the formation of electron dense deposits, again suggesting that humoral and cellular responses may be discordant [343].

Cellular Immune Mechanisms of Initiation of Glomerular Disease

The exciting possibility that T-lymphocytes may participate in the induction of glomerular injury in a delayed-type hypersensitivity (DTH) reaction is gaining momentum in the field of renal immunopathology. However, it must be cautioned at the outset that at the present time there is no direct proof that such mechanisms play a role in man. Historically it has been assumed that the integrity of the cellular immune system was necessary only because of the role it played in regulating the production of the antibodies that are involved in humorally mediated renal diseases. However, there are a variety of human glomerular diseases, particularly those of a primary and chronic nature, for which evidence of humorally mediated injury is completely lacking.

As long ago as 1951, Jones [219] concluded that invading mononuclear cells were present in the glomeruli of patients dying of acute post-streptococcal glomerulonephritis and that these cells actively participate in the renal damage. With the improvement in techniques available for the evaluation of tissue obtained from human renal biopsies, pathologists indeed have become impressed with the observation that glomerular hypercellularity is not entirely explained on the basis of the proliferation of endogenous cells but that it is partly accounted for by the infiltration of monuclear cells. This occasioned the need to critically evaluate the role of this cellular infiltrate and for the first time to consider the possibility that the glomerular influx of mononuclear cells could in some situations be the result of cell-mediated immune reactions, such as one sees in the dermis when a pre-sensitized lymphocyte is exposed to BCG antigen. The question has now been carried one step further, asking if sensitized T-lymphocytes themselves can be directly cytotoxic to the glomerulus, either in an antibody-dependent reaction (antibody-dependent cell-mediated cytotoxicity), antibody-independent fashion (cytotoxic T-cell mediated cytolysis), or through the release of toxic lymphokines.

Indirect evidence consistent with a role for lymphocytic involvement first appeared several years ago, beginning with the study of Bendixen in 1968 [34] designed to evaluate in vitro the reactivity of human peripheral blood lymphocytes to glomerular antigens. The basis of this and subsequent studies was the quantitation of either lymphocyte proliferation or the release of macrophage migration inhibition factor on exposure of lymphocytes to glomerular antigens. This approach led to the conclusion that cellular sensitization to GBM antigens was detectable in some patients with glomerulonephritis, especially those with anti-GBM antibodies but also in some patients thought to have immune complex glomerulonephritis. Patients with active renal disease or progressive proliferative glomerulonephritis had more significant cellular reactivity than patients with inactive disease, and, as reported by Fillet et al. [125], this reactivity was more apparent if the GBM had been chemically modified with glycosidase (perhaps analogous to GBM changes induced by inflammation) before its use as an antigen. However, these positive lymphocyte assays by no means prove that these cells contributed to glomerular damage in vivo, but they provided some of the background that led to studies designed to explore a possible role for DTH in experimental glomerulonephritis.

More direct evidence that cell-mediated mechanisms can induce glomerular inflammation was obtained in the experiments of Bhan et al. [37,38], in which small quantities of antigen at subnephritic doses of anti-GBM antibody or soluble immune complexes were passively administered and fixed within glomeruli, following which lymphocytes were transferred from syngeneic donor rats that had been presensitized to the same antigen. The glomerular binding of the initial "antigen" was shown not to produce detectable glomerular injury; subsequent to lymphocyte transfer, glomerular hypercellularity and occasional foci of necrosis developed. These authors concluded that the sensitized lymphocytes interacted with the foreign antigen planted in the glomerulus and initiated a DTH reaction leading to mononuclear cell infiltration. In more recent work, these authors suggested that the antigen need not actually be fixed within the glomerulus but may react with sensitized lymphocytes while it is still in the circulation, in which case the subsequent accumulation of cells within glomeruli might be induced by release of lymphokine [39].

In an avian model of experimental glomerulonephritis, Bolton et al. [49] eliminated humoral immunity almost completely by bursectomizing chickens with cyclophosphamide. Immunization with bovine GBM produced a severe proliferative glomerulonephritis, identical to that seen in chickens with an intact humoral immune system, even though the chickens failed to develop linear deposits of IgG along the GBM, as seen in the control animals. The bursectomized chickens were shown to have an intact cellular immune system, thus favoring the hypothesis that this was the mediator system responsible for the induction of glomerulonephritis. The components of this system were not fully characterized, but the authors were unable to demonstrate glomerular infiltration by monocytes or lymphocytes, thus suggesting that the glomerular hypercellularity represented proliferation of intrinsic glomerular cells. This study raises important questions regarding our current belief that the presence of antibodies along the GBM supports the conclusion that humoral mechanisms are responsible for the inflammatory changes observed.

A few additional observations suggest that T-lymphocytes could be involved in glomerular damage: Removal of T cells by total lymphoid irradiation [476] or short-term thoracic duct drainage [460] has beneficial effects in various types of glomerulonephritis; nude mice chronically injected with human GBM fail to develop the nephropathy seen in normal mice [47]; and cannulation of renal lymph in dogs injected with nephrotoxic serum reveals early changes in the lymphocyte population leaving the kidney, consisting of their enlargement and evidence of mitoses suggesting lymphocyte activation [146]. It seems most reasonable that many of the immune-mediated diseases are the result of collaboration between humoral and cell-mediated mechanisms.

The kidney has traditionally been considered an innocent bystander, suffering the consequences of various pathological immune reactions. There is reason to consider that this may be incorrect and that under certain circumstances cells resident within the glomerulus may demonstrate immune competence. Such a suggestion comes largely from the work of Schreiner et al. [431,432], who have demonstrated the presence of a second population of cells resident within the mesangium of normal rats that appear to represent bone marrow-derived mononuclear phagocytes of the glomerulus. This subpopulation accounts for 1% to 2% of the mesangial cells; bears Ia antigens, that is, membrane proteins encoded in the immune response gene region of the histocompatibility locus (counterpart of the HLA class II antigens in man); has phagocytic ability; and is able to stimulate sensitized syngeneic lymphocytes. Unfortunately, a similar cell population has not yet been identified in the normal human glomerulus, although here the evaluation is considerably more difficult due to the presence of Ia antigens on normal endothelial cells of the glomerular and peritubular capillaries [183,185,188,348].

In discussing the lines of evidence suggestive of DTH reactions in renal disease, it seems appropriate to end with a discussion of the idiopathic nephrotic syndrome in man. Although the pathogenesis of this disease is unknown, Shaloub [440] proposed in 1974 that it was a manifestation of T cell dysfunction that released a lymphokine toxic to "an immunologically innocent GBM." He proposed such a hypothesis based on several clinical observations, including that remissions can be induced by rubeola, which is known to suppress cell-mediated immunity; response to therapy with immunosuppressant drugs, including corticosteroids and alkylating agents; occurrence of the syndrome in Hodgkin's disease; and lack of evidence to support activation of humoral immunity. To this list can now be added the occurrence of minimal lesion nephrotic syndrome in two patients with thymoma [387,497] and five patients treated with recombinant leucocyte interferon A [18,258,439(a)]. Studies of peripheral blood lymphocytes obtained from these patients have shown a variety of immunological abnormalities (reviewed in 322). In addition, Bolton-Jones et al. cultured lymphocytes obtained from patients with nephrotic syndrome and infused the culture supernatant into the renal artery of rats, thereby producing partial fusion of epithelial cell podocytes and a decrease in glomerular anionic charge sites [55]. Nonetheless, at the present time there is still no conclusive evidence that cellular immune mechanisms play a role in the pathogenesis of idiopathic nephrotic syndrome.

Secondary Mediators of Renal Injury

Following the primary immunopathogenic event that initiates renal disease, a series of secondary mechanisms are activated that contribute directly to the process of glomerular inflammation. Proof that such pathways are critically involved in the generation of renal damage stems largely from observations in experimental animals who were made deficient or inactive with respect to the biological activity of the effector system in question. It should be noted that most of these models have been focused on the short-term effects of depletion, and less information is available for chronic disease.

Polymorphonuclear Leucocytes

The polymorphonuclear leucocyte (PMN) was the first cell given recognition for its role in the pathogenesis of glomerulonephritis. Studies of the heterologous phase of nephrotoxic serum nephritis demonstrated that glomerular hypercellularity and proteinuria could be abrogated by prior PMN depletion. In addition, the PMN accumulation required the presence of an intact complement cascade, with generation of chemotaxins from the cleavage of C3 and C5 thought to be responsible for the subsequent recruitment of PMN. As summarized in the section on nephrotoxic serum nephritis (acute or homologous phase), the PMN-complement dependent mechanisms of renal injury have gained wide acceptance. However, under certain experimental conditions it appears that PMN-complement independent mechanisms may be more directly responsible for the glomerular inflammation of nephrotoxic serum nephritis. The PMN has a role to play in the production of glomerular damage during the autologous phase of nephrotoxic serum nephritis and in the accelerated model in the rabbit (where their accumulation is independent of complement), but the PMN does not appear to contribute to renal injury in acute serum sickness or Heymann nephritis [63]. In fact, with the recent interest in the role of monocytes, there has been a relative decline in additional explorations of the actual role of the PMN. However, it should not be forgotten that in several forms of human glomerulonephritis the presence of PMNs within the glomeruli may be very conspicuous.

Monocytes

Substantial evidence has accumulated in the last few years, initially from the studies of human renal biopsies and more recently in experimental renal disease, that monocytes can accumulate within the glomerulus and contribute significantly to the hypercellularity of glomerulonephritis [126] (Fig. 13-15). Numerous reports are available in the recent literature reporting the presence of monocytes in several types of acute and chronic proliferative glomerulonephritis in man [15,16,184,219,221,266,293,294,337,338,373,

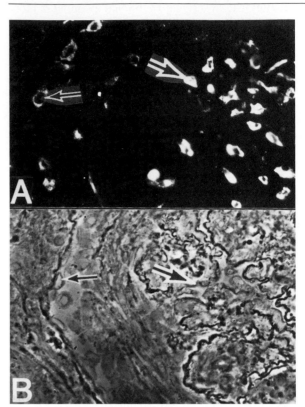

FIG. 13-15. *Immunofluorescence photomicrograph demonstrating the presence of monocytes infiltrating the glomerular tuft (large arrow) and crescent (small arrow) in a patient with acute post-streptococcal glomerulonephritis (A). The monocytes are identified by reactivity with monoclonal antibody MN-41, which identifies the CR3 receptor [112]. The phase contrast photomicrograph of the corresponding glomerulus helps to localize the reactive cells (B).*

417,423,442,451]. Using a variety of morphological, histochemical, and immunohistochemical techniques, monocytic accumulation has been impressive in the early phase of acute proliferative glomerulonephritis, in cryoglobulinemia, diffuse proliferative lupus glomerulonephritis, chronic proliferative glomerulonephritis (especially if associated with subendothelial deposits), and in early crescentic glomerulonephritis. In these studies, monocytes have been conspicuously absent in mesangiocapillary glomerulonephritis type I (with subendothelial deposits) and in IgA nephropathy. The detection of monocytes, however, does not in and of itself provide proof that they are important in the pathogenesis of damage. Indeed, even today there is considerable controversy as to whether the predominant role of the glomerular-bound monocyte is one of destruction or more of a phagocytic scavenger attempting to remove immune reactants, thus initiating a healing process.

Certain experimental evidence is convincing that monocytes can be injurious to the kidney and can help to initiate proteinuria, as first suggested by the work of Schreiner et al. in 1978 [430] in an accelerated model of nephrotoxic serum nephritis and Hunsicker et al. [203] in 1979 in acute serum sickness. Additional work supporting a role for monocytes in mediating glomerulonephritis was reviewed earlier in sections discussing anti-GBM nephritis and immune complex nephritis.

It should be remembered that monocytes have another vital function, namely the induction of immune responses by the processing and presentation of antigen to T-lymphocytes in a genetically restricted fashion. This limb of monocyte function has not been explored in detail with respect to renal disease, but a very recent observation in BXSB mice (murine SLE model) may prove interesting. These mice undergo a progressive and dramatic increase in their peripheral monocyte count beginning at two months of age, so that by six months more than 50% of the circulating mononuclear cells are monocytes and, in some animals, they account for 90% of this cell population [524]. A progressive monocytosis was not detected in the other murine models of SLE (NZB/NZW and MRL/1 mice), leading the authors to conclude that this change might be a clue to the fundamental defect initiating the autoimmune disease of the BXSB mice rather than a secondary effect of the autoimmune process.

Convinced of the potentially important role of monocytes, several important questions follow regarding the recruitment of monocytes and the way in which they induce renal damage. Although several options exist for this multifunctional cell, neither of these issues has been resolved. A variety of mechanisms may recruit monocytes into the glomerulus. (1) Monocytes carry surface receptors for various complement components, suggesting that they might bind to immune reactants that have fixed complement. However, in experimental models of anti-GBM nephritis (autologous phase) and serum sickness nephritis, monocyte accumulation was not affected by decomplementation [76,479]. Striker et al. [468] demonstrated in the model of passively induced immune complex nephritis that renal lesions of equal severity developed whether the complexes were prepared with either intact antibodies or reduced and alkylated antibodies that are unable to effectively fix complement.

(2) Monocyte surface receptors for the Fc fragment of IgG (FcR) could provide a basis for interaction with antibodies bound to the glomerulus. Studies by Holdsworth [194] using the F(ab')$_2$ fragment of sheep anti-rabbit GBM antibody in a passive model of the autologous phase of anti-GBM nephritis demonstrated that monocytic infiltration and the development of proteinuria were dependent on the availability of intact antibody carrying Fc fragments.

(3) Monocytic infiltration may be a nonspecific inflammatory response to cellular injury within the glomerulus. For example, monocytes bind in vitro to a variety of non-immune macromolecules, including fibronectin, collagen, and vimentin, all of which are present normally within the glomerulus and may potentially become exposed during the induction of glomerulonephritis [287]. Dubois et al. [107] demonstrated in vitro binding of rat monocytes to cultured normal mesangial cells in a reaction that suggested the involvement of Fc receptors and fibronectin. Monocyte surface adhesion molecules that mediate binding to matrix proteins are just now being defined. Other non-identified products of glomerular inflammation may prove to be chemotactic to monocytes. The recently described monocyte chemo attractant protein is one example. In studies of nephrotoxic nephritis by Thomson et al. [480], fibrin was shown to be involved in the recruitment of monocytes into crescents. The following sequence was observed by electron microscopy: Subsequent to the disruption of a capillary loop, fibrin appeared within Bowman's space, followed by migration of macrophages from the glomerular tuft into this space, where they were observed to phagocytose fibrin, transform into epitheloid cells, and assume residence within the developing crescent.

(4) As discussed in the previous section, monocytic infiltration may be a manifestation of cell-mediated immunity in a reaction driven by lymphokines that attract and activate monocytes. Recall that in the classical delayed-type hypersensitivity reaction observed in the skin, the cellular infiltrate is composed largely of mononuclear cells, of which a significant number have been identified as monocytes [383].

Unraveling the effector pathways of monocyte-associated renal injury is a challenging process since this cell has an enormous number of potential activities, including (1) release of a variety of enzymes, including collagenase, elastase, other proteases, lysosomal enzymes and protease inhibitors [433,473]; (2) secretion of certain coagulation and plasminogen activators; (3) synthesis of plasma proteins, including components of the complement cascade; (4) release of factors known to influence other cells, including platelet activating factor [381], angiogenesis factor responsible for the induction of endothelial proliferation [385], interferon, and interleukin-1 (the latter is a polypeptide that not only stimulates B and T lymphocytes but has been shown to enhance the proliferation of rat mesangial cells in culture), and peptide growth factors such as transforming growth factor beta, fibroblast growth factor, and platelet-derived growth factor [289]; (5) production of prostaglandins; (6) secretion of toxic free oxygen radicals (acute glomerular injury following the intrarenal administration of the anti-GBM antibody can be significantly reduced by the simultaneous injection of catalase, which converts H_2O_2 to O_2 and H_2O; although the oxygen radicals are most likely derived from PMNs in this particular model, monocytes can also release oxygen radicals, supporing a role for oxygen products as mediators of renal injury.) [395]; (7) release of a variety of cationic proteins with the potential for electrostatic binding to anionic glomerular charge sites [65]. Thus, it is reasonable to conclude that the infiltration of glomeruli by monocytes from the circulation is a significant component of the hypercellularity in many types of "proliferative" glomerulonephritis and is almost certainly a major factor in the pathogenesis of these diseases.

Resident Glomerular Cells

An adequate review of the role of resident glomerular cells in the mediation of glomerular injury is beyond the scope of this chapter. The reader is referred to an appended list of updated references at the end of this chapter.

The mesangial cell population expands in many varieties of proliferative glomerulonephritis. Not only the expansion of its volume but also its contractile capabilities may be detrimental to renal function by effecting a decrease in the capillary surface area available for filtration. In addition, evidence is slowly accumulating to suggest that activated mesangial cells have the potential to participate in an inflammatory process within the glomerulus. Mesangial cells in culture have been shown to synthesize prostaglandins, a variety of lysosomal enzymes, interleukin-1, and oxygen free radicals, and to have the ability to phagocytose certain macromolecules [27,62,95,261,288,418]. The recent detection of a small subpopulation of mesangial cells that appear to be immune-competent bone marrow-derived macrophages has been reviewed in an earlier section.

The visceral epithelial cells of the human glomerulus possess membrane receptors for C3b [149], possibly for the Fc fragment of IgG [335,434], and share antigenic determinants in common with lymphohemopoietic cells of the B-lymphocyte lineage [382]. The function and significance of these epithelial markers is unknown. Glomerular epithelial cells have demonstrated the ability to endocytose certain macromolecules [436] and are known to synthesize derivatives of arachadonic acid [261].

Studies of the functional potential of glomerular endothelial cells have been limited by the fact that these cells have been difficult to isolate and maintain in culture [469]. Human glomerular endothelial cells are known to possess membrane proteins encoded by the HLA-D locus of the histocompatibility complex (analogous to Ia antigens). Until recently endothelial cells were thought to play a passive role in glomerular injury, but newer studies strongly contradict this notion. As one example, it has recently been shown that following fixation of antibody (in a model of antibody-mediated hyperacute vascular rejection), platelet activating factor is rapidly released from the target endothelial cell, suggesting that under certain circumstances these cells may play a more active role in glomerular disease [211]. Aided by the ability to isolate and culture relatively pure subpopulations of glomerular cells, future studies will no doubt expand our understanding of their biological functions and help to clarify potential mechanisms that might contribute directly to glomerular injury.

Complement

Following the binding of an antibody to specific antigens, either fixed in tissues or present in the circulation, the complement system may be activated. The complement cascade is composed of 21 plasma proteins (13 components and eight regulatory proteins), which can be subdivided into three operational units—the classical and alternative recognition pathways that activate different early components and a common terminal unit leading to the generation of the membrane attack complex (summarized in Fig. 13-16) [247,340]. Immune complexes composed of IgG or IgM usually activate complement by way of the classical pathway; however, it has been shown that complexes of guinea pig IgG_1 or aggregates of human IgA or IgE may

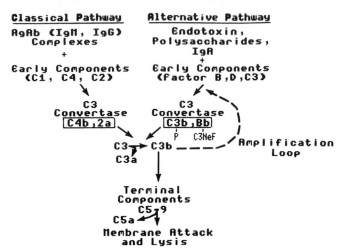

FIG. 13-16. Schematic representation of the complement cascade. The classical pathway is composed of 11 serum proteins (C1–C9) and is most commonly activated by immune complexes or aggregates of IgM or IgG. The alternative pathway bypasses the early components (C1, C4, C2) but involves the participation of two serum proteins, factors B and D. An additional component, properidin (P), stabilizes the alternative pathway convertase, thus playing an important role in the amplication loop of complement activation. The autoantibody C3 nephritic factor (C_3NeF) similarly reacts with and stabilizes the alternative pathway C3 convertase. The two pathways converge at C3 to share a common terminal effector pathway, which results in cell destruction. For simplicity, the regulatory proteins of the complement cascade are not illustrated. (Modified from Gilliland, In Harrison's Principles of Internal Medicine, 10th ed., 1982.)

trigger the alternative pathway. In certain situations the classical pathway may also be activated by antibody-independent substrates such as RNA tumor viruses, vesicular stomatitis virus, DNA, C-reactive protein, certain endotoxins, and monosodium urate crystals. In most situations the alternative pathway is activated independently of immunoglobulin by interaction with substances such as plant, fungal, or bacterial polysaccharides (endotoxin, zymosan, inulin, for example), and by some viruses and gram-negative bacteria.

At the present time the role of complement as a direct mediator of renal injury is somewhat controversial. On the one hand, there are several lines of evidence that the complement cascade may be activated during the course of glomerulonephritis, and certain experimental models of acute glomerulonephritis using decomplemented or genetically complement-deficient animals show significantly diminished glomerular pathology when compared to normocomplementemic controls, thus suggesting that complement can directly participate in the development of renal damage. On the other hand, the observation that patients have genetic deficiencies of complement, particularly of the early components, and have an increased incidence of immune-complex disease, including nephritis, has led others to conclude that the complement cascade is more important for the protection it affords against renal

disease. The considerable experimental data available documenting an important role for complement in the solubilization of immune complexes also have led to this conclusion. The evidence for these contrary points of view will be summarized in this section; for the present time, the role of complement as a mediator of renal disease should remain open.

COMPLEMENT-DEPENDENT GLOMERULONEPHRITIS

In most experimental models and human forms of glomerulonephritis that demonstrate glomerular deposition of immunoglobulin, glomerular accumulation of complement components is also seen. In most cases of presumed immune complex nephritis, the classical pathway appears to be activated with deposits of C1q, C4, C3, and the components of the membrane attack complex within the glomeruli. However, in hypocomplementemic mesangiocapillary glomerulonephritis, evidence may favor involvement of the alternative pathway, with deposits in the kidney containing C3 and properdin along with the membrane attack complex [120,241]. In this later situation evidence for immunoglobulin deposition within the glomeruli is often lacking (as in dense intramembranous deposit disease, for example). In this regard, it is interesting that preparations of intact GBM isolated from human kidneys have been shown in vitro to directly initiate activation of the human alternative complement pathway along its epithelial surface [514]. Furthermore, soluble enzyme digests of GBM have been shown to cause fluid phase consumption of alternative pathway components [264,265]. In addition to the presence of complement within the glomeruli, other observations have suggested that the human complement system is activated in various forms of glomerulonephritis: serum levels of some complement components may be depressed; complement cleavage products may become detectable in the plasma, and hypercatabolism of complement may be shown by studies of the survival of intravenously injected radiolabelled complement proteins [514].

Two mechanisms have been proposed to explain the way in which complement actually produces injury to the glomerulus, and each of these is illustrated in turn by the experimental models of the heterologous phase of nephrotoxic serum nephritis and passive Heymann nephritis respectively, the only two models providing direct evidence for a pathogenic role of complement.

Complement activation generates small peptides, including C4a, C3a, and C5a, which are collectively termed anaphylatoxins because of their smooth muscle-contracting activity and their capacity to induce mast cells to release mediators such as histamine [428]. C5a is uniquely important for its chemotactic activity, resulting in the recruitment and stimulation of leukocytes, leading to their appearance, adherence, and secretory activity. Thus, in this system complement produces inflammation indirectly by the influence it exerts on neutrophils similar to that observed in the classical Arthus reaction. Cobra venom factor (CVF) is a nonenzymatic non-toxic glycoprotein of 140,000 daltons that structurally resembles human C3 [501]. When injected into animals, CVF combines with factor B, forming a stable C3/C5 convertase that rapidly

consumes complement components to produce a state of profound complement deficiency that lasts approximately five days. Animals decomplemented with cobra venom factor prior to the injection of nephrotoxic serum are able to bind antibody to the GBM, but in the absence of complement fail to manifest neutrophilic infiltration or to develop proteinuria as seen in control animals [73,483]. The role of polymorphonuclear leucocytes is further confirmed by the observation that normocomplementemic animals fail to develop proteinuria during the heterologous phase of nephrotoxic serum nephritis if they have been pre-treated to eliminate neutrophils [489]. In a somewhat analogous situation, the systemic generation of C5a by injection of rats with CVF [481] or by exposure of circulatory complement to artificial membranes during hemodialysis [90] results in acute changes in the pulmonary microcirculation characterized by the deposition of C5a and recruitment of circulating neutrophils.

In a second experimental model, that of passive Heymann nephritis, the production of proteinuria requires an intact complement system, but the presence of neutrophils is not necessary [411]. Induction of membranous nephropathy in rats by either the passive administration of anti-Fx1A antibody or a variation of this model using subnephritic doses of sheep anti-Fx1A as a planted antigen, followed by transplantation of kidneys into rats presensitized to sheep IgG or subsequently injected with anti-sheep IgG, produced proteinuria that could be abrogated by decomplementation but was unaffected by depletion of neutrophils. Although the mechanism is not established by which complement, independent of cellular mediators, can induce proteinuria as observed in this experimental model, it has been proposed that the assembly of complement components C5b-9 to form the membrane attack complex (MAC) may produce glomerular cell injury in a fashion analogous to the disruptive effect this complex has on other cell membranes [41]. Using antisera to rat MAC neoantigens, Biesecker et al. [42] observed significant deposits in the glomeruli of rats during the active phase of injury in this model. However, during the later phase of more chronic disease, when the animals continued to have proteinuria, only minimal amounts of the MAC could be found in glomeruli. The glomerular deposition of terminal complement components has recently been confirmed in the models of passive [6] and active Heymann nephritis [93].

Although the precise mechanism whereby the MAC disrupts membrane barriers is not certain, two alternative theories have been proposed [41]. The well documented insertion of the MAC into the cell membrane may lead to a reorganization of the lipid bilayers, resulting in the formation of a transmembrane lipid channel or, alternatively, the entire MAC complex or its polymerized C9 subunit, arranged as a hollow, thin-walled cylinder, may itself form the walls of a transmembrane channel. Such channels would allow the passage of salt, water, and small proteins across the membrane to the cell's interior, associated with passive diffusion of water, cellular swelling, and, ultimately, membrane disruption. However, unlike erythrocytes, nucleated cells appear quite resistant to MAC-induced lysis. In these cells, insertion of MAC into the cell membrane likely activates intracellular signalling pathways resulting in alterations of cellular function(s).

Two recent studies of chronic serum sickness provide some indirect evidence in support of a role for the MAC in immune complex glomerulonephritis. Using an antisera to a neoantigen of the MAC, Koffler et al. [252] demonstrated that rats chronically injected with bovine serum albumin developed glomerulonephritis and proteinuria associated with immune complexes containing C3 and the MAC along the subepithelial aspect of the GBM. However, the distribution of the MAC was somewhat restricted in that significantly lesser amounts were detectable within the deposits present along the subendothelial aspect and scattered within the lamina densa of the GBM. Chronic serum sickness in rabbits induced by repeated injection of cationized bovine serum albumin appears to require the presence of the terminal components of the complement cascade for the production of proteinuria during the initial phase prior to the influx of inflammatory cells. Rabbits genetically deficient in C6 failed to develop the proteinuria detectable in normocomplementemic controls one week after daily injections of cationized BSA (animals were presensitized to BSA in adjuvant) [172]. However, coincident with the onset of glomerular hypercellularity at two weeks, the C6-deficient rabbits developed proteinuria and thereafter did not differ from controls. In a model of anti-GBM nephritis, C6 deficient rabbits had less proteinuria in the first 24 hours (heterologous phase) than the control rabbits [173]. These authors concluded, given that the only known biological action of C6 is the assembly of the MAC, that these observations supported a role for the MAC in the generation of immune injury and proteinuria.

Studies of the pathogenesis of hyperacute rejection using the model of cardiac allograft transplantation in presensitized rats also support a role for complement independent of inflammatory cells in the induction of immunological vascular injury. This severe form of rejection was ameliorated by complement depletion of the recipients prior to transplantation but was uninfluenced by the depletion of neutrophils or platelets [132,133]. In addition, hyperacute rejection of heart xenografts was delayed in C6-deficient recipient rabbits when compared to rabbits with an intact complement system [68].

Neoantigens expressed on the MAC or its polymerized C9 subunit can be demonstrated in a variety of human glomerular diseases where it may be found in association with C3 as reported for mesangiocapillary glomerulonephritis, IgA nephropathy, anaphylactoid purpura, and systemic lupus erythematosus; or it may be found in areas where C3 deposition is minimal, particularly in the glomerular regions of sclerosis in end-stage kidneys, hyalinization in hypertension, mesangial matrix PAS-positive material in diabetes, and thioflavin T-positive deposits in amyloidosis [40,117] (Fig. 13-17). Since the expression of these neoantigens is dependent upon complement activation, these observations strengthen the concept that complement is indeed activated within the kidney and not merely passively trapped as a secondary consequence of pre-existent glomerular pathology. The recent observation [118] that patients with active SLE have detectable serum levels of MAC not found in normal individuals or in SLE patients with inactive disease provides an additional basis for interest in the role of these components as a mediator system in immune-complex induced disease (Fig. 13-18).

It is possible, at least in theory, that complement may initiate pathological changes within the kidney in the absence of collaboration with cells, by mechanisms other than the formation of the membrane attack complex and its insertion into the phospholipid membranes of glomerular cells, although no direct data are currently available.

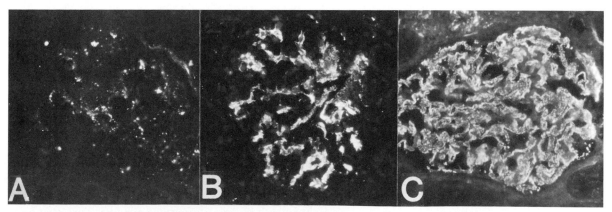

FIG. 13-17. *Glomerular deposition of the membrane attack complex (MAC) demonstrated by immunofluorescence microscopy of human kidneys stained with a monoclonal antibody to a neoantigen on the C9 portion of the MAC. The mesangium of the normal glomerulus (A) reacts weakly; mesangial deposits present in a patient with systemic lupus erythematosus (B) are strongly reactive; and the subepithelial deposits present in a patient with membranous nephropathy (C) correspond to the granular staining along the GBM. (Reprinted from Falk et al: J Clin Invest 72:560, 1983, with permission from the publisher.)*

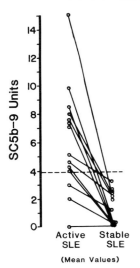

FIG. 13-18. *Detection of a neoantigen of the membrane attack complex (MAC) in the serum of patients with active systemic lupus erythematosus (SLE). With the use of a radioimmunoassay employing a monoclonal antibody to a neoantigen of MAC, 95% of normal individuals have serum levels below the dashed line similar to those observed in patients with clinically stable SLE. In contrast, during clinically active SLE, elevated serum levels are detectable. (Reproduced from Falk et al: N Engl J Med 312:1594, 1985, with permission from the publisher).*

For example, the generation of vasoactive fragments (C3a, C5a) may alter glomerular permeability; C1q may interact in the Hagemen factor—dependent systems, and activated C2 may affect permeability in a manner analogous to that seen in patients with hereditary angioedema [428].

AMELIORATION OF GLOMERULONEPHRITIS BY COMPLEMENT

Now turning to the counterpoint to discuss the beneficial effects of complement, it has been clearly shown that complement plays a role in the solubilization of immune complexes. Under physiological circumstances, individuals are constantly exposed to foreign antigens, leading to an antibody response and the generation of immune complexes. Under these circumstances it is proposed that components of the complement classical pathway play a role in maintaining these complexes in solution by interfering with their aggregation until they are eliminated by the mononuclear phagocytic system.

In mammals, an additional role for complement may exist at this stage, as the opsonization of antigen-antibody complexes by complement enables them to be taken up by C3b-receptors on erythrocytes whereafter they undergo rapid elimination by the liver [81]. Baboons decomplemented with cobra venom factor demonstrate decreased binding of immune complexes to erythrocytes, therefore higher levels of "free" circulating immune complexes that more rapidly disappear from the circulation [57]. This enhanced elimination reported in decomplemented baboons

was not due to increased hepatic or splenic uptake, raising the possibility that this resulted in increased deposition in organs vulnerable to immune-complex mediated injury. Thus, complement may have an important role to play in the afferent limb of immune complex elimination, not simply indirectly by virtue of its function in the maintenance of soluble, freely-circulating immune complexes, but more directly through its ability to bridge complexes to erythrocytes and leucocytes through surface receptors that are specific for activated complement proteins. The net effect of these complement-related activities should facilitate delivery to and elimination by the phagocytes fixed within the mononuclear phagocytic system. As discussed in the section dealing with immune complex nephritis, it has been observed by several groups of investigators that patients with systemic lupus erythematosus have decreased numbers of detectable erythrocyte C3b receptors. Although this decrease may be explained on the basis that these receptors are undetectable because they are hidden by or have been internalized along with the bound opsonized immune complexes, one group has provided evidence that this represents a primary, genetically determined decrease, thus suggesting a role for C3b-receptor deficiency in the pathogenesis of immune complex disease.

The alternative pathway of complement is not required during the early phase immediately following immune complex formation when the classical pathway plays an active role, keeping the complexes in solution apparently by preventing further complex aggregation and precipitation [424,425]. However, the alternative pathway has an established role in the resolubilization of antigen-antibody precipitates [91,331]. It has been proposed that this solubilization is the result of activation of the alternative pathway, which leads in sequence to the interposition of C3 molecules into the complex lattice, resulting in its rearrangement into smaller and therefore more soluble molecules (a reaction that is affected by antibody avidity). The concept that complement may similarly modify immune complexes deposited with glomeruli was first suggested by the observation that glomerular deposits of complement increased during the phase of resolution of acute serum sickness. Bartolotti et al. [25] demonstrated in an experimental model of acute serum sickness in rabbits that complement depletion by cobra venom factor significantly decreased the rate of disappearance of radiolabelled immune complexes bound to diseased glomeruli. The $T_{\frac{1}{2}}$ was 19.5 days as compared to 11.3 days in control animals, suggesting that complement may be important during the amelioration of immune-complex induced renal injury.

HUMAN COMPLEMENT DEFICIENCY SYNDROMES

Perhaps the most exciting human data supporting a protective role for complement against immune complex diseases comes from the observations of experiments of nature in man. Genetic complement deficiencies, particularly of the early components, are associated not only with an increased susceptibility to infections but also to certain immune disorders [388,409,435]. Such deficiencies are often seen associated with a lupus-like syndrome with or without nephritis, but also occasionally with various forms

Table 13-8. *Complement deficiencies and glomerulonephritis*

Complement component	Lupus-like syndrome	Other glomerulonephritis
C1q	6	1—Mesangial Proliferative GN
C1r	3	1—End-Stage
C2	10	6—MPGN
		3—Anaphylactoid Purpura
		2—Mesangial Proliferative GN
		1—Unknown
C1 Inhibiter Deficiency	1	3—Mesangial Proliferative GN
C4	2	
C3 (Homozygous)	—	2—MPGN
		2—Unknown
C3 (Partial)*	—	1—MPGN
		2—Unknown
C5	1	—
C6	—	3—MPGN
C7	1	1—Unknown
C8	2	—
H (B1H) Deficiency	—	3—IgA Nephropathy
		1—Hemolytic Uremic Syndrome

* 1 patient within family of 3 with homozygous deficiency, 1 associated with unusual C3 allotype (C3F), 1 abnormal synthesis
MPGN = Membranoproliferative glomerulonephritis
RPGN = Rapidly progressive glomerulonephritis
This table was prepared from information reviewed in references 35, 54, 79, 388.

of "primary" glomerulonephritis and anaphylactoid purpura nephritis. Epidemiological and statistical studies confirm that this association is definitely explained by more than chance alone.

Two types of genetic variations have been described for the human complement proteins. The first is a polymorphism described for components C4, C2, C3, factor B, and C6, and the second, a deficiency state that has now been described for almost every complement protein [388]. The genes for C2, factor B, and the C4 genes (C4A and C4B) are located in the major histocompatibility complex (HLA) of chromosome 6 situated between the HLA-B and HLA-D loci. The complement components encoded by these three genes are sometimes referred to as the HLA-class III proteins.

Taken as a group, patients with a wide variety of inherited complement deficiencies not only have an increased risk of autoimmune disease, but the diseases share in common many clinical and biological features (summarized in Table 13-8). Particularly remarkable is the increased risk of SLE and glomerulonephritis in individuals born with deficiencies of the early components, C1, C4, and C2, suggesting an important role for the classical complement pathway in the prevention of similar diseases in normal individuals. The most frequent complement deficiency is that of C2 deficiency, which affects approximately one in 10,000 individuals, the vast majority of whom are otherwise normal.

Four possibilities have been suggested to explain these associations [388]. First, complement deficiencies are associated with an increased risk of bacterial or viral infections, which may alter host immune defenses or initiate the formation of potentially pathogenic immune complexes. Secondly, as reviewed earlier, deficiency of complement may decrease the solubilization of immune complexes, thereby leading to a slower rate of elimination and enhanced precipitation in abnormal sites. Third, the deficiency of certain complement proteins, which have the potential ability to influence the activity of various components of the immune system, may conceivably induce an abnormal immune response. Finally, it is possible that a given deficiency of a complement protein is a genetic but not a biological marker. This is a particularly attractive hypothesis for the HLA-linked genetic deficiencies of C2, C4, and factor B, but fails to explain the relationship for other complement deficiencies that are not encoded by genes linked to the HLA-complex. However, it is conceivable that other immune response genes that are currently unknown may be closely linked to some of the other complement genes.

Another relative complement deficiency syndrome, that associated with C3 nephritic factor (C3NeF), is noteworthy [166,241,428]. This factor was first isolated from the serum of patients with mesangiocapillary glomerulonephritis and is detectable in 60% of patients with dense intramembranous deposit disease, 10% to 20% of patients with type I mesangiocapillary glomerulonephritis, occasionally in other acute glomerulonephridites, and in certain individuals with partial lipodystrophy unassociated with renal pathology. The C3 nephritic factor has been further characterized as an IgG autoantibody reactive with the alternative pathway C3 convertase, C3b,Bb (Fig. 13-16). Binding of this antibody to the convertase complex enhances enzyme activity leading to an accelerated rate of consumption of C3 and subnormal serum levels. Properdin exerts a similar stabilizing effect on C3b,Bb but unlike C3NeF, its action is normally held in check by the regulatory protein, Factor H (BIH).

The expression of certain complement phenotypes (polymorphisms) is associated with an increased risk of nephritis [388]. These genetically determined variants are identified by their differences in electrophoretic mobility, and by convention they are referred to as F (fast) and S (slow) for factor B; A, B, or C for C2; and by numbers for C4. These three HLA-linked complement alleles appear to be inherited as a single unit (complotype). The following are examples of an association between a particular complement allotype and nephritis. (1) Double silent or "null" genes (Q0) at the same C4 locus (i.e., homozygous C4A/Q0 or C4B/Q0) are present in 15% of patients with IgA nephropathy, 26% of patients with anaphylactoid purpura, and in only 3.9% of the normal population [317]. In addition, some of these allotypes show linkage disequilibrium with certain HLA groups. For example, the C4A/Q0 gene is almost always associated with the HLA-A1, B18, BR3 haplotype and C4B/Q0 with HLA-AW30, B18, BfFl, DR3. (2) A strong association has been reported between a rare C4B allele, C4B*2.9 and primary glomerulonephritis. The presence of this allele was noted in 25% of 59 unselected German individuals with primary glomerulonephritis, vs. 2% of the general population [506]. Expression of this allele was not found to be linked to a particular HLA haplotype; it was also found in higher frequency in patients with type I diabetes mellitus and in adults with rheumatoid arthritis. (3) A rare factor B allele, BfFl, was found in higher than normal frequency in patients with idiopathic membranous glomerulopathy and in Type I diabetes mellitus, where it showed strong linkage disequilibrium with HLA B18 and DRW3 [110]. (4) An increased frequency of the fast C3 variant has been reported in patients with type I mesangiocapillary glomerulonephritis [316].

Platelets

Although a role for platelets in the production of human glomerular injury was proposed by Kincaid-Smith more than two decades ago [242], platelets had been given little further consideration until recently. The key question, whether or not platelet activation contributes directly to glomerular injury, has yet to be answered. Platelets are observed in the glomerular capillaries in various forms of glomerulonephritis, and platelet membrane antigens or the contents of platelet granules are detectble by immunofluorescence even in the absence of identifiable platelets. Furthermore, there is considerable evidence that platelets are activated in vivo in patients with glomerulonephritis [332]. Platelet counts are usually within the normal range except in some patients with SLE. Platelet survival is often shortened, an observation that may be explained on the basis of increased consumption within the kidney. Increased aggregates of platelets have been detected in the plasma of patients with nephritis, even in the absence of nephrotic syndrome. Circulating platelets may be depleted of dense body amines (serotonin and ADP) and alpha-granule contents (platelet factor 4 and B-thromboglobulin) while the corresponding plasma levels may be elevated (lending support to the notion that platelets have been stimulated to release these contents) [64]. In vitro, platelets

obtained from certain patients with glomerulonephritis demonstrate augmented aggregation after exposure to ADP. Additional clinical studies are beginning to provide indirect evidence that platelets may contribute to certain types of glomerular injury. In a prospective controlled trial of type I mesangiocapillary glomerulonephritis, the combined use of the anti-platelet drugs aspirin and dipyridamole was associated with an improvement in renal function compared to the control, untreated group [99].

The mechanism of activation of platelets during the course of glomerulonephritis has yet to be defined. It may represent secondary activation following activation of the coagulation cascade, although direct platelet stimulation is at least theoretically possible. Hughes et al. [202] demonstrated that exposed tubular basement membrane and, to a lesser extent, glomerular basement membrane could induce platelet adhesion and aggregation similar to that occurring after exposure to collagen. Human platelets can bind immune complexes directly by way of membrane Fc receptors. Such complexes, particularly if insoluble, can cause platelets to aggregate and release their contents [70]. Platelet-activating factor (PAF-acether), a low molecular weight phospholipid (1100 daltons) can be released not only from basophils, monocytes, and granulocytes, but has recently been isolated from rat glomerular and medullary cells and from human and rabbit endothelial cells [526]. In many forms of glomerulonephritis, platelet turnover is accelerated while fibrinogen consumption is normal, supporting a primary role for platelets in intraglomerular coagulation [151].

Platelets possess a variety of activities that could be potentially injurious to the kidney, including several functions shared with leucocytes—not surprising when one recalls that they are all derived from a common precursor stem cell [64]. They contain vasoactive amines, including serotonin and ADP, and produce leukotrienes that may alter glomerular permeability, thereby exerting an influence on the glomerular deposition of immune complexes. Platelets release a variety of proteolytic enzymes (many strongly cationic), several prostanoids (including thromboxane A2, PGG2 and PGH2), and platelet-activating factor, which not only serves to further augment platelet aggregation but may also exert an effect on white blood cells. Additional platelet secretory products include platelet-derived growth factor and mitogenic proteins capable of stimulating proliferation of the myointimal cells of smooth muscle as well as cultured glomerular mesangial cells. The functions of two proteins specifically released from platelets have not been completely explored. The first, B-thromboglobulin, is known to inhibit prostacyclin production by endothelium. The second, platelet factor 4, not only plays an important role in the clotting cascade but is also chemotactic for monocytes and granulocytes. This is an anionic protein that can bind to heparan sulfate proteoglycan isolated from the human renal cortex, suggesting that it may bind and neutralize anionic sites along the GBM in vivo [526]. Platelets may interact with the complement system through their ability to activate C3 and C5.

The study of the role of platelets in experimental renal disease has not been optimal [63,64,332]. Platelet-depletion studies have been difficult because profound and sustained platelet depletion, if achieved, usually leads to death due to hemorrhage, while incomplete platelet depletion often leaves few but adequate numbers of platelets to maintain many of their functions so that no definitive conclusions can be made. Injection of antisera leading to platelet-destruction is associated with release of platelet amines that produce significant hemodynamic changes that could influence the deposition of immune complexes. Lavelle et al. [270] were unable to inhibit the development of the autologous phase of nephrotoxic serum nephritis using antiplatelet antisera. Knicker and Cochrane [248–250] demonstrated inhibition of glomerular deposition of immune complexes in rabbits depleted of platelets with antisera. Although a variety of drugs alter platelet function, they usually have a broad spectrum of activity. Furthermore, there are rather remarkable differences in the immunology and pharmacology of human platelets as compared to most laboratory animals, therefore making it difficult to draw conclusions from experimental observations [64]. For example, most animal platelets carry membrane receptors for C3b—human platelets lack these; the platelet amine content in rabbits is 20-fold to 30-fold higher than that of the human platelet. The results of use of antiplatelet drugs in experimental immune complex nephritis are summarized in Table 13-9.

In one recent study using a model of antibody and complement dependent renal injury, namely, that of hyperacute allograft rejection in presensitized rabbits, massive intravascular accumulation of platelets was observed within five minutes of revascularization, suggesting that platelets might be important in the early phase of immunological allograft destruction [211].

The Coagulation Factors

The coagulation system is convincingly involved in the genesis of glomerular injury seen in association with microangiopathy, such as observed in the hemolytic uremic syndrome, and in the pathogenesis of extracapillary proliferation to form glomerular crescents (see Chap. 14). However, in models of experimental renal disease and from observations of glomerulonephritis in man, the role of the coagulation mechanism is controversial. Evidence for participation of the coagulation cascade in human renal disease is derived from the following indirect observations: (1) morphological and immunohistochemical studies demonstrating the deposition of fibrin-related antigens and factor VIII; (2) histochemical changes in renal cortical plasminogen activator activity; (3) changes in serum levels of factor VIII, antiplasmins and antiactivators; (4) elevation of serum and urinary levels of fibrinogen and fibrin related antigens; and (5) radioisotope kinetic studies demonstrating shortened survival of fibrinogen and plasminogen [332].

The role of the coagulation system has been studied in experimental models of glomerulonephritis using pharmacological manipulations with agents such as anticoagulants, including heparin and warfarin or coumadin; ancrod, a defibrinating agent extracted from the Malayan pit venom; epsilon aminocapnoic acid (EACA), a fibrinolytic inhibiter; and streptokinase, a fibrinolytic agent. Fibrin appears to be important for the formation of crescents, and morphological studies suggest the following sequence of events. Associated with the formation of gaps in the GBM, fibrin deposits become detectable in Bowman's space; shortly thereafter, monocytes appear in Bowman's space, where they have been observed to phagocytose fibrin; thereafter, proliferation of the parietal epithelial cells lining Bowman's capsule begins [478,480]. At this early stage, factor VIII can be demonstrated in the crescent, while in the later stages it is present only in the periphery of the crescent [443]. It has thus been suggested that polymerization of fibrinogen during the generation of crescents may be triggered by both mechanisms dependent and independent of the intrinsic coagulation pathway. Platelets are remarkable for their absence in this process. Fibrin persists much longer in the crescents than within glomerular deposits, suggesting that fibrinolysis is less effective or less available to regions beyond the glomerular tuft. Crescent formation can be largely prevented in nephrotoxic serum nephritis by coumadin or ancrod but not by heparin [50,332]. Daily administration of ancrod has decreased crescent formation in chronic serum sickness in rabbits [478].

Although fibrin deposition may be prominent in experimental anti-GBM nephritis, anticoagulant therapy has not been uniformly successful. Its effectiveness appears to de-

TABLE 13-9. *Results of antiplatelet therapy in immune complex glomerulonephritis*

Investigator	Animal	Drugs or Antisera	Result
Kniker and Cochrane	Rabbit	Chlorpheneramine Maleate Methylsergide Maleate	Positive
Kniker and Cochrane	Rabbit	Antiplatelet Antiserum	Positive
Kniker and Cochrane	Rabbit	Cyproheptadine	Positive
Bolten et al	Rat	Cyproheptadine	Negative
Kupor et al	Rat	Aspirin	Negative
		Periactin	Negative
		Indomethicin	Negative
Wardle	Rabbit	Dipyridamole	Negative
		Salicyladoxime	Negative

This table was based on material reviewed by Miller [332].

TABLE 13-10. *Results of anticoagulant therapy in immune complex glomerulonephritis*

Investigator	Animal	Drugs	Result
Lee	Rabbit	Heparin	Positive
Baliah and Drummond	Rabbit	Warfarin	Negative
Border et al	Rabbit	Heparin	Negative
Thomson et al	Rabbit	Ancrod	Positive
McGiven	NZB/NZW Mice	Warfarin	Negative
Lambert	NZB/NZW Mice	Heparin	Positive

Table based on references 265(a), 312, 332.

TABLE 13-11. *Results of anticoagulant therapy in anti-GBM nephritis*

Investigator	Animal	Drugs	Results
Kleinerman	Rabbit	Heparin	Positive[a]
Halpern	Rabbit	Heparin	Positive
Vassalli and McCluskey	Rabbit	Warfarin	Positive
Briggs et al	Mice	Heparin Urokinase	Negative
Watanabe and Tanaka	Rabbit	Heparin	Positive
Borrero et al	Belgian hare	Warfarin	Positive
Naish et al	Rabbit	Ancrod	Positive
Thomson et al	Rabbit	Ancrod	Positive
Thomson et al	Rabbit	Heparin	Positive[b]
Thomson et al	Rabbit	Ancrod	Positive[c]
Bone et al	Rat	Heparin	Negative
Border et al	Rabbit	Heparin	Negative

[a] Negative result if heparin therapy is begun after nephrotoxic serum is administered.
[b] Dose of heparin necessary to be effective exceeds therapeutic levels in man.
[c] Ancrod begun during the autologous phase.
Information in this table modified from references 59, 332.

pend to some extent on the severity of the immunological injury as well as the type and adequacy of anticoagulation. Endothelial injury could directly activate coagulation by exposure of GBM surfaces to circulating coagulation proteins such as the Hageman factor, or infiltrated macrophages might promote coagulation following the release of their secretory products. As summarized in Table 13-10, early studies using heparin or warfarin in mild nephrotoxic serum nephritis seemed beneficial, although studies by Thomson et al. noted that the doses required would be therapeutically impossible in man [477a]. Recently, heparin was shown to be of little or no benefit in more severe models of glomerular injury [50]. Use of the defibrinating agent ancrod was shown to be protective provided that renal function was only mildly impaired. It has been suggested that the presence of glomerular fibrin in the face of therapeutic levels of heparin implies that fibrin deposition may occur through a thrombin-independent pathway.

Variable results of anticoagulation therapy have also been observed in experimental models of immune complex induced glomerular injury (summarized in Table 13-11). Thus, although no satisfactory conclusions can be made at this juncture regarding the efficacy of anticoagulation therapy in immunological renal disease, it must be considered that significant variability in response may exist between different species, making any generalizations inappropriate.

On the contrary, the demonstration that certain anticoagulants can ameliorate renal injury does not necessarily prove a role for the clotting system. For example, heparin has been reported to delay the progression of an experimental model of non-immunological renal disease, namely, the rat remnant kidney model, by mechanisms not fully defined [367]. Although its role as an anticogulant was shown to be important in that model, additional mechanisms were also entertained, including the effect of heparin on systemic blood pressure and intrarenal hemodynamics possibly mediated by inhibition of renal kallikrein), its inhibitory effect on glomerular hypertrophy, and the ability of polyanionic heparin to increase the negative electrostatic potential of the glomerular capillary wall.

THE HAGEMAN FACTOR RELATED PATHWAYS

The Hageman factor (M.W. 80,000) plays an important role as clotting factor XII capable of activating factor XI of the intrinsic coagulation cascade and factor VII of the extrinsic pathway. However, this protein is unique in that it is able to trigger additional reactions that may lead to tissue injury (Fig. 13-19). In fact, the complement proteins together with the Hageman factor contact system represent the major plasma protein systems with such functions. Studies over recent years have focused on the biochemistry

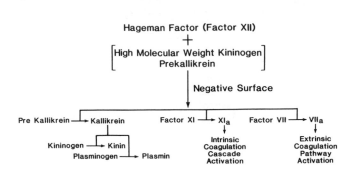

Hageman Factor (Factor XII)
+
[High Molecular Weight Kininogen
Prekallikrein]

Negative Surface

Pre Kallikrein → Kallikrein   Factor XI → XI$_a$ Factor VII → VII$_a$

Kininogen → Kinin   Intrinsic   Extrinsic
                                                    Coagulation   Coagulation
Plasminogen → Plasmin   Cascade   Pathway
                                                    Activation   Activation

FIG. 13-19. *Schematic summary of the Hageman factor related pathways. (Modified from Cochrane, In* Contemp Issues Nephrol, *3:106, 1979.)*

of this system, and while several observations suggest that the contact system is likely to play a role as a mediator of glomerular injury, this has yet to be confirmed [76,77]. The Hageman factor is activated upon exposure to negative surfaces but only if it simultaneously interacts with two other factors. The first of these, pre-kallikrein (M.W. 80,000) is an enzyme that not only interacts with and activates Hageman factor, but, in doing so, becomes simultaneously activated itself to generate kallikrein. The second required factor for contact activation is high molecular weight kininogen (M.W. 110,000), which is not enzymatic but possibly functions by bringing about surface binding of the other participating factors.

The activation of this system generates a cascade with several potential biological functions. Activated Hageman factor may increase vascular permeability, stimulate coagulation, and activate additional soluble prekallikrein. In fact, Hageman factor appears to be essential for the endogenous activation of plasma prekallikrein. Kallikrein is a peptidase that releases bradykinin and two lesser known kinins, kallidin and met-lys-bradykinin, from their precursor (kininogen), leading to effects such as increased vascular permeability, hypotensin, contraction of smooth muscle, and stimulation of phospholipase A2, resulting in increased prostaglandin synthesis. In addition, bradykinin plays an important role in the regulation of glomerular blood flow through its ability to decrease renal vascular resistance. Kallikrein also cleaves the fibrinolytic enzyme plasmin from its precursor, plasminogen. The action of plasmin on fibrinogen and fibrin may release smaller fragments capable of increasing vascular permeability and attracting granulocytes. Plasmin may interact with the complement cascade through its ability to activate components C1 and C3.

As yet there is no experimental evidence to confirm a role for the contact system in immune mediated glomerulonephritis. Hageman factor does bind to isolated GBM and becomes activated in the presence of kallikrein. The Hageman factor is activated in the kidney during anti-GBM nephritis in rabbits [77]. Furthermore, the urinary excretion of kallikrein has been shown to decrease in rats

with anti-GBM nephritis, suggesting a possible role for this mediator in the induction of proteinuria [164]. Now that the components of the Hageman factor-associated contact system have been isolated and better characterized, these three Hageman factor-dependent systems generating, respectively, kinins, fibrin, and fibrinolysins will no doubt be studied in greater detail for their potential roles as mediators in immunological renal disease.

Prostanoids

Prostanoids are a group of compounds synthesized from 20-carbon polyunsaturated membrane phospholipids, which are released from virtually every tissue in the body, including the kidney. These act as hormones, exerting their maximal biological effects locally at sites of production. Extensive work on the role of the renal prostaglandins (PG) has demonstrated that they participate in the regulation of many physiological activities, such as salt and water excretion, renal blood flow, and renin release [284]. In addition, prostanoids have been strongly implicated as promoters of inflammatory reactions [262]; more recently, prostaglandins primarily of the E series have demonstrated the ability to modulate inflammatory reactions in a manner that prevents rather than promotes tissue injury. Such opposing roles for different prostaglandins have been observed elsewhere. For example, vasodilation is induced by PGI_2 (prostacyclin), PGE_1, PGE_2, PGD_2, and PGA_2 (stable prostaglandins), whereas vasoconstriction follows exposure to PGG_2, PGH_2 (cyclic endoperoxides), and thromboxane A_2. Platelet aggregation is promoted by PGG_2, PGH_2, and thromboxane A_2, whereas PGI_2, PGE_1, PGE_2, and PGD_2 inhibit platelet aggregation.

Following the observation by Zurier et al. [534] in 1971 that adjuvant arthritis in rats could be suppressed by prostaglandin PGE_1, additional studies have suggested that PGE_1 (synthesized by cyclo-oxygenation of 8,11,14-eicosatrienoic acid) and PGE_2 (derived from arachidonic acid by cyclo-oxygenation) can also decrease the inflammatory response and reduce glomerular injury in several models of experimental glomerulonephritis (summarized in Table 13-12). These prostaglandins have numerous biological actions and likely modify immunologically induced renal disease by multiple mechanisms. For example, systemic administration of PGE_1 has been shown to block the increase in vascular permeability produced by vasoactive inflammatory mediators, an effect that could influence the renal deposition of immune reactants [119]. Renal plasma flow can be modified by the effects of prostaglandins on vascular resistance. It is most likely that the decline in the glomerular filtration rate and the reduction in proteinuria frequently observed in patients with various types of glomerular disease following the administration of cyclooxygenase inhibitors occurs on a hemodynamic basis [72,108,285]. However, the E series prostaglandins usually induce vasodilatation, which should increase renal plasma flow. Lianos et al. [282] reported an increase in glomerular production of thromboxane in rats with nephrotoxic serum nephritis, which was temporarily associated with a decline in GFR and correlated with the extent of proteinuria.

Table 13-12. *Effects of prostanoids on experimental glomerulonephritis*

Model	Prostanoid	Effect	Reference
A. *Murine SLE*			
1) NZB/W	PGE$_1$	Protective	Zurier [535]
2) NZB/W	PGE$_1$	Protective	Zurier [536]
	PGF$_{2\alpha}$	No effect	
3) NZB/W	PGE$_1$, PGE$_2$	Protective	Kelley [234]
4) NZB/W	PGE$_1$	Protective	Izui [215]
MRL/l	PGE$_1$	Protective	
BXSB	PGE$_1$	No effect	
5) MRL/l	PGE$_1$	Protective	Kelley [236]
6) NZB/W	Dietary EPA*	Protective	Prickett [389]
7) NZB/W	PGE$_1$	Protective	Winkelstein [523]
MRL/l	PGE$_1$	Protective	
8) MRL/l	PGE$_1$	Protective	Eastcott [111]
9) MRL/l	Dietary fish oil	Protective	Kelley [237]
B. *Murine Human Plasma-induced Nephritis*			
1) DBA/2J	PGE$_1$	Protective	Kelley [235]
	PGF$_{2\alpha}$	No effect	
C. *Murine Apoferritin-induced Nephritis*			
1) Swiss albino	PGE$_1$	Protective	McLeish [318]
2) Swiss albino	PGE$_1$, PGE$_2$	Protective	McLeish [319]
3) Swiss albino	PGE$_2$	Protective	McLeish [320]
D. *Rabbit BSA-induced Nephritis*			
1) NZW Rabbit	Thromboxane synthetase inhibitor	Protective	Saito [410]
E. *Anti-GBM Nephritis*			
1) Maxx rats	PGE$_1$	Protective	Kunkel [236]
2) Sprague-Dawley rats	Thromboxane synthetase inhibitor	GFR improved	Lianos [282]

* Eicosapentaenoic acid (precursor of prostanoid-3 series)

Pretreatment of animals with thromboxane synthetase inhibitors prevented the decline in GFR otherwise observed during the acute heterologous phase.

Prostaglandins may modify the activity of other mediators participating in glomerular injury [283]. It has been observed that the E series of prostaglandins decreases leukocyte chemotaxis, inhibits leukocyte lysosomal enzyme release, prevents IgE-induced release of histamine from basophils, and inhibits platelet aggregation. It is noteworthy that human peripheral blood monocytes can be stimulated to release significant quantities of prostaglandins.

The key question yet to be resolved in this field is whether prostaglandins can influence glomerular injury by directly modifying the immune response. There is in vitro evidence suggesting that the E series prostaglandins inhibit some lymphocyte functions, such as mitogen responsiveness, antibody synthesis, T-lymphocyte cytotoxicity, lymphokine secretion, and antibody-dependent cell-mediated cytotoxicity [170]. In mice, the PGE series also inhibits macrophage expression of Ia antigens, which could lead to an alteration in antigen processing [449].

Studies of experimental immune complex glomerulonephritis, performed largely in the murine model of SLE, provide some evidence to suggest that the E series of prostaglandins may preserve renal function by modifying the immune response. In these mice, not only are fewer immune complexes detected within the circulation (gp 70 anti-gp 70 complexes) and deposited within the peripheral capillary loops [215,253], but the MRL/1 strains do not develop lymphoid hyperplasia or the suppression of T-lymphocyte mitogen responses demonstrable in the untreated mice [111,236]. Circulating anti-DNA antibody levels appear not to be affected by such treatment [234,535,536]. In the murine model of nephritis induced by the administration of apoferritin, the amelioration of nephritis by PGE$_1$ is associated with decreased serum levels of anti-apoferritin antibodies [318,320]. Administration of PGE$_1$ to rats during nephrotoxic serum nephritis significantly reduced the degree of hypercellularity and proteinuria even though the binding of the anti-GBM antibody was not altered [263].

Since the products of arachidonate metabolism are so diverse and frequently oppositional in action, it is possible that either proinflammatory or anti-inflammatory effects might be observed, depending upon the predominant prostanoid released. For example, despite the apparent beneficial effect of exogenous prostaglandin E in several murine models of SLE, administration of dietary fish oil rich in eicosapentaenoic acid has been shown recently to prolong survival even though this therapy was associated with decreased endogenous production of cyclooxygenase metabolites including prostaglandin E2. Thus, it is probable that each of these therapies acts at different levels to alter the ultimate expression of autoimmune disease [237]. As a final word of caution, it is important to remember that these compounds are normally produced in vivo in very small quantities that act locally so that systemic administration of relatively high doses of prostaglandins may not be relevant to the usual sequence of events in vivo.

Human Leukocyte Antigens and Renal Disease

Following the discovery that communication between cells participating in immune responses is regulated by the products of genes encoded in the major histocompatibility complex (MHC), investigations began to address the possibility that this genetic region might directly influence factors in the host predisposing to immunologic disease [247]. Such a theory was particularly attractive as there are so many different alleles possible at each locus (each inherited in Mendelian codominant fashion) that the HLA system is in fact the most polymorphic genetic system known in man.

The human MHC, located on the short arm of chromosome 6, encodes for two major groups of cell surface glycoproteins (human leukocyte antigens). The class I molecules—the classical transplantation antigens (HLA-A, HLA-B, HLA-C)—are present on all nucleated cells, are serologically defined by alloantibodies, and are important for their role in the regulation of cytotoxic T-lymphocytes. By contrast, the class II molecules—the immune response region-associated antigens (Ia)—are less widely distributed, being expressed mainly on B lymphocytes, activated T cells, macrophages and epidermal Langerhans cells. The class II antigens—HLA-DR, DP, and DQ—are defined primarily by lymphocyte culture techniques. This second group of molecules regulates helper T-lymphocyte function and is essential for antigen presentation to helper T-lymphocytes by macrophages and for the subsequent collaboration between B cells and T cells.

Thus far, the numerous studies searching for evidence of linkage disequilibrium—here meaning that the presence within the same haplotype of alleles at separate genetic loci such as those at HLA loci and those regulating the expression of renal disease occurs more frequently than would be predicted by random association—have been disappointing for nephrologists. This by no means precludes the possibility that new immune response genes or loci or both will be determined in the future and prove more meaningful. One current limitation of many of the studies done to date is the difficulty in identifying homogenous populations of adequate size and of clearly defined genetic backgrounds. Thus, although the possibility that the genes governing the pathological immune reactions that induce renal injury might be linked to certain HLA antigens is an attractive hypothesis, this is presently more speculation than fact. This topic has recently been reviewed [394], and those associations consistently found are summarized in Table 13-13. With the introduction of the field of molecular genetics, new observations on the genetic basis of glomerular disease may be forthcoming.

Tubulo-Interstitial Nephritis

It has only been within the past 20 years that investigators interested in renal immunopathology have begun to focus attention on the tubulo-interstitial unit as an important participant in or victim of certain pathological immune processes. Indeed, it was following the first descriptions of experimental anti-tubular basement membrane (TBM) nephritis in guinea pigs that similar diseases began to be recognized in man. Increasingly apparent is the need for a healthy renal interstitium to maintain the normal process of glomerular filtration. Lessons from clinical experience, especially in renal transplantation, continually remind us of the devastating decline in renal function associated with inflammatory interstitial disease. In certain of the primary glomerulonephridites seen in man, the glomerular filtration rate actually correlates better with the concomitant tubulo-interstitial pathology than with the degree of glomerular disease. In this section, immune mechanisms of tubulo-interstitial injury, as observed by the study of specific animal models will be reviewed. It is anticipated that this field of knowledge will expand greatly within the next few years; at the present time our level of understanding lags behind that available for comparable mechanisms of glomerular damage.

Humoral Mechanisms

ANTIBODIES AGAINST INTRINSIC COMPONENTS OF THE TUBULAR BASEMENT MEMBRANE

The biochemical structure of TBM is similar in many respects to that of the GBM, sharing such constituents as type IV and V collagen, laminin, entactin, and heparan sulfate proteoglycan [304,392]. Visualized by electron microscopy, the TBM usually appears more homogeneous rather than being divided into electron-lucent and electron-dense zones. The actual structural arrangements of these macromolecules within the TBM is unknown. However, it is also apparent that each of these renal basement membranes (GBM and TBM) has its own unique features as well. For example, certain antibodies reactive with the TBM fail to bind to the GBM and visa versa [327]. In most situations the nature of the nephritogenic TBM antigen(s) is unknown, with perhaps the following exceptions: A tubular antigen isolated from trypsin-digested human TBM of MW 30,000 can induce tubulo-interstitial nephritis in goats and certain strains of mice [505]; Brown Norway rats immunized with bovine cortical TBM develop interstitial nephritis with antibodies to a 42,000 molecular weight antigen obtained from collagenase-solubilized TBM [531]; and a glycoprotein of 48,000 MW (3M-1) has been isoalted from rabbit TBM and its presence shown to be essential for the induction of interstitial nephritis in Brown Norway rats [71].

In human tubulo-interstitial diseases, evidence for participation of anti-TBM antibodies is infrequently found [310]. Such antibodies have been detected in as many as 70% of patients with anti-GBM nephritis (Goodpasture's syndrome) and in a few cases reports of presumed immune complex glomerulonephritis, including systemic lupus erythematosus, membranous nephropathy, post-streptococcal

Table 13-13. *HLA and human renal disease*

Renal disease	Associated HLA antigen	Weaker HLA association
1. Anti-GBM Nephritis		
—Caucasian (Europe, Australia, USA)	DR$_2$	B7*
2. Membranous Nephropathy		
—Caucasian (Europe, not USA)	DR3	B8, B18**
—Japanese	DR2	
3. IgA Nephropathy***		
—Japanese	DR4	
4. Minimal Lesion Nephrotic Syndrome		
—Caucasian (Europe, Australia)	DR7	B8
—Japanese	DR8	

* When inherited with HLA-B7 prognosis worse.
** Probably reflects linkage dysequilibrium with respective DR antigens.
*** Early reports in Caucasians of an association with DR4 and BW35 were not confirmed in later studies.
This table was prepared from information reviewed in reference 394.

glomerulonephritis, methicillin nephrotoxicity, and idiopathic tubulo-interstitial nephritis. Perhaps the most frequent human situation encountered is the development of anti-TBM antibodies following renal transplantation where it has been observed in two different environments—reacting with an antigen present on the allograft but not the native kidney and binding to both kidneys simultaneously [246,517]. One interesting patient has been described with intractable diarrhea, nephrotic syndrome, and kidney-eluted antibodies reactive with the basement membranes of renal tubules and the jejunum [519].

Exploration of the pathogenesis of tubulo-interstitial nephritis induced by anti-TBM antibodies, particularly in the guinea pig model but also in mice and rats, has just begun to unravel the interwoven complexities of this pattern of immunologically mediated renal injury. In particular, it is already apparent that a critical interplay exists between cellular and humoral mechanisms. In addition, the individual effector mechanisms producing anti-TBM nephritis vary depending upon the species under study. For this reason, each experimental model will be described separately, followed by an attempt to summarize the factors presently thought to influence the expression of anti-TBM disease, including genetic susceptibility and mediator systems such as humoral immunity, complement, polymorphonuclear leukocytes, monocytes, and lymphocytes.

Experimental Model of Anti-TBM Nephritis in Guinea Pigs

The first experimental model of tubulo-interstitial nephritis induced by antibodies reacting with TBM was described by Steblay and Rudofsky [458] in 1971 in guinea pigs immunized with a rabbit renal cortical basement membrane preparation. Lehman et al [272] produced a similar disease using bovine TBM as the immunogen, and it is now known that heterologous TBM from other sources, including human and murine TBM, may initiate tubulo-interstitial nephritis in guinea pigs while homologous TBM preparations have been ineffective. The renal lesions are fully developed by two weeks following injection and are characterized by cortical interstitial infiltration of mononuclear cells, for-

mation of multinucleated giant cells, and tubular destruction. Disease susceptibility is influenced by certain genetic factors. For example, guinea pig strain XIII is usually selected for study since it predictably develops severe disease. In contrast, strain II, which has a much weaker antibody response, fails to develop disease [204]. However, the lack of disease expression in strain II guinea pigs is not solely explained by the presence of low levels of anti-TBM antibodies, because the passive transfer of antibodies does not result in renal injury even though the nephritogenic antigen is present in the TBM, suggesting that secondary immune effector mechanisms are not appropriately triggered in the strain II animals. In these strains of guinea pigs, expression of disease susceptibility is linked to a locus on the major histocompatibility complex [205].

Humoral immunity obviously plays a vital role in the initiation of anti-TBM nephritis, although it is clear that the simple deposition of antibody on the TBM per se is not sufficient to produce inflammation (Fig. 13-20). Early in the study of experimental tubulo-interstitial nephritis it was shown that the passive transfer of anti-TBM antibody obtained from the circulation or eluted from the kidneys of nephritic animals could produce similar disease in naive susceptible strains [204,402,403,459,495]. In addition, serum antibody titers generally correlate with the extent of renal disease. Studies by Neilson and Philips [354] have shown that these anti-TBM antibodies obtained from nephritic guinea pigs can effectively participate in the antibody-dependent cellular cytoxicity reaction of natural killer cells as they were able to cause lysis of chicken RBC targets coated with guinea pig renal tubular antigens.

Studies of tubulo-interstitial nephritis produced passively in guinea pigs have suggested that the initial anti-TBM antibody response may not trigger an effector immune reaction until additional humoral mechanisms strengthen the antibody response. Hall et al. [180] demonstrated that the passive transfer of anti-TBM antibody of a single isotype (e.g., IgG$_1$) was associated with tubulo-interstitial disease and circulating levels of anti-TBM antibodies, not only of IgG$_1$ isotype found in titers higher than anticipated for the dose injected, but also of IgG$_2$ isotype, suggesting that the

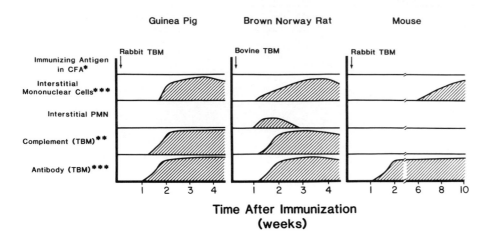

FIG. 13-20. *Schematic summary of the sequence of events observed in anti-TBM nephritis induced in three different experimental animals by immunization with preparations of heterologous TBM in Freund's complete adjuvant (*). Deposition of complement along the TBM has been detected in the majority of guinea pig studies although a few of the earlier studies were negative (**). The demonstration of complement deposition in the mouse model has been technically difficult and generally interpreted as negative. A key role for the anti-TBM antibody (humoral immunity) in the induction of disease is supported by the observation that the disease can be reproduced by passive transfer of the antibody in all three animal models. Although the role of cellular immunity has not yet been fully defined, immune cells passively transferred to naive susceptible stains of rats and mice have induced disease (***).*

passive transfer of antibody initiated additional antibody production by the recipient animal—a process referred to as "autoimmune amplification." It is unknown whether this process represents inactivation of mechanisms responsible for tolerance, production of anti-idiotypic antibodies, reaction to TBM antigens altered by the binding of the primary antibody, or other as yet undefined activities. It has recently been reported that the induction of anti-idiotypic antibodies, that is, antibodies reactive with unique determinants in the variable portion of the immunoglobulin chain close to the antigen-binding site, is involved in the regulation of expression of anti-TBM disease. Brown et al. [60] reported that guinea pigs pretreated with anti-idiotypic antibodies failed to develop anti-TBM nephritis following immunization with rabbit TBM. The suppression of the antibody response in this study was shown to be specific for TBM antigens, and, although the mechanism of suppression is unknown, currently it is thought to be more complex than the simple neutralization of antibodies by the formation of idiotype-anti-idiotype complexes and may represent clonal depletion of B cells or the production of suppressor T cells.

Depending upon the techniques employed, C3 is usually found with IgG, deposited along the TBM in a linear pattern. Decomplemented guinea pigs fail to develop disease while guinea pigs with a genetic deficiency of C4 develop tubulo-interstitial inflammation indistinguishable from that seen in animals with an intact complement cascade, suggesting that complement fixation is necessary and must proceed by way of the alternative pathway

[402,404]. This proposal is strengthened by the observation that factor B (C3 proactivator of the alternative pathway) can be demonstrated along the TBM with IgG and C3 [406]. However, the mechanism by which complement contributes to renal injury is at present not clear since there is no morphological evidence of infiltration of polymorphonuclear leucocytes in the early phase of the guinea pig model, although this is a universal feature of the initial tubulo-interstitial inflammation in the rat models. As discussed in the previous sections, complement plays a key role in the early inflammatory changes seen in anti-GBM nephritis due to its function as a chemotaxin resulting in the recruitment of polymorphonuclear leukocytes. It should be mentioned that a few investigators have been unable to detect complement deposition along the TBM even in guinea pigs with significant disease [180,204,495].

The histologic hallmark of acute tubulo-interstitial disease, namely, the infiltration of mononuclear cells, is suggestive of a cell-mediated immune reaction, although such a finding is not pathognomonic since these cells may predominate in certain antibody-mediated and non-immunological reactions as well. There is no question, based on the passive transfer studies, that humoral mechanisms are clearly implicated in the initiation of anti-TBM disease; however, the irradiation studies of Rudofsky et al [405] in 1975 demonstrated that a functioning bone marrow was essential for the actual development of disease. Guinea pigs that were irradiated prior to the passive transfer of anti-TBM antibodies fixed antibody and complement along the TBM but failed to manifest evidence of tubular injury.

Early attempts to transfer tubulo-interstitial disease by the passive administration of lymphocytes were largely unsuccessful, leading to the premature conclusion that sensitized lymphoid cells contribute minimally to tubular injury [495].

The extensive studies of the guinea pig model by Neilson and Phillips [351–354] now provide strong evidence that a significant population of lymphocytes becomes sensitized to tubular antigens early in the induction phase of anti-TBM disease and demonstrates the potential not only to participate in renal injury but also to provide a system to regulate disease activity. Evaluation of lymphocyte function following immunization of guinea pigs with TBM preparations has led to the following observations: (1) A subpopulation of lymphocytes has become sensitized to TBM antigens even before anti-TBM antibody production is detectable [351]. These cells can be identified in vivo by skin testing for delayed-type hypersensitivity reactions to tubular antigens and in vitro as lymphocyte proliferation induced by stimulation with similar antigens. At the same time, a nonspecific, polyclonal suppressor lymphocyte system is apparently activated, as suggested by in vitro mitogen stimulation assays. (2) A subpopulation of lymphocytes obtained from diseased animals appears to be primed to migrate to the kidney, whether it is diseased or normal, as demonstrated by tracing the route of radiolabeled lymphoid cells transferred from nephritic animals into a second recipient [352]. (3) Cytotoxic lymphocytes reactive in vitro with target kidney monolayers are present only in nephritic guinea pigs, suggesting that they may function in vivo, participating directly in cytotoxic reactions [352]. However, this cytotoxic activity may be held in check by the simultaneous activation of a population of lymphocytes (obtained experimentally from the spleens of nephritic animals) that have the ability to suppress this cytotoxic response. (4) The sensitized lymphocytes may participate indirectly in renal injury through the secretion of lymphokines or lymphotoxins. For example, normal guinea pig lymphocytes in culture secrete a soluble inhibitor of fibroblast proliferation and collagen synthesis whereas cultured lymphocytes obtained from nephritic guinea pigs produce a factor that enhances these activities [353]. (5) The natural surveillance provided by natural killer cells may directly participate in tubular cytoxicity by virtue of the ability of these cells to bind to TBM-bound antibodies and induce injury (demonstrated by the ability of natural killer cells isolated from normal guinea pig spleens to interact with anti-TBM antibodies obtained from the sera of nephritic animals and lyse target cells coated with tubular antigens) [354].

The role of monocytes and macrophages in the expression of anti-TBM disease has not been studied in detail, although in all animal models examined to date these cells can be identified in the interstitial inflammatory lesions, especially in the later stages where they occasionally participate in the formation of multinucleated giant cells. The irradiation studies of Rudofsky and Pollara [405] propose that the progression of interstitial nephritis in irradiated guinea pigs can be restored in animals rescued with bone marrow cells but not with spleen or lymph node cells, suggesting the need for monocytes in addition to lymphocytes [405].

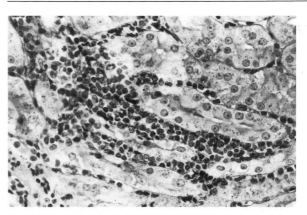

FIG. 13-21. *Light photomicrograph of the kidney obtained from a Brown Norway rat 13 days after immunization with heterologous (bovine) TBM in adjuvant demonstrates impressive infiltration of the renal interstitium with mononuclear cells and occasional polymorphonuclear leucocytes.*

Experimental Model of Anti-TBM Nephritis in Rats

Rats immunized with preparations of heterologous TBM may develop tubulo-interstitial disease similar to that observed in guinea pigs (Figs. 13-21, 13-22) with the notable exception that the lesions usually develop more slowly and are associated with an early phase of infiltration of polymorphonuclear leucocytes, which has not been reported in guinea pigs [273] (Fig. 13-20). Injection of rats with homologous kidney preparations may also induce tubulo-interstitial disease associated with the formation of anti-TBM antibodies although this protocol also produces the glomerular lesion of Heymann nephritis [360,470].

Under the various immunization protocols that have been employed, it has been consistently observed that only certain strains of rats develop tubulo-interstitial nephritis. This susceptibility to disease is under genetic control, which operates at a level different from that observed in guinea pigs. In rats, it is the expression or lack of expression of nephritogenic antigens along the TBM that differs between strains [273]. Rats immunized with bovine TBM produce antibodies cross-reactive with an alloantigen present in the TBM of their own proximal tubules. Lewis (LE), Wistar-Furth, and Maxx strains of rats lack this alloantigen, fail to bind the circulating nephritogenic antibody produced in response to heterologous TBM, and, hence, remain disease free. Transplantation of an antigen-positive kidney from a (LEx BN) F1 hybrid rat into a Lewis rat results in the development of tubulo-interstitial nephritis in the renal allograft. A collagenase-solubilized TBM antigen of 42,000 daltons isolated from bovine and Brown Norway (BN) rat TBM has been shown to be strongly reactive with antibodies eluted from the kidneys of rats with anti-TBM nephritis, supporting a role for this antigen in the development of anti-TBM nephritis [531]. More recently, a glycoprotein of 48,000 daltons (3M-1) has been isolated from collagenase-solubilized rabbit TBM. Immunization with this protein produces interstitial nephritis in

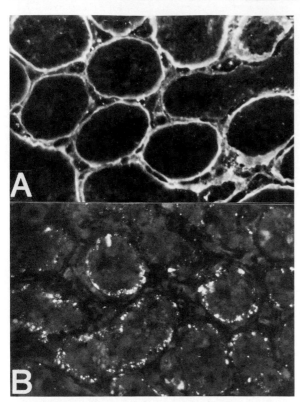

FIG. 13-22. *Immunofluorescence photomicrographs demonstrating two distinct patterns of immunological tubulointerstitial disease. Linear deposition of rat IgG is found along the TBM in Brown Norway rats with experimental anti-TBM nephritis produced by immunization with preparations of heterologous TBM suspended in Freund's adjuvant (A). Rabbits with chronic serum sickness induced by repetitive administration of bovine serum albumin may develop tubulointerstitial nephritis characterized by the granular deposition of antibodies and C3 along the TBM (B).*

susceptible rat strains [71]. The gene controlling expression of the TBM antigen is not linked to the major histocompatibility complex [378]. Other rat strains, including F344 and August, express the TBM-alloantigen but fail to develop disease due to the failure of production of anti-TBM antibodies following immunization with heterologous TBM. The genetic basis for this difference in anti-TBM response is unknown. It has been suggested that the development of secondary interstitial cellular infiltrates in rats is HLA-linked at the RT1 locus [357,358].

The timing of induction of interstitial inflammation and tubular injury in rats is somewhat variable depending upon the immunogen preparation. Complement deposition is frequently reported by nine to 14 days. Unique to this model is the transient infiltration of polymorphonuclear leukocytes, usually beginning in the second week and gone by the end of the third week [273,471].

Very little is known about the role of the mononuclear cells found invading the interstitium. A recent immunohistochemical study of anti-TBM nephritis in the rat employing monoclonal antibodies has characterized the mononuclear infiltrate as being composed largely of T-helper lymphocytes with smaller contributions by B-lymphocytes, T-suppressor lymphocytes, and monocytes, the latter participating primarily in the more advanced stages of disease [297]. Passive transfer studies have demonstrated that both anti-TBM antibody and immune cells can induce mild disease in susceptible rat strains [275,472]. The latter was suggested by the demonstration that peritoneal exudate cells elicited from rats with anti-TBM nephritis and injected under the renal capsule of normal recipients produced focal interstitial lesions. Neilson et al. [355,358] reported that rats immunized with heterologous TBM developed anti-TBM antibodies in association with renal disease, but failed to simultaneously produce anti-idiotypic antibodies directed against the new anti-TBM antibodies. They hypothesized that disease develops because immunization with TBM not only activates humoral immunity but also triggers a population of suppressor cells that block the anticipated anti-idiotype response. Unchallenged nephritogenic antibody was thus available to induce severe inflammation within the kidney. As with the guinea pig model, it has been demonstrated that pretreatment of rats with anti-idiotypic antiserum abrogates tubulo-interstitial disease associated with active TBM immunization [532]. Thus, the humoral afferent limb initiating tubulo-interstitial disease may be held in check by counter-regulatory mechanisms that tightly control its activity. As is so often the case when one attempts to dissect the pathways of immunologic injury, humoral and cellular mechanisms often converge, making it difficult to evaluate each pathway independently.

Experimental Model of Anti-TBM Nephritis in Mice

Anti-TBM antibodies have occasionally been noted to develop spontaneously in the murine models of SLE (NZB/W and MRL mice) [407]. The development of experimental anti-TBM associated tubulo-interstitial nephritis in mice was first studied in some detail by Rudofsky in 1980 [309,407,408]. Certain strains of mice immunized with heterologous preparations of TBM develop disease, although the damage is mild and late in onset, usually beginning six to ten weeks after immunization. The actual role of antibody in disease production has been challenged even though passive transfer studies have shown that the anti-TBM antibody does transfer disease. Although all strains of mice studied to date produce anti-TBM antibodies following active immunization, only certain strains subsequently develop tubulo-interstitial nephritis [407,408]. In fact, this susceptibility to disease appears to be influenced by gene products linked to the major histocompatibility complex at the H-2K locus [356]. Furthermore, once these antibodies bind to the TBM, a lag period of four to five weeks ensues before any signs of disease are notable.

It has been difficult to demonstrate a role for complement in the murine models. The renal deposition of C3 is difficult to determine convincingly since deposits are present in normal mice. Also, mice with a genetic deficiency of C5 develop disease similar to that seen in C5 sufficient mice [46,407].

Recent studies are beginning to point to the cellular

immune system as a probable key mediator of injury in this model. Identical disease can be induced in naive mice by the passive transfer of T-lymphocytes obtained from the lymph nodes or spleen of nephritic mice [530]. Disease expression in such studies has been linked to the transfer of cytotoxic T-lymphocytes (effector cells) identified by surface markers Thy-1.2, Lyt-1,2 in the absence of deposition of antibody and complement along the TBM, supporting the conclusion that cellular rather than humoral immunity induced the observed disease. Cell-counting studies employing monoclonal antibodies suggest that macrophages account for approximately 20% of the interstitial cellular infiltrate in mice. The role of these cells has not been explored [358].

ANTIBODIES AGAINST ANTIGENIC DETERMINANTS WITHIN THE TUBULAR CAPILLARY WALL (NON-TBM ANTIGENS)

The first description of the formation of immune complexes in situ within the tubular capillary wall was in rabbits injected with preparations of renal tissue or given repeated renal allografts [244,489]. Antibodies from these kidneys demonstrated specific reactivity with deposits in similarly diseased kidneys but also with the cytoplasm of the proximal tubules of normal rabbits, suggesting that the antigen involved in the formation of these complexes was a component normally found in proximal tubular epithelial cells.

The nephritogenic antigen of Heymann nephritis (Fx1A, gp 330) present along the brush border of proximal tubules has received relatively little attention as a potentially nephritic TBM antigen, as experimental interest has been more focused on the participation of an immunologically cross-reactive antigen present in the glomerulus in the induction of membranous nephropathy. However, following the detection of circulating anti-Fx1A antibodies, deposition of IgG along the luminal border of proximal tubules is observed [324,360]. Morphological studies suggest that these anti-brush border antibodies are cytotoxic to tubular epithelial cells, resulting in the destruction of microvilli and degeneration and proliferation of epithelial cells. Electron dense deposits may be observed much later in the course of Heymann nephritis along the subepithelial aspect of the TBM associated with the deposition of IgG and C3 [245,324]. Thus, it has been suggested that this antigen may play a dual role in antibody-initiated tubular injury: Firstly, as a TBM-bound ligand it couples the cytotoxic antibody present in the urine of proteinuric animals directly to the luminal surface of tubular epithelial cells, resulting in epithelial toxicity; secondly, in the more advanced states this antigen may be released from damaged cells and migrate toward the anti-luminal surface, where it again encounters antibody (delivered through the peritubular capillaries) and leads to the formation of immune complexes in situ along the TBM.

Tamm-Horsfall Protein Associated Nephritis
An antigen normally present on the surface of epithelial cells of the thick ascending limb of the loop of Henle, Tamm-Horsfall protein, may participate in tubulo-intersti-tial nephritis by the formation of immune complexes [199–201]. Tamm-Horsfall protein is a glycoprotein made exclusively in the kidney and excreted into the urine (approximately 50 mg/day in the adult man) where it forms the major constituent of urinary casts. It has been suggested that the extratubular deposition of this protein, which has been observed in the kidneys of patients suffering from a variety of diseases, including medullary cystic disease, obstructive uropathy, chronic pyelonephritis, idiopathic tubulo-interstitial nephritis, and renal allograft rejection, may play a role in these pathological conditions [78, 201,529].

Hoyer [200] reported that rats chronically immunized with Tamm-Horsfall protein develop tubulo-interstitial disease. This disease is characterized by the formation of circulating anti-Tamm-Horsfall antibodies, deposition of IgG and C3 along the epithelial aspect of the TBM in the medullary regions of the kidney associated with the ascending loops of Henle and early distal tubule (namely, the areas of the kidney where Tamm-Horsfall protein is normally found), and the presence of electron dense deposits in an extracellular position located between the basal cell membrane infoldings of the epithelial cells and the TBM [439]. Since similar lesions did not develop in the glomeruli and antibody deposition failed to occur along the luminal side of the epithelium, it was proposed that nephritis resulted from the interaction of Tamm-Horsfall protein present on the surface or released from within the specified tubular epithelial cells with antibodies delivered through the peritubular capillaries rather than with antibodies present in the glomerular filtrate (Fig. 13-23). This lesion can be passively transferred with high doses of anti-Tamm-Horsfall antisera, although the TBM deposits are rapidly removed following the elimination of circulating antibodies, as contrasted with the deposits formed during chronic active immunization, which may persist as long as 12 months following the final boost [139]. At the present time, the pathway of elimination of immune complexes formed within the tubular capillary unit is unknown, although migration through the renal lymphatics or backflow into the circulation through the peritubular capillaries seems more likely than the urinary route of excretion.

TBM DEPOSITION OF CIRCULATING IMMUNE COMPLEXES

In the evaluation of human renal diseases thought to be of immunological origin, immune deposits along the TBM are only rarely found, with the notable exception of systemic lupus erythematosus [58,274,369]. Although such deposits may be associated with significant tubulo-interstitial pathology, in some cases of SLE abundant deposits may be found without evidence of damage, which raises important unanswered questions regarding the pathogenicity of these deposits [278]. Immune complexes have been rarely found along the TBM in patients with Sjögren's syndrome, mesangiocapillary glomerulonephritis, membranous nephropathy, idiopathic crescentic nephritis, shunt nephritis, and mixed cryoglobulinemia or in renal allografts [310]. Experimentally, immune deposits along the TBM have been reported in the model of chronic serum sickness in rabbits

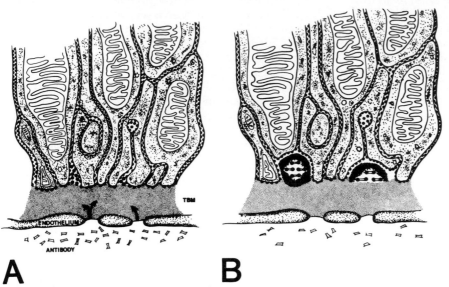

FIG. 13-23. *The mechanism of formation of immune complexes in situ along the TBM in animals immunized with a normal tubular antigen, Tamm-Horsfall protein (THP). THP is present along the surface of epithelial cells lining the thick ascending limb of the loop of Henle (represented by solid half circles) and within the subepithelial space between cells (solid circles). Antibodies to THP circulating within the peritubular capillaries of immunized animals diffuse across the TBM (shaded area) (A) to form electron dense immune deposits (large dark deposits) along the subepithelial aspect of the TBM (B). (Reprinted from Seiler MW, Hoyer JR, Lab Invest 45:321, 1981, with permission.)*

[56] (Fig. 13-22). Such deposits were most readily produced by multiple daily injections of BSA into rabbits with high titer antibody responses, suggesting that very elevated levels of circulating immune complexes developed, saturing sites within the mononuclear phagocytic system and glomerulus before deposition within the tubular capillary unit was detectable. These deposits were associated with interstitial infiltration of polymorphonuclear and mononuclear leucocytes, interstitial fibrosis, deposition of IgG, IgM, and C3 along the TBM, and electron dense deposits detectable along both the subendothelial and subepithelial aspects of the TBM. Renal interstitial deposits of immune complexes have been observed in the murine models of SLE [308,310]. Given the present assumption that the majority of human glomerulonephritis is initiated by the deposition of immune complexes from the circulation, it is indeed remarkable that these complexes are only rarely found within the tubulo-interstitial compartment of the kidney—an observation that is not well understood. Furthermore, it appears that the secondary mediators of immune injury may not always be accessible to deposits in these locations since tubulo-interstitial deposits have been observed in the absence of significant pathological changes.

Cellular Mechanisms of Tubulo-Interstitial Nephritis

As discussed in the previous section, recruitment of mononuclear cells appears to be the major mediator of tubulo-

interstitial injury initiated by the binding of antibodies to components of the TBM. What remains to be unraveled is whether cellular immune mechanisms can initiate tubulo-interstitial nephritis in the absence of antibody and immune complexes. In this area, so little experimental data are available that this theoretical mechanism must be considered speculative at the present time. A delayed-type hypersensitivity reaction can be elicited in the renal cortex of presensitized rats and guinea pigs subjected to intra-renal injections of aggregated bovine gamma globulin—a reaction that could be transferred with lymph node cells but not with serum [496].

Studies of a unique model of tubulo-interstitial nephritis in Lewis rats immunized with homologous TBM provide some support for a primary role of cellular immunity in interstitial nephritis [472]. Lewis rats injected with a renal homogenate in adjuvant obtained from normal Lewis rats developed a severe tubulo-interstitial nephritis by days ten to 14 in the absence of detectable IgG, C3, or immune deposits. The lesion was transferable to normal rats with lymph node or spleen cells but not with serum. More recently it has been reported that a similar lesion develops in Lewis rats immunized with a TBM preparation obtained from Brown-Norway rats [21a]. Recall from the previous section that the proximal tubules of Lewis rats lack the so-called "nephritogenic" tubular antigen present in several other rat strains. The passive transfer of cells but not serum produced interstitial nephritis in naive Lewis rats. In contrast, transfer of the same serum to tubular-antigen positive, normal Brown Norway rats resulted in the development of classical anti-TBM nephritis. In this model, in vitro lymphocyte proliferation studies showed evidence of sensitization of lymphocytes obtained from nephritic Lewis rats to tubular-antigen positive TBM but not to tubular-antigen negative TBM. Future studies are needed to determine whether or not a delayed-type hypersensitivity reaction can initiate disease within the renal interstitium.

References

1. Abrahamson DR, Caulfield JP: Proteinuria and structural alterations in rat glomerular basement membranes induced by intravenously injected anti-laminin immunoglobulin G. *J Exp Med* 156:128, 1982.
2. Abrass CK, Border WA, Glassock RJ: Circulating immune complexes in rats with autologous immune complex glomerulonephritis. *Lab Invest* 43:18, 1980.
3. Abrass CK, McVay J, Glassock RJ: Evaluation of homologous and isologous passive Heymann nephritis: Influence on endogenous antibody production. *J Immunol* 130:195, 1983.
4. Abrass CK: Autologous immune complex nephritis in rats. Influence of modification of mononuclear phagocyte system function. *Lab Invest* 51:162, 1984.
5. Adler S, Salant DJ, Dittmer JE, et al: Mediation of proteinuria in membranous nephropathy due to a planted glomerular antigen. *Kidney Int* 23:807, 1983.
6. Adler S, Baker PJ, Pritzl P, et al: Detection of terminal complement components in experimental immune glomerular injury. *Kidney Int* 26:830, 1984.
7. Agodoa LYC, Gauthier VJ, Mannik M: Precipitating antigen-antibody systems are required for the formation of subepithelial electron-dense immune deposits in rat glomeruli. *J Exp Med* 158:1259, 1983.
8. Albini B, Ossi E, Andres G: The pathogenesis of pericardial, pleural and peritonal effusions in rabbits with serum sickness. *Lab Invest* 37:64, 1977.
9. Albini B, Andres G: Autoimmune disease induced in rabbits by administration of mercuric chloride: Evidence suggesting a role for antigens of the connective tissue matrix. *In* Cummings NB, Michael AF, Wilson CB (eds): *Immune Mechanisms in Renal Disease.* New York, Plenum, 1983, p 249.
10. Alousi MA, Post RA, Heymann W: Experimental autoimmune nephrosis in rats. Morphogenesis of the glomerular lesion: Immunohistochemical and electron microscopic studies. *Am J Pathol* 54:47, 1969.
11. Andrews BS, Eisenberg RA, Theofilopoulos AN, et al: Spontaneous murine lupus-like syndromes. *J Exp Med* 148:1198, 1978.
12. Arend WP, Mannik M: Studies on antigen-antibody complexes. II. Quantification of tissue uptake of soluble complexes in normal and complement-depleted rabbits. *J Immunol* 107:63, 1971.
13. Arend WP, Mannik M: In vitro adherence of soluble immune complexes to macrophages. *J Exp Med* 136:514, 1972.
14. Arisz L, Noble B, Milgrom M, et al: Experimental chronic serum sickness in rats. A model of immune complex glomerulonephritis and systemic immune complex deposition. *Int Arch Allergy Appl Immunol* 60:80, 1979.
15. Atkins RC, Glasgow EF, Holdsworth SR, et al: The macrophage in human rapidly progressive glomerulonephritis. *The Lancet* 1:830, 1976.
16. Atkins RC, Holdsworth SR, Hancock WW, et al: Cellular immune mechanisms in human glomerulonephritis: The role of mononuclear leucocytes. *Springer Semin. Immunopathol.* 5:269, 1982.
17. Atkinson JP, Frank MM: The effect of bacillus Calmette-Guerin induced macrophage activation in the in vivo clearance of sensitized erythrocytes. *J Clin Invest* 53:1742, 1974.
18. Averbuch SD, Austin HA, Sherwin SA, et al: Acute interstitial nephritis with the nephrotic syndrome following recombinant leukocyte A interferon therapy for mycosis fungoides. *N Engl J Med* 310:32, 1984.
19. Banks KL, Henson JB, McGuire TC: Immunologically mediated glomerulitis of horses: I. Pathogenesis in persistent infection by equine infectious anemia virus. *Lab Invest* 26:701, 1972.
20. Banks KL, Henson JB: Immunologically mediated glomerulitis of horses: II. Antiglomerular basement membrane antibody and other mechanisms in spontaneous disease. *Lab Invest* 26:706, 1972.
21. Bannister KM, Hay J, Clarkson AR, et al: Fc-specific reticulo-endothelial clearance in systemic lupus erythematosus and glomerulonephritis. *Am J Kidney Dis* 3:287, 1984.
21a. Bannister KM, Ulrich TR, Wilson CB: Cell-mediated autoimmune tubulo-interstitial nephritis in the Lewis rat (abstr). *Kidney Int* 27:205, 1985.
22. Barabas AZ, Lannigan R: Induction of an autologous immune complex glomerulonephritis in the rat by intravenous injection of heterologous anti-rat kidney tubular antibody. I. Production of chronic progressive immune-complex glomerulonephritis. *Brit J Exp Pathol* 55:47, 1974.
23. Barcelli V, Rademacher R, Ooi YM, et al: Modification of glomerular immune complex deposition in mice by activation of the reticuloendothelial system. *J Clin Invest* 67:20, 1981.
24. Barnett EV, Bluestone R, Cracchiolo A, III, et al: Cryoglobulinemia and disease. *Ann Intern Med* 73:95, 1970.
25. Bartolotti SR, Peters DK: Delayed removal of renal-bound antigen in decomplemented rabbits with acute serum sickness. *Clin Exp Immunol* 32:199, 1978.
26. Batsford SR, Takamiya H, Vogt A: A model of in situ immune complex glomerulonephritis in the rat employing cationized ferritin. *Clin Nephrol* 14:211, 1980.
27. Baud L, Hagege J, Sraer J, et al: Reactive oxygen production by cultured rat glomerular mesangial cells during phagocytosis is associated with stimulation of lipoxygenase activity. *J Exp Med* 158:1836, 1983.
28. Baxter JH, Goodman HC: Nephrotoxic serum nephritis in rats: I. Distribution and specificity of the antigen responsible for the production of nephrotoxic antibodies. *J Exp Med* 104:467, 1956.
29. Becker CG: Demonstration of actinomycin in mesangial cells of the renal glomerulus. *Am J Pathol* 66:97, 1972.
30. Becker GJ, Hancock WW, Stow JL, et al: Involvement of the macrophage in experimental chronic immune complex glomerulonephritis. *Nephron* 32:227, 1982.
31. Benacerraf B, McCluskey RT, Patras D: Localization of colloidal substances in vascular endothelium. A mechanism of tissue damage: I. Factors causing the pathologic deposition of colloidal carbon. *Am J Pathol* 35:75, 1959.
32. Benacerraf B, Sebestyen M, Cooper NS: The clearance of antigen-antibody complexes from the blood by the reticuloendothelial system. *J Immunol* 82:131, 1959.
33. Bender BL, Jaffe R, Carlin B, et al: Immunolocalization of entactin, a sulfated basement membrane component, in rodent tissues, and comparison with GP-2 (laminin). *Am J Pathol* 103:419, 1981.

34. Bendixen G: Organ-specific inhibition of the in vitro migration of leucocytes in human glomerulonephritis. *Acta Med Scand* 184:99, 1968.

35. Berger M, Balaw JE, Wilson CB, et al: Circulating immune complexes and glomerulonephritis in a patient with congenital absence of the third component of complement. *N Engl J Med* 308:1009, 1983.

36. Bertani T, Remuzzi G, Poggi A, et al: Severe glomerular epithelial cell damage does not prevent passive Heymann nephritis in rats. *Clin Exp Immunol* 51:38, 1983.

37. Bhan AK, Schneeberger EE, Collins AB, et al: Evidence for a pathogenic role of a cell-mediated immune mechanism in experimental glomerulonephritis. *J Exp Med* 148:246, 1978.

38. Bhan AK, Collins AB, Schneeberger EE, et al: A cell-mediated reaction against glomerular-bound immune complexes. *J Exp Med* 150:1410, 1979.

39. Bhan AK, Schneeberger EE, Collins AB, et al: Systemic cell-mediated reactions in vivo. *Am J Pathol* 116:77, 1984.

40. Biesecker G, Katz S, Koffler D: Renal localization of the membrane attack complex in systemic lupus erythematosus nephritis. *J Exp Med* 154:1779, 1981.

41. Biesecker G: Biology of disease: Membrane attack complex of complement as a pathologic mediator. *Lab Invest* 49:237, 1983.

42. Biesecker G, Noble B, Andres GA, et al: Immunopathogenesis of Heymann's nephritis. *Clin Immunol Immunopathol* 33:333, 1984.

43. Blantz RC, Wilson CB: Acute effects of anti-glomerular basement membrane antibody on the process of glomerular filtration in the rat. *J Clin Invest* 58:899, 1976.

44. Blantz RC, Tucker BJ, Wilson CB: The acute effects of antiglomerular basement membrane antibody on the process of glomerular fibration in the rat. The influence of dose and complement depletion. *J Clin Invest* 61:910, 1978.

45. Bolton WK, Sturgill BC: Bovine serum albumen chronic serum sickness nephropathy in rats. *Br J Exp Pathol* 59:167, 1978.

46. Bolton WK, Benton FR, Sturgill BC: Autoimmune glomerulotubular nephropathy in mice. *Clin Exp Immunol* 33:463, 1978.

47. Bolton WK, Benton FR, Lobo PI: Requirement of functional T-cells in the production of autoimmune glomerulotubular nephropathy in mice. *Clin Exp Immunol* 33:474, 1978.

48. Bolton WK, Tucker FL, Sturgill BC: Experimental autoimmune glomerulonephritis in chickens. *J Clin Lab Immunol* 3:179, 1980.

49. Bolton WK, Tucker FL, Sturgill BC: New avian model of experimental glomerulonephritis consistent with mediation by cellular immunity. Nonhumorally mediated glomerulonephritis in chickens. *J Clin Invest* 73:1263, 1984.

50. Border, WA, Wilson CB, Dixon FJ: Failure of heparin to affect two types of experimental glomerulonephritis in rabbits. *Kidney Int* 8:140, 1975.

51. Border WA, Ward HJ, Kamil ES, et al: Induction of membranous nephropathy in rabbits by administration of an exogenous cationic antigen. *J Clin Invest* 69:451, 1982.

52. Border WA, Cohen AH: Role of immunoglobulin class in mediation of experimental mesangial glomerulonephritis. *Clin Immunol Immunopathol* 27:187, 1983.

53. Borel Y, Lewis RM, Andre-Schwartz J, et al: Treatment of lupus nephritis in adult (NZBxNZW) F_1 mice by cortisone-facilitated tolerance to nucleic acid antigens. *J Clin Invest* 61:276, 1978.

54. Borzy MS, Houghton D: Mixed-pattern immune deposit glomerulonephritis in a child with inherited deficiency of the third component of complement. *Am J Kidney Dis* 5:54, 1985.

55. Boulton-Jones JM, Tulloch I, Dore B, et al: Changes in the glomerular capillary wall induced by lymphocyte products and serum of nephrotic patients. *Clin Nephrol* 20:72, 1983.

56. Brentjens JR, O'Connell DW, Pawlowski IB, et al: Extraglomerular lesions associated with deposition of circulating antigen-antibody complexes in kidneys of rabbits with chronic serum sickness. *Clin Immunol Immunopathol* 3:112, 1974.

57. Brentjens JR, O'Connell DW, Albini B, et al: Experimental chronic serum sickness in rabbits that receive daily multiple and high doses of antigen: A systemic disease. *Ann New York Acad Sci* 254:603, 1975.

58. Brentjens JR, Sepulveda M, Baliah T, et al: Interstitial immune complex nephritis in patients with systemic lupus erythematosus. *Kidney Int* 7:342, 1975.

59. Briggs JD, Kwaan HC, Potter EV: The role of fibrinogen in renal disease. III. Fibrinolytic and anticoagulant treatment of nephrotoxic serum nephritis in mice. *J Lab Clin Med* 74:715, 1969.

60. Brown CA, Carey K, Colvin RB: Inhibition of autoimmune interstitial nephritis in guinea pigs by heterologous antisera containing anti-idiotype antibodies. *J Immunol* 123:2102, 1979.

61. Buchmeier MJ, Oldstone MBA: Virus-induced immune complex disease: Identification of specific viral antigens and antibodies deposited in complexes during chronic lymphocytic choriomeningitis virus infection. *J Immunol* 120:1297, 1978.

62. Camazine SM, Ryan GB, Unanue ER, et al: Isolation of phagocytic cells from the rat renal glomerulus. *Lab Invest* 35:315, 1976.

63. Cameron JS: Glomerulonephritis: Current problems and understanding. *J Lab Clin Med* 99:755, 1982.

64. Cameron JS: Platelets in glomerular disease. *Ann Rev Med* 35:175, 1984.

65. Camussi G, Tetta C, Segoloni G, et al: Localization of neutrophil cationic proteins and loss of anionic charges in glomeruli of patients with systemic lupus erythematosus glomerulonephritis. *Clin Immunol Immunopathol* 24:299, 1982.

66. Cattell V, Arlidge S: The origin of proliferating cells in the glomerulus and Bowman's capsule in nephrotoxic serum nephritis: effects of unilateral renal irradiation. *Br J Exp Path* 62:669, 1981.

67. Caulin-Glaser T, Gallo GR, Lamm ME: Nondissociating cationic immune complexes can deposit in glomerular basement membrane. *J Exp Med* 158:1561, 1983.

68. Chartrand C, O'Regan S, Robitaille P, et al: Delayed rejection of cardiac xenografts in C6-deficient rabbits. *Immunology* 38:245, 1979.

69. Chorvath D, Brozman M: Nephrotoxic and pneumotoxic antibodies and their acute action on lungs: I. Preparation, isolation and characterization of antibodies. *Exp Pathol (Jena)* 9:199, 1974.

70. Clark WF, Teraarwerk GJM, Bandali K, et al: Platelet aggregation and release associated with immune complex formation in pig plasma. *J Lab Clin Med* 96:654, 1980.

71. Clayman MD, Martinez-Hernandez A, Michaud L, et al: Isolation and characterization of the nephritogenic antigen producing anti-tubular basement membrane disease. *J Exp Med* 161:290, 1985.

72. Clive DM, Stoff JS: Renal syndromes associated with nonsteroidal antiinflammatory drugs. *N Engl J Med* 310:563, 1984.

73. Cochrane CG, Unanue ER, Dixon FJ: A role of polymorphonuclear leukocytes and complement in nephrotoxic nephritis. J Exp Med 122:99, 1965.

74. Cochrane CG, Hawkins D: Studies on circulating immune complexes: III. Factors governing the ability of circulating complexes to localize in blood vessels. J Exp Med 127:137, 1968.

75. Cochrane CG, Janoff A: The Arthus reaction: A model of neutrophil and complement mediated injury. In Zweifach BW, Grant L, McCluskey RT (eds): The Inflammatory Process (2nd ed.). New York, Academic, 1974, p 85.

76. Cochrane CG: Mediation systems in neutrophil-independent immunologic injury of the glomerulus. In Wilson CB (ed): Immunologic Mechanisms of Renal Disease. Contemporary Issues in Nephrology. New York, Churchill Livingstone, 1979, p 106.

77. Cochrane CG, Revak SD, Wiggins RC: The contact (Hageman factor) system in inflammation. In Cummings NB, Michael AF, Wilson CB (eds): Immune Mechanisms in Renal Disease. New York, Plenum, 1983, p 419.

78. Cohen AH, Border WA, Rafjer J, et al: Interstitital Tamm-Horsfall protein in rejecting renal allografts. Identification and morphologic pattern of injury. Lab Invest 50:519, 1984.

79. Coleman TH, Forristal J, Kosaka T, et al: Inherited complement component deficiencies in membranoproliferative glomerulonephritis. Kidney Int 24:681, 1983.

80. Cordonnier D, Martin H, Groslambert P, et al: Mixed IgG-IgM cryoglobulinemia with glomerulonephritis. Immunochemical, fluorescent and ultrastructural study of kidney and in vitro cryoprecipitate. Am J Med 59:867, 1975.

81. Cornacoff JB, Hebert A, Smead WL, et al: Primate erythrocyte-immune complex-clearing mechanism. J Clin Invest 71:236, 1983.

82. Costanza ME, Pinn V, Schwartz RS, et al: Carcinoembryonic antigen-antibody complexes in a patient with colonic carcinoma and nephrotic syndrome. N Engl J Med 289:520, 1973.

83. Courtoy PJ, Timpl R, Farquhar MG: Comparative distribution of laminin, type IV collagen and fibronectin in the rat glomerulus. J Histochem Cytochem 30:874, 1982.

84. Couser WG, Stilmant M, Lewis EJ: Experimental glomerulonephritis in the guinea pig. I. Glomerular lesions associated with antiglomerular basement membrane antibody deposits. Lab Invest 29:236, 1973.

85. Couser WG, Wagonfeld JB, Spargo BH, et al: Glomerular deposition of tumor antigen in membranous nephropathy associated with colonic carcinoma. Am J Med 57:962, 1974.

86. Couser WG, Stilmant MM, Jermanovich MB: Complement-independent nephrotoxic nephritis in the guinea pig. Kidney Int 11:170, 1977.

87. Couser WG, Steinmuller DR, Stilmant MM, et al: Experimental glomerulonephritis in the isolated perfused rat kidney. J Clin Invest 62:1275, 1978.

88. Couser WG, Jermanovich NB, Belok S, et al: Effect of aminonucleoside nephrosis on immune complex localization in autologous immune complex nephropathy in rats. J Clin Invest 61:561, 1978.

89. Couser WG, Salant DJ: In situ immune complex formation and glomerular injury. Kidney Int 17:1, 1980.

89a. Couser WG: What are circulating immune complexes doing in glomerulonephritis? N Engl J Med 304:1230, 1981.

90. Craddock PR, Fehr J, Dalmasso AP, et al: Hemodialysis leukopenia. Pulmonary vascular leukostasis resulting from complement activation by dialyzer cellophane membranes. J Clin Invest 59:879, 1977.

91. Czop J, Nussenzweig V: Studies on the mechanism of sol-

ubilization of immune precipitates by serum. J Exp Med 143:615, 1976.

92. Dang H, Harbeck R: A comparison of anti-DNA antibodies from the serum and kidney eluates of NZB x NZW F_1 mice. Arthritis Rheum 22:603, 1979.

93. deHeer E, Daha MR, Bhakdi S, et al: Possible involvement of terminal complement complex in active Heymann nephritis. Kidney Int 27:388, 1985.

94. Devey ME, Bleasdale K, Stanley C, et al: Failure of affinity maturation leads to increased susceptibility to immune complex glomerulonephritis. Immunology 52:377, 1984.

95. Dinarello CA: Interleukin-1 and the pathogenesis of the acute-phase response. N Engl J Med 311:1413, 1984.

96. Dixon FJ, Vazquez JJ, Weigle WO, et al: Pathogenesis of serum sickness. AMA Arch Pathol 65:18, 1958.

97. Dixon FJ, Feldman JD, Vazquez JJ: Experimental glomerulonephritis: The pathogenesis of a laboratory model resembling the spectrum of human glomerulonephritis. J Exp Med 113:899, 1961.

98. Dixon FJ: The role of antigen-antibody complexes in disease. Harvey Lect 58:21, 1963.

99. Donadio JV, Anderson CF, Mitchell JC, et al: Membranoproliferative glomerulonephritis: A prospective clinical trial of platelet-inhibitor therapy. N Engl J Med 310:1421, 1984.

100. Douglas MFS, Rabideau DP, Schwartz MM, et al: Evidence of autologous immune-complex nephritis. N Engl J Med 305:1326, 1981.

101. Downie, GH, Roholt OA, Jennings L, et al: Experimental anti-alveolar basement membrane antibody-mediated pneumonitis. II. Role of endothelial damage and repair, induction of autologous phase, and kinetics of antibody deposition in Lewis rats. J Immunol 129:2647, 1982.

102. Dressman GR, Germuth FG, Jr: Immune complex disease: IV. The nature of the circulating complexes associated with glomerulonephritis in the acute BSA-rabbit system. Johns Hopkins Med J 130:335, 1972.

103. Druet E, Sapin C, Gunther E, et al: Mercuric chloride-induced antiglomerular basement membrane antibodies in the rat. Genetic control. Eur J Immunol 7:348, 1977.

104. Druet E, Sapin C, Fournie G, et al: Genetic control of susceptibility to mercury-induced immune nephritis in various strains of rat. Clin Immunol Immunopathol 25:203, 1982.

105. Druet P, Letonturier P, Contet A, et al: Cryoglobulinaemia in human renal diseases. A study of seventy-six cases. Clin Exp Immunol 15:483, 1973.

106. Dubois CH, Foidart JB, Hautier MB, et al: Proliferative glomerulonephritis in rats: Evidence that mononuclear phagocytes infiltrating the glomeruli stimulate the proliferation of endothelial and mesangial cells. Eur J Clin Invest 11:91, 1981.

107. Dubois CH, Goffinet G, Foidart JB, et al: Evidence for a particular binding capacity of rat peritoneal macrophages to rat glomerular mesangial cells in vitro. Eur J Clin Invest 12:239, 1982.

108. Dunn MJ: Nonsteroidal antiinflammatory drugs and renal function. Ann Rev Med 35:411, 1984.

109. Dyck RK, Lockwood CM, Kershaw W, et al: Amyloid P component is a constituent of normal human glomerular basement membrane. J Exp Med 152:1162, 1980.

110. Dyer PA, Koula PT, Harris R, et al: Properidin factor B alleles in patients with idiopathic membranous nephropathy. Tissue Antigens 15:505, 1980.

111. Eastcott JW, Kelley VE: Preservation of T-lymphocyte activity in autoimmune MRL-lpr mice treated with prostaglandin. Clin Immunol Immunopathol 29:78, 1983.

112. Ebling F, Hahn BH: Restricted subpopulations of DNA antibodies in kidneys of mice with systemic lupus. *Arthritis Rheum* 23:392, 1980.

113. Eddy A, Newman SL, Cosio F, et al: The distribution of the CR3 receptor on human cells and tissue as revealed by a monoclonal antibody. *Clin Immunol Immunopathol* 31:371, 1984.

114. Edgington TS, Glassock RJ, Dixon FJ: Autologous immune complex pathogenesis of experimental allergic glomerulonephritis. *Science* 155:1432, 1967.

115. Edgington TS, Glassock RJ, Dixon FJ: Autologous immune complex nephritis induced with renal tubular antigen: I. Identification and isolation of the pathogenetic antigen. *J Exp Med* 127:555, 1968.

116. Engelfriet CP, von dem Borne AEG, Fleer FW, et al: In vivo RES function of erythrocytes by complement binding and non-complement binding antibodies. *In* Sandler SG, Nusbacher J, Schanfield MS (eds): *Immunobiology of the Erythrocyte.* New York, AR Liss, 1980, p 213.

117. Falk RJ, Dalmasso AP, Kim Y, et al: Neoantigen of the polymerized ninth component of complement. *J Clin Invest* 72:560, 1983.

118. Falk RJ, Dalmasso AP, Kim Y, et al: Radioimmunoassay of the attack complex of complement in sera from patients with systemic lupus erythematosus. *N Engl J Med* 312:1594, 1985.

119. Fantone JC, Kunkel SL, Ward PA, et al: Suppression by prostaglandin E_1 of vascular permeability induced by vasoactive inflammatory mediators. *J Immunol* 125:2591, 1980.

120. Fearon DT, Austen KF: The alternative pathway of complement. A system for host resistance to microbial infection. *N Engl J Med* 303:259, 1980.

121. Feenstra K, Lee RVD, Greben HA, et al: Experimental glomerulonephritis in the rat induced by antibodies directed against tubular antigens. I. The natural history: A histologic and immunohistologic study at the light microscopic and ultrastructural level. *Lab Invest* 32:235, 1975.

122. Feiner H, Gallo G: Ultrastructure in glomerulonephritis associated with cryoglobulinemia. A report of six cases and review of the literature. *Am J Pathol* 88:145, 1977.

123. Feldman JD: Electron microscopy of serum sickness nephritis. *J Exp Med* 108:957, 1958.

124. Fennell RH, Pardo VM: Experimental glomerulonephritis in rats. *Lab Invest* 17:481, 1967.

125. Fillit HM, Read SE, Sherman RL, et al: Cellular reactivity to altered glomerular basement membrane in glomerulonephritis. *N Engl J Med* 298:861, 1978.

126. Fillit HM, Zabriskie JB: Cellular immunity in glomerulonephritis. *Am J Pathol* 109:227, 1982.

127. Finbloom DS, Plotz PH: Studies of reticuloendothelial function in the mouse with model immune complexes. II. Serum clearance, tissue uptake, and reticuloendothelial saturation in NZB/W mice. *J Immunol* 123:1600, 1979.

128. Finbloom DS, Magilavy DB, Harford JB, et al: Influence of antigen on immune complex behavior in mice. *J Clin Invest* 68:214, 1981.

129. Fish AJ, Michael AF, Vernier RL, et al: Acute serum sickness nephritis in the rabbit (an immune deposit disease). *Am J Pathol* 49:997, 1966.

130. Fisher ER, Bark J: Effect of hypertension on vascular and other lesions of serum sickness. *Am J Pathol* 39:665, 1961.

131. Foidart JM, Bere EW, Yaar M, et al: Distribution and immunoelectron microscopic localization of laminin, a noncollagenous basement membrane glycoprotein. *Lab Invest* 42:336, 1980.

132. Forbes RDC, Guttmann RD, Kuramochi T, et al: Nonessential role of neutrophils as mediators of hyperacute cardiac allograft rejection in the rat. *Lab Invest* 34:229, 1976.

133. Forbes RDC, Pinto-Blonde M, Guttmann RD: The effect of anticomplementary cobra venom factor on hyperacute rat cardiac allograft rejection. *Lab Invest* 39:463, 1978.

134. Ford PM: The effect of manipulation of reticuloendothelial system activity on glomerular deposition of aggregated protein and immune complexes in two different strains of mice. *Br J Exp Path* 56:523, 1975.

135. Ford PM, Kosatka I: The effect of in situ formation of antigen-antibody complexes in the glomerulus on the subsequent glomerular localization of passively administered immune complexes. *Immunology* 39:337, 1980.

136. Frank MM, Shreiber AD, Atkinson JP, et al: Pathophysiology of immune hemolytic anemia. *Ann Intern Med* 87:210, 1977.

137. Frank MM, Hamburger MI, Lawley TJ, et al: Defective reticuloendothelial system Fc-receptor function in systemic lupus erythematosus. *N Engl J Med* 300:518, 1979.

138. Freire-Maia L, Lemos Fernandes AD, Azevedo AD, et al: Cardiovascular and respiratory changes during acute pulmonary edema produced by nephrotoxic serum in the rat. *Agents Actions* 3:326, 1973.

139. Friedman J, Hoyer JR, Seiler MW: Formation and clearance of tubulointerstitial immune complexes in kidneys of rats immunized with heterologous antisera to Tamm-Horsfall protein. *Kidney Int* 21:575, 1982.

140. Friend PS, Kim Y, Michael AF, et al: Pathogenesis of membranous nephropathy in systemic lupus erythematosus: possible role of nonprecipitating DNA antibody. *Br Med J* 1:25, 1977.

141. Friend PS: A unique antibody response associated with the development of membranous nephropathy in systemic lupus erythematosus. *Am Heart J* 95:672, 1978.

142. Fries LF, Mullins WW, Cho KR, et al: Monocyte receptors for the Fc portion of IgG are increased in systemic lupus erythematosus. *J Immunol* 132:695, 1984.

143. Gallo GR, Caulin-Glaser T, Lamm M: Charge of circulating immune complexes as a factor in glomerular basement membrane localization in mice. *J Clin Invest* 67:1305, 1981.

144. Gallo GR, Caulin-Glaser T, Emancipator SN, et al: Nephritogenicity and differential distribution of glomerular immune complexes related to immunogen charge. *Lab Invest* 48:353, 1983.

145. Gang NF, Mautner W, Kalant N: Nephrotoxic serum nephritis. II. Chemical, morphologic, and functional correlates of glomerular basement membrane at the onset of proteinuria. *Lab Invest* 23:150, 1970.

146. Garber SL, O'Morchoe PJ, O'Morchoe CCC: Effect of experimental glomerulonephritis on the cells in canine renal lymph with special reference to the veiled cell. *Clin Exp Immunol* 49:347, 1982.

147. Gauthier VJ, Mannik M, Striker GE: Effect of cationized antibodies in preformed immune complexes on deposition and persistence in renal glomeruli. *J Exp Med* 156:766, 1982.

148. Gauthier VJ, Striker GE, Mannik M: Glomerular localization of preformed immune complexes prepared with anionic antibodies or with cationic antigens. *Lab Invest* 50:636, 1984.

149. Gelfand MC, Frank MM, Green I: A receptor for the third component of complement in the human renal glomerulus. *J Exp Med* 142:1029, 1975.

150. Genin C, Cosio F, Michael AF: Macromolecular charge and reticuloendothelial function: comparison between the

kinetics of administered native and cationized ferritins and the corresponding immune complexes in the mouse. *Immunology* 51:225, 1984.

151. George CRP, Slichter SJ, Quadracoi LJ, et al: A kinetic evaluation of hemostasis in renal disease. *N Engl J Med* 291:111, 1974.

152. Germuth FG, Jr: Comparative histologic and immunologic study in rabbits of induced hypersensitivity of serum sickness type. *J Exp Med* 97:257, 1953.

153. Germuth FG, Flanagan C, Montenegro MR: The relationships between the chemical nature of the antigen, antigen dosage, rate of antibody synthesis and the occurrence of arteritis and glomerulonephritis in experimental hypersensitivity. *Johns Hopkins Med J* 101:149, 1957.

154. Germuth FG, Jr, Senterfit LB, Pollack AD: Immune complex disease. I. Experimental acute and chronic glomerulonephritis. *Johns Hopkins Med J* 120:225, 1967.

155. Germuth FG, Jr, Kelemen WA, Pollack AD: Immune complex disease. II. The role of circulatory dynamics and glomerular filtration in the development of experimental glomerulonephritis. *Johns Hopkins Med J* 120:252, 1967.

156. Germuth FG, Jr, Senterfit LB, Dreesman GR: Immune complex disease. V. The nature of the circulating complexes associated with glomerular alterations in the chronic BSA-rabbit system. *Johns Hopkins Med J* 130:344, 1972.

157. Germuth FG, Rodriguez E: *Immunopathology of the Renal Glomerulus.* Boston: Little, Brown, 1973.

158. Germuth FG, Rodriguez E, Diddiqui SY, et al: Immune complex disease. VII. Experimental mesangiopathic glomerulonephritis produced by chronic immunization with thyroglobulin. *Lab Invest* 38:404, 1978.

159. Germuth FG, Jr, Rodriguez E, Lorelle CA, et al: Passive immune complex glomerulonephritis in mice: Models for various lesions found in human disease. I. High avidity complexes and mesangiopathic glomerulonephritis. *Lab Invest* 41:360, 1979.

160. Germuth FG, Rodriguez E, Lorelle CA, et al: Passive immune complex glomerulonephritis in mice: Models for various lesions found in human disease. II. Low avidity complexes and diffuse proliferative glomerulonephritis with subepithelial deposits. *Lab Invest* 41:366, 1979.

161. Gewurz H, Pickering RJ, Moberg A, et al: Reactivities to horse anti-lymphocyte globulin II. Serum sickness nephritis with complement alterations in man. *Int Arch Allergy Appl Immunol* 39:210, 1970.

162. Gilliland BC: Clinical immunology. *In* Petersdorf RG, Adams RD, Braunwald E, et al (eds): *Harrison's Principles of Internal Medicine* (10th ed.), New York, McGraw-Hill, 1982, p 344.

163. Gitlin D, Latta H, Batchelor WH, et al: Experimental hypersensitivity in the rabbit: Disappearance rates of native and labeld heterologous proteins from the serum after intravenous injection. *J Immunol* 66:451, 1951.

164. Glasser RJ, Michael AF: Urinary kallikrein in experimental renal disease. *Lab Invest* 34:616, 1976.

165. Glassock RJ, Edgington TS, Watson JI, et al: Autologous immune complex nephritis induced with renal tubular antigen: II. The pathogenetic mechanism. *J Exp Med* 127:573, 1968.

166. Glassock RJ, Adler SG, Ward HJ, et al: Primary glomerular diseases. *In* Brenner BM, Rector FC (eds): *The Kidney* (4th ed.), Philadelphia, Saunders, 1991, p 1182.

167. Golbus SM, Wilson CB: Experimental glomerulonephritis induced by in situ formation of immune complexes in glomerular capillary wall. *Kidney Int* 16:148, 1979.

168. Golde D, Epstein W: Mixed cryoglobulins and glomerulonephritis. *Ann Intern Med* 69:1221, 1968.

169. Goldman M, Rose LM, Hochmann A, et al: Deposition of idiotype-anti-idiotype immune complexes in renal glomeruli after polyclonal B cell activation. *J Exp Med* 155:1385, 1982.

170. Goodwin JS, Webb DR: Regulation of the immune response by prostaglandins. *Clin Immunol Immunopathol* 15:106, 1980.

171. Greenspoon SA, Krakower CA: Direct evidence for the antigenicity of the glomeruli in the production of nephrotoxic serums. *AMA Arch Pathol* 49:291, 1950.

172. Groggel GC, Adler S, Rennke HG, et al: Role of the terminal complement pathway in experimental membranous nephropathy in the rabbit. *J Clin Invest* 72:1948, 1983.

173. Groggel GC, Salant DJ, Darby C, et al: Role of terminal complement pathway in the heterologous phase of anti-glomerular basement membrane nephritis. *Kidney Int* 27:643, 1985.

174. Grupe WE, Kaplan MH: A proximal tubular antigen in the pathogenesis of autoimmune nephrosis. *Fed Proc* 26:573, 1967.

175. Grupe WE, Kaplan MH: Demonstration of an antibody to proximal tubular antigen in the pathogenesis of experimental autoimmune nephrosis in rats. *J Lab Clin Med* 74:400, 1969.

176. Haakenstad AO, Mannik M: Saturation of the reticuloendothelial system with soluble immune complexes. *J Immunol* 112:1939, 1974.

177. Haakenstad AO, Case JB, Mannik M: Effect of cortisone on the disappearance kinetics and tissue localization of soluble immune complexes. *J Immunol* 114:1153, 1975.

178. Haakenstad AO, Striker GE, Mannik M: The glomerular deposition of soluble immune complexes prepared with reduced and alkylated antibodies and with intact antibodies in mice. *Lab Invest* 35:293, 1976.

179. Haakenstad AO, Striker GE, Mannik M: Removal of glomerular immune complex deposits by excess antigen in chronic mouse model of immune complex disease. *Lab Invest* 48:323, 1983.

180. Hall CL, Carey K, Colvin RB, et al: Passive transfer of autoimmune disease with isologous IgG1 and IgG2 antibodies to the tubular basement membrane in strain XIII guinea pigs. *J Exp Med* 146:1246, 1977.

181. Hamburger MI, Lawley TJ, Kimberly R, et al: A serial study of splenic reticuloendothelial system Fc receptor functional activity in systemic lupus erythematosus. *Arthrit Rheumat* 25:48, 1982.

182. Hammer DK, Dixon FJ: Experimental glomerulonephritis: II. Immunologic events in the pathogenesis of nephrotoxic serum nephritis in the rat. *J Exp Med* 117:1019, 1963.

183. Hancock WW, Kraft N, Atkins RC: The immunohistochemical demonstration of major histocompatibility antigens in the human kidney using monoclonal antibodies. *Pathology* 14:409, 1982.

184. Harry T, Bryant D, Coles GA, et al: The detection of monocytes in human renal biopsies: A prospective study. *Clin Nephrol* 18:29, 1982.

185. Hart DNJ, Fuggle SV, Williams KA, et al: Localization of HLA-ABC and DR antigens in human kidney. *Transplantation* 31:423, 1981.

186. Henson PM, Cochrane CG: Acute immune complex disease in rabbits: The role of complement and of a leukocyte-dependent release of vasoactive amines from platelets. *J Exp Med* 133:554, 1971.

187. Heymann W, Hackel DB, Harwood S, et al: Production of nephrotic syndrome in rats by Freund's adjuvants and rat kidney suspensions. *Proc Soc Exp Biol Med* 100:660, 1959.

188. Hinglais N, Kazatchkine MD, Charron DJ, et al: Immunohistochemical study of Ia antigen in the normal and diseased human kidney. *Kidney Int* 25:544, 1984.

189. Hoffsten PE: LCM virus infection and nephritis. *In* Cummings NB, Michael AF, Wilson CB (eds): *Immune Mechanisms in Renal Disease.* New York, Plenum, 1983, p 167.

190. Hogan BLM, Taylor A, Kurkinen M, et al: Synthesis and localization of two sulfated glycoproteins associated with basement membranes and the extracellular matrix. *J Cell Biol* 95:197, 1982.

191. Holdsworth SR, Thomson NM, Glasgow EF, et al: Tissue culture of isolated glomeruli in experimental crescentic glomerulonephritis. *J Exp Med* 147:98, 1978.

192. Holdworth SR, Neale TJ, Wilson CB: The participation of macrophages and monocytes in experimental immune complex glomerulonephritis. *Clin Immunol Immunopathol* 15:510, 1980.

193. Holdsworth SR, Neale TJ, Wilson CB: Abrogation of macrophage-dependent injury in experimental glomerulonephritis in the rabbit. *J Clin Invest* 68:686, 1981.

194. Holdsworth SR: Fc dependence of macrophage accumulation and subsequent injury in experimental glomerulonephritis. *J Immunol* 130:735, 1983.

195. Holdsworth SR, Neale TJ: Macrophage-induced glomerular injury. Cell transfer studies in passive autologous antiglomerular basement membrane antibody-initiated experimental glomerulonephritis. *Lab Invest* 51:172, 1984.

196. Holthofer H, Miettinen A, Lehto V-P, et al: Expression of vimentin and cytokeratin types of intermediate filament proteins in developing and adult human kidneys. *Lab Invest* 50:552, 1984.

197. Houser MT, Scheinman JI, Basgen J, et al: Preservation of mesangium and immunohistochemically defined antigens in glomerular basement membrane isolated by detergent extraction. *J Clin Invest* 69:1169, 1982.

198. Houssin D, Druet E, Hinglais N, et al: Glomerular and vascular IgG deposits in HgCl$_2$ nephritis: Role of circulating antibodies and of immune complexes. *Clin Immunol Immunopathol* 29:167, 1983.

199. Hoyer JR, Seiler MW: Pathophysiology of Tamm-Horsfall protein. *Kidney Int* 16:279, 1979.

200. Hoyer JR: Tubulointerstitial immune complex nephritis in rats immunized with Tamm-Horsfall protein. *Kidney Int* 17:284, 1980.

201. Hoyer JR, Friedman J, Seiler MW: Autoimmunity to Tamm-Horsfall protein. *In* Cummings NB, Michael AF, Wilson CB (eds): *Immune Mechanisms in Renal Disease.* New York, Plenum, 1983, p 295.

202. Hughes J, Mahieu P: Platelet aggregation induced by basement membranes. *Thromb Diath Haemorrh* 24:395, 1970.

203. Hunsicker LG, Shearer TP, Plattner SB, et al: The role of monocytes in serum sickness nephritis. *J Exp Med* 150:413, 1979.

204. Hyman LR, Colvin RB, Steinberg AD: Immunopathogenesis of autoimmune tubulointerstitial nephritis. *J Immunol* 116:327, 1976.

205. Hyman LR, Steinberg AD, Colvin RB, et al: Immunopathogenesis of autoimmune tubulointerstitial nephritis. II. Role of an immune response gene linked to the major histocompatability locus. *J Immunol* 117:1894, 1977.

206. Iida K, Mornaghi R, Nussenzweig V: Complement receptor (CR$_1$) deficiency in erythrocytes from patients with systemic lupus erythematosus. *J Exp Med* 155:1427, 1982.

207. Isaacs KL, Miller F: Role of antigen size and charge in immune complex glomerulonephritis. I. Active induction of disease with dextran and its derivatives. *Lab Invest* 47:198, 1982.

208. Isaacs KL, Miller F: Antigen size and charge in immune complex glomerulonephritis. II. Passive induction of immune deposits with dextran-anti-dextran immune complexes. *Am J Pathol* 111:298, 1983.

209. Iskandar SS, Jennette JC: Interaction of antigen load and antibody response in determining heterologous protein nephritogenicity in inbred mice. *Lab Invest* 48:726, 1983.

210. Iskander SS, Jennette JC: Influence of antibody avidity on glomerular immune complex localization. *Am J Pathol* 112:155, 1983.

211. Ito S, Camussi SIG, Tetta C, et al: Hyperacute renal allograft rejection in the rabbit. The role of platelet-activating factor and of cationic proteins derived from polymorphonuclear leukocytes and from platelets. *Lab Invest* 51:148, 1984.

212. Iwasaki Y, Porter KA, Amend JR, et al: The preparation and testing of horse antidog and antihuman antilymphoid plasma on serum and its protein fractions. *Surg Gynecol Obstet* 124:1, 1967.

213. Izui S, Lambert PH, Miescher PA: In vitro demonstration of a particular affinity of glomerular basement membrane and collagen for DNA: A possible basis for a local formation of DNA-anti-DNA complexes in systemic lupus erythematosus. *J Exp Med* 144:428, 1976.

214. Izui S, McConahey PJ, Theofilopoulos AN, et al: Association of circulating retroviral gp70-anti-gp70 immune complexes with murine systemic lupus erythematosis. *J Exp Med* 149:1099, 1979.

215. Izui S, Kelley VE, McConahey PJ, et al: Selective suppression of retroviral gp70-anti-gp70 immune complex formation by prostaglandin E$_1$ in murine systemic lupus erythematosus. *J Exp Med* 152:1645, 1980.

216. Jenis EH, Valeski JE, Calcagno PL: Variability of anti-GBM binding in hereditary nephritis. *Clin Nephrol* 15:111, 1981.

217. Jennings L, Roholt OA, Pressman D, et al: Experimental anti-alveolar basement membrane antibody-mediated pneumonitis. I. Role of increased permeability of the alveolar capillary wall induced by oxygen. *J Immunol* 127:129, 1981.

218. Jeraj K, Kim Y, Vernier RL, et al: Absence of Goodpasture's antigen in male patients with familial nephritis. *Am J Kidney Dis* 2:626, 1983.

219. Jones DB: Inflammation and repair of the glomerulus. *Am J Pathol* 27:991, 1951.

220. Jordan SC, Buckingham B, Sakai R, et al: Studies of immune complex glomerulonephritis mediated by human thyroglobulin. *N Engl J Med* 304:1212, 1981.

221. Jothy S, Sawka RJ: Presence of monocytes in lupus glomerulonephritis: Marker study and significance. *Arch Path Lab Med* 105:590, 1981.

222. Kajima M, Pollard M: Ultrastructural pathology of glomerular lesions in gnotobiotic mice with congenital lymphocytic choriomeningitis (LCM) virus infection. *Am J Pathol* 61:117, 1970.

223. Kanwar YS, Farquhar MG: Anionic sites in the glomerular basement membrane. In vivo and in vitro localization to the laminae rarae by cationic probes. *J Cell Biol* 81:137, 1976.

224. Kanwar YS, Farquhar MG: Presence of heparin sulfate in the glomerular basement membranes. *Proc Natl Acad Sci USA* 76:1303, 1979.

225. Kanwar YS, Farquhar MG: Isolation of glycosaminoglycans (heparin sulfate) from glomerular basement membranes. *Proc Natl Acad Sci USA* 76:4493, 1979.

226. Kanwar YS, Jakubowski ML, Rosenzweig LJ: Distribution of sulfated glycosminoglycans in the glomerular basement membrane and mesangial matrix. *Eur J Cell Biol* 31:290, 1983.

227. Kanwar YS: Biology of Disease. Biophysiology of glomerular filtration and proteinuria. *Lab Invest* 51:7, 1984.

228. Karesen R, Godal T: Induction of thyroiditis in guinea pigs by intravenous injection of rabbit anti-guinea pig thyroglobulin serum. I. Light microscopic study. *Immunology* 17:847, 1969.

229. Karesen R, Godal T: Induction of thyroiditis in guinea pigs by intravenous injection of rabbit anti-guinea pig thyroglobulin serum. II. Studies with fluorescent antibody technique. *Immunology* 17:863, 1969.

230. Karnovsky MJ: The ultrastructure of glomerular filtration. *Ann Rev Med* 30:213, 1979.

231. Katayama S, Chia D, Knutson DW, et al: Decreased Fc receptor avidity and degradative function of monocytes from patients with systemic lupus erythematosus. *J Immunol* 131:217, 1983.

232. Kay CF: The mechanism by which experimental nephritis is produced in rabbits injected with nephrotic duck serum. *J Exp Med* 72:559, 1940.

233. Kay CF: The mechanism of a form of glomerulonephritis. Nephrotoxic nephritis in rabbits. *Am J Med Sci* 204:483, 1942.

234. Kelley VE, Winkelstein A, Izui S: Effect of prostaglandin E on immune complex nephritis in NZB/W mice. *Lab Invest* 41:531, 1979.

235. Kelley VE, Winkelstein A: Effect of prostaglandin E₁ treatment on murine acute immune complex glomerulonephritis. *Clin Immunol Immunopathol* 16:316, 1980.

236. Kelley VE, Winkelstein A, Izui A, et al: Prostaglandin E₁ inhibits T cell proliferation and renal disease in MRL/1 mice. *Clin Immunol Immunopathol* 21:190, 1981.

237. Kelley VE, Ferretti A, Izui S, et al: A fish oil diet rich in eicosapentaenoic acid reduces cyclooxygenase metabolites and suppresses lupus in MRL-lpr mice. *J Immunol* 134:1914, 1985.

238. Kerjaschki D, Farquhar MG: The pathogenic antigen of Heymann nephritis is a membrane glycoprotein of the renal proximal tubule brush border. *Pro Natl Acad Sci USA* 79:5557, 1982.

239. Kerjaschki D, Farquhar MG: Immunocytochemical localization of the Heymann nephritis antigen (GP330) in glomerular epithelial cells of normal Lewis rats. *J Exp Med* 157:667, 1983.

240. Kerjaschki D, Sharkey DJ, Farquhar MG: Identification and characterization of podocalyxin—the major sialoprotein of the renal glomerular epithelial cell. *J Cell Biol* 98:1591, 1984.

241. Kim Y, Michael AF, Fish AJ: Idiopathic membranoproliferative glomerulonephritis. *In* Brenner BM, Stein JH (eds): *Contemporary Issues in Nephrology.* New York, Churchill Livingstone, 1982, p 237.

242. Kincaid-Smith P: Modification of the vascular lesions of rejection in cadaveric renal allografts by dipyridamole and anticoagulants. *Lancet* ii:920, 1969.

243. Klassen J, Milgrom F: Autoimmune concomitants of renal allografts. *Transplant Proc.* 1:605, 1969.

244. Klassen J, McCluskey RT, Milgrom F: Nonglomerular renal disease produced in rabbits by immunization with homologous kidney. *Am J Pathol* 63:333, 1971.

245. Klassen J, Sugisaki T, Milgrom F, et al: Studies on multiple renal lesions in Heymann nephritis. *Lab Invest* 25:577, 1971.

246. Klassen J, Kano K, Milgrom F, et al: Tubular lesions produced by autoantibodies to tubular basement membrane in human renal allografts. *Int Arch Allergy Applied Immunol* 45:675, 1973.

247. Klein J: *Immunology, The Science of Self-Nonself Discrimination.* New York, Wiley, 1982.

248. Kniker WT, Cochrane CG: Pathogenic factors in vascular lesions of experimental serum sickness. *J Exp Med* 122:83, 1965.

249. Kniker WT, Cochrane CG: The localization of circulating immune complexes in experimental serum sickness. *J Exp Med* 127:119, 1967.

250. Kniker WT, Cochrane CG: The localization of circulating immune complexes in experimental serum sickness: The role of vasoactive amines and hydrodynamic forces. *J Exp Med* 127:119, 1968.

251. Kobayashi Y, Shigematsu H, Tada T: Nephrogenic properties of nephrotoxic guinea pig antibodies. II. Glomerular lesions induced by F(ab')₂ fragments of nephrotoxic IgG' antibody in rats. *Virchows Arch. (Cell Pathol)* 15:35, 1973.

252. Koffler D, Biesecker G, Noble B, et al: Localization of the membrane attack complex (MAC) in experimental immune complex glomerulonephritis. *J Exp Med* 157:1885, 1983.

253. Kondo Y, Shigematsu H, Kobayashi Y: Cellular aspects of rabbit Masugi nephritis. *Lab Invest* 27:620, 1972.

254. Koss MN, Chenack WJ, Griswold WR, et al: The choroid plexus in acute serum sickness. Morphologic, ultrastructural and immunohistologic studies. *Arch Pathol* 96:331, 1973.

255. Koyama A, Niwa Y, Shigematsu H, et al: Studies on passive serum sickness: II. Factors determining the localization of antigen-antibody complexes in the murine renal glomerulus. *Lab Invest* 38:253, 1978.

256. Krakower CA, Greenspoon SA: Localization of the nephrotoxic antigen within the isolated renal glomerulus. *AMA Arch Pathol* 51:639, 1951.

257. Krakower CA, Greenspoon SA: The localization of the 'nephrotoxic' antigen(s) in extraglomerular tissues. *Arch Pathol* 66:364, 1958.

258. Kramer P, Bijnen AB, ten Kate FWJ, et al: Recombinant leucocyte interferon A induces steroid-resistant acute vascular rejection episodes in renal transplant recipients. *Lancet* 1:989, 1984.

259. Kreisberg JI, Wayne DB, Karnvosky M: Rapid and focal loss of negative charge associated with mononuclear cell infiltration early in nephrotoxic serum nephritis. *Kidney Int* 16:290, 1979.

260. Kreisberg JI: Contractile properties of the glomerular mesangium. *Federation Proc* 42:3053, 1983.

261. Kreisberg JI, Karnovsky MJ: Glomerular cells in culture. *Kidney Int* 23:439, 1983.

262. Kuehl FA, Jr, Egan RW: Prostaglandins, arachidonic acid, and inflammation. *Science* 210:978, 1980.

263. Kunkel SL, Zanetti M, Sapin C: Suppression of nephrotoxic serum nephritis in rats by prostaglandin E₁. *Am J Pathol* 108:240, 1982.

264. Lambert PH: Etude immunologique de glomerulonephrites spontanees. University of Liege. Thesis. 1970.

265. Lambert PH, Perrin LH, Mahieu P, et al: Activation of complement in human nephritis. *Adv Nephrol* 4:79, 1974.

265a. Lambert PH: Etude immunologique de glomerulonephrities spontanees. Universite de Liege. Thesis, 1970. *In* Hamburger J, Crosnier J, Maxwell MH (eds): *Advances in Nephrology,* Vol 1. Chicago, Year Book, 1971.

266. Laohapand T, Cattell V, Gabriel JRT: Monocyte infiltration in human glomerulonephritis: Alpha-1-antitrypsin as a marker for mononuclear phagocytes in renal biopsies. *Clin Nephrol* 19:309, 1983.

267. Latta H: Experimental hypersensitivity in the rabbit. Blood and tissue concentrations of foreign proteins labeled with radioactive iodine and injected intravenously. *J Immunol* 66:635, 1950.

268. Latta H, Maunsbach AB, Madden SC: The centrolobular region of the renal glomerulus studied by electron microscopy. *J Ultrastruct Res* 4:455, 1960.

269. Latta H, Johnson WH, Stanley TM: Sialoglycoproteins and filtration barriers in the glomerular capillary wall. *J Ultrastruct Res* 51:354, 1975.

270. Lavelle KJ, Ransdell BA, Kleit SA: The influence of selective thrombocytopenia on nephrotoxic nephritis. *J Lab Clin Med* 87:967, 1976.

271. Lavelle KJ, Durland BD, Yum MN: The effect of antimacrophage antiserum on immune complex glomerulonephritis. *J Lab Clin Med* 98:195, 1981.

272. Lehman DH, Marquardt H, Wilson CB, et al: Specificity of autoantibodies to tubular and glomerular basement membranes induced in guinea pigs. *J Immunol* 112:241, 1974.

273. Lehman DH, Wilson CB, Dixon FJ: Interstitial nephritis in rats immunized with heterologous tubular basement membrane. *Kidney Int* 5:187, 1974.

274. Lehman DH, Wilson CB, Dixon FJ: Extraglomerular immunoglobulin deposits in human nephritis. *Am J Med* 58:765, 1975.

275. Lehman DH, Wilson CB: Role of sensitized cells in antitibular basement membrane interstitial nephritis. *Int Archs Allergy Appl Immun* 51:168, 1976.

276. Lerner RA, Dixon FJ: Transfer of bovine experimental allergic glomerulonephritis (EAG) with serum. *J Exp Med* 124:431, 1966.

277. Lerner RA, Dixon FJ: The induction of acute glomerulonephritis in rabbits with soluble antigens isolated from normal homologous and autologous urine. *J Immunol* 100:1277, 1968.

278. Levy M, Guesry P, Loirat C, et al: Immunologically mediated tubulo-interstitial nephritis in children. *Interstitial Nephropathies* 16:132, 1979.

279. Lew AM, Steward MW: Glomerulonephritis: the use of grafted hybridomas to investigate the role of epitope density, antibody affinity and antibody isotype in active serum sickness. *Immunology* 52:367, 1984.

280. Lew AM, Staines NA, Steward MW: Glomerulonephritis induced by pre-formed immune complexes containing monoclonal antibodies of defined affinity and isotype. *Clin Exp Immunol* 57:413, 1984.

281. Lewis MG, Loughridge LW, Phillips TM: Immunological studies in nephrotic syndrome associated with extrarenal malignant disease. *Lancet* 2:134, 1971.

282. Lianos EA, Andres GA, Dunn MJ: Glomerular prostaglandin and thromboxane synthesis in rat nephrotoxic serum nephritis. *J Clin Invest* 72:1439, 1983.

283. Lianos EA: Biosynthesis and role of arachidonic acid metabolites in glomerulonephritis. *Nephron* 37:73, 1984.

284. Lifschitz MD, Stein JH: Renal vasoactive hormones. *In* Brenner BM, Rector FC (eds): *The Kidney* (2nd ed.), Philadelphia, Saunders, 1981, p 65.

285. Lifschitz MD: Renal effects of nonsteroidal anti-inflammatory agents. *J Lab Clin Med* 102:313, 1983.

286. Lindemann W: Sur la mode d'action de certains poisons renaux. *Ann Inst Pasteur* 14:49, 1900.

287. Linder E, Helin H, Chang C-M, et al: Complement-mediated binding of monocytes to intermediate filaments in vitro. *Am J Pathol* 112:267, 1983.

288. Lovett DH, Ryan JL, Kashgarian M, et al: Lysosomal enzymes in glomerular cells of the rat. *Am J Pathol* 107:161, 1982.

289. Lovett DH, Ryan JL, Sterzel RB: Stimulation of rat mesangial cell proliferation by macrophage interleukin 1. *J Immunol* 131:2830, 1983.

290. Lowry RP, Forbes RDC, Blackburn JH: Immune reactivity and immunosuppressive intervention (TLI) in experimental nephritis. I. Immunopathologic correlates in the accelerated autologous form of nephrotoxic serum nephritis. *J Immunol* 132:1001, 1984.

291. Lowry RP, Forbes RDC, Carpenter CB, et al: Immune reactivity and immunosuppressive intervention in experimental nephritis. II. Effect of TLI on the course of two models of nephritis in the inbred cat. *J Immunol* 132:1007, 1984.

292. Madaio MP, Salant DJ, Cohen AJ, et al: Comparative study of in situ immune deposit formation in active and passive Heymann nephritis. *Kidney Int* 23:498, 1983.

292a. Madaio MP, Salant DJ, Adler S, et al: Effect of antibody charge and concentration on deposition of antibody to glomerular basement membrane. *Kidney Int* 26:397, 1984.

293. Magil AB, Wadsworth LD, Loewen M: Monocytes and human renal glomerular disease. A quantitative evaluation. *Lab Invest* 44:27, 1981.

294. Magil AB, Wadsworth LD: Monocyte involvement in glomerular crescents. A histochemical and ultrastructural study. *Lab Invest* 47:160, 1982.

295. Makker SP, Moorthy B: In situ immune complex formation in isolated perfused kidney using homologous antibody. *Lab Invest* 44:1, 1981.

296. Makker SP, Singh AK: Characterization of the antigen (gp600) of Heymann nephritis. *Lab Invest* 50, 287, 1984.

297. Mampaso FM, Wilson CB: Characterization of inflammatory cells in autoimmune tubulointerstitial nephritis in rats. *Kidney Int* 23:448, 1983.

298. Mancilla-Jimenez R, Bellon B, Kuhn J, et al: Phagocytosis of heat-aggregated immunoglobulins by mesangial cells. An immunoperoxidase and acid phosphatase study. *Lab Invest* 46:243, 1982.

299. Mannik M, Arend WP: Fate of preformed immune complexes in rabbits and rhesus monkeys. *J Exp Med* 134:19s, 1971.

300. Mannik M, Arend WP, Hall AP, et al: Studies on antigen-antibody complexes. I. Elimination of soluble complexes from rabbit circulation. *J Exp Med* 133:713, 1971.

301. Mannik M, Striker GE: Removal of glomerular deposits of immune complexes in mice by administration of excess antigen. *Lab Invest* 42:483, 1980.

302. Mannik M, Agodoa LYC, David KA: Rearrangement of immune complexes in glomeruli leads to persistence and development of electron-dense deposits. *J Exp Med* 157:1516, 1983.

303. Martinez-Hernandez A, Miller EJ, Damjanov I, et al: Laminin-secreting yolk salk carcinoma of the rat. Biochemical and electron immunohistochemical studies. *Lab Invest* 47:247, 1982.

304. Martinez-Hernandez A, Amenta PS: The basement membrane in pathology. *Lab Invest* 48:656, 1983.

305. Masugi M: Uber das Wesen der Spezifischen Veranderungen der Niere und der Leber durch das Nephrotoxin bzw. das Hepatotoxin. *Beitr Pathol Anat Allg Pathol* 91:82, 1933.

306. Mauer SM, Sutherland DER, Howard RJ, et al: The glomerular mesangium. III. Acute immune mesangial injury:

A new model of glomerulonephritis. *J Exp Med* 137:533, 1973.

307. McCluskey RT, Benacerraf B, Miller F: Passive acute glomerulonephritis induced by antigen-antibody complexes solubilized in hapten excess. *Proc Soc Exp Biol Med* 111:764, 1962.

308. McCluskey RT, Brentjens JR, Andres GA: Tubular and interstitial renal diseases produced by immunological mechanisms. *La Ricerca. Clinica e in Laboratorio* 4:795, 1974.

309. McCluskey RT: Immunological mechanisms in glomerular disease. In Heptinstall RM (ed): *Pathology of the Kidney* (3rd ed.), Boston, Little, Brown, 1983.

310. McCluskey RT: Immunologically mediated tubulo-interstitial nephritis. In Cotran RS, Brenner BM, Stein JH (eds): *Contemporary Issues in Nephrology* (10), New York, Churchill Livingstone, 1983.

311. McCoy RC, Johnson HK, Stone WJ, et al: Absence of nephritogenic GBM antigen(s) in some patients with hereditary nephritis. *Kidney Int* 21:642, 1982.

312. McGiven AR: Blood coagulation and the effect of warfarin on renal disease in NZB/NZW mice. *Br J Exp Pathol* 48:552, 1967.

313. McIntosh RM, Kihara H, Kulvinskas C, et al: Chemical and immunological characteristics of a basement membrane-like glycoprotein in the rat. *Ann Rheum Dis* 30:631, 1971.

314. McIntosh RM, Koss MN, Chernack WB, et al: Experimental pulmonary disease and autoimmune nephritis in the rabbit produced by homologous and heterologous choroid plexus (experimental Goodpasture's syndrome). *Proc Soc Exp Biol Med* 147:216, 1974.

315. McIntosh RM, Griswold WR, Chernack WB, et al: Cryoglobulins. III. Further studies on the nature, incidence, clinical, diagnostic, prognostic and immunopathologic significance of cryoglobulins in renal disease. *Q J Med* 174:285, 1975.

316. McLean RH, Seigel NJ: Increased frequency of the C3 fast variant of the third component of complement C3 in patients with membrano-proliferative glomerulopnephritis (MPGN) on partial lipodystrophy (PLD). *Abs IVth Int Cong Immunol*, Paris, July, 1980.

317. McLean RH, Wyatt RJ, Julian BA: Complement phenotypes in glomerulonephritis: Increased frequency of homozygous null C4 phenotypes in IgA nephropathy and Henoch-Schonlein purpura. *Kidney Int* 26:855, 1984.

318. McLeish KR, Gohara AF, Gunning WT, III, et al: Prostaglandin E$_1$ therapy of murine chronic serum sickness. *J Lab Clin Med* 96:470, 1980.

319. McLeish KR, Gohara AF, Gunning WT, III: Suppression of antibody synthesis by prostaglandin E as a mechanism for preventing murine immune complex glomerulonephritis. *Lab Invest* 47:147, 1982.

320. McLeish KR, Gohara AF, Stelzer GT, et al: Treatment of murine immune complex glomerulonephritis with prostaglandin E$_2$: Dose-response of immune complex deposition, antibody synthesis, and glomerular damage. *Clin Immunol Immunopathol* 26:18, 1983.

321. McPhaul JJ, Jr: Cryoimmunoglobulinaemia in patients with primary renal disease and systemic lupus erythematosus. I. IgG- and DNA-binding assessed by co-precipitation. *Clin Exp Immunol* 31:131, 1978.

322. Melvin T, Sibley R, Michael AF: Nephrotic syndrome. In Tune BM, Mendoza SA, Brenner BM, et al (eds): *Contemporary Issues in Nephrology* (12). New York, Churchill Livingstone, 1983, p 191.

323. Melvin T, Kim Y, Michael AF: Selective binding of IgG4

324. Mendrick DL, Noble B, Brentjens JR, et al: Antibody mediated injury to proximal tubules in Heymann nephritis. *Kidney Int* 18:328, 1980.

325. Mendrick DL, Rennke HG, Cotran RS, et al: Methods in laboratory investigation. Monoclonal antibodies against rat glomerular antigens: Production and specificity. *Lab Invest* 49:107, 1983.

326. Michael AF, Keane WF, Raij L, et al: The glomerular mesangium. *Kidney Int* 17:141, 1980.

327. Michael AF, Yang J-Y, Falk RJ, et al: Monoclonal antibodies to human renal basement membranes: Heterogenic and ontogenic changes. *Kidney Int* 24:74, 1983.

328. Michael AF, Falk RJ, Platt JL, et al: Antigens of the human glomerular basement membrane. Fouser LS, Michael AF, eds. *Springer Seminars in Immunopathology* 9:317, 1987.

329. Miettinen A, Tornroth T, Tikkanen I, et al: Heymann nephritis induced by kidney brush border glycoproteins. *Lab Invest* 43:547, 1980.

330. Miller GW, Steinberg AD, Green I, et al: Complement-dependent alterations in the handling of immune complexes by NZB/W mice. *J Immunol* 114:1166, 1975.

331. Miller GW, Nussenzweig V: A new complement function: Solubilization of antigen-antibody aggregates. *Proc Natl Acad Sci (USA)* 72:418, 1975.

332. Miller K, Michael AF: Coagulation of the kidney. In McIntosh RM, Guggenheim SJ, Schrier RW (eds): *Hematologic and Vascular Aspects of Kidney Disease.* New York, Wiley, 1977, p 3.

333. Milliner DW, Pierides AM, Holley KE: Renal transplantation in Alport's syndrome. Anti-glomerular basement membrane glomerulonephritis in the allograft. *Mayo Clin Proc* 57:35, 1982.

334. Minota S, Terai C, Nojima Y, et al: Low C3b receptor reactivity on erythrocytes from patients with systemic lupus erythematosus detected by immune adherence hemagglutination and radioimmunoassays with monoclonal antibody. *Arth Rheumat* 27:1329, 1984.

335. Mizoguchi Y, Horiuchi Y: Localization of IgG-Fc receptors in human renal glomeruli. *Clin Immunol* 24:320, 1982.

336. Monaco AP, Wood ML, Russell PS: Some effects of purified heterologous anti-human lymphocyte serum in man. *Transplantation* 5:1106, 1967.

337. Monga G, Mazzucco G, Barbiano di Belgiojoso G, et al: The presence and possible role of monocyte infiltration in human chronic proliferative glomerulonephritis. Light microscopic, immunofluorescence, and histochemical correlations. *Am J Pathol* 94:271, 1979.

338. Monga G, Mazzucco G, Barbiano di Belgiojoso G, et al: Monocyte infiltration and glomerular hypercellularity in human acute and persistent glomerulonephritis. Light and electron microscopic, immunofluorescence, and histochemical investigation on twenty-eight cases. *Lab Invest* 44:381, 1981.

339. Morrison WI, Wright NB: Viruses associated with renal disease of man and animals. *Prog Med Virol* 23:22, 1977.

340. Muller-Eberhard HJ: Complement. *Ann Rev Biochem* 44:697, 1975.

341. Murphy-Ullrich JE, Oberley TD, Mosher DF: Glomerular and vascular injury in mice following immunization with heterologous and autologous fibronectin. *Virchows Arch (Cell Pathol)* 39:305, 1982.

342. Murphy-Ullrich JE, Oberley TD: Immune-mediated injury to basement membranes in mice immunized with murine laminin. *Clin Immunol Immunopathol* 31:33, 1984.

343. Nagle RB, Dong S, Janacek LL, et al: Glomerular accumulation of monocytes and macrophages in experimental glomerulonephritis associated with Trypanosoma rhodesiense infection. *Lab Invest* 46:365, 1982.

344. Naish PF, Thomson NM, Simpson IJ, et al: The role of polymorphonuclear leucocytes in the autologous phase of nephrotoxic nephritis. *Clin Exp Immunol* 22:102, 1975.

345. Nakamura RM, Weigle WO: Transfer of experimental autoimmune thyroiditis by serum from thyroidectomized donors. *J Exp Med* 130:263, 1969.

346. Naruse T, Kitamura K, Mujakawa Y, et al: Deposition of renal tubular epithelial antigen along the glomerular capillary walls of patients with membranous glomerulonephritis. *J Immunol* 110:1163, 1973.

347. Naruse T, Fukasawa T, Hirakawa N, et al: The pathogenesis of experimental membranous glomerulonephritis induced with homologous nephritogenic tubular antigen. *J Exp Med* 144:1347, 1976.

348. Natali PG, Martino CD, Marcellini M, et al: Expression of Ia-like antigens on the vasculature of human kidney. *Clin Immunol Immunopathol* 20:11, 1981.

349. Neale TJ, Wilson CB: Glomerular antigens in Heymann's nephritis: Reactivity of eluted and circulating antibody. *J Immunol* 128:323, 1982.

350. Neild GH, Ivory K, Hiramatsu M, et al: Cyclosporin A inhibits acute serum sickness nephritis in rabbits. *Clin Exp Immunol* 52:586, 1983.

351. Neilson EG, Phillips SM: Cell-mediated immunity in interstitial nephritis. I. T lymphocyte systems in nephritic guinea pigs: The natural history and diversity of the immune response. *J Immunol* 123:2373, 1979.

352. Neilson EG, Phillips SM: Cell-mediated immunity in interstitial nephritis. II. T lymphocyte effector mechanisms in nephritic guinea pigs: analysis of the renotropic migration and cytotoxic response. *J Immunol* 123:2381, 1979.

353. Neilson EG, Jimenez SA, Phillips SM: Cell-mediated immunity in interstitial nephritis. III. T lymphocyte-mediated fibroblast proliferation and collagen synthesis: An immune mechanism for renal fibrogenesis. *J Immunol* 125:1708, 1980.

354. Neilson EG, Phillips SM: Cell-mediated immunity in interstitial nephritis. IV. Anti-tubular basement membrane antibodies can function in antibody-dependent cellular cytotoxicity reactions: Observations on a nephritogenic effector mechanism acting as an informational bridge between the humoral and cellular immune response. *J Immunol* 126:1990, 1981.

355. Neilson EG, Phillips SM: Suppression of interstitial nephritis by auto-anti-idiotypic immunity. *J Exp Med* 155:1179, 1982.

356. Neilson EG, Phillips SM: Murine interstitial nephritis. I. Analysis of disease susceptibility and its relationship to pleiomorphic gene products defining both immune-response genes and a restrictive requirement for cytotoxic T cells at H-2K. *J Exp Med* 155:1075, 1982.

357. Neilson EG, Gasser DL, McCafferty E, et al: Polymorphism of genes involved in anti-tubular basement membrane disease in rats. *Immunogenetics* 17:55, 1983.

358. Neilson EG, McCafferty E, Phillips JM, et al: Antiidiotypic immunity in interstitial nephritis. II. Rats developing antitubular basement membrane disease fail to make an antiidiotypic regulatory response: the modulatory role of an RT7.1⁺, OX8-Suppressor T cell mechanism. *J Exp Med* 159:1009, 1984.

359. Nevins TE, Michael AF: Isolation of anionic sialoproteins from the rat glomerulus. *Kidney Int* 19:553, 1981.

360. Noble B, Mendrick DL, Brentjens JR, et al: Antibody-mediated injury to proximal tubules in the rat kidney induced by passive transfer of homologous anti-brush border serum. *Clin Immunol Immunopathol* 19:289, 1981.

361. Noble B, Van Liew JB, Andres GA, et al: Factors influencing susceptibility of LEW rats to Heymann nephritis. *Clin Immunol Immunopathol* 30:241, 1984.

362. Oite T, Batsford SR, Mihatsch MJ, et al: Quantitative studies of in situ immune complex glomerulonephritis in the rat induced by planted cationized antigen. *J Exp Med* 155:460, 1982.

363. Oldstone MBA, Dixon FJ: Lymphocytic choriomeningitis: Production of antibody by "tolerant" infected mice. *Science* 158:1193, 1967.

364. Oldstone MBA, Dixon FJ: Pathogenesis of chronic disease associated with persistent lymphocytic choriomeningitis viral infection. I. Relationship of antibody production to disease in neonatally infected mice. *J Exp Med* 129:483, 1969.

365. Oldstone MBA, Buchmeier MJ, Doyle MV, et al: Virus-induced immune complex disease; specific anti-viral antibody and C1q-binding material in the circulation during persistent lymphocytic choriomeningitis virus infection. *J Immunol* 124:831, 1980.

366. Olson DL, Anand SK, Landing DH, et al: Diagnosis of hereditary nephritis by failure of glomeruli to bind anti-glomerular basement membrane antibodies. *J Pediatr* 96:697, 1980.

367. Olson JL: Role of heparin as a protective agent following reduction of renal mass. *Kidney Int* 25:376, 1984.

368. O'Regan S, Fong JSC, Kaplan BS, et al: Thyroid antigen-antibody nephritis. *Clin Immunol Immunopathol* 6:341, 1976.

369. Orfilo C, Rakotoarivonz J, Durand D, et al: A correlative study of immunofluorescence, electron and light microscopy in immunologically mediated renal tubular disease in man. *Nephron* 23:14, 1979.

370. Ozawa T, Pluss R, Lacher J, et al: Endogenous immune complex nephropathy associated with malignancy. I. Studies on the nature and immunopathogenic significance of glomerular bound antigen and antibody. Isolation and characterization of tumor specific antigen and antibody and circulating immune complexes. *Q J Med* 68:523, 1975.

371. Palmer JM, Eversole SL, Stamey TA: Unilateral glomerulonephritis. Virtual absence of nephritis in a kidney with partial occlusion of the main renal artery. *Am J Med* 40:816, 1966.

372. Paronetto F, Koffler D: Autoimmune proliferative glomerulonephritis in monkeys. *Am J Pathol* 50:887, 1967.

373. Parra G, Platt JL, Falk RJ, et al: Cell populations and membrane attack complex in glomeruli of patients with post-streptococcal glomerulonephritis: Identification using monoclonal antibodies by indirect immunofluorescence. *Clin Immunol Immunopathol* 33:324, 1984.

374. Parris TM, Kimberly RP, Inman RD, et al: Defective Fc receptor-mediated function of the mononuclear phagocyte system in lupus nephritis. *Ann Intern Med* 97:526, 1982.

375. Passos HC, Siqueira M, Martinez OC, et al: Studies on the nephrotoxic activity of guinea-pig gamma-I and gamma-2 antibodies. *Immunology* 26:407, 1974.

376. Passwell JH, Steward MW, Soothill JF: Inter-mouse strain differences in macrophage function and its relationship to antibody responses. *Clin Exp Immunol* 17:159, 1974.

377. Patrick CC, Virello G, McManus JFA, et al: Induction of extraglomerular renal damage in experimental chronic serum sickness. *Lab Invest* 40:603, 1979.

378. Paul LC, Carpenter CB: Antigenic determinants of tubular basement membranes and Bowman's capsule in rats. *Kidney Int* 21:800, 1982.

379. Peress NS, Muller F, Palu W: The immunopathophysiological effects of chronic serum sickness on rat clonoid plexus, ciliary process and renal glomeruli. *J Neuropathol Exp Neurol* 36:726, 1977.

380. Pilia PA, Boackle RJ, Swain RP, et al: Complement-independent nephrotoxic serum nephritis in Munich Wistar rats. Immunologic and ultrastructural studies. *Lab Invest* 48:585, 1983.

381. Pirotzky E, Ninio E, Bidault J, et al: Biosynthesis of platelet-activating factor. VI. Precursor of platelet-activating factor and acetyltransferase activity in isolated rat kidney cells. *Lab Invest* 51:567, 1984.

382. Platt JL, LeBien TW, Michael AF: Stages of renal ontogenesis identified by monoclonal antibodies reactive with lymphohemopoietic differentiation antigens. *J Exp Med* 157:155, 1983.

383. Platt JL, Grant BW, Eddy AA, et al: Immune cell populations in cutaneous delayed-type hypersensitivity. *J Exp Med* 158:1227, 1983.

384. Ploth DW, Fitz A, Schnetzler D, et al: Thyroglobulin-antithyroglobulin immune complex glomerulonephritis complicating radioiodine therapy. *Clin Immunopathol* 9:327, 1978.

385. Polverini P, Cotran RS, Gimbrone MA, et al: Activated macrophages induce vascular proliferation. *Nature* 269:804, 1977.

386. Porush JG, Grishman E, Alter AA, et al: Paraproteinemia and cryoglobulinemia associated with atypical glomerulonephritis and the nephrotic syndrome. *Am J Med* 47:957, 1969.

387. Posner MR, Prout MN, Berk S: Trymona and nephrotic syndrome. *Cancer* 45:387, 1980.

388. Praz F, Halbwachs L, Lesavre P: Genetic aspects of complement and glomerulonephritis. In Bach J-F, Crosnier J, Funck-Brentano J-L, et al (eds): *Advances in Nephrology.* Chicago, Yearbook, 1984, p 271.

389. Prickett JD, Robinson DR, Steinberg AD: Dietary enrichment with the polyunsaturated fatty acid eicosapentaenoic acid prevents proteinuria and prolongs survival in NZB x NZW F_1 mice. *J Clin Invest* 68:556, 1981.

390. Raij L, Sibley RK, Keane WF: Mononuclear phagocytic system stimulation. Protective role from glomerular immune complex deposition. *J Lab Clin Med* 98:558, 1981.

391. Riaj L, Azar S, Keane W: Mesangial immune injury, hypertension and progressive glomerular damage in Dahl rats. *Kidney Int* 26:137, 1984 (Abstract).

392. Rand-Weaver M, Price RG: Renal basement membranes: Macromolecular associations, antigenicity, and variation in disease. *Biosci Rep* 3:713, 1983.

393. Rees AJ, Peters DK, Amos N, et al: The influence of HLA-linked genes on the severity of anti-GBM antibody-mediated nephritis. *Kidney Int* 26:444, 1984.

394. Rees AJ: The HLA complex and susceptibility to glomerulonephritis. *Plasma Ther Transfus Technol* 5:455, 1984.

395. Rehan A, Johnson KJ, Wiggins RC, et al: Evidence for the role of oxygen radicals in acute nephrotoxic nephritis. *Lab Invest* 51:396, 1984.

396. Rennke HG, Venkatachalam MA: Glomerular permeability: In vitro tracer studies with polyanionic and polycationic ferritins. *Kidney Int* 11:44, 1977.

397. Rich AR, Gregory JE: The experimental demonstration that periarteritis nodosa is a manifestation of hypersensitivity. *Bull Johns Hopkins Hosp* 72:65, 1943.

398. Richet G, Adam C, Morel-Maroger L: Cryoglobulinemia in glomerulonephritis exclusive of general diseases. *Adv Nephrol* 3:119, 1974.

398a. Roman-Franco AA, Turiello M, Albini B, et al: Anti-basement membrane antibodies and antigen-antibody complexes in rabbits injected with mercuric chloride. *Clin Immunol Immunopathol* 9:464, 1978.

399. Ross GD: Structure and function of membrane complement receptors. *Fed Proc* 41:3089, 1982.

400. Rother K, Rother U, Vassalli P, et al: Nephrotoxic serum nephritis in C6-deficient rabbits. I. Study of the second phase of the disease. *J Immunol* 98:965, 1967.

401. Rudofsky U, Steblay RW: Studies on autoimmune nephritis in sheep: II. Passive transfer of nephritis in sheep by plasma. *Fed Proc* 25:659, 1966.

402. Rudofsky UH, McMaster PRB, Ma W-S, et al: Experimental autoimmune renal cortical tubulointerstitial disease in guinea pigs lacking the fourth component of complement (C4). *J Immunol* 112:1387, 1974.

403. Rudofsky UH, Pollara B: Studies on the pathogenesis of experimental autoimmune renal tubulointerstitial disease in guinea pigs. I. Inhibition of tissue injury in leukocyte-depleted passive transfer recipients. *Clin Immunol Immunopathol* 4:425, 1975.

404. Rudofsky UH, Steblay RW, Pollara B: Inhibition of experimental autoimmune renal tubulointerstitial disease in guinea pigs by depletion of complement with cobra venom factor. *Clin Immunol Immunopathol* 3:396, 1975.

405. Rudofsky UH, Pollara B: Studies on the pathogenesis of experimental autoimmune renal tubulointerstitial disease in guinea pigs. II. Passive transfer of renal lesions by anti-tubular basement membrane autoantibody and nonimmune bone marrow cells to leukocyte-depleted recipients. *Clin Immunol Immunopathol* 6:107, 1976.

406. Rudofsky UH, Esposito LL, Dilwith RL, et al: Studies on the pathogenesis of experimental autoimmune renal tubulointerstitial disease in guinea pigs. 5. Deposition of C3PA on the tubular basement membranes. *Clin Immunol Immunopathol* 8:467, 1977.

407. Rudofsky UH: Spontaneous and induced autoantibodies to renal and nonrenal basement membranes in mice. *Clin Immunol Immunopathol* 15:200, 1980.

408. Rudofsky UH, Dilwith RL, Tung KSK: Susceptibility differences of inbred mice to induction of autoimmune renal tubulointerstitial lesions. *Lab Invest* 43:463, 1980.

409. Rynes RI: Inherited complement deficiency states and SLE. *Clinics in Rheumatic Dis* 8:29, 1982.

410. Saito H, Ideura T, Takeuchi J: Effects of a selective thromboxane A_2 synthetase inhibitor on immune complex glomerulonephritis. *Nephron* 36:38, 1984.

411. Salant DJ, Belok S, Madaio MP, et al: A new role for complement in experimental membranous nephropathy in rats. *J Clin Invest* 66:1339, 1980.

412. Salant DJ, Darby C, Couser WG: Experimental membranous glomerulonephritis in rats. Quantitative studies of glomerular immune deposit formation in isolated glomeruli and whole animals. *J Clin Invest* 66:71, 1980.

413. Salant DJ, Madaio MP, Adler S, et al: Altered glomerular permeability induced by $F(ab')_2$ and Fab' antibodies to rat renal tubular epithelial antigen. *Kidney Int* 21:36, 1981.

414. Salmon JE, Kimberly RP, Gibofsky A, et al: Defective mononuclear phagocyte function in systemic lupus erythematosus: Dissociation of Fc receptor-ligand binding and internalization. *J Immunol* 133:2525, 1984.

415. Sano M: Participation of monocytes in glomerulonephritis

in acute serum sickness of rabbits. *Act Pathol Jpn* 26:423, 1976.

416. Sapin C, Druet E, Druet P: Induction of anti-glomerular basement membrane antibodies in the Brown-Norway rat by mercuric chloride. *Clin Exp Immunol* 28:173, 1977.

417. Sarno EN, Gattass CR, Alvarenga FDE-BF, et al: Analysis of cell populations in crescentic glomerulonephritis. *Brazilian J Med Biol Res* 16:227, 1983.

418. Scharschmidt LA, Dunn ML: Prostaglandin synthesis by rat glomerular mesangial cells in culture. Effects of angiotensin II and arginine vaspressin. *J Clin Invest* 71:1756, 1983.

419. Scheinman JI, Fish AJ, Michael AF: The immunohistopathology of glomerular antigens: The glomerular basement collagen and actinomysin antigens in normal and diseased kidneys. *J Clin Invest* 54:1144, 1974.

420. Scheinman JI, Fish AJ, Brown DM, et al: Human glomerular smooth muscle (mesangial) cells in culture. *Lab Invest* 34:150, 1976.

421. Scheinman JI, Foidart J-M, Gehron-Robey P, et al: The immunohistology of glomerular antigens. IV. Laminin, a defined non-collagen basement membrane glycoprotein. *Clin Immunol Immunopathol* 15:175, 1980.

422. Scheinman JI, Foidart J-M, Michael AF: The immunohistology of glomerular antigens. V. The collagenous antigens of the glomerulus. *Lab Invest* 43:373, 1980.

423. Schiffer MS, Michael AF: Renal cell turnover studied by Y chromosome (Y body) staining of the transplanted human kidney. *J Lab Clin Med* 92:841, 1978.

424. Schifferli JA, Woo P, Peters DK: Complement mediated inhibition of immune precipitation. I. Role of the classical and alternative pathways. *Clin Exp Immunol* 47:563, 1982.

425. Schifferli JA, Peters DK: Complement, the immune-complex lattice, and the pathophysiology of complement-deficiency syndromes. *Lancet* ii:957, 1983.

426. Schneeberger EE, O'Brien A, Grupe WE: Altered glomerular permeability in Munich-Wistar rats and autologous immune complex nephritis. *Lab Invest* 40:227, 1979.

427. Schreiber AD, Frank MM: The role of antibody and complement in the immune clearance and destruction of erythrocytes. I. In vivo effects of IgG and IgM complement fixing sites. *J Clin Invest* 51:575, 1972.

428. Schreiber RD, Muller-Eberhard HJ: Complement and renal disease. *In* Wilson CB, Brenner BM, Stein JH (eds): *Immunologic Mechanisms of Renal Disease.* New York, Churchill Livingstone, 1979, p 67.

429. Schreiber RD: The chemistry and biology of complement receptors. *Springer Semin Immunopathol* 7:221, 1984.

430. Schreiner GF, Cotran RS, Pardo V, et al: A mononuclear cell component in experimental immunological glomerulonephritis. *J Exp Med* 147:369, 1978.

431. Schreiner GF, Kiely J-M, Cotran RS, et al: Characterization of resident glomerular cells in the rat expressing Ia determinants and manifesting genetically restricted interactions with lymphocytes. *J Clin Invest* 68:920, 1981.

432. Schreiner GF, Cotran RS: Localization of an Ia-bearing glomerular cell in the mesangium. *J Cell Biol* 94:483, 1982.

433. Schreiner GF, Cotran RS, Unanue ER: Macrophages and cellular immunity in experimental glomerulonephritis. *Springer Semin Immunopathol* 5:251, 1982.

434. Schrieber L, Penny R: Tissue distribution of IgG Fc receptors. *Clin Exp Immunol* 47:917, 1982.

435. Schur PH: Complement testing in the diagnosis of immune and autoimmune diseases. *Am J Clin Pathol* 68:647, 1977.

436. Schwartz MM, Sharon Z, Bidani AK, et al: Evidence for glomerular epithelial cell endocytosis in vitro. *Lab Invest* 44:502, 1981.

437. Schwartz RS: Immunologic and genetic aspects of systemic lupus erythematosus. *Kidney Int* 19:474, 1981.

438. Seegal BC, Loeb EN: The production of chronic glomerulonephritis in rats by the injection of rabbit anti-rat-placenta serum. *J Exp Med* 84:211, 1946.

439. Seiler MW, Hoyer JR: Ultrastructural studies of tubulointerstitial immune complex nephritis in rats immunized with Tamm-Horsfall protein. *Lab Invest* 45:321, 1981.

439a. Selby P, Kohn J, Raymond J, et al: Nephrotic syndrome during treatment with interferon. *Br Med J* 290:1180, 1985.

440. Shalhoub RJ: Pathogenesis of lipoid nephrosis: A disorder of T-cell function. *Lancet* 2:566, 1974.

441. Shibata S, Sakaguchi H, Nagasawa T: Exfoliation of endothelial cytoplasm in nephrotoxic serum nephritis: A study using antiserum against water soluble glycoprotein isolated from the glomerular basement membrane. *Lab Invest* 38:201, 1978.

442. Shigematsu H, Shishida H, Kuhara K, et al: Participation of monocytes in transient glomerular hypercellularity in poststreptococcal glomerulonephritis. *Virchows Arch (Cell Pathol)* 12:367, 1973.

443. Silva FG, Hoyer JR, Pirani CL: Sequential studies of glomerular crescent formation in rats with antiglomerular basement membrane-induced glomerulonephritis and the role of coagulation factors. *Lab Invest* 51:404, 1984.

444. Simpson IJ, Amos N, Evans DJ, et al: Guinea-pig nephrotoxic nephritis. I. The role of complement and polymorphonuclear leucocytes and the effect of antibody subclass and fragments in the heterologous phase. *Clin Exp Immunol* 19:499, 1975.

445. Sindrey M, Naish P: The mediation of the localization of polymorphonuclear leucocytes in glomeruli during the autologous phase of nephrotoxic nephritis. *Clin Exp Immunol* 35:350, 1979.

446. Sisson S, Dysart NK, Jr, Fish AJ, et al: Localization of the Goodpasture antigen by immunoelectron microscopy. *Clin Immunol Immunopathol* 23:414, 1982.

447. Skrifvars B, Tallquist G, Tornroth T: Renal involvement in essential cryoglobulinaemia. *Acta Med Scand* 194:229, 1973.

448. Smith RD, Wehner RW: Acute cytomegalovirus glomerulonephritis. *Lab Invest* 43:278, 1980.

449. Snyder DS, Beller DI, Unanue ER: Prostaglandins modulate macrophage Ia expression. *Nature* 299:163, 1982.

450. Soothill JF, Steward MW: The immunopathological significance of the heterogeneity of the antibody affinity. *Clin Exp Med* 9:193, 1971.

451. Stachura I, Si L, Madan E, et al: Mononuclear cell subsets in human renal disease. Enumeration in tissue sections with monoclonal antibodies. *Clin Immunol Immunopathol* 30:362, 1984.

452. Steblay RW: Glomerulonephritis reduced in sheep by injections of heterologous glomerular basement membrane and Freund's complete adjuvant. *J Exp Med* 116:253, 1962.

453. Steblay RW: Some immunologic properties of human and dog glomerular basement membranes. III. Production of glomerulonephritis in juxtamedullary glomeruli of neonatal pups with rabbit anti-human glomerular basement membrane sera. *Lab Invest* 12:432, 1963.

454. Steblay RW: Glomerulonephritis induced in monkeys by injections of heterologous glomerular basement membrane and Freund's adjuvant. *Nature* 197:1173, 1963.

455. Steblay RW, Rudofsky U: Further evidence for autoantibodies as mediators of experimental autoimmune nephritis in sheep. *J Lab Clin Med* 68:1021, 1966.

456. Steblay RW, Rudofsky U: Autoimmune glomerulonephritis

induced in sheep by injections of human lung and Freund's adjuvant. *Science* 160:204, 1968.

457. Steblay RW, Rudofsky U: In vitro and in vivo properties of autoantibodies eluted from kidneys of sheep with autoimmune glomerulonephritis. *Nature* 218:1269, 1968.

458. Steblay RW, Rudofsky U: Renal tubular disease and autoantibodies against tubular basement membrane induced in guinea pigs. *J Immunol* 107:589, 1971.

459. Steblay RW, Rudofsky U: Transfer of experimental autoimmune renal cortical tubular and interstitial disease in guinea pigs by serum. *Science* 180:966, 1973.

460. Stefoni S, Vangelista A, Costa AN, et al: Short-term thoracic duct drainage in drug resistant immunologically mediated glomerulonephritis. Evaluation of lymph and blood lymphocyte characteristics during drainage. *Clin Nephrol* 16:300, 1981.

461. Stein HD, Feddergreen W, Kashgarian M, et al: Role of angiotensin II-induced renal functional changes in mesangial deposition of exogenous ferritin in rats. *Lab Invest* 49:270, 1983.

462. Steinberg AD, Huston DP, Taurog JD, et al: The cellular and genetic basis of murine lupus. *Immunol Rev* 55:121, 1981.

463. Steinberg, AD, Raveche ES, Laskin CA, et al: Systemic lupus erythematosus: Insights from animal models. *Ann Intern Med* 100:714, 1984.

464. Stenglein B, Thoenes GH, Gunther E: Genetic control or susceptibility to autologous immune complex glomerulonephritis in inbred rat strains. *Clin Exp Immunol* 33:88, 1978.

465. Sterzel RB, Pabst R: The temporal relationship between glomerular cell proliferation and monocyte infiltration in experimental glomerulonephritis. *Virchows Arch (Cell Pathol)* 38:337, 1982.

466. Steward MW: Chronic immune complex disease in mice: The role of antibody affinity. *Clin Exp Immunol* 38:414, 1979.

467. Stilmant MM, Couser WG, Cotran RS: Experimental glomerulonephritis in the mouse associated with mesangial deposition of autologous ferritin immune complexes. *Lab Invest* 32:746, 1975.

468. Striker GE, Mannik M, Tung MY: The role of marrow-derived monocytes and mesangial cells in removal of immune complexes from renal glomeruli. *J Exp Med* 149:127, 1979.

469. Striker GE, Soderland C, Bowen-Pope DF, et al: Isolation, characterization, and propagation in vitro of human glomerular endothelial cells. *J Exp Med* 160:323, 1984.

470. Sugisaki T, Klassen J, Andres G, et al: Passive transfer of Heymann nephritis with serum. *Kidney Int* 3:66, 1973.

471. Sugisaki T, Klassen J, Milgrom F, et al: Immunopathological study of autoimmune tubular and interstitial renal disease in Brown Norway rats. *Lab Invest* 28:658, 1973.

472. Sugisaki T, Yoshida T, McCluskey RT, et al: Autoimmune cell-mediated tubulointerstitial nephritis induced in Lewis rats by renal antigens. *Clin Immunol Immunopathol* 15:33, 1980.

473. Takemaru R, Werb Z: Secretory products of macrophages and their physiological functions. *Am J Physiol* 246(Cell Physiol 15):C1, 1984.

474. Theofilopoulos AN, Andrews BS, Urist MM, et al: The nature of immune complexes in human cancer sera. *J Immunol* 119:657, 1977.

475. Theofilopoulos AN, McConahey PJ, Izui S, et al: A comparative immunologic analysis of several murine strains with autoimmune manifestations. *Clin Immunol Immunopathol* 15:258, 1980.

476. Theofilopoulos AN, Balderas R, Shawler DL, et al: Inhibition of T cell proliferation and SLE-like syndrome of MRL/1 mice by whole body or total lymphoid irradiation. *J Immunol* 125:2137, 1980.

477. Theofilopoulos AN, Dixon FJ: Etiopathogenesis of murine SLE. *Immunol Rev* 55:179, 1981.

477a. Thomson NM, Simpson IJ, Peters DK: A quantitative evaluation of anticoagulants in experimental nephrotoxic nephritis. *Ann Exp Immunol* 19:301, 1975.

478. Thomson NM, Moran J, Simpson IJ, et al: Defibrination with ancrod in nephrotoxic nephritis in rabbits. *Kidney Int* 10:343, 1976.

479. Thomson NM, Naish PF, Simpson IJ, et al: The role of C3 in the autologous phase of nephrotoxic nephritis. *Clin Exp Immunol* 24:464, 1976.

480. Thomson NM, Holdworth SR, Glasgow EF, et al: The macrophage in the development of experimental crescentic glomerulonephritis. *Am J Pathol* 94:223, 1979.

481. Till GO, Johnson KJ, Kunkel R, et al: Intravascular activation of complement and acute lung injury. Dependency on neutrophils and toxic oxygen metabolites. *J Clin Invest* 69:1126, 1982.

482. Tomino Y, Sakai H, Takaya M, et al: Solubilization of intraglomerular deposits of IgG immune complexes by human sera or gamma-globulin in patients with lupus nephritis. *Clin Exp Immunol* 58:42, 1984.

483. Unanue ER, Dixon FJ: Experimental glomerulonephritis: IV. Participation of complement in nephrotoxic nephritis. *J Exp Med* 119:965, 1964.

484. Unanue ER, Dixon FJ: Experimental glomerulonephritis. V. Studies on the interaction of nephrotoxic antibodies with tissues of the rat. *J Exp Med* 121:697, 1965.

485. Unanue ER, Dixon FJ: Experimental glomerulonephritis: VI. The autologous phase of nephrotoxic serum nephritis. *J Exp Med* 121:715, 1965.

486. Unanue ER, Dixon FJ: Experimental glomerulonephritis. Immunological events and pathogenetic mechanisms. *Adv Immunol* 6:1, 1967.

487. Unanue ER, Mardiney MR, Dixon FJ: Nephrotoxin serum nephritis in complement intact and deficient mice. *J Immunol* 98:609, 1967.

488. Unanue ER, Dixon FJ: Experimental allergic glomerulonephritis induced in rabbit with heterologous renal antigens. *J Exp Med* 125:149, 1967.

489. Unanue ER, Dixon FJ, Feldman JD: Experimental allergic glomerulonephritis induced in the rabbit with homologous renal antigens. *J Exp Med* 125:163, 1967.

490. Unanue ER, Benacerraf B: *Textbook of Immunology* (2nd ed.), Baltimore, Williams and Wilkins, 1984, p 260.

491. Valdes AJ, Senterfit LB, Pollack AD, et al: The effect of antigen excess on chronic immune complex glomerulonephritis. *Johns Hopkins Med J* 124:9, 1969.

492. Van Damme BJC, Fleuren GJ, Bakker WW, et al: Experimental glomerulonephritis in the rat induced by antibodies directed against tubular antigens. V. Fixed glomerular antigens in the pathogenesis of heterologous immune complex glomerulonephritis. *Lab Invest* 38:502, 1978.

493. van der Woude FJ, van der Geissen M, Kallenberg CGM, et al: Reticuloendothelial Fc receptor function in SLE patients. I. Primary HLA linked defect or acquired dysfunction secondary to disease activity? *Clin Exp Immunol* 55:473, 1984.

494. van der Woude FJ, Kallenberg CGM, Limburg PC, et al: Reticuloendothelial Fc receptor function in SLE patients. II. Associations with humoral immune response parameters in vivo and in vitro. *Clin Exp Immunol* 55:481, 1984.

495. Van Zwieten MJ, Bhan AK, McCluskey RT, et al: Studies

on the pathogenesis of experimental antitubular basement membrane nephritis in the guinea pig. *Am J Pathol* 83:531, 1976.

496. Van Zwieten MJ, Leber PD, Bhan AK, et al: Experimental cell-mediated interstitial nephritis induced with exogenous antigens. *J Immunol* 118:589, 1977.

497. Varsano S, Bruderman I, Bernheim JL, et al: Minimal-change nephropathy and malignant thymoma. *Chest* 77:695, 1980.

498. Vassalli P, McCluskey RT: The pathogenic role of fibrin deposition in immunologically induced glomerulonephritis. *Ann NY Acad Sci* 116:1052, 1964.

499. Venkatachalam MA, Rennke HG: The structural and molecular basis of glomerular filtration. *Circ Res* 43:337, 1978.

500. Vladutiu AO, Rose NR: Transfer of experimental autoimmune thyroiditis of the mouse by serum. *J Immunol* 106:1139, 1971.

501. Vogel C-W, Smith CA, Muller-Eberhard HJ: Cobra venom factor: Structural homology with the third component of human complement. *J Immunol* 133:3235, 1984.

502. Vogt A, Rohrbach R, Simizu F, et al: Interaction of cationized antigen with rat glomerular basement membrane: In situ immune complex formation. *Kidney Int* 22:27, 1982.

503. Vogt A: New aspects of the pathogenesis of immune complex glomerulonephritis: formation of subepithelial deposits. *Clin Nephrol* 21:15, 1984.

504. Von Pirquet CE: Allergy. *Arch Intern Med* 7:259, 1911.

505. Wakashin Y, Takei I, Ueda S, et al: Autoimmune interstitial disease of the kidney and associated antigen purification and characterization of a soluble tubular basement membrane antigen. *Clin Immunol Immunopathol* 19:360, 1981.

506. Wank R, O'Neill GJ, Held E, et al: Rare variant of complement C4 is seen in high frequency in patients with primary glomerulonephritis. *Lancet* i:872, 1984.

507. Waxman FJ, Hebert LA, Cornacoff JB, et al: Complement depletion accelerates the clearance of immune complexes from the circulation of primates. *J Clin Invest* 74:1329, 1984.

508. Weening JJ, Fleuren GJ, Hoedemaeker PJ: Demonstration of antinuclear antibodies in mercuric chloride-induced glomerulopathy in the rat. *Lab Invest* 39:405, 1978.

509. Weigle WO, Nakamura RM: Perpetuation of autoimmune thyroiditis and production of secondary renal lesions following periodic injections of aqueous preparations of altered thyroglobulin. *Clin Exp Immunol* 4:645, 1969.

510. Weislander J, Bygren P, Heinegard D: Isolation of the specific glomerular basement membrane antigen involved in Goodpasture syndrome. *Proc Natl Acad Sci (USA)* 81:1544, 1984.

511. Weksler ME, Carey T, Day N, et al: Nephrotic syndrome in malignant melanoma: Demonstration of melanoma antigen-antibody complexes in kidney. *Kidney Int* 6:112a, 1974.

512. Wick G, Muller PU, Timpl R: In vivo localization and pathological effects of passively transferred antibodies to type IV collagen and laminin in mice. *Clin Immunol Immunopathol* 23:656, 1982.

513. Wilens SL: Enhancement of serum sickness lesions in rabbits with pressor agents. *Arch Pathol* 80:590, 1965.

514. Williams JD, Czop JK, Abrahamson DR, et al: Activation of the alternative complement pathway by isolated human glomerular basement membrane. *J Immunol* 133:394, 1984.

515. Wilson CB, Dixon FJ: Antigen quantitation in experimental immune complex glomerulonephritis. I. Acute serum sickness. *J Immunol* 105:279, 1970.

516. Wilson CB, Dixon FJ: Quantitation of acute and chronic serum sickness in the rabbit. *J Exp Med* 134:7s, 1971.

517. Wilson CB, Lehman DH, McCoy RC, et al: Antitubular basement membranes after renal transplantation. *Transplantation* 18:447, 1974.

518. Wilson CB, Dixon FJ: Renal injury from immune reactions involving antigensin or out of the kidney. *In* Wilson CB, Brenner BM, Stein JH (eds): *Contemporary Issues in Nephrology*, Vol. 3. New York, Churchill Livingstone, 1979, p 35.

519. Wilson CB, Dixon FJ: The renal response to immunological injury. *In* Brenner BM, Rector FC (eds): *The Kidney* (2nd ed.), Philadelphia, Saunders, 1981.

520. Wilson JG, Wong WW, Schur PH, et al: Mode of inheritance of decreased C3b receptors on erythrocytes of patients with systemic lupus erythematosus. *N Engl J Med* 307:981, 1982.

521. Wilson JG, Fearon DT: Altered expression of complement receptors as a pathogenetic factor in systemic lupus erythematosus. *Arthritis Rheum* 27:1321, 1984.

522. Winfield JB, Faifermann I, Koffler D: Avidity of anti-DNA antibodies in serum and IgG glomerular eluates from patients with systemic lupus erythematosus. Association of high avidity antinative DNA antibody with glomerulonephritis. *J Clin Invest* 59:90, 1977.

523. Winkelstein A, Kelley VE: Effects of PGE_1 in murine models of SLE: Changes in circulating immune complexes. *Clin Immunol Immunopathol* 20:188, 1981.

524. Wofsy D, Kerger CE, Seaman WE: Monocytes in the BXSB model for systemic lupus erythematosus. *J Exp Med* 159:629, 1984.

525. Wright NG, Morrison WI, Thompson H, et al: Mesangial localization of immune complexes in experimental canine adenovirus glomerulonephritis. *Br J Exp Pathol* 55:458, 1974.

526. Wu V-Y, Cohen MP: Platelet factor 4 binding to glomerular microvascular matrix. *Biochimica Biophysica Acta* 797:76, 1984.

527. Yaar M, Foidart JM, Brown KS, et al: The Goodpasture-like syndrome in mice induced by intravous injections of anti-type IV collagen and anti-laminin antibody. *Am J Pathol* 107:79, 1982.

528. Yoshioka K, Michael AF, Fish AJ: Detection of hidden nephritogenic antigen determinants in human renal and non-renal basement membranes. (Submitted for publication).

529. Zager RA, Cotran RS, Hoyer JR: Pathologic localization of Tamm-Horsfall protein in interstitial deposits in renal disease. *Lab Invest* 38:52, 1978.

530. Zakheim B, McCafferty E, Phillips SM, et al: Murine interstitial nephritis. II. The adoptive transfer of disease with immune T lymphocytes produces a phenotypically complex interstitial lesion. *J Immunol* 133:234, 1984.

531. Zanetti M, Wilson CB: Characterization of anti-tubular basement membrane antibodies in rats. *J Immunol* 130:2173, 1983.

532. Zanetti M, Mampaso F, Wilson CB: Anti-idiotype as a probe in the analysis of autoimmune tubulointerstitial nephritis in the Brown Norway rat. *J Immunol* 131:1268, 1983.

533. Zanetti M, Wilson CB: Participation of auto-anti-idiotypes in immune complex glomerulonephritis in rabbits. *J Immunol* 131:2781, 1983.

534. Zurier RB, Quagliata F: Effect of prostaglandin E_1 on adjuvant arthritis. *Nature* 234:304, 1971.

535. Zurier RB, Damjanov I, Sayadoff DM, et al: Prostaglandin

E$_1$ treatment of NZB/NZW F$_1$ hybrid mice. *Arthritis Rheum* 20:1449, 1977.

536. Zurier RB, Damjanov I, Miller Pl, et al: Prostaglandin E$_1$ treatment prevents progression of nephritis in murine lupus erythematosus. *J Clin Lab Immunol* 1:95, 1978.

Bibliography

The following key references have been published since the preparation of this chapter.

Immune Mechanisms of Renal Injury: Reviews

Andres G, Brentjens JR, Caldwell PRB, et al: Biology of disease. Formation of immune deposits and disease. *Lab Invest* 55:510, 1986.

Bruijn JA, Hoedemaeker PJ, Fleuren GJ: Biology of disease. Pathogenesis of anti-basement membrane glomerulopathy and immune-complex glomerulonephritis: Dichotomy dissolved. *Lab Invest* 61:480, 1989.

Couser WG: Mediation of immune glomerular injury. *J Am Soc Nephrol* 1:13, 1990.

Dixon FJ, Wilson CB: The development of immunopathologic investigation of kidney disease. *Am J Kidney Dis* 16:574, 1990.

Goldman M, Baran D, Druet P: Polyclonal activation and experimental nephropathies. *Kidney Int* 34:141, 1988.

Oliveira DBG, Peters DK: Autoimmunity and the pathogenesis of glomerulonephritis. *Pediatr Nephrol* 4:185, 1990.

Wilson CB, Blantz RC: Nephroimmunopathology and pathophysiology. *Am J Physiol* 248:F319, 1985.

Glomerular Structure

GLOMERULAR BASEMENT MEMBRANE

Abrahamson DR: Recent studies on the structure and pathology of basement membranes. *J Pathol* 149:257, 1986.

Batsford SR, Rohrbach R, Vogt A: Size restriction in the glomerular capillary wall: Importance of lamina densa. *Kidney Int* 31:710, 1987.

Fouser LS, Michael AF: Antigens of the human glomerular basement membrane. *Springer Semin Immunopathol* 9:317, 1987.

Morita M, White RHR, Raafat F, et al: Glomerular basement membrane thickness in children. A morphometric study. *Pediatr Nephrol* 2:190, 1988.

Timpl R: Recent advances in the biochemistry of glomerular basement membrane. *Kidney Int* 30:293, 1986.

PODOCYTES AND PROTEOGLYCANS

Fries JWU, Rumpelt H-J, Thoenes W: Alterations of glomerular podocytic processes in immunologically mediated glomerular disorders. *Kidney Int* 32:742, 1987.

Keriaschki D, Poczewski H, Dekan G, et al: Identification of a major sialoprotein in the glycocalyx of human visceral glomerular epithelial cells. *J Clin Invest* 78:1142, 1986.

Schleicher ED, Wagner E-M, Olgemöller B, et al: Characterization and localization of basement membrane-associated heparan sulfate proteoglycan in human tissues. *Lab Invest* 61:323, 1989.

Stow JL, Sawada H, Farquhar MG: Basement membrane heparan sulfate proteoglycans are concentrated in the laminae rarae and in podocytes of the rat renal glomerulus. *Proc Natl Acad Sci USA* 82:3296, 1985.

Stow JL, Soroka CJ, MacKay K, et al: Basement membrane heparan sulfate proteoglycan is the main proteoglycan synthesized by glomerular epithelial cells in culture. *Am J Pathol* 135:637, 1989.

MESANGIUM

Kashgarian M: Mesangium and glomerular disease. *Lab Invest* 52:569, 1985.

Kriz W, Elger M, Lemley K, et al: Structure of the glomerular mesangium: A biomechanical interpretation. *Kidney Int* (suppl)38:S2, 1990.

Latta H, Fligiel S: Mesangial fenestrations, sieving, filtration, and flow. *Lab Invest* 52:591, 1985.

Humoral Mechanisms

NEPHROTOXIC SERUM NEPHRITIS

Blantz RC, Gabbai F, Gushwa LC, et al: The influence of concomitant experimental hypertension and glomerulonephritis. *Kidney Int* 32:652, 1987.

Boyce NW, Holdsworth SR: Anti-glomerular basement membrane antibody-induced experimental glomerulonephritis: Evidence for dose-dependent, direct antibody and complement-induced, cell-independent injury. *J Immunol* 135:3918, 1985.

Boyce NW, Holdsworth SR: Direct anti-GBM antibody induced alterations in glomerular permselectivity. *Kidney Int* 30:666, 1986.

Boyce NW, Holdsworth SR: Intrarenal hemodynamic alterations induced by anti-GBM antibody. *Kidney Int* 31:8, 1987.

Couser WG, Darby C, Salant DJ, et al: Anti-GBM antibody-induced proteinuria in isolated perfused rat kidney. *Am J Physiol* 249:F241, 1985.

Neugarten J, Kaminetsky B, Feiner H, et al: Nephrotoxic serum nephritis with hypertension: Amelioration by antihypertensive therapy. *Kidney Int* 28:135, 1985.

Schrijver G, Schalkwijk J, Robben JCM, et al: Antiglomerular basement membrane nephritis in beige mice. Deficiency of leukocytic neutral proteinases prevents the induction of albuminuria in the heterologous phase. *J Exp Med* 169:1435, 1989.

Schrijver G, Bogman MJJT, Assmann KJM, et al: Anti-GBM nephritis in the mouse: Role of granulocytes in the heterologous phase. *Kidney Int* 38:86, 1990.

Tucker BJ, Gushwa LC, Wilson CB, et al: Effect of leukocyte depletion on glomerular dynamics during acute glomerular immune injury. *Kidney Int* 28:28, 1985.

Weening JJ, Prins FA, Fransen JAM, et al: Ultrastructural localization and quantitation of nephritogenic antibodies in experimental glomerulonephritis. *Lab Invest* 55:372, 1986.

PULMONARY DISEASE

Queluz TH, Pawlowski I, Brunda MJ, et al: Pathogenesis of an experimental model of Goodpasture's hemorrhagic pneumonitis. *J Clin Invest* 85:1507, 1990.

Yamamoto T, Wilson CB: Binding of anti-basement membrane antibody to alveolar basement membrane after intratracheal gasoline instillation in rabbits. *Am J Pathol* 126:497, 1987.

IMMUNE RESPONSE TO GBM ANTIGENS (ANIMAL MODELS)

Abrass CK, Cohen AH: Characterization of renal injury initiated by immunization of rats with heparan sulfate. *Am J Pathol* 130:103, 1988.

Bygren P, Wieslander J, Heinegärd D: Glomerulonephritis induced in sheep by immunization with human glomerular basement membrane. *Kidney Int* 31:25, 1987.

Faaber P, Rijke TPM, van de Putte LBA, et al: Cross-reactivity of human and murine anti-DNA antibodies with heparan sulfate. The major glycosaminoglycan in glomerular basement membrane. *J Clin Invest* 77:1824, 1986.

Feintzeig ID, Abrahmson DR, Cybulsky AV, et al: Nephritogenic potential of sheep antibodies against glomerular basement membrane laminin in the rat. *Lab Invest* 54:531, 1986.

Makino H, Gibbons JT, Reddy MK, et al: Nephritogenicity of antibodies to proteoglycans of the glomerular basement membrane-1. *J Clin Invest* 77:142, 1986.

Makino H, Lelongt B, Kanwar YS: Nephritogenicity of proteoglycans. II. A model of immune complex nephritis. *Kidney Int* 34:195, 1988.

Makino H, Lelongt B, Kanwar YS: Nephritogenicity of proteoglycans. III. Mechanism of immune deposit formation. *Kidney Int* 34:209, 1988.

Matsuo S, Brentjens JR, Andres G, et al: Distribution of basement membrane antigens in glomeruli of mice with autoimmune glomerulonephritis. *Am J Pathol* 122:36, 1986.

Miettinen A, Stow JL, Mentone S, et al: Antibodies to basement membrane heparan sulfate proteoglycans bind to the laminae rarae of the glomerular basement membrane (GBM) and induce subepithelial GBM thickening. *J Exp Med* 163:1064, 1986.

Murphy-Ullrich JE, Oberley TD, Mosher DF: Serologic and pathologic studies of mice immunized with homologous fibronectin. *Am J Pathol* 125:182, 1986.

Saxena R, Bygren P, Butkowski R, et al: Entactin: A possible auto-antigen in the pathogenesis of non-Goodpasture anti-GBM nephritis. *Kidney Int* 38:263, 1990.

Wick G, Von der Mark H, Dietrich H, et al: Globular domain of basement membrane collagen induces autoimmune pulmonary lesions in mice resembling human Goodpasture disease. *Lab Invest* 55:308, 1986.

IMMUNE RESPONSE TO GBM ANTIGENS (HUMAN DISEASE)

Cederholm B, Wieslander J, Bygren P, et al: Patients with IgA nephropathy have circulating anti-basement membrane antibodies reacting with structures common to collagen I, II, and IV. *Proc Natl Acad Sci USA* 83:6151, 1986.

Fillit H, Damle SP, Gregory JD, et al: Sera from patients with poststreptococcal glomerulonephritis contain antibodies to glomerular heparan sulfate proteoglycan. *J Exp Med* 161:277, 1985.

Fivush B, Melvin T, Solez K, et al: Idiopathic linear glomerular IgA deposition. *Arch Pathol Lab Med* 110:1189, 1986.

Foidart J-M, Hunt J, Lapiere C-M, et al: Antibodies to laminin in preeclampsia. *Kidney Int* 29:1050, 1986.

Hudson BG, Wieslander J, Wisdom BJ Jr, et al: Biology of disease. Goodpasture syndrome: Molecular architecture and function of basement membrane antigen. *Lab Invest* 61:256, 1989.

Kefalides NA, Pegg MT, Ohno N, et al: Antibodies to basement membrane collagen and to laminin are present in sera from patients with poststreptococcal glomerulonephritis. *J Exp Med* 163:588, 1986.

Pusey CD, Dash A, Kershaw MJ, et al: A single autoantigen in

Goodpasture's syndrome identified by a monoclonal antibody to human glomerular basement membrane. *Lab Invest* 56:23, 1987.

Raidt H, Voss B, Lison AE, et al: Occurrence of antibodies against collagen type IV in a family with nail patella syndrome. *In* Lubec G, Hudson BG (eds): *Glomerular Basement Membrane.* International Symposium Proceedings. London, John Libbey, 1985, p 201.

Termaat RM, Brinkman K, Nossent JC, et al: Anti-heparan sulfate reactivity in sera from patients with systemic lupus erythematosus with renal or non-renal manifestations. *Clin Exp Immunol* 82:268, 1990.

Wieslander J, Kataja M, Hudson BG: Characterization of the human Goodpasture antigen. *Clin Exp Immunol* 69:332, 987.

HEREDITARY NEPHRITIS: IDENTIFICATION OF THE MISSING ANTIGEN

Brunner H, Schröder C, van Bennekom C, et al: Localization of the gene for X-linked Alport's syndrome. *Kidney Int* 34:507, 1988.

Butkowski RJ, Wieslander J, Kleppel M, et al: Basement membrane collagen in the kidney: Regional localization of novel chains related to collagen IV. *Kidney Int* 35:1195, 1989.

Desjardins M, Gros F, Wieslander J, et al: Heterogeneous distribution of monomeric elements from the globular domain (NC1) of type IV collagen in renal basement membranes as revealed by high resolution quantitative immunocytochemistry. *Lab Invest* 63:637, 1990.

Hostikka SL, Eddy RL, Byers MG, et al: Identification of a distinct type IV collagen α chain with restricted kidney distribution and assignment of its gene to the locus of X chromosome-linked Alport syndrome. *Proc Natl Acad Sci USA* 87:1606, 1990.

Jansen B, Tryphonas L, Wong J, et al: Mode of inheritance of Samoyed hereditary glomerulopathy: An animal model for hereditary nephritis in humans. *J Lab Clin Med* 107:551, 1986.

Jansen B, Thorner P, Baumal R, et al: Samoyed hereditary glomerulopathy (SHG). Evolution of splitting of glomerular capillary basement membranes. *Am J Pathol* 125:536, 1986.

Kashtan C, Fish AJ, Kleppel M, et al: Nephritogenic antigen determinants in epidermal and renal basement membranes of kindreds with Alport-type familial nephritis. *J Clin Invest* 78:1035, 1986.

Kashtan CE, Atkin CL, Gregory MC, et al: Identification of variant Alport phenotypes using an Alport-specific antibody probe. *Kidney Int* 36:669, 1989.

Kashtan CE, Butkowski RJ, Kleppel MM, et al: Posttransplant anti-glomerular basement membrane nephritis in related males with Alport syndrome. *J Lab Clin Med* 116:508, 1990.

Kashtan CE, Kleppel MM, Butkowski RJ, et al: Alport syndrome, basement membranes and collagen. *Pediatr Nephrol* 4:523, 1990.

Kashtan CE, Rich SS, Michael AF, et al: Gene mapping in Alport families with different basement membrane antigenic phenotypes. *Kidney Int* 38:925, 1990.

Kleppel MM, Michael AF, Fish AJ: Antibody specificity of human glomerular basement membrane type IV collagen NC1 subunits. Species variation in subunit composition. *J Biol Chem* 261:16547, 1986.

Kleppel MM, Kashtan CE, Butkowski RJ, et al: Alport familial nephritis. Absence of 28 kilodalton non-collagenous monomers of type IV collagen in glomerular basement membrane. *J Clin Invest* 80:263, 1987.

Kleppel MM, Kashtan C, Santi PA, et al: Distribution of familial nephritis antigen in normal tissue and renal basement membranes of patients with homozygous and heterozygous Alport familial nephritis. Relationship of familial nephritis and Goodpasture antigens to novel collagen chains and type IV collagen. *Lab Invest* 61:278, 1989.

Kleppel MM, Santi PA, Cameron JD, et al: Human tissue distribution of novel basement membrane collagen. *Am J Pathol* 134:813, 1989.

Melvin T, Kim Y, Michael AF: Amyloid P component is not present in the glomerular basement membrane in Alport-type hereditary nephritis. *Am J Pathol* 125:460, 1986.

Myers JC, Jones TA, Pohjolainen E-R, et al: Molecular cloning of α5(IV) collagen and assignment of the gene to the region of the X chromosome containing the Alport syndrome locus. *Am J Hum Genet* 46:1024, 1990.

Pihlajaniemi T, Pohjolainen E-R, Myers JC: Complete primary structure of the triple-helical region and the carboxyl-terminal domain of a new type IV collagen chain, α5(IV). *J Biol Chem* 265:13758, 1990.

Saus J, Wieslander J, Langeveld JPM, et al: Identification of the Goodpasture antigen as the α3(IV) chain of collagen IV. *J Biol Chem* 263:13374, 1988.

Savage COS, Pusey CD, Kershaw MJ, et al: The Goodpasture antigen in Alport's syndrome: Studies with a monoclonal antibody. *Kidney Int* 30:107, 1986.

Savage COS, Noel L-H, Crutcher E, et al: Hereditary nephritis: Immunoblotting studies of the glomerular basement membrane. *Lab Invest* 60:613, 1989.

Thorner P, Jansen B, Baumal R, et al: Samoyed hereditary glomerulopathy. Immunohistochemical staining of basement membranes of kidney for laminin, collagen type IV, fibronectin, and Goodpasture antigen, and correlation with electron microscopy of glomerular capillary basement membranes. *Lab Invest* 56:435, 1987.

Thorner P, Baumal R, Binnington A, et al: The NC1 domain of collagen type IV in neonatal dog glomerular basement membranes. Significance in Samoyed hereditary glomerulopathy. *Am J Pathol* 134:1047, 1989.

Thorner P, Baumal R, Valli VEO, et al: Abnormalities in the NC1 domain of collagen type IV in GBM in canine hereditary nephritis. *Kidney Int* 35:843, 1989.

MERCURIC-CHLORIDE INDUCED DISEASE

Pelletier L, Pasquier R, Hirsch F, et al: Autoreactive T cells in mercury-induced autoimmune disease: In vitro demonstration. *J Immunol* 137:2548, 1986.

Interaction of Antibodies with Glomerular (non-GBM) Antigens

HEYMANN NEPHRITIS

Camussi G, Brentjens JR, Noble B, et al: Antibody-induced redistribution of Heymann antigen on the surface of cultured glomerular visceral epithelial cells: Possible role in the pathogenesis of Heymann glomerulonephritis. *J Immunol* 135:2409, 1985.

Camussi G, Noble B, van Liew J, et al: Pathogenesis of passive Heymann glomerulonephritis: Chlorpromazine inhibits antibody-mediated redistribution of cell surface antigens and prevents development of the disease. *J Immunol* 136:2127, 1986.

Kamata K, Baird LG, Erikson ME, et al: Characterization of antigens and antibody specificities involved in Heymann nephritis. *J Immunol* 135:2400, 1985.

Kanalas JJ, Makker SP: Isolation of a 330-kDa glycoprotein from human kidney similar to the Heymann nephritis autoantigen (gp330). *J Am Soc Nephrol* 1:792, 1990.

Makker SP, Kanalas JJ: Course of transplanted Heymann nephritis kidney in normal host. Implications for mechanism of proteinuria in membranous glomerulonephropathy. *J Immunol* 142:3406, 1989.

Natori Y, Hayakawa I, Shibata S: Role of dipeptidyl peptidase IV (gp108) in passive Heymann nephritis. Use of dipeptidyl peptidase IV-deficient rats. *Am J Pathol* 134:405, 1989.

Pietromonaco S, Kerjaschki D, Binder S, et al: Molecular cloning of a cDNA encoding a major pathogenic domain of the Heymann nephritis antigen gp330. *Proc Natl Acad Sci USA* 87:1811, 1990.

Quigg RJ, Abrahamson DR, Cybulsky V, et al: Studies with antibodies to cultured rat glomerular epithelial cells. Subepithelial immune deposit formation after in vivo injection. *Am J Pathol* 134:1125, 1989.

Raychowdhury R, Niles JL, McCluskey RT, et al: Autoimmune target in Heymann nephritis is a glycoprotein with homology to the LDL receptor. *Science* 244:1163, 1989.

Ronco P, Neale TJ, Wilson CB, et al: An immunopathologic study of a 330-kD protein defined by monoclonal antibodies and reactive with anti-RTEα5 antibodies and kidney eluates from active Heymann nephritis. *J Immunol* 136:125, 1986.

Rydel JJ, Schwartz MM, Singh AK: Sequential localization of antibody to multiple regions of the glomerular capillary wall in passive Heymann nephritis. *Lab Invest* 60:492, 1989.

Salant DJ, Quigg RJ, Cybulsky AV: Heymann nephritis: Mechanisms of renal injury. *Kidney Int* 35:976, 1989.

INTERACTION WITH OTHER GLOMERULAR CELL ANTIGENS

Assmann KJM, Ronco P, Tangelder MM, et al: Involvement of an antigen distinct from the Heymann antigen in membranous glomerulonephritis in the mouse. *Lab Invest* 60:138, 1989.

Bagchus WM, Hoedemaeker PhJ, Rozing J, et al: Glomerulonephritis induced by monoclonal anti-thy 1.1 antibodies. A sequential histological and ultrastructural study in the rat. *Lab Invest* 55:680, 1986.

Bagchus WM, Jeunink MF, Elema JD: The mesangium in anti-thy-1 nephritis. Influx of macrophages, mesangial cell hypercellularity, and macromolecular accumulation. *Am J Pathol* 137:215, 1990.

Brentjens JR, Andres G: Interaction of antibodies with renal cell surface antigens. *Kidney Int* 35:954, 1989.

Fukatsu A, Yuzawa Y, Olson L, et al: Interaction of antibodies with human glomerular epithelial cells. *Lab Invest* 61:389, 1989.

Hogendoorn PCW, Bruijn JA, Broek LJCMVD, et al: Antibodies to purified renal tubular epithelial antigens contain activity against laminin, fibronectin, and type IV collagen. *Lab Invest* 58:278, 1988.

Matsuo S, Fukatsu A, Taub ML, et al: Glomerulonephritis induced in the rabbit by antiendothelial antibodies. *J Clin Invest* 79:1798, 1987.

Orikasa M, Matsui K, Oite T, et al: Massive proteinuria induced in rats by a single intravenous injection of a monoclonal antibody. *J Immunol* 141:807, 1988.

Yamamoto T, Wilson CB: Complement dependence of antibody-induced mesangial cell injury in the rat. *J Immunol* 138:3758, 1987.

Yamamoto T, Wilson CB: Quantitative and qualitative studies of antibody-induced mesangial cell damage in the rat. *Kidney Int* 32:514, 1987.

Verroust PJ: Kinetics of immune deposits in membranous nephropathy. *Kidney Int* 35:1418, 1989.

OTHER IN SITU MODELS

Agodoa LYC, Mannik M: Removal of subepithelial immune complexes with excess unaltered or cationic antigen. *Kidney Int* 32:13, 1987.

Cosio FG, Mahan JD, Sedmak DD: Experimental glomerulonephritis induced by antigen that binds to glomerular fibronectin. *Am J Kidney Dis* 15:160, 1990.

Feintzeig ID, Dittmer JE, Cybulsky AV, et al: Antibody, antigen, and glomerular capillary wall charge interactions: Influence of antigen location on in situ immune complex formation. *Kidney Int* 29:649, 1986.

Madaio MP, Carlson J, Cataldo J, et al: Murine monoclonal anti-DNA antibodies bind directly to glomerular antigens and form immune deposits. *J Immunol* 138:2883, 1987.

Matsuo S, Yoshida F, Yuzawa Y, et al: Experimental glomerulonephritis induced in rats by a lectin and its antibodies. *Kidney Int* 36:1011, 1989.

Mendrick DL, Rennke HG: Immune deposits formed in situ by a monoclonal antibody recognizing a new intrinsic rat mesangial matrix antigen. *J Immunol* 137:1517, 1986.

Salant DJ, Adler S, Darby C, et al: Influence of antigen distribution on the mediation of immunological glomerular injury. *Kidney Int* 27:938, 1985.

Glomerular Deposition of Circulating Immune Complexes

GLOMERULAR DEPOSITION AND IN SITU REARRANGEMENTS OF IMMUNE COMPLEXES

Apple RJ, Domen PL, Muckerheide A, et al: Cationization of protein antigens. IV. Increased antigen uptake by antigen-presenting cells. *J Immunol* 140:3290, 1988.

Barnes JL, Reznicek MJ, Radnik RA, et al: Anionization of an antigen promotes glomerular binding and immune complex formation. *Kidney Int* 34:156, 1988.

Cosio FG, Birmingham DJ, Sexton DJ, et al: Interactions between precipitating and nonprecipitating antibodies in the formation of immune complexes. *J Immunol* 138:2587, 1987.

Couser WG: Mechanisms of glomerular injury in immune-complex disease. *Kidney Int* 28:569, 1985.

Fries JWU, Mendrick DL, Rennke HG: Determinants of immune complex-mediated glomerulonephritis. *Kidney Int* 34:333, 1988.

Gauthier VJ, Mannik M: Only the initial binding of cationic immune complexes to glomerular anionic sites is mediated by charge-charge interactions. *J Immunol* 136:3266, 1986.

Gauthier VJ, Mannik M: A small proportion of cationic antibodies in immune complexes is sufficient to mediate their deposition in glomeruli. *J Immunol* 145:3348, 1990.

Kanwar YS, Caulin-Glaser T, Gallo GR, et al: Interaction of immune complexes with glomerular heparan sulfate-proteoglycans. *Kidney Int* 30:842, 1986.

Mannik M, Gauthier VJ, Stapleton SA, et al: Immune complexes with cationic antibodies deposit in glomeruli more effectively than cationic antibodies alone. *J Immunol* 38:4209, 1987.

Schifferli JA, Taylor RP: Physiological and pathological aspects of circulating immune complexes. *Kidney Int* 35:993, 1989.

Ward DM, Lee S, Wilson CB: Direct antigen binding to glomerular immune complex deposits. *Kidney Int* 30:706, 1986.

Zanetti M, Wilson CB: A role for antiidiotypic antibodies in immunologically mediated nephritis. *Am J Kidney Dis* 7:445, 1986.

COMPLEMENT AND FC-RECEPTOR DEPENDENT CLEARANCE OF IMMUNE COMPLEXES

Appay M-D, Kazatchkine MD, Levi-Strauss M, et al: Expression of CR1 (CD35) mRNA in podocytes from adult and fetal human kidneys. *Kidney Int* 38:289, 1990.

Birmingham DJ, Cosio FG: Chracterization of the baboon erythrocyte C3b-binding protein. *J Immunol* 142:3140, 1989.

Birmingham DJ, Hebert LA, Cosio FG, et al: Immune complex erythrocyte complement receptor interactions in vivo during induction of glomerulonephritis in nonhuman primates. *J Lab Clin Med* 116:242, 1990.

Clark MR, Liu L, Clarkson SB, et al: An abnormality of the gene that encodes neutrophil Fc receptor III in a patient with systemic lupus erythematosus. *J Clin Invest* 86:341, 1990.

Cosio FG, Xiao-Ping S, Hebert LA: Immune complexes bind preferentially to specific subpopulations of human erythrocytes. *Clin Immunol Immunopathol* 55:337, 1990.

Cosio FG, Xiao-Ping S, Birmingham DJ, et al: Evaluation of the mechanisms responsible for the reduction in erythrocyte complement receptors when immune complexes form in vivo in primates. *J Immunol* 145:4198, 1990.

Davies KA, Hird V, Stewart S, et al: A study of in vivo immune complex formation and clearance in man. *J Immunol* 144:4613, 1990.

Dorval BL, Cosio FG, Birmingham DJ, et al: Human erythrocytes inhibit complement-mediated solubilization of immune complexes. *J Immunol* 142:2721, 1989.

Hebert LA, Cosio FG: The erythrocyte-immune complex-glomerulonephritis connection in man. *Kidney Int* 31:877, 1987.

Hebert LA, Cosio FG, Birmingham DJ, et al: Experimental immune complex-mediated glomerulonephritis in the nonhuman primate. *Kidney Int* 39:44, 1991.

Kimberly RP, Edberg JC, Merriam LT, et al: In vivo handling of soluble complement fixing Ab/dsDNA immune complexes in chimpanzees. *J Clin Invest* 84:962, 1989.

Ross GD, Yount WJ, Walport MJ, et al: Disease-associated loss of erythrocyte complement receptors (CR$_1$, C3b receptors) in patients with systemic lupus erythematosus and other diseases involving autoantibodies and/or complement activation. *J Immunol* 135:2005, 1985.

Schifferli JA, Ng YC, Peters DK: The role of complement and its receptor in the elimination of immune complexes. *N Engl J Med* 315:488, 1986.

Schifferli JA, Ng YC, Estreicher J, et al: The clearance of tetanus toxoid/anti-tetanus toxoid immune complexes from the circulation of humans. *J Immunol* 140:899, 1988.

Waxman FJ, Hebert LA, Cosio FG, et al: Differential binding of immunoglobulin A and immunoglobulin G1 immune complexes to primate erythrocytes in vivo. Immunoglobulin A immune complexes bind less well to erythrocytes and are preferentially deposited in glomeruli. *J Clin Invest* 77:82, 1986.

Wilson JG, Wong WW, Murphy EE III, et al: Deficiency of the C3b/C4b receptor (CR1) of erythrocytes in systemic lupus erythematosus: Analysis of the stability of the defect and of a restriction fragment length polymorphism of the CR1 gene. *J Immunol* 138:2706, 1987.

Yeh CG, Marsh HC Jr, Carson GR, et al: Recombinant soluble human complement receptor type 1 inhibits inflammation in the reversed passive arthus reaction in rats. *J Immunol* 146:250, 1991.

Cellular Immune Mechanisms of Initiation of Glomerular Disease

T-LYMPHOCYTES IN EXPERIMENTAL NEPHRITIS

Bolton WK, Chandra M, Tyson TM, et al: Transfer of experimental glomerulonephritis in chickens by mononuclear cells. *Kidney Int* 34:598, 1988.

Boyce NW, Tipping PG, Hodsworth SR: Lymphokine (MIF) production by glomerular T-lymphocytes in experimental glomerulonephritis. *Kidney Int* 30:673, 1986.

Gibbs VC, Wood DM, Garovoy MR: The response of cultured human kidney capillary endothelium to immunologic stimuli. *Hum Immunol* 14:259, 1985.

Masuyama J, Minato N, Kano S: Mechanisms of lymphocyte adhesion to human vascular endothelial cells in culture. T lymphocyte adhesion to endothelial cells through endothelial HLA-DR antigens induced by gamma interferon. *J Clin Invest* 77:1596, 1986.

Neilson EG, Clayman MD, Haverty T, et al: Experimental strategies for the study of cellular immunity in renal disease. *Kidney Int* 30:264, 1986.

Parra G, Mosquera J, Rodríguez-Iturbe B: Migration inhibition factor in acute serum sickness nephritis. *Kidney Int* 38:1118, 1990.

Prud'homme GJ, Parfrey NA: Biology of disease. Role of T helper lymphocytes in autoimmune diseases. *Lab Invest* 59:158, 1988.

Tipping PG, Neale TJ, Holdsworth SR: T lymphocyte participation in antibody-induced experimental glomerulonephritis. *Kidney Int* 27:530, 1985.

T-LYMPHOCYTES AND LYMPHOKINES IN HUMAN GLOMERULAR DISEASE

Bolton WK, Innes DJ Jr, Sturgill BC, et al: T-cells and macrophages in rapidly progressive glomerulonephritis: Clinicopathologic correlations. *Kidney Int* 32:869, 1987.

Bakker WW, van Luijk WHJ: Do circulating factors play a role in the pathogenesis of minimal change nephrotic syndrome? *Pediatr Nephrol* 3:341, 1989.

Dabbs JD, Striker L, Mignon F, et al: Glomerular lesions in lymphomas and leukemias. *Am J Med* 80:63, 1986.

Levin M, Gascoine P, Turner MW, et al: A highly cationic protein in plasma and urine of children with steroid-responsive nephrotic syndrome. *Kidney Int* 36:867, 1989.

Nolasco FEB, Cameron JS, Hartley B, et al: Intraglomerular T cells and monocytes in nephritis: Study with monoclonal antibodies. *Kidney Int* 31:1160, 1987.

Schnaper HW, Aune TM: Identification of the lymphokine soluble immune response suppressor in urine of nephrotic children. *J Clin Invest* 76:341, 1985.

Schnaper HW, Aune TM: Steroid-sensitive mechanism of soluble immune response suppressor production in steroid-responsive nephrotic syndrome. *J Clin Invest* 79:257, 1987.

Schnaper HW: The immune system in minimal change nephrotic syndrome. *Pediatr Nephrol* 3:101, 1989.

Thomson NM, Kraft N: Normal human serum also contains the lymphotoxin found in minimal change nephropathy. *Kidney Int* 31:1186, 1987.

Polymorphonuclear Leukocytes

PMN RECRUITMENT AND ACTIVATION

Baggiolini M, Walz A, Kunkel SL: Neutrophil-activating peptide-1/interleukin 8, a novel cytokine that activates neutrophils. *J Clin Invest* 84:1045, 1989.

Camussi G, Tetta C, Bussolino F, et al: Effect of leukocyte stimulation on rabbit immune complex glomerulonephritis. *Kidney Int* 38:1047, 1990.

Falk RJ, Terrell RS, Charles LA, et al: Anti-neutrophil cytoplasmic autoantibodies induce neutrophils to degranulate and produce oxygen radicals in vitro. *Proc Natl Acad Sci USA* 87:4115, 1990.

Kallenberg CGM, Tervaert JWC, van der Woude FJ, et al: Autoimmunity to lysosomal enzymes: New clues to vasculitis and glomerulonephritis? *Immunol Today* 12:61, 1991.

Kincaid-Smith P, Nicholls K, Birchall I: Polymorphs infiltrate glomeruli in mesangial IgA glomerulonephritis. *Kidney Int* 36:1108, 1989.

Shah SV, Baricos WH, Basci A: Degradation of human glomerular basement membrane by stimulated neutrophils. Activation of a metalloproteinase(s) by reactive oxygen metabolites. *J Clin Invest* 79:25, 1987.

Terranova VP, DiFlorio R, Hujanen ES, et al: Laminin promotes rabbit neutrophil motility and attachment. *J Clin Invest* 77:1180, 1986.

Yoon PS, Boxer LA, Mayo LA, et al: Human neutrophil laminin receptors: Activation-dependent receptor expression. *J Immunol* 138:259, 1987.

PMN-DERIVED OXYGEN FREE RADICALS

Baud L, Ardaillou R: Reactive oxygen species: Production and role in the kidney. *Am J Physiol* 251:F765, 1986.

Boyce NW, Holdsworth SR: Hydroxyl radical mediation of immune renal injury by desferrioxamine. *Kidney Int* 30:813, 1986.

Farber JL, Kyle ME, Coleman JB: Biology of disease. Mechanisms of cell injury by activated oxygen species. *Lab Invest* 62:670, 1990.

Jasin HE: Oxidative cross-linking of immune complexes by human polymorphonuclear leukocytes. *J Clin Invest* 81:6, 1988.

Johnson RJ, Couser WG, Chi EY, et al: New mechanism for glomerular injury. Myeloperoxidase-hydrogen peroxide-halide system. *J Clin Invest* 79:1379, 1987.

Johnson RJ, Klebanoff SJ, Ochi RF, et al: Participation of the myeloperoxidase-H_2O_2-halide system in immune complex nephritis. *Kidney Int* 32:342, 1987.

Johnson RJ, Guggenheim SJ, Klebanoff SJ, et al: Morphologic correlates of glomerular oxidant injury induced by the myeloperoxidase-hydrogen peroxide-halide system of the neutrophil. *Lab Invest* 5:294, 1988.

Rehan A, Wiggins RC, Kunkel RG, et al: Glomerular injury and proteinuria in rats after intrarenal injection of cobra venom factor. Evidence for the role of neutrophil-derived oxygen free radicals. *Am J Pathol* 123:57, 1986.

Shah SV: Role of reactive oxygen metabolites in experimental glomerular disease. *Kidney Int* 35:1093, 1989.

Winterbourn CC: Myeloperoxidase as an effective inhibitor of hydroxyl radical production. Implications for the oxidative reactions of neutrophils. *J Clin Invest* 78:545, 1986.

Monocytes

MONOCYTE RECRUITMENT

Baud L, Sraer J, Delarue F, et al: Lipoxygenase products mediate the attachment of rat macrophages to glomeruli in vitro. *Kidney Int* 27:855, 1985.

Berliner JA, Territo MC, Sevanian A, et al: Minimally modified low density lipoprotein stimulates monocyte endothelial interactions. *J Clin Invest* 85:1260, 1990.

Boyce NW, Holdsworth SR: Macrophage-Fc-receptor affinity:

Role in cellular mediation of antibody initiated glomerulonephritis. *Kidney Int* 36:537, 1989.

Cook HT, Smith J, Cattell V: Isolation and characterization of inflammatory leukocytes from glomeruli in an in situ model of glomerulonephritis in the rat. *Am J Pathol* 126:126, 1987.

Eddy AA, McCulloch LM, Adams JA: Intraglomerular leukocyte recruitment during nephrotoxic serum nephritis in rats. *Clin Immunol Immunopathol* 57:441, 1990.

Fogelman AM, van Lenten BJ, Warden C, et al: Macrophage lipoprotein receptors. *J Cell Sci* 9S:135, 1988.

Horsburgh CR Jr, Clark RA -, Kirkpatrick CH: Lymphokines and platelets promote human monocyte adherence to fibrinogen and fibronectin in vitro. *J Leuk Biol* 41:14, 1987.

Kimura M, Nagase M, Hishida A, et al: Intramesangial passage of mononuclear phagocytes in murine lupus glomerulonephritis. *Am J Pathol* 127:149, 1987.

MONOCYTE-DERIVED INFLAMMATORY MEDIATORS

Arend WP, Joslin FG, Massoni RJ: Effects of immune complexes on production by human monocytes of interleukin 1 or an interleukin 1 inhibitor. *J Immunol* 134:3868, 1985.

Boyce NW, Tipping PG, Holdsworth SR: Glomerular macrophages produce reactive oxygen species in experimental glomerulonephritis. *Kidney Int* 35:778, 1989.

Cattell V, Cook T, Moncada S: Glomeruli synthesize nitrite in experimental nephrotoxic nephritis. *Kidney Int* 38:1056, 1990.

Cook HT, Smith J, Salmon JA, et al: Functional characteristics of macrophages in glomerulonephritis in the rat. O_2-generation, MHC class II expression, and eicosanoid synthesis. *Am J Pathol* 134:431, 1989.

Jennette JC, Tidwell RR, Geratz JD, et al: Amelioration of immune complex-mediated glomerulonephritis by synthetic protease inhibitors. *Am J Pathol* 127:499, 1987.

Martin J, Lovett DH, Gemsa D, et al: Enhancement of glomerular mesangial cell neutral proteinase secretion by macrophages: Role of interleukin 1. *J Immunol* 137:525, 1986.

Matsumoto K, Hatano M: Production of interleukin 1 in glomerular cell cultures from rats with nephrotoxic serum nephritis. *Clin Exp Immunol* 75:123, 1989.

Nakazawa M, Emancipator SN, Lamm ME: Removal of glomerular immune complexes in passive serum sickness nephritis by treatment in vivo with proteolytic enzymes. *Lab Invest* 55:551, 1986.

Nathan CF: Secretory products of macrophages. *J Clin Invest* 79:319, 1987.

Noble B, Ren K, Taverne J, et al: Mononuclear cells in glomeruli and cytokines in urine reflect the severity of experimental proliferative immune complex glomerulonephritis. *Clin Exp Immunol* 80:281, 1990.

Scher W: Biology of disease. The role of extracellular proteases in cell proliferation and differentiation. *Lab Invest* 57:607, 1987.

Tipping PG, Lowe MG, Holdsworth SR: Glomerular interleukin 1 production is dependent on macrophage infiltration in anti-GBM glomerulonephritis. *Kidney Int* 39:103, 1991.

Vissers MCM, Wiggins R, Fantone JC: Comparative ability of human monocytes and neutrophils to degrade glomerular basement membrane in vitro. *Lab Invest* 60:831, 1989.

Resident Glomerular Cells

ENDOTHELIAL CELLS

Brenner BM, Troy JL, Ballermann BJ: Endothelium-dependent vascular responses. Mediators and mechanisms. *J Clin Invest* 84:1373, 1989.

Cotran RS: New roles for the endothelium in inflammation and immunity. *Am J Pathol* 129:407, 1987.

Form DM, Pratt BM, Madri JA: Endothelial cell proliferation during angiogenesis. In vitro modulation by basement membrane components. *Lab Invest* 55:521, 1986.

Furchgott RF, Vanhouette PM: Endothelium-derived relaxing and contracting factors. *FASEB J* 3:2007, 1989.

Furcht LT: Critical factors controlling angiogenesis: Cell products, cell matrix, and growth factors. *Lab Invest* 55:505, 1986.

Marsden PA, Goligorsky MS, Brenner BM: Endothelial cell biology in relation to current concepts of vessel wall structure and function. *J Am Soc Nephrol* 1:931, 1991.

Sweeney C, Shultz P, Raij L: Interactions of the endothelium and mesangium in glomerular injury. *J Am Soc Nephrol* 1:S13, 1990.

Vane JR, Änggard EE, Botting RM: Regulatory functions of the vascular endothelium. *N Engl J Med* 323:27, 1990.

ENDOTHELIN AND THE GLOMERULUS

Edwards RM, Trizna W, Ohlstein EH: Renal microvascular effects of endothelin. *Am J Physiol* 259:F217, 1990.

Jaffer FE, Knauss TC, Poptic E, et al: Endothelin stimulates PDGF secretion in cultured human mesangial cells. *Kidney Int* 38:1193, 1990.

Kon V, Yoshioka T, Fogo A, et al: Glomerular actions of endothelin in vivo. *J Clin Invest* 83:1762, 1989.

Loutzenhiser R, Epstein M, Hayashi K, et al: Direct visualization of effects of endothelin on the renal microvasculature. *Am J Physiol* 258:F61, 1990.

Simonson MS, Dunn MJ: Endothelin-1 stimulates contraction of rat glomerular mesangial cells and potentiates β-adrenergic-mediated cyclic adenosine monophosphate accumulation. *J Clin Invest* 85:790, 1990.

Simonson MS, Dunn MJ: Endothelin peptides: A possible role in glomerular inflammation. *Lab Invest* 64:1, 1991.

Stacy DL, Scott JW, Granger JP: Control of renal function during intrarenal infusion of endothelin. *Am J Physiol* 258:F1232, 1990.

Zoja C, Orisio S, Perico N, et al: Constitutive expression of endothelin gene in cultured human mesangial cells and its modulation by transforming growth factor-β, thrombin, and a thromboxane A_2 analogue. *Lab Invest* 64:16, 1991.

EPITHELIAL CELLS

Appay M-D, Mounier F, Gubler M-C, et al: Ontogenesis of the glomerular C3b receptor (CR1) in fetal human kidney. *Clin Immunol Immunopathol* 37:103, 1985.

Fischer E, Appay M-D, Cook J, et al: Characterization of the human glomerular C3 receptor as the C3b/C4b complement type one (CR1) receptor. *J Immunol* 136:1373, 1986.

Gröne H-J, Walli AK, Gröne E, et al: Receptor mediated uptake of apo B and apo E rich lipoproteins by human glomerular epithelial cells. *Kidney Int* 37:1449, 1990.

Kasinath BS, Maaba MR, Schwartz MM, et al: Demonstration and characterization of C3 receptors on rat glomerular epithelial cells. *Kidney Int* 30:852, 1986.

Mendrick DL, Kelly DM, Rennke HG: Antigen processing and presentation by glomerular visceral epithelium in vitro. *Kidney Int* 39:71, 1991.

Minota S, Terai C, Nojima Y, et al: Correlative expression of C3b receptors in the glomerulus and on erythrocytes. *Clin Immunol Immunopathol* 38:85, 1986.

MESANGIAL CELLS

Brennan DC, Jevnikar AM, Takei F, et al: Mesangial cell accessory functions: Mediation by intercellular adhesion molecule-1. *Kidney Int* 38:1039, 1990.

Kreisberg JI, Venkatchalam M, Troyer D: Contractile properties of cultured glomerular mesangial cells. *Am J Physiol* 249:F457, 1985.

Mené P, Simonson MS, Dunn MJ: Physiology of the mesangial cell. *Physiol Rev* 69:1347, 1989.

Santiago A, Mori T, Satriano J, et al: Regulation of Fc receptors for IgG on cultured rat mesangial cells. *Kidney Int* 39:87, 1991.

Schlondorff D: The glomerular mesangial cell: An expanding role for a specialized pericyte. *FASEB J* 1:272, 1987.

Wasserman J, Santiago A, Rifici V, et al: Interactions of low density lipoprotein with rat mesangial cells. *Kidney Int* 35:1168, 1989.

Complement

COMPLEMENT IN RENAL DISEASE

Colten HR: Biology of disease. Molecular basis of complement deficiency syndromes. *Lab Invest* 52:468, 1985.

Falk RJ, Jennette JC: Immune complex induced glomerular lesions in C5 sufficient and deficient mice. *Kidney Int* 30:678, 1986.

Frank MM: Complement in the pathophysiology of human disease. *N Engl J Med* 316:1525, 1987.

Garcia-Estan J, Roman RJ, Lianos EA, et al: Effects of complement depletion on glomerular eicosanoid production and renal hemodynamics in rat nephrotoxic serum nephritis. *J Lab Clin Med* 114:389, 1989.

Sawtell NM, Hartman AL, Weiss MA, et al: C3 dependent, C5 independent immune complex glomerulopathy in the mouse. *Lab Invest* 58:287, 1988.

Zwirner J, Felber E, Herzog V, et al: Classical pathway of complement activation in normal and diseased human glomeruli. *Kidney Int* 36:1069, 1989.

GLOMERULAR INJURY INDUCED BY THE MEMBRANE ATTACK COMPLEX

Adler S, Baker PJ, Johnson RJ, et al: Complement membrane attack complex stimulates production of reactive oxygen metabolites by cultured rat mesangial cells. *J Clin Invest* 77:762, 1986.

Biesecker G: The complement SC5b-9 complex mediates cell adhesion through a vitronectin receptor. *J Immunol* 145:209, 1990.

Boyce NW, Holdsworth SR: Evidence for direct renal injury as a consequence of glomerular complement activation. *J Immunol* 136:2421, 1986.

Camussi G, Salvidio G, Biesecker G, et al: Heymann antibodies induce complement-dependent injury of rat glomerular visceral epithelial cells. *J Immunol* 139:2906, 1987.

Couser WG, Baker PJ, Adler S: Complement and the direct mediation of immune glomerular injury: A new perspective. *Kidney Int* 28:879, 1985.

Cybulsky AV, Quigg RJ, Salant DJ: The membrane attack complex in complement-mediated glomerular epithelial cell injury: Formation and stability of C5b-9 and C5b-7 in rat membranous nephropathy. *J Immunol* 137:1511, 1986.

Cybulsky AV, Rennke HG, Feintzeig ID, et al: Complement-induced glomerular epithelial cell injury. Role of the membrane attack complex in rat membranous nephropathy. *J Clin Invest* 77:1096, 1986.

Falk RJ, Dalmasso AP, Kim Y, et al: Radioimmunoassay of the attack complex of complement in serum from patients with systemic lupus erythematosus. *N Engl J Med* 312:1594, 1985.

Groggel GC, Salant DJ, Darby C, et al: Role of terminal complement pathway in the heterologous phase of antiglomerular basement membrane nephritis. *Kidney Int* 27:643, 1985.

Groggel GC, Terreros DA: Role of the terminal complement pathway in accelerated autologous anti-glomerular basement membrane nephritis. *Am J Pathol* 136:533, 1990.

Hänsch GM, Betz M, Günther J, et al: The complement membrane attack complex stimulates the prostanoid production of cultured glomerular epithelial cells. *Int Arch Allergy Appl Immun* 85:87, 1988.

Hinglais N, Kazatchkine MD, Bhakdi S, et al: Immunohistochemical study of the C5b-9 complex of complement in human kidneys. *Kidney Int* 30:399, 1986.

Imagawa DK, Osifchin NE, Ramm LE, et al: Release of arachidonic acid and formation of oxygenated derivatives after complement attack on macrophages: Role of channel formation. *J Immunol* 136:4637, 1986.

Kerjaschki D, Schulze M, Binder S, et al: Transcellular transport and membrane insertion of the C5b-9 membrane attack complex of complement by glomerular epithelial cells in experimental membranous nephropathy. *J Immunol* 143:546, 1989.

Lovett DH, Haensch G-M, Goppelt M, et al: Activation of glomerular mesangial cells by the terminal membrane attack complex of complement. *J Immunol* 138:2473, 1987.

Perkinson DT, Baker PJ, Couser WG, et al: Membrane attack complex deposition in experimental glomerular injury. *Am J Pathol* 120:121, 1985.

Pruchno CJ, Burns MW, Schulze M, et al: Urinary excretion of C5b-9 reflects disease activity in passive Heymann nephritis. *Kidney Int* 36:65, 1989.

Pruchno CJ, Burns MW, Schulze M, et al: Urinary excretion of the C5b-9 membrane attack complex of complement is a marker of immune disease activity in autologous immune complex nephritis. *Am J Pathol* 138:203, 1991.

Quigg RJ, Cybulsky AV, Jacobs JB, et al: Anti-Fx1A produces complement-dependent cytotoxicity of glomerular epithelial cells. *Kidney Int* 34:43, 1988.

Schulze M, Baker PJ, Perkinson DT, et al: Increased urinary excretion of C5b-9 distinguishes passive Heymann nephritis in the rat. *Kidney Int* 35:60, 1989.

Seeger W, Suttorp N, Hellwig A, et al: Noncytolytic terminal complement complexes may serve as calcium gates to elicit leukotriene B4 generation in human polymorphonuclear leukocytes. *J Immunol* 137:1286, 1986.

Suttorp N, Seeger W, Zinsky S, et al: Complement complex C5b-8 induces PGI$_2$ formation in cultured endothelial cells. *Am J Physiol* 253:C13, 1987.

Torbohm I, Schönermark M, Wingen A-M, et al: C5b-8 and C5b-9 modulate the collagen release of human glomerular epithelial cells. *Kidney Int* 37:1098, 1990.

COMPLEMENT REGULATORY PROTEINS IN RENAL DISEASE

Cosio FG, Sedmak DD, Mahan JD, et al: Localization of decay accelerating factor in normal and diseased kidneys. *Kidney Int* 36:100, 1989.

Eddy AA, Fritz IB: Localization of clusterin in the epimembranous deposits of passive Heymann nephritis. *Kidney Int* 39:247, 1991.

Falk RJ, Podack E, Dalmasso AP, et al: Localization of S protein and its relationship to the membrane attack complex of complement in renal tissue. *Am J Pathol* 127:182, 1987.

Lai KN, Lo STH, Lai FM-M: Immunohistochemical study of the

membrane attack complex of complement and S-protein in idiopathic and secondary membranous nephropathy. *Am J Pathol* 135:469, 1989.

Murphy BF, Kirszbaum L, Walker ID, et al: SP-40,40, a newly identified normal human serum protein found in the SC5b-9 complex of complement and in the immune deposits in glomerulonephritis. *J Clin Invest* 81:1858, 1988.

Quigg RJ, Nicholson-Weller A, Cybulsky AV, et al: Decay accelerating factor regulates complement activation on glomerular epithelial cells. *J Immunol* 142:877, 1989.

Platelets

PLATELET MEDIATION OF GLOMERULAR INJURY

Barnes JL, Venkatachalam MA: The role of platelets and polycationic mediators in glomerular vascular injury. *Semin Nephrol* 5:57, 1985.

Barnes JL, Camussi G, Tetta C, et al: Glomerular localization of platelet cationic proteins after immune complex-induced platelet activation. *Lab Invest* 63:755, 1990.

Henson PM: Interactions between neutrophils and platelets. *Lab Invest* 62:391, 1990.

Johnson RJ, Alpers CE, Pritzl P, et al: Platelets mediate neutrophil-dependent immune complex nephritis in the rat. *J Clin Invest* 82:1225, 1988.

Johnson RJ, Alpers CE, Pruchno C, et al: Mechanisms and kinetics for platelet and neutrophil localization in immune complex nephritis. *Kidney Int* 36:780, 1989.

Johnson RJ, Garcia RL, Pritzl P, et al: Platelets mediate glomerular cell proliferation in immune complex nephritis induced by anti-mesangial cell antibodies in the rat. *Am J Pathol* 136:369, 1990.

Johnson RJ, Pritzl P, Iida H, et al: Platelet-complement interactions in mesangial proliferative nephritis in the rat. *Am J Pathol* 138:313, 1991.

Poelstra K, Hardonk MJ, Koudstaal J, et al: Intraglomerular platelet aggregation and experimental glomerulonephritis. *Kidney Int* 37:1500, 1990.

PLATELET-ACTIVATING FACTOR

Badr KF, DeBoer DK, Takahashi K, et al: Glomerular responses to platelet-activating factor in the rat: Role of thromboxane A_2. *Am J Physiol* 256:F35, 1989.

Baldi E, Emancipator SN, Hassan MO, et al: Platelet activating factor receptor blockade ameliorates murine systemic lupus erythematosus. *Kidney Int* 38:1030, 1990.

Bertani T, Livio M, Macconi D, et al: Platelet activating factor (PAF) as a mediator of injury in nephrotoxic nephritis. *Kidney Int* 31:1248, 1987.

Camussi G: Potential role of platelet-activating factor in renal pathophysiology. *Kidney Int* 29:469, 1986.

Egido J, Ramirez F, Rodriguez M-J, et al: The role of platelet-activating factor in glomerular kidney disease. *In* Braquet P (ed): *New Trends in Lipid Mediators Research*, vol 2. Basel, Karger, 1988, p 167.

Lianos EA, Zanglis A: Glomerular platelet-activating factor levels and origin in experimental glomerulonephritis. *Kidney Int* 37:736, 1990.

Perico N, Delaini F, Tagliaferri M, et al: Effect of platelet-activating factor and its specific receptor antagonist on glomerular permeability to proteins in isolated perfused rat kidney. *Lab Invest* 58:163, 1988.

Schlondorff D, Neuwirth R: Platelet-activating factor and the kidney. *Am J Physiol* 251:F1, 1986.

Schlondorff D, Goldwasser P, Neuwirth R, et al: Production of platelet-activating factor in glomeruli and cultured glomerular mesangial cells. *Am J Physiol* 250:F1123, 1986.

Warren JS, Mandel DM, Johnson KJ, et al: Evidence for the role of platelet-activating factor in immune complex vasculitis in the rat. *J Clin Invest* 83:669, 1989.

Zanglis A, Linos EA: Platelet activating factor biosynthesis and degradation in rat glomeruli. *J Lab Clin Med* 110:330, 1987.

Coagulation Factors

Boucher A, Droz D, Adafer E, et al: Relationship between the integrity of Bowman's capsule and the composition of cellular crescents in human crescentic glomerulonephritis. *Lab Invest* 56:526, 1987.

Brentjens JR: Glomerular procoagulant activity and glomerulonephritis. *Lab Invest* 57:107, 1987.

Bergstein JM, Riley M, Bang NU: Analysis of the plasminogen activator activity of the human glomerulus. *Kidney Int* 33:868, 1988.

Cole EH, Glynn MFX, Laskin CA, et al: Ancrod improves survival in murine systemic lupus erythematosus. *Kidney Int* 37:29, 1990.

Holdsworth SR, Tipping PG: Macrophage-induced glomerular fibrin deposition in experimental glomerulonephritis in the rabbit. *J Clin Invest* 76:1367, 1985.

Kanfer A, de Prost D, Guettier C, et al: Enhanced glomerular procoagulant activity and fibrin deposition in rats with mercuric chloride-induced autoimmune nephritis. *Lab Invest* 57:138, 1987.

Takemura T, Yoshioka K, Akano N, et al: Glomerular deposition of cross-linked fibrin in human kidney diseases. *Kidney Int* 32:102, 1987.

Tannenbaum SH, Finko R, Cines DB: Antibody and immune complexes induce tissue factor production by human endothelial cells. *J Immunol* 137:1532, 1986.

Tipping PG, Holdsworth SR: The participation of macrophages, glomerular procoagulant activity, and factor VIII in glomerular fibrin deposition. Studies on anti-GBM antibody-induced glomerulonephritis in rabbits. *Am J Pathol* 124:10, 1986.

Tipping PG, Dowling JP, Holdsworth SR: Glomerular procoagulant activity in human proliferative glomerulonephritis. *J Clin Invest* 81:119, 1988.

Tipping PG, Lowe MG, Holdsworth SR: Glomerular macrophages express augmented procoagulant activity in experimental fibrin-related glomerulonephritis in rabbits. *J Clin Invest* 82:1253, 1988.

Tipping PG, Worthington LA, Holdsworth SR: Quantitation and characterization of glomerular procoagulant activity in experimental glomerulonephritis. *Lab Invest* 56:155, 1987.

Tsumangari T, Tanaka K: Effects of fibrinogen degradation products on glomerular mesangial cells in culture. *Kidney Int* 26:712, 1984.

Villamediana LM, Rondeau E, He C-J, et al: Thrombin regulates components of the fibrinolytic system in human mesangial cells. *Kidney Int* 38:956, 1990.

Wiggins RC, Glatfelter A, Brukman J: Procoagulant activity in glomeruli and urine of rabbits with nephrotoxic nephritis. *Lab Invest* 53:156, 1985.

Wiggins R, Glatfelter A, Kshirsagar B, et al: Lipid microvesicles and their association with procoagulant activity in urine and glomeruli of rabbits with nephrotoxic nephritis. *Lab Invest* 56:264, 1987.

Wohlwend A, Belin D, Vassalli J-D: Plasminogen activator-specific inhibitors produced by human monocytes/macrophages. *J Exp Med* 165:320, 1987.

Zoja C, Corna D, Macconi D, et al: Tissue plasminogen activator therapy of rabbit nephrotoxic nephritis. *Lab Invest* 62:34, 1990.

Hageman Factor Related Pathways

Scicli AG, Carretero OA: Renal kallikrein-kinin system. *Kidney Int* 29:120, 1986.

Vio CP, Figueroa CD: Subcellular localization of renal kallikrein by ultrastructural immunocytochemistry. *Kidney Int* 28:36, 1985.

Weinberg MS, Azar P, Trebbin WM, et al: The role of urinary kininogen in the regulation of kinin generation. *Kidney Int* 28:975, 1985.

Wiggins RC: Hageman factor in experimental nephrotoxic nephritis in the rabbit. *Lab Invest* 53:335, 1985.

Prostanoids

PROSTAGLANDINS

Bertani T, Benigni A, Cutillo F, et al: Effect of aspirin and sulindac in rabbit nephrotoxic nephritis. *J Lab Clin Med* 107:261, 1986.

Cattell V, Smith J, Cook HT: Prostaglandin E1 suppresses macrophage infiltration and ameliorates injury in an experimental model of macrophage-dependent glomerulonephritis. *Clin Exp Immunol* 79:260, 1990.

Kaizu K, Marsh D, Zipser R, et al: Role of prostaglandins and angiotensin II in experimental glomerulonephritis. *Kidney Int* 28:629, 1985.

Kunkel SL: The importance of arachidonate metabolism by immune and nonimmune cells. *Lab Invest* 58:119, 1988.

Lavelle KJ, Golichowski AM, Neff LC, et al: Effect of prostaglandins on immune complex interaction with glomerular cells in vitro. *Immunological Invest* 14:57, 1985.

Lianos EA: Eicosanoids and the modulation of glomerular immune injury. *Kidney Int* 35:985, 1989.

Patrono C, Dunn MJ: The clinical significance of inhibition of renal prostaglandin synthesis. *Kidney Int* 32:1, 1987.

Rahman MA, Emancipator SN, Dunn MJ: Immune complex effects on glomerular eicosanoid production and renal hemodynamics. *Kidney Int* 31:1317, 1987.

Rahman MA, Stork JE, Dunn MJ: The role of eicosanoids in experimental glomerulonephritis. *Kidney Int* 32:S40, 1987.

Rahman MA, Liu CN, Dunn MJ, et al: Complement and leukocyte independent proteinuria and eicosanoid synthesis in rat membranous nephropathy. *Lab Invest* 59:477, 1988.

Schlondorff D, Ardaillou R: Prostaglandins and other arachidonic acid metabolites in the kidney. *Kidney Int* 29:108, 1986.

Stahl RAK, Thaiss F: Eicosanoids: Biosynthesis and function in the glomerulus. *Renal Physiol* 10:1, 1987.

Stahl RAK, Adler S, Baker PJ, et al: Enhanced glomerular prostaglandin formation in experimental membranous nephropathy. *Kidney Int* 31:1126, 1987.

THROMBOXANE

Cybulsky AV, Lieberthal W, Quigg RJ, et al: A role for thromboxane in complement-mediated glomerular injury. *Am J Pathol* 128:45, 1987.

Kelley VE, Sneve S, Musinski S: Increased renal thromboxane production in murine lupus nephritis. *J Clin Invest* 77:252, 1986.

Patrono C, Ciabattoni G, Remuzzi G, et al: Functional significance of renal prostacyclin and thromboxane A₂ production in

patients with systemic lupus erythematosus. *J Clin Invest* 76:1011, 1985.

Pierucci A, Simonetti BM, Pecci G, et al: Improvement of renal function with selective thromboxane antagonism in lupus nephritis. *N Engl J Med* 320:421, 1989.

Salvati P, Ferti C, Ferrario RG, et al: Role of enhanced glomerular synthesis of thromboxane A₂ in progressive kidney disease. *Kidney Int* 38:447, 1990.

Sraer J, Wolf C, Oudinet J-P, et al: Human glomeruli release fatty acids which stimulate thromboxane synthesis in platelets. *Kidney Int* 32:62, 1987.

Stahl RAK, Thaiss F, Kahf S, et al: Immune-mediated mesangial cell injury—Biosynthesis and function of prostanoids. *Kidney Int* 38:273, 1990.

Takahashi K, Schreiner GF, Yamashita K, et al: Predominant functional roles for thromboxane A₂ and prostaglandin E₂ during late nephrotoxic serum glomerulonephritis in the rat. *J Clin Invest* 85:1974, 1990.

Thaiss F, Germann PJ, Kahf S, et al: Effect of thromboxane synthesis inhibition in a model of membranous nephropathy. *Kidney Int* 35:76, 1989.

Zoja C, Benigni A, Verroust P, et al: Indomethacin reduces proteinuria in passive Heymann nephritis in rats. *Kidney Int* 31:1335, 1987.

LEUKOTRIENES

Badr KF, Schreiner GF, Wassermann M, et al: Preservation of the glomerular capillary ultrafiltration coefficient during rat nephrotoxic serum nephritis by a specific leukotriene D₄ receptor antagonist. *J Clin Invest* 81:1702, 1988.

Fauler J, Wiemeyer A, Marx K-H, et al: LTB₄ in nephrotoxic serum nephritis in rats. *Kidney Int* 36:46, 1989.

Lianos EA: Synthesis of hydroxyeicosatetraenoic acids and leukotrienes in rat nephrotoxic serum glomerulonephritis. Role of anti-glomerular basement membrane antibody dose, complement, and neutrophiles. *J Clin Invest* 82:427, 1988.

Lianos EA, Noble B: Glomerular leukotriene synthesis in Heymann nephritis. *Kidney Int* 36:998, 1989.

Rahman MA, Nakazawa M, Emancipator SN, et al: Increased leukotriene B₄ synthesis in immune injured rat glomeruli. *J Clin Invest* 81:1945, 1988.

Spurney RF, Ruiz P, Pisetsky DS, et al: Enhanced renal leukotriene production in murine lupus: Role of lipoxygenase metabolites. *Kidney Int* 39:95, 1991.

Tubulointerstitial Nephritis

OVERVIEW

Kelly CJ: T cell regulation of autoimmune interstitial nephritis. *J Am Soc Nephrol* 1:140, 1990.

Wilson CB: Study of the immunopathogenesis of tubulointerstitial nephritis using model systems. *Kidney Int* 35:938, 1989.

Wilson CB: Nephritogenic tubulointerstitial antigens. *Kidney Int* 39:501, 1991.

Yoshioka K, Morimoto Y, Iseki T, et al: Characterization of tubular basement membrane antigens in human kidney. *J Immunol* 136:1654, 1986.

ANTI-TBM DISEASE IN RATS

Agus D, Mann R, Clayman M, et al: The effects of daily cyclophosphamide administration on the development and extent of primary experimental interstitial nephritis in rats. *Kidney Int* 29:635, 1986.

Alfrey AC, Froment DH, Hammond WS: Role of iron in the

tubulo-interstitial injury in nephrotoxic serum nephritis. *Kidney Int* 36:753, 1989.

Bannister KM, Wilson CB: Transfer of tubulointerstitial nephritis in the Brown Norway rat with anti-tubular basement membrane antibody: Quantitation and kinetics of binding and effect of decomplementation. *J Immunol* 135:3911, 1985.

Bannister KM, Ulich TR, Wilson CB: Induction, characterization, and cell transfer of autoimmune tubulointerstitial nephritis. *Kidney Int* 32:642, 1987.

Eddy AA: Tubulointerstitial nephritis during the heterologous phase of nephrotoxic serum nephritis. *Nephron* 59:304, 1991.

Kelly CJ, Silvers WK, Neilson EG: Tolerance to parenchymal self. Regulatory role of major histocompatibility complex-restricted, OX8+ suppressor T cells specific for autologous renal tubular antigen in experimental interstitial nephritis. *J Exp Med* 162:1892, 1985.

Kelly CJ, Clayman MD, Neilson EG: Immunoregulation in experimental interstitial nephritis: Immunization with renal tubular antigen in incomplete Freund's adjuvant induces major histocompatibility complex-restricted, OX8+ suppressor T cells which are antigen-specific and inhibit the expression of disease. *J Immunol* 136:903, 1986.

Ulich TR, Bannister KM, Wilson CB: Tubulointerstitial nephritis induced in the Brown-Norway rat with chaotropically solubilized bovine tubular basement membrane: The model and the humoral and cellular responses. *Clin Immunol Immunopathol* 36:187, 1985.

Ulich TR, Bannister KM, Wilson CB: Inhibition of the neutrophilic infiltrate of experimental tubulointerstitial nephritis in the Brown-Norway rat by decomplementation. *Clin Immunol Immunopathol* 42:288, 1987.

Yoshida H, Wakashin Y, Ueda S, et al: Detection of nephritogenic antigen from the Lewis rat renal tubular basement membrane. *Kidney Int* 37:1286, 1990.

ANTI-TBM NEPHRITIS IN MICE

Clayman MD, Martinez-Hernandez A, Michaud L, et al: Isolation and characterization of the nephritogenic antigen producing anti-tubular basement membrane disease. *J Exp Med* 161:290, 1985.

Clayman MD, Michaud L, Neilson EG: Murine interstitial nephritis. VI. Characterization of the B cell response in anti-tubular basement membrane disease. *J Immunol* 139:2242, 1987.

Kelly CJ, Korngold R, Mann R, et al: Spontaneous interstitial nephritis in kdkd mice. II. Characterization of a tubular antigen-specific, H-2K-restricted Lyt-2+ effector T cell that mediates destructive tubulointerstitial injury. *J Immunol* 136:526, 1986.

Kelly CJ, Neilson EG: Contrasuppression in autoimmunity. Abnormal contrasuppression facilitates expression of nephritogenic effector T cells and interstitial nephritis in kdkd mice. *J Exp Med* 165:107, 1987.

Kelly CJ, Mok H, Neilson EG: The selection of effector T cell phenotype by contrasuppression modulates susceptibility to autoimmune injury. *J Immunol* 141:3022, 1988.

Mann R, Zakheim B, Clayman M, et al: Murine interstitial nephritis. IV. Long-term cultured L3T4+ T cell lines transfer delayed expression of disease as I-A-restricted inducers of the effector T cell repertoire. *J Immunol* 135:286, 1985.

Neilson EG, McCafferty E, Mann R, et al: Murine interstitial nephritis. III. The selection of phenotypic (Lyt and L3T4) and idiotypic (RE-Id) T cell preferences by genes in Igh-1 and H-2K characterizes the cell-mediated potential for disease expression: Susceptible mice provide a unique effector T cell repertoire in response to tubular antigen. *J Immunol* 134:2375, 1985.

Neilson EG, Kelly CJ, Clayman MD, et al: Murine interstitial nephritis. VII. Suppression of renal injury after treatment with soluble suppressor factor TsF$_1$. *J Immunol* 139:1518, 1987.

TBM IMMUNE COMPLEX DISEASE

Fukatsu A, Yuzawa Y, Niesen N, et al: Local formation of immune deposits in rabbit renal proximal tubules. *Kidney Int* 34:611, 1988.

Ishidate T, Ward HJ, Hoyer JR: Quantitative studies of tubular immune complex formation clearance in rats. *Kidney Int* 38:1075, 1990.

Polypeptide Growth Factors/Cytokines as Mediators of Glomerular Injury

OVERVIEW

Cotran RS, Pober JS: Effects of cytokines on vascular endothelium: Their role in vascular and immune injury. *Kidney Int* 35:969, 1989.

Cotran RS, Pober JS: Cytokine-endothelial interactions in inflammation, immunity, and vascular injury. *J Am Soc Nephrol* 1:225, 1990.

Kujubu DA, Fine LG: Physiology and cell biology update: Polypeptide growth factors and their relation to renal disease. *Am J Kidney Dis* 14:61, 1989.

Pober JS: Cytokine-mediated activation of vascular endothelium. Physiology and pathology. *Am J Pathol* 133:426, 1988.

Segal R, Fine LG: Polypeptide growth factors and the kidney. *Kidney Int* 36:S2, 1989.

INTERLEUKINS

Bevilacqua MP, Pober JS, Wheeler ME, et al: Interleukin 1 acts on cultured human vascular endothelium to increase the adhesion of polymorphonuclear leukocytes, monocytes, and related leukocyte cell lines. *J Clin Invest* 76:2003, 1985.

Horii Y, Muraguchi A, Iwano M, et al: Involvement of IL-6 in mesangial proliferative glomerulonephritis. *J Immunol* 143:3949, 1989.

MacCarthy EP, Hsu A, Ooi YM, et al: Evidence for a mouse mesangial cell-derived factor that stimulates lymphocyte proliferation. *J Clin Invest* 76:426, 1985.

Ruef C, Budde K, Lacy J, et al: Interleukin 6 is an autocrine growth factor for mesangial cells. *Kidney Int* 38:249, 1990.

INTERFERON

Cockfield SM, Urmson J, Pleasants JR, et al: The regulation of expression of MHC products in mice. Factors determining the level of expression in kidneys of normal mice. *J Immunol* 144:2967, 1990.

Halloran PF, Urmson J, Ramassar V, et al: Increased class I and class II MHC products in mRNA in kidneys of MRL-1pr/1pr mice during autoimmune nephritis and inhibition by cyclosporine. *J Immunol* 141:2303, 1988.

Halloran PF, Urmson J, van der Meide PH, et al: Regulation of MHC expression in vivo. II. IFN-α/β inducers and recombinant IFN-α modulate MHC antigen expression in mouse tissues. *J Immunol* 142:4241, 1989.

Jacob CO, van der Meide PH, McDevitt HO: In vivo treatment of (NZB X NZW)F$_1$ lupus-like nephritis with monoclonal antibody to γ interferon. *J Exp Med* 166:798, 1987.

Madrenas J, Parfrey NA, Halloran PF: Interferon gamma-mediated renal MHC expression in mercuric chloride-induced glomerulonephritis. *Kidney Int* 39:273, 1991.

Martin M, Schwinzer R, Schellekens H, et al: Glomerular mesangial cells in local inflammation. Induction of the expression of MHC class II antigens by IFN-γ. *J Immunol* 142:1887, 1989.

COLONY-STIMULATING FACTORS

Budde K, Coleman DL, Lacy J, et al: Rat mesangial cells produce granulocyte-macrophage colony-stimulating factor. *Am J Physiol* 257:F1065, 1989.

Bussolino F, Ziche M, Wang JM, et al: In vitro and in vivo activation of endothelial cells by colony-stimulating factors. *J Clin Invest* 87:986, 1991.

Mori T, Bartocci A, Satriano J, et al: Mouse mesangial cells produce colony-stimulating factor-1 (CSF-1) and express the CSF-1 receptor. *J Immunol* 144:4697, 1990.

Wu M-C, Reuben PM: Granulocyte-macrophage colony-stimulating factor from cultured normal rat kidney cell line. *Exp Hematol* 12:267, 1984.

EPIDERMAL GROWTH FACTOR (EGF)

Adler S, Eng B: Reversal of inhibition of rat glomerular epithelial cell growth by growth factors. *Am J Pathol* 136:557, 1990.

Creely JJ, DiMari SJ, Howe AM, et al: Effects of epidermal growth factor on collagen synthesis by an epithelioid cell line derived from normal rat kidney. *Am J Pathol* 136:1247, 1990.

INSULINLIKE GROWTH FACTORS

Conti FG, Striker LJ, Elliot SJ, et al: Synthesis and release of insulinlike growth factor I by mesangial cells in culture. *Am J Physiol* 255:F1214, 1988.

PLATELET-DERIVED GROWTH FACTOR (PDGF)

Barnes JL, Hevey KA: Glomerular mesangial cell migration in response to platelet-derived growth factor. *Lab Invest* 62:379, 1990.

Shultz PJ, DiCorleto PE, Silver BJ, et al: Mesangial cells express PDGF mRNAs and proliferate in response to PDGF. *Am J Physiol* 255:F674, 1988.

Shultz PJ, Knauss TC, Mené P, et al: Mitogenic signals for thrombin in mesangial cells: Regulation of phospholipase C and PDGF genes. *Am J Physiol* 257:366, 1989.

TRANSFERRING GROWTH FACTOR BETA (TGFβ)

Border WA, Okuda S, Languino LR, et al: Suppression of experimental glomerulonephritis by antiserum against transforming growth factor β1. *Nature* 346:371, 1990.

Border WA, Okuda S, Languino LR, et al: Transforming growth factor-β regulates production of proteoglycans by mesangial cells. *Kidney Int* 37:689, 1990.

Coimbra T, Wiggins R, Noh JW, et al: Transforming growth factor-β production in anti-glomerular basement membrane disease in the rabbit. *Am J Pathol* 138:223, 1991.

Jaffer F, Saunders C, Shultz P, et al: Regulation of mesangial cell growth by polypeptide mitogens. Inhibitory role of transforming growth factor beta. *Am J Pathol* 135:261, 1989.

MacKay K, Kondaiah P, Danielpour D, et al: Expression of transforming growth factor-β1 and β2 in rat glomeruli. *Kidney Int* 38:1095, 1990.

MacKay K, Robbins AR, Bruce MD, et al: Identification of disulfide-linked transforming growth factor-β1-specific binding proteins in rat glomeruli. *J Biol Chem* 265:9351, 1990.

Okuda S, Languino LR, Ruoslahti E, et al: Elevated expression of transforming growth factor-β and proteoglycan production in experimental glomerulonephritis. Possible role in expansion of the mesangial extracellular matrix. *J Clin Invest* 86:453, 1990.

TUMOR NECROSIS FACTOR (TNF)

Boswell JM, Yui MA, Burt DW, et al: Increased tumor necrosis factor and IL-1 β gene expression in the kidneys of mice with lupus nephritis. *J Immunol* 141:3050, 1988.

Brennan DC, Yui MA, Wuthrich RP, et al: Tumor necrosis factor and IL-1 in New Zealand black/white mice. Enhanced gene expression and acceleration of renal injury. *J Immunol* 143:3470, 1989.

Jacob CO, McDevitt HO: Tumour necrosis factor-α in murine autoimmune 'lupus' nephritis. *Nature* 331:356, 1988.

Warren JS, Barton PA, Jones ML: Contrasting roles for tumor necrosis factor in the pathogenesis of IgA and IgG immune complex lung injury. *Am J Pathol* 138:581, 1991.

Wuthrich RP, Glimcher LH, Yui MA, et al: MHC class II, antigen presentation and tumor necrosis factor in renal tubular epithelial cells. *Kidney Int* 37:783, 1990.

Jerry M. Bergstein

14
Mechanisms of Renal Injury: Coagulation and Fibrinolysis

Several forms of kidney disease are associated with glomerular fibrin deposition. In diseases such as the hemolytic-uremic syndrome, thrombotic thrombocytopenic purpura, radiation nephritis, eclampsia, acute postpartum renal failure, and hyperacute renal transplant rejection, fibrin forms as intravascular glomerular thrombi. In diseases associated with crescent formation (the various types of rapidly progressive glomerulonephritis), fibrin formation is associated with extra-capillary crescents located in Bowman's space.

Activation of the coagulation system (Fig. 14-1) to form fibrin may be initiated by an "intrinsic" pathway that contains in solution in the blood all the coagulation factors necessary to activate coagulation factor X. The coagulation cascade also may be activated by an "extrinsic" pathway that requires the participation of tissue factor (thromboplastin) to activate factor X. Independent of the activation pathway, activation of factor X initiates a final common pathway leading to the formation of thrombin, a proteolytic enzyme that converts circulating fibrinogen to fibrin. The coagulation system also can be activated secondarily through pathways developed following complement or kinin activation [316].

In conjunction with activation of the clotting system, the fibrinolytic system is activated to remove vascular thrombi [78,192]. The fibrinolytic system is composed of a circulating inactive proenzyme plasminogen, which can be converted to the potent fibrinolytic enzyme plasmin by agents called plasminogen activators (Fig. 14-1). Two types of plasminogen activators have been defined in man: tissue plasminogen activator and urokinase [136]. Whereas the former was initially associated with vessel walls and the latter was originally found in the urine, both types of activators have now been detected in several locations, including endothelial cells [211] and human glomeruli [9,40]. Inhibitors of both plasminogen activators have recently been described [136]. The fibrinolysis of fibrin produces fibrin degradation products, digestion fragments of the fibrin thrombus.

The factors leading to glomerular fibrin deposition in human renal diseases are not clearly understood. However, several experimental models are available in which glomerular fibrin deposition may be studied. Understanding these animal models may allow insight into the role of coagulation in human renal disease.

Experimental Models of Glomerular Fibrin Deposition

Intravascular Thrombosis

The most thoroughly studied model of intravascular glomerular fibrin deposition is the generalized Shwartzman reaction. In rabbits, the reaction is produced by two intravenous injections of appropriate amounts [83] of endotoxin (lipopolysaccharide derived from the cell wall of gram-negative bacteria) approximately 24 hours apart [322]. After the second (provoking) injection of endotoxin, disseminated intravascular coagulation occurs, characterized by a dramatic decline in the levels of circulating leukocytes, platelets, coagulation factors V, VIII, and fibrinogen, and the development of generalized vascular thrombosis.

The renal lesion is characterized by massive intracapillary glomerular fibrin deposition (Fig. 14-2) as proved by immunohistologic (Fig. 14-3) and electron microscopic techniques [39,226,356]. Glomerular fibrin deposition can be prevented by anticoagulants such as sodium warfarin [294] and heparin [82], and by the production of severe hypofibrinogenemia with Arvin [an enzyme derived from the venom of Agkistrodon rhodostoma] [24], confirming that glomerular thrombosis is associated with activation of the coagulation system. The development of the glomerular fibrin depositions seems to occur in two phases [203,245, 247]. Initially, the coagulation system is activated, generating thrombin, which results in the formation of circulating soluble fibrin complexes. In the second phase, these complexes are deposited in the glomerular capillaries. Although the first phase can be prevented by anticoagulants, the second phase seems independent of the coagulation process.

Several mechanisms may be involved in the processes whereby endotoxin activates coagulation [243]. Circulating

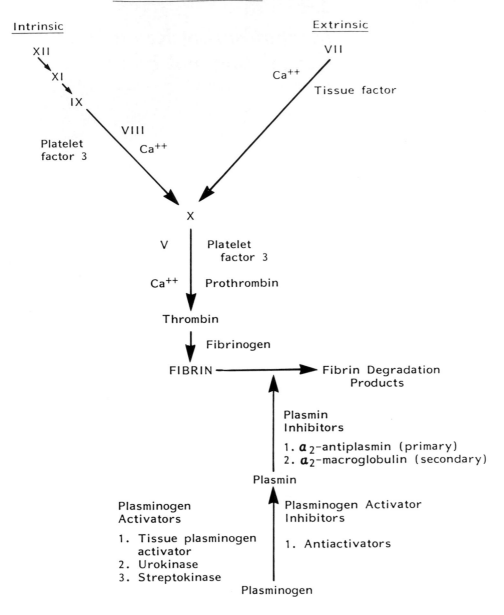

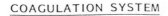

FIG. 14-1. *Pathways of the coagulation and fibrinolytic systems.*

endotoxin has been shown to injure (Fig. 14-4) vascular endothelial cells [115,117,225,305]; injury occurs despite granuloycte depletion [116] or anticoagulation with heparin [117], suggesting that endotoxin may be directly toxic to endothelial cells. This hypothesis is supported by the detection of endotoxin within vascular endothelial cells following intravenous infusion [284] and by the development of a unilateral Shwartzman reaction in the kidneys prepared with an infusion of endotoxin through the renal artery [276]. Direct endothelial cell injury could expose

the glomerular basement membrane, which can aggregate platelets [112,146,336], and/or the thrombogenic subendothelium, which contains the procoagulant tissue factor [358], thereby activating the coagulation process [260,292]. In addition, circulating endotoxin may also stimulate coagulation by activating the complement [157] and kinin [174] systems

In vitro, endotoxin both damages cultured bovine endothelial cells [131,132] and stimulates endothelial cell synthesis of tissue factor [290]. Increased levels of proco-

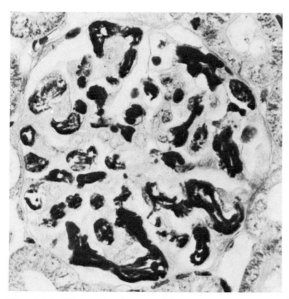

Fig. 14-2. *Glomerulus from a rabbit given two injections of endotoxin, demonstrating massive intracapillary fibrin deposition as typically seen in the generalized Shwartzman reaction. (Phosphotungstic acid-hematoxylin, ×210.) (From Bergstein JM, Michael AF Jr: Failure of Cobra venom factor to prevent the generalized Shwartzman reaction and loss of renal cortical fibrinolytic activity. Am J Pathol 74:19, 1974.)*

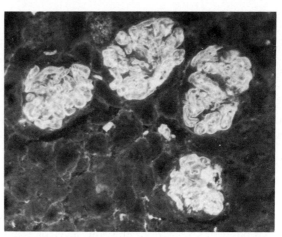

Fig. 14-3. *Immunofluorescent study of kidney from a rabbit given two injections of endotoxin, stained with goat antirabbit fibrinogen serum. The demonstration of large amounts of fibrin by immunofluorescence confirms the observations by light microscopy. (×72 before 75% reduction.) (From Bergstein JM, Michael AF Jr: Failure of Cobra venom factor to prevent the generalized Shwartzman reaction and loss of renal cortical fibrinolytic activity. Am J Pathol 74:19, 1974.)*

agulant activity have been detected in glomeruli of rabbits treated with endotoxin [58]. Endothelial cell synthesis of tissue factor may be stimulated by endotoxin-induced release of tumor necrosis factor and interleukin-1 from white blood cells, vascular endothelial cells, and mesangial cells [21,43,44,200,289,310]. Indeed, the intravenous infusion of tumor necrosis factor in rabbits produces a generalized Shwartzman-like reaction, strongly supporting the idea that tumor necrosis factor is an important mediator of endotoxin-induced glomerular injury [42]. Endotoxin, tumor necrosis factor, and interleukin-1 may also stimulate intravascular coagulation by (1) decreasing endothelial cell expression of thrombomodulin [239], a promoter of proteins C and S that inhibit thrombin formation and inactivate plasminogen activator inhibitor [288]; (2) stimulating endothelial cell production of plasminogen activator inhibitor [79,102,344]; (3) enhancing white blood cell and endothelial cell production of platelet activating factor [62], a mediator of inflammation and vascular injury; and (4) stimulating endothelial cell release of large multimers of von Willebrand factor [125], which promote the attachment of platelets to areas of endothelial injury.

Other factors, in conjunction with activation of the coagulation system, seem important in the genesis of the generalized Shwartzman reaction. Granulocytes are required for development of the reaction [46,109,141, 190,202,322], possibly through endotoxin stimulated granulocyte production and release of tissue factor, [178, 189,259] and neutral proteases or toxic oxygen radicals,

which may injure endothelial cells [133,278,342]. Platelets may be necessary for development of the reaction [218,219] although their exact role remains to be delineated [46,97, 179,202,244,246]. A platelet-derived inhibitor of glomerular fibrinolytic activity may play a role in the persistence of glomerular thrombi, promoting the development of renal cortical necrosis [30]. The sympathetic nervous system appears to be involved in the production of the reaction as infusion of norepinephrine promotes the reaction [227] while surgical [263] and chemical [47] sympathectomy and alpha-adrenergic blockage [227] prevent the reaction. Prostaglandins may also be involved in the generalized Shwartzman reaction as its development is suppressed by aspirin, indomethacin, and intravenous infusion of prostaglandins E_1 or I_2 [64,144,183,184,319].

The preparatory injection of endotoxin can be replaced by cortisone [185,323], Thorotrast (a colloidal suspension of thorium dioxide) [124,249], trypan blue [124], or carbon [304]. Although blockade of the reticuloendothelial system has been proposed as the the mechanism by which these agents substitute for endotoxin [188], substituting other colloidal and particulate materials does not prepare for the generalized Shwartzman reaction [124]. Several studies suggest that cortisone, Thorotrast, and trypan blue may act as preparatory agents by inhibiting renal cortical plasminogen activator activity [37,87,186,241,318,366].

The importance of inhibition of fibrinolysis in the pathogenesis of the generalized Shwartzman reaction was first suggested by the observations that epsilon aminocaproic acid, a potent inhibitor of fibrinolysis, can substitute for either the preparatory [204] or provoking [188] injection of endotoxin. Indeed, the unique sensitivity of the rabbit

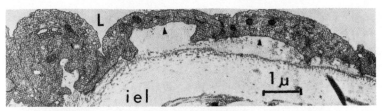

FIG. 14-4. *Electron micrograph of rabbit aorta following injection of endotoxin, demonstrating separation of endothelial cells (arrowheads) from the internal elastic lamina (iel). L = lumen. (From Spaet TH, et al: A vascular basis for the generalized Shwartzman Reaction.* Thromb Diath Haemorrh *[Suppl] 45:157, 1971.)*

to the reaction seems related to the low level of renal cortical plasminogen activator [103] and to the failure of endotoxin to activate the circulating fibrinolytic system [114]. Activation of fibrinolysis with streptokinase will both prevent and reduce glomerular fibrin deposition [80,177,282], and treatment with intravenous tissue plasminogen activator effectively removes glomerular fibrin deposits [31].

The precise mechanism whereby endotoxin inhibits glomerular plasminogen activator (fibrinolytic) activity is unknown. The failure of high concentrations of endotoxin to inhibit glomerular plasminogen activator activity in vitro [36] suggests that endotoxin inhibits the activator through the mediators. Although the complement system is activated in vivo by endotoxin [230,243] and may play a role in the development of the generalized Shwartzman reaction [107], it is not involved in the mechanism by which glomerular fibrinolysis is lost [38].

Platelets may be involved in the mechanism of endotoxin-induced inhibition of fibrinolysis. Platelets contain inhibitors of fibrinolysis [52,104,152,271] that may be released by the direct interaction of endotoxin with platelets [15,143,250]. Interestingly, anti-platelet antibody can be substituted for the preparatory injection of endotoxin in the generalized Shwartzman reaction, and animals made thrombocytopenic with anti-platelet antibody or endotoxin demonstrate decreased glomerular fibrinolytic activity in association with an inhibitor of glomerular fibrinolysis in the circulation [30]. In addition, fibrinolysis of normal glomeruli is inhibited in vitro by an agent that diffuses from washed normal platelets [30]. This suggests that platelet destruction, mediated by antibody or endotoxin, releases an inhibitor of fibrinolysis that plays a role in the development of the generalized Shwartzman reaction.

Endothelial cells may also be involved in the mechanism of endotoxin inhibition of fibrinolysis. In addition to the possibility of endotoxin-induced injury leading to diminished plasminogen activator production, endothelial cells produce plasminogen activator inhibitors [210,212,268] that may be released following exposure to endotoxin [79,84,97,129], thrombin [129,209], tumor necrosis factor [94,288,344], and interleukin-1 [102,288].

The important role of the fibrinolytic system in the development and subsequent fate of intravascular glomerular fibrin deposits is also suggested in other endotoxin-

mediated experimental models. Although normal rats are resistant to endotoxin [361], pregnant rats will develop the generalized Shwartzman reaction following a single injection of endotoxin [248,361]. The increased sensitivity to endotoxin may be explained by decreased renal cortical plasminogen activator activated during pregnancy [103].

In the rabbit, glomerular plasminogen activator activity is lost following endotoxin-induced glomerular fibrin deposition, resulting in cortical necrosis [36]. In the pregnant rat, however, glomerular plasminogen activator activity is retained following endotoxin-induced glomerular fibrin deposition with subsequent clearing (Fig. 14-5) of the fibrin deposits [33]. This confirms that glomerular plasminogen activator activity plays an important role in the removal of intravascular glomerular fibrin.

Intravascular glomerular fibrin deposits have also been produced in rabbits [188] and rats [220,308] following intravenous infusion of thrombin. In the absence of inhibition of fibrinolysis, glomerular thrombi clear spontaneously [188,217,308]. However, glomerular fibrin persists if the fibrinolytic system is inhibited during the thrombin infusion [25,220,308].

Immune Injury

The autologous phase of nephrotoxic serum nephritis (anti-glomerular basement membrane antibody disease) in rabbits is the most thoroughly studied model of glomerular fibrin formation associated with extra-capillary crescents. This phase of the disease is characterized by swelling and proliferation of the glomerular cells (Fig. 14-6), neutrophil and macrophage infiltration, basement membrane thickening, focal tuft necrosis, crescent formation (Fig. 14-7), glomerular sclerosis, and fibrin deposition within cells, along the glomerular basement membrane (Fig. 14-8), and within crescents (Fig. 14-9). In this model, animals anticoagulated with sodium warfarin on the day of antiserum injection develop little or no proliferation of glomerular cells [54,346,347]. Despite evidence that warfarin has no effect on the immune process, that neutrophil infiltration persists, and that proteinuria is no different between warfarin treated and untreated animals, fibrin does not develop, crescents do not appear, and sclerosis does not result. These studies suggest that the swelling and prolif-

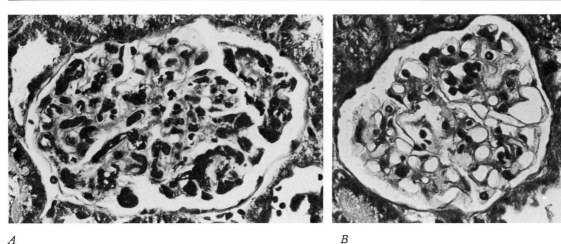

A   B

FIG. 14-5. A. Glomerular fibrin deposition in kidney from a pregnant rat obtained four hours after injection of endotoxin. B. Glomerulus from the same animal 24 hours after endotoxin, demonstrating absence of fibrin. (Phosphotungstic acid-hematoxylin, ×560 before 32% reduction.) (From Bergstein JM, et al: Glomerular fibrinolytic deposition in the pregnant rat. Am J Pathol 75:209, 1974.)

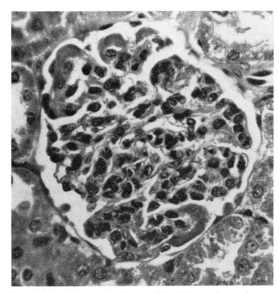

FIG. 14-6. Glomerulus from rabbit kidney obtained seven days after injection of sheep antirabbit kidney serum, demonstrating neutrophil infiltration, swelling and proliferation of glomerular cells, basement membrane thickening, and fibrinoid deposits. (H & E, ×400.) (From Vassilli P, McCluskey RT: The pathogenic role of the coagulation process in Masugi nephritis. Am J Pathol 45:653, 1964.)

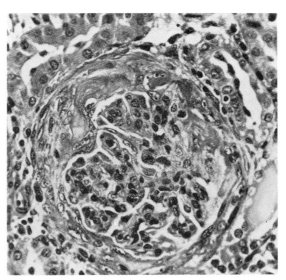

FIG. 14-7. Glomerulus from a rabbit 12 days after injection of nephrotoxic serum, demonstrating an epithelial cell crescent. (H & E, ×400.) (From Vassalli P, McCluskey R: The pathogenic role of the coagulation process in Masugi nephritis. Am J Pathol 45:653, 1964.)

eration of glomerular cells results from the phagocytosis of fibrin or other products formed during the coagulation process and that the intracellular material that stains with antifibrinogen serum in the absence of histologic fibrin represents incompletely polymerized fibrin. From these studies, it also appears that crescent formation results from

fibrin deposition in Bowman's space and that fibrin also plays a role in the development of glomerular sclerosis.

In rabbits, the induction of hypofibrinogenemia with Arvin at the time of and after the administration of nephrotoxic serum [252,254,326,328] decreases the severity of the glomerular changes, supporting the role of the coagu-

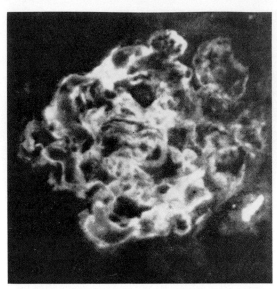

FIG. 14-8. *Glomerulus from a rabbit ten days after injection of nephrotoxic serum, demonstrating fibrin within cells and along the glomerular basement membrane. (Fluorescein-tagged guinea pig antirabbit fibrinogen serum, × 400.) (From Vassalli P, McCluskey RT: The pathogenic role of the coagulation process in Masugi nephritis. Am J Pathol 45:653, 1964.)*

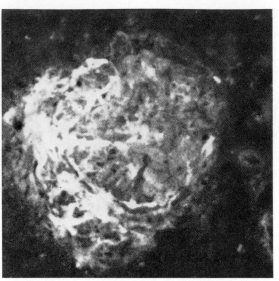

FIG. 14-9. *Fibrin within epithelial cell crescent. (Fluorescein-tagged guinea pig antirabbit fibrinogen serum, × 400.) (From Vassalli P, McCluskey RT: The pathogenic role of the coagulation process in Masugi nephritis. Am J Pathol 45:653, 1964.)*

lation process in the pathogenesis of the disease. In certain studies, anticoagulation with heparin at the time of [127,176,255,355] or shortly after [328] nephrotoxic serum administration also reduced the severity of the glomerular lesions. However, other investigators [53] were unable to demonstrate that heparin protects rabbits injected with horse or sheep antiglomerular basement membrane serum. The discrepancy between these results remains unexplained but may be related to differences in the nature or dose of the nephrotoxic antibody, the severity of the nephritis, or the amount of heparin administered. Heparin therapy appears to be of no benefit in nephrotoxic serum nephritis in mice [57] or rats [49], suggesting that glomerular fibrin deposition may not be a primary mediator of the pathogenic process in these species.

The mechanisms leading to activation of the coagulation process in the autologous phase of nephrotoxic serum nephritis in rabbits are incompletely understood. Platelets do not appear to be involved [187,303].

Recent studies suggest that macrophages play a central role in the formation of extra-capillary fibrin. Macrophages, which produce tissue factor procoagulant [274,333, 343], have been demonstrated in glomeruli of nephrotoxic serum treated rabbits prior to fibrin deposition and crescent formation [325,332,360]. Although the signal for macrophage attraction is unknown, macrophage accumulation in glomeruli is associated with a marked increase in glomerular procoagulant activity [139,334,360]. Prevention of macrophage accumulation with anti-macrophage serum [138] or mustine hydrochloride [139] dramatically reduces the severity of the histologic lesion and the degree of protein-

uria, whereas repletion of mononuclear inflammatory cells in mustine hydrochloride-treated animals restores glomerular macrophage accumulation and fibrin deposition [139]. In addition to the release of tissue factor, macrophages in glomeruli may promote coagulation by producing tumor necrosis factor, interleukin-1, and plasminogen activator inhibitior [10,233,333,350].

Thus, it seems likely that macrophages enter Bowman's space where they encounter plasma that exudes from the blood because of increased glomerular capillary wall permeability or gaps in the basement membrane [302]. The release of macrophage procoagulant activates the extrinsic coagulation system [334], producing fibrin deposits that stimulate the proliferation of the epithelial cells that line Bowman's capsule. Interestingly, warfarin, which is thought to reduce the severity of the autologous phase through its anticoagulant activity (see above), may also protect by reducing macrophage expression of tissue factor [100]. That the intrinsic coagulation system may also be involved in extra-capillary fibrin formation is suggested by the immunopathologic demonstration of fibrin and coagulation factor VIII in nephrotoxic serum induced crescents in rats [302] and in the latter stages of crescent formation in rabbits [332].

Intravascular fibrin formation in the rabbit model may be initiated by endothelial cell injury [300,302]. The fibrinolytic system may also be involved in the pathogenesis of rabbit nephrotoxic serum nephritis because glomerular and urinary fibrinolytic activity are diminished at the peak of the disease, inhibition of fibrinolysis enhances glomerular fibrin deposition, and treatment with fribrinolytic agents reduces fibrin deposition and crescent formation [2,317,331,355]. Indeed, the persistence of fibrin within crescents, which could play a role in the development of glomerular sclerosis, may be related to deficient extra-capillary fibrinolytic activity [10,302].

The role of the coagulation process in the development of experimental immune complex glomerulonephritis has not been adequately studied. Although macrophages [138,334] and platelets [66] may be involved in the mediation of immune complex injury, there is little evidence to suggest that this involves activation of coagulation. In rabbits given bovine serum to induce acute serum sickness, no improvement was detected in the glomerular lesions of animals anticoagulated with warfarin [18] or defibrinated with Arvin [254]. In chronic serum sickness in rabbits, heparin failed to alter the progression of the histologic lesion [53]; some protection was seen following defibrination [327].

Coagulation and Fibrinolysis in Human Renal Disease

Morphologic and Biochemical Observations

The histologic demonstration of fibrin-like material in glomeruli suggests that the coagulation process is involved in several forms of human renal disease [154]. However, fibrin-like material may be present in forms other than the usual cross-linked polymers seen in typical thrombi. The histologic stains used to detect fibrin by light microscopy react positively with urea-insoluble, cross-linked fibrin but fail to react with urea-soluble, non-cross-linked fibrin [120]. In several types of renal disease, fibrin may be detected by immunofluorescence but not by light [88,121] or electron microscopy [175,348], suggesting that, although antigenic determinants of fibrin (or fibrinogen) are present, cross-linked fibrin is absent. It seems likely that these antigenic determinants represent fibrin-fibrinogen degradation products that are formed in the kidney by plasminogen-dependent glomerular fibrinolytic activity or plasminogen-independent leukocyte protease fibrinolytic activity [111,270]. However, they could also represent trapped fibrinogen, fibrin monomers, or fibrin-fibrinogen degradation products derived from the circulation. The presence of fibrin degradation products in the kidney assumes increasing importance in light of the recent demonstrations that these products are chemotactic for neutrophils [228,309], increase vascular permeability [23,315], inhibit cell-mediated immune function [118], and are cytotoxic to endothelial [61,86,357] and mesangial [337] cells in tissue culture. Thus, the presence of fibrin-fibrinogen degradation products within the glomerulus might initiate additional mechanisms for further glomerular injury.

Following deposition in the glomerulus, the ultimate fate of fibrin is unclear. Fibrinolytic activity [35], mediated by the elaboration of tissue plasminogen activator and urokinase [9,40,180], has been demonstrated in the human glomerulus and may play a role in fibrin removal. As in the experimental model of nephrotoxic serum nephritis [348], fibrin and its degradation products may be phagocytized by glomerular cells or infiltrating macrophages [298]. Additionally, fibrin may be removed through the mesangium [231]. On the other hand, fibrin can persist in glomeruli and may lead to glomerular obsolescence [175], perhaps through organization into hyalin scars [348].

The demonstration of glomerular plasminogen activator activity suggests that fibrinolytic activity may be important in the removal of glomerular fibrin. Indeed, the level of this activity may be the limiting factor in determining the amount of glomerular injury resulting from fibrin deposition. The detection of fibrin degradation products in the blood and urine of patients with several forms of renal disease further supports the possible role of the fibrinolytic system in the pathogenesis of these diseases. Elevated levels of these products have been found in immune-related glomerulonephritis [3,5,48,72,75,81,95,101,126,135,155, 162,181,213,216,251,285,293,311,312,320, 341], pyelonephritis [293,341,359], vasculitis [5,48,75], minimal lesion nephrotic syndrome [5,75,101,126,311,341], hemolytic-uremic syndrome [5,16,101,135,169,213,312,320, 340], and renal homograft rejection [11,27,56,68,76,113, 135,147,213,253,291,293]. Although not clearly resolved, certain evidence suggests that elevated levels of fibrin degradation products may correlate with the immunofluorescent demonstration of glomerular fibrin [72,213,251,285]. In addition, these elevated levels seem to decline following successful treatment of glomerulonephritis [75,232] and homograft rejection [56,76,147]. However, it remains to be confirmed that elevated levels of blood and urine fibrin degradation products truly represent lysis of glomerular fibrin rather than resulting from decreased renal function and/or increased glomerular capillary wall permeability [90,126,156,175,208,320].

As yet, the site of enhanced fibrinolytic activity has not been determined. In fact, blood and urine fibrinolytic activity are frequently diminished in various forms of glomerulonephritis [17,123,242,296,354], nephrotic syndrome [7,12], and acute [12,159,221,296] and chronic [12,14,98,99,149,182,264,295,351] renal failure. Diminished blood fibrinolytic activity may result, at least in part, from elevated plasma levels of fibrinolytic inhibitors [12,26,149,159,324,354]. Elevated plasma levels of these inhibitors are often associated with proteinuria [7,12, 142,158,206,287,324]. Increased plasma levels of fibrinolytic inhibitors, coagulation factors V, VII, VIII, and fibrinogen, decreased plasma antithrombin III concentration, and increased platelet numbers and aggregability [1,4,7,150,229,281,339,349] may be responsible for the high risk of thromboembolic complications in patients having nephrotic syndrome [145,205].

Role of Platelets

Certain evidence suggests that platelets may be involved in several forms of human kidney disease although their precise role remains to be determined. Measurement of plasma levels of beta-thromboglobulin and platelet factor 4, two platelet specific proteins, seems to be the most reliable means of detecting in vivo platelet activation [165,368]. Elevated plasma levels of these proteins and serotonin and increased platelet aggregation have been found in several types of glomerulonephritis [8,20,265,

266,335,362,363], nephrotic syndrome [335,352], renal insufficiency [345], and renal allograft recipients [110]. Using immunofluorescent techniques, platelet antigens have been detected in glomeruli from patients having various forms of renal disease [67,90,92,233].

The means of platelet activation and aggregation may involve immune complexes, endothelial cell injury with resultant exposure of subendothelial collagen and high molecular weight von Willebrand factor, and the release of platelet activating factor from leukocytes and glomerular cells [8,65,168,321]. Platelet-induced glomerular injury may be mediated by the release of agents that increase vascular permeability and activate the inflammatory and coagulation systems [8,67,256,365].

Hemolytic-Uremic Syndrome

Although the precise pathogenesis of the hemolytic-uremic syndrome (HUS) is unknown, its development has been associated with bacterial, Bartonella, and viral infections and endotoxemia. Recently, outbreaks of HUS have been associated with verocytotoxin-producing strains of *Escherichia coli*, primarily serotype 0157:H7 [69,166,167,258, 262,277,307]. Verocytotoxin and a closely related toxin derived from certain Shigella species are cytotoxic to cultured Vero (African green monkey kidney cells) cell lines and may promote HUS by damaging endothelial cells [261,275]. Glycolipid receptors for verotoxin have been detected in human kidneys [55].

The syndrome has also been reported after the use of oral contraceptives, pyran copolymer (an inducer of interferon), cytotoxic drugs for cancer chemotherapy, and cyclosporin A to prevent graft rejection. In addition, an HUS-like state has been described in association with circulating anti-endothelial cell antibodies [191], disseminated intravascular coagulation, systemic lupus erythematosus, malignant hypertension, renal homograft rejection, pre-eclampsia, post-partum renal failure, and radiation nephritis. Genetic factors may also play a role in the predisposition to the disease.

Despite the multitude of factors that have been implicated in the pathogenesis of the syndrome, it remains probable that several of these may operate through a final common pathway—endothelial cell injury—which leads to localized intravascular coagulation. As in the Shwartzman reaction, endothelial cell injury may initiate coagulation by releasing tissue factor or exposing the thrombogenic subendothelium. However, in studies performed with Drs. Nils Bang and Stephen Zuckerman, we found no evidence of tumor necrosis factor or interleukin-1 in serum or plasma obtained from six children at the onset of HUS (unpublished observations).

Platelets may also be involved in the disease process. In HUS, platelet numbers and survival times are reduced [130], presumably due to adherence to intravascular thrombi or injured endothelium and to damage acquired during passage through the thrombosed microvasculature with subsequent removal from the circulation by the reticuloendothelial system. Adherent platelets may undergo the release reaction, inducing further platelet aggregation and

vasoconstriction through the release of thromboxanes. In vitro, platelet aggregation is reduced during the acute phase of HUS [108,163,267,353], suggesting that the remaining circulating platelets may have already undergone the release reaction. The presence of elevated plasma levels of beta-thromboglobulin, platelet factor 4 [13], serotonin [353], factors that aggregate platelets [235,238,353], and platelet-derived growth factors [194] in certain patients supports the hypothesis of intravascular platelet activation in HUS. Whether platelet activation is involved in the pathogenesis of the disease or results from the development of the disease remains to be determined.

Recent studies suggest that deficient vascular prostacyclin production may be important in the pathogenesis of HUS. Prostacyclin is a potent vasodilator and inhibitor of platelet aggregation, produced primarily by vascular endothelial cells [237]. Some patients with HUS seem to lack a plasma factor that stimulates endothelial cell prostacyclin production [71,92,153,193,313,338,353]; leukocyte prostacyclin production may also be reduced [89]. This has lead to the treatment of HUS with plasma infusion [207,280, 299,329] and/or plasmapheresis [19,22,29,70,106,119, 279,306], in hopes of replacing the missing plasma factor and/or removing potential circulating inhibitors of prostacyclin production. The value of such therapy remains to be determined. Interestingly, at least some patients with HUS show no deficiency in circulating prostacyclin levels [134,314,338].

Inhibition of glomerular fibrinolytic activity may play an important role in the pathogensis and outcome of HUS. Patients with this disease have a circulating inhibitor of glomerular fibrinolysis, and persistence of this inhibitor is associated with a poor outcome [34]. The inhibitor, which is a plasminogen activator inhibitor [32], is removed from

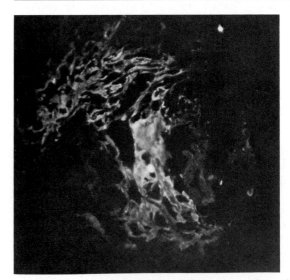

FIG. 14-10. *Fibrin within epithelial cell crescent in glomerulus from a patient with rapidly progressive glomerulonephritis. (Fluorescein-tagged rabbit antihuman fibrinogen serum, ×250 before 18% reduction.)*

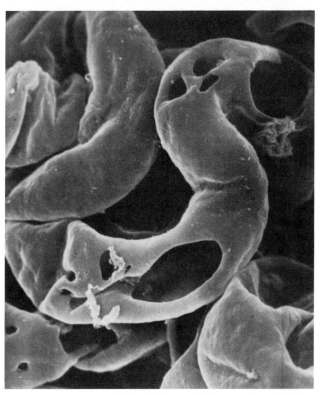

FIG. 14-11. Scanning electron micrograph depicting glomerular basement membrane defects in a glomerulus from a patient with necrotizing glomerulonephritis. (×2000) (From Bonsib SM: Glomerular basement membrane discontinuities. Am J Pathol 19:357, 1985.)

the circulation by peritoneal dialysis [34], which may account in part for the improved outcome reported by Kaplan and associates [164] in patients with HUS treated by early peritoneal dialysis.

Thrombotic Thrombocytopenic Purpura

Thrombotic thrombocytopenic purpura (TTP) is a rare disorder in childhood [28,41]. Its precise relationship to HUS in unclear. Like HUS, TTP may be associated with a microangiopathic hemolytic anemia, thrombocytopenia, renal failure, and neurologic manifestations. Unlike HUS, the disease occurs primarily in adults and may have widespread organ involvement, focal neurologic manifestations, absent renal involvement, purpura, intravascular platelet thrombi, and a poor prognosis in the absence of treatment [172,269].

Plasma from patients with TTP contains a platelet-aggregating factor, sometimes in association with large multimers of von Willebrand factor [148,170,171,196,197, 236,301]. Interestingly, plasma from these patients is cytotoxic for cultured endothelial cells; this toxicity seems to be related to the production of an IgG directed against endothelial cells [60]. In addition, the capacity of plasma proteins to bind prostacyclin is reduced in patients with TTP, decreasing the availability of prostacyclin for suppression of platelet aggregation [364].

The value of inhibitors of platelet aggregation in the treatment of TTP remains controversial. Some investigators suggest that such agents (aspirin, dipyridamole, dextran) may be beneficial [6,85,91,201]. Others indicate that such agents are ineffective [283], perhaps because they fail

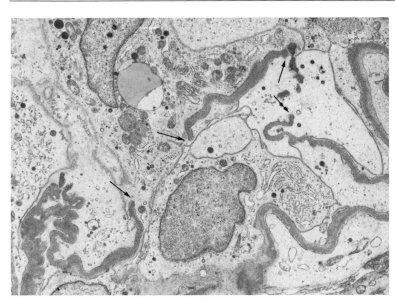

FIG. 14-12. Transmission electron micrograph demonstrating discontinuous fragments of glomerular capillary basement membrane (arrows) in renal tissue from patient with prominent crescent formation (×7100 before 25% reduction.) (From Morita T, et al: Structure and development of the glomerular crescent. Am J Pathol 72:249, 1973.)

to inhibit the platelet aggregating factor found in the plasma of these patients [199]. Plasma infusion or exchange seems beneficial in most patients [45,59,63,105,297], either through the removal of pathogenic agents or the contribution of substances such as non-specific adult IgG that inhibit the platelet aggregating factor [198].

Systemic Lupus Erythematosus

In addition to HUS and TTP, glomerular capillary thrombosis has recently been suggested to play a role in the pathogenesis of the focal and diffuse proliferative forms of lupus glomerulonephritis [161,272]. Immunologic events [161], increased monocyte procoagulant activity [77], intrarenal platelet consumption [74], and deficiency of a plasma factor that stimulates prostacyclin production [160] may be involved in the process of endothelial cell injury and activation of coagulation. Defibrination therapy may be helpful in such patients [93,173,273].

Rapidly Progressive Glomerulonephritis

The distinguishing characteristic of rapidly progressive glomerulonephritis, independent of the pathogenesis of the disorder, is glomerular crescent formation. Crescents form in Bowman's space and consist of the proliferating epithelial cells (parietal) that line Bowman's capsule, fibrin (Fig. 14-10), basement membrane-like material, and macrophages [73,128,140,151,195,215,286,367]. Although the precise stimulus for crescent formation is unclear, fibrin deposition in Bowman's space remains the best candidate. Presumably, plasma gains access to the urinary space through disruptions (Fig. 14-11) or gaps (Fig. 14-12) in the glomerular basement membrane, increased membrane permeability, necrosis of the capillary wall, or lysis of the mesangium [50,51,234,240]. As in the nephrotoxic serum nephritis model, tissue factor and interleukin-1 derived from macrophages may activate the coagulation process [222,257,330], resulting in fibrin formation.

Crescents appear to pass through three stages of development [240]. Fresh cellular crescents may resolve spontaneously [137,224], especially in poststreptococcal glomerulonephritis. In most other diseases, crescents progress through a fibrocellular stage to a fibrous state [240], perhaps due to the release of fibroblast mitogenic factors by macrophages [122] and the passage of inflammatory cells and mediators through gaps in Bowman's capsule [137].

References

1. Adler AJ, Lundin AP, Feinroth MV, et al: Beta-thromboglobulin levels in the nephrotic syndrome. *Am J Med* 69:551, 1980.
2. Akiba T, Tanaka K: Effects of fibrinolytic treatment on rabbit Masugi nephritis. *Acta Pathol Jpn* 33:773, 1983.
3. Alkjaersig NK, Fletcher AP, Lewis ML, et al: Pathophysiological response of the blood coagulation system in acute glomerulonephritis. *Kidney Int* 10:319,1976.
4. Alkjaersig NK, Fletcher AP, Narayanan M, et al: Course and resolution of the coagulopathy in nephrotic children. *Kidney Int* 31:722, 1987.
5. Amburs JL, Baliah T, Ambrus CL, et al: Fibrin-fibrinogen degradation products in children with renal disease. *NY State J Med* 7:1396, 1974.
6. Amorosi EL, Karpatkin S: Antiplatelet treatment of thrombotic thrombocytopenic purpura. *Ann Intern Med* 86:102, 1977.
7. Andrassy K, Ritz E, Bommer J: Hypercoagulability in the nephrotic syndrome. *Klin Wochenschr* 58:1029, 1980.
8. Andrassy K, Ritz E, Mauerhoff T, et al: What is the evidence for activated coagulation in glomerulonephritis? *Am J Nephrol* 2:293, 1982.
9. Angles-Cano E, Rondeau E, Delarue F, et al: Identification and cellular localization of plasminogen activators from human glomeruli. *Thromb Haemost* 54:688, 1985.
10. Antalis TM, Clark MA, Barnes T, et al: Cloning and expression of a cDNA coding for a human monocyte-derived plasminogen activator inhibitor. *Proc Natl Acad Sci USA* 85:985, 1988.
11. Antoine B, Neveu T, Ward PD: Fibrinuria during renal transplantation. *Transplantation* 8:98, 1969.
12. Aoki N: Natural inhibitors of fibrinolysis. *Prog Cardiovas Dis* 21:267, 1979.
13. Appiani AC, Edefonti A, Bettininelli A, et al: The relationship between plasma levels of the factor VIII complex and platelet release products (beta-thrombo-globulin and platelet factor 4) in children with the hemolytic-uremic syndrome. *Clin Nephrol* 17:195, 1982.
14. Asbeck F, Sistig E, Renner E, et al: Urokinase excretion in chronic renal diseases of different histological types. *Clin Nephrol* 1:46, 1973.
15. Ausprunk DH, Das J: Endotoxin-induced changes in human platelet membranes: Morphologic evidence. *Blood* 51:487, 1978.
16. Avalo JS, Vitacco M, Molinas F, et al: Coagulation studies in the hemolytic-uremic syndrome. *J Pediatr* 76:538, 1970.
17. Bachmann HJ, Haupt H: Investigation on fibrinolysis in children with inflammatory diseases of kidneys and urinary tract. *Z Kinderheilk* 109:300, 1971.
18. Baliah T, Drummond KN: The effect of anticoagulation on serum sickness nephritis in rabbits. *Proc Soc Exp Biol Med* 140:329, 1972.
19. Bambauer R, Jutzler GA, Hartman HG, et al: Hemolytic uremic syndrome successfully treated with plasma exchange. *In* Nose Y, Malchesky PS, Smith JD, et al (eds): *Plasmapheresis.* New York, Raven Press, 1983, p 379.
20. Bang NU, Trygstad CW, Schroeder JE, et al: Enhanced platelet function in glomerular renal disease. *J Lab Clin Med* 81:651, 1973.
21. Baud L, Oudinet JP, Bens M, et al: Production of tumor necrosis factor by rat mesangial cells in response to bacterial lipopolysaccharide. *Kidney Int* 35:1111, 1989.
22. Beattie, TJ, Murphy AV, Willoughby MLN, et al: Plasmapheresis in the haemolytic-uraemic syndrome in children, *Br Med J* 282:1667, 1981.
23. Belew M, Gerdin B, Lindeberg G, et al: Structure-activity relationships of vasoactive peptides derived from fibrin or fibrinogen degraded by plasmin. *Biochim Biophys Acta* 621:169, 1980.
24. Bell WR, Miller RE, Levin J: Inhibition of the generalized Shwartzman reaction by hypofibrinogenemia. *Blood* 40:697, 1972.
25. Beller FK, Mitchell PS, Gorstein F: Fibrin deposition in the rabbit kidney produced by protease inhibitors. *Thromb Diath Haemorrh* 17:427, 1967.

26. Bennett NB, Ogston D: Inhibitors of the fibrinolytic system in renal disease. *Clin Sci* 39:549, 1970.

27. Bennett NM, Bennett D, Holland NH, et al: Serum fibrin degradation products in the diagnosis of transplantation rejection. *Transplantation* 14:311, 1972.

28. Berberich FR, Cuene SA, Chard RL Jr, et al: Thrombotic thrombocytopenic purpura. *J Pediatr* 84:503, 1974.

29. Bergada E, Torras A, Puig L, et al: Plasmapheresis-dependent recovery from recurrent hemolytic-uremic syndrome. *Int J Artif Organs* 6:79, 1982.

30. Bergstein JM: Platelet inhibition of renal cortical fibrinolytic activity in the rabbit. *Lab Invest* 35:171, 1976.

31. Bergstein JM: Tissue plasminogen activator therapy of glomerular thrombi in the Shwartzman reaction. *Kidney Int* 35:14, 1989.

32. Bergstein JM, Bang NU: Plasminogen activator inhibitor-1 (PAI-1) is the circulating inhibitor of fibrinolysis (PAI-HUS) in the hemolytic-uremic syndrome (HUS). Abstract of The Am Soc Nephrol 22nd Annual Meeting, Washington, DC, December 3–6, 1989.

33. Bergstein JM, Hoyer JR, Michael AF Jr: Glomerular fibrinolytic activity following endotoxin-induced glomerular fibrin deposition in the pregnant rat. *Am J Pathol* 75:209, 1974.

34. Bergstein JM, Kuerderli U, Bang NU: Plasma inhibitor of glomerular fibrinolysis in the hemolytic-uremic syndrome. *Am J Med* 73:322, 1982.

35. Bergstein JM, Michael AF Jr: Cortial fibrinolytic activity in normal and diseased human kidneys. *J Lab Clin Med* 79:701, 1972.

36. Bergstein JM, Michael AF Jr: Renal cortical fibrinolytic activity in the rabbit following one or two doses of endotoxin. *Throm Diath Haemorrh* 29:27, 1973.

37. Bergstein JM, Michael AF Jr: The effect of Thorotrast and cortisone on renal cortical fibrinolytic activity in the rabbit. *Am J Pathol* 71:113, 1973.

38. Bergstein JM, Michael AF Jr: Failure of cobra venom factor to prevent the generalized Shwartzman reaction and loss of renal cortical fibrinolytic activity *Am J Pathol* 74:19, 1974.

39. Bergstein JM, Michael AF Jr: Generalized Shwartzman reaction in the rabbit. Immunopathologic findings in the kidney. *Arch Path* 97:230, 1974.

40. Bergstein JM, Riley M, Bang NU: Analysis of the plasminogen activator activity of the human glomerulus. *Kidney Int* 33:868, 1988.

41. Berman N, Finklestein JZ: Thrombotic thrombocytopenic purpura in childhood. *Scand J Haematol* 14:286, 1975.

42. Bertani T, Abbate M, Zoja C, et al: Tumor necrosis factor induces glomerular damage in the rabbit. *Am J Pathol* 134:419, 1989.

43. Bevilacqua MP, Pober JS, Majeau GR, et al: Recombinant tumor necrosis factor induces procoagulant activity in cultured human vascular endothelium: characterization and comparison with the action of interleukin-1. *Proc Natl Acad Sci USA* 83:4533, 1986.

44. Bevilacqua MP, Pober JS, Wheeler ME, et al: Interleukin-1 activation of vascular endothelium. *Am J Pathol* 121:393, 1985.

45. Blitzer JB, Granfortuna JM, Gottlieb AJ, et al: Thrombotic thrombocytopenic purpura: treatment with plasmapheresis. *Am J Hematol* 24:329, 1987.

46. Bohn E, Muller-Bergahus G: The effect of leukocyte and platelet transfusion on the activation of intravascular coagulation by endotoxin in granulocytopenic and thrombocytopenic rabbits. *Am J Pathol* 84:239, 1976.

47. Bolton WK, Atuk NO: Study of chemical sympathectomy in endotoxin-induced lethality and fibrin deposition. *Kidney Int* 13:263, 1978.

48. Bond RE, Donadio JV Jr, Holley KE, et al: Fibrinolytic split products. *Arch Intern Med* 132:182, 1973.

49. Bone MJ, Valdes AJ, Germuth FG Jr, et al: Heparin therapy in anti-basement membrane nephritis. *Kidney Int* 8:72, 1975.

50. Bonsib SM: Glomerular basement membrane discontinuities. *Am J Pathol* 119:357, 1985.

51. Bonsib SM: Glomerular basement membrane necrosis and crescent organization. *Kidney Int* 33:966, 1988.

52. Booth NA, Anderson JA, Bennett B: Platelet release protein which inhibits plasminogen activators. *J Clin Pathol* 38:825, 1985.

53. Border WA, Wilson CB, Dixon FJ: Failure of heparin to affect two types of experimental glomerulonephritis in rabbits. *Kidney Int* 8:140, 1975.

54. Borrero J, Todd ME, Becker CG, et al: Masugi nephritis: the renal lesion and the coagulation process. *Clin Nephrol* 1:86, 1973.

55. Boyd B, Lingwood C: Verotoxin receptor glycolipid in human renal tissue. *Nephron* 51:207, 1989.

56. Braun WE, Merril JP: Urine fibrinogen fragments in human renal allografts. *N Engl J Med* 278:1366, 1968.

57. Briggs JD, Kwaan HC, Potter EV: The role of fibrinogen in renal disease. III. Fibrinolytic and anticoagulant treatment of nephrotoxic serum nephritis in mice . *J Lab Clin Med* 74:715, 1969.

58. Brukman J, Wiggins RC: Procoagulant activity in kidneys of normal and bacterial lipopolysaccharide-treated rabbits. *Kidney Int* 32:31, 1987.

59. Bukowski RM, Hewlett JS, Reimer RR, et al: Therapy of thrombotic thrombocytopenic purpura: an overview. *Semin Thromb Hemost* 7:1, 1981.

60. Burns ER, Zuker-Franklin D: Pathologic effects of plasma from patients with thrombotic thrombocytopenic purpura on platelets and cultured vascular endothelial cells. *Blood* 60:1030, 1982.

61. Busch C, Gerdin B: Effect of low molecular weight fibrin degradation products on endothelial cells in culture. *Thromb Res* 22:33, 1981.

62. Bussolino F, Camussi G, Baglioni C: Synthesis and release of platelet-activating factor by human vascular endothelial cells treated with tumor necrosis factor or interleukin-1. *J Biol Chem* 263:11856, 1988.

63. Byrnes JJ: Plasma infusion in the treatment of thrombotic thrombocytopenic purpura. *Semin Thromb Hemost* 7:9, 1981.

64. Campos A, Kim Y, Azar SH, et al: Prevention of the generalized Shwartzman reaction in pregnant rats by prostacyclin infusion. *Lab Invest* 48:705, 1983.

65. Camussi G, Salvidio G, Tetta C: Platelet-activating factor in renal diseases. *Am J Nephrol* (suppl 1)9:23, 1989.

66. Camussi G, Tetta C, Deregibus MC, et al: Platelet-activating factor (PAF) in experimentally-induced rabbit acute serum sickness: role of basophil-derived PAF in immune complex deposition. *J Immunol* 128:86, 1982.

67. Camussi G, Tetta C, Mazzucco G, et al: Platelet cationic proteins are present in glomeruli of lupus nephritis patients. *Kidney Int* 30:355, 1986.

68. Carlsson S, Hedner U, Nilsson IM, et al: Kidney transplantation and fibrinolytic split products in serum and urine. *Transplantation* 10:366, 1970.

69. Carter AO, Borczyk AA, Carlson JAK, et al: A severe outbreak of *Escherichia coli* 0157:H7-associated hemorrhagic colitis in a nursing home. *N Engl J Med* 317:1496, 1987.

70. Cattran DC: Adult hemolytic-uremic syndrome: successful

treatment with plasmapheresis. *Am J Kidney Dis* 3:275, 1984.

71. Chamone DA, Proesmans WC, Monnens LA, et al: Reversible deficient prostacyclin release in child hemolytic uremic syndrome. *Int J Pediatr Nephrol* 3:13, 1982.

72. Chirawong P, Nanra RS, Kincaid-Smith P: Fibrin degradation products and the role of coagulation in persistent glomerulonephritis. *Ann Intern Med* 74:853, 1971.

73. Churg J, Morita T, Suzuki Y: Glomerulonephritis with fibrin and crescent formation. *In* Kincaid-Smith P, Mathew TH, Becker EL (eds): *Glomerulonephritis.* New York, Wiley, 1973, p 677.

74. Clark WF, Lewis ML, Cameron JS, et al: Intrarenal platelet consumption in the diffuse proliferative nephritis of systemic lupus erythematosus. *Clin Sci Mol Med* 49:247, 1975.

75. Clarkson AR, MacDonald MK, Petrie JJB, et al: Serum and urinary fibrin/fibrinogen degradation products in glomerulonephritis. *Br Med J* 3:447, 1971.

76. Clarkson AR, Morton JB, Cash JD: Urinary fibrin/fibrinogen degradation products after renal homotransplantation. *Lancet* 2:1220, 1970.

77. Cole EH, Schulman J, Urowitz M, et al: Monocyte procoagulant activity in glomerulonephritis associated with systmic lupus erythematosus. *J Clin Invest* 75:861, 1985.

78. Collen D: On the regulation and control of fibrinolysis. *Thromb Haemost* 43:77, 1980.

79. Colucci M, Paramo JA, Collen D: Generation in plasma of a fast-acting inhibitor of plasminogen activator in response to endotoxin stimulation. *J Clin Invest* 75:818, 1985.

80. Condie RM, Hong CY, Good RA: Reversal of the lesion of the generalized Shwartzman phenomenon by treatment of rabbits with streptokinase. *J Lab Clin Med* 50:803, 1957.

81. Conte J, Boneu B, Mignon-Conte M, et al: Exploration of intraglomerular phenomena by measurement of fibrin degradation products in the renal vein blood. *In* Kincaid-Smith P, Mathew TH, Becker EL (eds): *Glomerulonephritis.* New York, Wiley, 1973, p 915.

82. Corrigan JJ Jr: Effect of anticoagulating and nonanticoagulating concentrations of heparin on the generalized Shwartzman reaction. *Thromb Diath Haemorrh* 24:136, 1970.

83. Corrigan JJ, Abildgarrd CF, Vanderheiden JF, et al: Quantitative aspects of blood coagulation in the generalized Shwartzman reaction. *Pediatr Res* 1:39, 1967.

84. Crutchley DJ, Conanan LB: Endotoxin induction of an inhibitor of plasminogen activator in bovine pulmonary artery endothelial cells. *J Biol Chem* 261:154, 1986.

85. Cuttner J: Thrombotic thrombocytopenic purpura: a ten-year experience. *Blood* 56:302, 1980.

86. Dang CV, Bell WR, Kaiser D, et al: Disorganization of cultured vascular endothelial cell monolayers by fibrinogen fragment D. *Science* 227:1487, 1985.

87. Dano K, Reich E: Plasminogen activator from cells transformed by an oncogenic virus. *Biochim Biophys Acta* 566:138, 1979.

88. Davison AM, Thomson D, MacDonald MK: Identification of intrarenal fibrin deposition. *J Clin Pathol* 26:102, 1973.

89. Deckmyn H, Proesmans W, Vermylen J: Prostacyclin production by whole blood from children: impairment in the hemolytic uremic syndrome and excessive formation in chronic renal failure. *Thromb Res* 30:13, 1983.

90. Deguchi F, Tomura S, Yoshiyama N, et al: Intraglomerular deposition of coagulation-fibrinolysis factors and a platelet membrane antigen in various glomerular diseases. *Nephron* 51:377, 1989.

91. Del Zoppo GJ: Antiplatelet therapy in thrombotic thrombocytopenic purpura. *Semin Hematol* 24:130, 1987.

92. Donati MB, Misiani R, Marchesi D, et al: Hemolytic-uremic syndrome, prostaglandins, and plasma factors. *In* Remuzzi G, Mecca G, de Gaetano G (eds): *Hemostasis, Prostaglandins, and Renal Disease.* New York, Raven Press, 1980, p 283.

93. Dosekun AK, Pollak VE, Glas-Greenwalt P, et al: Ancrod in systemic lupus erythematosus with thrombosis. *Arch Intern Med* 144:37, 1984.

94. Dosne AM, Dubor F, Lutcher F, et al: Tumor necrosis factor (TNF) stimulates plasminogen activator inhibitor (PAI) production by endothelial cells and decreased blood fibrinolytic activity in the rat. *Thromb Res [Suppl]* 8:115, 1988.

95. Dotremont G, Vermylen J, Donati MB, et al: Urinary excretion of fibrinogen-fibrin-related antigen in glomerulonephritis. *In* Kincaid-Smith P, Mathew TH, Becker EL (eds): *Glomerulonephritis.* New York, Wiley, 1973, p 829.

96. Duffus P, Parbtani A, Frampton G, et al: Intraglomerular localization of platelet related antigens, platelet factor 4, and beta-thromboglobulin in glomerulonephritis. *Clin Nephrol* 17:288, 1982.

97. Eckhardt T, Muller-Berghaus G: The role of blood platelets in the precipitation of soluble fibrin by endotoxin. *Scand J Haematol* 14:181, 1975.

98. Edward N: Fibrinolysis in patients on regular hemodialysis. *Clin Nephrol* 1:97, 1973.

99. Edward N, Young DPG, MacLeod M: Fibrinolytic activity in plasma and urine in chronic renal disease. *J Clin Pathol* 17:365, 1964.

100. Edwards RL, Schreiber E, Brande W: The effect of sodium warfarin on rabbit monocyte tissue factor expression. *Thromb Res* 42:125, 1986.

101. Ekert H, Barratt TM, Chantler C, et al: Immunologically active equivalents of fibrinogen in sera and urine of children with renal disease. *Arch Dis Child* 47:90, 1972.

102. Emeis JJ, Kooistra T: Interleukin-1 and lipopolysaccharide induce an inhibitor of tissue-type plasminogen activator in vivo and in cultured endothelial cells. *J Exp Med* 163:1260, 1986.

103. Epstein MD, Beller FK, Douglas GW: Kidney tissue activator of fibrinolysis in relation to pregnancy. *Obstet Gynecol* 32:494, 1968.

104. Erickson LA, Ginsberg MH, Loskutoff DJ: Detection and partial characterization of an inhibitor of plasminogen activator in human platelets. *J Clin Invest* 74:1465, 1984.

105. Evans TL, Winkelstein A, Zeigler ZR, et al: Thrombotic thrombocytopenic purpura: clinical course and response to therapy in eight patients. *Am J Hematol* 17:401, 1984.

106. Feldhoff CM, Luboldt W, Bussmann K, et al: Plasma exchanges in frequently recurrent hemolytic-uremic syndrome in a child. *Int J Pediatr Nephrol* 4:239, 1983.

107. Fong JSC, Good RA: Prevention of the localized and generalized Shwartzman reactions by an anticomplementary agent, cobra venom factor. *J Exp Med* 134:642, 1971.

108. Fong JSC, Kaplan BS: Impairment of platelet aggregation in hemolytic-uremic syndrome: evidence for platelet "exhaustion." *Blood* 60:564, 1982.

109. Forman EN, Abildgaard CF, Bolger JF, et al: Generalized Shwartzman reaction: role of the granulocyte in intravascular coagulation and renal cortical necrosis. *Br J Haematol* 16:507, 1969.

110. Frampton G, Parbtani A, Marchesi D, et al: *In* vivo platelet activation with in vitro hyperaggregability to arachidonic acid in renal allograft recipients. *Kidney Int* 23:506, 1983.

111. Francis CW, Marder VJ: Degradation of cross-linked fibrin by human leukocyte proteases. *J Lab Clin Med* 107:342, 1986.

112. Freytag JW, Dalrymple PN, Maguire MH, et al: Glomerular basement membrane. Studies on its structure and interaction with platelets. *J Biol Chem* 253:9069, 1978.

113. Fukao K, Kashiwagi N, Kajiwara T, et al: Urine plasmin-like substances as an index of kidney allograft rejections. *Transplantation* 23:407, 1977.

114. Gans H, Krivit W: Effect of endotoxin on the clotting mechanism. II. On the variation in response in different species of animals. *Ann Surg* 153:453, 1961.

115. Gaynor E: Increased mitotic activity in rabbit endothelium after endotoxin. *Lab Invest* 24:318, 1971.

116. Gaynor E: The role of granulocytes in endotoxin-induced vascular injury. *Blood* 41:797, 1973.

117. Gaynor E, Bouvier C, Spaet TH: Vascular lesions: possible pathogenetic basis of the generalized Shwartzman reaction. 170:986, 1970.

118. Gerdin B, Saldeen T, Roszkowski W, et al: Immunosuppressive effect of vasoactive peptides derived from human fibrinogen. *Thromb Res* 18:461, 1980.

119. Gillor A, Bulla M, Roth B, et al: Plasmapheresis as a therapeutic measure in hemolytic-uremic syndrome in children. *Klin Wochenschr* 61:363, 1983.

120. Gitlin D, Craig JM: Variation in the staining characteristics of human fibrin. *Am J Pathol* 33:267, 1957.

121. Gitlin D, Craig JM, Janeway CA: Studies on the nature of fibrinoid in the collagen diseases. *Am J Pathol* 33:55, 1957.

122. Glassock RJ: The pathogenesis of crescentic glomerulonephritis in man. *In* Bertani T, Remuzzi G (eds): *Glomerular Injury 300 Years After Morgagni.* Milan, Wichtig Editore, 1983, p 195.

123. Goldschmidt B, Marosvari I: Blood fibrinolysis and the kidney. *Lancet* 2:48, 1968.

124. Good RA, Thomas L: Studies on the generalized Shwartzman reaction. II. The production of bilateral cortical necrosis of the kidneys by a single injection of bacterial toxin in rabbits previously treated with Thorotrast or trypan blue. *J Exp Med* 96:625, 1952.

125. Gralnick H, McKeown LP, Wilson OM, et al: von Willebrand factor release induced by endotoxin. *J Lab Clin Med* 113:118, 1989.

126. Hall CL, Pejhan N, Terry JM, et al: Urinary fibrin-fibrinogen degradation products in nephrotic syndrome. *Br Med J* 1:419, 1975.

127. Halpern B, Milliez P, Lagrue G, et al: Protective action of heparin in experimental immune nephritis. *Nature* 205:256, 1965.

128. Hancock WW, Atkins RC: Cellular composition of crescents in human rapidly progressive glomerulonephritis identified using monoclonal antibodies. *Am J Nephrol* 4:177, 1984.

129. Hanss M, Collen D: Secretion of tissue-type plasminogen activator and plasminogen activator inhibitor by cultured human endothelial cells: modulation by thrombin, endotoxin, and histamine. *J Lab Clin Med* 109:97, 1987.

130. Harker LA, Slichter SJ: Platelet and fibrinogen consumption in man. *N Engl J Med* 287:999, 1972.

131. Harlan JM, Harker LA, Reidy MA, et al: Lipopolysaccharide-mediated bovine endothelial cell injury in vitro. *Lab Invest* 48:269, 1983.

132. Harlan JM, Harker LA, Striker GE, et al: Effects of lipopolysaccharide on human endothelial cells in culture. *Thromb Res* 29:15, 1983.

133. Harlan JM, Killen PD, Harker LA, et al: Neutrophil-mediated endothelial injury in vitro. *J Clin Invest* 68:1394, 1981.

134. Hautekeete ML, Nagler JM, Cuykens JJ, et al: 6-keto-PGF1-alpha levels and prostacyclin therapy in 2 adult patients with hemolytic-uremic syndrome. *Clin Nephrol* 26:157, 1986.

135. Hedner U, Nilsson IM: Renal disease and fibrinogen degradation products. *Adv Nephrol* 3:241, 1974.

136. Hekman CM, Loskutoff DJ: Fibrinolytic pathways and the endothelium. *Semin Thromb Hemost* 13:514, 1987.

137. Hogg RJ: A clinico-pathologic study of crescentic glomerulonephritis in 50 children. *Kidney Int* 27:450, 1985.

138. Holdsworth SR, Neale TJ, Wilson CB: Abrogation of macrophage-dependent injury in experimental glomerulonephritis in the rabbit. *J Clin Invest* 68:686, 1981.

139. Holdsworth SR, Tipping PG: Macrophage-induced glomerular fibrin deposition in experimental glomerulonephritis in the rabbit. *J Clin Invest* 76:1367, 1985.

140. Hooke DH, Gee DC, Atkins RC: Leukocyte analysis using monoclonal antibodies in human glomerulonephritis. *Kidney Int* 31:964, 1987.

141. Horn RG, Collins RD: Studies on the pathogenesis of the generalized Shwartzman reaction. The role of granulocytes. *Lab Invest* 18:101, 1968.

142. Horne CHW, Briggs JD, Howie PW, et al: Serum alpha-macroglobulins in renal disease and preeclampsia. *J Clin Pathol* 25:590, 1972.

143. Horowitz HI, Des Pres RM, Hook EW: Effects of bacterial endotoxin on rabbit platelets. *J Exp Med* 116:619, 1962.

144. Howes EL Jr, Kwok MT, Mckay DG: The effects of indomethacin on the generalized Shwartzman reaction. *Am J Pathol* 90:7, 1978.

145. Hoyer PF, Gonda S, Barthels M, et al: Thromboembolic complications in children with nephrotic syndrome. *Acta Paediatr Scand* 75:804, 1986.

146. Hughes J, Mahieu P: Platelet aggregation induced by basement membranes. *Thromb Diath Haemorrh* 24:395, 1970.

147. Hulme B, Pitcher PM: Rapid latex-screening test for detection of fibrin/fibrinogen degradation products in urine after renal transplantation. *Lancet* 1:6, 1973.

148. Hussey CV, Hause LL, Gottschall JL, et al: A platelet aggregating factor in thrombotic thrombocytopenic purpura: Initial activity, fluctuations, and removal by plasma exchange. *Thromb Res* 44:355, 1986.

149. Ito T, Niwa T, Matsui E: Fibrinolytic activity in renal disease. *Clin Chim Acta* 36:145, 1972.

150. Jackson CA, Greaves M, Patterson AD, et al: Relationship between platelet aggregation, thromboxane synthesis and albumin concentration in nephrotic syndrome. *Br J Haematol* 52:69, 1982.

151. Jennette JC, Hipp CG: The epithelial antigen phenotype of glomerular crescent cells. *Am J Clin Pathol* 86:274, 1986.

152. Joist JH, Niewiarowski S, Nath N, et al: Platelet antiplasmin: its extrusion during the release reaction, subcellular localization, characterization, and relationship to antiheparin in pig platelets. *J Lab Clin Med* 87:659, 1976.

153. Jorgensen KA, Pedersen RS: Familial deficiency of prostacyclin production stimulating factor in the hemolytic uremic syndrome of childhood. *Thromb Res* 21:311, 1981.

154. Kamitsuji H, Kusumoto K, Taira K, et al: Localization of intrarenal cross-linked fibrin in children with various renal diseases. *Nephron* 35:94, 1983.

155. Kamitsuji H, Tani K, Taniguchi A, et al: Urinary fibrin-fibrinogen degradation products and intraglomerular fibrin-fibrinogen deposition in various renal diseases. *Thromb Res* 21:285, 1981.

156. Kamitsuji H, Whitworth JA, Dowling JP, et al: Urinary crosslinked fibrin degradation products in glomerular disease. *Am J Kidney Dis* 7:452, 1986.

157. Kane MA, May JE, Frank MM: Interactions of the classical and alternate complement pathway with endotoxin lipopolysaccharide. *J Clin Invest* 52:370, 1973.

158. Kanfer A, Kleinknecht D, Broyer M, et al: Coagulation studies in 45 cases of nephrotic syndrome without uremia. *Thromb Diath Haemorrh* 24:562, 1970.

159. Kanfer A, Vandewallele A, Beaufils M, et al: Enhanced antiplasmin activity in acute renal failure. *Br Med J* 4:195, 1975.

160. Kant KS, Dosekun AK, Chandran KGP, et al: Deficiency of a plasma factor stimulating vascular prostacyclin generation in patients with lupus nephritis and glomerular thrombi and its correction by ancrod: in-vivo and in-vitro observations. *Thromb Res* 27:651, 1982.

161. Kant KS, Pollak VE, Weiss MA, et al: Glomerular thrombosis in systemic lupus: prevalence and significance. *Medicine* 60:71, 1981.

162. Kanyerezi RR, Lwanga SK, Bloch KJ, et al: Fibrinogen degradation products in serum and urine of patients with systemic lupus erythematosus. *Arthritis Rheum* 14:267, 1971.

163. Kaplan BS, Fong JSC: Reduced platelet aggregation in hemolytic-uremic syndrome. *Thromb Hemost* 43:154, 1980.

164. Kaplan BS, Katz J, Krawitz S, et al: An analysis of the results of therapy of 67 cases of the hemolytic-uremic syndrome. *J Pediatr* 78:420, 1971.

165. Kaplan KL, Owen J: Plasma levels of beta-thromboglobulin and platelet factor 4 as indices of platelet activation in vivo. *Blood* 57:199, 1981.

166. Karmali MA, Petric M, Lim C, et al: The association between idiopathic hemolytic uremic syndrome and infection by verotoxin-producing *Escherichia coli*. *J Infect Dis* 151:775, 1985.

167. Karmali MA, Steele BT, Petric M, et al: Sporadic cases of haemolytic-uraemic syndrome associated with faecal cytotoxin and cytotoxin-producing *Escherichia coli* in stools. *Lancet* 1:619, 1983.

168. Kasai N, Parbtani A, Cameron JS, et al: Platelet-aggregating immune complexes and intraplatelet serotonin in idiopathic glomerulonephritis and systemic lupus. *Clin Exp Immunol* 43:64, 1981.

169. Katz J, Lurie A, Kaplan BS, et al: Coagulation findings in the hemolytic-uremic syndrome of infancy: similarity to hyperacute renal allograft rejection. *J Pediatr* 78:426, 1971.

170. Kelton JG, Moore JC, Murphy WG: Studies investigating platelet aggregation and release initiated by sera from patients with thrombotic thrombocytopenic purpura. *Blood* 69:924, 1987.

171. Kelton JG, Moore J, Santos A, et al: Detection of a platelet-agglutinating factor in thrombotic thrombocytopenic purpura. *Ann Intern Med* 101:589, 1984.

172. Kennedy SS, Zacharski LR, Beck JR: Thrombotic thrombocytopenic purpura: analysis of 48 unselected cases. *Semin Thromb Hemost* 6:341, 1980.

173. Kim S, Wadhwa NK, Kant KS, et al: Fibrinolysis in glomerulonephritis treated with ancrod: renal functional, immunologic and histopathologic effects. *Q J Med* 259:879, 1988.

174. Kimball HR, Melmon KL, Wolff SM: Endotoxin-induced kinin production in man. *Proc Soc Exp Biol Med* 139:1078, 1972.

175. Kincaid-Smith P: The role of coagulation in the obliteration of glomerular capillaries. *In* Kincaid-Smith P, Mathew TH, Becker EL (eds): *Glomerulonephritis*. New York, Wiley, 1973, p 871.

176. Kleinerman J: Effects of heparin on experimental nephritis in rabbits. *Lab Invest* 3:495, 1954.

177. Kliman A, McKay DG: The prevention of the generalized Shwartzman reaction by fibrinolytic activity. *Arch Pathol* 66:715, 1958.

178. Kociba GJ, Griesemer RA: Disseminated intravascular coagulation induced with leukocyte procoagulant. *Am J Pathol* 69:407, 1972.

179. Kramer W, Muller-Berghaus G: Effect of platelet antiserum on the activation of intravascular coagulation by endotoxin. *Thromb Res* 10:47, 1977.

180. Lacave R, Rondeau E, Ochi S, et al: Characterization of a plasminogen activator and its inhibitor in human mesangial cells. *Kidney Int* 35:806, 1989.

181. Lane DA, Ireland H, Knight I, et al: The significance of fibrinogen derivatives in plasma in human renal failure. *Br J Haematol* 56:251, 1984.

182. Larsson SO, Hedner U, Nilsson IM: On coagulation and fibrinolysis in conservatively treated chronic uremia. *Acta Med Scand* 189:433, 1971.

183. Latour J-G, Bernard F: Prevention by aspirin of the classic generalized Shwartzman reaction. *Am J Pathol* 91:595, 1978.

184. Latour J-G, Leger-Gauthier C: Prostaglandins in the pathogenesis of the generalized Shwartzman reaction. *Am J Obstet Gynecol* 135:577, 1979.

185. Latour J-G, Prejean JB, Margaretten W: Corticosteroids and the generalized Shwartzman reaction. *Am J Pathol* 65:189, 1971.

186. Laug WE: Glucocorticoids inhibit plasminogen activator production by endothelial cells. *Thromb Haemost* 50:888, 1983.

187. Lavelle KJ, Ransdell BA, Kleit SA: The influence of selective thrombocytopenia on nephrotoxic nephritis. *J Lab Clin Med* 87:967, 1976.

188. Lee L: Reticuloendothelial clearance of circulating fibrin in the pathogenesis of the generalized Shwartzman reaction. *J Exp Med* 115:1065, 1962.

189. Lerner RG, Goldstein R, Cummings G: Endotoxin induced disseminated intavascular coagulation: evidence that it is mediated by neutrophil production of tissue factor. *Thromb Res* 11:253, 1977.

190. Lerner RG, Rapaport SI, Spitzer JM: Endotoxin-induced intravascular clotting: the need for granulocytes. *Thromb Diath Haemorrh* 20:430, 1968.

191. Leung DY, Moake JL, Havens PL, et al: Lytic anti-endothelial cell antibodies in haemolytic-uraemic syndrome. *Lancet* 2:183, 1988.

192. Levin EG, Marzec U, Anderson J, et al: Thrombin stimulates tissue plasminogen activator release from cultured human endothelial cells. *J Clin Invest* 74:1988, 1984.

193. Levin M, Elkon KB, Nokes TJC, et al: Inhibitor of prostacyclin production in sporadic haemolytic uraemic syndrome. *Arch Dis Child* 58:703, 1983.

194. Levin M, Stroobant P, Walters MDS, et al: Platelet-derived growth factors as possible mediators of vascular proliferation in the sporadic haemolytic uraemic syndrome. *Lancet* 2:830, 1986.

195. Lewis EJ, Cavallo T, Harrington JT, et al: An immunopathologic study of rapidly progressive glomerulonephritis in the adult. *Hum Pathol* 2:185, 1971.

196. Lian EC-Y: Pathogenesis of thrombotic thrombocytopenic purpura. *Semin Hematol* 24:82, 1987.

197. Lian EC-Y: The role of increased platelet aggregation in TTP. *Semin Thromb Hemost* 6:401, 1980.

198. Lian EC-Y, Mui PTK, Siddiqui FA, et al: Inhibition of platelet-aggregating activity in thrombotic thrombocytopenic purpura plasma by normal adult immunoglobulin G. *J Clin Invest* 73:548, 1984.

199. Lian EC-Y, Savaraj N: Effects of platelet inhibitors on the platelet aggregation induced by plasma from patients with thrombotic thrombocytopenic purpura. Blood 58:354, 1981.

200. Libby P, Ordovas JM, Auger KR, et al: Endotoxin and tumor necrosis factor induce interleukin-1 gene expression in adult human vascular endothelial cells. Am J Pathol 124:179, 1986.

201. Lichtin AE, Schreiber AD, Hurwitz S, et al: Efficacy of intensive plasmapheresis in thrombotic thrombocytopenic purpura. Arch Intern Med 147:2122, 1987.

202. Lipinski B, Gurewich V: The effect of leukopenia versus thrombocytopenia on endotoxin induced intravascular coagulation. Thromb Res 8:403, 1976.

203. Lipinski B, Gurewich V, Nowak A, et al: The effect of heparin and dipyridamole on the deposition of fibrin-like material in rabbits infused with soluble fibrin monomer or fibrinogen. Thromb Res 5:343, 1974.

204. Lipinski B, Worowski K, Jeljaszewica J, et al: Participation of soluble fibrin monomer complexes and platelet factor 4 in the generalized Shwartzman reaction. Thromb Diath Haemorrh 20:284, 1968.

205. Llach F: Hypercoagulability, renal vein thrombosis, and other complications of nephrotic syndrome. Kidney Int 28:429, 1985.

206. Lohmann RC, Kendall AG, Dossetor JB, et al: The fibrinolytic system in the nephrotic syndrome. Clin Res 17:333, 1969.

207. Loirat C, Sonsino E, Hinglais N, et al: Treatment of the childhood haemolytic uraemic syndrome with plasma. Pediatr Nephrol 2:279, 1988.

208. Loschiavo C, Previato G, Valvo E, et al: Clinical significance of urinary fibrinogen degradation products in renal disease. Nephron 28:200, 1981.

209. Loskutoff DJ: Effect of thrombin on the fibrinolytic activity of cultured bovine endothelial cells. J Clin Invest 64:329, 1979.

210. Loskutoff DJ, Edgington TS: An inhibitor of plasminogen activator in rabbit endothelial cells. J Biol Chem 256:4142, 1981.

211. Loskutoff DJ, Mussoni L: Interactions between fibrin and plasminogen activators produced by cultured endothelial cells. Blood 62:62, 1983.

212. Loskutoff DJ, Van Mourik JA, Erickson LA, et al: Detection of an unusually stable fibrinolytic inhibitor produced by bovine endothelial cells. Proc Natl Acad Sci USA 80:2956, 1983.

213. Macdonald MK, Clarkson AR, Davison AM: The role of coagulation in renal disease. In Kincaid-Smith P, Mathew TH, Becker EL (eds): Glomerulonephritis. New York, Wiley, 1973, p 809.

214. Maggiore Q, Jovanovic B, Baldini G: Plasma fibrinolytic hyper-activity in children with acute post-streptococcal glomerulonephritis. Nephron 6:81, 1969.

215. Magil AB: Histogenesis of glomerular crescents. Am J Pathol 120:222, 1985.

216. Marchesi, SL, Aptekar RG, Steinberg AD, et al: Urinary fibrin split products in lupus nephritis. Arthritis Rheum 17:158, 1974.

217. Margaretten W, Csavossy I, McKay DG: An electron microscopic study of thrombin-induced disseminated intravascular coagulation. Blood 29:169, 1967.

218. Margaretten W, McKay DG: The role of platelet and leukocyte in disseminated intravascular coagulation caused by bacterial endotoxin. Thromb Diath Haemorrh [Suppl.] 36:151, 1969.

219. Margaretten W, McKay DG: The role of the platelet in the generalized Shwartzman reaction. J Exp Med 129:585, 1969.

220. Margaretten W, Zunker HO, McKay DG: Production of the generalized Shwartzman reaction in pregnant rats by intravenous infusion of thrombin. Lab Invest 13:552, 1964.

221. Markiewicz, A: Urokinase activity in acute renal failure. Pol Med J 10:54, 1971..

222. Matsumoto K, Dowling J, Atkins RC: Production of interleukin-1 in glomerular cell cultures from patients with rapidly progressive crescentric glomerulonephritis. Am J Nephrol 8:463, 1988.

223. Matsumoto K, Hatano M: Production of interleukin 1 in glomerular cell cultures from rats with nephrotoxic serum nephritis. Clin Exp Immunol 75:123, 1989.

224. McCluskey RT, Baldwin DS: Natural history of acute glomerulonephritis. Am J Med 35:213, 1963.

225. McGrath JM, Stewart GJ: The effect of endotoxin on vascular endothelium. J Exp Med 129:833, 1969.

226. McKay DG, Gitlin D, Craig JM: Immunochemical demonstration of fibrin in the generalized Shwartzman reaction. Arch Pathol 67:270, 1959.

227. McKay DG, Muller-Berghaus G, Cruse V: Activation of Hageman factor by ellagic acid and the generalized Shwartzman reaction. Am J Pathol 43:393, 1969.

228. McKenzi R, Pepper DS, Kay AB: The generation of chemotactic activity for human leukocytes by the action of plasmin on human fibrinogen. Thromb Res 6:1, 1975.

229. Mehls O, Andrassy K, Janti K, et al: Hemostasis and thromboembolism in children with nephrotic syndome: Differences from adults. J Pediatr 110:862, 1987.

230. Mergenhagen SE, Snyderman R, Gewurz H, et al: Significance of complement to the mechanism of action of endotoxin. Curr Top Microbiol Immunol 50:37, 1969.

231. Michael AF, Keane WF, Raij L, et al: The glomerular mesangium. Kidney Int 17:141, 1980.

232. Michielsen P, Roels L, Vanrenterghem Y, et al: Significance of urinary excretion of fibrin degradation products during treatment of glomerulonephritis. Clin Nephrol 5:106, 1976.

233. Miller K, Dresner IG, Michael AF: Localization of platelet antigens in human kidney disease. Kidney Int 18:472, 1980.

234. Min KW, Gyorkey F, Gyorkey P, et al: The morphogenesis of glomerular crescents in rapidly progressive glomerulonephritis. Kidney Int 5:47, 1974.

235. Moake JL, Byrnes JJ, Troll JH, et al: Abnormal VIII: von Willebrand factor patterns in the plasma of patients with the hemolytic-uremic syndrome. Blood 64:592, 1984.

236. Moake JL, Rudy CK, Troll JH, et al: Unusually large plasma factor VIII: von Willebrand factor multimers in chronic relapsing thrombotic thrombocytopenic purpura. N Engl J Med 307:1432, 1982.

237. Moncada S, Vane JR: Prostacyclin and blood coagulation. Drugs 21:430, 1981.

238. Monnens L, Van De Meer W, Langenhuysen C, et al: Platelet aggregating factor in the epidemic form of hemolytic-uremic syndrome in childhood. Clin Nephrol 24:135, 1985.

239. Moore KL, Esmon CT, Esmon NL: Tumor necrosis factor leads to internalization and degradation of thrombomodulin from the surface of bovine aortic endothelial cells in culture. Blood 73:159, 1989.

240. Morita T, Suzuki Y, Churg J: Structure and development of the glomerular crescent. Am J Pathol 72:349, 1973.

241. Moroz L: Inhibition of fibrinolytic activity of plasmin by suramin (antrypol) and trypan blue. Thromb Res 10:605, 1977.

242. Moroz LA, MacLean LD, Langleben D: Abnormalities in

the cellular phase of blood fibrinolytic activity in systemic lupus erythematosus and venous thromboembolism. *Thromb Res* 43:595, 1986.

243. Morrison DC, Ulevitch RJ: The effects of bacterial endotoxins on host mediation systems. *Am J Pathol* 93:527, 1978.

244. Muller-Berghaus G, Goldfinger D, Margaretten W, et al: Platelet factor 3 and the generalized Shwartzman reaction. *Thromb Diath Haemorrh* 18:726, 1967.

245. Muller-Berghaus G, Hocke M: Production of the generalized Shwartzman reaction in rabbits by Ancrod (Arvin) infusion and endotoxin injection. *Br J Haematol* 25:111, 1973.

246. Muller-Berghaus G, Kramer W: Effect of platelet antiserum on the precipitation of soluble fibrin by endotoxin. *Thromb Haemost* 35:237, 1976.

247. Muller-Berghaus G, Roka L, Lasch HG: Induction of glomerular microclot formation by fibrin monomer infusion. *Thromb Diath Haemorrh* 29:375, 1973.

248. Muller-Berghaus G, Schmidt-Ehry, B: The role of pregnancy in the induction of the generalized Shwartzman reaction. *Am J Obstet Gynecol* 114:847, 1972.

249. Muller-Berghaus G, Schneberger R: Hageman factor activation in the generalized Shwartzman induced by endotoxin. *Br J Haematol* 21:513, 1971.

250. Nagayama M, Zucker MB, Beller FK: Effects of a variety of endotoxins on human and rabbit platelet function. *Thromb Diath Haemorrh* 26:467, 1971.

251. Naish P, Evans DJ, Peters DK: Urinary fibrinogen derivative excretion and intraglomerular fibrin deposition in glomerulonephritis *Br Med J* 1:544, 1974.

252. Naish P, Penn GB, Evans DJ, et al: The effect of defibrination on nephrotoxic serum nephritis in rabbits. *Clin Sci* 42:643, 1972.

253. Naish P, Peters DK, Shackman R: Increased urinary fibrinogen derivatives after renal allotransplantation. *Lancet* 2:1280, 1973.

254. Naish PF, Evans DJ, Peters DK: The effects of defibrination with ancrod in experimental allergic glomerular injury. *Clin Exp Immunol* 20:303, 1975.

255. Nakamoto Y, Dohi K, Fujiike H, et al: Microangiographic evaluation of the effects of heparin on progressive Masugi nephritis. *Kidney Int* 13:297, 1978.

256. Nath KA: Platelet participation in renal diseases. *The Kidney* 20:1, 1987.

257. Neale TJ, Tipping PG, Carson SD, et al: Participation of cell-mediated immunity in deposition in fibrin in glomerulonephritis. *Lancet* 2:421, 1988.

258. Neill MA, Tarr PI, Clausen CR, et al: Escherichia coli 0157:H7 as the predominant pathogen associated with the hemolytic uremic syndome: A prospective study in the Pacific Northwest. *Pediatrics* 80:37, 1987.

259. Niemetz J: Coagulant activity of leukocytes. *J Clin Invest* 51:307, 1972.

260. Niemetz J, Marcus A: The stimulatory effect of platelets and platelet membranes on the procoagulant activity of leukocytes. *J Clin Invest* 54:1437, 1974.

261. Obrig TG, Del Vecchio PJ, Karmali MA, et al: Pathogenesis of haemolytic uraemic syndrome. *Lancet* 2:687, 1987.

262. Pai CH, Gordon R, Sims HV, et al: Sporadic cases of hemorrhagic colitis associated with *Escherichia coli* 0157:H7. *Ann Intern Med* 101:738, 1984.

263. Palmerio C, Ming SC, Frank E, et al: The role of the sympathetic nervous system in the generalized Shwartzman reaction. *J Exp Med* 115:609, 1962.

264. Panicucci F, Sagripanti A, Pinori E, et al: Comprehensive study of hemostasis in chronic uraemia. *Nephron* 33:5, 1983.

265. Parbtani A, Cameron JS: Platelet involvement in glomerulonephritis. In Remuzzi G, Mecca G, de Gaetano G (eds):

Hemostasis, Prostaglandins, and Renal Disease. New York, Raven Press, 1980, p 45.

266. Parbtani A, Frampton G, Cameron JS: Measurement of platelet release substances in glomerulonephritis: a comparison of beta-thromboglobulin (Beta-TG), platelet factor 4 (PF 4), and serotonin assays. *Thromb Res* 19:177, 1980.

267. Pareti FI, Capitanio A, Mannucci L, et al: Acquired dysfunction due to the circulation of "exhausted" platelets. *Am J Med* 69:235, 1980.

268. Philips M, Juul A, Thorsen S: Human endothelial cells produce a plasminogen activator inhibitor and a tissue-type plasminogen activator-inhibitor complex. *Biochim Biophys Acta* 802:99, 1984.

269. Pisciotta AV, Gottschall JL: Clinical features of thrombotic thrombocytopenic purpura. *Semin Thromb Hemost* 6:330, 1980.

270. Plow EF: The contribution of leukocyte proteases to fibrinolysis. *Blut* 53:1, 1986.

271. Plow EF, Collen D: The presence and release of alpha$_2$-antiplasmin from human platelets. *Blood* 58:1069, 1981.

272. Pollak VE, Dosekun AK: Evaluation of treatment in lupus nephritis: effects of prednisone. *Am J Kidney Dis* 2:170, 1982.

273. Pollak VE, Glueck HI, Weiss MA, et al: Defibrination with ancrod in glomerulonephritis: effects on clinical and histologic findings and on blood coagulation. *Am J Nephrol* 2:195, 1982.

274. Prydz H, Lyberg T, Deteix P, et al: In vitro stimulation of tissue thromboplastin (factor III) activity in human monocytes by immune complexes and lectins. *Thromb Res* 15:465, 1979.

275. Richardson SE, Karmali MA, Becker LE, et al: The histopathology of the hemolytic uremic syndrome associated with verocytotoxin-producing *Escherichia coli* infections. *Hum Pathol* 19:1102, 1988.

276. Raij L, Keane WF, Michael AF: Unilateral Shwartzman reaction: cortical necrosis in one kidney following in vivo perfusion with endotoxin. *Kidney Int* 12:91, 1977.

277. Ratnam S, March S, Ojah C, et al: Hemolytic-uremic syndrome associated with verotoxin-producing *Escherichia coli*. *Can Med Assoc J* 133:37, 1985.

278. Rehan A, Johnson KJ, Kunkel RG, et al: Role of oxygen radicals in phorbol myristate induced glomerular injury. *Kidney Int* 27:503, 1985.

279. Remuzzi G, Misiani R, Marchesi D, et al: Treatment of the hemolytic uremic syndrome with plasma. *Clin Nephrol* 12:279, 1979.

280. Rizzoni G, Claris-Appiani A, Edefonti A, et al: Plasma infusion for hemolytic-uremic syndrome in children: results of a multicenter controlled trial. *J Pediatr* 112:284, 1988.

281. Robert A, Olmer M, Sampol J, et al: Clinical correlation between hypercoagulability and thrombo-embolic phenomena. *Kidney Int* 31:830, 1987.

282. Rodriguez-Erdmann F: Studies on the pathogenesis of the generalized Shwartzman reaction. II. Role played by experimentally induced fibrinolysis. *Thromb Diath Haemorrh* 12:462, 1964.

283. Rosove MH, Ho WG, Goldfinger D: Ineffectiveness of aspirin and dipyridamole in the treatment of thrombotic thrombocytopenic purpura. *Ann Intern Med* 96:27, 1982.

284. Rubenstein HS, Fine J, Coons AH: Localization of endotoxin in the walls of the peripheral vascular system during lethal endotoxemia. *Proc Soc Exp Biol Med* 111:458, 1962.

285. Sakakibara K, Nagase M, Takada Y, et al: Relationship between urinary fibrinogen degradation products and various types of chronic nephritis. *Thromb Res* 45:403, 1987.

286. Salant DJ: Immunopathogenesis of crescentic glomerulonephritis and lung purpura. *Kidney Int* 32:408, 1987.
287. Scheinman J, Stiehm ER: Fibrinolytic studies in the nephrotic syndrome. *Pediatr Res* 5:206, 1971.
288. Schleef RR, Loskutoff DJ: Fibrinolytic system of vascular endothelial cells. *Haemostasis* 18:328, 1988.
289. Schorer AE, Kaplan ME, Rao GHR, et al: Interleukin-1 stimulates endothelial cell tissue factor production and expression by a prostaglandin-independent mechanism. *Thromb Haemost* 56:256, 1986.
290. Schorer AE, Rick PD, Swaim WR, et al: Structural features of endotoxin required for stimulation of endothelial cell tissue factor production: exposure of preformed tissue factor after oxidant-mediated endothelial cell injury. *J Lab Clin Med* 106:38, 1985.
291. Scott WL, Francis CW, Knutson DW, et al: Specific identification of urinary fibrinogen, fibrinogen degradation products, and cross-linked fibrin degradation products in renal diseases and after renal allotransplantation. *J Lab Clin Med* 107:534, 1986.
292. Semeraro N, Fumarola D, Mertens F, et al: Evidence that endotoxins enhance the factor X activator activity of washed human platelets. *Br J Haematol* 38:243, 1978.
293. Shah BC, Ambrus JL, Mink IB, et al: Fibrin degradation products in renal parenchymal disease states and renal transplant patients. *Transplantation* 14:705, 1972.
294. Shapiro SS, Mckay DG: The prevention of the generalized Shwartzman reaction with sodium warfarin. *J Exp Med* 107:377, 1958.
295. Sharma SD: Plasma fibrinolytic activity in chronic renal disease. *Indian Med Assoc J* 51:323, 1968.
296. Sharma SD, Chandler M: Fibrinolytic activity in acute renal failure. *Indian J Med Sci* 23:371, 1969.
297. Shepard KV, Bukowski RM: The treatment of thrombotic thrombocytopenic purpura with exchange transfusions, plasma infusions, and plasma exchange. *Semin Hematol* 24:178, 1987.
298. Sherman LA, Lee J: Specific binding of soluble fibrin to macrophages. *J Exp Med* 145:76, 1977.
299. Sheth KJ, Gill JC, Hanna J, et al: Failure of fresh frozen plasma infusions to alter the course of hemolytic uremic syndrome. *Child Nephrol Urol* 9:38, 1989.
300. Shibata S, Sakaguchi H, Nagasawa T: Exfoliation of endothelial cytoplasm in nephrotoxic serum nephritis. *Lab Invest* 38:201, 1978.
301. Siddiqui FA, Lian EC-Y: Novel platelet-agglutinating protein from a thrombotic thrombocytopenic purpura plasma. *J Clin Invest* 76:1330, 1985.
302. Silva FG, Hoyer JR, Pirani CL: Sequential studies of glomerular crescent formation in rats with antiglomerular basement membrane-induced glomerulonephritis and the role of coagulation factors. *Lab Invest* 51:404, 1984.
303. Sindrey M, Marshall TL, Naish P: Quantitative assessment of the effects of platelet depletion in the autologous phase of nephrotoxic serum nephritis. *Clin Exp Immunol* 36:90, 1979.
304. Smith RT, Thomas L, Good RA: Generalized Shwartzmann reaction. V. Intravenous injection of colloidal iron or carbon on response of rabbits to meningococcal toxin. *Proc Soc Exp Biol Med* 82:712, 1953.
305. Spaet TH, Gaynor E, Bouvier C: A vascular basis for the generalized Shwartzmann reaction. *Thromb Diath Haemorrh* [Suppl.] 45:157, 1971.
306. Spencer CD, Crane FM, Kumar JR, et al: Treatment of postpartum hemolytic uremic syndrome with plasma exchange. *JAMA* 247:2808, 1982.
307. Spika JS, Parsons JE, Nordenberg D, et al: Hemolytic uremic

308. Sraer JD, Delarue F, Dard S, et al: Glomerular fibrinolytic activity after thrombin perfusion in the rat. *Lab Invest* 32:515, 1975.
309. Stecher VJ, Sorkin E: The chemotactic activity of fibrin lysis products. *Int Arch Allergy Appl Immunol* 43:879, 1972.
310. Stern DM, Bank I, Nawroth PP, et al: Self-regulation of procoagulant events on the endothelial cell surface. *J Exp Med* 162:1223, 1985.
311. Stiehm ER, Kuplic LS, Uehling DT: Urinary fibrin split products in human renal disease. *J Lab Clin Med* 77:843, 1971.
312. Stiehm ER, Trygstad CW: Split products of fibrin in human renal disease. *Am J Med* 46:774, 1969.
313. Stuart MJ, Spitzer RE, Coppe D: Abnormal platelet and vascular prostaglandin synthesis in an infant with hemolytic uremic syndrome. *Pediatrics* 71:120, 1983.
314. Stuart MJ, Spitzer RE, Walenga RW, et al: Prostanoids in hemolytic uremic syndrome. *J Pediatr* 106:936, 1985.
315. Sueishi K, Nanno S, Tanaka K: Permeability enhancing and chemotactic activities of lower molecular weight degradation products of human fibrinogen. *Thromb Haemost* 45:90, 1981.
316. Sundsmo JS, Fair DS: Relationship among the complement, kinin, coagulation, and fibrinolytic systems. *Springer Semin Immunopathol* 6:231, 1983.
317. Suyama T, Matsumoto T, Hamano T, et al: Urokinase therapy of nephrotoxic nephritis (Masugi) in rabbits. In Tilsner V, Lenau H (eds): *Fibrinolysis and Urokinase—Serono Symposium No. 31.* London, Academic, 1980, p 405.
318. Szczepanski M, Lucer C: The influence of large doses of hydrocortisone on the generalized Shwartzman reaction in the rabbit. *Thromb Res* 8:71, 1976.
319. Szczepanski M, Lucer C, Staff-Zielinska E: Inhibitory effect of I.V. acetylsalicylic acid on the generalized Shwartzman reaction in the rabbit. *Thromb Res* 29:85, 1983.
320. Taira K, Matsunaga T, Kawahara S, et al: Fragments of urinary fibrin/fibrinogen degradation products and cross-linked fibrin degradation products in various renal diseases. *Thromb Res* 53:367, 1989.
321. Tannebaum SH, Rick ME, Shafer B, et al: Subendothelial matrix of cultured endothelial cells contains fully processed high molecular weight von Willebrand factor. *J Lab Clin Med* 113:372, 1989.
322. Thomas L, Good RA: Studies on the generalized Shwartzman reaction. I. General observations concerning the phenomenon. *J Exp Med* 96:605, 1952.
323. Thomas L, Good RA: The effect of cortisone on the Shwartzman reaction. *J Exp Med* 95:409, 1952.
324. Thomson C, Forbes CD, Prentice CRM, et al: Changes in blood coagulation and fibrinolysis in the nephrotic syndrome. *Q J Med* 43:399, 1974.
325. Thomson NM, Holdsworth SR, Glasgow EF, et al: The macrophage in the development of experimental crescentric glomerulonephritis. *Am J Pathol* 92:223, 1979.
326. Thomson NM, Moran J, Simpson IJ, et al: Defibrination with ancrod in nephrotoxic nephritis in rabbits. *Kidney Int* 10:343, 1976.
327. Thomson NM, Simpson IJ, Evans DJ, et al: Defibrination with ancrod in experimental chronic immune complex nephritis. *Clin Exp Immunol* 20:527, 1975.
328. Thomson NM, Simpson IJ, Peters DK: A quantitative evaluation of anticoagulants in experimental nephrotoxic nephritis. *Clin Exp Immunol* 19:301, 1975.
329. Thysell H, Oxelius V-A, Norlin M: Successful treatment of hemolytic uremic syndrome and thrombotic thrombocyto-

syndrome and diarrhea associated with *Escherichia coli* 0157:H7 in a day care center. *J Pediatr* 109:287, 1986.

penic purpura with fresh frozen plasma and plasma exchange. *Acta Med Scand* 212:285, 1982.

330. Tipping PG, Dowling JP, Holdsworth SR: Glomerular procoagulant activity in human proliferative glomerulonephritis. *J Clin Invest* 81:119, 1988.

331. Tipping PG, Holdsworth SR: Fibrinolytic therapy with streptokinase for established experimental glomerulonephritis. *Nephron* 43:258, 1986.

332. Tipping PG, Holdsworth SR: The participation of macrophages, glomerular procoagulant activity and factor VIII in glomerular fibrin deposition. *Am J Pathol* 124:10, 1986.

333. Tipping PG, Lowe MG, Holdsworth SR: Glomerular macrophages express augmented procoagulant activity in experimental fibrin-related glomerulonephritis in rabbits. *J Clin Invest* 82:1253, 1988.

334. Tipping PG, Worthington LA, Holdsworth SR: Quantitation and characterization of glomerular procoagulant activity in experimental glomerulonephritis. *Lab Invest* 56:155, 1987.

335. Tomura S, Ida T, Kuriyama R, et al: Activation of platelets in patients with chronic proliferative glomerulonephritis and the nephrotic syndrome. *Clin Nephrol* 17:24, 1982.

336. Ts'ao C-H: In vitro platelet reaction with isolated glomerular basement membrane. *Thromb Diath Haemorrh* 25:507, 1971.

337. Tsumagari T, Tanaka K: Effects of fibrinogen degradation products on glomerular mesangial cells in culture. *Kidney Int* 26:712, 1984.

338. Turi S, Beattie TJ, Belch JJF, et al: Disturbances of prostacyclin metabolism in children with hemolytic-uremic syndrome and in first degree relatives. *Clin Nephrol* 25:193, 1986.

339. Ueda N, Kawaguchi S, Niinomi Y, et al: Effect of corticosteroids on coagulation factors in children with nephrotic syndrome. *Pediatr Neprhol* 1:286, 1987.

340. Uttley WS: Serum levels of fibrin/fibrinogen degradation products in the haemolytic-uraemic syndrome. *Arch Dis Child* 45:587, 1970.

341. Uttley WS, Maxwell H, Cash JD: Fibrin/fibrinogen degradation products in children with renal disease. *Arch Dis Child* 49:137, 1974.

342. Vadanarayanan VV, Kaplan BS, Fong JSC: Neutrophil function in an experimental model of hemolytic uremic syndrome. *Pediatr Res* 21:252, 1987.

343. Van Ginkel CJW, Van Aken WG, Oh JIH, et al: Stimulation of monocyte procoagulant activity by adherence to different surfaces. *Br J Haematol* 37:35, 1977.

344. Van Hinsbergh VWM, Kooistra T, Van Den Berg EA, et al: Tumor necrosis factor increases the production of plasminogen activator inhibitor in human endothelial cells in vitro and in rats in vivo. *Blood* 72:1467, 1988.

345. Van Hulsteijn H, Van Es A, Bertina R, et al: Plasma beta-thromboglobulin and platelet factor 4 in renal failure. *Thromb Res* 24:175, 1981.

346. Vassali P, McCluskey RT: The pathogenic role of the coagulation process in rabbit Masugi nephritis. *Am J Pathol* 45:653, 1964.

347. Vassalli P, McCluskey RT: The pathogenic role of fibrin deposition in immunologically induced glomerulonephritis. *Ann NY Acad Sci* 116:1052, 1964.

348. Vassalli P, McCluskey RT: The pathogenic role of the co-

agulation process in glomerular diseases of immunological origin. *Adv Nephrol* 1:47, 1971.

349. Vaziri ND: Nephrotic syndrome and coagulation and fibrinolytic abnormalities. *Am J Nephrol* 3:1, 1983.

350. Vissers MCM, Fantone JC, Wiggins R, et al: Glomerular basement membrane-containing immune complexes stimulate tumor necrosis factor and interleukin-1 production by human monocytes. *Am J Pathol* 134:1, 1989.

351. Vreeken J, Boomgaard J, Deggeller K: Urokinase excretion in patients with renal diseases. *Acta Med Scand* 180:153, 1966.

352. Walter E, Deppermann D, Andrassy K, et al: Platelet hyperaggregability as a consequence of the nephrotic syndrome. *Thromb Res* 23:473, 1981.

353. Walters MDS, Levin M, Smith C, et al: Intravascular platelet activation in the hemolytic-uremic syndrome. *Kidney Int* 33:107, 1988.

354. Wardle EN, Menon IS, Rastogi SP: Study of proteins and fibrinolysis in patients with glomerulonephritis. *Br Med J* 2:260, 1970.

355. Watanabe T, Tanaka K: The role of coagulation and fibrinolysis in the development of rabbit Masugi nephritis. *Acta Pathol Jpn* 26:147, 1976.

356. Watanabe T, Tanaka K: Electron microscopic observations of the kidney in the generalized Shwartzman reaction. *Virchow's Arch [A]* 374:183, 1977.

357. Watanabe T, Tanaka K: Influence of fibrin, fibrinogen and fibrinogen degradation products on cultured endothelial cells. *Atherosclerosis* 48:57, 1983.

358. Weiss HJ, Turitto VT, Baumgartner HR, et al: Evidence for the presence of tissue factor activity on subendothelium. *Blood* 73:968, 1989.

359. Whitworth JA, Fairley KF, McIvor MA, et al: Urinary fibrin-degradation products and the site of urinary infection. *Lancet* 1:234, 1973.

360. Wiggins RC, Glatfelter A, Brukman J: Procoagulant activity in glomeruli and urine of rabbits with nephrotoxic nephritis. *Lab Invest* 53:156, 1985.

361. Wong TC: A study on the generalized Shwartzman in pregnant rats induced by bacterial endotoxin. *Am J Obstet Gynecol* 84:786, 1962.

362. Woo KT, Junor BJR, Salem H, et al: Beta-thromboglobulin and platelet aggregates in glomerulonephritis. *Clin Nephrol* 14:92, 1980.

363. Woo KT, Tan YO, Yap HK, et al: Beta-thromboglobulin in mesangial IgA nephritis. *Thromb Res* 24:259, 1981.

364. Wu KK, Hall ER, Rossi EC, et al: Serum prostacyclin binding defects in thrombotic thrombocytopenic purpura. *J Clin Invest* 75:168, 1985.

365. Wu V-Y, Cohen MP: Platelet factor 4 binding to glomerular microvascular matrix. *Biochim Biophys Acta* 797:76, 1984.

366. Wunschmann-Henderson B, Astrup T: Plasminogen activator production in organ cultures inhibited by cortisone. *Fed Proc* 32:313, 1973.

367. Yoshioka K, Takemura T, Akano N, et al: Cellular and non-cellular composition of crescents in human glomerulonephritis. *Kidney Int* 32:284, 1987.

368. Zahavi J, Kakkar VV: Beta-thromboglobulin—a specific marker of in-vivo platelet release reaction. *Thromb Haemost* 44:23, 1980.

Robin S. Goldstein
Jerry B. Hook

15
Biochemical Mechanisms of Nephrotoxicity

Mechanisms of Nephrotoxicity

The mechanisms by which chemicals produce toxicity are numerous and complex. Nephrotoxicity may result from either a cytotoxic lesion produced directly by a toxicant or an ischemic lesion mediated through circulatory disturbances. The first half of this chapter focuses on the general mechanisms of nephrotoxicity, the second half on the prerenal and intrarenal factors controlling the incidence and severity of chemically induced nephrotoxicity in the neonate and child.

Unique Susceptibility of the Kidney to Chemical Injury

Compared with other organs, the kidney is uniquely susceptible to chemical toxicity, partly because of its disproportionately high blood flow (25% of cardiac output). Thus, any blood-borne chemical will be delivered to the kidneys in significant amounts, resulting in increased exposure relative to that of most other organs. In addition, the unique anatomic and physiologic features of this multitubular organ predispose it to injury localized to specific cell types, e.g., in the proximal tubule [69]. This action may be a simple consequence of normal physiologic function. Potential toxicants can accumulate in high intracellular concentrations following their active transport by mechanisms unique to the proximal tubule (such as active secretion or reabsorption). Furthermore, most water reabsorption occurs in the proximal tubule, and changes brought about by concentrating a chemical within the tubular lumen would be expected to produce effects first at that site. There also appear to be differences in susceptibility to toxicity among the cell types within the proximal tubule. For example, the proximal convolution is the primary site of damage following exposure to chromium [6], whereas the pars recta is specifically affected by cisplatin [21].

The susceptibility of the renal medulla to toxicants may be related to a combination of its low blood flow and its countercurrent concentrating mechanism [33]. Chemicals that do reach this area may be trapped in the medulla, resulting in relatively high concentrations.

Biochemical Mechanisms of Toxicity

A significant advance in toxicology was made with the recognition that the offending (nephrotoxic) molecule may be a metabolite rather than the parent compound. On this basis, three different metabolic pathways are thought to mediate chemically induced renal damage:

1. the parent compound enters the renal cell and interferes directly with cellular function,
2. it enters the renal cell and is metabolized to a more reactive toxicant, and
3. an extrarenal metabolite damages the kidney either directly or following further intrarenal metabolism [70] (Fig. 15-1).

Once within the cell, a toxicant produces damage by disrupting essential metabolic and biochemical functions, viz., mitochondrial respiration, membrane transport and integrity, calcium flux, nuclear DNA metabolism, etc. Thus, the nephrotoxic potential of a chemical or drug is largely dependent on its ability to interfere with normal cellular function, which in turn may be influenced by (1) its metabolism to a reactive toxicant, (2) its reactivity with essential cellular constituents, and (3) the detoxification and repair capacity of the affected cellular constituents.

METABOLISM

The biotransformation of relatively inert chemicals to highly reactive metabolites, a phenomenon commonly termed "*metabolic activation*," is now recognized to be a primary event mediating the toxicity of many industrial, environmental, and therapeutic chemicals. Reactive metabolites and intermediates are generally electrophilic; i.e., they contain a single unpaired electron and seek out and react with electron-rich molecules (nucleophiles). Thus, reactive metabolites are chemically unstable and short-

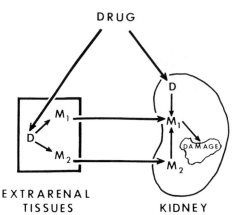

DRUG

EXTRARENAL
TISSUES   KIDNEY

Fig. 15-1. *Metabolic pathways mediating nephrotoxicity.* D_1, *parent drug;* M_1, *metabolite 1;* M_2, *metabolite 2.*

lived, and they potentially impair cellular function by reacting with cellular macromolecules.

The enzymes catalyzing the metabolic activation of xenobiotics often include the same family of enzymes responsible for detoxification, the cytochrome P-450-dependent mixed function oxidases (MFOs) [28]. The MFOs are localized in the endoplasmic reticulum of mammalian cells and catalyze the so-called phase I reactions of xenobiotic metabolism—those that include oxidation (removal of an electron), reduction (addition of an electron), and hydrolysis to produce more water-soluble and readily excreted metabolites [88]. Phase II metabolism, characterized by conjugation reactions, also results in the production of more water-soluble and excretable derivatives [88].

Although both phase I and II reactions are generally considered detoxification pathways, it appears that either type of reaction may contribute to the production of metabolites more cytotoxic than the parent compound. For example, the toxicities of many carcinogens are known to require oxidative metabolism to produce cellular damage, e.g., the polycyclic aromatic hydrocarbons [75], aromatic amines and aflatoxin [55]; industrial solvents, such as chloroform and carbon tetrachloride [65]; and drugs, such as acetaminophen [57]. Similarly, products of phase II reactions, such as sulfate, glucuronide, and glutathione conjugates, have been implicated in the toxicity of N-hydroxy-2-acetylaminofluorene (2-AAF), 1,2-dichloroethane, and hexachloro-1:3-butadiene [56,90].

Drug-metabolizing enzymes, including MFOs, have been identified in the kidney. Unlike MFO activity in the liver, renal MFOs are not uniformly distributed, but exhibit a corticopapillary gradient, with highest activity in the cortex [93]. Furthermore, MFOs within the cortex are not distributed equally among the different cell types; renal MFO activities and cytochrome P-450 concentrations appear to be located primarily in the S2 and S3 cells of the proximal tubule. For example, administration of 2,3,7,8 tetrachlorodibenzo-p-dioxin, an inducer of renal MFO activity, results in proliferation of smooth endoplasmic reticulum localized specifically in the S3 cells of rat kidneys

[25]. In untreated rabbit kidneys, cytochrome P-450 enzymes have been identified in both the S2 and S3 cells [20]. Thus, although renal MFO activity is quantitatively less than that of liver [27,50], the kidney may possess a higher specific enzymatic activity that is localized to the S2 and S3 cells. In addition to MFOs, other drug-metabolizing enzymes have been identified in the kidney, including prostaglandin endoperoxide synthetase, glutathione (GSH)-S-transferase, γ-glutamyltranspeptidase, aminopeptidase, N-acetyltransferase, sulfotransferase, and uridine diphosphate glucuronyltransferase [29,70].

The relationship between intrarenal metabolic activation and nephrotoxicity is best illustrated by chloroform, a common organic solvent capable of producing hepatic and renal injury in humans and experimental animals. The magnitude of chloroform nephrotoxicity varies with species, strain, and sex [14,17,23]. For example, chloroform produces both hepatic and renal necrosis in male mice, but only hepatic necrosis in female mice [17,23].

The concept that chloroform nephrotoxicity is mediated by a metabolite generated in the kidney is based on in vitro studies. Incubation with chloroform of renal cortical slices from male, but not female, mice results in a dose-related decrease in the accumulation of p-aminohippurate and tetraethylammonium [78]. This effect is blocked by carbon monoxide and cold exposure [76]. Furthermore, ^{14}C-CHCl$_3$ is metabolized by renal cortical microsomes from male mice and rabbits to a nephrotoxic metabolite, phosgene [3,11], and nephrotoxicity is enhanced in rabbits pretreated with an inducer of cytochrome P-450, phenobarbital [3]. Renal metabolism of chloroform requires oxygen and a nicotinamide-adenine dinucleotide phosphate (NADPH)-regenerating system, is dependent on incubation time, microsomal protein concentration, and substrate concentration, and is inhibited by carbon monoxide [76]. These data collectively indicate that renal metabolism is critical to the development of chloroform nephrotoxicity.

REACTIVITY WITH MACROMOLECULES

The exact initiating events and pathways leading to chemically induced cell injury are not well understood. However, at least two broad chemical reactions underlying toxicity have been proposed: covalent (alkylation or arylation) and peroxidative.

Covalent Reactions

The covalent binding of reactive intermediates to cellular macromolecules may disrupt normal cellular function and eventually cause cell damage or death. Alkylation or arylation of essential macromolecules may result from the reactions of electrophilic (electron-seeking) chemicals with the electron-rich atoms (nitrogen, oxygen, sulfur) of proteins, nucleic acids, and lipids to form more stable configurations through covalent bonds [55]. Thus, chemicals such as the nitrosoureas may react at critical sites within DNA to form adducts, which, if not excised and repaired, result in genotoxicity. In general, the extent of macromolecular covalent binding correlates with the degree of cell injury. However, macromolecular covalent binding per se does not necessarily induce cytotoxicity because sub-

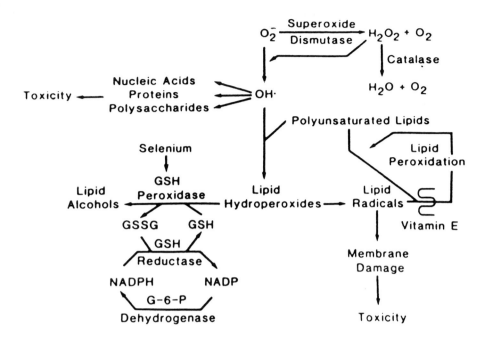

Fig. 15-2. *Biochemical defense mechanisms against activated oxygen toxicity. (From Bus JS, Gibson JE: Role of activated oxygen in chemical toxicity. In Mitchell JR, Horning MG [eds]: Drug Metabolism and Drug Toxicity. New York, Raven Press, 1984; with permission.)*

stantial covalent binding to tissue protein is not always accompanied by tissue necrosis [58].

Lipid Peroxidation

Another mechanism by which a chemical may produce damage is lipid peroxidation, a phenomenon characterized by the oxidative deterioration of polyunsaturated lipids. The initiation of lipid peroxidation in biologic tissues is mediated by singlet oxygen (a higher energy state of oxygen), hydroxy radicals, and other free radicals. Molecular oxygen is relatively inert; thus, metabolic activation is usually required for the mediation of peroxidative damage. Lipid peroxidation results from the reaction of singlet oxygen and free radicals with polyunsaturated lipids to form lipid free radicals and semistable hydroperoxides, which then promote free radical chain oxidations (Fig. 15-2). Unsaturated lipids are particularly susceptible to peroxidation, since the presence of a double bond weakens the adjacent carbon-hydrogen bond, facilitating abstraction of the hydrogen atom by initiators or free radicals. If unchecked, lipid peroxidation may destroy membrane architecture and degrade membrane bound enzymes.

Lipid peroxidation may play a role in the nephrotoxicity of certain chemicals. For example, administration of mercuric chloride [91] or cephaloridine [49] to rats increases the renal cortical concentration of conjugated dienes (products of lipid peroxidation). Similarly, in vitro exposure of renal cortical microsomes to mercuric chloride or

cephaloridine increases the formation of lipid peroxides, suggesting that lipid peroxidation contributes to or mediates the nephrotoxicity of these chemicals.

DEFENSE MECHANISMS

In the course of evolution, the mammalian cell has evolved several defense mechanisms against the harmful effects of reactive chemicals. Thus, intracellular accumulation of a toxicant does not necessarily result in cellular damage. For example, there are several mechanisms of antioxidant protection against lipid peroxidation. The first line of defense involves the destruction or interception of reactive oxygen radicals before their interaction with membrane lipids. This may be accomplished enzymatically by superoxide dismutase and catalase (see Fig. 15-2). If oxidants should be formed, a second line of defense involves the scavenging of free radicals by antioxidants. Two types of antioxidants function in vivo: water-soluble antioxidants (ascorbic acid and reduced glutathione) and lipid-soluble antioxidants (vitamin E and vitamin A). In general, antioxidants function by allowing a hydrogen to be abstracted from themselves rather than from the allylic hydrogen of unsaturated fatty acids. If lipid peroxidation is initiated despite these protective mechanisms, lipid hydroperoxides may be detoxified to lipid alcohols through enzymatic reduction by glutathione peroxidase (see Fig. 15-2).

In addition to playing a critical role in the detoxification of reactive oxygen intermediates, glutathione is also important to the detoxification of electrophiles. Glutathione acts as a strong nucleophile capable of reacting with electrophiles to yield glutathione conjugates. Glutathione is a polar molecule, conferring polarity to lipophilic xenobiotics and reducing the affinity of the xenobiotic with the lipid phase of cell membranes. The importance of glutathione in detoxification is strongly suggested by its universal occurrence in nature at relatively high concentrations (0.5–10 mM in mammalian cells) and its intracellular depletion following toxic insult [54].

The enzymatic activity of epoxide hydratase is also an important mechanism of detoxification. Metabolism of aromatic and olefinic compounds by cytochrome P-450 may result in the production of the corresponding epoxides, which are generally unstable and quite reactive. Epoxide hydratase catalyzes the conversion of these epoxides to the corresponding transdihydrodiol. Thus, epoxide hydratase plays an important role in the detoxification of reactive epoxides.

Finally, if interception or destruction of reactive molecules fails, the cell has evolved an exquisitely complex set of intracellular repair mechanisms that function primarily to restore the molecular integrity of DNA. The major repair mechanism operating before DNA replication is excision repair, a phenomenon involving the physical removal and replacement of the offending DNA adduct. This repair mechanism is thought to comprise a complex series of reactions, involving enzymes with varying degrees of specificity for certain types of DNA damage. Generally, the following processes are involved:

1. an endonuclease recognizes the lesion and introduces nick or break in a single strand,
2. an exonuclease excises the lesion as part of an oligonucleotide,
3. DNA replication is catalyzed by DNA polymerase, which inserts nucleotides complimentary to the opposite strand, and
4. DNA ligase covalently binds newly synthesized DNA with the nascent chain, yielding a repaired DNA molecule [68]. In this way, the ability of cells to excise and repair DNA adducts is important in protecting the DNA molecule from mutations.

Determinants of Nephrotoxic Potential

Balance Between Bioactivation and Detoxification

The induction and expression of chemically induced toxicity is ultimately dependent on the rates of reactions involved in both bioactivation and detoxification. For example, the chemically reactive hepatotoxic metabolites of acetaminophen are normal metabolic intermediates formed after the administration of nontoxic doses [39]. Appreciable macromolecular covalent binding of acetaminophen-related material occurs when the formation of reactive intermediates exceeds the capacity for conjugation with glutathione [66]. Similarly, bromobenzene hepatotoxicity

is thought to occur only when the production of toxic metabolites saturates the capacity for detoxification [38]. Thus, hepatotoxicity following acetaminophen or bromobenzene administration may be potentiated by inducing activation pathways, i.e., increase of cytochrome P-450-dependent MFOs, or by decreasing detoxification mechanisms, i.e., depletion of endogenous glutathione.

The balance between bioactivation and detoxification depends on intracellular enzymatic activity, which, in turn, is regulated by intracellular concentrations of substrates and cofactors. For example, the MFO system is multienzymatic in nature and is dependent on a continuous supply of reduced cofactor, NADPH [60]. Thus, MFO activity is intimately related to other cellular events involved in the generation of NADPH, i.e., activity of the pentosephosphate shunt [82]. Competition reactions for substrates and cofactors may therefore play a major role in determining the availability of NADPH for mixed function oxidation. Similarly, glucuronidation is dependent on the intracellular supply of substrate, uridine diphosphate glucuronic acid (UDPGA), and on the NAD+/NADH redox state. Since glucuronic acid is derived from glycogen and glucose, a major regulating factor for glucuronidation is the carbohydrate reserve. Thus, different nutritional and endocrine states that influence carbohydrate stores may affect intracellular UPDGA concentrations, the rate of glucuronidation, and possibly the balance between bioactivation and detoxification [67,82].

Prerenal Versus Intrarenal Factors

From the foregoing discussion, it is quite apparent that the susceptibility of the kidney to cellular injury is influenced by both prerenal and intrarenal events. Prerenal factors, such as absorption, distribution, hepatic xenobiotic metabolism, and protein binding, may profoundly affect the exposure of the kidney to potential toxicants.

Intrarenal mechanisms mediating chemically induced nephrotoxicity include the (1) delivery of a chemical to the kidney, i.e., glomerular filtration rate and renal plasma flow; (2) intracellular accumulation, i.e., active tubular secretion and reabsorption; (3) xenobiotic metabolism; and (4) concentrating mechanisms, i.e., countercurrent mechanisms. The contribution of prerenal and intrarenal events to chemically induced nephrotoxicity in the neonate and child are discussed in the following section.

Nephrotoxicity in the Neonate and Child

Prerenal Factors Influencing Nephrotoxicity

ABSORPTION

The delivery of a toxicant to the kidney is dependent on its systemic absorption following administration or exposure. Orally administered xenobiotics are absorbed via the same mechanisms that function in nutrient absorption: active transport, passive diffusion, pinocytosis, and lymphatic absorption. The major route of intestinal absorption in adults is passive diffusion, a process greatly influenced by the lipid solubility and ionization of unabsorbed chemicals.

Intestinal absorption of intact macromolecules, such as proteins and immunoglobulins, occurs only to a limited extent in adults. In neonates, however, intestinal absorption of intact macromolecules through pinocytosis is significant and may relate to the limited proteolytic enzyme activity of the immature GI tract [31]. Thus, any xenobiotic that is a macromolecule or can bind to dietary proteins may be absorbed readily through pinocytosis in the neonatal intestine. This route may be particularly important to the absorption of heavy metals in neonates.

Several ingested heavy metals, including cadmium, lead, and mercury, are known to be absorbed and retained more readily by young, immature animals than by adults [26,47,52]. Metabolic studies indicate that healthy male adults absorb only 10% of ingested lead, whereas healthy children (3 months to 8 years) absorb approximately 50% of ingested lead [1,42]. This enhanced absorption of lead in children may be a critical factor contributing to the increased incidence of acute lead nephropathy in children. Furthermore, these results are consistent with those of animal studies indicating enhanced GI absorption, retention, and toxicity of lead in suckling rats [47].

A higher intestinal absorption of several other cations in young animals has also been noted, e.g., cadmium, manganese, plutonium, and palladium. The milk diet of suckling animals appears to play an important role in the enhanced absorption of metals, inasmuch as feeding adult rats a milk diet increases metal absorption [47]. The mechanism by which milk enhances metal absorption is uncertain, although it may relate to binding of metals to milk proteins (and subsequent uptake by pinocytosis) or trace element deficiency in milk (and decreased competition for common mechanisms of absorption). Although intestinal absorption of metals is increased in the young, absorption of other chemicals or drugs may be less than or equal to that of adults.

DISTRIBUTION

Once absorbed, the delivery of a toxicant to the kidney is dependent on its pattern of distribution. Certain physiologic parameters, such as cardiac output and regional blood flow, and physicochemical properties of the toxicant, i.e., the ability to penetrate the cell membrane, are critical determinants of distribution. The latter is determined by the molecular size, lipid/water partition coefficient, and ionization constant of the toxicant, as well as by the extent to which it is protein bound. In general, cell membranes are relatively impermeable to water-soluble and strongly ionized molecules, although smaller molecules may diffuse through aqueous channels and pores.

The apparent volume of distribution is used to estimate the distribution of xenobiotic to certain major compartments of the body, e.g., total body water, extracellular fluid and plasma, and is defined as

$$Vd = Q/c$$

where Vd = apparent volume of distribution
  Q = total amount of chemical in body
  c = concentration of chemical in plasma

Toxicants may be sequestered or accumulated in tissue in higher concentrations than can be accounted for by diffusion equilibrium, a phenomenon that may be due to binding, active transport, or partitioning of the chemical into body fat. Such a phenomenon is characterized by an apparent volume of distribution that exceeds total body water or body weight, since the concentration of toxicant in the plasma is small compared with the total amount in the body. Although sequestration by fat and plasma proteins may serve as a protective mechanism by limiting access of the toxicant to the target organ, the chemical may be mobilized and released into the circulation following (1) excretion of the free chemical or (2) mobilization of stored fat for energy.

In infants, the apparent Vd for most xenobiotics tends to be higher in the newborn than in children or adults [61] and may limit renal exposure to toxicants. This age-related effect may be attributed, in part, to the neonate's increased total body water and extracellular fluid volume, both of which result in increased dilution of drug. On the other hand, the fractional plasma protein binding of xenobiotics is generally lower in infants than adults [61] and may result in increased delivery of the freely filterable toxicant to renal epithelium. For example, pharmacokinetic studies of gentamicin in children indicate a lower peak serum concentration, an increased half-life, and a correspondingly high Vd of gentamicin compared with those values in adults [22,74,92]. Since gentamicin is not significantly protein bound, it is unlikely that the renal epithelium of children is exposed to increased quantities of freely filterable drug. Rather, a decreased incidence of gentamicin nephrotoxicity in the young has been observed [13,51,81] and may be attributed to the immaturity of intrarenal mechanisms mediating gentamicin nephrotoxicity.

HEPATIC XENOBIOTIC METABOLISM

Hepatic metabolism of xenobiotics may be critical to the bioactivation and detoxification of nephrotoxicants. In general, both phase I and II relations of hepatic xenobiotic metabolism in laboratory animals are undetectable before birth and develop rapidly thereafter, reaching activities comparable with or greater than those of the adult within three to eight weeks of age [48,73]. Developmental patterns of MFO activities vary considerably with species, strain, sex, and metabolic substrate [37,46,48,59,73].

Human neonates exhibit a low overall hepatic monooxygenase activity, as indicated by decreased urinary metabolite concentrations of administered drugs (e.g., diphenylhydantoin, phenobarbital, caffeine, meperidine, chlorpromazine) [62]. In contrast, children two to eight years of age exhibit approximately twice the capacity of adults to metabolize antipyrene and phenylbutazone [2].

The hepatic microsomal metabolizing system of both immature and mature animals can be stimulated by pretreatment with chemicals that act as enzyme inducers. Young, rapidly growing animals are more sensitive to inducers of hepatic cytochrome P-450 than are adults. For example, induction of cytochrome P-450 by phenobarbital is maximal at 12 days of age in the rat and declines with age [5].

A similar phenomenon has been suggested to occur in

humans [87]. The toxicologic consequences of this enhanced induction of hepatic drug-metabolizing enzymes in the young may be profound and is ultimately dependent on the resulting balance between bioactivation and detoxification.

Intrarenal Factors Influencing Nephrotoxicity

The rates of renal elimination may be critical determinants in the half-life and total body retention of xenobiotics and are dependent on both extrarenal (protein binding, Vd, hepatic metabolism) and intrarenal factors. Although the increased Vd and decreased hepatic metabolism in the young would favor greater total body retention of a xenobiotic, decreased incidence and severity of chemically induced nephrotoxicity in neonates and children has been observed. This decreased susceptibility to nephrotoxicity in the young is attributable in part to the immaturity of those renal functions that normally render the adult kidney vulnerable to chemical toxicity. These underdeveloped functions include glomerular filtration, renal plasma flow, tubular transport, and concentrating ability, all of which are critical to the delivery, uptake, and concentration of toxicants in the renal epithelium.

ORGANIC ANION TRANSPORT (CEPHALORIDINE)

Cephaloridine, a broad-spectrum cephalosporin antibiotic, is a zwitterion and is actively transported by the renal organic anion system [12,83–87]. Although cephaloridine is actively accumulated within the proximal tubular cells in a manner similar to that of para-aminohippurate (PAH), it is not secreted into the tubular urine [12]. Consequently, high intracellular concentrations of cephaloridine are attained and appear to be critical to the development of nephrotoxicity, which is characterized by acute proximal tubular necrosis [84]. Several studies have indicated that inhibitors of the renal organic anion system, such as probenecid and PAH, significantly inhibit the renal cortical accumulation and nephrotoxicity of cephaloridine [83,86]. Furthermore, studies using a variety of different animal species have demonstrated a positive correlation between renal cortical accumulation of cephaloridine and nephrotoxicity; both uptake and nephrotoxicity of cephaloridine are greatest in the rabbit, intermediate in the guinea pig, and least in the rat and mouse [84]. These studies collectively indicate that transport of cephaloridine by organic anion transport pathways is requisite to the development of cephaloridine nephrotoxicity.

Renal organic anion transport is immature in human and other mammalian neonates, including rabbits and rats [32,34,43]. In laboratory animals, the in vitro accumulation of PAH in renal cortical slices is low at birth, increases rapidly to a peak at 4 weeks of age, and declines to an intermediate value in adulthood. Furthermore, treatment of young rats, rabbits, and dogs with substrates of organic anion transport (penicillin, PAH) enhances PAH accumulation by renal cortical slices [32]. This substrate stimulation occurs without any change in organic cation transport or in tissue ultrastructure. Substrate stimulation by

penicillin also enhances the extraction of PAH by the kidneys of newborn puppies [10].

Since organic anion transport is incompletely developed at birth, low intracellular accumulation of nephrotoxicants that are dependent on organic anion transport for renal uptake would be expected in newborns. Wold and coworkers tested this hypothesis by relating the maturation of the renal organic anionic transport system to cephaloridine nephrotoxicity. In these studies, cephaloridine produced a dose-related nephrotoxicity in adult and 30-day-old rabbits, but not in 5-day-old animals [89]. The increased susceptibility to cephaloridine nephrotoxicity with age paralleled maturation of the renal anionic transport system (Fig. 15-3). Furthermore, stimulation of this transport system by pretreatment with substrates of organic anion transport (e.g., PAH or penicillin) enhanced cephaloridine nephrotoxicity [89]. These results strongly indicate that cephaloridine nephrotoxicity is dependent on a fully functional anionic transport system for proximal tubular transport and subsequent intracellular accumulation. Thus, the absence of cephaloridine nephrotoxicity in the newborn results from immaturity of the organic anionic transport system.

GLOMERULAR FILTRATION AND RENAL BLOOD FLOW (AMINOGLYCOSIDES)

Aminoglycoside-induced nephrotoxicity is characterized by tubular necrosis of the convoluted and straight portions of the proximal tubule in both laboratory animals and humans. Ultrastructural studies have indicated that aminoglycoside treatment results in an increased number and size of secondary lysosomes, a decreased height and number of microvilli of brush border membranes, mitochondrial swelling, cytoplasmic vacuolization, and dilatation of the cisternae of rough endoplasmic reticulum [36]. Aminoglycosides accumulate within the renal cortex of laboratory animals and humans [4,35], and it is generally thought that the renal cortical accumulation of aminoglycoside, like that of cephaloridine, is intimately related to its nephrotoxicity. Indeed, for any given aminoglycoside, the incidence and severity of nephrotoxicity is directly related to its renal cortical concentration. For example, netilmicin is accumulated in the renal cortex at a concentration less than that of gentamicin [63], and the nephrotoxic potential of netilmicin is consequently significantly less than that of gentamicin [80].

The renal uptake of aminoglycosides is initially mediated by the binding of aminoglycosides to acidic phospholipid sites on the brush border membrane [71]. Furthermore, the extent of renal uptake correlates positively with the number of free amino groups on the aminoglycoside molecule [80]. Thus, binding between the aminoglycosides and membrane phospholipids is mediated by a charge interaction between the polybasic cationic aminoglycosides and the acidic anionic phospholipids. Following filtration and binding to the brush border membrane, the aminoglycosides are taken up by the cell through pinocytosis and are subsequently sequestered by lysosomes.

In contrast to the incidence of aminoglycoside nephrotoxicity in adults, which approximates 3% to 4% percent

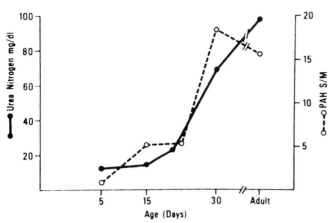

FIG. 15-3. *Relationship between maturation of PAH transport in untreated rabbits and susceptibility to cephaloridine nephrotoxicity. Treated rabbits were administered 900 mg/kg cephaloridine and BUN determined 48 hours later. (From Wold JS, Joost RR, Owen NV: Nephrotoxicity of cephaloridine in newborn rabbits: Role of the renal organic anion transport system. J Pharmacol Exp Ther 201:778, 1977; with permission.)*

[40], gentamicin nephrotoxicity in neonates and infants is rare. It has been suggested that these age-related differences in susceptibility relate to differences in the pharmacokinetics of gentamicin. Gentamicin readily distributes into the vascular compartment, resulting in distinct age-related differences in the apparent Vd; Vd is 40% to 60% of total body weight in newborns and decreases to 20% to 30% in infancy and early childhood [9]. Furthermore, the serum half-life of gentamicin averages 4 to 6 hours in newborns, decreasing to 1.4 to 2.0 hours in infants and children [9]. Since glomerular filtration rate in newborns is one-quarter of that of healthy adults, age-related changes in the serum half-life of gentamicin may reflect changes in both Vd and renal maturation. These results suggest that decreased glomerular filtration and, hence, decreased renal exposure and uptake of gentamicin may contribute to the decreased nephrotoxicity in the young.

Age-related susceptibility to aminoglycoside nephrotoxicity has also been reported in young rats, rabbits, and dogs [13,16,51]. Marre and coworkers attributed decreased nephrotoxicity to an inability of the immature renal cortex to accumulate gentamicin following treatment [51]. Supporting this concept, Cowan et al. detected less gentamicin in kidneys of treated puppies compared with adults [16]. Furthermore, the intrarenal distribution of gentamicin was affected by age, i.e., the ratio of gentamicin concentration (μg/g) in the outer/inner cortex averaged 0.67 in 10-day-old puppies and 2.84 in 30-day-old puppies [16] (Table 15-1). In newborn animals, nephrons in the juxtamedullary cortex received a major fraction of renal blood flow and manifested gentamicin toxicity earlier than did nephrons in the outer cortex; 10-day-old treated puppies exhibited an increased number and size of lysosomes in the juxtamedullary, but not the outer, cortex [16]. In contrast, 30-day-old puppy kidneys exhibited degeneration of tubular

epithelium of both the juxtamedullary and outer cortices. Since renal accumulation of gentamicin involves brush border uptake of filtered gentamicin, little if any accumulation would be expected in immature nonfiltering nephrons of the outer cortex of the neonatal kidney. Thus, the relative absence of gentamicin nephrotoxicity in the neonatal puppy may be attributed to the distribution of renal blood flow to the juxtamedullary nephrons at birth, a phenomenon that spares nonfiltering superficial nephrons from gentamicin accumulation and toxicity.

XENOBIOTIC METABOLISM (CHLOROFORM)

As previously indicated, the incidence and severity of chloroform ($CHCl_3$) nephrotoxicity in laboratory animals varies with species, strain, age, and sex; the last two variables are probably intimately related. For example, adult male mice, but not prepubertal (<27 days old) or castrated male mice, are susceptibile to $CHCl_3$ nephrotoxicity [17]. Furthermore, female mice and immature or castrated male mice treated with testosterone exhibit $CHCl_3$ nephrotoxicity comparable in severity with that of adult male mice [17].

Sex differences in susceptibility to $CHCl_3$ nephrotoxicity in mice are accompanied by similar sex differences in intrarenal metabolism of $CHCl_3$, suggesting a relationship between metabolism and toxicity [76,77]. Furthermore, the susceptibility of male and female mice to $CHCl_3$ nephrotoxicity appears to be related to differences in renal cytochrome P-450 concentrations and MFO activities [79]. Cytochrome P-450 concentrations and MFO activities are markedly lower in female than male mice and can be induced by testosterone and diminished by castration [79]. These data strongly suggest that the age-related differences (prepubertal versus adult male) in susceptibility to $CHCl_3$ nephrotoxicity in mice are mediated by androgen-dependent effects on renal drug-metabolizing enzymes.

MISCELLANEOUS (HEAVY METALS)

In mature animals, mercuric chloride treatment produces a dose-related nephrotoxicity characterized by selective injury to the proximal tubule, particularly to the pars recta [24,30,44]. Functional correlates of mercuric chloride nephrotoxicity include abnormalities in tubular transport (glycosuria, aminoaciduria), enzymuria, polyuria, anuria, and increased BUN and serum creatinine concentrations [53]. Ultrastructural abnormalities are characterized by loss of brush border, dispersion of ribosomes, cytoplasmic vacuolization, increased number and size of lysosomes, and mitochondrial swelling [24]. The fully developed lesion in both experimental animals and humans is often associated with acute renal failure. Although the exact biochemical mechanisms of mercuric chloride nephrotoxicity are not known, several hypotheses have been proposed, including the following:

1. impaired mitochondrial function,
2. altered plasma membrane function and integrity,
3. renal hemodynamic alterations mediated by the renin-angiotensin system or prostaglandins, and
4. lipid peroxidation [24,91].

TABLE 15-1. *Renal clearance and tissue accumulation of gentamicin from paired experiments*

Age (days)	Plasma Gentamicin		Clearance of Gentamicin (ml/min)	Gentamicin in Renal Cortex		
	Peak (µg/ml)	Trough (µg/ml)		Outer (µg/g)	Inner (µg/g)	Ratio outer/inner
10	4.41 ± 0.37*	0.22 ± 0.07	2.6 ± 0.6	91.1 ± 23.1	154.6 ± 31.2	0.67 ± 0.13
20	4.62 ± 0.98	0.35 ± 0.14	2.4 ± 0.8	752.3 ± 233.5†	486.0 ± 186.1	1.84 ± 0.27†
30	4.92 ± 0.41	0.21 ± 0.05	3.4 ± 1.0	811.5 ± 178.0†	367.2 ± 75.4	2.84 ± 0.81†

* Mean ± SE.
† Significantly different than 10-day-old animals.
From Cowan RH, Jukkola AF, Arant BS Jr, Pathophysiologic evidence of gentamicin nephrotoxicity in neonatal puppies. *Pediatr Res* 14:1204, 1980; with permission.

Results of several studies investigating mercuric chloride nephrotoxicity in young animals have been conflicting. Bidani et al. [8] reported that the degree of mercuric chloride nephrotoxicity was similar in young and older rats; however, renal functional recovery was delayed and mortality was higher in the younger animals. Furthermore, increased sodium intake had comparable protective effects in 3 to 4-week-old and 7 to 8-week-old rats [7]. In contrast to these studies, Datson et al. [18,19] reported that the rat neonatal kidney was less susceptible to the effects of mercuric chloride than older rat kidneys. Similarly, Kavlok [41] observed that postnatal administration of mercuric chloride did not affect relative kidney weight, basal or hydropenic urine osmolality, hydropenic urine volume or the histologic profile of the kidney. The nephrotoxicity of another heavy metal associated with acute renal failure, uranyl nitrate, has also been reported to be more profound in older dogs than in the young [64].

Kleinman [45] reported that administration of lead to young rats had a negligible effect on glomerular filtration rate, renal plasma flow, intrarenal blood flow distribution and tubular transport of phosphate and amino acids. However, further investigation revealed an impairment of proximal tubular reabsorption of sodium and water, a phenomenon that may be related to the observed decreased tubular sensitivity to antidiuretic hormone (ADH) and ADH-stimulated adenylate cyclase activity. Inasmuch as basal and ADH-stimulated adenylate cyclase activity is low in newborns [72], these results may suggest that lead interferes with the normal development of the tubular action of ADH.

References

1. Alexander FW: The uptake of lead by children in differing environments. *Environ Health Perspect* 7:155, 1974.
2. Alveres AP, Kapelner S, Sassa S, et al: Drug metabolism in normal children, lead-poisoned children and normal adults. *Clin Pharmacol Ther* 17:179, 1975.
3. Bailie MB, Smith JH, Newton JF, et al: Mechanism of chloroform nephrotoxicity. IV. Phenobarbital potentiation of in vitro chloroform metabolism and toxicity in rabbit kidneys. *Toxicol Appl Pharmacol* 74:285, 1984.
4. Barza M, Murray T, Hamburger RJ: Uptake of gentamicin by separated viable renal tubules from rabbits. *J Infect Dis* 141:510, 1980.
5. Basu TK, Dickerson JWT, Parke DVW: Effect of development on the activity of microsomal drug-metabolizing enzymes in rat liver. *Biochem J* 124:19, 1971.
6. Berndt WO: The effect of potassium dichromate on renal tubular transport processes. *Toxicol Appl Pharmacol* 32:40, 1975.
7. Bidani A, Churchill P: Effects of sodium intake and nephrotoxin dose on acute failure in the young rat. *Pediatr Res* 16:277, 1982.
8. Bidani A, Churchill P, Fleischmann, L, et al: HgCl$_2$-induced acute renal failure in the developing rat. *Pediatr Res* 14:183, 1979.
9. Blumer JL, Reed MD: Clinical pharmacology of aminoglycoside antibiotics in pediatrics. *Pediatr Clin North Am* 30:195, 1983.
10. Bond JT, Bailie MD, Hook JB: Maturation of renal organic acid transport in vivo: Substrate stimulation by penicillin. *J Pharmacol Exp Ther* 199:25, 1976.
11. Branchflower RV, Nunn DS, Highet RJ, et al: Nephrotoxicity of chloroform: Metabolism to phosgene by the mouse kidney. *Toxicol Appl Pharmacol* 72:159, 1984.
12. Child KJ, Dodds MG: Mechanism of urinary excretion of cephaloridine and its effects on renal function in animals. *Br J Pharmacol* 26:108, 1966.
13. Chonko A, Savin R, Stewart R, et al: The effects of gentamicin on renal function in the mature vs immature rabbit. *Clin Res* 27:664A, 1979.
14. Clemens TL, Hil RN, Bullick LP, et al: Chloroform toxicity in the mouse: Role of genetic factors and steroids. *Toxicol Appl Pharmacol* 48:117, 1979.
15. Cojocel C, Dociu N, Ceacmacudis E, et al: Nephrotoxic effects of aminoglycoside treatment on renal protein reabsorption and accumulation. *Nephron* 37:113, 1984.
16. Cowan RH, Jukkola AF, Arant BS Jr: Pathophysiologic evidence of gentamicin nephrotoxicity in neonatal puppies. *Pediatr Res* 14:1204, 1980.
17. Culliford D, Hewitt HB: The influence of sex hormone status on the susceptibility of mice to chloroform-induced necrosis of the renal tubules. *J Endocrinol* 14:381, 1957.
18. Datson GP, Gry JA, Carver B, et al: Toxicity of mercuric chloride to the developing rat kidney. II. Effect of increased dosages on renal function in suckling pups. *Toxicol Appl Pharmacol* 74:35, 1984.
19. Datson GP, Kavlock RJ, Rogers EH, et al: Toxicity of mercuric chloride to the developing rat kidney. I. Postnatal

ontogeny of renal sensitivity. *Toxicol Appl Pharmacol* 71:24, 1983.

20. Dees JH, Masters BS, Moller-Berhard, et al: Effect of 2,3,7,8-tetrachlorodibenzo-p-dioxin and phenobarbital on the occurrence and distribution of four cytochrome P-450 isozymes in rabbit kidney, lung and liver. *Cancer Res* 42:1423, 1982.

21. Dobyan DC, Levi J, Jacobs C, et al: Mechanism of cisplatinum nephrotoxicity. II. Morphologic observations. *J Pharmacol Exp Ther* 213:551, 1980.

22. Echeverria P, Siber GR, Paisley J, et al: Age-dependent dose response to gentamicin. *J Pediatr* 87:805, 1975.

23. Eschenbrenner AB, Miller E: Sex differences in kidney morphology and chloroform necrosis. *Science* 102:302, 1945.

24. Fowler BA: General subcellular effects of lead, mercury, cadmium and arsenic. *Environ Health Perspect* 22:37, 1978.

25. Fowler BA, Hook GER, Lucier GW: Tetrachlorodibenzo-p-dioxan induction of renal microsomal enzyme systems. Ultrastructural effects on pars recta (S3) proximal tubule cells of the rat kidney. *J Pharmacol Exp Ther* 203:712, 1977.

26. Fox MRS: Nutritional influences on metal toxicity: Cadmium as a model toxic element. *Environ Health Perspect* 29:95, 1979.

27. Fry JR, Wiebkin P, Kao, J, et al: A comparison of drug metabolizing capability in isolated viable hepatocytes and renal tubule fragments. *Xenobiotica* 8:113, 1978.

28. Gillette JR, Mitchell JR, Brodie BB: Biochemical mechanisms of drug toxicity. *Ann Rev Pharmacol* 14:271, 1974.

29. Goldstein RS, Kuo C-H, Hook JB: Biochemical mechanisms of xenobiotic induced nephrotoxicity. In Goldstein RS, Hewitt WR, Hook JB (eds): *Toxic Interaction*. San Diego, Academic Press, 1991, p 262.

30. Haagsma BH, Pound AW: Mercuric chloride induced renal tubular necrosis in the rat. *Br J Exp Pathol* 60:341, 1979.

31. Henning SJ: Development of feeding behavior and digestive function. *Banbury Report* 11:53, 1982.

32. Hirsch GH, Hook JB: Maturation of renal organic acid transport: Substrate stimulation by penicillin and PAH. *J Pharmacol Exp Ther* 17:103, 1970.

33. Hook JB: Mechanisms of renal toxicity. *In* Brown SS, Davies DS (eds): *Organ-Directed Toxicity-Chemical Indices and Mechanisms*. Oxford, Pergamon Press, 1981, p 45.

34. Hook JB, Hewitt WR: Development of mechanisms for drug excretion. *Am J Med* 62:497, 1977.

35. Hsu CH, Kurtz TW, Weller JM: In vitro uptake of gentamicin by rat renal cortical tissue. *Antimicrob Agents Chemother* 12:192, 1977.

36. Humes AD, Weinberg JM, Knauss TC: Clinical and pathophysiologic aspects of aminoglycoside nephrotoxicity. *Am J Kid Dis* 2:5, 1982.

37. James MO, Foureman GL, Law FC, et al: The perinatal development of epoxide-metabolizing enzyme activities in liver and extrahepatic organs of guinea pig and rabbit. *Drug Metab Dispos* 5:19, 1977.

38. Jollow DJ, Mitchell JR, Zampaglione N, et al: Bromobenzene-induced liver necrosis. Protective role of glutathione and evidence for 3,4, bromobenzene oxide as the hepatotoxic metabolite. *Pharmacology* 11:151, 1974.

39. Jollow DL, Thorgeirsson SS, Potter WZ, et al: Acetaminophen-induced hepatic necrosis. VI. Metabolic disposition of toxic and nontoxic doses of acetaminophen. *Pharmacology* 12:251, 1974.

40. Kahlmeter G, Dahlager JI: Aminoglycoside toxicity—a review of clincial studies published between 1975 and 1982. *J Antimicrob Chemother* (suppl A)13:9, 1984.

41. Kavlok RJ: The ontogeny of the hydropenia response in neonatal rats and its application in developmental toxicology studies. *Banbury Report* 11:175, 1982.

42. Kehoe RA: The metabolism of lead in man in health and disease. The Harber Lectures. J.R. Inst. *Public Health* 24:81, 1961.

43. Kim JK, Hirsch GH, Hook JB: In vitro analysis of organic ion transport in renal cortex of the newborn rat. *Pediatr Res* 6:600, 1972.

44. Kirschbaum BB, Oken DE: The effect of mercuric chloride on renal brush border membrane. *Exp Mol Pathol* 31:101, 1979.

45. Kleinman LI: The effect of lead on the maturing kidney. *Banbury Report* 11:153, 1982.

46. Klinger W, Muller D, Kleeberg U, et al: Peri- and postnatal development of phase I reactions. *In* Kimmel CA, Buelke-Sam J (eds): *Developmental Toxicology*. New York, Raven Press, 1981.

47. Kostial K, Kello D, Jugo S, et al: Influence of age on metal metabolism and toxicity. *Environ Health Perspect* 25:81, 1978.

48. Kuo C-H, Hook JB: Postnatal development of renal and hepatic drug metabolizing enzymes in male and female Fischer 344 rats. *Life Sci* 27:2433, 1980.

49. Kuo C-H, Maita K, Sleight SD, et al: Lipid peroxidation: A possible mechanism of cephaloridine-induced nephrotoxicity. *Toxicol Appl Pharmacol* 67:78, 1983.

50. Litterst CL, Mimnaugh EG, Reagan RL, et al: Comparison of in vitro drug metabolism by lung, liver and kidney of several common laboratory species. *Drug Metab Dispos* 3:259, 1975.

51. Marre R, Tarara N, Louton T, et al: Age-dependent nephrotoxicity and the pharmacokinetics of gentamicin in rats. *Eur J Pediatr* 13:25, 1980.

52. McCabe EB: Age and sensitivity to lead toxicity: A review. *Environ Health Perspect* 29:29, 1979.

53. McDowell EM, Nagle RB, Zalme RC, et al: Studies on the pathophysiology of acute renal failure. I. Correlation of ultrastructure and function on the proximal tubule of the rat following administration of mercuric chloride. *Virchows Arch [B]* 22:173, 1976.

54. Meister A, Anderson ME: Glutathione. *Ann Rev Biochem* 52:711, 1983.

55. Miller EC, Miller JA: Reactive metabolites as key intermediates in pharmacologic and toxicologic responses: Example from chemical carcinogenesis. *In* Snyder R, Parke DV, Kocsis JJ (eds): *Biological Reactive Intermediates. II. Chemical Mechanisms and Biological Effects, Part A*. New York, Plenum Press, 1982.

56. Miller JA: Carcinogenesis by chemicals: An overview. *Cancer Res* 10:163, 1970.

57. Mitchell JR, Jollow DJ, Potter WZ, et al: Acetaminophen-induced hepatic necrosis. I. Role of drug metabolism. *J Pharmacol Exp Ther* 187:185, 1973.

58. Mitchell JR, Smith CV, Lauterburg BH, et al: Reactive metabolites and the pathophysiology of acute lethal cell injury. *In* Mitchell JR, Horning MG (eds): *Drug Metabolism and Toxicity*. New York, Raven Press, 1984.

59. Mitchell SC: The development of drug metabolizing enzymes in the neonatal guinea-pig. *Xenobiotica* 13:453, 1983.

60. Neal RA: Metabolism of toxic substances. *In* Doull J, Klaassen CD, Amdur MO (eds): *Toxicology. The Basic Science of Poisons*. New York, Macmillan, 1980.

61. Neims AH: The effect of age on drug disposition and action. *Banbury Report* 11:529, 1982.

62. Neims AH, Warner M, Loughnan PM, et al: Developmental aspects of the hepatic cytochrome P450 monooxygenase system. *Annu Rev Pharmacol Toxciol* 16:427, 1976.

63. Pastoriza-Munoz E, Timmerman D, Kaloyanides GJ: Renal transport of netilimicin in the rat. *J Pharmacol Exp Ther* 228:65, 1984.

64. Pelayo JC, Andrews PM, Coffey AK, et al: The influence of age on acute renal toxicity of uranyl nitrate in the dog. *Pediatr Res* 17:985, 1983.

65. Pohl LR, Martin JL, Taburet AM, et al: Oxidative bioactivation of haloforms into hepatotoxins. *In* Coon MJ, Conney AH, Estabrook RW, et al (eds): *Microsomes, Drug Oxidations and Chemical Carcinogenesis.* New York, Academic, 1980.

66. Potter WZ, Thorgeirsson SS, Jollow DJ, et al: Acetaminophen-induced hepatic necrosis. V. Correlation of hepatic necrosis, covalent binding and glutathione depletion in hamsters. *Pharmacology* 12:129, 1974.

67. Price VF, Jollow DJ: Increased resistance of diabetic rats to acetaminophen-induced hepatotoxicity. *J Pharmacol Exp Ther* 220:504, 1982.

68. Roberts JJ: Cellular responses to carcinogen induced DNA damage and the role of DNA repair. *Br Med Bull* 36:25, 1980.

69. Rush GF, Hook JB: The kidney as a target organ for toxicity. *In* Cohen G (ed): *Target Organ Toxicity.* Boca Raton, Florida, CRC Press. Vol II, 1986, p 1.

70. Rush GF, Smith JH, Newton JF, et al: Chemically induced nephrotoxicity: Role of metabolic activation. *CRC Crit Rev in Toxicol* 13:99, 1984.

71. Sastrasinh M, Knauss TC, Weinberg JM, et al: Identification of the aminoglycoside binding site in rat renal brush border membranes. *J Pharmacol Exp Ther* 222:350, 1982.

72. Schlondorff D, Weber H, Trizna W, et al: Vasopressin responsiveness of renal adenylate cyclase in newborn rats and rabbits. *Am J Physiol* 234:F16, 1978.

73. Short CR, Maines MD, Westfall BA: Postnatal development of drug-metabolizing enzyme activity in liver and extrahepatic tissues of swine. *Biol Neonate* 21:54, 1972.

74. Siber GR, Echeverria P, Smith AL, et al: Pharmacokinetics of gentamicin in children and adults. *J Infect Dis* 132:637, 1975.

75. Sims P, Grover PL: Epoxides in polycyclic aromatic hydrocarbon metabolism and carcinogenesis. *Adv Cancer Res* 20:166, 1974.

76. Smith JH, Hook JB: Mechanism of chloroform nephrotoxicity. II. In vitro evidence for renal metabolism of chloroform in mice. *Toxicol Appl Pharmacol* 70:480, 1983.

77. Smith JH, Hook JB: Mechanism of chloroform nephrotoxicity. III. Renal and hepatic microsomal metabolism of chloroform in mice. *Toxicol Appl Pharmacol* 73:511, 1984.

78. Smith JH, Maita K, Sleight SD, et al: Mechanism of chloroform nephrotoxicity. I. Time course of chloroform toxicity in male and female mice. *Toxicol Appl Pharmacol* 70:467, 1983.

79. Smith JH, Maita K, Sleight SD, et al: Effect of sex hormone status on chloroform nephrotoxicity and renal mixed function oxidases in mice. *Toxicology* 30:305, 1984.

80. Soberon L, Bowman RL, Pasoriza-Munoz, E, et al: Comparative nephrotoxicities of gentamicin, netilimicin and tobramycin in the rat. *J Pharmacol Exp Ther* 210:334, 1979.

81. Tessin I, Bergmark J, Hiesche K, et al: Renal function of neonates during gentamicin treatment. *Arch Dis Child* 57:758, 1982.

82. Thurman RG, Kauffman FC: Factors regulating drug metabolism in intact hepatocytes. *Pharmacol Rev* 31:229, 1980.

83. Tune BM: Effect of organic acid transport inhibitors on renal cortical uptake and proximal tubular toxicity of cephaloridine. *J Pharmacol Exp Ther* 181:250, 1972.

84. Tune BM: Relationship between the transport and toxicity of cephalosporins in the kidney. *J Infect Dis* 132:189, 1975.

85. Tune BM, Fernholt M, Schwartz A: Mechanism of cephaloridine transport in the kidney. *J Pharmacol Exp Ther* 191:311, 1974.

86. Tune BM, Wu KY, Kempson RL: Inhibition of transport and prevention of toxicity of cephaloridine in the kidney. Dose-responsiveness of the rabbit and guinea pig to probenecid. *J Pharmacol Exp Ther* 202:466, 1977.

87. Vessell E: Dynamically interacting genetic and environmental factors that affect the response of developing individuals to toxicants. *Banbury Report* 11:107, 1982.

88. Wislocki PG, Miwa GT, Lu AYH: Reactions catalyzed by the cytochrome P-450 system. *In* Jakoby WB (ed): *Enzymatic Basis of Detoxification.* Vol 1. New York, Academic, 1980.

89. Wold JS, Joost RR, Owen NY: Nephrotoxicity of cephaloridine in newborn rabbits: Role of the renal organic anionic transport system. *J Pharmacol Exp Ther* 201:778, 1977.

90. Wolf CR, Berry PA, Nash JA, et al: Role of microsomal and cytosolic glutathione S-transferases in the conjugation of hexachloro-1:3-butadiene and its possible relevance to toxicity. *J Pharmacol Exp Ther* 228:202, 1984.

91. Yonaha M, Itoh E, Ohbayashi Y, et al: Induction of lipid peroxidation in rats by mercuric chloride. *Res Commun Chem Pathol Pharmacol* 28:105, 1980.

92. Zenk KE, Miwa L, Cohen JL, et al: Effect of body weight on gentamicin pharmacokinetics in neonates. *Clin Pharm* 3:170, 1984.

93. Zenser TV, Mattammal MB, Davis BB: Differential distribution of the mixed function oxidase activities in rabbit kidney. *J Pharmacol Exp Ther* 207:712, 1978.

DONALD E. OKEN

16
Acute Renal Failure

Vasomotor nephropathy is a condition characterized by an abrupt, sustained, and marked impairment of renal function that most frequently follows trauma, a transfusion reaction, sepsis, poisoning, shock, or an obstetrical accident. The mediators immediately responsible for the disorder remain unknown.

Formerly termed lower nephron nephrosis, this entity now is most commonly called acute tubular necrosis (ATN) or acute renal failure (ARF); the name "tubulointerstitial nephropathy" has found popularity in the Scandinavian literature [83]. None of these terms is universally accepted, since tubular injury is not confined to distal tubular segments, overt tubular necrosis is not essential to the syndrome, ARF occurs with totally unrelated diseases such as glomerulonephritis and lupus erythematosus, and a totally different entity, most commonly related to drug hypersensitivity, also is known as interstitial nephritis. Therefore, we have preferred the term *vasomotor nephropathy* (VMN), which avoids the many implications inherent in the other nomenclature and, as is shown in this chapter, calls attention to a critical pathogenetic feature that is found universally in this syndrome in humans. Here, however, we use the terms vasomotor nephropathy, acute renal failure, and acute tubular necrosis interchangeably.

Historical Considerations

The adverse effects of various poisons on the kidney were well known [59] and the renal consequences of massive hemolysis (e.g., blackwater fever) were recognized before the turn of this century [122]. In 1917, German pathologists called attention to distinct pathologic alterations of the renal architecture found in fatal battle casualties [43], but the functional significance of those changes appears not to have been fully recognized. Husfeldt and Bjering [54] reported on the relationship between trauma and the development of ARF in 1937, but this association first became widely appreciated early in World War II with the discovery of persistent oliguria and sustained renal failure in patients severely injured in the London "blitz" [20].

Pathophysiology

The immediate cause of this "new" syndrome became a subject for speculation. At autopsy, the glomeruli and renal vasculature were found on histologic examination to be normal, whereas the tubules often were severely injured. It thus was postulated that glomerular filtration was normal and that the filtrate formed was almost quantitatively absorbed across a tubular epithelial structure that could no longer serve as an effective barrier. This concept of pathogenesis was termed the *passive backflow theory.*

The presence of debris or heme pigment in tubular lumens gave rise to the alternative theory that renal failure is due largely to tubular outflow obstruction. The *obstruction theory* found particular support in early experimental studies of hemoglobinuria [122]; it was merged with the passive backflow theory by some who pointed out that obstruction, by raising intratubular pressure, also would increase the driving force for the leakage of filtrate. Others suggested that interstitial edema and tubular compression might also contribute to urinary outflow obstruction [88], but few believed that hemodynamic factors might be the essential feature [110].

Quite early, measurements of inulin and creatinine clearances suggested that the glomerular filtration rate (GFR) of subjects with ARF was very low [17,18]. To serve as a marker of glomerular filtration, however, the reference substance must be freely filterable and neither absorbed nor secreted to any significant extent. If filtered inulin or creatinine were to leak across damaged tubular epithelium, as suggested by the passive backflow theory, studies based on clearance measurements could not be relied on. Similarly, the use of para-aminohippurate or iodopyracet (Diodrast) clearances as a measure of renal blood flow (RBF) presupposes that tubular secretory capacity is reasonably intact and that the indicator substance, once secreted, will be quantitatively excreted in the urine. Because such preconditions could not be assumed with any degree of confidence in the presence of severe tubular injury, the very low values of RBF found universally in this syndrome also were suspect. Since then, however, newer techniques that do not

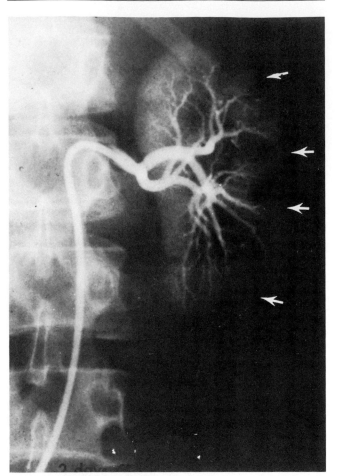

FIG. 16-1. *Selective renal arteriogram typical of that found in human vasomotor nephropathy. Narrowing of the arcuate arteries and the virtually total lack of filling of the outer cortical vessels signify the marked increase in renocortical (preglomerular) resistance characteristic of this disorder. The outer cortical margin, normally demarcated by contrast-filled vessels, is poorly seen (arrows).*

1. In patients with chronic renal disease and comparably reduced rates of blood flow, GFR may be far higher than that measured in patients with ARF [66];
2. There appears to be an imperfect correlation between the degree of cortical ischemia and the GFR in individual patients and between different patients with ARF [66];
3. Intra-arterial injections of renal vasodilators cause a marked increase in renocortical blood flow but little or no change in GFR [60]; and
4. RBF in virtually all models of murine ARF is normal or only modestly reduced (see following).

Each of these objections is considered in turn:

1. It is quite clear that both the histologic and the hemodynamic abnormalities in ARF are very different from those of chronic renal failure. Figure 16-1 illustrates the diffuse reduction in blood flow found throughout the renal cortex in ARF; in chronic renal failure, by contrast, perfused nephrons lie side by side with obsolescent ones in a bed of avascular scar tissue [16]. Thus, while whole kidney blood flow is grossly reduced in advanced chronic renal failure, blood flow to individual functioning nephrons is well maintained [16]. Extrapolation from the abnormalities of chronic renal failure to ARF thus may be inappropriate.
2. Nor would one necessarily expect that the GFR should correlate with cortical blood flow in a series of individuals or even in the same individual studied at different times, since RBF is a simple expression of blood pressure and total renovascular resistance. By contrast, GFR is determined by the relative resistances of the preglomerular and postglomerular vascular beds (the R_A-R_E ratio) as well as by the total vascular resistance and other factors to be described.
3. Vasodilator agents act largely on the postglomerular resistance [34], an effect that would raise the R_A-R_E ratio, further depress filtration pressure, and in no way help to support filtration in the presence of marked preglomerular vasoconstriction.
4. The determinants of glomerular dynamics in the normal rat appear to be distinctly different from those of humans [78], R_A being 1.5 to 2 times higher than R_E in the former, whereas R_E seems to be by far the larger resistance in the human kidney [78]. Mean blood pressure in humans is some 30 mm Hg lower and Bowman's space pressure is substantively higher than in the rat [78]. The response of the vascular beds in humans and rats to noxious stimuli thus might be quite dissimilar. As already noted, renal blood flow is greatly reduced in human subjects but remains normal in most models of murine ARF [24].

In addition to a 50% to 80% reduction in renocortical blood flow [17,49] and an inulin clearance that typically is well below 10% of normal [17,18], two other features stand out in human oliguric ARF:

1. Proximal tubular pressure, as judged by measurements of wedged renal venous pressure, is essentially normal [66]; and

require intact tubular secretory capacity and are independent of the permeability characteristics of the tubules have established that RBF is indeed massively reduced in all forms of VMN in humans, regardless of its etiology [17,49,50,60,66,89,113]. As shown in Fig. 16-1, arteriograms reveal marked narrowing of the arcuate arteries and the virtual disappearance of the distal cortical vessels in both toxin-induced and hemodynamically induced renal failure [49]. Because a vessel's resistance, estimated as the fourth power of the radius (Poiseuille's law), is extremely sensitive to even small changes in caliber (Fig. 16-2), a major reduction in the size of the preglomerular vessels, as seen in Fig. 16-1, presumably accounts for much (if not all) of the decrease in RBF found in this disorder.

The pathogenetic importance of this impressive reduction in renocortical blood flow has been questioned on various grounds:

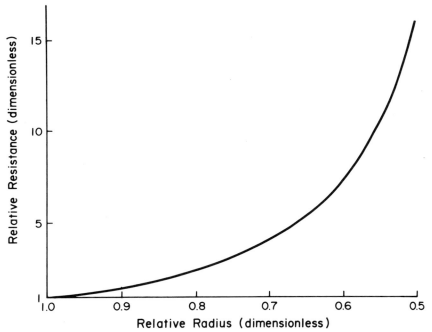

FIG. 16-2. *The effect of vasoconstriction on vascular resistance, assuming that resistance changes as a function of the fourth power of the radius (Poiseuille's law). It may be seen that a 15% decrease in radius (relative radius 0.85) results in a near doubling of resistance (relative resistance 1.92), whereas decreases of 25% to 50% increase vascular resistance 3.2-fold and 16-fold, respectively.*

2. Histologic abnormalities of the tubules are usually quite slight [83].

Because many of the kidneys of patients with ARF that were microdissected by Oliver, MacDowell, and Tracy [82] showed patchy and often extreme degrees of tubular injury, it is sometimes stated that ordinary histologic techniques conceal the existence of tubular lesions that are essential to the pathogenesis of renal failure. However, careful reading of the report on which that view is based [82] shows that ". . . even in severely damaged kidneys, not all nephrons are affected and, in the moderate example, only occasional ones." By that account as well as many other histologic reports in the literature [66,83,96], filtration failure in human vasomotor nephropathy can occur in the absence of widespread tubular necrosis.

The origins and the relative importance of hemodynamic factors, tubular leakage, and tubular obstruction in the genesis of this disorder are still debated.

Tubular Necrosis and Abnormal Tubular Permeability in Human Acute Renal Failure

The theory that ARF in humans reflects quantitative leakage of filtrate across necrotic and pathologically permeable tubular structures stemmed from the assumption that tubular necrosis is a constant feature of this syndrome. How-ever, Sevitt [96], Finckh et al. [36], Bohle et al. [13], Olsen [83], and other pathologists have emphasized the paucity of tubular degenerative changes in the kidneys of most patients with ARF. Sevitt [96] and Finckh et al. [36] reported that they could not find any specific tubular lesions in a given patient dying of ARF that necessarily set him or her apart from another dying without evident renal dysfunction. Both categories of patients showed tubular lesions, but these, for the most part, were considered neither constant nor diagnostic. More recently, Solez and Finckh [100] have reviewed again the pathologic material that served as the basis for the original report of Finckh, Jeremy, and Whyte [36], employing rigorous statistical methodology. Luminal pigmented casts, interstitial inflammatory changes, and nucleated cells in the vasa recta were found far more frequently in patients with ARF than in controls, but the pathogenetic implications of these abnormalities are uncertain. More germane to this discussion, distal tubular injury and signs of proximal and distal tubular regeneration were found more often in patients who had died in renal failure, although proximal tubular injury was not. Importantly, however, 20 of the 28 patients with ARF showed no evidence of proximal tubular injury at all, and a like number displayed either no (n = 12) or only 1+ distal tubular change (scored on a scale of 0 to 4+) (n = 13). This study thus did show that certain anatomic changes occur more frequently in the population of subjects with ARF than in controls. However, the coexistence of renal failure with slight or no evidence of tubular necrosis in the majority of patients does not support the concept of a freely permeable epithelium, which served as the basis for the passive backflow hypothesis. As noted by the authors [100], these findings in no way controvert the original conclusion that "tubular changes in this syndrome are inconstant, generally mild, and of unclear pathogenetic importance" [36].

In evaluating the passive backflow theory of ARF, the crucial question is not whether some degree of tubular leakage can or does occur in a given form of ARF but, rather, whether indiscriminate leakage of filtrate is either the sole abnormality accounting for the massively reduced GFR or an essential contributor without which renal function would be reasonably well maintained.

Myers et al. [69,70] reported on studies in which the possibility of tubular leakage in human ARF was examined by comparing the simultaneously derived clearances of inulin and polydisperse dextrans ranging in size from 18 to 42 Å, the dextran-inulin (D-I) clearance ratio. In half their patients, the D-I clearance ratio for one or more of the lowest molecular weight dextran moieties was somewhat higher than unity, and the clearance ratio for the larger dextrans was almost routinely higher than that of controls. These results were interpreted to reflect the leakage of some 20% to 42% of filtered inulin in individual patients with ARF [69]. The authors acknowledged, however, that the high D-I ratio for the large molecular weight dextrans might be explained in part by changes in the sieving properties of the glomerulus or altered glomerular hemodynamics or both [69]. Indeed, in a separate study, the same authors found the 40 Å D-I clearance ratio to be 60% higher than controls in patients with simple heart failure and, presumably, no intrinsic renal disease [71]. Here, however, we concern ourselves only with the implications to be drawn if 20% to 40% of all the filtered inulin truly does undergo passive absorption in human ARF.

The potential importance of tubular leakage in the genesis of renal failure can be assessed by comparing the measured GFR obtained at any assumed degree of inulin "leak" with that expected if no leakage were present. If inulin, the customary marker of filtration, is passively absorbed in either human or experimental acute renal failure, the degree to which the measured whole kidney filtration rate underestimates the true filtration rate can be estimated from the equation:

$$C_{in} = C_{in}^{True}(1 - Absn_{in}) \qquad (1)$$

where C_{in} is the measured inulin clearance, C_{in}^{True} is the true filtration rate and $Absn_{in}$ is the fraction of filtered inulin lost by leakage. With a normal filtration rate and leakage of 30%, 50%, or 70% of the filtered inulin, the measured filtration rate would fall correspondingly to 70%, 50%, or 30% of normal. This degree of leakage, at least, does not provide the 95% or greater decrease in inulin clearance expected in fully established oliguric renal failure. One thus would have to postulate a larger proportion of leakage or, in addition, a true decrease in the filtration rate.

Figure 16-3, based on Equation 1, shows the change in

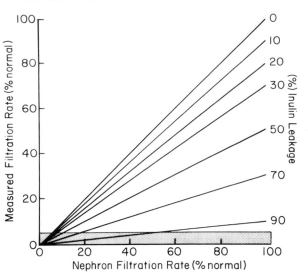

FIG. 16-3. *The relationship between the measured filtration rate and actual nephron filtration rate assuming different degrees of tubular inulin leakage. At measured filtration rates consistent with oliguric vasomotor nephropathy (stippled zone), the measured values of GFR minimally underestimate the true GFR, despite leakage of up to 50% of the inulin filtered.*

the GFR required to yield any given measured GFR when the latter is artifactually lowered by tubular leakage. If 30% of the inulin filtered escapes excretion because of tubular absorption, for example, a 95% reduction in the measured GFR can be attained only if the true filtration rate falls concomitantly by 93%. The decrease from normal of both measured and actual GFR values differs by a mere 2% despite this substantive inulin leakage.

The passive movement of a normally impermeant substance such as inulin across an imperfect tubular barrier is determined as a function of both the tubule's permeability and the driving force(s) available to produce that movement. Diffusional absorption of a molecule as large as inulin should be quite slow, limited as it is by the very low free diffusion coefficient of this molecule and the small inulin concentration difference between lumen and interstitium. Nor does the low net transtubular pressure difference promise brisk inulin movement by bulk fluid flow. Let us presume, nonetheless, that half of all the inulin filtered by patients with ARF is resorbed by this mechanism and conservatively assume that tubular fluid flow along the nephron is 20% of normal (a deliberate gross overestimate of the probable flow rate). Assuming that tubular permeability and the driving force for absorption are independent of the flow rate of fluid along the nephron, the reabsorptive loss of inulin per unit time also should be independent of the tubular flow rate. Figure 16-4 illustrates a model in which fluid containing a permeant solute (in this instance inulin) flows from a central reservoir into two identical side limbs, A and B, at different rates. The permeability-potential product permits the passive absorption of 5 arbitrary units/minute of fluid from each limb by convective transfer, but flow through limb A is set at the rate of 10 units/minute (ARF), while that in B is set at a normal rate of 50 units/minute. It may be seen that one-half of the inulin appearing at the absorption site is absorbed in limb A, whereas 90% emerges unabsorbed from limb B with the faster axial flow rate. By extrapolation, therefore, one cannot assume that the degree of inulin leakage found in a subject with ARF equals that which would be present when the GFR is normal. Thus, if as much as 50% of filtered inulin is absorbed when the GFR is 5 ml/minute or so, only 5% or less might be lost in the presence of a normal filtration rate. Leakage, per se, then would exert only a trivial effect on estimation of renal function. Any degree of inulin leakage will contribute to a measured decrease in filtration rate but, as seen in this example, the seeming importance of such leakage might be greatly exaggerated by the very existence of renal failure.

Glomerular Dynamics in Human Acute Renal Failure

Glomerular filtration is a passive phenomenon, driven by the net hydrostatic pressure gradient across the glomerular capillary wall and modulated by the surface area and hydraulic conductivity of the filtering surface. (Because they cannot be measured individually, the two latter variables are combined into a single term, the ultrafiltration coefficient, K_f). Thus:

$$SNGFR = K_f (P_g - P_{BS} - \overline{COP}) \qquad (2)$$

where SNGFR is the single nephron GFR, Pg represents glomerular capillary hydrostatic pressure, P_{BS} is the hydrostatic pressure in Bowman's space, and COP is the mean colloid osmotic pressure of plasma proteins exerted within the glomerular tuft. Of these variables, only K_f and P_{BS} are independent determinants of filtration, P_g being determined at any given arterial blood pressure by the set of the

vascular resistances before (R_A), within (R_{cap}), and after (R_E) the glomerular capillaries. (P_g also is influenced indirectly by K_f, P_{BS}, blood hematocrit, and serum protein concentration, insofar as these variables affect the volume of filtrate formed and thus the flow-related pressure drop across R_E [77]. This effect is relatively small, however.) P_{BS} is a complex function of SNGFR, tubular outflow resistance, and tubular compliance, while itself serving as a determinant of filtration.

It is evident from Equation 2 that filtration will be vanishingly low if the K_f becomes sufficiently small, if P_g falls toward a value equal to the sum (P_{BS} + COP), or if a large increase in P_{BS} raises this last term to a pressure that approaches that of P_g.

Although values for the individual determinants of glomerular filtration have been well established for the normal rat and dog in renal micropuncture studies, such is not the case for humans. Knowing RBF, whole kidney GFR, and the number of nephrons in the normal human kidney, however, we can estimate that the mean single nephron GFR is 60 to 65 nl/minute, glomerular blood flow (GBF) approximates 575 nl/minute, and the total vascular resistance per nephron is some 1.2×10^{10} dyne sec cm^{-5} [78]. As extrapolated from renal venous wedge pressures, Bowman's space pressure, P_{BS}, is taken to be 15 to 25 mm Hg [66,116], the higher value having been more recently obtained. Applying these values to network thermodynamic modeling and assuming a normal P_{BS} of 25 mm Hg, we have found previously that the normal preglomerular resistance in humans cannot exceed 40% and is very unlikely to be less than 25% of the total renal vascular resistance [78]. Preglomerular resistance thus lies somewhere between 0.32 and 0.48 $\times$ 10^{10} dyne sec cm^{-5}, postglomerular resistance correspondingly is 0.88 to 0.72 $\times$ 10^{10} dyne sec cm^{-5}, and the R_A-R_E ratio is set between possible upper and lower limits of 0.36 and 0.66. The former resistance values require ultrafiltration coefficient of some 4 nl/minute/mm Hg and the latter 18 nl/minute/mm Hg to provide a normal single nephron GFR value of 65 nl/minute [78]. Applying these limiting normal values to network ther-

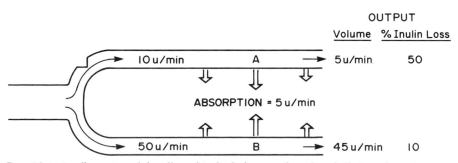

FIG. 16-4. An illustration of the effect of inulin leakage resulting from bulk flow absorption across injured epithelium. In limb A, where flow is set at 20% of normal, absorption of 5 arbitrary units of volume per minute results in a 50% inulin loss. With the same putative driving force and absorption rate but a normal axial flow rate, only 10% of the inulin is lost (see text).

modynamic modeling, we have estimated the degree of change in K_f, R_A, R_E, and P_{BS} that would be required to yield the typical single nephron GFR and blood flow values of human ARF [80].

In assigning an etiologic role to a pathologic finding, it is not enough merely to document its presence. Rather, one must be confident that the degree of abnormality is sufficiently marked to exert the effect envisioned. That decision is not always intuitively obvious in complex physiologic systems. One thus might attribute far too much or far too little importance to an experimental finding unless its quantitative significance is fully appreciated. Network thermodynamic modeling provides an excellent means of examining the importance of change in any of the several determinants of glomerular filtration in ARF [77]. This can be achieved prospectively by taking the normal values for each of the normal determinants of glomerular dynamics, changing the values for each in turn, and observing the effect on glomerular filtration, glomerular capillary pressure, and GBF. The practical importance of a single abnormal variable in ARF can be tested first by returning all other aberrant variables to normal while the entity in question is held at its pathologic value. If that variable is key to the development of renal failure, the SNGFR should remain distinctly subnormal. As a next step, that determinant is returned to normal while all other abnormalities are held at their experimental values. If the low filtration rate persists despite the abrogation of the determinant in question, that determinant cannot be contributing greatly to the maintenance of renal failure.

Role of Increased Bowman's Space Pressure

Figure 16-5 shows the predicted effect of an isolated change in Bowman's space pressure on the SNGFR at the putative maximum and minimum normal R_A-R_E ratios of 0.35 and 0.65, respectively. With the lowest acceptable normal R_A-R_E ratio, a SNGFR consistent with that expected in human ARF is not attained until P_{BS} is increased from the assumed normal pressure of 25 mm Hg to 37 mm Hg. At the highest probable R_A-R_E ratio, failed filtration requires a 22 mm Hg pressure rise, i.e., to 47 mm Hg. It seems unlikely that such large increases in pressure would have gone undetected in measurements of wedged renal venous pressure [66]. In the remainder of our analysis, therefore, we assume that Bowman's space pressure remains essentially normal in ARF.

Role of Decreased Ultrafiltration Coefficient

The effects of K_f on SNGFR at the putative upper and lower limits for the normal R_A-R_E ratio are shown in Fig. 16-6. With the preglomerular and postglomerular renovascular resistances held at any of these limiting normal values, an 80% fall in K_f would leave GFR significantly above one-third of normal, far above the GFR expected in ARF. The glomerular membrane must become almost totally impermeable (i.e., K_f approaching zero) before this factor alone could account for the customary filtration deficit.

In view of the greatly reduced blood flow found in ARF,

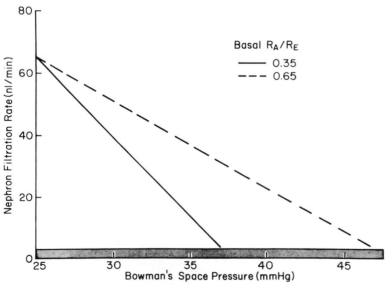

FIG. 16-5. *The effect of increased Bowman's space pressure on the nephron filtration rate of human kidney estimated by network modeling. Lines are shown for the theoretic normal maximal and minimal ratios of preglomerular and postglomerular resistance. The stippled area represents the nephron filtration rate in ARF.*

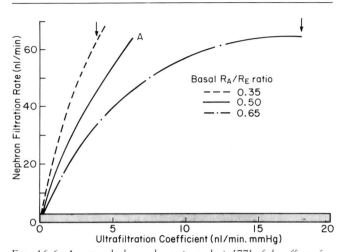

FIG. 16-6. *A network thermodynamic analysis [77] of the effect of a solitary change in the ultrafiltration coefficient (K_f) on glomerular filtration in humans. Curves are shown for the putative minimum and maximum basal values for the preglomerular (R_A) and postglomerular (R_E) resistances and for the intermediate value (line A, R_A-R_E = 0.5). Different normal, basal K_f values, shown with arrows, are required at each R_A-R_E ratio to provide a normal nephron GFR of 65 nl/minute. It may be seen that the K_f in humans must approach zero to lower filtration to the level expected in fully established vasomotor nephropathy (stippled area).*

it is clear that a change in K_f would not occur in isolation. What, then, is the potential effect of reducing the K_f in concert with increased preglomerular resistance? For ease of illustration, we have assumed an R_A-R_E ratio of 0.5, a value midway between the putative upper and lower limits, which requires a K_f of 6.5 nl/minute/mm Hg to provide a normal filtration rate. As may be seen in Fig. 16-7, R_A must be raised to 0.91×10^{10} dyne sec cm^{-5} in humans to reduce the filtration rate by 90% when K_f is held unchanged. A 77% reduction in K_f superimposed on this degree of change in R_A decreases the SNGFR by only 2% more, an effect with very little consequence for renal function. It appears, therefore, that an increase in K_f of even this magnitude makes very little difference to the filtration rate when superimposed on a primary change in R_A. A change in K_f of this magnitude also makes little difference to the degree of change in R_A required to cause filtration failure, the rise in R_A being only 5% higher than when the K_f remains entirely normal. Although not shown in Fig. 16-7, the effect of this degree of K_f change on SNGFR is no greater when introduced with concomitant changes in the preglomerular and postglomerular resistances or Bowman's space pressure [80]. Thus, although any reduction in K_f must lower filtration to some degree, change in this variable apparently can contribute importantly to the pathogenesis of ARF only if the glomerular membrane becomes virtually impermeable.

Role of Preglomerular and Postglomerular Resistance

Figure 16-8 illustrates the effect of an isolated increase in preglomerular vascular resistance on SNGFR in humans with all other glomerular dynamic parameters held at their normal values. It can be seen that frank filtration failure is obtained when R_A rises only twofold to threefold, the actual value depending on the basal R_A-R_E ratio assumed. With a presumed normal R_A-R_E ratio of 0.5 (see previously), however, this degree of change in R_A would reduce renal cortical blood flow by only some 30%. Indeed, modeling shows that a fourfold rise in R_A would be required to cause a 50% decrease in RBF and an eightfold rise is needed to reduce blood flow by 70% [80]. If, therefore, preglomerular vasoconstriction is the primary cause of renal ischemia in this disorder, it more than suffices to produce frank filtration failure as well.

The postglomerular vasculature cannot be visualized angiographically, and we do not know whether the marked preglomerular resistance change found in human ARF is accompanied by either constriction or relaxation of the postglomerular vascular segment. Postglomerular vascular relaxation would lower the degree of rise in preglomerular resistance needed to provide filtration failure, whereas concomitant constriction of the two vascular beds would have the converse effect. Figure 16-9 shows the fall in glomerular filtration predicted when the preglomerular and postglomerular resistances are raised proportionally over a wide range. The glomerular ultrafiltration coefficient and Bowman's space pressure are held at their normal values. It may be seen that doubling both resistances to reduce cortical blood flow by one-half would leave filtration at 52% to 67% of normal. Filtration would be maintained at 34% to 57% of normal with even the 3.3-fold rise in total vascular resistance required to produce a 70% fall in blood flow. Such a high GFR is not consistent with human ARF, and, if changes in the resistances of the preglomerular and postglomerular beds actually are matched in this disorder, the extremely low measured GFR could be accounted for only by superimposing a massive reduction in glomerular permeability or almost total leakage of all the filtrate formed. Because the preglomerular and postglomerular vessels do not appear to change resistance precisely equally in response to other known vasoconstrictor and vasodilator stimuli [34], however, there is no reason to believe that the tone of these two vascular beds should change in that manner in subjects with acute renal failure. Such a possibility cannot be formally excluded, but the mere 15% to 25% decrease in preglomerular vessel caliber that would accompany this smaller rise in preglomerular resistance (see Fig. 16-2) is not at all consistent with the very marked arterial attenuation found in this disorder.

Although precisely matched increases in preglomerular and postglomerular resistance alone cannot cause the extreme filtration deficit typical of ARF, failed filtration is readily attained with simultaneous changes in the two resistances, provided that the change in R_E is somewhat less than that in R_A. With cortical blood flow reduced by one-half, for instance, full filtration failure can be attained with

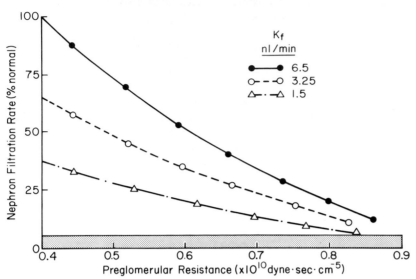

FIG. 16-7. *Network analysis [80] of the effect of combined changes in preglomerular resistance and the ultrafiltration coefficient (K_f) on nephron filtration rate in humans, using a putative normal R_A-R_E ratio of 0.5 and K_f of 6.5 nl/minute mm Hg. Raising R_A to 0.85 $\times$ 10^{10} dyne sec cm^{-5} with K_f held at its putative normal value (upper curve) lowers SNGFR toward the level expected in vasomotor nephropathy (shaded area). Reducing K_f by as much as 50% or 77% (lower curves) has only a small additional effect on filtration.*

failed filtration can occur with even a twofold increase in R_E [80]. In theory, then, renal failure can be induced in humans on a purely hemodynamic basis despite a very substantial increase in postglomerular resistance [80]. The actual contribution of the individual preglomerular and postglomerular vascular beds to the overall resistance change remains to be proved.

Micropuncture Studies of Acute Renal Failure in the Rat

The original micropuncture study of ARF in the rat [42] was undertaken to determine whether glomerular filtration in high dose mercury poisoning is well preserved (as postulated by the passive backflow theory) and, if not, whether tubular obstruction is essential to the development of filtration failure. That study showed the virtual absence of filtration with no evident tubular obstruction and no need to incriminate tubular leakage as an essential pathogenetic factor [42]. A number of studies performed since then have yielded similar results. Where discrepancies have appeared in different studies of a given model, some seem to reflect the different intervals between the induction of ARF and the time of study, whereas others relate to the use of different dosages of the inciting agent. Still others seem to be due as much to the interpretation of results as to differences in the results themselves. Certain models, however, stand apart and have distinctly different pathogenetic features from the rest.

Glomerular Filtration and Blood Flow in Murine Acute Renal Failure

Glomerular filtration in surface nephrons (SNGFR) is greatly reduced or totally lacking in fully established ARF induced by uranium, mercury, dichromate, glycerol, or methemoglobin[9,26,39,40,42,48,53,56,73,74,76,91,102, 107,117–120]. An essentially normal SNGFR has been reported in three studies of low dose mercury poisoning [6,28,40], possibly caused by an artifact of nephron venting. Blantz [11] found the SNGFR to be reduced by only 35% early in the course of uranyl nitrate poisoning, and well-maintained values of SNGFR have been found in the early phase of postischemic ARF [2,35,57,104–106]. It is important to note that in these two models of ARF in the rat, unlike other forms of ARF, proximal tubular pressure is very high [2,35,57,104–106], which should result in a low filtration rate. Tanner et al. [104] commented that the filtration rates may have been falsely raised by venting this excessive pressure. Conger et al. [27] have documented the effects of such pressure venting in the norepinephrine/acetylcholine model.

Hemodynamic Factors in the Pathogenesis of Acute Renal Failure in the Rat

Renal blood flow is essentially normal in high and low dose mercury poisoning [24,52], glycerol-induced myohemoglobinuria [24,51], methemoglobinemia [56], postischemic

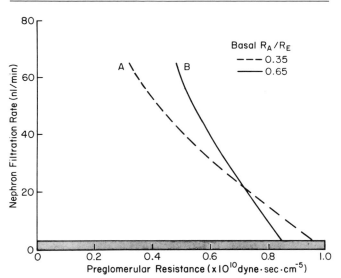

FIG. 16-8. *The effect of isolated change in preglomerular resistance on nephron filtration in humans at putative preglomerular to postglomerular resistance ratios of 0.35 (A) and 0.65 (B) in the control state. Filtration is seen to fall to the level expected in vasomotor nephropathy (shaded area) with only a 75% (curve E) to 2.8-fold increase in resistance (curve A) at the two limiting RA-RE ratios.*

ARF [2,24], and the norepinephrine model [27]. The early phase of glycerol-induced [4,22] and uranyl nitrate–induced ARF [11] and the late phase of postischemic ARF [23,57] are exceptions, RBF being considerably reduced. The essentially normal RBF found in most forms of murine ARF contrasts sharply with the marked renal ischemia found in humans (see previously).

Some authors have assumed that normal RBF necessarily equates with a reasonably normal GFR, and that tubular backleakage thus must be the cause of renal failure in the rat. That assumption is not warranted from a theoretic point of view, since normal blood flow can coexist with total filtration failure in the presence of reciprocal changes in preglomerular and postglomerular vascular resistance, increased Bowman's space pressure, or reduced glomerular permeability [79].

Network modeling [77] has shown that a solitary increase in preglomerular resistance large enough to decrease single nephron filtration in the rat by 90% would reduce GBF by approximately one-half [79]. A decrease in postglomerular resistance sufficient to produce this same impairment of filtration would cause a 20% to 25% increase in blood flow. Thus, a change in either resistance alone is indeed inconsistent with the normal blood flow values reported. On the other hand, modeling also has shown that a rise in R_A of as little as 26% would reduce filtration in the hydropenic rat to 10% of control if matched by a comparable decrease in R_E [44]; blood flow would be minimally changed. A 30% increase in R_A under the same circumstance would totally abolish filtration [79]. Experiments cited subse-

quently have documented such reciprocal changes in vascular resistance and normal blood flow in high dose mercury and glycerol-induced renal failure [119,120].

Glomerular Permeability in Murine Acute Renal Failure

Decreased glomerular capillary hydraulic conductivity would seem to be an attractive potential cause for failed filtration, particularly in models in which both RBF and proximal tubular pressure are essentially normal. In support of that view, Blantz [11] has reported a 74% reduction in K_f in uranium poisoned rats, and Baylis et al. [8] have found K_f reduced by 37% in animals given toxic doses of gentamicin. However, an entirely normal K_f has been documented in the partial ischemia model [30]; furthermore, the essentially normal SNGFR found after pressure venting of nephrons in ARF induced with folic acid [5], renal artery clamping [2], norepinephrine [27], and low doses of mercury [29] could not have been obtained if the K_f were significantly reduced.

It is difficult to assess the importance of any given change in K_f encountered experimentally without having some quantitative measure of the effect such as abnormality as would have on the SNGFR. Network thermodynamic modeling [77] has shown that the 37% fall in K_f reported for gentamicin poisoned rats [8] by itself would have decreased filtration by no more than 7%. Even the 74% reduction in K_f found early in the course of uranium poisoning should lower the SNGFR by only one-third [77], and that, in fact, was precisely the degree of change reported [11]. Thus, although changes in K_f of this magnitude might seem intuitively to be important to the genesis of filtration failure, the glomerulus would have to become almost totally impermeable before a reduced K_f by itself could provide for the degree of filtration failure found in most ARF models [78–80] (Fig. 16-10).

Tubular Obstruction as a Cause of Filtration Failure

Tubular obstruction has been assumed at times to play a key role in the development of both human and experimental ARF, on the basis of debris or "casts" found in tubular lumens. Hemoglobin casts are common in pigment-induced ARF; brush border "blebs" often fill the lumens of tubules with postischemic ARF; and luminal debris is found in abundance in mercury, uranium, and dichromate poisoning. Whether or not it obstructs tubular outflow, material present within tubular lumens at the time filtration stops has no way of escaping from the nephron until filtration is restored and flushes it from the kidney. The finding of luminal debris on histologic examination of the kidney thus gives no indication of its role in the genesis of ARF, and one must rely on measurements of proximal tubular pressure to determine whether such materials represent the cause or the result of failed filtration.

Obstruction to urine outflow can be assumed with con-

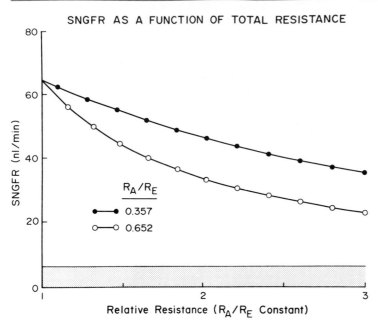

FIG. 16-9. *Network thermodynamic analysis of the effect of proportionally equal increases in R_A and R_E on glomerular filtration (SNGFR) in humans. The R_A-R_E ratios shown represent the apparent minimal and maximal limits consistent with normal glomerular function. Total vascular resistance is raised from its normal value (a relative resistance of 1) to a value that would reduce blood flow by some 66% (a relative resistance of 3). Even at this latter resistance, filtration is far above that expected in vasomotor nephropathy (stippled area). (From Oken DE: Hemodynamic basis for human acute renal failure [Vasomotor Nephropathy]. Am J Med 76. 702, 1984; with permission of the American Journal of Medicine.)*

fidence in any ARF model in which proximal tubular pressure is greatly increased. However, network modeling has shown that luminal pressure must rise some threefold to fourfold in the rat before this change by itself would depress filtration to the degree expected in fully established renal failure [79]. That degree of pressure change has been found repeatedly in the initial phase of postischemic and norepinephrine-induced ARF [2,27,104–106], although the pressure falls later in the course as complex hemodynamic abnormalities are superimposed [2,28,37,38].

Renal failure induced with large doses of folate [4] and globin [48] also is attended by a large rise in proximal tubular pressure, presumably as the result of the intratubular precipitation of these compounds when water absorption raises their concentration within the tubule. Proximal tubular pressure in these forms of ARF approximates the normal glomerular capillary pressure [2,104–106]. Because such massively elevated tubular pressures can be attained only when glomerular capillary pressure is normal or increased, it seems that hemodynamic factors play no immediate pathogenetic role in these particular models, at least in the early phase. With net filtration pressure virtually abolished by the high pressure in Bowman's space, moreover, any change in K_f that might be present could be of virtually no functional importance. Tubular outflow obstruction alone thus provides sufficient reason for filtration failure in these "obstructive" models.

A very large increase in proximal tubular pressure indicative of obstruction has been found also in the initial phase of uranium poisoning [11], but in this instance a comparable increase in glomerular capillary pressure left net filtration pressure unchanged. The raised proximal tubular pressure thus was not considered to play a significant role in the early phase of this form of ARF [11].

Almost all studies of fully established uranium, mercury, and dichromate poisoning as well as glycerol-induced myohemoglobinuric and methemoglobinuric ARF have shown an essentially normal or even decreased proximal tubular pressure [9,26,39,40,42,48,53,56,73,74,76,91, 102,107,117–120]. This finding by itself does not rule out the existence of tubular obstruction, because the proximal tubular pressure of otherwise normal rats with ureteral obstruction [3] and rats with postischemic ARF [2,105] falls spontaneously from a very high value to normal within 24 hours. An obstructive rise in proximal tubular pressure thus might be missed when the first measurements are made 24 hours or more after the onset of renal failure. However, that reservation does not apply to the mercury [42,118], methemoglobinuric [26,91], and glycerol [73,119] models in which serial measurements have shown low or essentially normal proximal tubular pressures during both the developmental and the established phases of renal failure. In these several models of murine renal failure, at least, failed filtration is not attributable to tubular obstruction.

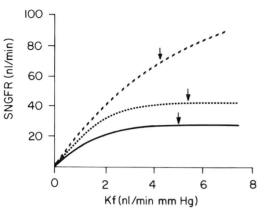

FIG. 16-10. *The effect of change in the glomerular ultrafiltration coefficient on nephron filtration rate in the "euvolemic" rat (dotted line), "hydropenic" rat (solid line), and dog (dashed line). Arrows signify the normal K_f and SNGFR with the different data bases. Note that, as in humans, the K_f must approach zero before the SNGFR falls below 10% of control.*

Tubular Fluid Absorption and Inulin Leakage

The severe tubular injury found in virtually all experimental models of ARF has led to the postulate that indiscriminate leakage of inulin is inevitable. An electron microscopic study of postischemic ARF reported by Donohoe et al. [33] has clearly shown the transtubular leakage of macromolecular markers. Histologic studies give no indication of the degree to which such leakage might contribute to the overall reduction in GFR, however, and glomerular filtration may fall markedly before tubular injury becomes evident [7,42,48,73,91,104]. Furthermore, rats given saline solution in place of tap water for several weeks before being challenged with mercury, dichromate, uranyl nitrate, or glycerol exhibit widespread tubular necrosis but maintain a near normal whole kidney GFR [32,40,48,92,107]. Animals recovering from either glycerol-induced or mercury-induced renal failure also are effectively protected from ARF after a second challenge with either agent, despite the recurrence of major tubular abnormalities [76]. The relationship between the development of renal failure and tubular histologic abnormalities thus is imperfect at best.

As judged from the tubular fluid-inulin concentration ratio in proximal and distal tubules, fractional water absorption is significantly decreased in several models of ARF [39,40,42,48,53,73,74,91,105]. When filtration has been too slow to permit such measurements, decreased water absorptive capacity has been demonstrated from the slow absorption of isotonic saline injected directly into the proximal tubules [9,39,40,42,48,73,74,104]. Such results are consistent with the decreased active sodium (and thus water) transport that might be anticipated in the presence of major tubular injury. On the other hand, stained solutions injected directly into the proximal tubule have sometimes been observed to leak from the lumen [9,53,104], and Huguenin et al. [53] have reported that fluid absorption

can be greatly augmented in the most severely damaged tubules of mercury poisoned rats by slightly increasing luminal hydrostatic pressure.

In some studies, reduced proximal tubule fractional water absorption has been associated with evidence of inulin leakage at some more distal site [11,29]. Thus, impaired salt and water absorption over most of the tubule's length and pathologic leakage of inulin from distal nephron segments at times may go hand in hand.

The role of tubular leakage in the pathogenesis of various models of murine ARF has been explored by direct intratubular injection of inulin [8,9,11,29,33,39,81,95,103, 104]. In these experiments, radiolabeled inulin is injected into single proximal tubules and the amount of inulin in urine recovered from the ipsilateral and contralateral kidneys is measured for a period of time thereafter. Major degrees of tubular permeability to inulin are effectively ruled out by the recovery of all or almost all the injected inulin in the urine produced by the injected kidney. Incomplete recovery of inulin from the injected kidney may reflect leakage, but it also could be caused by sequestration of the marker in tubules with virtually no flow to wash it out [81]. Any inulin injected into tubules of one kidney that appears in urine from the other must first have been absorbed into the blood stream, recirculated, and filtered before being excreted. This finding serves as proof of pathologic tubular permeability to inulin.

A certain amount of caution is appropriate in performing and interpreting inulin microinjection studies. The tubular epithelium is very friable in most forms of murine ARF [9,53,81], and there is thus the risk that insertion of a micropipet and injection of fluid might cause leakage that was not present in the undisturbed nephron [53]. The risk of leakage artifact seems to be greatest in those models that display both severe tubular injury and massively increased tubular pressure [61].

Of the several studies employing intratubular inulin injections to assess the presence and magnitude of tubular leakage, some have revealed little or no inulin loss from the injected kidney [7–9,27,28,30,37,38,81] and others have shown substantial or almost quantitative absorption of all the inulin injected [11,29,33,104]. Evidence of tubular leakage has been found routinely in the early phase of ARF produced by prolonged unilateral renal artery occlusion [33,81,104].

Blantz [11] reported on inulin leakage occurring in rats after the injection of uranyl nitrate. In most instances, most of the injected inulin was recovered from the injected kidney, providing evidence against, rather than for, tubular permeability as a major contributor to failed filtration.

Conger and Falk [29] reported that 18% of inulin injected into the tubules of one kidney was excreted by the opposite kidney within 20 minutes, despite GFR 10% of normal. Even when inulin is injected intravenously, however, one cannot recover 18% of the injectate from each kidney in only 20 minutes unless the measured GFR is essentially normal (unpublished observation).

In view of the numerous studies in which inulin leakage has not been found, it seems inappropriate to assume that abnormal tubular permeability is essential to the development of ARF. Even when inulin leakage is present in a given model of ARF, implications for renal function are the same as those discussed earlier for the human kidney (see Fig. 16-3), i.e., even massive tubular leakage could not account for the observed values of glomerular filtration in the absence of major hemodynamic changes.

Studies of Glomerular Dynamics in Experimental Acute Renal Failure

Studies of glomerular dynamics serve as the most direct means of investigating the abnormalities responsible for renal failure in the several murine models of ARF. Experiments of this type have now been performed in rats with gentamicin toxicity [8,95], partial renal ischemia [30], uranyl nitrate poisoning [11,12], low [29] and high dose mercury poisoning [119], and glycerol-induced myohemoglobinuria [120].

In the partial ischemia model, Daugharty et al. [30] found reduced filtration attributable exclusively to a modest decrease in GBF. Blantz [11] reported normal GBF, but a major decrease in K_f and leakage of the reduced volume of filtrate formed by rats studied in the first two hours after uranium injection. Baylis et al. [8] found a decreased K_f as the sole cause of the filtration deficit in gentamicin poisoned rats and detected no abnormality in tubular permeability to inulin. These three studies thus provide conflicting results. Nevertheless, since the GFR was depressed by only one-third to one-half, the applicability of those findings to models with fully established renal failure is uncertain.

As noted earlier, prolonged renal artery clamping results in a massive increase in proximal tubular pressure [2,87,105]. Glomerular capillary pressure is normal or increased and filtration is brisk when tubular pressure is vented. Presumably, therefore, K_f in these models is not substantively decreased [104].

Conger and Falk [29] have reported on the glomerular dynamics of ARF induced with low dose mercury poisoning. All the determinants of glomerular dynamics were entirely normal, as was the SNGFR; renal failure was attributed solely to pathologic tubular permeability.

Very different findings have been obtained in high dose mercury poisoning [119]. In this model, the superficial nephrons formed virtually no filtrate either before or after the insertion of a collecting pipette. Renocortical blood flow was normal, and Bowman's space pressure was not increased during either the development or the established phase of ARF. A major increase in preglomerular resistance and a reciprocal fall in postglomerular resistance reduced glomerular capillary hydraulic pressure to a degree that made filtration failure inevitable [119]. K_f could not be assessed in the absence of filtration, but, with virtually no driving force to promote filtration, even a massive reduction in this determinant would be of little practical importance. Deranged tubular permeability can be functionally significant only when a reasonable volume of filtrate is presented to the absorptive site. Because virtually no filtrate was formed, tubular leakage could not have contributed to the development of filtration failure. Similar

findings have been obtained in rats with glycerol-induced myohemoglobinuria [120].

Summary of Experimental Acute Renal Failure in the Rat

Because of the differing results obtained in various ARF models, views on the pathogenesis of murine ARF are sometimes considered controversial. However, the differences between studies seem far more closely related to the model employed than to the investigator performing the study. In fact, the various ARF models can be categorized into two general groups. One encompasses the mercury, uranyl nitrate, dichromate, methemoglobinuric, and myohemoglobinuric (glycerol) models, and the other contains the postischemic and norepinephrine models. Infusions of potentially obstructive doses of folic acid, Bence Jones protein, or globin produce abnormalities quite similar to those of the second group. That, however, is inevitable, since these latter models are destined by design to cause tubular obstruction.

In the first category, the majority of surface tubules are devoid of fluid and usually exhibit a normal or low luminal hydrostatic pressure from the very outset of renal failure. Filtration in these nephrons is grossly reduced or, at times, totally lacking. Greatly reduced glomerular capillary pressure has provided evidence that changes in vascular resistance play the key pathogenetic role. This group appears to fit the criteria for a "vasomotor nephropathy."

In the second group, proximal tubules are distended with fluid and have a remarkably high luminal pressure, which, by itself, is sufficient to stop filtration [2,104–106]. Nearly normal filtration rates are obtained after venting the excess pressure. These forms of ARF seem directly attributable to tubular obstruction, although complex hemodynamic alterations ensue later in the course of the disease [2,37,105]. The retained capacity to form large volumes of filtrate effectively rules out a major reduction in glomerular permeability as an important determinant in these models.

Some experimental models show a degree of overlap between the two major categories. In methemoglobinuria, for example, most nephrons manifest tubular collapse and low or normal tubular pressures, but a minority of tubules in the same kidney may be clearly obstructed [56]. In low dose mercury poisoning, spontaneous filtration is reported to be very scant and tubular pressures are not elevated [40]. Despite the normal proximal tubular pressure, however, a near normal SNGFR has been found after tubular venting [6,29,40]. This finding, which presently is not fully explained, seems to set low dose mercury somewhat apart from the other nephrotoxic models.

Mechanisms Underlying the Basic Abnormalities in Acute Renal Failure

Whether or not tubular injury is evident on histologic examination, tubular transport mechanisms are seriously impaired in both human and experimental ARF. The mechanisms immediately responsible for tubular injury in experimental models of ARF have been the subject of intense investigation in recent years [14,19,46,47,63,64, 86,93,99,108,109,114,115]. Most of these studies have been performed on tubules with a degree of injury far greater than that found in human ARF. Passive absorption of filtrate is not an essential feature of all ARF models, and renal function in humans would not be greatly improved if a tubular defect of the magnitude reported could be prevented or reversed. This, then, does not provide the essential relationship between impaired tubular transport capacity and filtration failure, which must be sought elsewhere.

Ischemic injury in the glycerol-damaged rat is attended by a fall in renal adenosine triphosphate (ATP) to approximately one-half its normal concentration [108]. The ATP activity rises spontaneously within hours, however, and may be normal during the phase of established renal failure [108]. Siegel et al. [97,98] have proposed that ATP depletion plays a major role in the pathogenesis of ARF in the rat. These authors and others [1] have reported that infusions of ATP with magnesium chloride offer substantial (but incomplete) protection of both renal function and renal histology in rats subjected to renal artery clamping. The mechanism by which such protection is mediated is unknown.

Although it is tempting to suggest that a product or products released from injured epithelium might be at least partly responsible for the hemodynamic abnormalities of ARF, the existence of such a factor has not yet been proved.

Adenosine is a potent renal vasoconstrictor with distinctly deleterious effects on both glomerular filtration and blood flow. In micropuncture studies of the effects of adenosine in the normal dog, Osswald et al. [84] found the SNGFR and glomerular plasma flow reduced by almost one-half. A large fall in glomerular capillary pressure was attributed to a doubling of preglomerular resistance with a slight increase in postglomerular resistance. The K_f was unchanged. It is intriguing and perhaps not merely coincidental that long-term salt loading, which is a highly effective means of preventing most nonobstructive forms of ARF in the rat, also minimizes the renal hemodynamic effects of adenosine [85].

Adenosine is present at measurable concentrations in normal rat kidney and rises some eightfold after only 10 minutes of renal arterial occlusion [25,86]. Theophylline and other methylxanthines reverse the general effects of adenosine [84], and Bidani and Churchill [10] and Bowmer et al. [15] have shown that these compounds provide significant protection of renal function in rats with glycerol-induced ARF. A distinct but lesser beneficial effect also has been found with theophylline [10], a considerably weaker adenosine blocker.

Hormonal Mediators of the Hemodynamic Aberrations of Acute Renal Failure

The control of renal and glomerular hemodynamics is assigned to the domains of the renin-angiotensin system, the prostaglandins, catecholamines, and kinins, all interacting in a complex fashion with neurogenic mechanisms. There is conflicting evidence regarding the possibility that the renin-angiotensin system plays a key pathogenetic role in ARF. The strongest support is found in the fact that long-term saline loading in the rat can almost totally prevent renal failure in a number of ARF models [32,48,107], a maneuver associated with maximal depletion of renal stores of renin. Administration of potassium chloride has a similar, although lesser, beneficial effect [41]. On the other hand, rats recovering from prior non-obstructive ARF also are highly refractory to a second ARF challenge [76], yet they have a normal renal renin content and release renin normally in response to either hemorrhage or isoproterenol injection [21]. The close interaction between angiotensin, catecholamines, prostaglandins, kinins, and adenosine on vascular reactivity makes interpretation of the salt loading experiments difficult. Treatment with captopril has yielded a degree of functional protection in studies of gentamicin [95] and uranium poisoning [12], and propranolol has been reported to ameliorate postischemic ARF modestly [55, 101].

On the negative side, active or passive immunization to renin and angiotensin [75] and captopril or saralasin treatment have been entirely ineffectual in preventing or reversing various forms of ARF in the rat.

Despite theoretic indications and early reports incriminating prostaglandin depletion in the pathogenesis of ARF, data that would firmly implicate such a mechanism in any form of renal failure have not yet appeared.

ARF occurs with some frequency in the totally denervated transplanted kidney in humans and persists in kidneys of rats with ARF after transplantation into normal recipients [98a]; thus, the renal nerves and other extrarenal factors do not appear to play an essential role in this disorder.

Comparison of Acute Renal Failure in Humans and Rats

With two or more distinctly different families of experimental ARF models, we cannot reasonably extrapolate from one model to the next, and it probably is inappropriate to assume that any murine model of ARF corresponds precisely to the disorder in humans.

Prolonged, total renal ischemia comparable to that produced in the ischemic and norepinephrine models rarely is seen in the setting for human renal failure. On the other hand, heavy metal poisoning is a well-known cause of human ARF, and methemoglobinuria bears some resemblance to the hemolytic diatheses. Similarly, the glycerol model shares many features with the crush syndrome and, when given to reduce cerebral edema, glycerol infusions have been documented to cause vasomotor nephropathy in humans [44]. The severe renocortical ischemia found in human vasomotor nephropathy is not duplicated in most murine models, however, and the human kidney rarely displays the extensive tubular necrosis found in the rat. Marked preglomerular vasoconstriction seems to provide sufficient cause for the virtual cessation of filtration in human ARF, but an increase or a decrease in postglomerular resistance may be present as well. Studies in the rat cannot prove the case in humans. Nonetheless, it is of some interest that this same abnormality has been found in the high dose mercury [119], dichromate (unpublished observation), and glycerol models [120], despite the maintenance of an essentially normal RBF. The thesis that at least some forms of ARF in the rat can have a purely "vasomotor" pathogenesis thus finds direct experimental support. The normal blood flow in these models is attained by coupling reciprocal changes in preglomerular and postglomerular resistance [119,120]. It is unknown whether postglomerular resistance might be reduced in human ARF but, if so, that change must be small relative to the degree of preglomerular vasoconstriction attained.

References

1. Andrews PM, Coffey AK: Protection of kidneys from acute renal failure resulting from normothermic ischemia. *Lab Invest* 49:87, 1983.
2. Arendshorst WJ, Finn WJ, Gottschalk CW: Pathogenesis of acute renal failure following temporary renal ischemia in the rat. *Circ Res* 37:558, 1975.
3. Arendshorst WJ, Finn WF, Gottschalk CW: Nephron stop-flow pressure response to obstruction for 24 hours in the rat kidney. *J Clin Invest* 53:1497, 1974.
4. Ayer G, Grandchamp A, Wyler T, et al: Intrarenal hemodynamics in glycerol-induced myohemoglobinuric acute renal failure in the rat. *Circ Res* 29:128, 1971.
5. Ayer G, Schmidt U, Truniger B: Intrarenal hemodynamics in two different models of acute renal failure (ARF) in the rat. Proc Fifth International Congress of Nephrology. Mexico City, 1972, p 165.
6. Bank N, Mutz BF, Aynedjian HS: The role of "leakage" of tubular fluid in anuria due to mercury poisoning. *J Clin Invest* 46:695, 1967.
7. Barenberg RL, Solomon S, Papper S, et al: Clearance and micropuncture study of renal function in mercuric chloride treated rats. *J Lab Clin Med* 42:473, 1968.
8. Baylis C, Rennke HR, Brenner BM: Mechanisms of the defect in glomerular ultrafiltration associated with gentamicin administration. *Kidney Int* 12:344, 1977.
9. Biber TUL, Mylle M, Baines AD, et al: A study by micropuncture and microdissection of acute renal damage in rats. *Am J Med* 44:664, 1968.
10. Bidani AK, Churchill PC: Aminophylline ameliorates glycerol-induced acute renal failure in rats. *Canad J Physiol Pharmacol* 61:567, 1983.
11. Blantz RC: The mechanism of acute renal failure after uranyl nitrate. *J Clin Invest* 55:621, 1975.
12. Blantz RC, Gushwa L: Amelioration of uranyl nitrate acute renal failure by converting enzyme inhibition and plasma volume expansion. *Kidney Int* 21:215, 1982.
13. Bohle A, Jahnecke J, Rauscher A: Vergleichende Histometrische untersungen an Bioptisch und Autopsisch gewonnenem Nierengewebe mit normaler Funktion und beim akuten Nierenversagen. *Klin Wochenschr* 43:1, 1964.
14. Bore PJ, Sehr PA, Chan L, et al: The importance of pH in renal preservation. *Transplant Proc* 13:707, 1981.
15. Bowmer CJ, Collis MG, Yates MS: Effect of the adenosine antagonist 8-phenyltheophylline on glycerol-induced acute renal failure in the rat. *Br J Pharmacol* 88:205, 1986.
16. Bricker NS: On the meaning of the intact nephron hypothesis. *Am J Med* 46:1, 1969.
17. Brun C, Crone C, Davidsen HG, et al: Renal blood flow in anuric human subject determined by use of radioactive krypton 85. *Proc Soc Exp Biol Med* 89:658, 1955.
18. Bull GM, Joekes AM, Lowe KG: Lesions of the kidney in acute tubular necrosis. *Clin Sci* 9:379, 1950.
19. Burke TJ, Schrier RW: Ischemic acute renal failure—pathogenetic steps leading to acute tubular necrosis. *Circ Shock* 11:255, 1983.
20. Bywaters EGL, Beall D: Crush injuries with impairment of renal function. *Br Med J* 1:427, 1941.
20a. Carrie BJ, Hilberman M, Schroeder JS, et al: Albuminuria and the permselective properties of the glomerulus in cardiac failure. *Kidney Int* 17:507, 1980.
21. Carvalho JS, Landwehr DM, Oken DE: Renin release and the refractoriness to acute renal failure of rats recovering from prior renal failure. *Nephron* 22:107, 1978.
22. Chedru MF, Baethke R, Oken DE: Renal cortical blood flow and glomerular filtration in myohemoglobinuric acute renal failure. *Kidney Int* 1:232, 1972.
23. Chevalier RL, Finn WF: Effects of propranolol on postischemic acute renal failure. *Nephron* 25:77, 1980.
24. Churchill S, Zarlengo MC, Carvalho JS, et al: Normal renocortical blood flow in experimental acute renal failure. *Kidney Int* 11:246, 1977.
25. Churchill PC, Bidani AK: Hypothesis: Adenosine mediates hemodynamic changes in renal failure. *Med Hypothesis* 8:275, 1982.
26. Cirksena WJ, Keller HI, Bernier G, et al: Pathogenetic studies in a model of pigment nephropathy in the rat. In Gessler U, Schroder K, Wedinger H (eds): *Pathogenesis and Clinical Findings with Renal Failure.* Georg Thieme Verlag, Stuttgart, 1971, p 105.
27. Conger JD, Robinette JB, Guggenheim SJ: Effect of acetylcholine on the early phase of reversible norepinephrine-induced acute renal failure. *Kidney Int* 19:399, 1981.
28. Conger JD, Robinette JB, Kelleher SP: Nephron heterogeneity in ischemic acute renal failure. *Kidney Int* 26:422, 1984.
29. Conger JD, Falk SA: Glomerular and tubular dynamics in mercuric-chloride-induced acute renal failure. *J Lab Clin Med* 107:281, 1986.
30. Daugharty TM, Ueki IF, Mercer PF, et al: Dynamics of glomerular ultrafiltration in the rat. V. Response to ischemic injury. *J Clin Invest* 53:105, 1974.
31. de Rougemont D, Oeschger A, Konrad L, et al: Gentamicin-induced acute renal failure in the rat. Effect of dehydration, DOCA-saline and furosemide. *Nephron* 29:176, 1981.
32. DiBona GF, McDonald FD, Flamenbaum W, et al: Maintenance of renal function in salt depleted rats despite severe tubular necrosis induced by HgCl$_2$. *Nephron* 8:205, 1971.
33. Donohoe JF, Venkatachalam MA, Bernard DB, et al: Tubular leakage and obstruction after renal ischemia: Structural-functional correlations. *Kidney Int* 13:208, 1978.
34. Edwards RM: Segmental effects of norepinephrine and angiotensin II on isolated renal microvessels. *Am J Physiol* 244:F526, 1983.
35. Eisenbach G, Steinhausen M: Micropuncture studies after temporary ischemia. *Pflueger Arch* 343:11, 1973.
36. Finckh ES, Jeremy D, Whyte HM: Structural renal damage and its relation to the clinical features in oliguric acte renal failure. *Quart J Med* 31:429, 1962.
37. Finn WF, Chevalier RL: Recovery from post-ischemic acute renal failure in the rat. *Kidney Int* 16:113, 1979.
38. Finn WF: Enhanced recovery from postischemic acute renal failure. Micropuncture studies in the rat. *Circ Res* 46:440, 1980.
39. Flamenbaum W, Huddleston ML, McNeil JS, et al: Uranyl

nitrate-induced acute renal failure in the rat: Micropuncture and renal hemodynamic studies. *Kidney Int* 6:408, 1974.

40. Flamenbaum W, McDonald FD, DiBona GF, et al: Micropuncture study of renal tubular factors in low dose mercury poisoning. *Nephron* 8:221, 1971.

41. Flamenbaum W, Kotchen TA, Nagle R, et al: Effect of potassium on the renin angiotensin system and HgCl$_2$-induced acute renal failure. *Am J Physiol* 224:305, 1973.

42. Flanigan WJ, Oken DE: Renal micropuncture study of the development of anuria in the rat with mercury-induced acute renal failure. *J Clin Invest* 44:449, 1965.

43. Hackradt A: Uber akute, todliche Vasomotorische Nephrose nach Verschuttung. Inaugural dissertation. Munich, 1917.

44. Hagnevik K, Gordon E, Lins LE, et al: Glycerol induced haemolysis with haemoglobinuria and acute renal failure. *Lancet* 1:75, 1974.

45. Hall JE, Granger JP: Renal hemodynamics and arterial pressure during chronic intrarenal adenosine infusion in conscious dogs. *Am J Physiol* 250:F32, 1986.

46. Hanson R, Johnson O, Lundstam S, et al: Effects of free radical scavengers on renal circulation after ischemia in the rabbit. *Clin Sci* 65:605, 1983.

47. Hems DA, Brosnan JT: Effect of ischemia on content of metabolites in rat liver and kidney in vivo. *Biochem J* 120:105, 1970.

48. Henry LN, Lane CE, Kashgarian M: Micropuncture studies of the pathophysiology of acute renal failure in the rat. *Lab Invest* 19:309, 1968.

49. Hollenberg NK, Epstein M, Rosen SM, et al: Acute oliguric renal failure in man. Evidence for preferential renal cortical ischemia. *Medicine* (Baltimore) 47:455, 1968.

50. Hollenberg NK, Adams DF, Oken DE, et al: Acute renal failure due to nephrotoxins. *N Engl J Med* 282:1329, 1970.

51. Hsu CH, Kurtz TW, Goldstein JR, et al: Intrarenal hemodynamics in acute myohemoglobinuric renal failure. *Nephron* 17:65, 1976.

52. Hsu CH, Kurtz TW, Rosenzweig J, et al: Renal hemodynamics in HgCl$_2$-induced acute renal failure. *Nephron* 18:326, 1977.

53. Huguenin M, Thiel G, Brunner FP: HgCl$_2$-induced acute renal failure studied by split drop micropuncture technique in the rat. *Nephron* 20:147, 1978.

54. Husfeldt E, Bjering T: Renal lesion from traumatic shock. *Acta Med Scand* 91:279, 1937.

55. Iaina A, Solomon S, Eliahou HE: Reduction in severity of acute renal failure by beta-adrenergic blockade. *Lancet* 2:157, 1975.

56. Jaenike JR: Micropuncture study of methemoglobin-induced acute renal failure in the rat. *J Lab Clin Med* 73:459, 1969.

57. Karlberg L, Kallskog O, Norlen BJ, et al: Nephron function in postischemic acute renal failure. *Scand J Urol Nephrol* 16:167, 1982.

58. Karlberg L, Norlen BJ, Ojteg G, et al: Impaired medullary circulation in post-ischemic acute renal failure. *Acta Physiol Scand* 118:11, 1983.

59. Kaufmann E: Neuer Beitrag zur Sublimatintoxikation nebst Bunerkungen Uber die Sublimatnure. *Virchow's Arch Path Anat* 117:227, 1889.

60. Ladefoged J, Winkler K: Hemodynamics in acute renal failure. The effect of hypotension induced by dihydralazine on renal blood flow, mean circulation time for plasma, and renal vascular volume in patients with acute oliguric renal failure. *Scand J Clin Lab Invest* 26:83, 1970.

61. Lorentz WB, Lassiter WE, Gottschalk CW: Renal tubular permeability during increased intrarenal pressure. *J Clin Invest* 51:484, 1972.

62. Mason J, Olbricht C, Takabatake T, et al: The early phase

63. Mergner WJ, Smith MW, Sahaphong S, et al: Studies on the pathogenesis of ischemic cell injury. VI. Accumulation of calcium by isolated mitochondria in ischemic rat kidney cortex. *Virchow's Arch Path (Cell Pathol)* 26:1, 1977.

64. Mergner WJ, Smith MA, Trump BF: Studies on the pathogenesis of ischemic cell injury. IV. Alteration of ionic permeability of mitochondria from ischemic rat kidney. *Exp Mol Pathol* 26:1, 1977.

65. Miller WL, Thomas RA, Berne RM, et al: Adenosine production in the ischemic kidney. *Circ Res* 43:390, 1978.

66. Munck O: Renal circulation in acute renal failure. Oxford: Blackwell, 1958.

67. Munck O, Ladefoged J, Pedersen F: Distribution of blood flow in the kidney in acute renal failure. *In* Gessler U, Schroder K, Weidinger H (eds): *Pathogenesis and Clinical Findings with Renal Failure.* Georg Thiem Verlag, Stuttgart, 1971, p 1.

68. Murray RD, Churchill PC: Effects of adenosine receptor agonists in the isolated, perfused rat kidney. *Am J Physiol* 247:H343, 1984.

69. Myers BD, Chui F, Hilberman M, et al: Transtubular leakage of glomerular filtrate in human acute renal failure. *Am J Physiol* 237:F319, 1979.

70. Myers BD, Hilberman M, Spencer RJ, et al: Glomerular and tubular function in non-oliguric acute renal failure. *Am J Med* 72:642, 1982.

71. Myers BD, Carrie BJ, Yee RR, et al: Pathophysiology of hemodynamically mediated acute renal failure in man. *Kidney Int* 18:495, 1980.

72. Neugarten J, Aynedjian HS, Bank N: Role of tubular obstruction in acute renal failure due to gentamicin. *Kidney Int* 24:330, 1983.

73. Oken DE, Arce ML, Wilson DR: Glycerol-induced hemoglobinuric acute renal failure in the rat. I. Micropuncture study of the development of oliguria. *J Clin Invest* 45:724, 1966.

74. Oken DE, DiBona GF, McDonald FD: Micropuncture studies of the recovery phase of myohemoglobinuric acute renal failure in the rat. *J Clin Invest* 49:730, 1970.

75. Oken DE, Cotes SC, Flamenbaum W, et al: Active and passive immunization to angiotensin in experimental acute renal failure. *Kidney Int* 7:12, 1975.

76. Oken DE, Mende CW, Taraba I, et al: Resistance to acute renal failure afforded by prior renal failure: Examination of the role of renal renin content. *Nephron* 15:131, 1975.

77. Oken DE, Thomas SR, Mikulecky DC: A network thermodynamic model of glomerular dynamics: Application in the rat. *Kidney Int* 19:359, 1981.

78. Oken DE: An analysis of glomerular dynamics in rat, dog, and man. *Kidney Int* 22:136, 1982.

79. Oken DE: Theoretical analysis of pathogenetic mechanisms in experimental acute renal failure. *Kidney Int* 24:16, 1983.

80. Oken DE: Hemodynamic basis for human acute renal failure (Vasomotor Nephropathy). *Am J Med* 76:702, 1984.

81. Olbricht C, Mason J, Takabatake T, et al: The early phase of experimental acute renal failure. II. Tubular leakage and the reliability of glomerular markers. *Pflugers Arch* 372:251, 1977.

82. Oliver J, MacDowell M, Tracy A: The pathogenesis of acute renal failure associated with traumatic and toxic injury. Renal ischemia, nephrotoxic damage and the ischemuric episode. *J Clin Invest* 30:1307, 1951.

83. Olsen TS: Ultrastructure of the renal tubules in acute renal insufficiency. *Acta Path Microbiol Scand* 71:203, 1967.

84. Osswald H, Spielman WS, Knox FG: Mechanism of aden-

osine mediated decrease in glomerular filtration rate in dogs. *Circ Res* 43:465, 1978.

85. Osswald H, Schmitz H-J, Heidenreich O: Adenosine response of the rat kidney after saline loading, sodium restriction and hemorrhagia. *Pflugers Arch* 357:323, 1975.

86. Osswald H, Schmitz H-J, Kemper R: Tissue content of adenosine, inosine and hypoxanthine in the rat kidney after ischemia and postischemic recirculation. *Pflugers Arch* 371:45, 1977.

87. Parekh N, Esslinger H-U, Steinhausen M: Glomerular filtration and tubular reabsorption during anuria in postischemic acute renal failure. *Kidney Int* 25:33, 1984.

88. Peters JT: Oliguria and anuria due to increased intrarenal pressure. *Ann Int Med* 23:221, 1945.

89. Reubi FC: The pathogenesis of anuria following shock. *Kidney Int* 5:106, 1974.

90. Reubi TC, Vorburger C, Tuckman J: Renal distribution volumes of indocyanine green, 51Cr-EDTA and 24Na in man during acute renal failure after shock. *J Clin Invest* 52:223, 1973.

91. Ruiz-Guinazu A, Coelho JB, Paz RA: Methemoglobin-induced acute renal failure in the rat. *Nephron* 4:257, 1967.

92. Ryan R, McNeil JS, Flamenbaum W, et al: Uranyl nitrate induced acute renal failure in the rat. Effect of varying doses and saline loading. *Proc Soc Exp Biol Med* 143:289, 1973.

93. Sastrasinh M, Weinberg JM, Humes DM: The effects of gentamicin on calcium uptake by renal mitochondria. *Life Sci* 30:2309, 1982.

94. Schmidt U, Huguenin M, Thiel G, et al: Pathogenesis of folic acid induced acute renal failure. Proc Int Congr Nephrol, Mexico, 1972.

95. Schor N, Ichikawa I, Rennke HG, et al: Pathophysiology of altered glomerular function in aminoglycoside-treated rats. *Kidney Int* 19:288, 1981.

96. Sevitt S: Pathogenesis of traumatic uremia—a revised concept. *Lancet* II:135, 1959.

97. Siegel NJ, Glazier WB, Chaudry IH, et al: Enhanced recovery from acute renal failure by the postischemic infusion of adenine nucleotides and magnesium chloride in rats. *Kidney Int* 17:338, 1980.

98. Siegel NJ, Avison MJ, Reilly H, et al: Enhanced recovery of renal ATP with postischemic infusion of ATP-MgCl$_2$ determined by ^{31}P-NMR. *Am J Physiol* 245:F530, 1983.

98a. Silber JS: Transplantation of rat kidneys with acute tubular necrosis into salt loaded and normal recipients. *Surgery* 77:487, 1975.

99. Smith MW, Collan Y, Kahng MW, et al: Changes in renal mitochondrial lipids of rat kidney during ischemia. *Biochem Biophys Acta* 618:192, 1980.

100. Solez K, Finckh ES: Is there a correlation between morphologic and functional changes in acute renal failure? The data of Finckh, Jeremy and White re-examined twenty years later. *In* Solez K, Whelton A (eds): *Acute Renal Failure. Correlations between morphology and function.* Marcel Dekker, New York, 1984, pp 3–12.

101. Solez K, Freshwater MF, Su CT: The effect of propranolol on postischemic acute renal failure in the rat. *Transplantation* 24:148, 1977.

102. Stein JH, Gottschall J, Osgood RW, et al: Pathophysiology of a nephrotoxic model of acute renal failure. *Kidney Int* 8:27, 1975.

103. Steinhausen M, Eisenbach GM, Helmstadter V: Concentration of lissamine green in proximal tubules of antidiuretic

and mercury poisoned rats and the permeability of these tubules. *Pfluegers Arch Ges Physiol* 311:1, 1969.

104. Tanner GA, Sloan KL, Sophasan S: Effects of renal artery occlusion on kidney function in the rat. *Kidney Int* 4:377, 1973.

105. Tanner GA, Sophasan S: Kidney pressures after temporary renal artery occlusion in the rat. *Am J Physiol* 230:1173, 1976.

106. Tanner GA, Steinhausen M: Tubular obstruction in ischemia-induced acute renal failure in the rat. *Kidney Int* 10:S65, 1976.

107. Thiel G, McDonald FD, Oken DE: Micropuncture studies of the basis for protection of renin depletion rats from glycerol-induced acute renal failure. *Nephron* 7:67, 1970.

108. Trifillis AL, Kahng MW, Trump BF: Metabolic studies of glycerol-induced acute renal failure in the rat. *Exp Mol Pathol* 35:1, 1981.

109. Trifillis AL, Kahng MW, Trump BF: Metabolic studies of HgCl$_2$-induced acute renal failure in the rat. *Exp Mol Pathol* 35:14, 1981.

110. Trueta J, Barclay AE, Daniel PM, et al: Studies of the Renal Circulation. Charles C Thomas, Springfield, Ill., 1947.

111. Tune BM, Wu KY, Fravtert D, et al: Effect of cephaloridine on respiration by renal cortical mitochondria. *J Pharmacol Exper Ther* 210:98, 1970.

112. Vanholder RC, Praet MM, Pattyn PA, et al: Dissociation of glomerular filtration and renal blood flow in HgCl-induced acute renal failure. *Kidney Int* 22:162, 1982.

113. Walker JG, Silva H, Lawson TR, et al: Renal blood flow in acute renal failure measured by renal arterial infusion of indocyanine green. *Proc Soc Exp Biol Med* 112:932, 1963.

114. Weinberg JM, Harding PG, Humes HD: Mechanisms of gentamicin-induced dysfunction of renal cortical mitochondria. II. Effects of mitochondrial monovalent cation transport. *Arch Biochem Biophys* 205:232, 1980.

115. Weinberg JM, Harding PG, Humes HD: Mitochondrial bioenergetics during the initiation of mercuric chloride induced renal injury: I. Direct effects of in vitro mercuric chloride on renal cortical mitochondrial injury. *J Biol Chem* 257:60, 1982.

116. Willassen Y, Ofstad J: Postglomerular vascular hydrostatic and oncotic pressures during saline volume expansion in normotensive man. *Scand J Lab Invest* 39:707, 1979.

117. Wilson DR, Thiel G, Arce ML, et al: Glycerol-induced hemoglobinuric acute renal failure in the rat. III. Micropuncture study of the effects of mannitol and isotonic saline on individual nephron function. *Nephron* 4:337, 1967.

118. Wilson DR, Thiel G, Arce ML, et al: The role of concentrating mechanisms in the development of acute renal failure: Micropuncture studies using diabetes insipidus rats. *Nephron* 6:128, 1969.

119. Wolfert AI, Laveri LA, Reilly KM, et al: Glomerular dynamics in mercury-induced acute renal failure. *Kidney Int* 32:246, 1987.

120. Wolfert AI, Oken DE: Glomerular dynamic abnormalities in established glycerol induced acute renal failure in the rat. *J Clin Invest* 84:1967, 1989.

121. Wolgast M, Harvig G, Kallskog O, et al: Impaired medullary circulation as the causative factor in acute renal failure. *Uppsala J Med Sci* 26:S76, 1979.

122. Yorke W, Nauss RW: The mechanism of the production of suppression of urine in blackwater fever. *Ann Trop Med* 5:287, 1911.

ROBERT L. CHEVALIER

17
Response of the Developing Kidney to Nephron Loss

Successful adaptation to congenital or acquired nephron loss has been recognized for centuries [107]. Mechanisms by which remaining nephrons respond to reduced renal mass have been intensively studied over the past half century, but the unique problem of maintenance of homeostasis with nephron loss during development has been investigated only during the last few years. A number of similarities and differences have been identified in comparing normal with compensatory renal growth, and many important questions remain unanswered. Because most of our current understanding of compensatory renal adaptation during development has come from animal studies, this information is reviewed first, followed by an overview of specific clinical problems.

Experimental Studies of Compensatory and Normal Renal Growth

In considering compensatory renal growth during development, two separate stimuli must be evaluated: (1) requirements for normal somatic growth and (2) reduction in renal mass. Increase in renal size following unilateral nephrectomy is proportionately greater in the newborn rat or guinea pig than in the adult animal [39,136]. Hayslett [64] has shown that compensatory renal growth of the weanling rat exceeds that of the adult even when 75% of the renal mass is removed (Fig. 17-1). It is tempting to postulate, therefore, that compensatory renal growth is simply an enhancement of the normal growth process that is operative in early development. However, in a series of ingenious and technically difficult experiments, Silber and co-workers [137,139-141] demonstrated distinguishing features of the two types of growth. Transplantation of a third kidney into normal rats resulted in no change in the growth rate of any of the three kidneys in either young or adult animals [137,141]. In addition, renal plasma flow (RPF) and glomerular filtration rate (GFR) two months after transplantation were approximately 50% greater than those of control two-kidney littermates [141]. However, transplantation of a kidney from a previously uninephrectomized rat to another previously uninephrectomized animal resulted in progressive reduction in renal size, GFR, and RPF to normal levels [141]. In addition, Provoost et al. [124]

have shown an augmented compensatory increase in GFR and estimated RPF following transplantation of a juvenile donor kidney into an adult nephrectomized rat and attenuation of the response of an adult donor kidney transplanted into a juvenile recipient. These results suggest that compensatory renal growth is reversible, unlike normal or "obligatory" renal growth, which continues at a fixed rate regardless of the extrarenal environment. The question thus remains as to why compensatory hypertrophy is more complete in the neonate than the adult.

The premise that compensatory renal growth is age-dependent has been contested. Because the ratio of kidney weight to body weight normally decreases with age [39,136], Hutson et al. [73] examined compensatory renal growth in the mouse using principles of allometry that mathematically account for changing proportionalities between organ weight and body weight. These authors concluded that compensatory renal growth is complete 15 days after uninephrectomy and that the amount of compensatory growth is not dependent on the age at operation [73].

Using a different mathematical model, Harsing et al. [62] concluded that following unilateral nephrectomy in the rat, the remaining kidney grows at the same rate as the combined normal kidneys, with resultant mass equal to 70% of the total normal mass. They suggested that these findings are in fact consistent with a common mechanism for both normal and compensatory renal growth [62]. Nevertheless, as discussed previously, there are distinguishing features between the two types of growth.

Changes in Nephron Number and Size During Renal Growth

GLOMERULAR NUMBER

The question whether the mammalian kidney can increase the number of glomeruli following postnatal reduction in renal mass has interested anatomists for over 100 years [14]. A number of studies originally suggested that unilateral nephrectomy in early development may result in formation of additional nephrons. Following a report by Arataki in 1926 [4], in which nephron number was shown not to increase following uninephrectomy in the rat re-

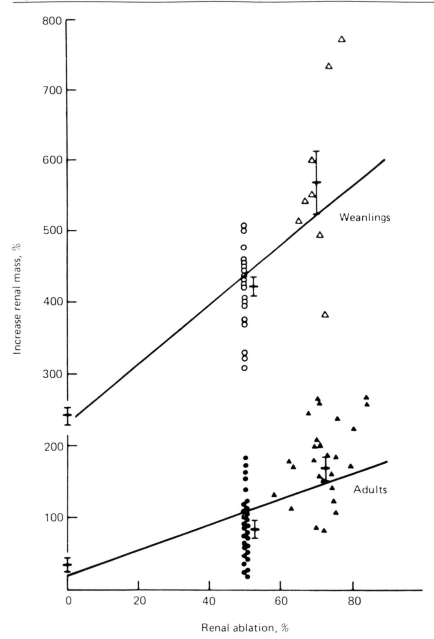

FIG. 17-1. *Compensatory renal growth in weanling and adult male Sprague-Dawley rats. The data show the percent increase in kidney mass 4 weeks following surgery in animals with varying degrees of surgical ablation. Bars represent mean ± SEM, in controls, after 50% nephrectomy (circles), and after approximately 70% nephrectomy (triangles). (From Hayslett JP: Effect of age on compensatory renal growth. Kidney Int 23:599, 1983; with permission.)*

gardless of age, the matter was thought to be settled. However, nearly 50 years later, Bonvalet et al. [15] reported compensatory nephrogenesis in the same species. Although in earlier studies glomeruli were counted in serial histologic sections, a tedious procedure limiting the number of animals examined, Bonvalet and co-workers counted glomeruli in acid digests of large numbers of rats [15]. The technique was further refined by Kaufman et al. [84] and Larsson et al. [92], who found no increase over normal in the number of glomeruli of rats uninephrectomized as early

as five days of life. Furthermore, careful histologic study failed to reveal nephrogenesis after the fifth postnatal day [92]. The apparent increase in the number of glomeruli reported by others was ascribed to artifacts resulting from overdigestion of the kidney or to accelerated development of pre-existing nephrons [92].

Additional studies were performed in the guinea pig, in which, like the human, nephrogenesis is completed before birth [22]. India ink was injected in vivo to identify perfused glomeruli, and glomeruli containing ink were counted

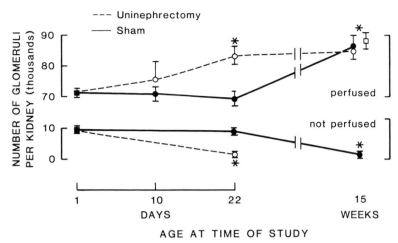

FIG. 17-2. *Number of glomeruli identified by India ink ("perfused," upper panel) and by Wright stain ("not perfused," lower panel). Uninephrectomy performed at birth (open circles) except group uninephrectomized at 12 weeks (open square). *P<0.01 vs. 1 day old. (From Chevalier RL. In Brodehl J, Ehrich JHH (eds): Paediatric Nephrology. Springer-Verlag, Berlin, 1984, p 56; with permission. Data originally from Reference 22.)*

in acid digests [22]. As shown in Figure 17-2, there was a 21% increase in the number of perfused glomeruli between three and 15 weeks of age in sham-operated animals. In animals uninephrectomized within the first 36 hours of life, the increase was apparent before 22 days of age, whereas uninephrectomy at birth or in adulthood had no effect on the number of perfused glomeruli at 15 weeks of age. At each age studied, the number of nonperfused glomeruli was inversely proportional to the number perfused (Fig. 17-2). This study suggests that during postnatal maturation of the guinea pig, up to 20% of glomeruli present at birth are not completely perfused until a later stage in maturation. This process is accelerated by uninephrectomy at birth but unaffected by uninephrectomy in adulthood when all glomeruli are perfused [22]. Since inhibition of angiotensin converting enzyme also accelerated complete glomerular perfusion [31], patchy vasoconstriction in early development may be mediated by angiotensin II.

GLOMERULAR AND TUBULAR SIZE

During normal growth of the rat, glomerular volume increases fourfold during the first five weeks of postnatal life [111]. During normal maturation of the dog from three to ten weeks of age, glomerular volume increases only 33% compared with an increase in nonglomerular volume of 235% [69]. Uninephrectomy in neonatal rats resulted in a sixfold increase in glomerular volume, which represents a 50% increment over normal growth [111]. Although there are no published studies of renal tubular growth following unilateral nephrectomy in the neonate, uninephrectomy in the adult rat resulted in a 35% increase in length and 96% increase in volume of the proximal convoluted tubule, with only a 25% increase in volume of the distal tubule [66]. Removal of 75% of renal mass resulted in a fivefold increase in proximal tubular volume, which enlarged even

further when the animal was given a high protein diet [110]. It is therefore likely that compensatory increase in renal mass during development is also due mainly to proximal tubular enlargement.

Changes in Cell Number and Size During Renal Growth

In a study of the effects of unilateral nephrectomy in the young rat, Rollason [128] noted hypertrophy of the proximal tubules as early as 24 hours after nephrectomy; this was followed by an increase in the number of mitoses throughout the kidney. Subsequent studies showed an increase in cellular RNA and protein content in the mouse within an hour of uninephrectomy [76]. The earliest detectable increase in cellular RNA content may represent slower degradation of rRNA, with enhanced rRNA synthesis occurring several days later [98].

Cellular hyperplasia measured by DNA synthesis peaked at approximately 48 hours after uninephrectomy in the adult mouse and accounted for only 25% of compensatory hypertrophy five days after operation [76]. In comparing the response of weanling and adult rats, Phillips and Leong [117] found that peak mitosis occurred at approximately 36 hours after uninephrectomy in both age groups, but the hyperplastic response was significantly higher in younger animals.

Because DNA was found to increase in rats uninephrectomized at four to five days of age but not as adults, other investigators concluded that hyperplasia occurs with compensatory renal hypertrophy only during early development, as an expression of augmented normal growth [39,79]. Celsi et al. [20] found that uninephrectomy in the rat at five days of age resulted in progressive increase in DNA content through adulthood, suggesting a primary hyperplastic response. However, in the guinea pig, a species characterized by renal maturation similar to the human, proportionately greater compensatory renal hypertrophy in neonatal animals was due to cellular hypertrophy rather than hyperplasia [136]. It therefore appears that compensatory renal growth results from a combination of increased cell number as well as increased cell size, with the relative contribution of each depending on the species under study.

Because compensatory renal hypertrophy is due mainly to increase in tubular mass, it is not surprising that the RNA-DNA ratio of renal cortical tubules increases as early as one day following uninephrectomy, while glomerular RNA content increases only slightly [147]. However, complex cellular changes take place in the glomerulus as well. The ratio of hypertrophy to hyperplasia is different for each glomerular cell type, with epithelial cells predominantly undergoing hypertrophy and endothelial and mesangial cells mainly hyperplasia [111].

Compensatory growth results in enhancement of the normal pattern of cellular hypertrophy and hyperplasia, which takes place uniformly throughout the cortical glomeruli [111]. Basement membrane surface area was found to increase 3.5-fold during normal growth with an additional 38% increase resulting from uninephrectomy of the young animal [111]. Of particular interest was an 11-fold increase in mesangial matrix during compensatory growth, double that occurring during normal maturation [111].

Changes in Cellular Metabolism During Renal Growth

Renal choline kinase activity is increased during normal postnatal development of the rat [9]. In the young rat, the initial cellular response of the remaining kidney to nephron loss includes an increase in choline kinase activity within two hours of uninephrectomy [9]. Because this enzyme is involved in cell membrane synthesis, its activation may initiate the compensatory hypertrophic response [9].

Although the signal for compensatory renal growth remains unidentified, cyclic nucleotides appear to be involved in the earliest response; cyclic adenosine monophosphate (cAMP) fell and cyclic guanosine monophosphate (cGMP) increased threefold within two hours of uninephrectomy in the adult rat [133]. In contrast, the cAMP-cGMP ratio increased during early postnatal development, and uninephrectomy at four to seven days of age prevented the normal rise [133].

Dicker [35] has postulated that a rise of cGMP and fall in cAMP within minutes of uninephrectomy may trigger compensatory renal hypertrophic changes after stimulation by a circulating humoral growth stimulating factor. However, the role of cyclic nucleotides in normal and compensatory renal growth is far from established and may be significantly influenced by experimental design [143].

Differences between compensatory and normal renal growth are also evident for the enzyme Na-K-ATPase, which increases in proportion to kidney weight in response to enhanced sodium resorption or potassium secretion during compensatory renal hypertrophy in the adult rat [46]. During normal renal growth, on the other hand, Na-K-

ATPase activity increases in proportion to protein content [118]. Compensatory growth of the remaining kidney following uninephrectomy in the weanling rat may result in changes in sodium reabsorption that are more similar to normal growth than to adaptive renal growth in the adult [46].

Stimuli for Compensatory Renal Growth

Considerable data have been generated to suggest that reduction in renal mass results in release of blood-borne renotropic factors (or suppression of circulating inhibitors of renal growth) [7]. The three major lines of evidence in support of the existence of renotropin are (1) cross-circulation studies showing hypertrophy in normal kidneys of parabiotic animals following reduction in renal mass of the partner; (2) demonstration of increased renal DNA synthesis following injection of plasma or serum from nephrectomized animals into normal animals; and (3) demonstration of increased DNA synthesis by in vitro systems after addition of plasma or serum from animals with decreased renal mass [7].

Persistence of the circulating renotropin may be required for maintenance of compensatory renal growth, since early biochemical changes as well as long-term increases in renal mass are reversed by removal of the stimulus [44,141]. Although circulating renotropin is probably not released from the kidneys themselves [61], a specific renal tissue factor may be required to activate the humoral one [121,122]. Interestingly, preliminary studies suggest that both serum and tissue factors from uninephrectomized young adult rats can increase thymidine incorporation into DNA of incubating rat renal slices, but sera and tissue extract from uninephrectomized older rats cannot [120]. In addition, Fine et al. [47] found that BSC-1 growth inhibitor (produced by monkey kidney epithelial cells) transformed a mitogenic stimulus into a hypertrophic stimulus for renal proximal tubular cells in culture. These investigators postulated that action of such an inhibitor may explain the predominantly hypertrophic pattern of compensatory renal growth in the mouse [47]. Of potential significance in this regard, a renal growth inhibitory factor could be extracted from the renal cortex of adult rats and mice, but not from kidneys of newborn animals [36]. Thus, enhanced compensatory renal hypertrophy during development may depend at least in part on quantitative or qualitative differences in specific growth factors and inhibitors.

Renotropins may be excreted in urine [61] and appear to be large molecules (12,000 to 25,000 daltons) [78,121]. Because renotropic factors have been shown to be heat stable [45,61], they are probably not proteins, although not all investigators agree [78].

An important question that remains to be answered is whether the circulating renotropins that have been characterized thus far represent factors that are actually involved in the hypertrophic response to reduced renal mass. It is now clear that the signal for release or activation of renotropins is not related to an increase in renal "work load," at least reflected by tubular sodium reabsorption [82]. Although bilateral ureteral ligation for 24 hours did not result in increased renal mass and cellular RNA content in normal kidneys of a parabiotic animal [108], reinfusion of half the urine output of an adult rat stimulated renal protein synthesis, increased DNA content, and accelerated growth [59-61]. Furthermore, unilateral ureteral ligation caused progressive increase in RNA-DNA ratio and mass of the contralateral kidney [38]. It is therefore likely that while increased solute load per nephron does not itself provide a stimulus for compensatory renal growth, the concomitant increase in the filtered load and reabsorption of renotropins may play important roles in this process [59-61].

In general, the response of the contralateral kidney to unilateral ureteral obstruction is similar to that observed in uninephrectomy and reflects the progressive atrophy of the affected kidney [150]. As with renal ablation, compensatory hypertrophy by the contralateral kidney appears to be proportionately greater in the newborn than the adult [71,145].

In addition to reduced renal mass and contralateral ureteral obstruction, a number of stimuli have been found to enhance renal growth. These include increased intake of protein, sodium, ammonium chloride, folic acid, and a variety of hormones, including thyroxine, testosterone, growth hormone, and mineralocorticoids [54]. Whether the mechanism of renal enlargement due to such stimuli differs from that due to reduced renal mass has not been generally established. However, the effect of growth hormone on renal growth appears to be stimulation of hyperplasia, whereas reduced renal mass results primarily in cellular hypertrophy [72].

Because RNA-protein ratio and DNA content of the remaining kidney increased following uninephrectomy but not with increased dietary protein, the biochemical effects of these stimuli also appear to differ [58]. Furthermore, the augmented hypertrophic response to uninephrectomy of young animals cannot be ascribed to a proportionately greater protein intake in early development [97]. It therefore appears that dietary protein and growth hormone, like age, may significantly modulate the hypertrophic response but are not its primary determinants.

The specific effect of dietary protein in adaptation of remaining nephrons to renal ablation is of particular interest because, although renal growth is initially enhanced by high protein intake [37], glomerular sclerosis and tubular atrophy also develop in an accelerated fashion [91,102]. As described subsequently, this progressive glomerular damage appears to be related to hyperfiltration of protein by remnant nephrons [70].

Functional Aspects of Compensatory Renal Growth

Acute Responses to Reduced Renal Mass During Development

The data regarding changes in renal blood flow (RBF) and GFR following acute reduction in renal mass are conflicting. Most studies have shown no change or a decrease in RBF following acute nephron loss [1,71,115,119]. However, Krohn et al. [90] found a 30% increase in RBF

immediately following uninephrectomy in the dog. More recently, Chevalier and Kaiser [30] reported that 30 minutes after right renal pedicle ligation in 30- to 40-day-old and three-month-old rats, left kidney RBF increased 13% to 22%. The reasons for these discrepancies are not clear, but probably relate to the technique of blood flow measurement. Clearance techniques are likely to obscure small acute changes in RBF, whereas use of a flow probe [30,90] reveals the earliest hemodynamic response to uninephrectomy.

Acute reduction in renal mass was found not to affect GFR by some investigators [1,71,115], but Potter et al. [119] observed an increase in filtration fraction and GFR 30 to 60 minutes after acute uninephrectomy in the adult rat, and Provoost and Molenaar [123] found a 25% increase in GFR of the remaining kidney four hours after contralateral nephrectomy. Fifteen hours after uninephrectomy in the adult rat, superficial single nephron GFR (SNGFR) increased 18% in the remaining kidney, although whole kidney GFR was found not to increase [40]. The increase in GFR in response to acute reduction in renal mass during early development has not been investigated but would probably be less than that of the adult, in view of the relative functional immaturity of superficial nephrons [144].

In contrast to changes in RBF and GFR, there is general agreement that urine flow and urinary sodium excretion increase promptly following reduction in renal mass [1,40,71,115,119]. This response has been termed "compensatory adaptation" by Peters [115], in contradistinction to "compensatory hyperfunction," which develops days or weeks after uninephrectomy [115,116].

Results of recent studies suggest that increased cation excretion following unilateral nephrectomy may relate to hemodynamic changes mediated by activation of a renorenal neural reflex [71,126]. Increased kaliuresis, which also results from acute uninephrectomy and is not dependent on renal innervation [126], may result from increased prostaglandin synthesis by the remaining kidney [63]. The role of these mechanisms in the response to acute reduction of renal mass during development remains to be investigated.

Chronic Responses to Reduced Renal Mass During Development

There is agreement that two weeks following reduction in renal mass, GFR has increased in remaining nephrons [64]. The time at which an increase is first measurable appears to vary between species, and is earlier in dogs [131] than in rats [119].

HEMODYNAMIC RESPONSES

In a study of renal ablation in the adult rat, Kaufman et al. [85] showed that the increase in the perfusion of remaining glomeruli was proportional to the amount of renal mass removed. Uninephrectomy resulted in a doubling of GBF, whereas 75% nephrectomy resulted in a 3.4-fold increase in flow 2 to 3 weeks after surgery [85]. Because RBF was found to increase proportionately more in the inner cortex than in the outer cortex, these investigators

Table 17-1. *Response of the canine puppy to loss of 75% of renal mass*

	Surgery at birth Study at 6 weeks			Surgery at 8 weeks Study at 14 weeks		
	Sham	75% NX†		Sham		75% NX
Renal plasma flow (ml/min/m²)	249.3 ±35.7	179.5 ±19.3		586.4 ±81.3	*	239.3 ±27.2
Glomerular filtration rate (ml/min/m²)	92.9 ± 7.8	80.0 ± 4.9		161.1 ±12.3	*	73.2 ± 9.0
N	7	14		4		3

Mean ± SEM.
* $P < 0.05$.
† ¾ Nephrectomy.
Data from Aschinberg LC, Koskimies O, Bernstein J, et al: The influence of age on the response to renal parenchymal loss. *Yale J Biol Med* 51:341, 1978.

R$_E$ raised by as little as 50%; with a 70% fall in blood flow, concluded that vasodilation resulting from renal ablation takes place predominantly in the deeper cortical areas [85].

In 14-week-old dogs studied six weeks after 75% renal ablation, RPF of the remaining kidney was less than 50% that of age-matched controls (Table 17-1), and increased glomerular perfusion was confined to deeper nephrons [6]. In eight-week-old animals subjected to 75% renal ablation at birth, however, RPF was not different from controls, and glomerular perfusion increased throughout the renal cortex [6]. These results indicate that hemodynamic adaptation to nephron loss is more complete in early development than later in life.

More recently, hemodynamic changes occurring within the first four weeks of life in guinea pigs uninephrectomized at birth have been compared with those of sham-operated littermates [23]. RBF more than doubled with normal growth from 10 to 20 days of age and increased an additional 70% as a result of uninephrectomy at birth [23]. Although the increase in RBF during development depended on both increasing cardiac output and falling renal vascular resistance (RVR) [23], the early compensatory rise in RBF in uninephrectomized neonatal guinea pigs was due solely to changes in RVR, which may be due in part to vasodilation of previously underperfused glomeruli [22].

Similar to the findings in puppies with 75% renal ablation [6], glomerular perfusion rate increased proportionately in all cortical levels during normal or compensatory renal growth in the neonatal guinea pig and was higher in outer and inner cortical thirds than in the middle cortex (Fig. 17-3). It appears, therefore, that hemodynamic responses of the newborn to renal growth are in most respects independent of the stimulus to increased renal function and that reduction in renal mass accelerates and amplifies the normal developmental pattern.

Renal hemodynamic function following uninephrectomy in early development does differ in some ways, however, from that resulting from normal growth. Although both normal and compensatory renal growth are characterized by vasodilation, the renal response to reduction in perfusion pressure varies with age. Autoregulation, whereby RBF is maintained constant during changes in perfusion pres-

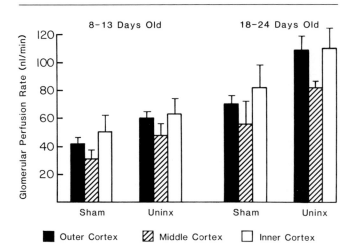

Fig. 17-3. *Glomerular perfusion rate related to cortical level sham-operated guinea pigs and animals uninephrectomized (Uninx) at birth. (Data from* Chevalier RL: Hemodynamic adaptation to reduced renal mass in early postnatal development. Pediatr Res 17:620, 1983.)

sure, takes place in the adult rat at pressures greater than 100 mm Hg [5,28], a range that includes normal mean arterial blood pressure [28]. In rats 30 to 40 days old, however, the autoregulatory range was found to be lower (Fig. 17-4) and encompasses normal arterial pressure at this age [28]. Uninephrectomy in the adult rat resulted in a 30% rise in RBF over the entire autoregulatory range, whereas uninephrectomy in the young animal resulted in a 35% rise in RBF at normal arterial pressure but only a 17% rise at a perfusion pressure of 70 mm Hg (Fig. 17-4).

It appears that the autoregulatory range shifts with increasing mean arterial pressure during normal growth and that autoregulation is reset to higher flows in the uninephrectomized adult but is impaired by uninephrectomy in the newborn rat. Because RVR rises more sharply at low perfusion pressures in the young animal than in the adult [28], the newborn kidney may be more susceptible to ischemic damage.

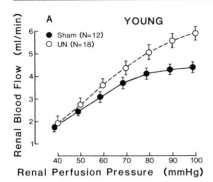

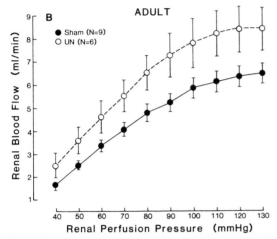

FIG. 17-4. *Relationship of renal blood flow to renal perfusion pressure for sham-operated rats and animals subjected to uninephrectomy (UN) 3 to 4 weeks previously. Upper panel (A) depicts young animals studied at 30 to 40 days of age; lower panel (B) shows adults studied at 3 months of age. Values are mean ± SE. (From Chevalier RL, Kaiser DL: Autoregulation of renal blood flow in the rat: Effects of growth and uninephrectomy. Am J Physiol 244:F483, 1983; with permission.)*

GLOMERULAR FILTRATION RATE

The compensatory increase in GFR following reduction in renal mass in the adult is generally less than the rise in RBF, such that filtration fraction is reduced [85,89,94]. Lack of change in filtration fraction following uninephrectomy in the developing guinea pig [23] indicates that in early stages of development forces favoring filtration balance decreased RVR.

The increase in GFR resulting from normal growth or renal ablation has been shown to be proportional to kidney weight [6,51] and appears to be unrelated to either cell number or size during hyperplasia and hypertrophy [118]. Increase in GFR following uninephrectomy can also be dissociated from cellular hypertrophy by using the RNA-DNA ratio [106]. These observations led Northrup and Malvin [106] to postulate that physiologic and biochemical adaptation to reduced renal mass may be under separate control systems. However, other investigators have found an increase in the ratio of GFR to kidney weight following

uninephrectomy [81,83] and a decrease following more severe renal ablation [83,85]. The latter is presumably due to compensatory increase in tubular mass after nephron number has been significantly reduced [83,110]. Because of the differing rates of growth of renal vascular volume, tubular volume, and cellular mass during normal and compensatory renal growth, factoring RBF or GFR by kidney weight may be misleading when comparing groups of different ages or degree of renal ablation.

Because increase in whole kidney GFR after reduction in renal mass is proportionally greater in early development than in later life (see Table 17-1), two possibilities exist: the sequence of normal physiologic maturation may be accelerated or augmented (as for RBF), or functional renal development may be altered by the added stimulus of nephron loss.

Adaptation by superficial and deeper nephrons must be considered separately since deep nephron function predominates during early postnatal maturation, with subsequent increasing contribution by more superficial nephrons. In a study of guinea pigs uninephrectomized at birth [21], compensatory increase in superficial SNGFR at ten days of age was found to be proportionally greater than that of deeper nephrons. This suggests that the centrifugal pattern of renal functional development is accelerated soon after nephron loss at birth. By 21 days of age, guinea pigs uninephrectomized at birth had achieved 90% of the GFR of sham-operated littermates, a process that may depend in part on earlier recruitment of glomeruli that normally remain underperfused until after three weeks of age [21,22]. It is interesting that whereas the normal centrifugal maturation of GFR is accelerated by nephron loss at birth, reduction of renal mass later in life results in equal compensatory increase in GFR of superficial and juxtamedullary nephrons [18,19,114].

For rats subjected to 70% to 85% renal ablation, SNGFR increases twofold to threefold compared with controls [83,114]. This may represent a limit to compensatory adaptation, as glomerular damage progresses rapidly in remaining nephrons when renal mass is reduced further [70].

Changes in glomerular dynamics that are responsible for the compensatory increase in SNGFR in the guinea pig uninephrectomized at birth have been studied by micropuncture in euvolemic animals [24]. Uninephrectomy resulted in a small increase in mean arterial blood pressure and glomerular capillary pressure and a fall in proximal intratubular hydrostatic pressure [24]. As a result of these changes, afferent effective filtration pressure (EFP_A) increased by 30%; no increase in EFP_A occurred during a comparable period of normal development [24]. Thus, in contrast to normal maturation [144], augmented pressure gradients for glomerular ultrafiltration contributed to early compensatory renal adaptation. In adult Wistar rats subjected to uninephrectomy, the compensatory increase in SNGFR was found to result from both increased glomerular plasma flow and transcapillary hydraulic pressure difference, but ultrafiltration coefficient (K_f) did not differ from that of control littermates [34]. However, in a study of uninephrectomy in adult Sprague-Dawley rats, EFP_A was unchanged, whereas K_f increased in the remaining kidney [48]. These discrepancies may be due to differences in strain, since filtration pressure equilibrium obtains in some Wistar rats but not in Sprague-Dawley rats [48].

Preliminary studies suggest that filtration pressure equilibrium is present in guinea pigs younger than 10 days [80], but data are not available for older animals with higher glomerular plasma flow rates. The relative contribution of glomerular plasma flow, EFP, and K_f to the increase in SNGFR following nephron loss in the neonatal guinea pig, therefore, remains to be established. However, increased glomerular perfusion and enhanced pressure gradients appear to play a significant role, whereas the rise in SNGFR with normal postnatal development may depend more on increasing surface area for glomerular filtration [75].

GLOMERULAR INJURY RESULTING FROM COMPENSATORY ADAPTATION

Studies suggest that increased glomerular capillary pressure and plasma flow resulting from extreme ablation of renal mass may result in glomerular injury by a number of processes [16,70]. These include increased protein filtration due to higher SNGFR and greater glomerular permeability to protein resulting from passage of larger molecules through the glomerular capillary wall, which also suffers a decrease in anionic charge-selective properties [70,112]. This phenomenon may be related to the increased uptake of injurious molecules by mesangial cells, whose function has been disrupted by nephron loss [57], and may be responsible for progressive mesangial sclerosis characteristic of more severe reduction in renal mass [121]. Activation of thrombotic mechanisms may also be involved in development of the glomerular lesion [125].

The cellular response of glomeruli undergoing compensatory growth ultimately depends on a delicate balance between residual renal mass, nephron GFR, and dietary protein intake [70]. The maladaptive responses are exaggerated by unrestricted dietary protein intake, such that protein restriction in uremic rats may actualy lead to improved somatic growth as well as preservation of GFR [88]. The specific mechanisms by which dietary excesses result in such adverse responses are not completely understood [87], and severe dietary restriction raises the risk of undernutrition, which would be particularly deleterious during early development [49].

TUBULAR FUNCTION

Limited data are available regarding tubular adaptation to reduced renal mass during development. In adult rats subjected to uninephrectomy, the reabsorptive rate of sodium per unit tubular volume remains constant in the proximal tubule and increases in the distal tubule, which undergoes proportionately less enlargement [66]. Proximal glomerulotubular balance is also maintained during normal and compensatory renal growth in the postnatal guinea pig, as shown by the linear relationship between the absolute rate of proximal tubular fluid reabsorption and superficial SNGFR (Fig. 17-5).

With greater than 50% reduction in renal mass, proximal glomerulotubular balance is disturbed. Studies of remnant kidneys of young rats indicate that distal sodium and water delivery are increased and fractional reabsorption by the terminal portion of the collecting duct is markedly

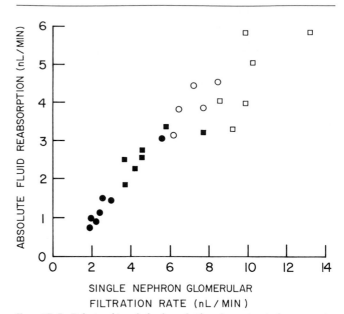

FIG. 17-5. Relationship of absolute fluid reabsorption in last accessible loop of superficial proximal tubules to single nephron glomerular filtration rate. Circles represent sham-operated guinea pigs; squares represent animals uninephrectomized at birth. Open symbols denote animals studied at 7 to 13 days of age; closed symbols, animals studied at 19 to 25 days of age. Correlation coefficients: sham, r = 0.98; uninephrectomy, r = 0.90. (From Chevalier RL: Functional adaptation to reduced renal mass in early development. Am J Physiol 242:F190, 1982; with permission.)

reduced [18]. Following 66% infarction of one kidney in young rats, the function of the surface nephrons of the remnant kidney was unaffected, whereas that of the deep nephrons was significantly altered [17]. Decreased fractional sodium delivery to the bend of the loop of Henle of deep nephrons results in impaired papillary solute deposition and lower urine osmolality [17]. However, uninephrectomy in adult rats has been shown to result in a concentrating ability exceeding that expected solely from doubling the filtered load of solute per nephron [132]. The effects of reduced renal mass on urinary concentration appear, therefore, to depend on the experimental model used and to be modulated by the stage of maturation at the time of the nephron loss.

Many important aspects of functional adaptation to reduced renal mass have not been investigated during early development, including response to volume expansion, potassium handling, calcium and phosphorus homeostasis, and acid excretion.

Clinical Aspects of Compensatory Renal Hypertrophy in the Infant and Child
Response to Uninephrectomy

In a study of renal growth of children who had undergone unilateral nephrectomy between 6 months and 13 years of age, Aperia et al. [2] found that renal size 1 to 20 years later was 68% to 82% of two normal kidneys. The ultimate size of the remaining kidney was inversely related to the age at the time of uninephrectomy. Somatic growth was normal in all patients [2]. GFR was proportional to renal size and averaged 75% of normal; bicarbonate threshold was normal. These data are in close agreement with a report of 27 patients who underwent unilateral nephrectomy between one month and 12 years of age and 17 to 33 years later had creatinine clearances averaging 74% of healthy controls with two kidneys [127].

In adult kidney donors examined 3 years after unilateral nephrectomy, renal area was found to be only 62% of that of both kidneys measured preoperatively, and the creatinine clearance was 77% of the preoperative value [42]. In both this and a previous study [109], compensatory increase in GFR was found to be inversely related to the age of the donor, but no effect of donor age on compensatory adaptation was detected in two other reports [13,113]. Boner et al. [12] have shown that the adaptive increase in GFR three weeks after nephrectomy in donors 21 to 63 years old is not influenced by age, sex, or previous GFR. However, four years later, donors under 40 years old had significantly greater compensatory increase in GFR than older subjects [12]. These data indicate that in the human, as in the experimental animal, compensatory adaptation to reduced renal mass is inversely related to age.

An issue of equal relevance is that of the hypertrophy of the transplanted kidney. Surprisingly, despite the surgical manipulation of the organ and the potential effects of nephrotoxic drugs, paired observations have revealed that the GFR of the single kidney increased to a similar extent in both donors and recipients, reaching about 77% of the preoperative GFR of the donor [45]. In an earlier study performed 2 to 4 years after transplantation, the GFR and estimated renal plasma flow of the donors and recipients were similar [109]. These studies indicated that the function of the transplanted kidney is limited by the capacity of the donor organ for compensatory adaptation.

Silber [138] examined the effects on renal growth of renal transplantation between adults and children. He found no increase in renal length of kidneys transplanted from adults to children, but a significant increase in length of kidneys transplanted from children to adults (Table 17-2). As expected, remaining kidneys of adult donors also showed compensatory hypertrophy [138]. The remarkable capacity of the infant kidney to undergo compensatory hypertrophy was illustrated by a 5-cm increase in renal

length six months after transplantation of a kidney from a 16-month-old into a 16-year-old recipient [74]. The authors postulate that the increase in GFR in the recipient was greater than the expected compensatory increment that would have followed uninephrectomy in the donor [74]. Provoost et al. [124] have found that three weeks following transplantation of adult kidneys into children, creatinine clearance (uncorrected for surface area) was lower in recipients under 12 years of age than in those older than 12 years. These observations suggest that compensatory adaptation is governed as much by stimuli present in the recipient as by endogenous characteristics of the donor kidney.

Exogenous insults may affect the capacity of the kidney to adapt. In a study of 108 children undergoing unilateral nephrectomy and radiation therapy for malignant disease, Mitus et al. [101] found that those receiving less than 1200 cGy had a greater creatinine clearance than those receiving more than 2400 cGy. Of 21 children eight months to six years of age with unilateral Wilms' tumor, 83% achieved "complete relative renal hypertrophy" 12 months after unilateral nephrectomy despite postoperative irradiation and dactinomycin therapy [95]. The compensatory hypertrophy was faster in patients over two years of age than in those under two years of age [95]. It is likely that younger children have a higher susceptibility to the nephrotoxic effects of radiation and chemotherapy than do older children.

Long-Term Effects of Reduced Renal Mass

Despite the apparent short-term adaptive advantage of infants and children compared with the adult deprived of functioning renal mass, their long-term outlook may actually be worse. Although unilateral renal agenesis had previously been regarded as a benign condition, it now appears that patients born with a single kidney carry a significant risk of developing focal segmental glomerulosclerosis, with evolution of hypertension, proteinuria, and renal insufficiency in adulthood [11,86].

Although adults may develop proteinuria 8 to 21 years following uninephrectomy for unilateral renal disease, hypertension and renal insufficiency usually are not observed, even when lesions of focal glomerulosclerosis are present [142,151]. There is increasing experimental evidence, described previously, suggesting that the adaptive increment in blood flow and filtration by remnant nephrons is re-

TABLE 17-2. *Longitudinal axis of kidneys (in cm) transplanted between adults and children*

	At time of transplant	4–6 weeks	5–9 weeks
Child's kidney transplanted into adult	10.5 ±0.3	12.7 ±0.6	13.4 ±0.2
		1 month	
Adult kidney transplanted into child	13.4 ±0.2	13.4 ±0.1	

Mean ± SD.
Data from Silber SJ. Renal transplantion between adults and children: Differences in renal growth. JAMA 228:1143, 1974.

sponsible for the lesions of focal glomerulosclerosis [70]. Because these functional changes are proportionately greater in early development, the infant and child may be at increased risk of progressive glomerular damage and onset of renal insufficiency [86]. Consistent with this hypothesis is the observation that patients with oligomeganephronia have less than 25% of the normal nephron number and develop renal failure in childhood [11,44].

Compensatory Renal Hypertrophy in the Fetus

Experimental Studies

Because homeostasis in the fetus is maintained almost entirely by placental function, it is not clear if decreased renal mass is a stimulus for compensatory renal hypertrophy before birth. Following maternal nephrectomy, there is an increase in the number of mitoses in the nephrogenic zone of fetal rats [129] but no increase in renal mass [53,129]. Unilateral nephrectomy in the 18½-day-old fetal rat resulted in increased mitosis in the remaining kidney; no renal enlargement was detected in this [130] and other studies [55]. Moore et al. [103] examined the response of the fetal lamb to unilateral nephrectomy during midgestation. Although these investigators found a significant increase in kidney weight 72 hours after operation, there

was no increase in GFR or para-aminohippuric acid (PAH) clearance [103]. Interpretation of the results is complicated by the use of single fetuses in the experimental group and twins in the controls [103]. Further studies are needed to resolve this issue.

Clinical Aspects

Laufer and Griscom [93] measured renal length in patients born with unilateral multicystic kidney, and normal contralateral kidney, a model of intrauterine unilateral nephrectomy. As shown in Figure 17-6, length of the normal kidney was not different from that of the kidneys of normal newborns, indicating that no compensatory hypertrophy had taken place in utero. However, rapid compensatory increase in renal length took place in the first 18 months of life, after which renal growth paralleled that of normal infants (Fig. 17-6). Estimated renal volume of the single functioning kidney at one year of age was equal to that of two normal kidneys, suggesting full adaptation in terms of compensatory renal growth [93].

Early functional adaptation of patients with unilateral renal agenesis also appears to be complete and exceeds that of children uninephrectomized in later childhood [3,134]. Compensatory increase in size of the single kidney takes place promptly after birth and may be detected sonographically as early as nine days of age [27].

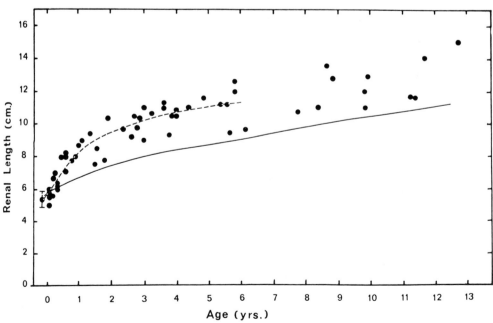

FIG. 17-6. Mean length of normal kidney measured from excretory urograms related to age of children born with unilateral multicystic renal dysplasia (interrupted line). Vertical line at zero years represents 24 measurements within the first month of life, with 1 SD being indicated. Beyond this age, the individual measurements are shown. Mean renal length for patients with two normal kidneys is represented by solid line. (From Laufer I, Griscom NT: Compensatory renal hypertrophy: Absence in utero and development in early life. Am J Roentgenol Rad Ther Nucl Med 113:464, 1971; with permission.)

Compensatory Growth Following Urinary Tract Obstruction

Experimental Studies

Growth of the kidney after unilateral ureteral obstruction differs in a number of respects from that of the contralateral kidney. Complete or severe partial ureteral obstruction results in renal enlargement due to dilatation of the pelvis, calyces, and tubules and proliferation of interstitial fibroblasts and mononuclear cells [29,104,150]. Increased cell turnover, detectable in the cortex and outer medulla within 24 hours of ureteral ligation, exceeds that of the contralateral kidney [105] and presumably constitutes a response to injury rather than compensatory growth. Unlike the contralateral kidney, initial growth of the obstructed kidney is due primarily to proliferation of mesenchymal cells (macrophages and fibroblasts) [150].

When partial ureteral obstruction is produced in the newborn period, impaired growth of the ipsilateral kidney is detectable by two to four weeks of age [29,145]. Furthermore, the magnitude of the compensatory hypertrophy of the contralateral kidney decreases progressively with age at the time when the unilateral ureteral constriction occurred [145]. Removal of the contralateral kidney at the time when the ureter was obstructed in the neonatal guinea pig resulted in compensatory hypertrophy of the obstructed

kidney, albeit of a lesser magnitude than that observed in a normal kidney [29]. Alterations in endogenous renotropins or growth inhibitors [121] presumably contribute to growth arrest of the obstructed kidney, and imposition of the entire excretory burden on the kidney with partial obstruction (by contralateral nephrectomy) may favor its continued growth.

Functional Responses to Urinary Tract Obstruction

Adaptation to nephron loss due to urinary tract obstruction differs from that due to removal of renal mass. Because acute ureteral obstruction does not result in nephron loss, only studies of chronic obstruction are considered here.

Congenital complete urinary tract obstruction results in a nonfunctional kidney, often with dysplastic changes [10,56]. In a colony of Wistar rats with mild unilateral congenital hydronephrosis, ipsilateral RBF and GFR were reduced by approximately 50% [50]. Partial unilateral ureteral obstruction in the newborn guinea pig resulted in a more profound reduction in GFR and tubular reabsorption of phosphate of the ipsilateral kidney than that observed with obstruction later in life [145]. The decrease in glomerular filtration in this model appeared to be consequent mainly to vasoconstriction (Fig. 17-7) associated with re-

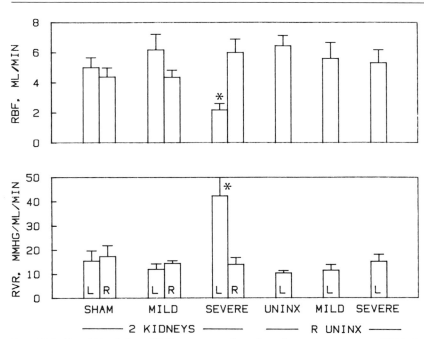

FIG. 17-7. Renal blood flow (RBF, upper panel) and renal vascular resistance (RVR, lower panel) for left (L) and right (R) kidneys of guinea pigs 18 to 30 days of age (mean ± SE). Animals were subjected to left partial ureteral obstruction within the first 2 days of life, resulting in "mild" (ureteral diameter < 3 mm) or "severe" (ureteral diameter ≥ 3mm) hydroureteronephrosis, and compared with sham-operated controls (2 kidneys). Contralateral nephrectomy (R Uninx) was performed in an additional group of animals at the time of ureteral constriction, and these animals were compared with those undergoing Uninx only. *P < 0.05 vs. sham control. (Data from Chevalier RL, Kaiser DL: Chronic partial ureteral obstruction in the neonatal guinea pig I: Influence of uninephrectomy or growth and hemodynamics. Pediatr Res 18:1266, 1984.)

distribution of RBF from inner to outer cortex [29]. Increased renal vascular resistance was due in part to the action of endogenous angiotensin II [31]. Removal of the contralateral kidney at the time of ureteral constriction prevented vasoconstriction (Fig. 17-7), and cortical RBF was redistributed toward deeper, more mature, glomeruli [29]. Recruitment of underperfused glomeruli, which normally occurs in the uninephrectomized newborn guinea pig [22], was not impaired by severe partial ureteral obstruction [29]. However, since filtration fraction was reduced during chronic partial ureteral obstruction in the newborn guinea pig regardless of the presence of the contralateral kidney [29], reduced RBF is not the only factor that results in decreased GFR. Increased proximal intratubular hydrostatic pressure and a lower ultrafiltration coefficient contribute significantly to the impaired renal function of newborn guinea pigs with severe chronic partial ureteral obstruction [26]. In contrast to the adaptation to renal ablation (which is more complete in early development than in the adult), the maturing kidney appears to be more susceptible than the adult to injury resulting from urinary tract obstruction. Prompt relief of the obstruction and preservation of functional renal mass consequently appear necessary to maintain homeostasis.

Clinical Aspects of Nephron Loss Due to Urinary Obstruction

Although a small kidney associated with vesicoureteral reflux had been viewed as "atrophic," implying progressive

contraction of renal mass, Lyon [96] suggested that renal growth is in fact arrested by the presence of reflux. Several reports have shown that surgical correction of reflux is associated with resumption of a normal growth rate of the affected kidney [96,99,148]. Wilton et al. [149] found that severe vesicoureteral reflux interfered with compensatory hypertrophy in response to a scarred contralateral kidney. Recurrent urinary tract infection, however, does not appear to affect compensatory hypertrophy of remaining nephrons [149].

In a group of 19 children with severe unilateral scarring associated with reflux, Bauer et al. [8] found that following ureteral reimplantation, the small scarred kidney grew at a normal rate regardless of the degree of contralateral renal hypertrophy. This observation lends further support to Silber's theory [127] that normal renal growth is predetermined, whereas compensatory renal growth is in some way controlled by total renal mass. Renal functional adaptation in children with unilateral hydronephrosis may depend on "counterbalance" between the two kidneys, resulting in constant functional renal mass [67]. Claesson et al. [32] have shown that compensatory hypertrophy of the contralateral normal kidney is directly proportional to the reduction in renal mass resulting from progressive scarring of the affected kidney (Fig. 17-8).

During development, the control mechanism may be particularly sensitive to stimuli. In the young child with unilateral ureteropelvic junction obstruction [100], compensatory hypertrophy of the contralateral kidney is detectable before significant hydronephrosis develops and becomes complete. By contrast, compensatory renal

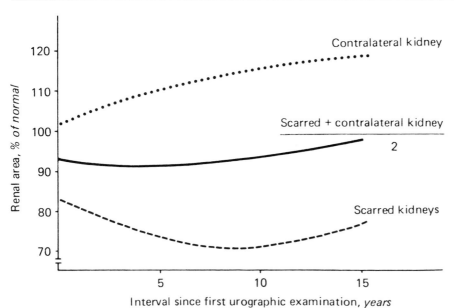

FIG. 17-8. *Renal parenchymal area in percent of normal in 26 children with unilateral scarring. The areas of the scarred and contralateral kidneys and the mean total area are given as function of time after the first investigation. (From Claesson I, Jacobsson B, Jodal U, et al: Compensatory kidney growth in children with urinary tract infection and unilateral renal scarring: An epidemiologic study. Kidney Int 20:759, 1981; with permission.)*

hypertrophy in adults with unilateral hydronephrosis is only partial [33,68,150].

Children and adults with reflux nephropathy may also develop focal glomerulosclerosis with proteinuria, renal insufficiency, or renal failure [146]. Although the decrease in GFR in children appears to parallel progressive loss of renal mass [149], adults may manifest declining renal function without significant change in renal size [146]. Radiologic monitoring of renal size in children with renal disease may lead to more timely surgical or medical intervention in a variety of disorders [43].

Congenital obstruction to urinary outflow results in significant impairment of renal growth and progressive parenchymal injury. Adaptation to urinary tract obstruction is largely dependent on the response of intact nephrons, which compensate more rapidly in the infant and child than in the adult.

References

1. Allison MEM, Lipham EM, Lassiter WE, et al: The acutely reduced kidney. *Kidney Int* 3:354, 1973.
2. Aperia A, Broberger O, Wikstad I, et al: Renal growth and function in patients nephrectomized in childhood. *Acta Paediatr Scand* 66:185, 1977.
3. Aperia A, Broberger O, Wilton P: Renal functional adaptation in the remnant kidney in patients with renal agenesis and in patients nephrectomized in childhood. *Acta Paediatr Scand* 67:611, 1978.
4. Arataki M: Experimental researches on the compensatory enlargement of the surviving kidney after unilateral nephrectomy (albino rat). *Am J Anat* 36:437, 1926.
5. Arendshorst WJ, Finn WF, Gottschalk CW: Autoregulation of blood flow in the rat kidney. *Am J Physiol* 228:127, 1975.
6. Aschinberg LC, Koskimies O, Bernstein J, et al: The influence of age on the response to renal parenchymal loss. *Yale J Biol Med* 51:341, 1978.
7. Austin H, Goldin H, Preuss HG, et al: Humoral regulation of renal growth. *Nephron* 27:163, 1981.
8. Bauer SB, Willscher MK, Zammuto PJ, et al: Dilemma of small pyelonephritic kidney associated with vesicoureteral reflux. *Urology* 15:466, 1980.
9. Bean GH, Lowenstein LM: Choline pathways during normal and stimulated renal growth in rats. *J Clin Invest* 21:1551, 1978.
10. Beck AD: The effect of intra-uterine urinary obstruction upon the development of the fetal kidney. *J Urol* 105:784, 1971.
11. Bhathena DB, Julian BA, McMorrow RG, et al: Focal sclerosis of hypertrophied glomeruli in solitary functioning kidneys of humans. *Am J Kid Dis* 5:226, 1985.
12. Boner G, Shelp WD, Newton M, et al: Factors influencing the increase in glomerular filtration rate in the remaining kidney of transplant donors. *Am J Med* 55:169, 1973.
13. Boner G, Sherry J, Rieselbach RE: Hypertrophy of the normal human kidney following contralateral nephrectomy. *Nephron* 9:364, 1972.
14. Bonvalet JP: Evidence of induction of new nephrons in immature kidneys undergoing hypertrophy. *Yale J Biol Med* 51:315, 1978.
15. Bonvalet JP, Champion M, Wanstok F, et al: Compensatory renal hypertrophy in young rats: Increase in the number of nephrons. *Kidney Int* 1:391, 1972.
16. Brenner BM, Meyer TW, Hostetter TH: Dietary protein intake and the progressive nature of kidney disease: The role of hemodynamically mediated glomerular injury in the pathogenesis of progressive glomerular sclerosis in aging, renal ablation, and intrinsic renal disease. *N Engl J Med* 307:652, 1982.
17. Buerkert J, Martin D: Deep nephron and collecting duct function after unilateral reduction in renal mass. *Mineral Electrolyte Metab* 9:137, 1983.
18. Buerkert J, Martin D, Prasad J, et al: Response of deep nephrons and the terminal collecting duct to a reduction in renal mass. *Am J Physiol* 236:F454, 1979.
19. Carriere S, Brunette MG: Compensatory renal hypertrophy in dogs: Single nephron glomerular filtration rate. *Can J Physiol Pharmacol* 55:105, 1977.
20. Celsi G, Jakobsson B, Aperia A: Influence of age on compensatory renal growth in rats. *Pediatr Res* 20:347, 1986.
21. Chevalier RL: Functional adaptation to reduced renal mass in early development. *Am J Physiol* 242:F190, 1982.
22. Chevalier RL: Glomerular number and perfusion during normal and compensatory renal growth in the guinea pig. *Pediatr Res* 16:436, 1982.
23. Chevalier RL: Hemodynamic adaptation to reduced renal mass in early postnatal development. *Pediatr Res* 17:620, 1983.
24. Chevalier RL: Reduced renal mass in early postnatal development: Glomerular dynamics in the guinea pig. *Biol Neonate* 44:158, 1983.
25. Chevalier RL: Functional adaptation to reduced renal mass in early postnatal development. *In* Brodehl J, Ehrich JHH (eds): *Paediatric Nephrology* Berlin: Springer-Verlag, 1984, p 56.
26. Chevalier RL: Chronic partial ureteral obstruction in the neonatal guinea pig II: Pressure gradients affecting glomerular filtration rate. *Pediatr Res* 18:1271, 1984.
27. Chevalier RL, Campbell F, Brenbridge ANAG: Nephrosonography and renal scintigraphy in evaluation of the newborn with renomegaly. *Urology* 24:96, 1984.
28. Chevalier RL, Kaiser DL: Autoregulation of renal blood flow in the rat: Effects of growth and uninephrectomy. *Am J Physiol* 244:F483, 1983.
29. Chevalier RL, Kaiser DL: Chronic partial ureteral obstruction in the neonatal guinea pig I: Influence of uninephrectomy on growth and hemodynamics. *Pediatr Res* 18:1266, 1984.
30. Chevalier RL, Kaiser DL: Effects of acute uninephrectomy and age on renal blood flow autoregulation in the rat. *Am J Physiol* 249:F672, 1985.
31. Chevalier RL, Peach MJ: Hemodynamic effects of enalapril on neonatal chronic partial ureteral obstruction. *Kidney Int* 28:891, 1985.
32. Claesson I, Jacobsson B, Jodal U, et al: Compensatory kidney growth in children with urinary tract infection and unilateral renal scarring: An epidemiologic study. *Kidney Int* 20:759, 1981.
33. Davies P, Roylance J, Gordon IRS: Hydronephrosis. *Clin Radiol* 23:312, 1972.
34. Deen WM, Maddox DA, Robertson CR, et al: Dynamics of glomerular ultrafiltration in the rat. VII. Response to reduced renal mass. *Am J Physiol* 227:556, 1974.
35. Dicker SE: Changes in renal cyclic nucleotides as a trigger to the onset of compensatory renal hypertrophy. *Yale J Biol Med* 51:381, 1978.
36. Dicker SE, Morris C: Renal control of kidney growth. *J Physiol* (Lond.) 241:20P, 1974.
37. Dicker SE, Shirley DG: Mechanism of compensatory renal hypertrophy. *J Physiol* 219:507, 1971.

38. Dicker SE, Shirley DG: Compensatory hypertrophy of the contralateral kidney after unilateral ureteral ligation. *J Physiol* 220:199, 1972.

39. Dicker SE, Shirley DG: Compensatory renal growth after unilateral nephrectomy in the new-born rat. *J Physiol* 228:193, 1973.

40. Diezi, J., Michoud P, Grandchamp A, et al: Effects of nephrectomy on renal salt and water transport in the remaining kidney. *Kidney Int* 10:450, 1976.

41. Dijkhuis CM, van Urk H, Malamud D, et al: Rapid reversal of compensatory renal hypertrophy after withdrawal of the stimulus. *Surgery* 78:476, 1975.

42. Edgren J, Laasonen L, Kock B, et al: Kidney function and compensatory growth of the kidney in living kidney donors. *Scand J Urol Nephrol* 10:134, 1976.

43. Effman EL, Ablow RC, Siegel NJ: Renal growth. *Radiol Clin North Am* 15:3, 1977.

44. Elema JD: Is one kidney sufficient? *Kidney Int* 9:308, 1976.

45. Enger E: Functional compensation of kidney function in recipients and donors after transplantation between related subjects. *Scand J Urol Nephrol* 7:200, 1973.

46. Epstein FH, Charney AN, Silva P: Factors influencing the increase in Na-K-ATPase in compensatory renal hypertrophy. *Yale J Biol Med* 51:365, 1978.

47. Fine LG, Holley RW, Nasri H, et al: BSC-1 growth inhibitor transforms a mitogenic stimulus into a hypertrophic stimulus for renal proximal tubular cells: Relationship to Na/H antiport activity. *Proc Natl Acad Sci* (USA) 82:6163, 1985.

48. Finn WF: Compensatory renal hypertrophy in sprague-dawley rats: glomerular ultrafiltration dynamics. *Renal Physiol* 5:222, 1982.

49. Friedman AL, Pityer R: Benefit of mild protein restriction on survival and growth in young rats with chronic renal insufficiency. *Pediatr Res* 20:450A, 1986.

50. Friedman J, Hoyer JR, McCormick B, Lewy JE: Congenital unilateral hydronephrosis in the rat. *Kidney Int* 15:56, 1979.

51. Galla JH, Klein-Robbenhaar T, Hayslett JP: Influence of age on the compensatory response in growth and function to unilateral nephrectomy. *Yale J Biol Med* 47:218, 1974.

52. Gaydos DS, Goldin H, Jenson B, et al: Partial characterization of a renotropic factor. *Renal Physiol* 6:139, 1983.

53. Goss RJ: Effects of maternal nephrectomy on foetal kidneys. *Nature* 198:1108, 1963.

54. Goss RJ, Dittmer JE: Compensatory renal hypertrophy: problems and prospects. *In* Nowinski WW, Goss RJ (eds): *Compensatory Renal Hypertrophy*. New York, Academic, 1969.

55. Goss RJ, Walker MJ: Compensatory renal hypertrophy in fetal rats. *J Urol* 106:360, 1971.

56. Griscom NT, Vawter GF, Fellers FX: Pelvoinfundibular atresia: The usual form of multicystic kidney: 44 unilateral and two bilateral cases. *Semin Roentgenol* 10:125, 1975.

57. Grond J, Schilthuis S, Koudstaal J, et al: Mesangial function and glomerular sclerosis in rats after unilateral nephrectomy. *Kidney Int* 22:338, 1982.

58. Halliburton IW: The effect of unilateral nephrectomy and of diet on the composition of the kidney. *In* Nowinski WW, Goss RJ (eds): *Compensatory Renal Hypertrophy*. New York, Academic, 1969.

59. Harris RH, Best CF: Circulatory retention of urinary factors as a stimulus to renal growth. *Kidney Int* 12:305, 1977.

60. Harris RH, Best CF: Slowly dialyzable stimulators of renal protein synthesis in urine. *Am J Physiol* 237:F299, 1979.

61. Harris RH, Hise MK, Best CF: Renotrophic Factors in urine. *Kidney Int* 23:616, 1983.

62. Harsing L, Baranyi K, Posch E: Pattern of renal growth and compensatory hypertrophy during development in rats: a mathematical approach. *Kidney Int* 22:398, 1982.

63. Hartupee DA, Weidner WJ: Influence of indomethacin on cation excretion after acute unilateral nephrectomy in dogs. *Prostag Med* 5:243, 1980.

64. Hayslett JP: Functional adaptation to reduction in renal mass. *Physiol Rev* 59:137, 1979.

65. Hayslett JP: Effect of age on compensatory renal growth. *Kidney Int* 23:599, 1983.

66. Hayslett JP, Kashgarian M, Epstein FH: Functional correlates of compensatory renal hypertrophy. *J Clin Invest* 47:774, 1968.

67. Hinman F: Renal counterbalance: An experimental and clinical study with reference to the significance of disuse atrophy. *J Urol* 9:289, 1923.

68. Hodson CJ, Craven JD: The radiology of obstructive atrophy of the kidney. *Radiology* 17:305, 1966.

69. Horster M, Kemler BJ, Valtin H: Intracortical distribution of number and volume of glomeruli during postnatal maturation in the dog. *J Clin Invest* 50:796, 1971.

70. Hostetter TH, Olson JL, Rennke HG, et al: Hyperfiltration in remnant nephrons: A potentially adverse response to renal ablation. *Am J Physiol* 241:F85, 1981.

71. Humphreys MH, Ayus JC: Role of hemodynamic changes in the increased cation excretion after acute unilateral nephrectomy in the anesthetized dog. *J Clin Invest* 61:590, 1978.

72. Hutson JM, Graystone JE, Egami K, et al: Compensatory renal growth in the mouse. II. The effect of growth hormone deficiency. *Pediatr Res* 15:1375, 1981.

73. Hutson JM, Holt AB, Egami K, et al: Compensatory renal growth in the mouse. I. Allometric approach to the effect of age. *Pediatr Res* 15:1370, 1981.

74. Ingelfinger JR, Teele R, Treves S, et al: Renal growth after transplantation: Infant kidney received by adolescent. *Clin Nephrol* 15:28, 1981.

75. John E, Goldsmith DI, Spitzer A: Quantitative changes in the canine glomerular vasculature during development: Physiologic implications. *Kidney Int* 20:223, 1981.

76. Johnson HA, Roman JMV: Compensatory renal enlargement: Hypertrophy versus hyperplasia. *Am J Pathol* 45:1, 1966.

77. Josephson S, Robertson B, Claesson G, et al: Experimental obstructive hydronephrosis in newborn rats. *Invest Urol* 17:478, 1980.

78. Kanetake H, Yamamoto N: Studies on the mechanism of compensatory renal hypertrophy and hyperplasia in a nephrectomized animal model. I. Evidence for a renotropic growth stimulating factor in uninephrectomized rabbit sera using tissue culture. *Invest Urol* 18:326, 1981.

79. Karp R, Brasel JA, Winick M: Compensatory kidney growth after uninephrectomy in adult and infant rats. *Am J Dis Child* 121:186, 1971.

80. Kaskel FJ, Kuman AM, Spitzer A: Dynamics of glomerular filtration in developing guinea pig. *Pediatr Res* 17:352A, 1983.

81. Katz AI, Epstein FH: Relation of glomerular filtration rate and sodium reabsorption to kidney size in compensatory renal hypertrophy. *Yale J Biol Med* 40:222, 1967.

82. Katz AI, Toback FG, Lindheimer MD: Independence of onset of compensatory kidney growth from changes in renal function. *Am J Physiol* 230:1067, 1976.

83. Kaufman JM, DiMeola HJ, Siegel NJ, et al: Compensatory adaptation of structure and function following progressive renal ablation. *Kidney Int* 6:10, 1974.

84. Kaufman JM, Hardy R, Hayslett JP: Age-dependent characteristics of compensatory renal growth. *Kidney Int* 8:21, 1975.

85. Kaufman JM, Siegel NJ, Hayslett JP: Functional and hemodynamic adaptation to progressive renal ablation. *Circ Res* 36:286, 1975.

86. Kiprov DD, Colvin RB, McCluskey RT: Focal and segmental glomerulosclerosis and proteinuria associated with unilateral renal agenesis. *Lab Invest* 46:275, 1982.

87. Klahr S, Buerkert J, Purkerson ML: Role of dietary factors in the progression of chronic renal disease. *Kidney Int* 24:579, 1983.

88. Kleinknecht C, Salusky I, Broyer M, et al: Effect of various protein diets on growth, renal function, and survival of uremic rats. *Kidney Int* 15:534, 1979.

89. Kolberg A, Kogan J: Renal function as influenced by compensatory growth after subtotal nephrectomy in dog. *J Med* 1:156, 1970.

90. Krohn AG, Peng BBK, Antell HI, et al: Compensatory renal hypertrophy: The role of immediate vascular changes in its production. *J Urol* 103:564, 1970.

91. Lalich JJ, Burkholder PM, Paik WCW: Protein overload nephropathy in rats with unilateral nephrectomy. *Arch Pathol* 99:72, 1975.

92. Larsson L, Aperia A, Wilton P: Effect of normal development on compensatory renal growth. *Kidney Int* 18:29, 1980.

93. Laufer I, Griscom NT: Compensatory renal hypertrophy: Absence in utero and development in early life. *Am J Roentgenol Rad Ther Nucl Med* 113:464, 1971.

94. Lopez-Novoa JM, Ramos B, Martin-Oar JE, et al: Functional compensatory changes after unilateral nephrectomy in rats. *Renal Physiol* 5:76, 1982.

95. Luttenegger TJ, Gooding CA, Fickenscher LG: Compensatory renal hypertrophy after treatment for Wilms' tumor. *Am J Roentgenol Rad Ther Nucl Med* 125:348, 1975.

96. Lyon RP: Renal arrest. *J Urol* 109:707, 1973.

97. MacKay EM, MacKay LL, Addis T: The degree of compensatory renal hypertrophy following unilateral nephrectomy. *J Exp Med* 56:255, 1932.

98. Malt RA: Macromolecular metabolism in compensatory renal hypertrophy. *Yale J Biol Med* 51:419, 1978.

99. McRae CU, Shannon FT, Utley WLF: Effect on renal growth of reimplantation of refluxing ureters. *Lancet* I:1310, 1974.

100. Miller M, Mortensson W: Size of the unaffected kidney in children with unilateral hydronephrosis. *Acta Radiol Diagn* 21:275, 1980.

101. Mitus A, Tefft M, Fellers FX: Long-term follow-up of renal functions of 108 children who underwent nephrectomy for malignant disease. *Pediatrics* 44:912, 1969.

102. Moise TS, Smith AH: The effect of high protein diet on the kidneys: an experimental study. *Arch Pathol* 4:530, 1927.

103. Moore ES, deLeon LB, Weiss LS, et al: Compensatory renal hypertrophy in fetal lambs. *Pediatr Res* 13:1125, 1979.

104. Nagle RB, Bulger RE: Unilateral obstructive nephropathy in the rabbit. II. Late morphologic changes. *Lab Invest* 38:270, 1978.

105. Nagle RB, Johnson ME, Jervis HR: Proliferation of renal interstitial cells following injury induced by ureteral obstruction. *Lab Invest* 35:18, 1976.

106. Northrup TE, Malvin RL: Cellular hypertrophy and renal function during compensatory renal growth. *Am J Physiol* 231:1191, 1976.

107. Nowinski WW: Early history of renal hypertrophy. In Nowinski, WW, Goss RJ (eds): *Compensatory Renal Hypertrophy.* New York, Academic, 1969.

108. Obertop H, Malt RA: Lost mass and excretion as stimuli to parabiotic compensatory renal hypertrophy. *Am J Physiol* 232:F405, 1971.

109. Ogden DA: Donor and recipient function 2 to 4 years after renal homotransplantation. *Ann Intern Med* 67:998, 1967.

110. Oliver J: New directions in renal morphology: A method, its results and its future. *Harvey Lect* 40:102, 1944.

111. Olivetti G, Anversa P, Melissari M, et al: Morphometry of the renal corpuscle during postnatal growth and compensatory hypertrophy. *Kidney Int* 17:438, 1980.

112. Olson JL, Hostetter TH, Rennke HG, et al: Altered glomerular permselectivity and progressive sclerosis following extreme ablation of renal mass. *Kidney Int* 22:112, 1982.

113. Orecklin JR, Craven JD, Lecky JW: Compensatory renal hypertrophy: A morphologic study in transplant donors. *J Urol* 109:952, 1973.

114. Pennell J, Bourgoignie JJ: Adaptive changes of juxtamedullary glomerular filtration in the remnant kidney. *Pflugers Arch* 389:131, 1981.

115. Peters G: Compensatory adaptation of renal functions in the unanesthetized rat. *Am J Physiol* 205:1042, 1963.

116. Peters G: Introduction: History and problems of compensatory adaptation of renal functions and of compensatory hypertrophy of the kidney. *Yale J Biol Med* 51:235, 1978.

117. Phillips TL, Leong GF: Kidney cell proliferation after unilateral nephrectomy as related to age. *Cancer Res* 27:286, 1967.

118. Potter D, Jarrah A, Sakai T, et al: Character of function and size in kidney during normal growth of rats. *Pediatr Res* 3:51, 1969.

119. Potter DE, Leumann EP, Sakai T, et al: Early responses of glomerular filtration rate to unilateral nephrectomy. *Kidney Int* 5:131, 1974.

120. Preuss HG: Compensatory renal growth symposium: An introduction. *Kidney Int* 23:571, 1983.

121. Preuss HG, Goldin H: A renotropic system in rats. *J Clin Invest* 59:94, 1976.

122. Preuss HG, Goldin H, Shivers M: Further studies of a renotropic system in rats. *Yale J Biol Med* 51:403, 1978.

123. Provoost AP, Molenaar JC: Changes in the glomerular filtration rate after unilateral nephrectomy in rats. *Pflugers Arch* 385:161, 1980.

124. Provoost AP, Wolff ED, de Keijzer MH, et al: Influence of the recipients size upon renal function following kidney transplantation. An experimental and clinical investigation. *J Pediatr Surg* 19:63, 1984.

125. Purkerson ML, Hoffsten PE, Klahr S: Pathogenesis of the glomerulopathy associated with renal infarction in rats. *Kidney Int* 9:407, 1976.

126. Ribstein J, Humphreys MH: Renal nerves and cation excretion after acute reduction in functioning renal mass in the rat. *Am J Physiol* 246:F260, 1984.

127. Robitaille P, Mongeau JG, Lortie L, et al: Long-term follow-up of patients who underwent unilateral nephrectomy in childhood. *Lancet* I:1297, 1985.

128. Rollason HD: Compensatory hypertrophy of the kidney of the young rat with special emphasis on the role of cellular hyperplasia. *Anat Rec* 104:263, 1949.

129. Rollason HD: Growth and differentiation of the fetal kidney following bilateral nephrectomy of the pregnant rat at 18½ days of gestation. *Anat Rec* 141:183, 1961.

130. Rollason HD: Mitotic activity in the fetal rat kidney following maternal and fetal nephrectomy. In Nowinski WW, Goss RJ (eds): *Compensatory Renal Hypertrophy.* New York, Academic, 1969.

131. Rous SN, Wakim KG: Kidney function before during and after compensatory hypertrophy. *J Urol* 98:30, 1967.

132. Sachtjen E, Rabinowitz L, Binkered PE: Renal concentrating ability in the uninephrectomized rat. *Am J Physiol* 233:F428, 1977.

133. Schlondorff D, Weber H: Evidence for altered cyclic nucleotide metabolism during compensatory renal hypertrophy and neonatal kidney growth. *Yale J Biol Med* 51:387, 1978.

134. Seipelt VH, Zoellner K, Grossmann P: Morphologische und funktionell studien bei einierigen kindern. *Z Urol Nephrol* 63:349, 1970.

135. Shimamura T, Morrison AB: A progressive glomerulosclerosis occurring in partial five-sixths nephrectomized rats. *Am J Pathol* 79:95, 1975.

136. Shirley DG: Developmental and compensatory renal growth in the guinea pig. *Biol Neonate* 30:169, 1976.

137. Silber SJ: Compensatory and obligatory renal growth in babies and adults. *Aust NZ J Surg* 44:421, 1974.

138. Silber SJ: Renal transplantation between adults and children: Differences in renal growth. *JAMA* 228:1143, 1974.

139. Silber SJ: Growth of baby kidneys transplanted into adults. *Surg Forum* 26:579, 1975.

140. Silber SJ, Crudup J: The three-kidney rat model. *Invest Urol* 11:466, 1974.

141. Silber S, Malvin RL: Compensatory and obligatory renal growth in rats. *Am J Physiol* 226:114, 1974.

142. Smith S, Laprad P, Grantham J: Long-term effect of uninephrectomy on serum creatinine concentration and arterial blood pressure. *Am J Kidney Dis* 6:143, 1985.

143. Solomon S, Wise PM, Sanborn C, et al: Cyclic nucleotide concentrations in relation to renal growth and hypertrophy. *Yale J Biol Med* 51:373, 1978.

144. Spitzer A, Brandis M: Functional and morphologic maturation of the superficial nephrons: Relationship to the total kidney function. *J Clin Invest* 53:279, 1974.

145. Taki M, Goldsmith DI, Spitzer A: Impact of age on effects of ureteral obstruction on renal function. *Kidney Int* 24:602, 1983.

146. Torres VE, Velosa JA, Holley KE, et al: The progression of vesicoureteral reflux nephropathy. *Ann Intern Med* 92:776, 1980.

147. Vancura P, Miller WL, Little JW, et al: Contribution of glomerular and tubular RNA synthesis to compensatory renal growth. *Am J Physiol* 219:78, 1970.

148. Willscher MK, Bauer SB, Zammuto PJ, et al: Renal growth and urinary infection following antireflux surgery in infants and children. *J Urol* 115:722, 1976.

149. Wilton P, Aperia A, Broberger O, et al: Compensatory hypertrophy in children with unilateral renal disease. *Acta Paediatr Scand* 69:83, 1980.

150. Zelman SJ, Zenser TV, Davis BB: Renal growth in response to unilateral ureteral obstruction. *Kidney Int* 23:594, 1983.

151. Zucchelli P, Cagnoli L, Casanova S, et al: Focal glomerulosclerosis in patients with unilateral nephrectomy. *Kidney Int* 24:649, 1983.

III
Evaluation for Disease

David I. Goldsmith
Antonia C. Novello

18
Clinical and Laboratory Evaluation of Renal Function

Evaluation of the child with potential renal disease includes examinations that confirm the existence and determine the nature of disease, as well as performance of studies that aid in defining renal functional status. The immunologic aspects of renal disease are discussed in Chap. 13. Radiologic, radioisotopic, and sonographic methods are discussed in Chap. 19.

The workup in patients with a specific disease or disorder is discussed in the chapter devoted to that entity; the evaluation of the infant or child with urinary tract infection, for example, is dealt with extensively in Chap. 91. This chapter is concerned with the general aspects of urinary examination and the performance and interpretation of tests of renal function. Since the physician caring for infants and children with renal disease must have an intimate knowledge of renal physiology, particularly of its developmental aspects, the reader is referred also to Chaps. 1 through 12.

Examination of the Urine
Collection

It is difficult to collect urine specimens from infants and children because of their unwillingness or inability to cooperate and to void on command. Catheterization for a routine urine specimen is not an acceptable alternative. Adequate samples of urine usually can be obtained from young infants by using a plastic bag applied to the perineum with adhesive. Careful supervision prevents loss or fecal contamination of the sample. A volume diuresis facilitates the procedure by increasing the frequency of voiding; however, important indexes of renal function, such as the ability to concentrate the urine, cannot be tested under that condition. Furthermore, abnormal rates of excretion of cells and casts may not be detected if expressed per unit volume rather than per unit time. Special procedures must be employed for urine collection if the specimen is to be examined bacteriologically. This is considered in Chap. 91.

Chemical and Physicochemical Examination
APPEARANCE

The freshly voided urine normally is clear, yet some turbidity may result from the precipitation of phosphates or urates, particularly in concentrated, chilled, or alkaline urine. A variety of pathologic conditions, such as urinary tract infection or chyluria, may also be associated with turbid or opalescent urine.

The color of the urine varies considerably during the course of the day and may range from pale yellow to deep amber. Changes in urine color of no pathologic significance may result from ingestion of certain foods and drugs or from the aerobic oxidation of urobilinogen. The urine is also unusually dark amber in the presence of bilirubin or excessive amounts of carotene. Changes in the color of the urine may reflect the presence of abnormal constituents such as blood or amino acids (Table 18-1).

ODOR

The urine normally is slightly aromatic, which can be modified by ingestion of certain foods, including asparagus and garlic. Bacterial infection often is associated with a fetid or ammoniacal odor. Several metabolic disorders may be suggested by noting particular odors of the urine. Phenylketonuria, maple syrup urine disease, isovaleric acidemia, methioninemia, and oast-house urine disease can be detected by the musty, sweet, sweaty-foot, fishy, and hops or malt odor, respectively.

URINARY PH

The urinary pH is usually measured by pH paper impregnated with colorimetric indicators, although a pH meter is required if a precise measurement is necessary. Urinary pH normally ranges from 4.5 to 7.5, depending on the patient's metabolic state, which must be known if the appropriateness of the urinary pH is to be assessed. It is essential that the pH be determined on a freshly voided specimen, since substantial changes may occur when the urine is exposed to air, through the diffusional loss of carbon dioxide, or in

Table 18-1. *Causes of abnormal coloration of the urine*

Red-burgundy-pink	Dark brown or black	Greenish-blue	Milky
Pathologic	Pathologic	Pathologic	Pathologic
Frankly bloody urine	Homogentisic aciduria	Obstructive jaundice	Nephrotic syndrome
Gross hematuria	Alkaptonuria	Blue diaper syndrome	Elephantiasis
Hemoglobinuria, hemolytic	Methemoglobinemia	Hepatitis	Chyluria
diseases	Melanin	Phenol poisoning	
Porphyria	Tyrosinosis		
Serratia marcescens	Phenol poisoning		
Myoglobinuria			
Physiologic and drug and food	Drug or food ingestion	Drug or food ingestion	
ingestion	Analine	Methylene blue	
Urates	Cascara	Indigo-carmine	
Anthrocyanin	Resorcinol	Resorcinol	
Rhodamine B (food	Senna	Tetrahydronaphthalene	
coloring)	Thymol	Methocarbamol	
Blackberries	Hydroxyquinone	Carotene	
Phenophthalein		Riboflavin	
Pyridium		Concentrated yeast	
Aminopyrine			
Phenytoin sodium			
Azo dyes			

the presence of bacterial contamination. The latter has an inconstant effect on pH. Certain microbial agents split urea and produce alkaline ammonium salts, whereas others render the urine increasingly acidic, due to their metabolic production of volatile and nonvolatile acids.

SPECIFIC GRAVITY AND OSMOLALITY

The solute of the urine contributes to both its weight (specific gravity) and its osmolality. In most instances the osmolality can be approximated from the specific gravity according to the following formula [27]:

$$\text{Osmolality} = (\text{specific gravity} - 1.000) \times 40,000$$

Several variations of this formula have been published with slight improvement in its accuracy [35]. The advantage of the newer formulas lies mainly in their ability to detect unusual urinary solutes.

The specific gravity of the urine ranges normally between 1.001 and 1.030 and has corresponding osmolalities ranging between 40 and 1200 mOsm/kg. Meaningful interpretation of the urinary solute content requires that additional clinical or laboratory data be known. The presence of certain solutes such as albumin, glucose, mannitol, or diatrizoate contributes more to the weight of the urine than to its osmolality and thus alters the relationship between weight and osmolality [34]. In these instances, osmolality is the preferred measurement, since it provides a better estimate than the specific gravity of the osmotic work performed by the kidney.

URINARY PROTEIN

Urinary protein is one of the most important indicators of renal disease in childhood (see Chap. 21). Richard Bright

was the first to associate the presence of renal disease with abnormal proteinuria. Heat coagulation of urinary protein, as used by Bright, has since been modified to chemical coagulation, and, as a result, it has been possible to develop semiquantitative and quantitative turbidometric procedures. Chemical precipitation of urinary protein is most commonly achieved by the addition of either 3% sulfosalicylic acid or ethanolic phosphotungstic acid as in the biuret method.

The utility of these turbidometric tests is limited by several physical and chemical characteristics of the urine. The urine may be turbid due to the precipitation of urate or phosphates before the addition of the protein precipitins; this obstacle may be overcome by filtering or centrifuging the urine before testing. Also, the chemical precipitins are not specific for protein, and turbidity may result from a variety of substances present in the urine, such as radiographic contrast media, penicillins, and metabolites of tolbutamide. It is of interest that the precipitation of urates by trichloroacetic acid gave rise to the claim that the urine of the newborn contains protein at concentrations usually considered to be pathologic. "Dip and read" (dipstick) colorimetric tests (e.g., Labstix or Albustix) overcome some of the problems associated with turbidometric determinations of urinary protein, are reliable, and are the simplest to perform.

The absolute amount of protein found in the urine of normal children is not well defined. DeLuna and Hulet [23] reported a mean urinary excretion of 240 mg/m^2/24 h in children ranging from 1 to 5 years of age. The use of these values is hazardous, however, since the method of protein determination was not reported. Arant [1] reported substantially lower values for protein excretion in neonates of gestational ages ranging from 28 to 40 weeks. In this study, 3% sulfosalicylic acid was used as the chemical precipitant, and the average protein excretion was 1.74 mg/m^2/h. There were minor differences in protein excretion among the various gestational age groups. Karlsson and Hellsing [38] reported mean urinary albumin concentrations of 1.08 mg/dl in neonates (at 0–4 weeks) and 0.28 mg/dl thereafter. The upper 95% confidence limit was 9.8 mg/dl in the neonates and ranged from 1.1 to 3.4 mg/dl in older children. It is important to note that these are values for urinary protein concentration and not protein excretion. As a result, they are subject to variations due to changes in the amount of water excreted. Nevertheless, after the neonatal period, the upper limit of normal urinary protein concentration in random specimens is below the level of detectability by semiquantitative methods, suggesting that any proteinuria detected by the usual methods may be abnormal in children. Data gathered from our laboratory on the rate of protein excretion in overnight collections tend to support this conclusion.

GLUCOSE AND OTHER REDUCING SUBSTANCES

The most widely used screening tests for glucosuria are semiquantitative and are based on either the oxidation of glucose by the specific catalytic enzyme glucose oxidase (e.g., Clinistix) or the reduction of copper in a hot alkaline solution (e.g., Clinitest). The urine normally does not contain sufficient quantities of either glucose or other reducing substances to be detectable by these tests. The most frequent cause of a positive test result for reducing substance in the urine is glucosuria. A positive test result for reducing substance and a negative glucose oxidase test result indicate mellituria or pseudomellituria.

The glucose oxidase test gives false-negative results if large quantities of reducing agents such as vitamin C, tetracyclines, or homogentisic acid are present in the urine. False-positive reactions have not been reported. The copper reduction tests are positive in the presence of a large variety of reducing substances of metabolic, dietary, or drug origin.

HEMOGLOBIN AND MYOGLOBIN

Examination of the urine with dipsticks can be used to detect the presence of occult blood. Dipsticks are sensitive to the presence of any heme prosthetic group, and thus positive results occur in the presence of either intact RBCs, hemoglobin, or myoglobin.

The high sensitivity of this method reduces the possibility of obtaining false-negative results. In a study of proteinuria and hematuria in school children, over 12,000 urine specimens were examined by dipstick and compared with the results obtained by microscopic analysis [24]. There were no false-negative results. Of the urine specimens with positive results by dipstick, 90% were found to have at least three to five RBCs per high-power field. Some of the apparently false-positive test results may have been due to the presence of free hemoglobin or myoglobin. True false-positive reactions may result from the presence of oxidizing materials such as hypochlorite or microbial peroxidase.

A urine specimen that is positive by dipstick should be examined microscopically to confirm the presence of RBCs.

If no cells or red cell ghosts are noted, and contamination has been excluded, the differentiation of hemoglobinuria from myoglobinuria can be accomplished with immunodiffusion techniques [54].

Microscopic Analysis

The microscopic examination of the urine is the least standardized procedure in clinical chemistry. Some of the factors that promote variability in the results are the volume of urine employed, the rate of centrifugation, the volume of fluid in which the pellet is resuspended, the magnification and breadth of field of the microscope, and the inconsistent use of a cover slip. Generally, a 15-ml specimen is centrifuged at 2000 rpm for five minutes; the pellet is then suspended in a volume of 0.25 ml and observed at a 0.35-mm, high-power field. The results are reported as the number of casts per low-power field and the number of RBCs and WBCs per high-power field. Standardization can be achieved by using a counting chamber and expressing the results as the number of cast or cells per milliliter.

In normal subjects, casts usually are not seen. Most investigators consider more than three to five WBCs or zero to one RBCs per high-power field abnormal. The upper limit of normal for concentration of white cells in urine [37,65] is 10 cells/mm^3 for boys and 50 cells/mm^3 for girls. Both sexes have less than five RBCs per cubic millimeter of urine [65].

Determination of the rate of excretion of formed elements in the urine was proposed by Addis, who recommended examination of a 12-hour specimen of urine after a 12-hour period of fluid restriction. An aliquot of the urine was counted in the hemocytometer. Lyttle [42] modified the procedure for use in children by reducing the period of fluid restriction. Edelmann et al. [27] modified the test further to eliminate the variation in rates of excretion that occurs as the result of activity. Fluid is restricted after lunch, and the child is provided with a dry supper. A few ice chips are given if extreme thirst occurs. The parent is instructed to have the child void before going to bed and to note the time; this specimen is discarded. On arising, the child voids into a clean receptacle and the time is again noted. If the child awakens during the night to void, the specimens are saved, refrigerated, and mixed with the first morning specimen before analysis. The specimen can be examined for protein content, specific gravity or osmolality, the presence of reducing substances, pH, and formed elements. The latter is accomplished by centrifugation of an aliquot equivalent to the volume excreted in 20 minutes at 1800 rpm for five minutes. The supernate is decanted, and the pellet is resuspended in 1.0 ml. Casts, red cells, and white cells are counted, under high power, in a volume of 0.9 mm^3 (all nine large squares of one side of a counting chamber). It is of utmost importance that the specimen be examined as soon as possible in order to limit dissolution of casts and crenation or lysis of cells. The number of each element counted is multiplied by 40,000 to determine the excretion rate per 12 hours.

The upper limit of normal for the rate of excretion of

RBCs is 240,000 per 12 hours; normal subjects may excrete as many as 500,000 or more WBCs in the same period [64]. The upper limit for the rate of excretion of casts is taken as 10,000 to 20,000.*

Once the presence of hematuria is established, it is important to localize the source of blood. The presence of casts, particularly RBC casts, suggests renal pathology. Since blood from the upper urinary tract is usually well mixed with urine by the time it is voided, examination of the early, midportion, and end of the urinary stream may be helpful. Varying amounts of blood in the three specimens suggests a lower tract origin of the bleeding.

Differentiation of glomerular and nonglomerular bleeding can frequently be achieved by examining the urine using noninvasive phase-contrast microscopy. To perform this test, 10 ml of a fresh urine sample is centrifuged for five minutes at 750 g, 9.5 ml is removed, and the pellet is resuspended in the remaining 0.5 ml. The sample is then examined in a Fuchs-Rosenthal chamber. By using this technique, bleeding caused by glomerular disease can be distinguished from other causes of hematuria. The diagnosis of glomerular bleeding is established when morphologic variations, i.e., dysmorphic RBCs, are found in the centrifuged sediment. When bleeding is from the lower urinary tract, conventional red cell morphology is found. The changes in RBC morphology are obvious enough to make it feasible for the physician to diagnose, quite accurately, in a single urine examination, glomerular versus lower tract bleeding [31].

Recent reports of the frequency of hematuria with hypercalciuria in otherwise asymptomatic children suggest that urinary calcium should be evaluated in all patients with unexplained hematuria [45,66]. A simple, noninvasive test ($U_{ca/cr}$) using a random voided urine calcium-creatinine concentration ratio (milligrams per millgram) can be used to screen for hypercalciuria [45]. The normal Ca/Cr ratio in this test is 0.06 ± 0.12 (mean $\pm$ 2 SD). Ratios greater than 0.18 should be followed and confirmed by quantitative urinary calcium excretion in one or more 24-hour urine collections.

The $U_{ca/cr}$ on the first day of life is 0.11 ± 0.06 in infants of less than 30-weeks' gestation [2]. This value decreases with the length of gestation to 0.3 ± 0.01 in full-term infants. In neonates, as contrasted to older children, the $U_{ca/cr}$ varies with fractional urine flow (V/GFR), gestational age, and the urinary excretion of phosphorus and sodium. Similarly, any factor that may increase urinary calcium excretion by increasing V/GFR (namely aggressive fluid therapy, high sodium intake, volume expansion, furosemide) may in turn further lower plasma calcium concentration and produce symptomatic hypocalcemia.

More precise measurement of urinary calcium excretion is best performed by the atomic absorption technique. For greater accuracy, a random urine specimen, not the first morning void, should be used. This should avoid a false-negative test result in subjects with absorptive hypercalciuria. As with the screening test, the creatinine excretion should be measured in the same voided specimen. Urine

for calcium excretion should be collected in an acidic environment (e.g., 10 ml, 6N HCL) or in the presence of thymol blue crystals in order to inhibit bacterial growth. Falsely low values of calcium excretion may be obtained if the urine is allowed to stand since the calcium may bind nonspecifically to the collection container.

Bacterial Examination

The evaluation of the child with suspected or known urinary tract infection is discussed in Chap. 91.

Examination of the Blood
Blood Urea

Urea is the predominant end product of protein-nitrogen catabolism. It is freely filtered at the glomerulus and reabsorbed by the tubule. Reabsorption occurs primarily in the proximal tubule, so that at normal rates of glomerular filtration, approximately one-half the filtered urea remains in the luminal fluid at the end of the accessible portion of this proximal segment. The renal handling of urea beyond the proximal tubule is flow-dependent. At high rates of flow, proximal fractional reabsorption is diminished and the fraction of filtered urea reabsorbed distally is minimal, leaving approximately 60% of the filtered urea in the urine (i.e., urea clearance is 60% of the glomerular filtration rate [GFR]). The fractional excretion of urea also increases as GFR falls because the load to each functional nephron increases. This increase in fractional excretion accounts for the fact that urea clearance approaches inulin clearance in patients with severe renal insufficiency.

The urea concentration of the blood, plasma, or serum is usually measured colorimetrically using automated techniques. On average, the concentration of urea in whole blood is 14% less than that in the plasma or serum. Normal values for plasma urea in children from 1 to 20 years of age were studied by Schwartz et al. [59], with means and standard deviations determined at yearly intervals. The average urea concentration varied from 4.23 to 6.23 mM, and the standard deviation ranged from 1.18 to 3.00. These values are equivalent to BUN concentrations of 10.2 and 15.0 mg/dl (plasma urea $\times$ 2.8 = plasma urea nitrogen, and plasma urea nitrogen $\times$ 0.86 = BUN). Girls and boys were found to have similar BUN values. The BUN concentration in infants is similar to that observed in older children, although in early infancy, values of BUN as low as 5 mg/dl may be observed in breast-fed infants.

The interpretation of BUN values must take into account factors that influence the metabolism of urea, including liver function (which influences production), urine flow rate, nonrenal clearance, and changes in the protein content of the diet.

Since alterations in GFR result in modifications in the BUN, the latter can be used as a coarse screening test for glomerular dysfunction. The relationship between BUN and GFR is hyperbolic, and, as a result, only a small absolute increase in the urea concentration occurs when

---

* Edelmann CM Jr: Unpublished data, 1967.

GFR is substantially reduced from a normal level, whereas large increments can be noted with minor decreases in a severely compromised filtration rate. It is important to note, however, that the relative change in urea concentration is inversely proportional to the relative change in GFR if diet and urine flow rates are constant and the patient is in a steady state condition. Thus, a 50% decrease from a normal GFR of 120 ml/min will be associated with a doubling of the BUN (e.g., from 15 mg/dl to 30 mg/dl, an increase of 15 mg/dl), whereas a 50% decrease in a severely compromised filtration rate of 20 ml/min will also result in a doubling of the BUN (e.g., from 60 mg/dl to 120 mg/dl, an increase of 60 mg/dl).

Creatinine

Creatinine results from the enzymatic degradation of creatine found in the skeletal muscle. Since muscle mass is proportional to body mass in the normally proportioned subject, and body mass is related to the cube of body length, it follows that the daily production of creatinine must be proportional to the cube of body length. The production of creatinine is influenced only slightly by day-to-day changes in the diet, and its excretion occurs principally through the urine. It is freely filtered by the glomerulus and secreted by the tubule. Tubular secretion is not, however, a simple rate-limited process. Goldman et al. [33] have demonstrated that the ratio of creatinine clearance to inulin clearance increases as plasma creatinine is raised, reaches a maximum of approximately 1.7, and decreases thereafter. Normally, the secretory component accounts for 10% to 30% of the excretion. Some antibiotics, probenecid, and H_2-blockers can inhibit the creatinine secretory process, raising the serum creatinine, and thus appear to reduce the level of the GFR [46].

Creatinine concentration of serum, plasma, and urine is usually measured with the alkaline picrate method described by Jaffe. In the Jaffe reaction, creatinine values in plasma or serum are overestimated due to the presence of other substances that react with alkaline picrate. The concentration of noncreatinine chromogens has been shown to be unrelated to age and to generate sufficient color to be interpreted as approximately 0.2 to 0.3 mg/dl of creatinine. In the normal adult this represents approximately 25% of the total chromogen content, but may be as much as 50% in the young child. The noncreatinine chromogens, unlike creatinine, have a low renal clearance and as a result are not present to a significant degree in the urine.

Normal values for plasma creatinine in children ranging from 1 to 20 years of age are shown in Table 18-2 [59]. The methodology used to determine creatinine concentration in this study employed a minor modification of the commonly used AutoAnalyzer technique. Since plasma creatinine varies with age, reference to a table or figure is required for interpretation. To overcome this difficulty, an estimate of the normal plasma creatinine for a child of a given size can be obtained from the following formula [12]:

Creatinine concentration = 0.004 × height (in cm)

TABLE 18-2. *Distribution of creatinine concentrations for boys and girls 1 to 20 years of age*

Age	Girls		Boys	
	$\bar{x}$	s	$\bar{x}$	s
1	0.35	0.05	0.41	0.10
2	0.45	0.07	0.43	0.12
3	0.42	0.08	0.46	0.11
4	0.47	0.12	0.45	0.11
5	0.46	0.11	0.50	0.11
6	0.48	0.11	0.52	0.12
7	0.53	0.12	0.54	0.14
8	0.53	0.11	0.57	0.16
9	0.55	0.11	0.59	0.16
10	0.55	0.13	0.61	0.22
11	0.60	0.13	0.62	0.14
12	0.59	0.13	0.65	0.16
13	0.62	0.14	0.68	0.21
14	0.65	0.13	0.72	0.24
15	0.67	0.22	0.76	0.22
16	0.65	0.15	0.74	0.23
17	0.70	0.20	0.80	0.18
18–20	0.72	0.19	0.91	0.17

Note: $\bar{x}$ = mean plasma creatinine concentration (mg/dl); s = standard deviation.
Modified from Schwartz GJ, Haycock GB, Spitzer A: Plasma creatinine and urea concentration in children: Normal values for age and sex. J Pediatr 88:830, 1976.

Measurement of serum creatinine is one of the methods most widely used to estimate the GFR. Its superiority over plasma urea is clear, considering the limited variation provoked by diet and rate of urine flow as compared with the major changes in urea clearance. Nevertheless, the inherent inaccuracy of the method due to the presence in plasma of noncreatinine chromogens, the wide variation in normal values, the large coefficient of variation of the creatinine method, and the changes that occur with age all limit its utility. In our laboratory we found a mean coefficient of variance of 7.44% ± 1.84% (SE) following quadruplicate determinations. This indicates that an approximate 15% change in plasma creatinine must occur before it can be detected at the 95% confidence level. Despite these limitations, serial measurements of plasma creatinine provide a useful and readily available method for evaluating renal function.

Clearance Studies
Clearance Concept and Methods

The assessment of renal function must take into consideration the mechanisms responsible for the formation of urine, namely, filtration, reabsorption, and secretion. The steady state is characterized by a precise balance between the amount of a substance excreted or used for growth and the amount that is produced by the body or acquired from the diet. As a result, excretory rates provide little insight into the level of renal function. The concept of clearance resolves this difficulty. *Clearance* is defined as the equivalent volume of plasma from which a substance would have to be totally removed to account for its excretion in urine per unit of time.

The renal clearance of a substance classically is calculated as

$$Clearance_s = \frac{U_s V}{P_s}$$

where U_s = urinary concentration of a substance, P_s = plasma concentration of the substance, and V = the urine flow rate (volume/time).

Since the clearance of a substance relates to its removal from the blood, it is also possible to determine the plasma clearance by infusing the substance at a constant rate until a steady state is achieved. The clearance can then be calculated from the rate of infusion and the concentration in plasma [20]:

$$Clearance = IR/P$$

where I = infusion concentration, R = infusion rate, and P = plasma concentration.

SINGLE INJECTION CLEARANCE TECHNIQUES

The renal clearance of a substance that is not metabolically produced or degraded and that is excreted from the body totally or almost totally in the urine can be calculated from compartmental analysis by noting its rate of disappearance from plasma following a single intravenous injection [57]. The rates of disappearance from plasma of substances useful in the estimation of GFR and renal plasma flow follow an exponential decay, representing equilibration with plasma and interstitial fluid and excretion by the kidney. The decay curve can be represented by two linear functions by plotting the log of the plasma concentration of the substance as a function of time and applying the standard technique of curve stripping. The terminal slow portion of the curve (Fig. 18-1, line A) is extrapolated back to zero time, and its Y-axis intercept (A) and half-time ($T_{1/2}A$) are noted. When the values along line A are subtracted from the original exponential, a second linear function (line B) can be constructed. Its Y-axis intercept (B) and half-time ($T_{1/2}B$) are also noted. The clearance of the substance, which is taken as the GFR if the substance has the usual properties of a marker of glomerular filtration, can be calculated as follows [57]:

$$Clearance = \frac{Dose \times 0.693}{(A \times T_{1/2}A) + (B \times T_{1/2}B)}$$

A number of radionuclides have been shown to be suitable for single injection clearance measurements, in addition to nonradioisotopic inulin (see Single Injection Clearance of Inulin Without Urine Collection). Several studies have demonstrated the validity and utility of these techniques in children [18,19,56,63], in whom they are particularly suited when quantitative collection of urine is difficult or impossible, such as in infants or children with major urologic abnormalities.

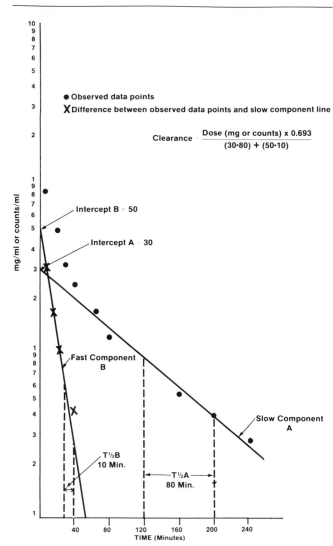

FIG. 18-1. *Double exponential decay curve usually encountered in clearance studies. See text for details of technique for stripping.*

Glomerular Filtration Rate

The maintenance of glomerular filtration is essential to the formation of urine and to normal homeostasis. It is the mechanism by which waste products are separated from particulate matter and large molecular weight proteins in the blood. It is the chief function affected by most kidney diseases and as such its measurement is essential whenever quantification of the remaining reserve is needed.

For the clearance of a substance to be used as an estimate of GFR, it must be filterable by the glomerular capillaries to the same extent as water, it must be neither secreted nor reabsorbed by the tubule, and it must not be metabolized or synthesized by the kidney. Substances that fulfill these requirements include inulin, diatrizoate, vitamin B_{12}, diethylenetriamine penta-acetic acid, iothalamate, and CrEDTA. Recent studies suggest that iothalamate and diatrizoate, because of tubular secretion, approximate the creatinine clearance rather than inulin clearance [46].

Inulin has been clearly shown to be freely filtered through the glomerular capillary in adult animals, but this has not been demonstrated to be true during development. The studies of Arturson et al. [7] suggest that the passage of molecules the size of inulin might be retarded. Barnett et al. [9] demonstrated that inulin is neither reabsorbed nor secreted by the tubules of premature infants, and micropuncture studies in newborn animals [41] have verified the lack of reabsorption. This latter study also demonstrated that molecules the size of mannitol (molecular weight of 180, in contrast to inulin, molecular weight of 5500) might be reabsorbed and indicates that erroneously low values may be obtained if small molecules are used to evaluate GFR in the young subject. Inulin has been shown to be metabolically inert and to be excreted rapidly and almost completely by the kidney, with only small amounts excreted in the bile. The other markers of glomerular filtration have been evaluated primarily by comparing their clearances with that of inulin.

INULIN CLEARANCE
Standard Clearance with Urine Collection
The patient is fasted overnight but permitted to drink water before the test. Food containing protein can raise the GFR [14], and ingestion of fruit juices containing fructose may interfere with the determination of inulin concentration. The patient's height and weight are carefully measured and surface area is calculated. The patient is made as comfortable as possible, and an attempt is made to relieve anxiety. In apparently normal patients, 0.9% or 0.45% saline is infused intravenously at a rate of 2 ml/m^2/min. An indwelling needle, attached to a heparin lock (25–30 U/ml), is placed in a second vein, and 30 to 60 minutes after the infusion is started, specimens of urine and blood are obtained for measurements of blank inulin concentration. A priming dose of 10% inulin, 0.5 ml/kg, is infused over one to two minutes, and a sustaining infusion of inulin is initiated. The volume of 10% inulin required to sustain the plasma concentration at approximately 20 mg/dl is calculated as 0.6 × estimated GFR and is added to a volume of saline calculated as 600 ml × surface area. This will provide an amount of solution sufficient for a five-hour test if the infusion rate is 2 ml/m^2/min.

After the inulin infusion is begun, a 45-minute equilibration period is allowed to elapse. A sample of blood is obtained then and at the end of each of three collections of urine.

The mean plasma concentration for each urine collection period is calculated as follows:

$$\frac{P_1 - P_2}{2.3 \log P_1/P_2}$$

Or the mean plasma concentration can be approximated by interpolation of a semilogarithmic plot of the plasma concentrations as a function of time. In practice, the constant infusion of inulin minimizes the changes in plasma concentration, and arithmetic means are sufficiently ac-

TABLE 18-3. Glomerular filtration in infants and children

Age	GFR (ml/min/1.73 m^2)	References
Preterm neonates at birth*		
28 weeks gestation	0.35	17
32 weeks gestation	0.50	17
36 weeks gestation	1.21	17
Full-term neonates at birth*	2.24	17
2–8 days	39 (17–60)[+]	22,43,51,55
4–28 days	47 (26–78)	9,10,43,55,67
37–95 days	58 (30–86)	10,67
1–6 months	77 (39–114)	51,55
6–12 months	103 (49–157)	55
12–19 months	127 (62–191)	55
2–12 years	127 (89–165)	11,51,55

*Milliliters per minute uncorrected for surface area.
[+]Numbers in parentheses show range.

curate. Clearance is calculated as UV/P. Values of GFR for infants and children of various ages using classic clearance techniques are shown in Table 18-3.

Constant Infusion Clearance of Inulin Without Urine Collection
The technique for measuring inulin clearance without urine collection is similar to that just described. However, blood is sampled at 45- to 60-minute intervals during an observation period of several hours. An aliquot of the infusate is retained for determination of inulin concentration, and the rate of infusion by the pump is calibrated after each clearance study. Two to three consecutive and stable plasma inulin concentrations indicate the steady state concentration.

Cole et al. [20] reported that constant plasma concentrations were achieved in most children by three hours, whereas a four-hour period is usually required in adults. In newborn infants, steady state concentrations may be achieved after only one to two hours [39,40].

Single Injection Clearance of Inulin Without Urine Collection
The patient is prepared for the clearance as previously discussed. A dose of 100 to 200 mg of inulin per kilogram of body weight is injected intravenously. Blood samples are obtained at 5, 10, 15, 30, 60, 90, 120, 150, and 180 minutes after injection. If the GFR is thought to be less than 40 ml/minute, additional samples at 240 and 270 minutes after injection are needed. The theory underlying this method and calculation of the clearance are discussed under Single Injection Clearance Techniques.

CREATININE CLEARANCE AND ESTIMATED FILTRATION RATE

In clinical practice, precise measurements of GFR are not usually necessary, and the renal clearance of creatinine rather than inulin is used commonly. Creatinine is secreted to a small extent by the renal tubule, and therefore its clearance is slightly greater than GFR. Tubular secretion increases the creatinine excretion and clearance by approximately 20% in a normal humans. In contrast, the clearance of total creatinine chromogen approximates GFR, due to the presence of chromogen in the plasma that is not excreted in the urine. Thus, the overestimate imposed by creatinine secretion is balanced by the chromogen present in the plasma.

The close relationship between creatinine clearance and GFR on the one hand, and creatinine production and muscle mass on the other, has suggested that estimates of GFR can be made from the plasma creatinine. Schwartz et al. [58] studied the relationship between plasma creatinine, GFR, and body size and empirically derived the formula

$$GFR = \frac{0.55\,L}{Pcr}$$

where GFR = glomerular filtration rate corrected to 1.73 m^2, L = height or length in centimeters, Pcr = plasma creatinine concentration in milligrams per deciliter, and 0.55, or K, is an empirically derived constant.

Counahan et al. [21] noted that GFR after the age of 2 years is proportional to body weight. Since weight is proportional to height, they reasoned that GFR/surface area would be proportional to length/Pcr. They found that GFR/1.73 m^2 = 0.43 height/Pcr. This formula differs from that derived by Schwartz et al. [58] only in the value of K, and the difference may lie in the fact that Schwartz et al. determined plasma creatinine chromogen concentration, whereas Counahan et al. [21] measured creatinine after removal of noncreatinine chromogen with an ion exchange resin. A second possible reason for the difference might be that Schwartz et al. defined GFR as the clearance of endogenous creatinine measured with urine collections, whereas Counahan et al. used the plasma disappearance of ^{51}CrEDTA. In either case, this approach appears to be a useful clinical guide to estimation of GFR. It is important to note, however, that this mode of GFR estimation might not apply to patients with marked disturbances in body proportions, since surface area is dependent on weight as well as length; and it might not apply to patients with reduced muscle mass or muscle disease, since the production of, and hence the excretion of, creatinine in these patients will not bear the same relationship to body weight as it does in normal patients. In addition, the relationship between muscle mass and body length changes with age.

In order to overcome this last limitation, Schwartz et al. have defined various values of K for different subsets of children, with lower values for full-term infants and higher values for muscular, adolescent boys [60,61]. However, the need to apply several different constants to less than optimally defined groups of patients limits the utility of this approach. For the newborn less than one week of age and

for the preterm neonate, it is doubtful that a valid formula for estimating GFR using only the plasma creatinine concentration can be defined [1]. The plasma creatinine concentration at birth, regardless of gestational age, equals the maternal value, and its rate of decrease has been shown to vary with gestational age [2]. Even in a healthy, full-term neonate, the plasma creatinine in the first day or two of extrauterine life is more a reflection of the mother's kidney function than the neonate's [52].

The problem of estimating GFR in the neonate underscores the implicit assumption made when using any relationship between body size and urinary creatinine excretion, namely that the patient is in a steady state, i.e., the rates of creatinine excretion and production are equal. This assumption is valid neither for the neonate nor for any acute change in renal function. In these circumstances there will be major discrepancies between the estimated GFR and the measured creatinine clearance. In patients with normal body proportions and muscle mass, these discrepancies can be used initially to differentiate acute from chronic renal insufficiency. Once acute changes in renal function are documented, the patient is best followed by noting the change in plasma creatinine rather than making daily or weekly estimates of GFR.

The reciprocal relationship between GFR and plasma creatinine has led some authors to advocate the use of plots of 1/Pcr versus time to follow the progression of renal disease and the effects of therapeutic maneuvers on GFR in adults [44], as well as in children in whom the accuracy of the method has been assumed exclusively from the high correlation coefficients observed [4,50]. However, theoretical and practical considerations suggest that caution should be exercised when using this model. First, progression of renal disease leads both to a reduction in the number of filtering nephrons and to an increase in the proportion of creatinine deriving from tubular secretion [62]. Thus, mathematically, a double reciprocal with two different coefficients would be needed to establish an accurate model. Second, as indicated previously, creatinine production is predominantly dependent on muscle mass. The use of a constant does not allow for consideration of the decrease in muscle mass consequent to malnutrition. In children, the problem is more complex because growth and increases in muscle mass are sustained when renal insufficiency is mild or moderate. Good growth and development in a patient with stable but compromised renal function could be erroneously interpreted as progression of renal insufficiency. Finally, from a practical point of view, the model has a wide predictive error that limits its application to individual patients [35].

Renal Plasma Flow

There is a general concordance between the blood flow to the kidney and the GFR. Diseases that primarily affect the glomerular basement membrane, in the long run, usually influence the renal plasma flow. However, in acute conditions such as acute tubular necrosis the renal blood flow may be well preserved in comparison to glomerular filtration. This preservation of renal plasma flow (RPF) is particularly important in the evaluation of post-transplantation oliguria. Clinically, scintiscanning of the kidney is often used to assess renal blood flow, GFR, and urinary excretion in order to make the distinction between acute tubular necrosis, acute or hyperacute rejection, and urinary tract obstruction. More traditional methods for measuring renal blood flow are usually limited to the clinical research laboratory.

PARA-AMINOHIPPURATE CLEARANCE

Wolf [72] proposed a modified formula for application of the Fick principle to the measurement of RPF:

$$RPF = \frac{(U_s - V_s) \cdot V}{A_s - V_s}$$

where V_s = venous concentration of substance s, A_s = arterial concentration, U_s = urinary concentration, and V = urine flow rate.

The Fick method for determination of RPF is limited in its clinical utility by the difficulty encountered in obtaining plasma from the renal vein; however, the principle is applicable for substances that are completely extracted from the blood in a single passage, in which case the V_s term is zero, and the plasma flow can be calculated from the usual clearance formula [72]. Many substances have been examined, but none is extracted completely. Iodopyracet (Diodrast) and several derivatives of hippurate are extracted to the extent of 90% to 95% in a single passage through the kidney of a normal adult human or dog. The clearance of para-aminohippurate (PAH) or iodohippurate is termed the *effective renal plasma flow* (ERPF), since it represents the plasma flow from which PAH can be extracted. In normal adults, the difference between ERPF and true RPF is reasonably small and the ratio ERPF-RPF is relatively constant. In the developing or diseased kidney, however, these relationships are not maintained.

Bradley et al. [15] have demonstrated that in end-stage renal failure, the extraction of PAH on one passage through the kidney may be as low as 14%. Calcagno and Rubin [17] found that renal PAH extraction in infants and children increased from about 60% in the first month of life to more than 90% after 1 year of age. These findings indicate the impossibility of accurately determining RPF in young children using the usual clearance technique without measurement of the PAH extraction ratio. In Calcagno and Rubin's [17] study, mean RPF in infants 8 days to 3 months of age was 68 ml/min/1.73 m^2, with a range of 50 to 86. Infants 5 to 10 months of age had a mean value of 91 ml/min/1.73 m^2, with a range of 79 to 109.

Method for Determination of Effective Renal Plasma Flow: Clearance Technique

The patient is prepared in a manner identical to that described for inulin clearance. The priming dose of PAH is 8 mg/kg of body weight, or 0.04 ml/kg of a 20% solution. This dose is sufficient to achieve a plasma concentration of 2 mg/dl; higher plasma concentrations should be avoided since they may result in incomplete extraction of PAH. The maximal rate of transport of PAH in normal adults is

about 80 mg/min/1.73 m^2, which is observed at a plasma concentration of 13 to 14 mg/dl. However, a decreased extraction ratio may be encountered in normal adults with plasma concentrations as low as 8 mg/dl. Plasma concentrations well below this value should be used for the calculation of effective RPF.

The sustaining dose of PAH is calculated from the following formula:

PAH (mg) = estimated ERPF (uncorrected for surface area) × 0.02 (mg/dl) × duration of the test (minutes)

A solution adequate for an infusion rate of 2 ml/m^2/min for five hours, to sustain a plasma PAH concentration of 2 mg/dl in a patient with normal renal function, can be prepared by mixing 10 ml of 20% PAH per square meter with 600 ml/m^2 saline. The amount of PAH should be reduced in proportion to the degree of renal insufficiency.

The single injection method for the determination of RPF is the same as that described for inulin, but the radiopharmaceutical is ^{131}I-hippuran. This is administered in a dose of 40 μCi/m^2.

Scintiscanning for Assessment of Renal Blood Flow or Glomerular Filtration Rate

An alternative method for the evaluation of renal function has made use of imaging technology. Radiorenography, first described in 1956, has gone through a complex development whereby numerous methods were devised for quantitative evaluation of the renogram [73], but precision has been largely abandoned because of the need to separate the kinetics of the excretory compartments from that of the parenchyma. Nevertheless, reasonable estimates of GFR and RPF can be made from radionuclide scans. An agent well suited for GFR measurement, technetium 99m DTPA, is associated with a low radiation dose and provides a clearance measurement that is 3% to 5% below the true GFR [13]. Gates [33] derived formulas from experimental data correlating 24-hour creatinine clearance values with renal activity following DTPA scans. These formulas are more simple to use than the rigorous mathematics required for precise determination of GFR from the renal uptake or disappearance of radiopharmaceuticals, and they eliminate the need for repeated blood sampling.

^{131}I-hippuran also permits imaging and is handled by the kidney in a manner similar to para-aminohippurate, but the ratio of hippuran clearance to PAH clearance is usually only about 0.8. The radiation effect of the high dose agent, because of the ^{131}I, is minimized clinically by using only small amounts of radioactivity, but this compromises the ability to obtain adequate estimates of renal blood flow. ^{123}I-hippuran has a much lower radiation dose, but its use is limited by its expense. Several new agents that chelate to diamide disulfur or to the monosulfur group are promising compounds for the assessment of renal blood flow with technetium 99m.

Diffusible Gas Indicators for the Measurement of Renal Blood Flow

If an inert gas is introduced into the kidney, it is possible to determine the renal blood flow from the rate at which the gas is washed out of the kidney. Only one study using this technique in children has been reported [36], and none of the children considered to have normal kidneys was under 2 years of age. Moreover, the authors did not evaluate mean renal blood flow and reported only the values for the most rapid and second most rapid exponentials of the disappearance curve. Autoradiographic studies in neonatal dogs have shown that these exponentials are derived from the blood flow to an outer cortical zone and a composite zone of inner cortex and outer medulla, respectively [8]. Due to the limits imposed by the methods, similar localization studies cannot be performed in humans.

Titration Studies

Both the maximal rate of tubular transport (Tm) and threshold can be measured in the course of a titration study. In essence, an inulin clearance is performed while the test substance is infused to gradually raise its concentration in the plasma. It is evident that if threshold is to be determined, the initial plasma concentration of the test substance must be sufficiently low so that it does not appear in the urine. It is also important to avoid extracellular fluid volume expansion, since its occurrence has been shown to depress Tm [49,53]. Urine and blood samples are analyzed for the concentration of the test substance, as well as for inulin. The amount filtered per unit time (the product of GFR and the plasma concentration) and the excretion rate are calculated; the difference is equal to the reabsorptive rate. The filtered loads, rates of excretion, and rates of reabsorption can be plotted on a single graph as a function of the plasma concentration [30]. The threshold is identified by the value at which the reabsorptive rate falls below the filtered load. Tm is taken as the ordinate value at which reabsorption remains constant despite an increasing filtered load.

Changes in GFR and tubular reabsorptive capacity that occur under different physiologic circumstances, as well as those that occur with growth and maturation, have pronounced effects on Tm; several authors have minimized the effect by expressing all values per deciliter of GFR. This has no influence on the value for threshold, since it is defined as a plasma concentration.

Bicarbonate Titration

Differentiation between the various types of renal tubular acidosis has both prognostic and therapeutic implications, and titration or loading studies are often necessary to fully evaluate the patient (Chap. 81). The ability of the proximal tubule to reabsorb bicarbonate is assessed by the bicarbonate titration, whereas the function of the distal tubule is assessed by acid loading. It should be emphasized that in order to confirm a low threshold for bicarbonate it is necessary to impose an acid load. For this reason the two tests are often done together.

According to the Henderson-Hasselbalch equation, a small but finite quantity of bicarbonate is present in the urine as long as the P_{CO_2} remains above zero. In addition,

certain patients, such as those with renal tubular acidosis, always have significant amounts of bicarbonate in the urine. As a result, the usual definition of threshold does not apply. Edelmann et al. [30] defined the threshold as the point at which urinary excretion of bicarbonate exceeded 0.01 to 0.02 mmol/dl GFR and was increasing rapidly; Oetliker and Rossi [47] used the criterion of a urinary pH above 6.8.

The test procedure is begun by obtaining a urine specimen for the measurement of pH. If the pH in this sample is below 5.8, little measurable bicarbonate is present, and the plasma bicarbonate is probably at or below the renal threshold. A baseline arterialized capillary blood sample is obtained for measurements of tCO_2, pH, and pCO_2.

An infusion of inulin is begun as described for the measurements of GFR; however, the rate is kept at or below 1 ml/m²/min to avoid expansion of the extracellular fluid volume. After collection of two or three control samples, the plasma bicarbonate concentration is raised approximately 2 mmol/L/h by infusing a solution of 7.5% sodium bicarbonate at a rate of 1.4 ml/kg body weight per hour. Once threshold is reached, as judged by a urine pH between 6.5 and 7.0, two or three additional collections of urine are obtained, and then the rate of bicarbonate administration is doubled in order to raise the plasma concentration by 4 mmol/L/h.

The filtered load of bicarbonate is calculated as the product of the plasma bicarbonate and GFR. Estimation of urine bicarbonate requires correction of the P_k for the cation concentration [B]. This is accomplished with the formula $P_k = 6.33 - 0.5$ [B], where [B] is estimated as the sum of the Na^+ and K^+ concentrations expressed in equivalents per liter and the solubility coefficient for carbon dioxide in urine is 0.0309. With these values, filtered, reabsorbed, and excreted bicarbonate can be calculated.

Glucose Titration

Glucose titration studies are now rarely performed outside the research environment and are included here for reference purposes. This test is used to establish the functional adequacy of the proximal tubule, with distinctions made between threshold and tubular maximal transport capacity.

Patients should be in the fasting state to ensure that the urine is free of glucose. The inulin prime is given, and the constant infusion using the slow flow rate described for the bicarbonate titration is started. After equilibration and collection of two control samples of urine, a glucose infusion is begun. We have found that adequate titration curves can be obtained by infusing a 30% solution at progressively increasing rates. The initial flow rate is adjusted to 1.6 ml/m²/min, and after a 20-minute equilibration period, two or three 15-minute collections of urine are obtained. The process is then repeated at flow rates of 3.3, 5.0, and 6.6 ml/m²/min. These flow rates provide glucose loads of 0.5, 1.0, 1.5, and 2.0 g/m²/min.

Brodehl et al. [16] reported values of Tm glucose in infants aged 2½ to 24 weeks of age to be 294±74 (SD) mg/dl GFR. The Tm in children aged 1½ to 13 years was 283±47 ml/dl GFR.

Table 18-4. *Urinary concentrating capacity*

Age	Urinary concentration	References
7–40 days	600–1100 mOsm/kg	26,28,48
2 months to 3 years	Osmolality (mOsm/kg) = 416 log (age in days) + 63	71
2–16 years	1089 (870–1309) mOsm/kg	27

Tests of Renal Concentrating Capacity

Damage to the renal tubules is frequently first reflected in the reduction of the ability to concentrate the urine. This may be the result of obstructive disorders, recurrent infections, or toxic insult to the tubule. The concentrating capacity is therefore one of the tests done early in the management of patients with renal disease.

The simplest method of assessing concentrating capacity is to measure urinary osmolality after an overnight thirst. We prefer to do this along with the Addis count. If frank diabetes insipidus is suspected, a prolonged period of water deprivation may result in dangerous degrees of dehydration, and it is wise to perform water deprivation tests under careful observation for a period of six to eight hours. A weight loss of 3% of the body weight indicates that the test should be terminated. If the weight loss is less than 3%, the patient can usually sustain the rigors of overnight thirsting.

A normal noon meal is given the day of the test, following which, except for a dry evening meal, the child goes without water and food until the test is completed. The bladder is emptied at bedtime, the time noted, and all urine passed between this time and the first morning specimen is collected, ending the Addis collection. The urine specimen is analyzed for osmolality. Values obtained in normal infants and children are shown in Table 18-4.

If a concentrating defect is demonstrated, the sensitivity of the kidney to exogenous hormone administration can be tested. This is easily performed by administering antidiuretic hormone or one of the synthetic analogues. Winberg [71] used Pitressin tannate in oil, 0.1 ml (0.5 units) per 5 kg body weight at 4 p.m. the evening before urine collection. No fluids were given after the normal dinner, and the urine was collected the following morning.

More recently, D-deamino (8-D-arginine) vasopressin has been used (desmopressin, DDAVP). Doses of 10 μg in infants and 20 μg in children, given intranasally, have been shown to result in maximal urinary osmolalities that compared well with those observed following water deprivation [5,70]. This drug has the advantage of rapid action, with the maximal effect seen two to fours hours after administration, and less vasopressor activity than Pitressin.

Acidification Tests
Acid Loading

Since the complexity and duration of the long, or five-day, acid loading test precludes its use in routine clinical evaluation of infants and children, we prefer to use the short loading test [29,30], which is described here (Table 18-5).

To ensure adequate urine flow, the patient is provided water by mouth (60 ml/m^2/h). After the collection of one or two control urine specimens, an acidifying agent is administered, in a dose of 75 to 150 mEq/m^2. In most cases this is ammonium chloride, but the use of arginine hydrochloride has been shown to yield a similar response. In either case, the dose should be sufficient to decrease the plasma bicarbonate concentration by at least several millimoles per liter. Urinary pH, ammonium, and titratable acid concentrations are determined in urine specimens collected in one-hour periods. The maximal response is generally noted at three to five hours after administration of the acidifying agent. Normal values are shown in Table 18-5.

Urine-Blood pCO$_2$

Recently, it has become apparent that the pathophysiologic mechanisms leading to type I (distal or classic) renal tubular acidosis vary according to the underlying etiology (Chap. 81). In addition to the well-recognized gradient defect, rate limitations due to either voltage dependency or secretory deficiencies have been shown to underlie distal renal tubular acidosis consequent to drugs, urinary tract

Table 18-5. *Renal response to administration of ammonium chloride* *

Age group	Urinary pH	Titratable acid (Eq/min/1.73 m^2)	Ammonium Eq/min/1.73m^2
Premature infants (1–3 weeks)	5.96 ± 0.05†	24.9 ± 13.4†	29.3 ± 6.4†
Full-term infants (1–3 weeks)	5.0 ± 0.15†	32.4 ± 8.2†	55.8 ± 8.8†
1–12 months	5.0	62 (43–111)‡	57 (42–79)‡
3–15 years	5.5	52 (33–71)‡	73 (46–100)‡

* Maximal response noted 3 to 5 hours after ingestion of ammonium chloride. [29,30,68,69]
† Mean ± SD.
‡ Mean and range.

obstruction, or inherited disease [6,25]. Clinically, the differences can be uncovered by measuring acid excretion under control conditions and following loading with sodium sulfate or bicarbonate. The provision of excess anion to the distal tubule allows the continued secretion of H^+ ion without developing a substantial pH gradient. If bicarbonate is used as the test agent, the test is substantially simplified because only the urinary and blood pCO_2 need to be measured. In the presence of a high bicarbonate delivery to the distal nephron, secreted hydrogen ions are trapped by forming H_2CO_3, which is dehydrated slowly due to the paucity of carbonic anhydrase in this segment, resulting in an increase in the pCO_2 of the urine. The test performed is similar to a bicarbonate titration with the additional measurement of pCO_2 in the blood and urine. Normal values for adults are approximately 70 mm Hg.

Although the specificity of the urinary pCO_2 has been debated, and is certainly affected by urine flow rate, buffer delivery, urinary concentration, and the ampholyte effect, the test is sufficiently reliable to provide insight into the underlying pathophysiology (see also Chap. 81).

References

1. Arant BS Jr: Developmental patterns of renal functional maturation compared in the human neonate. *J Pediatr* 92:705, 1978.
2. Arant BS Jr: Renal handling of calcium and phosphorus in normal human neonates. *Semin Nephrol* 3:94, 1983.
3. Arant BS Jr: Estimating glomerular filtration rate in infants. *J Pediatr* 104:890, 1984.
4. Arbus GS, Bacheyie GS: Method for predicting when children with progressive renal disease may reach high serum creatinine level. *Pediatrics* 67:871, 1981.
5. Aronson AS, Svenningsen NW: DDAVP test for estimation of renal concentrating capacity in infants and children. *Arch Dis Child* 49:654, 1974.
6. Arruda JAL, Kurtzman NA: Mechanisms and classifications of deranged distal urinary acidification. *Am J Physiol* 239:F515, 1980.
7. Arturson G, Groth T, Grotte G: Human glomerular membrane porosity and filtration pressure; dextran clearance analyzed by theoretical models. *Clin Sci* 40:137, 1971.
8. Aschinberg LC, Goldsmith DI, Olbing H, et al: Neonatal changes in renal blood flow distribution in puppies. *Am J Physiol* 228:1453, 1975.
9. Barnett HL, Hare WK, McNamara H, et al: Measurements of glomerular filtration rate in premature infants. *J Clin Invest* 32:691, 1948.
10. Barnett HL, Hare WK, McNamara H, et al: Influence of postnatal age on kidney function of premature infants. *Proc Soc Exp Biol Med* 69:55, 1948.
11. Barnett HL, McNamara H, Schultz S, et al: Renal clearance of sodium penicillin G, procaine penicillin G and inulin in infants and children. *Pediatrics* 3:418, 1949.
12. Barratt TM, Chantler C: Clinical assessment of renal function. *In* Rubin MI, Barratt TM (eds): *Pediatric Nephrology.* Baltimore, Williams & Wilkins, 1975, p 55.
13. Blaufox MD: The current status of renal radiopharmaceuticals. *Contrib Nephrol* 56:31, 1987.
14. Bosch JP, Saccaggi A, Lauer A, et al: Effect of protein intake on glomerular filtration rate. *Am J Med* 75:943, 1983.
15. Bradley SW, Bradley GP, Tyson CI, et al: Renal function in renal disease. *Am J Med* 9:766, 1950.
16. Brodehl J, Franken A, Gellissen K: Maximal tubular reabsorption of glucose in infants and children. *Acta Paediatr Scand* 61:413, 1972.
17. Calcagno PL, Rubin MI: Renal extraction of para-aminohippurate in infants and children. *J Clin Invest* 42:1632, 1963.
18. Chantler C, Garbett ES, Parson V, et al: Glomerular filtration rate measurement in man by the single injection method using ^{51}Cr-EDTA. *Clin Sci* 37:169, 1969.
19. Cohen MI, Smith FG, Mandell RS, et al: A simple reliable method of measuring glomerular filtration rate using single low dose sodium iothalamate I^{131}. *Pediatrics* 43:407, 1969.
20. Cole BR, Giangiacomo J, Ingelfinger JR, et al: Measurement of renal function without urine collection. *N Engl J Med* 287:1109, 1972.
21. Counahan R, Chantler C, Ghazali S, et al: Estimation of glomerular filtration rate from plasma creatinine concentration in children. *Arch Dis Child* 51:875, 1976.
22. Dean RFA, McCance RA: Inulin, diodone, creatinine, and urea clearances in newborn infants. *J Physiol (Lond)* 106:904, 1947.
23. DeLuna MB, Hulet WH: Urinary protein excretion in healthy infants, children, and adults. *Proceedings of the First Annual Meeting American Society of Nephrology,* 1967.
24. Dodge WF, West EF, Smith EH, et al: Proteinuria and hematuria in school children. Epidemiology and early natural history. *J Pediatr* 88:327, 1976.
25. DuBose TD Jr, Caflisch CR: Validation of the difference in urine and blood carbon dioxide tension during bicarbonate loading as an index of distal nephron acidification in experimental models of distal renal tubular acidosis. *J Clin Invest* 75:1116, 1985.
26. Edelmann CM Jr, Barnett HL: Role of the kidney in water metabolism in young infants. Physiologic and clinical considerations. *J Pediatr* 56:154, 1960.
27. Edelmann CM Jr, Barnett HL, Boichis H, et al: A standardized test of renal concentrating capacity in children. *Am J Dis Child* 114:639, 1967.
28. Edelmann CM Jr, Barnett HL, Troupkou V: Renal concentrating mechanisms in newborn infants. Effect of dietary protein and water content, role of urea, and responsiveness to antidiuretic hormone. *J Clin Invest* 39:1062, 1960.
29. Edelmann CM Jr, Boichis H, Rodriguez-Soriano J, et al: The renal response of children to acute ammonium chloride acidosis. *Pediatr Res* 1:452, 1967.
30. Edelmann CM Jr, Rodriguez-Soriano J, Boichis H, et al: Renal bicarbonate reabsorption and hydrogen ion excretion in infants. *J Clin Invest* 46:1309, 1967.
31. Fairley KF, Birch DF: Hematuria: A simple method for identifying glomerular bleeding. *Kidney Int* 21:105, 1982.
32. Gates GF: Glomerular filtration rate: Estimation from fractional renal accumulation of 99m Tc-DTPA (stannous). *Am J Radiol* 138:565, 1982.
33. Goldman R, Yadley RA, Nourok DS: Comparison of endogenous and exogenous creatinine clearances in man. *Proc Soc Exp Biol Med* 125:205, 1967.
34. Goldsmith DI, Martinez AB, Schwartz GJ: Identification of osmotically active solutes in urine. *Crit Care Med* 13:468, 1985.
35. Gretz N, Manz F, Strauch M: Predictability of the progression of chronic renal failure. *Kidney Int* (suppl 15)24:S2, 1983.
36. Gruskin AB, Auerback VH, Black IFS: Intrarenal blood flow in children with normal kidneys and congenital heart disease. Changes attributable to angiography. *Pediatr Res* 8:561, 1974.
37. Houston IB: Urinary white cell excretion in childhood. *Arch Dis Child* 40:313, 1965.

38. Karlsson FA, Hellsing K: Urinary protein excretion in early infancy. *J Pediatr* 89:89, 1976.

39. Leake RD, Trygstad CW: Glomerular filtration rate during the period of adaptation to extrauterine life. *Pediatr Res* 11:959, 1977.

40. Leake RD, Trygstad CW, Oh W: Inulin clearance in the newborn infant. Relationship to gestational and postnatal age. *Pediatr Res* 10:759, 1976.

41. Lockhart E, Spitzer A: Permeability characteristics of the renal tubule during maturation (abstr). *Pediatr Res* 8:181A, 1974.

42. Lyttle JD: The Addis count in normal children. *J Clin Invest* 12:87, 1933.

43. McCrory WW, Forman CW, McNamara H, et al: Renal excretion of phosphate in newborn infants. *J Clin Invest* 31:357, 1952.

44. Mitch WE, Walser M, Steinman TE, et al: The effect of a keto acid-amino acid supplement to a restricted diet on the progression of chronic renal failure. *N Engl J Med* 311:623, 1984.

45. Moore ES, Coe FL, McMann BJ, et al: Idiopathic hypercalciuria in children: Prevalence and metabolic characteristics. *J Pediatr* 92, 6:906, 1978.

46. Odlund B, Hallgren R, Sohtell M, et al: Is ^{125}I iothalamate an ideal marker for glomerular filtration? *Kidney Int* 27:9, 1985.

47. Oetliker O, Rossi E: The influence of extracellular fluid volume on the renal bicarbonate threshold. A study of two children with Lowe's syndrome. *Pediatr Res* 3:140, 1969.

48. Polacek E, Vocel J, Neugebauerova L, et al: The osmotic concentrating ability in healthy infants and children. *Arch Dis Child* 40:291, 1965.

49. Purkerson ML, Lubowitz H, White RW, et al: On the influence of extracellular fluid volume expansion on bicarbonate reabsorption in the rat. *J Clin Invest* 48:1754, 1969.

50. Reimold EW: Chronic progressive renal failure: Rate of progression monitored by change of serum creatinine concentration. *Am J Dis Child* 135:1039, 1981.

51. Richmond JB, Kravitz H, Segar W, et al: Renal clearance of endogenous phosphate in infants and children. *Proc Soc Exp Biol Med* 77:83, 1951.

52. Robson A: Pediatric perspectives. *Am J Kidney Dis* 4:207, 1984.

53. Robson AM, Srivastava PL, Bricker NS: The influence of saline loading on renal glucose reabsorption in the rat. *J Clin Invest* 47:329, 1968.

54. Rozman JM, Peterson JA, Adams EC: Differentiation of hemoglobin and myoglobin by immunochemical methods. *J Invest Urol* 1:518, 1964.

55. Rubin MI, Bruck E, Rapoport M: Maturation of renal function in childhood. *J Clin Invest* 28:1144, 1949.

56. Sakai T, Leumann EP, Holliday MA: Single injection clearance in children. *Pediatrics* 44:905, 1969.

57. Sapirstein LL, Viat DG, Mandel MJ, et al: Volume of distribution and clearances of intravenously injected creatinine in the dog. *Am J Physiol* 181:330, 1955.

58. Schwartz GJ, Haycock GB, Edelmann CM Jr, et al: A simple estimate of glomerular filtration rate in children derived from body length and plasma creatinine. *Pediatrics* 58:259, 1976.

59. Schwartz GJ, Haycock GB, Spitzer A: Plasma creatinine and urea concentrations in children; normal values for age and sex. *J Pediatr* 88:828, 1976.

60. Schwartz GJ, Langford DJ, Feld LG: A simple estimate of glomerular filtration rate in infants. *J Pediatr* 104:849, 1984.

61. Schwartz GJ, Gauthier B: A simple estimate of glomerular filtration rate in adolescent boys. *J Pediatr* 106:522, 1985.

62. Shemesh O, Myers BD: Tubular secretory vs. glomerular filtration rates of creatinine in primary glomerular disease (abstr). *Kidney Int* 27:250 1985.

63. Silkans GI, Jeck D, Earon J, et al: Simultaneous measurement of glomerular filtration rate and renal plasma flow using plasma disappearance curves. *J Pediatr* 83:749, 1973.

64. Snoke AW: The normal Addis count in children. *J Pediatr* 12:473, 1938.

65. Stansfield JM: The measurement and meaning of pyuria. *Arch Dis Child* 37:257, 1962.

66. Stapleton FB, Roy S, Noe HN, et al: Hypercalciuria in children with hematuria. *N Engl J Med* 310:1345, 1984.

67. Strauss J, Adamsons K Jr, James LS: Renal function of normal full-term infants in the first hours of extrauterine life. *Am J Obstet Gynecol* 91:286, 1965.

68. Sulyok E, Hein T: Assessment of maximal urinary acidification in premature infants. *Biol Neonate* 19:200, 1971.

69. Sulyok E, Hein T, Soltesz G, et al: Influence of maturity on renal control of acidosis in newborn infants. *Biol Neonate* 21:418, 1972.

70. Svenningsen NW, Aronson AS: Postnatal development of renal concentration capacity as estimated by DDAVP test in normal and asphyxiated neonates. *Biol Neonate* 25:230, 1974.

71. Winberg J: Determination of renal concentration capacity in infants and children without renal disease. *Acta Paediatr Scand* 48:318, 1959.

72. Wolf AV: Total renal blood flow at any urine flow or extraction fraction. *Am J Physiol* 133:469, 1941.

73. Zum Winkel K: Evaluation of renal function and morphology with radionuclides. *Eur J Nucl Med* 9:323, 1984.

Leonard E. Swischuk
C. Keith Hayden, Jr.

19
Imaging of the Urinary Tract

Plain Film and Intravenous Urogram

With the advent of ultrasonography, imaging of the urinary tract in children has taken on a totally new perspective. Ultrasonography has been shown to be capable of demonstrating almost every aspect of urinary tract pathology. To a great extent it has replaced the intravenous urogram (IVU), is possibly superior to the CT scan, and is complementary to nuclear medicine studies. Although none of these modalities has been abandoned, their roles have been altered significantly.

Plain Film

The plain film provides limited information regarding the urinary tract. It is often possible to see the kidneys and assess size, shape, and position; however, frequently the kidneys are obscured by overlying gas. Calcifications, either in the kidneys or the collecting systems, are relatively easily detected with the plain film. A variety of configurations ranging from diffuse nephrocalcinosis to individual stones can be seen (Fig. 19-1). Other than this, however, plain films provide little information.

Intravenous Urogram

For decades the IVU was the mainstay in the investigation of urinary tract disease in children. Together with the voiding cystourethrogram (VCU), it was used both to define renal anatomy and to give some indication of renal function. The latter, at best, was a rough approximation, and renal function now is far better assessed with nuclear medicine studies [74,79].

Standard contrast agents used for intravenous urography usually are hypertonic solutions of diatrizoate and meglumine salts, and as such they pose problems for neonates. Significant electrolyte disturbances may occur, and pulmonary edema can result from volume overload. In addition, precipitation of Tamm-Horsfall protein may lead to prolonged nephrograms and temporarily impaired renal function [11,84]. Nonetheless, these contrast agents are in wide use since these complications are relatively rare, and allergic or sensitivity reactions in children are almost nonexistent. However, it is likely that isotonic agents such as metrizamide will replace other contrast agents [67,80] because they are less injurious to the various body systems. Economic factors currently prohibit their widespread use.

In performing the IVU two films are obtained within 5 to 15 minutes after injection of contrast material. Oblique and lateral films are obtained only if an abnormality requires further delineation. In the past, such films usually were obtained primarily for assessment of suspected renal and ureteral displacement, but these findings now are more vividly demonstrated with ultrasonography and CT scanning.

The normal IVU usually allows one to assess the kidneys for number, location, size, and shape and remains one of the best ways to document renal scarring, small kidneys, clubbed calyces, and renal location (Fig. 19-2). One can derive some idea regarding renal function by noting the rapidity with which contrast material passes through the kidney (Fig. 19-3). The intravenous pyelogram also may localize the level of obstruction, but in any case, as hydronephrosis becomes more severe, the calyces become more dilated and blunted. Other causes of blunted, dilated calyces include pericalyceal abscess (diverticulum), papillary necrosis, and the condition known as congenital megacalyces. This last condition is of no clinical consequence but can be misinterpreted as hydronephrosis.

The IVU usually detects renal masses with ease except for very small ones. However, the IVU cannot determine whether the mass is tumor, cyst, or abscess (Fig. 19-4), and in some cases it is difficult to determine whether the mass is renal or extrarenal. Ultrasonography is much better at providing this type of information.

Voiding Cystourethrography

The VCU came into its own in the early 1960s, primarily as a detector of ureteral reflux [13,76–78]. It remains the main investigative procedure for this problem, but it should

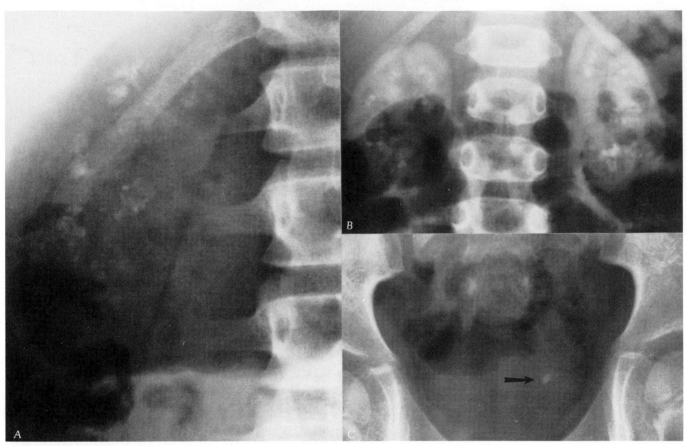

FIG. 19-1. Plain film calcifications. A. *Typical mottled irregular calcifications in renal tubular acidosis.* B. *Diffuse nephrocalcinosis with focal irregular calcifications in oxalosis.* C. *Calcified ureteral calculus* (arrow) *causing renal colic.*

be noted that reflux also can be demonstrated with nuclear medicine studies [15,57,60] and to some extent with ultrasonography [43,89]. The latter procedure, however, is not very sensitive in demonstrating mild degrees of reflux. Other information obtained from the VCU includes (1) rate and completeness of bladder emptying, (2) size and shape of the bladder, (3) presence of mucosal irregularities, (4) presence of intrinsic or extrinsic masses, (5) urethral configuration, and (6) presence of urethral obstruction.

When performing a VCU, the bladder is filled manually or by gravity drip. The latter method is preferred by most, although either method yields good results. The bladder must be fully distended so that the patient can void on command. During filling of the bladder, fluoroscopic observation is used to detect ureteral reflux. Transient episodes of reflux into the lower inch or two of the ureter when the bladder is fully distended probably are not significant; this is termed *high pressure* reflux. Reflux occurring before the bladder is fully distended is termed *low pressure reflux* and usually is more significant.

Reflux is graded from 1 to 4, or in a more recent classification 1 to 5 [52]. Grade 4 reflux in the first scheme

represents intrarenal reflux, the only form of reflux clearly associated with renal scarring [68] (Fig. 19-5). Intrarenal reflux occurs in infancy and is associated with inability of the collecting ducts to be totally occluded when the calyx is stretched and distended by the accumulation of urine [26,36,66]. Intrarenal reflux also occurs in neonates with severely dysplastic kidneys [63]. The more recent classification omits intrarenal reflux and establishes the grade on the basis of upper tract distention and ureteral tortuosity (Fig. 19-5b).

All grades of reflux are readily demonstrable with voiding cystourethrography (Fig. 19-6) and generally are associated with urinary tract infection. In addition, although all investigators do not agree [20], infection is believed to play an important role in the development of scarring in patients with ureteral reflux [23,36,65,66,75,81]. In a few instances, however, reflux of sterile urine is said to produce scarring [53,61,73,93].

Normally the ureters enter the bladder on a slant, tunneling submucosally, and as the bladder fills, the intramural ureter is compressed so that reflux does not occur. In most cases, ureteral reflux occurs because of alteration to a more

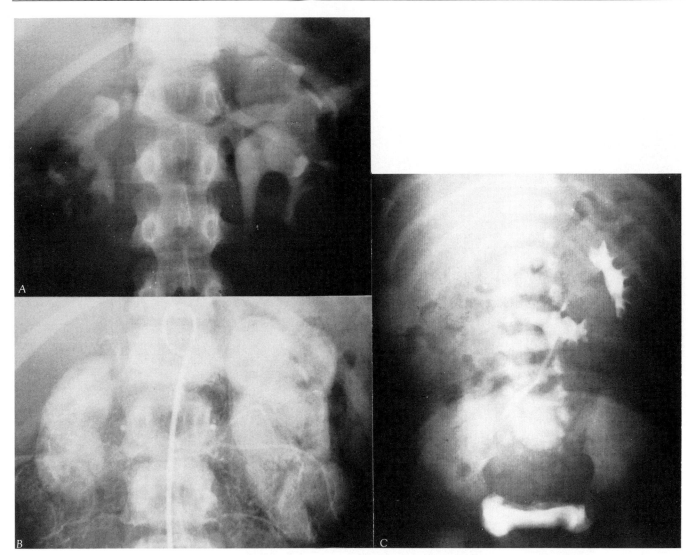

FIG. 19-2. Scarred kidneys—IVU findings. A. *Note small, scarred right kidney and slightly larger, but still scarred left kidney. Also note that the calyces are blunted and that the renal cortex is thin and sparse.* B. *Nephrogram, as part of an arteriogram, demonstrates the renal contours to better advantage.* C. *Abnormality of renal position; cross fused ectopia.*

horizontal insertion of the ureter on a congenital basis. With infection, the angle of insertion also is altered to a more horizontal configuration, and in either case as the bladder fills, the now horizontal ureter cannot be occluded. This permits reflux to occur, but with infection may disappear after therapy. It is important, therefore, not to perform the VCU during the early stages of an acute urinary tract infection, but to defer the study for 6 to 8 weeks. Other reasons for not performing the study when the patient is infected is that one can induce renal damage and sepsis secondary to intrarenal reflux of infected urine [55].

On a more chronic basis, persistent horizontal positioning of the distal ureter as it enters the urinary bladder is due to bladder wall thickening. This can occur with infec-

tion or obstruction. Reflux secondary to abnormal positioning of the distal ureter is seen also with the so-called "Hutch diverticulum." This diverticulum, occurring at the ureterovesical junction, can be seen on cystourethrography and is commonly associated with lower urinary tract obstruction (Fig. 19-7). On a congenital basis, reflux is due to inherent, horizontal positioning of the ureter. This is accompanied by the so-called golf hole ureteral orifice. Most of these cases are familial.

Generally speaking, voiding cystourethrography is performed after the first documented urinary tract infection in either a male or a female under the age of 2 to 4 years. In the older female one may prefer not to perform the study until after the second documented infection. In males, on

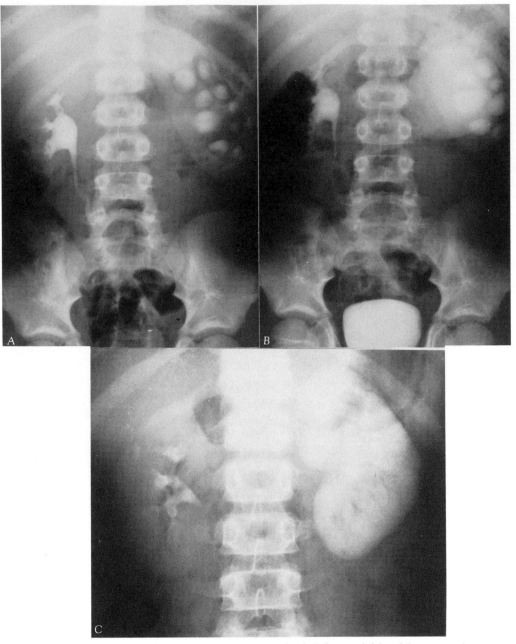

FIG. 19-3. IVU findings with obstruction. A. *Note normal right kidney and delayed function with early filling of dilated calyces on the left.* B. *Delayed film demonstrates classic ureteropelvic junction obstruction on the left.* C. *Another patient. Note the normal right kidney but slightly enlarged left kidney with a delayed and persistent nephrogram due to obstruction secondary to a renal stone.*

the other hand, performance of the study after the first infection is favored. The function of the VCU is twofold: (1) to detect the presence of obstruction and (2) to determine whether reflux is present.

Once reflux is documented, a repeat study should be performed to determine whether it has disappeared with appropriate therapy. A radionuclide cystogram is quite satisfactory for this purpose and in fact is desirable. The main

reason for performing a radiographic VCU as the initial study is that in addition to reflux, information regarding other anatomic abnormalities can be obtained. This is most important in males.

Size, shape, and configuration of the bladder are readily demonstrable with cystourethrography. Large, smooth bladders are seen with hypervolemic states such as Bartter's syndrome, diabetes insipidus, chronic water intoxication,

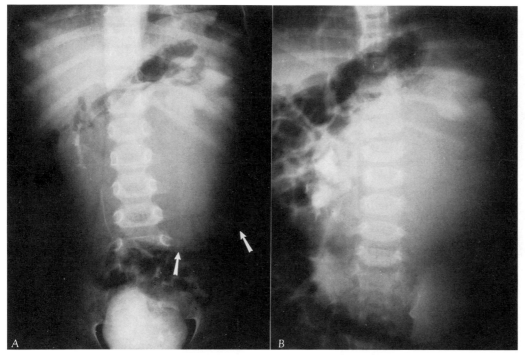

FIG. 19-4. IVU demonstration of a mass. A. *Note large mass (Wilms' tumor) on the left (arrows), producing upward displacement and dilatation of the calyces. B. Similar findings due to a renal cyst. For the ultrasonographic findings in this patient, see Fig. 19-19.*

FIG. 19-7.
row) *with*
ureter.

GRADES OF REFLUX

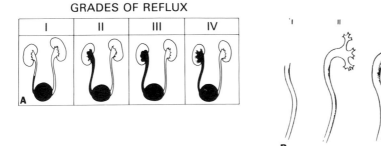

FIG. 19-5. Grading of reflux. A. *Grades I-V. Note that in grade III reflux the calyces are blunted and that in grade IV there is intrarenal reflux. B. Another system of grading. Beyond grade II reflux, the upper collecting systems become filled. The degree of distention separates grade II from grade III reflux, while with grade IV reflux calyceal blunting is present. With grade V reflux marked blunting along with tortuosity of the ureter is seen. (From Levitt SB: Medical versus surgical treatment of primary vesicoureteral reflux, report of the international reflux study committee. Pediatrics 67:392, 1981; with permission.)*

19-12b).
their uret
vaginal r
factors in
   Abnor
The mos
terior ur
called sa
19-13). 7
insertion
insert an
opening
the fused
opening
With th
exists, an
of urine.
with the
19-13). \

and the infrequent voider. Large, smooth bladders also are seen in some neurogenic states [3,25] and in the congenital megacystis-microcolon syndrome [4,9,45,47,64,85]. A small bladder is less common, and although slight degrees of smallness can be seen in normal individuals, small bladders usually are seen with severe bladder wall thickening and spasticity secondary to infection, inflammation, or neurogenic disease. In terms of the latter, the heavily

trabeculated, so-called Christmas tree bladder is typical (Fig. 19-8a).
   When assessing bladder wall trabeculation, it is important not to confuse slight, normal irregularity of the posterior wall of the bladder during voiding with true irregularity that persists when the bladder is filled to capacity (Fig. 19-8b). It should be noted that mucosal irregularity is seen normally during the emptying stage of the voiding

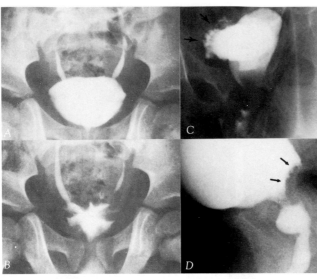

FIG. 19-9. Cystitis. A. *Patient with cyclophosphamide cystitis. With the bladder full the mucosa appears relatively smooth. Bilateral reflux is present. B. After voiding, the marked thickening and nodularity of the mucosa is noted. C. Another patient with focal cystitis causing deep trabeculation and cellule formation (arrow). D. Rhabdomyosarcoma (arrows) produces indentation and mucosal irregularity along the base of the bladder.*

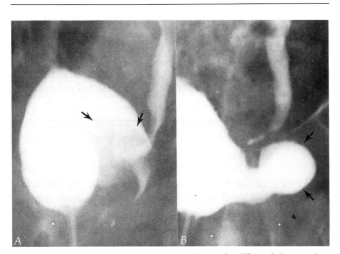

FIG. 19-10. Everting ureterocele. A. *Note the filling defect in the bladder (arrows) due to the ureterocele. Reflux is present. B. With voiding, the ureterocele everts to form a diverticulum (arrows). Note how this distorts the entrance of the ureter into the bladder.*

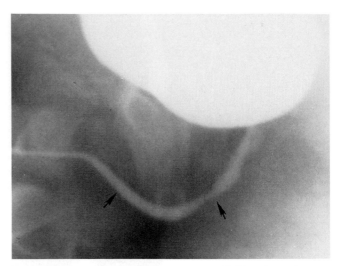

FIG. 19-11. Low flow pattern: neurogenic bladder. *Note that while anatomically the urethra (arrows) in this male appears normal, it is very thin, reflecting a low flow pattern secondary to impeded emptying of the bladder.*

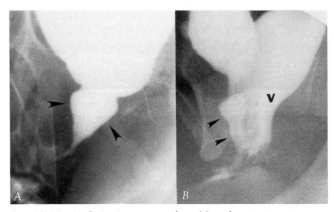

FIG. 19-12. A. Spinning top urethra. *Note the spinning top appearance of the urethra (arrows) in this female. B. Vaginal reflux. With voiding, the bladder empties and the urethra remains a little distended (arrows). Gross reflux has occurred into the vagina (V).*

Ultrasonographic, Computed Tomography, and Magnetic Resonance Imaging

Of these three modalities, ultrasonography has had the greatest impact on the investigation of renal disease in children, affording excellent visualization of the kidneys and perirenal structures. MRI can provide some additional data regarding abnormalities of renal parenchymal disease and tumors but probably will not displace ultrasonography. Currently it has little application in investigation of urinary tract disease in children except tumors.

With the development of newer-generation, high-reso-

suspected bladder neck or urethral trauma. With trauma it is important to perform the retrograde study before inserting a catheter into the bladder since the catheter may pass through a urethral tear. One looks for extravasation of contrast material and compression of the urethra and bladder by the adjacent collection of blood and fluid.

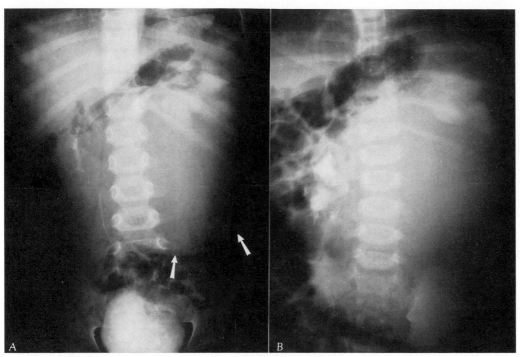

FIG. 19-4. IVU demonstration of a mass. A. *Note large mass (Wilms' tumor) on the left (arrows), producing upward displacement and dilatation of the calyces.* B. *Similar findings due to a renal cyst. For the ultrasonographic findings in this patient, see Fig. 19-19.*

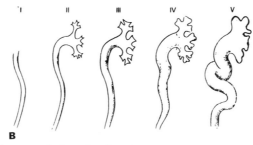

FIG. 19-5. Grading of reflux. A. *Grades I-V. Note that in grade III reflux the calyces are blunted and that in grade IV there is intrarenal reflux.* B. *Another system of grading. Beyond grade II reflux, the upper collecting systems become filled. The degree of distention separates grade II from grade III reflux, while with grade IV reflux calyceal blunting is present. With grade V reflux marked blunting along with tortuosity of the ureter is seen.* (From Levitt SB: Medical versus surgical treatment of primary vesicoureteral reflux, report of the international reflux study committee. Pediatrics 67:392, 1981; with permission.)

and the infrequent voider. Large, smooth bladders also are seen in some neurogenic states [3,25] and in the congenital megacystis-microcolon syndrome [4,9,45,47,64,85]. A small bladder is less common, and although slight degrees of smallness can be seen in normal individuals, small bladders usually are seen with severe bladder wall thickening and spasticity secondary to infection, inflammation, or neurogenic disease. In terms of the latter, the heavily

trabeculated, so-called Christmas tree bladder is typical (Fig. 19-8a).

When assessing bladder wall trabeculation, it is important not to confuse slight, normal irregularity of the posterior wall of the bladder during voiding with true irregularity that persists when the bladder is filled to capacity (Fig. 19-8b). It should be noted that mucosal irregularity is seen normally during the emptying stage of the voiding

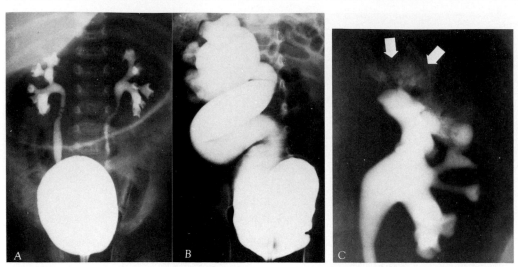

FIG. 19-6. Ureteral reflux. A. *The findings represent grade III or IV reflux depending on the method used.* B. *Grade V reflux by method B as demonstrated in Fig. 19-5.* C. *Grade IV, intrarenal reflux (arrows), as graded by method A in Fig. 19-5.*

study and is due to crinkling of the mucosa as the bladder contracts. Such crinkling is rather delicate and fine; when coarse and nodular, cystitis should be suspected (Fig. 19-9). With the bladder distended, this irregularity may be hidden.

Cystitis most often is of bacterial origin, but it can be secondary to viral infection or chemotherapeutic agents such as cyclophosphamide. Any of these conditions may cause focal irregularity of the bladder (Fig. 19-9c). Focal mucosal irregularity also can be seen with tumors (Fig. 19-9d). In addition, perivascular inflammatory disease such as an appendiceal or pelvic abscess and Crohn's disease can produce similar findings.

Other abnormalities demonstrable with cystourethrography include a variety of bladder diverticula and outpouchings. Numerous small outpouchings are seen with heavily trabeculated bladders (see Fig. 19-9b), but these are not true diverticula. The most common true diverticulum is the Hutch diverticulum, described previously (see Fig. 19-7). Other bladder diverticula can be quite large, and the patient may, in fact, void into the diverticulum. Urachal remnants, often small, are seen over the dome of the bladder. They can enlarge with any cause of bladder distension and often are quite large in the prune-belly syndrome. Bladder diverticula also are seen in the cutis laxa syndrome [42].

Filling defects in the bladder may be due to tumors, polyps, stones, blood clots, or ureteroceles. Tumors usually are contiguous with the bladder wall and project into the lumen from a broad base (Fig. 19-9d). Polyps may be seen to move or dangle; they are uncommon in children. Stones and blood clots may move with changes in position. Bladder stones are seen on plain films. Ureteroceles produce

round to oval filling defects in the bladder. The latter is most likely to occur with the ectopic ureterocele, whereas with simple ureteroceles a cobra-head deformity is more frequent (see Fig. 19-24e). Simple ureteroceles usually are seen with solitary kidneys and ectopic ureteroceles with duplicated kidneys. The latter tend to occur in females. The characteristic findings of renal displacement and an oval or round filling defect in the bladder are pathognomonic. These ureteroceles may be obstructed and under tension or relatively flaccid. When flaccid, they may be compressed during filling of the bladder and during voiding may evert to form a diverticulum [15] (Fig. 19-10).

Finally, during the voiding portion of the cystourethrogram one can obtain considerable information regarding rate of bladder emptying and configuration of the urethra. Most normal individuals empty their bladders completely, but infants may show small residual volumes. If the bladder is not emptied completely on repeated occasions, and more than a quarter of the contrast material remains, one should be suspicious of underlying pathology. For the most part, this means the presence of some form of neurogenic bladder or urethral obstruction. In either case, the urethra is of diminutive caliber, constituting the so-called low-flow pattern (Fig. 19-11).

Urethral obstruction from a congenital abnormality is almost nonexistent in the female. Rarely distal urethral stenosis is encountered, with widening of the proximal urethra, resulting in the so-called spinning top or carrot-shaped configuration [78,86,90] (Fig. 19-12a). A similar configuration is seen with spasm of the distal urethra associated with urinary tract infection.

Reflux of contrast material into the vagina is common during voiding and may be seen on the VCU (Fig.

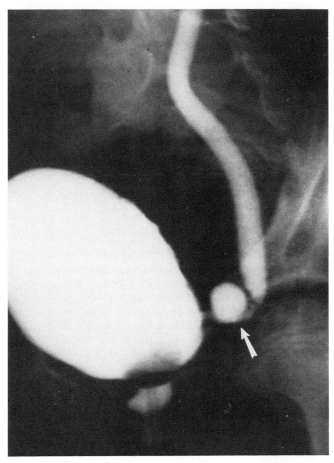

FIG. 19-7. Hutch diverticulum. *Typical Hutch diverticulum (arrow) with ureteral reflux and abnormal, horizontal insertion of the ureter.*

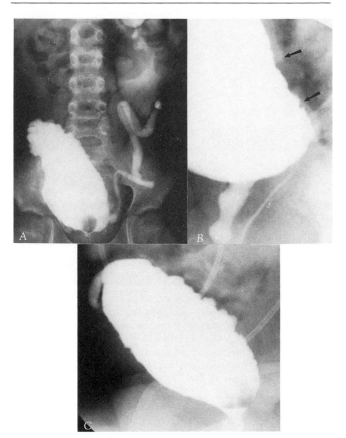

FIG. 19-8. Bladder trabeculation and irregularity. A. *Typical "Christmas tree" bladder secondary to neurogenic disease. Also note gross reflux into the left system.* B. *Localized irregularity along the posterior bladder wall (arrows), secondary to urinary tract infection.* C. *More pronounced trabeculation with cellule (pseudodiverticulum) formation. The outpouching over the dome is a normal urachal remnant.*

19-12b). It has been suggested that these patients have their urethral and vaginal orifices close together, permitting vaginal reflux to occur. This may be one of the underlying factors in urinary tract disease in young girls [8,89].

Abnormalities of the urethra are more frequent in boys. The most common lesion to cause obstruction is the posterior urethral valve. The most common type is the so-called sail valve; the other is the diaphragm valve (Fig. 19-13). The sail valve results from abnormal migration and insertion of the urethral vaginal folds. As a result, they insert anteriorly, fuse along the midline, and leave an opening posteriorly. As urine passes through the urethra, the fused folds dilate out in sail fashion and the posterior opening is inadequate to allow normal passage of urine. With the diaphragm valve, an actual diaphragm or iris exists, and the opening through it is restrictive to the flow of urine. Usually there is less posterior urethral dilatation with the diaphragm valve than with the sail valve (Fig. 19-13). With the sail valve commonly there is considerable

thickening of the bladder and bladder neck, marked reflux into grossly dilated ureters, and regurgitation of contrast material into the prostatic ducts, seminal vesicles, or both.

Other obstructing urethral lesions are much less common; they include iatrogenic stenosis, distal meatal stenosis, so-called anterior valves (actually diverticula), Cowper's gland remnants, and phimosis. The VCU serves to detect the site of obstruction and to suggest the most likely cause.

Congenital abnormalities of the urethra, such as double urethra and megalourethra, also are demonstrable on the VCU, although they are rare. In the prune, belly or Eagle-Barrett syndrome, the posterior urethra often is of a peculiar configuration; posterior urethral valves may be suggested (Fig. 19-14) [10,38,44,59,62].

Retrograde urethrography and cystography are performed when information cannot be obtained from a standard VCU. The study is used mainly to delineate a variety of stenoses and narrowings of the anterior urethra and in

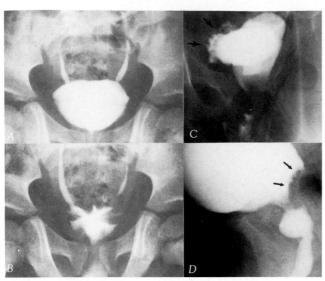

FIG. 19-9. Cystitis. A. *Patient with cyclophosphamide cystitis. With the bladder full the mucosa appears relatively smooth. Bilateral reflux is present.* B. *After voiding, the marked thickening and nodularity of the mucosa is noted.* C. *Another patient with focal cystitis causing deep trabeculation and cellule formation (arrow).* D. *Rhabdomyosarcoma (arrows) produces indentation and mucosal irregularity along the base of the bladder.*

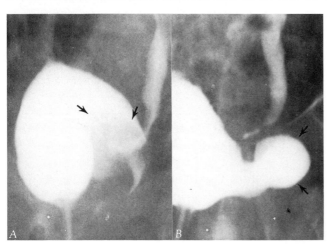

FIG. 19-10. Everting ureterocele. A. *Note the filling defect in the bladder (arrows) due to the ureterocele. Reflux is present.* B. *With voiding, the ureterocele everts to form a diverticulum (arrows). Note how this distorts the entrance of the ureter into the bladder.*

suspected bladder neck or urethral trauma. With trauma it is important to perform the retrograde study before inserting a catheter into the bladder since the catheter may pass through a urethral tear. One looks for extravasation of contrast material and compression of the urethra and bladder by the adjacent collection of blood and fluid.

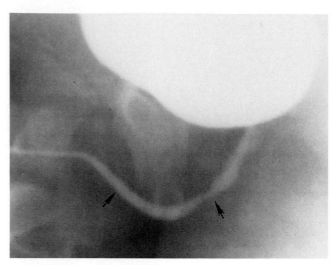

FIG. 19-11. Low flow pattern: neurogenic bladder. *Note that while anatomically the urethra (arrows) in this male appears normal, it is very thin, reflecting a low flow pattern secondary to impeded emptying of the bladder.*

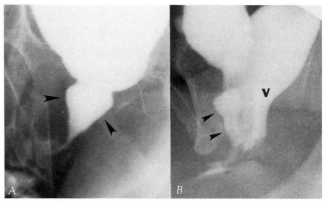

FIG. 19-12. A. Spinning top urethra. *Note the spinning top appearance of the urethra (arrows) in this female.* B. *Vaginal reflux. With voiding, the bladder empties and the urethra remains a little distended (arrows). Gross reflux has occurred into the vagina (V).*

Ultrasonographic, Computed Tomography, and Magnetic Resonance Imaging

Of these three modalities, ultrasonography has had the greatest impact on the investigation of renal disease in children, affording excellent visualization of the kidneys and perirenal structures. MRI can provide some additional data regarding abnormalities of renal parenchymal disease and tumors but probably will not displace ultrasonography. Currently it has little application in investigation of urinary tract disease in children except tumors.

With the development of newer-generation, high-reso-

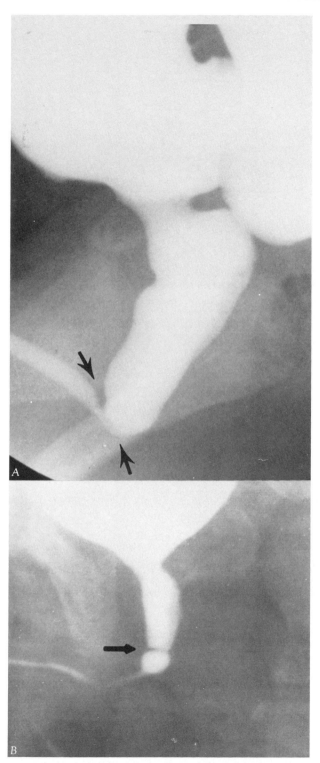

FIG. 19-13. Posterior urethral valves. a. *Typical sail valve producing obstruction at the level of the membranous urethra* (arrows). *The posterior urethra shows marked dilatation.* b. *Typical iris or diaphragm valve* (arrow).

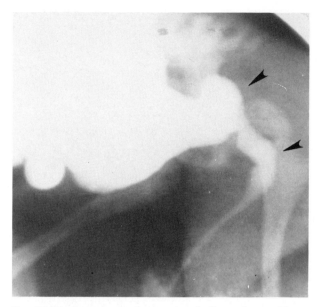

FIG. 19-14. Posterior urethra—prune-belly syndrome. *Note peculiar configuration of the bladder neck and posterior urethra* (arrows) *in this young male with prune-belly syndrome. The bladder is markedly dilated and enlarged.*

lution, real-time sector scanners, the use of ultrasonography in the pediatric patient has greatly expanded. The new equipment is ideally suited for the evaluation of the infant and young child. Sedation is virtually never required, and accurate information is available regarding almost any abnormality of the renal tract, including diffuse parenchymal disease.

It is important for the physician to appreciate that what is imaged on a sonogram is somewhat different from that seen with the IVU. With the IVU, the ureters, pelves, and calyceal structures as well as the renal outline and renal parenchyma are well defined. In contrast, the renal sonogram does not identify the renal pelvis, ureters, or calyceal structures to any great extent, unless they are abnormally dilated. However, corticomedullary differentiation is good, and consequently the renal cortex, renal pyramids, and renal sinus are routinely visualized (Fig. 19-15). The renal sinus is located centrally and is very echogenic because it contains peripelvic fat and fibrous tissue. This finding is a constant feature in older children, although often less well defined in the neonate (Fig. 19-15).

Sonographic characteristics of the renal cortex also are different in the neonate. In the older infant and child, as in the adult, the renal cortex is relatively sonolucent and far less echogenic than the adjacent liver or splenic parenchyma (Fig. 19-15). In the neonate and young infant, the renal cortex may be as echogenic as the adjacent liver parenchyma, although normally it is not more echogenic (Fig. 19-15).

This sonographic appearance usually changes to a more "adult-like" pattern between 2 and 3 months of age, and

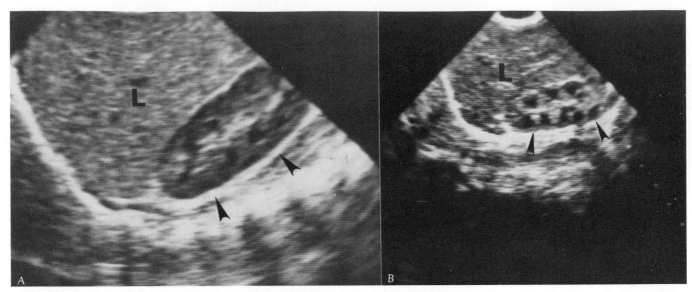

FIG. 19-15. Normal kidney—ultrasonography. A. *Older infant demonstrating anechoic outer renal parenchyma (arrows) and central echoes of the renal sinus. Note that the adjacent liver (L) is more echogenic than the renal parenchyma. B. In the neonate, the liver (L) and kidney (arrows) are of the same echogenicity. The small black areas suggesting cysts represent the normal ultrasonographic appearance of the medullary pyramids in the neonatal kidney.*

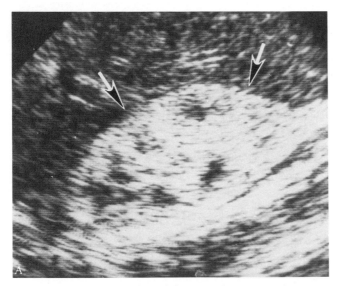

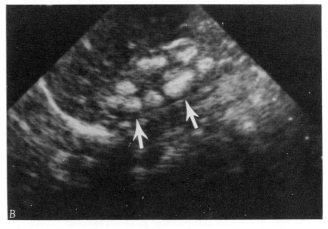

FIG. 19-16. Renal parenchymal disease—ultrasonography. A. *Note that the kidney (arrows) is more echogenic than the adjacent liver. This is characteristic of renal parenchymal disease. In this case corticomedullary definition is preserved. B. Nephrocalcinosis. Note numerous areas of focal echogenicity due to calcium deposition in the pyramids (arrows).*

by 4 months of age 90% of all normal infants demonstrate the adult features [32,35,40]. However, regardless of the age of the infant or child, the renal pyramids remain strikingly sonolucent in relationship to the renal cortex and

renal sinus. In the neonate, these ovoid or triangular sonolucent areas frequently were misinterpreted as renal cysts (Fig. 19-15b).

When renal parenchymal disease is present, the renal

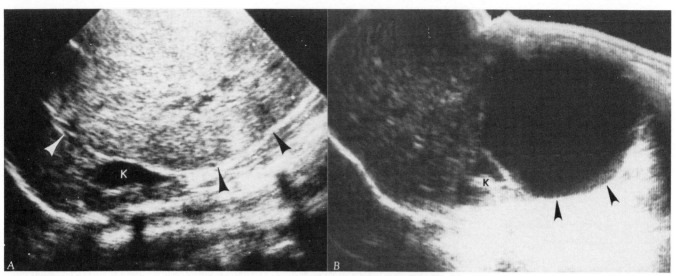

FIG. 19-17. Solid vs. cystic lesions—ultrasonography. A. *Note diffuse echogenicity throughout this large Wilms' tumor (arrows) causing hydronephrosis of the residual kidney (K). B. Large anechoic simple renal cyst (arrows). Ultrasonography quickly and precisely differentiates between solid and cystic lesions. Residual kidney (k). For the intravenous urograms in these patients see Fig. 19-4. K, Kidney; L, liver.*

cortex becomes more echogenic than normal (Fig. 19-16a), and, although the finding is nonspecific, it is easy to detect [35,46]. There is occasional loss of corticomedullary differentiation. The increase in cortical echogenicity associated with such renal parenchymal disease usually is secondary to glomerular and tubulointerstitial changes, such as fibrosis or glomerular sclerosis, but also can be seen with calcium deposition (Fig. 19-16b).

Edema of the kidney also may produce an increase in echogenicity, as in acute glomerulonephritis, renal vein thrombosis, and minimal lesion nephrotic syndrome [35,50,70]. Other causes of a hyperechoic renal parenchyma include infantile polycystic kidney disease, adult polycystic disease appearing in infancy, medullary cystic disease, and infiltration of the renal parenchyma with leukemia, lymphoma, and mucopolysaccaridoses. It should be noted that in leukemia and lymphoma the infiltration may be so intense and homogeneous that no acoustical interfaces are encountered. Consequently, the entire kidney or part of the kidney can appear relatively anechoic.

Tumor

The rapid and reliable differentiation of whether a renal mass is solid or cystic continues to be a very important role for ultrasonography. A cystic lesion produces one or more purely anechoic areas, whereas solid lesions produce homogeneous or irregular echogenicity (Fig. 19-17). In some of the solid lesions, in which malignant tissue growth is rapid, hemorrhagic-degenerative areas may produce inter-

spersed anechoic areas, leading to a so-called mixed pattern of echogenicity.

Wilms' tumor is encapsulated and clearly identified with ultrasonography (Fig. 19-18). Most often it is clearly identified as being intrarenal [41], but if there is doubt, MRI or enhanced CT scanning, may be required. However, CT [17,24,48], although very efficient in defining normal and abnormal anatomy, is no more, and probably even less, effective than ultrasonography when it comes to determining whether a lesion is intrarenal or extrarenal. This is especially true on the right side, where it may be impossible to determine whether a tumor is arising in the kidney and extending into the liver, or vice-versa. MRI may prove more helpful in this area.

With diagnosis of Wilms' tumor the contralateral kidney is examined by ultrasonography for additional lesions. Thereafter one should evaluate the inferior vena cava, looking for intracaval extension of the tumor [81] (Fig. 19-18c). If tumor or thrombus extends into the inferior vena cava, an area of intraluminal echogenicity is seen (Fig. 19-18d). In these cases, using the right lobe of the liver as an acoustic window, it is possible to examine the right atrium of the heart for extension of tumor.

Other tumors of the kidney, although less common than Wilms' tumor, have a similar echogenic pattern. These include the benign fetal renal hamartoma (mesenchymoma) and the odd renal cell carcinoma. The sonographic appearance of nephroblastoma differs in that a discrete mass is not identified. The kidney is riddled with numerous, small tumors and becomes enlarged. In the so-called cystic Wilms' tumor (i.e., multilocular cystic nephroma, benign

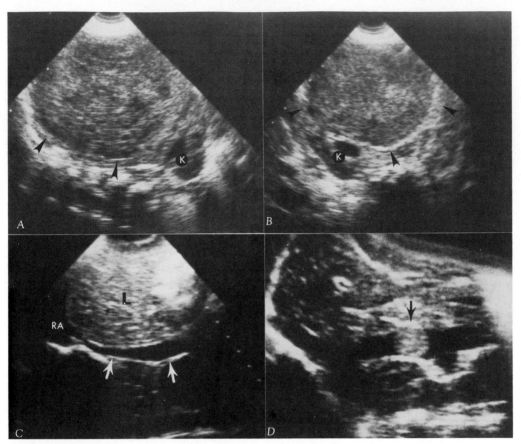

FIG. 19-18. Wilms' tumor—ultrasonographic findings. A. *Note the solid, diffusely echogenic tumor mass (arrows). The kidney (K) is displaced and compressed in this transverse view. B. Longitudinal view demonstrates the same tumor mass (arrows), and residual, displaced hydronephrotic kidney (K). C. View of the inferior vena cava (arrows) shows it to be normally anechoic and free of tumor extension. RA, right atrium; L, Liver. D. Note tumor thrombus (arrow) in the inferior vena cava of another patient. (Courtesy of T. Lobe, M.D.)*

epithelioblastoma, polycystic nephroma), a wide variety of patterns may be encountered, but usually one sees a multiloculated or multiseptated lesion, with an adjacent solid lesion (Fig. 19-19). Because of the complexity of these lesions, another study, such as CT or MRI, may be needed.

Cystic Disease

Simple renal cysts, although rare, are readily identified with ultrasonography, as is the classic multicystic dysplastic kidney (Fig. 19-20a). The latter entity produces multiple anechoic cavities, which do not connect with each other or an identifiable renal pelvis [30,72,83]. Renal parenchymal tissue and ureters cannot be identified despite the fact that almost all of these kidneys are the result of high-grade intrauterine, upper ureteric obstruction [21,28]. It is believed that a vascular insult early in fetal life produces hydronephrosis with subsequent dysplastic cystic change. The ureter is atretic. The vascular insult is believed to occur around the ureteropelvic junction, and consequently, the renal pelvis is atretic and not identified as a separate structure. This is most important in differentiating multicystic dysplastic kidneys from end stage hydronephrotic kidneys. With the latter, the renal pelvis is identified and the dilated calyces are seen to communicate with it (see Fig. 19-22a). If a renal pelvis persists in a multicystic dysplastic kidney, it may be difficult to differentiate it completely from classic ureteropelvic junction obstruction. In such cases, the final answer may come from nuclear scintography. With multicystic dysplastic kidney disease, there is no renal function, whereas in most cases of classic ureteropelvic junction obstruction some degree of renal function is present. Finally, it should be noted that although most cases of multicystic dysplastic kidney disease produce large kidneys, some produce small, atrophic kidneys. In these cases the cysts still are identifiable with

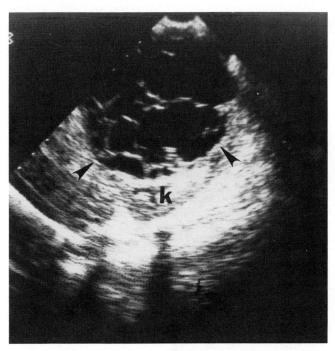

FIG. 19-19. Cystic Wilms' tumor—ultrasound. *Note the multi-loculated cystic appearance of this lesion (arrows). Residual renal parenchyma is seen in the inferior portion (K).*

ultrasonography, although the total renal mass is not very large.

Infantile polycystic kidney disease usually produces a nonspecific ultrasonographic pattern consisting of large kidneys with diffuse hyperechogenicity [12,30]. Renal architecture is totally lost and corticomedullary differentiation is poor or nonexistent. We have noted in one or two cases a relative sonolucent rim in these kidneys (Fig. 19-20b), possibly reflecting the outer rim of compressed cortex. Presumably, not enough cortical interfaces exist in this area to produce echos. However, an increase in echogenicity does occur throughout the remaining bulk of the kidney, which consists of dilated tubules. We are not certain as to how definitive this finding is, but believe it does have potential differential diagnostic value. In addition, some of these kidneys show small cysts or even tortuous, dilated tubules.

Adult polycystic disease presenting in the neonate appears similar to infantile polycystic disease, but the peripheral anechoic rim is not seen. The cysts at this early stage of the disease are too small to be recognized as individual structures, but there are so many of them that numerous acoustical interfaces exist and echogenicity is pronounced [21,34]. Indeed, one may have a very homogeneous pattern of increased echogenicity (Fig. 19-20c). Later in life, as some of the cysts become larger, multiple round to oval anechoic areas develop [87] (Fig. 19-20d).

With medullary cystic disease or familial nephronophthisis, the kidneys are small and hyperechoic and the

cysts are small. Cortical cysts, usually rather small, also are seen sporadically in conditions such as Zellweger's syndrome (Fig. 19-20e), and punctate epiphyseal dysplasia.

Hydronephrosis

The ultrasonographic findings in hydronephrosis are well described [19,23]. In minimal cases a slit-like anechoic area is seen in the region of the renal sinus (Fig. 19-21a). With greater degrees of hydronephrosis this area becomes larger (Fig. 19-21b) and the calyces are visualized (Fig. 19-21c). Eventually these structures all become large and, depending on the degree of hydronephrosis, show associated loss of renal cortex (Fig. 19-21c). Classically, the calyces are seen to communicate with the renal pelvis; depending on the level of obstruction, one may or may not see a dilated ureter (Fig. 19-22a). With more distal obstruction, of course, the dilated ureters are readily identified (Fig. 22b,c,d). Most often such ureters are dilated down to their insertion into the urinary bladder; consequently, it is not possible to determine whether the ureters are dilated because of obstruction or gross reflux.

Vesicoureteral Reflux

Reflux has been identified with ultrasonography and is relatively easy to demonstrate with grossly dilated ureters (Fig. 19-23). With filling of the bladder, turbulence and microbubble formation produce echogenic signals as the urine refluxes into the ureter [43,89]. The findings are more difficult to demonstrate with minimally dilated ureters and lesser degrees of reflux. Therefore, ultrasonography probably will not replace the VCU for the initial identification and characterization of this abnormality. However, color flow Doppler ultrasonography may have a more viable role in the future.

Ureter, Bladder, and Urethra

In evaluating dilated ureters, it should be noted that dilated loops of intestine, filled with fluid, can be misinterpreted for dilated ureters, as can the normal psoas muscle. Apart from these pitfalls, however, dilated ureters usually are readily identified.

With ureteral dilation the bladder is examined for lesions such as ectopic ureterocele [5,54,70] (Fig. 19-24a,b), simple ureterocele (Fig. 19-24c,d), and lesions of the bladder that might cause obstruction of the ureter.

Ultrasonography, CT, and MRI all provide information regarding the bladder and urethra. However, once again, because the bladder can be filled with fluid or urine, a perfect "window" for ultrasonography is provided. The bladder usually is identified in its entirety, and the intraluminal filling defects and bladder wall thickenings are well demonstrated (Fig. 19-25). Nothing has replaced the VCU for imaging the urethra, but the dilated posterior urethra can be visualized with ultrasonography in cases of posterior urethral valves and the prune-belly syndrome [27,56] (Fig.

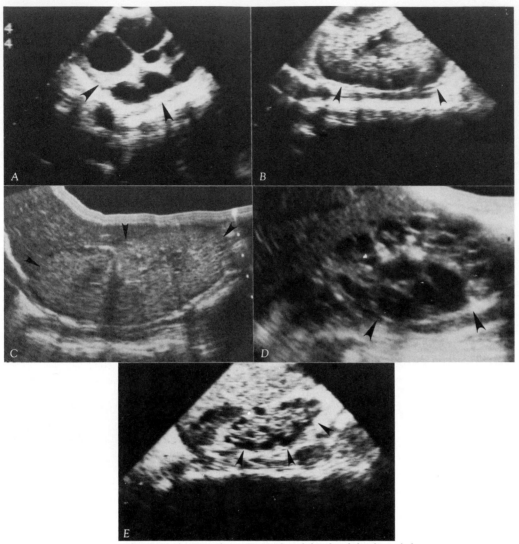

FIG. 19-20. Renal cystic disease—ultrasound. A. *Typical multiloculated dysplastic kidney* (arrows). B. *Kidney in an infant with infantile polycystic kidney disease. Note diffuse central echogenicity and a peripheral anechoic rim* (arrows). C. *Adult polycystic disease in the neonate. Note diffuse and extremely homogeneous hyperechogenicity of the enlarged kidney* (arrows). D. *Typical appearance of adult polycystic kidney disease in an adult* (arrows). e. *Small peripheral cortical cysts* (arrows) *in a small, hyperechoic kidney seen in Zellweger's syndrome.*

19-26). Otherwise the urethra is not well visualized with ultrasonography.

Urinary Tract Infection

The sonogram is not very useful in acute urinary tract infection. It can detect a renal abscess, which is uncommon in children. Acute lobar nephronia (acute focal pyelonephritis) shows rapid resolution in response to antibiotics after initially presenting as an area of focally increased echogenicity.

Focal scars and clubbed calyces can be demonstrated with ultrasonography but only when the changes are rather marked. With acute pyelonephritis the kidney may be enlarged and in some cases even hyperechoic. However, in most cases the kidneys appear normal. Ultrasonography's primary role, therefore, is to exclude surgically correctable lesions causing urinary tract obstruction.

Renal Size, Location, and Number

Ultrasonography can be used for determining renal size, location of the kidneys, and anomalies of kidney number

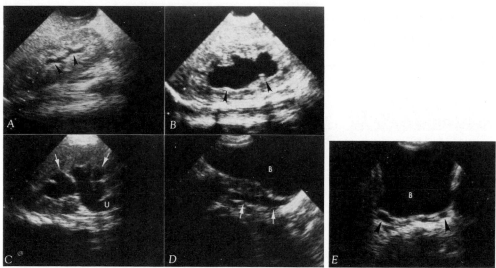

FIG. 19-21. Hydronephrosis—ultrasound. A. *Note minimal dilatation of the pelvis (arrows).* B. *More pronounced dilatation of the same structures (arrows).* C. *Gross hydronephrosis with calyceal dilatation (arrows) and visualization of the dilated ureter (U).* D. *Visualization of the dilated ureter (arrows) as it inserts into the bladder (B). This was a longitudinal scan.* E. *Cross-section of the bladder (B) demonstrates both ureters in this patient to be dilated (arrows).*

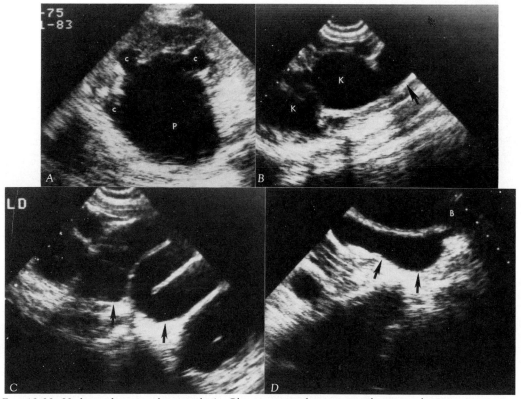

FIG. 19-22. Hydronephrosis—ultrasound. A. *Classic ureteropelvic junction obstruction demonstrating the dilated renal pelvis (P) and peripheral calyces (C). The ureter is not visualized.* B. *Another patient with gross hydronephrosis and visualization of the dilated upper collecting system (K) and a very tortuous, dilated ureter (arrow).* C. *Marked tortuosity of the ureter in the same patient as in B.* D. *The same patient, with longitudinal section through the bladder (B) demonstrating the large dilated ureter (arrows) inserting into the bladder. Same patient as in Fig. 4B.*

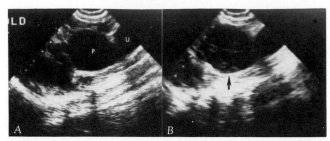

FIG. 19-23. Ureteral vesical reflux—ultrasound. A. *Note the dilated renal pelvis (P) and ureter (U) in this patient with gross hydronephrosis. B. Reflux produces multiple echoes in the dilated renal pelvis (arrow) due to the presence of microbubbles.*

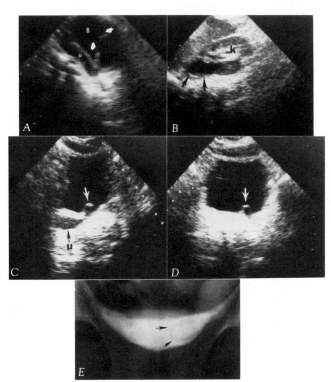

FIG. 19-24. Ureteroceles—ultrasound. A. *Typical, rounded appearance of ectopic ureterocele (arrows), projecting into the bladder (B). The dilated ureter (U) is seen below. B. Renal ultrasonogram demonstrates the normal lower kidney (K) and the dilated, hydroneprotic upper kidney (arrows). Same case as in Fig. 19-6. C. Simple ureterocele (arrow), longitudinal section of bladder. Note the dilated ureter (U). D. Cross-section of the bladder demonstrates the same simple ureterocele (arrow). E. IVU demonstrating simple ureterocele as the typical cobra-head deformity (arrow).*

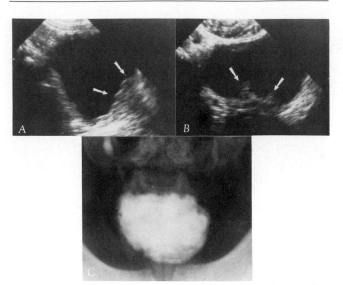

FIG. 19-25. Intraluminal and bladder wall defects—ultrasound. A. *Note increased echoes in this bladder wall tumor (arrows). B. Profound cystitis with papilliform extensions into the bladder (arrows). C. Cystogram in same patient.*

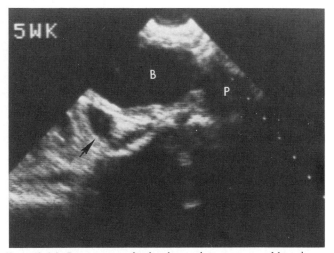

FIG. 19-26. Posterior urethral valve—ultrasonogram. *Note the bladder (B) and the dilated posterior urethra (P). The hypertrophied bladder neck is seen in between and the dilated ureter posteriorly (arrow).*

(Fig. 19-27). For renal measurements, scanning is accomplished in both the longitudinal and the cross-sectional planes, and accurate measurements are readily obtained with cursor placement (see subsequently). Small kidneys are readily visualized with ultrasonography (Fig. 19-28); many of these are scarred and hyperechoic.

CT scanning and MRI provide similar information. The advantage eventually may lean in favor of MRI since it requires no ionizing radiation. However, neither is likely to replace ultrasonography. Both CT and MRI are excellent in delineating geographic anatomy (Fig. 19-29), and are particularly useful in delineating tumor margins (Fig. 19-30). However, the studies are not always as effective as ultrasonography in distinguishing cystic from solid lesions.

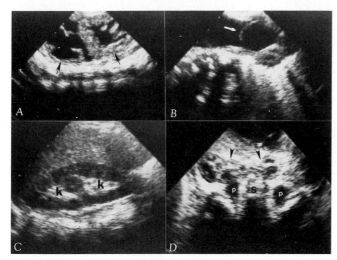

FIG. 19-27. Duplicated kidneys—ultrasound. A. *Note hydrone-phrosis of both parts of this duplicated kidney (arrows); more pronounced in the upper segment. B. Ectopic ureterocele (arrow), causing obstruction of the upper kidney. The dilated ureter caused secondary obstruction of the lower kidney. C. Duplicated normal kidney (K). D. Horseshoe kidney (arrows), lying over the spine (S) and psoas muscles (P).*

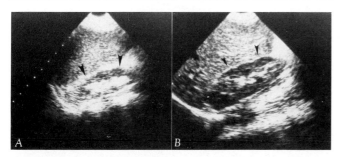

FIG. 19-28. Small fibrotic kidney—ultrasound. A. *Note increased echogenicity of the right kidney (arrows) and poor definition of its anatomy. The kidney is small. B. Normal kidney on the other side for comparison (arrows).*

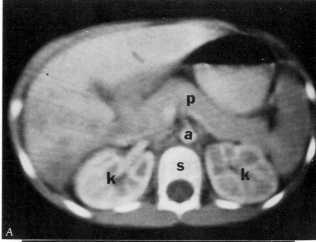

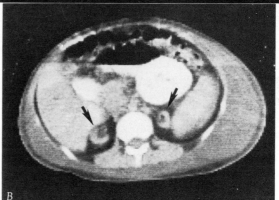

FIG. 19-29. Normal and small kidneys—CT. A. *Note the normal right and left kidneys (K) on this contrast-enhanced CT scan. This patient was being evaluated for pancreatitis and demonstrates an enlarged pancreas (P). In the kidneys, note the cortex (outer white rim), and the gray medullary pyramids. A, aorta; S, spine. B. Small atrophic kidneys (arrows) surrounded by perinephric fat.*

Trauma

CT is superior to ultrasonography in the evaluation of renal trauma (Fig. 19-31). Although in most cases, ultrasonography can readily identify intrarenal as well as perirenal collections of fluid, and in some instances actually identify renal lacerations, it does not provide the exquisite anatomic detail that CT does and does not pick up the minor degrees of trauma that CT is capable of identifying (Fig. 19-31). Most importantly, however, ultrasonography gives no information concerning renal function and does not provide the two most important pieces of information that the surgeon requires: (1) whether the renal pedicle has

been damaged and renal perfusion impaired and (2) whether there is a significant leak of urine. Indeed, in general CT scanning of the abdomen is favored over ultrasonography for intra-abdominal injuries, and also over the intravenous pyelogram.

Nephrocalcinosis and Nephrolithiasis

Diffuse calcification within the renal parenchyma characteristically produces hyperechogenicity [2,3], and the finding is not difficult to detect (see Fig. 19-16b). Identification of renal stones is often more fortuitous than definitive. When large, however, these stones are echogenic and produce acoustic impedance or shadowing (Fig. 19-32). Most renal stones are better detected with plain films and intravenous urography but also are readily demonstrable with CT scanning.

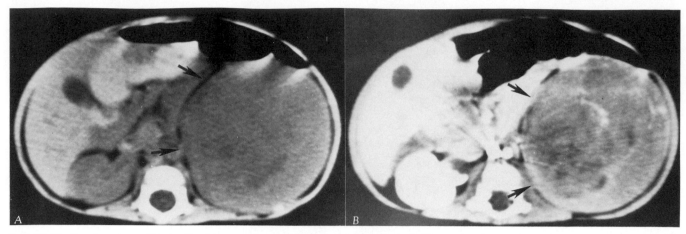

FIG. 19-30. Renal tumor—CT. A. On this non–contrast-enhanced scan note the well-delineated and relatively homogeneous Wilms' tumor (arrows). B. With contrast enhancement the disorganized nature of the tumor is more evident (arrows). (Courtesy of C. J. Fagan, M.D.)

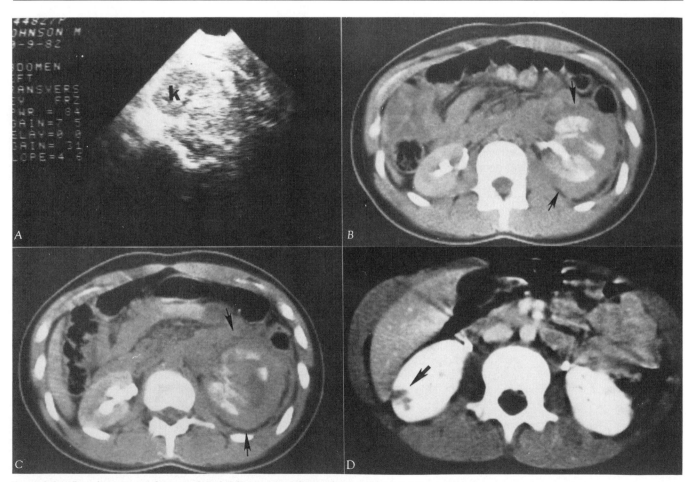

FIG. 19-31. Renal trauma—ultrasound and CT. A. Note the poorly visualized left kidney (K). A great deal of echo activity (hematoma) surrounds the kidney, and only the upper pole appears clearly visualized. B. CT demonstrates the completely fractured left kidney and perinephric hematoma (arrows). Compare with the normal right kidney. C. Slightly lower scan demonstrates the extensive nature of the injury and the accumulation of perinephric blood (arrows). D. Small contusion (arrow) in the right kidney. This would be difficult to detect with ultrasonography or intravenous pyelography.

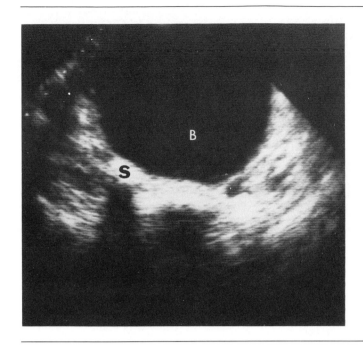

FIG. 19-32. Urinary tract calculi—ultrasound. *Note increased echoes in this renal stone (S), which produced obstruction of the distal ureter. Also note the fan-shaped, black area of acoustical impedance or shadowing distal to the stone. B, bladder.*

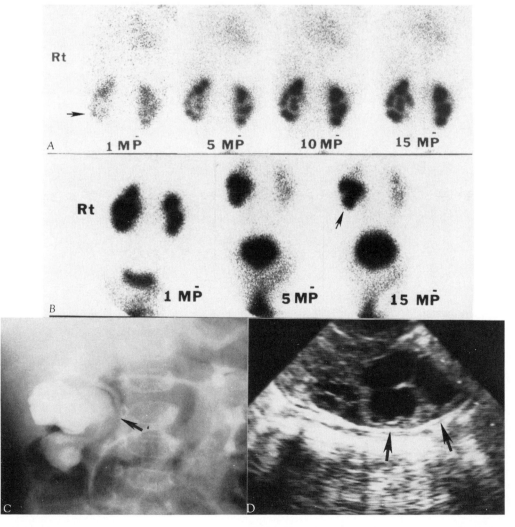

FIG. 19-33. Technetium DTPA study in obstructive uropathy. *A. Early phase demonstrates decreased function and filling of the calyces on the right, especially in the lower pole (arrow). B. With furosemide washout there is progressive decrease in isotope activity over the left kidney and over the right upper pole. However, there is failure of washout of the isotope from the lower pole (arrow). C. This is due to hydronephrosis (arrow) of the lower pole, secondary to a ureteropelvic junction obstruction. The upper pole of this partially duplicated kidney is slightly dilated due to secondary compression. D. Longitudinal sonogram demonstrates the marked hydronephrosis of the lower pole (arrows) and slight hydronephrosis of the upper pole.*

493

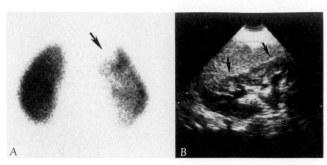

FIG. 19-34. ^{99m}Glucoheptanate scintigram. A. *Note the generally
decreased and irregular activity in the left kidney with a focal defect
in the upper pole* (arrow). B. *Ultrasonogram demonstrates a normal
appearing kidney.*

Nuclear Radiology

Prior to the early 1970s, few pediatric urologic radionuclide
studies were performed, primarily because of the high radiation exposure associated with the mercurial and io-
dinated radioisotopic compounds available for renal imaging. With the development of technetium compounds with
short half-lives, a larger amount of isotope could be injected and a better image obtained. In addition, the development of the gamma camera made possible dynamic
sequential imaging and thus the ability to evaluate renal
perfusion, function, and clearance. The addition of com-
puters to this technique has enabled even more sophisticated evaluation.

Currently, the renal radionuclide used most often in
pediatric nuclear medicine is technetium DTPA. Renal
clearance of this substance occurs primarily by way of glomerular filtration (95%), and there is no significant tubular
excretion or renal parenchymal retention. The initial transit of the isotope through the kidney reflects renal perfusion, while renal activity between 1 and 3 minutes after
injection is a measure of the functioning renal mass. Because the renal clearance is predominantly by glomerular
filtration, the rate of isotope clearance can be used as an
accurate measurement of glomerular filtration rate [79]. In
addition, the high concentration of isotope in the urine
allows relatively good visualization of the pelvicalyceal
structures, ureters, and bladder. In this way morphologic
information, roughly similar to that obtained with the
IVU, is available. The study often is augmented by administering a diuretic to produce a so-called washout study.
This is especially useful in detecting obstruction and demonstrating differential function from side to side (Fig.
19-33).

Two other renal imaging agents now are being used when
better visualization of renal anatomy is desired, particularly
if the primary concern is the evaluation of the renal cortex.
This becomes especially important in the evaluation of
acute pyelonephritis and renal scarring. Technetium 99m-
dimercaptosuccinic acid (DMSA) is used for this purpose
because 60% to 70% of the agent remains within the renal
cortex [58,72]. DMSA is tightly bound to the renal tubules
with only 2% to 5% being excreted in the urine. Because
of tubular binding, however, this agent is poor for studying
the pelvicalyceal system. With the other agent, technetium
99m-glucoheptonate, blood clearance is rapid, and thus
early in the course of the study there is moderately good

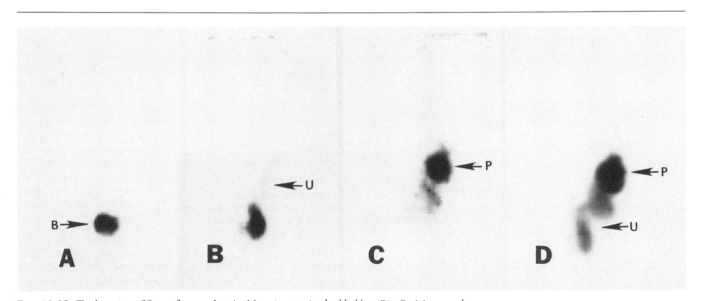

FIG. 19-35. Technetium 99m reflux study. A. *Note isotope in the bladder* (B). B. *Moments later
some isotope activity is seen refluxing into the ureter* (U). C. *and* D. *Later, the entire collecting system
is delineated with most of the isotope now being present in the dilated pelvis* (P) *and ureter* (U).
(*Courtesy of Dan Fawcett, M.D.*)

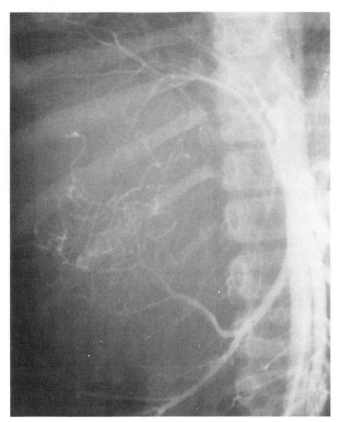

FIG. 19-36. Arteriography—Wilms' tumor. *Note numerous abnormal so-called tumor vessels extending into this large Wilms' tumor.*

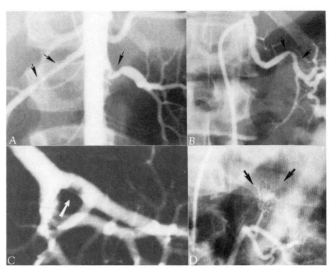

FIG. 19-37. Renal artery abnormalities—angiography. A. *Note focal stenosis of both the right and the left renal arteries (arrows). B. Corrugated appearance of the renal artery in fibromuscular hyperplasia (arrows). C. Focal defect in renal artery (arrows) in periarteritis nodosa. This probably represents an area of hyperplastic vasculitis. D. Focally abnormal intraparenchymal vessels (arrows) in patients with hypertension and neurofibromatosis.*

visualization of the pelvicalyceal collecting systems. At the same time, approximately 5% to 15% of the isotope is retained in the tubular cells, and, therefore, delayed imaging (2 hours or later) provides excellent visualization of the renal cortical anatomy (Fig. 19-34). This agent also appears to be advantageous over technetium DMSA in that it has a significantly lower renal radiation dose for the same cortical concentration.

A very important use of radionuclides is in the study of the urinary tract for vesicoureteral reflux. Technetium pertechnetate mixed with normal saline and introduced into the bladder through a catheter has proved to be an excellent method of studying vesicoureteral reflux (Fig. 19-35). This study should not be used for the initial investigation for reflux in boys because it does not provide the anatomic detail provided by the conventional cystourethrogram. However, the radioisotopic cystogram is well suited for girls and as a follow-up study in both sexes. It delivers a significantly lower radiation dose to the patient than the VCU.

Information regarding urinary tract obstruction, duplicated kidneys, ectopic kidneys, renal masses, and other lesions may be obtained with nuclear medicine studies. However, because anatomic detail is not available with these studies, they are seldom used for these purposes.

Arteriography

The role of renal arteriography is limited in pediatrics. It is almost never used for the evaluation of renal masses or infection and its complications. Although it is capable of demonstrating abnormal tumor vascularity (Fig. 19-36), this also is seldom required. Consequently its primary function now is relegated to the investigation of systemic hypertension, renal artery thrombosis, and the integrity of the renal artery and vein in renal trauma. By far, its greatest use lies with the investigation of systemic hypertension.

In evaluating hypertension, the renal arteriogram's main function is to detect areas of narrowing of the renal artery, intrarenal arteriovenous aneurysms, or other vascular abnormalities. Renal artery stenoses are relatively easy to demonstrate and assume a variety of configurations; some are focal, others multiple, and still others corrugated and characteristic of fibromuscular hyperplasia (Fig. 19-37). Most cases of renovascular hypertension are due to large vessel disease, but a few result from small, intraparenchymal vascular abnormalities [38] (Fig. 19-37d). Selective arterial studies with subtraction often are required to demonstrate these focal abnormalities. Nonsurgical dilatation of the renal artery is performed under fluoroscopic control.

Miscellaneous Problems
Renal Size

Renal size usually is adequately evaluated with the IVU, but very often linear tomography is employed to define the

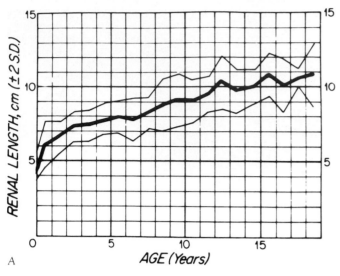

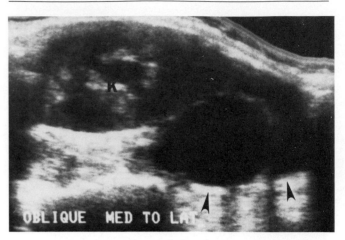

FIG. 19-39. Renal transplant with lymphocele. *Note the kidney (K) and the adjacent collection of fluid (arrows), representing a lymphocele.*

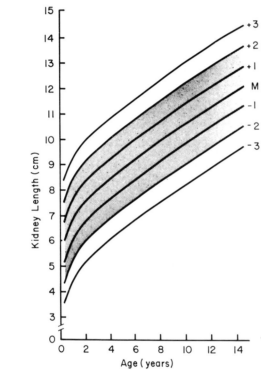

FIG. 19-38. Renal size determination. A. *Ultrasonographic measurement.* B. *Pyelographic measurements. (A. From Rosenbaum DM, Korngold E, Teele RL: Sonographic assessment of real length in normal children. AJR 142:467, 1984 with permission.); (B. from Currarino G, Williams B K; with permission.)*

Renal Transplant

The assessment of the renal transplant centers around function and obstruction. Function is best assessed with radionuclide studies, whereas obstruction lends itself best to ultrasonographic investigation. The functional changes are no different from those seen with any other cause of decreased function due to renal parenchymal disease. Ultrasonography can define hydronephrosis and also can demonstrate the presence of compressing perirenal fluid collections, such as lymphoceles and urinomas (Fig. 19-39). Arteriography occasionally is employed when renal arteriostenosis is suspected.

References

1. Adelman RD, Shapiro SR, Woerner S: Psychogenic polydipsia with hydronephrosis in an infant. *Pediatrics* 65:344, 1980.
2. Afschrift M, Nachtegaele P, Van Rattinghe R, et al: Nephrocalcinosis demonstrated by ultrasound and CT. *Pediatr Radiol* 13:42, 1983.
3. Alon U, Brewer WH, Chan JCM: Nephrocalcinosis: Detection by ultrasonography. *Pediatrics* 71:970, 1983.
4. Amoury RA, Fellows RA, Goodwin CD, et al: Megacystis-microcolon intestinal hypoperistalsis syndrome; a cause of intestinal obstruction in the newborn period. *J Pediatr Surg* 12:1063, 1977.
5. Athey PA, Carpenter RJ, Hadlock FP, et al: Ultrasonic demonstration of ectopic ureterocele. *Pediatrics* 71:568, 1983.
6. Bacopoulos C, Papahatzi-Kalmadi M, Karpathios T, et al: Renal-vertebral index in normal children. *Arch Dis Child* 56:390, 1981.
7. Baghdassarian-Gatewood OM, Glaser RJ, Van Houtte JD: Roentgen evaluation of renal size in pediatric age groups. *Am J Dis Child* 110:162, 1965.
8. Beale G: Intravaginal and intrauterine refluxing of urine in children; some postulates arising from these findings. *Australas Radiol* 19:194, 1975.

renal margins more clearly. In the older child, a normal kidney measures the length of four vertebral bodies and their intervening disc spaces. Numerous methods of measuring the kidneys have been devised, and tables of normal values for both pyelographic and ultrasonographic studies are available [6,7,16,18,36,39,69] (Fig. 19-38).

9. Berdon WE, Baker DH, Blanc WA, et al: Megacystis-micro-colon intestinal hypoperistalsis syndrome; new cause of intestinal obstruction in the newborn—report of radiologic findings in five newborn girls. *AJR* 126:959, 1976.

10. Berdon WE, Baker DH, Wigger HJ, et al: The radiologic and pathologic spectrum of the prune belly syndrome; the importance of urethral obstruction in prognosis. *Radiol Clin North Am* 1:83, 1977.

11. Berdon WE, Schwartz RH, Becker J, et al: Tamm-Horsfall proteinuria. *Radiology* 92:714, 1969.

12. Boad DK, Teele RL: Sonography of infantile polycystic kidney disease. *AJR* 135:575, 1980.

13. Clayton CB, Dee PM, Scott JES, et al: Micturating urethrogram in female children. *Br J Radiol* 39:771, 1966.

14. Conway JJ, Belman AB, King LR: Direct and indirect radionuclide cystography. *Semin Nucl Med* 4:197, 1974.

15. Cremin BJ, Funston MR, Aaronson IA: The intrauretic diverticulum, a manifestation of ureterocele intussusception. *Pediatr Radiol* 6:92, 1977.

16. Currarino G, Williams B, Dana K: Kidney length correlated with age: Normal values in children. *Radiology* 150:703, 1984.

17. Damgaard-Pedersen K: CT and IVU in the diagnosis of Wilms' tumour. A comparative study. *Pediatric Radiol* 9:207, 1980.

18. De Vries L, Levene MI: Measurement of renal size in preterm and term infants by real-time ultrasound. *Arch Dis Child* 58:145, 1983.

19. Diament MJ, Takasugi J, Kangarloo H: Hydronephrosis in childhood—reliability of ultrasound screening. *Pediatr Radiol* 14:31, 1984.

20. Dunbar JS, Nogrady MB: The calyceal crescent—a roentgenographic sign of obstructive hydronephrosis. *AJR* 110:520, 1970.

21. Fellows RA, Leonidas JC, Beatty EC: Radiologic features of "adult type" polycystic kidney disease in the neonate. *Pediatr Radiol* 4:87, 1976.

22. Felson B, Cussen LJ: The hydronephrotic type of unilateral congenital multicystic disease of the kidney. *Semin Roentgenol* 10:113, 1975.

23. Filly R, Friedland G, Govan DE, et al: Development and progression of clubbing and scarring in children with recurrent urinary tract infections. *Radiology* 113:145, 1974.

24. Fishman EK, Hartman DS, Goldman SM, et al: The CT appearance of Wilms' tumor. *J Comput Assist Tomogr* 7:659, 1983.

25. Friedland GW, Perkash I: Neuromuscular dysfunction of the bladder and urethra. *Semin Roentgenol* 18:255, 1983.

26. Funston MR, Cremin BJ: Intrarenal reflux—papillary morphology and pressure relationships in children's necropsy kidneys. *Br J Radiol* 51:665, 1978.

27. Gilanz V, Miller JH, Reid BS: Ultrasonic characteristics of posterior urethral valves. *Radiology* 145:143, 1982.

28. Griscom NT, Vawter GF, Fellers FX: Pelvoinfundibular atresia; the usual form of multicystic kidney; 44 unilateral and 2 bilateral cases. *Semin Roentgenol* 10:125, 1975.

29. Gross GW, Lebowitz RL: Infection does not cause reflux. *AJR* 137:929, 1981.

30. Grossman H, Rosenberg ER, Bowie JD, et al: Review. Sonographic diagnosis of renal cystic diseases. *AJR* 140:81, 1983.

31. Grossman H, Winchester PH, Colston WC: Neurogenic bladder in childhood. *Radiol Clin North Am* 6:155, 1968.

32. Haller JO, Berdon WE, Friedman AP: Increased renal cortical echogenicity: A normal finding in neonates and infants. *Radiology* 142:1, 173, 1982.

33. Hasch E: Ultrasound scanning for monitoring childhood hydronephrosis. *J Clin Ultrasound* 6:156, 1978.

34. Hayden CK Jr, Swischuk LE, Davis M, et al: Puddling: A distinguishing feature of adult polycystic kidney disease in the neonate. *AJR* 142:811, 1984.

35. Hayden CK Jr, Santa-Cruz FR, Amparo EG, et al: Ultrasonographic evaluation of the renal parenchyma in infancy and childhood. *Radiology* 1984.

36. Hodson CJ, Davies Z, Prescod A: Renal parenchymal radiographic measurement in infants and children. *Pediatr Radiol* 3:16, 1975.

37. Hodson CJ: Neuhauser Lecture. Reflux nephropathy: A personal historical review. *AJR* 137:451, 1981.

38. Hoffman EP, Salvatierra O Jr, Palubinskas AJ: Segmental kidney resection in children with small, hypertension-producing intrarenal vascular lesions. *Radiology* 143:683, 1982.

39. Holloway H, Jones TB, Robinson AE, et al: Sonographic determination of renal volumes in normal neonates. *Pediatr Radiol* 13:212, 1983.

40. Hricak H, Slovis TL, Callen CW, et al: Neonatal kidneys: Sonographic-anatomic correlation. *Radiology* 147:699, 1983.

41. Jaffe MH, White SJ, Silver TM, et al: Wilms' tumor ultrasonic features, pathologic correlation, and diagnostic pitfalls. *Radiology* 140:147, 1981.

42. Janik JS, Shandling B, Mancer K: Cutis laxa and hollow viscus diverticula. *J Pediatr Surg* 17:318, 1982.

43. Kessler RM, Altman DH: Real-time sonographic detection of vesicoureteral reflux in children. *AJR* 138:1033, 1982.

44. King CR, Prescott G: Pathogenesis of the prune belly anomalad. *J Pediatr* 93:273, 1978.

45. Kirtane J, Talwalker V, Dastur DK: Megacystis, microcolon, intestinal hypoperistalsis syndrome: Possible pathogenesis. *J Pediatr Surg* 19:206, 1984.

46. Krensky AM, Reddish JM, Teele RL: Causes of increased renal echogenicity in pediatric patients. *Pediatrics* 72:840, 1983.

47. Kroovand RL, Al-Ansari RM, Perlmutter AD: Urethral and genital malformations in prune belly syndrome. *J Urol* 127:94, 1982.

48. Kuhn JP, Berger PE: Computed tomography of the kidney in infancy and childhood. *Radiol Clin North Am* 19:445, 1981.

49. Lackman RS, Lindstrom RR, Hirose FM: The "septation sign" in multicystic dysplastic kidney. *Pediatr Radiol* 3:117, 1975.

50. Lam AH, Warren PS: Ultrasonographic diagnosis of neonatal renal venous thrombosis. *Ann Radiol (Paris)* 24:7, 1981.

51. LeVine M, Allen A, Stein KL, et al: Crescent sign. *Radiology* 81:971, 1963.

52. Levitt SB: Medical versus surgical treatment of primary vesicoureteral reflux, report of the international reflux study committee. *Pediatrics* 67:392, 1981.

53. Lewy PR, Belman AB: Familial occurrence of nonobstructive, noninfectious vesicoureteral reflux with renal scarring. *J Pediatr* 86:851, 1975.

54. Mascatello VJ, Smith EH, Carrera GF, et al: Ultrasonic evaluation of the obstructed duplex kidney. *AJR* 129:113, 1977.

55. McAlister WH, Caciarelli A, Shackleford GD: Complications associated with cystography in children. *Radiology* 111:167, 1974.

56. McAlister WH: Demonstration of the dilated prostatic urethra in posterior urethral valve patients. *J Ultrasound Med* 3:189, 1984.

57. Merrick MV, Uttley WS, Wild R: A comparison of two techniques of detecting vesico-ureteric reflux. *Br J Radiol* 52:792, 1979.

58. Merrick MV, Uttley WS, Wild SR: The detection of pyelonephritic scarring in children by radioisotope imaging. *Br J Radiol* 53:544, 1980.

59. Moerman P, Fryns J-P, Goddeeris P, et al: Pathogenesis of the prune-belly syndrome: A functional urethral obstruction caused by prostatic hypoplasia. *Pediatrics* 73:470, 1984.

60. Nasrallah PF, Nara S, Crawford J: Clinical applications of nuclear cystography. *J Urol* 128:550, 1982.

61. Newman L, Bucy JG, McAlister WH: Experimental production of reflux in the presence and absence of infected urine. *Radiology* 111:591, 1974.

62. Pagon RA, Smith DW, Shepard TH: Urethral obstruction malformation complex; a cause of abdominal muscle deficiency and the "prune belly." *J Pediatr* 94:900, 1979.

63. Pinckney LE, Currarino G, Weinberg AG: Parenchymal reflux in renal dysplasia. *Radiology* 141:681, 1981.

64. Puri P, Lake BD, Gorman F, et al: Megacystis-microcolon-intestinal hypoperistalsis syndrome: A visceral myopathy. *J Pediatr Surg* 18:64, 1983.

65. Roberts JA, Riopelle AJ: Vesicoureteral reflux in the primate. II. Maturation of the uretero-vesical junction. *Pediatrics* 59:566, 1977.

66. Roberts JA, Riopelle AJ: Vesicoureteral reflux in the primate. III. Effect of urinary tract infection on maturation of the ureterovesical junction. *Pediatrics* 61:853, 1978.

67. Robey G, Reilly BJ, Carusi PA, et al: Pediatric urography: Comparison of metrizamide and methylglucamine diatrizoate. *Radiology* 150:61, 1984.

68. Rolleston GL, Maling TMJ, Hodson CJ: Intrarenal reflux and the scarred kidney. *Arch Dis Child* 49:531, 1974.

69. Rosenbaum DM, Korngold E, Teele RL: Sonographic assessment of renal length in normal children. *AJR* 142:467, 1984.

70. Rose JS, McCarthy J, Yeh H: Ultrasound diagnosis of ectopic ureterocele. *Pediatr Radiol* 8:17, 1979.

71. Rosenberg ER, Trought WS, Kirks DR, et al: Ultrasonic diagnosis of renal vein thrombosis in neonates. *AJR* 134:35, 1980.

72. Sanders RC, Hartman DS: The sonographic distinction between neonatal multicystic kidney and hydronephrosis. *Radiology* 151:621, 1984.

73. Schmidt JD, Hawtrey CE, Flocks RH, et al: Vesicoureteral reflux; an inherited lesion. *JAMA* 220:821, 1972.

74. Senac MO Jr, Miller JH, Stanley P: Evaluation of obstructive uropathy in children: Radionuclide renography vs. the Whitake test. *AJR* 143:11, 1984.

75. Shah KJ, Robins DH, White RHR: Renal scarring and vesicoureteric reflux. *Arch Dis Child* 53:210, 1976.

76. Shopfner CE, Hutch JA: The normal urethrogram. *Radiol Clin North Am* 6:165, 1968.

77. Shopfner CE: Roentgen evaluation of distal urethral obstruction. *Radiology* 88:222, 1967.

78. Shopfner CE: Vesicoureteral reflux; five year reevaluation. *Radiology* 95:637, 1970.

79. Shore RM, Koff SA, Mentser M, et al: Glomerular filtration rate in children determination from the Tc-99m-DTPA renogram. *Radiology* 151:627, 1984.

80. Siegle RL, Davies P, Fullerton GD: Urography with metrizamide in children. *AJR* 139:927, 1982.

81. Slovis TL, Philippart AI, Cushing B, et al: Evaluation of the inferior vena cava by sonography and venography in children with renal and hepatic tumors. *Radiology* 140:767, 1981.

82. Smellie JM, Edwards D, Normand JCS, et al: Effect of vesicoureteric reflux on renal growth in children with urinary tract infection. *Arch Dis Child* 56:593, 1981.

83. Stuck KJ, Koff SA, Silver TM: Ultrasonic features of multicystic dysplastic kidney: Expanded diagnostic criteria. *Radiology* 143:217, 1982.

84. Swischuk LE: *Radiology of the Newborn and Young Infant*, 2nd ed. Baltimore, Williams & Wilkins, 1980, p 514.

85. Vinograd I, Mogle P, Lernau OZ, et al: Megacystic-microcolon-intestinal hypoperistalsis syndrome. *Arch Dis Child* 59:169, 1984.

86. Walker D, Richard GA: A critical evaluation of urethral obstruction in female children. *Pediatrics* 51:272, 1973.

87. Walker FC Jr, Loney LC, Root ER, et al: Diagnostic evaluation of adult polycystic kidney disease in childhood. *AJR* 142:1273, 1984.

88. Weissenbacher G, Wiltschke H: Chronic urinary tract infection and vulvitis in girls with high posterior commissures. *Padiatr Padol* 9L60, 1974.

89. Weitzel D: Ultrasonic diagnosis in children with vesico-ureteric reflux. *Ann Radiol (Paris)* 23:99, 1980.

90. Whitaker J, Johnston GS: Correlation of urethral resistance and shape in girls. *Radiology* 91:757, 1968.

91. Wikstad I, Aperia A, Broberger O, et al: Long-term effect of large vesicoureteral reflux with or without urinary tract infection. *Acta Radiol* 22:325 Fasc. 3B, 1981.

92. Woodhouse CRJ, Ransley PG, Innes-Williams D: Prune belly syndrome-report of 47 cases. *Arch Dis Child* 57:856, 1982.

93. Zel G, Retik AB: Familial vesicoureteral reflux. *Urology* 2:249, 1973.

Chester M. Edelmann, Jr.
Jacob Churg
Michael A. Gerber
Luther B. Travis

20

Renal Biopsy: Indications, Technique, and Interpretation

The systematic study of renal tissue obtained by biopsy has contributed enormously to the establishment of nephrology as a subspecialty of pediatrics and medicine [29]. Prior to the 1950s, only a few case reports had mentioned renal biopsy. In 1923, Gwyn [60] reported an open renal biopsy in a patient with nephrotic syndrome, and in 1934, Ball [9] performed the first closed-needle biopsy using an aspiration device. The first large series of biopsies was reported in 1951 by Iversen and Brun [67].

In 1954, Kark and Muehrcke [72] described the performance of percutaneous renal biopsy using an intravenous pyelogram to aid in localization of the kidney and the Franklin modification of the Vim-Silverman biopsy needle. This technique increased the yield of successful biopsies from 50% to greater than 90% and was associated with a low complication rate. The number of renal biopsies performed increased dramatically, so that by 1962, Slotkin and Madsen [117] were able to collect data on 5000 patients. In the same year Dodge et al. [38] collected reports of 450 biopsies in children, including 130 performed by Vernier et al. [128] and 205 of their own.

Percutaneous renal biopsy has been accepted as a safe and practical procedure in children. Several pediatric centers have performed more than 1000 renal biopsies [24,56]. Many modifications of the technique described by Kark have been described, including improved methods for localization of the kidneys and the development of biopsy needles specifically for use in children.

Several investigators [73,95,128] have compared the histologic findings on the small amount of tissue obtainable by percutaneous biopsy to those obtained at autopsy. A close correlation was found in diseases that diffusely affect the kidney, such as most of the glomerulopathies, whereas focal disease processes, such as neoplasms or pyelonephritis, showed a lower correlation. Thus, percutaneous renal biopsy enables the physician to evaluate most histopathologic processes in the kidney for the purposes of diagnosis, prognosis, and evaluation of response to therapy.

Indications

Evaluation of a renal biopsy specimen may be useful in establishing the diagnosis, evaluating the acuteness and severity of the disease process, and determining the degree of reversibility.

Clinical and laboratory evidence of glomerulonephropathy, either primary or secondary to systemic disease, is one of the most common indications for examination of renal tissue (Chap. 50) (Table 20-1). Biopsies are done, for example, to establish a histologic diagnosis in children with nephrotic syndrome [69] (Chap. 54), to establish a diagnosis in children with chronic glomerulonephritis, and to determine the nature of disease and the degree of renal injury in patients presenting clinically with acute glomerulonephritis (Chap. 52), particularly when severe. The indications for performance of renal biopsy in children with isolated hematuria [123] and proteinuria are discussed extensively in Chaps. 21 and 51. Although renal biopsy has been a useful investigative tool in patients with postural proteinuria, it adds little to the evaluation of a child in whom that diagnosis has been made (Chap. 21).

In patients with systemic disorders such as lupus erythematosus or Henoch-Schönlein syndrome, examination of renal tissue may be necessary to document involvement of the kidney and to provide information concerning the histologic type of disease and the magnitude of the renal injury.

Most authors agree that renal biopsy is of little value in the assessment of children with urinary tract infection. It has been applied only occasionally in the evaluation of cystic and dysplastic disorders. It is contraindicated when intrarenal neoplasm is suspected because the procedure may lead to intra-abdominal dissemination of tumor.

Biopsy may be indicated for patients with acute [96] or chronic renal failure of uncertain etiology (Chap. 50). Techniques not dependent on renal function, such as ultrasonography and radioisotopic scanning, should precede biopsy in an attempt to differentiate acute from chronic renal failure and to exclude extrarenal or urologic lesions such as obstruction.

Hypertension without other signs of renal involvement is not an indication for renal biopsy in children. The rate of serious complication of biopsy is increased in hypertensive individuals. If renal disease is suspected as the etiology of the hypertension and if a biopsy is to be performed, the hypertension must be well controlled prior to the procedure.

Table 20-1. *Indications for renal biopsy*

Syndrome	Agreed by most nephrologists	Controversial
Nephrotic Syndrome	Adult: at diagnosis Infant: onset up to 9–12 mo at diagnosis Child: (1) low C_3, at diagnosis 　　　　(2) after unresponsive to 4–6 wk cortico-steroid therapy 　　　　(3) relapsing with corticosteroids; consideration of cyclophosphamide or chlorambucil therapy	Child: 6–8 yr of age at time of diagnosis (particularly with hypertension, microscopic hematuria or impaired renal function)
Asymptomatic persistent proteinuria:		
Normal renal function	After 6–12 mo if microhematuria present and/or heavy proteinuria At diagnosis if suspicion of familial nephritis or SLE	At diagnosis if heavy proteinuria or microhematuria present After 6–12 months with isolated heavy proteinuria
Impaired renal function	At time of presentation if diagnosis uncertain, especially if microscopic hematuria present and/or hypertension	
Primary acute nephritic syndrome	As soon as possible if rapidly progressive GN suspected, or cause uncertain After 2–3 mo if hypertension, low C_3 and/or impaired renal function persists	At diagnosis for postinfectious GN with mild to moderate impairment of renal function (less indication in child than adult) and for Henoch-Schönlein nephritis
Systemic disorders with associated GN-vasculitis	At presentation: —SLE with proteinuria and/or abnormal sediment or impaired function —Suspected Wegener's granulomatosis, polyarteritis or hypersensitivity angiitis with evidence of renal involvement, but diagnosis uncertain	SLE with normal renal function and little or no proteinuria or abnormality of sediment; corticosteroids required for reasons primarily unrelated to kidney Diagnosis of vasculitic disorder established and decision to treat has been made
Acute renal failure	As soon as condition permits: —Rapidly progressive GN —Cause of acute renal failure obscure —Suspected acute interstitial nephritis if insufficient clinical evidence for diagnosis —After 3–6 wk if recovery has not commenced —Possible acute or chronic disorder	Suspected ATN, probable cause apparent Strong clinical evidence for hemolytic uremic syndrome or thrombotic thrombocytopenic purpura
Isolated gross hematuria	Suspected Berger's disease in adult Suspected familial nephritis	Suspected Berger's disease in child
Chronic renal failure	Diagnosis uncertain and kidneys no more than moderately reduced in size (avoid needle biopsy with very contracted kidneys)	Other situations
Transplant	Suspect recurrence of original disease in transplant, transplant rejection, or cyclosporine toxicity Seriously reduced renal function and cause uncertain	Other situations

SLE, systemic lupus erythematosus; GN, glomerulonephritis; ATN, acute tubular necrosis.
From Gault MH. Muehrcke RC: Renal biopsy: Current view and controversies. *Nephron* 34:1, 1983; with permission.

Prompt interpretation of biopsy tissue from renal allografts apparently undergoing acute rejection may aid in determining the correct therapy [6,11,40,46,105]. Biopsy may play a critical role also in the diagnosis of recurrent disease in renal transplants [59,90] and in determining the presence or absence of cyclosporine toxicity. The use of fine-needle biopsies has been advocated for the latter purpose [138a].

Other less common conditions in which renal biopsy may be indicated are included in Table 20-1.

Contraindications

Percutaneous renal biopsy is absolutely contraindicated in only a few circumstances (Table 20-2). Biopsy should be postponed in patients with a bleeding diathesis or in those who require anticoagulant therapy. Broyer [20] suggests that heparin be withheld for at least 10 days following biopsy, although Gotti et al. [54] reported successful biopsy in seven patients with acute renal failure and prolonged bleeding time in whom the bleeding time was brought to normal by use of washed red cell transfusions or administration of desmopressin (1-desamino-8-arginine vasopressin, DDAVP). Chodak et al. [26] claimed that by using an open biopsy technique and a cup biopsy forceps hemostasis could be obtained in patients with clotting disorders.

Open biopsy should be performed in children with a horseshoe kidney or other congenital abnormalities of position or fusion. The child with a solitary kidney who acquires another renal complication presents a unique problem for the pediatric nephrologist. Some have believed that the mere presence of a solitary kidney constitutes a contraindication to percutaneous renal biopsy, but, in the presence of an appropriate indication and with an experienced operator, a needle biopsy of the kidney carries less overall risk than does an open renal biopsy. Obviously, the many successful biopsies on solitary renal allografts have influenced this change in philosophy. Risk of dissemination contraindicates closed biopsy in children with a suspected renal tumor.

Relative contraindications to percutaneous renal biopsy are listed in Table 20-2. Blood pressure should be controlled prior to biopsy because a much higher incidence of major bleeding and arteriovenous fistula has been reported in hypertensive individuals [24,35,36,72]. Elective biopsy should be postponed if the child develops an acute respiratory or other febrile illness. The uncooperative patient is considered a relative contraindication for percutaneous biopsy with local anesthesia [107]. This might be thought to preclude biopsy in many young children. However, Sweet et al. [121b] have demonstrated that the risk of percutaneous renal biopsy is no greater than in older children and carries both a lower morbidity and cost than does an open renal biopsy. Experience with large numbers of children [24,41] has demonstrated that with adequate sedation and technical dexterity, biopsy in young children is as successful and has as low a complication rate as in older children and adults. Hypnosis has been used in children to avoid the need for general anesthesia [127].

Preparation for Biopsy

The child is usually admitted to the hospital on the day the biopsy is to be done. A complete history is obtained and a complete physical examination is performed to rule out clinical signs of acute infection or a bleeding diathesis and to ensure adequate control of hypertension. Routine examinations before the biopsy should include hematocrit, hemoglobin, platelet count, prothrombin time, and partial thromboplastin time. In some centers a blood specimen is sent to the blood bank to be typed and held in case transfusion is required. A urinalysis and urine culture are done to provide baseline information in case significant hematuria or infection should develop after biopsy. Other laboratory work planned for evaluation of the renal or systemic disease also can be obtained at this time.

The psychological preparation varies a great deal with each child and with the technique to be used. If the procedure is to be done under local anesthesia, and thus requires cooperation of the child, the child should be given

TABLE 20-2. *Contraindications to percutaneous renal biopsy*

Major
Bleeding diathesis
Anticoagulant therapy
Moderate to severe hypertension
Solitary kidney (controversial)
Intrarenal tumor

Minor
Hydronephrosis
Perinephric abscess
Acute intrarenal infection
Extensive nephrocalcinosis
Severe anemia
Small, contracted endstage kidney
Marked obesity

several opportunities to practice his or her role. If possible, the older child and the parents should be taken to the biopsy area and the equipment and procedure should be fully explained. Younger children may need simple reassurance, and arrangements to allow a parent to sleep in may considerably ease the child's anxiety.

Prebiopsy Preparation of Patient

Food and water are withheld for 8 hours for older children and 4 hours for infants to decrease the risk of vomiting and aspiration when sedation is required and when the stomach is compressed as the patient is placed in the proper position for biopsy. Cathartics or enemas are not employed.

Younger children and apprehensive older children should receive sedation 90 minutes prior to the procedure. Among the drugs found to be useful for prebiopsy sedation are meperidine, promethazine hydrochloride, chlorpromazine, and diazepam. The latter drug produces rapid, short-acting sedation and excellent amnesia, but it does impose a small risk of acute respiratory depression.

Renal Localization

Accurate localization of the kidney is the most important part of the biopsy procedure [134a]. The centrifugal arrangement of the glomeruli and the distance from major vessels, renal calyces, and other organs make the lower pole of the right kidney the preferred location for biopsy. Many nephrologists [20,24,38,50,89,95] still use intravenous pyelography and measurements from bony markers to approximate the location of the kidney, as originally described by Kark and Muehrcke [72] (Fig. 20-1). The placement of the biopsy needle by direct vision using fluoroscopy was first reported in 1956 by Lusted et al. [82]. By the mid-1960s, many centers had adopted this technique in adults [3,19,72] and in children [41]. Some authors have suggested the use of CT [61] or of radionuclide scan [47,91, 122,126] for localization, and several groups have recommended ultrasonography as the preferred technique for

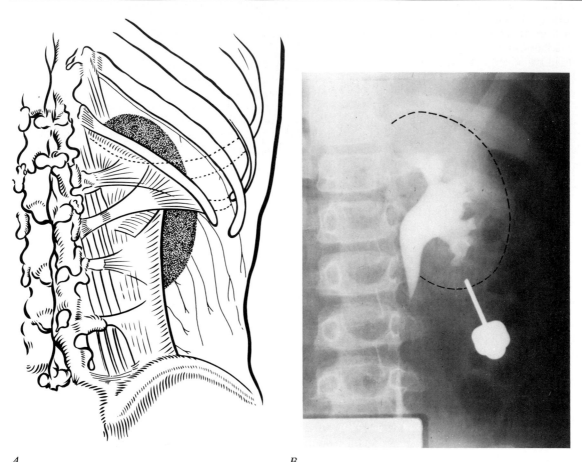

A   *B*

FIG. 20-1. A. *Anatomic relationships of the lower pole of the right kidney as seen from the back.*
(Redrawn from *Dodge WF, Daeschner CW, Brennan JC, et al: Percutaneous renal biopsy in chil-*
dren. I. General considerations. Pediatrics 30:287, 1962; *with permission.)* B. *Fluoroscopic image of*
the right kidney showing the position of a Franklin-Silverman needle in the renal capsule just prior to
obtaining a biopsy specimen.

renal localization [15,53,84,101,108,119,139]. In experienced hands [24,41,139], any of these techniques should yield successful biopsies in greater than 95% of children. Carvajal et al. [24] reported a higher complication rate in the first 6 months of the academic year when trainees are least experienced, emphasizing the importance of the skill and experience of the operator [42].

Many nephrologists still use the "blind" technique whereby, after the general position of the kidney is determined by either ultrasonography or abdominal flat-plate radiography, the kidney depth and lateral border are located by using an exploring (thin, spinal) needle. The biopsy needle is then passed along a similar tract to approximately the same depth. The kidney can usually be felt by the experienced examiner as the biopsy needle touches the renal cortex. Furthermore, the hub of the needle should always be seen to oscillate cephalad with the patient's inspiration. In the hands of experienced operators, the success rate and complication rate are as good as

all other techniques using various types of imaging for needle placement.

Bolton et al. [17] compared the accuracy and risks of various localization techniques with image intensification fluoroscopy. Radionuclide and ultrasound scans were as accurate as fluoroscopy in locating the lower pole of the kidney. The depth of the kidney found on ultrasonography correlated well with the actual depth found by the exploring needle at the time of biopsy. Pyelography gave a mean error of 3.9 cm in assessing renal length and 1.4 cm in estimating renal width. This distortion is attributed to projection error caused by the distance from the kidneys to the x-ray plate. In adults the absorbed radiation dose was calculated to be 4.4 cGy for a pyelogram, 3 cGy for 90 seconds of fluoroscopy, and 0.34 cGy of kidney and 0.01 cGy of gonadal exposure for the radionuclide scan [126]. These exposure levels are proportionately less in pediatric patients. Ultrasonography does not expose the patient to radiation or to contrast material and is not dependent on the level of renal function. Therefore, it appears to be the method of choice in renal failure or pregnancy. The major advantage of image intensification fluoroscopy is that it is the only method that allows the operator to follow the location of the biopsy needle during the procedure [41,42,62]. Current techniques to visualize the needle by ultrasonography during biopsy are less accurate [53].

Position

During localization the patient must be placed in exactly the same position as during the biopsy procedure. The patient is placed prone, and a sandbag or firmly rolled sheet is placed under the upper abdomen and lowermost ribs. This compresses and "fixes" the kidneys to the posterior abdominal wall, bringing the kidneys closer to the skin and limiting possible ballotment of the kidney by the biopsy needle.

Localization Using Fluoroscopy

A scout film of the abdomen is obtained to ensure proper radiologic technique. One to two ml/kg of 50% or 60% sodium diatrizoate (Hypaque) or diatrizoate meglumine (Renografin) compounds are given intravenously, as for an intravenous pyelogram. The larger doses are useful in smaller children, and up to 3 ml/kg may be necessary in an infant. The patient's back is cleansed and draped, and sterile technique is used throughout the remainder of the procedure. Additional sedation is given intravenously at this time if needed. A 3-minute film is obtained and checked for the presence and location of two functioning kidneys. Using the fluoroscope, a blunt radiopaque probe—for example, a long pair of Kelly forceps—is placed on the skin over the lower pole of the chosen kidney. This area is marked with a sterile indelible skin marker (e.g., methylene blue). The skin and subcutaneous tissue are infiltrated with a local anesthetic (2% lidocaine). This is often the most uncomfortable portion of the procedure, and the child may require assistance in remaining still.

An exploring needle (No. 20 or 22 gauge 3½-inch spinal needle) is advanced perpendicularly through the skin toward the kidney. At any time the operator may stop and compare the position of the needle with the fluoroscopic image of the lower pole of the kidney to make appropriate corrections in position and direction. Once the needle penetrates the renal capsule, the fluoroscopist will note that the needle tip moves in unison with the kidney (see Fig. 20-1) [41]. The operator will also note that the hub of the needle will swing cephalad-caudad with respiration. Arterial pulsations may be visibly transmitted by the needle hub. However, because the perirenal tissue as well as areas of the kidney undesirable for biopsy, such as near the large vessels or calyceal areas, will transmit the same movements [41], the position of the needle tip must be checked fluoroscopically. The ideal location for biopsy is 1 cm superior to the lower border of the lower pole.

When the operator is satisfied that the exploring needle

is placed properly in the renal capsule, the depth of insertion is noted with a measuring device or with a stop placed on the needle [135]. The trocar of the exploring needle is then withdrawn, and a small amount of local anesthetic is injected along the needle track as the needle is withdrawn.

A small skin incision is made with a No. 11 scalpel blade, and, during the pause following expiration, the biopsy needle is advanced into the renal capsule along the anesthetized track. The position of the biopsy needle is checked with the fluoroscope, just as was done for the exploring needle (see Fig. 20-1), and the depth is checked against the measurements made. Once a satisfactory position is obtained, the biopsy is taken (see following). A second or third core may be obtained using the same technique.

Postbiopsy vital signs should be checked, and a radiograph, CT, or ultrasound study [5,52] may be advisable to rule out gross extravasation of urine or acute development of a perirenal hematoma. The procedure, including injection of contrast material, usually requires about 30 minutes of time in the fluoroscopy room with 30 to 180 seconds of exposure.

Localization Using Pyelography

An intravenous pyelogram is obtained with the child prone in the biopsy position. The distance between the lateral border of the right kidney at the level of the lowest rib and the corresponding vertebral spinous process is measured on the pyelogram. A line representing the lateral border of the kidney is drawn on the skin this distance from and parallel to the spinous processes. This line, the lowest rib, and the border of the right paraspinal muscles form a triangle in which the puncture is made. In children more than 150 cm, the exploring needle is placed into the skin approximately 2.5 cm medial to the lateral line and 1.5 cm below the rib. In smaller children these distances are decreased appropriately. Dodge et al. [38] use a similar technique but rely primarily on anatomic landmarks rather than measurements.

The technique of localization with the exploring needle and the remainder of the biopsy procedure are identical to the technique described for fluoroscopy except that respiratory excursions and "feel" alone are used to estimate position and depth [20,38,72,95].

Localization Using Ultrasonography

The patient is positioned and prepared as for the fluoroscopic technique. The kidney to be biopsied is outlined using a commercial ultrasound scanner with a 2.25 or 3.5 MHz transducer. Body section images obtained along the plane of transducer motion are displayed electronically and photographed. Good contact between the transducer and the skin is ensured by using mineral oil or an aqueous coupling medium.

A series of transverse scans facilitates subsequent scanning along the true longitudinal axis of the kidney. The lower pole is identified on the longitudinal scan, and its limits are marked. If possible, all images should be obtained during the same phase of respiration to reduce respiratory excursion of the kidney. In uncooperative patients, adequate sedation may be sufficient to ensure minimal kidney motion during quiet breathing. Electronic markers may be superimposed on the resultant images so that the depth of the lower pole and the angle of needle entry may be determined readily (Fig. 20-2). The operator inserts the exploring needle with the knowledge of the measured depth, angle of entry, and location of the lower pole.

When a special biopsy transducer [53] is available, a sterile field is prepared before sonography and sterile mineral oil is used as the coupling agent. The biopsy needle is inserted through a predrilled hole in the center of the crystal while the transducer is held over the site of biopsy [15,53,84,101,119,139].

Localization Using Radioisotopic Scan

The full-sized child is given an intravenous injection of a technetium-labeled renal imaging agent such as Tc-Fe-ascorbic acid. An hour later the patient is placed in the biopsy position under the gamma camera. The oscilloscope is set in the store mode until the kidneys are clearly outlined, and the outline is drawn on the oscilloscope face with a wax pencil. The oscilloscope image is erased, and movable ^{57}Co markers are placed on the patient's back and moved until their image on the oscilloscope coincides with the location chosen for biopsy. This point on the back is marked with an indelible agent, and the operator may then proceed with the biopsy procedure as with intravenous pyelography [47,91,122,126].

Biopsy of the Renal Allograft

The transplanted kidney can usually be located using the description of its position in the operative note and direct palpation. Buselmeier et al. [23] approach the kidney either in a plane perpendicular to the lower pole or tangential to the lateral curvature of the allograft (Fig. 20-3). The biopsy needle is advanced without resistance until the fibrous capsule, which forms during the first 2 weeks after surgery, is reached. The needle is then inserted into the renal cortex and the biopsy is obtained [6,9,11,119]. Pillay and Kurtzman [99] report good results with fluoroscopic localization of the allograft using contrast agents.

Reeve et al. [105] have used a fine-gauge lumbar puncture needle and suction aspiration to prepare a cellular preparation of renal tissue, avoiding the trauma of a tissue biopsy.

Because the allograft is, in fact, a solitary kidney, some physicians prefer an open biopsy. If the kidney has been placed intraperitoneally, as in some small children, open biopsy is mandatory. If the kidney is not palpable because of its location or the presence of obesity, localization by fluoroscopy or ultrasonography or performance of an open biopsy is suggested.

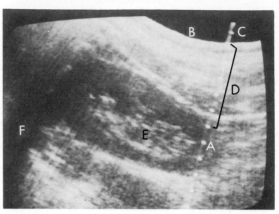

A

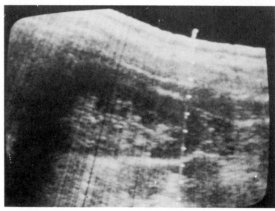

B

FIG. 20-2. A. *Longitudinal ultrasonogram demonstrating the relationship of the lower pole of the kidney (A) to the skin surface (B). The appropriate angle and depth (D) for correct needle placement can be determined from the centimeter gradations of the electronic marker (C). E, renal pelvis; F, rib shadow obscuring upper pole of kidney. B. The placement of a sandbag under the ribs and upper abdomen moves the lower pole of the kidney 1 cm closer to the skin surface.*

Use of the Biopsy Needle

The earliest percutaneous renal biopsies were done with an aspiration needle [67]. This instrument provided only a 50% success rate and was soon replaced by the Franklin modification of the Vim-Silverman needle, which is still one of the most commonly used instruments [72].

The needle, with stylet in place, is advanced to the area of the kidney chosen for biopsy. The renal capsule is punctured, and the stylet is replaced by the cutting prongs. Following an expiration, the cutting prongs are quickly inserted to their full depth into the kidney tissue. The needle is allowed to swing with respiration. During the next expiratory pause, the needle shaft is quickly and smoothly advanced over the prongs using a slight rotatory motion. The operator must be very careful not to move

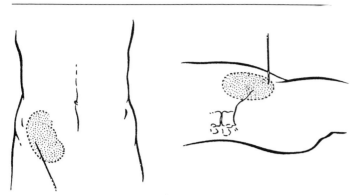

FIG. 20-3. *The allograft placed into the iliac fossa can be approached for biopsy in a plane (left) tangential to the lateral curvature or (right) perpendicular to the lower pole of the kidney. (From Buselmeier TJ, Schquer RM, Mauer SM, et al: A simplified method of percutaneous allograft biopsy. Nephron 16:318, 1976; with permission of the author and S. Karger AG, Basel.)*

the prongs. The entire instrument is then rapidly removed from the patient. Microscopic examination of the renal tissue is done to ensure that the specimen contains adequate numbers of glomeruli [63].

The procedure, from insertion of the cutting prongs into the kidney tissue to removal of the needle, ought to take 1 to 2 seconds and should be performed during the expiratory pause to diminish risk of tearing the kidney. Kark and Muehrcke [72] suggest practice of this technique on a piece of cheddar cheese to ensure rapid and reproducible procurement of adequate cores of tissue.

Modifications of the standard Franklin-Silverman needle for pediatric use include a stop to prevent cutting totally through the kidney [135] and short, lighter needles [92]. The cutting prongs of the Franklin-Silverman needle tend to compress the renal tissue, producing distortion of glomeruli on the edge of the core. Several investigators [70,136] report successful biopsies with less distortion with the disposable Tru-Cut needle (Travenol Laboratories, Baxter Scientific, Edison, NJ). With this instrument, after the central trocar is advanced into the kidney, the outer cannula is slid over the trocar, cleanly cutting off the piece of tissue. A pediatric version is manufactured. Success has been reported with the Biopty System, a spring-loaded, fine-caliber Tru-Cut needle with an automatic firing device [75a,132a].

Open Biopsy

Open biopsies [22,26,111,115] are performed in patients with anatomic malformations such as solitary or horseshoe kidney, small nonvisualizing kidneys, bleeding diatheses, hypertension, or marked obesity and in patients with allografts. The open biopsy gives less chance of bleeding and a 100% yield of tissue, compared with about 95% for the percutaneous techniques. The major disadvantages of open biopsy are the need for general anesthesia and the discom-

fort and risk of infection from the incision. Hospitalization is not necessarily prolonged [22].

A small superficial wedge of tissue is removed with a scalpel [115] or cup biopsy forceps [26] so that any bleeding points can be controlled. In biopsy of disease processes with pathognomonic histologic lesions limited to the juxtamedullary area (e.g., focal segmental sclerosis or nephronophthisis), the needle technique [22] may be preferable to avoid obtaining glomeruli only from the superficial regions of the cortex.

Postbiopsy Care

A heavy pressure dressing is placed over the biopsy site; in some programs this procedure is limited to patients with an allograft. The child is returned to his or her room accompanied by a nurse or physician in case of sudden bleeding. The child remains lying in bed. Blood pressure and pulse are checked every 15 minutes for 1 hour and hourly thereafter for 3 more hours. When the vital signs are stable and if there is no gross hematuria, pulse, blood pressure, and temperature should be checked subsequently every 4 hours. In some programs a hematocrit is obtained 4 and 12 hours after the procedure. Some authors [93] suggest encouragement of water intake following biopsy to decrease the risk of obstruction by clots. An aliquot of each urine passed should be saved to ascertain the degree of hematuria (see Complications).

The child is allowed out of bed the following day. If vital signs, hematocrit, and level of hematuria are satisfactory, the child is sent home. The child may return to school immediately, but for a week he or she should refrain from vigorous exercise, contact sports, or other activities such as diving that may traumatize the abdomen.

Complications

The incidence of complications following percutaneous renal biopsy is difficult to ascertain [3,4,36,66a] (Table 20-3). Microscopic hematuria or mild abdominal or flank pain that disappears within 24 to 48 hours is almost universal [41,110] and is generally not considered a complication. The incidence of more prolonged gross hematuria or passage of small clots has been reported to be 5% to 7% in two large series of biopsies in children, with transfusion required in 1% to 1.7% [24,38,41,92]. Hematomas that cause obstruction have been treated with urokinase. Perinephric hematomas that are recognizable clinically occur infrequently [38,117], but have been demonstrated with CT in more than half of biopsied adults [5,52,109].

Bleeding usually stops spontaneously with simple bed rest. Severe bleeding has been treated with Gelfoam embolization [44] and epsilon-aminocaproic acid [114]. Rarely, nephrectomy has been necessary to control bleeding.

The reported incidence of arteriovenous fistula in children is about 0.5% [24,41]. However, many small fistulas may go unreported or close spontaneously [35]. Improved techniques of localization, medical management of hem-

TABLE 20-3. *Complications of percutaneous renal biopsy*

Prolonged gross hematuria [1,24,35,38,41,68,70,92,117]
Perirenal hematoma [5,24,38,52,109,117,129]
Arteriovenous fistula [18,24,35,41,70,77]
Renal infection [70,112,117]
Severe back or flank pain [32,70]
Puncture of major renal vessel [107]
Renal infarction [38,92]
Renal colic secondary to passage of clots [70]
Ureteral obstruction [70,97]
Inadvertent biopsy of liver, spleen, bowel, pancreas, gallblad-
    der, adrenal gland; ileus, pneumothorax [62,70,117]
Sepsis [32,112]
Temporary loss of renal function [136a]

orrhage, and surgical repair of arteriovenous fistulas [35,77,86] have decreased the frequency of nephrectomy. A review of reports published from 1971 to 1976 of more than 1700 percutaneous renal biopsies in children [24,32,91,107,136,139] shows no nephrectomies or deaths associated with this procedure.

Interpretation of Renal Biopsies

The luxuriant growth of morphologic nephrology in the past 25 years has been due primarily to the widespread use of renal biopsy, which has allowed the nephrologist and pathologist to correlate the physiologic and clinical abnormalities with the histologic appearance of the kidney in the living patient. Renal tissue obtained by biopsy is vastly superior to autopsy material, which all too often represents an end stage of disease, devoid of specific morphologic features. The second contribution of importance has been the development of new histologic techniques. These include not only improved methods of cutting and staining tissues for light microscopy but also new procedures, such as electron microscopy and immunohistologic microscopy.

This section consists of three parts. The first examines the procedures for processing renal tissue and preparation of sections and slides for light, electron, and immunofluorescence microscopy. The second discusses methods of study of these preparations. The third is devoted to a brief review of the basic pathologic processes in the kidney.

Processing of Renal Biopsies

The renal (needle) biopsy specimen, when received by the pathologist, consists of a core of tissue about 1 to 2 mm in diameter and a few millimeters to 1 or even 2 cm in length. This piece has to be used for several procedures, including light, electron, and immunofluorescence microscopy. If possible, two cores should be obtained, particularly if additional procedures are planned, such as culture (in cases of suspected infections), freeze drying or freeze substitution (for autoradiography), or enzyme studies (histochemistry and microchemistry). These problems are, of course, greatly simplified if, instead of a needle biopsy, tissue from a wedge (open) biopsy is available. Under ideal circumstances, the pathologist or a specially trained technician is

present at the time of biopsy, to ensure that the tissue is handled properly and used to the greatest advantage.

In most instances, diagnosis can be established on light microscopy alone but much may be missed, even by an experienced pathologist. Whenever possible, light microscopy should be routinely supplemented by electron microscopy and immunofluorescence microscopy. The kidney tissue is gently removed from the biopsy needle, placed in a small Petri dish containing a small amount of cold saline (enough to cover the tissue), and examined under the dissecting microscope [63]. If glomeruli are present, the tissue is divided in such a manner that at least a few glomeruli are fixed for electron microscopy and a few are frozen for immunofluorescence; the remainder is fixed for light microscopy. To accomplish this, one can section the biopsy specimen longitudinally. However, this method tends to introduce mechanical artifacts, and it is better to cut off small pieces at the cortical end for election microscopy and for immunofluorescence. This division should be carried out with a sharp razor blade on a plate of dental wax. The tissue should be covered with a drop of saline to prevent drying.

Light Microscopy
Fixation

The four most useful fixatives for light microscopy are (1) alcoholic Bouin's (Duboscq-Brasil), (2) Helly's solution (Zenker-formol), (3) neutral or slightly acid-buffered formalin (concentrated formaldehyde [40%] diluted 1:10 in phosphate or acetate buffer), and (4) paraformaldehyde (47% in phosphate buffer, pH 7.2, 0.1 molar). Each of these fixatives has its advantages and disadvantages. Alcoholic Bouin's gives excellent cytoplasmic preservation, but the tissue is harmed by prolonged fixation. Zenker-formol requires long washing to get rid of mercury. Formaldehyde tends to produce pale hematoxylin and eosin stain and poorly differentiated trichrome stain unless sections are mordanted in acidified solution of mercuric bichloride; it is excellent for periodic acid-Schiff (PAS) and Jones' silver methenamine stains (PASM). Tissue may be left in formaldehyde for a considerable length of time without significant harm, and, in fact, overnight fixation provides the additional hardening necessary for the cutting of thin sections. The advantage of paraformaldehyde is that tissue can also be used for electron microscopy.

For certain purposes, special fixation is necessary. For example, to demonstrate crystals of cystine or uric acid, tissue should be fixed in absolute alcohol. Alcohol also preserves glycogen to the best advantage, although this material is partly preserved also with formalin and other fixatives. For demonstration of lipids one can use sections from the tissue frozen for immunofluorescence.

Embedding

The standard method of processing the tissue for light microscopy is by dehydrating it in graded alcohols and, after clearing, embedding in paraffin. Because renal biopsy specimens are so small, prolonged exposure to the dehydrating and clearing agents should be avoided. Renal specimens should not be processed together with other tissues but should be run separately (perhaps with other small biopsy specimens) in an automatic machine or by hand. The time in all solutions should be reduced to 15 to 30 minutes (instead of the usual 1 to 3 hours) to avoid excessive hardening of the tissue and consequent difficulties in cutting.

Embedding in plastic (glycol or butyl methacrylate) has been proposed [1]. This material permits cutting of very thin sections, on the order of 1 μ, which often produces superior images. It is also possible to cut 1-μ sections from osmium-fixed and Epon-embedded tissue (for electron microscopy). After proper pretreatment, such sections can be stained with PAS and PASM, but not too well with trichrome. However, the preferred method is to stain them with toluidine blue, which reveals very fine details of the glomerular structure and does not require any counterstain. Toluidine blue tends to fade after a relatively short time, and to obtain a permanent record, one has to resort to photomicrography.

Cutting

Thinness is a prerequisite of good renal biopsy sections. Standard histologic sections, which generally run 6 to 8 μ in thickness, are totally unsuitable. With proper processing, a good microtome, and a sharp knife, an experienced technician can routinely obtain sections 3 μ thick. It is frequently stated that renal biopsy sections should be cut at 2 μ. This indeed can be accomplished, but with a fair degree of difficulty. All too often, the attempt to set the microtome for 2-μ sections results in skipping, compression, and generally unsatisfactory preparations. Also, sections that are too thin stain too lightly; more satisfactory staining will be obtained with paraffin sections cut at 3 μ.

It is important not to lose any tissue by the usual method of trimming paraffin blocks. If the biopsy specimen is properly embedded and lies flat in the block, sections should be taken the moment the knife reaches the level of the tissue. Since a large number of sections is needed, some laboratories cut the entire block. In minimal change nephrotic syndrome, for example, the block should be cut entirely and sections searched for focal segmental glomerulosclerosis. Other laboratories are satisfied with preparing 10 to 20 slides. It is advisable to place no more than two to three sections on each slide. The slides should be numbered consecutively. We routinely stain slides 1,4,7, and 10 with hematoxylin and eosin, slides 2,5,8, and 11 with PAS, and slides 3 and so on with silver methenamine. Other stains and other combinations can be used. Special stains are used as necessary.

Staining

Most renal pathologists employ four routine stains: hematoxylin and eosin, PAS reagent, trichrome, and periodic acid-silver methenamine (PASM). Either PAS or trichrome (depending on the quality of the stain and individual preference) is used as the basic stain and the others serve as special stains. Hematoxylin and eosin is useful for the study of inflammatory infiltrates, red blood cells, the tubular cytoplasm, and glomerular "fibrinoid" deposits. Trichrome is also good for these purposes and for study of glomerular basement membranes. Periodic acid-Schiff with hematoxylin counterstain provides the greatest amount of information about the general structure of the glomerulus and the status of its basement membranes and mesangium. Silver methenamine is a superior stain for the details of the basement membrane structure. When used with a counterstain (hematoxylin and eosin, trichrome, or chromotrope), it also demonstrates deposits and other structural details. For the technical aspect of the various staining procedures, the reader is referred to standard textbooks of histologic techniques [10,80].

Electron Microscopy
Fixation for Electron Microscopy

Fixation for electron microscopy requires osmic acid (osmium tetroxide). The tissue may be placed directly in osmic acid in phosphate or collidin buffers, or it may be first prefixed in buffered glutaraldehyde or paraformaldehyde (see fixative for light microscopy). This prefixation allows better preservation of cytoplasmic proteins but somewhat obscures the glomerular structure. Both osmic acid and glutaraldehyde penetrate poorly, and for best fixation, tissue should be cut into small fragments, about 0.5 mm in diameter. Paraformaldehyde penetrates quite well and provides better visualization than does glutaraldehyde.

Preparation of Tissues

After fixation, the tissues are dehydrated in graded alcohols and embedded in a plastic medium such as Epon or Araldite. Preliminary sections 1 μ thick are cut from all the blocks and stained with toluidine blue or examined directly under the phase microscope, to select the best glomeruli or other areas of interest. As a routine, one should examine three glomeruli by electron microscopy, but sometimes one glomerulus will provide sufficient diagnostic information. Ultrathin sections are cut from selected blocks and examined under the electron microscope. Low-power and high-power photographs are taken and printed for detailed examination.

Immunofluorescence

The principle of immunofluorescence microscopy as introduced by Coons and Kaplan [33] is based on the specific binding of labeled antibody to tissue-bound antigen, so that identification of the label indicates the presence and localization of the particular antigen.

Preservation of Tissue

Preservation of tissue must be carried out carefully, since many antigens are easily degraded, resulting in loss of their antigenicity. Best results are obtained if the renal specimen is surrounded by a small amount of embedding medium, such as Tissue-Tek (Miles Diagnostic, Mishawaka, Indiana), and snap-frozen immediately in liquid nitrogen or a mixture of dry ice and isopentane, directly on the chuck of the microtome, and stored at a temperature of $-70°$ C. Paraffin-embedded tissue has been used for the immunoperoxidase technique, particularly if no or inadequate frozen tissue is available for immunofluorescence [21,64,121c]; however, some antigens, such as complement, are destroyed during routine histologic processing, while others, such as hepatitis B surface antigen [104] and carcinoembryonic antigen [103], are preserved. Immunohistochemistry on frozen sections represents the most sensitive and reproducible technique for the localization of extracellular immunoglobulins [116].

ANTISERA

Monoclonal and polyclonal antisera to all known human immunoglobulin classes, light and heavy chains of immunoglobulins, and a wide variety of plasma proteins, including fibrinogen and most components of the complement system, are commercially available. Alternatively, the antisera can be prepared in experimental animals by injection of purified antigens. The quality of the antisera, i.e., their potency and specificity, is of utmost importance and directly determines the reliability of the results obtained. Therefore, all antisera, including the commercial ones, should be tested before use in a system that has the same sensitivity as the technique employed. In this respect, agar gel double immunodiffusion and immunoelectrophoresis are inadequate to ensure specificity. Frozen sections of monoclonal plasma cells in myeloma tissue or agarose beads coated with the purified antigen [25] should be used. Second, the staining by the labeled antibody should be abolished by absorption with the purified antigen against which the antibody is directed. Blocking of the staining by the labeled antibody after prior incubation of tissue sections with unlabeled antibody is not sufficient to indicate the specificity of the antiserum. The importance of a good quality control program cannot be overemphasized [116].

Several labels are available to identify the bound antibody in tissue sections. Fluorescein isothiocyanate and rhodamine have been used most widely, but they fade with time, necessitating photographic documentation. They require a fluorescence microscope, preferably with epi-illumination. Products of enzyme reactions, particularly of peroxidase, have become very popular as labels, since they obviate the limitations that have been mentioned and provide better morphologic detail. Both fluorescein-labeled and peroxidase-labeled antisera are commercially available or can be prepared with relative ease [8,85].

Preparation of Tissue

The snap-frozen tissue is cut for examination in a closed cryostat. Frozen sections should be 2 to 4 μ thick. They are mounted on slides, desiccated, and fixed in acetone,

ether, or ethanol, or are used unfixed. After washing in phosphate-buffered saline (pH 7.2), they are incubated with the labeled antisera for 30 to 60 minutes at room temperature or for shorter periods at 37°C. Subsequently, they are washed and cover-slipped in a nonfluorescent embedding medium, such as Elvanol. If peroxidase-labeled antibodies are employed, they are developed in a mixture of diaminobenzidine and hydrogen peroxide [55]. In the indirect or sandwich method, which obviates the necessity of preparing labeled antibody for every antigen, unlabeled antiserum is applied first, followed after washing by labeled antibody to the first antiserum. This technique has the advantage of increasing the sensitivity of detection but the disadvantage of enhancing nonspecific staining. To detect technical failure, it is advisable to include with each staining procedure a renal specimen with known staining characteristics. One or two sections should be set aside for staining for light microscopy. This permits a direct comparison between the histologic and the immunohistochemical findings. To a large extent, immunoelectron microscopy remains a research technique [121a].

Light Microscopy

As a preliminary step, all the stained sections should be examined, to view the structures at several levels, compensating to some degree for the small amount of tissue available and increasing the chances of finding focal lesions. Several sections are selected for detailed examination. All glomeruli in the section are counted; after that, each glomerulus and the intervening tissue are examined under high magnification [100]. A high dry lens (40× or 60×) is often sufficient, but in many instances an oil immersion lens (100×) is necessary. Generally speaking, the glomerular count establishes the adequacy of the biopsy. A minimum of 10 to 15 glomeruli is considered necessary for the diagnosis, although with a diffuse lesion, even 5 glomeruli may be adequate. On the other hand, focal lesions producing clinical manifestations may affect 1% or fewer glomeruli and consequently may not be found in the available renal tissue. Occasionally, as in acute interstitial inflammation or in some cases of amyloidosis, diagnosis can be made even in the absence of glomeruli.

Examination of Glomeruli

Glomeruli are examined for the presence and the extent of abnormalities: enlargement, cellularity, mesangial expansion, thickening of capillary walls, deposits, thrombosis, necrosis, crescents, adhesions, sclerosis, and thickening of Bowman's capsule. These lesions may affect the whole glomerulus or only a part (segment) of it. Tubules may show epithelial changes (vacuolization, degeneration, necrosis), intraluminal casts, basement membrane thickening, and diffuse or focal atrophy. Within the interstitial tissue one may notice edema, fibrosis, and various types of inflammation. Arteries and arterioles may show sclerosis, hyalinization, narrowing of the lumen, thrombosis, necrosis, and inflammation.

Diagnosis

Sections should be examined by the pathologist without the knowledge of the clinical history. After thorough examination, the preliminary diagnosis or diagnoses can be written down and correlated with the clinical and laboratory data. It is best to discuss each case with the clinician in charge. The final diagnosis may be established at that time, or further studies, including electron microscopy and immunofluorescence, may need to be pursued. In addition to the specific diagnosis, the severity of the process and degree of tissue damage should be evaluated. Wherever possible, the character of the disease, whether acute and self-limited or chronic and progressive, should be determined.

Special Stains

For a complete diagnosis, special stains may be necessary. If amyloid is suspected, metachromatic stains (Crystal violet, Congo red, and thioflavine T) and, of course, electron microscopy are useful. Other special stains include those for hemoglobin, hemosiderin, fibrin, calcium, uric acid, and elastica.

Electron Microscopy

Although with experience many fine details of structure may be seen on light microscopy by means of the oil immersion lens, electron microscopy is extremely helpful in examination of the individual glomerular components. The changes in the capillary wall, often crucial to the understanding of the pathologic process, can be clearly visualized by the electron microscope: endothelial detachment, ingrowth or interposition of mesangium into the subendothelial space, thickening and splitting of the basement membrane, various types of deposits, and formation of basement membrane "spikes." Electron microscopy is also helpful in the study of the mesangium, indicating the presence and localization of deposits, from amyloid to immune complexes, changes in the amount and character of the mesangial matrix, and proliferation of cells. Special features revealed by the electron microscope may include the structure of deposits (crystals, organized patterns) or the presence of unusual constituents (myxovirus-like particles) in the cell cytoplasm.

Immunofluorescence Microscopy

Sections prepared for immunofluorescence microscopy should be examined soon after staining to avoid the effects of fading. For the same reason it is advisable to document the findings by microphotography. High-speed film will decrease the exposure time and thus diminish fading of the section during photography. The following points are noted:

1. The presence or absence of the specific substance examined for, e.g., immunoglobulin A, C3 (third component of complement), fibrinogen.
2. Intensity of staining. The intensity bears some relation to the amount of the substance but many other factors (thickness of section, fading, characteristics of the labeled antibody) also play a role, and it is dangerous to place too much reliance even on a semiquantitative evaluation.
3. Distribution: along the glomerular capillaries, in the mesangium, along the tubular basement membranes, in the interstitial vessels.
4. Form: granular, linear, pseudolinear, irregular ("lumpy," interrupted linear). *Pseudolinear* refers to numerous very fine granular deposits that produce the impression of a continuous line. Comparison with electron microscopy shows that most granular deposits are located between the basement membrane and the podocytes; irregular (lumpy, interrupted linear) deposits are located between the basement membrane and the endothelium. Linear deposits lie in the basement membrane and, unless of sufficient density, are often invisible by electron microscopy.

Basic Pathologic Processes in the Kidney
Glomerulus

Because glomerular changes are of crucial importance in many renal diseases and because they are easily examined by the currently available methods, these changes have been the major focus of attention in recent years. The significant glomerular changes are briefly mentioned under Examination of Renal Biopsy Sections. They are reviewed here in greater detail and to an extent related to specific diseases.

LIGHT MICROSCOPY
Enlargement
A glomerulus may be enlarged because of dilatation (and possibly an increase in number) of capillaries. This process is observed in compensatory hypertrophy of one kidney after removal of its mate. It is also seen in the better-preserved glomeruli in advanced chronic renal disease as well as in cyanotic congenital heart disease, chronic pulmonary disease, hepatic disease, and sickle cell anemia.

An increase in size may be caused by addition of cells or intercellular substances to the glomerular tuft or to Bowman's capsule. A conspicuous increase in the number of cells, both mononuclear and polymorphonuclear, in the mesangium and the capillary lumina will lead to the enlargement of the tuft (Fig. 20-4); proliferation of cells of Bowman's capsule will cause enlargement of the capsule and also marked narrowing of Bowman's space and compression of the capillaries (Fig. 20-5). These are typical changes of proliferative and of crescentic glomerulonephritis. Enlargement of the tuft may also be caused by

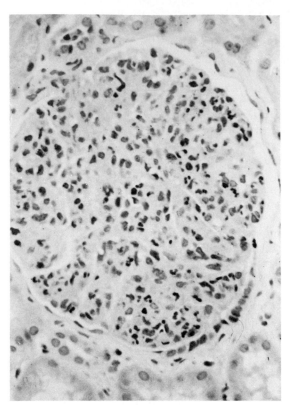

FIG. 20-4. *Glomerular enlargement due to proliferation and exudation in the tuft. Acute poststreptococcal glomerulonephritis. Large, very cellular glomerulus showing mesangial and endothelial proliferation and exudation of white blood cells. (×350) (From Churg J, Duffy JL: Classification of glomerulonephritis based on morphology. In Kincaid-Smith P, Mathew TH, Becker EL (eds): Glomerulonephritis. New York, Wiley, 1973; with permission.)*

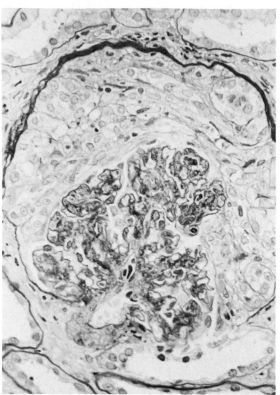

FIG. 20-5. *Glomerular enlargement due to crescent formation in the Bowman's space. Rapidly progressive extracapillary glomerulonephritis. The capillary tuft (on right side of picture) is collapsed. (×350) (From Churg J, Duffy JL: Classification of glomerulonephritis based on morphology. In Kincaid-Smith P, Mathew TH, Becker EL (eds): Glomerulonephritis. New York, Wiley, 1973; with permission.)*

edema of the endothelial and the mesangial cells, particularly in pre-eclamptic toxemia of pregnancy. Edema of the epithelial cell occurs typically in the nephrotic syndrome. Formation of various deposits, depending on their volume and location, may lead to the enlargement of the whole glomerulus or only of certain of its elements, such as the capillary wall or mesangium. The deposits often consist of—or, more accurately, contain—various immunoglobulins, elements of the complement cascade, fibrinogen and its derivatives, and other, poorly identified substances (e.g., those of hepatic glomerulosclerosis, probably lipid derived). Finally, enlargement of the whole glomerulus or its individual components may be caused by sclerosis, that is, an increase in the amount of mesangial matrix, as, for example, in diabetes or in certain forms of chronic glomerulonephritis (mesangiocapillary or lobular glomerulonephritis) (Fig. 20-6). Segmental enlargement caused by sclerosis occurs in so-called focal sclerosis associated with the nephrotic syndrome. This enlargement is caused by expansion of the mesangium, deposition of hyaline material, and simultaneous collapse of the pertinent capillaries. Such a segment may resemble a scar caused by

previous segmental inflammation or necrosis. However, it often can be distinguished by an increase in the mesangial cells and also by proliferation of podocytes covering the sclerotic segment.

Decrease in Size
The most frequent cause of decrease of the capillary tuft is ischemia brought about by narrowing of the blood vessels, especially of small arteries and arterioles. Such glomeruli have partially patent capillaries with distinctly wrinkled and apparently thickened capillary walls (Fig. 20-7). Prolonged and severe ischemia will eventually lead to atrophic sclerosis, in which the tuft is collapsed, acellular, and bloodless, and the whole glomerulus is small. It may consist of nothing more than a tangle of basement membranes, without the increase in mesangial matrix that characterizes most types of sclerosis. A similar picture prevails in the late stages of chronic glomerulonephritis (Fig. 20-8).

Simplification of Structure
Shrinkage of glomerular lobules caused by scarring, or, on the contrary, their expansion combined with enlargement of the glomerulus, accentuates the lobular architecture of

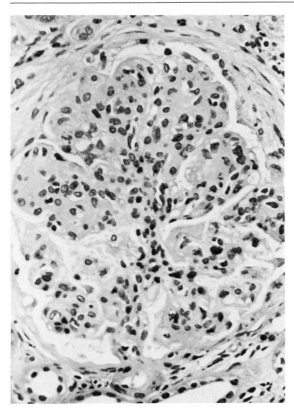

FIG. 20-6. *Glomerular enlargement caused by proliferation of mesangial cells and increase in mesangial matrix. There are also small fibrocellular crescents on the left side, top, and bottom. Lobular glomerulonephritis. (×350).*

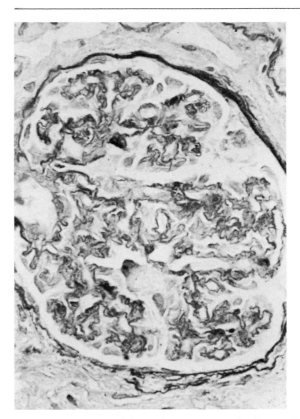

FIG. 20-7. *Decrease of glomerular size as a result of to capillary collapse. Note wrinkled capillary walls. Arteriolonephrosclerosis. (×350)*

the glomerulus. This is difficult to see under normal conditions because of overlapping of lobules.

Crescents and Adhesions

Proliferation of the cells of Bowman's capsule and formation of crescents were mentioned as one of the causes of glomerular cellularity. Crescents occur in numerous glomerular diseases and serve as an index of the severity of the process. Thus, one sees crescents in poststreptococcal glomerulonephritis, lupus nephritis, and malignant nephrosclerosis. Strikingly large (occlusive) crescents are typical of rapidly progressive glomerulonephritis (see Fig. 20-5). Small crescents, often composed mainly of podocytes, occur in focal glomerular sclerosis. Cellular crescents rapidly become organized and are converted into fibrocellular and, later, fibrous structures. Some crescents apparently may be absorbed. Fibrous crescents also arise by deposition of fibrous tissue on the inner aspects of Bowman's capsule. This ,is seen in ischemic collapse of glomeruli and in radiation nephritis. Adhesions may represent small fibrous crescents or may result from local damage to the epithelial cells, with formation of synechiae between the capillaries and Bowman's capsule (Fig. 20-9). Proliferation of the lining cells between the strands of fibrous tissue and the adhesions produces pseudotubules.

Changes of Capillary Lumens

Dilated capillary lumens may be overfilled with red blood cells, signifying severe congestion (so-called glomerular paralysis). True fibrin thrombi occur in the capillaries, often representing extension of thrombosis from the glomerular arteriole (Fig. 20-10). Small, nonoccluding collections of fibrin mixed with platelets are seen in a variety of glomerular diseases (e.g., glomerulonephritis, nephrotic syndrome). In other diseases, especially in systemic lupus erythematosus, thrombi have a hyaline appearance and consist mostly of proteins other than fibrin (Fig. 20-11). The exudative or insudative lesions, seen particularly in diabetes but also in many other chronic glomerular diseases, are hyaline thrombi containing a considerable proportion of lipid.

Necrosis

It is often difficult to distinguish primary capillary necrosis (Fig. 20-12) from that caused by thrombosis. Thrombosis causes obstruction of blood flow and eventual disintegration of capillary walls. However, primary necrosis undoubtedly occurs in diseases such as systemic lupus erythematosus. Its mechanism is unknown, but it is often accompanied by karyorrhexis and fragmentation of polymorphonuclear leukocytes.

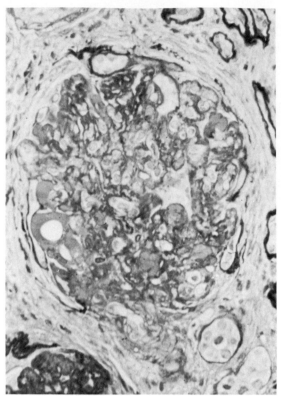

FIG. 20-8. *Decrease of glomerular size as a result of sclerosis and capillary obliteration. Chronic glomerulonephritis.* (×350.)

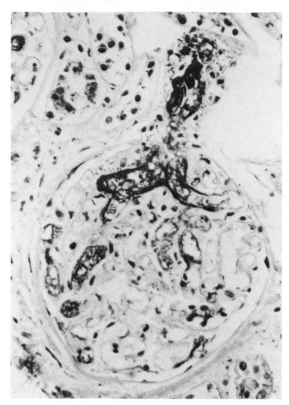

FIG. 20-10. *Fibrin deposition in the glomerular tuft. Fibrin thrombi in the afferent arteriole (on the left) extending into glomerular capillaries. Hemolytic-uremic syndrome.* (×350)

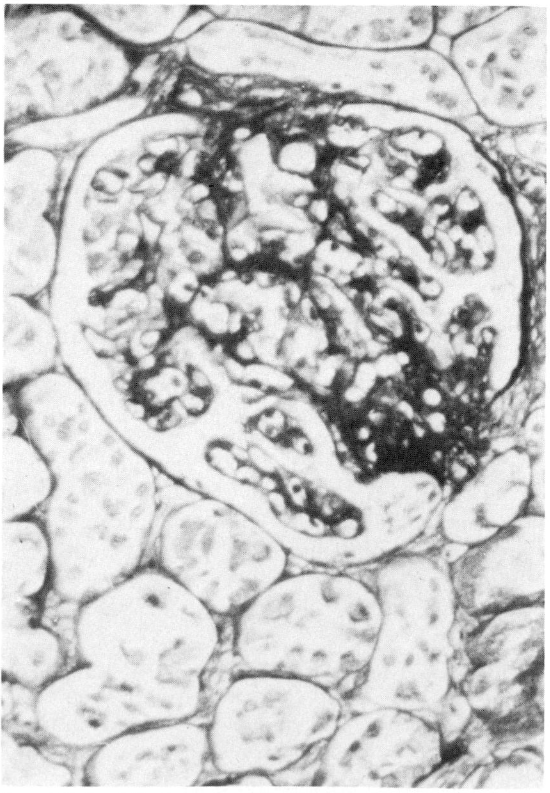

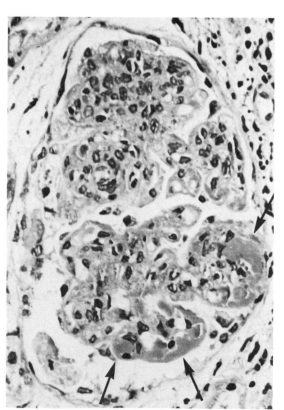

FIG. 20-9. *Adhesion of capillary tuft in Bowman's capsule (top center). Healed focal glomerulonephritis.* (×350)

FIG. 20-11. *Hyaline thrombi in glomerular capillaries (arrows). Lupus nephritis.* (×350)

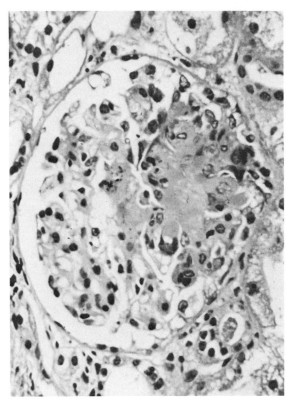

Fig. 20-12. *Segmental necrosis of glomerular tuft (near the top of the picture). Goodpasture's syndrome.* (×350)

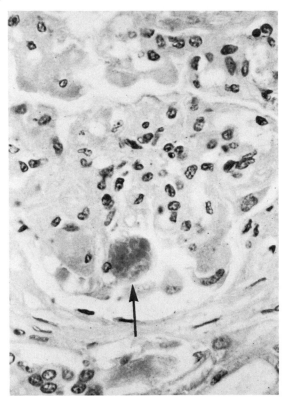

Fig. 20-13. *Hematoxylin body (arrow) in the glomerulus. Lupus nephritis.* (×560)

Special Features

Some diseases are identified by specific lesions. In lupus, "hematoxylin" bodies can be present in glomeruli (Fig. 20-13). These represent disintegrated nuclear material lying loose or in the cytoplasm of macrophages and various glomerular cells. Hematoxylin bodies are the tissue equivalent of the lupus erythematosus cell.

ELECTRON MICROSCOPY
Capillary Wall

Of all glomerular elements, electron microscopy is most useful for examination of the capillary walls [31]. The three layers of the wall, namely, the endothelium, basement membrane, and epithelium (podocytes), can be clearly distinguished (Fig. 20-14), and abnormalities affecting them can be detected.

The endothelium often undergoes swelling that is manifested by thickening and pallor of the cytoplasm and loss of fenestrations. Endothelial detachment, that is, separation from the basement membrane, is common and may be brought about by deposits, e.g., in lupus [27]; or it may be "primary" (radiation nephritis, transplant glomerulitis) [28,83], with subsequent subendothelial deposition of various substances such as fibrinogen and fibrin (hemolytic-uremic syndrome) [48,131] (Fig. 20-15). Mesangial cells and mesangial matrix frequently grow into the subendothelial space, producing the well-known mesangial inter-

position [29]. This is characteristically seen in mesangio-capillary glomerulonephritis (Fig. 20-16), but also occurs in a great variety of situations, from acute postinfectious glomerulonephritis to radiation nephritis.

In lupus, the endothelial cells often contain so-called myxovirus-like particles (Fig. 20-17), that is, fine arrays of interlacing tubules. This is not specific for lupus and may be present in other glomerular diseases, although less frequently.

The basement membrane is well preserved in many glomerular diseases or shows only slight irregularities, e.g., "mottling" in nephrotic syndrome. The membrane may become markedly attenuated because of dilatation of the capillaries or because of expansion of the mesangium by cellular proliferation. It may also be thin, without dilatation of capillaries, particularly in some forms of hereditary nephritis. Thickening of the basement membrane is a more common finding. It is invariably present in diabetes [34,98], sometimes very early in the disease, but is also seen in many advanced glomerular diseases in which it is a non-specific finding. The thickening observed in glomerular ischemia can be recognized on electron microscopy as mere wrinkling. Lesser degrees of thickening occur in hypothyroidism and scleroderma. Splitting of basement membranes is a characteristic feature of the Alport syndrome. The split layers are thin, generally parallel, and separated by pale structureless material interspersed with

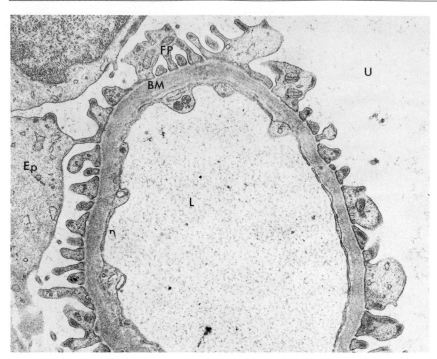

Fig. 20-14. *Normal glomerular capillary wall. Basement membrane (BM) is lined by thin endothelium on the luminal (L) side and by foot processes (FP) of the epithelial cells (Ep) on the urinary side (U). The connection between foot processes and cytoplasm of epithelial cells can be seen in some places.* (× 15,000)

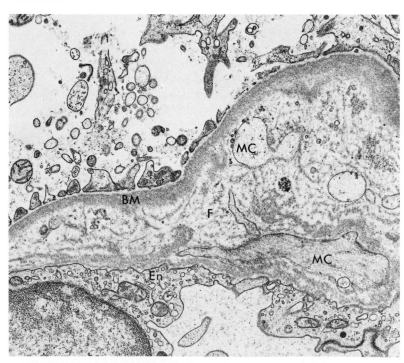

Fig. 20-15. *Abnormal glomerular capillary wall. Accumulation of pale, faintly fibrillar material (F) and cytoplasmic processes of mesangial cells (MC) between the endothelium (En) and the basement membrane (BM). Hemolytic-uremic syndrome.* (× 15,250)

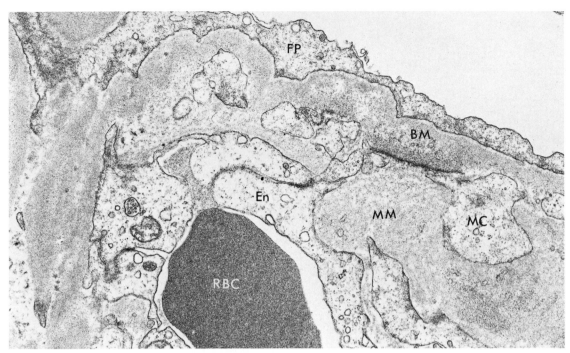

Fig. 20-16. *Accumulation of mesangial matrix (MM) and mesangial cell cytoplasm (MC) between the endothelium (En) and the basement membrane (BM). Epithelial foot processes (FP) are effaced. A red blood cell (RBC) lies in the capillary lumen. Membranoproliferative (mesangiocapillary) glomerulonephritis (×22,000)*

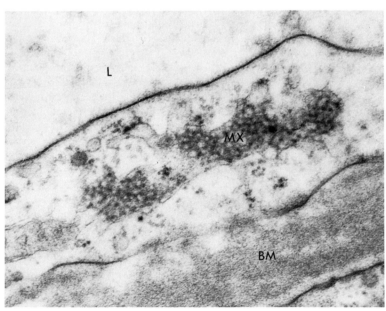

Fig. 20-17. *Myxovirus like particles (MX) (tubuloreticular structure) in the cytoplasm of an endothelial cell of glomerulus. L, capillary lumen; BM, basement membrane. (×51,3000)*

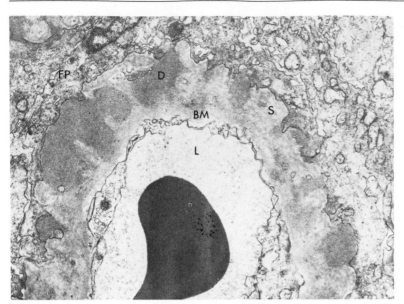

Fig. 20-18. *Membranous transformation. Subepithelial deposits (D) and spikes (S) cover the epithelial aspect of basement membrane (BM). The epithelial foot processes (FP) are "fused." L, capillary lumen. Membranous glomerulonephritis.* (×13,000)

dark granules [30,65,120]. Minor degrees of splitting occur in many glomerular diseases and are not diagnostic. In the nail-patella syndrome, collagen is present in the thickened basement membrane [12]. Although infrequent, actual breaks or gaps occur in the basement membrane in diseases varying from membranous glomerulonephritis to rapidly progressive glomerulonephritis [121]; they are particularly frequent in the latter and may be quite extensive in the areas of crescent formation [94]. A peculiar process called membranous transformation is seen in membranous glomerulonephritis, in a membranous form of lupus nephritis, and, rarely, in other nephritides. This process is characterized by projections (so-called spikes) on the epithelial side of the basement membrane, alternating with protein deposits [43] (Fig. 20-18). These spikes eventually form a new layer of basement membrane covering the deposits. Detached endothelial and epithelial cells are frequently capable of laying down a new layer of basement membrane, e.g., in radiation nephritis [83].

The most characteristic change of the visceral epithelial cells (podocytes) is effacement or "fusion" of their foot processes [7,45,125] (Fig. 20-19). This effacement is seen in nephrotic syndrome of various origins and also in other forms of glomerular damage, for example, in radiation nephritis. Foot-process effacement generally goes hand in hand with edema of the cell bodies, often with formation of numerous fine villi on the surfaces of the cells facing the urinary space. When severely damaged, epithelial cells become detached from the basement membrane and undergo necrosis. Alternatively, they recover to the point where they are apparently able to lay down multiple new layers of basement membrane, filling the space between the cell and the original membrane [57] (Fig. 20-20).

Epithelial cells also undergo hypertrophy, with increased number of organelles such as endoplasmic reticulum and ribosomes. In proteinuria or lipiduria the cell cytoplasm often contains vacuoles and droplets of protein or lipid. On rare occasions, protein crystals are noted. In some forms of glomerulonephritis, fibrils are present in large numbers. These fibrils resemble amyloid, but are considerably thicker (around 20 nm) and are probably related to immune deposits [39].

On electron microscopy the character and the location of the deposits in the capillary wall can be readily established. Protein deposits, particularly those containing immune complexes or immunoglobulins, are generally denser than the basement membrane. Deposits of fibrin are also dense and sometimes show the characteristic periodic structure, but some fibrinogen derivatives are, on the contrary, very light and fluffy [131] (see Fig. 20-15). Deposits in hepatic glomerulosclerosis consist of very fine, dark granules [113]. So-called dense deposits are almost black on electron microscopy and are characteristically found within the basement membrane [14] (Fig. 20-21). Some of the immune deposits may also lie within the basement membrane, e.g., deposits of kappa or lambda light chains, but more often they are seen under the endothelium, as in lupus nephritis (Fig. 20-22), in the subendothelial mesangium (in mesangiocapillary glomerulonephritis), or on the epithelial side of the basement membrane ("humps" of postinfectious glomerulonephritis [see Fig. 20-23] and deposits of membranous glomerulonephritis [see Fig. 20-18]). The pale deposits of fibrinogen derivatives invariably lie on the endothelial side of the basement membrane as in the hemolytic-uremic syndrome. When deposits are of the same density as the basement membrane, they are ex-

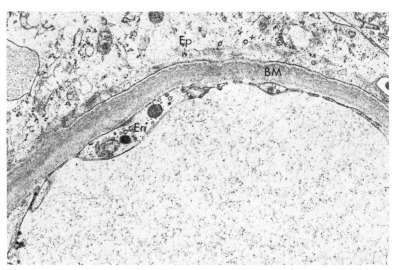

FIG. 20-19. *Complete loss, or effacement, of epithelial foot processes. The epithelial cytoplasm (Ep) rests directly on the basement membrane (BM). The endothelium (En) is preserved. Lipoid nephrosis—minimal change disease.* (×15,250)

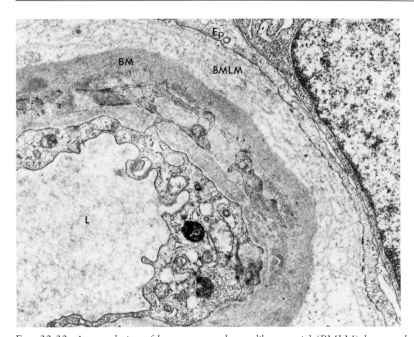

FIG. 20-20. *Accumulation of basement membrane–like material (BMLM) between basement membrane (BM) and detached epithelial cytoplasm (Ep). L, capillary lumen. Focal sclerosis.* (×14,200)

tremely difficult to recognize. Generally, the deposits are finely granular, but some are coarse, resembling to a degree the structure of viruses. Some deposits show organized patterns ("fingerprints" in lupus) [58]; others have a crystalline structure [102]. Amyloid deposits are fibrillar; they may be found in any location: under the endothelium, in the basement membrane, under the epithelium, and even in the urinary space.

Mesangium

Although the cells lying in the mesangium are readily seen by light microscopy, small amounts of matrix are difficult to see without the electron microscope. The character of the matrix varies with the disease. In acute processes such as acute glomerulonephritis and the hemolytic-uremic syndrome, the matrix may be swollen and reticulated. In diabetes the strands are thick, with a tendency to "layer-

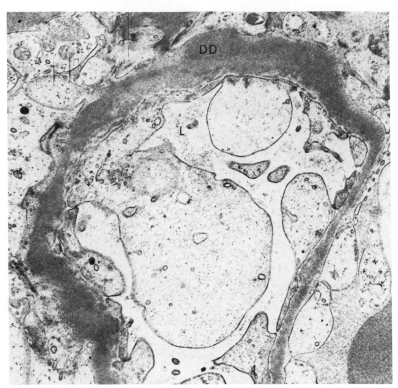

FIG. 20-21. Very dark, irregular deposits (DD) in the basement membrane. L, capillary lumen. Dense deposits disease. (×16,500)

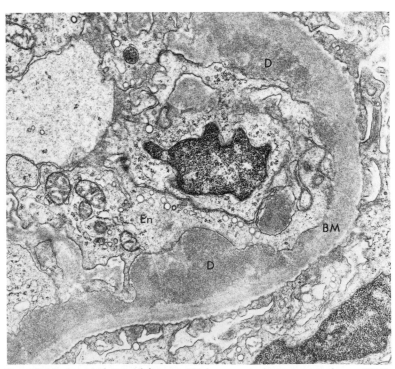

FIG. 20-22. Accumulation of deposits (D) between the basement membrane (BM) and swollen endothelium (En). Lupus nephritis. (×23,000)

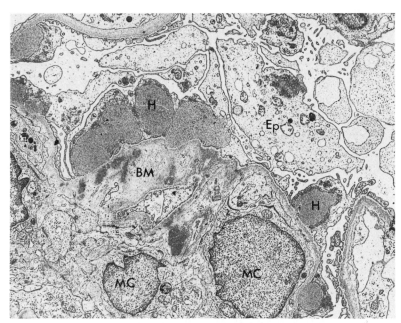

FIG. 20-23. *Subepithelial deposits ("humps") (H) between the basement membrane (BM) and the epithelial cells (Ep). There is proliferation of mesangial cells (MC) at the bottom of the picture. Poststreptococcal glomerulonephritis. (×7,100)*

ing," whereas in chronic glomerulonephritis the strands are at first thin and markedly irregular and do not form layered structures. The same type of deposits found in the capillary wall may also be present in the mesangium: protein deposits of various densities (e.g., immune deposits), amyloid, and deposits of hepatic glomerulosclerosis. They lie between the cell cytoplasm and the strands of matrix and often tend to accumulate along the basement membrane covering the mesangium. Often, the deposits actually infiltrate and partly replace the mesangial matrix (e.g., in amyloidosis, mesangiocapillary glomerulonephritis, and other diseases).

IMMUNOFLUORESCENCE MICROSCOPY

The main value of immunofluorescence microscopy lies in identification of glomerular deposits [137]. It is less useful than electron microscopy for their localization, although a distinction can usually be made between those along the capillary wall and those in the mesangium.

The deposition of immunoglobulins, complement, and fibrinogen has been well documented in a variety of immunologically mediated human glomerular diseases. Granular accumulation of immunoglobulins, predominantly IgG and IgM, and of complement along the glomerular capillary walls is suggestive of immune complex nephritis, such as acute poststreptococcal glomerulonephritis, nephritis associated with infections (e.g., bacterial endocarditis) or with anaphylactoid purpura and lupus nephritis [37,138]. Immunofluorescence is helpful in the differentiation of lipoid nephrosis (nil or minimal disease) from focal sclerosis (progressive lipoid nephrosis with focal glomerulosclerosis) and from membranous nephropathy. The latter shows gran-

ular accumulation of immunoglobulins and complement diffusely along the glomerular capillary walls (Fig. 20-24), and focal sclerosis shows segmental accumulation, mainly in the sclerotic areas [87] (Fig. 20-25). Irregular deposits of the third and late-acting components of complement without detectable immunoglobulins or early-acting components suggest activation of the alternative complement pathway, particularly if properdin is also present, as seen in mesangiocapillary (membranoproliferative) glomerulonephritis with hypocomplementemia [130] (Fig. 20-26). These findings distinguish it from acute diffuse proliferative glomerulonephritis. Mesangial accumulation of IgA is characteristic of IgA nephropathy; lesser amounts of IgG and sometimes of IgM may also be present [13,33a,43a, 133]. Complement and various immunoglobulins occur in the mesangium in the mesangial form of lupus nephritis [74] (Fig. 20-27).

Much less is known about different antigens presumed to be present in the immune complexes. In the minority of cases, often only after elution of the bound antibody, antigens have been identified in the diseased glomeruli, such as DNA in lupus nephritis [8], streptococcal antigen in poststreptococcal glomerulonephritis [12], malarial antigen in malarial nephropathy [134], and hepatitis B antigen [51] and tumor antigens [79] in some cases of membranous glomerulonephritis.

The second major category of immunologically mediated glomerular disease, i.e., antiglomerular basement membrane disease, is considerably less common than immune complex disease. Linear deposits of immunoglobulin and complement in glomeruli are characteristic of antiglomerular basement membrane antibodies as seen in rapidly

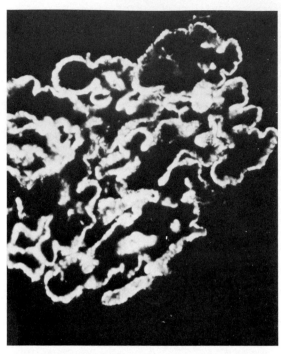

A

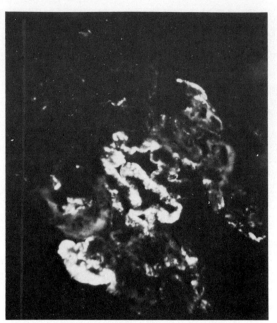

FIG. 20-25. *Focal granular deposition of IgG in a glomerulus. Focal glomerular sclerosis.* (×350)

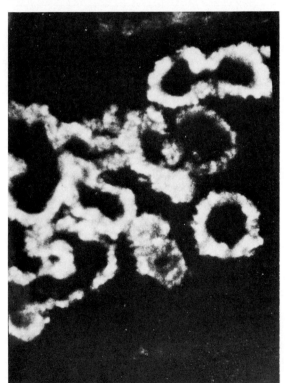

B

FIG. 20-24. *Immunofluorescence microscopy. a. Granular deposition of IgG along the glomerular capillary walls. Heavy deposits lead to a pseudolinear appearance in some areas.* (×350) *b. Higher magnification of A. showing definite granular appearance of deposits. Membranous glomerulonephritis.* (×560)

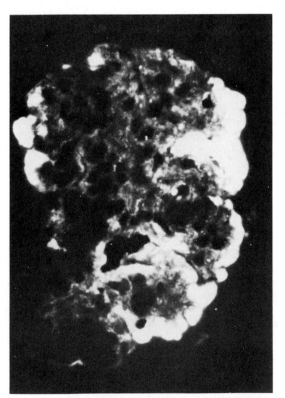

FIG. 20-26. *Granular and "lumpy" deposition of complement in periphery of glomerular capillary loops (mesangiocapillary) glomerulonephritis.* (×350)

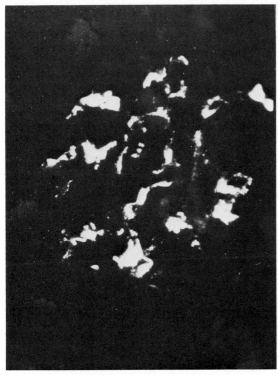

FIG. 20-27. *Mesangial deposition of complement. Systemic lupus erythematosus. (×350)*

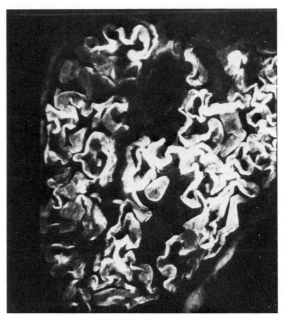

FIG. 20-28. *Linear accumulation of IgG along the glomerular capillary walls. Goodpastures syndrome. (×350)*

progressive or extracapillary glomerulonephritis and in patients with Goodpasture's syndrome [78] (Fig. 20-28).

Recent discoveries have modified the concept of two basic forms of glomerular disease and have revealed that granular immune deposits in glomeruli can also be formed in situ [5a, 20a].

Tubules

CELLS

A variety of changes can be found in tubular cells, often secondary to glomerular abnormalities or vascular ischemia. These changes can be classified under traditional headings such as degeneration, necrosis, or atrophy. With electron microscopy, however, more subtle abnormalities can be observed in the cellular cytoplasm.

Degeneration

Several forms of degeneration are described by pathologists, such as fatty, vacuolar, and hyaline-droplet degeneration. Sometimes these changes are truly indicative of considerable disturbance in the function of the tubular cells, but often they merely represent an overload of normally functioning cells due to excessive absorption from the tubular fluid. Thus, cytoplasmic vacuoles after intravenous administration of sugars (glucose, sucrose, mannitol), dextran, or polyvinylpyrrolidone are examples of cellular overload, whereas vacuoles in potassium deficiency [118] or after

administration of ethylene glycol represent vacuolar degeneration. Hyaline droplets usually indicate excessive protein absorption (Fig. 20-29) but may represent degeneration, as in severe ischemia. Accumulation of lipid droplets may also be due to excessive absorption or result from cellular malfunction. Glycogen in the cells occurs in metabolic diseases affecting carbohydrates. Other substances accumulate as the result of normal or abnormal metabolic activity, e.g., lipofuscin in the atrophic cells, iron in cases of hematuria or hemoglobinuria, or calcium in hypercalcemia [49]. On the electron-microscopic level, degeneration may be limited to a circumscribed area of the cytoplasm, in a process known as focal cytoplasmic degradation [66]. The affected area becomes enclosed by membranes and undergoes digestion by lysosomal enzymes. Other ultrastructural changes include loss of the apical portion and the brush border of the cell (potocytosis) and loss of basal infoldings.

Necrosis

Necrosis occurs in two forms. Liquefaction necrosis is similar to hydropic degeneration but much more severe. On electron microscopy it is manifested by the presence of large vacuoles, edema of mitochondria, mitochondrial and cytoplasmic densification, and nuclear lysis or pyknosis [106]. The affected cell becomes detached from the basement membrane, or it may break up at the apex, spilling the contents into the tubular lumen.

Coagulation necrosis progresses directly to the stage of mitochondrial and nuclear pyknosis and cytoplasmic densification [132]. The necrotic cell shrinks and either separates from the basement membrane or is retained in situ and is gradually absorbed.

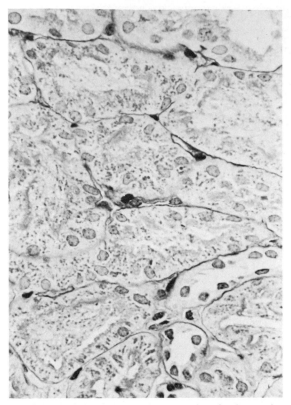

FIG. 20-29. *Tubular abnormalities. Hyaline droplets in the cytoplasm of tubular cells. Nephrotic syndrome. ($\times$350)*

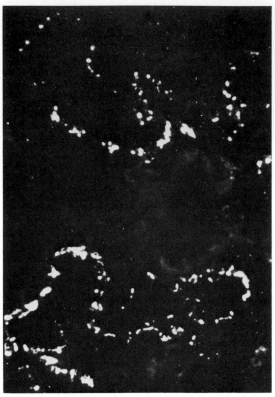

FIG. 20-30. *Granular deposits of IgG along tubular basement membranes. Lupus nephritis. ($\times$350)*

Regeneration

Regenerating cells arise from their better-preserved neighbors or from remnants of cells in the necrotic area. At first, they are flat and contain very few organelles. With maturation the cells increase in height, develop organelles at a rapid pace, and also develop microvilli and basal unfoldings. Functional maturation usually lags considerably behind the structural restitution.

Atrophy

Atrophy is most often caused by interference with blood supply secondary to glomerular or vascular disease. It may also follow direct injury to the tubules. The cells decrease in size, become cuboidal or flattened, and lose their basal infoldings and most of their microvilli as well as many of their organelles. Subnuclear lipid droplets and increased number of cytosomes are often noted. A very characteristic diffuse tubular atrophy with "clear" cells and only slight glomerular changes accompanies narrowing of major renal arteries (so-called endocrine kidney).

BASEMENT MEMBRANES

Thickening of tubular basement membranes is often seen in diabetes and in light chain deposition disease and is characteristically present in atrophic tubules in various renal diseases. The membranes may not only be thickened

but also split. Splitting is best seen by electron microscopy and should not be confused with the layered structure of some of the normal basement membranes, particularly around the collecting tubules. Protein deposits may be present in or around tubular basement membranes, for example, in dense deposit disease [14] and in light chain deposition disease (see Chapter 70). Some of the deposits are of an immune nature. In lupus, immune complexes are seen around the tubules and in the interstitial connective tissue. By immunofluorescence, they are granular in appearance and contain immunoglobulins and complement [76] (Fig. 20-30). Other immunologically mediated tubular and interstitial renal diseases [88] may or may not be associated with glomerular disease. In addition to immune complex deposits, there are also cases of linear immune deposits along the tubular basement membrane, presumably representing anti-tubular basement membrane disease.

TUBULAR LUMENS

Collections of material in the lumens are usually called casts. They may be hyaline, representing mainly protein, or granular, consisting of degenerated and fragmented tubular cells. In some instances (e.g., in multiple myeloma or in hemoglobinuria of various origins), casts have an injurious effect on the tubules, inducing the formation of giant cells. In renal hemorrhage, red blood cell casts may be present and, in infection, white blood cell casts. Crystals in the tubules are formed by a variety of substances, among them uric acid and urates, oxalates, and calcium (either as crystals of apatite or as amorphous calcifications of other types of casts). Administration of poorly soluble drugs, such as certain sulfonamides, may be the cause of crystalline casts.

Interstitial Tissue

Interstitial inflammation may be primary (pyelonephritis, drug induced nephritis, allergic reaction) or secondary to glomerular disease, tubular degeneration, or vascular embarrassment. In the acute stages, polymorphonuclear leukocytes usually predominate, particularly in cases of infection or necrosis. In allergic or hypersensitivity reactions, eosinophils may be found. However, the dominant cells, even in the acute stage, are mononuclear: lymphocytes, monocytes, and plasma cells. In severe inflammation, red blood cells are occasionally present in the interstitial tissue. Inflammation is accompanied by edema, but the latter also occurs without inflammation, for example, in renal vein thrombosis. Fibrosis follows unresolved inflammation or may be secondary to tubular atrophy. In contrast to edema, it is characterized by increased density of the interstitial tissue. Various deposits occur in the interstitial spaces; some, such as lipid, are usually located within interstitial

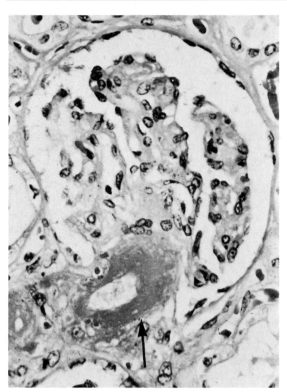

FIG. 20-32. *Fibrinoid necrosis of afferent arteriole* (arrow). *Malignant hypertension.* (× 350)

macrophages, but others, such as amyloid, lie loose in the connective tissue.

Blood Vessels

As a rule, only small and medium-sized arteries, arterioles, and corresponding venous structures can be seen in the biopsy section. Sclerosis of arteries, mainly intimal fibrosis, and arteriolar hyalinization are encountered in hypertension and also in diabetes mellitus and may accompany glomerular and interstitial disease. Myxoid or onion peel–layered thickening of the intima occurs in malignant hypertension but is also seen in scleroderma, with or without hypertension, and in the hemolytic-uremic syndrome. True arteritis with fibrinoid necrosis usually represents part of generalized periarteritis nodosa but may also occur in cryoglobulinemia. In such instances, immunofluorescence may show deposits of immunoglobulins, complement, and fibrinogen or fibrin in the affected wall. In systemic lupus erythematosus, small arteries and arterioles often contain immune complexes (Fig. 20-31) similar to those seen in the glomeruli. In untreated malignant hypertension, in scleroderma, and in the hemolytic-uremic syndrome, arterioles often undergo fibrinoid necrosis (Fig. 20-32). In the latter disease as well as in thrombotic thrombocytopenic purpura, aneurysms sometimes form at the entry of the arterioles into the glomerulus. Thrombosis is a frequent accompaniment of arterial inflammation and necrosis. Ve-

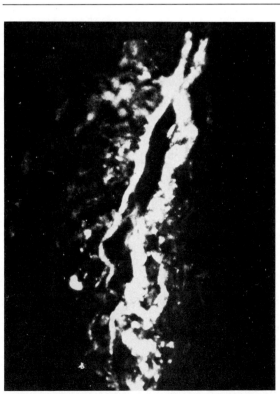

FIG. 20-31. *Vascular abnormalities. Deposition of IgG in intima and media of medium-sized renal artery. Lupus nephritis.* (× 350)

nous thrombi are seldom seen in biopsies. When present, they may be limited to small-caliber vessels or may represent the roots of thrombi of larger veins.

References

1. Ackerman GL, Lipsmeyer EA: Prolonged hematuria after renal biopsy. J Urol 97:790, 1968.
2. Agodoa LCY, Striker GE, Chi E: Glycol methacrylate embedding of renal biopsy specimens for light microscopy. Am J Clin Pathol 64:655, 1975.
3. Almkuist RD, Buckalew VM Jr: Techniques of renal biopsy. Urol Clin North Am 6:503, 1979.
4. Altebarmakian VK, Guthinger WP, Yacub YU, et al: Percutaneous renal biopsy. Complications and their management. Urology 18:118, 1981.
5. Alter AJ, Zimmerman S, Kirachaiwanich C: Computerized tomographic assessment of retroperitoneal hemorrhage after percutaneous renal biopsy. Arch Intern Med 140:1323, 1980.
5a. Andres G, Yuzawa Y, Cavalot F: Recent progress in renal immunopathology. Hum Pathol 19:1132, 1988.
6. Appel GB, Saltzman MJ, King DL, et al: Use of ultrasound for renal allograft biopsy. Kidney Int 19:471, 1981.
7. Arakawa M: A scanning electron microscope study of the human glomerulus. Am J Pathol 64:457, 1971.
8. Avrameas S: Coupling of enzymes to proteins with glutaraldehyde. Use of conjugates for the detection of antigens and antibodies. Immunochemistry 6:43, 1969.
9. Ball RP: Needle (aspiration) biopsy. J Tenn Med Assoc 27:203, 1934.
10. Bancroft JD, Stevens A: Histopathological Stains and Their Diagnostic Uses. Edinburgh, London, New York, Churchill-Livingstone, 1975.
11. Banfi G, Imbasciati A, Ponticelli C: Prognostic value of renal biopsy in acute rejection of kidney transplantation. Nephron 28:222, 1981.
12. Ben-Bassat M, Cohen L, Rosenfeld J: The glomerular basement membrane in the nail-patella syndrome. Arch Pathol 92:350, 1971.
13. Berger J: IgA glomerular deposits in renal disease. Transplant Proc 1:939, 1969.
14. Berger J, Galle P: Depots denses au sein des basales du rein. Presse Med 71:2351, 1963.
15. Berlyne GM: Ultrasonics in renal biopsy—an aid to determination of kidney position. Lancet 2:750, 1961.
16. Birnholz JC, Kasinath BS, Corwin HL: An improved technique for ultrasound guided percutaneous renal biopsy. Kidney Int 27:80, 1985.
17. Bolton WK, Tully RT, Lewis ET, et al: Localization of the kidney for percutaneous biopsy: A comparative study of methods. Ann Intern Med 81:159, 1974.
18. Bookstein JJ, Goldstein HM: Successful management of post-biopsy arteriovenous fistula with selective arterial embolization. Radiology 109:535, 1973.
19. Bretland PM, Hoffbrand BI: Kidney biopsy. Br Med J 5:281, 619, 1980.
20. Broyer M: Technique of needle biopsy of the kidney. In Royer P, Habib R, Mathieu H, et al (eds): Pediatric Nephrology. Philadelphia, Saunders, 1974, p 434.
20a. Bruijn JA, Hoedemaeker PJ, Fleuren GJ: Pathogenesis of anti-basement membrane glomerulopathy and immune-complex glomerulonephritis: Dichotomy dissolved. Lab Invest 61:480, 1989.
21. Burns J, Hambridge M, Taylor CR: Intracellular immunoglobulins. A comparative study on three standard tissue processing methods using horseradish peroxidase and fluorochrome conjugates. J Clin Pathol 27:548, 1974.
22. Burrington JD: Technique and results of 55 open renal biopsies in children. Surg Gynecol Obstet 140:613, 1975.
23. Buselmeier TJ, Schquer RM, Mauer SM, et al: A simplified method of percutaneous allograft biopsy. Nephron 16:318, 1976.
24. Carvajal HF, Travis LB, Srivastava RN, et al: Percutaneous renal biopsy in children: An analysis of complications in 890 consecutive biopsies. Tex Rep Biol Med 29:253, 1971.
25. Case JB, Lussier LM, Mannick M: Evaluation of immunological specificity of fluorescein conjugated antisera with agarose-antigen sections. Infect Immun 11:415, 1975.
26. Chodak GW, Gill WB, Wald V, et al: Diagnosis of renal parenchymal diseases by a modified open kidney biopsy technique. Kidney Int 24:804, 1983.
27. Churg J, Grishman E: Ultrastructure of glomerular disease: A review. Kidney Int 7:254, 1975.
28. Churg J, Grishman E: Electron microscopy of glomerulonephritis. In Grundmann E, Kirsten WH (eds): Current Topics in Pathology. Vol 61. Berlin-Heidelberg, Springer, 1976, p 107.
29. Churg J, Grishman E, Goldstein MH, et al: Idiopathic nephrotic syndrome in adults. A study and classification based on renal biopsies. N Engl J Med 272:165, 1965.
30. Churg J, Sherman RL: Pathologic characteristics of hereditary nephritis. Arch Pathol 95:374, 1973.
31. Churg J, Spargo BH, Sakaguchi H, et al: Diagnostic electron microscopy of renal diseases. In Trump BF, Jones RT (eds): Diagnostic Electron Microscopy. Vol 3. New York, Wiley, 1980.
32. Colodny AH, Reckler JM: A safe, simple, and reliable method for percutaneous (closed) renal biopsies in children: Results in 100 consecutive patients. J Urol 113:222, 1975.
33. Coons AH, Kaplan HM: Localization of antigen in tissue cells. J Exp Med 91:1, 1950.
33a. Croker BP, Dawson DV, Sanfilippo F: IgA nephropathy. Correlation of clinical and histologic features. Lab Invest 48:19, 1983.
34. Dachs S, Churg J, Matuner W, et al: Diabetic nephropathy. Am J Pathol 44:155, 1964.
35. DeBeukelaer MM, Schreiber MH, Dodge WF, et al: Intrarenal arteriovenous fistulas following needle biopsy of the kidney. J Pediatr 78:266, 1971.
36. Diaz-Buxo JA, Kopen DF, Donadio JV: Renal allograft arteriovenous fistula following percutaneous biopsy. J Urol 112:577, 1974.
37. Dixon FJ, Feldman JD, Vazquez JT: Experimental glomerulonephritis. The pathogenesis of a laboratory model resembling the spectrum of human glomerulonephritis. J Exp Med 113:899, 1961.
38. Dodge WF, Daeschner CW, Brennan JC, et al: Percutaneous renal biopsy in children. I. General considerations. Pediatrics 30:287, 1962.
39. Duffy JL, Khurana E, Susin M, et al: Fibrillary deposits and nephritis. Am J Pathol 113:279, 1983.
40. Durand D, Segonds A, Orfila C, et al: Transplant biopsies and short-term outcome of cadaveric renal allografts. Adv Nephrol 12:309, 1983.
41. Edelmann CM Jr, Greifer I: A modified technique for percutaneous needle biopsy of the kidney. J Pediatr 70:81, 1967.
42. Editorial. Techniques of renal biopsy. Lancet 2:1368, 1967.
43. Ehrenreich T, Churg J: Pathology of membranous nephropathy. In Sommers SC (ed): Pathology Annual 1968. Vol 3. New York, Appleton-Century-Crofts, 1968, p 145.

43a. Emancipator SN, Lamm ME: IgA nephropathy: Pathogenesis of the most common form of glomerulonephritis. *Lab Invest* 60:168, 1989.

44. Farmer CD, Diaz-Buxo JA, Chandler JT, et al: Control of post renal biopsy hemorrhage by gelfoam embolization. *Nephron* 28:149, 1981.

45. Farquhar MG, Vernier RL, Good RA: An electron microscopic study of the glomerulus in nephrosis, glomerulonephritis, and lupus erythematosus. *J Exp Med* 106:649, 1975.

46. Finkelstein FO, Siegel NJ, Booth C, et al: Kidney transplant biopsies in the diagnosis and management of acute rejection reactions. *Kidney Int* 10:171, 1976.

47. Forland M, Gottschalk A, Spargo BH, et al: Renal localization for percutaneous biopsy by scanning with technetium-99m-iron complex. *Pediatrics* 39:872, 1967.

48. Franklin WA, Simon NM, Potter EW, et al: The hemolytic-uremic syndrome. *Arch Pathol* 94:230, 1972.

49. Ganote CE, Philipsborn DS, Chen E, et al: Acute calcium nephrotoxicity. *Arch Pathol* 99:650, 1975.

50. Gault MH, Muehrcke RC: Renal biopsy: Current view and controversies. *Nephron* 34:1, 1983.

51. Gerber MA, Paronetto F: Hepatitis B antigen in human tissues. *In* Schaffner F, Sherlock S, Leevy CM (eds): *The Liver and Its Diseases.* New York, Intercontinental Medical Book, 1974, p 54.

52. Ginsberg JC, Fransman SL, Singer MA, et al: Use of computerized tomography to evaluate bleeding after renal biopsy. *Nephron* 26:240, 1980.

53. Goldberg BB, Pollack HM, Kellerman F: Ultrasonic localization for renal biopsy. *Radiology* 115:167, 1975.

54. Gotti E, Mecca G, Valentino C, et al: Renal biopsy in patients with acute renal failure and prolonged bleeding time: A preliminary report. *Am J Kidney Dis* 6:397, 1985.

55. Graham RC Jr, Karnovsky MJ: The early stages of absorption of injected horseradish peroxidase in the proximal tubules of mouse kidney: Ultrastructural cytochemistry by a new technique. *J Histochem Cytochem* 14:291, 1966.

56. Greifer I: Personal communication, 1977.

57. Grishman E, Churg J: Focal glomerulosclerosis in nephrotic patients: An electron microscopic study of glomerular podocytes. *Kidney Int* 7:111, 1975.

58. Grishman E, Porush JG, Rosen SM, et al: Lupus nephritis with organized deposits in the kidneys. *Lab Invest* 16:717, 1967.

59. Grizzle WE, Johnson KH: Membranous nephropathy in a renal allograft. *Arch Pathol Lab Med* 105:71, 1981.

60. Gwyn NB: Biopsies and the completion of certain surgical procedures. *Can Med Assoc J* 13:820, 1923.

61. Haaga JR, Alfidi RJ: Precise biopsy localization by computed tomography. *Radiology* 118:603, 1976.

62. Haddad JK, Mani RL: Percutaneous renal biopsy. *Arch Intern Med* 119:157, 1967.

63. Hefter LG, Brennan GG: Transillumination of renal biopsy specimens for rapid identification of glomeruli. *Kidney Int* 20:411, 1981.

64. Heron I: A paraffin embedding method in kidney immunofluorescent studies. *Acta Pathol Microbiol Immunol Scand [B]* 78:444, 1970.

65. Hinglais N, Grunfeld J-P, Bois E: Characteristic ultrastructural lesion of the glomerular basement membrane in progressive hereditary nephritis (Alport's syndrome). *Lab Invest* 27:473, 1972.

66. Hruban Z, Spargo B, Swift H, et al: Focal cytoplasmic degradation. *Am J Pathol* 42:657, 1963.

66a. Huraib S, Goldberg H, Katz A, et al: Percutaneous needle biopsy of the transplanted kidney: Technique and complications. *Am J Kidney Dis* 14:13, 1989.

67. Iversen P, Brun C: Aspiration biopsy of the kidney. *Am J Med* 11:324, 1951.

68. Karafin L, Kendall AR, Fleisher DS: Urologic complications in percutaneous renal biopsy in children. *J Urol* 103:332, 1970.

69. Kassirer JP: Is renal biopsy necessary for optimal management of the idiopathic nephrotic syndrome? *Kidney Int* 24:561, 1983.

70. Kark RM: Renal biopsy. *JAMA* 205:220, 1968.

71. Kark RM, Buenger RE: Television monitored fluoroscopy in percutaneous renal biopsy. *Lancet* 1:904, 1966.

72. Kark RM, Muehrcke RC: Biopsy of the kidney in prone position. *Lancet* 1:1047, 1954.

73. Kellow WF, Cotsonas NJ, Chomet B, et al: Evaluation of the adequacy of needle-biopsy specimens of the kidney: An autopsy study. *Arch Intern Med* 104:353, 1959.

74. Koffler D, Agnello V, Carr RI, et al: Variable patterns of immunoglobulin and complement deposition in the kidneys of patients with systemic lupus erythematosus. *Am J Pathol* 56:305, 1969.

75. Koffler D, Schur PH, Kunkel HG: Immunological studies of systemic lupus erythematosus. *J Exp Med* 126:607, 1967.

75a. Komaiko MS, Jordan SC, Querfeld U, et al: A new percutaneous renal biopsy device for pediatric patients. *Pediatr Nephrol* 3:191, 1989.

76. Lehman DH, Wilson CB, Dixon FJ: Extraglomerular immunoglobulin deposits in human nephritis. *Am J Med* 58:765, 1975.

77. Leiter E, Gribetz D, Cohen S: Arteriovenous fistula after percutaneous needle biopsy-surgical repair with preservation of renal function. *N Engl J Med* 287:971, 1972.

78. Lerner RA, Glassock RJ, Dixon FJ: The role of antiglomerular basement membrane antibody in the pathogenesis of human glomerulonephritis. *J Exp Med* 126:989, 1967.

79. Lewis MG, Loughbridge LW, Phillips TM: Immunological studies on a patient with the nephrotic syndrome associated with malignancy of non-renal origin. *Lancet* 2:134, 1971.

80. Lillie RD: *Histopathologic Technic and Practical Histochemistry,* 4th ed. New York, McGraw-Hill, 1976.

81. Lindeman RD: Percutaneous renal biopsy. *Kidney* 7:1, 1974.

82. Lusted LB, Mortimore GE, Hopper J: Needle renal biopsy under image amplifier control. *Am J Roentgenol Radi Ther Nucl Med* 75:953, 1956.

83. Madrazo A, Suzuki Y, Churg J: Radiation nephritis: Acute changes following high dose of radiation. *Am J Pathol* 54:507, 1969.

84. Mailloux LU, Mossey RT, McVicar MM, et al: Ultrasonic guidance for renal biopsy. *Arch Intern Med* 138:438, 1978.

85. Marshall JD, Eveland WC, Smith CW: Superiority of fluorescein isothiocyanate (Riggs) for fluorescent-antibody technique with modification of its application. *Proc Soc Exp Biol Med* 98:898, 1958.

86. Marshall FF, White RI, Kaufman SL, et al: Treatment of traumatic renal arteriovenous fistulas by detachable silicon balloon embolization. *J Urol* 122:237, 1979.

87. McCluskey RT: Evidence for immunologic mechanisms in several forms of human glomerular disease. *Bull NY Acad Med* 46:769, 1970.

88. McCluskey RT, Klassen J: Immunologically mediated glomerular, tubular and interstitial renal disease. *N Engl J Med* 288:564, 1973.

89. McGonigle R, Sharpstone P: Kidney biopsy. *Br Med J* 280:547, 1980.

90. McPhaul JJ, Lorden R, Thompson AL, et al: Nephritogenic immunopathologic mechanisms and human renal transplants: The problem of recurrent glomerulonephritis. *Kidney Int* 10:135, 1976.

91. McVicar M, Nicastri AD, Gauthier B: Improved renal biopsy technique in children. *NY State J Med* 74:830, 1974.

92. Metcoff J: Needles for percutaneous renal biopsy in infants and children. *Pediatrics* 46:788, 1970.

93. Moncrieff MW: Percutaneous renal biopsy in childhood. *Postgrad Med J* 48:427, 1972.

94. Morita T, Suzuki Y, Churg J: Structure and development of the glomerular crescent. *Am J Pathol* 72:349, 1973.

95. Muehrcke RC, Kark RM, Pirani CL: Biopsy of the kidney in the diagnosis and management of renal disease. *N Engl J Med* 753:537, 1955.

96. Mustonen J, Pasternak A, Helin H, et al: Renal biopsy in acute renal failure. *Am J Nephrol* 4:27, 1984.

97. Oettinger CW, Clark R: Transient obstruction uropathy complicating percutaneous renal biopsy. *Arch Intern Med* 135:1607, 1975.

98. Osterby R, Lundbaek K: The basement membrane morphology in diabetes mellitus. *In* Ellenberg M, Rifkin H (eds): *Diabetes Mellitus*. New York, McGraw-Hill, 1970, p 178.

99. Pillay, VK, Kurtzman NA: Percutaneous biopsy of the transplanted kidney. *JAMA* 226:1561, 1973.

100. Pirani CL, Salinas-Madrigal L: Evaluation of percutaneous renal biopsy. *In* Sommers SC (ed): *Pathology Annual 1968*. Vol 3. New York, Appleton-Century-Crofts, 1968, p 249.

101. Pollack HM, Goldberg BB, Kellerman E: Ultrasonically guided renal biopsy. *Arch Intern Med* 138:355, 1978.

102. Porush JG, Grishman E, Alter AA, et al: Paraproteinemia and cryoglobulinemia associated with atypical glomerulonephritis and the nephrotic syndrome. *Am J Med* 47:957, 1969.

103. Primus FJ, Wang H, Sharkey M, et al: Detection of carcinoembryonic antigen in tissue sections by immunoperoxidase. *J Immunol Methods* 8:267, 1975.

104. Ray MB, Desmet VJ: Immunofluorescent detection of hepatitis B antigen in paraffin-embedded liver tissue. *J Immunol Methods* 6:283, 1975.

105. Reeve RS, Cooksey G, Wenham PW, et al: A comparison of fine needle biopsy aspiration cytology and tru-cut tissue biopsy in the diagnosis of acute renal allograft rejection. *Nephron* 42:68, 1986.

106. Reimer KA, Ganote CE, Jennings RB: Alterations in renal cortex following ischemic injury. III. Ultrastructure of proximal tubules after ischemia or autolysis. *Lab Invest* 26:347, 1972.

107. Robson AM, Kissane JM, Manley CB, et al: Renal biopsy: Its place in the management of renal disease. *Clin Pediatr* 10:96, 1971.

108. Rose DH, Burden RP, Davies PE, et al: Kidney biopsy. *Br Med J* 5:281, 945, 1980.

109. Rosenbaum R, Hoffsten PE, Stanley RJ, et al: Use of computerized tomography to diagnose complications of percutaneous renal biopsy. *Kidney Int* 14:87, 1978.

110. Roy LP: Percutaneous renal biopsy in childhood. *Aust Paediatr J* 5:8, 1969.

111. Ruggieri G, Tata MV, Ventola FR, et al: A modified needle kidney biopsy: An open technique. *Nephron* 41:367, 1985.

112. Sagar SJ, Kaye MB: Systemic infection after needle biopsy of the kidney. *J Urol* 109:930, 1973.

113. Sakaguchi H, Dachs S, Grishman E, et al: Hepatic glomerulosclerosis. An electron microscopic study of renal biopsies in liver diseases. *Lab Invest* 14:533, 1965.

114. Savdic E, Mahoney JF, Storey BG: Control of bleeding after renal biopsy with epsilon-aminocaproic acid. *Br J Urol* 50:8, 1978.

115. Schmidt A, Baker R: Renal biopsy in children: Analysis

116. of 61 cases of open wedge biopsy and comparison with percutaneous biopsy. *J Urol* 116:79, 1976.

116. Sheibani K, Tubbs RR: Enzyme immunohistochemistry: Technical aspects. *Sem Diag Pathol* 1:235, 1984.

117. Slotkin EA, Madsen PO: Complications of renal biopsy: Incidence in 5000 reported cases. *J Urol* 87:13, 1962.

118. Spargo BH: Renal changes with potassium depletion. *In* Becker EL (ed): *Structural Basis of Renal Diseases*. New York, Hoeber Medical Division, Harper & Row, 1968, p 565.

119. Spear G, Slusser RJ: Alport's syndrome: Emphasizing electron microscopic studies of the glomerulus. *Am J Pathol* 69:213, 1972.

120. Spigos D, Capek V, Jomasson O: Percutaneous biopsy of renal transplants using ultrasonographic guidance. *J Urol* 117:699, 1977.

121. Stejskal J, Pirani CL, Okada M, et al: Discontinuities (gaps) of the glomerular capillary wall and basement membrane in renal disease. *Lab Invest* 28:149, 1973.

121a. Stirling JW: Immuno- and affinity probes for electron microscopy: A review of labeling and preparation techniques. *J Histochem Cytochem* 38:145, 1990.

121b. Sweet M, Brouhard BH, Ramirez-Seijas F, et al: Percutaneous renal biopsy in infants and young children. *Clin Nephrol* 26:192, 1986.

121c. Taylor CR: Monoclonal antibodies and "routine" paraffin sections. *Arch Pathol Lab Med* 109:115, 1985.

122. Telfer N, Ackroyd AE, Stock SL: Radioisotope localization for renal biopsy. *Lancet* 1:132, 1964.

123. Trachtman H, Weiss RA, Bennett B, et al: Isolated hematuria in children: Indications for a renal biopsy. *Kidney Int* 25:94, 1984.

124. Treser G, Semar M, McVicar M, et al: Antigenic streptococcal components in acute glomerulonephritis. *Science* 163:676, 1969.

125. Trump BF, Benditt EP: Electron microscopic studies of human renal disease: Observations of normal visceral glomerular epithelium and its modification in disease. *Lab Invest* 11:753, 1962.

126. Tully RJ, Stark VJ, Hoffer PB, et al: Renal scan prior to renal biopsy—a method of renal localization. *J Nucl Med* 13:544, 1972.

127. Usberti M, D'Auria CG, Borghi M, et al: Usefulness of hypnosis for renal needle biopsy in children. *Kidney Int* 26:351, 1984.

128. Vernier RL, Farquhar MG, Brunson JG, et al: Chronic renal disease in children. *Am J Dis Child* 96:306, 1958.

129. Vernier RL, Good RA: Renal biopsy in children. *Pediatrics* 22:1033, 1958.

130. Verroust PJ, Wilson CB, Cooper NR, et al: Glomerular complement components in human glomerulonephritis. *J Clin Invest* 53:77, 1974.

131. Vitsky BH, Suzuki Y, Strauss L, et al: The hemolytic-uremic syndrome: A study of renal pathologic alterations. *Am J Pathol* 57:627, 1969.

132. Wachstein M, Besen M: Electron microscopy of renal coagulative necrosis due to DL-serine, with special reference to mitochondrial pyknosis. *Am J Pathol* 44:383, 1964.

132a. Wahlberg J, Andersson T, Busch C, et al: The biopty biopsy technique: A major advance in the monitoring of renal transplant recipients. *Transplant Proc* 20:419, 1988.

133. Wallace AC: IgA nephropathy. *Pathology* 13:401, 1981.

134. Ward PA, Kibukamusoke JW: Evidence for soluble immune complexes in the pathogenesis of the glomerulonephritis of quartan malaria. *Lancet* 1:283, 1969.

134a. Welch TJ, Reading CC: Imaging-guided biopsy. *Mayo Clin Proc* 64:1295, 1989.

135. White RHR: A modified Silverman biopsy needle for use in children. *Lancet* 1:673, 1962.

136. White RHR, Jivani SKM: Evaluation of a disposable needle for renal biopsy in children. *Clin Nephrol* 2:120, 1974.

136a. Wijeyesinghe ECR, Richardson RMA, Uldall PR: Temporary loss of renal function: An unusual complication of perinephric hemorrhage after renal biopsy. *AM J Kidney Dis* 10:314, 1987.

137. Wilson CB, Yamamoto T, Ward DM: Renal diseases. *In* Stites DP, Stobo JD, Wells JV (eds): *Basic and Clinical Immunology.* Los Altos, Lange Medical Publications, 1987, p 495.

138. Wilson CB, Dixon FJ: The importance of immunologic mechanisms in the pathogenesis of glomerular disease. *In* Ingelfinger FJ, Ebert RV, Finland M, et al (eds): *Controversy in Internal Medicine.* Philadelphia, Saunders, 1974, p 685.

138a. Yussim A, Shapira Z, Shmueli D, et al: Use of modified fine needle aspiration for study of glomerular pathology in human kidneys. *Kidney Int* 37:812, 1990.

139. Zeis PM, Spigos DS, Samayoa C, et al: Ultrasound localization for percutaneous renal biopsy in children. *J Pediatr* 89:263, 1976.

IV
Manifestations of Renal Disease and Renal Insufficiency

V. Matti Vehaskari
Alan M. Robson

21
Proteinuria

Protein Handling by the Kidney

Contrary to earlier beliefs, it is now known that normal urine contains small amounts of a large number of proteins. Many of these proteins are derived from plasma. Indeed, most plasma proteins can be detected in urine by using sensitive methods [14,76,175]. Other proteins found in urine originate from various tissues, including the urinary tract. With few exceptions, an abnormally high urinary protein excretion is the result of an increase in one or more of the normal urinary constituents.

The protein composition of the final urine in both health and disease is the net result of three functions: (1) glomerular filtration of proteins present in plasma, (2) tubular reabsorption of the filtered protein, and (3) addition or "secretion" of protein into urine throughout the genitourinary tract. To provide a background for understanding different pathophysiologic perturbations leading to proteinuria, each of these mechanisms will be reviewed.

Glomerular Filtration of Protein

FUNCTION AND STRUCTURE OF GLOMERULAR CAPILLARY WALL

The peripheral or "loop" portion of the glomerular capillary wall is the filter across which both fluid and solutes must traverse to gain entry into the primary urine in Bowman's space; no filtration is believed to take place across the mesangial region. The three layers of the peripheral capillary wall are, from proximal to distal (Fig. 21-1), (1) the endothelial cell layer, (2) the glomerular basement membrane, and (3) the epithelial cell layer.

The *endothelial cell layer* possesses discrete fenestrae about 400 to 800 Å in diameter (see Fig. 21-1) [56,92] and thus would appear an unlikely site for restricting the passage of plasma proteins, most of which have an effective radius smaller than 100 Å. In carefully prepared specimens, a thin diaphragm, not seen in most routine electron micrographs, has, however, been described bridging the fenestrae [92]; whether this acts as a filtration barrier is not known. Most experimental studies with electron-dense tracers have demonstrated no restriction to molecules up to 61 Å at the level of the endothelium [37,56,158]. An exception is a study in which renal blood flow was preserved during the initial fixation of specimens; under these circumstances albumin was found to be confined to the capillary lumen, not crossing the endothelial fenestrae [176]. From these results it was suggested that an additional functional filtration barrier, consisting of large plasma proteins trapped between the endothelium and the basement membrane or in the inner aspect of the basement membrane, exists in vivo, but is rapidly dissipated when blood flow is interrupted [176].

The *glomerular basement membrane* is a morphologically continuous acellular structure between the endothelium and the epithelium; no pores, gaps, or discontinuities can be seen with the electron microscope. It has an electron-dense central layer, the lamina densa, sandwiched between two less dense, thinner layers, the lamina rara interna and lamina rara externa (see Fig. 21-1). The exact functional and chemical difference between the layers is not known. The identified components of the glomerular basement membrane include type IV collagen, glycoproteins (laminin, fibronectin, and entactin), and a proteoglycan, heparan sulfate [54,120]. The collagen is probably arranged in a very fine mesh in the lamina densa [53,120], which makes this network, embedded in a gel-like permeable matrix, a potential primary filter for macromolecules. In support of such a role, protein [56,158] and dextran [37] molecules of varying size have been shown to be retarded at the level of the basement membrane in ultrastructural tracer studies. Most investigators agree that the glomerular basement membrane provides the major barrier to macromolecular filtration.

The *visceral epithelial cell layer* consists of specialized epithelial cells. The main cell body sends out numerous arm-like processes from which smaller extensions, so-called foot processes or podocytes, branch to envelop the glomerular capillary wall (see Fig. 21-1). Thus, the peripheral capillary wall is totally covered by the foot processes on its outer aspect, with the exception of the narrow spaces between the adjacent foot processes. These spaces measure 250 to 600 Å in width, depending on the method of fixation, and they are bridged by a thin membrane called the filtration

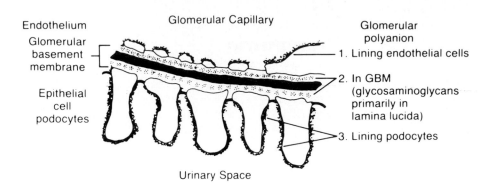

FIG. 21-1. *Diagram of the peripheral glomerular capillary wall. The three main layers are listed on the left, the components of the glomerular polyanion on the right. (From Schnaper HW, Robson AM: Nephrotic syndrome: Minimal change disease, focal glomerulosclerosis, and related disorders. In Schrier RW, Gottschalk CW (eds): Diseases of the Kidney. Boston, Little, Brown, 1988, with permission.)*

slit diaphragm. The fine structure of the slit diaphragm has been described as a central filament running parallel to the slit and connected to the foot processes on each side by regularly spaced cross-bridges. Rectangular "pores" with approximate dimensions of 40 × 140 Å exist between the cross-bridges [169]. There is some evidence to suggest that the slit diaphragms may function as filtration barriers to small molecules that penetrate the basement membrane [63,158]; other workers have rejected such a role [37]. Endocytotic protein-containing droplets can be seen within the epithelial cell cytoplasm in heavy proteinuria [55], but there is no evidence to indicate that under normal circumstances protein filtration takes place across the cell cytoplasm.

Although the glomerular capillary wall behaves like a porous membrane, restricting solute filtration according to the size of the molecule, it has become clear that additional properties of the capillary wall must affect the sieving of macromolecules, especially that of proteins. It is now accepted that interactions between electric charges play a prominent role, forming a *charge-selective barrier* to macromolecular filtration. Using specialized staining techniques, the glomerular capillary wall has been shown to contain negatively charged sites, the glomerular polyanion (see Fig. 21-1) [20,91,106,154]. These probably consist of sialic acid residues on the endothelial and epithelial cell surfaces as well as on the filtration slit diaphragms [106,133,154] and in the basement membrane of negatively charged proteoglycans, most prominently heparan sulfate [93,94,154]. The ability of systemically administered electron-dense tracers, visualized by electron microscopy, to traverse the glomerular capillary wall is highly dependent on the electric charge of the macromolecule; the more negatively charged the molecule, the poorer the penetrance across the capillary wall (Fig. 21-2) [158]. From these studies emerged the concept that electric repulsion between the negative charges of the macromolecular species on one hand and those in the glomerular filter (the glomerular

polyanion) on the other hand serves to decrease filtration below that seen with neutral molecules of similar size. Clearance studies using charged and uncharged polydisperse dextran preparations confirm the existence of a charge barrier. When dextran clearance is expressed as a fraction of inulin clearance and plotted against molecular size, the resulting permeability curve varies depending on molecular charge (Fig. 21-3) [21,28,38]. For any effective molecular radius between 18 Å and 40 Å, the glomerular permeability to the anionic species is lower than to the neutral species. Cationic dextran molecules penetrate the glomerular filter even more than the neutral molecules; this has been attributed to enhanced filtration by charge interaction. Clearance studies with native and charge-modified proteins have yielded similar results [17,157]. Although most evidence indicates that the anionic sites within the glomerular basement membrane form an important charge barrier [16,95,206], other layers of the capillary wall may contribute to this barrier as well [156].

Many plasma proteins are negatively charged at pH 7.4, but the charge-dependent restriction of albumin is quantitatively of greatest importance. The size of the albumin molecule (36 Å) would allow considerable amounts to be filtered if it were neutral (see Fig. 21-3), but because of the low isoelectric point (2.6), albumin is highly negatively charged at pH 7.4, and consequently only small quantities are normally filtered.

OTHER DETERMINANTS OF PROTEIN FILTRATION

The permeability of the glomerular capillary wall is only one of the determinants of macromolecular filtration. Others include the total surface area of the filtering membrane, the electrochemical and physical forces acting across the membrane, and both the shape and deformability of the molecule being filtered.

The filtering surface area obviously increases as the size

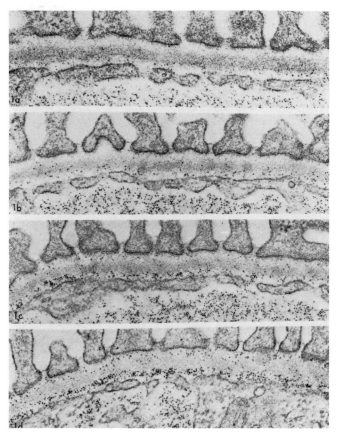

Fig. 21-2. Penetration of ferritin molecules (molecular radius approximately 60 Å) with different isoelectric points into glomerular capillary wall after systemic injection. The electric charge of the molecules changes from highly negative (pI 4.1 to 4.7) in the top panel to approximately neutral (pI 6.3 to 8.4) in the bottom panel. Very little penetration beyond the endothelial cell layer into the lamina rara interna is seen with the most anionic species (top panel). Penetration increases with increasing isoelectric point; the most cationic species are seen across the basement membrane and even adjacent to the epithelial cell foot processes (bottom panel). (From Rennke HG, Venkatachalam MA: Glomerular permeability: In vivo tracer studies with polyanionic and polycationic ferritins. Kidney Int 11:44, 1977, with permission.)

of the glomeruli increase with the growth of the child and his kidneys. This is the major reason for the increase in the absolute amount of urinary protein with age; when correlated to body size, there is very little change during childhood [131]. It is possible that acute changes occur in the filtering surface area under physiologic conditions. All glomerular capillaries may not be patent at all times; a collapse of some capillaries could result from arteriolar vasoconstriction or contraction of mesangial cells. The exact role of these mechanisms in protein excretion is not known.

Solute movement across the capillary wall can be divided into two components, convective and diffusive. Fluid moving across a membrane carries solute with it; this *convective* solute flux depends on the rate of fluid movement and on the restrictive properties of the membrane (i.e., restriction by molecular size and charge). Thus, the convective solute flux is secondarily affected by forces determining water flux, namely the hydrostatic and oncotic pressure differences across the capillary wall. Convective solute movement can take place in the absence of an electrochemical gradient. *Diffusion* of a solute occurs independently of fluid movement down the electrochemical gradient and is determined by the membrane characteristics and the magnitude of the concentration gradient. Indirectly, however, diffusion across the glomerular capillary wall is also affected by the determinants of fluid flux. This is the case because the intracapillary concentration of any solute whose diffusion is restricted by the capillary wall will increase along the length of the capillary, from afferent end to efferent end, as fluid moves out by ultrafiltration; the greater the ultrafiltration rate, the steeper the rise in concentration gradient.

An ideal mathematical model describing the macromolecular filtration across the glomerular capillary would have to include the membrane characteristics (surface area, restriction by size and charge, hydraulic conductivity), the hemodynamic variables determining fluid flux, and the plasma concentration of the macromolecule at the afferent end of the glomerular capillary. Although none of the proposed models has been able to accurately describe all these variables, these models have greatly advanced our understanding of the glomerular filtration process. The thermodynamic equations of Kedem and Katchalsky have been modified for calculating macromolecular filtration across the glomerular barrier at a random point as follows [39]:

$$J_s = wRT\Delta C_s + J_v(1-\delta)\overline{C_s}$$

where J_s is the solute flux; J_v is the volume flux; w is the solute permeability parameter; R is the universal gas constant; T is the absolute temperature; ΔC_s is the transcapillary solute concentration difference, and $\overline{C_s}$ is the log mean solute concentration at the point in question; and δ is the reflection coefficient. The term $wRT\Delta C_s$ describes the diffusive component, and the term $J_v(1-\delta)\overline{C_s}$ describes the convective component of filtration. It can easily be seen that the diffusion of protein depends, in addition to the membrane characteristics (w), directly on the local concentration gradient ΔC_s, which in turn depends on both the initial (systemic) plasma protein concentration and the filtration fraction in the segment of the capillary preceding the point in question. The higher the filtration fraction, the higher the local capillary protein concentration. Convection, or amount of solute (protein) carried by the volume flux, depends, of course, on the magnitude of the volume flux, J_v, the mean concentration of the solute, and the membrane characteristics (δ). Thus, this equation clearly illustrates the coupling of protein filtration not only to the membrane characteristics and plasma protein concentration but also to the hydrostatic and oncotic pressures governing fluid filtration. The coupling has been verified under various experimental conditions. For clinical purposes it is important to recognize that a hemodynamic perturbance leading to an increase in single-nephron filtra-

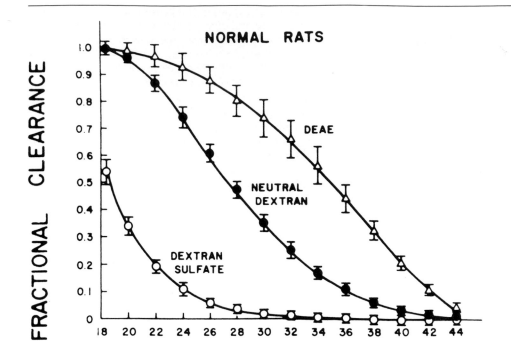

FIG. 21-3. *Glomerular permeability curves for neutral dextran, anionic dextran (dextran sulfate), and cationic dextran (DEAE). Clearance of each species is plotted as a fraction of inulin clearance against the molecular radius. See text for details. (From Bohrer MP, Baylis C, Humes HD, et al: Permselectivity of the glomerular capillary wall: Facilitated filtration of circulating polycations. J Clin Invest 61:72, 1978, with permission.)*

tion fraction, with or without an increase in single-nephron filtration rate, may increase protein filtration by virtue of increasing protein diffusion; and that an increase in single-nephron filtration rate may increase protein filtration via increased convection. Both of these mechanisms are illustrated in Figure 21-4.

Early micropuncture studies suggested that the protein concentration in normal glomerular filtrate may be as high as 10 mg/dl [34,48,107], but contamination of the samples with serum albumin probably made the results unreliable [140]. More recent observations have found albumin concentrations to be less than 1 mg/dl and perhaps as low as 0.1 mg/dl [50,139,140]. Thus, with a normal plasma albumin concentration of 4000 mg/dl, the sieving coefficient (ratio of concentration in glomerular filtrate to that in plasma) for albumin is less than 0.00025. A mean albumin concentration in the glomerular filtrate of 0.1 mg/dl translates into the transglomerular passage of about 150 mg of albumin per day in an adolescent or adult.

Because of very low concentrations, measurements of other plasma proteins in glomerular filtrate have been unreliable. The filtration of the larger plasma proteins, such as intact globulin molecules, appears to be negligible. In contrast, smaller molecules such as peptide hormones, e.g., insulin and growth hormone, or immunoproteins, e.g., β_2-microglobulin and light chains, can penetrate the glomer-

ular barrier with relative ease. They have sieving coefficients above 0.5 so that their concentrations in the glomerular filtrate are more than 50% of the plasma concentrations.

INCREASED PROTEIN FILTRATION AS A CAUSE OF PROTEINURIA

Causes of glomerular proteinuria are listed in Table 21-1 by the mechanism of increased protein filtration. Marked proteinuria most often results from diseases that increase glomerular permeability to protein. The increased filtered load of protein overwhelms tubular reabsorptive capacity, and most of the increment in filtered load is lost in the urine. Acute and chronic glomerulonephritides represent the most common causes for persistent severe proteinuria. These diseases are characterized by obvious pathologic abnormalities in the glomeruli, which are postulated to result in an increase in the glomerular "effective pore size." Both albumin and globulins appear in the urine in increased amounts, and the proteinuria is defined as nonselective.

In contrast, there is no obvious histologic injury to account for the proteinuria in minimal-change nephrotic syndrome of childhood. It is now believed that in this disease [29,167,181] and in congenital nephrotic syndrome of Finnish type [207], reduction or loss of glomerular charge

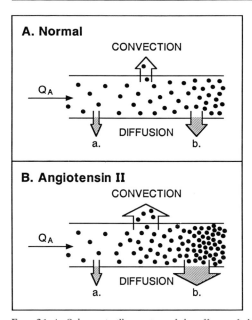

FIG. 21-4. *Schematic illustration of the effects of glomerular hemodynamics on protein filtration.* Q_A, *single nephron plasma flow. Solid dots symbolize protein molecules. Under normal circumstances (panel A), fluid ultrafiltration across the capillary wall (open arrow) carries protein molecules with it by convection. Because less protein than water leaves the capillary lumen this way, the intracapillary concentration of protein molecules increases from the afferent end to the efferent end. This rise in the electrochemical gradient along the capillary results in greater diffusion (shaded arrows) close to the efferent end (point b) than at the afferent end (point a). An increase in single-nephron filtration rate without a change in Q_A may result from a perturbation of glomerular microcirculation, exemplified by angiotensin II effect (panel B). Increased ultrafiltration is accompanied by increased convection of protein. In addition, the electrochemical gradient along the capillary rises steeper than under normal conditions, and the diffusion of protein at the efferent end is also increased. Consequently, both components of net protein filtration, convection and diffusion, are increased as a result of increased filtration fraction.*

TABLE 21-1. *Causes of increased glomerular filtration of protein*

I. *DEFECT IN GLOMERULAR CAPILLARY WALL*
   1. Acquired structural defect
      Immunologic injury (glomerulonephritides)
      Focal segmental glomerulosclerosis
      Hemolytic-uremic syndrome
   2. Loss of glomerular charge barrier
      Minimal-change nephrotic syndrome
      Congenital nephrotic syndrome of Finnish type
      (Focal segmental glomerulosclerosis)
      (Some glomerulonephritides)
   3. Abnormal composition of glomerular basement membrane
      Alport syndrome
      Diabetes mellitus
      Several inherited syndromes
II. *INCREASED FILTRATION THROUGH NORMAL GLOMERULAR CAPILLARY WALL*
   1. Altered glomerular microcirculation
      Angiotensin-induced proteinuria
      ? Orthostatic proteinuria
      Early diabetes mellitus
      Reduced number of functioning nephrons
      Congestive heart failure
      Hypertension
   2. Increased plasma protein level
      Plasma or albumin infusions
      Dysproteinemias
      Various tissue proteins

Hemodynamic factors, without any structural glomerular abnormality, may cause proteinuria as discussed above. Decreased number of functioning nephrons, which leads to increased single-nephron filtration rate in the remaining glomeruli, is associated with increased macromolecular filtration [168]. This mechanism may be responsible for the mild to moderate proteinuria in patients with advanced nonglomerular renal disease and in renal transplant donors. Early diabetic "microalbuminuria" may also be the result of glomerular hyperfiltration [46]. Increased filtration fraction explains the proteinuria observed with high levels of angiotensin [22,50] and may contribute to orthostatic proteinuria [212].

Another cause of increased glomerular filtration of protein is increased plasma protein level. The glomerular function is usually unperturbed; increased filtration results from the increased concentration gradient of the protein across the glomerular filtration barrier. Rarely, plasma protein level is sufficiently increased to lead to frank "overflow proteinuria." Repeated transfusions of albumin or plasma occasionally cause albuminuria [127]. Dysproteinemias are seldom seen in children. More commonly, a single or a few marker proteins are involved in very low concentrations, and the total urinary protein excretion is not significantly increased. Using sensitive assays, many such tissue proteins can be used for diagnostic purposes; e.g., tumor antigens, antigens of infectious agents, antigens released from tissue injury, and abnormal metabolites in metabolic disease can be detected in urine. The list of clinically useful markers is rapidly expanding and is beyond the scope of this text (see reference 171 for review).

barrier increases glomerular permeability to the highly anionic albumin molecule. The proteinuria, consisting almost entirely of albumin, is termed selective. There is, however, a slight increase in urine globulin content, both in these conditions and in experimental models of charge barrier loss [15]. Thus, it is possible that the glomerular polyanion is important for structural integrity of the glomerular basement membrane, and that loss of the negative charge sites leads to secondary disruption of the size-selective barrier. The charge barrier may also be perturbed in focal segmental glomerulosclerosis and some types of glomerulonephritis, but its role is quantitatively unimportant in the pathogenesis of the proteinuria. Obviously, abnormal chemical composition may lead to altered glomerular basement membrane structure and to increased permeability. This is the probable cause of proteinuria in some inherited conditions, e.g., in nail-patella syndrome.

Tubular Reabsorption of Protein

NORMAL FUNCTION

Quantitatively, only a small portion of the proteins and polypeptides filtered through the glomerulus is excreted in the urine. Under normal circumstances, the bulk of the filtered protein is reabsorbed by the proximal convoluted tubule [42,116,195]; no protein is reabsorbed beyond this segment. Protein reabsorption in the tubular epithelial cells is dependent on cell energy and takes place by endocytosis through the luminal cell membrane [42,116,122]. The initial step consists of binding of the protein to the glycocalyx surface of the cell membrane, the exact nature of this binding being unknown [115,116]. The protein migrates down the brush border to be concentrated in apical tubular invaginations that form between the microvilli. Here vesicles containing tubular fluid and protein are pinched off and enter the cytoplasm of the epithelial cell. Small vesicles fuse to form large vesicles and acquire hydrolytic enzymes by fusion with cytoplasmic lysozymes [41,42,122]. Intact protein molecules are not released from the tubular cells. Instead, proteins appear to be hydrolyzed by the lysosomal enzymes and returned to the body pool as amino acids or small polypeptides [83,90,101,141]. There is some evidence that the brush border contains enzymes capable of hydrolyzing some polypeptides prior to endocytosis; the formed fragments of the proteins are subsequently either reabsorbed or excreted in urine [144,193]. Consequently, all protein filtered through the glomerulus is lost from the body protein pool, by either tubular cell catabolism or urinary excretion. Uptake of certain proteins by basolateral endocytosis from the peritubular environment has been described, but quantitatively its role is minimal [25,137].

The kinetics of tubular protein reabsorption are not well understood. For most proteins studied, there seems to be a large difference between the threshold and transport maximum; some protein appears in the urine even with very small filtered loads, but the maximum reabsorptive capacity is not reached until a much greater amount is delivered to the proximal tubule [116]. For small proteins the reabsorptive mechanism operates normally well below the transport maximum [116]. At filtered loads below the transport maximum, the fractional excretion (portion of filtered load excreted in final urine) of a small protein is relatively constant, a characteristic that can be used to determine whether the reabsorptive function is intact.

As discussed above, the measured albumin concentrations in the glomerular filtrate range from 0.1 to 2 mg/dl or greater, the higher values probably representing contamination by plasma [140]. If a concentration of 0.1 mg/dl is correct, then the maximum daily filtered load in a normal adult is roughly 150 mg. A considerable portion of this, about 15 mg, appears in urine, reflecting a fractional reabsorption of only 90%, in contrast to the fractional reabsorption of small proteins, which in many cases exceeds 98% [52,195]. Thus, it has been argued that albumin reabsorption normally operates at or near transport maximum and that with increased filtered load the increment is almost quantitatively excreted in urine.

Proximal tubular microperfusion experiments have shed some new light on tubular albumin handling. In these in vitro experiments, the reabsorption mechanism appeared to possess a high capacity for albumin in comparison to the physiologic filtered load, but the affinity for the protein was low [141]. This model, too, is consistent with clinical observations. Glomerular damage and increased filtration of albumin would result in significantly increased albuminuria despite the simultaneously increased tubular reabsorption; fractional reabsorption would be little affected.

It has been proposed that larger plasma proteins such as albumin and IgG are reabsorbed by a common mechanism, with competition between the individual proteins. Increasing the filtered load of one protein would consequently decrease the reabsorption and increase the urinary excretion of all of the competing proteins [73]. Because urinary excretion of polypeptides and protein molecules smaller than albumin does not seem to be affected even by severalfold increases in filtered load of albumin, e.g., in nephrotic syndrome, it has been further postulated that a separate mechanism exists for the reabsorption of low-molecular-weight (LMW) proteins [69,74,145]. Conversely, tubular disorders in which urinary LMW protein excretion is greatly increased as a result of impaired reabsorption do not lead to significant albuminuria [145]. In support of two separate mechanisms, it was shown by microinjection techniques that, with similar proximal tubular fluid concentrations, two small proteins, insulin and ribonuclease, were reabsorbed more efficiently than albumin [44].

The nonselective nature of tubular reabsorption of small proteins has been seriously questioned [18,144,195]. Electric charge of the protein molecule seems to be one determinant of uptake by the proximal tubular cells. Microperfusion studies have shown that cationic proteins compete for the absorption process, but that there is a lack of competition between cationic and anionic proteins [195]. Other factors besides charge, however, must play a role because transport capacity and affinity vary even among proteins of similar molecular charge and size [195]. The exact nature of these factors is currently unknown but may include more specific brush border receptors since any selectivity of the endocytotic process beyond the initial binding is difficult to visualize. It should be emphasized, however, that in clinical situations in which a tubular disorder leads to LMW proteinuria, the measured excretion of most LMW proteins is increased and any of several LMW proteins can be used for diagnostic purposes.

The nonselectivity of large plasma protein reabsorption has also been challenged. For instance, modified ferritin molecules (MW 480,000) of varying charge are taken up at different rates by the proximal tubules, the most cationic molecules being reabsorbed most avidly [40]. Similarly, albumin molecules modified to carry a positive net charge are reabsorbed at much higher rates than native anionic albumin [141]. Whether true competition between large proteins, e.g., albumin and IgG, exists remains to be demonstrated.

For proteins and polypeptides with high sieving coefficients, the kidney is an important site of catabolism because the reabsorbed protein is catabolized in the tubular cells [194]. Significant proportions of growth hormone [90], insulin [98,173], parathyroid hormone [83,101], and luteinizing hormone-releasing hormone [193] have been shown to be removed from the body pool this way. Consequently, severely reduced renal function or bilateral nephrectomy will reduce the catabolic rate of these hormones and may raise their plasma levels [82,121,178,209,210]; the functional consequences of the elevated hormone levels are not fully understood. In contrast, the kidney contributes only minimally to the catabolism of albumin under normal circumstances [100], but in glomerular disease with heavy proteinuria, the renal elimination of albumin and other large plasma proteins through catabolism and urinary excretion becomes significant [62,99,209].

There probably are no major differences in renal tubular protein handling between children and adults. The exception is the neonatal period and early infancy. During the first month of life, urine protein excretion in full-term infants is twice as high as in later infancy, and it is even higher during the first days of life [96,97,131]. Even greater amounts are excreted by premature infants [131]. The quantity of urinary LMW proteins is increased much more than that of urinary albumin, leading to the conclusion that the higher protein excretion results from less complete tubular reabsorption [96,131]. In preterm infants up to 35 gestational weeks of age, the fractional excretion of LMW proteins such as β_2-microglobulin (MW 11,800) is said to correlate with gestational age, reflecting renal tubular maturation [9,10,12]. Others have been unable to confirm this correlation [51,200].

DISORDERS OF TUBULAR PROTEIN REABSORPTION

Failure of the proximal tubules to reabsorb protein results in only mild to moderate proteinuria (less than 1 g per day), owing to the fact that the protein content of the glomerular filtrate is low. Table 21-2 lists some of these conditions. It is unclear whether any disorders selectively affect tubular protein reabsorption without having an effect on other tubular functions. Rare cases of isolated defects in the reabsorption of LMW proteins have been described [58,197], but the LMW proteinuria may only have been the first clinically detectable sign of multiple tubular dysfunction [197]. In contrast, many types of tubular injury or dysfunction lead to impaired reabsorption of protein along with other disruptions in tubular functions. Typically, the reabsorption of albumin and larger proteins is only minimally, if at all, affected, while the urinary excretion of small proteins (MW 5,000 to 50,000) is increased many-fold [145,209]. In many conditions, the LMW proteinuria is variable and may not be present in early stages of the disease. In contrast, LMW protein excretion in a few conditions is so strikingly and consistently elevated that it is of diagnostic significance. In generalized Fanconi syndrome, whether idiopathic or secondary to systemic metabolic disease, impaired tubular protein reabsorption is part of the spectrum [13,209]. LMW proteinuria is also always associated with acute tubular necrosis of toxic or ischemic etiology [70,132,161,200]. The discrimination between lower and upper urinary tract infections by urine protein pattern is not absolute [2,129]. Some patients with

TABLE 21-2. *Tubular disorders with increased excretion of low-molecular-weight proteins*

I. *TUBULAR DISEASES*
   1. PRIMARY RENAL TUBULAR DISORDERS
      Isolated tubular proteinuria
      Idiopathic Fanconi syndrome
      Renal tubular acidosis
      Nephrogenic diabetes insipidus
      Bartter's syndrome
   2. TUBULAR DISORDERS SECONDARY TO SYSTEMIC DISEASE
      Cystinosis
      Glycogen storage disease
      Galactosemia
      Primary hyperoxaluria
      Hypercalciuria
      Wilson's disease
      Tyrosinemia
      Hereditary fructose intolerance
      Oculo-cerebro-renal syndrome (Lowe's syndrome)
      Cytochrome c oxidase deficiency
      Dysproteinemias
      Sickle cell disease
      Diabetes mellitus
II. *TUBULAR TOXINS*
   1. DRUGS
      Aminoglycosides
      Penicillins
      Polymyxins
      Outdated tetracycline
      Cephalothin
      Cisplatin
      6-Mercaptopurine
      Azathiaprine
   2. OTHER
      Heavy metals
      Free hemoglobin and myoglobin
      Uric acid
III. *ISCHEMIC TUBULAR INJURY*
      Neonatal asphyxia
      Hypovolemic shock
      Cardiogenic shock
      Endotoxemia
      Open-heart surgery
IV. *ACQUIRED TUBULOINTERSTITIAL DISEASE*
      Interstitial nephritis
      Pyelonephritis
      Glomerulonephritis with tubulointerstitial involvement
      Balkan nephropathy
      Hypokalemic nephropathy
V. *MISCELLANEOUS*
      Obstructive uropathy
      Medullary cystic disease/nephronophthisis
      Polycystic kidney disease
      Renal transplant rejection

primary glomerular disease exhibit LMW proteinuria as a sign of tubulointerstitial involvement [151], but quantitatively the tubular proteinuria is usually overshadowed by albuminuria. Recent evidence has suggested that early "microalbuminuria" in diabetes may not be entirely glomerular in origin but may be accompanied by LMW proteinuria as a sign of proximal tubular injury [59].

Proteins Originating from the Urinary Tract

A number of proteins are added to the urine along the urinary tract. These may be secreted, result from normal turnover of urogenital tissue, or be released following tissue injury. Under physiologic circumstances, Tamm-Horsfall mucoprotein is quantitatively the most important one, accounting for about 50% of normal urinary protein [64,125]. Tamm-Horsfall protein is a large glycoprotein with a molecular weight of 28×10^6, but smaller subunits can be found in the urine as well. It has a high content of sialic acid and a very low isoelectric point, which may be functionally important. Tamm-Horsfall protein can be localized by immunomorphologic techniques to the luminal membranes of the cells of the thick ascending loop of Henle, and it is probably synthesized by these cells [80,81]. Tamm-Horsfall protein has been postulated to play an important physiologic role in the very low water permeability of this segment of the nephron [80]. It is a major constituent of urinary casts and has been implicated in the pathophysiology of acute renal failure with tubular obstruction by casts [143]. Extraluminal entrapment of Tamm-Horsfall protein-containing casts, possibly leading to tubulointerstitial injury, has been described in human renal disease [159,213]. In healthy persons the excretion of Tamm-Horsfall protein appears to be fairly constant but may be temporarily increased after exercise [142]. Other conditions in which moderately increased urinary excretion has been described include nephrotic syndrome [125], cystic fibrosis [123], urolithiasis [26], acute renal failure [184], and renal allograft rejection [185].

Minute quantities of other proteins originating from the genitourinary tract can be found in normal urine. These include tubular brush border antigens [182], proteins from accessory sex glands [172], and antigens from the ureter, bladder, and urethra [65]. Because of their very low concentrations, detection of these antigens requires sensitive immunologic assays. Disorders of the genitourinary tract may result in increased excretion of some of these proteins in the urine. Increased quantities of tubular antigens have been demonstrated in urine from patients with various types of tubular injuries [6,86], renal transplant rejection [5,180], and severe glomerulonephritis [4,8,60]. In the latter, the glomerular disease presumably leads to secondary damage to corresponding tubules. Several of the renal antigens released into urine in response to injury are enzymes; lactic dehydrogenase [170], acid phosphatase [183], glutamine oxalacetic transaminase [183], alanine aminopeptidase [155], glutamyl transpeptidase [155], and alkaline phosphatase [155] have been found in urine in increased quantities.

Characterization of Proteinuria
Methods for Quantitation

Semiquantitative methods are usually employed for initial screening of urine samples for proteinuria. Dipsticks, all of which are based on the same principle of "protein error of indicators," are commonly used for their convenience and rapidity. Because the detection of protein is pH-dependent, extremely alkaline urine may show a false positive reading. Detergents may cause false positive results and should therefore be carefully rinsed off the perineum before the urine collection. The dipsticks are more sensitive to albumin than to other proteins, such as gammaglobulins, Bence-Jones protein, or Tamm-Horsfall protein. Their sensitivity is also affected by other qualities of the urine sample, such as specific gravity and presence of chromogens. A 1+ dipstick reading reflects urine protein concentration of at least 20 to 30 mg/dl [3,67]. Other semiquantitative methods include the turbidometric methods, which are based on the principle that proteins are insoluble at an acid pH. Sulfosalicylic acid, trichloracetic acid, and sodium sulfate can be used to precipitate the proteins. Radiographic contrast materials, metabolites of tolbutamide and sulfonamides, high levels of cephalosporins, and penicillin analogues can result in false positive tests.

For more accurate quantitation of urine protein concentration, the Lowry and biuret methods have traditionally been used and have proved adequate for clinical purposes, especially when modified to avoid errors due to the presence of peptides and amino acids. Recently, they have been largely replaced by dye-binding methods. The use of Coomassie brilliant blue has been best documented [27,112,124]. The method offers the advantage of improved precision and sensitivity over the older techniques and is relatively easy and rapid to perform [112,124]. It is not, however, equally sensitive for all proteins [27]. Its sensitivity is therefore dictated by the standard employed; using albumin as a standard, it is best suited for measuring glomerular proteinuria where the bulk of the urinary protein is albumin.

Normal Values

TIMED URINE COLLECTIONS

Because urinary total protein excretion is mainly determined by glomerular filtration and not greatly affected by urine flow rate, protein content in a timed urine collection is considered the gold standard for protein quantitation. A 12- or 24-hour urine collection is most frequently used. A protein excretion rate of less than 150 mg in 24 hours is considered normal in adults [14,186,202]. In children the information is limited, and the published figures for the upper limit of normal vary from 60 mg to 288 mg in 24 hours [131,208]. Only some of the variation can be explained by differences in assay methods. The method of calculating the upper limit is important. Urine protein excretion rate in the normal population does not follow standard distribution but is heavily skewed [76,84,202]; the customary mean + 2 SD is therefore not appropriate as the upper limit unless logarithmic transformation or other normalization of the data is first performed.

A determinant that is often ignored is the size of the child. Because a large portion of the normal urinary protein is filtered through the glomerulus, and the total glomerular filtering area increases as the child grows, there is a cor-

TABLE 21-3. *24-Hour urine protein excretion at different ages*

Age	Protein concentration (range, mg/L)	Protein in 24 hours (mg)	Protein/m² BSA in 24 hours (mg)
Premature 5–30 days	88–845	29 14–60	182 88–377
Full-term	94–455	32 15–68	145 68–309
2–12 months	70–315	38 17–85	109 48–244
2–4 years	45–217	49 20–121	91 37–223
4–10 years	50–223	71 26–194	85 31–234
10–16 years	45–391	83 29–238	63 22–181

BSA, body surface area. Except for protein concentration, the figures are expressed as mean and 95% confidence limits calculated from log transformed data. (Modified from Miltényi M: Urinary protein excretion in healthy children. *Clin Nephrol* 12:216, 1979, with permission)

relation between body size and protein excretion. Protein excretion rate factored by body surface area is therefore a more accurate and physiologic way of measuring proteinuria. Expressed this way, there is little variation between values from different age groups, as shown in Table 21-3. The neonatal period is the exception; infants less than 30 days old excrete relatively higher amounts of protein in the urine, the highest values being observed in the premature group.

A very important factor is diurnal variation of protein excretion. In a typical 24-hour period, most healthy persons excrete protein at higher rates during the day than at night [47,164,202]. This is due to an increased excretion rate induced by upright posture and physical activity [84,164], but some type of circadian rhythm may also be involved [134]. The greater variation in daytime protein excretion results in a much wider range of normal values, as illustrated in Figure 21-5 for albumin excretion in recumbent and supine positions. The wide variation in daytime protein excretion is reflected as a wide range in the total 24-hour urine protein excretion. Because of this, we believe that measurement of 24-hour protein excretion during uncontrolled physical activity and posture does not discriminate between normal and abnormal as well as when timed urine collected at rest is measured.

For quantitative measurement of protein excretion, we use timed 12-hour overnight urine collections with the child at rest. This is particularly helpful in evaluating the significance of unexplained proteinuria, since most children with postural or other benign intermittent proteinuria will have normal excretion rates at night, whereas the excretion rates of those children with proteinuria of renal disease probably vary little from day to night. We use 4 mg/m²/hour or 48 mg/m²/12 hours as the upper limit for normal, except in neonates, in whom the values may be as high as 150 mg/m²/12 hours.

Most of the filtered protein, both in health and glomerular disease, is albumin. Some authors therefore recommend measuring albumin instead of total protein for quantitation of proteinuria. Urinary albumin excretion is a more precise index of glomerular function because the role of proteins originating in the postglomerular urinary tract is eliminated. In early juvenile diabetes mellitus, determination of urinary albumin has become the norm for detecting minor increase in glomerular protein filtration ("microalbuminuria"). Davies et al. [47] measured albumin excretion in healthy schoolchildren using a sensitive ELISA technique. The approximate normal limits from their study are 15 mg/m²/24 hours in boys and 23 mg/m²/24 hours in girls. There was a slight increase in the excretion rate with age, and more than two-thirds of the albumin was excreted during the day.

RANDOM URINE SPECIMENS

Measuring protein concentration in random urine samples is the most common way of checking for proteinuria. Although this is adequate for routine screening, it should be recognized that urine concentration and dilution have a great influence on the measured urine protein concentration. Urine protein concentration of 15 mg/dl (trace on a dipstick) reflects an excretion rate of 3 mg/hour (normal for older children) if the urine flow rate is 20 ml/hour but is equal to 30 mg/hour (definitely abnormal) if the urine flow rate is 200 ml/hour.

To overcome the problem without timed urine collections, the protein concentration can be related to a marker of glomerular filtration, usually creatinine, thus negating the effect of urinary concentration and dilution. The protein-to-creatinine ratio in a random urine specimen has been shown to correlate well with 24-hour protein excretion rate [61,78,186]. Using the Coomassie blue dye–binding method, Houser et al. [78,79] have determined protein-to-creatinine ratios in daytime urine specimens from healthy children. In children older than 2 years, a ratio less than 250 (μg/mg) should be considered normal; a higher limit of 500 (μg/mg) applies to infants from 6 to 24 months of age. Much higher values have been obtained in infants less than 6 months of age, albeit using a different protein assay [96]. Analogously, the urine albumin-to-creatinine ratio has been advocated for the determination of

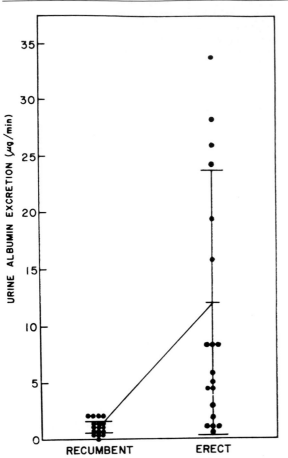

FIG. 21-5. *Urine albumin excretion in healthy nonproteinuric young men in the erect and recumbent postures. Brackets indicate one standard deviation. (From Robinson RR, Glenn WG: Fixed and reproducible orthostatic proteinuria. IV. Urinary albumin excretion by healthy human subjects in the recumbent and upright postures. J Lab Clin Med 64:717, 1964, with permission.)*

glomerular proteinuria. In the study of Davies et al. [47], the approximate upper limit for albumin-to-creatinine ratios (μg/mg) during the day was 31 in boys and 65 in girls; at night it was 15 in both sexes. Apart from variations in methodology, the protein-to-creatinine and albumin-to-creatinine ratios have inherent limitations as an estimate of protein excretion rate. First, creatinine concentration in serum and urine depends on muscle mass; two individuals with identical urine protein excretion rates but different muscle masses therefore do not have identical urine protein-to-creatinine ratios. This is a clinically significant problem only in children with severe nutritional problems. Second, the method has not been validated in children with very low glomerular filtration rates in whom tubular creatinine secretion may be responsible for a large proportion of urine creatinine content. Third, a random urine protein-to-creatinine ratio cannot reflect 12- or 24-hour protein excretion rates in conditions with wide fluctuations in protein excretion rate during the course of the day. Very high ratios may be obtained in children with orthostatic

proteinuria despite normal 24-hour protein excretion. For most clinical situations, however, the protein-to-creatinine ratio is useful and always more informative than urine protein concentration alone in a random urine.

Qualitative Aspects of Proteinuria

COMPOSITION OF NORMAL URINE

Table 21-4 depicts the relative contribution of several proteins to the total urinary protein content. Most proteins are excreted in approximately the same proportions in older children and adults. Transferrin, IgM, IgA, and immunoglobulin light chain excretion has been reported to be significantly lower in children than in adults [76]. In infants, information is only available for a few proteins. The excretion of LMW proteins is generally much higher, suggesting that these are not efficiently reabsorbed by the renal tubules in this age group [96,97,131]. The relative excretion of albumin may also be slightly higher during the first days of life [96].

SELECTIVITY OF PROTEINURIA

Heavy proteinuria can be assumed to be of glomerular origin. Albumin, because of its high plasma concentration, is always the most abundant protein in the urine when glomerular permeability to macromolecules is increased. Comparison of the relative clearances of different plasma proteins has been advocated for identifying the nature of the glomerular damage, based on the concept that more severe injury leads to a higher functional pore size in the glomerular filter and thus to relatively higher clearances of larger molecules. This technique, called protein selectivity, was first described using several intermediate to large (MW 40,000 to 1,300,000) proteins [19,33]. The relative clearances, expressed as a fraction of the clearance of one of the proteins, were plotted against the molecular weights on a double logarithmic scale (Fig. 21-6). The points fell approximately on a straight line, the slope of which was termed the selectivity angle; the steeper the slope, the

TABLE 21-4. *Protein composition of normal urine in children*

	Percentage of total
Proteins from the Urinary Tract	
Tamm-Horsfall protein	50
Large Plasma Proteins	
Albumin	20
IgG (including some fragments)	10
IgA	1
IgM	0.5
α_1-Acid-glycoprotein	2
Transferrin	2
Haptoglobin	0.3
Small Plasma Proteins	
Light chains	7
Lysozyme	0.5
β_2-Microglobulin	0.07

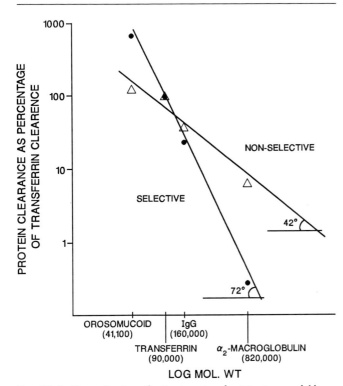

FIG. 21-6. *Determination of urine protein selectivity in two children with nephrotic syndrome. Clearance of each of four proteins is plotted as a percentage of transferrin clearance against the molecular size on a double logarithmic scale. Dots represent results from a 6-year-old child with steroid-responsive nephrotic syndrome (minimal-change disease) and highly selective proteinuria (selectivity angle 72°); triangles represent results from an 8-year-old child with steroid-resistant nephrotic syndrome (focal glomerulosclerosis) and nonselective proteinuria (selectivity angle 42°).*

DIFFERENTIATION BETWEEN GLOMERULAR AND TUBULAR PROTEINURIA

If in doubt whether mild to moderate proteinuria is the result of glomerular or tubular injury, the pattern of proteinuria can be used to distinguish between the two. Because of the predominant effect on the reabsorption of small proteins, disorders with tubular injury are associated with an increased excretion of proteins smaller than albumin (LMW proteinuria). This can be demonstrated by urinary protein electrophoresis, which shows increased intensity of LMW bands [69,209]. More accurately, specific proteins can be quantitatively measured. The ratio of albumin to a LMW protein in urine has been shown to differentiate between glomerular and tubular proteinuria [145]. β_2-Microglobulin (MW 11,800) is the LMW protein most commonly used for this purpose. It is a ubiquitous protein present on cell membranes and involved in cell recognition as part of the major histocompatibility complex. Because of its small size, it is filtered virtually unrestricted through the glomerulus. Plasma levels of β_2-microglobulin are affected not only by changes in glomerular filtration rate, but also by changes in the production rate. Neoplastic, inflammatory, and immunologic disorders resulting in increased turnover of immune cells may increase plasma levels, but this rarely causes practical diagnostic problems. The ratio of albumin to β_2-microglobulin (mg/mg) is approximately 30–200 in normal urine, 1,000–15,000 in glomerular proteinuria, and less than 300 in tubular proteinuria [114,145]. In primary glomerular disease, increased excretion of β_2-microglobulin [151] or an intermediate albumin to β_2-microglobulin ratio [114] indicates secondary tubular involvement.

DIAGNOSIS OF TUBULAR DYSFUNCTION

Even in the absence of quantitative proteinuria, increased excretion of small proteins is a sensitive indicator of proximal tubular injury or dysfunction. β_2-Microglobulin [9,11,43,66,70,72,151,152,200] and lysozyme [13,75], as well as LMW band on urinary electrophoresis [69,132,209], are most commonly employed. Simple determination of urine concentration of a specific LMW protein, e.g., β_2-microglobulin, is often sufficient. Urine β_2-microglobulin concentration should not exceed 0.4 mg/liter after 3 months of age [96,145]. The level may be as high as 4 mg/liter in the normal newborn [96,200]. There appears to be no transport maximum for tubular reabsorption of β_2-microglobulin within the physiologic or pathophysiologic range of filtered load [71,151]; a constant fraction is absorbed by intact proximal tubules. The determination of fractional excretion (ratio of β_2-microglobulin clearance to creatinine clearance) is theoretically superior because it eliminates potential problems due to urine concentration and dilution, low glomerular filtration rates, or high plasma levels. Fractional excretion can be conveniently calculated from simultaneous plasma and urine samples using the standard formula $(U_{\beta 2} \times P_{Cr})/(P_{\beta 2} \times U_{Cr})$. Although the reference values are not firmly established, fractional excretion of less than 12% in the full-term newborn [12,51] and less than 0.4% in the older child [72, Robson AM:

larger the proportion of small proteins and the more selective the proteinuria. Simplified versions of the selectivity test, using the ratios or relative clearances of only two proteins, were later introduced. The only practical use the selectivity measurements gained was for differentiating steroid-responsive nephrotic syndrome from other types of nephrotic syndromes. In children, a selectivity angle of greater than 50° (using five proteins with MW 40,000 to 840,000) [110] or a ratio of IgG (MW 160,000) to transferrin (MW 90,000) clearances of less than 0.2 [32] indicates high selectivity and a probable steroid-responsive condition. The only reported steroid-nonresponsive condition with selective proteinuria is congenital nephrotic syndrome of Finnish type [85]. Because the selectivity principle ignores the role of shape and charge of the protein molecules, it is not surprising that the discriminating power of the test is not absolute; there is considerable overlap between steroid-sensitive and other types of nephrotic syndrome. Because of this limitation, in addition to the requirement for immunologic determinations of plasma and urine protein concentrations, the selectivity indices are not widely used in clinical practice.

unpublished observations] should be considered normal. A clinically significant proximal tubule injury or dysfunction results in a several-fold increase in the fractional excretion and usually poses no problems in interpretation. Table 21-2 lists conditions in which LMW protein excretion may be increased. Usually all LMW protein reabsorption is affected; none of the proteins reflects any specific cause.

Asymptomatic Proteinuria

Proteinuria is the hallmark of many renal diseases. It is particularly prominent in nephrotic syndrome and various nephritides, but low-grade proteinuria may result on occasion from a tubular or lower urinary tract disorder. Proteinuria secondary to an abnormally high plasma concentration of a protein is rare in the pediatric age group. In many children with proteinuria, the type of underlying disorder is obvious from associated signs and symptoms. It is not our purpose to discuss in detail the differential diagnosis of all diseases causing proteinuria, as many of them will be presented in detail in other chapters of this book. Rather, we will focus on asymptomatic proteinuria without a readily identifiable cause, commonly discovered as a chance finding.

Epidemiology

The high prevalence of proteinuria in school-age children and adolescents has been well documented in a number of studies [49,128,153,187,188,204,208]. Figure 21-7 depicts the prevalence of proteinuria obtained from three studies. Obviously, the prevalence figures vary according to the definitions of proteinuria used. It is clear that the proteinuria in most cases is transient or intermittent, probably varying from void to void during the same day. Consequently, the greater the number of urine specimens examined, the greater the chance that proteinuria will be detected in any given individual. It can be safely assumed that at least 10% of children in this age group will at some time have a urine protein concentration in excess of 25 mg/dl [153,204,208]. In our survey of approximately 9,000 children, in which four urine specimens were collected from each child, proteinuria was documented in at least one of the four specimens in 10.7% of the subjects, but protein was found in all four specimens in only 0.1%. When 272 children with confirmed isolated proteinuria were followed with daily morning and evening urine samples collected for one week, none had protein in all specimens, and in 67 children no further proteinuria was recorded during that period [204].

In both sexes, the prevalence is highly dependent on age. As illustrated in Figure 21-7, there is a rise in prevalence from preteen years to adolescence. In boys the rise seems to lag behind that of girls by approximately 3 years; the peak, which in girls is reached at 13 years of age and in boys at 16 years of age, is followed by a decline [208]. In many adolescents, proteinuria disappears by adulthood, as evidenced by the lower prevalence figures in young adults [23,108,189]; yet in others, proteinuria may continue into middle age even in the absence of a demonstrable renal

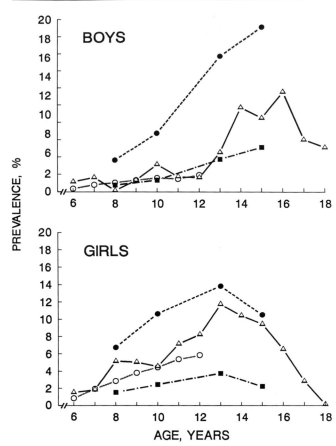

FIG. 21-7. *Prevalence of proteinuria in school-age children in three surveys. Closed circles are derived from data in reference 204, with proteinuria defined as dipstick 1+ or more in at least 1 of 4 specimens; closed squares are also derived from reference 204, with proteinuria defined as dipstick 1+ or more in at least 2 of 4 specimens; triangles are derived from reference 208, with proteinuria defined as dipstick 1+ or more in a single specimen; open circles are derived from reference 49, with proteinuria defined as 10 mg/dl or more in at least 2 of 3 specimens.*

disease [109,192,201]. In infants and preschoolers, proteinuria probably occurs less commonly than in older children [89,153,187,188]. Several studies have shown a higher overall prevalence of proteinuria in girls [49, 187,188,208], whereas other studies revealed no differences between the sexes [89,153,204]. In girls, contamination of urine by vaginal secretions may play a role in the higher figures reported.

Isolated Proteinuria

From both epidemiologic figures and clinical studies [126,203,204], it is clear that the majority of asymptomatic children found to have proteinuria do not have a progressive renal disease. Since any associated symptoms or findings will increase the likelihood that there is a serious underlying disease, it is important to distinguish patients with true isolated proteinuria from those in whom proteinuria is associated with other abnormalities. Isolated proteinuria can be defined as an abnormally high level of protein in the urine of an individual who feels perfectly well and has grown and developed normally, and in whom simple clinical and laboratory evaluation does not reveal additional abnormalities. In some children presenting with "asymptomatic" proteinuria, a careful history may reveal associated, overlooked symptoms and give a clue to the underlying cause; in others, abnormal clinical or laboratory findings become immediately apparent.

Contrary to popular belief, benign isolated proteinuria in adolescents is not always mild or borderline when examined in random urines. We have determined semiquantitative protein concentrations in 443 abnormal urine specimens from 199 schoolchildren with benign proteinuria; although the protein concentrations in the majority of the samples were only moderately elevated, 10% of the samples had a protein concentration of 3+ to 4+ (approximately 300 mg/dl or greater) (Vehaskari VM, unpublished observations).

Isolated proteinuria has been categorized with terms such as "cyclic," "functional," "constant," "persistent," "transient," and "orthostatic" or "postural." Since the categories are not necessarily mutually exclusive and the mechanism of proteinuria in most cases is obscure, they contribute little to our understanding of the proteinuria and should not be viewed as separate specific entities. Recognizing persistent proteinuria, however, has important prognostic implications. Another frequently used prognostic indicator is the orthostatic or postural pattern.

PERSISTENT PROTEINURIA

Persistent proteinuria, defined as proteinuria present at all times, is typical of nephrotic syndrome and many cases of glomerulonephritis. The coexisting abnormalities suggest the underlying cause. Persistent isolated proteinuria is probably overdiagnosed if only random urine specimens collected during office visits are evaluated. A true persistent pattern of isolated proteinuria is rare in children when carefully determined by a large number of urine samples, including samples taken while the child is recumbent [153,204]. As discussed above, in a group of 272 carefully studied schoolchildren with isolated asymptomatic proteinuria, not a single one was found to have persistent proteinuria [204].

Only a few detailed studies on isolated persistent proteinuria in children are available, most reporting on renal biopsy findings. At least three studies failed to find any diagnostic alterations in renal biopsies; the light microscopic picture was normal or showed mild mesangial proliferation [57,126,138,203], and electron microscopy revealed nonspecific ultrastructural changes, including basement membrane irregularities and thickening [138, 203]. In contrast, 10 cases of focal glomerulosclerosis were found in a series of 65 biopsies from children with apparently persistent isolated proteinuria [68], and another study reported several cases of diffuse endocapillary proliferation and/or glomerular sclerosis among 16 biopsies [211]. None of the investigators have reported sufficiently long follow-up periods to indicate the ultimate prognosis for these children. Proteinuria disappeared over the course of several

years in only a minority of these patients; on the other hand, most of them retained normal renal function during the same period [68,126,138,203,211].

Studies on adult patients provide some evidence that the long-term prognosis may not be as favorable as the relatively short observation periods in children would suggest. Morphologic investigations have demonstrated a serious disease in a considerable portion of adult subjects with persistent proteinuria [7,111,135,146,147,189], and some of the subjects have progressed into chronic renal failure [7,109]. It is not clear, however, whether all the patients in these reports had strictly isolated proteinuria.

Protein excretion rate in isolated persistent proteinuria in children may vary from less than 1 g to 6 g or more in 24 hours [126,138,203]. Heavy proteinuria should make one suspect a latent phase of nephrotic syndrome. For example, steroid-responsive minimal-change nephrotic syndrome may be present in some children and even spontaneously remit and relapse long before the appearance of symptoms. We have observed four totally asymptomatic children who had heavy proteinuria with hypoproteinemia for a prolonged period and only minimal changes in renal biopsy; two of them responded to steroid treatment with disappearance of proteinuria and normalization of serum proteins, and the other two continue to excrete large amounts of protein without any change in their clinical status. Such unresponsive cases may represent early stages of focal glomerulosclerosis; the diagnosis may be missed because of sampling error in the renal biopsy, or proteinuria may precede the typical morphologic changes. Isolated persistent proteinuria in a young infant suggests congenital nephrotic syndrome. If proteinuria is mild, severely reduced functioning renal mass, tubular disorders, and, in the younger child, structural abnormalities should be kept in mind as possible causes.

Children with unexplained persistent proteinuria clearly form a heterogeneous group. Until more information and long-term studies are available, the prognosis should be viewed with caution, particularly since unremitting proteinuria per se, irrespective of cause, may lead to progressive glomerular sclerosis [105]. Whether some of these children compose a specific entity with protein leakage associated with an inherent abnormality of the glomerular basement membrane, as has been suggested [126,203], remains hypothetical.

ORTHOSTATIC PROTEINURIA

The best characterized type of isolated proteinuria is orthostatic (postural) proteinuria, which may account for more than 50% of cases of symptomless proteinuria [49,102,165,189,204]. It is defined as an abnormally high protein excretion in upright posture only. Protein excretion must not exceed the normal limits when the subject is recumbent; patients with a proteinuric renal disease may further increase the degree of proteinuria on assuming an upright posture [103]. Some individuals with an otherwise typical orthostatic pattern will, however, continue to have proteinuria for some time after orthostasis [204]. Documenting orthostatic proteinuria is further complicated by the fact that only some of the subjects will have "fixed and reproducible" orthostatic proteinuria, i.e., respond with

proteinuria to every orthostatic challenge; in the rest, upright position will induce proteinuria inconsistently [165]. Thus, *ruling out* orthostatic proteinuria may in some cases be extremely difficult and not practically feasible. Upright posture with exaggerated lordosis is sometimes used to provoke proteinuria. This maneuver has been reported to produce proteinuria in 77% of adolescents [31]; the proteinuria may therefore be a more physiologic phenomenon and should not be equated with orthostatic proteinuria. Proteinuria associated with heavy exercise should also be distinguished from orthostatic proteinuria (see below).

Urine protein concentrations and protein excretion rates can, on occasions, reach very high values in orthostatic proteinuria, or they may be only slightly above the normal limits. Concentrations up to 100 mg/dl and excretion rates up to 400 mg/m²/hour have been measured in 2-hour urine collections [204]. The total protein excretion during a 24-hour period, however, rarely exceeds 1 g in children [204,208]. Most of the increased protein in the urine consists of large plasma proteins, predominantly albumin [164,198]. The excretion of LMW proteins is very little affected [198].

When studied by clearances of inert exogenous macromolecular markers, the permeability of the glomerular filter in individuals with orthostatic proteinuria appears normal [118]; whether this is true at the time of increased protein excretion during upright posture is not known. Urine protein selectivity in orthostatic proteinuria has been reported to be low, as in normal subjects [118,174], in contrast to the high selectivity in minimal-change nephrotic syndrome.

Most authors agree that orthostatic proteinuria is the result of excessive glomerular filtration of protein because of the "glomerular" pattern of urinary proteins, but a leakage of lymph into the urine has also been proposed [113]. Several theories have been suggested to explain the association of upright posture with proteinuria. The most widely held concept is that increased glomerular filtration of plasma proteins is secondary to an altered renal hemodynamic response to orthostasis. Since the forces responsible for macromolecular filtration across the glomerular barrier cannot be directly measured in humans, this remains speculative. Earlier studies in humans [31] and animals [199] suggested that partial obstruction of the renal vein in upright position might be responsible for the proteinuria. This explanation has been recently resurrected when radiographic and ultrasound studies were found to visualize a relative stenosis in renal veins of subjects with orthostatic proteinuria [30,186a]. A recent micropuncture study in rats confirms that renal vein obstruction may lead to significant proteinuria that is mediated mainly by changes in glomerular microcirculation [212].

An argument against hemodynamic factors as the sole cause of orthostatic proteinuria can be based on the following observations: First, the measurable renal hemodynamic changes that occur on assuming an upright position have been reported to be the same in subjects with orthostatic proteinuria and in control subjects [104,166]. Second, urinary albumin excretion in individuals with orthostatic proteinuria is higher than in controls even in recumbency [164]. Despite the statistically significant dif-

ference, however, it is still low enough to be regarded as normal. Third, renal biopsies in both adults [24,165,189] and children [37,203,204] with orthostatic proteinuria have shown subtle structural alterations or immune deposits in a considerable portion. Fourth, in postural proteinuria the increment in protein excretion on assuming upright position may reach values much higher [204] than those achieved by experimental maneuvers [212].

A tentative hypothesis for the pathophysiologic mechanism can be based on the currently available evidence, accounting for both the hemodynamic and morphologic data. Circulating immune complexes are not infrequently formed in humans in response to infections and other events [1]. Most of them are cleared from the circulation by the reticuloendothelial system, but at times the glomerular mesangium participates in the uptake and reabsorption [130]. Trapping of immune complexes in the glomeruli probably occurs commonly without any evidence of renal disease [196]. A transient accumulation of such complexes of low pathogenicity in the glomeruli may cause enough injury to lead to a slightly increased glomerular permeability, as reflected by a mildly increased baseline albumin excretion. Either the *normal* hemodynamic response to orthostasis, as suggested by Robinson [163], an *abnormal* hemodynamic response, or some other functional stress could then play a permissive role, allowing increased protein filtration across the damaged glomerular barrier and resulting in frank proteinuria.

Common clinical impression dictates that children with orthostatic proteinuria have a benign prognosis. A generalization that they have absolutely no increased risk of developing chronic renal disease cannot presently be based on hard facts because of lack of long-term prospective studies in children. The absence of definitive disease entities in renal biopsy material, however, indirectly supports the impression of a benign disorder [203,204]. Additional reassurance can be obtained from data on young adults with orthostatic proteinuria. In a 20-year prospective follow-up of 36 men with fixed and reproducible orthostatic proteinuria, not one subject developed renal impairment or additional signs of kidney disease [192]. Proteinuria was still demonstrable in 17% of the subjects. Retrospective studies with an observation period of up to 50 years have failed to show any increase in renal mortality or morbidity [109,177].

Thus, the available evidence, although not entirely conclusive for children, strongly suggests a uniformly benign prognosis in isolated orthostatic proteinuria. A clear distinction should, however, be made between isolated and nonisolated orthostatic proteinuria. The combination of orthostatic proteinuria and microscopic hematuria, for instance, can be a sign of serious underlying renal disease.

OTHER INTERMITTENT OR TRANSIENT PROTEINURIA

Although persistent proteinuria and orthostatic proteinuria are the two best characterized types of isolated proteinuria, a number of children with proteinuria do not fit either definition [49,204]. Some of them excrete increased amounts of protein in the urine during the day unrelated to posture; others have proteinuria even at night. The protein excretion rate is usually only modestly elevated [204]. Although intermittent proteinuria may occasionally be associated with chronic glomerulonephritis, for instance Berger's disease, as a rule it is accompanied in such cases by hematuria or other signs.

Very few studies have focused on intermittent proteinuria other than orthostatic proteinuria, partly because this is an ill-defined condition and the proteinuria is not reproducible in any consistent manner. Although some early morphologic studies in adults suggested a poor prognosis in some of the cases [135,136], this has not been the general clinical experience, especially in children. A retrospective long-term follow-up study in adults, which did not separate orthostatic and other intermittent proteinurias, reported no increase in mortality in intermittent proteinuria [109]. No similar data are available in children, but the reported benign morphology [204] supports the widely held belief that this condition does not carry any less favorable outlook than does orthostatic proteinuria.

A special category of transient benign proteinuria is the proteinuria associated with physical exercise. A number of vigorous athletic activities, including football [45], long-distance running [149], cross-country skiing [36], and bicycling [148], have been reported to induce proteinuria in adults. In children, bicycling [84] and various organized school sports [79] have been documented to cause an increase in urine protein level. Urine protein excretion rate and protein concentration are only modestly elevated [36,45,79,84,149,150], reaching their peak by 30 minutes after cessation of the exercise [150] and returning to normal by the next day [149]. The increase in protein excretion consists mainly of albumin and other larger plasma proteins, suggesting increased glomerular filtration [36,84, 149], although impaired tubular reabsorption of filtered protein has also been implicated [148,150]. Associated changes in urinary sediment are sometimes noted [36]. The benign nature of exercise-induced proteinuria is obvious. It should be stressed, however, that the published reports deal with strenuous physical exercise; proteinuria associated with usual daily activities or children's play should not be dismissed as exercise proteinuria.

Other factors believed to be associated with transient proteinuria include low ambient temperature [179] and strong emotional stimuli, but these associations are not as well documented. Theoretically, such proteinuria could result from changes in renal hemodynamics, and be mediated by autonomous nervous system or vasoactive substances such as angiotensin II or prostaglandins.

Nonisolated Proteinuria

PROTEINURIA COMBINED WITH OTHER MANIFESTATIONS OF RENAL DISEASE

Associated signs in a child presenting with asymptomatic proteinuria are easily overlooked but, if present, may denote a serious underlying condition. *Hematuria* is the most common and most important of these. Although proteinuria and hematuria may exist as an apparently benign combination, the presence of gross or microscopic hematuria greatly increases the likelihood of underlying disease

[189,204,211]. Almost any renal parenchymal disease may present with the combination of persistent or intermittent proteinuria and hematuria. In addition, low-grade proteinuria may accompany microscopic hematuria in urinary tract infections, malformations, obstruction, stones, and nephrocalcinosis.

Edema may at times be very subtle or elicited by history only. If renal in origin, it reflects either an increase in extracellular volume, as in acute glomerulonephritis, or a decrease in plasma oncotic pressure, as in nephrotic syndrome. We have experience with several children who presented with minimal-change nephrotic syndrome and who by history had a waxing and waning mild edema over several months to two years before the onset of frank symptoms.

High blood pressure and proteinuria typically indicate the presence of some type of glomerulonephritis, although hematuria is usually present as well. Hyperreninemia as the cause for both hypertension and proteinuria is much less common. Rarely, proteinuria is the presenting sign of *chronic renal failure*. Other manifestations, which are not always obvious, include fatigue, growth failure, osteodystrophy, and an inability to concentrate and dilute urine maximally. *Primary tubular disorders* do not usually present as symptomless proteinuria, but mild proteinuria of tubular pattern may coexist with other signs of tubular dysfunction (see Table 21-2).

PROTEINURIA IN NON-RENAL DISEASE

Although not truly asymptomatic, transient proteinuria occurring during an intercurrent non-renal illness may cause diagnostic problems. Mild to moderate proteinuria has been described in adults and children with various acute illnesses, including infections with and without fever [77,88,119,162,190] and seizures [119,160]. Many of these patients have been reported to have proteinuria of the tubular type, with high excretion of LMW proteins, and some kind of tubular injury has been implicated [77,88,162]. An alternative explanation is that many of these conditions lead to immune complex formation with deposition in glomeruli (and perhaps tubules), resulting in glomerular injury and proteinuria [88,190].

The excretion of albumin may be mildly increased in congestive heart failure [35,160]. Interestingly, the fractional excretion of albumin is increased to a greater extent than that of neutral dextran of similar size [35]. Increased protein excretion has also been reported in congenital heart disease without congestive failure [87,191]. Urinary protein excretion has been shown to be increased for several days after major surgery [117].

Evaluation for Asymptomatic Proteinuria

Because of the high prevalence of proteinuria, many children and adolescents are found to be proteinuric on routine health examinations or during the course of unrelated evaluations. It is clear that not all of this vast number of children should be submitted to extensive testing; the evaluation should be proportional to the estimated risk of serious renal disease. Fortunately, in most cases any serious

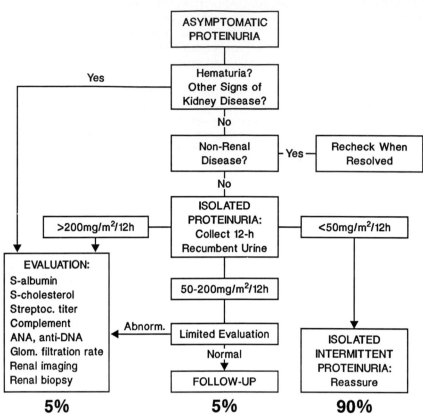

FIG. 21-8. *Algorithm for evaluating a child with asymptomatic proteinuria. Limited evaluation includes BUN, creatinine, and complement levels; antistreptococcal titer; lupus serologies in selected cases; renal imaging; and an index of tubular proteinuria. See text for details. Following the algorithm, 90% of children with asymptomatic proteinuria will require only one visit for the evaluation and can be reassured of a good prognosis.*

condition can be ruled out by a relatively simple set of studies. We believe that for most children with asymptomatic proteinuria, a good prognosis can be established by meeting two criteria: (1) that proteinuria is isolated and (2) that proteinuria is intermittent. The great majority of children with asymptomatic proteinuria fulfill these criteria [204,205]. The *isolated nature of proteinuria* is confirmed when other abnormalities are excluded by thorough history and physical examination and by excluding the presence of hematuria and other sediment abnormalities in a concentrated urine specimen. The *intermittency of proteinuria* can be demonstrated by testing a number of urine samples, including first morning urine samples, for protein. Alternatively, a 12-hour overnight urine sample at rest can be collected. If proteinuria is persistent, it usually results in protein excretion of more than 200 mg/m²/12 hours [126,203], while in intermittent proteinuria the excretion rate usually is much lower [204]. Intermittent proteinuria, whether orthostatic or not, probably carries no increased risk of serious renal disease. Since orthostatic proteinuria is better documented than other types of intermittent proteinuria, however, some physicians feel more comfortable

in reassuring the family if proteinuria can be shown to be associated with upright posture only.

The algorithm in Figure 21-8 presents a step-by-step approach to the investigation of a child found to have proteinuria on routine examination. A child in whom additional symptoms or signs of renal disease are immediately detected, or one who is found to have hematuria on urine sediment examination, usually requires thorough evaluation. The presence of a non-renal illness that might cause proteinuria, such as acute infection, requires rechecking the urine when the child has recovered. In the remaining group, proteinuria can be characterized by measuring protein excretion in a 12-hour urine sample collected with the child recumbent. (We prefer the timed urine collection to having multiple urine samples checked by dipstick at home because it gives a quantitative measurement and eliminates the effect of urine concentration and dilution as well as problems due to interpretation of the dipstick color change by unexperienced readers.) Depending on the circumstances, some physicians may want to determine BUN or serum creatinine concentration at the initial visit as well. Except for the urine collection, which can be done the same evening and returned the next morning, up to this point the evaluation takes place during a single visit; hence the frustrations and noncompliance often associated with prolonged evaluation with multiple visits can be avoided. If the initial evaluation is normal, including a normal protein excretion in the 12-hour urine sample taken with the child at rest (<50 mg/m²/12 hours), the child and the family can be reassured of the benign nature of the proteinuria. The great majority of proteinuric children, including those with orthostatic proteinuria, will fall into this category of isolated intermittent proteinuria. We do not believe a continuing follow-up, apart from normal health care visits, is indicated for this large number of children (as many as 10% of the adolescent population).

If analysis of the 12-hour urine collection shows abnormal protein excretion, suggesting persistent proteinuria, further evaluation at the subspecialty level is indicated (see Fig. 21-8). With moderate to heavy proteinuria at rest (> 200 mg/m²/12 hours), the evaluation includes determination of serum protein or albumin, serum cholesterol, complement levels, and streptococcal antibody titer, as well as renal imaging. In selected cases, lupus serologies, plasma renin activity, and more detailed characterization of urinary proteins for tubular proteinuria are warranted. Ultimately, renal biopsy is necessary in patients with glomerular proteinuria unless minimal-change nephrotic syndrome or acute postinfectious glomerulonephritis is strongly suspected.

Few proteinuric children will have borderline to mild proteinuria in the 12-hour urine collection at rest (50 to 200 mg/m²/12 hours). The prognostic significance of this finding is uncertain, but the yield of renal biopsy is small if no additional findings are present. A more limited evaluation, excluding the albumin and cholesterol levels and renal biopsy, is therefore appropriate. Because this degree of proteinuria may result from tubular dysfunction, an index of tubular proteinuria should be included. If the limited evaluation is normal, follow-up visits at infrequent intervals as long as the proteinuria continues are indicated to determine the ultimate prognosis.

References

1. Abuelo JG, Druet P: Circulating immune complexes in the general hospital population and in patients who have renal disease. Am J Pathol 73:547, 1980.
2. Alt JM, Jaenig H, Schurek HJ, et al: Study of renal protein excretion in chronic pyelonephritis. Contrib Nephrol 16:37, 1979.
3. Altman KA, Stellate R: Variation of protein content of urine in a 24-hour period. Clin Chem 9:63, 1963.
4. Antoine B, Neveu T: Pathological urinary excretion of tissue macromolecules (histuria). J Lab Clin Med 71:101, 1968.
5. Antoine B, Neveu T, Leski M, et al: Histuria during renal transplantation. Transplantation 8:110, 1969.
6. Antoine B, Patte D, Gourdin MF: Protein originating in the kidney in the urine of patients with hypokalemia. Am J Clin Pathol 54:53, 1970.
7. Antoine B, Symvoulidis A, Dardenne M: La stabilité évolutive des étas de protéinurie permanente isolée. Nephron 6:526, 1969.
8. Antoine B, Ward PD: Histuria and fibrinuria in cases of systemic lupus erythematosus. Clin Exp Immunol 6:153, 1970.
9. Aperia A, Broberger O: Beta-2-microglobulin, an indicator of renal tubular maturation and dysfunction in the newborn. Acta Paediatr Scand 68:669, 1979.
10. Aperia A, Broberger O, Elinder G, et al: Postnatal development of renal function in pre-term and full-term infants. Acta Paediatr Scand 70:183, 1981.
11. Assadi FK, Chow-Tung E: Renal handling of Beta-2-microglobulin in neonates treated with gentamicin. Nephron 49:114, 1988.
12. Assadi FK, John EG, Justice P, et al: Beta-2-microglobulin clearance in neonates: Index of tubular maturation. Kidney Int 28:153, 1985.
13. Barratt TM, Crawford R: Lysozyme excretion as a measure of renal tubular dysfunction in children. Clin Sci 39:457, 1970.
14. Berggård, I: Plasma proteins in normal human urine. In Manuel Y, Revillard JP, Betuel H (eds): Protein in Normal and Pathological Urine. Basel, S Karger, 1970, p 7.
15. Bertolatus JA, Abuyousef M, Hunsicker LG: Glomerular sieving of high molecular weight proteins in proteinuric rats. Kidney Int 31:1257, 1987.
16. Bertolatus JA, Foster SJ, Hunsicker LG: Stainable glomerular basement membrane polyanions and renal hemodynamics during hexadimethrine-induced proteinuria. J Lab Clin Med 103:632, 1984.
17. Bertolatus JA, Hunsicker LG: Glomerular sieving of anionic and neutral bovine albumins in proteinuric rats. Kidney Int 28:467, 1985.
18. Bienenstock J, Poortmans J: Renal clearance of 15 plasma proteins in renal disease. J Lab Clin Med 75:297, 1970.
19. Blainey JD, Brewer DB, Hardwicke J, et al: The nephrotic syndrome. Q J Med 29:235, 1960.
20. Blau EB, Haas JE: Glomerular sialic acid and proteinuria in human renal disease. Lab Invest 28:477, 1973.
21. Bohrer MP, Baylis C, Humes HD, et al: Permselectivity of the glomerular capillary wall: Facilitated filtration of circulating polycations. J Clin Invest 61:72, 1978.
22. Bohrer MP, Deen WM, Robertson CR, et al: Mechanism of angiotensin II-induced proteinuria in the rat. Am J Physiol 233:F13, 1977.
23. von Bonsdorff M, Koskenvuo K, Salmi HA, et al: Prevalence and causes of proteinuria in 20-year-old Finnish men. Scand J Urol Nephrol 15:285, 1981.
24. von Bonsdorff M, Törnroth T, Pasternack A: Renal biopsy findings in orthostatic proteinuria. Acta Pathol Microbiol Immunol Scand [A], 90:11, 1982.
25. Bourdeau JE, Carone FA: Contraluminal serum albumin uptake in isolated perfused renal tubules. Am J Physiol 224:399, 1973.
26. Boyce WH: Proteinuria in kidney calculous disease. In Manuel Y, Revillard JP, Betuel H (eds): Protein in Normal and Pathological Urine. Basel, S. Karger, 1970, p 235.
27. Bradford MM: A rapid and sensitive method for the quantitation of microgram quantities of protein utilizing the principle of protein-dye binding. Anal Biochem 72:248, 1976.
28. Brenner BM, Hostetter TH, Humes HD: Glomerular permselectivity: Barrier function based on discrimination of molecular size and charge. Am J Physiol 234:F455, 1978.
29. Bridges CR, Meyrs BD, Brenner BM, et al: Glomerular charge alterations in human minimal change nephropathy. Kidney Int 22:677, 1982.
30. Buchanec J, Kliment J, Javorka K, et al: X-ray changes in

the kidneys of children with orthostatic proteinuria. *Int Urol Nephrol* 15:3, 1983.

31. Bull GM: Postural proteinuria. *Clin Sci* 75:77, 1948.

32. Cameron JS, Blandford G: The simple assessment of selectivity in heavy proteinuria. *Lancet* 2:242, 1966.

33. Cameron JS, White RHR: Selectivity of proteinuria in children with the nephrotic syndrome. *Lancet* 1:463, 1965.

34. Carone FA, von Haam EVH: Micropuncture study of protein excretion in normal and proteinuric rats. *Clin Res* 13:302, 1965.

35. Carrie BJ, Hilberman M, Schroeder JS, et al: Albuminuria and the permselective properties of the glomerulus in cardiac failure. *Kidney Int* 17:507, 1980.

36. Castenfors J, Mossfeldt F, Piscator M: Effect of prolonged heavy exercise on renal function and urinary protein excretion. *Acta Physiol Scand* 70:194, 1967.

37. Caulfield JP, Farquhar MG: The permeability of glomerular capillaries to graded dextrans. *J Cell Biol* 63:883, 1974.

38. Chang RLS, Deen WM, Robertson CR, et al: Permselectivity of the glomerular capillary wall. III. Restricted transport of polyanions. *Kidney Int* 8:212, 1975.

39. Chang RLS, Robertson CR, Deen WM, et al: Permselectivity of the glomerular capillary wall to macromolecules. I. Theoretical considerations. *Biophys J* 15:861, 1975.

40. Christensen EI, Carone FA, Rennke HG: Effect of molecular charge on endocytic uptake of ferritin in renal proximal tubule cells. *Lab Invest* 44:351, 1981.

41. Christensen EI, Maunsbach AB: Intralysosomal digestion of lysozyme in renal proximal tubule cells. *Kidney Int* 6:396, 1974.

42. Christensen EI: Rapid protein uptake and digestion in proximal tubule lysosomes. *Kidney Int* 10:301, 1976.

43. Cole JW, Portman RJ, Lim Y, et al: Urinary β_2-microglobulin in full-term newborns: Evidence for proximal tubular dysfunction in infants with meconium-stained amniotic fluid. *Pediatrics* 76:958, 1985.

44. Courtney MA, Sawin LL, Weiss DD: Renal tubular protein absorption in the rat. *J Clin Invest* 49:1, 1970.

45. Coye RD, Rosandich RR: Proteinuria during the 24-hour period following exercise. *J Appl Physiol* 15:592, 1960.

46. Dahlquist G, Aperia A, Broberger O, et al: Renal function in relation to metabolic control in children with diabetes of different duration. *Acta Paediatr Scand* 72:903, 1983.

47. Davies AG, Postlethwaite RJ, Price DA, et al: Urinary albumin excretion in school children. *Arch Dis Child* 59:625, 1984.

48. Dirks JH, Clapp JR, Berliner R: The protein concentration in the proximal tubule of the dog. *J Clin Invest* 43:916, 1964.

49. Dodge WF, West EF, Smith EH, et al: Proteinuria and hematuria in schoolchildren. *J Pediatr* 88:327, 1976.

50. Eisenbach GM, van Liew JB, Boylan JW: Effect of angiotensin on the filtration of protein in the rat kidney: A micropuncture study. *Kidney Int* 8:80, 1975.

51. Engle WD, Arant BS Jr: Renal handling of beta-2-microglobulin in the human neonate. *Kidney Int* 24:358, 1983.

52. Evrin PE, Wibell L: The serum levels and urinary excretion of β_2-microglobulin in apparently healthy subjects. *Scand J Clin Lab Invest* 29:69, 1972.

53. Farquhar MG: Structure and function in glomerular capillaries. Role of basement membrane in glomerular filtration. *In* Kefalides N (ed): *Biology and Chemistry of Basement Membranes*. New York, Academic Press, 1978, p 43.

54. Farquhar MG, Courtoy PJ, Lemkin MC, et al: Current knowledge of the functional architecture of the glomerular basement membrane. *In* Kuehn K, Schoene H, Timpl R (eds): *New Trends in Basement Membrane Research*. New York, Raven Press, 1982, p 9.

55. Farquhar MG, Palade GE: Glomerular permeability. II. Ferritin transfer across the glomerular capillary wall in nephrotic rats. *J Exp Med* 114:699, 1961.

56. Farquhar MG, Wissig SL, Palade GE: Glomerular permeability. I. Ferritin transfer across the normal glomerular capillary wall. *J Exp Med* 113:47, 1961.

57. Gaillard L, Salle B, Manuel Y, et al: Ponction biopsie rénale et électrophoreses des protéines urinaires dans la classification des protéinuries apparemment isolées de l'enfant. *Pediatrie* 25:703, 1970.

58. Geary DF, Dillon MJ, Gammon K, et al: Tubular proteinuria in children without other defects of renal function. *Nephron* 40:329, 1985.

59. Gibb DM, Tomlinson PA, Dalton NR, et al: Renal tubular proteinuria and microalbuminuria in diabetic patients. *Arch Dis Child* 64:129, 1989.

60. Gillman G: Urinary proteins: The appearance of kidney protein in the urine of some cases of severe chronic glomerular nephritis. *J Urol* 34:727, 1935.

61. Ginsberg JM, Chang BS, Matarese RA, et al: Use of single voided urine samples to estimate quantitative proteinuria. *N Engl J Med* 309:1543, 1983.

62. Gitlin D, Janeway CA, Farr LE: Studies on the metabolism of plasma proteins in the nephrotic syndrome. I. Albumin, gammaglobulin, and iron-binding globulin. *J Clin Invest* 35:44, 1956.

63. Graham RC, Karnovsky MJ: Glomerular permeability: Ultrastructural cytochemical studies using peroxidases as protein tracers. *J Exp Med* 124:1123, 1966.

64. Grant AM, Baker LRI, Neuberger A: Urinary Tamm-Horsfall glycoprotein in certain kidney diseases and its content in renal and bladder calculi. *Clin Sci* 44:377, 1973.

65. Grant GH: The proteins of normal urine. II. From the urinary tract. *J Clin Pathol* 12:510, 1959.

66. Gutteberg TJ, Strømme P, Saebø-Larsen J, et al: Unilateral vesicoureteral reflux in children. *Eur Urol* 13:390, 1987.

67. Guyre WL: Comparison of several methods for semiquantitative determination of urinary protein. *Clin Chem* 23:876, 1977.

68. Habib R, Loirat C: The major syndromes. Proteinuria. *In* Royer P, Habib R, Mathieu M, et al (eds): *Pediatric Nephrology*. Philadelphia, WB Saunders, 1974, p 247.

69. Hall CL, Hardwicke J: Low molecular weight proteinuria. *Annu Rev Med* 30:199, 1979.

70. Hall PW: β_2-Microglobulin in the differential diagnosis of renal disorders. *In* Anderstem A (ed): β_2-*Microglobulin in Renal Diseases*. Uppsala, Sweden, Pharmacia Diagnostics AB, 1979, p 39.

71. Hall PW, Chung-Park M, Vacca CV, et al: The renal handling of β_2-microglobulin in the dog. *Kidney Int* 22:156, 1982.

72. Hall PW III, Ricanati ES: Renal handling of beta-2-microglobulin in renal disorders; with special reference to hepatorenal syndrome. *Nephron* 27:62, 1981.

73. Hardwicke J, Squire JR: The relationship between plasma albumin concentration and protein excretion in patients with proteinuria. *Clin Sci* 14:509, 1955.

74. Harrison JF, Blainey JD: Low molecular weight proteinuria in chronic renal disease. *Clin Sci* 33:381, 1967.

75. Harrison JF, Lunt GS, Scott P, et al: Urinary lysozyme, ribonuclease and low molecular weight protein in renal disease. *Lancet* 1:371, 1968.

76. Hemmingsen L, Skaarup P: The 24-hour excretion of plasma proteins in the urine of apparently healthy subjects. *Scand J Clin Lab Invest* 35:347, 1975.

77. Hemmingsen L, Skaarup P: Urinary excretion of ten plasma proteins in patients with febrile diseases. *Acta Med Scand* 201:359, 1977.

78. Houser M: Assessment of proteinuria using random urine samples. *J Pediatr* 104:845, 1984.

79. Houser MT, Jahn MF, Kobayashi A, et al: Assessment of urinary protein excretion in the adolescent: Effect of body position and exercise. *J Pediatr* 109:556, 1986.

80. Hoyer JR, Seiler MW: Pathophysiology of Tamm-Horsfall protein. *Kidney Int* 16:279, 1979.

81. Hoyer JR, Sissons S, Vernier RL: Tamm-Horsfall glycoprotein; ultrastructural immunoperoxidase localization in rat kidney. *Lab Invest* 41:168, 1979.

82. Hruska KA, Kopelman R, Rutherford WE, et al: Metabolism of immunoreactive parathyroid hormone in the dog. *J Clin Invest* 56:39, 1975.

83. Hruska KA, Martin K, Mennes P, et al: Degradation of parathyroid hormone and fragment production by the isolated perfused dog kidney. *J Clin Invest* 60:501, 1977.

84. Huttunen NP, Käär ML, Pietilainen M, et al: Exercise-induced proteinuria in children and adolescents. *Scand J Clin Lab Invest* 41:583, 1981.

85. Huttunen NP, Savilahti E, Rapola J: Selectivity of proteinuria in congenital nephrotic syndrome of Finnish type. *Kidney Int* 8:255, 1975.

86. Iesato K, Wakashin M, Wakashin Y, et al: Renal tubular dysfunction in Minamata disease: Detection of renal tubular antigen and beta-2-microglobulin in the urine. *Ann Intern Med* 86:731, 1977.

87. Ingelfinger JR, Kissane JM, Robson AM: Glomerulomegaly in a patient with cyanotic congenital heart disease. *Am J Dis Child* 120:69, 1970.

88. Jensen H, Henriksen K: Proteinuria in non-renal infectious diseases. *Acta Med Scand* 196:75, 1974.

89. Johnson A, Heap GJ, Hurley BP: A survey of bacteriuria, proteinuria and glycosuria in five-year-old schoolchildren in Canberra. *Med J Aust* 2:122, 1974.

90. Johnson V, Maack T: Renal extraction, filtration, absorption, and catabolism of growth hormone. *Am J Physiol* 233:F185, 1977.

91. Jones DB: Mucosubstances of the glomerulus. *Lab Invest* 21:119, 1969.

92. Jørgensen F: *The Ultrastructure of the Normal Human Glomerulus.* Copenhagen, Ejnar Munksgaard, 1966.

93. Kanwar YS, Farquhar MG: Anionic sites in the glomerular basement membrane. In vivo and in vitro localization to the laminae rarae by cationic probes. *J Cell Biol* 81:137, 1979.

94. Kanwar YS, Farquhar MG: Isolation of glycosaminoglycans (heparan sulfate) from glomerular basement membranes. *Proc Natl Acad Sci USA* 76:4493, 1979.

95. Kanwar YS, Linker A, Farquhar MG: Increased permeability of the glomerular basement membrane to ferritin after removal of glycosaminoglycans (heparan sulfate) by enzyme digestion. *J Cell Biol* 86:688, 1980.

96. Karlsson FA, Hardell L-I, Hellsing K: A prospective study of urinary proteins in early infancy. *Acta Paediatr Scand* 68:663, 1979.

97. Karlsson FA, Hellsing K: Urinary protein excretion in early infancy. *J Pediatr* 89:89, 1976.

98. Katz AI, Rubenstein AH: Metabolism of proinsulin, insulin, and C-peptide in the rat. *J Clin Invest* 52:1113, 1973.

99. Katz J, Bonorris G, Sellers AL: Albumin metabolism in aminonucleoside nephrotic rats. *J Lab Clin Med* 62:910, 1963.

100. Katz J, Rosenfeld S, Sellers AL: Role of the kidney in plasma albumin catabolism. *Am J Physiol* 198:814, 1960.

101. Kau ST, Maack T: Transport and catabolism of parathyroid hormone in isolated rat kidney. *Am J Physiol* 233:F445, 1977.

102. King SE: Patterns of protein excretion by the kidneys. *Ann Intern Med* 42:296, 1955.

103. King SE: Postural adjustments and protein excretion by the kidney in renal disease. *Ann Intern Med* 46:360, 1957.

104. King SE, Baldwin DS: Renal hemodynamics during erect lordosis in normal man and subjects with orthostatic proteinuria. *Proc Soc Exp Biol Med* 86:634, 1954.

105. Klahr S, Schreiner G, Ichikawa I: The progression of renal disease. *N Engl J Med* 318:1657, 1988.

106. Latta H, Johnston WH, Stanley TM: Sialoglycoproteins and filtration barriers in the glomerular capillary wall. *J Ultrastruct Res* 51:354, 1975.

107. Leber PD, Marsh DJ: Micropuncture study of concentration and fate of albumin in rat nephron. *Am J Physiol* 219:358, 1970.

108. Leonard CD, Dempsey JG, Hall RD, et al: Proteinuria screening and kidney disease questionnaire in an industrial population. *Industrial Med Surg* 42:27, 1973.

109. Levitt JI: The prognostic significance of proteinuria in young college students. *Ann Intern Med* 66:685, 1967.

110. Lines DR: Selectivity of proteinuria in childhood nephrotic syndrome. *Arch Dis Child* 44:461, 1969.

111. Lornoy W, Beaufils H, Legrain M: Interet de la biopsie renale dans l'etude des proteinuries isolees ou associees a une hypertension. *Acta Clin Belg* 29:41, 1974.

112. Lott JA, Stephan VA, Pritchard KA Jr: Evaluation of the Coomassie Brilliant Blue G-250 method for urinary protein. *Clin Chem* 29:1946, 1983.

113. Löwgren E: Studies on benign proteinuria. *Acta Med Scand* (Suppl)300:151, 1955.

114. Lubega J: β_2 Microglobulin and analytical characterization of proteinuria. *Med Lab Sci* 39:129, 138, 1982.

115. Maack T: Renal handling of low molecular weight proteins. *Am J Med* 58:57, 1975.

116. Maack T, Johnson V, Kau ST, et al: Renal filtration, transport, and metabolism of low-molecular-weight proteins: A review. *Kidney Int* 16:251, 1979.

117. Macbeth WAAG, Pope GR: Effect of abdominal operation upon protein excretion in man. *Lancet* 1:215, 1968.

118. MacLean PR, Petrie JJB, Robson JS: Glomerular permeability to high molecular weight dextrans in acute ischaemic renal failure and postural proteinuria. *Clin Sci* 38:93, 1970.

119. Marks MI, McLaine PN, Drummond KN: Proteinuria in children with febrile illnesses. *Arch Dis Child* 45:250, 1970.

120. Martin GR, Rohrbach DH, Terranova VP, et al: Structure, function, and pathology of basement membranes. In Wagner BM, Fleischmajer R, Kaufman N (eds): *Connective Tissue Diseases.* Baltimore, Williams & Wilkins, 1983, p 16.

121. Martin TJ, Melick RA, DeLuise M: The effect of nephrectomy on the metabolism of labelled parathyroid hormone. *Clin Sci* 37:137, 1969.

122. Maunsbach AB: Absorption of I^{125}-labeled homologous albumin by rat kidney proximal tubule cells. *J Ultrastruct Res* 15:197, 1966.

123. Maxfield M, Wolins W: A molecular abnormality of urinary mucoprotein in cystic fibrosis of the pancreas. *J Clin Invest* 41:455, 1962.

124. McElderry LA, Tarbit IF, Cassells-Smith AJ: Six methods for urinary protein compared. *Clin Chem* 28:356, 1982.

125. McKenzie JK, Patel R, McQueen EG: The excretion rate of Tamm-Horsfall urinary mucoprotein in normals and in patients with renal disease. *Aust Ann Med* 13:32, 1964.

126. McLaine PN, Drummond KN: Benign persistent symptomatic proteinuria in childhood. *Pediatrics* 46:548, 1970.

127. McLaine PN, Marks MI, Baliah T, et al: Hyperproteinemic proteinuria induced by plasma infusion. *Pediatr Res* 3:597, 1969.

128. Meadow SR, White RHR, Johnston NM: Prevalence of

symptomless urinary tract disease in Birmingham school-children. *Br Med J* 3:81, 1969.

129. Mengoli C, Lechi A, Arosio E, et al: Contribution of four markers of tubular proteinuria in detecting upper urinary tract infections. *Nephron* 32:234, 1982.

130. Michael AF, Keane WF, Raij L, et al: The glomerular mesangium. *Kidney Int* 17:141, 1980.

131. Miltényi M: Urinary protein excretion in healthy children. *Clin Nephrol* 12:216, 1979.

132. Miltényi M, Pohlandt F, Boka G, et al: Tubular proteinuria after perinatal hypoxia. *Acta Paediatr Scand* 70:399, 1981.

133. Mohos SC, Skoza L: Glomerular sialoprotein. *Science* 164:1519, 1969.

134. Montagna G, Buzio C, Calderini C, et al: Relationship of proteinuria and albuminuria to posture and to urine collection period. *Nephron* 35:143, 1983.

135. Morel-Maroger L, Leoroux-Robert C, Richet G: Renal histology in 30 cases of isolated proteinuria. *Isr J Med Sci* 3:98, 1967.

136. Muth RG: Asymptomatic mild intermittent proteinuria. *Arch Intern Med* 115:569, 1965.

137. Nielsen JT, Christensen EI: Basolateral endocytosis of protein in isolated perfused proximal tubules. *Kidney Int* 27:39, 1985.

138. Okada T, Okawa K, Wada H, et al: Symptomless persistent proteinuria in childhood. *Acta Med Biol* 24:1, 1976.

139. Oken DE, Flamenbaum W: Micropuncture studies of proximal tubule albumin concentration in normal and nephrotic rats. *J Clin Invest* 50:1498, 1971.

140. Oken DE, Kirschbaum BB, Landwehr DM: Micropuncture studies of the mechanism of normal and pathologic albuminuria. *Contrib Nephrol* 24:1, 1981.

141. Park CH, Maack T: Albumin absorption and catabolism by isolated perfused proximal convoluted tubules of the rabbit. *J Clin Invest* 73:767, 1984.

142. Patel R: Urinary casts in exercise. *Aust Ann Med* 13:170, 1964.

143. Patel R, McKenzie JL, McQueen EG: Tamm-Horsfall urinary mucoprotein and tubular obstruction by casts in acute renal failure. *Lancet* 1:457, 1964.

144. Peterson DR, Oparil S, Flouret G, et al: Handling of angiotensin II and oxytocin by renal tubular segments perfused in vitro. *Am J Physiol* 232:F319, 1977.

145. Peterson PA, Evrin P-E, Berggård I: Differentiation of glomerular, tubular, and normal proteinuria: Determinations of urinary excretion of β_2-microglobulin, albumin, and total protein. *J Clin Invest* 48:1189, 1969.

146. Phillippi PJ, Reynolds CJ, Yamauchi H, et al: Persistent proteinuria in asymptomatic individuals: Renal biopsy studies in 50 patients. *Milit Med* 131:1311, 1966.

147. Pollak VE, Pirani CL, Muehrcke RC, et al: Asymptomatic persistent proteinuria: Studies by renal biopsies. *Guy's Hosp Rep* 107:353, 1958.

148. Poortmans JR, Brauman H, Staroukine M, et al: Indirect evidence of glomerular/tubular mixed-type postexercise proteinuria in healthy humans. *Am J Physiol* 254:F277, 1988.

149. Poortmans JR, Haralambie G: Biochemical changes in a 100 km run: Proteins in serum and urine. *Eur J Appl Physiol* 40:245, 1979.

150. Poortmans JR, Vancalck B: Renal glomerular and tubular impairment during strenuous exercise in young women. *Eur J Clin Invest* 8:175, 1978.

151. Portman RJ, Kissane JM, Robson AM: The use of β_2 microglobulin to diagnose tubular injury in pediatric renal disease. *Kidney Int* 30:91, 1986.

152. Prischl F, Gremmel F, Schwabe J, et al: Beta-2-microglobulin for differentiation between cyclosporin A nephrotox-

icity and graft rejection in renal transplant recipients. *Nephron* 51:330, 1989.

153. Randolph MF, Greenfield M: Proteinuria. *Am J Dis Child* 114:631, 1967.

154. Reeves WH, Kanwar YS, Farquhar MG: Assembly of the glomerular filtration surface. Differentiation of anionic sites in glomerular capillaries of newborn rat kidney. *J Cell Biol* 85:735, 1980.

155. Reitinger W, Mondorf AW, Scherberich JE, et al: Das Auftreten tubularer Zellmembranantigene im Harn bei akuter und chronischer Glomerulonephritis. *Verh Dtsch Ges Inn Med* 80:771, 1974.

156. Rennke HG, Cotran RS, Venkatachalam MA: Role of molecular charge in glomerular permeability: Tracer studies with cationized ferritins. *J Cell Biol* 67:638, 1975.

157. Rennke HG, Patel Y, Venkatachalam MA: Glomerular filtration of proteins: Clearance of anionic, neutral, and cationic horseradish peroxidase in the rat. *Kidney Int* 13:324, 1978.

158. Rennke HG, Venkatachalam MA: Glomerular permeability: In vivo tracer studies with polyanionic and polycationic ferritins. *Kidney Int* 11:44, 1977.

159. Resnick JL, Sissons S, Vernier RL: Tamm-Horsfall protein: Abnormal localization in renal disease. *Lab Invest* 38:550, 1978.

160. Reuben DB, Wachtel TJ, Brown PC, et al: Transient proteinuria in emergency medical admissions. *N Engl J Med* 306:1031, 1982.

161. Revillard JP, Manuel Y, Francois R, et al: Renal diseases associated with tubular proteinuria. *In* Manuel Y, Revillard JP, Betuel H (eds): *Proteins in Normal and Pathological Urine*. Basel, S Karger, 1970, p 209.

162. Richmond JM, Sibbald WJ, Linton AM, et al: Patterns of urinary protein excretion in patients with sepsis. *Nephron* 31:219, 1982.

163. Robinson RR: Isolated proteinuria. *Contrib Nephrol* 24:53, 1981.

164. Robinson RR, Glenn WG: Fixed and reproducible orthostatic proteinuria. IV. Urinary albumin excretion by healthy human subjects in the recumbent and upright postures. *Lab Clin Med* 64:717, 1964.

165. Robinson RR, Glover SN, Phillippi PJ, et al: Fixed and reproducible orthostatic proteinuria. I. Light microscopic studies of the kidney. *Am J Pathol* 39:291, 1961.

166. Robinson RR, Lecocq FR, Phillippi PJ, et al: Fixed and reproducible orthostatic proteinuria. III. Effect of induced renal hemodynamic alterations upon urinary protein excretion. *J Clin Invest* 42:100, 1963.

167. Robson AM, Giangiacomo J, Kienstra RA, et al: Normal glomerular permeability and its modification by minimal change nephrotic syndrome. *J Clin Invest* 54:1190, 1974.

168. Robson AM, Mor J, Root ER, et al: Mechanism of proteinuria in nonglomerular renal disease. *Kidney Int* 16:416, 1979.

169. Rodewald R, Karnovsky MJ: Porous structure of the glomerular slit diaphragm in the rat and mouse. *J Cell Biol* 60:423, 1974.

170. Rosalski SB, Wilkinson JH: Urinary lactic dehydrogenase in renal disease. *Lancet* 2:327, 1959.

171. Rosenmann E, Boss JH: Tissue antigens in normal and pathologic urine samples: A review. *Kidney Int* 16:337, 1979.

172. Rosenmann E, Dishon T, Boss JH: Excretion of accessory genital gland specific antigens in the urine of healthy male rats. *J Lab Clin Med* 74:31, 1969.

173. Rubenstein AH, Spitz I: Role of the kidney in insulin metabolism and excretion. *Diabetes* 17:161, 1968.

174. Ruckley VA, MacDonald MK, MacLean PR, et al: Glo-

merular ultrastructure and function in postural proteinuria. *Nephron* 3:153, 1966.

175. Rudman D, Chawla RK, Nixon DW: The specific proteinuria of cancer patients. *Trans Assoc Am Physicians* 91:229, 1978.

176. Ryan GB, Karnovsky MJ: Distribution of endogenous albumin in the rat glomerulus: Role of hemodynamic factors in glomerular barrier function. *Kidney Int* 9:36, 1976.

177. Rytand DA, Spreiter S: Prognosis in postural (orthostatic) proteinuria: Forty to fifty-year follow-up of six patients after diagnosis by Thomas Addis. *N Engl J Med* 305:618, 1981.

178. Samaan N, Freeman RM: Growth hormone levels in severe renal failure. *Metabolism* 19:102, 1970.

179. Sargent F, Johnson RE: The effects of diet on renal function in healthy men. *Am J Clin Nutr* 4:466, 1956.

180. Scherberich J, Mondorf W, Fassbinder W, et al: Tubular histuria and serum proteinuria following kidney allotransplantation. *Kidney Int* 10:199, 1976.

181. Schnaper HW, Robson AM: Nephrotic syndrome: Minimal change disease, focal glomerulosclerosis, and related disorders. *In* Schrier RW, Gottschalk CW (eds): *Diseases of the Kidney*. Boston, Little, Brown, 1988, p 1949.

182. Schoenfeld LS, Glassock RJ: Renal tubular antigen excretion in normal human urine. I. Immunochemical identification. *Kidney Int* 3:309, 1973.

183. Schoenfeld MR, Gulotta S: Renal tubular acidosis, hypokalemia and acid phosphatase. *Ann Intern Med* 65:1258, 1966.

184. Schwartz RH, Lewis RA, Schenk EA: Tamm-Horsfall mucoprotein. III. Potassium dichromate-induced renal tubular damage. *Lab Invest* 27:214, 1972.

185. Schwartz RH, van Ess JD, May AG, et al: Tamm-Horsfall glycoproteinuria and renal allograft rejection. *Transplantation* 16:83, 1973.

186. Shaw AB, Risdon P, Lewis-Jackson JD: Protein, creatinine and Albustix in assessment of proteinuria. *Br Med J* 287:929, 1983.

186a. Shintaku N, Takahashi Y, Akaishi K, et al: Entrapment of left renal vein in children with orthostatic proteinuria. *Ped Nephrol* 4:324, 1990.

187. Silverberg DS: City-wide screening for urinary abnormalities in schoolboys. *Can Med Assoc J* 111:410, 1974.

188. Silverberg DS, Allard MJ, Ulan RA, et al: City-wide screening for urinary abnormalities in schoolgirls. *Can Med Assoc J* 109:981, 1973.

189. Sinniah R, Law CH, Pwee HS: Glomerular lesions in patients with asymptomatic persistent and orthostatic proteinuria discovered on routine medical examination. *Clin Nephrol* 7:1, 1977.

190. Sølling J, Sølling K, Mogensen CE: Patterns of proteinuria and circulating immune complexes in febrile patients. *Acta Med Scand* 212:167, 1982.

191. Spear GS: Implications of the glomerular lesions of cyanotic congenital heart disease. *J Chronic Dis* 19:1083, 1966.

192. Springberg PD, Garret LE, Thompson AL, et al: Fixed and reproducible orthostatic proteinuria: Results of a 20-year follow-up study. *Ann Intern Med* 97:516, 1982.

193. Stetler-Stevenson MA, Flouret G, Peterson DR: Handling of luteinizing hormone-releasing hormone by renal proximal tubular segments in vitro. *Am J Physiol* 241:F117, 1981.

194. Strober W, Waldmann TA: The role of the kidney in the metabolism of plasma proteins. *Nephron* 13:35, 1974.

195. Sumpio BE, Maack T: Kinetics, competition, and selectivity of tubular absorption of proteins. *Am J Physiol* 243:F379, 1982.

196. Sutherland JC, vann Markham R Jr, Mardiney MR Jr: Subclinical immune complexes in the glomeruli of kidneys postmortem. *Am J Med* 57:536, 1974.

197. Suzuki Y, Okada T, Higuchi A, et al: Asymptomatic low molecular weight proteinuria: A report on 5 cases. *Clin Nephrol* 23:249, 1985.

198. Suzuki Y, Shimao S, Okada T, et al: Quantitative determination of urinary protein components of children with postural proteinuria. *Eur J Pediatr* 140:268, 1983.

199. Swann GH, Wilson PC: A study of the proteinurias following manipulation of the renal blood vessels. *Am J Med Sci* 246:153, 1963.

200. Tack ED, Perlman FM, Robson AM: Renal injury in sick newborn infants: A prospective evaluation using urinary β_2-microglobulin concentrations. *Pediatrics* 81:432, 1988.

201. Thompson AL, Durrett RR, Robinson RR: Fixed and reproducible orthostatic proteinuria. VI. Results of a 10-year follow-up evaluation. *Ann Intern Med* 73:235, 1970.

202. Tidstrøm B: Quantitative determination of protein in normal urine. *Scand J Clin Lab Invest* 15:167, 1963.

203. Urizar RE, Tinglof BO, Smith FG Jr, et al: Persistent asymptomatic proteinuria in children. *Am J Clin Pathol* 62:461, 1974.

204. Vehaskari VM, Rapola J: Isolated proteinuria: Analysis of a school-age population. *J Pediatr* 101:661, 1982.

205. Vehaskari VM, Rapola J, Koskimies O, et al: Microscopic hematuria in schoolchildren: Epidemiology and clinicopathologic evaluation. *J Pediatr* 95:676, 1979.

206. Vehaskari VM, Root ER, Germuth FG Jr, et al: Glomerular charge and urinary protein excretion: Effects of systemic and intrarenal polycation infusion in the rat. *Kidney Int* 22:127, 1982.

207. Vernier RL, Klein DJ, Sissons SP, et al: Heparan sulfate-rich anionic sites in the human glomerular basement membrane. Decreased concentrations in congenital nephrotic syndrome. *N Engl J Med* 309:1001, 1983.

208. Wagner MG, Smith FG, Tinglof BO, et al: Epidemiology of proteinuria. *J Pediatr* 73:825, 1968.

209. Waldmann TA, Strober W, Mogielnicki RP: Renal handling of low molecular weight proteins. *J Clin Invest* 51:2162, 1972.

210. Wallace ALC, Stacy BD: Disappearance of ^{125}I-labelled rat growth hormone in nephrectomized and sham operated rats. *Horm Metab Res* 7:135, 1975.

211. Yoshikawa N, Uehara S, Yamana K, et al: Clinicopathological correlations of persistent asymptomatic proteinuria in children. *Nephron* 25:127, 1980.

212. Yoshioka T, Mitarai T, Kon V, et al: Role of angiotensin II in an overt functional proteinuria. *Kidney Int* 30:538, 1986.

213. Zager RA, Cotran RS, Hoyer JR: Pathologic localization of Tamm-Horsfall protein in interstitial deposits in renal disease. *Lab Invest* 38:52, 1978.

ALOK KALIA
LUTHER B. TRAVIS

22

Hematuria, Leukocyturia, and Cylindruria

Hematuria

The discovery of hematuria in a child is one of the common problems for which the pediatric nephrologist is consulted, either for help in establishing an etiologic diagnosis or for suggestions on management.

The etiology of hematuria is sometimes easy to determine from the clinical data and simple laboratory tests. Often, however, it is not. This is particularly true in children who appear to be "well" and in whom the urinalysis reveals the presence of blood but is otherwise normal. This is not an uncommon situation; in a study involving almost 12,000 schoolchildren [21], 4% were found to have an abnormally high number of red blood cells (RBCs) in at least one of four urine collections. Obviously, all these children did not have significant renal or urologic disease. The prevalence of hematuria is high, but the outcome is benign in the vast majority of children. There are exceptions, however, and in an occasional child blood in the urine may be a sign of serious disease. This dichotomy mandates that the physician caring for a child with hematuria have an understanding of the causes and clinical spectrum of hematuria as well as the prognosis for children in whom it is the sole abnormality. It is important to be able to decide when to engage in invasive investigations and when to "leave well enough alone."

Urinary Red Blood Cell Excretion

An occasional RBC can be found in the urine of most people. In his pioneering studies, Addis [2] found an average of 65,750 cells (range 0 to 425,000) in eighty-two 12-hour urine collections obtained from 74 medical students. The distinction between normal and abnormal RBC excretion, however, is not clear. This ambiguity exists not only because of differences in the methods used for microscopic examination of the urine but also because the concentration of the urine, and therefore the number of cells contained per unit volume, is variable and any random sample technique will at best be semiquantitative.

The most convenient screening test for hematuria is the reagent-impregnated strip test, which utilizes the peroxidase-like activity of hemoglobin to catalyze the reaction of cumene hydroperoxide and tetramethylbenzidine, resulting in a color change. The test is capable of detecting 5 to 20 intact RBCs per cubic millimeter of urine and is slightly more sensitive to free hemoglobin [37]. The sensitivity of the strip test is decreased if the urine is of high specific gravity or contains ascorbic acid in a concentration greater than 5 mg/dl. A false positive reaction may occur in the presence of other oxidizing agents such as bleach (hypochlorite), commonly used for cleaning urinals. A positive dipstick test should always be followed by microscopic examination of the urine sample, not only to distinguish hematuria from hemoglobinuria (Table 22-1) and myoglobinuria but also to look for other formed elements such as leukocytes, casts, and crystals.

Most laboratories use one of two microscopic techniques for semiquantitative estimation of urinary RBC excretion. In the first, urine is centrifuged using a standardized technique. The sediment is examined and the number of RBCs per high-power field (HPF) is reported. Although the presence of up to four cells per HPF was considered normal by Dodge [21], it is unusual to find more than one or two RBCs per HPF in most specimens. The second method entails counting the number of cells in 0.9 mm^3 of fresh unspun urine in a counting chamber. Using this technique, Vehaskari considered the presence of more than 5 cells/mm^3 to be abnormal [86]. In our laboratory every specimen of urine is examined by both techniques. We have found the ratio between the number of cells counted by the first method and that by the second to be approximately 1:3.

Many investigators have attempted to eliminate the variability inherent in such semiquantitative methods by estimating the number of RBCs in a timed urine collection (excretion of RBCs/unit time). Somewhat surprisingly, the results have been disparate. Whereas Addis determined the mean 12-hour RBC excretion to be 65,750 [2], Lyttle, in children 4 to 12 years of age, recorded a mean 12-hour excretion of 15,181, with a range of 0 to 129,000 [46]. Snoke [74] estimated the mean 12-hour urinary RBC ex-

TABLE 22-1. *Causes of hemoglobinuria*

Diseases
Hemolytic anemias
Hemolytic uremic syndrome
Paroxysmal nocturnal hemoglobinuria

Drugs and Chemicals
Aspidium
Betanapthol
Carbolic acid
Carbon monoxide
Chloroform
Fava beans
Poisonous mushrooms
Naphthalene
Pamaquine
Phenylhydrazine
Potassium chlorate
Quinine
Snake venom
Spider venom
Sulfonamides

Miscellaneous
Cardiopulmonary bypass
Freshwater drowning
Mismatched blood transfusion

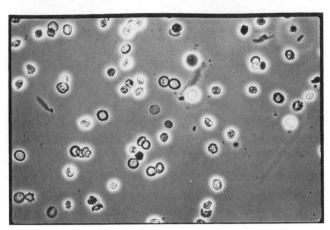

FIG. 22-1. *Phase contrast microscopy of urinary sediment from a child with IgA nephropathy who had gross hematuria following flank trauma. The majority of RBCs are dysmorphic; a few isomorphic cells are also present.*

cretion in 202 children to be 81,600 (range 0 to 800,000), while Edelman [22] suggests that the upper limit of normal is 240,000. At least some of this variation can be attributed to differences in methodology, and the test should ideally be standardized by each laboratory. Quantitative estimation of urinary RBC excretion has been used to monitor the activity of certain nephritides [31,47,66]. It is rarely used as a diagnostic tool, since the combination of the reagent strip and microscopic examination of the urine leaves little doubt about the presence or absence of hematuria.

Hematuria may originate either from the glomerulus or from a postglomerular site. The mechanism of glomerular hematuria is not known. Structural damage to the glomerulus with physical disruption of the glomerular capillary wall can be demonstrated in many diseases, and it may be surmised that erythrocytes are pushed through the gaps by the hydraulic pressure in the capillary lumen. However, normal humans also excrete RBCs in the urine, as do individuals with renal diseases in which discontinuity of the capillary wall is not apparent. That an RBC can squeeze through a break in the membrane much smaller than its own diameter has been demonstrated [45], and electron micrographs of erythrocytes migrating through disruptions in the glomerular basement membrane (GBM) less than 2 μ across have been published [53].

Microscopic examination of the urinary sediment is helpful in distinguishing glomerular hematuria from postglomerular bleeding. The presence of RBC casts in the sediment is prima facie evidence of glomerular bleeding, although failure to detect casts obviously does not exclude it. Casts tend to aggregate at the edge of the film of sediment on the slide. Centrifugation of two successive aliquots of urine in the same tube doubles the amount of

material available for examination. An assiduous search is often required to locate RBC casts, but the effort is well worth the time if a diagnosis can be established without resorting to more extensive or invasive testing.

Examination of the urinary sediment using the phase contrast microscope may help to distinguish glomerular hematuria from postglomerular bleeding. It is hypothesized that red cells that traverse the glomerular basement membrane to enter Bowman's space become distorted and may rupture; in contrast, those originating from a site lower down in the urinary tract maintain a relatively normal architecture. The difference in morphology is discernible with phase contrast microscopy (Fig. 22-1). This technique was pioneered by Fairley and Birch [9,23]. Urine from 55 of 58 patients with histologically confirmed glomerular disease contained only dysmorphic cells; the other three had a mixed picture, with a majority of cells displaying dysmorphic features. Dysmorphic cells were not found in the urine of 30 patients with nonglomerular hematuria. A subsequent prospective study [10] involving 117 consecutive patients with hematuria yielded similar results. The usefulness of this technique in children has also been documented [18,62].

The range of morphologic variations in the RBCs has been elegantly demonstrated with the scanning electron microscope [24]. The cell volume of urinary RBCs, measured in an automated counter, has been shown to provide similar information, with dysmorphic cells being smaller [17,72]. Evidence has also been provided that dysmorphic RBCs can be differentiated from isomorphic cells under ordinary brightfield microscopy [75].

The presence of more than 80% of isomorphic or dysmorphic cells appears reliably to indicate the site of origin, but, on occasion, one will find a mixed population of cells of uncertain predictive value [18,25,58,87]. Recent reports also indicate that the relationship between dysmorphic RBCs and a glomerular site of origin may not be absolute. A diminished RBC volume, indicative of glomerular bleed-

Table 22-2. *Causes of discolored urine suggesting hematuria*

Pink, Red, Coke-Colored, Burgundy
Associated with disease
    Hemoglobinuria
    Myoglobinuria
    Porphyrinuria
Associated with food or drug ingestion
    Aminopyrine
    Anthrocyans
    Azo dyes
    Beets
    Blackberries
    Chloroquine
    Desferrioxamine
    Ibuprofen
    Methyldopa
    Nitrofurantoin
    Phenazopyridine
    Rifampin
    Rhodamine B
    Sulfasalazine
    Urates
Dark Brown or Black
Associated with disease
    Alkaptonuria
    Homogentisic aciduria
    Melanin
    Methemoglobinuria
    Tyrosinosis
Associated with food or drug ingestion
    Alanine
    Cascara
    Resorcinol
    Thymol

ing, has been described in patients with cystitis [72]. In another study, the proportion of dysmorphic RBCs in the urine samples taken before and after a renal biopsy in individuals with glomerular disease did not differ in spite of the increase in hematuria following the procedure [58]. The authors speculate that dysmorphic cells may indicate a renal, not just a glomerular, site of origin. In the same study, even though patients with lower-tract bleeding had a significantly smaller percentage of dysmorphic cells than patients with proved glomerulonephritis (49% vs. 66%), there was a considerable overlap.

It should be noted that red or brown coloration of the urine does not invariably indicate the presence of blood. Conditions that may mimic hematuria or hemoglobinuria are listed in Table 22-2.

The Clinical Spectrum of Hematuria

Hematuria is generally an isolated finding in a child who is otherwise considered normal. Less often, it is accompanied by other markers of pathology, such as proteinuria or a depressed serum C3 level; even more infrequently it occurs in conjunction with obvious clinical indicators of disease such as edema and hypertension. Since the management, and often the prognosis, is influenced by the presentation and associated findings, it is useful to assign children with hematuria into two groups: those in whom hematuria appears to be the only abnormality—isolated hematuria—and those in whom it is found to be associated with other clinical or laboratory aberrations.

ISOLATED HEMATURIA

The phenomenon of isolated hematuria was described in 1839 by Rayer [61], who wrote, "Finally, there are a certain number of hematurias that cannot be attributed to a lesion of the urinary apparatus or to a determined malady; these one designates as essential hematurias." Baehr, in 1926, described 14 patients [6] with clinical presentations compatible with isolated hematuria and noted the apparently benign prognosis. That hematuria may persist for years without the development of clinical or laboratory evidence of disease was subsequently confirmed by a number of other investigators [4,84,89].

The term *isolated hematuria* appears to best describe the occurrence of hematuria as the sole abnormality on the urinalysis in an individual in whom neither the history nor the physical examination provides any indication of a systemic disorder or of renal or urologic disease. This definition includes both gross and microscopic hematuria and makes no assumptions about the site of origin of the blood, the presence or absence of subclinical disease, or the prognosis. It considers isolated hematuria to be a symptom, not a diagnosis. Terms that have been used in a similar, but not identical, context include *primary hematuria, idiopathic hematuria, essential hematuria, benign hematuria,* and *recurrent focal nephritis*. The *histologic* term *focal nephritis* is confusing, since it was used in the past to describe a *clinical* syndrome. According to Ross [64], "it is not a well-defined entity, but is diagnosed when hematuria, proteinuria, and urinary casts are observed at the height of an infection without oedema, hypertension or impairment of renal function." Ross described the histologic findings in 5 patients with recurrent gross hematuria and termed the condition *recurrent focal nephritis* with a clinical—not a histologic—connotation. The term, although no longer in use, is common in older literature concerning hematuria.

A measure of diversity still exists regarding one aspect of the definition of isolated hematuria. Ideally, the patient with microhematuria who has more than a trace amount of protein in the urine should not be labeled as having isolated hematuria. Children who have a combination of urinary findings probably have a different prognosis and require a different clinical approach from those with isolated hematuria. In spite of the fact that this distinction has not always been strictly applied, recent studies on hematuria in children have helped to define the prevalence, persistence, clinical patterns, and prognosis of isolated hematuria.

Isolated hematuria is not uncommon in children. Two elegant studies—one by Dodge and associates [21] in Galveston county, Texas, and the other by Vehaskari's group [86] in Finland, have helped to define the prevalence of this condition. The Galveston study involved more than 12,000 children in the first, second, and third grades, who were tested for the presence of blood in the urine at least once a year for five consecutive years. A total of 6070 children were studied for all five years. The presence of five or more RBCs per HPF was considered a positive result. All children who were found to have blood on the initial examination were retested twice, generally within a week. *Half the children who had a positive result for the initial specimen did not have signs of hematuria on the second and third examinations.* The prevalence of hematuria, if defined as the presence of blood in at least two of three specimens, was 1% in girls and 0.5% in boys. The rate of disappearence of hematuria was 30% per year. None of the children with persistent isolated hematuria had clinical or laboratory evidence of renal disease.

In the Finnish study [86], 8954 children aged 8 to 15 years participated. The presence of 6 or more RBCs/mm³ of urine or of more than 100,000 RBCs per hour in an Addis collection was considered abnormal. Four specimens were obtained from each child. On analysis, 364 (4%) had blood in at least one collection; 59 of these had both blood and protein. Of the remaining 305 children, *222 had blood in only one of four collections.* Of the 83 children with more than one positive specimen, one was discovered to be bleeding from a covert menstrual disturbance, four were known to have hematuria and had been previously investigated (normal biopsy, benign familial hematuria, healing postinfectious nephritis, and chronic urinary infection with reflux), and follow-up data were not available in six. The remaining 72 were reexamined 1 month later; only 43 still had hematuria, and this number dropped to 27 at 4 to 6 months. Examination of the renal histology in this group revealed that two children had IgA nephropathy, and one had basement membrane findings suggestive of Alport's disease. In this study, the prevalence of hematuria, if defined as the presence of blood in at least two collections, was 1.1%.

The two studies are in agreement that the incidental discovery of blood in the urine of an apparently healthy child is not an uncommon event, but, in the majority of such children, this is a transient phenomenon that resolves spontaneously in a few days to a few months. It is also evident that the presence of significant renal histologic abnormalities in children with persistent isolated hematuria is the exception, not the rule. Furthermore, none of the children in whom histologic abnormalities were detected had a disease in which therapeutic intervention is known to affect the outcome.

A number of other studies have helped to elucidate the renal histology in children with isolated hematuria [52,57,82,83,91,92]. Examination of the biopsy will usually reveal one of the following patterns on immunofluorescent (IF) or electron microscopy (EM): (1) normal histology, (2) diffuse attenuation of the glomerular basement membrane (GBM), (3) IgA nephropathy, (4) changes typical of Alport's syndrome, or (5) vascular C3 staining, the significance of which is unknown [52,57, 82,83,86,91,92]. On light microscopy, the tissue may appear to be normal or show changes ranging from minimal mesangial hypercellularity to diffuse global and segmental sclerosis, crescent formation, and areas of tubular atrophy. Significant involvement demonstrable on light microscopy should always be a cause for concern regardless of the findings on IF or EM examination [52].

The pattern of bleeding in children with isolated hematuria can often be used as an indicator not only of the prognosis but also of the renal histology. The majority of children with intermittent or continuous microhematuria, or intermittent gross hematuria with *complete clearing between episodes,* who have no proteinuria or other clinical or laboratory abnormalities (and no family history of hematuria, proteinuria, neurosensory deafness, or renal insufficiency), will have entirely normal renal histology by all modalities of examination, have a good chance of spontaneously clearing their urine, and have an excellent prognosis [52,83,92]. An occasional child may have IgA nephropathy, diffuse thinning or even lamellation of the GBM [57], or vascular C3 staining [52]. In none of the studies cited here or later in this section has there been a systematic effort to differentiate glomerular from nonglomerular bleeding, and it is likely that at least some of the children in this first group have nonglomerular hematuria.

Persistent microhematuria interspersed with episodes of gross bleeding is of greater concern. In one study [83], 79% of such children had abnormal renal histology, with 13 of 19 children having Alport's syndrome or IgA nephropathy. The fact that this combination may indicate a less favorable prognosis has been confirmed in another report [52]. Persistent hematuria with proteinuria also signifies a poor prognosis; in addition to the acquired nephritides, new mutations of Alport's disease may present in this manner [92]. As discussed above, however, this is not isolated hematuria.

A detailed review of the family history may be the single most useful exercise when investigating a child with isolated hematuria. Familial hematurias appear to run a similar course in successive generations, and the outcome in a child can often be predicted from that in an older relative. One of two patterns can usually be recognized. In the first, a child with hematuria will have relatives in one or more older generations (parents, grandparents, aunts, uncles, etc.) with isolated hematuria but *without neurosensory deafness or a tendency to progress to renal insufficiency.* This has been termed *benign familial hematuria* or *thin basement membrane disease,* and kindreds have been reported with up to four generations with hematuria and persistently normal renal function [63]. These children have diffuse attenuation of the GBM and lamina densa on EM [83,91,92], although the presence of areas of lamellation of the GBM has also been described [57]. The prognosis for maintaining normal renal function is good.

In the second group are children with hematuria and a family history of one or more of the following: (1) hematuria and proteinuria, (2) neurosensory deafness, and (3) renal insufficiency. These are indicative of Alport's syndrome and may bode a poor prognosis. There is evidence to indicate that all components may not be present in every affected individual [91]. The age at which the EM changes of this disease (lamellation of the GBM with a "basket weave" appearence) develop is also variable [34,35]. Typical alterations have been described in children less than 5 years of age [35] but may not occur until late in the course of the disease [5]. Habib et al. have also reported on patients with a clinical picture compatible with Alport's syndrome, who show only diffuse attenuation of the GBM [35] with no evidence of lamellation. Conversely, a strong association between familial thin base-ment membrane disease and abnormalities on careful au-diologic evaluation has also been reported [29]. It appears that Alport's syndrome lies at one end of the spectrum of hereditary nephritis, the other end being occupied by be-nign familial hematuria. The prognosis appears to depend more on the degree of clinical expression in other members of the family and less on the histologic findings.

HEMATURIA ASSOCIATED WITH CLINICAL OR BIOCHEMICAL ABNORMALITIES

Renal Hematuria of Glomerular Origin

Glomerular hematuria is often accompanied by proteinuria. This serves as a marker for the site of origin of the blood, since microscopic hematuria arising from a site lower down in the urinary tract is not associated with proteinuria. Grossly bloody urine, of course, will always contain protein regardless of its site of origin.

Postinfectious nephritis is the most common nonsup-purative renal disease of childhood (Table 22-3). Subclin-ical cases probably outnumber those with obvious disease [21], and hematuria may persist up to a year [19]. This entity is probably the most common cause of glomerular hematuria and proteinuria. IgA nephropathy and Alport's syndrome present primarily as hematuria; any of the other nephritides may also do so, including mesangiocapillary glomerulonephritis, lupus nephritis, the nephritis of Hen-och-Schönlein purpura, and focal segmental glomerulo-sclerosis, although the urinalysis usually reveals some pro-teinuria. In the International Study of Kidney Disease in Children, 23% of patients with minimal-lesion nephrotic syndrome were found to have microscopic hematuria [40]. Hematuria is a feature of the nephritis of chronic bacte-remia—the so-called shunt nephritis. Glomerular hema-turia may also be the result of vascular disease such as polyarteritis nodosa and nephrosclerosis. In the majority of these conditions, clinical or laboratory findings will be present that invalidate a diagnosis of isolated hematuria.

Renal Hematuria of Tubular Origin

The term *tubulointerstitial nephropathy* (interstitial nephritis) encompasses a variety of conditions, some of which can result in hematuria (Chap. 72). Prominent among these is the nephropathy caused by methicillin and related peni-cillins. This may present as isolated hematuria or be part of a triad that includes fever and rash [28]. Hematuria may also be seen in pyelonephritis, where it is often accompa-nied by other urinary findings such as pyuria and leukocyte casts. A history of urinary infection, present or past, can usually be obtained.

Tubulointerstitial nephropathy resulting from metabolic disorders (uric acid, oxalate, and hypercalcemic nephrop-athy) can result in hematuria. This may occur acutely, for example, during treatment of lymphoid neoplasia (uric acid), ethylene glycol ingestion (oxalate), or vitamin D intoxication (hypercalcemia). It can also develop insidi-ously and present with symptoms of nephrolithiasis or uri-nary infection. Hematuria occurs during the course of acute tubular necrosis and may persist after the serum creatinine level has returned to normal.

TABLE 22-3. *Causes of hematuria*

Renal
Glomerular
1. Glomerulonephritis, proliferative
   Postinfectious
   IgA nephropathy
   Mesangiocapillary
   Mesangial proliferative
   Lupus glomerulonephritis
   Nephritis of anaphylactoid purpura
   Rapidly progressive glomerulonephritis
2. Glomerulopathy, nonproliferative
   Hereditary progressive nephritis
   Benign familial hematuria
   Focal glomerulosclerosis (global and segmental)
   Minimal-lesion nephrotic syndrome
   Membranous nephropathy
   Nephrosclerosis (hypertensive, other)
   Vasculitic injury (microangiopathy, cortical necrosis)

Nonglomerular
1. Tubulointerstitial nephropathy
   Infectious (pyelonephritis, tuberculosis)
   Metabolic (uric acid, oxalate, nephrocalcinosis)
   Allergic vasculitis
   Drug or poison induced (analgesics, antimicrobials)
   Acute tubular necrosis
2. Vascular
   Renal venous thrombosis
   Hemoglobin S nephropathy
   Malformations (hemangioma, aneurysm, arteriovenous fistula)
3. Tumors
   Wilms'
   Renal cell carcinoma
   Angiomyoma, cortical rests, etc.
4. Developmental
   Polycystic renal disease
   Simple cysts

Renal Pelvic and Ureteral
   Urolithiasis
   Trauma
   Vascular malformations
   Papillary necrosis
   Hydronephrosis
   Infections
   Vasculitis

Vesical
   Infection/inflammation (any cause)
   Obstruction/dilatation (any cause)
   Stones
   Drugs (cyclophosphamide)
   Trauma
   Tumors
   Vascular malformations

Urethral
   Infection/inflammation
   Trauma

Other
   Prostatic and epididymal infection
   Factitious

Undefined
   Hypercalciuria
   Exercise-induced hematuria

Other Causes of Renal Hematuria

In a child with persistent hematuria the specter of a renal tumor is often raised. Wilms' tumor is by far the most common malignant renal tumor in children. Hematuria does occasionally occur with Wilms' tumor but almost never without the simultaneous presence of a palpable renal mass; the latter is present at the time of diagnosis in about 95% of the cases [33]. Hematuria can occasionally be the initial manifestation of renal cell carcinoma, but this tumor is extremely rare in children [14]. A few reports of benign tumors such as angiomyoma [54] and renal hemangiomas [11] presenting as gross or microscopic hematuria in young adults can be found in the literature, as can reports of renal bleeding occurring from embryonic cortical cell rests [32] and endometriosis of the kidney [36].

Hematuria in hemoglobin S disorders (SS, SA, SC, and S-thalassemia) is well documented [3] (Chap. 64) and in heterozygous individuals may be the only significant pathologic consequence of the hemoglobinopathy [69]. In any child with unexplained hematuria and an African heritage, investigation for the presence of hemoglobin S is mandatory. The precise etiology and site of origin of the bleeding is uncertain. It is hypothesized that a combination of the low oxygen tension, sluggish blood flow, low pH, and high osmolality in the renal medulla induces sickling and sludging of erythrocytes even in heterozygous individuals, resulting in areas of infarction and hemorrhage [13,15].

Both intrarenal and extrarenal vascular abnormalities can result in renal bleeding. Renal venous thrombosis results in hematuria, a large kidney, and thrombocytopenia (Chap. 88). It is rare but should be suspected in newborns and children with nephrosis who develop hematuria after experiencing an episode of dehydration or hypotension [43,51,60]. The "loin pain–hematuria" syndrome [1,55] described in young women is associated with abnormalities of interlobar, arcuate, and interlobular arteries. Small areas of infarction are sometimes seen. Compression of the left renal vein between the aorta and the superior mesenteric artery—the "nut-cracker" syndrome [88]—and circumaortic position of the left renal vein [59] have both been reported to cause hematuria, presumably by inducing intrarenal varicosities.

Renal tuberculosis, simple cysts, and polycystic kidney disease are uncommon causes of hematuria in children.

Post-renal Hematuria

Bacterial infections can cause bleeding, accounting for as many as 26% of all cases of gross hematuria in one retrospective series [39]. All these children had clinical features suggestive of urinary infection, but not all had microbiologic documentation. In our experience, infection not complicated by hypercalciuria or urolithiasis is an uncommon cause of gross hematuria. Urethritis and meatitis are occasional causes of hematuria; prostatitis or epidydimitis are rarely seen in children. Adenoviral hemorrhagic cystitis is known to cause gross hematuria [56]. The urine contains numerous RBCs and leukocytes. Gross hematuria usually disappears within a week.

Hematuria commonly accompanies urolithiasis (Chap. 93). Occasionally, the stone will obstruct not only the flow of urine but also the flow of blood, and the urinalysis may remain normal until the obstruction is relieved. Dilatation of the urinary tract from any cause increases the tendency to hemorrhage; a hydronephrotic kidney may bleed after minimal trauma [70]. In addition, a dilated tract is subject to infection, which also may lead to hematuria.

As many as 30% of patients with appendicitis, with or without a ruptured appendix, may have microscopic hematuria [7,68]. In the majority of these, the appendix lies in a pelvic position in close proximity to the ureter.

Malignant tumors of the bladder or prostate, such as rhabdomyosarcoma, may result in hematuria, but these tumors are rare in children. Another unusual cause of postrenal hematuria is hereditary hemorrhagic telangiectasia involving the bladder [16]. Hematuria produced by external trauma to the kidney or urinary tract is easy to diagnose, but bleeding resulting from insertion of objects into the urethra or bladder should also be considered in the differential diagnosis of hematuria. Hemorrhagic cystitis used to be a feared complication of cyclophosphamide administration. It results from stasis of the drug and its metabolites in the bladder urine at night. Once the etiology of the condition was determined and it became customary to administer the drug only in the morning, the problem disappeared. Ticarcillin and other penicillins are also known occasionally to cause hemorrhagic cystitis [49].

Hematuria With an Undefined Site of Origin

Hypercalciuria without urolithiasis has recently been described as a cause of asymptomatic gross and microscopic hematuria [42,65]. The sine qua non of this condition is the subsidence of hematuria with anticalciuric therapy. Most patients have a family history of urolithiasis. The prevalence of hypercalciuric hematuria is unknown, but Stapleton [80] found 23 of 83 consecutive patients with isolated hematuria to be hypercalciuric. Hematuria resolved in all but three patients when measures were taken to reduce urinary calcium excretion. The disease appears to be uncommon in blacks [78]. The site of origin of the blood has not yet been defined but is unlikely to be the glomerulus. RBC casts are not usually found, and renal histology results in children who have undergone a biopsy have been normal or minimally abnormal [42,65]. Estimation of the urinary excretion of calcium should be performed in every child with isolated hematuria. The normal upper limit of daily excretion is 4 mg/kg [30], but estimation of the calcium-to-creatinine ratio in a "spot" urine (upper limit of normal, 0.2) is a useful screening procedure [79].

The mechanism and site of origin of exercise-induced hematuria are also unclear [44]. Reports concerning this phenomenon have become more common since jogging and long-distance running achieved their present popularity, but it has also been reported after other forms of exercise [12]. In one study, hematuria, but no RBC casts, was found in 9 of 50 men after a marathon run [71], but in another study [26], in which 33 of 44 runners had an abnormally high rate of RBC excretion, the cells were found to be dysmorphic by phase contrast microscopy. Hematuria disappears within 24 to 48 hours. It is believed to be benign, and extensive investigation is not recommended.

An Approach to the Child with Hematuria

Hematuria has a multiplicity of associations. It is usually a transient phenomenon of little significance but may sometimes be the harbinger of serious disease. This diversity of possible outcomes necessitates the use of a systematic, step-by-step approach to every child with this problem.

Because hematuria is often evanescent, urinalysis should be repeated two or three times at intervals of a few days. The presence of blood in more than one specimen of urine is an indication for proceeding with clinical and, if necessary, laboratory investigation.

A detailed family history, up to and including second-degree relatives, should be obtained and urinalysis performed where applicable. As was mentioned earlier, presence of stable hematuria in an older relative often bodes a good prognosis. On the other hand, heavy proteinuria, renal insufficiency and neurosensory deafness—singly or in combination—are suggestive of Alport's syndrome and are strong indicators of a serious outcome. Many other conditions associated with hematuria have a familial component. A common example is hypercalciuric hematuria, where a history of urolithiasis in a first- or second-order relative is often present; some other examples are listed in Table 22-4.

Precipitating factors should be looked for. Impetigo or a pharyngeal infection often precede poststreptococcal glomerulonephritis. Occurrence of gross hematuria during or a few days after an upper respiratory infection is strongly suggestive of IgA nephropathy or preexisting glomerulonephritis. The nephropathy of Henoch-Schönlein purpura may be preceded by an incomplete expression of the syndrome, with only one or two of the components being prominent. Abdominal pain or colic preceding or accompanying hematuria is suggestive of Henoch-Schönlein purpura, urolithiasis, pyelonephritis, cystitis, hydronephrosis, polycystic kidney disease, sickle cell nephropathy, or the loin pain–hematuria syndrome. Colic may also occur during the passage of a blood clot. Diffuse abdominal pain occasionally occurs in children with poststreptococcal glo-

TABLE 22-4. *Hematuria with familial association*

Renal
Glomerular
  Alport's syndrome
  Benign familial hematuria
  Collagen vascular disease
  Microangiopathic vasculitis
Nonglomerular
  Metabolic (uric acid, oxalosis, cystinuria)
  Hypercalciuria
  Vascular malformations
  Polycystic renal disease (adult type)
  Tumors

Post-renal
  Vesicoureteral reflux (primary)
  Vascular malformations
  Urolithiasis

merulonephritis, and nonspecific abdominal discomfort is sometimes experienced by children with hypercalciuric hematuria. Joint pain may occur in Henoch-Schönlein purpura or collagen vascular disease. Drugs such as methicillin or anticoagulants can precipitate hematuria, as can strenuous exercise.

Measurement of the growth parameters is an essential part of the physical examination, since failure to grow often accompanies a chronic reduction in renal function. Hypertension is another strong indicator of renal disease, and the blood pressure must be obtained regardless of the age of the child. If it is found to be high, the elevation should not be ascribed merely to the child being in a stressful setting of the physician's office; arrangements should be made for measurement of the blood pressure at home or in school. Presence of severe pallor or edema is easily ascertained, but rashes, petechiae, ecchymoses, and hemangiomas may not be visible in a clothed child. Abdominal examination should include a search for a mass as well as for costovertebral angle and suprapubic tenderness. The external genitalia should be examined for bleeding, infection, or trauma. A rectal examination for prostatitis should be performed in older boys. A formal examination for neurosensory hearing loss is a must in any child with isolated glomerular hematuria.

The next step in the evaluation should be examination of the urine to determine the site of origin of the RBCs. The presence or absence of leukocytes, leukocyte casts, and crystals should also be established. If protein is present, a 12- or 24-hour urine collection should be obtained for its quantitation. The urinary calcium-to-creatinine ratio should be determined in all children with isolated hematuria. In those with nonglomerular bleeding without an obvious cause, a urine culture is also indicated.

At this stage one will be able to:

1. Make a tentative etiologic diagnosis and decide on the specific investigations necessary for its confirmation (Alport's syndrome, IgA nephropathy, post-streptococcal nephritis, hypercalciuria, urinary infection, etc.), or
2. Determine that the clinical or laboratory evidence (growth failure, hypertension, edema, significant proteinuria, etc.) indicates the need for further investigation and proceed accordingly, or
3. Establish that neither "1" nor "2" is applicable.

If the third alternative is true, the child has isolated hematuria. Isolated hematuria almost never indicates the presence of a condition in which therapeutic intervention would affect the outcome. Furthermore, stable isolated hematuria, that is, when there is no evidence of either a change in the pattern of hematuria or of development of additional signs, is unlikely to lead to a serious outcome. No further investigation should be undertaken at this time. A period of observation is likely to pay the maximum dividends, although it is sometimes difficult to convince anxious parents that this is the appropriate course of action. The child needs to be monitored for the appearance of new clinical signs such as hypertension; changes in the pattern or severity of hematuria (appearance of gross hematuria or the association of hematuria with upper respiratory infections); and for the emergence of proteinuria. The frequency of follow-up visits will initially depend on the level of anxiety of the physician and the parents, but if there is no change in the first year, observation at yearly intervals is probably adequate.

One of three outcomes is possible during this period:

1. The hematuria will disappear. If this happens, the child should be reexamined a year later; if the clinical examination and the urine are normal, no further follow-up is required. This is the expected outcome in the majority of children.
2. New evidence will emerge on clinical examination or urinalysis, indicating the need for further investigation (the hematuria will no longer be "isolated").
3. Hematuria will persist. Follow-up should be continued at yearly intervals, with reassessment of the history, a complete physical examination, and urinalysis being performed at each visit. To allay anxiety, the serum level of creatinine may also be determined yearly.

Children who continue to have hematuria for many years may need investigation, including a renal biopsy, to establish the absence of a progressive renal or urologic disease to the satisfaction of life insurance companies and prospective employers and occasionally for genetic counseling.

The discovery of hematuria in a child provokes anxiety both in the parents and the physician. A systematic, deliberate approach based on a knowledge of the causes, significance, and natural history of hematuria will help in separating the many children in whom this phenomenon is of no consequence from the few in whom it may be an omen of disease.

Leukocyturia

The rate of excretion of leukocytes in the urine is variable, and the distinction between normal and abnormal excretion is not well defined. The rate appears to vary with the sex and the age of the child. White blood cells (WBCs) are also present in other secretions (prostatic, vaginal, vulvar) that may mix with the urine and elevate the count. Stansfield and Webb [77] found <10 WBCs/mm^3 of uncentrifuged urine in 98% of 1142 specimens from 359 boys; the majority had 0 to 1 WBC/mm^3. Urine collections from female infants demonstrated similarly low counts. In contrast, older girls may have a somewhat higher concentration of leukocytes in the urine; of 1067 specimens obtained from 273 girls, 16% had more than 10 WBCs/mm^3. It appears that the higher counts obtained in females result from contamination of the urine by other secretions, since 98 of 100 specimens obtained from girls by *catheterization* contained <10 WBCs/mm^3. Mabeck [48] found similar urinary leukocyte counts in adult females without obvious urinary infection. Thus, the evidence appears to indicate that the presence of 10 or more leukocytes/mm^3 of urine should be viewed with suspicion. On the basis of the relationship between the counts obtained in uncentrifuged

specimens and those reported as "cells per HPF" in centrifuged specimens (3:1), more than 3 WBCs per HPF in a randomly obtained clean-catch specimen should be considered abnormal. Quantitative estimation of the urinary leukocyte excretion was used for the diagnosis of urinary infection prior to the development of bacteriologic criteria [38,76] and was also considered to be of use in tracking the activity of glomerular disease [31,47]. The urinary leukocyte excretion rate has diminished in significance as an investigative tool in recent years.

Granulocytes are the most common type of WBCs found in the urine. Leukocytes survive for 48 hours or longer in acidic urine but are rapidly destroyed at a pH of 8 or more [76,85]. Survival is also shortened in hypotonic urine. Under high power, these cells can be seen as granular spheres approximately 10 to 12 μ across or about one and a half times the size of an RBC. The nucleus is lobulated or segmented. The Sternheimer-Malbin stain [81] facilitates evaluation of cellular morphology, especially for the novice. Granulocyte nuclei stain reddish-purple, whereas the granules take on a violet hue. RBCs, on the other hand, either remain unstained or may appear a light pink color. "Glitter" cells are granulocytes that are larger than usual; they take up stain poorly, either remaining unstained or changing to a pale blue color. The granules exhibit brownian movement. The mechanism of formation of glitter cells as well as their significance has been the subject of controversy [41,81]. They were originally felt to be pathognomonic of pyelonephritis. It is now known that formation of glitter cells is encouraged by, and may be dependent on, low urine tonicity [8]. Stamey and Kindrachuk believe that these are "fresh" leukocytes that resist the entry of stain and are indicative of injury to the urinary tract without being specific for any particular site [75]. They have also been found in normal prostatic and vaginal secretions [8].

The most common cause of leukocyturia is infection of the renal parenchyma or of the urinary tract. With parenchymal infection, the urine contains not only leukocytes but also epithelial cell and leukocyte casts. The presence of bacterial infection is easy to determine, but chlamydial, viral (especially adenovirus), and trichomonal infections are also occasional causes of leukocyturia in children. Urinary infection is not invariably accompanied by leukocyturia; this is especially true for recurrent infections and asymptomatic bacteriuria. On the other hand, tuberculosis of the kidney may present with "sterile" pyuria, since the bacterium does not grow on the usual culture media.

Leukocyturia is commonly found with inflammatory and proliferative glomerular disease, such as postinfectious nephritis or lupus nephritis. Rarely, it accompanies urolithiasis and renal or urinary tract tumors if mucosal erosion has occurred. It may also be caused by inflammation of structures contiguous with the urinary tract, for example, if an inflamed appendix lies across the ureter. Cellular rejection of a renal allograft is accompanied by the presence of lymphocytes, granulocytes, and plasma cells in the urine. However, in conditions other than infection of the urinary tract, leukocyturia is usually considered an incidental finding without much diagnostic or prognostic significance.

Cylindruria

Urinary casts provide a unique glimpse into the kidney. The constituents of a cast can reveal the presence of inflammatory or anoxic injury to the renal tubules or the glomeruli. Casts, in a sense, transport a sampling of the microenvironment of the kidney to the outside world.

The shape of the cast reflects the architecture of the tubule in which it was formed. The matrix of a urinary cast is formed by precipitation or "gelling" of Tamm-Horsfall protein in the renal tubules [50,67]. Precipitation of the protein is facilitated in the presence of a concentrated, acid urine [73]; casts dissolve rapidly in alkaline urine. The usual sites of formation of casts are the distal tubule and the collecting duct. An exception to this rule is seen in patients with multiple myeloma in whom the high concentration of Bence Jones protein allows casts to be formed in the proximal tubule. If erythrocytes, leukocytes, or epithelial cells are present in the tubule during the formation of a cast, they are incorporated into the matrix. Particulate material and fat globules may also be trapped in casts. The typical cast has parallel sides, rounded blunt ends, and a distinct outline.

The classification of casts is based on the presence and type of inclusions.

1. Hyaline casts are clear and colorless. They are characterized by the absence of inclusions and are difficult to visualize with brightfield microscopy. Hyaline casts are found in the urine of normal individuals. An increase in the number of hyaline casts is seen after strenuous exercise. In the presence of renal disease, they are seen in conjunction with other types of casts.
2. Granular casts contain coarse or fine particles embedded in the hyaline matrix. The inclusions are felt to be either precipitated plasma proteins [67] or cells in various stages of disintegration. Granular casts may be seen after exercise in normal individuals, but their presence may be indicative of renal disease. They are also seen in chronic lead intoxication [73]. "Waxy" casts are believed to result from complete disintegration of inclusions present in granular casts. These are homogeneous but, in contrast to hyaline casts, are easy to see because they are highly refractile.
3. Leukocyte casts can be identified if the cells are well preserved and typical multilobed granulocyte nuclei are visible. They are common in inflammatory glomerular diseases such as postinfectious or mesangiocapillary glomerulonephritis and may also be found with renal parenchymal inflammation, for example, in pyelonephritis, interstitial nephritis, and renal transplant rejection.
4. Epithelial cell casts are difficult to distinguish from leukocyte casts, especially in unstained urine. These casts indicate tubular damage and are most often seen in pyelonephritis. They are also present in other types of tubulointerstitial nephropathies, such as methicillin-induced interstitial nephritis, ethylene glycol intoxication, and renal allograft rejection.
5. RBC casts may contain intact or partly degenerated erythrocytes and are golden yellow or light brown in color. In stained preparations the erythrocytes remain unstained or appear a light pink color. RBC casts indicate glomerular disease. Complete disintegration of the erythrocytes results in the formation of hemosiderin or hematin casts.
6. Pigment casts are seen in conditions that result in hemoglobinuria or myoglobinuria. They are also seen in cholestatic jaundice.
7. Fatty casts are formed by incorporation of lipid droplets or fat-laden tubular cells into the hyaline matrix. They are seen in hyperlipidemic conditions such as the nephrotic syndrome.

Casts may also contain bacterial or crystalline inclusions. In alkaline urine, clumps of phosphate crystals may simulate casts, but these do not have a clearly delimited margin. They disappear when a drop of acid is added to the specimen. "Broad" casts are two to five times the diameter of ordinary casts. They are often waxy in appearence and are believed to originate in dilated tubules. Broad casts indicate chronic renal parenchymal disease and are considered a poor prognostic sign.

The presence of casts is often indicative of glomerular or tubular injury. A diligent search for casts is an inexpensive exercise that provides valuable information and should be an integral part of every urinalysis.

References

1. Aber GM, Higgins PM: The natural history and management of the loin pain/hematuria syndrome. Br J Urol 54:613, 1982.
2. Addis T: The number of formed elements in the urinary sediment of normal individuals. J Clin Invest 2:409, 1925–1926.
3. Asnes RS, Migel PF, Wisotsky DH: Massive hematuria in a young adolescent with sickle cell trait. Clin Pediatr (Phila) 22:150, 1983.
4. Ayoub EM, Vernier RL: Benign recurrent hematuria. Am J Dis Child 109:217, 1965.
5. Beathard GA, Granholm NA: Development of the characteristic ultrastructural lesion of hereditary nephritis during the course of the disease. Am J Med 62:751, 1977.
6. Baehr G: Benign and curable form of hemorrhagic nephritis. JAMA 86:1001, 1926.
7. Berger M, Travis LB, Tyson KR, et al: Ruptured appendix: An unusual cause of gross hematuria. J Pediatr 83:502, 1973.
8. Berman LB, Schreiner GE, Feye JO: Observations on the glitter-cell phenomenon. N Eng J Med 255:989, 1956.
9. Birch DF, Fairley KF: Hematuria: Glomerular or non-glomerular? Lancet 2:845, 1979.
10. Birch DF, Fairley KF, Whitworth JA, et al: Urinary erythrocyte morphology in the diagnosis of glomerular hematuria. Clin Nephrol 20:78, 1983.
11. Bishop AF, Stanley RJ, Kissane JM: Spontaneous hematuria and left renal enlargement in a young man. Urol Radiol 4:52, 1982.
12. Boileau M, Fuchs E, Barry JM, et al: Stress hematuria: Athletic pseudonephritis in marathoners. Urology 15:471, 1980.
13. Buckalew VM, Someren A: Renal manifestations of sickle cell disease. Arch Intern Med 133:660, 1974.
14. Chan HSL, Daneman A, Gribbin M, et al: Renal cell car-

cinoma in the first two decades of life. *Pediatr Radiol* 13:324, 1983.

15. Chaplin H: Hematuria in hemoglobin S disorders. *Arch Intern Med* 140:1573, 1980.

16. Cos LR, Rabinowitz R, Bryson MF, et al: Hereditary hemorrhagic telangiectasia of bladder in a child. *Urology* 20:302, 1982.

17. deCaestecker MP, Hall CL, Basterfield PT, et al: Localization of hematuria by red cell analysers and phase contrast microscopy. *Nephron* 52:170, 1989.

18. DeSanto NG, Nuzzi F, Capodicasa G, et al: Phase contrast microscopy of the urine sediment for the diagnosis of glomerular and nonglomerular bleeding—data in children and adults with normal creatinine clearance. *Nephron* 45:35, 1987.

19. Dodge WF, Spargo BF, Travis LB: Occurrence of acute glomerulonephritis in sibling contacts of children with sporadic acute glomerulonephritis. *Pediatrics* 40:1029, 1967.

20. Dodge WF, Spargo BF, Travis LB, et al: Poststreptococcal glomerulonephritis. A prospective study in children. *N Engl J Med* 286:273, 1972.

21. Dodge WF, West EF, Smith EH, et al: Proteinuria and hematuria in schoolchildren: Epidemiology and early natural history. *J Pediatr* 88:327, 1976.

22. Edelman CM: Unpublished observations, 1967.

23. Fairley KF, Birch DF: Hematuria: A simple method for identifying glomerular bleeding. *Kidney Int* 21:105, 1982.

24. Fassett RG, Horgan B, Gove D, et al: Scanning electron microscopy of glomerular and non-glomerular red blood cells. *Clin Nephrol* 20:11, 1983.

25. Fasset RG, Horgan B, Mathew TD: Detection of glomerular bleeding by phase-contrast microsccopy. *Lancet* 1:1432, 1982.

26. Fassett RG, Owen JE, Fairley J, et al: Urinary red-cell morphology during exercise. *Br Med J* 285:1455, 1982.

27. Gaboardi F, Edefonti A, Imbasciati E, et al: Alport's syndrome. Progressive hereditary nephritis. *Clin Nephrol* 2:143, 1974.

28. Galpin JE, Shinaberger JH, Stanley TM, et al: Acute interstitial nephritis due to methicillin. *Am J Med* 65:756, 1978.

29. Gauthier B, Trachtman H, Frank R, et al: Familial thin basement membrane nephropathy in children with asymptomatic microhematuria. *Nephron* 51:502, 1989.

30. Ghazali S, Barratt TM: Urinary excretion of calcium and magnesium in children. *Arch Dis Child* 49:97, 1974.

31. Giles MD: The Addis count in the prognosis of acute nephritis in childhood. *Arch Dis Child* 22:232, 1947.

32. Gittes RF, Elliot ML: Renal cortical rest and chronic hematuria: A syndrome treated by mid-kidney partial nephrectomy. *J Urol* 109:14, 1973.

33. Greenwood MF, Holland P: Clinical and biochemical manifestations of Wilms' tumor. *In* Pochedly C, Baum S (eds): *Wilms' Tumor: Clinical and Biological Manifestations.* New York, Elsevier, 1984, p 11.

34. Gubler M, Levy M, Broyer M, et al: Alport's syndrome: A report of 58 cases and a review of the literature. *Am J Med* 70:493, 1981.

35. Habib R, Gubler MC, Hinglais N, et al: Alport's syndrome: Experience at Hospital Necker. *Kidney Int* 21:5, 1982.

36. Hajdu SI, Koss LG: Endometriosis of the kidney. *Am J Obstet Gynecol* 106:314, 1970.

37. Henry JB: *Clinical Diagnosis and Management by Laboratory Methods,* 16th ed, Philadelphi, WB Saunders, 1979, p 569.

38. Houston JB: Urinary white cell excretion in childhood. *Arch Dis Child* 40:313, 1965.

39. Ingelfinger JR, Davis AE, Grupe EW: Frequency and etiology of gross hematuria in a general pediatric setting. *Pediatrics* 59:557, 1977.

40. International Study of Kidney Disease in Children. The nephrotic syndrome in children: Prediction of histopathology from clinical and laboratory characteristics at the time of diagnosis. *Kidney Int* 13:159, 1978.

41. Jackson JF: Cytology of degenerating leukocytes. *J Lab Clin Med* 43:227, 1954.

42. Kalia A, Travis LB, Brouhard BH: The association of idiopathic hypercalciuria and asymptomatic gross hematuria in children. *J Pediatr* 99:716, 1981.

43. Kaufman HJ: Renal vein thrombosis. *Am J Dis Child* 95:377, 1958.

44. Kincaid-Smith P: Hematuria and exercise related hematuria. *Br Med J* 285:1595, 1982.

45. Lin JT, Wada H, Maeda H, et al: Mechanism of hematuria in glomerular disease. *Nephron* 35:68, 1983.

46. Lyttle JD: The Addis sediment count in normal children. *J Clin Invest* 12:87, 1933.

47. Lyttle JD: The Addis sediment count in scarlet fever. *J Clin Invest* 12:95, 1933.

48. Mabeck CE: Studies in urinary tract infections. IV. Urinary leukocyte excretion in bacteriuria. *Acta Med Scand* 186:193, 1969.

49. Marx CM, Alpert SE: Ticarcillin induced cystitis. *Am J Dis Child* 138:670, 1984.

50. McQueen EG: Composition of urinary casts. *Lancet* 1:397, 1966.

51. Miller HC, Benjamin JA: Acute idiopathic renal vein thrombosis in infants. *Pediatrics* 30:247, 1962.

52. Miller PFW, Spiers NI, Aparicio SR, et al: Long-term prognosis of recurrent hematuria. *Arch Dis Child* 60:420, 1985.

53. Mouradian JA, Sherman RL: Passage of an erythrocyte through a glomerular basement membrane gap. *N Engl J Med* 293:940, 1975.

54. Neih PT, Conant JK, Zablow BC, et al: Episodic flank pain and gross hematuria in a young woman. *J Urol* 131:99, 1984.

55. Nicholls AJ, Muirhead N, Edward N, et al: Loin pain and hematuria in young women: Diagnostic pitfalls. *Br J Urol* 54:209, 1982.

56. Numazaki Y, Kumasaka T, Yano N, et al: Further study on acute hemorrhage cystitis due to adenovirus Type II. *N Engl J Med* 289:344, 1973.

57. Piel CF, Biava CG, Goodman JR: Glomerular basement membrane attenuation in familial nephritis and "benign" hematuria. *J Pediatr* 101:358, 1982.

58. Pollock C, Liu PL, Gyory AZ, et al: Dysmorphism of urinary red blood cells—value in diagnosis. *Kidney Int* 36:1045, 1989.

59. Positano N, Nadalini VF, Bruttini GP: Hematuria due to circumaortic left renal vein. *Urology* 16:73, 1980.

60. Rasoulpour M, McLean RH: Renal venous thrombosis in neonates. *Am J Dis Child* 134:276, 1980.

61. Rayer PF: *Traite des Malades de Reins.* Paris, JB Bailliere, 1839, p 326.

62. Rizzoni G, Braggion F, Zacchello G: Evaluation of glomerular and non-glomerular hematuria by phase-contrast microscopy. *J Pediatr* 103:370, 1983.

63. Rogers PW, Kurtzman NA, Bunn SM, et al: Familial benign essential hematuria. *Arch Intern Med* 131:257, 1973.

64. Ross JH: Recurrent focal nephritis. *Q J Med* 29:391, 1960.

65. Roy S III, Stapleton BJ, Noe HN, et al: Hematuria preceding renal calculus formation in children with hypercalciuria. *J Pediatr* 99:712, 1981.

66. Ruben MI, Rapoport M, Waltz AD: A comparison of routine urinalysis, Addis count and blood sedimentation rate as criteria of activity in acute glomerulonephritis. *J Pediatr* 20:32, 1942.

67. Rutecki GJ, Goldsmith C, Schreiner GE: Characterization of proteins in urinary casts. *N Engl J Med* 284:1049, 1971.

68. Scott JH, Amin M, Harty JI: Abnormal urinalysis in appendicitis. *J Urol* 129:1015, 1983.
69. Sears DA: The morbidity of sickle-cell trait. *Am J Med* 64:1021, 1978.
70. Seerup A, Rasmussen OS: Blunt trauma to hydronephrotic kidneys. *Fortschr Rontgenstr* 138:621, 1983.
71. Seigel AJ, Hennekens CH, Solomon HS, et al: Exercise related hematuria: Findings in a group of marathon runners. *JAMA* 241:391, 1979.
72. Shichiri M, Hosoda K, Nishio Y, et al: Red-cell volume distribution curves in diagnosis of glomerular and non-glomerular hematuria. *Lancet* 1:908, 1988.
73. Shuman GB: *Urine Sediment Examination.* Baltimore, Williams & Wilkins, 1980.
74. Snoke AW: The normal Addis count in children. *J Pediatr* 12:473, 1938.
75. Stamey TA, Kindrachuk RW: *Urinary Sediment and Urinalysis.* Philadelphia, WB Saunders, 1985, p 54.
76. Stansfield JM: The measurement and meaning of pyuria. *Arch Dis Child* 37:257, 1962.
77. Stansfield JM, Webb JKG: Observations on pyuria in children. *Arch Dis Child* 28:386, 1953.
78. Stapleton FB: Idiopathic hypercalciuria: Association with isolated hematuria and risk for urolithiasis in children. A Report of the Southwest Pediatric Nephrology Study Group. *Kidney Int* 37:807, 1990.
79. Stapleton FB, Noe HN, Jerkins G, et al: Urinary excretion of calcium following an oral calcium loading test in healthy children. *Pediatrics* 69:594, 1982.
80. Stapleton FB, Roy S III, Noe HN, et al: Hypercalciuria in children with hematuria. *N Engl J Med* 310:1345, 1984.
81. Sternheimer R, Malbin B: Clinical recognition of pyelonephritis with a new stain for urinary sediments. *Am J Med* 11:338, 1951.
82. Tina L, Jenis E, Jose P, et al: The glomerular basement membrane in benign familial hematuria. *Clin Nephrol* 17:1, 1982.
83. Trachtman H, Weiss RA, Bennett B, et al: Isolated hematuria in children: Indications for a renal biopsy. *Kidney Int* 25:94, 1984.
84. Travis LB, Daeschner CW, Dodge WF, et al: "Idiopathic" hematuria. *J Pediatr* 60:24, 1962.
85. Triger DR, Smith JWG: Survival of urinary leukocytes. *J Clin Pathol* 19:443, 1966.
86. Vehaskari VM, Rapola J, Koskimies O, et al: Microscopic hematuria in school children: Epidemiology and clinicopathologic evaluation. *J Pediatr* 95:676, 1979.
87. Venkat Raman G, Pead L, Lee HA, et al: A blind controlled trial of phase-contrast microscopy by two observers for evaluating the source of hematuria. *Nephron* 44:304, 1986.
88. Weiner SN, Bernstein RG, Morehouse H, et al: Hematuria secondary to left peripelvic and gonadal vein varices. *Urology* 22:81, 1983.
89. Wyllie GC: Hematuria in children. *Proc R Soc Med* 48:1113, 1955.
90. Yoshikawa N, Ito H, Matsuyama S, et al: Hereditary nephritis in children with and without characteristic glomerular basement membrane alterations. *Clin Nephrol* 30:122, 1988.
91. Yoshikawa N, White RHR, Cameron AH: Familial hematuria: Clinicopathological correlations. *Clin Nephrol* 17:172, 1982.
90. Yoshikawa N, Ito H, Matsuyama S, et al: Hereditary nephritis in children with and without characteristic glomerular basement membrane alterations. *Clin Nephrol* 30:122, 1988.
92. Yum M, Bergstein JM: Basement membrane nephropathy: A new classification for Alport's syndrome and asymptomatic hematuria based on ultrastructural findings. *Hum Pathol* 14:996, 1983.

Bradley S. Dixon
Tomas Berl

23

Pathogenesis of Edema in Renal Disease

Edema is the cardinal manifestation of an excess in total body salt and water. The term derives from the Greek *etymon oidema*, meaning to swell. Depending on the specific cause of the swelling, either local or generalized forms of edema can occur. Local edema results most commonly from isolated obstruction of a peripheral vein or lymphatic channel, producing edema localized distal to the site of obstruction. Generalized edema, on the other hand, is typically symptomatic of severe cardiac, hepatic, or renal dysfunction. Characteristically, the swelling occurs in the most dependent parts of the body such as the legs or presacral region (in a bedfast patient). However, the swelling may occur in other locations, such as periorbital, intraperitoneal (ascites), or intrapulmonary, offering clues as to its specific pathogenesis. Edema represents an important symptom of an abnormal pathologic process leading to either localized or generalized retention of salt and water.

This chapter reviews the pathogenesis of edema in the setting of renal disease. It must be recognized, however, that all generalized edema ultimately depends on the capacity of the kidney to retain salt and water and thereby promote further edema formation. To foster a better understanding of the pathophysiologic processes involved, a brief overview is presented of both the dynamics of transcapillary fluid exchange (Starling forces) and volume regulation (sodium balance).

Transcapillary Fluid Exchange

At the tissue level edema formation must ultimately be determined by an imbalance in forces determining transcapillary fluid exchange [77]. These factors, which control the direction and rate of fluid movement across the capillary wall, are those defined by Starling in the mid-1890s [154]. Symbolically the familiar equation relating them is written as follows:

$$J = K[(P_c - P_i) - \delta(\pi_c - \pi_i)]$$

where J = the net fluid flux, K = the total hydraulic conductance (a product of specific hydraulic conductance and surface area), P_c and P_i = the hydrostatic pressures, π_c and π_i = the protein osmotic pressures, the subscripts c and i denote the capillary and interstitial spaces, respectively, and δ = the protein reflection coefficient, usually assumed to be near unity. Representative values are shown in Figure 23-1. Increases in interstitial fluid are promoted by conditions that increase the hydrostatic pressure difference driving fluid out of the capillary or decrease the oncotic pressure difference opposing this filtration. Furthermore, increase in either the capillary hydraulic or oncotic permeability enhances transcapillary fluid egress into the interstitium. If a sufficient imbalance of the forces promoting filtration over those promoting reabsorption persists, an expansion of the interstitial space occurs and clinical edema may be observed [77,120].

It is important to remember that this is not a static process. Figure 23-1 demonstrates that the balance of forces operative near the precapillary sphincter favors filtration, whereas reabsorption is generally favored toward the venous end of the capillary bed. Filtration exceeds reabsorption and would expand the interstitial compartment were it not for several modulating processes [77]. Most important is the lymphatic conduit, which siphons off excess fluid and returns it centrally to the intravascular compartment. It is estimated that under normal circumstances 2 to 4 liters of fluid per day are transported by this system [69]. In edematous states this amount can increase several-fold, providing considerable protection against an overexpansion of the interstitial compartment.

In addition to the lymphatic system, three factors contribute to the defense against an excessive accumulation of interstitial fluid [77]. Processes that increase filtration across the semipermeable capillary wall tend to dilute the interstitium by replacing the lymphatic fluid with fluid of a lower protein content, reducing interstitial oncotic pressure and partially offsetting the increased filtration [132,138]. The second factor that protects against edema is the compliance of the interstitium. Although poorly understood, the mechanical characteristics of the elastic gel-like substance of the interstitium impart a stiffness that varies from tissue to tissue. For a given perturbation in Starling forces, stiffer tissues (lower compliance) swell less

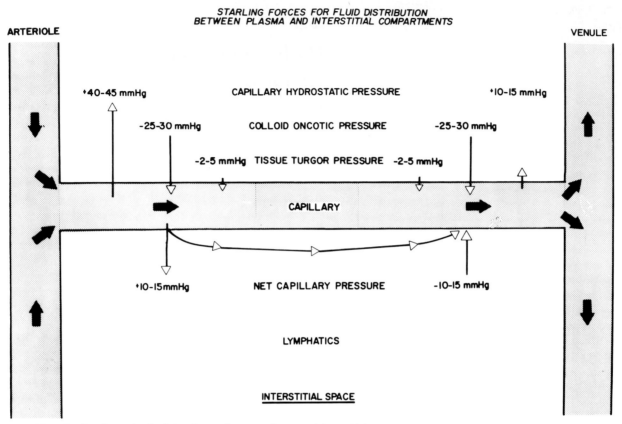

Fig. 23-1. *Starling forces for fluid distribution between plasma and interstitial compartments.*

than looser tissues. For instance, subcutaneous tissue is less compliant than the renal interstitium and generally swells less with comparable changes in transcapillary driving forces [77]. Third, the hydraulic permeability of the capillary wall determines the susceptibility of a given tissue to edema formation. Other factors being constant, leakier tissues accumulate interstitial fluid more readily than those with a tight endovascular barrier.

Volume Regulation

Although altered Starling forces are the immediate cause of interstitial accumulation of fluid, clinically overt edema does not appear without an associated retention of salt and water. If this did not occur, depletion of the intravascular compartment and subsequent vascular collapse would result. Enhanced renal retention of salt and water may be either primary or secondary, depending on whether the stimulus for enhanced salt reabsorption is intrinsic or extrinsic to the kidney. Although this distinction is important from a pathophysiologic and therapeutic standpoint, as we shall see, it remains a controversial issue in several edematous conditions. Regardless, edema formation is inextricably associated with an altered sodium balance and volume regulation. A brief overview of volume regulation and renal sodium handling is presented in this section.

More detailed reviews are provided by Skorecki and Brenner [150], Licht and Danovitch [110], Navar [129], and Meyer and Brenner [127] (see also Chap. 5).

Maintenance of volume homeostasis requires an afferent sensor, capable of detecting perturbations in extracellular volume, and an activating (or inhibiting) efferent effector able to rectify the displacement [150]. A central processing unit, located in the CNS, probably integrates and modulates the input from afferent sensors before it enters the efferent effector pathway. This model represents an oversimplification of a complex, interwoven, and only partially understood cybernetic system. An example is the set point for volume (sodium) homeostasis. It is still unknown whether sodium balance is regulated with reference to a single value of total body sodium [86] or to multiple values that depend on the particular physiologic state existing at the time of measurement [19]. Despite this complexity, some general insights can be gleaned by considering a simple system of afferent (sensory) and efferent (effector) limbs.

Control of Extracellular Fluid Volume

Sodium, as the major osmotic agent in the extracellular fluid, controls the size of the extravascular compartment. Control of sodium balance thus involves sensors that respond to changes in extracellular fluid volume. Although input from multiple sensors present in both the vascular and interstitial compartments of all vascular beds are integrated to determine the total extracellular fluid volume, certain compartments are predominant over others. In particular, the intrathoracic vascular compartment appears to be of central importance [150].

Considerable data have accumulated supporting the existence of both high [53,63] and low pressure receptors [54,63] located in and about the heart and great vessels. Low pressure volume receptors appear to be located in the cardiac atria and perhaps the right ventricle [63,76]. These receptors are sensitive to atrial stretch, increased distention leading to natriuresis and diuresis, and vice versa [139]. Epstein et al [54] showed that water immersion, which translocates fluid from the periphery into the central vascular compartment, results in a marked natriuresis and diuresis. These effects are probably mediated through neural reflexes traveling through the vagus nerve that alter the release of renin and antidiuretic hormone and also modulate sympathetic discharge to the kidneys [150]. In addition to direct renal effects, the sympathetic activity and hormonal release may alter the ratio of precapillary to postcapillary resistance and thus affect capillary ultrafiltration and interstitial volume in all vascular beds [153]. Recent evidence also indicates that in response to increased cardiac filling there is release of atrial natriuretic factor, which influences the vascular tone and elicits natriuresis [117]. A multiplicity of efferent limbs regulating sodium balance can thus be modulated by changes in atrial stretch.

High pressure baroreceptors are located on the arterial side of the circulation, particularly in the aortic and carotid sinuses [81]. These receptors also respond to stretch, sensing the adequacy of arterial filling. Neurally mediated hormone release and sympathetic activity ensue, as observed with atrial stretch [93]. The relevance of these baroreceptors to volume regulation in humans is demonstrated by the occurrence of natriuresis on closure of atrioventricular fistulas [53]. This maneuver increases blood pressure and arterial fullness while decreasing right atrial and intrapulmonary distention and leaving unchanged glomerular filtration rate and renal plasma flow.

Another well-established sensor of volume status is the kidney itself. The kidney is sensitive to changes in intravascular and perhaps interstitial volume. Renin release by the kidney is modulated by transmural pressure within the afferent arteriole as well as the rate of electrolyte delivery past the macula densa [61]. Furthermore, increased renal perfusion pressure alone can result in a so-called pressure natriuresis, although sensor and effector are indistinguishable in this setting [80]. Finally, evidence has been presented that saline loading stimulates release of a natriuretic substance from the kidney [73,110]. This substance has potent inhibitory effects on Na^+-K^+-ATPase and thus might inhibit renal sodium reabsorption [110]. At least one and possibly two other natriuretic factors probably exist. One is the atrial natriuretic factor, which is a polypeptide hormone, and the other is a low molecular weight substance with some digitalis-like properties [110]. This latter substance (or perhaps a precursor) may be the antinatriuretic factor released from the kidney.

There is growing evidence that supports the existence of volume sensors located outside the vascular system. Specifically, mechanoreceptors in the CNS, liver, and pulmonary interstitium have been postulated to exist [150]. Because of the unique constraints imposed by the calvarium on volume changes in the CNS, it is not surprising that volume receptors might exist there. Alterations of the sodium concentration of the cerebrospinal fluid may alter thirst and sodium appetite as well as modulate the release of antidiuretic hormone [4]. In addition, natriuretic hormone(s) has been allegedly isolated from various CNS tissues [110]. Undoubtedly, future work will reveal an increasing number and complexity of volume-sodium sensitive sensors that modulate sodium balance.

Control of Sodium Balance

The sodium excreted in the urine represents the difference between the amount filtered and that reabsorbed. In the normal state approximately 20,000 mEq of sodium are filtered per day while 200 mEq/d (1%) is excreted in the urine. Clearly, small changes in glomerular filtration or tubular reabsorption could result in massive alterations in sodium balance [37,129].

Approximately 50% to 70% of the initial filtrate is reabsorbed isotonically in the proximal convoluted and straight tubules. The absolute reabsorption varies with (1) the filtered load (so-called glomerulotubular balance), (2) alterations in peritubular physical forces (Starling forces) [103], (3) hormones (e.g., angiotensin II stimulates sodium reabsorption in rabbit proximal tubule) [147], and (4) sympathetic stimulation (adrenergic agents can directly increase tubular sodium and water reabsorption) [41].

The sodium that escapes reabsorption in the proximal tubule flows into the descending limb of Henle's loop where water is extracted into the hypertonic interstitium, concentrating the intratubular sodium. Subsequent ascent in the relatively sodium-permeable but water-impermeable thin limb allows for passive sodium diffusion into the interstitium. Washout of medullary tonicity could thus impair sodium reabsorption and result in natriuresis, particularly by the juxtamedullary nephrons [135]. In the thick ascending limb, active transport of sodium without water produces a hypotonic fluid that is delivered to the distal convoluted tubule. The thick ascending limb possesses considerable transport reserve, producing a fluid of nearly constant sodium concentration irrespective of variations in sodium delivery. Consequently, the major alterations in urinary sodium excretion occur in the more distal segments of the nephron [127].

Generally, 5% to 10% of the filtered sodium is delivered into the distal convoluted tubule where sodium reabsorption continues, but passive water reabsorption keeps the hypotonicity of the fluid nearly constant. Major changes in sodium concentration do occur, however, within the collecting duct [90,155]. The tight epithelium of this portion of the nephron is generally impermeable to salt and water. Yet, if stimulated by antidiuretic hormone or aldosterone, selective reabsorption of water or sodium ensues, thus allowing for fine tuning of the salt content and osmolality of the urine. Although only 2% to 3% of the filtered sodium is usually delivered into the collecting tu-

Table 23-1. *Efferent factors controlling sodium balance*

	Prominent site of action
Glomerular filtration rate	G
Renal perfusion pressure	?
Peritubular physical forces	P,(D)
Capillary hydrostatic, oncotic and interstitial pressures, and capillary epithelial permeability	
Nonelectrolyte composition of tubular fluid (e.g., glucose)	P
Transepithelial concentration gradients	P
Hormones	
Aldosterone	D
Angiotensin	G,P,D?
Antidiuretic hormone	G,D
Prostaglandins	G,D
Natriuretic factors(s)	G,P?,D
Sympathetic nervous system (catecholamines)	G,P,D

Abbreviations: G = glomerulus; P = proximal nephron; D = distal nephron.

bule, this is sufficient for the overall control of sodium balance [90,155].

Major factors that affect sodium excretion are listed in Table 23-1. Some general comments are in order. First, variations in glomerular filtration rate may substantially alter the filtered load of sodium, but its effect on renal sodium excretion is limited by glomerulotubular balance [129,156]. A somewhat analogous situation exists in primary, isolated alterations in peritubular factors affecting proximal sodium handling: tubulotubular balance blunts their impact on sodium excretion [129]. Factors that affect several nephron sites, such as adrenergic activity, renal hormones, or intrarenal distribution of blood flow, are potentially more potent in influencing sodium excretion. Yet, even with changes in these factors, secondary protective counterforces may intervene. For instance, after several days of sodium retention due to chronic infusion of aldosterone or angiotensin II, sodium escape occurs, perhaps related to the development of a compensatory pressure natriuresis [82,83]. This is another effector mechanism that probably represents a combination of several of the factors listed in Table 23-1.

The considerable data that exist apply to each of the factors that modify sodium excretion, studied singly, rather than to the hierarchy of complexity that develops when these factors are allowed to interact as they normally do. It is these interactions (or lack of them) that make understanding the pathophysiology of edema in renal diseases so difficult.

Pathogenesis of Edema in the Nephrotic Syndrome

The nephrotic syndrome comprises a diverse spectrum of conditions that share the clinical characteristics of marked proteinuria, hypoproteinemia, and edema (Chap. 54) [67]. Histopathologically, pathogenetically, and even clinically these diseases are heterogeneous. Yet, the mechanism of edema formation formally was considered to be basically the same for all. The marked proteinuria was thought to engender hypoproteinemia and consequently a reduced plasma colloid oncotic pressure. This, in turn, would alter transcapillary Starling forces, promoting increased flux of fluid into the interstitium and a decrease in blood volume. The decrement in plasma volume would then stimulate renal salt and water retention. This sequence of events is depicted in Figure 23-2 (left panel).

Because of its primary focus on the state of functional hypovolemia, this pathogenetic scheme was designated the underfilling hypothesis. The apparent simplicity of this scheme has led to its wide use as a pedagogic paradigm. Recent studies have brought into question the central role of vascular underfilling and have suggested instead that edema is a consequence of vascular overfilling brought about by a primary defect in renal salt and water excretion [44,45,64,65,88]. This alternative pathogenetic sequence is depicted in Figure 23-2 (right panel). The cause for the primary renal salt and water retention in the overfilling hypothesis is unknown. Current support for this hypothesis rests on the failure to demonstrate the existence of hypovolemia, coupled with the demonstration of renal salt retention in animal models of nephrotic syndrome [64,88].

It must be noted that a unitary pathophysiology of edema in nephrotic syndrome has come into question. Preliminary evidence suggests the existence of subsets of patients, some underfilled (minimal change disease) and others overfilled (nephrotic syndrome associated with other histologic forms) [65,84,125].

Systemic Factors in the Pathogenesis of Edema

BLOOD VOLUME

Central to the issue of the pathogenesis of edema in the nephrotic syndrome is the adequacy of the vascular volume, particularly as it affects renal perfusion and afferent stimuli for salt and water retention. This adequacy has been assessed by a number of different methods. Some of these approaches are listed in Table 23-2 along with the expected finding in underfilling or overfilling states. The interpre-

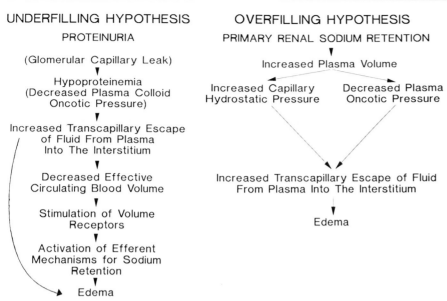

FIG. 23-2. *Underfilling and overfilling hypotheses for development of edema in nephrotic syndrome.*

TABLE 23-2. *Expected clinical and laboratory correlates of the underfilling and overfilling hypotheses*

	Underfilling	Overfilling
1. Plasma/blood volumes	↓	↑ normal
2. Hormones		
Norepinephrine	↑	↓ normal
Renin/aldosterone	↑	↓ normal
Antidiuretic hormone	↑	↓ normal
3. Plasma volume expansion	Diuresis (edema)	No diuresis (edema unchanged)
4. Hemodynamic measurements		
BP	↓	↑
Arterial pressure	↓	↑
5. Orthostatic changes	Present	Absent

tation of these measurements, however, requires some consideration.

Technical Considerations in Measurements of Blood Volume in the Nephrotic Syndrome

The most direct method to assess vascular volume is the indicator dilution technique based on the homogeneous distribution of a marker presumably limited to the vascular space [170]. The vascular space is composed of a fluid phase and a cellular phase, each of which can vary independently of the other (within obvious limits). No single marker can accurately and simultaneously measure both of these spaces. Consequently, the simultaneous assessment of vascular or blood volume (BV) has to depend on the use of two markers: one for plasma volume (PV, by ^{131}I-albumin) and another for RBC volume (RCV, by ^{51}Cr-labeled RBC).

A commonly used shortcut involves the measurement of only one of these spaces (either PV or RCV) from which the BV is calculated by a formula requiring the F-cell ratio (whole body hematocrit/venous hematocrit). This ratio corrects for the known disparity between the calculated whole body hematocrit and the peripheral venous hematocrits (that which is usually measured). The normal value of the ratio is around 0.85 to 0.90, but there is some variation even in normal subjects [8,121,170]. Problems arise, however, when the normal ratio is assumed to apply to disease states in which wide variations in F ratio have been shown to occur [95]. Thus, an accurate determination of BV must be based on the simultaneous measurement of PV and RCV.

Other factors affecting the determination of BV by the indicator dilution technique have been addressed elsewhere [170]. The alteration in albumin distribution and metabolism that occurs in nephrotic syndrome due to the increased transcapillary escape and hypercatabolism of albumin is important [64,67]. If not accounted for, these variables cause an overestimation of BV. Correction can be made by plotting ^{131}I-labeled albumin concentration as a function of time on semilog paper (assumes first order decay) and then determining the PV by extrapolating isotope concentration at time zero. BV must also be corrected for deviations in weight from the normal lean body mass.

Measurements of Blood Volume

From a historical perspective, the measurements of blood volume in nephrotic syndrome have left a legacy of confusing and conflicting results. PVs before and after resolution of the nephrotic syndrome have been reported to be increased, decreased, or unchanged [52,133]. This allowed one reviewer to state that PV is reduced in nephrotic syndrome [152] and another that this is a controversial issue [23]. Perhaps more than anything, these early data underscored the need for careful attention to the technical aspects of these measurements.

A survey of five articles published within the last decade comprising 117 patients with nephrotic syndrome (Table 23-3) suggests that only 5% of them have reduced BV [27,43,64,105,125]. Furthermore, in only 3 of 18 episodes of nephrotic syndrome (including 3 relapses) for which serial measurements are available did PV or BV increase after remission.

To date the most thorough analysis of this issue is the one by Dorhout-Mees et al. [44]. In their study, measurements of plasma and red cell volumes were simultaneously performed and BVs were corrected for lean body mass. These authors also corrected for transcapillary escape of albumin, which was found to be twice normal but to account only for a 1% overestimation in PV [44]. Only one nephrotic subject out of 88 fell below the 95% confidence limit for normal blood volume, whereas 13 were above their expected BVs. Thus, the evidence appears to favor a normal or expanded BV in most edematous patients with the nephrotic syndrome [44].

Although as a group patients with nephrotic syndrome appear to have high-to-normal BVs, there is some stratification between the various pathologic subgroups. In agreement with an earlier study [125], a more recent one

[65] revealed a tendency toward lower PV in patients with minimal changes than among those with other lesions.

Since BV measurements by themselves do not define fully the adequacy of vascular filling, an assessment of other systemic hemodynamic factors is important.

SYSTEMIC HEMODYNAMICS

Shapiro et al [148] have examined systemic hemodynamics by inserting Swan-Ganz catheters in nine edematous patients with nephrotic syndrome. Only one patient had minimal change disease. In addition to confirming a normal PV they found that mean arterial pressure, cardiac index, left and right atrial pressures, and systemic vascular resistance were not different in the nephrotic and normal subjects.

Earlier studies suggested that excessive orthostatic hypotension, occasionally with fainting, occurs with some frequency in patients with nephrotic syndrome [172]. Presumably, excessive transcapillary leak caused decreased BV on standing. This was assumed to promote renal salt and water retention in addition to hypotension [51]. A study by Dorhout-Mees et al. revealed that the decrease in PV on standing was indeed larger in nephrotic than in normal subjects [44], and that the diastolic BP rose more with standing in nephrotic syndrome than in normal subjects, suggesting increased peripheral resistance. However, neither orthostatic hypotension nor tachycardia was observed in either group.

HYPOPROTEINEMIA

Hypoproteinemia has been assumed to play a primary role in the pathogenesis of edema in nephrotic syndrome [49,152]. This was supported by the fact that experimentally induced hypoproteinemia by repeated plasmapheresis produced edema and occasionally ascites in dogs [166]. However, although sodium retention was noted throughout plasmapheresis, edema did not become manifest until the serum albumin level decreased below 1.5 to 1.0 g/dl. Furthermore, an adequate salt intake was necessary for its development. One dog that did not eat failed to develop edema despite comparably reduced serum albumin concentration. Edema occurred also in protein malnourished dogs

TABLE 23-3. Measurements of blood volume in patients with nephrotic syndrome

| | | Number of patients | |
Reference	Total	Low blood volume (<90% nl)	High blood volume (>110% nl)
Meltzer et al. (125)	5*	1	4
Dorhout Mees et al. (43)	13*	0	4
Brown et al. (26,27)	12	3	3
Krishna and Danovitch et al. (105)	9	1	4
Geers et al. (64)	88	1†	13†
Total	127	6	28

* Paired measurements: blood volume determined during the edematous phase and again during remission.
† Values above or below the 95% confidence limits.

at higher levels of serum albumin (1.5–2.0 g/dl) and without as marked a dependence on sodium intake [166] as in normally nourished dogs, thereby suggesting a possible role for protein starvation in the pathogenesis of edema of nephrosis.

Although severe hypoproteinemia can produce edema, patients with nephrotic syndrome often have only moderately reduced serum protein levels and no evidence of protein malnutrition. Furthermore, a number of subjects with congenital analbuminemia had no evidence of edema [10,96]. In these unusual patients salt and water homeostasis was achieved in spite of a reduced oncotic pressure by maintaining a near normal glomerular filtration rate (due to increased filtration fraction) and reducing tubular sodium reabsorption [10,96].

Reduction in plasma protein concentration triggers various compensatory factors that minimize the tendency to edema. The fall in plasma oncotic pressure initially results in an increased filtration flux that dilutes and expands the interstitium. In response to this, there is an increased lymphatic flow that removes excess fluid and protein from the interstitium, reducing the interstitial oncotic pressure and tending to restore the normal transcapillary fluid balance [132,169]. Clearly, limits exist to this compensatory mechanism, but in minimal-to-moderate hypoproteinemia a balance can be achieved.

One consequence of this adaptation to hypoproteinemia is relative protection of intravascular volume. Studies by Manning and Guyton [122] in plasmapheresis-induced hypoproteinemic dogs support this conclusion. A 33% decrease in plasma protein (to about 5 g/dl) increased the sodium space by 11% but did not affect the BV or PV. A 68% decrease in plasma protein (to 2.4 g/dl) resulted in a marked decrease in PV and BV (about 65% of control) and a substantial increase in plasma renin activity. Blockade of the alpha-sympathetic and angiotensin systems failed to affect BV homeostasis during moderate hypoproteinemia (33% decrease in plasma proteins). Interpretation of these results is complicated by a decrease in mean arterial pressure during hypoproteinemia that might have influenced the salt and water balance. Overall, the results suggest that moderate degrees of hypoproteinemia may not be associated with a decreased BV and that marked renal salt and water retention must be due to other factors [121,122,169].

Thus, hypoproteinemia by itself is rarely the cause of edema in nephrotic syndrome. Yet, its presence reduces the protective reserve that exists against edema formation [92a]. Mechanisms that normally induce escape from excessive sodium accumulation (i.e., increased renal perfusion pressure [83]) may be affected by the low oncotic pressure, resulting in an overflow into the interstitial compartment and thus in edema formation.

HORMONAL FACTORS

A number of hormones, including angiotensin II, aldosterone, and catecholamines, have been considered to be functional indices of volume status [123], at least in normal subjects. This reflects their role in the regulation of systemic and renal hemodynamics and in the tubular control of salt and water excretion by the kidney. Considerable interest, therefore, has centered on hormone levels in nephrotic syndrome, both as mediators of the observed renal avidity for salt and water as well as a gauge of the effective circulating volume.

Aldosterone and Plasma Renin Activity

Early studies revealed the presence of excess amounts of a sodium-retaining corticoid in the urine of children with nephrotic syndrome [116]. This hormone was later identified as aldosterone. Subsequent studies have demonstrated increased, normal, or decreased aldosterone levels in both plasma and urine of such patients [3,27,32,84,134]. Similarly, high, normal, or low levels of plasma renin have been found [18,27,32,84,125]. Interpretation of these results is difficult because almost all studies have been done during the established phase of nephrotic syndrome in patients with varying degrees of urinary sodium retention and oral sodium intake. The use of steroids, diuretics, and other treatment modalities, as well as the variability in the nature of the nephrotic syndrome and in the extent of alterations in glomerular hemodynamic and renal tubular functions, obscure further relevant associations.

A survey of studies published from 1977 through 1984 highlights the continued controversy in the field. Chonko et al. [32] sodium loaded 10 adult patients with nephrotic syndrome who had high plasma renin, eight of whom also had high plasma aldosterone levels. In only two of these patients was the plasma renin suppressed by the ingestion of a sodium supplement of 300 mEq/d. Meltzer et al. [125] studied 16 adult patients with nephrotic syndrome of various etiologies, in clinical circumstances ranging from untreated edema and avid sodium retention to the diuretic phase, either spontaneous or treatment induced. Based on the result of renin profiling (relative to sodium excretion), these authors proposed the existence of two pathophysiologic forms of edema in the nephrotic syndrome: (1) the classic form, characterized by high renin and aldosterone levels secondary to hypovolemia, seen primarily in patients with the minimal change lesion, and (2) a form characterized by low plasma renin and aldosterone levels, associated with hypervolemia and hypertension, presumed due to a primary defect in renal sodium excretion. The majority of these patients presumably had histologic lesions other than minimal change. Remission was associated with a return of the hormonal profile to normal in both groups. In contrast, Dorhout-Mees et al. [43] found normal or reduced plasma renin activities (corrected for sodium intake) in 10 adult patients with steroid-responsive (minimal change) nephrotic syndrome. During 11 episodes of remission (one relapse included), the plasma renin increased in eight and decreased in only three. Furthermore, the patients tended to have hypertension and normal to elevated BVs, which decreased after remission. A subsequent study of 27 patients with diverse histologic forms of nephrotic syndrome, including some of the patients in the earlier group, revealed normal or suppressed plasma renin activity for the level of sodium intake in 24 of the patients (89%) and elevated plasma renin in only three (11%), all of whom had minimal change disease. Plasma renin substrate was also studied and found to be low in 8% and normal or elevated in 92% of the patients, suggesting that substrate limitation is not a cause for the normal or low renin levels [18].

A somewhat different picture, supporting the observations of Meltzer et al., emerged from the study by Ammenti et al. [3] of 24 children (18 with minimal change disease) during relapse. In addition to plasma renin and aldosterone, they examined the urinary excretion of aldosterone precursors and of products of aldosterone metabolism, including urinary free aldosterone, aldosterone-18 glucuronide, and tetra-hydroaldosterone. Whereas only 22% of the nephrotic children, all with edema, had elevated basal levels of plasma aldosterone, the proportion of patients with elevated excretion of free aldosterone and aldosterone precursors and metabolites was 44%. There was a strong inverse correlation between the urinary excretion of sodium and aldosterone. A weaker inverse correlation was noted between plasma albumin and urinary aldosterone excretion, indicating that the low serum albumin stimulated the secretion of aldosterone, presumably through hypovolemia. The authors suggested that increased aldosterone levels are necessary for edema formation in patients with nephrotic syndrome.

Two studies in adults have also revealed an indirect correlation between sodium excretion and plasma aldosterone [65,140]. In addition, one study showed a weak indirect correlation between serum albumin and plasma aldosterone [65]. However, this study revealed no significant correlation between BV and either plasma renin activity, aldosterone, or serum albumin levels. However, when only patients with minimal change disease were considered, an indirect correlation between BV and plasma aldosterone was noted. These findings are generally supported by two other studies [27,134]. In rats with nephrotic syndrome induced by aminonucleoside of puromycin, a model of human lipoid nephrosis [36,88,91], adrenalectomy, followed by constant replacement doses of aldosterone and corticosterone, prevented the development of edema. Administration of aldosterone in a dose sufficient to raise the plasma aldosterone concentration to that observed in intact nephrotic rats resulted in edema [91]. Thus, hyperaldosteronism, ostensibly secondary to hypovolemia, was presumably the primary cause of renal salt and water retention. It must be noted, however, that increased aldosterone levels were not needed for edema formation if the animals were on a high sodium diet [91].

Both captopril, an angiotensin-converting enzyme inhibitor, and saralasin, a competitive blocker of angiotensin II with weak agonist properties, have been used in an attempt to blunt edema formation [27,28,46]. Administration of captopril to eight adult patients for 5 days during 10 episodes of fluid retention revealed no marked effect on renal sodium excretion [28]. The expected effects of increased plasma renin activity and decreased aldosterone were documented. However, careful inspection of the data reveals that over half of the patients with low initial urinary sodium excretion and high plasma renin activity had a mild but definite natriuretic response. Several and possibly all of these patients had minimal change disease. Furthermore, the documented drop in BP during captopril administration may have limited a more impressive natriuresis.

Acute intravenous administration of saralasin to six patients with nephrotic syndrome (unspecified histology) failed to produce a natriuresis [46]. Declining glomerular filtration rates and unchanged or increased plasma aldosterone levels complicated the interpretation of the results. Finally, suppression of renin and aldosterone by acute hyperoncotic albumin infusion (3 days) produced only small and inconsequential natriuresis [26,101].

In summary, we can state that average plasma renin activity and aldosterone levels are not significantly elevated when measured in a heterogeneous sample of patients with nephrotic syndrome. However, stratification suggests higher values in patients with minimal change disease and lower levels in those with other histologic lesions [65,84,125], thus supporting the presence of functional hypovolemia in minimal change disease but not in other forms of nephrotic syndrome.

Catecholamines

Kelsch et al. [94] showed elevated plasma norepinephrine levels in children with edema and avid sodium retention. Dorhout-Mees et al. [44] noted normal levels in supine adults but an exaggerated elevation on standing. Criticism was directed at the former investigators for performing the measurements at a 30 degree tilt. Differences in the histology of nephrotic syndrome between children and adults may account for the inconsistency of the findings.

Vasopressin

Plasma vasopressin has been measured in patients with nephrotic syndrome (8 of 16 subjects with minimal change disease). In spite of mild hyponatremia, the levels were not significantly higher than those of control subjects [158]. Failure to suppress vasopressin by a water load correlated with decreased BV.

Natriuretic Factor

Volume expansion with saline has been shown to stimulate a natriuretic factor(s) in both animals and humans [29,30,56,58,92,110]. The resulting natriuresis is independent of glomerular filtration rate or levels of mineralocorticoids [40,56,92]. Given the marked extracellular volume expansion present in nephrotic syndrome, the natriuretic factor should be elevated. However, several investigators [21,71] have failed to reveal natriuretic activity in either plasma or urine of patients with nephrotic syndrome. This was in contrast to non-nephrotic patients with chronic renal failure. Favre and Gourjon [57] have found that in normal rats, but not in nephrotic rats, saline expansion stimulated natriuretic activity of kidney extract. However, nephrotic rats demonstrated a natriuretic response equal to that of normal rats when injected with natriuretic factor extracted from human urine. This suggests that the production, release, and/or activation of this natriuretic factor is impaired in nephrotic syndrome.

In summary, renin, aldosterone, norepinephrine, and antidiuretic hormones appear low or normal in nephrotic syndrome with histologic lesions other than minimal change but elevated in patients with the minimal change lesion. Yet, correlations between BV and hormonal levels are often absent or weak, pointing toward the existence of confounding factors controlling the release and metabolism of these hormones [123]. No information is available about renal hormones, such as prostaglandins [62].

The role of the hormones in the pathogenesis of salt and water retention in nephrotic syndrome remains unsettled. Isolated primary hyperaldosteronism does not result in edema formation, due to the escape mechanisms [5,83, 102]. Yet, in nephrotic syndrome many studies have revealed a correlation between sodium excretion or serum albumin and plasma aldosterone levels, suggesting some, although not necessarily a cause and effect, relationship.

VOLUME EXPANSION

Both intravascular volume expansion with hyperoncotic solutions and head-out water immersion produce a diuresis and natriuresis in some edematous patients with nephrosis [12,46,89,105,114,115,126,148]. This observation has been used as support for the underfilling hypothesis. In 1945 Thorn et al. [157] demonstrated a satisfactory diuresis by daily infusion of a 10% albumin solution to edematous adult patients with glomerulonephritis. Subsequent studies confirmed these findings in both children and adults [49,89,114,115,126]. The response to hyperoncotic infusion consisted of an early diuresis followed by a natriuresis. Although in some patients glomerular filtration rate went up with the infusion, this was inconsistent. Altered tubular sodium reabsorption was postulated to play the prominent role, due to the suppression of aldosterone and antidiuretic hormone by volume expansion [115,126]. Unfortunately, this therapy was successful mostly in patients with modest hypoproteinemia and high rates of glomerular filtration.

Two recent studies have indicated that PV expansion evokes only minimal natriuresis [26,101]. The reports describe 15 attempts to expand BV and produce a natriuresis in 13 adult patients with nephrotic syndrome (eight with minimal change histology). In spite of reduction of renin and aldosterone levels into the low normal range and elevation of BVs, only a small natriuresis was observed. Continued infusion tended to produce increasing natriuresis in two of three patients so studied. No patient was said to have exhibited a negative sodium balance while on an intake of 100 to 180 mEq sodium per day.

Head-out water immersion, in which peripheral venous and subcutaneous fluid is hydrostatically compressed toward the thorax, results in central BV expansion. Diuresis and natriuresis follow, in both normal subjects and in patients with nephrotic syndrome [12,105,148]. The natriuresis was positively correlated with baseline plasma volume [105] and with inulin clearance [148].

Intrarenal Factors in the Pathogenesis of Edema in the Nephrotic Syndrome

RENAL HEMODYNAMICS

In view of the marked variability in underlying pathology, it is not surprising that in patients with the nephrotic syndrome the glomerular filtration rate is also variable. In one study [148] glomerular filtration rate measured by inulin clearance was found to range from 10 to nearly 100 ml/min with an average of 55 ml/min. The clearance of para-aminohippurate was also reduced, but not to the same degree as the inulin clearance. Hence, filtration fraction was less than normal in all patients. Similar findings have been reported by others [11,65,140]. In general, patients

with minimal change nephrotic syndrome maintain normal rates of glomerular filtration, whereas those with other histologic lesions do not. The reduced filtration fraction in the face of hypoproteinemia (which should increase filtration fraction) suggests a decrease in the glomerular capillary permeability coefficient. A number of studies have revealed a direct correlation between fractional sodium excretion and inulin clearance in patients with nephrotic syndrome [49,140,148]. However, glomerular filtration rate is often normal or supranormal in patients with nephrotic syndrome, suggesting that sodium retention is due to other variables.

TUBULAR FACTORS

A decrease in filtration fraction should result in decreased proximal tubular reabsorption and adequate salt and water excretion unless excessive distal reabsorption occurs. Earley and collaborators [78] demonstrated a markedly decreased proximal fractional sodium reabsorption by inducing distal blockade with chlorthiazide and ethacrynic acid in five patients with nephrotic syndrome. By contrast, Koomans et al [101] found increased proximal sodium reabsorption during water diuresis. Both studies, however, showed increased distal sodium reabsorption. This was confirmed by studies of experimental nephrosis. Bernard et al [13] assessed sodium handling by micropuncture techniques in a model of nephrosis similar to membranous nephropathy (autologous immune complex nephropathy), in which glomerular filtration is well maintained. Compared with control animals, proximal sodium reabsorption was reduced although distal delivery was the same. Sodium reabsorption was unaltered in the loop of Henle and distal convoluted tubule. The fraction of sodium appearing in the urine was significantly lower in the nephrotic than in control rats, suggesting enhanced reabsorption in the collecting duct or a population of deep nephrons. Some problems arise in interpreting their data since the animals were volume expanded, which may by itself alter proximal tubular function. Also unaccounted for are possible changes in renal interstitial pressure [7,111].

Ichikawa et al [88] used a unilateral infusion of puromycin aminonucleoside to induce nephrosis in one kidney while avoiding the systemic effects of hypoproteinemia. Fractional reabsorption of sodium was higher in the infused than in the contralateral kidney. Although glomerular filtration rate was moderately reduced, sodium delivery to the distal tubule was normal, and the sodium retention appeared to occur at a site beyond the distal convoluted tubule. Administration of saralasin increased glomerular filtration rate but failed to increase sodium excretion. Thus, there were alterations in sodium handling in this model of nephrotic syndrome that were independent of systemic hemodynamic or hormonal influence.

Pathogenesis of Edema in Glomerulonephritis

Edema in acute glomerulonephritis, although hardly ever as severe as in the nephrotic syndrome, is, nevertheless, quite common [31,85,107–109]. Characteristically, it is periorbital and facial but occasionally is generalized, particularly if excessive salt intake is allowed [131]. Interestingly, patients with rapidly progressive glomerulonephritis appear to have a lower incidence of edema despite the severity of the disease [118,128,130].

Systemic Factors in the Pathogenesis of Edema in Glomerulonephritis

In contrast to the classical picture of hypovolemia in the nephrotic syndrome, the acute nephritic syndrome presents with signs and symptoms of vascular congestion. Indeed, acute glomerulonephritis is often associated with hypertension and occasionally with severe pulmonary congestion and congestive heart failure [31,85,107,109,131,143]. This vascular congestion in the setting of a reduced glomerular filtration rate, enhanced tubular reabsorption of sodium, and often normal serum protein concentration suggests a primary renal cause for salt and water retention. Hence, nephritic edema appears to result from a vascular overflow that makes the transcapillary forces favoring filtration exceed those promoting reabsorption. Interstitial fluid volume and pressures thus rise until the Starling forces reach a new balance.

In general, clinical studies have supported this pathophysiologic scheme. As noted previously, hypertension and symptoms of congestive heart failure are common. Over two-thirds of patients hospitalized with poststreptococcal glomerulonephritis have hypertension (up to 90% in some reports), which correlates loosely with the presence of edema [31,47,109,131,142,143].

The hypertension is considered to be volume mediated, although the evidence is circumstantial. BP was found to correlate directly with fluid retention [142], and the plasma renin levels were found to be low [15,137]. Moreover, plasma renin and aldosterone concentrations were reported to be appropriately suppressed for the degree of fluid retention [142]. Finally, sodium restriction appears to ameliorate the hypertension [131].

Evidence of congestive heart failure with pulmonary edema and elevated venous pressure occurs in approximately 10% to 20% of patients with acute poststreptococcal glomerulonephritis [85,109,131], although considerably higher frequencies have been reported [31,131]. Cases of acute glomerulonephritis with congestive symptoms in the absence of hypertension have also been reported [75]; thus, hypertension may play little more than a contributory role [131]. Myocarditis, described in some of adult patients with acute glomerulonephritis [75], is practically nonexistent among children [31].

The overwhelming preponderance of studies indicate that primary sodium and water retention is the proximate cause of high output cardiac failure in acute glomerulonephritis. Blood volume is elevated in patients with acute poststreptococcal glomerulonephritis even without symptoms of congestion or obvious cardiac failure, suggesting that the expansion of the intravascular volume precedes the circulatory congestion [42,50]. Moreover, hemodynamic evaluation performed during circulatory congestion has revealed elevated cardiac index, stroke volume, and both left and right filling pressures [39]. An elevated oxygen consumption and reduced arteriovenous oxygen differ-

ence were also observed. With exercise there is an appropriate increase in cardiac index, suggesting the existence of adequate cardiac reserve [14]. These findings are characteristic of high output cardiac failure, apparently due to salt and water retention.

An elevated capillary hydraulic pressure secondary to sodium retention appears to be the main cause of edema in acute glomerulonephritis. Hypoproteinemia is usually lacking or is of such modest degree that a reduced plasma oncotic pressure plays only a minimal role. There is no alteration in capillary permeability leading to interstitial transudation of protein and fluid [164], although this may be a factor in acute glomerulonephritis associated with systemic vasculitis. Changes in interstitial hydraulic and oncotic pressures are probably compensatory rather than primary.

Renal Mechanisms of Sodium Retention in Glomerulonephritis

As is evident from the foregoing discussion, an increase in the renal reabsorption of sodium is central to the retention of fluid seen in glomerulonephritis. Although glomerular filtration rate is consistently depressed in patients with acute glomerulonephritis, this is unlikely by itself to lead to edema [156]. There is no evidence from clinical studies of an abnormality in proximal tubular function [47]. On the other hand, there is a blunted response to a saline load [17], which is not due to the decrease in glomerular filtration rate (GFR) [48] or to aldosterone excess [137,142].

Experimental models of acute glomerulonephritis have also been used in an attempt to elucidate the mechanism of solute and water retention. Nephrotoxic serum nephritis (antiglomerular basement membrane glomerulonephritis) is an animal model of acute glomerulonephritis that mimics human antiglomerular basement membrane disease [171]. In this model basal fractional sodium excretion is low and natriuresis in response to isotonic saline volume expansion is subnormal [16,167]. Clearance studies have revealed a 30% to 40% decrease in GFR with relatively normal renal blood flow, suggesting a reduced filtration fraction. The reduced filtered load of sodium in the presence of a normal proximal glomerulotubular balance resulted in a reduction in absolute proximal resorption [87]. Despite the reduction in proximal tubular reabsorption, distal sodium and water deliveries were low. The low fractional sodium excretion was presumed to result both from decreased absolute distal delivery as well as enhanced distal fractional sodium reabsorption [163]. Similar findings were reported in both unilateral and bilateral nephrotoxic nephritis [138].

Kuroda et al. [106] employed micropuncture to examine sodium reabsorption in this model of acute glomerulonephritis. They found increased proximal tubular reabsorption associated with increased proximal tubular hydrostatic pressure and dilated tubules, suggesting that tubular obstruction, possibly by proteinaceous casts, increased resistance to flow and thus increased proximal tubular reabsorption and decreased salt and water excretion. There was a substantial decrease in glomerular filtration rate in this model (40% decrement from normal) associated with a proportional reduction in the clearance of sodium. As sodium clearance is preserved with this degree of decrease in glomerular filtration rate, the authors postulated that the tubular obstruction they observed must have caused the decreased sodium clearance.

Godon [70] reported that rats in the delayed phase of autologous nephrotoxic nephritis had a reduced basal fractional sodium excretion and impaired natriuresis in response to hypertonic saline infusion. This was allegedly due to an altered glomerulotubular balance [72], induced by the absence of a natriuretic substance produced by cortical tubular cells [71,73].

A number of studies of delayed autologous nephrotoxic nephritis are in general disagreement with the findings of Godon [1,113,124,141,162]. In particular, a normal or increased basal fractional sodium excretion was observed, associated with relatively well-preserved glomerulotubular balance [87,159], but an impaired natriuresis in response to acute saline loading [163]. There is no clear explanation for the discrepancy between the result obtained by Godon and those obtained by others. Presumably, some nuances in the methods of producing the autologous nephrotoxic nephritis account for the divergent results.

Pathogenesis of Edema in Chronic Renal Failure

Chronic, progressive decrements in glomerular filtration rate impose an increasing impediment on the maintenance of a normal sodium balance. Assuming a constant sodium intake, every 50% reduction in glomerular filtration rate (and thus filtered sodium load) requires a compensatory two-fold increase in fractional sodium excretion. This has been referred to as the magnification phenomenon [24,25]. The mechanisms involved depend on the primary cause of renal insufficiency, but, in general, as the absolute filtered load of sodium falls, a geometric decrease in fractional renal tubular sodium reabsorption must occur. Failure of this homeostatic mechanism will lead to progressive sodium retention, circulatory congestion, and edema. The relative infrequency of these clinical signs underscores the remarkable adequacy of this mechanism. In fact, the presence of clinical edema in chronic renal failure (in the absence of the nephrotic syndrome) often suggests progression to a critically low glomerular filtration rate or intercurrent secondary causes of edema formation, such as congestive heart failure or cardiac tamponade.

Considering for a moment the determinants of transcapillary fluid flux, it would seem likely that the pathogenesis of edema in chronic renal failure would be similar to that of acute glomerulonephritis, namely an increase in capillary hydrostatic pressure due to impaired salt excretion. Yet, despite the frequent occurrence of hypertension [34,123], elevated PVs [17,98,136], and the potential presence of a uremic myocardiopathy [104], edema is distinctly uncommon. Clearly, a remarkable adaptation in sodium handling must occur to limit sodium retention and edema formation. Although the major adaptation concerns renal sodium excretion (to be discussed in the following section), several

studies suggest that changes in the compliance of the interstitium may also occur.

Koomans et al [97,98] have reported that patients with moderate-to-severe chronic renal failure manifest a high sensitivity to salt, which results in an inappropriate rise in BP during intravenous saline infusion. From measurements of extracellular volume and PV they concluded that, for a given sodium load, there is an inverse correlation between creatinine clearance and the expansion in PV relative to interstitial volume. This suggests an altered transcapillary fluid distribution in severe chronic renal failure. Although a subsequent study has raised doubts about this conclusion [99], the presence of increased salt sensitivity has important implications. For instance, for a given salt intake, patients with chronic renal failure may have greater increases in BP than subjects with normal renal function. This may activate afferent volume sensors, leading to enhanced renal sodium excretion. In addition, the high BP may by itself induce increased renal sodium excretion [80].

In general, sodium homeostasis is well regulated in chronic renal failure, as virtually all patients come into sodium balance when placed on either very low or very high salt intake. However, the reduction in sodium intake needs to be very gradual in order for this balance to be achieved [35]. A progressive decrease in glomerular filtration rate is associated with increasing fractional excretion of sodium that results in the maintenance of external sodium balance [24,25,151]. Acute saline loading of patients with chronic renal failure results in an appropriate decrease in fractional sodium reabsorption, the magnitude of which is inversely proportional to the baseline glomerular filtration rate [79,151].

Clearance studies have suggested that both decreased proximal and distal reabsorption contribute to the natriuresis [100]. This decreased fractional reabsorption of sodium was found to occur independent of acute alterations in glomerular filtration rate or serum aldosterone levels [146,151,168]. DeWardener et al. [29,33,40] have suggested that this response is mediated by a natriuretic factor, which was demonstrated in patients with chronic renal failure and studied in laboratory animals [21,30,58,60]. The substance was uniformly found in patients with chronic renal failure who demonstrated the appropriate adaptation in fractional sodium excretion [20]. Yet, patients with nephrotic syndrome and animals in which sodium intake was reduced in proportion to the decrease in glomerular filtration rate failed to demonstrate either the natriuretic factor or increased fractional sodium excretion [21,144].

In addition, the diseased kidney possesses intrinsic adaptive mechanisms. Gutmann and Rieselbach [79] have demonstrated in humans and dogs that, even in the absence of a uremic environment or apparent volume expansion, the diseased kidney is more reactive to an acute saline load than its normal counterpart. A subsequent study suggested that this effect was mediated in part by acute alterations in peritubular Starling forces to which the diseased kidney appears to be more sensitive than the normal organ [160].

An enhanced responsiveness of the diseased kidney to natriuretic factor has also been noted by Fine et al [59,60]. In contrast to Gutmann and Rieselbach [79], however, they found an enhanced end-organ response to natriuretic factor only in the diseased kidneys functioning in a uremic environment. In addition to the peritubular factors mentioned, saline loading also lowers hematocrit, increases glomerular filtration rate, and alters volume-sensitive hormone release, including natriuretic factor [129]. This combination of factors probably elicits the enhanced sodium excretion of diseased kidneys in the nonuremic environment.

It must be noted that patients with chronic renal failure are not a homogeneous group. Hypertension and sodium retention are more frequent in the glomerular than the tubulointerstitial type of chronic renal failure [74,123]. Further differences characterize these two categories of chronic renal failure at the single nephron level.

When studied by micropuncture, experimental chronic glomerulonephritis is found to be associated with a generalized decrease in single nephron glomerular filtration rate [1,141,162] and a normal glomerulotubular balance [1,113,161,162]. If sodium balance is to be maintained, large decreases in fractional sodium resorption must occur in the distal nephron.

The experimentally produced pyelonephritic or remnant kidney serves as a model for the tubulointerstitial form of chronic renal failure. The prominent feature of these models is a normal (pyelonephritis) or elevated (remnant kidney) single nephron glomerular filtration rate, with wide variability in individual values [2,112,145,165]. The increase in single nephron glomerular filtration rate is attributable to increases in glomerular plasma flow and glomerular hydrostatic pressure [38]. Assuming constancy of proximal glomerulotubular balance [6,25], the absolute distal sodium delivery per nephron must be normal or high. Yet, the absolute delivery for the entire kidney is significantly reduced due to a lower number of nephrons. Hence, as in experimental glomerulonephritis, in experimental nonglomerular chronic renal failure distal fractional sodium resorption must be decreased in order to maintain external sodium balance. Thus, in each of these models of chronic renal failure the distal tubule serves as the major site for the modulation of sodium reabsorption [25].

While sodium balance is maintained in chronic renal failure, the rapidity with which adjustments can occur appears to be diminished. Bourgoignie et al. [22] acutely administered a saline load to dogs with a remnant kidney and moderate chronic renal insufficiency. Urine collected over the next 5 hours was found to contain much less of the sodium load than in normal animals. This was associated with a hemodilution of circulating proteins, suggesting intravascular volume expansion. A subsequent period of 24 hours was required to restore sodium balance.

Fluid retention might be the stimulus for adaptation. Bricker et al. [146,151] offer a dissenting opinion. Rats with remnant kidneys and moderate chronic renal failure were found to excrete a sodium load as well as normal rats. These investigators suggested that adaptation occurred independently of chronic extracellular fluid volume expansion.

Although all the previously mentioned studies convey the view that the diseased kidney is capable of maintaining sodium balance over a wide range of sodium intakes, it must be noted that this adaptation is by no means as wide as it is in normal subjects. Flexibility decreases with decreasing renal function. If sodium intake exceeds excretory capacity of the kidney, positive sodium balance and edema ensue. The positive sodium balance frequently plays an important role in the pathogenesis of the hypertension seen in advanced renal insufficiency; the increase in systemic pressure, in turn, can accelerate the deterioration in renal function. It is important therefore to ensure that neither positive nor negative sodium balance occurs in these patients.

References

1. Allison MEM, Wilson CB, Gottschalk CW: Pathophysiology of experimental glomerulonephritis in rats. J Clin Invest 53:1402, 1974.
2. Allison MEM, Lipham EM, Lassiter WE, et al: The acutely reduced kidney. Kidney Int 3:354, 1973.
3. Ammenti A, Muller-Wiefel DE, Scharer K, et al: Mineralocorticoids in the nephrotic syndrome of children. Clin Nephrol 14:238, 1980.
4. Andersson B, Ledsell LG, Rundgren M: Regulation of body fluids: Intake and output. In Staub NC, Taylor AE (eds): Edema. New York, Raven Press, 1984.
5. August JT, Nelson DH, Thorn GW: Response of normal subjects to large amounts of aldosterone. J Clin Invest 37:1549, 1958.
6. Bank N, Aynedjian HS: Individual nephron function in experimental bilateral pyelonephritis. I. Glomerular filtration rate and proximal tubular sodium, potassium, and water reabsorption. J Lab Clin Med 68:713, 1966.
7. Bank N, Aynedjian HS: Failure of changes in intracapillary pressures to alter proximal fluid reabsorption. Kidney Int 26:275, 1984.
8. Bauer JH, Brooks CS: Body-fluid composition in normal and hypertensive man. Clin Sci 62:43, 1982.
9. Bennett M, Thompson GR, Glassock RJ: Sodium homeostasis in acute glomerulonephritis. Miner Electrolyte Metab 2:63, 1979.
10. Bennhold H, Klaus D, Scheurlen PG: Volume regulation and renal function in analbuminaemia. Lancet 2:1169, 1960.
11. Berg U, Bohlin AB: Renal hemodynamics in minimal change nephrotic syndrome in childhood. Int J Pediatr Nephrol 3:187, 1982.
12. Berlyne GM, Brown C, Adler A, et al: Water immersion in nephrotic syndrome. Arch Intern Med 141:1275, 1981.
13. Bernard DB, Alexander EA, Couser WG, et al: Renal sodium retention during volume expansion in experimental nephrotic syndrome. Kidney Int 14:478, 1978.
14. Binak K, Sirmaci N, Ucak D, et al: Circulatory changes in acute glomerulonephritis at rest and during exercise. Br Heart J 37:833, 1975.
15. Birkenhager WH, Schalekamp MADH, Schalenkamp-Kuyken MPA, et al: Interrelations between arterial pressure, fluid-volumes, and plasma-renin concentration in the course of acute glomerulonephritis. Lancet 1:1086, 1970.
16. Blantz RC, Wilson CB: Acute effects of antiglomerular basement membrane antibody on the process of glomerular filtration in the rat. J Clin Invest 58:899, 1976.
17. Blumberg A, Nelp WB, Hegstrom RV, et al: Extracellular volume in patients with chronic renal disease treated for hypertension by sodium restriction. Lancet 2:69, 1967.
18. Boer P, Roos JC, Geyskes GG, et al: Observations on plasma

renin substrate in the nephrotic syndrome. *Nephron* 26:121, 1980.

19. Bonventre JV, Leaf A: Sodium homeostasis: Steady states without a set point. *Kidney Int* 21:880, 1982.

20. Bourgoignie JJ, Hwang KH, Espinel C, et al: A natriuretic factor in the serum of patients with chronic uremia. *J Clin Invest* 51:1514, 1972.

21. Bourgoignie JJ, Hwang KH, Ipakchi E, et al: The presence of a natriuretic factor in urine of patients with chronic uremia: The absence of the factor in nephrotic uremic patients. *J Clin Invest* 53:1559, 1974.

22. Bourgoignie JJ, Kaplan M, Gavellas G, et al: Sodium homeostasis in dogs with chronic renal insufficiency. *Kidney Int* 21:820, 1982.

23. Bradley SE, Tyson CJ: The "nephrotic syndrome." *N Engl J Med* 238:260, 1948.

24. Bricker NS, Fine LG, Kaplan M, et al: "Magnification phenomenon" in chronic renal disease. *N Engl J Med* 299:1287, 1978.

25. Bricker NS: Sodium homeostasis in chronic renal disease. *Kidney Int* 21:886, 1982.

26. Brown EA, Sagnella GA, Jones BE, et al: Evidence that some mechanism other than the renin system causes sodium retention in nephrotic syndrome. *Lancet* 2:1237, 1982.

27. Brown EA, Markandu ND, Roulston JE, et al: Is the renin-angiotensin-aldosterone system involved in the sodium retention in the nephrotic syndrome. *Nephron* 32:102, 1982.

28. Brown EA, Markandu ND, Sagnella GA, et al: Lack of effect of captopril on the sodium retention of the nephrotic syndrome. *Nephron* 37:43, 1984.

29. Brown PR, Koutsaimanis KG, DeWardener HE: Effect of urinary extracts from salt-loaded man on urinary sodium excretion by the rat. *Kidney Int* 2:1, 1972.

30. Buckalew VM Jr, Nelson DB: Natriuretic and sodium transport inhibitory activity in plasma of volume-expanded dogs. *Kidney Int* 5:12, 1974.

31. Burke FG, Ross S: Acute glomerulonephritis. A review of ninety cases. *J Pediatr* 30:157, 1947.

32. Chonko AV, Bay WH, Stein JH, et al: The role of renin and aldosterone in the salt retention of edema. *Am J Med* 63:881, 1977.

33. Clarkson EM, Raw SM, DeWardener HE: Two natriuretic substances in extracts of urine from normal man when salt-depleted and salt-loaded. *Kidney Int* 10:381, 1976.

34. Danielsen H, Kornerup HJ, Olsen S, et al: Arterial hypertension in chronic glomerulonephritis. An analysis of 310 cases. *Clin Nephrol* 19:284, 1983.

35. Danovitch GM, Bourgoignie J, Bricker NS: Reversibility of the "salt-losing" tendency of chronic renal failure. *N Engl J Med* 296:14, 1977.

36. Gupta DD, Kalant N, Giroud CJP: Experimental aminonucleoside nephrosis (II): Effect of adrenalectomy of fluid retention of aminonucleoside nephrosis. *Proc Soc Exp Biol Med* 100:602, 1957.

37. Daugharty TM, Ueki IF, Nicholas DP, et al: Renal response to chronic intravenous salt loading in the rat. *J Clin Invest* 52:21, 1973.

38. Deen WM, Maddox DA, Robertson CR, et al: Dynamics of glomerular ultrafiltration in the rat. VII. Response to reduced renal mass. *Am J Physiol* 227:556, 1974.

39. DeFazio V, Christensen RC, Regan TJ, et al: Circulatory changes in acute glomerulonephritis. *Circulation* 20:190, 1959.

40. DeWardener HE, Mills IH, Clapham WF, et al: Studies on the efferent mechanism of the sodium diuresis which follows the administration of intravenous saline in the dog. *Clin Sci* 21:249, 1961.

41. DiBona GF: Neurogenic regulation of renal tubular sodium reabsorption. *Am J Physiol* 233:73, 1977.

42. Dodge WF, Travis LB, Haggard ME, et al: Studies of physiology during the early stage of acute glomerulonephritis in children. In Metcoff J (ed): *Acute Glomerulonephritis.* Boston, Little, Brown, 1967.

43. Dorhout Mees EJ, Roos JC, Boer P, et al: Observations on edema formation in the nephrotic syndrome in adults with minimal lesions. *Am J Med* 67:378, 1979.

44. Dorhout Mees EJ, Geers AB, Koomans HA: Blood volume and sodium retention in the nephrotic syndrome: A controversial pathophysiological concept. *Nephron* 36:201, 1984.

45. Dorhout Mees EJ: Edema formation in the nephrotic syndrome. *Contrib Nephrol* 43:64, 1984.

46. Dusing R, Vetter H, Kramer HJ: The renin-angiotensin-aldosterone system in patients with nephrotic syndrome: Effects of 1-sar-8-ala-angiotensin II. *Nephron* 25:187, 1980.

47. Earle KP, Farber SJ, Alexander JD, et al: Renal function and electrolyte metabolism in acute glomerulonephritis. *J Clin Invest* 30:421, 1951.

48. Earley LE, Daugharty TM: Sodium metabolism. *N Engl J Med* 281:72, 1969.

49. Eder HA, Lauson HD, Chinard FP, et al: A study of the mechanisms of edema formation in patients with the nephrotic syndrome. *J Clin Invest* 33:636, 1954.

50. Eisenberg S: Blood volume in patients with acute glomerulonephritis as determined by radioactive chromium tagged red cells. *Am J Med* 27:241, 1959.

51. Eisenberg S: Postural changes in plasma volume in hypoalbuminemia. *Arch Intern Med* 112:544, 1963.

52. Eisenberg S: Blood volume in persons with the nephrotic syndrome. *Am J Med Sci* 225:320, 1968.

53. Epstein FH, Post RS, McDowell M: The effect of an arteriovenous fistula on renal hemodynamics and electrolyte excretion. *J Clin Invest* 32:233, 1953.

54. Epstein M: Cardiovascular and renal effects of head-out water immersion in man: Application of the model in the assessment of volume homeostasis. *Circ Res* 39:619, 1976.

55. Farber SJ: Physiologic aspects of glomerulonephritis. *J Chronic Dis* 5:87, 1957.

56. Favre H, Hwang KH, Schmidt RW, et al: An inhibitor of sodium transport in the urine of dogs with normal renal function. *J Clin Invest* 56:1302, 1975.

57. Favre H, Gourjon M: Absence of production of natriuretic factor following acute saline expansion in nephrotic rats. *Clin Sci* 63:317, 1982.

58. Favre H: Role of the natriuretic factor in the disorders of sodium balance. *Adv Nephrol* 11:3, 1982.

59. Fine LG, Bourgoignie JJ, Weber H, et al: Enhanced end-organ responsiveness of the uremic kidney to the natriuretic factor. *Kidney Int* 10:364, 1976.

60. Fine LG, Bourgoignie JJ, Hwang KH, et al: On the influence of the natriuretic factor from patients with chronic uremia on the bioelectric properties and sodium transport of the isolated mammalian collecting tubule. *J Clin Invest* 58:590, 1976.

61. Fray JCS: Stimulus-secretion coupling of renin: Role of hemodynamic and other factors. *Circ Res* 47:485, 1980.

62. Garin EH, Sausvill PJ, Richard GA: Plasma prostaglandin E_2 concentration in nephrotic syndrome. *J Pediatr* 103:253, 1983.

63. Gauer OH, Henry JP, Behn C: The regulation of extracellular fluid volume. *Ann Rev Physiol* 32:547, 1970.

64. Geers AB, Koomans HA, Boer P, et al: Plasma and blood volumes in patients with the nephrotic syndrome. *Nephron* 38:170, 1984.

65. Geers AB, Koomans HA, Roos JC, et al: Functional rela-

baroreceptors respond at levels of about 30 mmHg higher. Baroreceptor impulses go to the medullary vasoconstrictor center and inhibit it and excite the vagal center. The result is a decrease in heart rate, vasodilatation, and decrease in myocardial contractility, resulting in lowering of blood pressure. Baroreceptors are probably important in control of blood pressure during positional changes. Chemoreceptors located in the carotid and aortic bodies are richly innervated and vascularized and concerned primarily with blood gas homeostasis; secondarily they may affect vasomotor and respiratory centers. If stimulated, they increase systemic blood pressure.

Additional receptors in the left atrium, ventricle, pulmonary artery, and pulmonary vein may affect changes in heart rate and peripheral resistance when stimulated by stress or various drugs [110,113,218]. Furthermore, an increase in stretch in the atria releases atrial natriuretic factor, which results in natriuresis and diuresis and affects blood pressure [30].

Hormonal Factors in Blood Pressure Control

Renin–Angiotensin System

The role of the renin–angiotensin system (RAS) in blood pressure control has been recognized since the early 1930s, when Goldblatt and colleagues demonstrated that renal artery constriction could cause chronic blood pressure elevation [67]. The research stimulated by that seminal experiment has resulted in the identification of multiple components of the renin–angiotensin–aldosterone system, clarified its role in regulation of blood pressure as well as salt and water balance, and in recent years resulted in the elucidation of the molecular biology of this system [24,34–42,45,60,83,156]. In addition, there is abundant evidence that components of the RAS are present in many tissues and may have local functions distinct from blood pressure regulation.

Renin is secreted by the renal juxtaglomerular apparatus, which is located in the wall of the afferent arteriole and adjoining macula densa portion of the distal tubule. Renin is an acid protease related to other acid proteases, such as cathepsin D and pepsin, and has a half-time in the circulation of 20 to 60 minutes. Its amino acid composition and gene structure have been determined.

The prohormone prorenin is also secreted by the kidney but is present even in anephric individuals [15,36,171]. Prorenin makes up the major portion of total plasma renin and is present in especially high levels in anephric individuals, during pregnancy, and in abnormal conditions such as long-standing diabetes. The function of circulating prorenin remains to be delineated, although activation of prorenin in the circulation undoubtedly occurs. The mechanism of activation is not clear, but acidification, prolonged storage at cold temperatures, and exposure to proteolytic enzymes such as trypsin may activate it.

Renin in the circulation acts on the protein substrate angiotensinogen, which is synthesized in the liver [45,156] as a glycoprotein with a molecular weight of about 65,000. Angiotensinogen release is stimulated by angiotensin II (AII), estrogens, and adrenocortical steroids [25,141,191].

Plasma levels of angiotensinogen may be important, since its concentration is a determinant of the rate of angiotensin formation.

Angiotensinogen has been shown by molecular biologic techniques to be present in numerous other tissues, including the kidney, brain, and adrenal glands [25,141]. The role of this substrate in local tissue renin–angiotensin systems and its interaction with blood pressure homeostatic mechanisms remain to be elucidated.

Renin cleaves angiotensinogen to form a decapeptide, angiotensin I (AI). Within the lungs, but also in other organs, angiotensin-converting enzyme (ACE; dipeptidylcarboxypeptidase) cleaves angiotensin I by removing the carboxy terminal His-Leu to produce an octapeptide, AII. This potent vasoconstrictor is also a stimulus for aldosterone production and, in turn, for increased angiotensinogen production by the liver. Angiotensin appears to be the prime mover in the physiologic effects of the RAS, although both angiotensin I and smaller fragments of angiotensins may themselves have direct physiologic effects. Figure 24-1 shows the primary components of the circulating RAS in humans.

Angiotensin II has actions other than as a vasoconstrictor: it stimulates aldosterone and catecholamine production by the adrenal medulla [47,101,148,149,210], it causes sympathetic vasomotor discharge within the CNS, and it stimulates norepinephrine synthesis and release at adrenergic nerve endings [8,9,90,121,122]. Other effects of angiotensin II, such as the CNS induction of thirst [50,109,172], the possible induction of follicle maturation in the ovary [65,92], and sodium–hydrogen exchange in the kidney [76,105,166], have led to a variety of hypotheses suggesting the interaction of the RAS system with processes other than blood pressure homeostasis.

CONTROL OF RENIN SECRETION

Renin synthesis and release are influenced by multiple variables, including sympathetic nervous system stimulation, vasoactive hormones such as AII, vasopressin, prostaglandins, atrial natriuretic peptide, plasma electrolyte concentrations such as potassium and calcium, and macula densa and baroreceptor mechanisms.

Beta-adrenergic receptor stimulation promotes renin release by increasing both renin secretion and renin mRNA synthesis, constituting a major way in which the sympathetic nervous system interacts with the RAS. The effects of beta-adrenergic stimulation presumably are mediated by cyclic AMP [2,167,216]. Increased sympathetic nerve traffic may be responsible for the increase in plasma renin activity with exercise or stress [13,28,33,93,106,126,142,153,196].

Angiotensin [26,54,136], vasopressin [200], and probably atrial natriuretic factor [21,77] inhibit renin secretion. Prostaglandins may mediate renin release, whereas prostaglandin inhibitors such as nonsteroidal anti-inflammatory agents may inhibit it [10,52,55,62,86,104,173]. Increased potassium concentration in plasma may inhibit renin secretion, but the effect in humans is unclear [174].

Alterations in the net flux of calcium in juxtaglomerular cells may be a final pathway for renin release. Decreased intracellular calcium promotes renin release, and increased

renin substrate in the nephrotic syndrome. *Nephron* 26:121, 1980.

19. Bonventre JV, Leaf A: Sodium homeostasis: Steady states without a set point. *Kidney Int* 21:880, 1982.

20. Bourgoignie JJ, Hwang KH, Espinel C, et al: A natriuretic factor in the serum of patients with chronic uremia. *J Clin Invest* 51:1514, 1972.

21. Bourgoignie JJ, Hwang KH, Ipakchi E, et al: The presence of a natriuretic factor in urine of patients with chronic uremia: The absence of the factor in nephrotic uremic patients. *J Clin Invest* 53:1559, 1974.

22. Bourgoignie JJ, Kaplan M, Gavellas G, et al: Sodium homeostasis in dogs with chronic renal insufficiency. *Kidney Int* 21:820, 1982.

23. Bradley SE, Tyson CJ: The "nephrotic syndrome." *N Engl J Med* 238:260, 1948.

24. Bricker NS, Fine LG, Kaplan M, et al: "Magnification phenomenon" in chronic renal disease. *N Engl J Med* 299:1287, 1978.

25. Bricker NS: Sodium homeostasis in chronic renal disease. *Kidney Int* 21:886, 1982.

26. Brown EA, Sagnella GA, Jones BE, et al: Evidence that some mechanism other than the renin system causes sodium retention in nephrotic syndrome. *Lancet* 2:1237, 1982.

27. Brown EA, Markandu ND, Roulston JE, et al: Is the renin-angiotensin-aldosterone system involved in the sodium retention in the nephrotic syndrome. *Nephron* 32:102, 1982.

28. Brown EA, Markandu ND, Sagnella GA, et al: Lack of effect of captopril on the sodium retention of the nephrotic syndrome. *Nephron* 37:43, 1984.

29. Brown PR, Koutsaimanis KG, DeWardener HE: Effect of urinary extracts from salt-loaded man on urinary sodium excretion by the rat. *Kidney Int* 2:1, 1972.

30. Buckalew VM Jr, Nelson DB: Natriuretic and sodium transport inhibitory activity in plasma of volume-expanded dogs. *Kidney Int* 5:12, 1974.

31. Burke FG, Ross S: Acute glomerulonephritis. A review of ninety cases. *J Pediatr* 30:157, 1947.

32. Chonko AV, Bay WH, Stein JH, et al: The role of renin and aldosterone in the salt retention of edema. *Am J Med* 63:881, 1977.

33. Clarkson EM, Raw SM, DeWardener HE: Two natriuretic substances in extracts of urine from normal man when salt-depleted and salt-loaded. *Kidney Int* 10:381, 1976.

34. Danielsen H, Kornerup HJ, Olsen S, et al: Arterial hypertension in chronic glomerulonephritis. An analysis of 310 cases. *Clin Nephrol* 19:284, 1983.

35. Danovitch GM, Bourgoignie J, Bricker NS: Reversibility of the "salt-losing" tendency of chronic renal failure. *N Engl J Med* 296:14, 1977.

36. Gupta DD, Kalant N, Giroud CJP: Experimental aminonucleoside nephrosis (II): Effect of adrenalectomy of fluid retention of aminonucleoside nephrosis. *Proc Soc Exp Biol Med* 100:602, 1957.

37. Daugharty TM, Ueki IF, Nicholas DP, et al: Renal response to chronic intravenous salt loading in the rat. *J Clin Invest* 52:21, 1973.

38. Deen WM, Maddox DA, Robertson CR, et al: Dynamics of glomerular ultrafiltration in the rat. VII. Response to reduced renal mass. *Am J Physiol* 227:556, 1974.

39. DeFazio V, Christensen RC, Regan TJ, et al: Circulatory changes in acute glomerulonephritis. *Circulation* 20:190, 1959.

40. DeWardener HE, Mills IH, Clapham WF, et al: Studies on the efferent mechanism of the sodium diuresis which follows the administration of intravenous saline in the dog. *Clin Sci* 21:249, 1961.

41. DiBona GF: Neurogenic regulation of renal tubular sodium reabsorption. *Am J Physiol* 233:73, 1977.

42. Dodge WF, Travis LB, Haggard ME, et al: Studies of physiology during the early stage of acute glomerulonephritis in children. *In* Metcoff J (ed): *Acute Glomerulonephritis.* Boston, Little, Brown, 1967.

43. Dorhout Mees EJ, Roos JC, Boer P, et al: Observations on edema formation in the nephrotic syndrome in adults with minimal lesions. *Am J Med* 67:378, 1979.

44. Dorhout Mees EJ, Geers AB, Koomans HA: Blood volume and sodium retention in the nephrotic syndrome: A controversial pathophysiological concept. *Nephron* 36:201, 1984.

45. Dorhout Mees EJ: Edema formation in the nephrotic syndrome. *Contrib Nephrol* 43:64, 1984.

46. Dusing R, Vetter H, Kramer HJ: The renin-angiotensin-aldosterone system in patients with nephrotic syndrome: Effects of 1-sar-8-ala-angiotensin II. *Nephron* 25:187, 1980.

47. Earle KP, Farber SJ, Alexander JD, et al: Renal function and electrolyte metabolism in acute glomerulonephritis. *J Clin Invest* 30:421, 1951.

48. Earley LE, Daugharty TM: Sodium metabolism. *N Engl J Med* 281:72, 1969.

49. Eder HA, Lauson HD, Chinard FP, et al: A study of the mechanisms of edema formation in patients with the nephrotic syndrome. *J Clin Invest* 33:636, 1954.

50. Eisenberg S: Blood volume in patients with acute glomerulonephritis as determined by radioactive chromium tagged red cells. *Am J Med* 27:241, 1959.

51. Eisenberg S: Postural changes in plasma volume in hypoalbuminemia. *Arch Intern Med* 112:544, 1963.

52. Eisenberg S: Blood volume in persons with the nephrotic syndrome. *Am J Med Sci* 225:320, 1968.

53. Epstein FH, Post RS, McDowell M: The effect of an arteriovenous fistula on renal hemodynamics and electrolyte excretion. *J Clin Invest* 32:233, 1953.

54. Epstein M: Cardiovascular and renal effects of head-out water immersion in man: Application of the model in the assessment of volume homeostasis. *Circ Res* 39:619, 1976.

55. Farber SJ: Physiologic aspects of glomerulonephritis. *J Chronic Dis* 5:87, 1957.

56. Favre H, Hwang KH, Schmidt RW, et al: An inhibitor of sodium transport in the urine of dogs with normal renal function. *J Clin Invest* 56:1302, 1975.

57. Favre H, Gourjon M: Absence of production of natriuretic factor following acute saline expansion in nephrotic rats. *Clin Sci* 63:317, 1982.

58. Favre H: Role of the natriuretic factor in the disorders of sodium balance. *Adv Nephrol* 11:3, 1982.

59. Fine LG, Bourgoignie JJ, Weber H, et al: Enhanced end-organ responsiveness of the uremic kidney to the natriuretic factor. *Kidney Int* 10:364, 1976.

60. Fine LG, Bourgoignie JJ, Hwang KH, et al: On the influence of the natriuretic factor from patients with chronic uremia on the bioelectric properties and sodium transport of the isolated mammalian collecting tubule. *J Clin Invest* 58:590, 1976.

61. Fray JCS: Stimulus-secretion coupling of renin: Role of hemodynamic and other factors. *Circ Res* 47:485, 1980.

62. Garin EH, Sausvill PJ, Richard GA: Plasma prostaglandin E_2 concentration in nephrotic syndrome. *J Pediatr* 103:253, 1983.

63. Gauer OH, Henry JP, Behn C: The regulation of extracellular fluid volume. *Ann Rev Physiol* 32:547, 1970.

64. Geers AB, Koomans HA, Boer P, et al: Plasma and blood volumes in patients with the nephrotic syndrome. *Nephron* 38:170, 1984.

65. Geers AB, Koomans HA, Roos JC, et al: Functional rela-

tionships in the nephrotic syndrome. *Kidney Int* 26:324, 1984.

66. Glassock RJ: Sodium homeostasis in acute glomerulonephritis and the nephrotic syndrome. *Contrib Nephrol* 23:181, 1980.

67. Glassock RJ, Cohen AH, Bennett CM: Primary glomerular diseases. *In* Brenner BM, Rector FC (eds): *Kidney.* Philadelphia, WB Saunders, 1981, p 1351.

68. Glassock RJ, Bennett C, Kayser B, et al: Glomerular hemodynamics in nephrotoxic serum nephritis. *Kidney Int* 14:725, 1978.

69. Gnepp DR: Lymphatics. *In* Staub NC, Taylor AE (eds): *Edema.* New York, Raven Press, 1984, p 263.

70. Godon JP: Sodium and water retention in experimental glomerulonephritis. *Kidney Int* 2:271, 1972.

71. Godon JP: The oedematous phase of human glomerulonephritis is related to the disappearance of a natriuretic factor which reappears during recovery. *Proc EDTA* 12:330, 1975.

72. Godon JP: Evidence of increased proximal sodium and water reabsorption in experimental glomerulonephritis: Role of a natriuretic factor of renal origin. *Nephron* 21:146, 1978.

73. Godon JP, Cambrier P, Nizet A: Renal origin of a natriuretic material. *Proc EDTA* 15:424, 1978.

74. Gonick HC, Maxwell MH, Rubini ME, et al: Functional impairment in chronic renal disease. I. Studies of sodium-conserving ability. *Nephron* 3:137, 1966.

75. Gore I, Saphir O: Myocarditis associated with acute and subacute glomerulonephritis. *Am Heart J* 36:390, 1948.

76. Goetz KL, Bond GC, Bloxham DD: Atrial receptors and renal function. *Physiol Rev* 55:157, 1975.

77. Granger HJ, Laine GA, Barnes GE, et al: Dynamics and control of transmicrovascular fluid exchange. *In* Staub NC, Taylor AE (eds): *Edema.* New York, Raven Press, 1984, p 189.

78. Grausz H, Lieberman R, Earley LE: Effect of plasma albumin on sodium reabsorption in patients with nephrotic syndrome. *Kidney Int* 1:47, 1972.

79. Gutmann FD, Rieselbach RE: Disproportionate inhibition of sodium reabsorption in the unilaterally diseased kidney of dog and man after an acute saline load. *J Clin Invest* 50:422, 1971.

80. Guyton AC, Coleman TG, Cowley AW Jr, et al: Arterial pressure regulation: Overriding dominance of the kidneys in long-term regulation and in hypertension. *Am J Med* 52:584, 1972.

81. Guyton AC: *Textbook of Medical Physiology,* 5th ed. Philadelphia, WB Saunders, 1976, p 265.

82. Hall JE, Granger JP, Hester RL, et al: Mechanisms of escape from sodium retention during angiotensin II hypertension. *Am J Physiol* 246:F627, 1984.

83. Hall JE, Granger JP, Smith MJ Jr, et al: Role of renal hemodynamics and arterial pressure in aldosterone "escape." *Hypertension* 1:1, 1984.

84. Hammond TG, Whitworth JA, Saines D, et al: Renin-angiotensin-aldosterone system in nephrotic syndrome. *Am J Kidney Dis* 4:18, 1984.

85. Hinglais N, Garcia-Torres R, Kleinknecht D: Long-term prognosis in acute glomerulonephritis: The predictive value of early clinical and pathologic features observed in 65 patients. *Am J Med* 56:52, 1974.

86. Hollenberg NK: Set point for sodium homeostasis: Surfeit, deficit, and their implications. *Kidney Int* 17:423, 1980.

87. Ichikawa I, Hoyer JR, Seiler MW, et al: Mechanism of glomerulotubular balance in the setting of heterogeneous glomerular injury: Preservation of a close functional linkage between individual nephrons and surrounding microvasculature. *J Clin Invest* 69:185, 1982.

88. Ichikawa I, Bennke HG, Hoyer JR, et al: Role for intrarenal mechanisms in the impaired salt excretion of experimental nephrotic syndrome. *J Clin Invest* 71:91, 1983.

89. James J, Gordillo G, Metcoff J: Effects of infusion of hyperoncotic dextran in children with the nephrotic syndrome. *J Clin Invest* 33:1346, 1954.

90. Jamison RL, Sonnenberg H, Stein JH: Questions and replies: Role of the collecting tubule in fluid, sodium, and potassium balance. *Am J Physiol* 237:F247, 1979.

91. Kalant N, Das Gupta D, Despointes R, et al: Mechanisms of edema in experimental nephrosis. *Am J Physiol* 202:91, 1962.

92. Kaloyanides GJ, Azer M: Evidence for a humoral mechanism in volume expansion natriuresis. *J Clin Invest* 50:1603, 1971.

92a. Kaysen GA, Paukert TT, Menke DJ, et al: Plasma volume expansion is necessary for edema formation in the rat with Heymann nephritis. *Am J Physiol* 17:F247, 1985.

93. Keeler R: Natriuresis after unilateral stimulation of carotid receptors in unanesthetized rats. *Am J Physiol* 226:507, 1974.

94. Kelsch RC, Light GS, Oliver WJ: The effect of albumin infusion upon plasma norepinephrine concentration in nephrotic children. *J Lab Clin Med* 79:516, 1972.

95. Kirch KA, Johnson RF, Gorter RJ: The significance of total body hematocrit in measurements of blood compartments. *J Nucl Med* 12:17, 1971.

96. Klaus D, Rossler R: Reninsekretion bei analbuminamie. *Klin Wochenschr* 51:969, 1973.

97. Koomans HA, Geers AB, Boer P, et al: A study on the distribution of body fluids after rapid saline expansion in normal subjects and in patients with renal insufficiency: Preferential intravascular deposition in renal failure. *Clin Sci* 64:153, 1983.

98. Koomans HA, Roos JC, Boer P, et al: Salt sensitivity of blood pressure in chronic renal failure: Evidence for renal control of body fluid distribution in man. *Hypertension* 4:190, 1982.

99. Koomans HA, Geers AB, Boer P, et al: Plasma volumes, noradrenaline levels and renin activity during posture changes in end-stage renal failure. *Clin Physiol* 4:103, 1984.

100. Koomans HA, Roos JC, Boer P, et al: Salt handling in patients with chronic renal insufficiency. *Miner Electrolyte Metab* 7:134, 1982.

101. Koomans HA, Geers AB, vd Meiracker AH, et al: Effects of plasma volume expansion on renal salt handling in patients with the nephrotic syndrome. *Am J Nephrol* 4:227, 1984.

102. Knox FG, Burnett JC Jr: Mechanism of mineralocorticoid escape. *In* Lichardus B, Schrier R, Ponec J (eds): *Hormonal Regulation of Sodium Excretion.* New York, Elsevier, 1980, p 19.

103. Knox FG, Mertz JI, Burnett JC Jr, et al: Role of hydrostatic and oncotic pressures in renal sodium reabsorption. *Circ Res* 52:491, 1983.

104. Kreusser W, Mann J, Rambausek M, et al: Cardiac function in experimental uremia. *Kidney Int* 24 (Suppl 15):S-83, 1983.

105. Krishna GG, Danovitch GM: Effects of water immersion on renal function in the nephrotic syndrome. *Kidney Int* 21:395, 1982.

106. Kuroda S, Aynedjian HS, Bank N: A micropuncture study of renal sodium retention in nephrotic syndrome in rat: Evidence for increased resistance to tubular fluid flow. *Kidney Int* 16:561, 1979.

107. Lemieux MDG, Cuvelier AA, Lefebvre R: The clinical spectrum of renal insufficiency during acute glomerulonephritis in the adult. *J Can Med Assoc* 96:1129, 1967.

108. Leonard CD, Nagle RB, Striker GE, et al: Acute glomeru-

lonephritis with prolonged oliguria. *Ann Intern Med* 73:703, 1970.

109. Lewy JE, Salinas-Madrigal L, Herdson PB, et al: A correlation between renal functions, morphologic damage and clinical course of 46 children with acute poststreptococcal glomerulonephritis. *Medicine* 50:453, 1971.

110. Licht A, Danovitch GM: Sodium metabolism and volume regulation. *Cur Nephrol* 6:283, 1983.

111. Lowenstein J, Schacht RG, Baldwin DS: Renal failure in minimal change nephrotic syndrome. *Am J Med* 70:227, 1981.

112. Lubowitz H, Purkerson ML, Sugita M, et al: GFR per nephron and per kidney in chronically diseased (pyelonephritic) kidney of the rat. *Am J Physiol* 217:853, 1969.

113. Lubowitz H, Mazumdar DC, Kawamura J, et al: Experimental glomerulonephritis in the rat: Structural and functional observations. *Kidney Int* 5:356, 1974.

114. Luetscher JA Jr, Hall AD, Kremer VL: Treatment of nephrosis with concentrated human serum albumin. I. Effects on the proteins of body fluids. *J Clin Invest* 28:700, 1949.

115. Luetscher JA Jr, Hall AD, Kremer VL: Treatment of nephrosis with concentrated human serum albumin. II. Effects on renal function and on excretion of water and some electrolytes. *J Clin Invest* 29:896, 1950.

116. Luetscher JA Jr, Johnson BB: Chromatographic separation of the sodium-retaining corticoid from the urine of children with nephrosis, compared with observations on normal children. *J Clin Invest* 33:276, 1954.

117. Maack T, Marion DN, Camargo MJF, et al: Effects of auriculin (atrial natriuretic factor) on blood pressure, renal function, and the renin-aldosterone system in dogs. *Am J Med* 77:1069, 1984.

118. McLeish KR, Yum MN, Luft FC: Rapidly progressive glomerulonephritis in adults: Clinical and histologic correlations. *Clin Nephrol* 10:43, 1978.

119. Maddox DA, Bennett CM, Deen WM, et al: Control of proximal tubule fluid reabsorption in experimental glomerulonephritis. *J Clin Invest* 55:1315, 1975.

120. Manning RD Jr, Guyton AC: Dynamics of fluid distribution between the blood and interstitium during overhydration. *Am J Physiol* 238:H645, 1980.

121. Manning RD Jr, Guyton AC: Control of blood volume. *Rev Physiol Biochem Pharmacol* 93:69, 1982.

122. Manning RD Jr, Guyton AC: Effects of hypoproteinemia on fluid volumes and arterial pressure. *Am J Physiol* 245:H284, 1983.

123. Maxwell MH, Weidmann P: The renin-angiotensin-aldosterone system in parenchymal kidney disease. *Adv Nephrol* 5:301, 1975.

124. Mazumdar DC, Crosson JT, Lubowitz H: Glomerulotubular relationships in glomerulonephritis. *J Lab Clin Med* 85:292, 1975.

125. Meltzer JI, Keim HJ, Laragh JH, et al: Nephrotic syndrome: Vasoconstriction and hypervolemic types indicated by renin-sodium profiling. *Ann Intern Med* 91:688, 1979.

126. Metcoff J, Janeway CA: Studies on the pathogenesis of nephrotic edema. *J Pediatr* 58:640, 1961.

127. Meyer TW, Brenner BM: Physiological and pharmacological considerations in the renal excretion of salt and water. *In* Staub NC, Taylor AE (eds): *Edema*. New York, Raven Press, 1984, p 441.

128. Morrin PAF, Hinglais N, Nabarra B, et al: Rapidly progressive glomerulonephritis: A clinical and pathologic study. *Am J Med* 65:446, 1978.

129. Navar LG: Renal regulation of body fluid balance. *In* Staub NC, Taylor AE (eds): *Edema*. New York, Raven Press, 1984, p 319.

130. Neild GH, Cameron JS, Ogg CS, et al: Rapidly progressive glomerulonephritis with extensive glomerular crescent formation. *Q J Med* (New Series) II(207):395, 1983.

131. Nissenson AR, Baraff LJ, Fine RN, et al: Poststreptococcal acute glomerulonephritis: Fact and controversy. *Ann Intern Med* 91:76, 1979.

132. Noddeland H, Riisnes SM, Fadnes HO: Interstitial fluid colloid osmotic and hydrostatic pressures in subcutaneous tissue of patients with nephrotic syndrome. *Scand J Clin Lab Invest* 42:139, 1982.

133. Oliver WJ: Physiologic responses associated with steroid-induced diuresis in the nephrotic syndrome. *J Lab Clin Med* 62:449, 1963.

134. Oliver WJ, Owings CL: Sodium excretion in the nephrotic syndrome. *Am J Dis Child* 113:352, 1967.

135. Osgood RW, Reineck HJ, Stein JH: Further studies on segmental sodium transport in the rat kidney during expansion of the extracellular fluid volume. *J Clin Invest* 62:311, 1978.

136. de Planque BA, Mulder E, Dorhout Mees EJ: The behavior of blood and extracellular volume in hypertensive patients with renal insufficiency. *Acta Med Scand* 186:75, 1969.

137. Powell HR, Rotenberg H, Williams AL, et al: Plasma renin activity in acute poststreptococcal glomerulonephritis and the haemolytic uraemic syndrome. *Arch Dis Child* 48:802, 1974.

138. Reed RK: Interstitial fluid volume, colloid osmotic and hydrostatic pressures in rat skeletal muscle. Effect of hypoproteinemia. *Acta Physiol Scand* 112:141, 1981.

139. Reinhardt HW, Eisele R, Kaezmarczyk G, et al: The control of sodium excretion by reflexes from the low pressure system independent of adrenal activity. *Pflugers Arch* 384:171, 1980.

140. Reubi FC, Weidmann P, Gluck Z: Interrelationships between sodium clearance, plasma aldosterone, plasma renin activity, renal hemodynamics and blood pressure in renal disease. *Klin Wochenschr* 57:1273, 1979.

141. Rocha A, Marcondes M, Malnic G: Micropuncture study in rats with experimental glomerulonephritis. *Kidney Int* 3:14, 1973.

142. Rodriguez-Iturbe B, Baggio B, Colina-Chourio J, et al: Studies on the renin-aldosterone system in the acute nephritic syndrome. *Kidney Int* 19:445, 1981.

143. Roy S III, Pitcock JA, Etteldorf JN: Prognosis of acute poststreptococcal glomerulonephritis in childhood: Prospective study and review of the literature. *Adv Pediatr* 23:35, 1976.

144. Schmidt RW, Bourgoignie JJ, Bricker NS: On the adaptation in sodium excretion in chronic uremia: The effects of "proportional reduction" of sodium intake. *J Clin Invest* 53:1736, 1974.

145. Schultze RG, Weisser F, Bricker NS: The influence of uremia on fractional sodium reabsorption by the proximal tubule of rats. *Kidney Int* 2:59, 1972.

146. Schultze RG, Shapiro HS, Bricker NS: Studies on the control of sodium excretion in experimental uremia. *J Clin Invest* 48:869, 1969.

147. Schuster VL, Kokko JP, Jacobson HR: Angiotensin II directly stimulates sodium transport in rabbit proximal convoluted tubules. *J Clin Invest* 73:507, 1984.

148. Shapiro M, Nicholls K, Schrier R: Mechanism of impaired water excretion in nephrotic syndrome. *Kidney Int* 27:154, 1985.

149. Shapiro MS, Mendoza E, Grunberger M, et al: The magnified natriuresis per nephron in CRD: On the role of chronic ECF volume expansion and of a preexisting state of Na adaptation. *Kidney Int* 27:219, 1983.

150. Skorecki KL, Brenner BM: Body fluid homeostasis in man: A contemporary overview. *Am J Med* 70:77, 1981.

151. Slatopolsky E, Elkan IO, Weerts C, et al: Studies on the characteristics of the control system governing sodium excretion in uremic man. *J Clin Invest* 47:521, 1968.

152. Squire JR: The nephrotic syndrome. *Adv Intern Med* 7:201, 1955.

153. Sparks HV Jr, Korthuis RJ, Scott JB: Pharmacology of hemodynamic factors in fluid balance. *In* Staub NC, Taylor AE (eds): *Edema.* New York, Raven Press, 1984, p 425.

154. Starling EH: On the absorption of fluids from the connective tissue spaces. *J Physiol* 19:312, 1895.

155. Stein JH, Kirschenbaum MA, Bay WH, et al: Role of the collecting duct in the regulation of sodium balance. *Circ Res* 36–37 (Suppl I):I-119, 1975.

156. Surtshin A, Rolf D, White HL: Constancy of sodium excretion in the presence of chronically altered glomerular filtration rate. *Am J Physiol* 165:429, 1951.

157. Thorn GW, Armstrong SH, Davenport VD, et al: Chemical, clinical, and immunological studies on the products of human plasma fractionation. XXX. The use of salt-poor concentrated human serum albumin solution in the treatment of chronic Bright's disease. *J Clin Invest* 24:802, 1945.

158. Usberti M, Federico S, Meccariello S, et al: Role of plasma vasopressin in the impairment of water excretion in nephrotic syndrome. *Kidney Int* 25:422, 1984.

159. Van Liew JB, Von Baeyer HR: Proximal tubule volume reabsorption in anti-GBM nephritic rats. *The Physiologist* 17:348, 1974.

160. Wagnild JP, Gutmann FD, Rieselbach RE: Influence of hydrostatic and oncotic pressure on sodium reabsorption in the unilateral pyelonephritic dog kidney. *Clin Sci Mol Med* 47:367, 1974.

161. Wagnild JP, Gutmann FD, Rieselbach RE: Functional characterization of chronic unilateral glomerulonephritis in the dog. *Kidney Int* 5:422, 1974.

162. Wagnild JP, Gutmann FD: Functional adaptation of nephrons in dogs with acute progressing to chronic experimental glomerulonephritis. *J Clin Invest* 57:1575, 1976.

163. Wagnild JP, Wen S: Sodium transport in dogs with acute remnant and glomerulonephritic kidneys. *J Lab Clin Med* 91:911, 1978.

164. Warren JV, Stead EA Jr: The protein content of edema fluid in patients with acute glomerulonephritis. *Am J Med Sci* 208:618, 1944.

165. Weber H, Lin K, Bricker NS: Effect of sodium intake on single nephron glomerular filtration rate and sodium reabsorption in experimental uremia. *Kidney Int* 8:14, 1975.

166. Weech AA, Snelling CE, Goettsch E: The relation between plasma protein content, plasma specific gravity and edema in dogs maintained on a protein inadequate diet and in dogs rendered edematous by plasmapheresis. *J Clin Invest* 12:193, 1935.

167. Wen S, Wagnild JP: Acute effect of nephrotoxic serum on renal sodium transport in the dog. *Kidney Int* 9:243, 1976.

168. Willassen Y, Oestad J: Intrarenal pressure and sodium excretion in hypertension of chronic glomerulonephritis in humans. *Hypertension* 5:375, 1983.

169. Wraight EP: Capillary permeability to protein as a factor in the control of plasma volume. *J Physiol* 237:39, 1974.

170. Wright RR, Tono M, Pollycove M: Blood volume. *Semin Nucl Med* 5:63, 1975.

171. Wilson CB, Dixon FJ: The renal response to immunologic injury. *In* Brenner GM, Rector FC (eds): *The Kidney.* Philadelphia, WB Saunders, 1981, p 1237.

172. Yamauchi H, Hopper J Jr: Hypovolemic shock and hypotension as a complication in the nephrotic syndrome. *Ann Intern Med* 60:242, 1964.

Julie R. Ingelfinger

24
Hypertension

Numerous physical, hemodynamic, hormonal, and neural factors modulate arterial blood pressure control [38,73, 145]. Some of these factors, such as baroreceptors, chemoreceptors, the CNS ischemic response, and stress relaxation may be set into action within minutes after a sudden change in arterial pressure, as, for example, with hemorrhage. Other factors such as the renin–angiotensin system and other vasoactive hormones begin to have an effect within minutes. Within an hour following a sudden change in arterial pressure, still other factors, including fluid shifts and nonvascular modulation due to exogenous fluid administration, become involved. Renal and blood volume–pressure control mechanisms as well as aldosterone effect take many hours to a day to exert their effects. This chapter examines the individual contributions of these various humoral, hemodynamic, and neural variables with respect to blood pressure control and refers the reader to more detailed reviews and primary works.

Hemodynamic Factors in Blood Pressure Control

Mean arterial pressure is the product of cardiac output and total peripheral resistance [22,56–58,61,73,85,160,176, 190]. Total peripheral resistance (TPR) may be calculated from pressure and flow differences within a vessel. For instance, if blood flow in a vessel is 1 ml per second and the difference in pressure from one end of the vessel to the other is 1 mmHg, the resistance might be said to be 1 peripheral resistance unit (PRU). In the basal state, blood flow in humans is about 100 ml per second, and the difference in the pressure of systemic arteries to veins is close to 100 mmHg. Thus, TPR is about 1 PRU. In general, TPR varies from about 0.2 PRU in vasodilatation to 4 PRU in vasoconstriction. Various factors both actively and passively alter flow resistance, and TPR measures or delineates the sum of all the interacting vascular beds and parallel circuits.

Cardiac output [32,40,97,184,206] is defined as stroke volume times the heart rate per minute. The amount of blood ejected per heart beat is defined as stroke volume

and is determined by venous return to the heart (preload, a function of intravascular volume) and arterial resistance (afterload, defined by smooth vascular tone).

Multiple factors, including sympathetic tone, determine the heart rate. Ranges in cardiac contractile force are determined by a multiplicity of factors, including beta-adrenergic stimulation, positive inotropes, negative inotropes, and the state of the myocardium per se. Thus, venous return, the status of extracardiac neural activity, circulating substances, and myocardial contractility together determine cardiac output.

Systemic blood pressure is determined by direct measurement or by indirect measurement over the arteries [22,56,73,85,176]. The pressure in small and large arteries, as well as in the aorta, tends to be comparable; the pressure in arterioles, capillaries, venules, small veins, and large veins drops off considerably. The lowest pressure is reached at diastole, and the peak of systole is equivalent to the height of arterial pressure. The mean area of pulsatile pressure is the area of pressures above and below the actual true mean. Clinically one can rapidly estimate mean arterial pressure by subtracting diastolic pressure from systolic and adding one-third of this difference to the diastolic pressure. Thus, a person with a blood pressure of 110/70 has a mean pressure of 83 (110 minus 70 equals 40; 40 divided by 3 is 13.3; 70 plus 13 is 83).

Chemoreceptors, Baroreceptors, and Cardiac Reflexes

Short-term blood pressure control is regulated by chemoreceptors, baroreceptors, and cardiovascular reflexes [110, 113, 218]. Special stretch receptors are located within arterial walls and are concentrated in high density in the carotid sinus and aortic arch regions. They respond most quickly during rapid blood pressure changes. When pressure is rising, the rate of firing is greater than when it is falling. For instance, carotid baroreceptors respond with increasing frequency above the level of 60 mmHg but do not respond between 0 and 60 mmHg; the maximum response is reached at a pressure of 180 mmHg. Within the aorta, baroreceptors respond at levels of about 30 mmHg higher. Baroreceptor impulses go to the medullary vasoconstrictor center and inhibit it and excite the vagal center. The result is a decrease in heart rate, vasodilatation, and decrease in myocardial contractility, resulting in lowering of blood pressure. Baroreceptors are probably important in control of blood pressure during positional changes. Chemoreceptors located in the carotid and aortic bodies are richly innervated and vascularized and concerned primarily with blood gas homeostasis; secondarily they may affect vasomotor and respiratory centers. If stimulated, they increase systemic blood pressure.

Additional receptors in the left atrium, ventricle, pulmonary artery, and pulmonary vein may affect changes in heart rate and peripheral resistance when stimulated by stress or various drugs [110,113,218]. Furthermore, an increase in stretch in the atria releases atrial natriuretic factor, which results in natriuresis and diuresis and affects blood pressure [30].

Hormonal Factors in Blood Pressure Control

Renin–Angiotensin System

The role of the renin–angiotensin system (RAS) in blood pressure control has been recognized since the early 1930s, when Goldblatt and colleagues demonstrated that renal artery constriction could cause chronic blood pressure elevation [67]. The research stimulated by that seminal experiment has resulted in the identification of multiple components of the renin–angiotensin–aldosterone system, clarified its role in regulation of blood pressure as well as salt and water balance, and in recent years resulted in the elucidation of the molecular biology of this system [24,34–42,45,60,83,156]. In addition, there is abundant evidence that components of the RAS are present in many tissues and may have local functions distinct from blood pressure regulation.

Renin is secreted by the renal juxtaglomerular apparatus, which is located in the wall of the afferent arteriole and adjoining macula densa portion of the distal tubule. Renin is an acid protease related to other acid proteases, such as cathepsin D and pepsin, and has a half-time in the circulation of 20 to 60 minutes. Its amino acid composition and gene structure have been determined.

The prohormone prorenin is also secreted by the kidney but is present even in anephric individuals [15,36,171]. Prorenin makes up the major portion of total plasma renin and is present in especially high levels in anephric individuals, during pregnancy, and in abnormal conditions such as long-standing diabetes. The function of circulating prorenin remains to be delineated, although activation of prorenin in the circulation undoubtedly occurs. The mechanism of activation is not clear, but acidification, prolonged storage at cold temperatures, and exposure to proteolytic enzymes such as trypsin may activate it.

Renin in the circulation acts on the protein substrate angiotensinogen, which is synthesized in the liver [45,156] as a glycoprotein with a molecular weight of about 65,000. Angiotensinogen release is stimulated by angiotensin II (AII), estrogens, and adrenocortical steroids [25,141,191].

Plasma levels of angiotensinogen may be important, since its concentration is a determinant of the rate of angiotensin formation.

Angiotensinogen has been shown by molecular biologic techniques to be present in numerous other tissues, including the kidney, brain, and adrenal glands [25,141]. The role of this substrate in local tissue renin–angiotensin systems and its interaction with blood pressure homeostatic mechanisms remain to be elucidated.

Renin cleaves angiotensinogen to form a decapeptide, angiotensin I (AI). Within the lungs, but also in other organs, angiotensin-converting enzyme (ACE; dipeptidylcarboxypeptidase) cleaves angiotensin I by removing the carboxy terminal His-Leu to produce an octapeptide, AII. This potent vasoconstrictor is also a stimulus for aldosterone production and, in turn, for increased angiotensinogen production by the liver. Angiotensin appears to be the prime mover in the physiologic effects of the RAS, although both angiotensin I and smaller fragments of angiotensins may themselves have direct physiologic effects. Figure 24-1 shows the primary components of the circulating RAS in humans.

Angiotensin II has actions other than as a vasoconstrictor: it stimulates aldosterone and catecholamine production by the adrenal medulla [47,101,148,149,210], it causes sympathetic vasomotor discharge within the CNS, and it stimulates norepinephrine synthesis and release at adrenergic nerve endings [8,9,90,121,122]. Other effects of angiotensin II, such as the CNS induction of thirst [50,109,172], the possible induction of follicle maturation in the ovary [65,92], and sodium–hydrogen exchange in the kidney [76,105,166], have led to a variety of hypotheses suggesting the interaction of the RAS system with processes other than blood pressure homeostasis.

CONTROL OF RENIN SECRETION

Renin synthesis and release are influenced by multiple variables, including sympathetic nervous system stimulation, vasoactive hormones such as AII, vasopressin, prostaglandins, atrial natriuretic peptide, plasma electrolyte concentrations such as potassium and calcium, and macula densa and baroreceptor mechanisms.

Beta-adrenergic receptor stimulation promotes renin release by increasing both renin secretion and renin mRNA synthesis, constituting a major way in which the sympathetic nervous system interacts with the RAS. The effects of beta-adrenergic stimulation presumably are mediated by cyclic AMP [2,167,216]. Increased sympathetic nerve traffic may be responsible for the increase in plasma renin activity with exercise or stress [13,28,33,93,106,126,142, 153,196].

Angiotensin [26,54,136], vasopressin [200], and probably atrial natriuretic factor [21,77] inhibit renin secretion. Prostaglandins may mediate renin release, whereas prostaglandin inhibitors such as nonsteroidal anti-inflammatory agents may inhibit it [10,52,55,62,86,104,173]. Increased potassium concentration in plasma may inhibit renin secretion, but the effect in humans is unclear [174].

Alterations in the net flux of calcium in juxtaglomerular cells may be a final pathway for renin release. Decreased intracellular calcium promotes renin release, and increased

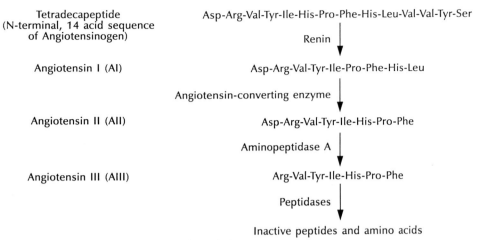

Tetradecapeptide (N-terminal, 14 acid sequence of Angiotensinogen)	Asp-Arg-Val-Tyr-Ile-His-Pro-Phe-His-Leu-Val-Val-Tyr-Ser
	↓ Renin
Angiotensin I (AI)	Asp-Arg-Val-Tyr-Ile-Pro-Phe-His-Leu
	Angiotensin-converting enzyme ↓
Angiotensin II (AII)	Asp-Arg-Val-Tyr-Ile-His-Pro-Phe
	Aminopeptidase A ↓
Angiotensin III (AIII)	Arg-Val-Tyr-Ile-His-Pro-Phe
	Peptidases ↓
	Inactive peptides and amino acids

FIG. 24-1. *The renin-angiotensin cascade in the human.*

intracellular calcium inhibits it [49,75,147,150,203]. There is an inverse correlation between calcium and calcium-regulatory hormones in humans with hypertension [117,118,135,158].

Sodium load perceived by the macula densa also regulates renin secretion [163,193,194,199]. There is controversy concerning how sodium signals are perceived, with variables such as tubular load of sodium chloride and sodium chloride flux and gradient across tubular epithelium being considered [138,163,164,192–194,199,213,214]. Decrease in sodium load perceived by the macula densa may stimulate renin release, which might explain how volume depletion is associated with increase of renin release. On the other hand, an acute increase in sodium chloride concentration in the distal tubule, such as that induced by a diuretic, also increases renin release. It may be that the glomerular tubular feedback mechanism for the RAS may act as a local mediator or "gate" between the signal perceived at the macula densa and the hemodynamic response in the glomerulus. Peripheral plasma renin activity may not reflect the intrarenal milieu, which may explain some of the differing experimental results.

A reduction of stretch or transmural pressure occurs when arterial pressure at the juxtaglomerular apparatus drops, which increases renin release [7,53,195]. This so-called baroreceptor mechanism does account for renin release whenever arterial pressure decreases, whether it be related to systemic hypotension or to localized intrarenal hypotension. The AII that is generated from baroreceptor-mediated renin release also stimulates aldosterone. Aldosterone then secondarily increases tubular reabsorption of sodium, thus gradually increasing plasma volume. Aldosterone secretion is controlled not only by interaction with the RAS but by ACTH and by plasma levels of sodium and potassium as well. Angiotensin II directly stimulates the zona glomerulosa of the adrenal cortex, thus increasing the conversion of mineralocorticoid precursors to aldosterone [79,157].

ANGIOTENSIN II RECEPTORS

Plasma membrane angiotensin II (AII) receptors are present in vascular smooth muscle [37,71], the adrenal gland [66,197], renal glomeruli [18,179], hepatocytes [31], the proximal tubule of the kidney [17], and certain CNS nuclei [177]. Whether there are multiple AII receptor types is unknown. AII receptor binding is enhanced by magnesium, manganese, and calcium and is reduced by guanine nucleotides (GTP) [11,215]. It is known that mesangial cells have AII receptors, which, when activated, may cause glomerular contraction, decrease in glomerular capillary surface area, and decrease in ultrafiltration [51,72]. Activation of proximal tubular AII receptors may increase sodium–hydrogen exchange and bicarbonate resorption [76,105,166].

ANGIOTENSIN-CONVERTING ENZYME

Angiotensin-converting enzyme (ACE) is present not only in the lung [178,187], but also in other tissues, including the kidney [23,35,154,217]. ACE within the kidney may be involved in both intrarenal modulation of renal hemodynamics and tubular function.

THE RENIN–ANGIOTENSIN SYSTEM IN PATHOPHYSIOLOGIC STATES

It has been recognized for some time that plasma renin activity is increased or decreased in many clinically important conditions (Table 24-1) [43,69,88,123,143,161, 165,180].

The RAS plays an important and well-recognized role in the initiation of hypertension in renovascular disease (Chapter 87). For instance, in models of renovascular hypertension, such as two-kidney, one-clip hypertension or one-kidney, one-clip hypertension, there are initially acute increases in plasma renin activity and angiotensin as well as a rapid increase in blood pressure, alterations in intra-

TABLE 24-1. *Plasma renin activity (PRA) and plasma aldosterone (PA) levels in various disease states*

	Normal or low blood pressure	Hypertension

PRA and PA increased	Bartter's syndrome
	Diuretic abuse
	Vomiting
	Hepatic disease
	Idiopathic nephrotic syndrome
	Hemorrhage
	Pregnancy
	Renal unresponsiveness to mineralo-
	   corticoids
		Renovascular disease
		Reninoma
		High-renin essential hypertension
		Malignant hypertension
		Chronic renal disease
		Coarctation of the aorta
		Hypertensive patients on diuretics,
		   vasodilators

PRA increased; PA decreased	Addison's disease (primary) Congenital adrenal hyperplasia Adrenal insufficiency in the severely ill patient	
PRA decreased; PA increased		Primary aldosteronism (Conn's syn- drome)
PRA decreased; PA normal		Low-renin essential hypertension
PRA and PA decreased		Excess mineralocorticoids other than aldosterone Liddle's syndrome Licorice ingestion Carbenoxolone ingestion Hypereninemic hypoaldosteronism

This table lists conditions in which plasma renin activity (PRA) and plasma aldosterone (PA) are altered.

renal hemodynamics, and an increase in aldosterone secretion [84]. AII antagonists, converting enzyme inhibitors, and renin-specific antibody normalize blood pressure in these models of experimental hypertension, indicating a causal relationship [5,44,127,146]. Pre-treatment with pharmacologic blockers before surgery can also prevent acute hypertension. Aldosterone secretion and hemodynamic shifts in these models, which have clinical correlates, enhance sodium reabsorption. The result is a second, more chronic phase of hypertension in which renin activity declines toward normal or actually reaches normal. Subsequently, depending on the sodium state, plasma renin activity in both clinical and experimental renovascular disease will vary.

In individuals with essential hypertension, plasma renin may be elevated, normal, or low [4,19,100]. In young people with essential hypertension, high plasma renin activity and its correlation with a particular type of essential hypertension are not clearly understood. In adults with "high renin" essential hypertension, it is felt that AII-induced vasoconstriction is responsible for blood pressure elevation. These individuals do not respond to plasma volume reduction or diuretic therapy and are not "salt sensitive." However, salt-sensitive individuals or "nonmodulators" may have an abnormal response to AII [39,211]. Although peripheral renin activity measurement has been suggested as a reasonable "screen" for hypertension, there are clear overlaps in values, even of AI levels,

in various groups of adults, and this phenomenon is even more marked in adolescents with primary hypertension.

MEASUREMENT OF RENIN ACTIVITY

Indirect radioimmunoassay is the usual manner in which plasma renin activity is clinically determined [70,74,170]. Direct radioimmunoassays are now available for measuring both active and inactive (prorenin) renin in the human although these assays are not generally clinically available [170]. Measurement of AII is accomplished by radioimmunoassay [112], but the technique is difficult because there are many angiotensinases present in plasma. Clinical measurement of angiotensinogen is difficult and not generally performed [14,78]. In the future, the RAS may be assessed by restriction enzyme analysis of genomic DNA or antibody-mediated testing, but these methods are not clinically available at present.

Another technique for measuring or assessing activity of the RAS clinically consists of pharmacologic interference of the RAS, as with competitive antagonists such as saralasin or teprotide [46,185]. Converting enzyme inhibition may also be helpful [103]. Drugs and other substances that may increase or decrease plasma renin activity are listed in Table 24-2. Again, in interpreting the situation, it is important to know whether a patient is receiving any agents that affect the RAS, as well the sodium chloride intake and balance of the individual. Furthermore, the RAS with

TABLE 24-2. *Drugs and other substances affecting renin release*

Stimulatory
Diuretics
Aldosterone antagonists
Diazoxide
Prazosin
Phenoxybenzamine
Phentolamine
Nitroprusside
Hydralazine
Minoxidil
Converting enzyme inhibitors (PRA by blocking AII production)
AII competitive antagonists
Beta-agonists
PGE_2, PGI_2
Prostacyclin
Histamine
Glucagon
PTH
Kallikrein
ACTH
Estrogen

Inhibitory
Nonsteroidal anti-inflammatory agents
Clonidine
Ganglionic blockers
Reserpine
Oxymetazoline
Alpha-methylodopa
Alpha-agonists
Beta-antagonists (nonselective more effective than selective B_1), e.g., propranolol, pindolol, timolol, nadolol, acebutolol
Angiotensin II
Vasopressin
Atrial natriuretic factor
K^+, Ca^{2+}

its various components does change with age, and it is important to know the normative data for a child of any given age group prior to interpreting clinical information, as discussed in the next section.

THE RENIN–ANGIOTENSIN SYSTEM IN DEVELOPMENT

The RAS is active during fetal life, and the human kidney is able to produce renin by the twentieth week of gestation [95]. Other components of the RAS, for example AII and aldosterone, are expressed in high levels in the fetus and the newborn. In fact, the RAS appears to be turned on and expressing its component parts at a higher level in the newborn than at any other time in life, although reasons for this are unclear [3,16,63,94,95,130,152,162,182,186, 198,201] (Chapter 11). The role of the RAS in the transition from fetal to extrauterine life may be substantial, with changes in flow and pressure in various vascular beds, changes in sodium balance, and the adaptations of kidney function to extrauterine life all interacting with the RAS. Because levels of renin, AI, and AII vary during life, age-

appropriate normative data must be used in interpreting values clinically.

Atriopeptin and Blood Pressure Regulation

Atriopeptins, a family of peptide hormones produced primarily in cardiac atria and derived in humans from a 151-amino acid precursor, have potent diuretic and natriuretic effects and appear to affect systemic blood pressure [6,29,30,99,108,139,140]. The high-molecular-weight parent compound is stored in cardiac atrial granules, and smaller forms are released with volume expansion or increase in right atrial pressure (as with pharmacologic agents and water immersion). The principal circulating form contains 28 amino acids and is referred to as atrial natriuretic protein (ANP).

Atriopeptins may be involved in blood pressure homeostasis via (1) vascular and cardiac effects; (2) renal effects, such as natriuresis and diuresis, as well as inhibition of renin release; (3) hormonal effects, such as decrease in aldosterone synthesis and secretion; and (4) inhibition of both vasopressin release and its peripheral actions. Vascular and cardiac effects of ANP include vasodilation, which may be mediated via atriopeptin-specific receptors, and subsequent stimulation of guanylate cyclase [48–80,212]. Cardiac output generally decreases in response to ANP, perhaps largely due to venodilation [29]. In humans, a variety of studies have shown that exogenous ANP leads to natriuresis and diuresis. ANP levels in humans vary with position and activity. For instance, levels are increased in children with volume overload or hypertension. However, conditions of different studies vary, making interpretation difficult.

Efforts to understand the role of atriopeptins in blood pressure homeostasis and hypertension are ongoing in multiple laboratories using several models of hypertension. Exogenous ANP lowers blood pressure, and a number of studies suggest the involvement of ANP in hypertensive states.

Prostaglandins

It has been known for some time that endogenous renal prostaglandins such as E_1 and E_2 increase renin secretion, whereas others such as prostaglandin F_2 do not have consistent effects [82,181,184]. Renal prostaglandins may be local mediators or modulators of other hormones affecting blood pressure regulation and secondarily may control blood pressure. Because angiotensin-converting enzyme, or kininase II, interacts both with angiotensin conversion and prostaglandin metabolism, complex interactions almost certainly occur. An example would be that intrarenal prostaglandins antagonize the action of antidiuretic hormone, which affects both water and sodium excretion at the same time as they might change renin secretion.

Prostaglandins and fatty acid metabolites of arachidonic acid may influence blood pressure regulation by a variety of modes, including primary intrinsic vasomotor responses, the capacity to modulate vasoconstrictor response to pressor hormones as previously described, the ability to change sodium balance (prostaglandins being natriuretic), the modulation of renin release in adrenergic nerve transmission, and the positive inotropic effect on the heart [107,131,155,184].

There is increasing evidence that abnormalities in prostaglandin and thromboxane metabolism contribute to the pathophysiology of hypertension. In primary hypertension there may be diminished endogenous synthesis of vasodilator prostaglandins and enhanced production of vasoconstrictor thromboxane [1,189,204]. Clinically, the use of nonsteroidal anti-inflammatory agents known to inhibit prostaglandin synthesis may make blood pressure control difficult [185]. Enhancing the synthesis of certain endogenous vasodilatory prostaglandin metabolites may provide a new means to control blood pressure [107,131,155,184].

Much remains to be learned about the role of prostaglandins in primary and secondary hypertension, but it would appear that enhancing synthesis by providing polyunsaturated fatty acid substrate might be clinically helpful.

Kinins

Kallikrein is an enzyme that forms kinins and acts on its substrate of kininogen to produce lysyl-bradykinin, which is a powerful vasodilator [27,81,102,115,125,129,137, 169]. Kallikrein affects water and electrolyte metabolism and is probably secondarily involved with arterial pressure regulation. It would appear that there is familial aggregation of kallikrein levels that may segregate with blood pressure levels. Whether therapeutic maneuvers designed to change kallikrein excretion rates and kinin levels within the kidney will be found to be clinically important remains to be determined.

Vasopressin

Vasopressin induces calcium flux and cellular contraction in vascular smooth muscle cells. Such cellular action may be mediated by cyclic AMP. In general, vasopressin maintains blood pressure secondarily because it causes renal water resorption. However, the direct association with any abnormality in vasopressin secretion and hypertension is unclear at this time [20,64,91,96,144,159,175,188].

Various models of hypertension, including desoxycorticosterone acetate (DOCA)-salt hypertension, renal artery hypertension (both one- and two-kidney), and essential hypertension (as in SHR rats), display increased secretion of vasopressin. In these models antivasopressin antisera have been reported to lower blood pressure, providing evidence that vasopressin does have an influence on blood pressure. Certain findings in clinical hypertension also suggest a role for vasopressin. For example, vasopressin has been reported to be decreased in primary aldosteronism and elevated in some patients with accelerated hypertension. A number of studies purport to show increases or decreases in plasma vasopressin activity with postural changes in patients with primary hypertension. Further studies are needed before it can be stated with assurance that vasopressin secretion plays a significant role in human hypertension.

Renomedullary Hormones

A dialyzable, low molecular weight peptide or substance (K_D <4500) appears to lower blood pressure experimentally [111,133,134]. This "renomedullary" substance appears to be derived from interstitial cells within the renal medulla. It appears to be distinct from renal prostaglandins and may prove to be a blood pressure–lowering substance with physiologic importance.

Glucocorticoids and Blood Pressure

It has long been known that an excess of glucocorticoids, whether from endogenous Cushing's syndrome or caused by administration of steroids, is associated with blood pressure elevation [151]. A variety of studies has led to the theory that steroid hormones raise blood pressure by a "hypertensinogenic" action distinct from the classic mineralocorticoid and glucocorticoid actions. Steroids possibly bind to some sort of receptor, perhaps in the CNS. In addition, the sodium-retaining, volume-expanding aspects of glucocorticoids also may contribute to the hypertension. Furthermore, cortisol potentiates pressor effects of epinephrine and may interact with prostaglandins, altering their synthesis. Changes in membrane transport also occur in response to steroids. Within the kidney, corticosteroids increase individual glomerular capillary flow and may contribute to glomerular hypertension and thus secondarily to systemic hypertension.

Parathyroid Hormone

That calcium is important in vascular smooth muscle contraction is supported by a large body of data [12,89, 116,147]. Decrease in ionized calcium in the plasma has been demonstrated to be a feature of essential hypertension in certain individuals. Furthermore, intracellular platelet calcium is high in many patients with essential hypertension. Such studies, stemming from information concerning adults, have yet to be performed in children and adolescents. Elevated total calcium and ionized calcium as in hyperparathyroidism and calcium poisoning (milk–alkali syndrome) are associated with the hypertension described in these conditions. Correlation with parathyroid hormone and other calcium metabolic hormones remains to be further elucidated.

Prolactin

Prolactin has been demonstrated to cause salt and water retention and may modify the responsiveness of the peripheral vasculature to depressor agents [114,128]. These effects may be mediated by prostaglandins. The role of prolactin in human hypertension is unsettled. During stress, prolactin secretion occurs in brief surges; its relationship to labile hypertension and stress-induced hypertension remains to be elucidated.

Blood Pressure and Sympathetic Nervous System Tone

Primary hypertension has been considered by some as a disorder of noradrenergic neurons since the discovery that norepinephrine is a pressor agent. In essential hypertension, certain patients have increased nervous system tone as reflected by mild increases in plasma catecholamines. Metabolites such as dopamine beta-hydroxylase have been studied as a means of identifying individuals with essential hypertension [98]. Nonetheless it has been difficult to demonstrate a consistent role for catecholamines in primary hypertension [120,132,202,207].

Norepinephrine, the major humoral transmitter, binds to specific alpha- and beta-adrenergic receptors. Nerve impulses traveling distally via adrenergic neurons reach blood vessels, the heart, and the kidneys, releasing norepinephrine, which then binds to these receptors. In general, stimulation of alpha-adrenergic receptor sites leads to arteriolar and venous vasoconstriction, whereas beta-adrenergic receptor stimulation promotes peripheral vasodilatation and increased heart rate as well as increased myocardial contractility. Beta-adrenergic stimulation also releases renin. Catecholamines are synthesized in multiple tissues in sympathetic nerve endings, the brain, and chromaffin tissue. Multiple interactions with hormonal systems occur, so that a straightforward interaction with blood pressure regulation is difficult to predict. The role of nerves in renal-mediated hypertension and other forms of hypertension remains a fertile area of hypertension investigation [68,87]. At the present time, the only definite form of hypertension known to be catecholamine related is that seen with neural crest tumors, such as pheochromocytoma [124,183].

Endothelin

Endothelium-dependent vasoconstriction mediated by the release of soluble factors and by direct cell to cell communications via gap junctions modulates vascular tone. One such factor, endothelin, a 21 amino-acid polypeptide, was isolated and described by Yanigasawa et al. in 1988 [216a]. This substance, more potent than any heretofore described vasoconstrictor, has potent systemic and renal effects [92a]. When administered intravenously, endothelin causes a biphasic pressure response, first lowering and then raising blood pressure. It increases renal vascular resistance, lowers renal blood flow, and may affect glomerular filtration rate variably. As endothelin receptors are present on numerous cell types, the substance is likely both an autocrine and paracrine mediator of blood pressure. How it is involved as a circulating modulator of blood pressure is as yet unknown. Its role in clinical hypertension and its interaction with other vasoactive substances is an area of active research.

ENDOTHELIUM-DERIVED VASOACTIVE SUBSTANCES

Endothelial cells synthesize and release a variety of vasoactive substances [107a]. In addition to angiotensin II (which may be taken up from the circulation or produced de novo) and a variety of prostanoids, endothelial-derived relaxing factor (EDRF) has been demonstrated in most mammalian species. Nitric oxide, NO, has been suggested as identical with EDRF; but other substances such as activators of Na^+,K^+-ATPase may also act as EDRF. Endothelial-derived constricting factors (EDCF) are also present, some not fully characterized. In addition to endothelin (described above), a nonprostanoid EDCF as well as a prostanoid EDCF appear to exist. The interaction of such factors are no doubt of importance in regulation of peripheral vascular resistance.

References

1. Abe K, Kasujima M, Chiba S, et al: Effect of furosemide on urinary excretion of prostaglandin E in normal volun-

teers and patients with essential hypertension. *Prostaglandins* 14:513, 1977.

2. Allison DJ, Tanigawa H, Assaykeen TA: The effects of cyclic nucleotides on plasma renin activity and renal function in dogs. *Adv Exp Med Biol* 17:33, 1972.

3. Aperia A, Broberger O, Henn P, et al: Sodium excretion in relation to sodium intake and aldosterone excretion in newborn pre-term and full-term infants. *Acta Paediatr Scand* 68:813, 1977.

4. Atlas SA, Case DB: Renin in essential hypertension. *Clin Endocrinol Metab* 10:537, 1981.

5. Atlas SA, Niarchos AP, Case DB: Inhibitors of the renin-angiotensin system. Effects on blood pressure, aldosterone secretion and renal function. *Am J Nephrol* 3:118, 1983.

6. Ballerman BJ, Brenner BM: Biologically active atrial peptides. *J Clin Invest* 76:2041, 1985.

7. Barajas L: The juxtaglomerular apparatus: Anatomical considerations in feedback control of glomerular filtration rate. *Fed Proc* 40:78, 1981.

8. Bell C: Mechanism of enhancement by angiotensin II of sympathetic adrenergic transmission in the guinea pig. *Circ Res* 31:348, 1972.

9. Benelli G, DellaBella D, Gandini A: Angiotensin and peripheral sympathetic nerve activity. *Br J Pharmacol* 22:211, 1964.

10. Blackshear JL, Spielman WS, Knox FG, et al: Dissociation of renin release and renal vasodilation by prostaglandin synthesis inhibitors. *Am J Physiol* 237:F20, 1979.

11. Blanc EB, Sraer J, Sraer JD, et al: Ca^{+2} and Mg^{+2} dependence of angiotensin II binding to isolated rat renal glomeruli. *Biochem Pharmacol* 25:517, 1978.

12. Blaustein MP, Hamlyn JM: Sodium transport inhibition, cell calcium, and hypertension. The natriuretic hormone/Na^+-Ca^{2+} exchange/hypertension hypothesis. *Am J Med* 77(4a):45, 1984.

13. Bonelli J, Waldhausl W, Magometchnigg D, et al: Effect of exercise and of prolonged oral administration of propranolol on hemodynamic variables, plasma renin concentration, plasma aldosterone and cAMP. *Eur J Clin Invest* 7:337, 1977.

14. Bouhnik J, Clauser E, Gardes J, et al: Direct radioimmunoassay of rat angiotensinogen and its application to rats in various endocrine states. *Clin Sci* 62:355, 1982.

15. Boyd GW: An inactive higher molecular weight renin in normal subjects and hypertensive patients. *Lancet* 1:215, 1977.

16. Broughton-Pipkin F, Smales ORC, O'Callaghan MJ: Renin and angiotensin levels in children. *Arch Dis Child* 56:298, 1981.

17. Brown G, Douglas J: Angiotensin II binding sites in rat and primate isolated renal tubular basolateral membranes. *Endocrinology* 112:2007, 1983.

18. Brown GP, Doublas JG, Krontiris-Litowitz J: Properties of angiotensin II receptors of isolated rat glomeruli: Factors influencing binding affinity and comparative binding of angiotensin analogs. *Endocrinology* 106:1923, 1980.

19. Brunner HR, Sealey JE, Laragh JH: Renin as a risk factor in essential hypertension: More evidence. *Am J Med* 55:295, 1973.

20. Bunag RD, Page IH, McCubbin JW: Inhibition of renin release by vasopressin and angiotensin. *Cardiovasc Res* I:67, 1967.

21. Burnett JC Jr, Granger JP, Opgenorth TJ: Effects of synthetic atrial natriuretic factor on renal function and renin release. *Am J Physiol* 247:F863, 1986.

22. Burton AC: *Physiology and Biophysics of the Circulation*, 2nd ed. Chicago, Year Book Medical Publishers, 1972.

23. Caldwell PRB, Seegal BC, Hsu KC, et al: Angiotensin-converting enzyme: Vascular endothelial localization. *Science* 191:1050, 1976.

24. Campbell DJ: The site of angiotensin production. *J Hypertens* 3:199, 1985.

25. Campbell DJ, Habener JF: Angiotensinogen gene is expressed and differentially regulated in multiple tissues of the rat. *J Clin Invest* 78:31, 1986.

26. Carey RM, Vaughn ED Jr, Peach MJ, et al: Activity of {des-aspartyl}-angiotensin II and angiotensin II in man. Differences in blood pressure and adrenocortical responses during normal and low sodium intake. *J Clin Invest* 62:20, 1978.

27. Carretero OA, Scicli AG: Possible role of kinins in circulatory homeostasis. State of the art review. *Hypertension* 3(Suppl I)I-5, 1981.

28. Clamge DM, Sanford CS, Vander AJ, et al: Effects of psychosocial stimuli on plasma renin activity in rats. *Am J Physiol* 231:1290, 1976.

29. Cole BR: The involvement of atriopeptins in blood pressure regulation. *Pediatric Nephrology* 1:109, 1987.

30. Cole BR, Needleman P: Atriopeptins: Volume regulatory hormones. *Clin Res* 33:389, 1985.

31. Crane JK, Campanile CP, Garrison C: The hepatic angiotensin II receptor. *J Biol Chem* 257:4959, 1982.

32. Culpepper WS: Cardiac anatomy and function in juvenile hypertension. *Am J Med* 99:57, 1983.

33. Dampney R, Stella AL, Golin R, et al: Vagal and sinoaortic reflexes in postural control of circulation and renin release. *Am J Physiol* 237:H146, 1979.

34. Deboben A, Iragami T, Ganten D: Tissue renin. *In* Genest J, Kuchel O, Hamet P, et al (eds): *Hypertension: Physiopathology and Treatment.* New York, McGraw-Hill, 1982, p 194.

35. Depierre D, Bargetzi JP, Roth M: Dipeptidyl carboxypeptidase from human seminal plasma. *Biochim Biophys Acta* 523:469, 1978.

36. Derkx FHM, Gool J, Wenting GJ, et al: Inactive renin in human plasma. *Lancet* 2:496, 1976.

37. Devynck MA, Pernollet MG, Meyer P, et al: Angiotensin receptors in smooth muscle cell membrane. *Nature (New Biol)* 245:55, 1973.

38. DeWardener HE, MacGregor GA: Blood pressure and the kidney. *In* Schrier RW, Gottschalk CW (eds): *Diseases of the Kidney*, 4th ed. Boston, Little, Brown, 1988, p 1543.

39. Dluhy RG, Bavli SZ, Leung FK, et al: Abnormal adrenal responsiveness and angiotensin II dependency in high renin essential hypertension. *J Clin Invest* 64:1270, 1979.

40. Dow P: Estimates of cardiac output and central blood volume by dye dilution. *Physiol Rev* 36:77, 1956.

41. Dzau VJ: Significance of vascular renin-angiotensin pathway. *Hypertension* 8:553, 1986.

42. Dzau VJ, Burt D, Pratt RE: The molecular biology of the renin-angiotensin system. *American J Physiol* 255:P F563, 1988.

43. Dzau VJ, Colucci WS, Hollenberg NK, et al: Relation of the renin-angiotensin-aldosterone system to clinical state in congestive heart failure. *Circulation* 63:645, 1981.

44. Dzau VJ, Kopelman RI, Barger AC, et al: Comparison of renin-specific IgG and antibody fragments in studies of blood pressure regulation. *Am J Physiol* 246:H404, 1984.

45. Dzau VJ, Pratt RE: Renin-angiotensin system: Biology, physiology and pharmacology. *In* Haber E, Morgan H, Katz A, et al (eds): *Handbook of Experimental Cardiology.* New York, Raven Press, 1986, p 1631.

46. Favre L, Boerth RC, Braren V, et al: Angiotensin II blockade by saralasin in the evaluation of hypertension in children. *Kidney Int* 15(Suppl 9):75, 1979.

47. Feldberg W, Lewis GP: The action of peptides on the adrenal medulla. Release of adrenaline by bradykinin and angiotensin. *J Physiol (Lond)* 171:98, 1964.

48. Fiscus RR, Rapoport RM, Waldman SA, et al: Atriopeptin II elevates cyclic GMP, activates cyclic GMP-dependent protein kinase and causes relaxation in rat thoracic aorta. *Biochim Biophys Acta.* 846:179, 1985.

49. Fishman MC: Membrane potential of juxtaglomerular cells. *Nature* 260:542, 1976.

50. Fitzsimmons JT: The physiologic basis of thirst. *Kidney Int* 10:3, 1976.

51. Foidart J, Sraer J, Delarue F, et al: Evidence for mesangial glomerular receptors for angiotensin II linked to mesangial cell contractility. *FEBs Lett* 121:333, 1980.

52. Francisco LL, Osborn JL, DiBona CF: Prostaglandins in renin release during sodium deprivation. *Am J Physiol* 243:F537, 1982.

53. Fray JGS: Stretch receptor model for renin release with evidence from perfused rat kidney. *Am J Physiol* 23:936, 1976.

54. Freeman RH, Dais JO, Lohmeier TE: Des-I-Asp-angiotensin II. Possible intrarenal role in homeostasis in the dog. *Circ Res* 37:30, 1975.

55. Freeman RH, Davis JO, Villareal R: Role of renal prostaglandins in the control of renin release. *Circ Res* 54:1, 1984.

56. Freis ED: Hemodynamics of hypertension. *Physiol Rev* 40:27, 1960.

57. Frohlich ED: The heart in hypertension. *In* Genest J, Kuchel O, Hamet P, et al (eds): *Hypertension*, 2nd ed. New York, McGraw-Hill, 1983, p 791.

58. Frohlich Ed: Hemodynamics of hypertension. *In* Genest J, Koiw E, Kuchel O (eds): *Hypertension: Pathophysiology and Treatment*. New York, McGraw-Hill, 1977, p 15.

59. Frolich JC, Hollifield JW, Michelakis AM, et al: Reduction of plasma renin activity by inhibition of the fatty acid cyclooxygenase in human subjects. *Circ Res* 44:81, 1979.

60. Ganten D, Schelling P, Vecsei P, et al: Iso-renin of extrarenal origin. The tissue angiotensinogenase systems. *Am J Med* 60:760, 1976.

61. Genest J, Tarazi RC: The hemodynamics of hypertension. *In* Genest J, Kuchel O, Hamet P, et al (eds): *Hypertension*, 2nd ed. New York, McGraw-Hill, 1983, p 15.

62. Gerber JG, Nies AS, Olsen RD: Control of canine renin release: Macula densa requires prostaglandin synthesis. *J Physiol* 319:419, 1981.

63. Giovannelli G: Plasma renin activity in normal children. *J Pediatr* 91:847, 1977.

64. Glanzer K, Prubing B, Dusing R, et al: Hemodynamic and hormonal responses to 8-arginine-vasopressin in healthy man. *Klin Wochenschr* 60:1234, 1982.

65. Glorioso N, Atlas SA, Laragh JH, et al: Prorenin high concentration in human ovarian follicular fluid. *Science* 233:1422, 1986.

66. Glossmann H, Baukal AJ, Catt KJ: Properties of angiotensin II receptors in the bovine and rat adrenal cortex. *J Biol Chem* 249:825, 1974.

67. Goldblatt H, Lynch J, Hanzal RF, et al: Studies in experimental hypertension. I. The production of persistent elevation of systolic blood pressure by means of renal ischemia. *J Exp Med* 59:347, 1934.

68. Goldstein DS: Plasma norepinephrine in essential hypertension: A study of studies. *Hypertension* 3:48, 1981.

69. Gottshall RW, Davis JO, Shade RE, et al: Effects of renal denervation on renin release in sodium-depleted dogs. *Am J Physiol* 225:344, 1973.

70. Gould AB, Skeggs LT, Kahn JR: Measurement of renin and substrate concentrations in human serum. *Lab Invest* 15:1802, 1966.

71. Gunther S, Gimbrone MA Jr, Alexander RW: Identification and characterization of the high affinity vascular angiotensin II receptor in rat mesenteric artery. *Circ Res* 47:278, 1980.

72. Gunther S, Gimbrone MA Jr, Alexander RW: Regulation by angiotensin II of its receptors in resistance blood vessels. *Nature* 287:230, 1980.

73. Guyton AC: *Arterial Pressure and Hypertension.* Philadelphia, WB Saunders, 1981.

74. Haber E, Loerner T, Page LB, et al: Application of radioimmunoassay for angiotensin I to the physiologic measurements of plasma renin activity in normal human subjects. *J Clin Endocrinol Metab* 29:1349, 1969.

75. Harada E, Lester GE, Rubin RP: Stimulation of renin secretion from the intact kidney and from isolated glomeruli by the calcium ionophore A23187. *Biochim Biophys Acta* 583:20, 1979.

76. Harris PJ, Navar LG: Tubular transport responses to angiotensin. *Am J Physiol* 248:F621, 1985.

77. Henrich W, McAllister L, Smith P, et al: Direct effects of atriopeptin (AP) in renin release. *Clin Res* 33:528A, 1986.

78. Hidaka H, Itoh T, Sato R, et al: A new direct radioimmunoassay for human renin substrate and heterogeneity of human renin substrate in pathological states. *Jpn Circ J* 44:375, 1980.

79. Himathongkam T, Dluhy RG, Williams GH: Potassium-aldosterone-renin interrelationships. *J Clin Endocrinol Metab* 41:153, 1975.

80. Hirata Y, Masahiro T, Hiroki Y, et al: Specific receptors for atrial natriuretic factor (ANF) in cultured vascular smooth muscle cells of rat aorta. *Biochem Biophys Res Commun* 125:562, 1984.

81. Holland OB, Chud JM, Braunstein H: Urinary kallikrein excretion in essential and mineralocorticoid hypertension. *J Clin Invest* 65:347, 1980.

82. Iaconi JM, Dougherty RM, Puska P: Reduction of blood pressure associated with dietary polyunsaturated fat. *Hypertension* 4(Suppl III):III-34, 1982.

83. Inagami T, Murakami K: Pure renin: Isolation from hog kidney and characterization. *J Biol Chem* 252:2978, 1977.

84. Ingelfinger JR: Experimental models of hypertension. *In* Ingelfinger JR: *Pediatric Hypertension.* Philadelphia, WB Saunders, 1982, p 269.

85. Ingelfinger JR: Hemodynamics and blood pressure. *In* Ingelfinger JR: *Pediatric Hypertension.* Philadelphia, WB Saunders, 1982, p 64.

86. Jackson EK, Herzer WA, Zimmerman JB, et al: Effects of indomethacin on beta-adrenoreceptor-stimulated renin release in the dog. *J Pharmacol Exp Ther* 222:414, 1982.

87. Jose P: Adrenergic regulation of blood pressure. *In* Loggie JMH, Horan MJ, Gruskin AB, et al (eds): *NHLBI Workshop on Juvenile Hypertension.* New York, Biomedical Information Corporation, 1984, p 205.

88. Kaplan NM, Kem DC, Holland B, et al: The intravenous furosemide test: A simple way to evaluate renin responsiveness. *Ann Intern Med* 84:639, 1976.

89. Kesteloot H, Geboers J: Calcium and blood pressure. *Lancet* 1:813, 1982.

90. Khairallah PA: Action of angiotensin on adrenergic nerve endings: Inhibition of norepinephrine uptake. *Fed Proc* 31:1351, 1972.

91. Khokhar AM, Hough C, Slater JDH: Increased urine vasopressin concentration in essential hypertension. *Clin Sci Molec Med* 47:9P, 1974.

92. Kim S-J, Shinjo M, Tada M, et al: Ovarian renin gene

expression is regulated by follicle stimulating hormone. *Biochem Biophys Res Commun* 146:989, 1987.

92a. King AJ, Marsden PA, Brenner BM: Endothelin: A potent vasoactive peptide of endothelial origin. *In* Laragh JH, Brenner BM (eds): Hypertension: Pathophysiology, diagnosis and management. New York, Raven Press (eds): 1990, p 649.

93. Kopp WG, DiBona GF: Interaction between neural and nonneural mechanisms controlling renin secretion rate. *Am J Physiol* 246:F620, 1984.

94. Kotchen TA, Strickland AL, Rice TW, et al: A study of the renin-angiotensin system in newborn infants. *J Pediatr* 80:938, 1972.

95. Kowarski A, Katz H, Migeon CJ: Plasma aldosterone concentration in normal subjects from infancy to adulthood. *J Clin Endocrinol Metab* 38:489, 1974.

96. Krakoff LR, Elijovich F, Barry C: The role of vasopressin in experimental and clinical hypertension. *Am J Kidney Dis* 5:A40, 1985.

97. Kronik G, Slany J, Mossbacher H: Comparative value of eight M-mode echocardiographic formulas for determining left ventricular stroke volume: A correlative study with thermodilution and left ventricular single plan cinecardiography. *Circulation* 60:1308, 1979.

98. Lake CR, Ziegler MG, Coleman M, et al: Lack of correlation of plasma norepinephrine and dopamine beta hydroxylase in hypertensive and normotensive subjects. *Circ Res* 41:865, 1977.

99. Laragh JH: Atrial natriuretic hormone, the renin aldosterone axis, and blood pressure-electrolyte homeostasis. *N Engl J Med* 313:1330, 1985.

100. Laragh JH: Vasoconstriction-volume analysis for understanding and treating hypertension: The use of renin and aldosterone profiles. *Am J Med* 55:261, 1973.

101. Laragh JH, Angers M, Kelly WG, et al: Hypotensive agents and pressor substances: The effect of epinephrine, norepinephrine, angiotensin II, and others on the secretory rate of aldosterone in man. *JAMA* 174:234, 1960.

102. Lawton WJ, Fitz AE: Urinary kallikrein in normal renin essential hypertension. *Circulation* 56:856, 1977.

103. Levenson DJ, Dzau VJ: Effects of angiotensin-converting enzyme inhibition on renal hemodynamics in renal artery stenosis. *Kidney Int* 31(S20:S-173, 1987.

104. Lin CS, Iwao H, Puttkammer S, et al: Prostaglandins and renin release in vitro. *Am J Physiol* 240:E609, 1981.

105. Liu FY, Cogan MG: Angiotension II: A potent regulator of acidification in the rat early proximal convoluted tubule. *J Clin Invest* 80:273, 1987.

106. Loeffer JR, Stockigt JR, Ganong WF: Effect of alpha and beta adrenergic blocking agents on the increase in renin secretion produced by stimulation of the renal nerves. *Neuroendocrinology* 10:129, 1972.

107. Lorenz R, Spengler U, Fischer S, et al: Platelet function, thromboxane formation, and blood pressure control during supplementation of the Western diet with cold liver oil. *Circulation* 67:504, 1983.

107a. Luscher TF, Diederich D, Buhler FR, et al: Interactions between platelets and the vessel wall. Role of endothelium-derived vasoactive substances. *In* Laragh JH, Brenner BM (eds): Hypertension: Pathophysiology, diagnosis and management. New York, Raven Press (eds): 1990, p 637.

108. Maack T, Camargo MJF, Kleinert HD, et al: Atrial natriuretic factor: Structure and functional properties. *Kidney Int* 27:607, 1985.

109. Malvin RL: Possible role of the renin-angiotensin system in the regulation of anti-diuretic hormone secretion. *Fed Proc* 30:1382, 1971.

110. Mancia G, Mark AL: Arterial baroreflexes in humans. *In* Shepherd JT, Abboud FM (eds): *Handbook of Physiology, Section 2, The Cardiovascular System.* American Physiological Society. Baltimore, Williams & Wilkins, 1983, p 755.

111. Manger WM, VanPraag D, Weiss RJ, et al: Effect of transplanting renomedullary tissue into spontaneously hypertensive rats (SHR) *Fed Proc* 35:556, 1976.

112. Margolis SA, Konash PL: The high-performance liquid chromatographic analysis of diastereomers and structural analogs of angiotensins I and II. *Anal Biochem* 134:163, 1983.

113. Mark AL, Marcia E: Cardiopulmonary basoreflexes in humans. *In* Shepherd JT, Abboud FM (eds): *Handbook of Physiology, Section 2, The Cardiovascular System.* American Physiological Society. Baltimore, Williams & Wilkins, 1983, p 795.

114. Mati JK, Mugambi M, Odipo WS, et al: Prolactin and hypertension. *Am J Obstet Gynecol* 127:616, 1977.

115. Mayfield RK, Margolius HS: Renal kallikrein-kinin-system. Relation to renal function and blood pressure. *Am J Nephrol* 3:145, 1983.

116. McCarron DA: Calcium in the pathogenesis and therapy of human hypertension. *Am J Med* 78(Suppl 2B):27, 1985.

117. McCarron DA: Low serum concentrations of ionized calcium in patients with hypertension. *N Engl J Med* 307:226, 1982.

118. McCarron DA, Morris DA, Cole C: Dietary calcium in human hypertention. *Science* 217:267, 1982.

119. McCarron DA, Pingree PA, Rubin RJ, et al: Enhanced parathyroid function in essential hypertension: A homeostatic response to a urinary calcium leak. *Hypertension* 2:162, 1980.

120. McCrory WW, Klein AA, Rosenthal RA: Blood pressure, heart rate and plasma catecholamines in normal and hypertensive children and their siblings at rest and after standing. *Hypertension* 4:507, 1982.

121. McCubbin JW: Peripheral effects of angiotensin on the autonomic nervous system. *In* Page IH, Bumpus FM (eds): *Angiotensin.* New York, Springer-Verlag, 1974, p 417.

122. McCubbin JW, Page IH: Renal pressor system and neurogenic control of arterial pressure. *Circ Res* 12:553, 1963.

123. Medina A, Davies DL, Brown JJ, et al: A study of the renin-angiotensin system in the nephrotic syndrome. *Nephron* 12:233, 1974.

124. Mendlowitz M: Neural crest tumors of sympathetic or chromaffin origin (pheochromocytoma, ganglioneuroma and neuroblastoma). *In* Genest J, Koiw K, Kuchel O (eds): *Hypertension.* New York, McGraw-Hill, 1977, p 781.

125. Mersey JH, Williams GH, Emanuel R, et al: Plasma bradykinin levels and urinary kallikrein excretion in normal renin essential hypertension. *J Clin Endocrinol Metab* 48:642, 1979.

126. Michelakis AM, McAllister RG: The effect of chronic adrenergic receptor blockade on plasma renin activity in man. *J Clin Endocrinol Metab* 34:386, 1972.

127. Mimran A, Jover B, Casellas D: Renal adaptation to sodium deprivation. Effect of captopril in the rat. *Am J Med* 76:14, 1984.

128. Modlinger RS, Gutkin M: Plasma prolactin in essential and renovascular hypertension. *J Lab Clin Med* 91:693, 1978.

129. Mohring J, Mohring B, Petri M, et al: Plasma vasopressin concentration and effects of vasopressin antiserum in blood pressure in rats with malignant two-kidney Goldblatt hypertension. *Circ Res* 42:17, 1978.

130. Molteni A, Rahil WJ, Koo JH: Evidence for a vasopressor substance (renin in human fetal kidneys). *Lab Invest* 30:115, 1974.

131. Moncada S, Vane JR: Arachidonic acid metabolites and their interactions between platelet and blood-vessel walls. *N Engl J Med* 300:1142, 1979.

132. Mongeau JG, deChamplain J, Davignon A: Study of sympathetic activity in adolescents suffering from essential hypertension: Preliminary data on plasma catecholamines. *In* Giovanelli G, New MI, Gorini S (eds): *Hypertension in Children and Adolescents.* New York, Raven Press, 1981, p 152.

133. Muirehead EE: Renomedullary system of blood pressure control. *Hypertension* 8(Suppl I):I-38, 1986.

134. Muirehead EE, Rightsel WA, Leach BE, et al: Reversal of hypertension by transplants and lipid extracts of cultured renomedullary interstitial cells. *Lab Invest* 35:162, 1977.

135. Naftilan AJ, Oparil S: The role of calcium in the control of renin release. *Hypertension* 4:670, 1982.

136. Naftilan AJ, Oparil S: Inhibition of renin release from rat kidney slices by the angiotensins. *Am J Physiol* 235:F62, 1978.

137. Nasjletti A, Malik KU: Renal kinin-prostaglandin relationship. Implications for renal function. *Kidney Int* 19:860, 1981.

138. Navar LG, Rosivall L: Contribution of the renin-angiotensin system to the control of intrarenal hemodynamics. *Kidney Int* 25:857, 1984.

139. Needleman P, Adams SP, Cole BR, et al: Atriopeptins as cardiac hormones. *Hypertension* 7:469, 1985.

140. Needleman P, Greenwald JE: Atriopeptin: A cardiac hormone intimately involved in fluid, electrolyte, and blood-pressure homeostasis. *N Engl J Med* 314:828, 1986.

141. Ohkubo H, Nakayama K, Tamaka T, et al: Tissue distribution of rat angiotensinogen mRNA and structural analysis. *J Biol Chem* 261:319, 1986.

142. O'Malley K, Velasco M, Wells J, et al: Control of plasma renin activity and changes in sympathetic tone as determinants of minoxidil-induced increase in plasma renin activity. *J Clin Invest* 55:230, 1975.

143. Oparil S, Vassaux C, Sanders CA, et al: Role of renin in acute postural homeostasis. *Circulation* 41:89, 1970.

144. Padfield PL, Brown TJ, Lever AF, et al: Changes of vasopressin in hypertension: Cause or effect? *Lancet* 1:1255, 1976.

145. Page IH: Some regulatory mechanisms of renovascular and essential arterial hypertension. *In* Genest J, Koiw E, Kuchel O (eds): *Hypertension.* New York, McGraw-Hill, 1977, p 576.

146. Paller MS, Linas SL: Role of angiotensin II, β-adrenergic system and arginine vasopressin on arterial pressure in the rat. *Am J Physiol* 246:H25, 1984.

147. Park CS, Malvin RL: Calcium in the control of renin release. *Am J Physiol* 235:F22, 1978.

148. Peach MJ, Ackerly JA: Angiotensin antagonists and the adrenal cortex and medulla. *Fed Proc* 35:2502, 1976.

149. Peach MJ, Bumpus FM, Khairallah PA: Release of adrenal catecholamines by angiotensin I. *J Pharmacol Exp Ther* 176:366, 1971.

150. Peart S, Quesada T, Tenyi I: Effects of EDTA and EGTA and renin secretion. *Br J Pharmacol* 59:247, 1977.

151. Perera A: Cortisone and blood pressure. *Proc Soc Exp Biol Med* 76:583, 1951.

152. Pernollet MG, Devynck MA, Macdonald GJ, et al: Plasma renin activity and adrenal angiotensin II receptors in fetal, newborn, and pregnant rabbits. *Biol Neonate* 36:119, 1979.

153. Peytremann A, Favre L, Valloton B: Effect of cold pressor test and 2-deoxy-D-glucose infusion on plasma renin activity in man. *Eur J Clin Invest* 2:432, 1972.

154. Phillips MI: New evidence for brain angiotensin and for its role in hypertension. *Fed Proc* 42:2667, 1983.

155. Puska P, Nissinen A, Vartiainen E, et al: Controlled, randomized trial of the effect of dietary fat on blood pressure. *Lancet* 1:1, 1983.

156. Rauh W: Renin-angiotensin system. *In* Holliday MA, Barratt TM, Vernier RL (eds): *Pediatric Nephrology,* 2nd ed. Baltimore, Williams & Wilkins, 1987, p 227.

157. Reid IA, Ganong WF: Control of aldosterone secretion. *In* Genest J, Koiw E, Kuchel O (eds): *Hypertension.* New York, McGraw-Hill, 1977, p. 265.

158. Resnick LM, Laragh JH, Sealey JE, et al; Divalent cations in essential hypertension—relations between serum ionized calcium, magnesium, and plasma renin activity. *N Engl J Med* 309:888, 1983.

159. Rocha E, Silva M Jr, Rosenberg M: Release of vasopressin in response to hemorrhage and its role in the mechanisms of blood pressure regulation. *J Physiol* 202:535, 1969.

160. Safar ME, London GM, Simon AC, et al: Volume factors, total exchangeable sodium nd potassium in hypertensive disease. *In* Genest J, Kuchel O, Hamet P, et al (eds): *Hypertension,* 2nd ed. New York, McGraw-Hill, 1983, p 42.

161. Sancho J, Re R, Burton J, et al: The role of the renin-angiotensin-aldosterone system in cardiovascular homeostasis in normal human subjects. *Circulation* 53:400, 1976.

162. Sassard J, Sann L, Vincent M, et al: Plasma renin activity in normal subjects from infancy to puberty. *J Clin Endocrinol Metab* 40:524, 1975.

163. Schnermann J, Briggs J: Concentration-dependent sodium chloride transport as the signal in feedback control of glomerular filtration rate. *Kidney Int* 22(Suppl 12)S82, 1982.

164. Schnermann J, Ploth DW, Hermle M: Activation of tubuloglomerular feedback by chloride transport. *Pflugers Arch* 362:229, 1976.

165. Schroeder ET, Anderson GH, Goldman SH, et al: Effects of blockade of angiotensin II on blood pressure, renin and aldosterone in cirrhosis and ascites. *Kidney Int* 9:511, 1976.

166. Schuster VL, Kokko JP, Jacobsen HR: Angiotension II directly stimulates sodium transport in rabbit proximal convoluted tubules. *J Clin Invest* 73:507, 1984.

167. Schwertschlag U, Hackerthal E: Forskolin stimulates renin release from the isolated perfused rat kidney. *Eur J Pharmacol* 84:111, 1982.

168. Scoggins BA, Coghlan JP, Denton DA, et al: "How do adrenocortical steroid hormones produce hypertension?" *Clin Exp Hypertens* A6:315, 1984.

169. Sealey JE, Atlas SA, Laragh JH: Human urinary kallikrein converts inactive to active renin and is a possible physiological activator of renin. *Nature* 275:144, 1978.

170. Sealey JE, Laragh JH: How to do a plasma renin assay. *Cardiovascular Medicine.* 2:1079, 1977.

171. Sealey JE, Moon C, Laragh JH, et al: Plasma prorenin: Cryoactivation and relationship to renin substrate in normal subjects. *Am J Med* 61:731, 1976.

172. Severs WB, Daniels-Severs AE: Effects of angiotensin on the central nervous system. *Pharmacol Rev* 25:415, 1973.

173. Seymour AA, Zehr JE: Influence of renal prostaglandin synthesis on renin control mechanisms in the dog. *Circ Res* 45:13, 1979.

174. Shade RE, Davis JO, Johnson JA, et al: Effects of renal arterial infusion of sodium and potassium on renin secretion in the dog. *Circ Res* 31:719, 1972.

175. Share L, Crofton JT: The role of vasopressin in hypertension. *Fed Proc* 43:103, 1984.

176. Shkhvatsabaya LK, Erina E, Almusavi AI: Venous tone in essential hypertension. *Cor Vasa* 19:184, 1977.

177. Sirett NJ, McLean AB, Bray JJ, et al: Distribution of angiotensin II receptors in rat brain. *Brain Res* 122:299, 1977.

178. Skeggs LT, Kahn JR, Shumway NP: The preparation and function of the hypertensin-converting enzyme. *J Exp Med* 103:295, 1956.

179. Skorecki KL, Ballermann BJ, Rennke GH, et al: Angiotensin II receptor regulation in isolated renal glomeruli. *Fed Proc* 42:3064, 1983.

180. Skorecki KL, Brenner BM: Body fluid homeostasis in congestive heart failure and cirrhosis with ascites. *Am J Med* 72:323, 1982.

181. Smith MC, Dunn MJ: The role of prostaglandins in human hypertension. *Am J Kidney Dis* 5:A32, 1985.

182. Spitzer A: The role of the kidney in sodium homeostasis during maturation. *Kidney Int* 21:539, 1982.

183. Stackpole RH, Melicow MM, Uson AC: Pheochromocytoma in children: Report of 9 cases and review of the first 100 published cases with follow-up studies. *J Pediatr* 63:315, 1963.

184. Stoff JS: Prostaglandins and hypertension. *Am J Med* 80(Suppl 1A):56, 1986.

185. Streeter HP, Anderson GH, Freiberg JM, et al: Use of the angiotensin II antagonist saralasin in the recognition of "angiotensinogenic" hypertension. *N Engl J Med* 292:657, 1975.

186. Sulyok E, Nemeth M, Tenyi IF, et al: Relationship between maturity, electrolyte balance and the function of the renin-angiotensin-aldosterone system in newborn infants. *Biol Neonate* 35:60, 1979.

187. Sweet CS, Blaine EH: Angiotensin-converting enzyme and renin inhibitors. *In* Antonaccio M (ed): *Cardiovascular Pharmacology.* New York, Raven Press, 1984, p 119.

188. Szczepanska-Sadowska E: Hemodynamic effects of a moderate increase in the plasma vasopressin level in conscious dogs. *Pflugers Arch* 338:313, 1973.

189. Tan SY, Bravo E, Mulrow PJ: Impaired renal prostaglandin E₂ biosynthesis in human hypertensive states. *Prostaglandins Leukotrines Med* 1:76, 1978.

190. Tarazi AC: Introduction: Recent perspectives on hypertension and the heart. *Am J Cardiol* 44:845, 1979.

191. Tewksbury DA, Frome WL, Dumas ML: Characterization of human angiotensinogen. *J Biol Chem* 253:3817, 1978.

192. Thurau K, Gruner A, Mason J, et al; Tubular signal for the renin activity in the juxtaglomerular apparatus. *Kidney Int* 22(Suppl 12):S-55, 1982.

193. Thurau K, Mason J: The internal function of the juxtaglomerular apparatus. MTP-International Review of Science, Physiology Series. 1:6. *In* Thurau K (ed): *Kidney and Urinary Tract Physiology* London, Butterworth, 1974, p 357.

194. Thurau K, Schnermann J: Die Natrium-Konzentration an den Maculadensa-Zellen als reguherender Faktor für das Glomerulumfiltrat. *Klin Wochenschr* 43:410, 1965.

195. Tobian L, Tomboulian A, Janecek J: The effect of high perfusion pressure on the granulation of juxtaglomerular cells in an isolated kidney. *J Clin Invest* 38:605, 1959.

196. Torreti J: Sympathetic control of renin release. *Annu Rev Pharmacol Toxicol* 22:167, 1982.

197. Vallotton MB, Capponi AM, Grillet C, et al: Characterization of angiotensin receptors on bovine adrenal fasiculata cells. *Proc Natl Acad Sci USA* 78:592, 1981.

198. vanAcker KJ, Scharpe SL, Deprettere AJR, et al: Renin-angiotensin-aldosterone system in the healthy infant and child. *Kidney Int* 16:196, 1979.

199. Vander AJ: Control of renin release. *Physiol Rev* 47:359, 1967.

200. Vandongen R: Inhibition of renin secretion in the isolated rat kidney by antidiuretic hormone. *Clin Sci Mol Med* 49:73, 1975.

201. Vincent M, Dessart Y, Annat G, et al: Plasma renin activity, aldosterone and dopamine-β-hydroxylase activity as a function of age in normal children. *Pediatr Res* 14:894, 1980.

202. Vlachakis ND: Blood pressure and catecholamine responses to sympathetic stimulation in normotensive and hypertensive subjects. *J Clin Pharmacol* 19:458, 1979.

203. Watkins BE, Davis JO, Lohmeier TE, et al: Intrarenal site of action of calcium on renin secretion in dogs. *Circ Res* 39:847, 1976.

204. Weber PC, Scherer B, Held B, et al: Urinary prostaglandins and kallikrein in essential hypertension. *Clin Sci* 57:2595, 1979.

205. Weidmann P, Beretta-Piccoli C, Ziegler WH, et al: Age versus urinary sodium for judging renin, aldosterone, and catecholamine levels: Studies in normal subjects and patients with essential hypertension. *Kidney Int* 14:619, 1978.

206. Weisel RD, Berger RL, Hechtman HB: Current concepts in measurement of cardiac output by thermodilution. *N Engl J Med* 292:682, 1975.

207. Whitworth JA: Mechanisms of glucocorticoid-induced hypertension. *Kidney Int* 31:1213, 1987.

208. Whitworth JA, Connell JMC, Lever AF, et al: Pressor responsiveness in steroid induced hypertension in man. *Clin Exp Pharmacol Physiol* 13:353, 1986.

209. Whitworth JA, Connell JMC, Lever AF, et al: Haemodynamic and metabolic effects of oral hydrocortisone administration in man (abstract). *Proc Int Union Physiol Soc* XVI:600, 1986.

210. Williams GH, Dluhy RG: Aldosterone biosynthesis. Interrelationship of regulatory factors. *Am J Med* 53:595, 1972.

211. Williams GH, Hollenberg NK, Moore TJ, et al: The adrenal receptor for angiotensin II is altered in essential hypertension. *J Clin Invest* 63:419, 1979.

212. Winquist J, Faison EP, Waldman SA, et al: Atrial natriuretic factor elicits an endothelium-independent relaxation and activates particulate guanylate cyclase in vascular smooth muscle. *Proc Natl Acad Sci USA* 81:7661, 1984.

213. Wright FS, Briggs JP: Feedback control of glomerular blood flow, pressure, and filtration rate. *Physiol Rev* 59:958, 1979.

214. Wright FS, Schnermann J: Interference with feedback control of glomerular filtration rate by furosemide, triflocin and cyanide. *J Clin Invest* 53:1695, 1974.

215. Wright GB, Alexander RW, Ekstein LS, et al: Sodium divalent cations and guanine nucleotide regulate the affinity of the rat mesenteric artery angiotensin II receptor. *Circ Res* 50:462, 1982.

216. Yamamoto K, Okahara T, Abe Y, et al: Effects of cyclic AMP and dibutyryl cyclic AMP on renin release in vivo and in vitro. *Jpn Circ J* 37:1271, 1973.

216a. Yanigasawa M, Kurihara H, Kimura S, et al: A novel potent vasoconstrictor peptide produced by vascular endothelial cells. *Nature* 332:411, 1988.

217. Yokayama M, Hiwada K, Kokubu T, et al: Angiotensin converting enzyme in human prostate. *Clin Chim Acta* 100:253, 1980.

218. Zanchetti A: Overview of cardiovascular reflexes in hypertension. *Am J Cardiol* 44:912, 1979.

KARL SCHÄRER
GIULIO GILLI

25
Growth Retardation in Kidney Disease

Growth is a complex process that depends on the interaction of many hormonal and nonhormonal factors. In children with chronic renal disease this process can be slowed or even totally halted. The link between renal disease and growth disturbance has been recognized for almost a century. However, only with the advances in the treatment of terminal uremia made during the past two decades has this relationship been fully appreciated [13,28,68,80,93,108,123,128,136].

Short stature has a significant impact on the daily life of children, not only by imposing physical limitations, but also by affecting psychosocial adjustment. Growth retardation and failure to attain optimal adult stature are major hindrances to full rehabilitation of children and adolescents with chronic nephropathies.

Evaluation of Body Growth

The accurate assessment of growth in a child with renal disease requires a carefully taken history, precise measurements of body size, and a correct expression and analysis of growth data [4,111a]. The history should include data on prenatal events, birth weight and length, subsequent physical development, and past illnesses. A detailed alimentary history is essential in determining the relative importance of nutrient deficiency. The use of steroids or other drugs affecting growth should be investigated. Although measurements performed by different observers and with different equipment are often of limited value, whenever possible information should be obtained from health records to establish the pattern of growth as well as pubertal development before and during the illness. Height and weight of parents and siblings also should be recorded.

Measurement of Growth

Inaccurate measurements may lead to erroneous conclusions about the actual rate of growth, especially when growth increments are minimal over a long period of time.

Therefore, measurements should be obtained according to strict rules [22,107,111a,118]:

1. All measurements should be obtained by skilled observers and not be delegated to untrained personnel. To minimize variability, measurements should be obtained by the same observer when possible. Skeletal age is best assessed by an independent observer to reduce inherent bias.
2. Measurements should be carried out according to internationally recognized and standardized techniques and procedures.
3. Measurements should be done with accurate equipment, such as the Harpenden range of anthropometric instruments.

Measurements should be obtained at least every 6 months. They should be repeated at any major change in the mode of treatment, e.g., when a new drug is introduced, at initiation of dialysis, or at transplantation. The onset and the course of puberty should be recorded.

A minimal set of anthropometric measurements in children with renal diseases includes height, weight, skinfold thicknesses, upper arm circumference, and stage of puberty. Techniques of measurement have been detailed elsewhere [128].

Stature is measured as recumbent length or as standing height. Length measurements are recommended for children up to 24 to 36 months of age and height measurements thereafter. At transitional ages, both measurements should be performed to avoid erroneous interpretations of the height velocity. The use of an infantometer for measurement of length and of a stadiometer for measurement of height is recommended.

Weight should be measured under standard conditions, e.g., in the morning or, in dialyzed children, at the end of the dialysis session. The presence of edema should be recorded. Scales should be accurate to at least 0.1 kg.

Skinfold thickness is measured at the triceps site (at the midpoint between the acromion and the olecranon) and at the subscapular site (below the angle of the scapula).

Conventionally these measurements are taken on the left side. The use of a skinfold caliper with jaws exerting a constant pressure is required.

Upper arm circumference is measured on the left side at the same level as the measurement of the triceps skinfold thickness. A metallic tape is required and linen tapes should be avoided. Combined measurements of skinfold thickness at the triceps site and of upper arm circumference can be used to estimate body fat and muscle mass [50,61].

The *stage of puberty* is determined according to the Tanner maturity ratings [137]. Testicular size is an important measurement because its increase is the first physical sign of puberty [152]. The age at menarche and the pattern of subsequent menstruation should be recorded accurately.

Skeletal maturity is assessed from radiographs of the left hand and wrist or of the left knee. For the hand-wrist method, the scoring method of Tanner et al (TW 2) is recommended [140]. Alternatively, the method of Greulich and Pyle can be used [58]; with this method, skeletal age is best assessed as the median among bone-specific skeletal ages [117]. For the knee method, the Roche-Wainer-Thissen (RWT) method is suggested [119]. Comparability and reliability of the RWT method are about the same as that of the TW 2 method, but positioning of the subject is more difficult and a computer is needed for calculation of skeletal age.

Adult height can be predicted from the hand-wrist skeletal age in combination with actual height, weight, and midparental height [117,140]. Although these methods have been applied mainly to healthy children, they are also sufficiently reliable to estimate ultimate height of children with chronic renal disease [53,54].

Expression of Growth Data

Growth data obtained in a child with renal disease must be compared with suitable reference data [63,142]. Comprehensive sets of anthropometric reference data are limited, but reference standards for height and weight have been developed for most populations. Such data allow the selection of any individual who falls outside a predetermined level of growth performance. Differentiation between normal and abnormal growth is a matter of convention, but growth retardation usually is defined as a body height corresponding to 2 standard deviations (SD) or more below the reference mean for sex and chronologic age, or height that is below the third centile (i.e., -1.88 SD). Because skeletal maturation often is retarded in children with renal disease, some authors prefer to relate body height to skeletal age rather than to chronologic age. Although this approach may be biologically relevant, it should be noted that normal ranges of height for bone age are not available and are possibly not the same as for chronologic age. Therefore, we recommend the use of chronologic age for plotting growth data.

Because *malnutrition* can be a feature of chronic renal disease, it may be of interest to compare weight with height. Generally, this is done by comparing the patient's weight to the expected weight for the patient's height.

Charts of weight for height can also be used [63]. Both methods assume that the relationship between weight and height is age-independent, but this is true only between 1 and 5 years of age. Alternatively, the relationship of weight to height can be expressed by comparing the standard deviation scores (SDS) for weight and height or by indicating both weight and height as a fraction of the 50th centile for age [33].

Growth rate or *velocity* is calculated from longitudinal (serial) measurements by comparing the SDS of height (or of weight) at the beginning and at the end of a given observation period. This calculation provides the best mathematical description of relative loss or gain (in SDS/year). However, it should be emphasized that the physiologic fluctuations in SDS of growth variables are unknown. Growth velocity can also be calculated in cm/year and plotted on velocity charts. Such charts have been developed for normal British children [139,142], but can be used with sufficient accuracy for other populations, at least up to the onset of puberty.

Errors in Evaluation of Growth

Inaccurate collection of growth data and errors in expressing them may lead to erroneous conclusions. Measurements performed by different observers, with inadequate equipment, and without standardized techniques affect a proper assessment of growth. Reference data can be a further source of error, if they do not fit the population under study or if patients from different populations are compared with a single set of reference data.

Another pitfall in the assessment of growth can arise when body height is related to skeletal age rather than to chronologic age, and increments in height are related to increments in skeletal age. As growth can proceed without apparent increase in bone age, small gains in height may be misinterpreted as examples of catch-up growth.

Errors can arise also from the misuse of growth velocity charts [142]. It should be stressed that these charts represent standards calculated for one year and do not apply if observation periods are shorter or longer. Therefore, one should be cautious in extrapolating very short periods of observation to a whole year. It should also be kept in mind that the growth pattern of an individual healthy child looks different when it is plotted on a velocity chart rather than a longitudinal growth chart. In the latter, the child tends to follow the same channel throughout, a deviation of more than one channel being exceptional before puberty. However, on the velocity chart it is usual to observe that the velocity plots of the child are scattered both above and below the 50th centile line, with a tendency to compensate from one year to the next by crossing over this line [142]. Such changes in growth rate do not necessarily reflect the effect of disease or of therapeutic intervention.

It should be remembered that at adolescence a child's growth can temporarily deviate by one or two centile lines from the prepubertal level. This is explained by the fact that the *individual* adolescent growth spurt is more marked than the *mean* height increment at adolescence, since the latter is drawn from cross-sectional data and not centered on peak height velocity. Therefore, an increase in growth velocity above the 50th centile at the time of puberty should not be misinterpreted as an improvement in growth rate.

In recent years, many authors have made use of the so-called "growth velocity index" (GVI), the ratio between the increment in height observed during a given time interval and that expected for a normal child matched for sex and bone age and growing at the 50th centile. However, this index is based on a number of incorrect assumptions and is not adequate to assess growth. Its use should be rejected.

"Catch-up growth" is the term used when a child with growth retardation overcomes the growth deficit when the conditions disturbing growth are removed or ameliorated. The original description implies that "at the end of a period of growth retardation consequent to illness or starvation the child grows more rapidly than usual so that he catches up toward or into his original growth curve" [110]. This process, which is characterized by a sharp increase in the growth velocity above normal, is followed by a progressive deceleration until the original growth channel is reached. Another type of catch-up growth is described as delayed maturation, with a prolonged period of growth, without an above-normal increase in growth velocity. Catch-up growth can be complete or partial, depending on whether or not the original growth centile is regained. It is rarely complete if the growth-depressing factor is not removed until later childhood, as usually occurs in renal failure [138]. In most reports dealing with children with chronic renal disease, the pattern of growth does not fulfill the definition of catch-up growth.

Growth in Tubular and Interstitial Disorders
Tubular Disorders

A number of congenital tubular disorders interfere with normal growth [86,151]. The most severe forms of growth retardation have been observed in renal tubular acidosis, nephrogenic diabetes insipidus, chronic hypokalemia of tubular origin, idiopathic hypercalciuria, familial hypophosphatemic rickets, and complex tubular disorders, especially cystinosis.

In both the proximal and the distal types of *renal tubular acidosis*, growth retardation is frequent and often severe (see Chap. 81). It appears to be related to the metabolic acidosis, to the associated loss of cations, and to malnutrition. An impressive increase in growth rate usually is observed when acidosis is corrected with alkali therapy [14,87,100]. Growth is not impaired if patients with renal tubular acidosis are treated adequately from the first year of life [99].

Growth retardation occurs in about one-half of children with *nephrogenic diabetes insipidus* [70] (see Chap. 80). If hypernatremia and volume contraction are corrected, catch-up growth usually is observed within 2 years [101]. Exceptions occur mainly in infancy, when it may be diffi-

cult to maintain normal hydration and sufficient caloric intake. The introduction of indomethacin will probably further reduce growth retardation and malnutrition in some of these children.

In *chronic hypokalemia* due to renal potassium loss (Bartter's syndrome and similar disorders), growth failure is the rule and frequently the first sign leading to consultation [132] (see Chap. 86). In a subgroup of this condition, low birth weight indicates that growth has been inhibited in utero [130]. Both bone maturation and the pubertal growth spurt seem to be delayed in Bartter's syndrome, but the ultimate height usually is in the normal range, even when therapy is neglected [132]. Catch-up growth is difficult to obtain simply by supplementation with potassium and the use of spironolactone. The introduction of indomethacin has contributed to improved growth. It is not clear how long the medical treatment should be continued. There is no apparent relationship between growth rate and maintenance of normal serum potassium levels, since normal growth may occur in the presence of persistent hypokalemia [132].

Idiopathic hypercalciuria is another disorder frequently associated with failure to thrive, explained by the negative calcium balance with subsequent demineralization of the skeleton (see Chap. 75). Treatment with hydrochlorothiazide or indomethacin may improve the growth rate [14,143].

A number of other congenital tubular disorders affecting a single transport system may be associated with growth retardation, including familial hypophosphatemia (see Chap. 82) [135], pseudohypoaldosteronism (see Chap. 86), pseudohypoparathyroidism (see Chap. 82), dicarboxylic aminoaciduria, and dibasic hyperaminoaciduria (see Chap. 84).

From the observations cited it can be assumed that *complex tubular disorders* comprising multiple, congenital defects of proximal and distal tubular function are frequently accompanied by retardation of growth. This is most severe in the infantile form of nephropathic *cystinosis;* the onset of growth failure usually coincides with the manifestations of tubular dysfunction [18]. In contrast, patients with the rare adolescent form of cystinosis in which tubular function is not severely impaired usually show a normal growth pattern (see Chap. 85).

In a collaborative study of 209 children with nephropathic cystinosis, it was demonstrated that the loss of SDS in height is most severe in the second year of life when glomerular function is normal or only slightly reduced [10,81]. At the age of two years the mean SDS of height corresponded to slightly more than -2 SD Despite early and adequate replacement of electrolyte losses, the growth rates remained abnormal. When related to the level of serum creatinine, median SDS of height declined from -3.0 SD when a value of 0.75 mg/dl was exceeded to -4.0 SD at a value of 2 mg/dl. At the time of renal death median height was -4.3 SD (range -9.0 to -1.3).

Chronic dialysis and renal transplantation rarely are able to increase the rate of growth in patients with cystinosis, although sometimes moderate catch-up is observed [10,18]. In a multicenter study, 34 of 37 cystinotic children treated for various periods by dialysis or transplantation had a height less than 4 SD below the mean for healthy children [16]. However, adult height only exceptionally exceeds 55 inches (140 cm). Interestingly, siblings affected by cystinosis may have quite different growth curves, even when renal death occurs at a similar age.

Other complex tubular disorders that cause growth retardation include hereditary fructose intolerance [98], hepatorenal glycogenosis, Lowe syndrome, and idiopathic de Toni-Debre-Fanconi syndrome [12,99] (see Chap. 85).

Interstitial Disease

Body growth has rarely been investigated in renal disorders characterized by interstitial changes. Uttley et al. [146] found a significant correlation between height and maximal urinary concentration in children with urinary tract infection or hydronephrosis. Smellie et al. [133] analyzed growth in 114 girls receiving long-term, low-dose prophylactic treatment with co-trimoxazole for recurrent urinary infection. Growth velocity was not significantly different from normal children in those with or without vesicoureteral reflux, whether on or off antimicrobial therapy. It should be noted, however, that in a prior study a growth spurt was noted following successful antireflux surgery [95].

Growth in Glomerular Disorders

Retardation of growth is a frequent feature in children with long-standing *nephrotic syndrome*. A paper published shortly before the introduction of steroid therapy suggested that the nephrotic state per se was responsible for growth retardation [5a]. In a number of subsequent reports, inhibition of growth in children with nephrotic syndrome was found to vary considerably from child to child but to be closely related to the dose and duration of corticosteroids [30,78,145]. In addition, it was suggested that an alternate-day schedule of steroid administration reduced growth velocity less than daily administration [111]. However, in a study of 80 British patients with steroid-sensitive nephrotic syndrome, followed for 5 to 24 years, there was no correlation between total steroid dose and final height [49a]. Although many had growth suppression early in childhood, those who were adult and had completed growth had a mean height standard deviation score of 0.22, which is equivalent to a height on the 40th centile.

We examined body height and bone maturation of 61 pediatric patients with steroid-sensitive or steroid-resistant nephrotic syndrome from the time of onset of disease until the achievement of adult height [129]. Among those with steroid-sensitive nephrotic syndrome, girls had a lower capacity for catch-up growth after withdrawal of steroids, a greater advance in bone maturation, and a relatively lower score for adult height. However, even among those who had received large doses of steroids, permanent stunting was rare in both girls and boys (Fig. 25-1). In some boys the centile for adult height exceeded the original centile observed at the onset of disease, especially when low total

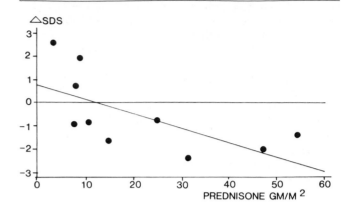

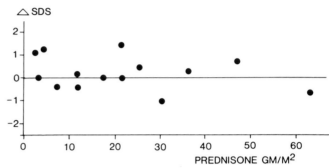

FIG. 25-1. *Adult height of 17 male patients (upper panel) and 11 female patients (lower panel) with steroid-sensitive nephrotic syndrome related to total dose of prednisone. The difference in SDS of adult height compared with that at the start of the disease is indicated on the ordinate. In contrast to males, the majority of female patients showed a loss in SDS. A significant relationship between SDS of height and total dose of prednisone was found only in female patients (r = 0.62, P < 0.05).*

doses of steroids were given. We speculated, therefore, that in contrast to general belief, low-dose steroids might have a growth-stimulating effect. This was also suggested by following the growth of individual patients longitudinally.

With regard to *bone maturation*, a phenomenon similar to catch-up growth was observed after removal of steroids, i.e., a transient retardation of skeletal age during steroid therapy, compensated for subsequently when steroid treatment was discontinued [129]. When growth or bone maturation had been stimulated during steroid therapy, this effect was lost after withdrawal of the drug. It appears, therefore, that the physiologic mechanisms regulating growth are operative in the nephrotic child.

In many children with *steroid-resistant* nephrotic syndrome, growth appears to be progressively depressed. It is noteworthy that this occurs even before glomerular filtration rate (GFR) declines (Fig. 25-2). It is disturbing that pari passu with the decline in growth rate there is a progressive reduction in predicted adult height. In the example given in Fig. 25-2, predicted adult height dropped by about 15 cm over a period of 10 years, whereas GFR fell only to 60 ml/minute/1.73 m².

It is of interest that in steroid-resistant nephrotic syn-

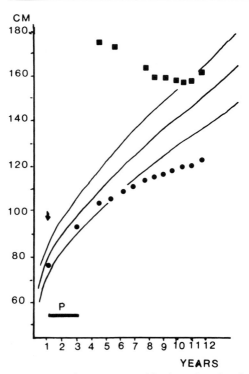

FIG. 25-2. *Changes in actual height and predicted adult height in a boy with steroid-resistant nephrotic syndrome associated with focal segmental glomerulosclerosis. Predictions of adult height according to the TW_2 method [140]. Serial assessments of inulin clearance gave normal values except for the last measurement at the age of 11 years (60 ml/minute/1.73 m²). With active disease the deviation of height from the normal mean increased and predicted adult height decreased.*
P = Prednisone treatment. ■ *= Predicted adult height.* ● = *Height*

drome a close correlation exists between growth velocity and serum total protein and albumin levels [129]. This suggests that protein malnutrition may play an important role. This problem is difficult to combat by presently available treatment.

It should be mentioned that some authors have alleged that *hypertension* is responsible for growth retardation [14]. It is difficult to evaluate this because in most instances high blood pressure is associated with other conditions known to interfere with growth, such as malnutrition and renal insufficiency.

Growth in Chronic Renal Insufficiency

Growth is retarded in many children prior to the onset of end-stage renal failure, even with minimal reduction of GFR. About one-third of children with chronic renal insufficiency (CRI) receiving conservative treatment are below the third centile for height [51]. On the other hand, growth may continue to be normal in patients with CRI for many years.

Depression of growth usually begins earlier and is more severe in children with congenital nephropathies than in those with acquired kidney disorders [30,125]. The most severe degrees of growth failure are found in cystinosis [18], followed by renal hypoplasia, nephronophthisis, and other hereditary nephropathies [125]. It seems, however, that retardation of growth is better related to the duration of renal disease than to either the type of nephropathy or the degree of glomerular dysfunction. Patients with very early onset and a long course of CRI are especially prone to develop growth retardation [7,13]. In children with congenital nephropathies, growth velocity is usually retarded in the first 2 to 3 years of life, but subsequently may proceed at a normal or even an increased rate [75]. Growth during the first years of life, therefore, is critical for maintaining normal height at a later age.

Effect of Long-Term Dialysis

Growth in children on *hemodialysis* has been reported mainly from European pediatric centers, where this mode of treatment is often maintained over longer periods of time than in the United States [20,51,62]. According to an early report from the Pediatric Registry of the European Dialysis and Transplant Association (EDTA), 39% of patients below 15 years of age at the start of dialysis had a body height below the third percentile for chronologic age [126]. Growth rates during the year preceding and during the first year on hemodialysis were similar; catch-up growth rarely was observed [51].

Growth velocity on long-term hemodialysis is reduced in the majority of children when related either to chronologic or to bone age, both before and during puberty [27,41,126]. In *prepubertal* patients treated by hemodialysis for more than 4 years, the SDS for height worsened at a mean rate of 0.43 SD/year [42]. In a single center study dealing with 51 prepubertal children on hemodialysis for more than 1 year, the mean relative loss of body height was similar (−0.38 SD/year) [74]. When long-term hemodialysis continues over years, growth velocity (which is usually below normal) remains more or less constant, leading to a progressive fall in the height centile [74,113,126]. After 5 years or more on hemodialysis prepubertal children have lost an average of 2.4 SD in height, compared with only 0.4 SD 5 years after transplantation [26].

During *puberty*, growth in dialyzed patients appears to be less retarded than in prepubertal children, based on an analysis of SDS for height [41,42]. Growth retardation in the pubertal age group is more severe in dialyzed boys, with a decrease of SDS for height about twice that observed in girls [42,126]. The pubertal growth spurt of children on hemodialysis or after transplantation is often delayed and of lesser magnitude than in normals [74,115,121b,126]. Even though growth continues in some adolescents on hemodialysis or after transplantation up to age 20 years and beyond [115,121b,128], this usually does not compensate completely for the height potential previously lost.

Skeletal maturation in children on hemodialysis and after transplantation is delayed to a degree similar to growth rate; however, mean growth rate per year advance in bone age is lower in dialyzed than in transplanted children [41,62,74].

All studies have failed to find a significant relationship between growth velocity and dialysis strategies, such as time on hemodialysis per week, the type of dialyzer, or the efficiency of dialysis, with the exception that growth rate was better in prepubertal boys on three hemodialysis sessions per week compared with two [26,74,126]. The degree of renal function had no appreciable effect [26], but concomitant hypertension appeared to be associated with a reduced growth rate [25].

Initial data suggested that growth of children on continuous ambulatory peritoneal dialysis (CAPD) was better than on hemodialysis [3,13]; however, subsequent studies yielded conflicting results, some authors claiming that growth rate was normal in the majority of CAPD patients [47,77], whereas others found that growth on CAPD was similar to or even lower than that observed on hemodialysis [5,15,37,120,147].

Effect of Renal Transplantation

Early reports of children followed after *renal transplantation* described normal [30] or decreased growth rates [59,104, 126]. More recent studies are difficult to compare because of differences in methodology and in patient selection [17,25,84,111b,115,116,123,127]. Most authors stress that growth is better following transplantation than during long-term dialysis [17,25,123], and this has been confirmed in a selected group of prepubertal children [26,27,41]. These studies also demonstrated that the growth of individual children is greater following transplantation than while on dialysis.

Factors that influence the growth rate of children following renal transplantation include chronologic age at the time of transplantation, level of skeletal maturation, dose and mode of steroid therapy, level of allograft function, and body height prior to transplantation.

Prepubertal and especially *very young children* grow better than pubertal patients following transplantation [11, 39,47,71,97]. In one series, 7 of 11 children below 7 years of age at the time of grafting had a growth rate above the mean and reached a normal height. In contrast, in 16 children between age 7 and 11 years, only one achieved normal height [71]. The better rate of growth of younger children may be related to a more severe degree of growth retardation at onset [11].

After *puberty* has begun it is difficult to differentiate the physiologic growth spurt from an increase in growth rate due to improved renal function or to manipulation of the immunosuppressive regimen. It is possible also that improved gonadal endocrine function contributes to the increased growth.

The degree of *skeletal maturation* at the time of transplantation is a critical factor for post-transplant growth. Bone age velocity after transplantation, at least before puberty, is usually not faster than height velocity [11,41]; therefore, a further loss of growth potential probably does not occur. Fine et al. [48] have observed that growth is minimal after attainment of a critical bone age of 12 years, a finding not confirmed by others [11,17,62].

There is no doubt that growth rate in transplanted children is determined to a large degree by the amount of *corticosteroids* given for immunosuppression (see Growth in Glomerular Disorders). Although there is not complete agreement, it appears that post-transplant growth is usually suppressed when the daily dose of prednisone exceeds 0.5 mg/kg/day [41,109,121]. Most centers have reported that growth is better on an alternate-day than on an every day schedule [11,17,26,46,65,71,109,115,121], but controlled studies are lacking. Peak height velocity in pubertal girls seems to be higher with alternate-day than daily steroid therapy. It appears that the use of cyclosporin as the main immunosuppressive agent results in improved growth rates [49,103].

Good *allograft function* appears to be an important precondition to allow normal growth after a transplantation [17,84,104,115]. Even a very moderate reduction of GFR (around 60 ml/minute/1.73 m^2) may reduce the growth rate in both prepubertal and pubertal children [11,17]. Other graft-related factors, such as the source of the kidney, have no significant influence on growth rate [39,71,84]. Studies support the concept that poor growth *before* transplantation has a greater influence on final height than post-transplant growth [11].

Adult Height of Pediatric Patients with Chronic Renal Disease

Despite the general concern about growth of children with chronic renal disease, there is scanty and conflicting information on the height ultimately achieved by these patients. In a study of 49 patients with CRI of variable duration and severity, only 14% attained adult heights more than 2 SD below the reference mean [54]. However, only 16% exceeded the mean, and the distribution of all adult scores was definitely shifted toward the lower percentiles (Fig. 25-3). A more recent study from our institution has largely confirmed these results [121a].

Although adult heights were not significantly correlated with the mode of treatment, the most marked stunting was observed in patients who were on hemodialysis at the completion of growth. No difference was noted between boys and girls, but patients with congenital kidney disease were shorter than those with acquired nephropathies. Interestingly, in most patients actual adult height was less than predicted at the time the children entered the study. These data suggest that final stunting is infrequent in CRI, although even patients with adult heights within the range of normal do not seem to reach their genetic potential. This has been confirmed by a report of the adult height of 44 uremic patients from central southern Italy. Most ended up below their target heights (as predicted from parental height) and were significantly smaller than their adult healthy siblings [Gilli G, de Santo N: Unpublished results].

The ability to predict adult height accurately has important implications for the management of children with chronic renal disease. In the presence of severe stunting it

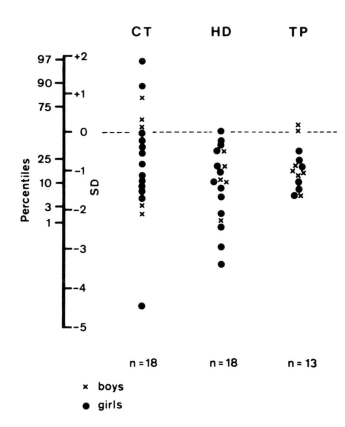

FIG. 25-3. Distribution of adult heights in 49 pediatric patients with chronic renal insufficiency. Patients are subdivided according to treatment at completion of growth: conservative treatment (CT), hemodialysis (HD), or transplantation (TP). Adult height is expressed in centiles (left of the vertical bar) and SD scores (right). Boys are indicated by crosses, girls closed circles. Note the almost even distribution of patients on CT, whereas only one patient on HD exceeds the 50th centile, and all transplanted children have adult heights within the normal range.

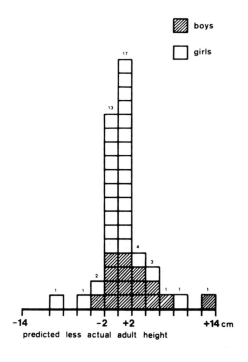

FIG. 25-4. Errors of prediction of adult height in 44 children with chronic renal insufficiency. Errors are expressed as predicted less actual adult height. Prediction was made at the time of the first observation by using Tanner's method [141]. Prediction was within ± 2 cm in 30 patients (68%). However, actual adult height was below the level of prediction in 61% (27 of 44), particularly with regard to grossly inaccurate predictions (10 of 14).

would be helpful in determining the choice for therapy. The accuracy of the original Tanner method [141] for predicting adult height has been tested in 22 pediatric patients with CRI who were followed until completion of growth [53]. Prediction was accurate within ±2 cm in 59% of patients, and the mean prediction error was 2.7 cm. In a subsequent study of 44 children with CRI different methods of prediction were compared [55]. Adult height was more accurately predicted by the method originally proposed by Tanner (Fig. 25-4) than by its subsequent modification [140] or by the Bayley-Pinneau and the RWT methods [117]. The Tanner method provided the most accurate prediction of adult height also in children with the nephrotic syndrome, although the errors of prediction were larger [129] than in patients with CRI [53]. All methods have shown that the actual adult heights of children with renal failure tend to fall below the level of earlier prediction [55].

Pathogenesis of Growth Retardation in Renal Disease

Growth retardation in children with kidney disease may be due to associated nonrenal disorders, such as Turner's syndrome, myelomeningocele [57], and various malformation syndromes [51a]. However, in most instances, abnormalities directly related to the underlying renal disorder appear to be of major importance.

The mechanisms leading to growth retardation in chronic renal disease are poorly understood. In recent years a number of experimental investigations have helped to elucidate the pathogenesis of renal dwarfism, especially in the presence of renal insufficiency [13,29,76,94]. However, animal experiments do not accurately reflect the biology of the growing child. For example, young rats made chronically uremic by subtotal nephrectomy differ from children with CRI in many ways, including their relative immaturity, absence of haversian systems in bone, failure to require vitamin D (when intake of calcium and phosphorus is optimal), incomplete catch-up growth following correction of malnutrition in the first 3 months of life, and absence of epiphyseal closure after maturation. Furthermore, the various species-specific influences in congenital and ac-

Table 25-1. *Pathogenic factors leading to growth retardation in renal disease*

Disturbances of water and electrolyte metabolism
    Hyposthenuria
    Depletion of sodium, potassium, phosphate, calcium,
        magnesium
    Metabolic acidosis
Bone disease
    Osteomalacia
    Osteofibrosis
    Osteoporosis
    Renal osteodystrophy
Hormonal alterations
    Reduced activity of somatomedin, growth hormone
        resistance
    Thyroid insufficiency
    Reduced production of testosterone, estrogen (?)
Metabolic changes related to uremia
    Accumulation of uremic toxins
    Protein-calorie malnutrition
    Deficiency of other nutrients (vitamins, trace minerals)

quired renal diseases in humans cannot be reproduced in the animal model. It seems, therefore, that the investigation of defective growth mechanisms in renal disorders must rely primarily on careful clinical observations from the first manifestation of renal disease until attainment of adult height.

Table 25-1 summarizes the major factors that are believed to influence growth rate in children with various nephropathies.

Water and Electrolyte Metabolism

Disturbances of water and electrolyte metabolism appear to be important mainly in the congenital and hereditary nephropathies characterized by tubular loss of these substances, resulting in alterations of the internal environment. *Hyposthenuria* with hyperosmolality of blood, an isolated feature in nephrogenic diabetes insipidus, is closely related to growth retardation, especially in young children. Its correction is followed by catch-up growth. Reduced capacity to concentrate the urine may also contribute to growth failure in other disorders affecting the distal tubule, such as nephronophthisis, hypoplasia/dysplasia, and obstructive uropathy [69,145].

Renal loss of electrolytes leading to depletion of intracellular and extracellular minerals occurs in many chronic kidney disorders. In most instances several electrolytes are lost in combination, so that the specific effect of an individual mineral deficiency is difficult to evaluate. Renal *potassium* loss is frequent in a number of tubular disorders, notably in Bartter's syndrome. However, as outlined previously, potassium supplements are unable to correct growth retardation in this condition [132]. Intracellular potassium, as determined by measurement of total body potassium, is reduced in children with chronic renal failure. Although this reduction is related to growth retardation [147], the mechanism is unknown.

Sodium deficiency has been shown to cause growth retardation in experimental animals [35,145a]. Salt wasting is prominent in some renal disorders associated with growth retardation, such as malformations of the urinary tract or nephronophthisis. It sometimes occurs in a hidden form, unaccompanied by hyponatremia. The exact mechanism by which sodium depletion or mild dehydration affects growth is unknown, but it is of interest that growth of connective tissue and cartilage is inhibited by contraction of the extracellular volume.

Phosphate depletion may be responsible for growth retardation in nephropathies that affect proximal tubular function, such as Fanconi syndrome or after transplantation. Phosphate depletion may be produced by administration of excessive amounts of antacids in patients with renal failure. The positive influence of phosphate supplementation on growth is best demonstrated in familial vitamin D–resistant rickets [56].

Calcium deficiency has long been postulated as a cause of growth retardation in idiopathic hypercalciuria as well as in chronic renal failure (which is often accompanied by reduced intestinal absorption of calcium). It is of interest that in uremic rats, but not in control animals, dietary calcium is a rate-limiting factor for growth [90].

Depletion of other electrolytes or trace elements, such as magnesium and zinc [43], may contribute to growth retardation in some patients.

Metabolic acidosis was recognized by West and Smith [149] as an important single component responsible for growth retardation in children with renal insufficiency. Cooke et al. [34] questioned the exclusive role of acidosis for growth retardation, because rats made acidotic by administration of acetazolamide showed normal growth. However, subsequent experimental studies using NH_4Cl or HCl confirmed the growth-depressing effect of acidosis [13,100].

In children the role of acid–base balance for growth is well demonstrated by the rapid catch-up growth noted after alkali treatment of renal tubular acidosis [87]. In more complex tubular disorders, e.g., cystinosis, or in chronic renal failure associated with acidosis, the growth promoting effect of alkali treatment is more difficult to evaluate [74]. Experimental studies indicate that important, but perhaps not exclusive, mechanisms responsible for acidosis-related growth retardation are the associated depletion of cations and the inhibition of $1,25(OH)_2D_3$ production [36]. Two clinical observations suggest that acidosis per se is not the decisive factor responsible for growth retardation: (1) children with chronic renal failure can grow normally in the presence of chronic acidosis [136], and (2) chronic acidosis resulting from exogenous dietary hydrogen ion overload, such as produced in phenylketonuria, is not associated with reduced growth [83].

Bone Disease

Most children with chronic renal disease have abnormalities of the *skeleton*, either osteomalacia, osteofibrosis, or osteoporosis, all of which may be associated with retarded growth (see Chap. 28). The role of vitamin D as a regulator of bone metabolism and therefore of growth is well established. Renal osteodystrophy is thought to be an important cause of growth failure in uremia; however, it is not clear at what stage and to what extent it contributes to stunting [88]. According to Hodson et al. [66] it affects height mainly in children with congenital kidney disease and when the GFR has fallen below 20 ml/minute/1.73 m^2.

It is well known that in uremia production of $1,25(OH)_2D_3$ is reduced and vitamin D metabolites are lost in urine. However, the influence of vitamin D therapy on growth in renal failure remains controversial. Some authors report a favorable effect of vitamin D analogs on growth in moderate degrees of renal insufficiency and in the presence of severe bone disease [23,32,79], whereas others have questioned a growth promoting effect of vitamin D metabolites [21,88]. In CAPD patients, high-dose $1,25(OH)_2D_3$ therapy failed to influence the rate of growth in spite of evident improvement of bone lesions [120]. In uremic rats growth was improved but not normalized by vitamin D or $1,25(OH)_2D_3$ [52,92].

It is not established if hyperparathyroidism as a second component of uremic bone disease contributes to growth retardation by destroying the architecture of the growth zone [88]. In some children with renal failure, parathyroidectomy was followed by acceleration of growth, which, however, was only transient and may have been due in part to correction of lower limb deformities [74].

Skeletal maturation may be delayed in chronic renal disorders, mainly in congenital tubulopathies, nephrotic syndrome, and CRI. This retardation seems most frequently related to concomitant bone disease, malnutrition, or preceding steroid therapy. In renal insufficiency, the delay in bone maturation is commensurate to that of body height, whether in the preterminal or in the terminal stage [41,53,66,72,74,126]. Some authors observed that after initiation of dialysis bone maturation proceeds at a rate similar to that of body growth [41,74,126], whereas others reported more rapid skeletal maturation, leading to a decrease of future growth potential [9]. It is unclear to what degree osteodystrophy contributes to retardation of bone maturation in uremia. Some studies suggested that during vitamin D therapy growth potential may improve by a less rapid maturation of bone compared with growth rate [74,79]. Long-term studies are required before this concept can be validated.

Endocrine Abnormalities

A number of *hormonal disturbances* have been alleged to contribute to reduced growth rate in chronic renal disease, but their precise role rarely has been documented [112, 123] (see Chap. 34). Early studies demonstrated that in renal failure there is no lack of growth hormone and that plasma levels are increased. In contrast, *somatomedin* (IGF-1) (insulin-like growth factor 1) levels have been found to be reduced when measured by bioassay [104,121] or protein-binding assay, although not when measured by radioreceptor assay [2,134]. During hemodialysis, somatomedin

activity in blood is increased, probably by removal of low-molecular-weight inhibitors [106]. Following transplantation somatomedin activity increases to normal levels and correlates with improved growth rate [105]. Growth hormone resistance and reduced somatomedin activity may be related to an excess of insulin-like growth factor binding proteins [144]. Growth of uremic rats can be stimulated by injections of supraphysiologic doses of porcine growth hormone [94a], suggesting end-organ unresponsiveness.

Thyroid insufficiency associated with renal failure or with severe proteinuria may contribute to growth retardation. There is no agreement as to whether the various hormonal alterations in uremia actually represent a hypothyroid state [112]. Recent studies confirm earlier suggestions that most children with renal insufficiency as well as with nephrotic syndrome are euthyroid [38,45]. However, characteristic clinical and laboratory findings of hypothyroidism are found in many children with infantile cystinosis [18] and congenital nephrotic syndrome [85]. Long-term studies are needed to prove that thyroxine promotes growth in these conditions.

In normal male puberty the rapid increase of *testosterone* production is the main factor responsible for the adolescent growth spurt. In boys with chronic renal failure, either before or after initiating dialysis, plasma testosterone levels are low both before and after stimulation with human chorionic gonadotropin [102,124]. It must be assumed that insufficient androgen production contributes to the flattened and delayed pubertal growth spurt frequently encountered in these patients. It seems possible that a similar depression in estrogen production interferes with pubertal growth in uremic girls.

Metabolic Changes of Uremia

It has long been postulated that accumulation of waste products in uremia may impair growth. Polyamines, substances known to accumulate in uremia, possibly have a specific toxic effect on growth because high concentrations of spermine inhibit incorporation of ^{3}H-thymidine into growth cartilage of uremic rats [90]. Early studies indicated that the degree of azotemia did not correlate with the rate of growth [6,149]. Although subsequent studies in patients on long-term dialysis showed an inverse correlation between growth rate and serum levels of creatinine [75], urea, urate [13], and inorganic phosphate, a multicenter study failed to find similar correlations [40].

The exact relationship between GFR and body growth in preterminal renal failure is not established. According to Betts and Magrath [7], growth is usually reduced when GFR drops below 25 ml/minute/1.73 m^2. In children with acquired kidney disease, Hodson et al. [66] observed a fall in growth rate when GFR fell below 50 ml/minute/1.73 m^2. Kleinknecht et al. [75] found that height loss was less in children with a GFR greater than 25 ml/minute/1.73 m^2 than in those with a value of less than 12 ml/minute/1.73 m^2, although the difference was not significant. These authors concluded that reduction of GFR is not a primary cause for reduced growth velocity in renal insufficiency as long as a limit of 5 ml/minute/1.73 m² is not reached. However, other clinical [66] and experimental data [76,89] sustain the concept that the degree of renal dysfunction is critical for growth failure in uremia.

Protein-calorie malnutrition has long been suggested as a cause of growth retardation in chronic renal disease [28,67,76,93,149]. This concept is sustained by a number of experimental studies that demonstrate a correlation between growth retardation and reduced overall food intake [91,122]. *Anorexia* is a frequent complaint in children with renal disease, especially in those with congenital tubular disorders, nephrotic syndrome, renal hypertension, and renal insufficiency. It can be attributed to many factors, including altered taste perception and compulsive drinking due to hyposthenuria or psychological stress, and often leads to severe reduction of nutrients.

A number of clinical and laboratory findings indicate that many children with chronic renal failure suffer from protein-calorie malnutrition: diminished body weight-to-height ratio in presence of stunted height [19,42,73,149], reduction in body cell mass [44,73,148], and signs of protein depletion as indicated by a decreased ratio of essential to nonessential aminoacids and various alterations at the cellular level [96]. It must be stressed, however, that no study has proved that these changes observed in uremic children are the direct result of reduced calorie or protein intake [90].

It has been postulated that in the uremic state the *requirements* of *energy* and *protein* for growth are increased [24,29]. In fact, at a given protein intake, the conversion of body protein is less efficient in uremic rats than in pair-fed control animals [91], and both decreased synthesis and increased catabolism of protein contribute to reduced gain in body protein [64]. The efficiency by which dietary protein is converted to body protein declines as the protein intake increases and, at the same time, more protein is used as a source of energy [90].

In 1972 Simmons et al. [131] reported an increase of growth velocity in some children undergoing long-term hemodialysis after receiving daily *energy supplements*. This study, which has been criticized because of the short period of dietary assessment, resulted in a widespread use of oral calorie supplementation in uremic children. It was soon recognized, however, that it is difficult to maintain high energy intake in children with chronic renal failure over long periods and that when the supplementation is maintained the increase in growth rate is not persistent [8]. Further studies showed that in dialyzed children, caloric and protein intakes were similar during periods of relatively poor and good growth [47], and that no correlation existed between caloric intake and growth rate in a mixed group of nondialyzed and dialyzed children, who partly received calorie supplements [8,89]. On the other hand, children with renal insufficiency with a low caloric intake (less than 75% RDA) and poor growth responded with increased growth rate following caloric supplementation [1].

The contribution of *protein intake* to growth of children with chronic kidney disease is controversial. As already discussed, in patients with persistent nephrotic syndrome a close relationship exists between serum protein levels and growth rate, suggesting that increased supply of protein in this disorder may promote growth [129]. In children with renal failure, signs of protein malnutrition were frequently observed in the early 1970s when prescribed dietary regimens were very low in protein content; nowadays such malnutrition is rare except in the presence of high urinary protein loss. In children on chronic hemodialysis, restriction of protein intake to 75% RDA was found to be associated with better growth when compared with children who were allowed a higher intake [74]. However, a correlation between protein intake and growth rate was demonstrated neither in the preterminal stage of renal failure nor during dialysis therapy [89]. On the other hand, in the multicenter study reported by the EDTA, the 1-year growth rate in prepubertal children was significantly less with unrestricted protein intake compared with children receiving 100% of RDA, whereas that of protein restricted patients showed intermediate values [40]. Obviously methodological problems in assessing dietary intake are difficult to overcome, especially in multicenter studies. However, clinical and experimental studies sustain the view that in advanced renal failure an optimal protein intake exists above which uremic toxicity depresses growth and below which malnutrition contributes to growth retardation [76].

It must be assumed that besides minerals, calories, and proteins *other nutritional factors* influence growth in children with chronic renal disease, similar to malnourished children. Among these, vitamins and trace minerals appear to be the most important. Vitamin D is known to have an anabolic effect, in addition to its various organ specific effects [92].

Treatment and Prevention

From the considerations outlined guidelines can be developed for the prevention and treatment of growth retardation, although the results often remain disappointing. Conditions that may respond to adequate dietary or drug therapy include metabolic acidosis, water and electrolyte depletion, rickets and osteodystrophy, urinary protein loss, and malnutrition (see Chap. 38). Correction of acidosis, hyperosmolality, and electrolyte losses are important, especially in congenital tubular disorders, although their value is sometimes limited, as demonstrated by the poor results in infantile cystinosis [18,81]. Guidelines for a comprehensive treatment of inherited tubular disorders are given in the section Tubular Disorders [82]. Substitution therapy seems to be important also for promoting growth in other forms of congenital nephropathies, especially those leading to early renal failure.

In avoiding growth retardation in children with renal disease, studies emphasize that the first 2 years of life are the most vital [75,114]. Therefore, one should not hesitate to introduce gastric feeding (by nasogastric tube or gastric fistula) in young anorectic children [60], although this may sometimes lead to poor appetite in later life. Transient intravenous feedings may be required, especially in infants, to allow adequate water, electrolyte, and caloric intake.

The results of such rigid treatment on overall growth, however, await further evaluation.

For combating *anorexia* and therefore protein-calorie malnutrition, the renal dietician should try to adapt the nutritional demands to the child's taste. Unacceptable salt-free diets can be avoided by the use of diuretics. In general, however, oral administration of drugs should be kept to a minimum, since they may depress appetite further. This applies especially to calcium salts and phosphate binders.

In advanced stages of renal failure it is questionable if any dietary therapy can increase growth rate except in cases of obvious malnutrition due to insufficient intake of calories or protein. There is not much point in using energy supplements if there is no evidence of malnutrition and if energy intake is already adequate, as documented by dietary records [24]. According to a study in nondialyzed children, an increase in growth rate may be expected if the total energy intake is below 78% of RDA [1]. Supplementation should be avoided if it produces anxiety and tension. Recently, diets with a relatively low protein content have been advocated in order to delay the progression of CRF. It remains to be demonstrated if this approach is also successful in children, without compromising statural growth [150].

Oral amino acids may be indicated if severe protein losses cannot be replaced by spontaneous protein intake, e.g., in persistent nephrotic syndrome or in patients treated by CAPD. Anabolic steroids have been used little in uremic children; they do not appear to improve growth rate in the long-term [113].

Recently, the use of recombinant human growth hormone applied as subcutaneous injections (4 $\mu/m^2/day$) has been demonstrated to increase the growth ratio by a factor of about 2 in growth retarded prepubertal children with preterminal CRF, on dialysis treatment or after transplantation [144]. In pubertal children the results were less consistent. Up to now no serious side effects have been noted. Studies are in progress to further delineate the indications of this therapy. The importance of close specialized *pediatric care* for promoting growth in renal patients has been emphasized by the results of the EDTA Registry, which reported that prepubertal children on dialysis treatment had a significantly higher growth rate when treated in specialized pediatric, as compared with nonspecialized (adult), centers [42]. Although the reason for this difference has not been elucidated, it might be related to better dietary surveillance, stricter treatment of osteodystrophy, and more adequate dialysis in pediatric centers.

Better growth after *transplantation* is an important argument in favor of this mode of treatment over long-term dialysis. The best guarantee for normal growth in a transplanted child seems to be offered by maintaining good graft function. Posttransplant growth may also be improved by modifying immunosuppressive therapy. After grafting, the daily dose of corticosteroids should be reduced rapidly and replaced by an alternate-day schedule as soon as kidney function becomes stable [109]. It seems that growth in grafted children is also improved by concomitant use of the immunosuppressive agent cyclosporin A [49,103]. There is no doubt that post-transplant growth of prepuber-

tal children has improved in recent years, whereas that of children treated by regular dialysis has remained unchanged [40].

In the management of children with growth retardation, *psychosocial factors* should not be neglected. The importance attributed to normal body growth and development varies among patients and depends on the severity and stress induced by other manifestations of chronic kidney disease, on personal achievements, and on the social background. In many children it might be wise not to try too hard to attain "normal height" if the price is neglect of other therapeutic goals.

References

1. Arnold WC, Danford D, Holliday MC: Effects of calorie supplementation on growth in children with uremia. *Kidney Int* 24:205, 1983.
2. Arnold WC, Uthne K, Spencer EM, et al: Somatomedin in children with chronic renal insufficiency. Relationship to growth rate and energy intake. *Int J Ped Nephrol* 4:29, 1983.
3. Balfe JW: Peritoneal dialysis. *In* Holliday MA, Barratt TM, Vernier RL (eds): *Pediatric Nephrology*. Baltimore, Williams & Wilkins, 1987, p 814.
4. Barratt TM, Broyer M, Chantler C, et al: Assessment of growth. *Am J Kidney Dis* 7:340, 1986.
5. Baluarte HJ, Morgenstern BZ, Kaiser BA, et al: Clinical aspects of continuous ambulatory peritoneal dialysis in children. *Dial Transpl* 14:18, 1985.
5a. Bauer H: Nephrosesyndrom und Körperwachstum. *Helv Paed Acta* 9:127, 1954.
6. Bergström WH, de Leon AS, van Gemund JJ: Growth aberrations in renal disease. *Pediat Clin North Am* 11:563, 1964.
7. Betts PR, Magrath G: Growth pattern and dietary intake of children with chronic renal insufficiency. *Br Med J* 2:189, 1974.
8. Betts PR, Magrath G, White RHR: Role of dietary energy supplementation in growth of children with chronic renal insufficiency. *Br Med J* 1:416, 1977.
9. Betts PR, White RHR: Growth potential and skeletal maturity in children with chronic renal insufficiency. *Nephron* 16:325, 1976.
10. Böhringer B: Wachstum bei Patienten mit nephropathischer Zystinose. *Doctoral Thesis*, University of Heidelberg, 1983.
11. Bosque M, Munian A, Bewick M, et al: Growth after renal transplants. *Arch Dis Child* 58:110, 1983.
12. Brodehl J: The Fanconi syndrome. *In* Edelmann CM (ed): *Pediatric Kidney Disease*. Boston, Little, Brown, 1978, p 995.
13. Broyer M: Growth in children with renal insufficiency. *Pediat Clin North Am* 29:991, 1982.
14. Broyer M: Croissance et néphropathies. *In* Royer P, Habib R, Mathieu H, et al (ed): *Néphrologie Pédiatrique* (3ème édition). Paris, Flammarion, 1983, p 441.
15. Broyer M, Donckerwolcke RA, Brunner FP, et al: Combined report on regular dialysis and transplantation of children in Europe XII, 1982. *Proc EDTA* 20:76, 1983.
16. Broyer M, Donckerwolcke RA, Brunner FP, et al: Combined report on regular dialysis and transplantation of children in Europe, 1980. *Proc EDTA* 18:60, 1981.

17. Broyer M, Guest G: Growth after kidney transplantation: a single-center experience. *In* Schärer K (ed): Growth and endocrine changes in children and adolescents with chronic renal failure. *Pediatr Adolesc Endocrinol.* Basel, Karger 20, 1989, p 36.

18. Broyer M, Guillot M, Gubler MC, et al: Infantile cystinosis: a reappraisal of early and late symptoms. *Adv Nephrol* 10:137, 1981.

19. Broyer M, Kleinknecht C, Gagnadoux MF, et al: Growth in uremic children. *In* Strauss J (ed): *Pediatric Nephrology,* Vol 4. New York, Garland STPM Press, 1978, p 185.

20. Broyer M, Kleinknecht C, Loirat C, et al: Growth in children treated with long-term hemodialysis. *J Pediat* 84:642, 1974.

21. Bulla M, Stock GJ, Delling G: Einfluβ der Vitamin D₃—Therapie auf die renale Osteodystrophie im Kindesalter. *Klin Wochenschr* 58:237, 1980.

22. Cameron N, Marshall WA, Goldstein H, et al: *The Measurement of Human Growth.* London and Sidney, Croom Hehn, 1984.

23. Chan JCM, Kodroff MB, Landwehr DM: Effects of 1.25-dihydroxy vitamin D₃ renal function and growth in children with severe chronic renal failure. *Pediatrics* 68:559, 1981.

24. Chantler C: Nutritional assessment and management of children with renal insufficiency. *In* Fine RN, Gruskin AB: *End-Stage Renal Disease in Children.* Philadelphia, Saunders, 1984, p 193.

25. Chantler C, Carter JE, Bewick M, et al: 10 years' experience with regular haemodialysis and renal transplantation. *Arch Dis Child* 55:435, 1980.

26. Chantler C, Donckerwolcke RA, Brunner FP, et al: Combined report on regular dialysis and transplantation of children in Europe, 1978. *Proc EDTA* 16:74, 1979.

27. Chantler C, Donckerwolcke RA, Brunner FP, et al: Combined report on regular dialysis and transplantation of children in Europe, 1976. *Proc EDTA* 14:70, 1977.

28. Chantler C, Holliday MA: Growth in children with renal disease with particular reference to the effects of calorie malnutrition: A review. *Clin Nephrol* 1:230, 1973.

29. Chantler C, Lieberman E, Holliday MA: A rat model for the study of growth failure in uremia. *Pediatr Res* 8:109, 1974.

30. Chantler C, Schärer K, Gilli G, et al: Dialysis and renal transplantation of children in Europe; 1975. *Acta Paediatr Scand* 67:5, 1978.

31. Chesney RW, Mazess RB, Rose PG, et al: Effect of prednisone on growth and bone mineral content in childhood glomerular disease. *Am J Dis Childh* 132:768, 1978.

32. Chesney RW, Moorthy AV, Eismann JA: Increased growth after long-term oral 1-alpha-25-vitamin D₃ in childhood renal osteodystrophy. *N Engl J Med* 298:238, 1978.

33. Cole TJ: A method for assessing age-standardized weight-for-height in children seen cross-sectionally. *Ann Hum Biol* 6:249, 1979.

34. Cooke RE, Boyden DG, Haller E: The relationship of acidosis and growth retardation. *J Pediatr* 57:326, 1960.

35. Cuisinier-Gleizes P, Debore F, Mathieu H: Experimental osteoporosis in growing rats. *In* Frame B, Duncan H, Parfitt AM (eds): *Clinical Aspects of Metabolic Bone Disease.* Amsterdam, Excerpta Medica, 1973, p 344.

36. Cunningham J, Avioli LV: Systemic accidosis and the bioactivation of vitamin D. *In* Norman AW, Schaefer K, v. Herrath D, Grigoleit HG (eds): *Vitamin D, Chemical, Biochemical and Clinical Endocrinology of Calcium Metabolism.* Berlin, New York, Walter de Gruyter, 1982, p 443.

37. De Santo NG, Capodicasa G, Gilli G, et al: Metabolic aspects of continuous ambulatory peritoneal dialysis with reference to energy-protein input and growth. *Int J Ped Nephrol* 3:279, 1982.

38. De Santo NG, Fine RN, Carella C, et al: Thyroidal status in uremic children. *Kidney Int.* 28(Suppl 17):S-166, 1985.

39. De Shazo CV, Simmons PL, Bernstein DM, et al: Results of renal transplantation in 100 children. *Surgery* 76:461, 1974.

40. Donckerwolcke RA, Broyer M, Brunner FP, et al: Combined report on regular dialysis and transplantation of children in Europe; XI, 1981. *Proc EDTA* 19:61, 1982.

41. Donckerwolcke RA, Chantler C, Broyer M, et al: Combined report on regular dialysis and transplantation of children in Europe; 1979. *Proc EDTA* 17:87, 1980.

42. Donckerwolcke RA, Chantler C, Brunner FP, et al: Combined report on regular dialysis and transplantation of children in Europe, 1977. *Proc EDTA* 15:77, 1978.

43. Eggert JV, Siegler RL, Edomkesmalee E: Zinc supplementation in chronic renal failure. *Int J Ped Nephrol* 3:21, 1982.

44. El Bishti M, Burke J, Gill D, et al: Body composition in children on regular hemodialysis. *Clin Nephrol* 15:53, 1981.

45. Etling N, Fonque F: Effect of prednisone on serum and urinary thyroid hormone levels in children during nephrotic syndrome. *Helv Paediat Acta* 37:257, 1982.

46. Feldhoff C, Goldmann AI, Najavarian JS, et al: A comparison of alternate day and daily steroid therapy in children following renal transplantation. *Int J Ped Nephrol* 5:11, 1984.

47. Fennell RS, Orak JK, Hudson T, et al: Growth in children with various therapies for end-stage renal disease. *Am J Dis Child* 138:28, 1984.

48. Fine RN, Malekzadeh MH, Pennisi AJ, et al: Long-term results of renal transplantation in children. *Pediatrics* 61:641, 1978.

49. Flechner SM, Conley SB, van Buren CT, et al: Impact of cyclosporine on renal function and growth in pediatric renal transplant recipients. *Transpl Proc* 17:1284, 1985.

49a. Foote KD, Brocklebank JT, Meadow SR: Height attainment in children with steroid-responsive nephrotic syndrome. *Lancet* 2:917, 1985.

50. Frisancho AR: New forms of upper limb fat and muscle areas for assessment of nutritional status. *Am J Clin Nutr* 34:2540, 1983.

51. Gilli G: Therapie der Wachstumsstörung bei chronischer Niereninsuffizienz. *Mschr Kinderheilk* 123:772, 1975.

51a. Gilli G, Berry AC, Chantler C: Syndromes with a renal component. *In* Holliday MA, Barratt TM, Vernier RL: *Pediatric Nephrology.* Baltimore, Williams & Wilkins, 1987, p 384.

52. Gilli G, Mehls O, Ritz E: Wirkung von Vitamin D₂ und 1.25(OH)₂D₃ auf das Wachstum bei Niereninsuffizienz. *Nieren- und Hochdruckkrankh* 10:259, 1981.

53. Gilli G, Mehls O, Wallstein B, et al: Prediction of adult height in children with chronic renal insufficiency. *Kidney Int* 24(Suppl 15):48, 1983.

54. Gilli G, Schärer K, Mehls O: Adult height in paediatric patients with chronic renal failure. *Proc EDTA* 21:830, 1984.

55. Gilli G, Schärer K, Mehls O: Adult height and its prediction in children with chronic renal insufficiency. *Ann Hum Biol* 12 (Suppl) 1:73, 1985.

56. Glorieux FH, Scriver CR, Reade TM, et al: Use of phosphate and vitamin D to prevent dwarfism and rickets in X linked hypophosphatemia. *N Engl J Med* 287:481, 1972.

57. Greene SA, Frank M, Zachmann M, et al: Growth and

sexual development in children with meningomyelocele. *Eur J Pediatr* 144:146, 1985.

58. Greulich WW, Pyle SI: *Radiographic Atlas of Skeletal Development of the Hand and Wrist.* 2nd ed. Stanford, Stanford University Press, 1959.
59. Grushkin CM, Fine RN: Growth in children and adolescents following renal transplantation. *Am J Dis Child* 121:514, 1973.
60. Guillot M, Broyer M, Cathelineau L: Nutrition entérale à débit constant en néphrologie pédiatrique. *Arch Franc Péd* 37:497, 1980.
61. Gurney JM, Jeliffe DB: Arm anthropometry in nutritional assessment. Normogram for rapid calculation of muscle circumference and cross-sectional muscle and fat areas. *Am J Clin Nutr* 26:912, 1973.
62. Gusmano R, Gilli G, Perfumo F: Valutazione critica dei resultati del trattamento emodialitico in età pediatrica. *Minerva Nefrol* 19:60, 1972.
63. Hamill PVV: NCHS growth curves for children, birth—18 years, United States DHEW Publication No(PHS) 78-1960. Hyattsville, U.S. Department of Health, Education, and Welfare, 1977.
64. Harter HE, Birge SJ, Martin KJ, et al: The effects of vitamin D metabolites on protein catabolism of muscle from uremic rats. *Kidney Int* 23:465, 1983.
65. Hoda Q, Hasinoff DJ, Arbus GS: Growth following renal transplantation in children and adolescents. *Clin Nephrol* 3:6, 1975.
66. Hodson EM, Shaw PF, Evans RA, et al: Growth retardation and renal osteodystrophy in children with chronic renal failure. *J Pediatr* 103:735, 1983.
67. Holliday MA: Calorie deficiency in children with uremia. *Pediatrics* 50:591, 1972.
68. Holliday MA, Chesney RW (eds): Growth in children with renal disease. A symposium. *Am J Kidney Dis* 7:255, 1986.

69. Holliday MA, Egan TJ, Morris RC, et al: Pitressin resistent hyposthenuria in renal disease. *Am J Med* 42:378, 1967.
70. Imura H, Matsumoto K, Ogata E, et al: "Hormone receptor diseases" in Japan: A nation-wide survey for testicular feminization syndromes, pseudohypoparathyroidism, nephrogenic diabetes insipidus, Bartter's syndrome and congenital adrenocortical unresponsiveness to ACTH. *Acta Endocrinol Jap* 56:1031, 1983.
71. Ingelfinger JR, Grupe WE, Harmon WE, et al: Growth acceleration following renal transplantation in children less than 7 years of age. *Pediatrics* 68:255, 1981.
72. Johannsen A, Nielsen HE, Hansen HE: Bone maturation in children with chronic renal failure: Effect of 1-α-hydroxy vitamin D₃ and renal transplantation. *Acta Radiol Diag* 20:193, 1979.
73. Jones RWA, Rigden SP, Barratt TM, et al: The effects of chronic renal failure in infancy on growth, nutritional status and body composition. *Pediatr Res* 16:784, 1982.
74. Kleinknecht C, Broyer M, Gagnadoux MF, et al: Growth in children treated with long-term dialysis. A study of 76 patients. *Adv Nephrol* 9:133, 1980.
75. Kleinknecht C, Broyer M, Hout D, et al: Growth and development of non-dialysed children with chronic renal failure. *Kidney Int* 24(Suppl 15):40, 1983.
76. Kleinknecht C, Laouari D, Broyer M, et al: Contribution of experimental studies on the nutritional management of children with chronic renal failure. *Pediatr Nephrol* 5:487, 1991.
77. Kohaut EC: Growth of the patient on CAPD. In Fine RN, Schärer K, Mehls O (eds): *CAPD in Children.* Berlin, Springer Verlag, 1985, p 106.

78. Lam CN, Arneil GC: Long-term dwarfing effects of corticosteroid treatment for childhood nephrosis. *Arch Dis Childh* 43:589, 1968.
79. Langman CB, Mazur AT, Baron R, et al: 25-hydroxy vitamin D₃ (calcifediol) therapy of juvenile renal osteodystrophy: Beneficial effect on linear growth velocity. *J Pediatr* 100:815, 1982.
80. Lewy JE, New MI: Growth in children with renal failure. *Am J Med* 58:65, 1975.
81. Manz F, Gretz N, Böhringer B, et al: Growth in cystinosis. *Ann Hum Biol* 12(Suppl 12):73, 1985.
82. Manz F, Schärer K: Long-term management of inherited renal tubular disorders. *Klin Wochenschr* 60:1115, 1982.
83. Manz F, Schmidt H, Schärer K, et al: Acid-base status in dietary treatment of phenylketonuria. *Pediatr Res* 11:1084, 1977.
84. Martin LW, McEnery PT, Rosenkrantz JG, et al: Renal homotransplantation in children. *J Ped Surg* 14:571, 1979.
85. McLean RH, Kennedy TL, Rosoulpour M, et al: Hypothyroidism in congenital nephrotic syndrome. *J Pediatr* 101:72, 1982.
86. McCrory WW: Growth disorders associated with renal disease. *J Pediatr* 57:5, 1960.
87. McSherry E: Acidosis and growth in nonuremic renal disease. *Kidney Int* 14:349, 1978.
88. Mehls O: Renal osteodystrophy in children: Etiology and clinical aspects. *In* Fine RN, Gruskin AB: *End-stage Renal Disease in Children.* Philadelphia, Saunders, 1984, p 227.
89. Mehls O, Gilli G, Schärer K: Analysis of growth and food intake in uremic children (abstr). *Kidney Int* 24(Suppl 16):344, 1983.
90. Mehls O, Ritz E: Skeletal growth in experimental uremia. *Kidney Int* 24 (Suppl. 15):53, 1983.
91. Mehls O, Ritz E, Gilli G, et al: Nitrogen metabolism and growth in experimental uremia. *Int J Ped Nephrol* 1:34, 1980.
92. Mehls O, Ritz E, Gilli G, et al: Effects of vitamin D on growth in experimental uremia. *Am J Clin Nutr* 31:1927, 1978.
93. Mehls O, Ritz E, Gilli G, et al: Growth in renal failure. *Nephron* 21:237, 1978.
94. Mehls O, Ritz E, Gilli G, et al: Skeletal changes and growth in experimental uremia. *Nephron* 18:288, 1977.
94a. Mehls O, Ritz E, Hunziker EB, et al: Improvement of growth and food utilizing human recombinant growth hormone in experimental uremia. *Kidney Int* 33:45, 1988.
95. Merrell RW, Mowad JJ: Increased physical growth after successful antireflux operation. *J Urol* 122:523, 1979.
96. Metcoff J, Fürst P, Schärer K, et al: Energy production, intracellular amino acid pools, and protein synthesis in chronic renal disease. *Am Coll Nutr* 8:271, 1989.
97. Miller LC, Book GH, Lum CT, et al: Transplantation of the adult kidney into the very small child: Long-term outcome. *J Pediatr* 100:675, 1982.
98. Mock DM, Perman JA, Thaler MM, et al: Chronic fructose intoxication after infancy in children with hereditary fructose intolerance. A cause of growth retardation. *N Engl J Med* 309:764, 1983.
99. Morris RC, Sebastian AS: Renal tubular acidosis and Fanconi syndrome. *In* Stanbury JB, Wyngaarden JB, Frederickson DS (eds): *The Metabolic Basis of Inherited Disease.* 3rd ed. New York, McGraw-Hill, 1983, p 1808.
100. Nash MA, Torrado AD, Greifer I, et al: Renal tubular acidosis in infants and children. *J Pediatr* 80:738, 1972.
101. Niaudet P, Dechaux M, Trivin C, et al: Nephrogenic diabetes insipidus. Clinical and pathophysiological aspects. *Adv Nephrol* 13:247, 1983.

102. Oertel PJ, Lichtwald K, Häfner S, et al: Hypothalamo-pituitary-gonadal axis in children with chronic renal failure. *Kidney Int* 24(Suppl 15):S-34, 1983.

103. Offner G, Aschendorff C, Brodehl J: Growth after renal transplantation: an update. *Pediatr Nephrol* 5:472, 1991.

104. Pennisi AJ, Costin C, Phillips LS, et al: Linear growth in long-term renal allograft recipients. *Clin Nephrol* 8:415, 1977.

105. Pennisi AJ, Costin C, Phillips LS, et al: Somatomedin and growth hormone studies in pediatric renal allograft recipients who receive daily prednisone. *Am J Dis Child* 133:950, 1979.

106. Philips LS, Kopple JD: Circulating somatomedin activity and sulfate level in adults with normal and impaired renal function. *Metabolism* 30:1091, 1981.

107. Potter DE, Broyer M, Chantler C, et al: Measurement of growth in children with renal insufficiency. *Kidney Int* 14:378, 1978.

108. Potter DE, Greifer I: Statural growth of children with renal disease. *Kidney Int* 14:334, 1978.

109. Potter DE: Alternate-day versus daily corticosteroid therapy in transplanted children. *In* Schärer K (ed): Growth and endocrine changes in children and adolescents with chronic renal failure. *Pediatr Adolesc Endocrinol.* Basel, Karger 20, 1989, p 126.

110. Prader A, Tanner JM, von Harnack GA: Catch-up growth following illness or starvation: An example of developmental canalization in men. *J Pediatr* 62:646, 1963.

111. Preece MA: The effect of administered corticosteroids on growth of children. *Postgrad Med J* 52:625, 1976.

111a. Preece MA: Statural growth and maturation. *In* Holliday MA, Barratt TM, Vernier R (eds): *Pediatric Nephrology.* 2nd ed, Baltimore, Williams & Wilkins, 1987, p 14.

111b. Ramirez JA, Fine RN: Factors affecting accelerated growth following renal transplantation. *In* Schärer K (ed): Growth and endocrine changes in children and adolescents with chronic renal failure. *Pediatr Adolesc Endocrinol.* Basel, Karger 20, 1989, p 46.

112. Rauh W, Oertel PJ: Endocrine function in children with end-stage renal disease. *In* Fine RN, Gruskin AB (eds): *End-stage Renal Disease in Children.* Philadelphia, Saunders, 1984, p 296.

113. Rigden SPA, Haycock GB, Chantler C: Growth in children on long-term hemodialysis. *Int J Ped Nephrol* 5:108, 1984.

114. Rizzoni B, Basso T, Setari M: Growth in children with chronic renal failure on conservative treatment. *Kidney Int* 26:52, 1984.

115. Rizzoni G, Broyer M, Brunner FP, et al: Combined report on regular dialysis and transplantation of children in Europe, XIII, 1983. *Proc EDTA* 23:69, 1984.

116. Rizzoni G, Malekzadeh MH, Pennisi AJ, et al: Renal transplantation in children less than 5 years of age. *Arch Dis Child* 55:532, 1980.

117. Roche AF: *Predicting Adult Stature for Individuals.* Basel, Karger, 1975.

118. Roche AF: Growth assessment in abnormal children. *Kidney Int* 14:369, 1978.

119. Roche AF, Wainer H, Thissen D: *Skeletal Maturity: The Kneejoint as a Biological Indicator.* New York, Plenum, 1975, p 91.

120. Salusky JB, Fine RN, Kangerloo H: "High-dose" calcitriol for control of renal osteodystrophy in children on CAPD. *Kidney Int* 32:89, 1987.

121. Saenger P, Wiedemann E, Schwartz E, et al: Somatomedin and growth after renal transplantation. *Pediatr Res* 8:163, 1974.

121a. Schaefer F, Gilli G, Schärer K: Pubertal growth and final height in chronic renal failure. *In* Schärer K (ed): Growth and endocrine changes in children and adolescents with chronic renal failure. *Pediatr Adolesc Endocrinol.* Basel, Karger 20, 1989, p 59.

121b. Schaefer F, Seidel C, Binding A, et al: Pubertal growth in chronic renal failure. *Pediatr Res* 28:5, 1990.

122. Schalch DS, Burstein PJ, Tewel SJ: The effect of renal impairment on growth in the rat: Relationship to malnutrition and serum somatomedin levels. *Endocrinology* 108:1653, 1981.

123. Schärer K, Mehls O (eds): Proceedings of the International Symposium on Growth, Nutrition and Endocrine Changes in Children with Chronic Renal Failure. *Pediatr Nephrol* 5:438, 1991.

124. Schärer K, Broyer M, Vescei P, et al: Damage to testicular function in chronic renal failure of children. *Proc EDTA* 17:725, 1980.

125. Schärer K, Chantler C, Brunner FP, et al: Combined report on regular dialysis and transplantation of children in Europe; 1974. *Proc EDTA* 12:65, 1975.

126. Schärer K, Chantler C, Brunner FP, et al: Combined report on regular dialysis and transplantation of children in Europe; 1975. *Proc EDTA* 13:59, 1976.

127. Schärer K, Dreikorn K, Mehls O, et al: Spätprognose der Nierentransplantation bei Kindern. *Z, Kinderchirur* 40:260, 1985.

128. Schärer K, Gilli G: Growth in children with chronic renal insufficiency. *In* Fine RN, Gruskin AB (eds): *End-stage Renal Disease in Children.* Philadelphia, Saunders, 1984, p 271.

129. Schärer K, Gilli G, Wagner A, et al: Growth pattern and adult height in idiopathic nephrotic syndrome (abstr) *Ann Hum Biol.* 12(Suppl 1):72, 1985..

130. Seyberth HJ, Rascher W, Schweer H, et al: Congenital hypokalemia with hypercalciuria in preterm infants: A hyperprostaglandinuric tubular syndrome different from Bartter syndrome. *J Pediatr* 107:694, 1985.

131. Simmons JM, Wilson CJ, Potter DE, et al: Relation of calorie deficiency to growth failure in children on hemodialysis and the growth response to calorie supplementation. *N Engl J Med* 285:653, 1971.

132. Simopoulos AP: Growth characteristics in patients with Bartter's syndrome. *Nephron* 23:130, 1979.

133. Smellie JM, Preece MA, Paton AM: Normal somatic growth in children receiving low-dose prophylactic co-trimoxazole. *Eur J Pediatr* 140:301, 1983.

134. Spencer EM, Uthne K, Arnold WC: Growth impairment with elevated somatomedin levels in children with chronic renal insufficiency. *Acta Endocrinol* (Kbn) 91:36, 1979.

135. Steendijk R, Herweijer TJ: Height, sitting height and leg length in patients with hypophosphatemic rickets. *Acta Paediatr Scand* 73:181, 1984.

136. Stickler GB: Growth failure in renal disease. *Pediatr Clin North Am* 23:885, 1976.

137. Tanner JM: *Growth at Adolescence.* Oxford, Blackwell, 1962.

138. Tanner JM: Catch-up growth in man. *Br Med Bull* 37:233, 1981.

139. Tanner JM, Whitehouse RH: Clinical longitudinal standards for height, weight, height velocity, weight velocity and stages of puberty. *Arch Dis Child* 51:170, 1976.

140. Tanner JM, Whitehouse RH, Cameron N, et al: *Assessment of Skeletal Maturity and Prediction of Adult Height (TW2 Method),* 2nd ed. London, Academic, 1983.

141. Tanner JM, Whitehouse RH, Marshall WA, et al: Prediction of adult height from weight, bone age and occurrence

of menarche at ages 4–16 years with allowance for midparent height. *Arch Dis Childh* 50:14, 1975.

142. Tanner JM, Whitehouse RH, Takaishi M: Standards from birth to puberty for height, weight, height velocity and weight velocity. *Arch Dis Childh* 41:454, 1966.

143. Tieder M, Stark H: Forme familiale d'hypercalciurie idiopathique avec nanisme, atteinte osseuse et rénale chez l'enfant. *Helv Paediat Acta* 34:359, 1979.

144. Tönshoff B, Schaefer F, Mehls O: Disturbance of growth-hormone-insulin-like growth factor axis in uremia. *Pediatr Nephrol* 4:654, 1990.

145. Travis LB, Chesney R, McEnery P, et al: Growth and glucocorticoids in children with kidney disease. *Kidney Int* 14:365, 1978.

146. Uttley WS, Paxton J, Thistlethwaite D: Urinary concentrating ability and growth failure in urinary tract disorders. *Arch Dis Childh* 47:436, 1972.

147. von Lilien T, Gilli G, Salusky JB: Growth in children undergoing continuous or cycling peritoneal dialysis. *In* Schärer K (ed): Growth and endocrine changes in children and adolecents with chronic renal failure. *Pediatr Adolesc Endocrinol.* Basel, Karger 20, 1989, p 27.

147a. Wassner SJ: The effect of sodium repletion on growth and protein turnover in sodium-depleted rats. *Pediatr Nephrol* 5:501, 1991.

148. Weber HP, Michalk D, Rauh W, et al: Total body potassium in children with chronic renal failure. *Int J Ped Nephrol* 1:42, 1980.

149. West CD, Smith WC: An attempt to elucidate the cause of growth retardation in renal disease. *Am J Dis Child* 91:460, 1956.

150. Wingen A-M, Fabian-Bach C, Mehls O: Low protein diet in children with chronic renal failure—1 year results. European study group for nutritional treatment of chronic renal failure in childhood. *Pediatr Nephrol* 5:496, 1991.

151. Worthen HG: Growth failure due to diseases of the proximal tubule. *J Pediatr* 57:14, 1960.

152. Zachmann M, Prader A, Kind HP, et al: Testicular volume during adolescence: cross-sectional and longitudinal studies. *Helv Paediat Acta* 29:61, 1974.

rectal mucosa of patients with renal insufficiency, colonic potassium secretion was found to be increased in patients with GFR less than 30 ml/min [97,127].

Renal excretion of potassium is a major determinant of steady state serum potassium [202]. The persistent capacity to maintain external potassium balance [190] and normal serum potassium until extreme degrees of chronic renal insufficiency is presumably due to progressive single nephron kaliuresis [95]. This increase in renal potassium secretion per nephron is similar to the adaptive response of the normal kidney to chronic potassium loading [170]. Indeed, the amount of potassium secreted can exceed the filtered load for potassium at very low levels of GFR.

Micropuncture studies in both normal and uremic rats have shown that potassium reabsorption appears to be nearly complete when tubular fluid reaches the distal tubule [6,25]. Thus, the kaliuresis results predominantly from an increased potassium secretion by distal nephron segments [95]. The cortical collecting tubule is the primary nephron segment responsible for this secretion [78,170]. Collecting tubules from uremic rabbits given a high potassium diet were able to secrete potassium at more than six times the normal rate [77]. The secretory rate was normal if the dietary potassium intake was reduced in proportion to the decreased GFR.

The adaptive mechanisms that permit excretion following an acute potassium load have not been fully characterized. In normal humans nearly 50% of an acute load is excreted in the urine over a six-hour period. The ability of patients with CRF to tolerate an acute potassium challenge is limited [83,201]. Most studies have pointed to an impaired extrarenal potassium uptake [15,108]. Following a potassium load, no difference in plasma potassium or urinary excretion was reported between patients with glomerular versus tubulointerstitial disease [77]. Furthermore, peak potassium plasma levels in both groups were not significantly different from control subjects, providing support for a major role of extrarenal uptake of potassium. In contrast, Kahn et al. [108] reported significant increases in plasma potassium in patients with CRF, compared with normal controls, four hours after an oral load of 25 mEq of potassium. A 24-hour urinary excretion of potassium was the same in the two groups.

Recently, Perez et al. [142,143] reported that patients with tubulointerstitial disease exhibited a defect in renal potassium excretion and that the defect was more severe in patients who also had hypoaldosteronism. Similarly, Bourgoignie et al. [25] showed a blunted kaliuresis and more severe hyperkalemia in dogs with CRF receiving a potassium load. The higher plasma potassium levels and aldosterone responses apparently helped increase potassium excretion during the remainder of the day, because the 24-hour potassium balance was normal. Insulin and glucagon showed no regulatory role in these studies.

In adrenalectomized dogs with a remnant kidney, the provision of a low, fixed dose of mineralocorticoid hormone permits the same degree of potassium adaptation as in animals given pharmacologic doses of mineralocorticoids [170]. Potassium adaptation in chronic uremia is independent of sodium, hydrogen ion, and phosphorus balance [69]. It occurs following production of GFR by renal artery

constriction, thus eliminating a direct role for the filtered load of potassium [170].

The rate of potassium secretion is blunted in the absence of normal plasma levels of aldosterone [95]. Patients with moderate renal insufficiency and hypoaldosteronism commonly present with hyperkalemia, which can be corrected by exogenous administration of mineralocorticoids. In addition, spironolactone (an aldosterone antagonist) decreases urinary potassium excretion, resulting in an increased circulating plasma potassium concentration [171]. Although aldosterone levels are often elevated in severe renal failure [100], some patients are able to maintain several-fold increases in potassium excretion per nephron at normal plasma aldosterone levels, and there is no direct relationship between fractional potassium excretion and aldosterone levels in many normal and pathologic circumstances [190].

The relationship of renal potassium excretion and the renin-aldosterone axis in children with CRF has been studied by Rodriguez-Soriano et al. [159]. Of 23 children with CRF, resulting from dysplasia and hypoplasia or various glomerular diseases, three were hyperkalemic and were shown to have hyporeninemic hypoaldosteronism.

Sodium delivery and/or tubular fluid flow rate in the distal tubule, as well as uptake of potassium at the peritubular membrane, can have a marked impact on potassium excretion rates [101]. Changes in serum potassium rapidly affect active peritubular uptake, which results in proportional changes in the intracellular potassium stores and rates of potassium secretion from cell to tubular lumen. Also, acid-base equilibrium or anionic composition of the tubular fluid can offset potassium excretion. Alkalosis enhances whereas acidosis decreases the peritubular uptake of potassium [81,82,113].

One of the factors proposed as a primary determinant of potassium adaptation in uremia is the activity of Na^+-K^+-ATPase. This enzyme is increased in the remnant kidney [78,163] and the normal cortical collecting tubule by potassium loading [65,173]. The adaptation for potassium secretion is intrinsic to the nephron [77,174]. Both transepithelial potential difference and aldosterone contributed to the adaptation in the cortical collecting tubule from uremic rabbits [77], but neither factor fully accounted for the phenomenon. Both aldosterone levels and transepithelial potential difference across the isolated collecting tubule were greater in uremia than in normal rabbits fed a diet rich in potassium. However, both factors were similar in normal and uremic patients fed a normal potassium diet, even though the fractional potassium excretion was significantly greater in the uremic rabbits. In the same studies, the intracellular potassium content per unit tubule length was increased in the uremic rabbit as a result of the increased size of cortical collecting tubule cells (hypertrophy). However, the intracellular potassium content was found to be similar in equally hypertrophied uremic rabbit tubules adapted from a normal to a high potassium diet. Although, as stated earlier, in intact animals fed a high potassium diet and in animals with CRF, the enhanced secretion of potassium has been attributed to an increased Na^+-K^+-ATPase activity of the outer medullary tissue [78,163], potassium adaptation by the cortical collecting tubule can occur without a measurable increase in Na$^+$-K$^+$-ATPase activity.

Water Balance

The kidney plays a major role in the maintenance of water balance through its ability to elaborate either concentrated or dilute urine. The control system regulating water excretion has been well defined and is discussed elsewhere (Chap. 8). Although abnormalities in total body water and the distribution of water have been described in both children and adults, it appears that the chronic malnutrition characteristic of CRF bears primary responsibility for these findings.

The principal elements in the water control system are ECF osmolality (signal element), hypothalamic osmoreceptors (detector), vasopressin or antidiuretic hormone (ADH) (effector-transmitter), and the collecting tubule (sensitive end-organ). Nonosmotic stimuli for ADH release are also important and include volume depletion, hypoxia, pain, and emotional stress. These appear to act through parasympathetic afferent pathways emanating from volume sensors in various vascular beds. ADH is released from the posterior hypophysis into the systemic circulation. On binding to receptors in the basolateral membrane of the collecting tubule it exerts its action on water excretion through a chain of intracellular events involving AMP formation and, ultimately, changes in the luminal permeability to water [1].

Basal plasma vasopressin levels in children with CRF have been found to be elevated above control values, a finding also reported in adults [103,150]. Less clear is the relationship between the increased vasopressin and serum osmolality. In one study in children [150] a lack of correlation between plasma osmolality and vasopressin levels was reported. Nonosmotic factors such as blood volume, stress, and BP may play an important modulating role in these patients [151,166]. Urea itself does not contribute to effective tonicity because it diffuses directly into cells and does not alter cell osmolality [164]. Thus, even though each increase in BUN of approximately 3 mg/dl adds 1 mOsm/kg to plasma osmolality, no effect on plasma vasopressin levels is observed. The role of secondary hyperparathyroidism in uremic patients as a mediator of calcium-stimulated vasopressin secretion has been reported [92].

Water balance is usually maintained until renal failure is in the advanced stage. Tubular adaptation for water excretion occurs, and, within a certain range of intake, water excretion by surviving nephrons increases progressively, thus preserving balance until the terminal stages of uremia. Nonetheless, as renal function decreases, a gradual and progressive limitation in the range of water excretion ensues. During this process, both diluting and concentrating ability are progressively decreased [75,95]. Urinary tonicity becomes fixed and deviates little from isotonicity.

Brodehl reported on a group of 41 children, aged 2 to 16 years, with variable degrees of renal insufficiency, and compared water and solute excretion with 28 age-matched normal controls [157]. All children received 20 ml/kg body weight as a water load and continuous oral and intravenous

water to maintain the diuresis. Children with GFR 10% or less of control had lower maximal urinary volume and minimum urinary osmolalities higher than controls. Free water clearance was significantly decreased, whereas total solute excretion remained unchanged. As expected, solute excretion per 100 ml GFR increased dramatically, whereas free water excretion per 100 ml GFR did not.

This loss of range for water excretion can be understood if one appreciates the constraints placed on the surviving nephron by the obligatory excretion of dietary solute and the available GFR with which to perform the osmolar excretion. To illustrate this point one may compare the fractional water excretion between a normal child with a GFR of 55 ml/min and a child with a GFR of 1.4 ml/min. If excretion of a given solute load in isotonic form requires excretion of 750 ml of urine, this would represent less than 1% of filtered water in the normal child but almost 40% in the uremic subject.

The decrease in functioning nephron mass in CRF requires that each remaining nephron unit excrete larger amounts of solute. The result of this process implies that each surviving nephron will be subjected to a solute diuresis that will of necessity limit the range of water excretion. Total osmolar excretion thus is a major determinant of urine volume in CRF, and urea excretion may play the most important role in determining output [75] (Fig. 26-3).

In advanced CRF the volume of fluid filtered and delivered to the diluting segment is of utmost importance to the renal capacity to excrete water and dilute urine. Thus, even though the qualitative ability to dilute urine persists in CRF [34,112,139], the quantitative capacity of the diseased kidney to excrete free water decreases progressively with advancing disease, and a severe limitation in urinary volume occurs when GFR is markedly depressed. If water

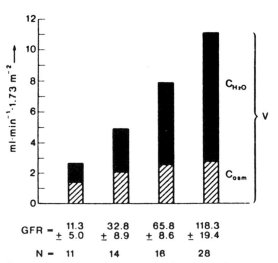

Fig. 26-3. *Urinary flow rate (V), free water clearance (CH$_2$O), and osmolar clearance (Cosm) for different degrees of CRF in children. N = number of patients. GFR in ml/min/1.73 m^2 body surface area.*

ingestion exceeds the capacity for excretion as a result of severely decreased GFR, water retention and hyponatremia will result.

By contrast, the inability to form a maximally concentrated urine and to excrete a minimal volume is characteristic of early renal insufficiency [173]. This loss of concentrating capacity, when assessed by maximal urinary osmolality, correlates well with the degree of renal insufficiency [5]. When GFR decreases below 20 ml/min/1.73 m², even maximal doses of vasopressin are associated with persistently hypotonic urine [185], i.e., the defect in concentrating ability is vasopressin resistant. Thus, CRF can be considered a form of acquired nephrogenic diabetes insipidus. Nocturia, polyuria, and polydipsia are typical symptoms.

The pathogenesis of the impairment of renal concentrating capacity in CRF is probably multifactorial [95]. The reduction of dietary sodium in chronically uremic rats reportedly improved their concentrating capacity [70]. The reduced number of functioning nephrons obligates them to excrete an increased solute load per nephron and thus to increase the fractional excretion of filtered solute and water [145]. A solute diuresis even in normal humans can result in isotonic urine in the presence of maximal amounts of vasopressin [185]. Even if the ability to generate negative free water clearance (T^CH_2O) were to remain normal at 6 ml/100 ml GFR, the total amount of water removed from 770 ml of isoosmotic urine would be only 120 ml/d at a

GFR of 3 ml/min/1.73 m². However, values for T^CH_2O/GFR do not remain normal in severe CRF [64], and the observed reduction in maximal urine osmolality cannot be accounted for merely by the increased solute and water diuresis per nephron [95,165].

Anatomic alterations in the renal medulla resulting in an impairment in sodium chloride transport in the thick ascending limb of Henle, or disruption of the countercurrent disposition of the loops of Henle, vasa recta, and collecting ducts, could render the medullary interstitium isotonic rather than hypotonic [95,165]. Indeed, patients with medullary cystic disease and adult polycystic kidney disease often appear to develop a concentrating defect early in their course [128]. However, available data fail to distinguish patients with nonglomerular disease from those with glomerulopathies [5]. Remnant kidney models also provide ample evidence for the defect in concentrating ability associated with CRF of any etiology [76]. Fine et al. [76] showed that the hydroosmotic response to a maximal dose of vasopressin was extensively attenuated in isolated cortical collecting tubules from uremic rabbits compared with collecting tubules from nonuremic animals (Fig. 26-4). Furthermore, maximal stimulation of collecting tubule adenylate cyclase by vasopressin was significantly decreased. In the uremic rabbit, circulating vasopressin levels were markedly increased, suggesting that downregulation of the vasopressin receptor had occurred [76]. Thus, the limitation in the maximal achievable urine osmolality

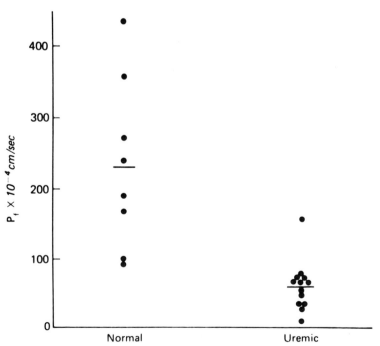

FIG. 26-4. *Transepithelial osmotic water permeability coefficient, p_f, of normal and uremic cortical collecting tubules exposed to a maximal concentration of vasopressin. (From Fine, LG, Schlondorff D, Trizna W, et al: Functional profile of the isolated uremic nephron. Impaired water permeability and adenylate cyclase responsiveness of the cortical collecting tubule to vasopressin. J Clin Invest 61: 1519, 1978, with permission.)*

found in CRF is due to a combination of nephron loss and impaired concentrating ability in the residual nephrons [131]. As a result of the isosthenuria, the circadian rhythm of urine formation is disturbed, with nocturia being an early sign of renal insufficiency.

References

1. Abramow M, Beauwens R, Cogan E: Cellular events in vasopressin action. Kidney Int 32:5, 1987.
2. Allison ME, Wilson CB, Gottschalk CW: Pathophysiology of experimental glomerulonephritis in rats. J Clin Invest 53:1402, 1974.
3. Altsheler P, Klahr S, Rosenbaum R, et al: Effects of inhibitors of prostaglandin synthesis on renal sodium excretion in normal dogs and dogs with decreased renal mass. Am J Physiol 235:F338, 1978.
4. Appel GB, Siegel NJ, Appel AS, et al: Studies on the mechanism of non-oliguric experimental acute renal failure. Yale J Biol Med 54:273, 1981.
5. Baldwin DS, Berman HJ, Heinemann HO, et al: The elaboration of osmotically concentrated urine in renal disease. J Clin Invest 34:800, 1955.
6. Bank N, Aynedjian HS: A micropuncture study of potassium excretion by the remnant kidney. J Clin Invest 52:1480, 1973.
7. Bank N, Aynedjian HS: Individual nephron function in experimental bilateral pyelonephritis. I. Glomerular filtration rate and proximal tubular sodium, potassium and water reabsorption. J Lab Clin Med 68:713, 1966.
8. Bastl C, Hayslett JP, Binder HJ: Increased large intestinal secretion of potassium in renal insufficiency. Kidney Int 12:9, 1977.
9. Battle D, Arruda J, Kurtzman N: Hyperkalemic distal renal tubular acidosis associated with obstructive uropathy. N Engl J Med 304:373, 1981.
10. Bergstrom J, Alvestrand A, Furst P, et al: Muscle intracellular electrolytes in patients with uremia. Kidney Int 24:S16, 1983.
11. Bergstrom J, Hultman E: Muscle composition in chronic renal failure. Minerva Nefrol 16:35, 1969.
12. Berl T, Katz FH, Henrich WL, et al: Role of aldosterone in the control of sodium excretion in patients with advanced chronic renal failure. Kidney Int 14:228, 1978.
13. Berlyne GM, Van Laethem L, Ben Ari J: Exchangeable potassium and renal potassium handling in advanced chronic renal failure in men. Nephron 8:264, 1971.
14. Better OS, Chaimowitz C, Gellei B, et al: Salt losing nephropathy. J Pediatr 75:872, 1969.
15. Bia M, DeFronzo RA: Extrarenal potassium homeostasis. Am J Physiol 240:F257, 1981.
16. Bilbrey GL, Carter NW, White MG, et al: Potassium deficiency in chronic renal failure. Kidney Int 4:423, 1973.
17. Blaine EH, Davis JO, Witty RT: Renin release after hemorrhage and after suprarenal aortic constriction in dogs without sodium delivery to the macula densa. Circ Res 27:1081, 1970.
18. Blainey JD, Hilton DD: The composition of the body in renal failure. Ann R Coll Surg Engl 47:45, 1970.
19. Blantz RC, Pelayo JC: A functional role for the tubuloglomerular feedback mechanism. Kidney Int 25:739, 1984.
20. Bolte HD, Reicker G, Rohl D: Measurements of membrane potential of individual muscle cells in normal men and patients with renal insufficiency, in Proceedings of the 2nd

International Congress of Nephrology, International Congress Series 78. Amsterdam, Excerpta Medica, 1964.
21. Bourgoignie JJ, Hwang KH, Espinel C, et al: A natriuretic factor in the serum of patients with chronic uremia. J Clin Invest 51:1514, 1972.
22. Bourgoignie JJ, Hwang KH, Ipakchi E, et al: The presence of a natriuretic factor in urine of patients with chronic uremia. The absence of the factor in nephrotic uremic patients. J Clin Invest 53:1559, 1974.
23. Bourgoignie JJ, Jacob AI, Sallman AL, et al: Water electrolyte and acid-base abnormalities in chronic renal failure. Semin Nephrol 1:91, 1981.
24. Bourgoignie JJ, Kaplan M, Gavellas G, et al: Sodium homeostasis in dogs with chronic renal insufficiency. Kidney Int 21:820, 1982.
25. Bourgoignie JJ, Kaplan M, Pincus J, et al: Renal handling of potassium in dogs with chronic renal insufficiency. Kidney Int 20:482, 1981.
26. Bourgoignie JJ, Klahr S, Bricker NS: Inhibition of transepithelial sodium transport in the frog skin by a low molecular weight fraction of uremic serum. J Clin Invest 50:303, 1971.
27. Brennan BL, Yasumura S, Letteri JM, et al: Total body electrolyte composition and distribution of body water in uremia. Kidney Int 17:364, 1980.
28. Bricker NS: On the pathogenesis of the uremic state. An exposition of the "trade-off hypothesis." N Engl J Med 286:1093, 1972.
29. Bricker NS: Sodium homeostasis in chronic renal disease. Kidney Int 21:886, 1982.
30. Bricker NS, Fine LG: The pathophysiology of chronic renal disease. In Maxwell MH, Kleeman CR (eds): Clinical Disorders of Fluid and Electrolyte Metabolism. New York, McGraw-Hill, 1980, p 799.
31. Bricker NS, Fine LG: The renal response to progressive nephron loss. In Brenner BM, Rector FC (eds): The Kidney, 2nd ed. Philadelphia, WB Saunders, 1981, p 1056.
32. Bricker NW, Fine LG: The trade-off hypothesis: Current status. Kidney Int (suppl 8)13:S-5, 1978.
33. Bricker NS, Fine LG, Kaplan M, et al: "Magnification phenomenon" in chronic renal disease. N Engl J Med 299:1287, 1978.
34. Bricker NS, Klahr S, Lubowitz H, et al: Renal function in chronic renal disease. Medicine 44:263, 1965.
35. Bricker NS, Lichet A: Natriuretic hormone: Biologic effects and progress in identification and isolation. In Lichardus B, Schrier RW, Ponec J (eds): Hormonal Regulation of Sodium Excretion, Proceedings of the Symposium on Regulation of Renal Sodium Excretion. Amsterdam, Elsevier/North Holland Biomedical Press, 1980.
36. Bricker NS, Schmidt RW, Favre H, et al: On the biology of sodium excretion: The search for a natriuretic hormone. Yale J Biol Med 48:293, 1975.
37. Bricker NS, Slatopolsky E, Liebowitz H, et al: Nephron alterations in renal failure: A model for study of the control system of sodium excretion. In Brest, AN (ed): Hahnemann Symposium. Philadelphia, JB Lippincott, 1967.
38. Briggs JP, Steipe B, Schubert G, et al: Micropuncture studies of the renal effects of atrial natriuretic substance. Pflugers Arch 395:271, 1982.
39. Brown RS: Potassium homeostasis and clinical implications. Am J Med 77(5A):3, 1984.
40. Brown PR, Koutsaimanis KG, de Wardener HE: Effect of urinary extracts from salt-loaded man on urinary sodium excretion by the rat. Kidney Int 2:1, 1972.
41. Burnell JM, Villamil MF, Uyeno BT, et al: The effect in humans of extracellular pH change on the relationship

between serum potassium concentration and intracellular potassium. *J Clin Invest* 35:935, 1956.

42. Casson IF, Lee MR, Brown JAM, et al: Failure of renal dopamine response to salt loading in chronic renal disease. *Br Med J* 286:503, 1983.

43. Cameron JS, Vick RM, Ogg CS, et al: Plasma C₃ and C₄ concentration in the management of glomerulonephritis. *Br Med J* 3:668, 1973.

44. Coles GA: Body composition in chronic renal failure *Q J Med* 41:25, 1972.

45. Comty CM: A longitudinal study of body composition in terminal uremics treated by regular hemodialysis. I. Body composition before treatment. *Can Med Assoc J* 98:482, 1968.

46. Carriere S, Wong NLM, Dirks JH: Redistribution of renal blood flow in acute and chronic reduction of renal mass. *Kidney Int* 3:364, 1973.

47. Chantler C, Holliday MA: Growth in children with renal disease with particular reference to the effects of calorie malnutrition. *Clin Nephrol* 1:230, 1973.

48. Cheek DB, Habicht JP, Berall J, et al: Protein-calorie malnutrition and the significance of cell mass relative to body length. *Am J Clin Nutr* 30:851, 1977.

48a. Cogan MG: Atrial natriuretic factor can increase renal solute excretion primarily by raising glomerular filtration. *Am J Physiol* (Renal Fluid Electrolyte Physiol 19) 250:F22, 1986.

48b. Cogan MG: Atrial natriuretic peptide. *Kidney Int* 37:1148, 1990.

49. Cole CH, Balfe JW, Welt LG: Induction of ouabain-sensitive ATPase defect by uremic plasma. *Trans Assoc Am Physicians* 81:213, 1968.

50. Coleman AJ, Arias M, Carter NW, et al: The mechanism of salt wastage in chronic renal disease. *J Clin Invest* 45:1116, 1966.

51. Cope CL, Pearson J: Aldosterone secretion in severe renal failure. *Clin Sci* 25:331, 1963.

52. Cotton JR, Woodard T, Carter N, et al: Resting skeletal muscle membrane potential as an index of uremic toxicity. *J Clin Invest* 63:501, 1979.

53. Cox M, Sterns RH, Singer I: The defense against hyperkalemia: The roles of insulin and aldosterone. *N Engl J Med* 299:525, 1978.

54. Currie MG, Geller DM, Cole BR, et al: Purification and sequence analysis of bioactive atrial peptides (atriopeptins). *Science* 223:67, 1984.

55. Danovitch GM, Bourgoignie JJ, Bricker NS: Reversibility of the "salt-losing" tendency of chronic renal failure. *N Engl J Med* 296:14, 1977.

56. Davis JO, Freeman RH: Mechanisms regulating renin release. *Physiol Rev* 56:1, 1976.

57. deBold AJ, Flynn TG: Cardionatrin I—a novel heart peptide with potent diuretic and natriuretic properties. *Life Sci* 33:297, 1983.

58. De Wardener HE, Clarkson EM: The natriuretic hormone: Recent developments. *Clin Sci* 63:415, 1982.

59. DiBona GF: Renal neural activity in hepatorenal syndrome. *Kidney Int* 25:841, 1984.

60. DiBona GF: The function of the renal nerves. *Rev Physiol Biochem Pharmacol* 94:75, 1982.

61. Dirks, JH, Wong NLM: Homeostatic adaptation of renal tubular transport of calcium and sodium in chronic renal failure. Athens, *Proceedings of the VIII International Congress of Nephrology*, 255, 1981.

62. Dodge WF, Spargo BH, Travis LB, et al: Poststreptococcal glomeruonephritis. A prospective study in children. *N Engl J Med* 286:273, 1972.

63. Dolislager D, Tune B: The hemolytic uremic syndrome.

Spectrum of severity and significance of prodrome. *Am J Dis Child* 132:55, 1978.

64. Dorhout Mees EJ: Role of osmotic diuresis in impairment of concentrating ability in renal disease. *Br Med J* 1:1156, 1959.

65. Doucet A, Katz AI: Renal potassium adaptation: Na-K-ATPase activity along the nephron after chronic potassium loading. *Am J Physiol* 238:F380, 1980.

65a. Dunn BR, Ichikawa I, Pfeffer JM, et al: Renal and systemic hemodynamic effects of synthetic atrial natriuretic peptide in the anesthetized rat. *Circ Res* 59:237, 1986.

66. El-Bishti M, Burke J, Gill D, et al: Body composition in children on regular hemodialysis. *Clin Nephrol* 15:53, 1981.

67. Epstein M: Cardiovascular and renal effects of head-out water immersion in man: Application of the model in the assessment of volume homeostasis. *Circ Res* 39:619, 1976.

68. Epstein M, Bricker NS, Bourgoignie JJ: The presence of a natriuretic factor in urine of normal men undergoing water immersion. *Kidney Int* 13:152, 1978.

69. Espinel CH: Effect of proportional reduction of sodium intake on the adaptive increase in glomerular filtration rate/nephron and potassium and phosphate excretion in chronic renal failure in the rat. *Clin Sci Mol Med* 49:193, 1975.

70. Espinel CH, Flora RE, Sprinkel M: Increased urinary concentration capacity in experimental chronic renal failure by proportional reduction of dietary salt and protein. *Clin Res* 25:430A, 1977.

71. Favre H, Hwang KH, Schmidt RW, et al: An inhibitor of sodium transport in the urine of dogs with normal renal function. *J Clin Invest* 56:1302, 1975.

72. Feldman D, Funder JW, Edelmann IS: Subcellular mechanisms in the action of adrenal steroids. *Am J Med* 53:545, 1972.

73. Feld LG, Springate JE, Fildes RD: Acute renal failure. I. Pathophysiology and diagnosis. *J Pediatr* 109:401, 1986.

74. Fildes RD, Springate JE, Feld LG: Acute renal failure. II. Management of suspected and established disease. *J Pediatr* 109:567, 1986.

75. Fine LG, Salehmoghaddam S: Water homeostatis in acute and chronic renal failure. *Semin Nephrol* 4:289, 1984.

76. Fine LG, Schlondorff D, Trizina W, et al: Functional profile of the isolated uremic nephrons. Impaired water permeability and adenylate cyclase responsiveness of the cortical collecting tubule to vasopressin. *J Clin Invest* 61:1519, 1978.

77. Fine LG, Yanagowa N, Schultze RG, et al: Functional profile of the isolated uremic nephron: Potassium adaptation in the rabbit cortical collecting tubule. *J Clin Invest* 64:1033, 1979.

78. Finkelstein FO, Hayslett JP: Role of medullary Na-K-ATPase in renal potassium adaptation. *Am J Physiol* 229:524, 1975.

79. Fitzhugh FW Jr, McWhorter RL Jr, Estes EH Jr, et al: The effect of application of tourniquets to the legs on cardiac output and renal function in normal human subjects. *J Clin Invest* 32:1163, 1953.

80. Fong JS, de Chadarevian JP, Kaplan BS: Hemolytic-uremic syndrome. Current concepts and management. *Pediatr Clin North Am* 29:835, 1982.

81. Gabow PA, Peterson LN: Disorders of potassium metabolism. *In* Schrier RW (ed): *Renal and Electrolyte Disorders*. Boston, Little, Brown, 1986, p 200.

82. Giebisch G, Stanton B: Potassium transport in the nephron. *Annu Rev Physiol* 41:241, 1979.

83. Gonick HC, Kleeman CR, Rubini ME, et al: Functional impairment in chronic renal disease: 3. Studies of potassium excretion. *Am J Med Sci* 261:281, 1971.

84. Gonick FC, Kleeman CR, Rubini ME, et al: Functional

impairment in chronic renal disease. II. Studies of acid-excretion. *Nephron* 6:28, 1969.

85. Gonick HC, Maxwell MJ, Rubini ME, et al: Functional impairment in chronic renal disease. I. Studies on sodium conserving ability. *Nephron* 3:137, 1966.

86. Gordon JA, Kim J, Petersen L, et al: Renal concentration defect (RCD) following nonoliguric acute renal failure (ARF) (abstr). *Kidney Int* 19:201, 1981.

87. Gottschalk CW: Function of the chronically diseased kidney: The adaptive nephron. *Circ Res* (suppl 2)28:1, 1971.

88. Graham JA, Lawson DH, Linton AL: Muscle biopsy water and electrolyte contents in chronic renal failure. *Clin Sci* 38:583, 1970.

89. Grantham JJ, Edwards RM: Natriuretic hormones: At last, bottled in bond? *J Lab Clin Med* 103:333, 1984.

90. Gribefz I, Ritter S, Grand MJH: Salt losing nephritis. *Am J Dis Child* 96:191, 1958.

91. Gruber KA, Whitaker JM, Buckalew VM Jr: Endogenous digitalis-like substance in plasma of volume-expanded dogs. *Nature* 287:743, 1980.

92. Hammer M, Ladefoged J, Madsen S, et al: Calcium-stimulated vasopressin secretion in uremic patients: An effect mediated via parathyroid hormone? *J Clin Endocrinol Metab* 51:1078, 1980.

93. Hampers CL, Zollinger RM Jr, Skillman JJ, et al: Hemodynamic and body composition changes following bilateral nephrectomy in chronic renal failure. *Circulation* 40:367, 1969.

94. Hayes CP, McLeod ME, Robinson RR: An extrarenal mechanism for the maintenance of potassium balance in severe chronic renal failure. *Trans Assoc Am Physicians* 80:207, 1967.

95. Hayslett JP: Functional adaptation to reduction in renal mass. *Physiol Rev* 59:137, 1979.

96. Hayslett JP, Kashgarian M, Epstein FH: Functional correlates of compensatory renal hypertrophy. *J Clin Invest* 47:774, 1968.

97. Hayslett JP, Myketey N, Bender HJ, et al: Mechanism of increased potassium secretion in potassium secretion in potassium loading and sodium deprivation. *Am J Physiol* 239:F378, 1980.

98. Hayslett JP, Kashgarian M, Epstein FH: Mechanisms of change in the excretion of sodium per nephron when renal mass is reduced. *J Clin Invest* 48:1002, 1969.

99. Heijden AJVD, Versteegh FGA, Wolff ED, et al: Acute tubular dysfunction in infants with obstructive uropathy. *Acta Paediatr Scand* 74:589, 1985.

100. Hene RJ, Boer P, Koomans HA, et al: Plasma aldosterone concentrations in chronic renal disease. *Kidney Int* 21:98, 1982.

101. Hene RJ, Koomans HA, Boer P, et al: Relation between plasma aldosterone concentration and renal handling of sodium and potassium, in particular in patients with chronic renal failure. *Nephron* 37:94, 1984.

102. Hene RJ, Boer P, Koomans HA, et al: Sodium potassium ATPase activity in human rectal mucosa with and without renal insufficiency. *Am J Kidney Dis* 5:177, 1985.

103. Horky K, Sramkova J, Lachmanova J, et al: Plasma concentration of antidiuretic hormone in patients with chronic renal insufficiency on maintenance dialysis. *Horm Metab Res* 11:241, 1979.

104. Hughes JM: Salt losing nephritis: A case report and a review. *Arch Intern Med* 114:190, 1964.

105. Jamison RL, Myers BD: Residual renal function in nonoliguric acute renal failure (abstr). *Kidney Int* 19:204, 1981.

106. Jamison RL, Sonnenberg H, Stein JH: Questions and replies: Role of the collecting tubule in fluid, sodium, and potassium balance. *Am J Physiol* 237:F247, 1979.

107. Jones RW, Rigden SP, Barratt TM, et al: The effects of chronic renal failure in infancy on growth, nutritional status and body composition. *Pediatr Res* 16:784, 1982.

108. Kahn T, Kaji DM, Nicolis G, et al: Factors related to potassium transport in chronic stable renal disease in man. *Clin Sci Mol Med* 54:661, 1978.

109. Kaplan MA, Bourgoignie JJ, Rosecan J, et al: The effects of the natriuretic factor from uremic urine on sodium transport, water and electrolyte content and pyruvate oxidation by the isolated toad bladder. *J Clin Invest* 53:1568, 1974.

110. Katz AI: Renal Na-K-ATPase: Its role in tubular sodium and potassium transport. *Am J Physiol* 242:F207, 1982.

111. Klahr S, Rodriguez HJ: Natriuretic hormone. *Nephron* 15:387, 1975.

112. Kleeman CR, Adams DA, Maxwell MH: An evaluation of maximal water diuresis in chronic renal disease. I. Normal solute intake. *J Lab Clin Med* 58:169, 1961.

113. Kliger AS, Hayslett JP: Disorders of potassium balance. *In* Brenner BM, Stein JH (eds): *Contemporary Issues in Nephrology*. Vol 2. *Acid-Base and Potassium Homeostasis*. New York, Churchill-Livingstone, 1978, p 168.

114. Kobayashi T: Extra-renal adaptation of sodium and potassium in renal failure. *In* Murakarmi K, Murakami K, Kitagawa T, et al (eds): *Recent Advances in Pediatric Nephrology*. New York, Elsevier, 1987, p 223.

115. Kon V, Ichikawa I: Research Seminar: Physiology of acute renal failure. *J Pediatr* 105:351, 1984.

116. Kopple JD, Coburn JW: Metabolic studies of low protein diets in uremia. I. Nitrogen and potassium. *Medicine (Baltimore)* 52:583, 1973.

117. Kramer HJ, Gospodinov D, Kruck F: Functional and metabolic studies on red blood cell sodium transport in chronic uremia. *Nephron* 16:344, 1976.

118. Lewy JE, Salinas-Madrigal L, Herdson PB, et al: Clinicopathologic correlations in acute poststreptococcal glomerulonephritis: A correlation between renal functions, morphologic damage and clinical course of 46 children with acute poststreptococcal glomerulonephritis. *Med* 50:453, 1971.

119. Lubowitz H, Mazumdar DC, Kawamura J, et al: Experimental glomerulonephritis in the rat: Structural and functional observations. *Kidney Int* 5:356, 1974.

120. Ludens JH, Fanestil DD: The mechanism of aldosterone function. *Pharmacol Ther* 2:371, 1976.

121. Luft FC, Aronoff GR, Sloan RS, et al: Intra- and interindividual variability in sodium intake in normal subjects and in patients with renal insufficiency. *Am J Kidney Dis* 7:375, 1986.

122. Luft FC, Sterzel RB, Lang RE, et al: Atrial natriuretic factor determinations and chronic sodium homeostasis. *Kidney Int* 19:1004, 1986.

123. Maddox DA, Bennett CM, Deen WM, et al: Control of proximal tubule fluid reabsorption in experimental glomerulonephritis. *J Clin Invest* 55:1315, 1975.

124. Maddox DA, Bennett CM, Deen WM, et al: Determinants of glomerular filtration in experimental glomerulonephritis in the rat. *J Clin Invest* 55:305, 1975.

125. Malnic G, Klose RM, Giebisch G: Micropuncture study of renal potassium excretion in the rat. *Am J Physiol* 206:647, 1964.

126. Marin-Grez M, Schubert F, Briggs JP, et al: Inhibition of haloperidol of the natriuresis induced by atrial natriuretic factor (atrim) (abstr). *Kidney Int* 27:261, 1985.

127. Martin RS, et Panere S, Virginillo M, et al: Increased secretion of potassium in the rectum of humans with chronic renal failure. *Am J Kidney Dis* 81:105, 1986.

128. Martinez-Maldonado M, Yium JJ, Eknoyan G, et al: Adult

polycystic kidney disease: Studies of the defect in urine concentration. *Kidney Int* 2:107, 1972.

129. Mason J, Moore LC: A new way of investigating tubuloglomerular feedback: The closed-loop mode. *Kidney Int* 22:S-151, 1982.

130. Miller PD, Krebs RA, Neal BJ, et al: Polyuric prerenal failure. *Arch Intern Med* 140:907, 1980.

131. Mitch WE, Wilcox CS: Disorders of body fluids, sodium and potassium in chronic renal failure. *Am J Med* 72:536, 1982.

132. Moss NG: Renal function and renal afferent and efferent nerve activity. *Am J Physiol* (Renal Fluid Electrolyte Physiol 12) 243:F425, 1982.

133. Nakayama N, Ohkubo H, Hirose T, et al: M RNA sequence for human cardiodilatin—atrial natriuretic precursor and regulation of precursor in M RNA in rat atria. *Nature* 310:699, 1984.

134. Navar LG: Renal autoregulation: Perspectives from whole kidney and single nephron studies. *Am J Physiol* (Renal Fluid Electrolyte Physiol 3) 234:F357, 1978.

135. Navar LG, Rosivall L: Contribution of the renin-angiotensin system to the control of intrarenal hemodynamics. *Kidney Int* 25:857, 1984.

136. Olgaard K, Madsen S, Ladefoged J, et al: Plasma aldosterone during extracellular fluid volume expansion in patients on regular hemodialysis. *Eur J Clin Invest* 7:61, 1977.

137. Osborn JL, Holdaas H, Thames MD, et al: Renal adrenoceptor mediation of antinatriuretic and renin secretion responses to low frequency renal nerve stimulation in the dog. *Circ Res* 53:298, 1983.

138. Osgood RW, Reineck HJ, Stein JH: Further studies on segmental sodium transport in the rat during expansion of the extracellular fluid volume. *J Clin Invest* 62:311, 1978.

139. Pabico RC, McKenna BA, Freeman RB: Renal function before and after unilateral nephrectomy in renal donors. *Kidney Int* 8:166, 1975.

140. Patrick J, Jones NF: Cell sodium, potassium and water in uraemia and the effects of regular dialysis as studied in the leucocyte. *Clin Sci Mol Med* 46:583, 1974.

141. Patrick J, Jones NF, Bradford B, et al: Leucocyte potassium in uraemia: Comparisons with erythrocyte potassium and total exchangeable potassium. *Clin Sci Mol Med* 43:669, 1972.

142. Perez GO, Kem DC, Oster JR, et al: Effect of acute metabolic acidosis on the renin-aldosterone system. Mechanisms of increases in plasma aldosterone in dogs infused with lactic acid. *J Lab Clin Med* 96:371, 1980.

143. Perez GO, Pelleya R, Oster JR, et al: Blunted kaliuresis after an acute potassium load in patients with chronic renal failure. *Kidney Int* 24:656, 1983.

144. Platt R: Structural and functional adaptation in renal failure. *Br Med J* 1:1372, 1952.

145. Platt R: Structural and functional adaptation in renal failure. *Br Med J* 1:1313, 1952.

146. Pollock DM, Banks RO: Effect of atrial extract on renal function in the rat. *Clin Sci* 65:47, 1983.

147. Porter G, Bennett W: Nephrotoxin-induced ARF. *In* Brenner B, Stein J (eds): *ARF. Contemporary Issues in Nephrology*. New York, Churchill-Livinstone, 1980, p 123.

148. Powell HR, Rotenberg E, Williams AL, et al: Plasma renin activity in acute poststreptococcal glomerulonephritis and the haemolytic-uraemic syndrome. *Arch Dis Child* 49:802, 1974.

149. Rascher W, Tulassay T, Lang RE: Atrial natriuretic peptide in plasma of volume overloaded children with chronic renal failure. *Lancet* 2:303, 1985.

150. Rauh W, Hund E, Sohl G, et al: Vasoactive hormones in children with chronic renal failure. *Kidney Int* 24:S-27, 1983.

151. Rauh W, Rascher W, Huber KH, et al: Nonosmotic factors in the regulation of antidiuretic hormone (ADH) in childhood (abstr). *Eur J Pediatr* 138:98, 1982.

152. Robertson CR, Deen WM, Troy JL, et al: Dynamics of glomerular ultrafiltration in the rat. III. Hemodynamics and autoregulation. *Am J Physiol* 223:1191, 1972.

153. Robinson RR, Murdaugh HV, Peschel E: Renal factors responsible for the hypermagnesemia of renal disease. *J Lab Clin Med* 53:572, 1959.

154. Rocha A, Marcondes M, Malnic G: Micropuncture study in rats with experimental glomerulonephritis. *Kidney Int* 5:356, 1974.

155. Rodriguez-Iturbe B: Epidemic poststreptococcal glomerulonephritis. *Kidney Int* 25:129, 1984.

156. Rodriguez-Iturbe B, Baggio B, Colina-Chourio J, et al: Studies on the renin-aldosterone system in the acute nephritic syndrome. *Kidney Int* 19:445, 1981.

157. Rodriguez-Soriano J, Arang BS, Brodehl J, et al: Fluid and electrolyte imbalances in children with chronic renal failure. *Am J Kidney Dis* 7:268, 1985.

158. Rodriguez-Soriano J, Vallo A, Bilbao F, et al: Different functional characteristics of residual nephrons in infantile vs. adult diffuse cortical necrosis. *Int J Pediatr Nephrol* 3:71, 1982.

159. Rodriguez-Soriano J, Vallo A, Sanquro P, et al: Hyporeninemic hypoaldosterone. *J Pediatr* 109:476, 1986.

160. Rosa RM, Silva P, Young JB, et al: Adrenergic modulation of extrarenal potassium disposal. *N Engl J Med* 302:431, 1980.

161. Saxenhofer H, Gnadinger MP, Weidmann P, et al: Plasma levels and dialysance of atrial natriuretic peptide in terminal renal failure. *Kidney Int* 32:554, 1987.

162. Schmidt RW, Bourgoignie JJ, Bricker NS: On the adaptation in sodium excretion in chronic uremia: The effects of "proportional reduction" of sodium intake. *J Clin Invest* 53:1736, 1974.

163. Schon DA, Silva P, Hayslett JP: Mechanism of potassium excretion in renal insufficiency. *Am J Physiol* 227:1323, 1974.

164. Schrier RW, Berl T: Disorders of water metabolism. *In* Schrier RW (ed): *Renal and Electrolyte Disorders*. Boston, Little, Brown, 1980.

165. Schrier RW, Berl T: Nonosmolar factors affecting renal water excretion. *N Engl J Med* 292:141, 1975.

166. Schrier RW, Berl T, Anderson RJ: Osmotic and nonosmotic control of vasopressin release. *Am J Physiol* (Renal Fluid Electrolyte Physiol 5) 236:F321, 1979.

167. Schrier RW, Regal EM: Influence of aldosterone on sodium, water and potassium metabolism in chronic renal disease. *Kidney Int* 1:156, 1972.

168. Schultze RG, Shapiro HS, Bricker NS: Studies on the control of sodium excretion in experimental uremia. *J Clin Invest* 48:869, 1969.

169. Schultze RG, Nissenson AR: Potassium: Physiology and pathophysiology. *In* Maxwell MH, Kleeman CR (eds): *Clinical Disorders of Fluid and Electrolyte Metabolism*. New York, McGraw-Hill, 1980, p 113.

170. Schultze RG, Taggart DD, Shapiro H, et al: On the adaptation in potassium excretion associated with nephron reduction in the dog. *J Clin Invest* 50:1061, 1971.

171. Schwartz GJ, Burg MB: Mineralocorticoid effects on cation transport by cortical collecting tubules in vitro. *Am J Physiol* (Renal Fluid Electrolyte Physiol 4) 235:F576, 1978.

172. Silva P, Charney AN, Epstein FH: Potassium adaptation

and Na-K-ATPase activity in mucosa of colon. *Am J Physiol* 229:1576, 1975.

173. Silva P, Hayslett JP, Epstein FH: The role of Na-K-activated adenosine triphosphatase in potassium adaptation. *J Clin Invest* 52:2665, 1973.

174. Silva P, Ross BD, Charney AN, et al: Potassium transport by the isolated perfused kidney. *J Clin Invest* 56:862, 1975.

175. Skorecki KL, Brenner BM: Body fluid homeostasis in man. *Am J Med* 70:77, 1981.

176. Slatopolsky E, Elkan IO, Weerts C, et al: Studies on the characteristics of the control system governing sodium excretion in uremic man. *J Clin Invest* 47:521, 1968.

177. Smith S, Anderson S, Ballerman BJ, et al: Role of atrial natriuretic peptide in the adaptation of sodium excretion with reduced renal mass. *J Clin Invest* 77:1395, 1986.

178. Sonnenberg H, Cupples WA, de Bold AJ, et al: Intrarenal localization of the natriuretic effect of cardiac atrial extract. *Can J Physiol Pharmacol* 60:1149, 1982.

179. Stanton B, Giebisch G: Mechanism of urinary potassium excretion. *Miner Electrolyte Metab* 5:100, 1981.

180. Steele TH, Wen SF, Evenson MA, et al: The contribution of the chronically diseased kidney to magnesium homeostasis in man. *J Lab Clin Med* 71:455, 1968.

181. Steiner RW: Interpreting the fractional excretion of sodium. *Am J Med* 77:699, 1984.

182. Sterns RH, Spital A: Disorders of internal potassium balance. *Semin Nephrol* 7:206, 1987.

183. Strauss MB: Acute renal insufficiency due to lower-nephron nephrosis. *N Engl J Med* 239:693, 1948.

184. Szekely K: Thorn's syndrome in the pediatric age group. Pseudo-Addison-disease as a result of nephropathy. *Helv Paediatr Acta* 15:94, 1960.

185. Tannen RL, Regal EM, Dunn MJ, et al: Vasopressin-resistant hyposthenuria in advanced chronic renal disease. *N Engl J Med* 280:1135, 1969.

186. Thibault G, Garcia R, Cantin M, et al: Atrial natriuretic factor. Characterization and partial purification. *Hypertension* (suppl I)5:I–75, 1983.

187. Thorn GW, Koeph GF, Clinton M Jr: Renal failure simulating adrenocortical insufficiency. *N Engl J Med* 231:76, 1944.

188. Travis LB, Dodge WF, Beathard GA, et al: Acute glomerulonephritis in children. A review of the natural history with emphasis on prognosis. *Clin Nephrol* 1:169, 1973.

189. Uribarri J, Oh MS, Carroll HJ: Salt-losing nephropathy. Clinical presentation and mechanisms. *Am J Nephrol* 3:193, 1983.

190. van Ypersele de Strihou C: Potassium homeostasis in renal failure. *Kidney Int* 11:491, 1977.

191. Walker WB, Jost LJ, Johnson JR, et al: Metabolic observations on salt wasting in a patient with renal disease. *Am J Med* 39:505, 1965.

192. Weber H, Lin K, Bricker NS: Effect of sodium intake on single nephron glomerular filtration rate and sodium reabsorption in experimental uremia. *Kidney Int* 8:14, 1975.

193. Weber HP, Michalk D, Rauh W, et al: Total body potassium in children with chronic renal failure. *Int J Pediatr Nephrol* 1:42, 1980.

194. Weidmann P, Maxwell MH, De Lima J, et al: Control of aldosterone responsiveness in terminal renal failure. *Kidney Int* 7:351, 1975.

195. Weinberg JM, Humes HD: Renal tubular cell integrity in mercuric chloride and gentamicin nephrotoxicity. *In* Solez K, Whelton A (eds): *Acute Renal Failure: Correlation between Morphology and Function.* New York, Marcel Dekker, 1984, p 179.

196. Weiner MW, Weinman EJ, Kashgarian M, et al: Accelerated reabsorption in the proximal tubule produced by volume depletion. *J Clin Invest* 50:1379, 1971.

197. Welt LG, Sachs JR, McManus TJ: An ion transport defect in erythrocytes from uremic patients. *Trans Assoc Am Physicians* 77:169, 1964.

198. Welt LG: Membrane transport defect: The sick cell. *Trans Assoc Am Physicians* 80:217, 1967.

199. Wen SF, Wong NL, Evanson RL, et al: Micropuncture studies of sodium transport in the remnant kidney of the dog. The effect of graded volume expansion. *J Clin Invest* 52:386, 1973.

200. Williams GH, Bailey GL, Hampers CL, et al: Studies on the metabolism of aldosterone in chronic renal failure and anephric man. *Kidney Int* 4:280, 1973.

200a. Windus DW, Stokes TJ, Morgan JR, et al: The effects of atrial peptide in humans with chronic renal failure. *Am J Kidney Dis* 13:477, 1989.

201. Winkler AW, Hoff HE, Smith PK: The toxicity of orally administered potassium salts in renal insufficiency. *J Clin Invest* 20:119, 1941.

202. Wright FS: Renal potassium handling. *Semin Nephrol* 7:174, 1987.

203. Zarich S, Fang LST, Diamond JRF: Fractional excretion of sodium. Exceptions to its diagnostic value. *Arch Intern Med* 145:108, 1985.

204. Zusman J, Brown D, Nesbit M: Hyperphosphatemia, hyperphosphaturia, and hypocalcemia in acute lymphoblastic leukemia. *N Engl J Med* 289:1335, 1983.

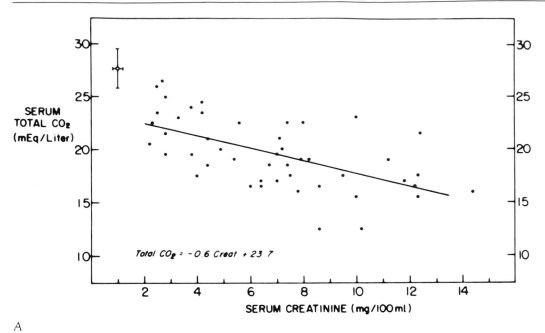

A

FIG. 27-1. A. *Relationship between serum total CO_2 and serum creatinine in patients with normal renal function (open circle) and in patients with various degrees of renal failure (closed circles). B. Relationship between serum unmeasured anion concentration and serum creatinine in patients with normal renal function (open circle) and in patients with various degrees of renal failure (closed circles). (From Widmer B, Gerhardt RE, Harrington JT, et al: Serum electrolyte and acid base composition. The influence of graded degrees of chronic renal failure. Arch Intern Med 139:1099, 1979, with permission.)*

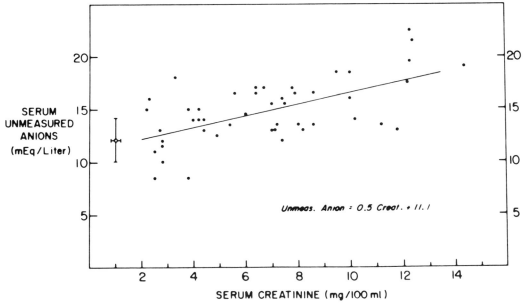

B

and Na-K-ATPase activity in mucosa of colon. *Am J Physiol* 229:1576, 1975.

173. Silva P, Hayslett JP, Epstein FH: The role of Na-K-activated adenosine triphosphatase in potassium adaptation. *J Clin Invest* 52:2665, 1973.

174. Silva P, Ross BD, Charney AN, et al: Potassium transport by the isolated perfused kidney. *J Clin Invest* 56:862, 1975.

175. Skorecki KL, Brenner BM: Body fluid homeostasis in man. *Am J Med* 70:77, 1981.

176. Slatopolsky E, Elkan IO, Weerts C, et al: Studies on the characteristics of the control system governing sodium excretion in uremic man. *J Clin Invest* 47:521, 1968.

177. Smith S, Anderson S, Ballerman BJ, et al: Role of atrial natriuretic peptide in the adaptation of sodium excretion with reduced renal mass. *J Clin Invest* 77:1395, 1986.

178. Sonnenberg H, Cupples WA, de Bold AJ, et al: Intrarenal localization of the natriuretic effect of cardiac atrial extract. *Can J Physiol Pharmacol* 60:1149, 1982.

179. Stanton B, Giebisch G: Mechanism of urinary potassium excretion. *Miner Electrolyte Metab* 5:100, 1981.

180. Steele TH, Wen SF, Evenson MA, et al: The contribution of the chronically diseased kidney to magnesium homeostasis in man. *J Lab Clin Med* 71:455, 1968.

181. Steiner RW: Interpreting the fractional excretion of sodium. *Am J Med* 77:699, 1984.

182. Sterns RH, Spital A: Disorders of internal potassium balance. *Semin Nephrol* 7:206, 1987.

183. Strauss MB: Acute renal insufficiency due to lower-nephron nephrosis. *N Engl J Med* 239:693, 1948.

184. Szekely K: Thorn's syndrome in the pediatric age group. Pseudo-Addison-disease as a result of nephropathy. *Helv Paediatr Acta* 15:94, 1960.

185. Tannen RL, Regal EM, Dunn MJ, et al: Vasopressin-resistant hyposthenuria in advanced chronic renal disease. *N Engl J Med* 280:1135, 1969.

186. Thibault G, Garcia R, Cantin M, et al: Atrial natriuretic factor. Characterization and partial purification. *Hypertension* (suppl I)5:I–75, 1983.

187. Thorn GW, Koeph GF, Clinton M Jr: Renal failure simulating adrenocortical insufficiency. *N Engl J Med* 231:76, 1944.

188. Travis LB, Dodge WF, Beathard GA, et al: Acute glomerulonephritis in children. A review of the natural history with emphasis on prognosis. *Clin Nephrol* 1:169, 1973.

189. Uribarri J, Oh MS, Carroll HJ: Salt-losing nephropathy. Clinical presentation and mechanisms. *Am J Nephrol* 3:193, 1983.

190. van Ypersele de Strihou C: Potassium homeostasis in renal failure. *Kidney Int* 11:491, 1977.

191. Walker WB, Jost LJ, Johnson JR, et al: Metabolic observations on salt wasting in a patient with renal disease. *Am J Med* 39:505, 1965.

192. Weber H, Lin K, Bricker NS: Effect of sodium intake on single nephron glomerular filtration rate and sodium reabsorption in experimental uremia. *Kidney Int* 8:14, 1975.

193. Weber HP, Michalk D, Rauh W, et al: Total body potassium in children with chronic renal failure. *Int J Pediatr Nephrol* 1:42, 1980.

194. Weidmann P, Maxwell MH, De Lima J, et al: Control of aldosterone responsiveness in terminal renal failure. *Kidney Int* 7:351, 1975.

195. Weinberg JM, Humes HD: Renal tubular cell integrity in mercuric chloride and gentamicin nephrotoxicity. *In* Solez K, Whelton A (eds): *Acute Renal Failure: Correlation between Morphology and Function*. New York, Marcel Dekker, 1984, p 179.

196. Weiner MW, Weinman EJ, Kashgarian M, et al: Accelerated reabsorption in the proximal tubule produced by volume depletion. *J Clin Invest* 50:1379, 1971.

197. Welt LG, Sachs JR, McManus TJ: An ion transport defect in erythrocytes from uremic patients. *Trans Assoc Am Physicians* 77:169, 1964.

198. Welt LG: Membrane transport defect: The sick cell. *Trans Assoc Am Physicians* 80:217, 1967.

199. Wen SF, Wong NL, Evanson RL, et al: Micropuncture studies of sodium transport in the remnant kidney of the dog. The effect of graded volume expansion. *J Clin Invest* 52:386, 1973.

200. Williams GH, Bailey GL, Hampers CL, et al: Studies on the metabolism of aldosterone in chronic renal failure and anephric man. *Kidney Int* 4:280, 1973.

200a. Windus DW, Stokes TJ, Morgan JR, et al: The effects of atrial peptide in humans with chronic renal failure. *Am J Kidney Dis* 13:477, 1989.

201. Winkler AW, Hoff HE, Smith PK: The toxicity of orally administered potassium salts in renal insufficiency. *J Clin Invest* 20:119, 1941.

202. Wright FS: Renal potassium handling. *Semin Nephrol* 7:174, 1987.

203. Zarich S, Fang LST, Diamond JRF: Fractional excretion of sodium. Exceptions to its diagnostic value. *Arch Intern Med* 145:108, 1985.

204. Zusman J, Brown D, Nesbit M: Hyperphosphatemia, hyperphosphaturia, and hypocalcemia in acute lymphoblastic leukemia. *N Engl J Med* 289:1335, 1983.

MICHAEL A. LINSHAW

27
Acid–Base Disturbances

The kidney plays a major role in acid excretion [101]. Henderson and Palmer [91–93] at the turn of the century reported that nonvolatile acids were excreted by the kidney, but thought that renal acid excretion occurred primarily in the form of titratable acid, the ammonia acting mainly to substitute for other bases in the urine, thereby conserving the body buffer base as the kidney excreted acid as monobasic phosphate. Acid excretion subsequently was found to be reduced in the acidosis of renal disease [222]. Ammonium excretion had already been related to the conservation of body stores of bicarbonate [157], and investigators came to realize that depletion of base (acidosis) in renal disease was due principally to the kidneys' decreased ability to excrete ammonium [93,157,164,222].

The remaining intact nephrons of the diseased kidney show remarkable adaptation to maintain body homeostasis [27,162] and to excrete acid at a rate per nephron that is several times normal [26,27]. The onset of acidosis, therefore, reflects a failure of total glomerular and tubular function to meet the body's need for bicarbonate reabsorption, net acid excretion, or both [168,185]. Persistent and relatively stable metabolic acidosis is a consistent characteristic of advanced chronic renal failure.

The degree of renal insufficiency that is reached before acidosis develops varies from patient to patient. A significant though mild degree of acidosis occurs long before glomerular filtration rate (GFR) is severely reduced and obvious signs and symptoms of uremia are present [229]. Marked acidosis usually is not observed until the GFR is less than 20% to 25% of normal [6,56,175].

The acidosis of chronic renal failure tends to stabilize at a moderately severe level, with serum bicarbonate concentrations usually not dropping below 15 mEq/L. This is illustrated in Fig. 27-1A, which relates total serum carbon dioxide to serum creatinine, comparing normal patients with those with varying degrees of renal insufficiency. Patients with mild-to-moderate degrees of renal insufficiency have a noticeable reduction in serum total carbon dioxide, averaging about 5 to 6 mEq/L below normal. With this degree of acidemia, as shown in Fig. 27-1B, the anion gap is not appreciably changed and there is mild hyperchloremia. As the serum creatinine increases, the total serum

carbon dioxide decreases progressively, and there is a gradual, concomitant increase in the anion gap. The acidosis of more severe renal insufficiency is characterized by a normal serum chloride concentration and a markedly elevated anion gap, reflecting the retention of phosphate and unmeasured anions (e.g., SO_4) [87].

The acidosis of uremia tends to be stable [185,229] in the absence of extrarenal complications such as sepsis, diarrhea, hypercatabolism, hypoxia, or ketoacidosis [71,168]. In the steady state of uremic metabolic acidosis, the hydrogen ion is eliminated from the blood at the same rate at which it is generated. Although the diseased kidney cannot excrete net hydrogen ion at a rate that is sufficient to maintain zero hydrogen ion balance, the stable degree of acidemia is maintained in the face of positive hydrogen balance by buffering of acid with alkaline salts derived from bone (see Extrarenal Buffering).

General Metabolic Considerations

The development and magnitude of acidosis in renal disease depend on a variety of factors, including (1) the acid load of the diet and the rate of production of acid from endogenous sources, (2) the extent of renal damage and loss of functional renal tissue (limiting acid excretion), and (3) other metabolic disturbances that may affect acid–base balance (such as the loss of acid from vomiting or nasogastric drainage and the loss of base from diarrhea or upper intestinal [nongastric] secretions). In catabolic states such as sepsis, fever, the use of steroids, or the postoperative period, the degree of acidosis may be significantly augmented, as it may be if other causes of acidosis, such as diabetic ketoacidosis, lactic acidosis, or ingestion of salicylate, are superimposed on primary renal insufficiency.

Endogenous Production of Acid and Base

The major endogenous sources of acid and alkali are the metabolic products of various dietary components. The neutral diet precursors that are converted to acids or bases

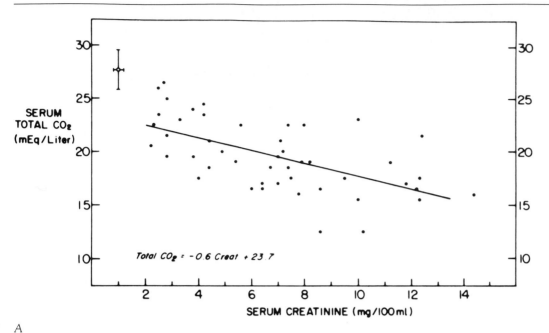

A

FIG. 27-1. A. Relationship between serum total CO_2 and serum creatinine in patients with normal renal function (open circle) and in patients with various degrees of renal failure (closed circles). B. Relationship between serum unmeasured anion concentration and serum creatinine in patients with normal renal function (open circle) and in patients with various degrees of renal failure (closed circles). (From Widmer B, Gerhardt RE, Harrington JT, et al: Serum electrolyte and acid base composition. The influence of graded degrees of chronic renal failure. Arch Intern Med 139:1099, 1979, with permission.)

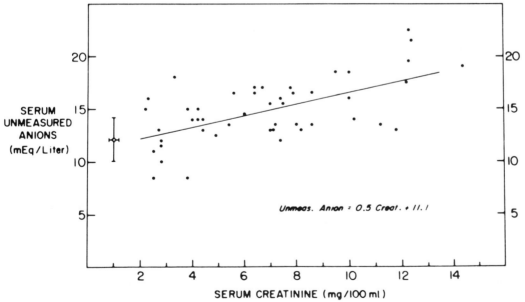

B

are summarized in Table 27-1. Acid derives primarily from sulfur-containing amino acids, organic substances that yield organic acid, and organic cations that on oxidation yield hydrogen ion and phospholipid. Sources of alkali include organic anions that combine with hydrogen ion when oxidized and dibasic phosphoester salts that combine with hydrogen ion when hydrolyzed (e.g., phosphoprotein) [71, 97,123,125,126,170].

In general, when completely oxidized, a primarily vegetable diet yields an alkaline ash, whereas a diet high in protein (meat, fish, and eggs) yields an acid ash. Carbohydrates and fats are metabolized almost completely to carbon dioxide and water. Carbonic acid is dehydrated to carbon dioxide and is rapidly excreted by the lungs, leaving no hydrogen ion to accumulate in body fluids. However, to the extent that the metabolism of carbohydrate and fat is incomplete (e.g., producing excess lactic acid), the ash analysis of a given diet cannot accurately measure the effect on acid–base balance [71,194]. Moreover, the acidity or alkalinity of the ash of a given diet appears to have little relationship to the urinary excretion of acid, apart from the sulfur content of the diet [97].

The average western diet generates about 1 mEq of acid per kilogram body weight per day in the adult [88,125] and between 1.5 and 2.5 mEq/kg body weight per day in the child [103,177]. Vegetarian diets may produce a net alkaline load, since such diets contain little sulfur. Dietary acid rather than actual loss of renal function is paramount in the pathogenesis of uremic acidosis, which is evident from the observation that ruminants such as cattle, ingesting a dietary alkaline load, develop metabolic *alkalosis* when made uremic by urethral ligation [192].

General Review of Acid Handling by the Kidney

Bicarbonate Reabsorption

The conservation of filtered bicarbonate occurs primarily in the proximal tubule, where 80% to 90% is reabsorbed and returned to the extracellular fluid. A variety of factors influence this reabsorption (Table 27-2). Bicarbonate reabsorption in this segment takes place without large lumen-to-blood pH gradients [109]. Hydrogen ion secretion occurs by an electrically neutral Na^+-H^+ exchanger in the brush border membrane, driven by the lumen-to-cell concentration gradient for sodium. Any maneuver that decreases this gradient interferes with H^+ secretion. Removing sodium from the luminal fluid of perfused isolated tubules largely inhibits bicarbonate reabsorption [19,109,140,182]. Intracellular pH is important in regulating Na^+-H^+ exchange and bicarbonate reabsorption since the rate of hydrogen secretion by the cell varies inversely with intracellular pH [23,24].

Although bicarbonate reabsorption appears to occur primarily in the proximal convoluted tubule, the proximal straight tubule also clearly participates in this resorptive process [70], and there is evidence that bicarbonate reabsorption continues along the ascending thick limb of Henle [75,79]. In the distal convoluted tubule and the collecting

TABLE 27-1. *Sources of endogenous acid and alkali**

Endogenous acids

1. Oxidation of sulfhydryl groups yielding sulfuric acid:

$$\left. \begin{array}{l} \text{Methionine} \\ \text{Cysteine} \end{array} \right\} \xrightarrow{O_2} CO_2 + H_2O + urea + H_2SO_4$$

2. Hydrolysis of phosphoester acid yielding phosphoric acid:

a.
$$R{-}O{-}\overset{\overset{\displaystyle O}{\|}}{\underset{\underset{\displaystyle OH}{|}}{P}}{-}OH \xrightarrow{H_2O} ROH + H_3PO_4$$

b.
$$R_1{-}O{-}\overset{\overset{\displaystyle O}{\|}}{\underset{\underset{\displaystyle OH}{|}}{P}}{-}O{-}R_2 \xrightarrow{2H_2O} R_1OH + R_2OH + H_3PO_4$$

c.
$$R{-}O{-}\overset{\overset{\displaystyle O}{\|}}{\underset{\underset{\displaystyle OH}{|}}{P}}{-}O{-}\overset{\overset{\displaystyle O}{\|}}{\underset{\underset{\displaystyle OH}{|}}{P}}{-}OH \xrightarrow{2H_2O} ROH + 2H_3PO_4$$

3. Oxidation of neutral dietery precursors yielding organic acids:

a. Glucose $\xrightarrow{O_2}$ lactic acid/pyruvic acid

b. Triglyceride $\xrightarrow{O_2}$ acetoacetic acid/3-OH butyric acid

c. Nucleoprotein $\xrightarrow{O_2}$ uric acid

4. Oxidation of organic cations yielding hydrogen ions:

$$R - NH_3 \xrightarrow{O_2} CO_2 + H_2O + urea + H^+$$

Endogenous alkali

1. Oxidation of organic anions yielding bicarbonate:

$$R{-}\overset{\overset{\displaystyle O}{\|}}{C}{-}O^- + H_2CO_3 \xrightarrow{O_2} CO_2 + H_2O + urea + HCO_3^-$$

2. Hydrolysis of phosphoester salts yielding bicarbonate:

$$R{-}O{-}\overset{\overset{\displaystyle O}{\|}}{\underset{\underset{\displaystyle O^-}{|}}{P}}{-}O^- + H_2CO_3 \xrightarrow{H_2O} ROH + H_2PO_4^- + HCO_3^-$$

* *Adapted from* Lennon EJ, Lemann J, Litzow JR: The effects of diet and stool composition on the net external acid balance of normal subjects. *J Clin Invest* 45:1601, 1966 as adapted by Gennari FJ, Cohen JJ, Kassirer JP: Determinants of plasma bicarbonate concentration and hydrogen ion balance. *In* Cohen JJ, Kassirer JP (eds): *Acid-Base.* Little, Brown, Boston, 1982, p 55.

duct, the rate of bicarbonate reabsorption is much less than in the proximal tubule, but tubular fluid nevertheless becomes increasingly more acid. Secretion of H^+ across the luminal membrane is driven by an electrogenic H^+ pump, using ATP, against an electrochemical gradient [109].

The collecting duct reabsorbs or secretes bicarbonate, depending on the prevailing acid–base status [109,141, 142]. Active electrogenic H^+ secretion in this segment can occur independent of luminal Na^+, K^+, and Cl^- [108,

Table 27-2. *Factors regulating proximal bicarbonate reabsorption*

Factors known to increase bicarbonate reabsorption	Factors known to decrease bicarbonate reabsorption
Major	*Major*
Volume contraction	Volume expansion
Increased filtered load of bicarbonate[a]	Decreased filtered load of bicarbonate[a]
Hypercapnia[b]	Hypocapnia[b]
Acidemia[b]	Alkalemia[b]
Hypokalemia	Hyperkalemia
	Carbonic anhydrase inhibition
Minor	
	Minor
Hypercalemia	
PTH deficiency	PTH excess
Vitamin D	Hypocalcemia
Thyroid hormone	Phosphate depletion
Glucose	Vitamin D deficiency
	Hypothyroidism
	Basic amino acids (lysine, arginine)
	Maleic acid

[a] The effect of filtered load of bicarbonate, rather than the effects of its two factors (i.e., GFR and bicarbonate), is listed, although both GFR and bicarbonate may have independent effects on bicarbonate reabsorption.
[b] Effects likely mediated by parallel changes in cell pH.

109,117,212]. Inhibition of carbonic anhydrase blocks bicarbonate reabsorption. Several other factors affect bicarbonate reabsorption or acid excretion:

1. Removing luminal sodium or adding amiloride or ouabain reduces bicarbonate reabsorption [108,109,117] perhaps because of an effect on potential difference.
2. Aldosterone increases acidification of the urine by stimulating sodium reabsorption, thus increasing the potential difference, i.e., becoming more negative across the luminal membrane [108,109].
3. A low urinary pH inhibits net tubular hydrogen secretion [109], which cannot occur against a urinary pH below 4.0 to 4.5 [71,184,211].

In the cortical and outer medullary collecting duct, proton secretion is believed to be accomplished by intercalated cells present in these segments. Bicarbonate reabsorption also can be demonstrated in rat inner medullary collecting ducts, including the terminal portions that do not contain intercalated cells [226]. Bicarbonate reabsorption (H^+ secretion) in this nephron segment is increased in response to both desoxycorticosterone and systemic loading with NH_4Cl and therefore appears to be regulated by similar factors affecting net acid excretion in other collecting duct segments. The specialized inner medullary collecting duct cells of this segment seem to lack carbonic anhydrase [33,133] as well as the proton translocating ATPase [32] that are characteristic of intercalated cells.

Excretion of Acid

TITRATABLE ACID

Titratable acid is composed mostly of phosphate, though other buffers, including citrate, acetate, creatinine, and

uric acid contribute to a lesser extent [71]. At extracellular fluid pH of 7.4, about 80% of inorganic phosphate exists as HPO_4^{2-}. In the distal tubular segments, where the tubular fluid pH falls below 6.8, the filtered dibasic phosphate is titrated to the monobasic form $H_2PO_4^-$. Based on a pK of 6.8, 99% of phosphate is in this monobasic or acid form at a urinary pH of 4.8. Phosphate that is filtered as $HPO_4^=$ and is excreted in the urine as $H_2PO_4^-$ results in the net excretion of H^+ or the net production of HCO_3^- by the kidney. Conversely, phosphate filtered in the form of $H_2PO_4^-$ cannot contribute to net hydrogen excretion. About half of the approximately 30 mmol of phosphate that is absorbed and excreted each day is in the monobasic form [83].

Under most circumstances, the capacity to excrete titratable acid is limited by the amount of buffer that is delivered to the distal tubule. Since this is not under physiologic control related to acid–base balance, the increase in excretion of titratable acid that occurs during acidosis is limited. Titratable acid is reduced almost to zero in states of severe phosphate depletion, due to the absence of phosphate in the urine [161,203]. Conversely, in states of high serum and urinary phosphate, there may be an increase in titratable acid [74,82].

EXCRETION OF AMMONIA
General Considerations
The majority of renal bicarbonate generation (or acid secretion) is accomplished by the production and urinary excretion of ammonium ions. According to the classic formulation of Pitts [158], glutamine is the major amino precursor for renal ammonia, the glutamine being metabolized to glutamic acid and NH_3. The lipid-soluble NH_3 rapidly traverses the lipoprotein membrane, in contrast to NH_4^+, which is water soluble, restricted to aqueous chan-

nels, and considerably less permeant. Once in the lumen, NH_3 binds to H^+, trapping it in tubular fluid, thereby providing a relatively nonpermeant vehicle (NH_4^+) for excretion of that proton [160,161] (Fig. 27-2). Though the pK of ammonia is 9.2 to 9.3, and at cell pH almost all of the ammonia exists as NH_4^+, Pitts considered that the very small amount of highly diffusible NH_3 would move to a site of lower concentration (lower pNH_3) in the tubular lumen, the tubular fluid acting as an NH_3 sink. The countercurrent exchange mechanism maintains a high level of interstitial ammonia in the renal medulla [78,79,173,213]. Pitts suggested that ammonia enters the medullary interstitium by absorption from the descending loop of Henle. Absorption is facilitated by the abstraction of water from the descending limb by the hypertonic medullary interstitium, which concentrates the luminal bicarbonate, increases the luminal pH, favors the formation of NH_3 over NH_4^+, and thus promotes NH_3 movement into the interstitium [159,161].

Ammonia Cycling in the Kidney

Ammonium excreted in the urine is derived almost exclusively from renal synthesis, primarily in the proximal convoluted and straight tubules [76,78]. Although this occurs mainly in the cortex, where a high rate of blood flow tends to return substances to the circulation, a large portion of the synthesized ammonia does nevertheless appear in the urine. Most of the ammonia produced in proximal tubule cells enters the early part of the proximal tubule lumen,

but a substantial portion, perhaps a third, is reabsorbed in the late proximal tubule. In states of chronic metabolic acidosis, ammonia secretion is stimulated so that secretion increases twofold in the early proximal convoluted tubule, and secretion continues even in the late portion of this nephron segment [77]. Some 40% to 80% of ammonia delivered to the loop of Henle is absorbed before reaching the distal tubule, primarily in the ascending limb [34,78,79,176] (Table 27-3). The ammonia can recycle to the descending limb and to deeper portions of the medulla. There is little net secretion of ammonia across the distal convoluted tubule, but substantial secretion in the collecting duct, probably in both the cortical and medullary segments [78,86,100,106,107,195,205,226]. The low rate of blood flow in the deep medulla allows ammonia to remain in the interstitium for collecting duct secretion. Metabolic acidosis, by stimulating proximal tubular synthesis of ammonia, increases the delivery of ammonia to the thick ascending limb where increased reabsorption and accumulation in the interstitium and increased secretion in the collecting duct facilitate acid excretion [78]. In the cortical collecting tubule, ammonia secretion appears to occur primarily by nonionic diffusion [86,106], though permeability to ammonia is low compared with the proximal convoluted tubule, and diffusion is significantly restricted [86]. Ammonia *secretion* is augmented in the acidotic state, particularly in the cortical collecting duct [34,176], but ammonia *synthesis* in this segment appears to be low and is not stimulated by metabolic acidosis [76,78].

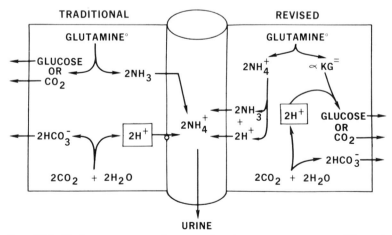

PATHWAY OF AMMONIUM EXCRETION

FIG. 27-2. *Hydrogen ion removal associated with ammonium excretion. The traditional view of ammonium excretion is outlined on the left side of the figure. The excretion of ammonium is described as the process by which hydrogen ions are eliminated as they bind to ammonia in the tubular lumen to form ammonium ion. In the adjusted view depicted on the right side, it is emphasized that ammonium ion (NH_4^+) and not ammonia (NH_3) is the product of glutamine and glutamate metabolism. Hydrogen ions are actually removed when alpha-ketoglutarate is metabolized to neutral end products. In acid–base terms, ammonium ion excretion prevents hydrogen ion formation in the liver (urea + H^+ synthesis). (From Halperin ML, Jungas RL: Metabolic production and renal disposal of hydrogen ions. Kidney Int 24:709, 1983, with permission.)*

Table 27-3. Percent of excreted ammonia delivered to various nephron sites

Nephron site	Control rats	Acidotic rats
Late PCT (superficial)	105*	82*
	112[†]	84[†]
Tip of Henle's loop (deep nephrons)	160[†]	124[†]
Distal tubule (superficial)	21*	32*
	71*	45*
Outer medullary collecting duct	53*	82*
Papillary collecting duct		
Base	93[†]	99[†]
Tip	100	100

Control rats: normal, nondiuretic rats. Acidotic rats given 0.17 to 0.30 M NH_4CL to drink for 4 to 5 days before experiments. Absolute total ammonia excretion rates were: control, 0.15 to 0.40 μmol/min/kidney and acidotic, 1.0 to 1.4 μmol/min/kidney.
Abbreviation: PCT = proximal convoluted tubule.
* *Data from* Sajo IM, Goldstein MB, Sonnenberg H, et al: Sites of ammonia addiction to tubular fluid in rats with chronic metabolic acidosis. *Kidney Int* 20:353, 1981.
† *Data from* Buerkert J, Martin D, Trigg D: Ammonium handling by superficial juxtamedullary nephrons in the rat. *J Clin Invest* 70:1, 1982.
From Good DW, Knepper MA: Ammonia transport in the mammalian kidney. *Am J Physiol* 248:F459, 1985, with permission.

Ammonia Transport

Traditionally, ammonia transport was thought to be accomplished primarily by movement of the permeant species NH_3, and current studies are consistent with this view [69,70,113]. However, recently this view has been challenged [78,174]. NH_4^+ is transported across membranes of lower life forms such as fungi, bacteria, plants, and fish gills, and across membranes from a variety of other tissues [4,22–25,73,105,146–148,174,183,218] including mammalian kidney [79]. NH_4^+ probably crosses cell membranes via carriers or through channels in the aqueous phase of the membrane rather than across the lipid phase [78]. In several tissues, including rabbit proximal straight tubules [68] NH_4^+ can substitute for potassium, supporting the hydrolysis of ATP by Na^+-K^+-ATPase [116,163,172,198] and increasing oxygen consumption [111,112,204]. NH_4^+ can replace either H^+ or Na^+ ions on the Na^+-H^+ exchanger of apical membrane vesicles of rabbit proximal tubules [5,104], and NH_4^+ appears to permeate K^+ and Na^+ channels of frog nerve tissue [94,95] and K^+ channels of frog skin [233]. Thus, NH_4^+ can cross membranes, enter channels of other ions, substitute for other ions on cation exchangers, and activate Na^+-K^+-ATPase. Secretion of ammonia along the medullary collecting duct may occur by nonionic diffusion [86,106] and depends on its medullary interstitial concentration.

Role of Ammonium Ion in Acid Transport

Good and Knepper [78] suggested that transepithelial secretion of NH_4^+ can lead to luminal acidification. As depicted in Fig. 27-3, NH_3 is protonated in the interstitium and transported as NH_4^+ across the basolateral membrane. NH_4^+ concentration increases in the cell and drives the formation of NH_3 and H^+. When NH_3 efflux and NH_4^+ influx across the basolateral membrane are in equilibrium, H^+ is available for apical membrane transport. In this view, H^+ secretion is accomplished without ammonia secretion into the lumen.

Halperin and Jungas [83] point out that although NH_3 theoretically could be produced by the kidney and diffuse

into the tubular fluid, combining with hydrogen ion to form NH_4^+, ammonia is present almost exclusively as NH_4^+ at physiologic pH. Thus, excretion of NH_4^+ per se would not accomplish the excretion of protons generated elsewhere and therefore would not affect net acid–base balance. These authors emphasize that glutamine is converted by hydrolysis at neutral pH to alpha-ketoglutarate plus NH_4^+ rather than to glutamic acid and NH_3 [150,151]. The metabolism of alpha-ketoglutarate, which contains two negative charges (two carboxyl groups), consumes two H^+ (generates bicarbonate) as glucose or carbon

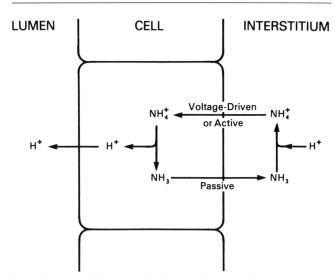

Fig. 27-3. *Possible means of carbonic anhydrase independent luminal acidification by basolateral ammonia recycling. At steady state net NH_4^+ influx and net NH_3 efflux are equal, providing continuous influx of protons to cell from interstitium for transport across apical membrane.* (From Good DW, Knepper MA: Ammonia transport in the mammalian kidney. *Am J Physiol* 248:F459, 1985, with permission.)

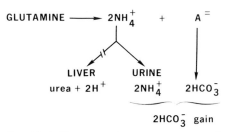

FIG. 27-4. *Excretion of ammonium is equivalent to addition of bicarbonate to the renal venous blood. Renal metabolism results in the conversion of the electroneutral glutamine into NH_4^+ plus the anion 2-oxoglutarate. To add bicarbonate to the renal venous blood, the anion must be metabolized, removing protons (which is equivalent to generating bicarbonate), and the NH_4^+ must be excreted in the urine (otherwise it will return through the renal vein to the liver and result in urea + proton formation). (From Halperin ML, Goldstein MB, Stinebaugh BJ, et al: Biochemistry and physiology of ammonium excreation. In Seldi DW, Giebisch G (eds): The Kidney: Physiology and Pathophysiology. New York, Raven Press, 1985, chap 64, p 1471, with permission.)*

dioxide or both are formed. The NH_4^+ produced is excreted in the urine, conserving cation and preventing the recycling of NH_4^+ in the liver, where formation of urea would consume bicarbonate (generate H^+) and thereby offset the consumption of H^+ as NH_4^+ was formed (Fig. 27-4).

General Pathophysiology of Acidosis in Chronic Renal Failure

Acidosis can result from excessive production or deficient excretion of hydrogen ion or both. On the basis of numerous metabolic balance studies, it has been established that production is not excessive, and that excretion (as suspected) is deficient in the face of a normal rate of production. When renal mass becomes reduced, residual intact nephrons adapt as attempts are made to minimize changes in systemic acid–base balance. In the remnant kidney model of renal failure, the proximal tubule increases its absolute reabsorption of bicarbonate [36,129,230] and quantitatively probably contributes more to the adaptive

changes. However, the distal tubule also appears to increase its proton secretion and may help maintain acid–base balance [110]. Acidosis occurs with progressive loss of renal tissue as the residual nephrons become unable to excrete the net acid load. The major factors to consider are (1) bicarbonate reabsorption, (2) urinary acidification (generation of titratable acid), and (3) urinary excretion of ammonium.

Bicarbonate Reabsorption

The administration of bicarbonate to uremic subjects to correct acidosis was shown to increase urinary pH and the rate of excretion of bicarbonate in urine [185]. These findings were reversed and urinary pH and plasma bicarbonate levels decreased rapidly when bicarbonate therapy was stopped. Although these observations were interpreted to indicate an intrinsic defect in tubular reabsorption of bicarbonate (renal bicarbonate leak), subsequent studies indicated that bicarbonate reabsorption was not impaired in renal insufficiency [129,171,201].

When the extracellular fluid volume is expanded, bicarbonate reabsorption is depressed in both normal subjects and uremics [114]. A true bicarbonate leak, however, rarely contributes to the acidosis of chronic renal failure in the absence of extracellular fluid volume expansion.

In micropuncture studies, bicarbonate delivered to the end of both proximal and distal tubules was substantially increased in rats made uremic by surgically reducing their renal mass about 70% [34]. However, bicarbonate reabsorption per nephron is actually increased in chronic renal failure in both humans and laboratory animals [9,11,165, 179,180,230]. Arruda et al. [11] found no evidence of a decrease in bicarbonate reabsorption relative to filtration rate, even though the extracellular fluid volume (as estimated by fractional chloride excretion) was higher than in normal subjects (Table 27-4 and Fig. 27-5). Moreover, as uremia increased in severity, these patients reabsorbed bicarbonate out of proportion to (i.e., in excess of) sodium [11]. Therefore, although factors such as volume expansion, hyperfiltration of residual nephrons, osmotic diuresis, or secondary hyperparathyroidism, all of which can occur in uremia, could impair bicarbonate reabsorption, the ability of residual nephrons to reabsorb bicarbonate appears largely intact. Any tendency to lose bicarbonate would appear to be related to increased delivery of filtered bicar-

TABLE 27-4. *Effect of chronic renal failure on bicarbonate reabsorption*

Subjects (number)	GFR (ml/min)	FE_{Cl} (%)	$TmHCO_3$/GFR (mmol/LGFR)	Absolute HCO_3^- reabsorption / Absolute Na reabsorption (%)
Normal (6)	140.7	2.1	28.6	21.1
Renal failure (8)	18.7	11.9	27.2	22.5

Mean values. FE_{Cl} = fractional chloride excretion.
Data from Arruda JAL, Nascimento L, Arevalo G, et al: Bicarbonate reabsorption in chronic renal failure studies in man and the rat. Pflugers Arch 376:193, 1978, with permission.

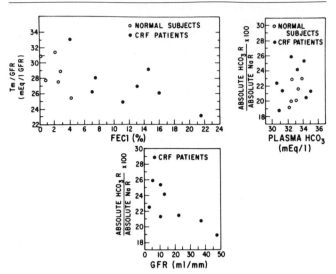

Fig. 27-5. *Bicarbonate reabsorption, expressed as Tm/GFR (left panel) and as the ratio of absolute bicarbonate reabsorption/absolute sodium reabsorption (right upper panel), is plotted against plasma bicarbonate in normal subjects and in patients with chronic renal failure. The lower panel shows the ratio of absolute bicarbonate reabsorption/absolute sodium reabsorption plotted against the GFR in patients with chronic renal failure. (From Arruda JAL, Nascimento L, Arevalo G, et al: Bicarbonate reabsorption in chronic renal failure studies in man and the rat. Pflugers Arch 376:193, 1978, with permission.)*

bonate beyond the proximal and distal reabsorptive sites [36,228].

Since parathyroid hormone (PTH) can depress bicarbonate reabsorption [12,53], and secondary hyperparathyroidism is associated with renal failure, it has been suggested that PTH contributes to the acidosis of uremia [149].

However, removing the parathyroid glands does not alter bicarbonate reabsorption in uremic animals [9]. Thus, PTH probably does not play an important role in bicarbonate reabsorption in the uremic state and does not *worsen* acidosis. The major effect of PTH in modifying the acidosis of renal failure is its *ameliorating* effect regarding extrarenal buffering [6,56,175], as discussed in a subsequent section (see Parathyroid Hormone).

Urinary pH

The chronically diseased kidney retains its ability to maximally acidify the urine [50,74,152,185]. Seldin et al. [190] found that control subjects had lowered urinary pH and nearly tripled net acid excretion after receiving an infusion of Na_2SO_4 along with salt-retaining hormones. In uremic, *nonacidotic* patients, the infusion led to increased urinary pH and urinary excretion of bicarbonate. However, if serum bicarbonate levels were low, the uremic patients showed a marked decrease in urinary pH after infusion of Na_2SO_4 and a modest increase in net acid excretion (Table 27-5). Thus, no intrinsic tubular defect in urinary acidification could be demonstrated [190].

Excretion of Acid

TITRATABLE ACID

Earlier measurements in chronic renal disease revealed that the excretion of titratable acid was reduced, generally to a modest degree, but that the ratio of ammonia to titratable acid was markedly decreased when compared with normal subjects [58,152,168,185,190,196,222,231]. Seldin et al. [190] (see Table 27-5) found that patients with chronic renal disease had rates of excretion of titratable acid close to that of controls and were able to generate a modest increase in titratable acid when challenged by Na_2SO_4. Simpson [196] showed that the urinary excretion of titrat-

TABLE 27-5. *Effect of Na_2SO_4 infusion on urinary pH and acid excretion in normal subjects and patients with chronic renal insufficiency with and without acidosis*

Subjects (number)	Period	GFR (ml/min)	Plasma CO_2 (mmol/L)	pH	Titratable acid (μEq/min)	Ammonium (μEq/min)	HCO_3^- (μEq/min)	Net acid (μEq/min)
					Urine			
Normal (6)	Control	108	27	6.05	20	25.2	12	33
	Na_2SO_4		25.7	4.32	38.2	43.8	0	82
Patients without acidosis (10)	Control	13.3	26.8	6.17	7	4.7	4.7	7
	Na_2SO_4		26.4	6.80	6	5.2	19.7	−8.4
Patients with acidosis (10)	Control	15.8	15.3	5.17	15.2	9.4	2	23
	Na_2SO_4		14.8	4.83	21.6	11.7	1	32.5

Values are mean. GFR = creatinine clearance; Net acid = titratable acid + ammonia − HCO_3.
Data from Seldin DW, Coleman AJ, Carter NW, et al: The effect of Na_2SO_4 on urinary acidification in chronic renal disease. *J Lab Clin Med* 69:893, 1967, with permission.

TABLE 27-6. *Comparison of acid excretion in normal and in acidotic patients with renal failure*

Subjects (number)	GFR (ml/min)	Plasma HCO₃⁻ (mEq/L)	Urine excretion						
				mEq/d			μEq/ml/GFR		
			pH	TA	NH₄⁺	H⁺	TA	NH₄⁺	H⁺
Normal (11)	120	28.2	6.17	23.0	36.5	56.0	0.13	0.21	0.32
Patients (10)	14.4	18.9	5.99	17.5	17.1	32.7	1.07	0.81	1.88

Values are mean. GFR = creatinine clearance; TA = titratable acid; NH₄⁺ = ammonium; H⁺ = hydrogen. Calculations are from individual patient data.
From Simpson DP: Control of hydrogen ion hemostasis and renal acidosis. *Medicine* 50:503, 1971, with permission.

able acid by uremic subjects was nearly equal to that of controls, although expressed as excretion relative to glomerular filtration, the rate of excretion of titratable acid was sixfold higher in the uremic patients (Table 27-6).

The quantity of titratable acid produced depends on the urinary pH and on the type and amount of anion buffer available. Once urinary pH is maximally depressed, the magnitude of the increase in titratable acid depends on the rate of excretion of buffer, which in turn depends on dietary metabolism. Phosphate depletion limits phosphate excretion [203], and thereby limits formation of titratable acid. In contrast, the diseased kidney as well as that of normal subjects can increase the rate of excretion of titratable acid in response to an increase in phosphate intake [30,74]. Considering that serum phosphate levels are often elevated in uremia, and secondary hyperparathyroidism has an inhibiting effect on renal phosphate reabsorption [200], it is not surprising that sufficient phosphate is available to maintain urine titratable acid excretion during renal insufficiency.

AMMONIA
General Concepts
The primary factor leading to acidosis in chronic renal failure is defective ammoniagenesis [28,29,55,58,66,74, 93,158,168,185,196,222,231], which results from a decrease in nephron mass rather than an intrinsic defect in ammonia production.

In micropuncture studies, Buerkert and colleagues evaluated the excretion of acid and ammonia in rats made uremic by renal ablation. While the rats acidified their urine, they drastically decreased net acid excretion, and the reduction in acid excretion could be accounted for by a decrease in net ammonium excretion [36]. Seldin et al. [190] found a negligible increase in ammonium excretion in patients with renal failure following infusion of Na₂SO₄ (see Table 27-5). Simpson [196] showed that uremic subjects had a rate of excretion of ammonia that was less than half that of controls. In general clinical terms, the adaptive increase in production of renal ammonia by residual intact nephrons is insufficient to meet the need to excrete all the acid produced in daily metabolism, and an overall decrease in absolute production of renal ammonia results. However, as emphasized by Warnock, the production of renal am-

monia can increase four- to fivefold so that a limitation in net acid excretion does not become evident until glomerular filtration has decreased below about 20% of normal [228]. In the study by Simpson, ammonium excretion in the uremic patients was actually increased per unit of nephron function (see Table 27-6).

Dorhout-Mees and colleagues [55] compared ammonium excretion of the normal dog kidney (stage 1), the pyelonephritic kidney in the presence of the normal contralateral kidney (stage 2), and the pyelonephritic kidney after the normal kidney was removed (stage 3) (Table 27-7), permitting the diseased kidney to be evaluated in the absence (stage 2) and presence (stage 3) of uremia. Although GFR and absolute rates of excretion of NH₄⁺ and titratable acid decreased in the experimental kidney in stage 2, all values increased in stage 3, demonstrating the reserve capacity of even the uremic kidney. There was a marked increase in ammonium excretion per 100 ml GFR in both stages 2 and 3. Thus, although total ammonium excretion was decreased in the uremic state, the ammonium excretion per functional nephron was actually increased.

Maclean and Hayslett [213] found that ammonium excretion per nephron in uremic rats increased threefold, and titratable acid excretion increased about ninefold. The ammonia production rate tended to parallel the ammonium excretion rate. By factoring the rate of production of ammonia by the DNA content of renal tissue (as a measure of cell number), the authors concluded that the increase in ammonium excretion per nephron was probably due to an increase in the number of cells rather than to a greater production rate of ammonia per cell. Similar findings were reported by Schoolwerth et al. [181].

Glutamine Metabolism
Generally, the chronic metabolic acidosis of chronic renal insufficiency is associated with increased utilization of glutamine and synthesis of ammonia [158,160,197], permitting nephrons to maintain greater H⁺ consumption. However, Simpson [196] suggested that ammonia formation is limited by the degree of renal failure. In some patients, an elevation of blood glutamine levels was not associated with an augmented renal utilization of glutamine [196], raising the possibility that the ability to produce ammonia from glutamine was already maximally stimulated and could not

TABLE 27-7. Effect of chronic renal insufficiency on titratable acid and ammonium excretion in the experimental kidney of the dog

Experimental stage	GFR (ml/min)	Titratable acid excretion		Ammonium excretion	
		Absolute (μEq/min)	per GFR (μEq/100 ml GFR)	Absolute (μEq/min)	per GFR (μEq/100 ml GFR)
1	41.5	45.4	110	53.1	133
2	15.3	21.5	122	24.7	172
3	20.3	38.5	194	43.9	226

Values are mean.
Data from Dorhout-Mees EJ, Machado M, Slatopolsky E, et al: The functional adaptation of the diseased kidney. III. Ammonium excretion. J Clin Invest 45:289, 1966.

TABLE 27-8. Effect of acidosis and chronic renal insufficiency on renal glutamine extraction and NH_4^+ production in humans

Subjects (number)	Glutamine extracted (μmol/min)	NH_4^+ produced (μmol/min)
Normal (6)	34.8 ± 2.2	50.3 ± 1.8
6 days NH_4CL acidosis (6)	109.6 ± 16.5	149.0 ± 21.8
Chronic renal insufficiency (6)	2.7 ± 1.3*	22.4 ± 3.9*

Mean ± SEM; * = significantly different from normal subjects and with NH_4Cl acidosis by $p < 0.001$.
Data from Tizianello A, DeFerrari G, Garibotto G, et al: Effects of chronic renal insufficiency and metabolic acidosis on glutamine metabolism in man. Clin Sci Mol Med 55:391, 1978.

be increased further, or, alternatively, the rate of ammonium excretion was limited by a relative impairment in the rate of ammonia synthesis in the cortex. (It should be noted, however, that despite low total ammonium excretion rates in these patients, their NH_4^+ excretion rate per milliliter GFR was still greater than normal.)

Tizianello et al. [57,219] found significant alterations in glutamine metabolism in several organs in patients with chronic renal insufficiency and metabolic acidosis. Normal subjects with ammonium chloride-induced acidosis showed no change in arterial levels of glutamine, but demonstrated a threefold increase in glutamine extraction and ammonia production (ratio unchanged). However, in acidotic patients with renal insufficiency, arterial glutamine levels were significantly increased, but utilization of glutamine (renal extraction) was negligible. The amount of ammonia produced was reduced, however, to a much lesser extent than glutamine extraction (ratio increased) (Table 27-8), suggesting that there was considerable ammoniagenesis from nonglutamine sources. In other studies designed to evaluate net amino acid and ammonia metabolism in subjects with chronic uremia, Tizianello et al. [220] found the following: (1) in uremic patients, total ammonium excretion was reduced by nearly 60% and renal glutamine extraction was reduced, but ammonia production in μmol/min/100 ml GFR actually increased more than threefold and the rate of glutamine extraction by the kidneys per unit of GFR was not different from control; (2) uremia was associated with an increased renal extraction of citrulline and an increased renal release of alanine, arginine, and tyrosine; (3) although the amount of glutamine extracted from the blood in control subjects was sufficient to account

for all the ammonia produced, in uremic patients only about 35% of ammonia produced could be accounted for by the amount of glutamine extracted from arterial blood; and (4) in the uremic patients, the total amount of nitrogen released was more than twice the total amount of nitrogen extracted or taken up by the kidneys. These findings taken together were interpreted to indicate that in uremia, residual functioning renal tissue does not extract enough glutamine (or adequately use it) to account for the observed ammonia production, and perhaps half of the ammonia produced comes from precursors made available from protein and peptide degradation within the kidney, not from glutamine or other amino acids supplied to the kidney from arterial blood. Simpson [196] also found that glutamine extraction in uremic patients was reduced modestly, whereas ammonia production per nephron increased substantially. Tizianello et al. [57,219] suggested that a uremic toxin may inhibit glutaminase or glutamine transport into the mitochondrion. They point out that methylguanidine depresses ammonia production from glutamine in rat renal cortex slices and inhibits renal phosphate-independent glutaminase activity [1].

Stimulus for Ammoniagenesis
The signal stimulating renal ammoniagenesis is unclear, although not specifically related to blood pH [184,216]. The relationship between the renal handling of salt and ammoniagenesis has recently been evaluated by Halperin et al. [85]. These investigators had previously suggested that since renal glutamine metabolism and synthesis of ammonia leads to ATP production, the maximal rate of renal glutamine metabolism or ammonia formation might

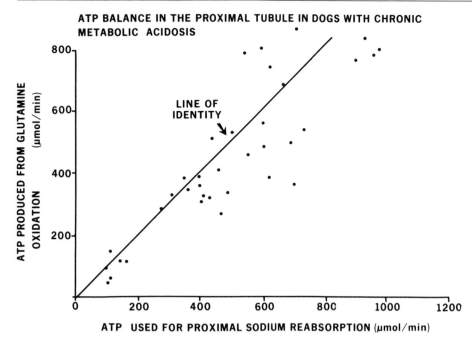

ATP BALANCE IN THE PROXIMAL TUBULE IN DOGS WITH CHRONIC METABOLIC ACIDOSIS

FIG. 27-6. *ATP balance in proximal tubules of dogs with chronic metabolic acidosis. Each point represents mean value for triplicate observations in the control period of individual dogs. ATP required for proximal sodium reabsorption is shown on the abscissa and was calculated using two assumptions: (1) 60% of sodium reabsorption occurs in the proximal convoluted tubule and (2) this segment pumps a net of 4.6 sodium ions per ATP. Ordinate shows quantity of ATP formed during glutamine oxidation. Glutamine conversion to ATP was calculated as follows. Glutamine extraction was measured by A-V difference × the renal blood flow. Alanine and aspartate outputs were assumed to be derived from glutamine and yield nine ATPs per amino acid released. Remainder of glutamine should be oxidized to CO_2 yielding 27 ATPs per glutamine. Solid line is line of identity for these two parameters. (From Halperin ML, Vinay P, Gougoux A, et al: Regulation of the maximal rate of renal ammonia genesis in the acidotic rat. Am J Physiol 248:F607, 1985, with permission.)*

be limited by the rate of ATP consumption [84]. Renal ATP production, estimated from oxygen consumption and used primarily for proximal tubular sodium reabsorption, was found to correlate closely with ammonium synthesis (Fig. 27-6). A decrease in reabsorbed sodium was associated with a proportional decrease in renal ammoniagenesis. Since the GFR and therefore sodium reabsorption is decreased in chronic renal disease, the reduced rate of ATP hydrolysis associated with reduction of renal mass could limit the maximum rate of ATP production. Thus, ATP balance and sodium reabsorption might be important overall regulators of ammoniagenesis in chronic renal failure.

This relationship between NH_4^+ produced and ATP used for sodium reabsorption is of particular interest in light of earlier data published by Steinmetz et al. [206]. Acid excretion per kidney was determined separately in patients with unilateral renal disease. Inulin clearance, and thus sodium filtered, in the diseased kidney was one-third to one-half that of the contralateral kidney. Total excretion of NH_4^+ was significantly decreased in the diseased kidney. However, when expressed per milliliter of GFR, the excretion rates of NH_4^+ by the diseased and contralateral kidney correlated very closely (Fig. 27-7).

Corticomedullary Ammonia Gradient

The ability of the kidney to concentrate ammonia in the medullary interstitium appears critical to maintaining high rates of ammonium excretion. Stern et al. [207] found in acidotic rats that both ammonium excretion and production were increased. In the control state, vasa recta ammonia, a measure of medullary content, was nearly 100-fold greater than renal vein ammonium, a measure of cortical content, both values approximately doubling during acidosis. Furthermore, net movement of ammonium into the inner medullary collecting duct was substantially increased during acidosis when (1) medullary ammonium was high and (2) ammonium production and secretion were stimulated. Infusion of mannitol in acidotic animals eliminated the rise in medullary content of ammonium, dissipated the corticomedullary gradient, and resulted in no appreciable addition of ammonium to the collecting duct.

Buerkert et al. [36] provided evidence that the accumulation and subsequent re-entrapment of medullary ammonium is impaired in chronic renal disease. These investigators induced renal insufficiency in rats by partial infarction of one kidney and subsequent contralateral nephrectomy. In the uremic animals, ammonium excretion

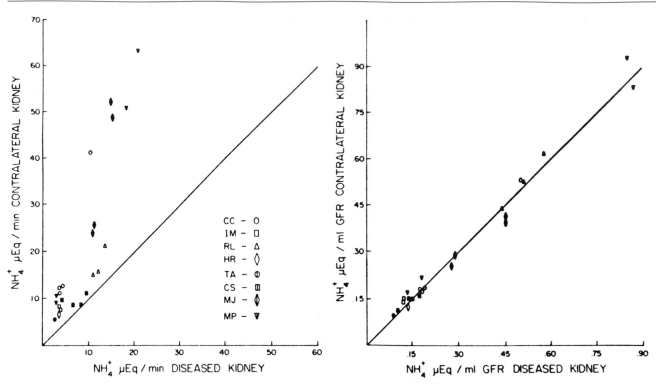

FIG. 27-7. *Comparison of ammonium excretion in the two kidneys of eight patients with unilateral renal disease. In the frame on the left total excretion rates are plotted and in the frame on the right excretion rates per unit of GFR. (From Steinmetz PR, Eisinger RP, Lowenstein J: The excretion of acid in unilateral renal disease in man. J Clin Invest 44:582, 1965, with permission.)*

decreased by about 50%, although there was a threefold increase in delivery of ammonium to the end of the proximal tubule of superficial nephrons [36]. Compared with the end of the proximal tubule, ammonium delivery to the distal tubule decreased in control animals, indicating reabsorption along the loop. While reabsorption along the loop appeared to also occur in the remnant kidney, delivery of ammonium out of the distal tubule was nearly threefold greater in the remnant kidney. Since this occurred in the face of decreased net ammonium excretion, ammonium absorption would seem to be enhanced at sites even more distal in the nephron and entry to distal luminal fluid would appear to be impaired. The increase in NH_4^+ at the bend of Henle's loop in deep nephrons was much less in these remnant kidneys (Table 27-9) than in kidneys from chronically acidotic nonuremic animals [34,35]. In remnant kidney nephrons, ammonium entry along the collecting duct was reduced, as was the papillary interstitial NH_4^+ concentration, the urinary osmolality of loop fluid, and the concentration gradient for NH_4^+ between the end proximal tubule and bend of the loop. Estimates for interstitial medullary ammonium content in the remnant kidney were less than one-half that of control. High rates of tubular flow in the loop of deep remnant nephrons may have contributed to this finding. The osmotic diuresis of the uremic state thus may contribute to the reduction in renal acid excretion by limiting the medullary accumulation of

ammonium and its transfer to the collecting duct. In any event, the intrarenal accumulation of ammonium was not normal in this model of chronic renal insufficiency.

Histologic Findings

Zalups et al. [232] studied the intercalated cells (the acid-secreting cells) of the cortical collecting tubule in a remnant kidney model. They reported an increase in the surface area of the luminal membrane and a significant reduction in the number of vesicles in the apical cytoplasm (Fig. 27-8). The basolateral membrane of the intercalated cells did not appear to be affected. Although the cell area did not change, the surface density of the luminal membrane nearly doubled, as did the boundary length of this membrane. Similar changes were not observed along the distal convoluted tubule. Although there was variation in the ultrastructure of intercalated cell types, the authors found an increase in the number of intercalated cells with abundant microplicae.

It has been suggested that amplification of the apical membrane of the intercalated cells is related to insertion of hydrogen ion pumps, which promote acidification of the tubular fluid [208]. Such changes have been previously observed in intercalated cells of medullary collecting tubules during other states of acidosis [134,135] as well as

TABLE 27-9. *Effect of acidosis and reduction of renal mass on ammonium delivery to proximal and distal tubules of superficial nephrons, bend of Henle's loop of deep nephrons, and base and tip of papillary collecting ducts in rats*

	GFR (nl/min)	Absolute NH_4^+ delivery (pmol/min)	Fractional NH_4^+ delivery (%)	Tubular NH_4^+ secretion (pmol/min)
		Superficial nephrons		
Control				
End proximal	14.7	18.4	1052	16.6
End distal	13.3	10.7	655	−9.1
Acidotic				
End proximal	10.7	21.5	1197	20.3
End distal	9.5	9.4	642	−12.2
Remnant				
End proximal	27.8	66.2	1823	62.3
End distal	28.0	29.3	941	−38.2
		Deep nephrons: bend Henle's loop		
Control	23.8	45.6	1567	40.8
Acidotic	19.4	54.6	1780	51.7
Remnant	35.9	70.2	1400	65.1
				Tubule fluid NH_4^+ concentration (nmol/L)
		Papillary collecting duct		
Control			902	105
Base			862	142
Tip				
Acidotic			1415	196
Base			1431	246
Tip				
Remnant			1323	60
Base			1335	74.6
Tip				

Data are mean.
Data from Buerkert J, Martin D, Trigg D, et al: Effect of reduced renal mass on ammonium handling and net acid formation by the superficial and juxtamedullary nephron of the rat. *J Clin Invest* 71:1661, 1983 and Buerkert J, Martin D, Trigg D, et al: Ammonium handling by superficial and juxtamedullary nephrons in the rat. *J Clin Invest* 70:1, 1982.

after chronic dietary potassium depletion [209]. These histologic changes may be related to the increase in single nephron acid secretion in states of chronic renal insufficiency [36,232].

Hyperchloremic Metabolic Acidosis

Although most patients with advanced renal disease have normochloremic metabolic acidosis, patients with moderate renal failure occasionally develop hyperchloremic acidosis [6,46,48,51,56,156, 229]. This state may result from volume depletion, aldosterone deficiency, or from a distal nephron acidification defect, and may be associated with hyperkalemia despite only modest reduction in renal function [6,10,46,48,51,178,187]. Hyperchloremic renal acidosis associated with interstitial nephropathy occurs occasionally in association with proximal tubular dysfunction [45,46]. Fanconi syndrome or type II renal tubular acidosis may develop along with progressive renal disease from

heavy metal exposure (lead) or genetic defects such as cystinosis [46,48].

Hyperchloremic acidosis may occur with moderate renal failure of any etiology; it is thought to be most common in patients with tubulointerstitial forms of nephropathy, whereas a high anion gap, normochloremic acidosis is thought more likely in glomerular or vascular diseases. However, recent studies have not confirmed this correlation [61,227,229]. The acidosis of tubulointerstitial nephropathy may be more severe than in patients with glomerular disease and comparable degrees of renal insufficiency [41,118].

Hyperchloremic metabolic acidosis is not uncommon in adult patients with mild renal insufficiency and hyperkalemia [51] who have hyporeninemic hypoaldosteronism, probably the result of damage to the juxtaglomerular apparatus. This form of hyperchloremic metabolic acidosis may be the result of extensive damage to the renal medulla with salt wasting and a significant defect in ammonia production or secretion, related perhaps to the inhibitory ef-

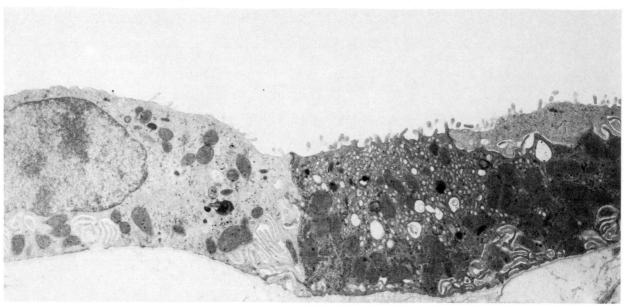

A

FIG. 27-8. A. *Principal cell (PC) and intercalated cell (IC) of an initial cortical collecting tubule from a sham operated rat (× 8400). B. Principal cell (PC) and intercalated cell (IC) of an initial cortical collecting tubule from a 75% nephrectomized rat. Note that the basolateral membrane of the principal cell is considerably greater than that of the principal cell in A. The size of the cell is also greater. The luminal membrane of the intercalated cell is substantially greater than that of the intercalated cell in A, but the number of vesicles in the apical cytoplasm is markedly reduced (× 8400). (From Zalups RK, Stanton BA, Wade JB, et al: Structural adaptation in initial collecting tubule following reduction in renal mass. Kidney Int 27:636, 1985, with permission.)*

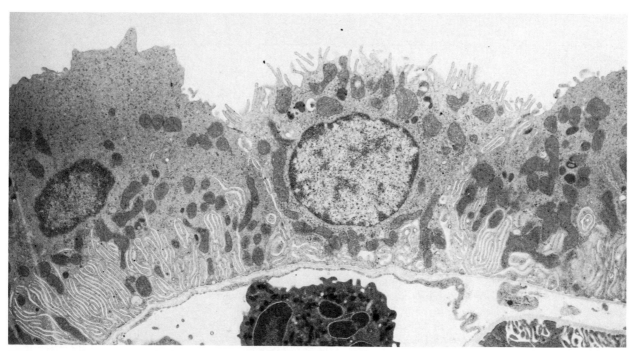

B

fect that hyperkalemia may have on ammoniagenesis [217].

A potassium-secreting defect as well as sodium wasting may be present [46,48,51]. Tissue damage may be direct, such as in methicillin-induced interstitital nephritis [47] or, more commonly, mediated by damage to the juxtaglomerular apparatus with defective release of renin leading to hyporeninemic hypoaldosteronism [46,48,51,156]. The characteristic hyperkalemic (type IV) renal tubular acidosis is associated with a variety of illnesses, such as diabetes [51], sickle cell disease [52], obstructive uropathy [14], and polycystic kidney disease [67] (Chap. 81). The salt loss may lead to volume contraction, which, in the absence of the provision of bicarbonate, leads to enhanced reabsorption of sodium chloride [6,48,56,175]. Since the normal ratio of plasma Na^+ to Cl^- is approximately 1.4:1, if the extracellular fluid volume is expanded with NaCl on a 1:1 basis, hyperchloremia will develop. It also may indicate the presence of aldosterone deficiency or a defect in distal acidification. Its importance is that if it represents volume contraction in a patient with moderate renal failure, the patient will continue to lose sodium with unreabsorbed anions and remain volume contracted if salt restricted, and the hyperchloremia will worsen. Although a high anion gap metabolic acidosis would be expected in end-stage renal disease patients who accumulate sulfate and phosphate, dialysis patients, in fact, were found to have a high anion gap acidosis only about 30% of the time [49]. In these studies, a mixed high anion gap and hyperchloremic or relatively pure hyperchloremic acidosis occurred 46% and 24% of the time, respectively. After standard acetate dialysis, the pattern shifted toward a pure hyperchloremic acidosis (48%) or mixed acidosis (33%), with a relatively pure high anion gap acidosis observed only 19% of the time. Acetate from the dialysate is converted to bicarbonate, but the net increase in serum bicarbonate will depend on the predialysis bicarbonate level. The greater likelihood of a hyperchloremic or mixed acidosis following dialysis was thought to reflect the removal of unmeasured anions at a faster rate than the bicarbonate deficit could be corrected [49].

Extrarenal Buffering

Extracellular bicarbonate provides approximately half the buffer response to an acid load, the rest of the buffering occurring within cells and bone [2,7,20,65,71,127,186, 214]. In adult uremic subjects, daily net acid excretion is about 10 to 20 mEq less than the daily endogenous acid production [80], and there is a close inverse correlation between calcium balance and hydrogen balance [103, 121,122], suggesting buffering of retained hydrogen ions by alkaline salts of bone. Bone provides a large potential source for buffering in the form of carbonate and phosphate salts of calcium and sodium, perhaps as much as 35,000 to 50,000 mEq of carbonate being available in the adult [120,121,128]. Direct analysis has revealed a loss of bone carbonate during experimental metabolic acidosis [37,155].

It is noteworthy that acidosis can cause bone resorption independent of changes in parathyroid hormone or calci-

tonin [56]. Acidosis causes calcium efflux from cells, and bone mobilization seems to depend primarily on hydrogen ion concentration [17,39,54,166]. The titration of alkaline bone salts appears to contribute to a major degree to the renal osteodystrophy that complicates renal failure [124].

Parathyroid Hormone

PTH has several effects that could alter acid–base homeostasis: PTH decreases proximal tubular reabsorption of bicarbonate and suppresses secretion of H^+ [145]. However, a sustained increase in PTH secretion, such as occurs in primary hyperparathyroidism, seems to have little effect on acid–base equilibrium [96]. Variations in PTH levels probably do not exert a major influence on acid–base equilib-

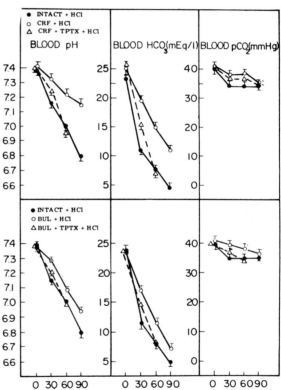

FIG. 27-9. *Upper panel shows blood pH, bicarbonate, and P_{CO_2} in rats with chronic renal failure (CRF) with (open circles) and without (open triangles) parathyroid glands. Data of control rats shown for comparison are represented by filled circles. Rats with CRF and parathyroid glands have significantly higher blood pH and bicarbonate than controls and rats with CRF who have been thyroparathyroidectomized. Lower panel displays similar data in rats with bilateral ureteral ligation in the presence (open circles) and absence (open triangles) of parathyroid glands. Blood pH and bicarbonate were significantly higher in rats with bilateral ureteral ligation and parathyroid glands than in controls and rats with bilateral ureteral ligation who had also been thyroparathyroidectomized. (From Arruda JAL, Alla V, Rubenstein H, et al: Parathyroid hormone and extrarenal acid buffering. Am J Physiol 239:F533, 1980, with permission.)*

TABLE 27-10. *Extrarenal buffering capacity in experimental conditions associated with altered parathyroid hormone activity*

Maneuver	Mechanism of action	Effect on extrarenal buffering
Thyroparathyroidectomy	Removed PTH	Decreases [7,61,105]
Phosphate depletion	↓ PTH, ↑ bone resorption [16]	Enhances [8,56]
Colchicine	↑ PTH release [40,81]	Enhances
Diphosphonates	Inhibit bone resorption [198]	No change, but mortality increases
Ethylenediaminetetra-acetic acid	↓ plasma calcium ↑ PTH release [40]	Enhances
Acetazolamide	Inhibits carbonic anhydrase: inhibits PTH-mediated bone resorption [125,201,202]	Decreases
Vasopressin	↑ adenylate cyclase; PTH-like effect in high doses [13,99,121]	Enhances
Vitamin D	Mobilizes bone buffer [181]	Enhances
Calcitonin	Inhibits bone resorption [147]	Decreases

From Sabatini S: The acidosis of chronic renal failure. *Med Clin North Am* 67:845, 1983, with permission.

rium in normal subjects, but in patients with uremic acidosis, PTH appears to be of major importance, primarily because of the osteoclastic stimulatory effect of this hormone [7,154].

Fraley and Adler [65] showed that PTH was needed to mediate the extrarenal buffering of hydrogen ion following acute acid loads. Rats and dogs that had been thyroparathyroidectomized (TPTX) and given an acute acid load all died; intact, animals given the same acid load survived. PTH administration restored the buffering capacity of the TPTX animals to that of the controls.

Arruda et al. [7] studied rats with acute or chronic renal failure; half of the animals underwent TPTX two hours before acid infusion (Fig. 27-9). Acidotic animals were first treated with sodium bicarbonate to normalize plasma HCO_3^- and serum pH and then were infused with HCl. Both intact animals and TPTX animals in acute renal failure developed profound acidosis, less severe in those with intact parathyroid glands. Similar results were reported in animals with chronic renal failure. In bilaterally nephrectomized rats, severe acidosis was associated with higher mortality when the parathyroid glands were removed; the acidosis could be substantially reduced by administering PTH [7,65]. Moreover, maneuvers designed to block the action of PTH on bone (such as acetazolamide to block carbonic anhydrase or calcitonin to inhibit bone resorption) decreased the extrarenal buffering capacity in acidosis (Table 27-10), whereas maneuvers designed to increase the release or activity of PTH or bone buffers (such as ethylenediaminetetra-acetic acid or colchicine) enhanced the extrarenal buffering capacity [175].

Secondary hyperparathyroidism in chronic renal disease appears to minimize changes in systemic pH, and abnormalities in bone histology can be identified relatively early in renal insufficiency [137]. It is known that patients with chronic renal failure demonstrate positive hydrogen balance for a prolonged period of time before developing overt acidosis [87,121] and that uremic acidosis is not progressive. Therefore, it is of interest that hyperparathyroidism with the attendant elevated levels of circulating PTH also occurs long before alterations are appreciated in serum calcium and phosphorus and before there are clinically detectable bone abnormalities [199]. The increased PTH may not only help stabilize the acidosis of well-advanced renal disease but also may help mask or minimize the acidosis early in the course of the illness.

Therapy

Although the acidosis of chronic renal failure tends to be moderate, treatment should be instituted and follow-up should be sufficient to ensure stable and reasonably normal serum bicarbonate levels. Persistent acidosis contributes to growth failure (Chap. 25) as well as to the generation of renal osteodystrophy (Chap. 28). Table 27-11 lists several clinical systemic derangements associated with acidosis.

Not only do patients feel better when acidosis is treated, but there is considerably more leeway in the overall management if serum bicarbonate levels are high enough so that extrarenal complications (e.g., sepsis or diarrhea) are less likely to result in severe acidosis. Therapy with alkali may improve nitrogen balance [21,130,153] and offset the hypercalciuric effect of acidosis [43,138].

Standard therapy for acidosis is provision of sodium bicarbonate or sodium citrate. Caution should be used with patients who are edematous or have hypertension; in this case sodium bicarbonate appears to be better tolerated [99]. In general, however, if sodium intake is high, supplementation with $NaHCO_3$ should be accompanied by restriction of NaCl to maintain sodium balance and minimize the effects of sodium overload [56,98].

Often 1 or 2 mEq/kg/d of bicarbonate is sufficient to maintain serum bicarbonate near normal, although dosages as high as 3 to 6 mEq/kg/d may be needed.

Hyperkalemia probably contributes to the acidosis of chronic renal disease and may develop in some patients with only moderate renal failure. The metabolic acidosis may be ameliorated by correcting hyperkalemia. Mineralocorticoids and furosemide augment the excretion of both

Table 27-11. *Clinical complications of metabolic acidosis*

System or function	Mechanism and/or manifestation
Pulmonary	Central stimulation: hyperventilation, especially depth rather than rate [60,91]
CNS	Cerebral vasodilation: headache, confusion, disorientation, stupor, coma [59,60]
GI	Nausea, anorexia, vomiting, diarrhea [78]
Cardiac	Potentiates ventricular fibrillation (decreases threshold) [31,65,103,188]. Increases risk for bradyarrhythmias [57]
Vascular	Arteriolar-vasodilation: if severe acidosis, decreased catecholamine responsiveness, and shock may occur [38,57]
	Venous-constriction: increases central blood volume with pulmonary edema [58,72,80,173]
Metabolic	
Oxygen	Acute acidosis: O_2 dissociation curve shifts to right and increases O_2 release from hemoglobin [18,171]
	Chronic acidosis: more than 6–8 hours, decreases RBC [2,3] diphosphoglycerate and shifts curve back [126]
Glucose	Suppresses glycolysis, interferes with action of insulin [149]
Potassium	Cellular ion shift: hyperkalemia with an appropriate increase of serum (K^+) of 0.6 mEq/l/0.1 unit drop in pH. Not seen with organic metabolic acidosis [3,36]
Calcium	Reduced calcium reabsorption and increased calcium excretion. Loss of bone carbonate [35,104–106]
Nitrogen	Adverse effect on nitrogen balance in uremia; bicarbonate therapy improves nitrogen balance and induces decrease in blood and urine urea nitrogen [133]

Data from Harrington JT, Cohen JJ: Metabolic acidosis, in Cohen JJ, Kassirer JP (eds): *Metabolic Acidosis.* Boston, Little, Brown, 1982, p 121; and Emmett M, Seldin DW: Clinical syndromes of metabolic acidosis and metabolic alkalosis. *In* Seldin DW, Giebisch G (eds): *The Kidney: Physiology and Pathophysiology.* New York, Raven Press, 1985, p 1567.

renal hydrogen and potassium [188,189,215], and cation exchange resins such as sodium polystyrene sulfonate bind potassium, hydrogen, ammonium, and calcium [223]. Moreover, cation exchange resins appear to decrease net acid production by chelating calcium and freeing bicarbonate and other organic anions to be absorbed in the intestine [223].

Furosemide may reduce acidosis when used alone, and particularly when used in combination with mineralocorticoid (fludrocortisone) in patients with and without hypoaldosteronism [189]. Hyperkalemia per se contributes significantly to the acidosis of chronic renal insufficiency [136]. Extrarenal and renal mechanisms both appear to contribute to the acidosis.

References

1. Acquarone N, Tizianello A, DeFerrari G, et al: Inibizione della glutaminasi. Fosfato-indipendente da parte della metilguanidina e sue ripercussioni sull'ammoniogenesi renale. *Minerva Nephrologica* 24:341, 1977.
2. Adler S, Roy A, Relman AS: Intracellular acid-base regulation. 1. The response of muscle cells to changes in CO_2 tension or extracellular bicarbonate concentration. *J Clin Invest* 44:8, 1965.
3. Adrogue HJ, Madias NE: Changes in plasma potassium concentration during acute acid-base disturbances. *Am J Med* 71:456, 1981.
4. Aickin CC, Thomas RC: Micro-electrode measurement of the intracellular pH and buffering power of mouse soleus muscle fibres. *J Physiol (Lond)* 267:791, 1977.
5. Aronson PS: Mechanisms of active H^+ secretion in the proximal tubule. *Am J Physiol* 245:F647, 1983.
6. Arruda JAL: Acidosis of renal failure. *Semin Nephrol* 1:275, 1981.
7. Arruda JAL, Alla V, Rubenstein H, et al: Parathyroid hormone and extrarenal acid buffering. *Am J Physiol* 239:F533, 1980.
8. Arruda JAL, Alla V, Rubenstein H, et al: Metabolic and hormonal factors influencing extrarenal buffering of an acute acid load. *Miner Electrolyte Metab* 8:36, 1982.
9. Arruda JAL, Carrasquillo T, Cubria A, et al: Bicarbonate reabsorption in chronic renal failure. *Kidney Int* 9:481, 1976.
10. Arruda JAL, Kurtzman NA: Mechanisms and classification of deranged distal acidification defects. *Am J Physiol* 239:F515, 1980.
11. Arruda JAL, Nascimento L, Arevalo G, et al: Bicarbonate reabsorption in chronic renal failure studies in man and the rat. *Pflugers Arch* 376:193, 1978.
12. Arruda JAL, Nascimento L, Westenfelder C, et al: Effect of parathyroid hormone on urinary acidification. *Am J Physiol* 232:F429, 1977.
13. Arruda JAL, Stipanuk S, Walter R, et al: Effect of vasopressin administration on sodium excretion and plasma phosphate concentration. *Proc Soc Exp Biol Med* 155:308, 1977.
14. Batlle DC, Arruda JAL, Kurtzman NA: Hyperkalemic distal renal tubular acidosis associated with obstructive uropathy. *N Engl J Med* 304:373, 1981.
15. Batlle DC, Kurtzman NA: Renal regulation of acid-base homeostasis: Integrated response. *In* Seldin DW, Giebisch G (ed): *The Kidney: Physiology and Pathophysiology.* New York, Raven Press, 1985, chap 67, p 1539.
16. Baylink D, Wergedal J, Stauffer M: Formation, mineralization, and resorption of bone in hypophosphatemic rats. *J Clin Invest* 50:2519, 1971.
17. Beck N, Webster SK: Effects of acute metabolic acidosis on parathyroid hormone action and calcium mobilization. *Am J Physiol* 230:127, 1976.
18. Bellingham AJ, Detter JC, Lenfant C: Regulatory mechanisms of hemoglobin oxygen affinity in acidosis and alkalosis. *J Clin Invest* 50:700, 1971.

19. Berry CA, Warnock DG: Acidification in the in vitro perfused tubule. *Kidney Int* 22:507, 1982.

20. Bettice JA, Gamble JL Jr: Skeletal buffering of acute metabolic acidosis. *Am J Physiol* 229:1618, 1975.

21. Blom Van Assendelft PM, Dorhout-Mees EJ: Urea metabolism in patients with chronic renal failure: Influence of sodium bicarbonate or sodium chloride administration. *Metabolism* 19:1053, 1970.

22. Boron WF: Intracellular pH transients in giant barnacle muscle fibers. *Am J Physiol* 233:C61, 1977.

23. Boron WF, Boulpaep EL: Intracellular pH regulation in the renal proximal tubule of the salamander: Na-H exchange. *J Gen Physiol* 81:29, 1983.

24. Boron WF, Boulpaep EL: Intracellular pH regulation in the renal proximal tubule of the salamander: Basolateral HCO_3^- transport. *J Gen Physiol* 81:53, 1983.

25. Boron WF, DeWeer P: Intracellular pH transients in squid giant axons caused by CO_2, NH_3 and metabolic inhibitors. *J Gen Physiol* 67:91, 1976.

26. Bricker NS, Fine LG: The renal response to progressive nephron loss. *In* Brenner B, Rector FC (eds): *The Kidney.* Vol 2. Philadelphia, WB Saunders, 1981, p 1056.

27. Bricker NS, Morrin PAF, Kime SW: The pathological physiology of chronic Bright's disease. An exposition of the "intact nephron hypothesis." *Am J Med* 28:77, 1960.

28. Briggs AP: The acidosis of nephritis. *Arch Intern Med* 49:56, 1932.

29. Briggs AP, Findley T: Normal acid-base regulations and derangements in fixed anion acidosis. *Metabolism* 16:697, 1967.

30. Briggs AP, Waugh WH, Harms WS, et al: Pathogenesis of uremic acidosis as indicated by urinary acidification on a controlled diet. *Metabolism* 10:749, 1961.

31. Brooks DK, Feldman SA: Metabolic acidosis. *Anaesthesia* 17:161, 1962.

32. Brown D, Hirsch S, Gluck S: Localization of a proton pumping ATPase in rat kidney. *J Clin Invest* 82:2114, 1988.

33. Brown D, Kumpulainen T, Roth J, et al: Immunohistochemical localization of carbonic anhydrase in postnatal and adult rat kidney. *Am J Physiol* (Renal Fluid Electrolyte Physiol 14) 245:F110, 1983.

34. Buerkert J, Martin D, Trigg D: Ammonium handling by superficial and juxtamedullary nephrons in the rat. *J Clin Invest* 70:1, 1982.

35. Buerkert J, Martin D, Trigg D: Segmental analysis of the renal tubule in buffer production and net acid formation. *Am J Physiol* 244:F442, 1983.

36. Buerkert J, Martin D, Trigg D, et al: Effect of reduced renal mass on ammonium handling and net acid formation by superficial and juxtamedullary nephron of the rat. *J Clin Invest* 71:1661, 1983.

37. Burnell JM, Teubner E: Changes in bone sodium and carbonate in metabolic acidosis and alkalosis in the dog. *J Clin Invest* 50:327, 1971.

38. Burnell JM, Villamil MF, Myeno BT, et al: The effect in humans of extracellular pH change on the relationship between serum potassium concentration and intracellular potassium. *J Clin Invest* 35:935, 1956.

39. Bushinsky DA, Krieger NS, Geisser DI, et al: Effects of pH on bone calcium and proton fluxes in vitro. *Am J Physiol* 245:F204, 1983.

40. Bygdeman S: Vascular reactivity in cats during induced changes in acid-base balance of the blood. *Acta Physiol Scand* [Suppl]221:1, 1963.

41. Carroll HJ, Farber SJ: Hyperkalemia and hyperchloremic acidosis in chronic pyelonephritis. *Metabolism* 13:808, 1964.

42. Chanard J, Black R, Purkerson M, et al: Effects of colchicine and vinblastine on parathyroid hormone secretion in the rat. *Endocrinology* 101:1792, 1977.

43. Cochran M, Bulusu L, Horsman A, et al: Hypocalcemia and bone disease in renal failure. *Nephron* 10:113, 1973.

44. Cochran M, Nordin BEC: The causes of hypocalcemia in chronic renal failure. *Clin Sci* 40:305, 1971.

45. Cogan MG: Disorders of proximal nephron function. *Am J Med* 72:275, 1982.

46. Cogan MG: Classification and patterns of renal dysfunction. *In* Cotran RS, Brenner BM, Stein JH (eds): *Tubulo-interstitial Nephropathies.* New York, Churchill-Livingstone, 1983, p 35.

47. Cogan MG, Arieff A: 1. Sodium wasting, acidosis and hyperkalemia induced by methicillin interstitial nephritis. Evidence for selective distal tubular dysfunction. *Am J Med* 64:500, 1978.

48. Cogan MG, Rector FC Jr, Seldin DW: Acid-base disorders. *In* Brenner BM, Rector FC Jr (eds): *The Kidney,* 2nd ed. Philadelphia, WB Saunders, 1981, chap 27, p 841.

49. Cohen E, Liu K, Batlle DC: Patterns of metabolic acidosis in patients with chronic renal failure: Impact of hemodialysis. *Int J Artif Organs* 11:440, 1988.

50. Davies HEF, Wrong O: Acidity of urine and excretion of ammonium in renal disease. *Lancet* 2:625, 1957.

51. DeFronzo RA: Nephrology forum: Hyperkalemia and hyporeninemic hypoaldosteronism. *Kidney Int* 17:118, 1980.

52. DeFronzo RA, Taufield PA, Black H, et al: Impaired renal tubular potassium secretion in sickle cell disease. *Ann Intern Med* 90:310, 1979.

53. Diaz-Buxo JA, Ott CE, Cuche JL, et al: Effects of extracellular fluid volume contraction and expansion on the bicarbonaturia of parathyroid hormone. *Kidney Int* 8:105, 1975.

54. Dominquez JH, Raisz LG: Effects of changing hydrogen ion, carbonic acid and bicarbonate concentrations on bone reabsorption in vitro. *Calcif Tissue Int* 29:7, 1979.

55. Dorhout-Mees EJ, Machado M, Slatopolsky E, et al: The functional adaptation of the diseased kidney. III. Ammonium excretion. *J Clin Invest* 45:289, 1966.

56. Dubose TD Jr: Acid-base physiology in uremia. *Artif Organs* 6:363, 1982.

57. Editorial. Renal failure, acidosis and glutamine metabolism in man. *Nutr Rev* 37:224, 1979.

58. Elkington JR: Hydrogen ion turnover in health and in renal diseae. *Ann Intern Med* 57:660, 1962.

59. Emmett M, Goldfarb S, Agus ZS, et al: The pathophysiology of acid-base changes in chronically phosphate depleted rats. Bone-kidney interactions. *J Clin Invest* 59:291, 1977.

60. Emmett M, Seldin DW: Clinical syndromes of metabolic acidosis and metabolic alkalosis. *In* Seldin DW, Giebisch G (eds): *The Kidney: Physiology and Pathophysiology.* New York, Raven Press, 1985, p 1567.

61. Enia G, Catalano C, Zoccali C, et al: Hyperchloremia: A nonspecific finding in chronic renal failure. *Nephron* 41:189, 1985.

62. Enson Y, Harvey RM, Lewis ML, et al: Hemodynamic effects of metabolic acidosis in cholera: Implications for fluid repletion in severe burns. *Ann NY Acad Sci* 150:577, 1968.

63. Fencl V, Miller TB, Pappenheimer JR: Studies on the respiratory response to disturbances of acid-base balance, with deductions concerning the ionic composition of cerebral interstitial fluid. *Am J Physiol* 210:459, 1966.

64. Fencl V, Vale JR, Broch JA: Respiration and cerebral blood flow in metabolic acidosis and alkalosis in humans. *J Appl Physiol* 27:67, 1969.

65. Fraley DS, Adler S: An extrarenal role for parathyroid hor-

mone in the disposal of acute acid loads in rats and dogs. *J Clin Invest* 63:985, 1979.

66. Gamble JL, Blackfan KD, Hamilton B: A study of the diuretic action of acid producing salts. *J Clin Invest* 1:359, 1925.

67. Gardner KD Jr: Medullary cystic diseases. The nephron-ophthisis-cystic renal medulla complex and medullary sponge kidney. *In* Earley LE, Gottschalk CW (eds): *Strauss and Welt's Disease of the Kidney*, 3rd ed. Boston, Little, Brown, 1979, p 1147.

68. Garvin JL, Burg MB, Knepper MA: Ammonia replaces potassium in supporting sodium transport by the Na-K-ATPase of renal proximal straight tubules. *Am J Physiol* 249:F785, 1985.

69. Garvin JL, Burg MB, Knepper MA: NH_3 and NH_4^+ transport by rabbit renal proximal straight tubules. *Am J Physiol* (Renal Fluid Electrolyte Physiol 21) 252:F232, 1987.

70. Garvin JL, Knepper MA: Bicarbonate and ammonia transport in isolated perfused rat proximal straight tubules. *Am J Physiol* (Renal Fluid Electrolyte Physiol 22) 253:F277, 1987.

71. Gennari FJ, Cohen JJ, Kassirer JP: Determinants of plasma bicarbonate concentration and hydrogen ion balance. *In* Cohen JJ, Kassirer JP (eds): *Acid Base*, 1st ed. Boston, Little, Brown, 1982, p 55.

72. Gerst PH, Fleming WH, Malm JR: Increased susceptibility of the heart to ventricular fibrillation during metabolic acidosis. *Circ Res* 19:63, 1966.

73. Goldstein L, Claiborne JB, Evans DE: Ammonia excretion by the gills of two marine teleost fish: The importance of NH_4^+ permeance. *J Exp Zool* 219:395, 1982.

74. Gonick HC, Kleeman CR, Rubini ME, et al: Functional impairment in chronic renal disease. II. Studies of acid excretion. *Nephron* 6:28, 1969.

75. Good DW: Adaptation of HCO_3^- and NH_4^+ transport in rat MTAL: Effects of chronic metabolic acidosis and Na^+ intake. *Am J Physiol* (Renal Fluid Electrolyte Physiol 27) 258:F1345, 1990.

76. Good DW, Burg MB: Ammonia production by individual segments of the rat nephron. *J Clin Invest* 73:602, 1984.

77. Good DW, Dubose TD Jr: Ammonia transport by early and late proximal convoluted tubules of the rat. *J Clin Invest* 79:684, 1987.

78. Good DW, Knepper MA: Ammonia transport in the mammalian kidney. *Am J Physiol* 248:F459, 1985.

79. Good DW, Knepper MA, Burg MB: Ammonia and bicarbonate transport by thick ascending limb of rat kidney. *Am J Physiol* 247:F35, 1984.

80. Goodman AD, Lemann J Jr, Lennon EJ, et al: Production, excretion and net balance of fixed acid in patients with renal acidosis. *J Clin Invest* 44:495, 1965.

81. Greenough WB III, Hirschhorn N, Gordon RS Jr, et al: Pulmonary oedema associated with acidosis in patients with cholera. *Trop Geogr Med* 28:86, 1976.

82. Hall PW: Factors limiting hydrogen ion excretion in renal disease. *J Lab Clin Med* 58:823, 1961.

83. Halperin ML, Jungas RL: Metabolic production and renal disposal of hydrogen ions. *Kidney Int* 24:709, 1983.

84. Halperin ML, Jungas RL, Pickette C, et al: A quantitative analysis of renal ammoniagenesis and energy balance: A theoretical approach. *Can J Physiol Pharmacol* 60:1431, 1982.

85. Halperin ML, Vinay P, Gougoux A, et al: Regulation of the maximal rate of renal ammoniagenesis in the acidotic dog. *Am J Physiol* 248:F607, 1985.

86. Hamm LL, Trigg D, Martin D, et al: Transport of ammonia

in the rabbit cortical collecting tubule. *J Clin Invest* 75:478, 1985.

87. Harrington JT, Cohen JJ: Metabolic acidosis. *In* Cohen JJ, Kassirer JP (eds): *Metabolic Acidosis*. Boston, Little, Brown, 1982, p 121.

88. Harrington JT, Lemann JR Jr: The metabolic production and disposal of acid and alkali. *Med Clin North Am* 54:1543, 1970.

89. Harvey RM, Enson Y, Lewis ML, et al: Hemodynamic effects of dehydration and metabolic acidosis in Asiatic cholera. *Trans Assoc Am Physicians* 79:177, 1966.

90. Heath DA, Palmer JS, Aurbach GD: The hypocalcemic action of colchine. *Endocrinology* 90:1589, 1972.

91. Henderson LJ: A critical study of the process of acid excretion. *J Biol Chem* 9:403, 1911.

92. Henderson LJ, Palmer WW: On the several factors of acid excretion. *J Biol Chem* 17:305, 1914.

93. Henderson LJ, Palmer WW: On the several factors of acid excretion in nephritis. *J Biol Chem* 21:37, 1915.

94. Hille B: The permeability of the sodium channel to organic cations in myelinated nerve. *J Gen Physiol* 58:599, 1971.

95. Hille B: Potassium channels in myelinated nerve. Selective permeability to small cations. *J Gen Physiol* 61:669, 1973.

96. Hulter HN, Peterson JC: Acid-base homeostasis during chronic PTH excess in humans. *Kidney Int* 28:187, 1985.

97. Hunt JN: The influence of dietary sulphur on the urinary output of acid in man. *Clin Sci* 15:119, 1956.

98. Husted FC, Nolph KD: $NaHCO_3$ and NaCl tolerance in chronic renal failure 11. *Clin Nephrol* 7:21, 1977.

99. Husted FC, Nolph KD, Maher JF: $NaHCO_3$ and NaCl tolerance in chronic renal failure. *J Clin Invest* 56:414, 1975.

100. Jaeger P, Karlmark B, Giebisch G: Ammonium transport in rat cortical tubule: Relationship to potassium metabolism. *Am J Physiol* 245:F593, 1983.

101. Kassirer JP: Historical perspective. *In* Cohen JJ, Kassirer JP (eds): *Acid-Base*, 1st ed. Boston, Little, Brown, 1982, p 449.

102. Kety SS, Polis BD, Nadler CS, et al: The blood flow and oxygen consumption of the human brain in diabetic acidosis and coma. *J Clin Invest* 27:500, 1948.

103. Kildeberg P, Engel K, Winters RW: Balance of net acid in growing infants. *Acta Paediatr Scand* 58:321, 1969.

104. Kinsella JL, Aronson PS: Interaction of NH_4^+ and Li^+ with the renal microvillus membrane Na^+-H^+ exchanger. *Am J Physiol* 241:C220, 1981.

105. Kleiner D: The transport of NH_3 and NH_4^+ across biological membranes. *Biochim Biophys Acta* 639:41, 1981.

106. Knepper MA, Good DW, Burg MB: Ammonia and bicarbonate transport by rat cortical collecting ducts perfused in vitro. *Am J Physiol* (Renal Fluid Electrolyte Physiol 18) 249:F870, 1985.

107. Knepper MA, Good DW, Burg MB: Mechanism of ammonia secretion by cortical collecting ducts of rabbits. *Am J Physiol* (Renal Fluid Electrolyte Physiol 16) 247:F729, 1984.

108. Koeppen BM, Helman SI: Acidification of luminal fluid by the rabbit cortical collecting tubule perfused in vitro. *Am J Physiol* 242:F521, 1982.

109. Koeppen BM, Steinmetz PR: Basic mechanisms of urinary acidification. *Med Clin North Am* 67:753, 1983.

110. Kunau RT Jr, Walker KA: Distal tubular acidification in the remnant kidney. *Am J Physiol* (Renal Fluid Electrolyte Physiol 27) 258:F69, 1990.

111. Kurtz I, Balaban R: Metabolic evidence for active ammonium uptake by Na^+-K^+-ATPase in proximal kidney tubule cells (abstr). *Biophys J* 47:152a, 1985.

112. Kurtz I, Balaban R: Ammonium as a substrate for Na^+-K^+-

ATPase in rabbit proximal tubules. *Am J Physiol* (Renal Fluid Electrolyte Physiol 19) 250:F497, 1986.

113. Kurtz I, Star R, Balaban RS, et al: Spontaneous luminal disequilibrium pH in S3 proximal tubules: Role in ammonia and bicarbonate transport. *J Clin Invest* 78:989, 1986.

114. Kurtzman NA: Regulation of renal bicarbonate reabsorption by extracellular volume. *J Clin Invest* 49:586, 1970.

115. Kurtzman NA, Rogers PW, Boonjarern S, et al: Effect of infusion of pharmacologic amounts of vasopressin on renal electrolyte excretion. *Am J Physiol* 228:890, 1975.

116. Landon EJ, Norris JL: Sodium and potassium dependent adenosine triphosphatase activity in a rat-kidney endoplasmic reticulum fraction. *Biochim Biophys Acta* 71:266, 1963.

117. Laski ME, Kurtzman NA: Characterization of acidification in the cortical and medullary collecting tubule of the rabbit. *J Clin Invest* 72:2050, 1983.

118. Lathem W: Hyperchloremic acidosis in chronic pyelonephritis. *N Engl J Med* 258:1031, 1958.

119. Ledingham IM, Norman JN: Acid-base studies in experimental circulatory arrest. *Lancet* 2:967, 1962.

120. Lemann J Jr, Lennon EJ: Role of diet, gastrointestinal tract and bone in acid base homeostasis. *Kidney Int* 1:275, 1972.

121. Lemann J Jr, Litzow JR, Lennon EJ: The effects of chronic acid loads in normal man: Further evidence for the participation of bone mineral in the defense against chronic metabolic acidosis. *J Clin Invest* 45:1608, 1966.

122. Lemann J Jr, Litzow JR, Lennon EJ: Studies of the mechanism by which chronic metabolic acidosis augments urinary calcium excretion in man. *J Clin Invest* 46:1318, 1967.

123. Lemann J Jr, Relman AS: The relation of sulfur metabolism to acid-base balance and electrolyte excretion: The effects of DL-methionine in normal man. *J Clin Invest* 38:2215, 1959.

124. Lennon EJ: Metabolic acidosis. A factor in the pathogenesis of azotemic osteodystrophy? *Arch Intern Med* 124:557, 1969.

125. Lennon EJ, Lemann J Jr, Litzow JR: The effects of diet and stool composition on the net external acid balance of normal subject. *J Clin Invest* 45:1601, 1966.

126. Lennon EJ, Lemann J Jr, Relman AS: The effect of phosphoproteins on acid balance in normal subjects. *J Clin Invest* 41:637, 1962.

127. Levitt MF, Turner LB, Sweet AY, et al: The response of bone, connective tissue and muscle to acute acidosis. *J Clin Invest* 35:98, 1956.

128. Litzow JR, Lemann J Jr, Lennon EJ: The effect of treatment of acidosis on calcium balance in patients with chronic azotemic renal disease. *J Clin Invest* 46:280, 1967.

129. Lubowitz M, Purkerson ML, Rolf DB, et al: Effect of nephron loss on proximal tubular bicarbonate reabsorption in the rat. *Am J Physiol* 220:457, 1971.

130. Lyon DM, Dunlop DM, Stewart CP: The alkaline treatment of chronic nephritis. *Lancet* 2:1009, 1931.

131. Maclean AJ, Hayslett JP: Adaptive change in ammonia excretion in renal insufficiency. *Kidney Int* 17:595, 1980.

132. Maddox DA, Horn JF, Famiano FC, et al: Load dependence of proximal tubular fluid and bicarbonate reabsorption in the remnant kidney of the Munich-Wister rat. *J Clin Invest* 77:1639, 1986.

133. Madsen KM, Clapp WL, Verlander JW: Structure and function of the inner medullary collecting duct. *Kidney Int* 34:441, 1988.

134. Madsen K, Tisher CC: Cellular response to acute respiratory acidosis in rat medullary collecting duct. *Am J Physiol* 245:F670, 1983.

135. Madsen K, Tisher CC: Response of intercalated cells of rat

in the outer medulla collecting duct to chronic metabolic acidosis (MA). *Lab Invest* 51:268, 1984.

136. Maher T, Schambelan M, Kurtz I, et al: Amelioration of metabolic acidosis by dietary potassium restriction in hyperkalemic patients with chronic renal insufficiency. *J Lab Clin Med* 103:432, 1984.

137. Malluche HH, Ritz E, Lange HP, et al: Bone histology in incipient and advanced renal failure. *Kidney Int* 9:355, 1976.

138. Marone CC, Wong NLM, Sutton RAL, et al: Acidosis and renal calcium excretion in experimental chronic renal failure. *Nephron* 28:294, 1981.

139. Martinez-Maldonado M, Eknoyan G, Suki WN: Natriuretic effects of vasopressin and cyclic AMP: Possible site of action in the nephron. *Am J Physiol* 220:2013, 1971.

140. McKinney TD, Burg MB: Bicarbonate and fluid absorption by renal proximal straight tubules. *Kidney Int* 12:1, 1977.

141. McKinney TD, Burg MB: Bicarbonate secretion by rabbit cortical collecting tubules in vitro. *J Clin Invest* 61:1421, 1978.

142. McKinney TD, Burg MB: Bicarbonate absorption by rabbit cortical collecting tubules in vitro. *Am J Physiol* 234:F141, 1978.

143. Minkin C, Jennings JM: Carbonic anhydrase and bone remodeling: Sulfonamide inhibition of bone resorption in organ culture. *Science* 176:1031, 1972.

144. Mitchell JH, Wildenthal K, Johnson RL Jr: The effects of acid-base disturbances of cardiovascular and pulmonary function. *Kidney Int* 1:375, 1972.

145. Mizgala CL, Quamme GA: Renal handing of phosphate. *Physiol Rev* 65:431, 1985.

146. Moody W Jr: Appearance of calcium action potentials in crayfish slow muscle fibres under conditions of low intracellular pH. *J Physiol (Lond)* 302:335, 1980.

147. Moody WJ Jr: Ionic mechanism of intracellular pH regulation in crayfish neurones. *J Physiol (Lond)* 316:293, 1981.

148. Mossberg SM, Ross G: Ammonia movement in the small intestine: Preferential transport by the ileum. *J Clin Invest* 46:490, 1967.

149. Muldowney FP, Donohoe JF, Carrol DV, et al: Parathyroid acidosis in uremia. *Q J Med* 41:321, 1972.

150. Oliver J, Bourke E: Interrelationship of urea and ammonia excretion in metabolic acidosis. *Ir J Med Sci* 144:129, 1975.

151. Oliver J, Bourke E: Adaptations in urea ammonium excretion in metabolic acidosis in the rat: A reinterpretation. *Clin Sci and Mol Med* 48:515, 1975.

152. Palmer WW, Henderson LJ: A study of the several factors of acid excretion in nephritis. *Arch Intern Med* 16:109, 1915.

153. Papadoyannakis NJ, Stefanidis CJ, McGeown M: The effect of the correction of metabolic acidosis on nitrogen and potassium balance of patients with chronic renal failure. *Am J Clin Nutr* 40:623, 1984.

154. Parfitt AM: The actions of parathyroid hormone on bone. Relation to bone remodeling and turnover, calcium homeostasis, and metabolic bone diseases. II. PTH and bone cells: Bone turnover and plasma calcium regulation. *Metabolism* 25:909, 1976.

155. Pellegrino ED, Blitz RM: The composition of human bone in uremia. *Medicine* 44:397, 1965.

156. Perez GO, Oster JR, Vaamonde CA: Renal acidosis and renal potassium handling in selective hypoaldosteronism. *Am J Med* 57:809, 1974.

157. Peters JP: Acid base equilibrium and salt and water exchange. *Yale J Biol Med* 2:183, 1930.

158. Pitts RF: The renal excretion of acid. *Federation Proc* 7:418, 1948.

159. Pitts RF: Renal production and excretion of ammonia. *Am J Med* 36:720, 1964.

160. Pitts RF: Control of renal production of ammonia. *Kidney Int* 1:297, 1972.
161. Pitts RF: *Physiology of the kidney and body fluids*, 3rd ed. Chicago, Yearbook Medical Publishers, 1974, p 198.
162. Platt R: Structural and functional adaptation in renal failure. *Br Med J* 1:1313, 1372, 1952.
163. Post RL, Jolly PC: Linkage of sodium, potassium, and ammonium active transport across human erythrocyte membrane. *Biochim Biophys Acta* 25:118, 1957.
164. Rabinowitch IM: The origin of urinary ammonia. *Arch Intern Med* 33:394, 1924.
165. Rademacher DR, Arruda JAL, Kurtzman NA: On the quantitation of bicarbonate reabsorption. *Miner Electrolyte Metab* 1:21, 1978.
166. Raisz LG: Bone resorption in tissue culture: Factors influencing the response to parathyroid hormone. *J Clin Invest* 44:103, 1965.
167. Rasmussen H, Anast C, Arnaud C: Thyrocalcitonin, EGTA and urinary electrolyte excretion. *J Clin Invest* 46:746, 1967.
168. Relman AS: Renal acidosis and renal excretion of acid in health and disease. *Adv Intern Med* 12:295, 1964.
169. Relman AS: Metabolic consequences of acid-base disorders. *Kidney Int* 1:347, 1972.
170. Relman AS, Lennon EJ, Lemann J Jr: Endogenous production of fixed acid and the measurement of the net balance of acid in normal subjects. *J Clin Invest* 40:1621, 1961.
171. Roberts KE, Randall HT, Vanamee P, et al: Renal mechanisms involved in bicarbonate absorption. *Metabolism* 5:404, 1956.
172. Robinson JD: Interactions between monovalent cations and the $(Na^+ + K^+)$ ATPase dependent adenosine triphosphatase. *Arch Biochem Biophys* 139:17, 1970.
173. Robinson RR, Owen EE: Intrarenal distribution of ammonia during diuresis and antidiuresis. *Am J Physiol* 208:1129, 1965.
174. Roos A, Boron WF: Intracellular pH. *Physiol Rev* 61:296, 1981.
175. Sabatini S: The acidosis of chronic renal failure. *Med Clin North Am* 67:845, 1983.
176. Sajo IM, Goldstein MB, Sonnenberg H, et al: Sites of ammonia addition to tubular fluid in rats with chronic metabolic acidosis. *Kidney Int* 20:353, 1981.
177. Salcedo JR, Jackson ML, Coleman TN, et al: Endogenous net acid production in infants, children and adults. *Pediatr Res* 10:443, 1976.
178. Schambelan M, Sebastian A, Hulter H: Mineralocorticoid excess and deficiency syndromes. *In* Brenner BM, Stein JM (eds): *Acid-base and potassium homeostasis. Contemporary Issues in Nephrology* 2:232. New York, Churchill-Livingstone, 1978.
179. Schmidt RW, Bricker NS, Gavellas G: Renal bicarbonate reabsorption in the dog with experimental uremia. *Kidney Int* 10:287, 1976.
180. Schmidt RW, Gavellas G: Bicarbonate reabsorption in dogs with experimental renal disease: Effects of proportional reduction of sodium or phosphate intake. *Kidney Int* 12:393, 1977.
181. Schoolwerth AC, Sandler RS, Hoffman PM, et al: Effects of nephron reduction and dietary protein content on renal ammoniagenesis in the rat. *Kidney Int* 7:397, 1975.
182. Schwartz GJ: Na^+-dependent H^+ efflux from proximal tubule: Evidence for reversible Na^+-H^+ exchange. *Am J Physiol* 241:F380, 1981.
183. Schwartz JH, Tripolone M: Characteristics of NH_4^+ and NH_3 transport across the isolated turtle urinary bladder. *Am J Physiol* 245:F210, 1983.
184. Schwartz WB, Cohen JJ: The nature of the renal response to chronic disorders of acid-base equilibrium. *Am J Med* 64:417, 1978.
185. Schwartz WB, Hall PW, Hays RM, et al: On the mechanism of acidosis in chronic renal disease. *J Clin Invest* 38:39, 1959.
186. Schwartz WB, Jenson RL, Relman AS: The disposition of acid administered to sodium depleted subjects: The renal response and the role of the whole body buffers. *J Clin Invest* 33:587, 1954.
187. Sebastian A, Hulter NH, Kurtz I, et al: Disorders of distal nephron function. *Am J Med* 72:289, 1982.
188. Sebastian A, Schambelan M, Lindenfeld S, et al: Amelioration of metabolic acidosis with fludrocortisone therapy in hyporeninemic hypoaldosteronism. *N Engl J Med* 297:576, 1977.
189. Sebastian A, Schambelan M, Sutton JM: Amelioration of hyperchloremic acidosis with furosemide therapy in patients with chronic renal insufficiency and type 4 renal tubular acidosis. *Am J Nephrol* 4:287, 1984.
190. Seldin DW, Coleman AJ, Carter NW, et al: The effect of Na_2SO_4 on urinary acidification in chronic renal disease. *J Lab Clin Med* 69:893, 1967.
191. Severinghaus JW: Oxyhemoglobin dissociation curve correction for temperature and pH variation in human blood. *J Appl Physiol* 12:485, 1958.
192. Sharma SN, Singh J, Kumar R, et al: Acid-base status and blood gas alterations following experimental uremia in cattle. *Am J Vet Res* 42:333, 1981.
193. Sharpey-Schafer EP, Semple SJG, Halls RW, et al: Venous constriction after exercise; its relation to the acid-base changes in venous blood. *Clin Sci* 29:397, 1965.
194. Sherman HC, Gettler AO: The balance of acid-forming and base forming elements in foods and its relation to ammonia metabolism. *J Biol Chem* 11:323, 1912.
195. Simon E, Martin D, Fritsch J, et al: Distal tubule ammonia entry (abstr). *Kidney Int* 25:283, 1984.
196. Simpson DP: Control of hydrogen ion homeostasis and renal acidosis. *Medicine* 50:503, 1971.
197. Simpson DP, Sherrard DJ: Regulation of glutamine metabolism in vitro by bicarbonate ion and pH. *J Clin Invest* 48:1088, 1969.
198. Skou JC: Further investigations on a $Mg^{++} + N^+$-activated adenosine triphosphatase, possibly related to the active linked transport of Na^+ and K^+ across the nerve membrane. *Biochim Biophys Acta* 42:6, 1960.
199. Slatopolsky E, Bricker NS: The role of phosphorus restriction in the prevention of secondary hyperparathyroidism in chronic renal disease. *Kidney Int* 4:141, 1973.
200. Slatopolsky E, Cagler S, Pennell JP, et al: On the pathogenesis of hyperparathyroidism in chronic experimental renal insufficiency in the dog. *J Clin Invest* 50:492, 1971.
201. Slatopolsky E, Hoffsten P, Purkerson M, et al: On the influence of extracellular fluid volume expansion and of uremia on bicarbonate reabsorption in man. *J Clin Invest* 49:988, 1970.
202. Slatopolsky E, Hruska K, Rutherford WT: Current concepts of parathyroid hormone and vitamin D metabolism. Perturbations in chronic renal disease. *Kidney Int* 7:S90, 1975.
203. Slatopolsky E, Robson AM, Elkan I, et al: Control of phosphate excretion in uremic man. *J Clin Invest* 47:1865, 1968.
204. Soltoff SP, Mandel LJ: Active ion transport in renal proximal tubule. II. Ionic dependence of the Na pump. *J Gen Physiol* 84:623, 1984.
205. Star RA, Burg MB, Knepper MA: Luminal disequilibrium pH and ammonia transport in outer medullary collecting duct. *Am J Physiol* (Renal Fluid Electrolyte Physiol 21) 252:F1148, 1987.
206. Steinmetz PR, Eisinger RP, Lowenstein J: The excretion of

acid in unilateral renal disease in man. *J Clin Invest* 44:582, 1965.

207. Stern L, Backman KA, Hayslett JP: Effect of cortical-medullary gradient for ammonia on urinary excretion of ammonia. *Kidney Int* 27:652, 1985.

208. Stetson DL, Steinmetz PR: Role of membrane fusion in CO_2 stimulation of proton secretion by turtle bladder. *Am J Physiol* 245:C113, 1983.

209. Stetson D, Wade JB, Giebisch G: Morphological alterations in the rat medullary collecting duct following potassium depletion. *Kidney Int* 17:45, 1980.

210. Stewart JSS, Stewart WK, Gillies HC: Cardiac arrest and acidosis. *Lancet* 2:964, 1962.

211. Stine KC, Linshaw MA: The use of furosemide in the evaluation of renal tubular acidosis. *J Pediatr* 107:559, 1985.

212. Stoner LC, Burg MB, Orloff J: Ion transport in cortical collecting tubule: Effect of amiloride. *Am J Physiol* 227:453, 1974.

213. Sullivan LP: Ammonium excretion during stopped flow: A hypothetical ammonium countercurrent system. *Am J Physiol* 209:273, 1965.

214. Swan RC, Pitts RF: Neutralization of infused acid by nephrectomized dogs. *J Clin Invest* 34:205, 1955.

215. Szylman P, Better OS, Chaimowitz C, et al: Role of hyperkalemia in the metabolic acidosis of isolated hypoaldosteronism. *N Engl J Med* 294:361, 1976.

216. Tannen RL: Ammonia metabolism. *Am J Physiol* 235:F265, 1978.

217. Tannen RL, Wedell E, Moore R: Renal adaptation to a high potassium intake: The role of hydrogen ion. *J Clin Invest* 52:2089, 1973.

218. Thomas RC: Intracellular pH of snail neurones measured with a new pH-sensitive glass microelectrode. *J Physiol (Lond)* 238:159, 1974.

219. Tizianello A, DeFerrari G, Garibotto G, et al: Effects of chronic renal insufficiency and metabolic acidosis on glutamine metabolism in man. *Clin Sci and Mol Med* 55:391, 1978.

220. Tizianello A, DeFarrari G, Garibotto G, et al: Renal metabolism of amino acids and ammonia in subjects with normal renal function and in patients with chronic renal insufficiency. *J Clin Invest* 65:1162, 1980.

221. Trechsel U, Schenk R, Bonjour JP, et al: Relation between bone mineralization, Ca absorption and plasma Ca in phosphonate-treated rats. *Am J Physiol* 232:E298, 1977.

222. Van Slyke DD, Linder GC, Hiller A, et al: The excretion of ammonia and titratable acid in nephritis. *J Clin Invest* 2:255, 1926.

223. Van Ypersele De Strihou C: Importance of endogenous acid production in the regulation of acid-base equilibrium: The role of the digestive tract. *In* Hamburger J, Maxwell MG (eds): *Advances in Nephrology.* Chicago, Year Book Medical Publishers, 1980, p 367.

224. Waite LC: Carbonic anhydrase inhibitors, parathyroid hormone and calcium metabolism. *Endocrinology* 91:1160, 1972.

225. Waite LC, Volkert WA, Kenny AD: Inhibition of bone resorption by acetazolamide in the rat. *Endocrinology* 87:1129, 1970.

226. Wall SM, Sands JM, Flessner MF, et al: Net acid transport by isolated perfused inner medullary collecting ducts. *Am J Physiol* (Renal Fluid Electrolyte Physiol 27) 258:F75, 1990.

227. Wallia R, Greenberg A, Piraino B, et al: Serum electrolyte patterns in end-stage renal disease. *Am J Kidney Dis* 8:98, 1986.

228. Warnock DG: Uremic acidosis. *Kidney Int* 34:278, 1988.

229. Widmer B, Gerhardt RE, Harrington JT, et al: Serum electrolyte and acid base composition. The influence of graded degrees of chronic renal failure. *Arch Intern Med* 139:1099, 1979.

230. Wong NLM, Quamme GA, Dirks JH: Tubular handling of bicarbonate in dogs with experimental renal failure. *Kidney Int* 25:912, 1984.

231. Wrong O, Davies HEF: The excretion of acid in renal disease. *Q J Med* 28:259, 1959.

232. Zalups RK, Stanton BA, Wade JB, et al: Structural adaptation in initial collecting tubule following reduction in renal mass. *Kidney Int* 27:636, 1985.

233. Zeiske W, Van Driessche W: The interaction of "K^+-like" cations with the apical K^+ channel in frog skin. *J Membr Biol* 76:57, 1983.

Russell W. Chesney
Louis V. Avioli

28
Childhood Renal Osteodystrophy

The first well-documented association between renal disease and skeletal deformities in adolescents was presented by Lucas [231] in 1883. He described four male patients who ranged in age from 12 to 16 years and shared a common syndrome characterized by albuminuria and rachitic skeletal deformities. Three of the four young men were treated with "phosphate of iron and cod liver oil," and two appeared to respond dramatically. Subsequent to this classic essay, the association of skeletal lesions and chronic renal disease was well established in children, adolescents, and adults, and descriptive terms such as renal rickets and renal osteodystrophy were applied to the syndrome [31,79].

Chronic renal failure in children is characterized by profound alterations in the orderly metabolic sequences that normally guarantee cellular integrity and metabolic homeostasis [84]. Hormonal imbalances that contribute to these acquired defects include abnormal growth hormone secretory patterns; elevations in plasma aldosterone and glucagon; decreases in circulating somatomedin, testosterone, and thyroid hormone; and defective biologic degradation of cortisol and insulin. These hormonal imbalances, coupled with blunted end-organ response to hormonal stimulation, lead ultimately to disturbances in acid-base balance and in carbohydrate and lipid metabolism, as well as to defective synthesis and catabolism of structural and enzymatic proteins [84].

Since the kidney also normally occupies a pivotal role in the regulation of calcium, inorganic phosphate, parathyroid hormone, calcitonin, and vitamin D metabolism, one would anticipate that in children progressive loss of normal renal parenchyma would lead ultimately to derangements in mineral and bone metabolism with resultant alterations in skeletal growth and remodeling [257,260]. These changes, which are initially reflected by hypophosphatemia or mild hyperphosphatemia and occasional hypocalcemia, progress insidiously to a syndrome characterized by bone pain and recurrent skeletal fractures; malabsorption of calcium; parathyroid gland overactivity; cutaneous, vascular, and visceral calcification; and an impairment in the biologic activation of vitamin D. So-called renal osteodystrophy or renal rickets subsequently becomes

resistant to vitamin D therapy, in that the dose of the vitamin required for effective biologic response is increased when compared to dosages used in simple nonuremic forms of vitamin D deficiency [78].

The Composition and Structure of Bone
The Mineral Phase

In order to fully appreciate the nature of the skeletal defects that are acquired during the progression of the uremic state, it seems appropriate to delineate certain well-established principles that normally condition the formation and maturation of skeletal tissue. Calcium in the solid mineral phase of bone is usually considered to be a variant of purely crystalline hydroxyapatite, $Ca_{10}(PO_4)_6$ $^-(OH)_2$, containing small but significant amounts of carbonate (4%–6% by weight) and lesser amounts (<15%) of other ions such as Na^+, K^+, Mg^{++}, and Cl^-. X-ray diffraction, infrared spectrophotometry, and electron spin resonance spectroscopic measurements of fresh, whole bone tissue reveal that the mineral moiety of bone is composed of crystals of varying sizes. There appears to be two distinct phases other than hydroxyapatite: brushite and a β-tricalcium calcium phosphate [78]. No temporal relationship has been established in the nonapatitic and apatitic phase of bone, nor is there presently any evidence that nonapatitic phases are precursors of a final apatitic phase in bone [22].

The Organic Phase

Fully mineralized bone consists, approximately 65% to 70% by weight, of inorganic mineral complexes and 30% to 35% of organic material. Although the fibrous protein collagen represents only 23% of the total dry weight of bone, it comprises 90% to 95% of the organic matrix. Collagen fibers in bone are spatially oriented, highly organized in interlacing bundles and layers, and embedded in a gelatinous mucopolysaccharide substance consisting primarily of glucosoaminoglycans and hyaluronic acid. It has been well established that mature collagen fibers can act as nucleation centers for the precipitation of calcium phosphates from supersaturated solutions of calcium and phosphate salts [149]. The spatial orientation of the collagen fibers within the organic bone matrix is considered essential to the process of phase transformation and heterogeneous nucleation that normally initiates the deposition of microcrystalline material within and on the fibrillar bone matrix [148], since only collagen fibers of bones and teeth normally calcify, despite the fact that extracellular fluids are normally supersaturated with respect to calcium and inorganic phosphate. The specific orientation of the collagen fibrils within the bone matrix and their spatial relationship to the crystalline phase also impart structural integrity to the skeleton and the mechanical properties of a two-phase system, the latter conditioning the breaking strength and elasticity of bone. Biochemical cross-linkages within collagen subunits and between individual helical polypeptidic units [149] are established as part of the complex biochemical and physiochemical reactions that attend skeletal maturation and remodeling. These cross-links determine, to a large extent, the properties of the intact, mature, fibrous, collagenous protein in bones [264].

The amino acid hydroxyproline accounts for about 14% of the amino acid residues in collagen, whereas its concentration in the closely related fibrous protein elastin approximates 2% of the constituent amino acids. Hydroxyproline conditions the formation of the peptide subunits within the osteoblast (see below) as well as their ultimate secretion in the extracellular matrix. The hydroxyproline of the collagen molecule is derived by an in situ hydroxylation of proline during the early stages of collagen biosynthesis within the bone cell and is not derived from dietary sources. When bone collagen is degraded, hydroxyproline is released either as the free amino acid or in peptidic form. Since the free form is not reutilized for collagen synthesis, it is either degraded by the liver [21] or excreted in the urine as a small percentage (2%) of the total hydroxyproline component. A fraction of the excreted hydroxyproline (5%–10%) is also present in nondialyzable peptides with molecular weights of 4500 to 10,000 [165,212]. The nondialyzable oligopeptide (or retentate) fraction reflects rapid degradation of newly synthesized immature collagen, while the remaining (or dialyzable) hydroxyproline-containing peptides reflect degradation of more mature collagen [139,165] and are characteristically elevated in uremia and in clinical disorders in which bone resorption is accelerated [165].

Hydroxylysine is an amino acid found exclusively in collagen; like hydroxyproline, it is not derived from a circulating free amino acid pool but rather from the hydroxylation of lysine after the latter has been incorporated into the peptide chain within the osteoblast. Hydroxylysine contributes to the molecular structure of the collagen molecule by participating in the cross-links that serve to stabilize the molecule and in the carbohydrate linkages that exist in skin and bone collagen. One-third of all the hydroxylysine residues are glycosylated in these tissues, but the relative amounts of the glycosylated hydroxylysines differ in skin and bone. Glycosylgalactosyl-hydroxylysine (Hyl-Glu-Gal) predominates in skin, and galactosyl-hydroxylysine (Hyl-Gal) predominates in bone [304]. Chil-

dren with disease known to increase bone turnover (e.g., hyperthyroidism, hyperparathyroidism) excrete more Hyl-Gal than Hyl-Glu-Gal in their urine, whereas those with extensive skin necrosis due to thermal burns excrete predominantly Hyl-Glu-Gal [305,343].

Two mature cross-linking amino acids of the 3-hydroxypyridinium family have also been used as biochemical markers of bone turnover. Hydroxylysyl-pyridinoline (HP) and lysylpyridinoline (LP) are intermolecular cross-linking compounds of collagen that are only present in its mature form. In contrast to the wide distributions of type I and type III, collagens HP and LP do not exist in skin ligament and fascia; their primary sources are bone and cartilage [161]. Urinary excretion of HP and LP reflect only collagen degradation occurring during osteoclastic bone resorption and not degradation of newly synthesized collagen [370]. Since the predominant collagen in bone is type I collagen, changes in the blood levels of the carboxy-terminal extension peptides of type I procollagen (pColl-C) also correlate with changes in bone collagen synthesis [349].

Other important constituents of the organic matrix of bone are represented by glycosoaminoglycans, proteoglycans, osteonectin, and a bone gla protein (osteocalcin). Although their exact role in bone maturation and mineralization is still incompletely understood, the polyanion-charged glycosoaminoglycans and proteoglycans are capable of binding calcium ions and inhibiting the precipitation of calcium and phosphate [49,56]. Their potential significance in biological calcification is exemplified by the mucopolysaccharidoses, a family of inherited disorders of children characterized by a deficiency of specific lysosomal enzymes that normally function to degrade glycosoaminoglycans in bone [56]. The resulting accumulation of glycosoaminoglycans leads to defective skeletal mineralization, osteopenia, and fractures.

The Cellular Phase

The metabolic functions of bone are controlled primarily by the cellular component, which comprises a very small proportion of its total mass. These cells appear to form a syncytium over the bone surfaces, separating them from the general extracellular space [185], and as such they are probably active in regulating mineral homeostasis [250]. The bone cell population is composed of osteoblasts, osteocytes, and osteoclasts. Osteoblasts are matrix- or collagen-synthesizing cells that cover surfaces actively undergoing bone formation. In the growing skeleton, they are found on the endosteal, haversian, and periosteal surfaces. With cessation of growth, however, they do not normally exist on the periosteal surface except in states of abnormal skeletal remodeling, such as in uremic children. Reflecting their role as protein synthesizers, osteoblasts contain abundant ribonuclear protein and hence are basophilic. They are also rich in enzymes, particularly alkaline phosphatase [240], illustrating the important role these cells play in mineralization as well as synthesis of bone matrix.

While characteristic osteoblasts are typically columnar, most bone surfaces, particularly those not undergoing bone synthesis, are lined by flat, membranous-appearing cells.

The function of these cells, which variously have been called inactive osteoblasts or osteoprogenitor cells, is unknown, although they communicate with typical osteoblasts and osteocytes and therefore are part of the bone cell syncytium [186]. With progressive matrix synthesis, osteoblasts are incorporated into bone matrix to form osteocytes. These cells are located within lacunae and anatomically communicate with each other and surface bone cells by canaliculi. While they have been classically viewed as relatively inactive, osteocytes are actually capable of both perilacunar bone formation [29] and resorption [30]. The significance of the contribution that osteocytic activity makes to mineral homeostasis, however, remains controversial [225].

Osteoclasts are large, usually multinucleated cells responsible for skeletal resorption. They are characteristically located juxtaposed to a scalloped bone surface known either as a resorptive bay or a Howship's lacuna. A variety of agents stimulate osteoclastic bone resorption. Those of most immediate concern in renal osteodystrophy are parathyroid hormone and vitamin D (including vitamin D metabolites). Osteoclasts that are actively resorbing bone are best identified by the presence of convoluted infoldings of their "bone-abutting" cell membrane, known as a ruffled border. This feature can be accurately appreciated only by electron microscopy. Resorptive stimuli promote the appearance of osteoclastic ruffled borders, while agents such as calcitonin, which inhibit resorption, suppress their appearance [200,240]. Osteoclastic bone resorption almost always requires the presence of mineralized bone matrix. As is discussed later, this has important implications in uremic osteodystrophy. Furthermore, the resorptive process probably entails lysosomal activity, reflecting the large concentration of phosphatase in the osteoclasts [374].

Skeletal Development

Because the unique features of childhood renal osteodystrophy relate to distinctions between the growing and fully grown skeleton [79], an appreciation of bone development is fundamental to the understanding of the uremic bone disease that attends the uremic syndrome of prepubescent children. Fetal bone development begins with clusters of mesenchymal cells that differentiate into chondroblasts or osteoblasts. If chondroid differentiation occurs, as is characteristic of long and tubular bone development, a small cartilaginous model of the adult bone is formed that is eventually replaced by osseous tissue. Hence the process is known as endochondral ossification. When, on the other hand, mesenchymal cells differentiate into osteoblasts, as commonly occurs in the flat bones (e.g., skull), osseous tissue is synthesized directly in a process known as intramembranous ossification.

Endochondral ossification occurs in those bones in which development requires a predominance of longitudinal growth. The process is achieved by an interplay of the distinct physical properties of the cartilaginous model and the bone that replaces it. In long bones, this replacement first occurs in the diaphysis and is characterized by chondrocyte hypertrophy and ingrowth of blood vessels. Simul-

taneously, the adjacent perichondrium differentiates into periosteum, which in turn forms a collar of bone about the middle of the shaft. This bone gradually encroaches on and replaces the diaphyseal cartilage.

A similar but not identical process to diaphyseal ossification takes place at the proximal and distal ends of the bone. Chondrocyte hypertrophy and ultimate atrophy, followed by osseous encroachment, occur within the ends of the cartilaginous models but do not involve differentiation of the adjacent perichondrium into periosteum. As such, a collar of cartilage surrounds these ossification centers that form the epiphyseal bone. The cartilage between the ossification center and the joint space eventuates into articular cartilage, while that separating the epiphyseal and diaphyseal bone forms the growth plate. This plate differentiates into four distinct zones, the development of which relates closely to longitudinal growth. The means by which this is achieved involves interstitial expansion of the growth plate by chondrocytes in zones juxtaposed to the epiphyseal ossification center.

Interstitial growth, a property unique in the skeleton to cartilage, implies expansion of tissue mass from within by replication of cells that have been incorporated into the interstices of the structure and matrix synthesis by these internalized cells. Therefore, the epiphyseal plate can increase in mass despite the absence of a free cartilaginous surface on which to layer additional cartilage. As the epiphyseal cartilage ages and moves toward the metaphysis, vascular invasion of the tissue occurs, resulting in oxygenation and death. The most mature part of the growth plate, known as the zone of provisional calcification, is characterized by mineralization of the cartilaginous matrix and its subsequent chondroclastic resorption. Those spicules of mineralized cartilage that remain serve as a scaffolding for the deposition of bone matrix. Consequently, in normal endochondral ossification there is an integral anatomic relationship between the primary bony trabeculae and the epiphyseal growth plate. This relationship has important implications in childhood renal osteodystrophy. With normal growth the trabeculae are actively resorbed, resulting in a diaphysis composed entirely of cortical bone. Therefore, longitudinal growth is accomplished by internal expansion of the growth plate and simultaneous resorption of the mineralized epiphyseal cartilage. The width of the epiphyseal plate consequently remains unchanged until growth ceases, at which time cartilaginous resorption exceeds formation, resulting in its gradual obliteration.

As opposed to endochondral growth, intramembranous ossification is entirely appositional. This type of bone development occurs predominantly in flat bones and, similar to its endochondral counterpart, originates with an accumulation of mesenchymal cells. However, in intramembranous ossification, these cells differentiate directly into osteoblasts that form a spicule containing immature woven collagen. Continued apposition and appropriate resorption results in a bone that is shaped similarly to its adult counterpart. During the third trimester and in the first few years of life, virtually all woven bone is resorbed and replaced by its mature lamellar counterpart. Periosteal growth and modeling ceases coincidentally with epiphyseal closure. While strictly speaking, expansion of the width of long bones is considered a component of endochondral ossification, the process in fact does not involve replacement of a cartilaginous model. This process occurs by matrix apposition at the periosteal surface and, in a sense, is more closely akin to intramembranous bone formaton. With epiphyseal closure, periosteal bone synthesis also normally ceases, although it is reactivated by diffuse or local pathologic processes.

The pathogenesis of childhood renal osteodystrophy can be best appreciated with an understanding of the four generic morphologic functions of osteoblasts and osteoclasts. The functions are *growth*, which involves the increase in skeletal mass; *modeling*, the process by which the small bones of a fetus are shaped into their adult counterparts; *remodeling*, the process intimately related to mineral homeostasis; and *repair*, the prototype of which is fracture healing. Those processes that are unique to the growing skeleton are growth and modeling. The fact that these activities function independently is illustrated by diseases that affect one to the exclusion of the others. For example, hypopituitary dwarfism is a growth dysfunction, while diaphyseal dysplasia or osteopetrosis may involve only modeling. If one considers the growing long bone a prototype, the functional distinction between growth and modeling becomes apparent. As longtitudinal growth progresses, the metaphysis, which is characteristically a wide area of bone, must be funnelled into the diaphysis. This requires resorption and formation at specific foci necessary to sculpture the bone. If modeling fails, the bone often assumes a tubular character, with little distinction between the diaphysis and metaphysis.

Remodeling, on the other hand is a process that occurs throughout life and is abnormal in both the uremic child and adult. The quintessential feature of this process is the cybernetic coupling between osteoblastic and osteoclastic activity [144]; that is, where osteoclastic resorption has occurred, osteoblastic bone formation invariably follows. While normal remodeling leaves residual histologic traces within relatively short periods of time, it does not normally affect the gross architecture of the bone. However, since with time the rate of bone resorption normally eventually exceeds that of formation, senescence is characterized by progressive loss of bone and an increased propensity to skeletal fracture [18].

Hormonal Control of Skeletal Metabolism

Osseous tissue is continually being deposited and resorbed, primarily as a result of the activity of the connective tissue cells covering its surfaces. Changes in bone resorption are not simply a consequence of changes in the activity of existing cell machinery; they depend on the continuous transformation of resting undifferentiated cells to osteocytes, osteoblasts, and osteoclasts. Osteoclastic and osteocytic response to parathyroid hormone represents one of the singular most effective control mechanisms available to facilitate the resorption of bone. This regulating action of parathyroid hormone is normally accomplished through continuous secretion, which is inversely related to ionized calcium concentration in the extracellular fluid. In contrast

to the action of parathyroid hormone on bone, the inhibition of bone resorption is the principal, if not sole, function of calcitonin. It is noteworthy that normally the resorptive activity of osteoclasts decreases in response to calcitonin. Relative to parathyroid hormone, the biologic response to calcitonin is rapid and short-lived. Parathyroid hormone and calcitonin constitute a dual proportional control system that effectively maintains a constant extracellular calcium concentration. In addition, vitamin D, through its biologically active metabolites, regulates the intestinal absorption of calcium and the responsiveness of bone to both parathyroid hormone and calcitonin, so that alterations in bone resorption serve the needs of skeletal growth and remodeling as well as calcium homeostasis.

Parathyroid Hormone

Parathyroid hormone has as its primary role the maintenance of the normal level of circulating calcium and inorganic phosphate. The parathyroid glands also synthesize precursor hormones (preproparathormone and proparathormone) that are immunologically different and higher in molecular weight than the circulating form [162,234]. It has also been demonstrated that circulating hormonal fragments are smaller than the 84-amino-acid hormone peptide secreted by the glands, as a result of peripheral metabolism of the intact hormone. Parathyroid hormone regulates calcium and phosphate homeostasis by exerting its effect on three independent end organs: bone, renal tubule, and intestinal mucosa. The hormone normally stimulates osteocytic and osteoclastic osteolysis, the latter probably resulting from the effect of parathyroid hormone or osteoblasts. The end result is mineral mobilization and degradation of both newly synthesized and mature collagen [185]. The skeletal demineralization and lysis of collagenous matrix observed following parathyroid hormone administration occur almost simultaneously. Parathyroid hormone also activates calcium transport across the intestinal mucosa and renal tubule. The renal effects occur within minutes and the bone effects within hours, whereas the intestinal response, achieved indirectly by way of stimulated bioactivation of vitamin D, requires days or even weeks to become apparent [39].

In the absence of vitamin D, parathyroid hormone regulation of either the intestinal absorption of calcium or the mobilization of skeletal calcium is blunted [15,279]. In contrast, the renal tubular effects of parathyroid hormone [320] seem to be independent of vitamin D. The so-called permissive role of vitamin D for parathyroid-induced bone resorption possibly involves a change in the availability of calcium to bone cells, since calcium administration in the absence of vitamin D mimics its effect [16]. In this regard, magnesium ion also appears to be permissive for maximal parathyroid hormone activity, since the blunted or limited skeletal and renal response to parathyroid hormone and hypocalcemia, often associated with clinical hypomagnesemia, can be reversed by magnesium administration [8,88,125,276]. Parathyroid hormone also stimulates hepatic glycogenolysis and gluconeogenesis [271], events that probably are mediated through cyclic adenosine 3',5'-cyclic phosphate (AMP) [61]. Accumulated evidence of Muldowney et al. [274,275] also suggests that systemic acid-base balance may be at least partially controlled by parathyroid hormone-regulated bicarbonate reabsorption by the kidney.

Developments in hormonal isolation, purification, and accurate quantitation by specific radioimmunoassay procedures, based on the ability of the hormones to competitively inhibit the binding of ^{131}I labeled hormone to specific antibody, have contributed not only to a verification of the existing hypothesis that circulating ionized calcium is the primary physiologic determinant of parathyroid hormone secretion, but also to the demonstration that magnesium may also control its synthesis and its release [8]. It has also been shown that parathyroid hormone is rapidly degraded with a plasma half-time of 8 minutes, has a volume of distribution equivalent to 30% of the body weight, and has a diurnal secretory rhythm with peak plasma levels occurring in the early morning hours [198]. Finally, it appears that parathyroid hormone is secreted continuously at normal plasma calcium levels and that the kidneys and liver play a permissive role in its biologic degradation [60,162,242,263].

Although the observations made with radioimmunoassay procedures are consistent with earlier in vitro studies in animals regarding parathyroid-calcium-bone homeostasis, there are a variety of conflicting reports concerning the quantity of parathyroid hormone found in the plasma of normal subjects or in patients with chronic uremia and apparent disagreements with respect to control of hormone secretion in primary and secondary hyperparathyroid states [13,14,15,134,348]. When one considers that the normal fragment or fragments present in blood may be detected by one antiserum but not by a second and that the fragments may be cleared from the circulation at rates that differ from that for the intact, recently secreted hormone, then entirely different impressions could be gathered concerning not only absolute concentrations of hormone, but also rates of hormonal disappearance. Thus, interpretation of data that concern the control of hormonal secretion and metabolism may depend on the characterization of the particular antiserum used in the radioimmunoassay [342].

The stimulation of skeletal resorption, intestinal calcium transport, and renal tubular calcium reabsorption collectively raises the calcium ion concentration in extracellular fluid and as such represents an appropriate response to the feedback-controlled release of parathyroid hormone by hypocalcemia. On the other hand, the physiologic importance of the phosphaturic response to the hormone is still ill-defined. Parathyroid hormone does stimulate adenyl cyclase activity in bone and kidney, leading to an increased concentration of cyclic AMP, an important regulator of hormone action [72,73,118,276]. Since adenyl cyclase is usually considered an integral part of the plasma membrane, the possibility exists that the observed skeletal and renal effects of the hormone simply reflect different end results of the same activated enzyme or membrane system. Chemical modifications of the hormone that destroy biologic activity inhibit both the skeletal and renal effects. These observations provide further evidence that the subcellular systems activated by the hormone in both bone and kidney are similar.

Calcitonin

Calcitonin, a hormone isolated from the human thyroid gland, is a single-chain 32-amino-acid polypeptide with a molecular weight of 3600. Salmon, bovine, ovine, eel, and porcine calcitonin have also been isolated in homogeneous forms, and their complete amino acid sequence has been determined [45]. Although all the calcitonins isolated to date contain 32 amino acids, only nine positions are homologous. Bovine calcitonin sequence differs from the porcine, bovine, or human preparations. The high biologic potency in vivo of salmon calcitonin may result from its relative resistance to metabolic degradation or the fact that skeletal and renal receptors for calcitonin have a high apparent affinity for salmon calcitonin [241,244].

Calcitonin is produced by the mitochondria-rich parafollicular or C cells of the thyroid and is secreted in response to elevations in circulating ionized calcium levels. Unlike parathyroid hormone secretion, which may also be stimulated by alterations in circulating magnesium, vitamin D, cortisol, and catecholamines, factors known to influence the rate of calcitonin excretion include glucagon and other gastrointestinal hormones [31,62,63,107,175]. Parafollicular C cells have been demonstrated to migrate embryologically from the ultimobranchial body, an endodermally derived structure. In lower animals, the thyroid is the primary source of the hormone, whereas in man, ectopic C cells containing calcitonin are present also in the parathyroid and thymus tissue. It should also be noted parenthetically that in the mature pig the adrenal medulla contains 7% to 28% as much calcitonin-like activity per gram as is found in the thyroid.

Although varied responses such as inhibition of intestinal phosphate absorption, increased magnesium excretion, calciuria, phosphaturia, and natriuresis have been attributed to calcitonin [1,11,37,364], the major and perhaps sole site of calcitonin activity is on bone, where it acts primarily to inhibit resorption. The degree to which calcitonin can inhibit bone resorption is dependent on the prevailing rate of bone resorption. The mechanism(s) whereby calcitonin acts on bone are presently uncertain. It has been established, however, that calcitonin acts neither by inhibiting parathyroid hormone-induced bone resorption nor by affecting the synthesis of cellular ribonucleic acid. It appears that the effects of calcitonin on bone, like those of parathyroid hormone, are mediated by cyclic AMP [241]. The two hormones act on different adenyl cyclases, probably in different types of bone cells [241]. Following calcitonin administration, the number of osteoclasts in bone decreases and the number of osteoblasts increases. Since the hypocalcemic action of the hormone is immediate, factors other than those affecting cell differentiation probably account for its acute effect.

The significance of calcitonin on calcium homeostatis of humans is not as well established as that of parathyroid hormone [153,217,315]. Human calcitonin is inactivated primarily in the kidney and to some extent in muscle or bone or both [241,350]. In normal human adults, the hypocalcemic effect of injected calcitonin is small. Available radioimmunoassay techniques are sensitive enough to detect the elevated calcitonin levels of patients with medullary carcinoma and normal individuals. Divergent findings of various investigators regarding age and sex-related changes in calcitonin secretion may be explained both by the heterogeneity of endogenous human calcitonin and by the varying affinity of different antibodies for binding sites on the human calcitonin molecule [64].

The hypocalcemic activity of exogenously administered calcitonin is maximal in young growing animals and in pathologic conditions in children characterized by increased bone turnover, such as juvenile Paget's disease [123], and hypercalcemia resulting from 25 OHD$_3$ treatment [255]. Although the physiologic role of calcitonin in children or adolescents is unclear, it may condition skeletal remodeling in the growing child by modulating the rate of bone resorption and thereby the supply of calcium from bone to extracellular fluids. In this regard, it should be noted that glucocorticoid suppression of longitudinal growth in children is associated with decreased circulating calcitonin levels. There is also some evidence, albeit still controversial, which suggests that inadequate calcitonin excretion and/or a "blunted" skeletal response to the hormone may also contribute to the pathogenesis of uremic bone disease [177].

Vitamin D

Before a reasonable analysis can be made of the nature of vitamin D resistance observed clinically in children or adolescents with end-stage renal failure, a review of recent developments relating to the biologic activation of vitamin D and the nature of its biologic effect(s) seems warranted. It is now well established that the metabolic activation of vitamin D is essential to its biologic expression in both animals and man. In fact, the term *vitamin D* may for all practical purposes be inappropriate, since the endogenous production of vitamin D$_3$ by the skin, its distribution by the bloodstream to kidney, liver, intestine, and bone, its biomolecular action through stimulated protein synthesis, and the negative feedback regulative control of its metabolism all resemble hormonal rather than dietary vitamin activity.

Vitamin D$_3$ is normally produced in the epidermal layer of skin nearest the capillary but just beneath the epidermal-dermal junction when ultraviolet irradiation is absorbed by the provitamin 7-dehydroxycholesterol (7-DHC) [320] (Fig. 28-1). A photochemical regulation mechanism of vitamin D production also exists in the skin. In fair-skinned individuals, exposure to sunlight for longer than 15 minutes results in increased conversion of 7-DHC to biologically inactive lumisterols and tachysterols. The rate of 7-DHC conversion to vitamin D$_3$ also depends on skin pigmentation. The endogenous production rate of vitamin D$_3$ in man is unknown, but it must be at least equivalent to the minimal vitamin D dietary dose of 200 to 400 IU daily essential to cure vitamin-D-deficiency rickets, since it has been observed that ultraviolet skin irradiation alone is curative in this regard [80].

Following the photochemical conversion of 7-DHC to vitamin D$_3$, the preformed vitamin D$_3$ is absorbed into the subepidermal microcirculation and transported in plasma

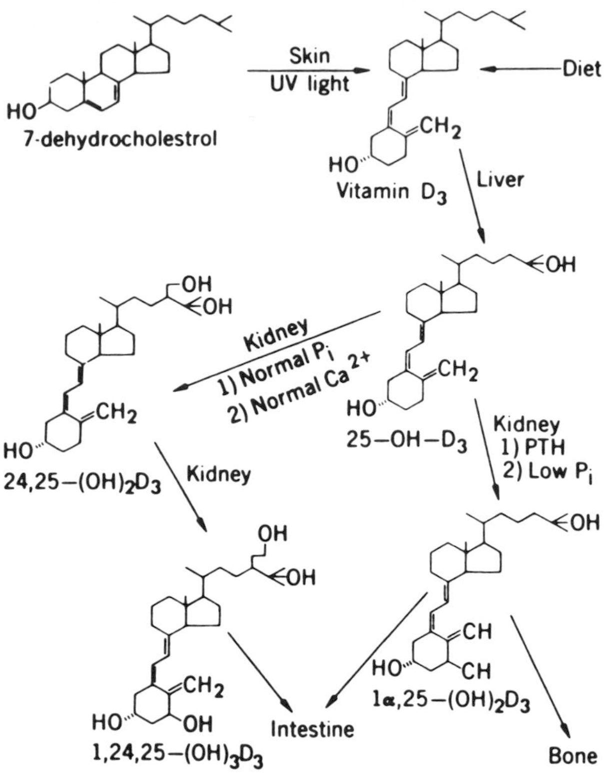

Fig. 28-1. *Metabolism of vitamin D. PTH, parathyroid hormone; Pi, inorganic phosphate. (Courtesy of H.F. DeLuca).*

to the liver and target organs bound to a specific globulin with a molecular weight of 52,000.

Dietary vitamin D$_3$ (cholecalciferol) or vitamin D$_2$ (ergocalciferol) is absorbed primarily from the duodenum and jejunum into lymphatic channels, with both bile salts and intraluminal lipids permissive in this regard. Although lipoproteins are not quantitatively important for the transport of vitamin D$_3$ in plasma, most of the vitamin absorbed from the intestine of animals and man is transported in lymph by chylomicrons [114]. The site of transfer of vitamin D$_3$ from chylomicrons to its specific plasma transport protein has not been established, although it appears likely that the liver is fundamental for this transformation. The absorbed vitamin D$_2$ or vitamin D$_3$ then admixes with endogenously synthesized vitamin D$_3$ and is either sequestered into storage depots such as adipose tissue and muscle by specific tissue-binding proteins or is metabolically transferred by the liver [114]. It seems likely that these tissue-binding proteins also play a role in the regulation of the metabolism of vitamin D and its metabolites [35,166,167, 191]. In human beings, circulating vitamin D (vitamin D$_3$ plus vitamin D$_2$) levels normally range between 8 and 45 nanograms per milliliter [20]. Whereas at normal plasma concentrations vitamin D disappears with a biologic half-life of 19 to 25 hours, its metabolic disposal is conditioned by the state of vitamin D nutrition and plasma concentrations, with high and low circulating levels resulting in a decrease and increase, respectively, in the plasma disappearance rate.

Endogenously synthesized and dietary vitamin D_3 and dietary vitamin D_2 are subsequently metabolized by the liver to their respective 25-hydroxylated derivatives (i.e., 25-hydroxycholecalciferol [25-OHD$_3$] and 25-hydroxyergocalciferol [25-OHD$_2$]) [187,290] (see Fig. 28-1). The enterohepatic circulation of vitamin D is negligible. Insignificant amounts of oral vitamin D are excreted in bile as 25-OHD. Most of the vitamin D is converted to highly polar (primary glucuronides) substances that are biologically inactive. Although it has been demonstrated that the hepatic 25-hydroxylation of vitamin D is substrate-specific, and to some extent feedback-regulated by the reaction product, the exact nature of the servocontrol mechanism is still controversial, as is its function in preventing the toxic effects of vitamin D overdosage. The hydroxylated vitamin D metabolites 25-OHD$_2$ and 25-OHD$_3$ also circulate bound to a globular protein that is indistinguishable from that which binds the parent vitamin D. The biologic half-life of 25-OHD (25-OHD$_2$ and 25-OHD$_3$) is 12 days [167].

Circulating levels of 25-OHD in normal subjects living in the United States [166] range between 15 and 30 nanograms per milliliter (Fig. 28-2). Reported lower mean circulating 25-OHD levels to 15 to 16 nanograms per milliliter in adults from the British Isles [27,311] and seasonal as well as age-related variations in serum levels of healthy individuals [253,311] presumably reflect both the higher dietary intake of vitamin D and the greater sunshine exposure in the United States because of its more southerly latitudes. A direct correlation does appear to exist between circulating maternal and fetal 25-OHD [116]; individual plasma levels of 25-OHD, vitamin D intake, timed exposure to sunlight (see Fig. 28-2), and total serum calcium values also correlate. Not only do 25-OHD$_2$ and 25-OHD$_3$ represent the major circulating forms of vitamin D, but they (i.e., 25-OHD$_3$) have been demonstrated to concentrate in skeletal tissue [383], to stimulate calcium absorption, and also to increase bone resorption without further structural modification [317,318]. It also has been demonstrated that 25-OHD$_3$ increases the proximal renal tubular reabsorption of calcium, sodium, and phosphate; and that its control of phosphate excretion is antagonistic to the phosphaturic effect of parathyroid hormone [306,313].

Whereas the metabolic fate of 25-OHD$_3$ in intestine, bone, and storage depot sites (i.e., adipose tissue and muscle) is ill-defined, it is further hydroxylated by the kidney to either 1,25-dihydroxycholecalciferol [1,25(OH)$_2$D$_3$] or 24,-25-dihydroxycholecalciferol [24,25(OH)$_2$D$_3$] (see Fig. 28-1). The control of 1,25(OH)$_2$D$_3$ production by the kidney is indeed complex, with intracellular concentrations of potassium, calcium, inorganic phosphate, prostaglandins, and cyclic AMP, as well as parathyroid hormone, sex hormones, calcitonin, and pH all functioning as controlling factors [27,36,37,38,118,139]. Preliminary observations suggest that the conversion of 25-OHD$_3$ to 1,25(OH)$_2$D$_3$ is regulated primarily by a sensitive servocontrol mechanism modulated by circulating calcium, parathyroid hormone, calcitonin, and the inorganic phosphate content of renal cortical cells. A theory coordinating these varied experimental observations would hold that hypocalcemia acts as a stimulus for parathyroid hormone

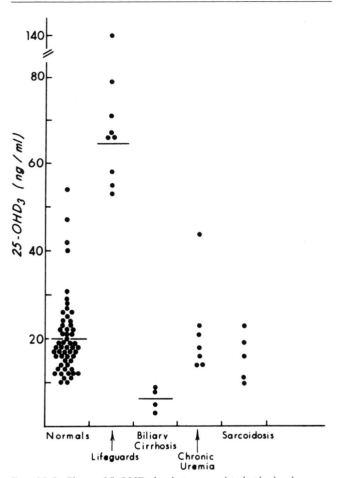

FIG. 28-2. *Plasma 25-OHD$_3$ levels in normal individuals, those subjected to excessive sunlight exposure (lifeguards), and others with documented disorders in calcium absorption.*

secretion; the latter, either directly or by depleting renal cortical inorganic phosphate concentration (or both), stimulates the hydroxylation of 25-OHD$_3$ to 1,25(OH)$_2$D$_3$, which in turn completes the negative feedback of hormonal control by stimulating the intestinal absorption and bone resorption of calcium [20]. As a consequence, the circulating ionized calcium levels are raised to normal and parathyroid hormone secretion returns to the basal state. On the other hand, hypercalcemia, while decreasing the rate of parathyroid hormone release, also stimulates calcitonin release from the parafollicular cells of the thyroid gland. In accordance with this unified homeostatic hypothesis, a rise in circulating calcitonin levels, either directly or indirectly by increasing renal cortical inorganic phosphate concentration (or both), results in a suppression of 1,25(OH)$_2$D$_3$ production, with a decrease in both bone resorption and intestinal reduction in calcitonin secretion by the thyroid gland.

Recently it has been demonstrated that 1,25(OH)$_2$D$_3$ also plays an integral role in the renal metabolism of 25-OHD$_3$, since 1,25(OH)$_2$D$_3$ administration to animals reduces the renal production of 1,25(OH)$_2$D$_3$ and stimulates the production of 24,25(OH)$_2$D$_3$ [363,365]. In contrast,

24,25(OH)$_2$D$_3$ appears to exert no effect on the conversion of 25-OHD$_3$ to 1,25(OH)$_2$D$_3$. Once synthesized by the kidney, 1,25(OH)$_2$D$_3$ is either subsequently degraded to a metabolite with unknown biologic activity [217] or converted to 1,24,25-trihydroxyvitamin D, 1,24,25-(OH)$_3$D$_3$ [208]. The kidney can also convert 24,25-dihydroxycholecalciferol, which circulates at a concentration of 1.68 ± 0.82 nanogram per milliliter in normal adults [366], to 1,24,25-(OH)$_3$D$_3$ (see Fig. 28-1). Evidence has also been produced demonstrating the formation of 1,24,25-(OH)$_3$D$_3$ from 25-OHD$_3$. It has reported that 1,24-25-trihydroxyvitamin D$_3$ is 60% as active as vitamin D$_3$ in curing rickets in animals and is less active on a weight basis than 1,25(OH)$_2$D$_3$ in stimulating and sustaining the intestinal absorption of calcium and bone resorption [184]. Presently, 1,24-25-(OH)$_3$D$_3$ is considered to exert its biologic activity preferentially on promoting the intestinal absorption of calcium [44].

Although the biologic significance of 24,25-(OH)$_2$D$_3$ is presently unknown, it has been shown to increase bone resorption in vitro [268,299], as well as intestinal calcium absorption, when administered to vitamin D deficient animals [44,219]. The intestinal effect probably results from the conversion of 24,25(OH)$_2$D$_3$ to a more polar metabolite [44].

It has been found that 1,25-dihydroxycholecalciferol [i.e., 1,25(OH)$_2$D$_2$ plus 1,25(OH)$_2$D$_3$] circulates with a biologic half-life of 24 hours at concentrations of 25 to 33 picograms per milliliter in adults [121,170,189]. Preliminary studies suggest that normal children have higher plasma levels, i.e., 49 to 66 picograms per milliliter [121]. It seems well established that the 1,25-hydroxylated vitamin D$_3$ derivation is the metabolic or hormonal form of vitamin D$_3$ that controls the intestinal transport of calcium, since it is some four to 13 times as effective as vitamin D$_3$ and over twice as effective as 25-OHD$_3$ in this regard. The renal tubular reabsorption of phosphate is also affected by 1,25(OH)$_2$D$_3$ [204], which possesses significant bone resorptive properties with an in vivo effectiveness some 100-fold that of the parent 25-OHD$_3$ [174]. The preferential accumulation of 1,25(OH)$_2$D$_3$ in the nucleus of bone cells and the subcellular skeletal distribution pattern of other vitamin D$_3$ metabolites suggest a mechanism of 1,25(OH)$_2$D$_3$ action in bone similar to that proposed for the control of calcium translocation across the intestinal cell [51]. Another vitamin D$_3$ diol metabolite, 25,26-dihydroxycholecalciferol, has been isolated from plasma and structurally identified with minimal biologic activity in intestine and bone [299]. There is rather substantial evidence that this dihydroxyl vitamin D metabolite is not a by-product of renal tubular or intestinal cellular metabolism of either 25-OHD$_3$, 1,25(OH)$_2$D$_3$, 24,25-(OH)$_2$D$_3$, or 1,24,25(OH)$_3$D$_3$. Thus, on the basis of experimental evidence obtained in man and a variety of animal species, the current working hypothesis depicts vitamin D$_3$ primarily as an inert reservoir substance; 25-OHD$_3$ as the major circulating biologically active metabolite; and 1,25(OH)$_2$D$_3$ as the metabolite with maximal biologic activity, which, together with parathyroid hormone and calcitonin, normally regulates the intestinal absorption of calcium and the growth and remodeling of bone [114].

Growth Hormone, Somatomedin, Thyroid Hormone, Estrogens, and Androgens

In order to appreciate the extent to which hormonal imbalance may interfere with normal remodeling maturation, and longitudinal growth of the childhood and adolescent skeleton, the age-related influence of pituitary, ovarian, thyroid, and testicular hormone and of somatomedin (IGF-I and IGF-II) on bone development must also be considered. This is discussed in some detail elsewhere in this volume [Chap. 34].

Pathogenesis of the Skeletal Changes in Pediatric Osteodystrophy

Although the pathogenesis and therapy of renal osteodystrophy in adults has been the subject of numerous reports and reviews [22,232,358,359], systematic analysis of the underlying hormonal and metabolic effects that initiate and perpetuate the skeletal abnormalities in growing uremic children are relatively few. As noted repeatedly in the past for adults with chronic renal failure, intestinal absorption of calcium is often (but not always) decreased [53,101,226,294,322,357] and circulating immunoreactive parathyroid hormone levels are usually elevated [41, 326,328] (Fig. 28-3) in uremic children; hypocalcemia,

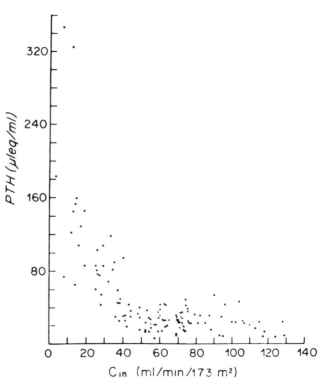

FIG. 28-3. *Relationship between renal clearance of inulin (Cin) and serum immunoreactive parathyroid hormone (PTH). Significant increments in hormone levels are noted at inulin clearance values below 40 ml/min. (From Arnaud CD: Hyperparathyroidism and renal failure. Kidney Int 4:89, 1973, with permission.)*

hypophosphatemia or hyperphosphatemia or hyperphosphatasia, and acidosis also attend the uremic syndrome (Fig. 28-4). In children the level of circulating alkaline phosphatase may be inappropriately low (Fig. 28-5). However, for the degree of skeletal involvement, circulating levels of calcium and phosphate bear little relationship to the histologic defects noted on bone biopsy specimens [387]. As noted earlier for adults, serum immunoreactive parathyroid hormone (iPTH) may be elevated in uremic children without radiologic evidence of bone disease, as well as in over 90% of those with clinically detectable skeletal lesions [326,328]. Although compensatory parathyroid overactivity (so-called secondary hyperparathyroidism) appears to be more severe in children with longstanding, clinically demonstrable bone disease, plasma immunoreactive parathyroid hormone returns to normal much sooner following renal transplantation in children than it does in adults [326]. Observations that the incidence of renal osteodystrophy in children and adolescents is higher than that reported for adults are consistent with the fact that the normally growing and rapidly remodeling young skeleton with a high rate of osteoclastic activity (i.e., high bone turnover) is much more susceptible to the alterations in circulating parathyroid hormone, 25-OHD$_3$, 1,25(OH)$_2$D$_3$, somatomedin, etc., that are acquired during the course of progressive renal insufficiency.

There are presently a limited number of recorded observations in children regarding the effect of end-stage renal disease on circulating 25-OHD$_3$ and 1,25(OH)$_2$D$_3$, although normal, low, and high plasma 25-OHD$_3$ values have been reported for adults with renal failure [233,344] (see Fig. 28-2; Fig. 28-6), and decreased 1,25-(OH)$_2$D$_3$ has been documented when glomerular filtration rates fall below 40 to 50 milliliter per minute [50,121,170]. In one study it was noted that renal 1-hydroxylation of 25-OHD$_3$, relatively deficient in two 10-year-old uremic children with severe end-stage renal disease, returned to normal as early as eight days following successful homotransplantation [301].

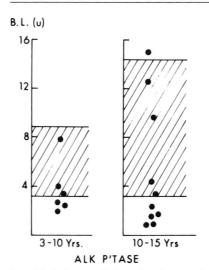

FIG. 28-5. Serum alkaline phosphatase of uremic children three to 15 years of age. Shaded areas represent normal values. (From a combination of data reported by Fine RN, Isaacson AS, Vaughn P et al: J Pediatr 80:243, 1972, with permission, and the authors' experience.)

The growing skeleton is extremely sensitive to vitamin D depletion, since the vitamin (and/or its biologically active metabolites) is essential for skeletal remodeling and endochondral bone formation at epiphyseal sites. The greater frequency with which florid azotemic rickets has been reported in the past in children from European and Asian communities [231,357] may reflect relatively lower circulating levels of 25-OHD$_3$ documented for normal individuals in these same geographical areas [311,355]. Without sunlight exposure or sufficient vitamin D intake (i.e., at least 400 IU/day), vitamin D deficiency ultimately develops in growing children. Moreover, in industrial cities with temperate climates, children may not receive sufficient exposure to ultraviolet light because of the combination of climatic conditions and atmospheric smog. Even on sunny days, smog absorbs most of the sun's short-wave ultraviolet light radiation, which is essential for the photoconversion of epidermal 7-dehydrocholesterol to vitamin D$_3$. In this regard, it should be mentioned that in North America the incidence of radiographic osteosclerosis [173] and osteitis fibrosa [326,327] is much greater than the incidence of renal rickets in uremic children.

General Pathologic Features of Uremic Bone

Despite significant differences in the pathology of adult and childhood uremic osteodystrophy, many similarities do exist. Therefore, it is appropriate to discuss the features of uremic bone disease that are common to skeletons of all ages prior to identifying lesions unique to children. Those involved in the study of uremic osteodystrophy are presently witness to the relatively simultaneous identifications of the biochemical and histopathologic lesions that characterize this group of disorders. Among the experimental

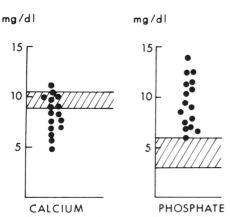

FIG. 28-4. Serum calcium and phosphate of uremic children three to 15 years of age. Shaded areas represent normal ranges. (From a combination of data reported by Fine RN, Isaacson AS, Vaughn P, et al: J. Pediatr 80:243, 1972, with permission, and the authors' experience.)

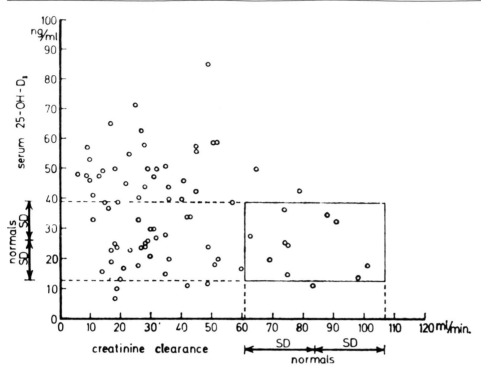

FIG. 28-6. *Serum concentrations of 25-OHD₃ in 81 nondialyzed patients with chronic renal failure.*
(From Lund B, Sorensen OH, Nielsen SP, et al: Lancet 2:372, 1975, with permission.)

studies most important in defining the biochemical abnormalities acquired by bone as the uremic state advances are those of Russell and coworkers [329–332] (Fig. 28-7), in which maturational defects of both the organic and inorganic components of uremic bone have been described. Since these studies were performed in the young growing rat, they may have particular significance as regards childhood renal osteodystrophy and its response to therapy. Furthermore, the parallel acquisition of morphologic and biochemical information has resulted in correlations of both variables in uremic bone [54]. For example, uremic bone magnesium, which characteristically is increased [33], is directly related to skeletal osteoid content [367] and most probably contributes to the mineralization defect in uremic bone [5]. In addition, in the bone of uremic patients there is an inverse relationship between skeletal osteoid and calcium [367]. These data are consistent with the observations that in chronic uremia, diminished total body calcium, as measured by neutron activation analysis, is usually associated with osteomalacia [115].

The skeletal morphology of virtually all chronically uremic patients is abnormal [177] despite normal radiographs in those with early osteodystrophy. However, the histologic spectrum of renal osteodystrophy is wide and is modified by therapeutic intervention. For example, the degree of uremic bone disease appears to be less in those patients treated with vitamin D in whom reasonable phosphate control is achieved. On the other hand, individuals with significant bone disease often have skeletal complications, including soft tissue calcification, which is often the most disabling component of their uremia [206].

Most patients have combinations of the basic histologic components of uremic bone disease, namely osteitis fibrosa, osteomalacia, and osteosclerosis. Osteoporosis, defined as a decreased mass of normally mineralized bone, is extremely unusual in chronic uremia. This is particularly true as regards younger patients, in whom an increase in bone mass usually attends progressive renal failure [57,124,173]. As osteitis fibrosa usually represents the skeletal effects of excess parathyroid hormone, it is an extremely common component of renal osteodystrophy. This condition may be radiologically diagnosed from hand films (see Fig. 28-7), in which the characteristic feature is subperiosteal resorption of the phalanges. Resorption of the calvaria, distal clavicles, and lamina dura also occurs. The histologic features of osteitis fibrosa reflect the role of parathyroid hormone as a general stimulator of bone cell activation [321,384]. There is proliferation of osteoclasts and osteoblasts (Fig. 28-8). The abundance of the bone-forming cells reflects the ability of parathyroid hormone to accelerate bone formation. As this hormone produces murine osteopetrosis, particularly in younger animals [374], its bone-stimulating properties may be responsible for the increase in bone mass and osteosclerosis commonly encountered in uremic children (Figs. 28-9, 28-10). Marrow fibrosis occurs in varying quantities in osteitis fibrosa. It probably represents bone osteoprogenitor cell activity and may be distinguished from idiopathic myelofibrosis by its peritrabecular location.

The excessive osteoid that accompanies uremic osteitis fibrosis is of questionable origin. While Sherrard and coworkers [346] attribute the hyperosteoidosis of renal osteitis

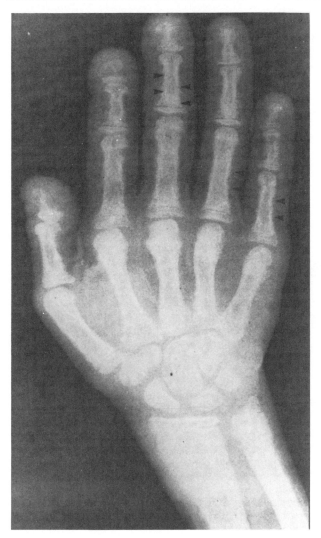

Fig. 28-7. *Subperiosteal resorption (arrows) in a 16-year-old boy with chronic renal disease. Note the extensive resorption of the distal phalangeal tufts producing pseudoclubbing of overlying soft tissue.*

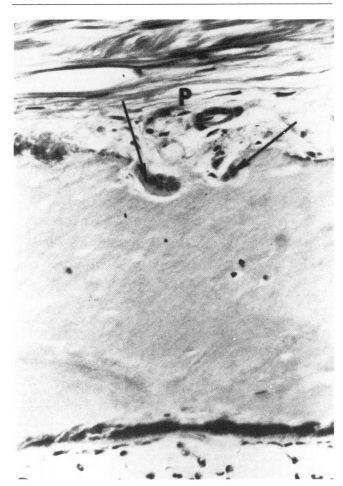

Fig. 28-8. *Subperiosteal resorption microscopically. Osteoclasts (arrows) are present in resorptive bays (Howship's lacunae) in approximation to the periosteum (P). (undecalcified, Goldner; × 100 before 9% reduction.)*

fibrosa to an absolute increase in skeletal collagen synthesis, other investigators [192,337] note a virtual universal decrease in the rate of bone formation with uremia. The excess osteoid of uremic osteodystrophy is most likely related to a mineralization defect, regardless of accompanying histopathologic manifestation.

Woven bone collagen is another characteristic feature of osteitis fibrosis in uremia (Fig. 28-11). In our experience, when woven bone collagen is in abundance it is a manifestation of relatively advanced disease. Krempien and co-workers [214,260] have demonstrated that uremic woven bone collagen represents all stages of a fluent transition from lamellar bone. Furthermore, they have found lamellar bone and woven collagen in the same bone remodeling unit, indicating that a single clone of osteoblasts is capable of synthesis of both forms of bone.

The histologic sine qua non of uremic osteomalacia is hyperosteoidosis (Fig. 28-12). One encounters both an increase in osteoid seam thickness and extent of bone surface covered by non-mineralized matrix. There is characteristically a relative paucity of osteoblasts on osteoid seams, and the osteoid-mineralized bone interface is more commonly smooth than serrated. It should be appreciated that while radiographic evidence of pseudofractures is pathognomonic of osteomalacia, this is a relatively unusual radiologic manifestation of uremic bone disease in North America. In reality, the term pseudofracture is a misnomer, as the entity represents a true fracture with no radiographic evidence of mineralized callus formation. This finding is due to the inability of the osteomalacic skeleton to mineralize reparative bone matrix.

Hyperosteoidosis per se is not pathognomonic of osteomalacia. Consequently, fluorescent tetracycline labeling is necessary to make the diagnosis with certainty [144]. The presence of increased quantities of osteoid with a decrement in the rate of mineralization, as measured by time-spaced tetracycline markers, is essential for the diagnosis of osteomalacia (Fig. 28-13). Probably due to the delay in uremia in maturation of amorphous calcium phosphate to

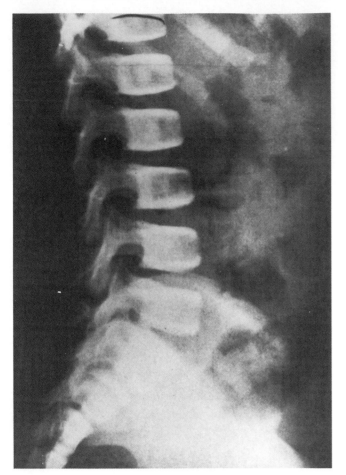

FIG. 28-9. *Vertebral osteosclerosis in a child with chronic renal disease. Note the characteristic increased density of upper and lower cortical plates separated by the less dense central portion of the vertebral process. This so called rugger-jersey sign resembles the horizontally striped shirts of Rugby football players.*

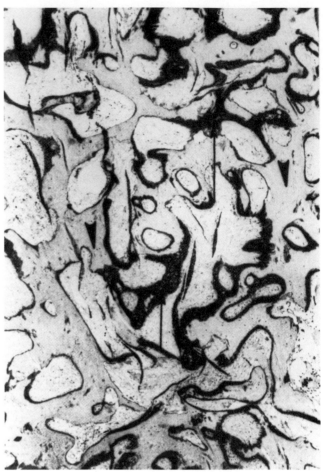

FIG. 28-10. *Histologic section of osteosclerotic uremic bone. A characteristic feature is increased mineralized bone matrix per total value of trabecular bone. Osteoid content (arrows) is also increased. (Undecalcified, Goldner; ×40.)*

its crystalline phase, a single tetracycline label is characteristically diffuse and irregular in the osteomalacic bone of uremic subjects. In addition, entire osteons often fluoresce in bone biopsies in uremic patients so labeled. Furthermore, in these patients in whom there is inhibition of bone mineral deposition, many osteoid-mineralized-bone interfaces fail to assume a tetracycline label.

Osteosclerosis, which is an increased quantity of bone matrix per unit skeletal volume, is not uncommon in uremia. The pathognomonic radiographic feature of osteosclerosis is the so-called rugger-jersey spine, which is characterized by alternating bands of increased and normal bone density. Histologically, osteosclerosis is characterized by loss of distinction between cortical and trabecular bone. This is due not only to an augmented cancellous bone mass but also to increased porosity of the cortex. The radiographic counterpart of this feature is medullary sclerosis and decreased cortical width of the phalanges of the osteosclerotic uremic patient. As the manifestations of osteitis fibrosa usually progress in tandem with osteosclerosis [104], histologic evidence of subperiosteal resorption contributes

to the increased porosity of cortical bone. In addition, extremely wide osteoid seams are common in osteosclerosis [147], usually representing associated osteomalacia. Osteosclerosis is generally a manifestation of long-standing renal disease. Its relationship to declining renal function has been documented by Malluche and coworkers [238]. As advanced uremia is usually associated with decrements in the rates of bone formation [192,337] and resorption [194], it is likely that osteosclerosis is due not to accelerated osteoblastic activity but to markedly decreased osteoclastic function.

The Specifics of Childhood Renal Osteodystrophy

All manifestations of renal osteodystrophy that occur in the adult may appear in childhood. The age at which symptoms develop is usually five to 10 years, although occasionally clinical findings are evident within the first few years of life, particularly if the child has congenital

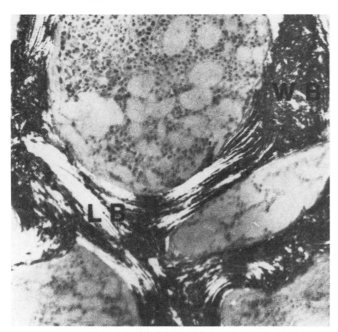

FIG. 28-11. *Bone of a uremic adult as seen under polarized light. The lamellar bone (LB) of a normal adult consists of parallel refractile collagen fibers. Woven bone (WB) reflects accelerated bone turnover and is always abnormal in the adult. The collagen fibers of woven bone are randomly arranged. (H&E, polarized; ×40.)*

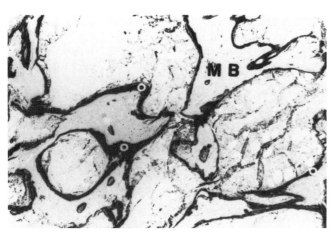

FIG. 28-12. *Uremic osteodystrophy exhibiting a predominance of osteomalacia as manifested by extensive osteoid (o) with minimal osteitis fibrosa. MB, mineralized bone. (Undecalcified, Goldner; ×40.)*

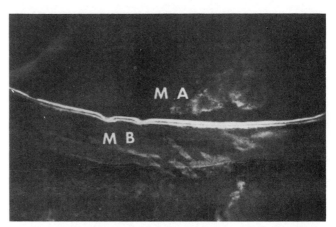

FIG. 28-13. *Time-spaced (double) fluorescent tetracycline labels in normal bone. Note the linear, smooth appearance of the fluorescent bands. MA, bone marrow; MB, mineralized bone. (Undecalcified, unstained fluorescent micrograph; ×100).*

obstructive uropathy with azotemia. Although variable in degree, inhibition of longitudinal growth occurs in the vast majority of uremic children (see Chap. 25). A variety of factors contribute to the growth arrest in these patients, including anorexia, chronic protein and calorie malnutrition, anemia, acidosis, and severe rachitic-form lesions. Another contributing factor to the short stature syndrome of uremic children is low plasma somatomedin. The relationship of this abnormality to growth failure in uremia is suggested by the correlation between increased growth velocity and rising blood somatomedin levels following renal transplantation [333]. Although radiologic evidence of rickets has been associated with severe growth retardation, severe dwarfism may occur without clinical or radiographic evidence of rickets.

Not only is skeletal growth per se inhibited by renal failure but attendant delay in bone maturation also occurs, with the retarded bone age usually reflecting the child's physiologic rather than chronologic age. The most severe examples of delayed bone maturation exist in patients in whom renal failure develops early in childhood [34]. Following variable periods of retardation, the rates of maturity characteristically parallel chronology, resulting in a constant degree of inhibited bone maturation for a given child. The acquired delay in bone maturation may in fact prove beneficial to children undergoing therapy who have significant growth potential [222]. It is unlikely that renal transplantation, for example, will result in significant growth in children with a bone age greater than 12 years, whereas it is often beneficial in patients with immature skeletons, regardless of their chronologic age [159]. This is of particular signficance, since bone age will progresss despite complete growth arrest, and it speaks for early therapeutic intervention.

Apart from those involving the epiphyseal regions, pathologic differences between adult and juvenile uremic skeletons are few. Osteosclerosis, osteoclastosis, and osteitis fibrosa are common in younger individuals [57], as is severe cancellization of the cortex [215], resulting in loss of distinction between trabecular and compact bone. Radiographic abnormalities in the region of the growth plate in childhood renal osteodystrophy (Figs. 28-14, 28-15), although occasionally presenting as those characteristically seen in nutritional rickets, may often be quite distinct. In the past, these changes have been inappropriately characterized as rachitic and were believed to be histologically indistinguishable from those of nutritional rickets [23]. The histopathology of classic rickets due to vitamin D or phos-

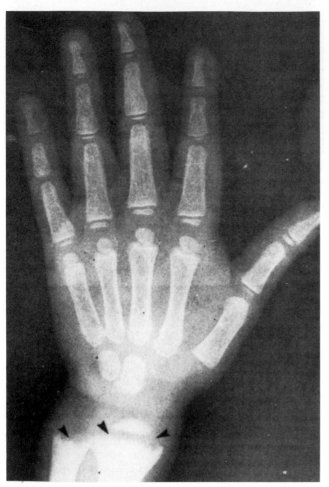

Fig. 28-14. *Epiphyseal abnormalities (arrows) in a young child with end-stage renal disease. Also note the diffuse demineralization of the metacarpals.*

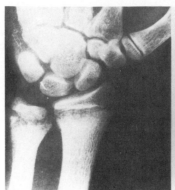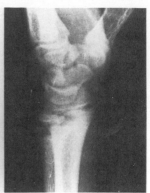

Fig. 28-15. *Slipped epiphysis in a 16-year-old boy with juvenile nephronophthisis and a serum creatinine of 7.8 mg per deciliter. Incipient displacement of radial epiphysis of left forearm. A. Dorsovolar view. B. Lateral view. Incipient displacement of radial epiphysis into ulnar (A) and dorsal (B) direction. There is a narrow growth plate with irregular outlines. Note the woolly, disorganized structure of upper metaphysis with large, irregularly outlined defects. There is a zone of subperiosteal resorption at the ulnar cortex and console formation at the ulnar side of the radial metaphysis. Dense, coarse trabeculae are present in the lower metaphysis. (Courtesy of Dr. E. Ritz)*

phate deficiency centers about abnormalities of the growth plate. The characteristic features include failure of chondrocytes of the zones of hypertrophy to form well-arranged columns and deficiencies in the development of the zone of provisional calcifications. As a result, the width of the growth plate increases, and its architecture becomes disarrayed. However, despite the failure of mineralization of the devitalized cartilage bordering on the metaphysis, woven bone collagen is deposited on these cores, resulting in formation of primary spongiosa and its cartilaginous cores. There is failure of modeling, and the cartilage persists within the deep metaphyseal bone. These phenomena result in the radiographic changes of a wide, overriding epiphysis with an irregular border and absence of a line of provisional calcification. Despite radiograph similarities to the rachitic epiphysis, the uremic growth plate, in contrast, is generally not increased in longitudinal width and is actually focally narrow [253] (see Figs. 28-14, 28-15). However, its horizontal diameter is generally expanded, contributing to overriding of the lateral border of the metaphysis. Full-thickness rupture of the growth plate may also occur [215].

Histologically, the chondrocytes of the uremic epiphyseal plate are arranged in grape-like clusters, and their longitudinal orientation is lost [215]. The disarrayed cartilage is reabsorbed and therefore does not function as a lattice on which bone is deposited. The attendant hyperparathyroidism also results in metaphyseal fibrosis immediately beneath the growth plate, which has been postulated by Krempien and coworkers to interfere with vascular invasion of the epiphyseal cartilage and hence its normal maturation [215]. As such, in the uremic child there is failure of development of the primary spongiosa. The formation of metaphyseal trabeculae occurs in a dysplastic fashion as spicules of woven osteoid within the subepiphyseal fibrous tissue. This area is radiolucent and is usually misinterpreted as representing the increased growth plate width characteristic of vitamin-D-deficiency rickets or so-called "renal rickets."

In some patients a bony "disk" develops between the epiphyseal plate and metaphysis, resulting in growth arrest [215]. As a result of these changes, there is loss of an interlocking connection between the growth plate and metaphyseal bone. These metaphyseal lesions form the basis for the increased incidence of genu valgum and the slipped epiphysis syndrome [215] in children and adolescents with chronic renal disease. These skeletal deformities are generally more severe in children with renal, rather than nutritional rickets, as the former are usually older and hence heavier and more ambulatory. Genu valgum and slipped femoral capital epiphyses that result from hyperparathyroid erosion of bone are also relatively more common in adolescents (i.e., 12 to 16 years of age) and seem to be precipitated by puberty. Of note in this regard are observations documenting severe secondary hyperparathyroidism in growing children with endemic genu valgum [351].

The availability of long-term maintenance hemodialysis in children has resulted in an increasing number of individuals with renal osteodystrophy [133,310,387]. Controversy exists, however, as to how dialysis per se influences the course of uremic bone disease. For example, although there is poor growth of adolescents on hemodialysis [32], there are also reports of the salutory effects of dialysis on the course of their skeletal lesions [104,323], even in the absence of supplemental vitamin D therapy [137]. Of particular significance is the markedly reduced incidence of slipped capital femoral epiphyses in dialyzed compared to nondialyzed uremic children and the markedly beneficial effect dialysis may have on the rachitic-like lesions. The variability of the influence of dialysis on the skeleton may reflect differences in therapeutic approach. Factors such as heparin; duration and frequency of hemodialysis; as well as dialysate magnesium, calcium, and fluoride concentrations; dietary phosphate control; and the dosage of vitamin D may all influence the course of bone disease. In addition, in some instances dialysis may reduce skeletal resistance to parathyroid hormone and as such stimulate the development of osteitis fibrosis [40,245,286].

Soft Tissue Calcification

Similar to their adult counterparts, children with renal failure develop extraosseous calcification. When extensive, this complication may be the most disabling component of the uremic syndrome. Furthermore, as maintenance hemodialysis has become available to children and resulted in increased longevity of those with end-stage renal disease, soft tissue and periarticular calcification are becoming increasingly common.

Extraskeletal mineralization in general is either metastatic or dystrophic. Metastatic calcification is the result of systemic alterations that predispose toward deposition of mineral in extraskeletal sites. In uremia, these predisposing factors include elevation of the circulating Ca X P product [206,300] and perhaps hypermagnesemia [106] and pyrophosphatemia [6,7,113]. On the other hand, dystrophic calcification reflects the influence of local alterations such as tissue necrosis. Since hypertension commonly attends uremia, vascular mineralization may be a form of dystrophic calcification, as may renal tubular calcification or nephrocalcinosis.

The frequency of specific organ system involvement by soft tissue mineralization in uremic children is probably similar to that occurring in adults, except perhaps there is a greater frequency of tumoral calcification in younger patients. The most commonly involved site is the vascular system, specifically the media [206,294]. Because of the nonluminal distribution of the mineral deposits, vascular compromise and dense gangrene are unusual [143]. On the other hand, advanced vascular calcification may result in difficulty in preparation of dialysis shunts. Furthermore, arterial calcification is more likely than other forms of extraskeletal mineralization to be refractory to therapeutic subtotal parathyroidectomy [120]. The lung [167] is another site of uremic soft tissue calcification, especially in adolescents with severe bone disease [120]. Corneal calcification may be appreciated by slit lamp examination, and

when severe, grossly apparent band keratopathy develops. Conjunctival calcification may become clinically evident with injection and tearing (red eye syndrome). Articular chondrocalcinosis and calcific periarthritis often result in skeletal disability. In some children, acute synovitis may often mimic the clinical gout syndrome of adults. Dermal calcification, which is often associated with agonizing intractable pruritis, does on occasion respond to subtotal parathyroidectomy [206] or low-phosphate dietary regimens.

Due to its general clinical quiescence until relatively advanced, the true incidence of visceral calcification in uremia is not appreciated. When clinical manifestations of pulmonary or myocardial mineralization occur, the prognosis is guarded, and respiratory insufficiency, cardiac arrhythmias, or both may occur. Often, a major concern is evidence of nephrocalcinosis in the child with early renal failure, because progression of this lesion may hasten the need for dialytic intervention. This is currently of particular significance because renal homotransplantation and therapy with the newly synthesized analogues of vitamin D, which hold great promise for the treatment of renal osteodystrophy, may result in hypercalcemia and potentially exaggerate preexisting nephrocalcinosis. However, despite the higher incidence of osteitis fibrosa in children and the liberal use of vitamin D when compared to adult uremic populations, the overall incidence of metastatic calcification appears to be low in the pediatric population.

Specific Features Requiring Therapy

Growth retardation is one of the principal consequences of renal insufficiency in children, occurring before and during dialysis (Table 28-1). Impairment of renal function during infancy or early in life appears to have a more deleterious effect on linear growth than does its development at an older age [3,231]. Growth failure is often present despite the absence of overt skeletal deformities, and a decrease in growth velocity rate may be found in children whose glomerular filtration rate (GFR) has only fallen to $25 \text{ ml/min}/1.73\text{m}^2$ [221]. Several factors are classically felt to cause this retarded growth: malnutrition [71], secondary to anorexia and chronic protein and calorie deficiencies; chronic metabolic acidosis [245,256]; impaired intestinal absorption of calcium [101,102]; somatomedin deficiency [333,334]; and osteodystrophy [257]. Fully 30% to 50% of children with "preterminal" renal failure have abnormally low growth velocity rates [259]. Hemodialysis and chronic

TABLE 28-1. *Characteristics of childhood renal osteodystrophy*

Growth retardation
Epiphyseal slipping
Pathologic fractures
Bone pain
Skeletal deformities
Myopathy
Osteomalacia in transplantation
Aluminum-related osteomalacia
Sharp angled bowing of extremities

peritoneal dialysis does not seem to improve the abnormalities of growth [176,210].

Epiphyseal slipping is the most dramatic and probably the most crippling manifestation of renal osteodystrophy on the growing skeleton [257]. Slippage was present in 10 of 33 (30%) non-dialyzed uremic children and in one of 82 undergoing dialysis. It is a late manifestation and clearly is more frequent in children with congenital forms of renal disease, who experience a longer duration of their renal failure. Hyperparathyroidism and hypocalcemia define these children [236]. In adolescents, the rate of epiphyseal slipping may accelerate after the onset of puberty [150]. The pattern of slipping of the epiphyses is age-related, with upper and lower femoral epiphyseal slipping in young children and upper femoral and/or radial and ulnar epiphyses in school-age children.

Older adolescent patients show forearm epiphyseal involvement. Gross skeletal deformities and impaired ambulation are frequent. Pathologic fractures appear to occur more frequently in patients with osteomalacia than in children with pure osteitis fibrosa cystica and may occur after seizures. However, fractures are still less frequent than in adults [257]. These fractures need to be distinguished from Looser's zones (pseudofractures). The stresses of weight bearing coupled with vitamin D deficiency can cause Looser's zones to extend across the full width of the bone and form a true fracture. These fractures tend to heal slowly, particularly if vitamin D deficiency goes untreated.

Bone pain can develop and progress slowly until the patient becomes nonambulatory. The type of bone histologic lesion does not influence the development of pain. This pain is often vague and may be located in the lower back, hips, legs, or knees. Frequently, it may suggest acute arthritis. In dialysis patients, with a predominance of osteomalacia, pain is sometimes restricted to the axial skeleton, with numerous fractures of the ribs; rib tenderness is a typical physical sign [386]. This syndrome is particularly prominent in the aluminum burdened patient [382]. Indeed, the incidence of aluminum burden disease may be as high as 20% to 30% of children on dialysis [262].

The skeletal features of advanced nutritional rickets, rosary ribs, Harrison's groove, and knob-like enlargement of the wrists and ankles, are present in small children with renal insufficiency, but the bizarre bowing of the diaphysis of long bones is usually not found since skeletal deformities of the extremities occur at the metaphysis. Unless renal failure develops during the first year of life, craniotabes and bossing do not occur.

Childhood osteodystrophy is often associated with a myopathy that characteristically affects proximal muscle groups [236] (see Table 28-1). Myopathic children present with difficulties in climbing stairs or rising from a sitting position and they develop a waddling gait. This uremic myopathy is indistinguishable from that evident in nutritional vitamin D deficiency or as the result of other causes [80,340]. This myopathy is often improved after treatment with various vitamin D analogs.

Although renal transplantation usually results in a gradual and steady improvement in renal bone disease, hypophosphatemic osteomalacia has been found since body phosphate stores can become depleted because of (1) the use of antacids, (2) hyperphosphaturia due to residual para-thyroid hyperplasia or to glucocorticoid induced phosphaturia, or (3) an acquired tubular phosphate leak that is independent of parathyroid hormone (PTH) [269]. Further, the prolonged use of glucocorticoids appears to result in a progressive decline in bone mineral content, as measured by single beam photon absorptiometry [83].

Role of Phosphate Retention

Hyperphosphatemia appears to play a pivotal role in the development and maintenance of secondary hyperparathyroidism in uremia by influencing the plasma concentrations of ionized calcium. Phosphate retention can be clearly demonstrated after the GFR declines by 70% to 80% [205]. Slatopolsky et al. [352] have postulated that there may be transient but imperceptible increases in serum phosphate levels early in renal failure, which could be responsible for a decreased ionized calcium level and enhanced secretion of PTH. Considerable evidence from clinical studies has shown that even in early uremia an intolerance to oral phosphate load occurs, which usually produces a prolonged hyperphosphatemia with subsequent elevation of iPTH levels [205]. The postulated role of phosphate retention in young children, who are hyperphosphatemic relative to adults under normal circumstances, has not been shown by clinical studies. In addition, hyperphosphatemia theoretically will reduce the rate of conversion of 25-hydroxyvitamin D_3 to 1,25-dihydroxyvitamin D_3 [87,362]. The low $1,25(OH)_2D_3$ may lead to the skeletal resistance to the action of PTH. Recent evidence from Portale et al. [308] suggests that phosphate retention at a GFR of 30–50 ml/$1.75m^2$ will impair $1,25(OH)_2D_3$ synthesis.

Experimental studies show that the restriction of dietary phosphorus in uremic dogs in proportion to the reduction in GFR prevents the occurrence of secondary hyperparathyroidism [352]. In adults, Maschio et al. [243] and Llach et al. [228] have shown that early dietary phosphate restriction was associated with a decrease in PTH levels and some amelioration of the bone disease.

Phosphate intake largely depends on dietary content of meat, legumes, soft drinks, and dairy products. In mild renal insufficiency, the dietary phosphorus intake can be reduced by about 50% to 60% by strict adherence to low-protein diets [211]. However, as renal failure becomes more advanced the use of phosphate-binding gels becomes mandatory to maintain a serum phosphate between 4.0 and 5.0 mg/dl. The aluminum-containing compounds employed to bind phosphorus in the gastrointestinal tract include aluminum hydroxide and aluminum carbonate. These agents are available in liquid, capsule, or tablet form. Magnesium-containing antacids are not usually recommended since hypermagnesemia often develops in renal insufficiency, even without the ingestion of these magnesium-containing compounds.

Restriction of phosphate is indicated not only since it causes hypocalcemia and secondary hyperparathyroidism but also since the rate of decline in renal function may be influenced by hyperphosphatemia [243]. This rapid decline in renal function may relate to intrarenal calcium phosphate precipitates [190]. In an uncontrolled study in adults with moderate renal insufficiency, the decline in renal function was forestalled by dietary phosphate (and protein) restriction [190,269].

At least five important factors severely limit the ability of a physician to strictly reduce the intake of phosphate: (1) the fear of hypophosphatemic osteomalacia; (2) important concerns over dietary protein restriction in growing children; (3) the pervasiveness of dairy products in the diet of children; (4) concerns about the aluminum content of most binding agents [262]; and (5) the use of vitamin D analogs that enhance gastrointestinal phosphate absorption [4,9,10,25,79,180,310,339]. Each of these items is discussed separately.

It is important to avoid reducing the serum phosphate to subnormal levels to prevent depletion. The resulting hypophosphatemia is associated with anorexia, weakness, bone pain, and osteomalacia [230].

Reduction of dietary protein to the levels used in adults undergoing hemodialysis severely limits growth [132,158]. Although the level of protein intake needed to permit optimal growth has not been established, levels as high as 2.5 g/kg/24 hr have been suggested, particularly in children undergoing chronic ambulatory peritoneal dialysis [132]. Children with chronic renal insufficiency due to congenital obstructive uropathy and/or renal dysplasia or hypoplasia frequently are salt cravers [79]. Dairy products such as milk, cheese, and yogurt appear to be preferred foods in these children, and parents are frequently loathe to limit the intake of dairy products.

Aluminum hydroxide has numerous side effects. Most patients experience constipation, and many report nausea and vomiting after ingesting this compound, making compliance difficult. Furthermore, there is mounting evidence that aluminum, previously felt to be impermanent in the intestine, can be absorbed by the gut [4]. Increased tissue concentrations of aluminum have been described in patients with encephalopathy and renal osteodystrophy [25], and aluminum toxicity is discussed below. Guillot et al. [160] suggest the use of magnesium-containing phosphate binders in uremic patients on hemodialysis in addition to aluminum-containing gels to control hyperphosphatemia, as long as the serum magnesium concentration is maintained below 4.5 mEq/L.

Special attention should be paid to the effect of the administration of vitamin D analogs in renal insufficiency. These compounds increase not only the intestinal absorption of calcium but also of phosphorus [377], thus increasing the serum phosphate. Their use of the hyperphosphatemia may be hazardous because of concerns over metastatic calcifications and the worsening of secondary hyperparathyroidism. By contrast $1,25(OH)_2D_3$ or other active metabolites may suppress directly secondary hyperparathyroidism, thus reducing bone resorption, permitting mineral deposition into osteoid, and leading to healing of osteomalacia (see below). Thus, one may actually find a fall in serum phosphorus and a decreased need for phosphate binders during the first months of treatment.

ALUMINUM TOXICITY

Acute aluminum toxicity has been recognized in human beings since the 1920s, but its peculiar hazard to the individual with reduced renal function has been appreciated

for less than two decades [4]. The studies of Coburn's group have shown that in addition to dialysis dementia [101–103], chronic aluminum use is associated with a form of bone disease that has a predilection for the axial skeleton—ribs, vertebrae, and hips [178,311]. Bone histologic analysis reveals aluminum both by specific stains [178,387] and by direct analysis [112]. A similar form of crippling bone disease has been experienced in patients on long-term total parenteral nutrition (TPN) who have aluminum contamination of the solutions that are infused [207]. In both dialysis-induced and TPN-induced disease, little evidence for osteitis is present, and osteomalacia with low bone turnover rates is evident [379,381].

Since the kidneys are responsible for the excretion of aluminum, renal functional impairment is associated with aluminum retention. Hence, any aluminum that is absorbed cannot be adequately excreted, and this metal appears to be deposited in bone and other tissue-bound sites [293,296]. Although aluminum contamination of hemodialysis solutions appeared to be a major cause of both dialysis dementia and osteomalacic bone disease in certain units in Canada, South Africa, the United States, and the United Kingdom [267,312,378], aluminum-induced bone disease is common in children who have never undergone hemodialysis or peritoneal dialysis [9,10,341]. Hence the notion that a water-borne agent is responsible for this bone disease [4] is incorrect, and one can invoke aluminum containing antacids as the main etiologic factor [9,10, 128,341]. Several studies in children have strongly led to the suggestion, which remains as yet unproved, that the intestine of infants and younger children may be more permeable to oral aluminum and that younger children are at greater risk for aluminum-induced encephalopathy and bone disease [25,136,157,278]. At present, the prevalence of aluminum-induced bone disease is unknown, particularly since factors such as compliance with antacid therapy, duration, dose, and frequency are variable [303].

The pathogenesis of aluminum-induced bone disease is uncertain, despite the finding of higher serum and bone aluminum values. Aluminum staining of bone is common in osteomalacic forms of renal osteodystrophy, and bone opposition rate appears to be low [292]. The aluminum is often, but not always, found at the interface of osteoid and mineralized bone [112,341]. These observations suggest that aluminum may directly impair the process of mineralization. An alternative and equally plausible hypothesis is that the deficiency of PTH found in aluminum-burdened patients contributes to low bone turnover osteomalacia [213,324]. A hypocalcemic stimulus in patients with dialysis osteomalacia is not followed by the usual rise in iPTH values [213]. An alternative hypothesis indicates that circulating PTH may actually enhance intestinal aluminum absorption [252]. This enhancement of aluminum absorption also appears to result in increased bone, brain, and gray matter aluminum levels. To further confuse this issue, aluminum may impair the basal and isoproterenol-stimulated values of cyclic AMP in cultured bovine parathyroid gland cells [252]. In adult patients with renal osteodystrophy, an inverse correlation between serum iPTH and bone aluminum can be found [179]. The accepted pathogenic sequence would involve PTH-induced absorption of aluminum with moderate renal failure, followed by a decline in PTH secretion as whole body aluminum increases, with the ultimate finding of low PTH, low bone turnover rate osteomalacia [262]. Those patients with advanced dialysis osteomalacia [181], who are easily recognized, clearly have diminished PTH secretion, but little is known about the early stages of this disorder.

Finally, aluminum may induce changes in vitamin D metabolism [152]. The short-term infusion of aluminum into dogs reduces bone formation, impairs PTH secretion, and results in lower $1,25(OH)_2D$ concentrations. As indicated previously, chronic TPN therapy can be associated with osteomalacia, reduced iPTH levels, and low levels of $1,25(OH)_2$ vitamin D [208] in general, in both man and animals, aluminum does not alter the serum values for $25(OH)$ vitamin D or $24,25(OH)_2$ vitamin D [69,208]. Studies of full vitamin D metabolite profiles in aluminum-burdened children are currently lacking.

Regardless of pathogenesis, three approaches can be taken to avoid aluminum-induced osteopenia. First, reverse osmosis is mandatory to avoid aluminum contamination of dialysate [4,25]. Second, aluminum-containing phosphate binding agents should be used with great caution, aiming at a maximal dose of 30 to 50 milligrams aluminum hydroxide kg/day [84]. The reports of extremely high aluminum levels in bone and plasma associated with oral aluminum hydroxide preparations are coincident with aluminum hydroxide intake levels exceeding 100 mg/kg/day [9,10,136,157,336,341]. It has been shown that calcium carbonate ($CaCO_3$) can function as an effective gut phosphate binding agent in children, whereas studies demonstrate its efficacy in preventing hyperphosphatemia [335]. The doses of calcium carbonate required to block phosphate absorption may be associated with hypercalcemia and

may be impossible to use if children are also receiving vitamin D analogs. Calcium carbonate should be ingested with meals [336]. Finally, aluminum can be removed from bone, with improvement in bone histologic status after treatment with the chelating agent desferrioxamine (DFO) [48]. Preliminary studies in children indicate the DFO at a dose of 40 mg/kg may enhance aluminum removal from tissue and loss into dialysate [335]. With a fuller appreciation of the problem of aluminum in uremic children, ongoing research may indicate a more effective means of preventing hyperphosphatemia [336].

Vitamin D Analogs

Abnormalities of mineral homeostasis resulting in crippling bone disease are frequent manifestations of renal insufficiency in childhood. Central to the occurrence of renal osteodystrophy is the failure of vitamin D, in usual doses, to prevent the hypocalcemia, osteopenia, and secondary hyperparathyroidism in patients with advanced renal insufficiency [19,232]. Resistance to vitamin D is indicated by intestinal malabsorption of calcium [103] (Fig. 28-16), by reduced total body calcium [115], and by a diminution of bone mineral content of the long bones and the spine [92,253]. Intestinal calcium absorption can be enhanced by the administration of vitamin D_2 (a plant product) [310], vitamin D_3 (a mammalian product) [232], or by the synthetic vitamin D analog, dihydrotachysterol (DHT) [108,109,110,117,226], at doses that would ordinarily induce hypercalcemia and hypercalciuria in healthy individuals. An explanation of this vitamin D resistance as evidenced by calcium malabsorption and by negative calcium

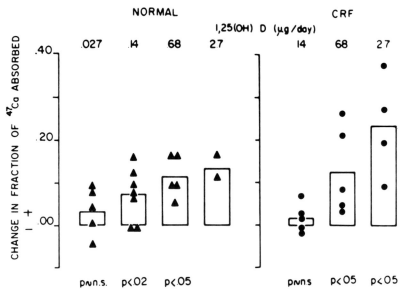

FIG. 28-16. *Changes in the fraction of 47Ca absorbed in individual subjects after the early administration of varied quantities of $1,25(OH)_2D_3$ for 6 to 7 days. Each symbol represents a separate subject. The heights of the columns indicate mean values. p values indicate significant changes from control. CRF, chronic renal failure. (From Brickman AS, et al: Ann Intern Med 80:161, 1974, with permission.)*

balance, despite normal serum antirachitic activity [19,232] comes from the almost simultaneous discovery by Fraser and Kodicek [143]; Norman et al. [283] and Gray, Boyle, and DeLuca [153] that the kidney is the site for the synthesis of the most active metabolite of vitamin D in terms of intestinal calcium absorption—1,25 dihydroxyvitamin D or $1,25(OH)_2D$ [114].

This vitamin D metabolite is not ordinarily detected in the blood of anephric patients [83,114]. The provision of only a fraction of a microgram of $1,25(OH)_2D$ increases serum calcium concentration and intestinal calcium absorption and decreases fecal calcium [46], thus strongly suggesting that "defective renal production of $1,25(OH)_2D$ in uremia" accounts for the "vitamin D resistance of uremia" [47]. It is also possible to show that serum $1,25(OH)_2D$ values are significantly lower with advanced renal failure in both adults [99,121,122,171,245,287,345, 353] and children [86,245]. At clearance values less than 50 ml/min corrected for surface area, a significant inverse relationship is found between creatinine or insulin clearance and serum $1,25(OH)_2D$ concentrations [86,99,197, 309] (Fig. 28-17). Reduced values of serum $1,25(OH)_2D$ are evident in patients with clearance values between 20

and 50 $ml/min/1.73m^2$ [7,309] (Fig. 28-18). In addition, the age-related variations in serum $1,25(OH)_2D$ values, being elevated in infancy and in adolescence, are not perceived in uremic children [86,96,197,309].

Renal tissue is also the major location of the synthesis of another metabolite of vitamin D, termed 24,25-dihydroxyvitamin D or $24,25(OH)_2D$ [114,171]. The potential therapeutic value of this metabolite is assessed below (Table 28-2), but the serum concentrations of this compound are reduced in uremic or anephric human beings [86,197,220,287,309,345]. The circulating value of $24,25(OH)_2D$ in children is 1–4 ng/ml of sera in comparison to a value for $1,25(OH)_2D$ of 20–80 pg/ml, the latter being roughly 10% of the former on a weight per weight basis [47,86]. The values for $24,25(OH)_2D$ and $1,25(OH)_2D$ in uremic children with a clearance under 15 $ml/min/1.73m^2$ is 0.6 ng/ml and 10 pg/ml, respectively [245,309]. The main circulating form of vitamin D in man is 25-hydroxyvitamin D or 25(OH)D [114,171]: it circulates at 20–60 ng/ml in children from North America and somewhat lower in European and British children [77]. The concentration of this metabolite is usually normal in uremic children [86,221], indicating the 25(OH)D defi-

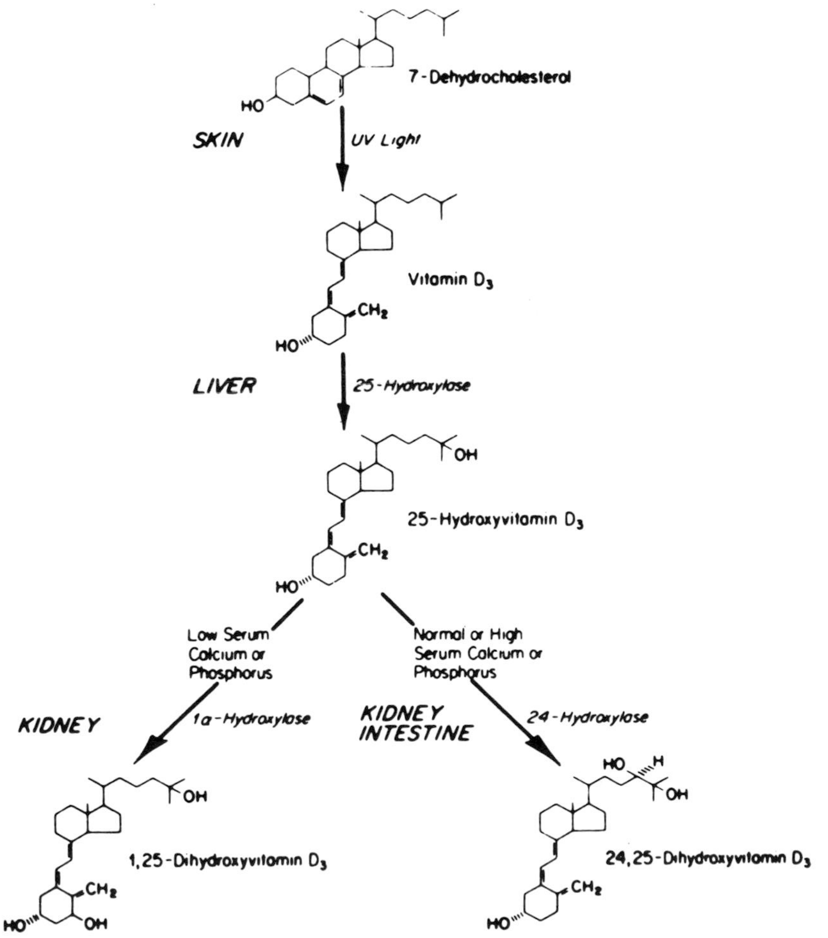

FIG. 28-17. *Vitamin D metabolism in man. (From Kumar R, Riggs, BL: Vitamin D in the therapy of disorders of calcium and phosphorus metabolism. Mayo Clin Proc 56:327, 1981.)*

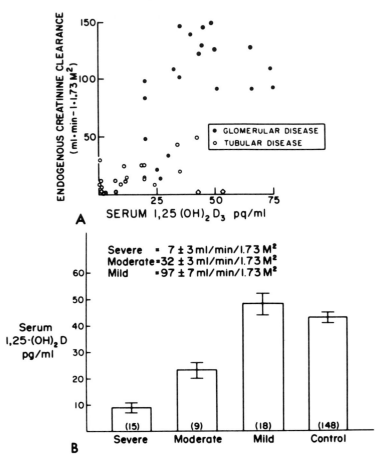

FIG. 28-18. A, Serum 1,25(OH)$_2$D vs. endogenous creatinine clearance. Note prevalence of tubulointerstitial disease in children with a clearance of less than 50 ml/min/1.73 M^2. B, Serum 1,25(OH)$_2$D values at several levels of renal function.

ciency is not usually evident in renal osteodystrophy and that the considerable alterations in bone and mineral homeostasis described previously in this chapter occur despite normal 25(OH)$_2$D values in the serum [18,75].

Therapy of childhood uremic osteodystrophy is focused at the provision of sufficient doses of whichever vitamin D analog is used to heal bone disease and, yet, still be safe. Hypercalcemia, hypercalciuria and the reduction in renal function that is evident with hypervitamin D should be a major concern [57]. Numerous clinical trials have clearly shown that no analog of vitamin D is safe if the potential for hypercalcemia is forgotten and if serum calcium values are not frequently evaluated [248,262,282].

This section reviews some of the recent studies that have evaluated the administration of the seven principal vitamin D analogs to uremic children: the natural vitamin D analogs, vitamin D$_2$ or ergocalciferol; vitamin D$_3$ or cholecalciferol; 25(OH)D or calcifediol; 1,25(OH)$_2$D or calcitriol; 24,25(OH)$_2$D, and the synthetic analogs DHT and 1-hydroxyvitamin D, or "1-alpha," [79,81] (Fig. 28-19).

Several general comments are in order. Unfortunately, most therapeutic trials in children are uncontrolled, and the vitamin D status of children prior to treatment is often not indicated. Few studies comparing the various vitamin

D analogs against one another have been reported, particularly with random selection of patients. No published reports on the therapeutic use of 24, 25(OH)$_2$D in children have appeared. Many studies are short-term, leaving the long-term effects of these agents unevaluated. Accordingly, it is difficult to clearly ascertain that any single vitamin D analog is superior in terms of its therapeutic efficacy, particularly when appropriate doses of the D analogs are given. However, since the kidney produces the most active vitamin D metabolite—1,25(OH)$_2$D—and because the serum concentrations of this metabolite are so clearly reduced in uremia despite concomitant hypocalcemia and elevated iPTH concentrations, there exists a rational basis for the use of 1,25(OH)$_2$D and the other 1-alpha-like agents—1α(OH)D and dihydrotachysterol (DHT)—in the correction of the derangements of relevant mineral metabolism and of bone [249,261].

Vitamin D

Since vitamins D$_2$ and D$_3$ are not converted to 1,25(OH)$_2$D [113], they must be given in fairly massive doses to overcome the resistance to vitamin D action found

TABLE 28-2. *Review of studies describing the role of 24,25(OH)$_2$D in renal osteodystrophy*

1. Made predominantly in kidney, thus reduced levels in uremia (0.7 vs. 3–4 ng/ml) [345].
2. Produced in cartilage and calvaria of *rats* [146].
3. Promotes normal ossification of bone when calcium and phosphate are supersaturated in bone ECF in *chicks* [291].
4. Reduces iPTH secretion in *dogs* when given IV or PO [58].
5. Blunts PTH resorption of bone in vitro in *rats* [223].
6. In uremic *human beings* [201]:
   a. Increases CA^{2+} absorption
   b. No rise in serum Ca^{2+}
   c. Suggests deposition in bone
7. Reversal of "skeletal resistance to PTH" in uremic human beings by 1,25 and 24,25 [248].
8. Combination of 25 and 1,25 or 24,25 and 1,25 best heals osteomalacia in human beings [319].
9. PTH is not always suppressed using 24,25(OH)$_2$D [353].
10. Difluoro-24,25(OH)$_2$D acts the same as 25(OH)D, casting doubts on the role of 24,25(OH)$_2$D [114].
11. Inconsistent results in clinical trials [126,273].

Conclusion: Unique biologic role unclear, but may be useful in combination with 1,25. Normal human beings have 25 to 24,25 to 1,25 in 1000/100/1 ratio, and uremia changes this relationship.

See text for large body of negative results.

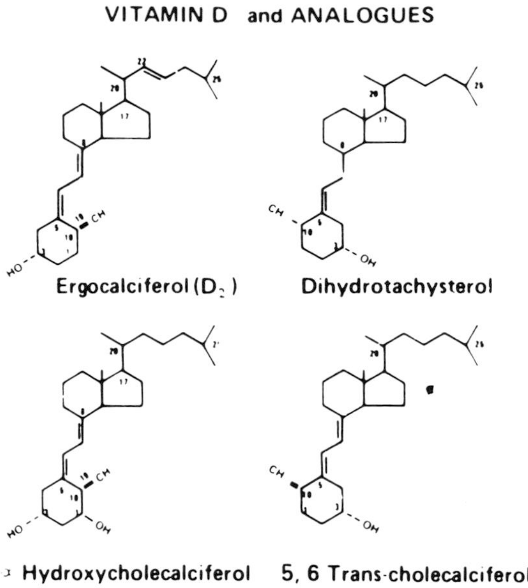

VITAMIN D and ANALOGUES

Ergocalciferol (D$_2$)   Dihydrotachysterol

1 α Hydroxycholecalciferol   5, 6 Trans-cholecalciferol

FIG. 28-19. *The structure of several vitamin D analogs including DHT. The 3β-OH group on the A-ring can rotate to form a 1α-hydroxyl group. (From Root AW, Harrison HE: Recent advances in calcium metabolism. J Pediatr 88:1, 1982.*

in uremia [92,103,115,232,310,373]. Potter et al. [310] employed vitamin D$_2$ at doses ranging from 32,000 to 57,000 IU (800–1425 μg) daily in six patients and demonstrated radiologic healing of bone lesions in three patients and hypercalcemia lasting from one to five weeks postcessation of vitamin D and conjunctival calcification in three patients each. Skin calcification did not appear to be increased. Bulla et al. [52], in a multicenter, carefully controlled study of children on hemodialysis in West Germany, employing both vitamin D$_3$ and 1,25(OH)$_2$D, reported a normalization of serum calcium, a reduction of iPTH values and reversal of osteitis fibrosa cystica with vitamin D$_3$ therapy at 10,000 to 50,000 IU (250–1250 μg) daily. The latency period, after vitamin D$_3$ administration, was no longer than after 1,25(OH)$_2$D, and when hypercalcemia occurred, it persisted significantly longer after cessation of vitamin D$_3$ after using the 1α-hydroxylated analog. In these patients, serum 25(OH)D values increased from 15 ± 6 ng/ml to a level of 100 to 300 ng/ml after beginning vitamin D$_3$ therapy. The studies of Bouillon et al. [43] also demonstrated an increase in serum calcium concentration and a fall in PTH values after vitamin D$_3$ treatment at 20,000–240,000 U/day.

As outlined in a recent review [373] and in a recent study by Hodson et al. [183] that examined bone histology before and after treatments, high dose vitamin D$_2$ can be used to effectively heal a large proportion of cases of bone disease. The main advantage of the use of these precursor metabolites is their low cost. Factors against their use are uncertainty of dose, slow onset of action, long biologic half-life, and the finding that hypercalcemia may persist for weeks to months, since these precursors are stored in fat and slowly released [114]. In addition, Bulla et al. [52] did not find healing of the endosteal osteomalacia found

in some bone biopsies, whereas more patients did respond to 1,25(OH)$_2$D. Vitamin D$_3$ is not an approved drug in the United States, despite the fact that the dairy industry often uses this metabolite to supplement milk at 400 IU (10 μg) per quart. These analogs should be used sparingly in treating uremic osteodystrophy for the reason given. However, they are generally useful in disorders of vitamin D in which renal function is normal such as nutritional rickets and anticonvulsant rickets [78].

25-Hydroxyvitamin D

Produced by the liver [113], 25-hydroxyvitamin D has been used in three trials in children [63,235,387]. A dose of 1–2 ng/kg/day has been shown to be effective in reversing hypocalcemia, in reducing PTH levels, in increasing linear growth, and promoting bone-healing, as demonstrated by improvement in histologic evidence of both endosteal osteomalacia and osteitis fibrosa and x-ray appearance [26,63,235]. Serum 25(OH)D concentrations of more than 250 ng/ml have been obtained using a mean dose of 1.6 ng/kg [83,221], and it is established that 25(OH)D is not metabolized to 1,25(OH)$_2$D in the patients, [83,106,197] (see Fig. 28-18).

This metabolite is not stored in fat to any extent and, thus its half-life is quite short, being 14 to 16 days [107]. The fact that 25(OH)D itself improves bone disease, and is not dependent on conversion to 1,25(OH)$_2$D, demonstrates that this analog in pharmacologic doses can improve calcium balance even in anephric man [63,67]. Although far more studies have been reported in adults—including studies comparing 25(OH)D with 1,25(OH)$_2$D [138], the available studies in children indicate improvement in osteomalacia, as well as in osteitis fibrosa [26,221,235,387]. However, as with all metabolites, neither osteomalacia nor osteitis fibrosa are completely healed in each patient. In one study an increase in growth velocity was reported, but no catch up growth was found [221].

Reports from France have reported a high incidence in osteomalacia in patients with uremic osteodystrophy [107,138,140,387], which possibly reflects the relatively low circulating 25(OH)D values found in individuals from Western Europe. It may be wise to employ 25(OH)D in patients living in Europe if these patients have any indication of 25(OH)D deficiency [245].

One benefit of 25(OH)D therapy that we have noticed in several young children is its relatively long half-life as compared to 1,25(OH)$_2$D [74]. Thus, if a patient is poorly compliant, plasma 25(OH)D values are unlikely to be influenced by missing an occasional dose [93]. By contrast, the use of 1,25(OH)$_2$D with its short half-life of four to six hours, means that patients must take all doses to avoid vitamin D deficiency. However, since 25(OH)D has a half-life of 14 to 16 days, the resolution of hypercalcemia may require as long as four weeks [113].

Nephrotic patients lose 25(OH)D in their urine and demonstrate very low circulating levels of this metabolite [91,151,338], since vitamin D-binding protein, which has a molecular weight identical to that of albumin, is spilled into the urine in large amounts [338]. The concentration of both 1,25(OH)$_2$D and 24,25(OH)$_2$D in serum also may be reduced [91,151]. Since 25(OH)D administration raises serum 25(OH)D values in nephrotic patients [151] there may be a role for this analog in treating nephrotic children, but this has not been shown in a controlled trial.

Dihydrotachysterol

Despite a small number of studies on the use of dihydrotachysterol (DHT) in children, this synthetic agent has been used widely in the treatment and prevention of renal osteodystrophy in both children and adults and appears to have more predictable efficacy than vitamin D$_2$ or D$_3$ [373]. DHT lacks the 10-19-diene on the A-ring of the vitamin D secosterol molecule, hence the A-ring is free to rotate. In DHT, the hydroxyl group responsible for its main biologic activity is a 3β-OH that appears to rotate to form a pseudo-1α-hydroxyl group [41,172,386] (see Fig. 28-3). Absorbed DHT also undergoes a hepatic 25-hydroxylation to form 25(OH)-DHT [169]. This compound can then most probably combine with intestinal receptors to increase active transcellular calcium uptake without the necessity for further renal metabolite conversion.

The now classical studies of Liu and Chu performed in Peking, China and reported in 1943 [226] indicated that the malabsorption of calcium causing high fecal calcium content could be overcome by administration of AT-10, composed of several vitamin D metabolites of which DHT is the active component [36]. Employing crystalline DHT, Malekzadeh et al. [236] demonstrated that uremic osteodystrophy could be treated at doses of 0.125 to 1.5 mg each day. The variability in the dosage needed to reverse

hypocalcemia is much less than that for vitamin D$_2$ or D$_3$, and the onset of action is shorter than that found using either vitamin D$_2$ or 25(OH)D [296]. Cordy [107,108, 109], in several uncontrolled studies found evidence of bone histologic improvement following the use of DHT and no accelerations in the rate of deterioration of renal function.

1α-Hydroxyvitamin D and 1,25-Dihydroxyvitamin D

Since renal tissue is the site of the 1α-hydroxylation of 25(OH)D, the use of 1α-hydroxy-vitamin D metabolites to improve calcium malabsorption and treat bone disease appears logical and "physiologic" doses of these 1α-hydroxy-metabolties can be employed. In 1972, Brickman et al. [47] reported enhanced intestinal calcium absorption and correction of hypocalcemia in a study performed only three years after the discovery of the pivotal role of the kidney in the metabolism of vitamin D. Numerous studies have examined the short-term or long-term use of either 1α-(OH)D or 1,25(OH)$_2$D in the treatment of childhood uremic bone disease [24,52,65–68,85,94,97,174,203, 280,281,302,321]. All of these studies compare therapy with the 1α-hydroxy-metabolite to prior treatment with other analogs—usually vitamin D$_2$ or D$_3$ or DHT—except for the controlled study of Bulla et al. [52]. Bone histomorphometry is not usually included, but it is reported in at least seven studies [52,73,74,199,262,280,302,325]. The clinical and laboratory findings induced by 1α-(OH) vitamin D analogs in all these studies are so similar that they can be reported as a group.

Following initiation of oral 1α-(OH)D at 1–2 μg/day and 1,25(OH)$_2$D at 10–50 pg/kg/day, hypocalcemia is normalized within one to two weeks. The first noticeable change is a dramatic reversal of the myopathy of uremia and is followed by improvement in gait disturbances and bone pain.

Serum phosphate may rise since these analogs increase intestinal phosphate absorption. This hyperphosphatemia usually responds to higher doses of phosphate-binding agents. Serum immunoreactive PTH values fall, but rarely into the completely normal range [24,66,67,68,73,94,97, 174,203]. Alkaline phosphatase values usually fall into the normal range within six months, at a time when an improvement in the radiologic appearance of the bones is apparent. Of all vitamin D metabolites used, the rise in serum calcium and the fall in alkaline phosphatase occurs most rapidly when the 1α-OH metabolites are used. It is interesting that the reversal of gait disturbance, bone pain, and myopathy precedes often by weeks to months these radiologic improvements. After the serum alkaline phosphatase level and bone radiologic appearance have normalized, hypercalcemia occurs in approximately 30% to 40% of cases. Because of the short half-life of these agents [four hours for 1,25(OH)$_2$D], hypercalcemia can be rapidly reversed following cessation of these compounds for a few days [67,91,94,203,280,325]. Hypercalcemia is usually mild [<11.5 mg/dl]; however, serum calcium should be measured frequently because of the potency of the 1α-hydroxy-metabolites in terms of intestinal calcium absorption.

The potential for renal damage following use of these analogs has been emphasized [99,259], but an examination of the reciprocal to the serum creatinine concentrations, both before and after therapy, usually does not show any change in the slope of the lines [67,75,325] (Fig. 28-20). These findings suggest that there is little or no acceleration in the rate of deterioration of GFR in treated patients if hypercalcemia is avoided. A few patients in these studies may have even demonstrated improved renal function for reasons that are unclear but that may relate to reduced phosphate intake. Hypercalciuria is not usually a problem [67,75,85] (Fig. 28-21). It cannot be overemphasized that careful avoidance of hypercalcemia usually prevents a rise in serum creatinine that is typical with high calcium concentrations.

As indicated from numerous studies in adults, children with renal osteodystrophy demonstrate osteomalacia, osteitis fibrosa, or a mixed lesion [26,65,203,280,302, 325,387]. The 1α-hydroxy analogs almost always improve or heal pure osteitis fibrosa, which is biochemically shown by the reduction in iPTH and alkaline phosphatase values. The effect on osteomalacia is variable [62,325] but, in general, the osteomalacia is not completely healed. As emphasized previously [4,324,336], widened osteoid seams with evidence of aluminum deposition is an osteomalacic lesion that is very difficult to treat. Trials employing DFO have been previously mentioned [48].

Several studies have indicated a dramatic improvement in growth over the first 12 to 18 months of therapy [65,85,94,176,325] (Fig. 28-22), but other studies have failed to show this acceleration of growth [65,237]. Pre-

dialysis patients who are young appear to show this accelerated growth rate. This acceleration of growth rate is not found in all patients [67,94,325], and sustained catch-up growth probably does not occur. Furthermore, marked growth failure in conjunction with renal osteodystrophy is found mainly in patients with congenital tubulointerstitial disease and in children under the age of 2 to 3 years [94,183,221]. Hodson et al. [183] have made the important observation that older children with the same degree of histologic abnormalities may not experience growth failure. Thus the older notion that osteodystrophy equals growth failure must be seriously questioned.

The major problems encountered on using the 1α-hydroxy compounds are (1) their incredible potency in terms of calcium absorption and (2) the short half-life of the drug. The smallest currently available oral dosage form of 1,25(OH)₂D is a 0.25-μg capsule, which is almost impossible to use in infants and small children. In children who weigh up to 12 kg, this high dose may be associated with hypercalcemia and is difficult to administer, particularly since children tend not to swallow capsules. Although these capsules can be opened or dissolved in milk, this is not recommended, and the precise dose administered cannot be known with certainty. Intravenous 1,25(OH)₂D₃ is commercially available, but little has been used in children [262]. Until a drop dosage form is available, it will be difficult to treat young children with oral 1,25(OH)₂D, which is unfortunate, since children of this age may have the severest form of bone disease. The inherent problem with the short half-lives of these compounds is that poorly compliant patients may have long periods of relative vitamin D deficiency, which can be avoided using compounds with longer half-lives. In our own experience, patients who are not receiving 1α-hydroxy analogs on a routine basis

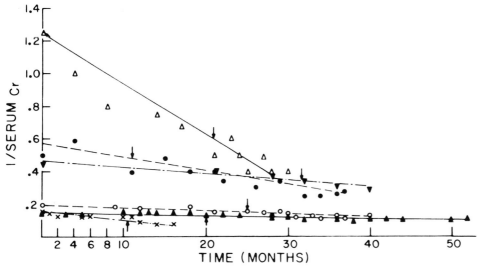

Fig. 28-20. *The reciprocal of serum creatinine (1/Scr) vs. time in six children with chronic renal failure. The arrow denotes the onset of 1,25 (OH)₂D therapy. (From Chesney RW, et al: Vitamin D metabolites in renal insufficiency and other vitamin D disorders of children. Kidney Int (suppl 15)24:563, 1983, with permission.)*

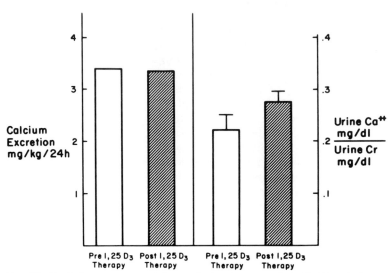

FIG. 28-21. *Calcium excretion before and after therapy with 1,25(OH)$_2$D showing no difference. (From Chesney RW, et al: Influence of long-term oral 1,25-dihydroxyvitamin D in childhood renal osteodystrophy. Contrib Nephrol 18:55, 1980, with permission.)*

appear to develop worse bone disease, which usually improves after using DHT or 25(OH)D [93,235].

The basic therapeutic strategy is to initiate 1,25(OH)$_2$D at 0.25 μg each day and to increase the dose at intervals every two weeks until normocalcemia is acheived. A twice-daily dosage schedule is logical, since the half-life of the compound is 4 to 6 hours; however, no controlled studies showing greater efficacy using this increased dosage schedule have been published.

24,25-Dihydroxyvitamin D

Recent studies in animals have raised the possibility that 24,25(OH)$_2$D may act as a mineralizing hormone [42,58, 59,78,90,147,201,202,223,227,248,291,319], but this point is not widely accepted. The evidence in support of a role for 24,25(OH)$_2$D is summarized in Table 28-2 and indicates that 24,25(OH)$_2$D decreases PTH secretion in some studies and may be important in the healing of osteomalacia of vitamin D. More recent direct information in human beings indicates that 24,25(OH)$_2$D may not be of clear benefit in terms of bone mineralization or reversal of hyperparathyroidism [289,339,347]. When a difluoro compound of vitamin D [24,25-difluoro-25(OH)D] is assessed, it has the same biologic activity as either 25(OH)D or vitamin D$_3$ [288,289,339,347]. This shows that vitamin D compounds, which cannot be 24-hydroxylated, evoke no disorder in bone mineralization and do not have a clear benefit in uremic osteodystrophy [289].

Clinical trials of 24,25(OH)$_2$D have been almost exclusively carried out in adults [127,273,347]. Patients have to also be treated with 1,25(OH)$_2$D in conjunction with 24,25(OH)$_2$D since patients do not respond to 24,25(OH)$_2$D alone. Sherrard et al. [347] treated 44 pa-

tients, 43 of whom had been on dialysis, who had "refractory osteomalacia," and hypercalcemia, a condition that is related to high bone aluminum content [179,180,182]. The addition of 24,25(OH)$_2$D permitted the use of higher 1,25(OH)$_2$D doses and resulted in the amelioration of hypercalcemia. Symptomatic improvement occurred in 21 of 36 patients, eight patients were unchanged, and seven had further deterioration, thus indicating a mixed response. Patients with secondary hyperparathyroidism were more likely to deteriorate, and in patients with paired biopsies, half showed improvement and 30% showed deterioration [347]. In other reports, 24,25(OH)$_2$D alone had no effect, and in combination with 1,25(OH)$_2$D failed to heal osteomalacia or osteitis fibrosa any more than did 1,25(OH)$_2$D alone [126,273]. No studies in children have been published.

The failure of 1,25(OH)$_2$D or 25(OH)D alone to fully correct the osteomalacia of uremia has been disappointing and has often led investigators to anticipate that the role of 24,25(OH)$_2$D in the treatment of this osteomalacia is to completely mineralize bone. Thus, the results of the reported clinical trials are discouraging [126,273,347]. Other factors such as parathyroid ablation [130] leading to dead bone disease, and bone aluminum [112,179,376] are probably more relevant in the failure of matrix mineralization. To further complicate interpretation, the metabolic clearance of 24,25(OH)$_2$D in human beings is very slow [204], so that it is very hard to compare the effects of 1,25(OH)$_2$D and 24,25(OH)$_2$D on bone, particularly in bone culture situations. Finally, the finding that 24,24-difluoro-25(OH)D administration to vitamin D-deficient rats results in no differences in bone histologic parameters from those found using 25(OH)D further indicates that this metabolite is unlikely to have an important role in bone modeling and mineralization.

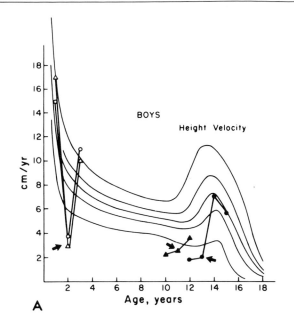

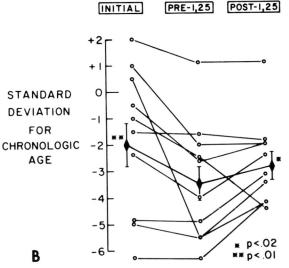

Fig. 28-22. A, *Growth velocity before and after 1,25(OH)₂D therapy. Arrow indicates the onset of therapy. Note the increase in growth velocity. (From Chesney RW, et al: N Engl J Med 298:238, 1978.) B, Long-term therapy (more than 30 months) of juvenile renal osteodystrophy indicating a significant increase in growth velocity but no evidence of prolonged catch-up growth. (From Chesney RW, et al: Vitamin D metabolites in renal insufficiency and other vitamin D disorders of children. Kidney Int (suppl 15)24:563, 1983, with permission.)*

Therapeutic Value of Parathyroidectomy

Medical management usually controls the manifestations of secondary hyperparathyroidism in uremia, especially with the use of the newer analogs of vitamin D. However, when conservative management fails, parathyroidectomy becomes a therapeutic option (Table 28-3). It should only

TABLE 28-3. *Possible indications for subtotal parathyroidectomy*

1. Marked secondary hyperparathyroidism (not responsive to medical management):
   a. increased iPTH
   b. bony erosions
   c. osteitis fibrosa cystica on bone biopsy
2. In association with:
   a. hypercalcemia
   b. progressive extraskeletal calcifications
   c. intractable pruritis
   d. severe bone pain, fractures through known tumors or epiphyseal slipping in children
   e. calciphylaxis

be considered when there is ample proof of secondary hyperparathyroidism as manifested by elevated levels of iPTH, bony erosions of osteitis fibrosa cystica on bone biopsy, or in association with several conditions [131,307]. The first is hypercalcemia, particularly if it is symptomatic, since patients may develop vomiting, nausea, or ulcer disease as a result of elevated calcium levels. There are some uremics who develop hypercalcemia in the absence of secondary hyperparathyroidism, in whom parathyroidectomy should not be performed. A second indication is progressive extraskeletal calcifications occurring in conjunction with Ca × P solubility product that is consistently greater than 70 to 80, despite phosphate restriction and the extensive use of phosphate-binding gels. Third, is intractable pruritis unresponsive to aggressive dialysis. Before considering surgical intervention, intravenous lidocaine and/or ultraviolet light should be tried. Fourth, is severe and progressive skeletal pain, fractures through known brown tumors, and epiphyseal slipping in children [134]. Since at times the bone disease may progress rapidly, parathyroidectomy may be the only option to halt and eventually reverse debilitating disease. Fifth, the appearance of calciphylaxis [148] is an indication. Rare in childhood uremia, it is a condition characterized by progressive necrosis of the digits, occurring at the fingertips and distal end of the toes in long-term dialysis patients or in renal transplant recipients, even despite normal renal function. This condition is rapidly progressive, and many patients may die due to gangrene and infections. Parathyroidectomy appears to arrest its progression and ameliorate the disease and, thus, is absolutely indicated when faced with a noncompliant patient who has severe bone disease and secondary hyperparathyroidism. Parathyroidectomy improves this bone disease. However, the complication of excess PTH secretion tends to recur if postoperative medical treatment and dietary restriction are again ignored.

In the past, a subtotal parathyroidectomy has been recommended. The surgeon usually identifies the presence of four parathyroid glands and excises 3¾ glands. The remnant gland is then marked by a metal clip or a long black silk suture to identify it should a repeat neck exploratory surgery be required. Generally, if only three glands are identified, they are all removed, assuming that the fourth one is present, even though it may not be seen. Ultrasonic examination of the neck can sometimes identify the enlarged glands [224,262].

Because the remnant tissue undergoes hyperplasia with recurrence of secondary hyperparathyroidism, and since a second surgical procedure has risks, some experts have advised that these patients undergo a total parathyroidectomy [361,382]. The excised parathyroid glands are cryopreserved and can potentially be later autotransplanted in the brachioradialis muscle under local anesthesia, usually without any sequelae. The main advantage of this technique is the accessibility of parathyroid tissue, if and when hyperplasia recurs. The "take rate" of the autotransplants in some studies is more than 90% [272]. In one study, only one patient of 16 had to have a second transplantation of cryopreserved autologous parathyroid tissue, which was successful. It should be noted that parathyroid hormone is important in bone remodeling and mineral accretion [295], indicating the significance of avoiding hypoparathyroidism secondary to these surgical maneuvers. More important, complete removal of all parathyroid tissue will lead to "dead bone disease," incapable of turnover and mineralization [381].

Postoperatively, it is essential to control the serum calcium. Hypocalcemia with seizures and tetany tend to develop in the presence of severe bone erosions. These can usually be averted by prior treatment with $1,25(OH)_2D_3$ and oral and/or intravenous calcium supplements. After remineralization of so-called "hungry" bones, serum calcium rises while alkaline phosphatase falls, necessitating the reduction or discontinuation of vitamin D analogs and calcium supplements as noted previously. Further, with the postoperative decline in serum phosphate, the dose of aluminum-containing gels is usually decreased or discontinued in order to maintain a serum phosphate level of 3.0 to 4.5 mg/dl. Both hypophosphatemia and hyperphosphatemia should be avoided.

The effects of parathyroidectomy, whether subtotal or total with subsequent autotransplantation, are stated to be good. In one study [360], 75% of the patients had symptomatic relief of bone pain. There was a decrease in the level of iPTH and improvement in the radiologic manifestations of renal osteodystrophy. However, no current study comparing aggressive management with 1α-hydroxy or 25(OH)D with the results obtained using this surgical approach has been reported. Weinstein [380] indicates that osteomalacia may occur despite the reduction of osteitis fibrosa cystica. Hypophosphatemia may have played a role in its evolution, or this may indicate dead bone disease [380,381]. Finally, a decline in renal function has been reported following parathyroidectomy, possibly associated with hypercalcemia [70].

In general, the benefits of this surgical procedure depend on the patient's compliance with medical treatment and diet [262].

Effect of Dialysis

Dialysis can potentially improve bone disease; however, the response is not uniform, and renal osteodystrophy worsens with poor or prolonged hemodialysis. Controlling the manifestations of secondary hyperparathyroidism before starting maintenance hemodialysis becomes necessary and is of particular importance in children, since they present for dialysis with hypocalcemia, hyperphosphatemia, and elevated iPTH levels.

Ample evidence suggests that the concentration of calcium in the dialysate plays a key role in the evolution of renal osteodystrophy. The dialysate calcium should be set so that the ionized calcium level remains normal and that postdialysis hypercalcemia is avoided. Various calcium concentrations in the bath have been evaluated (5.0–9.0 mg/dl) [196]. When a patient is normocalcemic or slightly hypocalcemic, the total plasma calcium concentration increases during dialysis, regardless of dialysate calcium concentration of 8.0 mg/dl or higher, hypercalcemia invariably occurs manifest by headache, pruritis, nausea, vomiting, and metastatic calcification whenever hyperphosphatemia is present. By contrast, dialysate levels of 5.0 mg/dl or less do not change the plasma calcium concentrations and these patients maintain a negative calcium balance because of fecal losses. As noted previously, jejunal absorption of calcium tends to be linear when intraluminal calcium is greater than 5.0 mg/dl. After intake of larger quantities of calcium (either from oral supplementation or by increased dialysate calcium), fecal losses do not increase proportionately and, hence, one can achieve a positive calcium balance [102,199].

Current recommendations favor a calcium concentration in the bath of 7.0 mg/dl. Studies indicate a decrease in iPTH levels and some improvement in the osteitis fibrosa cystica [195]. It is apparent, however, that parathyroid hyperplasia rarely involutes following the use of a high calcium-containing dialysate, particularly in children [257]. As discussed previously, vitamin D analogs result in a more dramatic decline in circulating iPTH values, probably due to specific parathyroid gland receptors for $1,25(OH)_2D$.

Phosphorus is poorly dialyzable and is sequestered in body tissues within a small volume of distribution. Hemodialysis and all types of peritoneal dialysis do not seem to alter serum phosphorus concentration. Despite dietary restrictions, many patients are hyperphosphatemic, requiring extensive use of aluminum-containing gels or calcium carbonate to maintain serum phosphorus levels between 4.0 and 5.0 mg/dl. It should be pointed out that hypophosphatemia is as detrimental as hyperphosphatemia, since it results in osteomalacia, and thus overzealous treatment with aluminum hydroxide should be avoided. Finally, a rare patient has been reported who develops hypophosphatemia without taking aluminum hydroxide and who needs phosphate supplementation [2]. These patients usually complain of weakness and develop osteomalacia and bone pain.

Many dialysis patients are magnesium overloaded [105], with the most common underlying cause being ingestion of magnesium-containing antacids. The impact of this overload on the course of renal osteodystrophy is unknown. However, it has been shown in a few studies that hypomagnesemia [264] and hypermagnesemia [305] tend to suppress PTH secretion. Consequently, the current recommendation is that dialysate magnesium content should be 1.5–2.0 mg/dl, which is slightly higher than normal serum levels.

The incidence of hyperparathyroid bone disease increases with the duration of renal failure [310], as well as with the duration of dialysis, particularly if the calcium concentration in the dialysate is less than 5.6 mg/dl [139]. Potter et al. [310] indicated an incidence of 47% in children on hemodialysis after a maximum of 17 months, which tends to confirm previous reports [134] that the incidence of overt bone disease is greater in children than in adults. However, for unknown reasons the frequency of epiphyseal slipping in dialyzed children is markedly reduced, which is extremely puzzling considering the fact that the secondary hyperparathyroidism persists [261]. The reduction in epiphyseal slipping could be related to positive calcium balance and to improved mineralizaton of woven bone in the metaphysis, or to a reduction in elevated iPTH, or to both. Moreover, some degree of secondary hyperparathyroidism is present in almost all patients with end-stage renal disease, with or without bone disease [156].

Most of this discussion has been limited to hemodialysis. With the advent of continuous ambulatory peritoneal dialysis (CAPD) and continuous cyclic peritoneal dialysis (CCPD), more patients with end-stage renal diseases are treated in this way [176,336]. However, information about the effect of this therapy on childhood renal osteodystrophy is limited [335,336]. In a study of adults [55], serum calcium remained unchanged, despite a negative peritoneal calcium balance, which may reflect the efficiency of compensatory mechanisms either by increasing intestinal absorption of calcium or by increasing bone resorption and osteitis fibrosa cystica. However, the osteomalacia seemed to respond to CAPD better than to vitamin D, in that fractures rapidly healed and no hypercalcemia was reported. It is postulated that CAPD may contribute to the maturation of collagen, thus facilitating its calcification by removing unidentified middle molecular weight substances that are not removed by hemodialysis.

In a study of 15 children undergoing CAPD for 0.3 to 2.4 years, no consistent healing of bone disease was evident [336]. Hyperparathyroid bone disease both appeared in patients without evidence of this lesion on skeletal radiographic studies, and pre-existing disease either healed, remained constant, or worsened. Hyperparathyroidism was reversed in only one patient, and hyperphosphatemia was a problem. A more recent study indicating that children receiving CAPD are at risk to develop elevated serum aluminum levels correlates with oral aluminum intake and inversely with body weight [193]. These data indicate that young children are most likely at greater risk to develop aluminum overload.

Is Early Treatment Warranted?

Early therapy has two distinct meanings. It can indicate aggressive therapy, including phosphate restriction and vitamin D analogs, at relatively moderate degrees of renal insufficiency or the initiation of treatment at an early age in children with chronic renal insufficiency. Since secondary hyperparathyroidism begins at creatinine clearance values as high as 50–60 ml/min/1.73m^2 [284] or higher [262], and since serum 1,25(OH)$_2$D concentrations are signifi-

cantly reduced at clearance values between 20 and 50 ml/min/1.73m^2 [86,202,309], treatment of patients with moderate renal insufficiency is indicated on a theoretical basis.

Several cogent arguments can be raised against such treatment:

1. renal disease may not be progressive during childhood;
2. phosphate restriction may worsen osteomalacia and prevent bone mineralization and growth;
3. the doses of vitamin D analogs [25(OH)D and 1,25(OH)$_2$D] that can be used may result in hypercalcemia;
4. this hypercalcemia may be associated with a progressive decline in renal function; and
5. until the other less clear factors contributing to uremic osteodystrophy—such as adequate nutrition, means of correcting osteomalacia, and reversing the defects in protein synthesis—can be adequately corrected, the role of early vitamin D and phosphate restriction therapy is questionable.

At present, only DHT can be successfully used in very young children, since drop preparations of 25(OH)D and 1,25(OH)$_2$D are not currently available.

The role of early treatment—either in the course of renal failure or in young children with congenital renal disease—may be important, but this is still an unproved assumption that only future studies can affirm or dispel [82]. It is important that pediatric nephrologists understand this lacunae in our knowledge before embarking on therapeutic misadventures.

Therapeutic Response: Its Assessment

The child with advanced renal osteodystrophy, slipped epiphyses, gait disturbance and myopathy is easy to assess in terms of the effectiveness of treatment [67,94,347]. Children with less marked osteodystrophy require assessment techniques that can detect more subtle changes [67, 75,94,174] (Table 28-4). Serial determinations of serum calcium, phosphate, alkaline phosphatase activity, iPTH level, and magnesium concentrations are needed. Unfortunately, iPTH is often a confusing and unrewarding indicator of the status of renal osteodystrophy, particularly if the antibody employed detects the C-terminal portion of the PTH molecule. As mentioned previously [75], the kidney is a major site of C-terminal PTH catabolism and, thus, the concentration of this molecule is high in the sera of uremic subjects even though this peptide has little or none of its biologic activity [97]. Since antibodies directed toward the N-terminal, or active portion of the molecule, are more problematic, the accurate measurement of bioactive PTH in uremia is only now being addressed, and long-term clinical studies in children are needed [262].

Although one can examine the serum Ca × PO$_4$ solubility product in a serial fashion, no pathologic values have been established in children, in whom there exists large variability in the serum phosphate for age. For instance, the normal neonate having a serum calcium of 10 mg/dl

TABLE 28-4. *Ways to assess the response to a given therapy in childhood renal osteodystrophy*

1. *Clinical status:*
   a. gait
   b. muscle strength
   c. appetite
   d. bone pain
   e. ability to run or ride a bicycle
2. *Biochemical profile*
   a. calcium
   b. phosphate
   c. alkaline phosphatase
   d. iPTH (N-terminal preferable)
   e. magnesium
   f. creatinine
   g. Ca × PO$_4$ solubility product
3. *Radiologic evaluation:*
   a. hand films using nongrid cassette or industrial-grade film that allows one to readily see subperiosteal erosions
   b. knee and wrist films to estimate epiphyseal slippage and metaphyseal lesions
   c. long bone films to assess bowing
4. *Photon absorptiometry:*
   a. Used to measure bone mineral content and bone density
5. *Bone histomorphometry:*
   a. to define the type of lesions—osteomalacia vs. osteitis fibrosa vs. mixed
   b. to define the rate of mineralization with double time-spaced tetracycline labeling
   c. to define the change in osteoid volume, mineral apposition rate, and cellular turnover after therapy
6. *Vitamin D metabolite values:*
   a. to assess the degree of deficiency of 25(OH)D

and phosphate of 7.0 mg/dl has a product of 70. It is unclear at what value for this product the patient is endangered in terms of soft tissue calcifications. However, calcium deposits at the limbus of the eye may be found following treatment with vitamin D analogs [65].

The radiologic appearance of renal osteodystrophy following treatment may show gross changes in bone appearance, but for the assessment of subtle changes a technique such as photon absorptiometry is useful [92]. The use of this technique detects improvement or decline in bone mineral content over time [89] and indicates changes as small as 2% to 3% with accuracy. Bone histology, histomorphometry, particularly after employment of a time-spaced tetracycline labeling process, is the most direct means of evaluating changes in bone after treatment [65,126,273,325,347]. The greatest difficulty encountered in employing this technique is its inherent invasiveness and the need for serial biopsies. However, this method is particularly useful in evaluating bone aluminum status and the effect of combination therapy [1,25(OH)$_2$D plus 24,25(OH)$_2$D].

Several groups have employed the measurement of vitamin D metabolite concentrations [86,220,228,244,308] to indicate the level of renal function at which values of 1,25(OH)$_2$D and 24,25(OH)$_2$D decline. These studies

have also indicated the influence of therapy on vitamin D metabolite values and suggest that therapeutic 25(OH)D values should be at least seven to ten times normal [220]. As these assays become more readily available, their use will be increased and their full utility appreciated. They can also be used to assess patient compliance.

The Goals of a Therapeutic Approach to Childhood Renal Osteodystrophy

The classical caveat that "therapy must be individualized" is especially relevant in childhood renal failure (see Table 28-4). The goals of therapy are to ensure adequate calcium intake, to raise intestinal calcium absorption, to remineralize bone, to reduce phosphate intake, to anticipate and correct acidosis, and to reduce PTH secretion. Oral calcium salts are usually necessary, but if used in conjunction with the 1α-hydroxyvitamin D metabolites, the amount of calcium administered should be lowered [67,75,94]. Calcium lactate and carbonate are notably useful, because one can also reverse acidosis with these compounds.

The choice of a phosphate binding agent is important because children often abhor the chalky taste [79]. Aluminum hydroxide-containing capsules can be swallowed by older children but are too large for younger children. Although aluminum hydroxide-containing cookies are available, children often complain of their gritty consistency [75,79]. Younger patients should probably continue to use low-phosphate formulas or formulas with a high calcium/phosphate ratio and avoid aluminum altogether.

The form of vitamin D chosen should be an individual decision and, as stressed above, a poorly compliant patient should receive a compound with a relatively long half-life such as vitamin D$_2$, 25(OH)D, or DHT. The main advantage of the 1α-hydroxylated vitamin D metabolites is their relatively short half-life, so that hypercalcemia or an elevated Ca × PO$_4$ solubility product is managed with greater ease.

The value of parathyroidectomy has changed since our understanding of vitamin D metabolites and their role in the suppression of PTH secretion has increased [114] and also since these metabolites are now freely available for therapeutic administration. Moreover, newer methods of PTH suppression—such as β-adrenergic blocking agents and antihistaminic agents [193]—have been suggested. The role of propranolol and cimetidine in the long-term suppression of secondary hyperparathyroidism is probably negligible, since not all investigators can document effective suppression after employing these drugs [144].

The early detection of renal osteodystrophy is a concern of all pediatric nephrologists. By use of one or more techniques, one can often demonstrate "early" osteodystrophy. The measurement of circulating iPTH levels shows that changes in calcium homeostasis occur at clearance values of 50 ml/min/1.73m^2 [283] or higher [260]. In addition, an elevation of the nephrogenous cyclic AMP (cAMP) has been shown parallel to these changes in iPTH [216]. Bone biopsy often reveals osteomalacia or osteitis fibrosa at clearance values of 30–50 ml/min/1.73m^2 [76]. Photon absorptiometry can also be used as a diagnostic tool [92,155], but bone scans do not appear to provide therapeutically useful information [181]. Serum chemical determinations of calcium, phosphate, and alkaline phosphatase have little utility in the detection of early osteodystrophy [98,283,308]. Since children with congenital renal disease [92,283] or obstructive uropathy [92,380] are at major risk for developing end-stage renal failure, this population should be assessed, possibly on a semi-annual basis. After the detection of changes in the measured parameters, therapy should be carefully instituted as outlined above in order to specifically prevent the progression of renal osteodystrophy.

References

1. Adachi I, Abe K, Tanaka M, et al: Phosphaturic effect of I.V. administered calcitonin in man. Endocrinol Jpn 21:317, 1974.
2. Ahmed KY, Varghese Z, Wills MR, et al: Persistent hypophosphatemia and osteomalacia in dialysis patients not on oral phosphate binders: Response to dihydrotachysterol therapy. Lancet 2:439, 1976.
3. Albright F, Drake TG, Sulkowitch HW: Renal osteitis fibrosa cystica: Report of a case with discussion of metabolic aspects. J Hopkins Med J 60:377, 1937.
4. Alfrey AC, Le Gendre GR, Kaehny WD: The dialysis encephalopathy syndrome: Possible aluminum intoxication. N Engl J Med 294:184, 1976.
5. Alfrey AC, Miller NL: Bone magnesium pools in uremia. J Clin Invest 52:3019, 1973.
6. Alfrey AC, Solomons CC, Circillo J, et al: Extraosseous calcification: Evidence for abnormal pyrophosphate metabolism in uremia. J Clin Invest 57:697, 1976.
7. Alfrey AC, Solomons CC: Bone pyrophosphate in uremia and its association with extraosseous calcification. J Clin Invest 57:700, 1976.
8. Anast CS, Mohs JM, Kaplan SL, et al: Evidence for parathyroid failure in magnesium deficiency. Science 177:606, 1972.
9. Andreoli S, Bergstein JM, Sherrard DJ: Elevated serum aluminum (Al) levels and osteomalacia in non-dialyzed (ND) uremic children due to oral aluminum hydroxide (AH). Pediatr Res 17:344A, 1983.
10. Andreoli S, Bergstein JM, Sherrard DJ: Aluminum intoxication from aluminum-containing phosphate binders in children with azotemia not undergoing dialysis. N Engl J Med 310:1079, 1984.
11. Ardaillou R, Fillastre JP, Milhaud G, et al: Renal excretion of phosphate, calcium and sodium during and after a prolonged thyrocalcitonin infusion in man. Proc Soc Exp Biol Med 131:56, 1969.
12. Arnaud CD: Hyperparathyroidism and renal failure. Kidney Int 4:89, 1973.
13. Arnaud CD: Immunochemical heterogeneity of circulating parathyroid hormone in man: Sequel to an original observation by Berson and Yalow. Mt Sinai J Med (NY) 40:422, 1973.
14. Arnaud CD, Goldsmith RS, Bordier PJ, et al: Influence of immunoheterogeneity of circulating parathyroid hormone on results of radioimmunoassays of serum in man. Am J Med 57:43, 1967.
15. Arnaud C, Rasmussen H, Anast C: Further studies on the interrelationship between parathyroid hormone and vitamin D. J Clin Invest 45:1955, 1966.
16. Au WYW, Raisz LG: Restoration of parathyroid respon-

siveness in vitamin D-deficient rats by parenteral calcium or dietary lactose. J Clin Invest 46:1572, 1967.
17. Avioli LV: Collagen metabolism, uremia and bone. Kidney Int 4:105, 1973.
18. Avioli L: Senile and post-menopausal osteoporosis. In Stollerman, GH (ed): Advances in Internal Medicine, vol 21. Chicago, Year Book Medical Publishers, 1976, p 391.
19. Avioli LV: Renal osteodystrophy and vitamin D. Dialysis and Transplant 7:244, 1978.
20. Avioli LV, Haddad JG: Vitamin D: Current concepts. Metabolism 22:507, 1973.
21. Avioli LV, Scharp C, Birge SJ: Catabolism of free hydroxyproline in chronic uremia. Am J Physiol 217:536, 1964.
22. Avioli LV, Teitelbaum S: Renal osteodystrophy. In Brenner B, Rector F (eds): Renal Osteodystrophy in the Kidney. Philadelphia, Saunders, 1976, p 1542.
23. Ball J: Diseases of bone. In Harrison CV (ed): Recent Advances in Pathology, 7th ed., London, Churchill Livingstone, 1960, p 293.
24. Balsan S, Gueris J, Levy D, et al: Suppressive effect of 1-hydroxyvitamin D$_3$ on the hyperparathyroidism of children on maintenance hemodialysis. Metab Bone Dis & Rel Res 1:15, 1978.
25. Baluarte HJ, Gruskin AB, Hiner LB, et al: Encephalopathy in children with chronic renal failure. Proc Clin Dial Transplant Forum 7:95, 1977.
26. Baron R, Norman M, Mazur A, et al: Bone histomorphometry in children with early chronic renal failure treated with 25(OH)D$_3$. In Norman AW, Schaefer K, Herrath D von, et al (eds): Vitamin D: Basic Research and Its Clinical Application. Berlin, Walter de Gruyter & Co, 1979, p 847.
27. Baxter LA, DeLuca HF: Stimulation of 25-hydroxyvitamin D$_3$-1α-hydroxylase by phosphate depletion. J Biol Chem 254:3158, 1976.
28. Bayard F, Bec P, Ton That H, et al: Plasma 25-hydroxycholecalciferol in chronic renal failure. Eur J Clin Invest 3:447, 1973.
29. Baylink D, Wergedal J: Bone formation and resorption by osteocytes: In Nichols GV, Wasserman RH (eds): Cellular Mechanisms for Calcium Transfer and Homeostasis. New York, Academic, 1971, p 257.
30. Belanger LF: Osteocytic osteolysis. Calcif Tissue Res 4:1, 1969.
31. Bell NH: Further studies on the regulation of calcitonin release in vitro. Horm Metab Res 7:77, 1975.
32. Bergstrom WH, deLeon AS, Van Gemund JJ: Growth aberrations in renal disease. Pediatr Clin North Am 11:563, 1964.
33. Berlyne GM, Ben-Air J, Szwarcberg J, et al: Increase in bone magnesium content in renal failure in man. Nephron 9:90, 1972.
34. Betts PR, White RHR: Growth potential and skeletal maturity in children with chronic renal insufficiency. Nephron 16:325, 1976.
35. Bijovet OLM, Van der Sluys Veer J, DeVries HR, et al: Natriuretic effect of calcitonin in man. N Engl J Med 284:681, 1971.
36. Bikle DD, Murphy EW, Rasmussen H: The ionic control of 1,25-dihydroxyvitamin D$_3$ synthesis in isolated chick renal mitochondria. J Clin Invest 55:299, 1975.
37. Bikle DD, Rasmussen H: The metabolism of 25-hydroxycholecalciferol by isolated renal tubules in vitro as studied by new chromatographic technique. Biochim Biophys Acta 362:425, 1974.
38. Bikle DD, Rasmussen H: The ionic control of 1,25-dihydroxyvitamin D$_3$ production in isolated chick renal tubules. J Clin Invest 55:292, 1975.

39. Birge SJ, Peck WA, Whedon GD, et al: Study of calcium absorption in man: A kinetic analysis and physiologic model. *J Clin Invest* 48:1705, 1969.

40. Bordier PJ, Arnaud C, Hawker C, et al: Relationship between serum iPTH, osteoclastic and osteocytic bone resorptions and serum calcium in primary hyperparathyroidism and osteomalacia. *In* Frame B, Parfitt AM, Duncan H (eds): *Clinical Aspects of Metabolic Bone Diseases* (International Congress Series No. 270). Amsterdam, Excerpta Medica, 1973, p 222.

41. Bordier PJ, Marie PJ, Arnaud CD: Evolution of renal osteodystrophy: Correlation of bone histomorphometry and serum mineral and immunoreactive parathyroid hormone values before and after treatment with calcium carbonate or 25-hydroxycholecalciferol. *Kidney Int* 7:S102, 1975.

42. Bordier P, Zingraff J, Gueris J, et al: The effect of 1-(OH)D₃ and 1,25(OH)₂D₃ on the bone in patients with renal osteodystrophy. *Am J Med* 64:101, 1978.

43. Bouillon R, Verberckmoes R, de Moor P: Influence of dialysate calcium concentration and vitamin D on serum parathyroid hormone during repetitive dialysis. *Kidney Int* 7:422, 1975.

44. Boyle IT, Omdahl JL, Gray RW, et al: The biological activity and metabolism of 24,25-dihydroxyvitamin D₃. *J Biol Chem* 248:4174, 1973.

45. Brewer HB Jr, Schlueter RJ, Aldred JP: Isolation and characterization of bovine thyrocalcitonin. *J Biol Chem* 245:4232, 1970.

46. Brickman AS, Coburn JW, Massry SG, et al: 1,25-dihydroxyvitamin D₃ in normal man and patients with renal failure. *Ann Intern Med* 80:161, 1974.

47. Brickman AS, Coburn JW, Norman AW: Action of 1,25-dihydroxycholecalciferol, a potent, kidney-produced metabolite of vitamin D₃, in uremic man. *N Engl J Med* 287:891, 1972.

48. Brown DJ, Ham KN, Dawborn JK, et al: Treatment of dialysis osteomalacia with desferrioxamine. *Lancet* 1:343, 1982.

49. Browness JM: Present concepts of the role of ground substance in calcification. *Cin Orthop* 59:223, 1968.

50. Brumbaugh PF, Haussler DH, Haussler R, et al: Radioreceptor assay for 1α-25 dihydroxyvitamin D₃. *Science* 183:1089, 1974.

51. Brumbaugh PF, Haussler MR: 1α-25-dihydroxycholecalciferol receptors in intestine. *J Biol Chem* 249:1251, 1974.

52. Bulla M, Delling G, Offermann G, et al: Renal bone disorder in children: Therapy with vitamin D₃ or 1,25-dihydroxycholecalciferol (1,25-DHCC). *In* Norman AW, Schaefer K, Herrath D von, et al (eds): *Vitamin D: Basic Research and Its Clinical Applications*. Berlin, Walter de Gruyter & Co, 1979, p 853.

53. Burke EC, Stickler GB, Rosevear JW: Renal osteodystrophy in two siblings. *Am J Dis Child* 105:90, 1963.

54. Burnell JM, Teubner E, Wergedal JE, et al: Bone crystal maturation in renal osteodystrophy in humans. *J Clin Invest* 53:52, 1974.

55. Calderaro V, Oreoporilos DG, Meema HE, et al: The evolution of renal osteodystrophy in patients undergoing continuous ambulatory peritoneal dialysis (CAPD). *Proc Eur Dial Trans Assoc* 17:533, 1980.

56. Campo RD: Protein-polysaccharides of cartilage in health and disease. *Clin Orthop* 68:182, 1970.

57. Campos C, Arata RO, Mautalen CA: Parathyroid hormone and vertebral osteosclerosis in uremic patients. *Metabolism* 25:495, 1976.

58. Canterbury JM, Bourgoignie JJ, Gavellas G, et al: Metabolic consequences of oral administration of 24,25(OH)₂D₃ to uremic dogs. *J Clin Invest* 65:571, 1980.

59. Canterbury JM, Lerman S, Claflin AJ, et al: Inhibition of parathyroid hormone secretion by 25-hydroxycholecalciferol and 24,25-dihydroxycholecalciferol in the dog. *J Clin Invest* 61:1375, 1978.

60. Canterbury JM, Levey GS, Reiss E: Activation of renal cortical adenylate cyclase by circulating immunoreactive parathyroid hormone fragments. *J Clin Invest* 52:524, 1973.

61. Canterbury JM, Levy G, Ruiz E, et al: Parathyroid hormone activation of adenylate cyclase in liver. *Proc Soc Exp Biol Med* 147:366, 1974.

62. Care AD, Bates RFL, Bruce JB, et al: Stimulation of calcitonin secretion by gastro-intestinal hormones. *J Endocrinol* 52:1, 1971.

63. Care AD, Bates RFL, Swaminathan R, et al: The role of gastrin as a calcitonin secretagogue. *J Endocrinol* 51:735, 1971.

64. Carter WB, Heath H III: Clinically useful calcitonin assays. *TEM* July/August:288, 1990.

65. Chan JCM, DeLuca HF: Growth velocity in a child on prolonged hemodialysis: Beneficial effect of 1-hydroxyvitamin D₃. *JAMA* 238:2053, 1977.

66. Chan JCM, DeLuca HF: Calcium and parathyroid disorders in children: Chronic renal failure and treatment with calcitriol. *JAMA* 241:1242, 1979.

67. Chan JCM, Kodroff MB, Landwehr DM: Effects of 1,25-dihydroxyvitamin D₃ on renal function, mineral balance and growth in children with severe chronic renal failure. *Pediatrics* 68:559, 1981.

68. Chan JCM, Young RB, Alon U, et al: Hypercalcemia in children with disorders of calcium and phosphorus metabolism during long-term treatment with 1,25-dihydroxyvitamin D₃. *Pediatrics* 72:225, 1983.

69. Chan Y-L, Alfrey AC, Posen S, et al: Effect of aluminum on normal and uremic rats: Tissue distribution, vitamin D metabolites, and quantitative bone histology. *Calcif Tissue Int* 35:344, 1983.

70. Chan YL, Posen S, Savdie E, et al: Total parathyroidectomy and renal function in patients with chronic renal failure. *Miner Electrolyte Metab* 9:57, 1983.

71. Chantler C, Holliday MA: Growth in children with renal failure, with special reference to the effects of caloric malnutrition. *Clin Nephrol* 1:230, 1973.

72. Chase LR, Aurbach GD: Parathyroid function and the renal excretion of 3'5'-adenylic acid. *Proc Nat Acad Sci USA* 58:518, 1967.

73. Chase LR, Fedak SA, Aurbach GD: Activation of skeletal adenyl cyclase by parathyroid hormone *in vitro*. *Endocrinology* 84:761, 1969.

74. Chesney: Personal Observation.

75. Chesney RW: 1,25-dihydroxyvitamin D₃ in the treatment of juvenile renal osteodystrophy. *In* Gruskin AB, Norman ME (eds): *Pediatric Nephrology*. The Hague, Martinus Nijhoff, 1980, p 209.

76. Chesney RW: Does uremic bone disease warrant early treatment with calcitriol? *Arch Intern Med* 140:1016, 1980.

77. Chesney RW: Current clinical applications of vitamin D metabolite research. *In* Urist MR (ed): *Clinical Orthopaedics and Related Research*. Philadelphia, JB Lippincott, 1981, p 285.

78. Chesney RW: Modified vitamin D compounds in the treatment of certain bone diseases. *In* Spiller G (ed): *Current Topics in Nutrition and Disease*. Vol 4. *Nutritional Pharmacology*. New York, Alan R Liss, 1981, p 147.

79. Chesney RW: Treatment of calcium and phosphorus ab-

normalities in childhood renal osteodystrophy. *Dialysis & Transplantation* 12:270, 1983.

80. Chesney RW: Metabolic bone disease. *Pediatr in Review* 5:227, 1984.

81. Chesney RW: Renal osteodystrophy in children. *In* Cummings NB, Klahr S (eds): *Chronic Renal Disease Causes, Complications and Treatment.* New York, Plenum Press, 1985, p 321.

82. Chesney RW, Dabbagh S, Uehling DF, et al: The importance of early treatment of renal bone disease in children. *Kidney Int* 28:575, 1985.

83. Chesney RW, DeLuca HF, Dabbagh S, et al: Vitamin D metabolism in longstanding nephrotic syndrome and chronic renal insufficiency. *In* Brodehl J, Ehrich JHH (eds): *Proceedings of 6th International Pediatric Nephrology Symposium.* Berlin, Springer-Verlag, 1984, p 393.

84. Chesney RW, Friedman AL: The medical management of chronic renal failure. *In* Brenner BM, Stein JH (eds): *Contemporary Issues in Nephrology.* Vol 12. *Pediatric Nephrology.* New York, Churchill Livingstone, 1984, p 321.

85. Chesney RW, Hamstra A, Jax DK, et al: Influence of long-term oral 1,25-dihydroxyvitamin D in childhood renal osteodystrophy. *Contrib Nephrol* 18:55, 1980.

86. Chesney RW, Hamstra AJ, Mazess RB, et al: Circulating vitamin D metabolite concentrations in childhood renal diseases. *Kidney Int* 21:65, 1982.

87. Chesney RW, Hamstra AJ, Phelps M, et al: Vitamin D metabolites in renal insufficiency and other vitamin D disorders of children. *Kidney Int* (suppl 15)24:563, 1983.

88. Chesney RW, Haughton PB: Tetany following phosphate enemas in chronic renal disease. *Am J Dis Child* 127:584, 1974.

89. Chesney RW, Shore RM: The noninvasive determination of bone mineral content by photon absorptiometry. *Am J Dis Child* 136:578, 1982.

90. Chesney RW, Mazess RB, Hamstra AJ, et al: Demineralization in hypophosphatemic rickets with normal 24,25-dihydroxyvitamin D and subnormal 1,25-dihydroxyvitamin D levels. *Clin Res* 27:653A, 1979.

91. Chesney RW, Mazess RB, Hamstra AJ, et al: Subnormal serum 1,25-dihydroxyvitamin D levels in children with glomerular disease treated with corticosteroids. *In* Norman AW, Schaefer K, Herrath D von, et al (eds): *Vitamin D: Basic Research and Its Clinical Application.* Berlin, Walter de Gruyter & Co, 1979, p 935.

92. Chesney RW, Mazess RB, Rose P, et al: Bone mineral status measured by direct photon absorptiometry in childhood renal disease. *Pediatrics* 60:864, 1977.

93. Chesney RW, Mehls O, Anast CS, et al: Renal osteodystrophy in children: The role of vitamin D, phosphorus and parathyroid hormone. *Am J Kidney Dis* 7:275, 1986.

94. Chesney RW, Moorthy AV, Eisman JA, et al: Increased growth after long-term oral 1,25-vitamin D₃ in childhood renal osteodystrophy. *N Engl J Med* 298:238, 1978.

95. Chesney RW, Rose PG, Mazess RB: Persistence of diminished bone mineral content following renal transplantation in childhood. *Pediatrics* 73:459, 1984.

96. Chesney RW, Rosen JF, Hamstra AJ, et al: Serum 1,25-dihydroxyvitamin D levels in normal children and in vitamin D disorders. *Am J Dis Child* 134:135, 1980.

97. Chesney RW, Rosen JF, Hamstra AJ, et al: The use of serum 1,25-dihydroxyvitamin D (calcitriol) concentrations in the clinical assessment of demineralizing disorders in children. *In* Cohn D, Talmage RV, LesMatthews J, et al (eds): *Hormonal Control of Calcium Metabolism.* Rotterdam, Excerpta Medica, 1981, p 252.

98. Chesney RW, Zimmerman J, Hamstra AJ, et al: The circulating levels of vitamin D metabolites in vitamin D deficiency: Are calcitriol levels normal? *Fifth Vitamin D Workshop,* February 19, 1982, Williamsburg, VA.

99. Christiansen C, Christensen MS, Melsen F, et al: Mineral metabolism in chronic renal failure with special reference to serum concentrations of 1,25(OH)₂D and 24,25(OH)₂D. *Clin Nephrol* 15:18, 1981.

100. Christiansen C, Rodbro P, Christensen MS, et al: Deterioration of renal function during treatment of renal failure with 1,25-dihydroxycholecalciferol. *Lancet* 2:700, 1978.

101. Coburn JW, Hartenbower DL, Massry SG: Intestinal absorption of calcium and the effect of renal insufficiency. *Kidney Int* 4:96, 1973.

102. Coburn JW, Koppel MH, Brickman AS, et al: Study of intestinal absorption of calcium in patients with renal failure. *Kidney Int* 3:264, 1973.

103. Coburn JW, Sherrard DJ, Ott SM, et al: Bone disease in uremia: A reappraisal. *In* Norman AW, Schaefer K, Herrath D von, et al (eds): *Vitamin D: Chemical, Biochemical and Clinical Endocrinology of Calcium Metabolism.* Berlin, Walter de Gruyter & Co, 1982, p 827.

104. Cohen MEL, Cohen GF, Ahad V, et al: Renal osteodystrophy in patients on chronic haemodialysis: A radiological study. *Clin Radiol* 21:124, 1970.

105. Contiguglia SR, Alfrey AC, Miller N, et al: Total-body magnesium excess in chronic renal failure. *Lancet* 1:1300, 1972.

106. Contiguglia SR, Alfrey AC, Miller NL, et al: Nature of soft tissue calcification in uremia. *Kidney Int* 4:229, 1973.

107. Cooper CW, Schwesinger WH, Ontjes DA, et al: Stimulation of secretion of pig thyrocalcitonin by gastrin and related hormonal peptides. *Endocrinology* 91:1079, 1972.

108. Cordy PE: Treatment of bone disease in patients on chronic haemodialysis with dihydrotachysterol. *Trans Amer Soc Artif Int Organs* 22:60, 1976.

109. Cordy PE: Treatment of bone disease with dihydrotachysterol in patients undergoing long-term hemodialysis. *CMA Journal* 117:766, 1977.

110. Cordy PE: The early detection and treatment of renal osteodystrophy. *In* Norman AW, Schaefer K, Herrath D von, et al (eds): *Vitamin D: Basic Research and Its Clinical Application.* Berlin, Walter de Gruyter & Co, 1979, p 775.

111. Cordy PE, Hodsman AB: Effect of treatment with dihydrotachysterol on renal function in patients with chronic renal failure. *Miner Electrolyte Metab* 10:281, 1984.

112. Cournot-Witmer G, Zingraff J, Plachot JJ, et al: Aluminum localization in bone from hemodialyzed patients: Relationship to matrix mineralization. *Kidney Int* 20:375, 1981.

113. David DS, Sakai S, Granda J, et al: Role of pyrophosphate in renal osteodystrophy. *Trans Am Soc Artif Intern Organs* 19:440, 1973.

114. DeLuca HF: The vitamin D system in the regulation of calcium and phosphorus metabolism. W.O. Atwater Memorial Lecture. *Nutr Rev* 37:161, 1979.

115. Denny JD, Sherrard DJ, Nelp WB, et al: Total body calcium and long time calcium balance in chronic renal disease. *J Lab Clin Med* 82:226, 1973.

116. Dent CE, Gupta MM: Plasma 25-hydroxyvitamin D levels during pregnancy in Caucasians and in vegetarian and non-vegetarian Asians. *Lancet* 2:1057, 1975.

117. Dent CE, Harper C, Philpott GR: The treatment of renal glomerular osteodystrophy. *Q J Med* 30:1, 1961.

118. DiBella FP, Dousa TP, Miller SS, et al: Parathyroid hormone receptors of renal cortex: Specific binding of biologically active ¹²⁵I-labeled hormone and relationship to aden-

ylate cyclase activation. *Proc Natl Acad Sci USA* 71:723, 1974.

119. Dominguez JH, Gray RW, Lemann J Jr: Dietary phosphate deprivation in women and men: Effects on mineral and acid balances, parathyroid hormone and the metabolism of 25-OH-Vitamin D. *J Clin Endocrinol Metab* 43:1056, 1976.

120. Eisenberg E, Bartholomew PV: Reversible calcinosis cutis: Calciphylaxis in man. *N Engl J Med* 268:1216, 1963.

121. Eisman JA, Hamstra AJ, Kream BE, et al: A sensitive, precise and convenient method for determination of 1,25 dihydroxyvitamin D in human plasma. *Anal Biochem Biophys* 80:298, 1976.

122. Eisman JE, Hamstra AJ, Kream BE, et al: 1,25-dihydroxy-vitamin D in biological fluids: A simplified and sensitive assay. *Science* 193:1021, 1976.

123. Elders MJ, Winfield BS, McNatt ML, et al: Glucocorticoid therapy in children. *Am J Dis Child* 129:1393, 1975.

124. Ellis HA, Peart KM: Azotemic renal osteodystrophy: A quantitative study on iliac bone. *J Clin Pathol* 26:83, 1973.

125. Estep H, Shaw WA, Watlington C, et al: Hypocalcemia due to hypomagnesemia and reversible parathyroid hormone unresponsiveness. *J Clin Endocrinol Metab* 29:842, 1969.

126. Evans RA, Hills E, Wong SYP, et al: The use of 24,25-dihydroxycholecalciferol alone and in combination with 1,25-dihydroxycholecalciferol in chronic renal failure. *In* Norman AW, Schaefer K, Herrath D von, et al (eds): *Vitamin D: Chemical, Biochemical and Clinical Endocrinology of Calcium Metabolism.* Berlin, Walter de Gruyter & Co, 1982, p 835.

127. Evans RA, Somerville PJ: The use of high calcium dialysate in the treatment of renal osteomalacia. *Aust N Z J Med* 6:10, 1976.

128. Feest TG, Ward MK, Ellis HA, et al: Osteomalacic dialysis osteodystrophy: A trial of phosphate-enriched dialysis fluid. *Br Med J* 1:18, 1978.

129. Felsenfeld AJ, Gutman RA, Llach F, et al: Osteomalacia in chronic renal failure: A syndrome previously reported only with maintenance dialysis. *Am J Nephrol* 2:147, 1982.

130. Felsenfeld AJ, Harrelson JM, Gutman RA, et al: Osteomalacia after parathyroidectomy in patients with uremia. *Ann Intern Med* 96:34, 1982.

131. Finch T, Jacobs JK: Indications for parathyroidectomy in patients with chronic renal failure. *Am Surg* 40:40, 1974.

132. Fine RN, Gruskin A: Treatment of end-stage renal disease in children. Philadelphia, WB Saunders, 1984.

133. Fine RN, Isaacson AS, Payne V, et al: Renal osteodystrophy in children: The effect of hemodialysis and renal homotransplantation. *J Pediatr* 80:243, 1972.

134. Firor HV, Moore ES, Levitsky LL, et al: Parathyroidectomy in children with chronic renal failure. *J Pediatr Surg* 7:535, 1972.

135. Fischer JA, Binswanger U, Dietrich FM: Human parathyroid hormone: Immunological characterization of antibodies against a glandular extract and the synthetic amino-terminal fragments 1–12 and 1–34 and their use in the determination of immunoreactive hormone in human sera. *J Clin Invest* 54:1382, 1974.

136. Foley CM, Polinsky MS, Gruskin AB, et al: Encephalopathy in infants and children with chronic renal disease. *Arch Neurol* 38:656, 1981.

137. Follis RH Jr.: Renal rickets and osteitis fibrosa in children and adolescents. *Bull Johns Hopkins Hosp* 87:593, 1950.

138. Fournier A, Bordier P, Gueris J, et al: Comparison of 1-hydroxycholecalciferol and 25-hydroxycholecalciferol in the treatment of renal osteodystrophy: Greater effect of 25-hydroxycholecalciferol on bone mineralization. *Kidney Int* 15:196, 1979.

139. Fournier AE, Johnson WJ, Taves DR, et al: Etiology of hyperparathyroidism and bone disease during chronic hemodialysis. I. Association of bone disease with potentially etiologic factors. *J Clin Invest* 50:592, 1971.

140. Fournier A, Sebert JL, Moriniere P, et al: Renal osteodystrophy: Pathophysiology and treatment. *Horm Res* 20:44, 1984.

141. Fraser DR, Kodicek E: Unique biosynthesis by kidney of a biologically active vitamin D metabolite. *Nature* 228:764, 1970.

142. Fraser DR, Kodicek E: Regulation of 25-hydroxycholecalciferol-1-hydroxylase activity in kidney by parathyroid hormone. *Nature [New Biol]* 241:163, 1973.

143. Friedman SA, Novak S, Thomson GE: Arterial calcification and gangrene in uremia. *N Engl J Med* 280:1392, 1969.

144. Frost HM: Tetracycline-based histological analysis of bone remodeling. *Calcif Tissue Res* 3:211, 1969.

145. Fuchs JE, von Herrath D, Kraft D, et al: The influence of 24,25(OH)$_2$-vitamin D$_3$, beta-blockers and cimetidine on the course of experimental renal osteodystrophy in rats. *In* Norman AW, Schaefer K, Herrath D von, et al (eds): *Vitamin D: Chemical, Biochemical and Clinical Endocrinology of Calcium Metabolism.* Berlin, Walter de Gruyter & Co, 1982, p 183.

146. Garabedian M, Liebenherr M, Corvol MT, et al: Cellular location and regulation of the 24,25-dihydroxyvitamin D$_3$ formation in cultured cells from bone and cartilage. *In* Norman AW, Schaefer K, Herrath D von, et al (eds): *Vitamin D: Basic Research and Its Clinical Application.* Berlin, Walter de Gruyter & Co, 1979, p 391.

147. Garner A, Bell J: Quantitative observations on mineralized and unmineralized bone in chronic renal azotemia and intestinal malabsorption syndrome. *J Pathol Bacteriol* 91:545, 1966.

148. Gipstein RH, Coburn JW, Adams DA, et al: Calciphylaxis in man: A syndrome of tissue necrosis and vascular calcification in 11 patients with chronic renal disease. *Arch Intern Med* 136:1273, 1976.

149. Glimcher MJ, Krane SM: The organization and structure of bone and the mechanism of calcification, vol 2B. *In* Gould BS (ed): *Treatise in Collagen.* New York, Academic, 1968, p 67.

150. Goldman AB, Lane JM, Salvate E: Slipped capital femoral epiphyses complicating renal osteodystrophy: A report of three cases. *Radiology* 126:333, 1978.

151. Goldstein DA, Haldimann B, Sherman D, et al: Vitamin D metabolites and calcium metabolism in patients with nephrotic syndrome and normal renal function. *J Clin Endocrinol Metab* 52:116, 1981.

152. Goodman WG, Henry DA, Horst R, et al: Parenteral aluminum administration in the dog. II. Induction of osteomalacia and effect on vitamin D metabolism. *Kidney Int* 25:370, 1984.

153. Gray R, Boyle I, DeLuca HF: Vitamin D metabolism: The role of kidney tissue. *Science* 172:1232, 1971.

154. Gray TK, Ontjes DA: Clinical aspects of thyrocalcitonin. *Clin Orthop* 111:238, 1975.

155. Griffiths HJ, Zimmerman R, Bailey G, et al: The use of photon absorptiometry in the diagnosis of renal osteodystrophy. *Radiology* 109:277, 1973.

156. Griffiths HJ, Zimmerman RE, Lazarus M, et al: The long-term follow-up of 195 patients with renal failure; a preliminary report. *Radiology* 122:643, 1977.

157. Griswold WR, Reznik V, Mendoza SA, et al: Accumulation of aluminum in a nondialyzed uremic child receiving aluminum hydroxide. *Pediatrics* 71:56, 1983.

158. Grupe WE, Harmon WE, Spinozzi NS: Protein and energy

requirements in children receiving chronic hemodialysis. *Kidney Int* (Suppl 15)24:S-6, 1983.

159. Grushkin CM, Fine RN: Growth in children following renal transplantation. *Am J Dis Child* 125:514, 1973.

160. Guillot AP, Hood VL, Runge CF, et al: The use of magnesium-containing phosphate binders in patients with end-stage renal disease on maintenance hemodialysis. *Nephron* 30:114, 1982.

161. Gunja-Smith Z, Boucek RJ: Collagen cross-linking compounds in human urine. *Biochem J* 197:759, 1981.

162. Habener JF, Mayer GP, Dee PC, et al: Metabolism of amino- and carboxylsequence immunoreactive parathyroid hormone in the bovine: Evidence for peripheral cleavage of hormone. *Metabolism* 25:385, 1976.

163. Habener JF, Potts JT Jr, Rich A: Preproparathyroid hormone: Evidence for an early biosynthetic precursor of proparathyroid hormone. *J Biol Chem* 251:3893, 1976.

164. Haddad JG Jr, Birge SJ: Widespread specific binding of 25-hydroxycholecalciferol in rat tissues. *J Biol Chem* 250:299, 1975.

165. Haddad JG Jr, Couranz S, Avioli LV: Non-dialyzable urinary hydroxyproline as an index for bone collagen formation. *J Clin Endocrinol Metab* 30:282, 1970.

166. Haddad JG Jr, Kyung JC: Competitive protein-binding radio-assay for 25-hydroxycholecalciferol. *J Clin Endocrinol Metab* 22:992, 1971.

167. Haddad JG Jr, Rojanasathit S: Acute administration of 25-hydroxycholecalciferol in man. *J Clin Endocrinol Metab* 42:284, 1976.

168. Haddad JG Jr, Walgate J: 25-hydroxyvitamin D transport in human plasma: Isolation and partial characterization of calcifediol-binding protein. *J Biol Chem* 254:4803, 1976.

169. Hallick MF, DeLuca HF: 25-hydroxydihydrotachysterol: Biosynthesis *in vivo* and *in vitro*. *J Biol Chem* 246:5733, 1971.

170. Haussler MR, Baylink DJ, Hughes MR, et al: The assay of 1α,25-dihydroxyvitamin D_3: Physiologic and pathologic modulation of circulating hormone levels. *Clin Endocrinol* 5:151S, 1976.

171. Haussler MR, Brickman AS: Vitamin D: Metabolism, actions and disease states. *In* Alvioli LV (ed): *Disorders of Mineral Metabolism*, vol 2. New York, Academic, 1982, p 359.

172. Haussler MR, Cordy PE: Metabolites and analogues of vitamin D: Which for what? *JAMA* 247:841, 1982.

173. Haust MD, Landing BH, Holmstrand K, et al: Osteosclerosis of renal disease in children: Comparative pathologic and radiographic studies. *Am J Pathol* 44:141, 1964.

174. Henderson RG, Russell RGG, Ledingham JGG, et al: Effects of 1,25-dihydroxycholecalciferol on calcium absorption, muscle weakness and bone disease in chronic renal failure. *Lancet* 1:379, 1974.

175. Hennessy JF, Wells SA Jr, Ontjes DA, et al: A comparison of pentagastrin injection and calcium infusion as provocative agents for the detection of medullary carcinoma of the thyroid. *J Clin Endocrinol Metab* 39:487, 1974.

176. Hewitt IK, Stefandis C, Reilly BJ, et al: Renal osteodystrophy in children undergoing continuous ambulatory peritoneal dialysis. *J Pediatr* 103:729, 1984.

177. Heynen G, Kanis JA, Oliver D, et al: Evidence that endogenous calcitonin protects against renal bone disease. *Lancet* 2:1322, 1976.

178. Hibberd KA, Norman AW: Comparative biological effects of vitamin D_2 and D_3 and dihydrotachysterol₂ and dihydrotachysterol₃ in the chick. *Biochem Pharmacol* 18:2347, 1969.

179. Hodsman AB, Sherrard DJ, Alfrey AC, et al: Bone alumi-

num and histomorphometric features of renal osteodystrophy. *J Clin Endocrinol Metab* 54:539, 1982.

180. Hodsman AB, Sherrard DJ, Alfrey AC, et al: Preliminary trials with 24,25 dihydroxyvitamin D_3 in dialysis osteomalacia. *Am J Med* 74:407, 1983.

181. Hodsman AB, Sherrard DJ, Wong EGC, et al: Vitamin-D-resistant osteomalacia in hemodialysis patients lacking secondary hyperparathyroidism. *Ann Intern Med* 94:629, 1981.

182. Hodson EM, Howman-Giles RB, Evans RA, et al: The diagnosis of renal osteodystrophy: A comparison of Technetium-99m-pyrophosphate bone scintigraphy with other techniques. *Clin Nephrol* 16:24, 1981.

183. Hodson EM, Shaw PF, Evans RA, et al: Growth retardation and renal osteodystrophy in children with chronic renal failure. *J Pediatr* 103:735, 1983.

184. Holick MF, Kleiner-Bossaller A, Schnoes HK, et al: 1,24,25-trihydroxyvitamin D_3. *J Biol Chem* 248:6691, 1973.

185. Holtrop JE, Raisz LG, Simmons HA: The effects of parathyroid hormone, colchicine, and calcitonin on the ultrastructure and the activity of osteoclasts in organ culture. *J Cell Biol* 60:346, 1974.

186. Holtrop ME, Weinger JM: Ultrastructural evidence for a transport system in bone. *In* Talmage RV, Munson PL (eds): *Calcium, Parathyroid Hormone and the Calcitonins* (International Congress Series No. 243). Amsterdam, Excerpta Medica, 1972, p 365.

187. Horsting M, DeLuca HF: *In vitro* production of 25-hydroxycholecalciferol. *Biochem Biophys Res Commun* 36:251, 1969.

188. Horwith M, Nunez EA, Krook L, et al: Hereditary bone dysplasia with hyperphosphatasia. Response to synthetic human calcitonin. *Clin Endocrinol* 5:341S, 1976.

189. Hughes MR, Baylink DJ, Jones PG, et al: Radioligand receptor assay for 25-hydroxyvitamin D_2/D_3 and 1α,25-dihydroxyvitamin D_2/D_3: Application to hypervitaminosis D. *J Clin Invest* 58:61, 1976.

190. Ibels LS, Alfrey AC, Haut L, et al: Preservation of function in experimental renal disease by dietary restriction of phosphate. *N Engl J Med* 298:122, 1978.

191. Imawari M, Kida K, Goodman DS: The transport of vitamin D and its 25-hydroxy metabolite in human plasma. *J Clin Invest* 58:514, 1976.

192. Ireland AW, Cameron DA, Steward DH, et al: Quantitative histology of bone in advanced renal failure. *Calcif Tissue Res* 4:282, 1969.

193. Jacob AL, Lanier D Jr, Canterbury J, et al: Reduction by cimetidine of serum parathyroid hormone levels in uremic patients. *N Engl J Med* 302:671, 1980.

194. Jaworski ZFG, Lok E, Wellington JL: Impaired osteoclastic function and linear bone erosion rate in secondary hyperparathyroidism associated with chronic renal failure. *Clin Orthop* 107:298, 1975.

195. Johnson JW, Hatter RS, Hampers CL, et al: Effects of hemodialysis on secondary hyperparathyroidism in patients with chronic renal failure. *Metabolism* 21:18, 1972.

196. Johnson WJ: Optimum dialysate calcium concentration during maintenance hemodialysis. *Nephron* 17:241, 1976.

197. Johnson WJ, Kumar R: Use of vitamin D analogues in renal failure. *In* Kumar R (ed): *Vitamin D: Basic and Clinical Aspects*. Berlin, Martinus Nijhoff, 1984, p 641.

198. Jubiz W, Canterbury JM, Reiss E, et al: Circadian rhythm in serum parathyroid hormone concentration in human subjects: Correlation with serum calcium, phosphate, albumin, and growth hormone levels. *J Clin Invest* 51:2040, 1972.

199. Juttmann JR, Hagenouw-Taal JCW, Lanmeyer LDF, et al: A longitudinal study of bone mineral content and intestinal

calcium absorption in patients with chronic renal failure. *Metabolism* 28:1114, 1979.

200. Kallio DM, Garant RR, Minkin C: Ultrastructural effects of calcitonin on osteoclasts in tissue culture. *J Ultrastruct Res* 39:205, 1972.

201. Kanis JA, Cundy T, Bartlett M, et al: Is 24,25-dihydroxycholecalciferol a calcium-regulating hormone in man? *Br Med J* 1:1382, 1978.

202. Kanis JA, Cundy T, Smith R, et al: Possible function of different renal metabolites of vitamin D in man. *Contrib Nephrol* 18:192, 1980.

203. Kanis JA, Henderson RG, Heynen G, et al: Renal osteodystrophy in nondialysed adolescents: Long-term treatment with 1-hydroxycholecalciferol. *Arch Dis Child* 52:473, 1977.

204. Kanis JA, Taylor CM, Douglas DL, et al: Effects of 24,25-dihydroxyvitamin D_3 on its plasma level in man. *Metab Bone Dis & Rel Res* 3:155, 1981.

205. Kaplan MA, Canterbury J, Jaffe D, et al: Effect of dietary phosphorus in the phosphaturic and calcemic response to parathyroid hormone in the uremic dog. *Kidney Int* 12:457, 1977.

206. Katz AI, Hampers CL, Merrill JP: Secondary hyperparathyroidism and renal osteodystrophy in chronic renal failure. *Medicine* 48:333, 1969.

207. Klein GL, Alfrey AC, Miller NL, et al: Aluminum loading during total parenteral nutrition. *Am J Clin Nutr* 35:1425, 1982.

208. Klein GL, Horst RL, Norman AW, et al: Reduced serum levels of 1,25-dihydroxyvitamin D during long-term total parenteral nutrition. *Ann Intern Med* 94:638, 1981.

209. Kleiner-Bossaller A, DeLuca HF: Formation of 1,24,25-trihydroxyvitamin D_3 from 1,25-dihydroxyvitamin D_3. *Biochim Biophys Acta* 338:489, 1974.

210. Kleinknect C, Broyer M, Gasnadoux MF, et al: Growth in children treated with long-term dialysis: A study of 76 patients. *Adv Nephrol* 9:133, 1980.

211. Kopple JD, Coburn JW: Metabolic studies of low protein diets in uremia. II. Calcium, phosphorus and magnesium. *Medicine* 52:597, 1973.

212. Krane SM, Munoz AJ, Harris ED: Urinary polypeptides related to collagen synthesis. *J Clin Invest* 49:716, 1970.

213. Kraut JA, Shinaberger JH, Singer FR, et al: Parathyroid gland responsiveness to acute hypocalcemia in dialysis osteomalacia. *Kidney Int* 23:725, 1983.

214. Krempien B, Geiger G, Ritz E: Alteration of bone tissue structure in secondary hyperparathyroidism: A scanning electron microscopical study. *In* Norman AW, Schaefer K, Grigoleit HG, et al (eds): *Vitamin D and Problems Related to Uremic Bone Disease.* Berlin, Walter de Gruyter & Co, 1975, p 157.

215. Krempien B, Mehls O, Ritz E: Morphological studies on pathogenesis of epiphyseal slipping in uremic children. *Virchows Arch [A]* 362:129, 1974.

216. Krensky AM, Harmon WE, Ingelfinger JR, et al: Elevated nephrogenous cyclic adenosine monophosphate to monitor early renal osteodystrophy. *Clin Nephrol* 16:245, 1981.

217. Kual DN, Hadji-Georgopoulos A, Foster, GV: Evidence for physiological importance of calcitonin in the regulation of plasma calcium in rats. *J Clin Invest* 55:72, 1975.

218. Kumar R, Harnden D, DeLuca HF: Metabolism of 1,25-dihydroxyvitamin D_3: Evidence for side-chain oxidation. *Biochemistry* 15:2420, 1976.

219. Lam H, Schnoes HK, DeLuca HF: 24,25-dihydroxyvitamin D_3: Synthesis and biological activity. *Biochemistry* 12:4851, 1973.

220. Lambert PW, Stern PH, Avioli RC, et al: Evidence for

extrarenal production of 1,25-dihydroxyvitamin D in man. *J Clin Invest* 69:722, 1982.

221. Langman CG, Mazur AT, Baron R, et al: 25-hydroxyvitamin D_3 (calcifediol) therapy of juvenile renal osteodystrophy: Beneficial effect on linear growth velocity. *J Pediatr* 100:815, 1982.

222. Lewy JE, New MI: Growth in children with renal failure. *Am J Med* 58:65, 1975.

223. Liebenherr M, Garabedian M, Guillozo H, et al: Interaction of 24,25-dihydroxyvitamin D_3 and parathyroid hormone on bone enzymes *in vitro*. *Calcif Tissue Int* 27:47, 1979.

224. Lilien T von, Mehls O, Dietrich RB, et al: Visualization of parathyroid glands by ultrasound in dialyzed children. *Kidney Int* 28:246, 1985.

225. Liu CC, Baylink DJ, Wergedal J: Vitamin D-enhanced osteoclastic bone resorption at vascular canals. *Endocrinology* 95:1011, 1974.

226. Liu SH, Chu HI: Studies of calcium and phosphorus metabolism with special reference to the pathogenesis and effect of dihydrotachysterol (AT 10) and iron. *Medicine (Baltimore)* 22:103, 1943.

227. Llach F, Brickman AD, Singer FR, et al: 24,25-dihydroxycholecalciferol, a vitamin D sterol with qualitatively unique effects in uremic man. *Metab Bone Dis & Rel Res* 2:11, 1979.

228. Llach F, Massry SG, Koffler A, et al: Secondary hyperparathyroidism in early renal failure: Role of phosphate retention. *Kidney Int* 12:459, 1977.

229. Loirat C, Danan JL, Nguyen Dai D, et al: 1(OH)D_3 and 1,25(OH)$_2D_3$ plus (1,25) therapy in hemodialyzed children with reference to plasma concentration of 1,25. *In* Norman AW, Schaefer K, Herrath D von, et al (eds): *Vitamin D: Chemical, Biochemical, and Clinical Endocrinology of Calcium Metabolism.* Berlin, Walter de Gruyter & Co, 1982, p 893.

230. Lotz M, Zisman E, Bartter FC: Evidence for a phosphorus-depletion syndrome in man. *N Engl J Med* 278:409, 1968.

231. Lucas RC: On a form of late rickets associated with albuminuria, rickets of adolescents. *Lancet* 1:933, 1883.

232. Lumb GA, Mawer EB, Stanbury SW: The apparent vitamin D resistance of chronic renal failure: A study of the physiology of vitamin D in man. *Am J Med* 50:421, 1971.

233. Lund B, Helmer Sorensen O, Pors Nielsen S, et al: 25-hydroxycholecalciferol in chronic renal failure. *Lancet* 2:372, 1975.

234. MacGregor RR, Chu LLH, Cohn DV: Conversion of proparathyroid hormone to parathyroid hormone by a particulate enzyme of the parathyroid gland. *J Biol Chem* 251:6711, 1976.

235. Mahan J, Kim YK, Fallon J, et al: Influence of 25 hydroxycholecalciferol therapy in anephric dialysis dependent children. *Pediatr Nephrol* (in press).

236. Malekzadeh M, Stanley P, Ettenger R, et al: Treatment of renal osteodystrophy in children on haemodialysis with dihydrotachysterol. *In* Norman AW, Schaefer K, Herrath D von, et al (eds): *Vitamin D: Biochemical, Chemical and Clinical Aspects Releated to Calcium Metabolism.* Berlin, Walter de Gruyter & Co, 1977, p 681.

237. Malekzadeh MH, Ettenger RB, Pennisi AJ, et al: Treatment of renal osteodystrophy in children with 1,25(OH)$_2D_3$. *In* Norman AW, Schaefer K, Herrath D von, et al (eds): *Vitamin D: Chemical, Biochemical, and Clinical Endocrinology of Calcium Metabolism.* Berlin, Walter de Gruyter & Co, 1982, p 200.

238. Malluche HH, Ritz E, Lang HP, et al: Bone histology in incipient and advanced renal failure. *Kidney Int* 9:355, 1976.

239. Martin BF, Jacoby F: Diffusion phenomenon complicating the histochemical reaction for alkaline phosphatase. *J Anat* 83:351, 1949.

240. Martin K, Hruska K, Grenwalt A, et al: Selective uptake of intake parathyroid hormone by the liver. *J Clin Invest* 58:781, 1976.

241. Marx SJ, Woodward CJ, Aurbach GD: Calcitonin receptors of kidney and bone. *Science* 178:999, 1972.

242. Marx SJ, Woodward CJ, Aurbach GD, et al: Renal receptors for calcitonin. *J Biol Chem* 248:4797, 1973.

243. Maschio G, Tessitore N, D'Angelo A, et al: Early dietary phosphorus restriction and calcium supplementation in the prevention of renal osteodystrophy. *Am J Clin Nutr* 33:1546, 1980.

244. Mason RS, Lissner D, Wilkinson M, et al: Vitamin D metabolites and their relationship to azotaemic osteodystrophy. *Clin Endocrinol* 13:375, 1980.

245. Massry S, Coburn JW, Popvtzer MM, et al: Secondary hyperparathyroidism in chronic renal failure: The clinical spectrum in uremia during hemodialysis and after renal transplantation. *Arch Intern Med* 124:431, 1969.

246. Massry SG: Requirements of vitamin D metabolites in patients with renal disease. *Am J Clin Nutr* 33:1530, 1980.

247. Massry SG, Goldstein DA: Is calcitriol (1,25(OH)₂D₃) harmful to renal function? *JAMA* 242:1875, 1979.

248. Massry SG, Turna S, Dua S, et al: Reversal of skeletal resistance to parathyroid hormone in uremia by vitamin D metabolites: Evidence for the requirement of 24,25(OH)₂D₃. *J Lab Clin Med* 94:152, 1979.

249. Matthews JL, Martin JH: Intracellular transport of calcium and its relationship to homeostasis and mineralization: An electron microscopic study. *Am J Med* 50:589, 1971.

250. Mawer EB, Backhouse J, Taylor CM, et al: Failure of formation of 1,25-dihydroxycholecalciferol in chronic renal insufficiency. *Lancet* 1:626, 1973.

251. Mayor GH, Burnatowska-Hledin MA: Impaired renal function and aluminum metabolism. *Federation Proc* 42:2979, 1983.

252. Mazess RB, Peppler WW, Lange TA, et al: Total body and regional bone mineral by dual-photon absorptiometry in metabolic bone disease. *Calcif Tissue Int* 36:8, 1984.

253. McLaughlin M, Fairney A, Lester E, et al: Seasonal variations in serum 25-hydroxycholecalciferol in healthy people. *Lancet* 1:536, 1974.

254. McSherry E: Acidosis and growth in non-uremic renal disease. *Kidney Int* 14:349, 1978.

255. McSherry E, Morris RC: Attainment and maintenance of normal status with alkali therapy in infants and children with classic renal tubular acidosis (RTA). *J Clin Invest* 61:509, 1978.

256. Mehls O, Eberhard R, Kreusser W, et al: Renal osteodystrophy in uremic children. *J Clin Endocrinol Metab* 9:151, 1980.

257. Mehls O, Krempien B, Ritz E, et al: Renal osteodystrophy in children on maintenance hemodialysis. *Proc Eur Dial Trans Assoc* 10:197, 1973.

258. Mehls O, Ritz E: Renal osteodystrophy. In Holliday MA, Barratt TM, Vernier RL (eds): *Pediatric Nephrology.* Baltimore, Williams & Wilkins, 1986.

259. Mehls O, Ritz E, Gilli G, et al: Growth in renal failure. *Nephron* 21:237, 1978.

260. Mehls O, Ritz E, Krempien B, et al: Roentgenological signs in the skeleton of uremic children: An analysis of the anatomical principles underlying the roentgenological changes. *Pediatr Radiol* 1:183, 1973.

261. Mehls O, Ritz E, Krempien B, et al: Slipped epiphyses in renal osteodystrophy. *Arch Dis Child* 50:545, 1975.

262. Mehls O, Salusky IB: Recent advances and controversies in childhood renal osteodystrophy. *Pediatr Nephrol* 1:212, 1987.

263. Melick RA, Martin TJ: Parathyroid hormone metabolism in man: Effect of nephrectomy. *Clin Sci* 37:667, 1969.

264. Mennes P, Rosenbaum R, Martin K, et al: Hypomagnesemia and impaired parathyroid hormone secretion in chronic renal failure. *Ann Intern Med* 88:206, 1978.

265. Miller EJ, Matukas VJ: Biosynthesis of collagen. *Fed Proc* 33:1198, 1974.

266. Miller SC, Halloran BP, DeLuca HF, et al: Studies on the role of 24-hydroxylation of vitamin D in the mineralization of cartilage and bone of vitamin D-deficient rats. *Calcif Tissue Int* 33:489, 1981.

267. Milne FJ, Sharf B, Bell P, et al: The effect of low aluminum water and desferrioxamine on the outcome of dialysis encephalopathy. *Clin Nephrol* 20:202, 1983.

268. Miravet L, Redel J, Carre M, et al: The biological activity of synthetic 25,26-dihydroxycholecalciferol and 24,25-dihydroxycholecalciferol in vitamin D-deficient rats. *Calcif Tissue Res* 21:145, 1976.

269. Mitch WE, Walser M, Steinman TI, et al: The effect of a keto acid-amino acid supplement to a restricted diet on the progression of chronic renal failure. *N Engl J Med* 311:623, 1984.

270. Moorhead JF, Wills MR, Ahmed KY, et al: Hypophosphatemic osteomalacia after cadaveric renal transplantation. *Lancet* 1:694, 1974.

271. Moxley MA, Bell NH, Wagle SR, et al: Parathyroid hormone stimulation of glucose and urea production in isolated liver cells. *Am J Physiol* 227:1058, 1974.

272. Mozes MF, Soper WD, Jonasson O, et al: Total parathyroidectomy and autotransplantation in secondary hyperparathyroidism. *Arch Surg* 115:378, 1980.

273. Muirhead N, Adami S, Sandler LM, et al: Long-term 24,25(OH)₂D₃ in the treatment of renal osteodystrophy. In Norman AW, Schaefer K, Herrath D von, et al (eds): *Vitamin D: Chemical, Biochemical and Clinical Endocrinology of Calcium Metabolism.* Berlin, Walter de Gruyter & Co, 1982, p 187.

274. Muldowney FP, Carroll DV, Donohoe JF, et al: Correction of renal bicarbonate wastage by parathyroidectomy. *Q J Med* 40:a487, 1971.

275. Muldowney FP, Donohoe JF, Freaney R, et al: Parathormone-induced renal bicarbonate wastage in intestinal malabsorption and in chronic renal failure: *Ir J Med Sci* 3:221, 1970.

276. Muldowney FP, McKenna TJ, Kyle LH, et al: Parathormone-like effect of magnesium replenishment in steatorrhea. *N Engl J Med* 218:61, 1970.

277. Nagata N, Rasmussen H: Parathyroid hormone and renal cell metabolism. *Biochemistry* 7:3728, 1968.

278. Nathan E, Pedersen SE: Dialysis encephalopathy in a non-dialysed uraemic boy treated with aluminum hydroxide orally. *Acta Paediatr Scand* 69:793, 1980.

279. Ney RL, Kelly G, Bartter FC: Actions of vitamin D independent of the parathyroid glands. *Endocrinology* 82:760, 1968.

280. Nielsen HE, Melsen F, Christensen MS, et al: 1-hydroxycholecalciferol treatment of long-term hemodialyzed patients: Effects on mineral metabolism, bone mineral content and bone morphometry. *Clin Nephrol* 8:429, 1977.

281. Nielsen SP, Binderup E, Godtfredsen WO, et al: 1-hydroxycholecalciferol: Long-term treatment of patients with uraemic osteodystrophy. *Nephron* 16:359, 1976.

282. Nordin BEC: Vitamin D analogs and renal function. *Lancet* 2:1259, 1978.

283. Norman AW, Midgett RJ, Myrtle JF, et al: Studies on calciferol metabolism. I. Production of vitamin D metabolite

4B from 25-OH-cholecalciferol by kidney homogenates. *Biochem Biophys Res Commun* 42:1082, 1971.

284. Norman ME, Mazur AT, Borden S IV, et al: Early diagnosis of juvenile renal osteodystrophy. *J Pediatr* 97:226, 1980.

285. Norman ME, Taylor A: Interrelationship of serum 25(OH)D₃ and 1,25(OH)₂D₃ levels in juvenile renal osteodystrophy during therapy with 25(OH)D₃. *Calcif Tissue Int* 33:340A, 1981.

286. O'Riordan JLH, Page J, Kerr KNS, et al: Hyperparathyroidism in chronic renal failure and dialysis osteodystrophy. *Q J Med* 39:359, 1970.

287. Ogura Y, Kawaguchi Y, Sakai S, et al: Plasma levels of vitamin D metabolites in renal diseases. *Contrib Nephrol* 22:18, 1980.

288. Okamoto S, Tanaka Y, DeLuca HF, et al: 24-difluoro-25-hydroxyvitamin D₃-enhanced bone mineralization in rats: Comparison with 25-hydroxyvitamin D₃ and vitamin D₃. *Arch Biochem Biophys* 206:8, 1981.

289. Olgaard K, Rothstein M, Arbelaez M, et al: Does 24,25(OH)₂D₃ have a beneficial effect in uremia? In Norman AW, Schaefer K, Herrath D von, et al (eds): *Vitamin D: Chemical, Biochemical and Clinical Endocrinology of Calcium Metabolism*. Berlin, Walter de Gruyter & Co, 1982, p 139.

290. Olson EB Jr, Knutson JC, Bhattacharyya MH, et al: The effect of hepatectomy on the synthesis of 25-hydroxyvitamin D₃. *J Clin Invest* 57:1213, 1976.

291. Ornoy A, Goodwin D, Noff D, et al: 24,25-dihydroxyvitamin D is a metabolite of vitamin D essential for bone formation. *Nature* 276:517, 1978.

292. Ott SM, Maloney NA, Coburn JW, et al: The prevalence of bone aluminum deposition in renal osteodystrophy and its relation to the response to calcitriol therapy. *N Engl J Med* 307:709, 1982.

293. Ott SM, Maloney NA, Klein GL, et al: Aluminum is associated with low bone formation in patients receiving chronic parenteral nutrition. *Ann Intern Med* 98:910, 1983.

294. Parfitt AM: Soft tissue calcification in uremia. *Arch Intern Med* 124:544, 1969.

295. Parfitt AM: The actions of parathyroid hormone on bone: Relation to bone remodelling and turnover calcium homeostasis and metabolic bone disease. *Metabolism* 25:909, 1976.

296. Parfitt AM, Frame B: Treatment of rickets and osteomalacia. *Semin Drug Treat* 2:83, 1972.

297. Parker RF, Vergne-Marini P, Hull AR, et al: Jejunal absorption and secretion of calcium in patients with chronic renal disease on hemodialysis. *J Clin Invest* 54:358, 1974.

298. Peacock M, Gallagher JC, Nordin BEC: Action of 1α-hydroxyvitamin D₃ on calcium absorption and bone resorption in man. *Lancet* 1:385, 1974.

299. Peacock M, Taylor GA, Redel J: The action of two metabolites of vitamin D₃; 25,26-dihydroxycholecalciferol (25,26(OH)₂D₃) and 24,25-dihydroxycholecalciferol (24,25(OH₂)D₃) on bone resorption. *FEBS Lett* 62:248, 1976.

300. Pendras JP: Parathyroid disease in long term maintenance hemodialysis. *Arch Intern Med* 124:312, 1969.

301. Piel CF, Roof BS, Avioli LV: Metabolism of tritiated 25-hydroxycholecalciferol in chronically uremic children before and after successful renal homotransplantation. *J Clin Endocrinol Metab* 37:944, 1973.

302. Pierides AM, Ellis HA, Dellagrammatikas H, et al: 1,25-dihydroxycholecalciferol in renal osteodystrophy: Epiphysiolysis-anticonvulsant therapy. *Arch Dis Child* 52:464, 1977.

303. Pillion G, Loirat C, Blum C, et al: Aluminum encephalopathy: A potential risk of aluminum gels in children with chronic renal failure. *Int J Pediatr Nephrol* 2:29, 1981.

304. Pinnel SR, Fox R, Krane SM: Human collagens: Differences in glycosylated hydroxylysines in skin and bone. *Biochim Biophys Acta* 229:119, 1971.

305. Pletka P, Bernstein DS, Hampers CL, et al: Relationship between magnesium and secondary hyperparathyroidism during long-term hemodialysis. *Metabolism* 23:619, 1974.

306. Popovtzer MM, Robinette JB, DeLuca HF, et al: The acute effect of 25-hydroxycholecalciferol on renal handling of phosphorus. *J Clin Invest* 53:913, 1974.

307. Popowniak KL, Esselstyn CB Jr, Nakamoto S: Parathyroidectomy for the treatment of renal osteodystrophy and tertiary hyperparathyroidism: Progress report. *Surg Clin North Am* 54:325, 1974.

308. Portale AA, Booth BE, Halloran BP, et al: Effect of dietary phosphorus on circulating concentrations of 1,25-dihydroxyvitamin D and immunoreactive parathyroid hormone in children with moderate renal insufficiency. *J Clin Invest* 73:1580, 1984.

309. Portale AA, Boothe BE, Tsai HC, et al: Reduced plasma concentration of 1,25-dihydroxyvitamin D in children with moderate renal insufficiency. *Kidney Int* 21:627, 1982.

310. Potter DE, Wilson CJ, Ozonoff MB: Hyperparathyroid bone disease in children undergoing long-term hemodialysis. Treatment with vitamin D. *J Pediatr* 85:60, 1974.

311. Preece MA, Tomlinson S, Ribot CA, et al: Studies of vitamin D deficiency in man. *Q J Med* 44:575, 1975.

312. Prior JC, Cameron EC, Knickerbocker WJ, et al: Dialysis encephalopathy and osteomalacic bone disease. *Am J Med* 72:33, 1982.

313. Puschett JB, Fernandez PC, Boyle IT, et al: The acute tubular effects of 1,25-dihydroxycholecalciferol. *Proc Soc Exp Biol Med* 141:379, 1972.

314. Puschett JB, Moranz K, Kurnick WS: Evidence for a direct action of cholecalciferol and 25-hydroxycholecalciferol on the renal transport of phosphate, sodium and calcium. *J Clin Invest* 51:373, 1972.

315. Queener SF, Bell NH: Calcitonin: A general survey. *Metabolism* 24:555, 1975.

316. Raisz LG: Inhibition of actinomycin D of bone resorption induced by parathyroid hormone or vitamin D. *Proc Soc Exp Biol Med* 119:614, 1965.

317. Raisz LG, Trummel CL, Holick MF, et al: 1,25-dihydroxycholecalciferol: A potent stimulator of bone resorption in tissue culture. *Science* 175:768, 1972.

318. Raisz LG, Trummel CL, Simmons H: Induction of bone resorption in tissue culture: Prolonged response after brief exposure to parathyroid hormone on 25-hydroxycholecalciferol. *Endocrinology* 90:744, 1972.

319. Rasmussen H, Bordier P: Evidence that different vitamin D sterols have qualitatively different effects in man. *Contrib Nephrol* 18:184, 1980.

320. Rasmussen H, DeLuca H, Arnaud C, et al: The relationship between vitamin D and parathyroid hormone. *J Clin Invest* 42:1940, 1963.

321. Rauschkolb EW, Davis HW, Fenimore DC, et al: Identification of vitamin D₃ in human skin. *J Invest Dermatol* 53:289, 1969.

322. Recker RR, Saville PD: Calcium absorption in renal failure: Its relation to blood urea nitrogen, dietary calcium intake, time on dialysis and other variables. *J Lab Clin Med* 78:380, 1971.

323. Ritz E, Franz HE, Jahns E: The course of secondary hyperparathyroidism during chronic hemodialysis. *Trans Am Soc Artif Intern Organs* 14:385, 1962.

324. Robertson JA, Felsenfeld AJ, Haygood CC, et al: Animal model of aluminum-induced osteomalacia: Role of chronic renal failure. *Kidney Int* 23:327, 1983.

325. Robitaille P, Marie PJ, Delvin EE, et al: Renal osteodystrophy in children treated with 1,25-dihydroxycholecalciferol (1,25(OH)$_2$D$_3$): Histologic bone studies. *Acta Paediatr Scand* 73:315, 1984.

326. Roof BS, Gordan GS, Goldman L, et al: Berson and Yalow's radioimmunoassay for parathyroid hormone (PTH): A clinical progress report. *Mt Sinai J Med (NY)* 40:433, 1973.

327. Roof BS, Piel CF, Carpenter BJ, et al: Natural course of secondary hyperparathyroidism after successful renal transplantation. *Proc Clin Dial Transplant Forum* 2:166, 1972.

328. Roof BS, Piel CF, Rames L, et al: Parathyroid function in uremic children with and without osteodystrophy. *Pediatrics* 53:404, 1974.

329. Russell JE, Avioli LV: Alterations of cartilaginous aerobic glycolysis in the chronic uremic state. *Kidney Int* 7:S333, 1975.

330. Russell JE, Avioli LV, Mechanic G: The nature of the collagen cross-links in bone in the chronic uraemic state (short communications). *Biochem J* 145:119, 1975.

331. Russell JE, Termine JD, Avioli LV: Abnormal bone mineral maturation in the chronic uremic state. *J Clin Invest* 52:2848, 1973.

332. Russell JE, Termine JD, Avioli LV: Experimental renal osteodystrophy: The response to 25-hydroxycholecalciferol and dichloromethylene diphosphate therapy. *J Clin Invest* 56:548, 1975.

333. Saenger P, Wiedemann E, Korth-Schutz S, et al: Role of somatomedin and renal function in growth after renal transplantation. *Pediatr Res* 7:411, 1973.

334. Saenger P, Wiedemann E, Schwartz E, et al: Somatomedin and growth after renal transplantation. *Pediatr Res* 8:163, 1974.

335. Salusky IB, Coburn JW, Foley J, et al: Effect of oral calcium chloride on control of serum phosphorus and changes in plasma aluminum levels after discontinuation of aluminum-containing gels in children receiving dialysis. *J Pediatr* 108:767, 1986.

336. Salusky IB, Coburn JW, Paunier L, et al: Role of aluminum hydroxide in raising serum aluminum levels in children undergoing continuous ambulatory peritoneal dialysis (CAPD). *J Pediatr* 105:717, 1984.

337. Sarnsethsiri P, Jaworski ZF, Shimizu AG, et al: Tissue-level bone formation rates in chronic renal failure, measured by means of tetracycline bone labeling. *Can J Physiol Pharmacol* 48:824, 1970.

338. Sato KA, Gray RW, Lemann J Jr: Urinary excretion of 25-hydroxyvitamin D in health and the nephrotic syndrome. *J Lab Clin Med* 99:325, 1982.

339. Schnoes HK, DeLuca HF: Recent progress in vitamin D metabolism and the chemistry of vitamin D metabolites. *Fed Proc* 39:2723, 1980.

340. Schott GD, Wills MR: Muscle weakness in osteomalacia. *Lancet* 1:626, 1976.

341. Sedman AB, Miller NL, Warady BA, et al: Aluminum loading in children with chronic renal failure. *Kidney Int* 26:201, 1984.

342. Segre GV: Advances in techniques for measurement of parathyroid hormone. *TEM* May/June:243, 1990.

343. Segrest JP, Cunningham LW: Variations in human urinary 0-hydroxylsyl glycoside levels and their relationships to collagen metabolism. *J Clin Invest* 49:1497, 1970.

344. Shen FH, Baylink DJ, Sherrard DJ, et al: Serum immunoreactive parathyroid hormone and 25-hydroxyvitamin D in patients with uremic bone disease. *J Clin Endocrinol Metab* 40:1009, 1975.

345. Shepard RM, Horst RL, Hamstra AJ, et al: Determination of vitamin D and its metabolites in plasma from normal and anephric man. *Biochem J* 182:55, 1979.

346. Sherrard DJ, Baylink DJ, Wergedal JE, et al: Quantitative histological studies on the pathogenesis of uremic bone disease. *J Clin Endocrinol Metab* 39:119, 1974.

347. Sherrard DJ, Ott SM, Maloney NA, et al: The use of 24,25(OH)$_2$-vitamin D in the refractory osteomalacia form of renal osteodystrophy. *In* Norman AW, Schaefer K, Herrath D von, et al (eds): *Vitamin D: Chemical, Biochemical and Clinical Endocrinology of Calcium Metabolism.* Berlin, Walter de Gruyter & Co, 1982, p 169.

348. Silverman R, Yalow RS: Heterogeneity of parathyroid hormone: Clinical and physiologic implications. *J Clin Invest* 52:1958, 1973.

349. Simon LS, Slovick DM, Neer RM, et al: Changes in serum levels of Type I and III procollagen extension peptides during infusion of human parathyroid hormone (1–34). *J Bone Min Res* 3:241, 1988.

350. Singer FR, Habener JF, Greene E, et al: Inactivation of calcitonin by specific organs. *Nature [New Biol]* 237:269, 1972.

351. Sivakumar B, Krishnamachari KAVR: Circulating levels of immunoreactive parathyroid hormone in endemic genu valgum. *Horm Metab Res* 8:317, 1976.

352. Slatopolsky E, Caglar S, Gradowska L, et al: On the prevention of secondary hyperparathyroidism in experimental chronic renal disease using "proportional reduction" of dietary phosphorus intake. *Kidney Int* 2:147, 1972.

353. Slatopolsky E, Gray R, Adams ND, et al: Low serum levels of 1,25(OH)$_2$D$_3$ are not responsible for the development of secondary hyperparathyroidism in early renal failure. *Kidney Int* 14:733, 1978.

354. Snapper I: *Medical Clinics in Bone Disease.* New York, Interscience, 1943.

355. Stamp TCB, Round JM, Rowe DJF, et al: Plasma levels and therapeutic effect of 25-hydroxycholecalciferol in epileptic patients taking anticonvulsant drugs. *Br Med J* 4:9, 1972.

356. Stanbury SW: The treatment of renal osteodystrophy. *Ann Intern Med* 65:1133, 1966.

357. Stanbury SW: Bone disease in uremia. *Am J Med* 44:714, 1968.

358. Stanbury SW, Lumb GA: Metabolic studies of renal osteodystrophy. I. Calcium, phosphorus and nitrogen metabolism in rickets, osteomalacia and hyperparathyroidism complicating chronic uremia and in the osteomalacia of adult Fanconi syndrome. *Medicine* 41:1, 1952.

359. Stanbury SW, Lumb GA: Parathyroid function in chronic renal failure: A statistical survey of the plasma biochemistry in azotemic renal osteodystrophy. *Q J Med* 35:1, 1966.

360. Swanson MR, Biggers JA, Remmers AR Jr, et al: Results of parathyroidectomy for autonomous hyperparathyroidism. *Arch Intern Med* 139:989, 1979.

361. Talwalkar YB, Puri HC, Hawker CC, et al: Parathyroid autotransplantation in renal osteodystrophy. *Am J Dis Child* 133:901, 1979.

362. Tanaka Y, DeLuca HF: The control of 24-hydroxyvitamin D metabolism by inorganic phosphorus. *Arch Biochem Biophys* 159:566, 1973.

363. Tanaka Y, DeLuca HF: Stimulation of the 24,25-dihydroxyvitamin D$_3$ production of 1,25-dihydroxyvitamin D$_3$. *Science* 183:1198, 1974.

364. Tanzer FS, Navia JM: Calcitonin inhibition of intestinal phosphate absorption. *Nature [New Biol]* 242:221, 1973.

365. Taylor CM, Hughes SE, de Silva P: Competitive protein binding assay for 24,25-dihydroxycholecalciferol. *Biochem Biophys Res Commun* 70:1243, 1976.

366. Taylor CM, Mawer EB, Wallace JE, et al: The absence of

24,25-dihydroxycholecalciferol in anephric patients. *Clin Sci Mol Med* 55:541, 1978.

367. Teitelbaum SL, Russell JE, Avioli LV: The relationship of biochemical and histometric determinants of uremic bone. *Arch Pathol* 103:228, 1979.

368. Termine JD: Mineral chemistry and skeletal biology. *Clin Orthop* 85:207, 1972.

369. Termine JD, Posner AS: Morphous/crystalline interrelationships in bone mineral. *Calcif Tissue Res* 1:8, 1967.

370. Uebelhart D, Gineyts E, Chapery M-C, et al: Urinary excretion of pyridinium crosslinks: A new marker of bone resorption in metabolic bone disease. *Bone Miner* 8:87, 1990.

371. Upjohn Company Bulletin: The role of calderol capsules (calcifediol) in the management of renal osteodystrophy: Report of a Clinical Conference, 1981.

372. Velentzas C, Meindok H, Ozeoporilos DG, et al: Detection and pathogenesis of visceral calcification in dialysis patients and patients with malignant disease. *Can Med Assoc J* 118:45, 1978.

373. Voigts AL, Felsenfeld AJ, Llach F: The effects of calciferol and its metabolites on patients with chronic renal failure. *Arch Intern Med* 143:960, 1983.

374. Walker DG: The induction of osteopetrotic changes in hypophysectomized, thyroparathyroidectomized and intact rats of various ages. *Endocrinology* 89:1389, 1971.

375. Walker DG: Enzymatic and electron microscopic analysis of isolated osteoclasts. *Calcif Tissue Res* 9:296, 1972.

376. Walker GS, Aaron JE, Peacock M, et al: Dialysate aluminum concentration and renal bone disease. *Kidney Int* 21:411, 1982.

377. Walling MW, Kimberg DV: Effects of 1-alpha, 25-dihydroxyvitamin D_3 and Solanum glaucophyllum on intestinal calcium and phosphate transport and on plasma Ca, Mg and P levels in the rat. *Endocrinology* 97:1567, 1975.

378. Ward MK, Ellis HA, Feest TG, et al: Osteomalacic dialysis osteodystrophy: Evidence for a water-borne etiological agent, probably aluminum. *Lancet* 1:841, 1978.

379. Warshaw BL, Edelbrock HH, Ettenger RB, et al: Progression to end-stage renal disease in children with obstructive uropathy. *J Pediatr* 100:183, 1982.

380. Weinstein RS: Decreased mineralization in hemodialysis patients after subtotal parathyroidectomy. *Calcif Tissue Int* 34:16, 1982.

381. Weinstein RS, Sappington LJ: Qualitative bone defect in uremic osteosclerosis. *Metabolism* 31:805, 1982.

382. Wells SA Jr, Gunnells JC, Shelburn JD: Transplantation of parathyroid glands in man: Clinical indications and results. *Surgery* 78:34, 1975.

383. Wezeman FH: 25-hydroxyvitamin D_3: Autoradiographic evidence of sites of action in epiphyseal cartilage and bone. *Lancet* 2:1069, 1976.

384. Wilde CD, Jaworski ZF, Villaneuva AR, et al: Quantitative histological measurements of bone turnover in primary hyperparathyroidism. *Calcif Tissue Res* 12:137, 1973.

385. Wills MR, Savory J: Aluminum poisoning: Dialysis encephalopathy, osteomalacia, and anemia. *Lancet* 1:29, 1983.

386. Wing RM, Okamura WH, Pirio MR, et al: Vitamin D in solution: Conformations of vitamins D_3, 1,25-dihydroxyvitamin D_2 and dihydrotachysterol. *Science* 186:939, 1974.

387. Witmer G, Margolis A, Fontaine O, et al: Effects of 25-hydroxycholecalciferol on bone lesions of children with terminal renal failure. *Kidney Int* 10:395, 1976.

FRANK G. BOINEAU
JAMES W. FISHER

29

Hematologic Abnormalities in Renal Disease

Anemia

Anemia is a cardinal feature of chronic renal failure in children, the severity being proportional to the degree of renal insufficiency. Anemia is almost invariably present when end-stage renal disease (ESRD) develops. Characteristically, the reduction in hemoglobin is proportional to the reduction in hematocrit. Erythrocytes appear normochromic and normocytic. The reticulocyte response is inadequate for the degree of anemia [15]. Anemia in children is usually more severe than in adults [11].

Children with creatinine clearances of 5 to 100 ml/min/1.73 m^2 were studied to determine the level of renal function at which anemia begins to develop [20,35]. The hematocrits ranged from 17% to 50%. There was a direct correlation between creatinine clearance and hematocrit (Fig. 29-1), and anemia usually was evident at a creatinine clearance less than 35 ml/min/1.73 m^2, despite a wide scatter of hematocrit values at any level of renal function.

Our knowledge of the effects of anemia in children with ESRD is incomplete. When severe, anemia contributes to fatigue, limited exercise tolerance, and increased cardiac demand. Its severity does not, however, correlate with the growth rate of children with ESRD who are on dialysis [11].

Ulmer and colleagues [61] reported on cardiovascular impairment and physical work in children with mild to severe renal insufficiency, including a group on hemodialysis. Physical work capacity was measured using a cycle ergometer. The work capacity of all subjects was compared to a group of normal children. Children whose serum creatinine was below 2 mg/dl had normal work capacity. In those with more severe renal insufficiency, the physical work capacity was inversely correlated to the serum creatinine. There was also a significant correlation between physical work capacity and the degree of anemia, which was described by an exponential relationship. Work capacity of children whose serum creatinine was above 5 mg/dl was slightly better in those on hemodialysis. When work capacity was measured before and after a hemodialysis session, it was found to be worse immediately after hemodialysis [61].

The cause of the anemia of ESRD is undoubtedly multifactorial. The model proposed by Fisher and colleagues [22] may serve as a useful conceptual guide to review this problem. Important mechanisms of the origin of the anemia of ESRD include the following:

1. Relative deficiency in the level of erythropoietin (Epo);
2. Accumulation in the serum of toxins that are inhibitors of erythropoiesis;
3. Decreased erythrocyte life span;
4. Blood loss from the gastrointestinal tract and other sites of bleeding; blood loss through dialysis;
5. Deficiency of iron, folic acid, or other nutrients.

Normal Maturation of Red Blood Cells

The normal maturation of red blood cells and the influence of Epo are shown in Fig. 29-2 [21]. Pluripotent stem cells in the bone marrow give rise to several cell lines. The stem cell is called colony-forming unit-spleen (CFU-S) because it gives rise to granulocytic, erythrocytic, and megakaryocytic colonies in the spleen of irradiated mice. The relationship between the myeloid and lymphoid stem cells is highly conjectural. Presumably, the lymphoid lines diverge at an early stage, but they appear to share a common ancestry with the myeloid line. The pluripotent stem cells become differentiated into progenitor cells committed to either granulocytic/myelocytic (CFU-GM), erythrocytic (BFU-E, CFU-E), or megakaryocytic (CFU-M) progenitors. The earliest cell that can be identified as an erythroid progenitor is called the burst-forming unit-erythroid (BFU-E), which differentiates into the CFU-E. This late BFU-E may be responsive to high concentrations of Epo (see Fig. 29-2), but its proliferation and differentiation is controlled by a burst-promoting factor. More mature BFU-Es become increasingly responsive to Epo. They subsequently evolve into CFU-Es, which are the primary target cells for Epo [21]. High concentrations of Epo may also directly stimulate the recognizable nucleated erythroid cell compartment to increase its numbers and may stimulate the marrow to release reticulocytes into the circulation

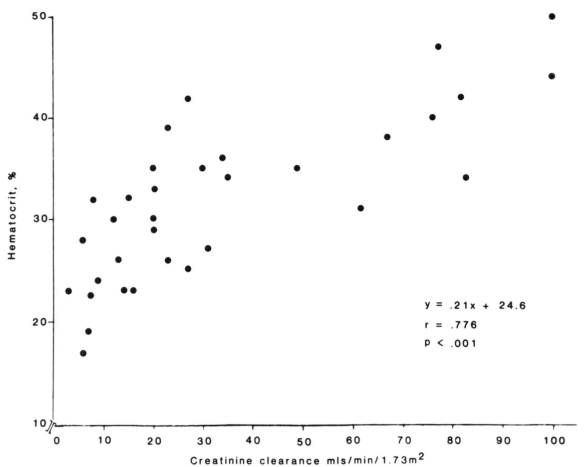

FIG. 29-1. *Relationship between creatinine clearance and hematocrit levels in children with normal renal function and varying degrees of anemia due to chronic renal insufficiency. (Based on data from McGonigle RJS, Boineau F, Beckman B, et al: Erythropoietin and inhibitors of in vivo erythropoiesis in the development of anemia in children with renal disease. J Lab Clin Med 105:449, 1985. Revised for presentation in Glassock and Massry, Textbook of Nephrology, 1988.*

when there is an extreme demand for new red blood cells [58].

Assay of Erythropoietin

For many years both clinical and basic fundamental research has been markedly hampered by the lack of a sensitive, specific, and reliable assay for Epo. At the present time the exhypoxic or hypertransfused polycythemic mouse assay for Epo is the international reference standard assay by which all in vitro and in vivo assay methods should be standardized using the International Reference Preparation Erythropoietin. Most clinical laboratories cannot use the polycythemic mouse assay as a standard because it is very expensive and time-consuming and requires highly skilled and experienced technical personnel. A radioimmunoassay for Epo has been developed with the availability of either the purified native hormone from human urine or recombinant Epo from transfected cells. With the availability of a commercial radioimmunoassay for Epo (SKF Biosciences,

St. Louis, MO), the determination of Epo levels in sera of patients with polycythemia vera or secondary polycythemias related to inappropriate production of Epo by tumors from the kidney, liver, and cerebellum, as well as studies in patients with anemia of renal failure, should be possible.

Renal Sites of Erythropoietin Production

It seems most likely that the cells within the kidney that produce Epo are localized in the kidney cortex. Epo has been demonstrated in extracts of both renal glomeruli and tubules.

Early studies using fluorescence microscopy reported the localization of Epo in the glomerular tuft of the anemic human kidney, the hypoxic dog kidney, and the anemic sheep kidney. Studies also indicate that the mesangial cells in the glomerular tuft are the site of production of Epo and that they respond to an oxygen deficit to elaborate small to moderate quantities of both prostaglandins and Epo. Using a highly specific antibody to a peptide fragment of

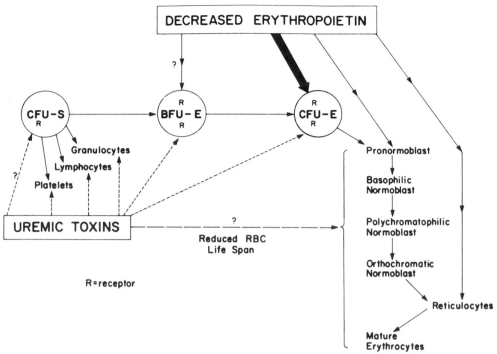

FIG. 29-2. Model for mechanism of anemia of chronic renal failure. R, receptor.

Epo, the localization of Epo in the glomerular epithelial cells of the human and the rat kidney has been shown in vitro. Using these immunocytochemical methods, no staining was found in the juxtaglomerular cells or renal tubules. Additional renal immunocytochemical studies using some of the more sophisticated cDNA probes for Epo are needed to dissociate trapping from cellular synthesis in the renal glomerular cells.

Koury et al. [27] and Lacombe et al. [29] have reported Epo mRNA in interstitial peritubular endothelial cells in the mouse kidney using an Epo mouse cDNA probe. No Epo has been found in these cells using immunocytochemical methods, however. Therefore, the question still arises as to whether Epo is translated in these cells.

CONTROL OF ERYTHROPOIETIN PRODUCTION BY THE NORMAL KIDNEY

Our model for kidney production of Epo postulates that hypoxia (hypobaric, anemic, or ischemic) produces oxygen deprivation to a critical renal sensor cell, which initiates a cascade of events leading to increased biosynthesis or secretion of Epo or both [21] (Fig. 29-3). Neither the physiologic nor the pathophysiologic control of kidney production of Epo is clearly understood, but hypoxia is considered to be the fundamental stimulus for the secretion of both renal and extrarenal Epo. The primary oxygen-sensing reaction of the kidney is initiated by a decrease in ambient partial pressure of oxygen (high altitude, hypobaria); interrupted gas exchange in the lung (obstructive lung diseases); diminished oxygen-carrying capacity of hemoglobin (anemia); molecular deprivation of oxygen (cobalt); and a

decrease in renal blood flow (ischemia due to arteriosclerosis, thrombosis, or renal artery constriction).

Adenosine production by the kidney is significantly increased very early following ischemic hypoxia. The primary oxygen-sensing reaction continues by triggering secondary biochemical changes, such as a decrease in cellular ATP, increase in ADP and NADH, or stimulation of adenosine and hypoxanthine. Two subclasses of cell membrane adenosine receptors have been proposed. These receptors have been characterized physiologically and pharmacologically. A_1-adenosine receptors exhibit high affinity in binding studies (nanomolar) and are coupled to and inhibit adenylate cyclase. On the other hand, A_2-adenosine receptors exhibit lower affinity (micromolar) and are coupled to and stimulate adenylate cyclase.

Adenosine could stimulate Epo production at high concentrations through adenosine A_2-receptor activation and inhibit Epo production at lower concentrations through adenosine A_1-receptor activation. A_1-receptor stimulation may lead to the production of an inhibitory G protein that reduces the activity of adenylate cyclase, whereas adenosine A_2 activation may stimulate a G protein that increases adenylate cyclase. When adenylate cyclase activity increases, this leads to the generation of AMP, which activates protein kinase A, leading to the phosphorylation of nuclear proteins that may be important in the transcriptional and/or the translational stage of Epo biosynthesis in the kidney [32]. These phosphoproteins generated may also be important in the release of Epo from the cell.

Dibutyrl cAMP also produces increased Epo secretion in Epo-producing renal carcinoma cells in culture and an increase in red cell mass when injected into mice. An

whereas plasma volume relative to body weight fell only slightly.

Effect of Erythropoietin on the Anemia of End-Stage Renal Disease

Favorable results of Epo on the anemia of ESRD in both animals and humans have been published. Eschbach and Adamson [16] showed that infusion of Epo-rich plasma obtained from chronically anemic sheep with normal renal function into sheep with chronic renal failure caused the hematocrits of the uremics to increase to normal levels.

Winearls and colleagues [65] administered recombinant Epo to 10 patients with chronic renal failure maintained on hemodialysis, including 4 who were anephric. The patients received Epo intravenously at the end of dialysis three times a week. All patients had a rise in hemoglobin, the mean level reaching 10.3 g/dl. Eschbach and colleagues [17] administered recombinant Epo to 25 anemic patients with ESRD three times a week. Doses of 50 U/kg/dose regularly increased hematocrits. In 2 of 5 patients treated with 50 U/kg/dose and in 9 of 10 patients treated with 150 or 500 U/kg/dose, the hematocrit increased to 35% or greater. Recombinant human Epo may reduce or eliminate the need for red blood cell transfusion.

Leukopoiesis

The leukocyte count in children with chronic renal failure is either normal or moderately decreased; the neutrophil count in untreated patients is either normal or moderately increased [9]. Several studies have examined the development of granulocytic-monocytic cells and the effect of sera from uremic patients on the early development and maturation of this series of cells. McGonigle and colleagues [37] studied granulopoiesis in patients with varying degrees of renal insufficiency, varying degrees of anemia without renal insufficiency, and normal subjects. The effect of serum on in vitro granulocytic progenitor cells was evaluated using an in vitro granulocyte colony-forming technique. Using cells cultured from human bone marrow, the researchers tested inhibition of growth of cells with 10% normal serum or serum from patients with either renal insufficiency or varying degrees of anemia. The overall inhibition of granulopoiesis by sera from normal subjects was significantly higher than that of the sera from patients with varying degrees of renal insufficiency. No colony-stimulating activity was detectable in the sera from 15 patients with renal insufficiency or the sera from 9 normal subjects.

Ponassi and colleagues [47] studied the in vitro growth of granulocyte-macrophage progenitor cells, leukocyte colony stimulating activity, differentiation and proliferation of granuloblasts, and the effect of uremic serum on the growth of normal granulocyte-macrophage progenitor cells. The concentration of granulocyte-macrophage progenitor cells and leukocyte colony stimulating activity in patients with chronic uremia were not significantly different from controls.

It was recently reported by Pavlovic-Kentera [45], who used the mouse bone marrow CFU-E system, that 34 of 35 hemodialysis patients with ESRD produced inhibitors of CFU-E, whereas none of these sera inhibited CFU-GM. In a study by Delwiche and colleagues [13] uremic serum was used to determine if it had an effect on erythroid, granulocyte-macrophage, and megakaryocytic colony formation in murine bone-marrow cultures. These authors found that normal human serum at concentrations of 5%, 10%, or 15% added to the in vitro cell system increased granulocyte-macrophage colony growth relative to controls. A dose-dependent inhibition of granulocyte-macrophage growth was observed when uremic serum was added in similar concentrations. The higher the percent of uremic serum, the greater the decrease in colony growth.

Weinstein and colleagues [64] found no differences in granulocyte-macrophage colony formation bone marrow cells obtained by aspiration biopsy from eight healthy volunteers and those from eight patients on hemodialysis. In a separate group of experiments, sera from normals or chronic renal failure patients were placed in the cultured media, and the formation of granulocyte-macrophage colonies from normal bone marrow was evaluated. Sera from chronic renal failure patients actually stimulated the growth of granulocyte-macrophage colonies compared with sera from normal patients.

Platelet Function and Coagulation in Renal Insufficiency

In the previously cited study by Delwiche and colleagues [13] varying concentrations of sera from 8 normal controls and predialysis sera from 10 patients with chronic renal failure were tested for their effect on mouse megakaryocyte colony stimulation. Normal human serum produced a dose-dependent decrease in megakaryocyte colonies. Sera from patients with renal disease did not demonstrate dose dependency but caused a 60% decrease in megakaryocyte colony formation.

Although the platelet count in patients with chronic renal failure is usually below normal, the level cannot account for the abnormal bleeding that is observed in chronic renal failure [54]. The most important defect appears to be platelet dysfunction.

Certain substances that are known to accumulate in chronic renal failure, mainly urea, creatinine, guanidinosuccinic acid, and phenol, have been shown experimentally to be associated with platelet dysfunction, most often problems of platelet aggregation. The release of platelet factor III, which is important in platelet function, has been impaired by phenolic acid in concentrations found in chronic renal failure and inhibited by guanidinosuccinic acid. Adequate dialysis, which lowers the concentrations of these substances, does not correct the abnormal bleeding time, suggesting that the uremic environment contributes to the bleeding tendencies of patients with chronic renal failure, but other nondialyzable factors must play equally important roles in platelet dysfunction.

An abnormal platelet–vessel wall interaction also may be important in promoting bleeding. Prostacyclin has potent antiaggregatory and vasodilatory activity. Venous tissue from patients with severe renal failure generated a significantly higher prostacyclin activity than specimens from healthy controls [52]. Platelet-poor plasma from uremic patients showed an enhanced capability to increase the synthesis and the release of prostacyclin from cultured endothelial cells, suggesting that the derangement of prostaglandin metabolism in uremia is likely to be mediated by a plasma factor. The resulting increased level of prostacyclin would significantly contribute to the bleeding tendency of uremic patients, even when controlled by regular dialysis [12].

The observation that the prolonged bleeding time of uremic patients can be corrected with the administration of cryoprecipitate or desmopressin suggests that altered factor VIII, or von Willebrand's factor, may be a contributing factor. There is evidence that the red blood cell per se also plays an important role in platelet adhesion and thrombus formation. Its deformability influences the rheology of blood and modifies transport mechanisms [8,53]. Evidence is accumulating that the reaction between platelets and vessel wall is intermediate in degree between simple collision and permanent adhesion and aggregation. Like adhesion, detachment of platelets from the vessel wall is also influenced by the shear rate and, consequently, rheologic factors. An increase in the red cell concentration in flowing blood is accompanied by increased platelet adhesion to subendothelial segments of rabbit aorta.

On the basis of an early observation by Hellem and colleagues [25] that the prolonged bleeding time of anemic patients was corrected by transfusions of washed red cells, Livio and colleagues [33] studied the relationship between bleeding time and packed red cell volume in patients with uremia or anemia from other causes. They found a significant negative correlation between bleeding time and packed cell volume in uremic and nonuremic patients, but bleeding times were significantly shorter at comparable packed cell volumes in nonuremic patients. A reduction of very prolonged bleeding time was observed in uremic patients with red cell transfusions as soon as the packed cell volume rose over 30%. Because transfusions improved (at least in some patients) platelet retention on glass beads without affecting platelet count, prothrombin consumption, serum thromboxane production, and intraplatelet AMP content, it was hypothesized that red cells enhance the hemostasis of uremic patients by a favorable effect on platelet–vessel wall interaction. The negative correlation between packed cell volume and bleeding time values has been subsequently confirmed by Fernandez and colleagues [19] in patients with chronic renal failure on hemodialysis and in patients with severe renal failure on conservative treatment. The authors also confirmed the therapeutic value of red cell transfusions. The results obtained by both studies strongly support the concept that anemia contributes to abnormal hemostasis of uremia and give important information for the management of uremic bleeding.

References

1. Akmal M, Telfer N, Ansari AN, et al: Erythrocyte survival in chronic renal failure: Role of secondary hyperparathyroidism. *J Clin Invest* 76:1695, 1985.
2. Amair P, Khanna R, Leibele B, et al: Continuous ambulatory peritoneal dialysis in diabetics with end-stage renal disease. *N Engl J Med* 306:625, 1982.
3. Baum M, Powell D, Calvin S, et al: Continuous ambulatory peritoneal dialysis in children: Comparison with hemodialysis. *N Engl J Med* 307:1537, 1982.
4. Beckman BS, Brookins JW, Shadduck RK, et al: Effect of different modes of dialysis on serum erythropoietin levels in pediatric patients. *Pediatric Nephrology* 2:436, 1988.
5. Beckman BS, Brookins JW, Garcia MM, et al: Measurement of erythropoietin in anephric children. *Pediatric Nephrology* 3:75, 1989.
6. Bell JD, Kincaid WR, Morgan RG, et al: Serum ferritin assay and bone-marrow iron stores in patients on maintenance hemodialysis. *Kidney Int* 17:242, 1980.
7. Bergstrom J, Furst P: Uremic toxins. *Kidney Int* 8:59, 1978.
8. Born GVR, Berqvist D, Arfors K-E: Evidence for inhibition platelet activation in blood by drug effect on erythrocyytes. *Nature* 259:233, 1976.
9. Callen IR, Limarzi LR: Bone and bone marrow studies in renal disease. *Am J Clin Pathol* 20:3, 1950.
10. Caro J, Brown S, Miller O, et al: Erythropoietin levels in uremic nephric and anephric patients. *J Lab Clin Med* 93:449, 1979.
11. Combined report on regular dialysis and transplantation of children in Europe, 1979. *Proc EDTA* 17:87, 1980.
12. Defreyn G, Vergara DM, Machin SJ, et al: A plasma factor in uremia which stimulates prostacyclin release from cultured endothelial cells. *Thromb Res* 19:695, 1980.
13. Delwiche F, Segal GM, Eschbach JW, et al: Hematopoietic inhibitors in chronic renal failure: Lack of in vitro specificity. *Kidney Int* 29:641, 1986.
14. Dunn CDR, Trent D: The effect of parathyroid hormone on erythropoiesis in serum free cultures of fetal mouse liver cells. *Proc Soc Exp Biol Med* 166:556, 1981.
15. Erslev AJ, Shapiro SS: Hematologic aspects of renal failure. *In* Earley LE, Gottschalk CW (eds): *Strauss and Welts Diseases of the Kidney*, 2nd ed. Boston, Little, Brown, 1979.
16. Eschbach JW, Adamson JW: Anemia of end stage renal disease (ESRD). *Kidney Int* 28:1, 1985.
17. Eschbach JW, Egrie JC, Downing MR, et al: Correction of the anemia of end-stage renal disease with recombinant human erythropoietin. *N Engl J Med* 316:73, 1987.
18. Eschbach JW, Mladenovic J, Garcia JF, et al: The anemia of chronic renal failure in sheep: Response to erythropoietin-rich plasma in vivo. *J Clin Invest* 74:434, 1984.
19. Fernandez F, Goudable C, Sie P, et al: Low hematocrit and prolonged bleeding time in uraemic patients: Effect of red cell transfusions. *Br J Haematol* 59:139, 1985.
20. Fisher JW: Erythropoietin. *In* Glassock RJ, Massry SG (eds): *Textbook of Nephrology*, 2nd ed. Baltimore, Williams & Wilkins, 1988, p 175.
21. Fisher JW: Regulation of erythropoietin production. *In* Windhager EE, Giebish GH (eds): *Handbook in Renal Physiology*, Washington, American Physiological Society, 1988.
22. Fisher JW, Radtke HW, Rege AB: Mechanism of the anemia of chronic renal failure. *In* Dunn CDR (ed): *Current Concepts in Erythropoiesis*. Sussex, England, Wiley, 1983.
23. Fukushima Y, Fukuda M, Yoshida K, et al: Serum erythropoietin levels and inhibitors of erythropoiesis in patients with chronic renal failure. *Tohoku J Exp Med* 150:1, 1986.
24. Grahl WA, Changus JW, Pitot AC: The effect of spermine and spermidine on proliferation in vitro of fibroblasts from normal and cystic fibrosis patients. *Pediatr Res* 12:531, 1976.
25. Hellem AJ, Borchgrevink CF, Ames SB: The role of red cells in haemostasis: The relation between haematocrit, bleeding time and platelet adhesiveness. *Br J Haematol* 7:42, 1961.
26. Joske RA, McAlister JM, Prankerd TAJ: Isotope investiga-

tion of red cell production and destruction in chronic renal disease. *Clin Sci* 15:511, 1956.

27. Koury ST, Bondurant MC, Koury MJ: Localization of erythropoietin, synthesizing cells in murine kidneys by in situ hybridization. *Blood* 71:524, 1988.

28. Lacke C, Senekjian HO, Knight TF, et al: Twelve months' experience with continuous ambulatory and intermittent peritoneal dialysis. *Arch Intern Med* 141:187, 1981.

29. Lacombe C, DaSilva JL, Bruneval P, et al: Peritubular cells are the site of erythropoietin synthesis in the murine hypoxic kidney. *J Clin Invest* 81:620, 1988.

30. Lertora J, Dargon JL, Rege AB, et al: Studies on a radioimmunoassay for human erythropoietin. *J Lab Clin Med* 86:140, 1975.

31. Levi JH, Bessler H, Hirsch I, et al: Increased RNA and heme synthesis in mouse erythroid precursors by parathyroid hormone. *Acta Haematol (Basel)* 61:125, 1979.

32. Lin FK, Suggs S, Lin CH, et al: Cloning and expression of the human erythropoietin gene. *Proc Natl Acad Sci USA* 82:7580, 1985.

33. Livio M, Marchesi D, Remuzzi G, et al: Uraemic bleeding: Role of anaemia and beneficial effect of red cell transfusion. *Lancet* 2:1013, 1982.

34. Loge JP, Lange RD, Moore CV: Characterization of the anemia associated with chronic renal insufficiency. *Am J Med* 24:4, 1958.

35. McGonigle RJS, Boineau FG, Beckman B, et al: Erythropoietin and inhibitors of in vitro erythropoiesis in the development of anemia in children with renal disease. *J Lab Clin Med* 105:449, 1985.

36. McGonigle RJS, Wallin JD, Husserl F, et al: Potential role of parathyroid hormone as an inhibitor of erythropoiesis in the anemia of renal failure. *J Lab Clin Med* 104:1016, 1984.

37. McGonigle RJS, Wallin JD, Shadduck RK, et al: Erythropoietin deficiency and inhibition of erythropoiesis in renal insufficiency. *Kidney Int* 25:437, 1984.

38. Meytes D, Bogin E, Ma A, et al: Effect of parathyroid hormone on erythropoiesis. *J Clin Invest* 67:1263, 1981.

39. Mladenovic J, Eschbach JW, Garcia JF, et al: The anemia of chronic renal failure in sheep: Studies in vitro. *Br J Haematol* 58:491, 1984.

40. Moriyama Y, Fisher JW: Effects of erythropoietin on erythroid colony formation in urmeic rabbit. *Blood* 45:659, 1975.

41. Nelson PK, Brookins J, Fisher JW: Erythropoietic effects of prostacyclin (PGI$_2$) and its metabolite 6-keto-prostaglandin (PG) E$_1$. *J Pharmacol Exp Ther* 226:493, 1983.

42. Nolph KD: Comparison of continuous ambulatory peritoneal dialysis and hemodialysis. *Kidney Int* 33(Suppl 24):S-123, 1988.

43. Ohno Y, Fisher JW: Inhibition of bone marrow erythroid colony forming cells (CFU-E) by serum from chronic anemic uremic rabbits. *Proc Soc Exp Biol Med* 156:56, 1977.

44. Ohno Y, Rege AB, Fisher JW, et al: Inhibitors of erythroid colony-forming cells (CFU-E and BFU-E) in sera of azotemic patients with anemia of renal disease. *J Lab Clin Med* 92:916, 1978.

45. Pavlovic-Kentera V: The inhibitors of erythropoiesis. *In* Najuran A, Giugon M (eds): Colloque, INSERM, Vol 162. City, John Libby Eurotext Ltd, 1987, p 133.

46. Podjarny E, Rathaus M, Korzets Z, et al: Is anemia of chronic renal failure related to secondary hyperparathyroidism? *Arch Intern Med* 141:453, 1981.

47. Ponassi A, Morra L, Gurreri G, et al: Alterations of granulopoiesis in chronic uremic patients treated with intermittent hemodialysis. *Acta Haematol (Basel)* 77:220, 1987.

48. Radtke HW, Claussner A, Erbes PM, et al: Serum erythropoietin concentration in chronic renal failure: Relationship to degree of anemia and excretory renal function. *Blood* 54:877, 1979.

49. Radtke HW, Frei U, Erbes PM, et al: Improving anemia by hemodialysis: Effect on serum erythropoietin. *Kidney Int* 17:382, 1980.

50. Radtke HW, Rege AB, Lamarche MB, et al: Identification of spermine as an inhibitor of erythropoiesis in patients with chronic renal failure. *J Clin Invest* 67:1623, 1981.

51. Radtke HW, Scheuermann EH, Desser H: Polyamine induced in vivo and in vitro suppression of erythropoiesis in uremia. *Haematologia (Budap)* 1983.

52. Remuzzi G, Cavenaghi AE, Mecca G, et al: Prostacyclin-like activity and bleeding in renal failure. *Lancet* 2:1195, 1977.

53. Remuzzi A, Languino LR, Costantini V, et al: Platelet adhesion to subendothelium: Effects of shear rate, hematocrit and platelet count on the dynamic equilibrium between platelets adhering to and detaching from the surface. *Thromb Haemost* 54:857, 1985.

54. Remuzzi G, Pusineri F: Coagulation defects in uremia. *Kidney Int* 33(Suppl 24):S13, 1988.

55. Saito A, Takagi T, Chung TG, et al: Serum levels of polyamines in patients with chronic renal failure. *Kidney Int* 24(Suppl 16):S-234, 1983.

56. Saltissi D, Coles GA, Napier JAF, et al: The hematological response to continuous ambulatory peritoneal dialysis. *Clin Nephrol* 22:21, 1984.

57. Shaw AB: Hemolysis in chronic renal failure. *Br Med J* 2:213, 1967.

58. Spivak JL: The mechanism of action of erythropoietin. *Int J Cell Cloning* 4:139, 1986.

59. Spragg BP, Hutchings AD: High performance liquid chromatographic determination of putrescine, spermidine and spermine after derivitisation with 4-Fluro-3-Nitrobenzotrifluoride. *J Chromatog Biomed Appl* 258:289, 1983.

60. Swendseid M, Panaque M, Kopple JD: Polyamine concentrations in red cells and urine of patients with chronic renal failure. *Life Sci* 26:533, 1980.

61. Ulmer HE, Greiner H, Schuler HW, et al: Cardiovascular impairment and physical work capacity in children with chronic renal failure. *Acta Paediatr Scand* 67:43, 1978.

62. Van Stone JC, Max P: Effect of erythropoietin on anemia of peritoneally dialyzed anephric rats. *Kidney Int* 15:370, 1979.

63. Wallner SF, Kwinick JE, Ward HP, et al: The anemia of chronic renal failure and chronic diseases: In vitro studies of erythropoiesis. *Blood* 47:561, 1976.

64. Weinstein T, Fishman P, Cline B, et al: Effect of cimetidine on granulocyte-macrophage colony formation by normal and chronic renal failure bone marrow cells. *Kidney Int* 26:741, 1984.

65. Winearls CG, Peppard MJ, Downing MR, et al: Effect of human erythropoietin derived from recombinant DNA on the anemia of patients maintained by chronic hemodialysis. *Lancet* 2:1175, 1986.

66. Zappacosta AR, Caro J, Erslev A: Normalization of hematocrit in patients with end-stage renal disease on continuous ambulatory peritoneal dialysis. *Am J Med* 72:53, 1982.

67. Zevin D, Levi J, Bessler H, et al: Effect of parathyroid hormone and 1,25-dihydroxyvitamin D$_3$ on RNA and heme synthesis by erythroid precursors. *Miner Electrolyte Metab* 6:125, 1981.

68. Zingraff J, Druke T, Marie P, et al: Anemia and secondary hyperparathyroidism. *Arch Intern Med* 138:1650, 1978.

Joseph H. French
Isabelle Rapin
Walter C. Martinez

30
Neurologic Complications of Renal Failure and Their Treatment

Acute or chronic renal failure produces many metabolic and vascular derangements that alter nervous system function. To evaluate the pathogenetic mechanisms responsible for these changes, this chapter discusses both those due to renal failure per se (encephalopathies, neuromuscular disorders) as well as those due to the complications of its management with drugs, dialysis, and transplantation [38a, 96a,109,151,203,230,253,261,267,302,316,335]. The last section of this chapter examines some known or suspected biochemical mechanisms that may be fundamental to the neurologic complications of renal failure.

Neurologic and renal dysfunction may coexist as consequences of multisystem diseases and genetic disorders with both renal and cerebral expressions (Table 30-1). Neither these disorders nor those associated with abnormalities of the eye and ear [204] will be reviewed here because they are discussed elsewhere in this volume (Chap. 45 and 60–71).

Uremic Encephalopathy
Clinical Features

The earliest sign of uremic encephalopathy is a nonspecific depression of cerebral function (Table 30-2). The child appears fatigued, listless, and drowsy in the daytime, restless and sleepless at night. His attention span is reduced. Characteristically, periods of well-being and good performance alternate with periods of lethargy.

Children with renal failure are frequently subject to mild headache that is usually vague in character and poorly localized. Headache is common during performance of dialysis but usually does not require treatment. It may indicate the presence of hyperosmolarity (hypernatremia), which is associated with brain shrinkage, or water intoxication (hyponatremia), which causes brain swelling. Uremia without hypertension is rarely associated with severe headache. Severe headache is infrequent in the absence of hypertensive encephalopathy; it may indicate the presence of increased intracranial pressure severe enough to require treatment or of a central nervous system hemorrhage.

As renal function deteriorates and glomerular filtration

falls below 5 ml/min/1.73 m^2 [253], the signs of toxic encephalopathy become more pronounced, especially if azotemia is acute. The child complains of generalized weakness and anorexia. Muscle cramps, fasiculations, twitching, and asterixis may appear. Speech is often slow and slurred. Disorientation, confusion, and memory deficits occur. Striking swings of confusion and mental lucidity are common. The child may develop a frank psychosis with delusions and hallucinations [314]; this psychosis can mimic many types of psychiatric illness [273].

Asterixis is a frequent physical finding in uremic encephalopathy [333]. It consists of a flap or sudden drop of the outstretched hand, commonly followed by two or three other flaps in quick succession. This postural lapse is associated with a silent period in the electromyogram (EMG). Asterixis is a nonspecific phenomenon that is seen in metabolic encephalopathies other than those associated with renal disease. It appears to reflect a supranuclear inhibition of motor neurons and is considered by some to be a "negative" myoclonus, with inhibitory rather than excitatory discharges affecting anterior horn cells. With further progression of renal failure, myoclonic jerks, convulsions, stupor, and, finally, coma, often associated with decorticate posture, appear. Convulsions, which constitute a medical emergency and require specific treatment, are discussed later in this chapter.

In addition to suffering from an impairment of alertness and of higher cortical functions, children with renal failure may develop transient focal neurologic deficits, such as temporary loss of vision (uremic amaurosis). Occasionally, they may have cranial nerve signs, such as abducens nerve palsy, loss of hearing, and nystagmus [213,335]. Other transient focal findings include unsteadiness of gait, frank cerebellar ataxia, tremor, and motor deficits such as monoplegia or hemiplegia. Their pathogenesis is often unclear. Many permutations and combinations of signs and symptoms may occur in a single child as the severity of the renal disease fluctuates. Longer lasting focal deficits may indicate focal ischemia in hypertensive encephalopathy, an embolic or thrombotic stroke [128], or, less often, intracranial hemorrhage.

Encephalopathies other than those caused by progressive

TABLE 30-1. *Diseases with renal and neurologic manifestations*

Systemic Diseases
Diabetes mellitus
Collagen—vascular diseases
Coagulopathies, e.g., hemolytic uremic syndrome thrombotic
　　thrombocytopenic purpura
Primary hyperparathyroidism
Coarctation of the aorta
Hydrocephalus with atrial shunt nephritis

Genetic—Metabolic Disorders
Sickle cell anemia
Tuberous sclerosis
von Hippel-Lindau disease
Polycystic kidneys with cerebral aneurysm
Lowe's syndrome [351]
Fabry's disease [278]
Nephrosialidosis [193]
Zellweger syndrome
Lesch-Nyhan syndrome
Acute intermittent porphyria
Mitochondrial cytopathies [84]
Renal tubular acidosis with hearing loss [69,79,305]

TABLE 30-2. *Uremic encephalopathy**

Early Signs
Nonspecific depression of cerebral function
Fatigue, listlessness, drowsiness
Sleep disturbance
Poor concentration, short attention span
Alteration of memory
Characteristically, periods of alertness alternating with periods
　　of depression

Late Signs
Weakness, anorexia
Muscle cramps, asterixis
Slow and slurred speech
Increasing confusion and memory deficits
Frank psychosis, delusions, hallucinations
Myoclonus, seizures, progressive lethargy
Coma with decorticate posture

* Usually more severe if azotemia is acute.

renal failure are discussed in subsequent sections. They include hypertensive encephalopathy, the encephalopathy of the dialysis disequilibrium syndrome, aluminum-related encephalopathies, acute rejection encephalopathy, and some complications resulting from drug administration.

Pathology

Olsen [236] examined the brains of 104 patients who died of renal failure. In the absence of hypertensive encephalopathy, chronic hypertension, and other complications of renal failure and its treatment, the findings were nonspecific and rather unimpressive. There was no brain edema. Constantinides [67] described swelling of astrocytes and separation of myelin lamellae in the brains of patients who died in renal failure, but Lumsden [186] attributed these findings to hypertensive encephalopathy and its attendant vascular damage. Neuronal degeneration was common but

had no characteristic distribution, with the possible exception of the sensory nuclei of the brain stem, the reticular formation, and the granular cells of the cerebral cortex. Neuronal loss was more severe in cases of longstanding renal failure and is presumed to be responsible for the brain atrophy seen in the computed tomographic (CT) scans of some of these patients [243,246,298].

Pathophysiology

The neurophysiologic and neurochemical changes that occur as a consequence of renal failure are complex and poorly understood. In general, there is lack of correlation between the occurrence and severity of signs of neurologic dysfunction and the level of any one chemical constituent of the blood (see the section on Potential Neuroscience Correlates).

Disorders of hydrogen ion homeostasis, water and electrolyte balance (including calcium and trace metal constituents), osmolal regulation, and vascular permeability are common. Brain swelling, causing increased intracranial pressure, may be the result of hypertensive encephalopathy, water intoxication, or prolonged seizures.

The success of dialysis in ameliorating the neurologic manifestations of uremia suggests that dialyzable compounds (uremic toxins) that accumulate in the body fluids are in some way responsible for the neurotoxic features of renal failure. Toxic substances that accumulate in uremia because of decreased excretion or altered metabolism tend to be metabolic end products, predominantly of proteins [184,185,214]. Patients with severe uremic symptoms have increased concentrations of urea, creatinine, urates, and other organic and inorganic acids in their serum. Attempts to reproduce the neurologic symptoms of renal failure by injecting any one of these substances have been unsuccessful, however.

The introduction of recent biochemical methods has revealed the presence of low, middle, and high molecular weight compounds in the plasma and dialysis fluid of patients with renal failure. Some of these compounds, notably parathyroid hormone (PTH) [97], are peptide hormones that may act as neuromodulators in the brain [310]. PTH is increased in both acute [69,117] and chronic [14] renal failure and has been implicated as a uremic neurotoxin. An electroencephalographic (EEG) pattern resembling that of renal failure has been produced in dogs by the administration of PTH; the animals also had increased amounts of calcium in the brain [117]. Similar observations have been made in patients with hyperparathyroidism with or without renal failure [63].

In chronic renal failure, cerebral energy consumption is reduced by variable degrees [295,337]. This alteration in cerebral metabolism cannot be attributed to decreased cerebral circulation, which, in fact, has been shown to be either normal or greater than normal in uremia [133,295]. Thus, these data suggest a derangement of neuronal metabolism. It seems plausible that alterations in cellular energy conservation may be responsible for some of the clinical manifestations of uremic encephalopathy.

Normal brain function requires energy-dependent ion pumps to maintain neuronal excitability, neuronal conduction, and water distribution. Aluminum, which may accumulate in brain as a result of dialysis and oral intake of phosphate binding agents [8,286], may interfere with hexose metabolism in neural tissue [349]. Children with renal failure since infancy and with aluminum intoxication may suffer from a progressive, at times fatal, encephalopathy [26,281], microcephaly, mental deficiency [25,253], and osteomalacia with muscle weakness [11,286].

Children with renal failure frequently manifest deficient somatic growth, as well as deficient growth of the brain [281]. Their somatic growth deficiency may, in part, reflect hypothalamic-pituitary dysfunction [298]. A complicated process such as growth has multiple controls, however, including caloric intake, availability of essential nutrients, nonneural hormonal factors, and responsivity of multiple tissues to these factors at a given stage of development. Thus, while altered neural control of pituitary function [104,195,232] is implicated in the delayed [191] or precocious [104] puberty of some uremic children, its precise role as regards growth failure is speculative.

Fishman and Raskin [93,94] have demonstrated that experimental uremic encephalopathy is characterized by complex changes in the permeability of the blood-brain barrier. Maintenance of osmotic gradients across the blood-brain barrier requires energy-consuming transport mechanisms and integrity of specialized cerebral vascular endothelial cells. Arterial hypertension [157] and altered plasma osmolality [148] may exceed the adaptive capability of these endothelial cells, thus leading to breakdown of the blood-brain barrier. This breakdown would be expected to alter the synaptic availability and function of neurohumors (proven and putative neurotransmitters and neuropeptides). The resulting modified activities of functionally coupled neurons could contribute to some of the behavioral derangements of uremia.

The multiplicity and complexity of metabolic derangements resulting from renal failure explain our frequent inability to find a specific cause for the encephalopathy of a given child. In general, the level of plasma electrolytes, urea, and creatinine do not correlate well with the mental status of the child. In assessing a child's neurologic status, it is more helpful in practice to consider trends over time rather than absolute levels of blood constituents.

Diagnostic Evaluation

Cerebral imaging techniques have done away with much of the uncertainty in interpreting focal defects observed in some patients with renal failure. The transaxial cranial CT scan is a sensitive test for visualizing intracranial hemorrhage and, after several days, the focal low density of ischemic cerebral infarction. Acute edema is not always apparent by CT and may be more easily visualized by magnetic resonance imaging (MRI) [172]. CT and MRI will also detect subdural hemotomas, brain abscesses, and neoplasms.

Diffuse brain swelling produces narrowing of the ventricles and extracerebral cisterns, as well as decreased density of the white matter. Transient lucency of the white matter following intermittent hemodialysis has been documented by CT [161]; this may represent brain edema or restitution

of water to brain that was dehydrated by chronic renal failure [75]. A common finding in patients with longstanding renal failure, especially those on dialysis, is atrophy of either the gray or white matter or both [243,246,281,299]. Evaluation of the functional significance of these structural changes is complicated by the likelihood that some of these patients have had progressive aluminum encephalopathy.

Comparison of psychological test results in adults before and after dialysis disclose short-term fluctuation of attention, fine-motor coordination, memory, and cognitive skills according to some studies [240] but not others [263]; chronic renal failure usually produces only mild if any permanent intellectual impairment in adults [40,129]. Although the depressed performance IQ of school-age children improves within a month of transplantation [92,260], children with early onset renal failure remain at cognitive disadvantage [331], even in the absence of aluminum intoxication [36,103a,253,254,281]. Malnutrition, uremic toxins, and environmental deprivation, as the result of chronic illness, may be responsible for the disability of such children.

No EEG pattern can be considered pathognomonic of renal failure. The EEG mirrors the patient's level of consciousness [109,253,267,335]; in adults, at least, the degree of EEG slowing and level of impaired performance on psychometric tests are correlated [325]. In the early stages of renal failure, the EEG is usually normal, or it may show low voltage with increased fast activity. As uremia increases, the normal alpha rhythm disappears and is replaced by diffuse slowing with a tendency for bursts of paroxysmal sharp waves, most notably in the frontoparietal-parasagittal areas [140,154,335]. The EEG may become severely and diffusely slow in stuporous or comatose patients. Asymmetric persistence of slow background rhythms in infants with chronic renal failure and cognitive impairment may reflect differential detrimental effects on maturation of the two cerebral hemispheres [36].

No reliable correlation can be made between the EEG and the level of any blood constituent, although there is a rough correlation between quantitative measures of EEG frequency and severity of renal failure [325]. Dramatic alterations in the EEG may occur without obvious clinical or laboratory changes, and vice versa [325]. Deterioration of the EEG occurs in about 75% of patients during dialysis; it usually returns to the predialysis level in 10 to 24 hours [124].

Patients in whom seizures develop tend to have a diffusely slow record, with or without paroxysmal activity. Sensitivity to photic stimulation is common in patients who have had seizures or who are in the recovery phase from acute renal failure. Persistent spike foci suggest a preexisting chronic convulsive disorder.

Evoked potential studies are useful for investigating the efficiency of conduction along central sensory pathways. Brain stem auditory evoked potentials provide an objective test of auditory sensitivity and can help localize pathology to the cochlea, auditory nerve, or relays of the central auditory pathway. Pattern-reversal visual evoked responses are more sensitive for detecting uremic encephalopathy than flash evoked potentials [279]. Latencies of visual and somatosensory cortical evoked potentials are increased and amplitudes are decreased in uremia, which indicates slowing and desynchronization of central conduction velocities [174,280,325].

Renal transplantation may reverse these changes, but dialysis does not; in fact, Kuba et al. [162] found more marked changes in dialyzed than chronically uremic patients, which suggests that the changes may not be transient functional ones. Although there is no clear correlation between any one blood constituent and the latency of evoked responses, there does seem to be a coupling between the severity of the renal failure and increase in latency [122]. Long latency (P300) cortical evoked potentials associated with the detection of a rare ("oddball") tone in a train of repeated tones were found to be delayed in some patients with renal failure, reflecting either decreased attentiveness or cognitive inefficiency [65].

Management

The preferred management of uremic encephalopathy is initiation of a treatment that effectively reverses the underlying renal disease (if possible); dialysis or transplantation are alternatives when this is not possible. Management of uremic seizures is discussed in the section on convulsions.

The neurologic signs and symptoms that arise in the course of renal failure deserve careful attention and management because they often contribute significantly to the child's disability. Acute behavioral changes due to uremic encephalopathy usually are short-lived and subside with adequate dialysis and control of the blood pressure within hours or in one to two days. Such changes associated with the dialysis disequilibrium syndrome are similarly transient. Drugs such as diazepam and the phenothiazines must be used sparingly, because they may accumulate and produce an iatrogenic encephalopathy or abnormal involuntary movements at unexpectedly low doses [320]. Tyler [335] cautions that half of an adult patient cohort with uremic encephalopathy also manifested drug toxicity.

Chronic renal disease, with its discomforts, curtailment of activity, dietary limitation, multiple hospitalizations, and other demands on the child and the family, is likely to result in major stresses [344]. Because there is evidence that renal failure present since early life has deleterious cognitive effects in at least some children [36,92, 96,103a,260,281,331], dialysis and transplantation should not be delayed unduly. Clearly, children and their families need ongoing help and support, and parents need advice on how to avoid overprotecting and infantilizing their child as well as to avoid making unrealistic demands on him or her.

Hypertensive Encephalopathy
Clinical Features

Hypertensive encephalopathy represents a serious neurologic complication of accelerated hypertension [356,357]. It is the most common cause of cerebral symptoms in children with acute glomerulonephritis and may be its presenting symptom [138].

The diagnosis of hypertensive encephalopathy should be considered in any child with severe or recent hypertension who vomits, complains of headache, or is drowsy, apprehensive, or confused. If untreated, hypertensive encephalopathy may progress to stupor, focal or generalized convulsions, coma, and death. Short-lived focal neurologic deficits are common. They may include focal weakness, reflex asymmetry, Babinski signs, nystagmus, oculomotor palsies, and transient visual obscurations. Visual disturbances may progress to visual field defects and cortical blindness [143]. The optic fundi may be normal or may show varying degrees of papilledema and arteriolar narrowing, as well as retinal hemorrhages and exudates [27,294].

The cerebrospinal fluid (CSF) pressure may be normal or high and is of little help in diagnosis as it is often mildly increased in hypertensive patients who do not have signs of an encephalopathy [61]. Hypertensive encephalopathy can be associated with severe brain swelling and with sufficiently increased CSF pressure to require therapy [336]. The CSF protein may be normal or moderately elevated and the fluid mildly xanthochromic. The EEG is usually abnormal, with suppression of alpha activity and the appearance of rhythmic, slow delta waves in the occipital leads [267,335]. Focal EEG abnormalities are common.

Although hypertensive encephalopathy is sometimes responsible for recent onset focal neurologic deficits, their cause most often is uremia, cerebral infarction, and subarachnoid or intracerebral hemorrhage [357]. Other diagnostic possibilities, including neoplasm, brain abscess, subdural hematoma, and pseudotumor cerebri, should be considered but are even less likely.

Pathology

The hallmark of hypertensive encephalopathy is a necrotizing arteriolitis, the same process that gives rise to papilledema and hemorrhages and exudates in the retina [2]. Disruption of the blood-brain barrier results in patchy brain swelling, petechial hemorrhages (especially in the gray matter), and perivascular exudates. Necrosis of blood vessel walls may occur, leading to infarctions or larger hemorrhages. The breakdown of the blood-brain barrier that results in brain edema is responsible for the increase in CSF protein that is observed in hypertensive encephalopathy. Rupture of large vessels, producing a major hemorrhagic stroke, is uncommon in the absence of a coagulopathy or of coexisting vascular disease, such as periarteritis or lupus erythematosus.

Pathophysiology

Much of our understanding of hypertensive encephalopathy is based on the work of Byrom [47], who studied its development in rats with renal ischemia, and Meyer et al. [206,207], who extended the observations to primates. These investigators observed three vascular abnormalities in the brain and in the retina: arterial vasoconstriction, focal increase in vascular permeability, and arteriolar necrosis. Focal or generalized constriction of cerebral arteries was a constant finding in the rat with hypertensive encephalopathy. It resulted in diminished cerebral blood flow, which contributed to the clinical manifestations, and in brain swelling. Injection of trypan blue and diffusion of the dye into the parenchyma of the brain documented breakdown of the blood-brain barrier and increased permeability of the cerebral vasculature. Areas of focal brain edema corresponded to areas of breakdown in blood vessel walls. In the later stages of the disease, diffuse brain swelling was a common finding. Less often, necrosis of the walls of arterioles resulted in parenchymal hemorrhages.

More recent studies indicate that the breakdown in the blood-brain barrier is associated with loss of unique tight junctions between endothelial cells of cerebral vessels [144,157]. Reversible opening of this barrier occurs during hyperosmolar stress [259]. CT scans suggest transiently increased water content immediately following dialysis [75,161].

Management

The best management of hypertensive encephalopathy is to prevent its occurrence by anticipating its development. When it does occur, its treatment is three-pronged: (1) Reduce the hypertension, (2) control seizures, and (3) reduce brain swelling. In addition, consideration must be given to the possible development of hemorrhagic complications of hypertension, which may confuse the neurologic picture and require further investigation by CT. Occasionally, neurosurgic intervention is indicated.

REDUCTION OF HYPERTENSION AND CONTROL OF SEIZURES

Reducing hypertension is the major goal in treating hypertensive encephalopathy. The principles of treatment and the drugs of choice to reduce hypertension rapidly and safely are discussed in Chap. 87. The control of seizures is attempted by intravenous administration of rapidly acting anticonvulsants (see the section on management of acute seizures). Prolonged therapy with anticonvulsants is not required unless there is evidence of persistent epileptogenic brain dysfunction or the patient is a known epileptic.

REDUCTION OF BRAIN SWELLING

The treatment of raised intracranial pressure is to decrease the volume of one of the three intracranial compartments—the brain parenchyma, CSF spaces, or vascular bed. In cases where the pressure is markedly increased and the brain is diffusely swollen (narrowing of the ventricles and obliteration of the cisterns on CT or MRI), it may be advisable to monitor intracranial pressure with a subarachnoid bolt or with an intraventricular catheter (which can also be used to decompress the ventricles) [336]. Intubation and hyperventilation and keeping the head of the patient elevated 30° shrink the vascular compartment. Hyperosmolar agents and steroids are used to reduce brain swelling. In addition, avoiding seizures and maintaining normothermia protect the already compromised brain against increased metabolic demands.

Following is a discussion of agents found most useful in reducing cerebral edema.

Hyperosmolar Agents

Mannitol is the most effective agent to reduce increased intracranial pressure rapidly. It is administered as a 20% solution, in a dose of 5 to 10 ml/kg (1 to 2 g/kg) by IV infusion over 20 minutes. This dose can be repeated every 4 to 6 hours if needed, but mannitol is rarely used for more than a few days. Glycerol, 1.5 to 2 g/kg/day, is administered by mouth or nasogastric tube. The daily amount is diluted with an equal amount of water or orange juice and is given in four daily doses. Its IV use has also been advocated [205].

Corticosteroids

The mechanism of corticosteroid action on brain edema is still uncertain, but it appears that at least one of the effects of corticosteroids is to stabilize the vascular wall [114,282]. Dexamethasone, 0.4 mg/kg/day, is the drug of choice. One half of the total dose is given rapidly IV, followed by one fourth of the dose IV or IM every 6 hours. The oral route can be used if long-term administration is required.

Convulsions
Clinical Features

Myoclonic jerks, focal seizures, and generalized tonic-clonic seizures, including status epilepticus, occur frequently in renal failure, especially in hypertensive encephalopathy [109,199b,261,267,335]. They may occur as a complication of uremia, malignant hypertension, or treatment with drugs or dialysis. Characteristics of the EEG in patients with seizures and renal failure have been described in an earlier section.

Myoclonic jerks are sudden, nonrhythmical muscle contractions that are of sufficient amplitude to move a body part. They may be symmetrical or asymmetric, and occasionally are generalized and difficult to differentiate from clonic seizures, of which they may be the harbingers. Myoclonic jerks have no localizing value and may reflect the unbridled discharge of brain stem as well as cortical neurons [55]. Myoclonus may be stimulus-sensitive, notably to somatosensory input from contracting muscles (action myoclonus) or to light. Uremic myoclonus may respond to clonazepam. Coarse myoclonus may also occur as a complication of treatment with meperidine [136,319] and its analogues during renal failure. Myoclonus is a prominent and early sign of aluminum encephalopathy [26,96,103, 253,254].

Seizures are most likely to be associated with rapid metabolic changes in blood pH, calcium, and other electrolytes; hyponatremia (e.g., following excessive water ingestion or administration to correct a hyperosmolar state) and a rapid fall in blood urea levels are common antecedents (see the section on dialysis disequilibrium syndrome). The brain is intolerant of rapid changes in solute gradients [244] because of lags in equilibration between brain and plasma owing to the presence of the blood-brain barrier. This intolerance may be a precipitating cause of seizures in patients with renal failure. Children with preexisting convulsive disorders are more likely than others to develop seizures during renal dysfunction and do so with less drastic metabolic provocation. Seizures occur occasionally as a complication of the administration of drugs (see Table 30-5). In renal failure, the absorption, plasma binding, metabolic conversion, and elimination of drugs may be altered, and drugs may accumulate in toxic amounts in the brain and CSF [35,335].

In acute renal failure, a seizure or series of seizures may occur just prior to, or shortly after, the onset of diuresis [180]. Seizures may signal the presence of hypertensive encephalopathy, or they may be the presenting sign of poststreptococcal glomerulonephritis [138].

Seizures usually occur late in the course of chronic renal failure. The probability of their occurrence correlates poorly with the degree of uremia. Many of the affected children are hypertensive as well as uremic, so it may be very difficult or impossible to determine which derangement is responsible for the seizure. Uremic seizures are usually generalized or myoclonic. Focal seizures suggest a focal brain lesion or preexisting pathology, the epileptic potential of which is triggered by the metabolic derangement. CT is helpful in such cases. Rarely, uremic patients have persistent focal seizures for which no anatomic lesion can be demonstrated at postmortem examination [299].

Management of Acute Seizures

EVALUATION

Most seizures are self-limited and usually stop before any specific medical treatment is given. Whenever possible, treatment should be directed toward the precipitating cause. Causes for seizures are implied in the following questions, which should be asked systematically:

1. Is the child hypertensive? Is he or she suffering from hypertensive encephalopathy?
2. Does the child have a fever? Does he or she have a bleeding tendency? After the seizure, does he or she complain of a severe headache? Is there a focal neurologic deficit or signs of meningeal irritation? Is the child becoming progressively lethargic? Positive answers point to the development of an intracranial hemorrhage or may suggest meningitis, brain abscess, or encephalitis.
3. Has the child received drugs, for example, massive doses of penicillin or other potential convulsants in the face of curtailed renal function (see Table 30-5). Is the child immunocompromised?
4. Has the sodium level fallen precipitously to below 125 mEq/L?
5. Is the child hypocalcemic or alkalotic?
6. Is he or she hypoglycemic?
7. Is the child severely hyperglycemic? We have observed a child with chronic renal failure, who developed chronic pancreatitis with secondary hyperglycemia and whose seizures probably reflected a hyperosmolar state (blood sugar 1400 mg/dl). Nonketotic hyperosmolar coma may develop in diabetic patients, including those on steroids, and in those dialyzed with hypertonic glucose-containing solutions [253].

Brief seizures probably do not have long-term effects on brain function. Single short seizures that develop during periods of metabolic shifts are usually self-limited and need not be treated with anticonvulsants. Prolonged seizures markedly increase oxygen utilization by the brain at a time when the child may be hypoxic and may have expended his glycogen stores, raised his body temperature, and developed a lactic acidosis. Prolonged status epilepticus rarely may cause permanent sequellae [3] because of the autodestruction of hyperexcited neurons that oxidize their fixed structural components in order to meet increased energy demands [330]. Permanent sequelae occur only infrequently in children who have experienced status epilepticus that is adequately treated [199a]; thus, the occurrence of status epilepticus does not automatically mandate the institution of chronic anticonvulsant therapy.

A child with prolonged or recurrent seizures who does not recover consciousness between attacks must be considered to be in status epilepticus and should be treated vigorously to prevent sequellae. Maintainence of an adequate airway and prevention of hyperthermia, as well as administration of oxygen and glucose to meet the increased metabolic needs of neurons during seizures, are essential steps in the management of status epilepticus.

ANTICONVULSANT THERAPY

Following are general principles that govern the acute treatment of children with renal failure and prolonged or repeated seizures.

With rare exceptions, anticonvulsants are administered intravenously. Levels of anticonvulsants in the serum should be monitored daily during the acute stage and periodically during long-term treatment to avoid reaching toxic levels. Measurement of anticonvulsant concentrations in the blood [10,101,164,187,215] enables one to administer an appropriate dosage in the face of varying degrees of renal insufficiency (see the discussion of complications of drug therapy). If the child has received adequate doses of anticonvulsants, "twitches" and "jerks" of short duration may be safely ignored.

Diazepam

Intravenous diazepam is one of the drugs of choice for the treatment of status epilepticus [216]. It is a rapidly acting anticonvulsant, faster than phenobarbital or phenytoin. In experimental studies, high levels were detected in the brain within minutes, especially in the gray matter. A rapid decline occurs in the serum concentration in the first 30 minutes, however [155,196]. This short half-life necessitates the administration of a second, longlasting drug in order to ensure that the attacks will not recur. The administration of diazepam is not recommended in children who have already received parenteral barbiturates or other hypnotic agents because of the danger of precipitating serious hypotension and respiratory arrest.

Diazepam is water insoluble and precipitates rapidly when mixed with normal saline or dextrose solutions. Therefore, injection through the plastic tubing of an ongoing infusion must be avoided. Because the dose needed to produce the desired effect is variable, the child is given repeated injections until all seizures are controlled or the maximum safe dose has been given. For children up to three years of age, a 0.5-mg (0.1-ml) bolus is given every 15 to 20 seconds, with a maximum dose of 5 mg. For children three years of age and older, a 1-mg (0.2-ml) bolus is given every 15 to 20 seconds, with a maximum of 10 mg. If the seizures are controlled, a longer acting agent is then administered intravenously.

Lorazepam

Intravenous lorazepam has a much longer half-life than diazepam; its anticonvulsant effect may last several hours, opposed to less than one hour for diazepam. It may suffice as a single agent to treat status epilepticus effectively. The dose is one tenth that of diazepam and is administered intravenously over the same time span after taking identical precautions, i.e., the immediate ability to intubate and ventilate the child if needed. A second dose may be given if the first is ineffective, followed by intravenous phenytoin and, if required, phenobarbital in refractory cases.

Phenobarbital

Phenobarbital is the barbiturate of choice and, administered intravenously, is widely used to control status epilepticus. The recommended dose in nonuremic children is 15 to 20 mg/kg; infants usually require the larger amount in order to achieve a therapeutic level of approximately 16 μg/ml [239]. There are no published guidelines as to dosage adjustment in patients with renal failure. We recommend two thirds of the nonuremic dose in order to avoid excessive sedation. In general, short-acting barbiturates such as amobarbital, thiopental, and secobarbital should be avoided because of their potential side effects, including laryngeal spasm and respiratory depression.

Phenobarbital is not a fast-acting anticonvulsant [41,198]. Shortly after its administration intravenously, it is present in high concentration in the more vascular organs, with the notable exception of the brain [256]. Consequently, it is necessary to wait at least 20 minutes to judge its effectiveness. If status epilepticus persists, it is our practice to administer parenteral phenytoin. Rarely, we ask an anesthesiologist to administer a centrally active inhalant rather than take the risk of overmedicating the child with long-acting drugs that depress vital functions.

In nonuremic patients, phenobarbital is metabolized slowly, primarily in the liver, while 11% to 25% appears unchanged in the urine. Both processes are slow, and its half-life ranges from 53 to 140 hours in adults [256] and from 37 to 98 hours in infants and children [241]. In a controlled study encompassing a span of seven days, Fabre et al. [89] found no difference between the phenobarbital levels in serum of normal and uremic patients. Few other quantitative data are available concerning the toxicity of phenobarbital in patients with renal disease. Caution should be exercised, however, because these patients may be more sensitive than normal subjects to a given level in blood [41,89,183,256], in part because of decreased binding to serum proteins [39].

Phenytoin

Phenytoin enters the brain rapidly when given intravenously because of its high lipid solubility [347]. It reaches a peak level in 15 minutes (more rapidly than phenobar-

bital). Concentrations in brain and plasma decline rapidly, however, as a result of its binding to serum albumin and storage in other tissues [353], and the neurophysiologic effects of the drug disappear. With continuous administration, these other tissues and the brain become saturated, but it takes four to five days to reach a steady-state level [353]. Rapid saturation has been obtained in adults with a large loading dose, in the range of 1000 mg. We use 15 to 20 mg/kg intravenously as a loading dose in the treatment of status epilepticus for nonuremic children under the age of 10 years. This dose is administered at a rate of infusion that should not exceed 50 mg/min, with monitoring of the blood pressure and electrocardiogram (ECG). This same loading dose is appropriate for patients with renal failure. It is followed 12 hours later with one-half of the 5 to 7 mg/kg daily maintenance dose. Phenytoin, because of its long half-life (average 22 hours), is used in adults in a single daily dose. The half-life is shorter in young children, and the drug is usually given in two divided doses.

Phenytoin is metabolized primarily in the liver, and only 5% appears unchanged in the urine [353]. On entering the circulation of nonuremic subjects, 90% of phenytoin is rapidly and reversibly bound to albumin. Only the unbound 10% is pharmacologically active [353] and can be measured conveniently in saliva [35a]. Albumin-binding has been reported to be unusually low in uremic patients [171,270]. Therefore, uremic patients respond favorably to phenytoin sodium at relatively low total plasma concentrations (4–8 μg/ml); conversely, they may experience toxicity at levels in plasma usually considered to be nontoxic. It is essential to monitor plasma levels closely, if possible including levels of the unbound fraction, because the pharmacokinetics of phenytoin are altered in a complex manner in renal failure (see the section on complications of drug therapy).

Parenteral phenytoin is highly alkaline and suitable only for intravenous administration. Intramuscular administration is ineffective and harmful; the drug is poorly absorbed [348] and causes muscle necrosis. Administration by mouth or nasogastric tube is satisfactory except in status epilepticus and in the presence of vomiting or other gastrointestinal problems.

Pediatricians should be aware of the possible idiosyncratic reaction to phenytoin, consisting of a morbilliform rash that may progress to an exfoliative dermatitis or the Stevens-Johnson syndrome. It usually occurs after several days and rarely later than a few weeks after starting administration of the drug. It is not dose-related and necessitates immediate cessation of the drug. Treatment of such reactions may require corticosteroid administration.

Paraldehyde

Paraldehyde is no longer available in the United States but is discussed nevertheless for readers in other parts of the world. It has been found to be particularly helpful in controlling status epilepticus due to metabolic causes, which often responds poorly to the more commonly used anticonvulsants. When used in large doses, however, one of paraldehyde's toxic effects is metabolic acidosis [119], an effect that may be especially undesirable in children with renal insufficiency.

Paraldehyde can be administered rectally as a retention enema, 0.3 ml/kg mixed with an equal or double amount of olive or mineral oil. It may be repeated every two to four hours. Because of its irritating effect on the rectal mucosa, prolonged rectal administration must be avoided. The same dose can be given by gavage.

Paraldehyde can be given intravenously in a dose of 0.15 ml/kg. The paraldehyde solution must be fresh and not discolored. Each milliliter of paraldehyde should be diluted in 10 ml glucose or saline solution and infused over 30 minutes. The rate of infusion is titrated according to the clinical response, until the appropriate lowest dose is found that will control the seizures. The maximum dose is 0.3 ml/kg/hr. It is important to use a glass syringe and to change the plastic intravenous tubing frequently. Phlebitis is a common complication, and the site of infusion needs to be changed frequently. Intramuscular injections are painful and are not recommended; they may give rise to sterile abscesses and necrosis of the overlying skin and fat.

Because paraldehyde is excreted primarily by the lungs, its use is not recommended in patients with acute pulmonary disease. Respiratory depression, hypotension, metabolic acidosis, and pulmonary damage have been reported in patients who receive toxic amounts.

Other

Lidocaine [261] and promazine [335] have been advocated as treatments of status epilepticus in uremic subjects. The authors have no personal experience with their use.

Management of Chronic Convulsive Disorders

Prolonged therapy with anticonvulsants is not required in most patients who have had a single seizure during an episode of renal failure. It may be indicated if the child is suffering from a chronic convulsive disorder or if there is evidence of persistent epileptogenic brain dysfunction manifested by a paroxysmal EEG. Frequent determination of anticonvulsant levels in blood is essential to guide management and avoid toxic reactions. The drugs used most frequently are phenobarbital [241] in young children, and phenytoin [353] and carbamazepine [137] in older children. Valproic acid is also acceptable [43,239]. There is no extensive experience with other anticonvulsants in uremic children.

Myoclonus is probably best not treated unless it is disabling. In nonuremic patients, clonazepam and valproic acid are the drugs of choice, although their efficacy is limited. The possibility that myoclonus represents the side effect of a drug taken by the patient should not be overlooked (see Table 30-5).

Peripheral Neuropathy
Clinical Features

Peripheral neuropathy is a common manifestation of chronic renal failure, especially in males; it has been reported in 13% to 86% of patients, depending on the stage of the disease and the author's clinical definition of neuropathy [24,29,68,224,226,261,267,293,324,327,335]. Few of the described cases were teenagers, and even fewer were below 10 years of age. Reported overt clinical neu-

ropathy in children is rare even though their nerve conduction velocities may be prolonged [1a,12].

In adults, the earliest clinical manifestation of uremic neuropathy is usually the *restless leg syndrome* [48], characterized by peculiar creeping, prickling, and tingling sensations in the lower limbs. The symptoms are worse at rest, especially at night, and characteristically are relieved by movement.

A marked hypersensitivity to touch and a burning feeling in the feet, the *burning feet syndrome,* may follow or occur independently of the restless leg syndrome. These initial manifestations may be followed by a progressive neuropathy that involves sensory, motor, and even sympathetic fibers, although the burning feet syndrome does not always progress to paralysis and sensory loss [335].

Neuropathy usually develops gradually over a period of many weeks, although occasionally it may appear rather suddenly over a few days [20]. It is predominantly distal and usually symmetrical. The arms are involved only in patients with severe involvement of the legs. Examination may reveal distal loss of strength as well as the sensations of vibration, position, touch, and pain, notably in the toes. Wasting may develop, and the tendon stretch reflexes may be abolished, especially the ankle jerks. Motor involvement may progress from a footdrop to paraplegia with inability to walk. As in alcoholic neuropathy, pressure palsies are quite common [38,326]. Involvement of autonomic fibers may be responsible for decreased sweating, postural hypotension, hiccups, and an abnormal response to the Valsalva maneuver in some patients with acute and chronic renal failure [23,152,173,230].

An elevated CSF protein is common in patients with advanced renal failure. It is not clear whether it is higher in those who have a neuropathy than in those who do not.

CRANIAL NERVES

Papilledema and hypertensive retinopathy occur regularly in malignant hypertension with encephalopathy. Occasionally, papilledema is said to persist in uremic patients after their hypertension has been controlled [27]. Papilledema enlarges the blind spot but does not impair visual acuity unless it has been so chronic as to produce secondary optic atrophy. *Uremic amaurosis* refers to sudden loss of vision that develops over minutes to hours and usually recedes over several days. Uremic amaurosis is attributed to focal swelling in the optic nerves or, more often, in the central visual pathways [335], in which case pupillary light responses are spared.

Abducens palsy usually occurs in the context of increased intracranial pressure. Uremic ophthalmoparesis, facial weakness, and miosis, with or without nystagmus, are usually transient. Nystagmus should suggest the possibility of drug intoxication, especially with barbiturate or other anticonvulsants [108,183]. Saccadic eye movements and facial myoclonus are characteristics of early aluminum dementia [96].

Hearing loss in association with renal failure [33] is often caused by a genetic disorder, such as Alport syndrome [218,237] or renal tubular acidosis [66,79,305] affecting both the ear and the kidney. Fluctuating hearing loss occurs in dialyzed patients [145] and disappears with transplantation [213]. Whereas in some patients hearing loss may be a direct consequence of renal failure, one should always consider the possibility that hearing loss reflects the use of an ototoxic drug such as furosemide, kanamycin, or another aminoglycoside antibiotic. Both vestibular and cochlear function may be affected [345].

Pathology

Uremic neuropathy is characterized by distal-to-proximal degeneration of axons (dying-back neuropathy) [20,81, 293,327]. Affected fibers are shrunken; their Schwann's cells degenerate [78], with resultant secondary segmental demyelination. Evidence of remyelination and Schwann's cell proliferation includes a decreased distance between nodes of Ranvier as well as onion bulb formation. Thinned axons contain fewer neurofilaments; it is not clear whether this change is due to decreased synthesis of neurofilaments in the perikaryon or to defective axon transport of neurofilaments [24,335] and other cytoskeletal components because of impaired axoplasmic flow [231]. Whereas medium and small sensory fibers are affected selectively, in severe cases large fibers and unmyelinated autonomic fibers may also be damaged. Proximal nerves and those of the arms are less severely involved than those of the leg and foot; the spinal roots are spared. Denervation in muscle predominates in type 2 fibers [289].

Pathophysiology

Several mechanisms contribute to the distal axonopathy of renal failure. Deficient energy metabolism, which has been shown to play a role in the pathogenesis of uremic encephalopathy, is a likely contributor [81]. Energy deficiency impairs both energy-dependent pumping mechanisms across cell membranes and synthetic metabolic reactions in the perikaryon; it might explain dysfunction of both neurons and Schwann's cells [225]. Defective axon transport [231] would be another expected consequence.

Uremic toxins also play a pathogenetic role. Peripheral neuropathy tends to be less troublesome in uremic patients treated with peritoneal dialysis than in those treated with hemodialysis [288]. This observation has been interpreted as evidence for neurotoxicity of middle or large molecular weight substances, because peritoneal dialysis clears them more efficiently than hemodialysis [76]. For example, elevated levels of PTH in serum correlate significantly with decrements in peroneal nerve conduction velocities [22].

In some patients, vitamin and other nutritional deficiencies may contribute to the development of neuropathy [167]. Lesions in the vasa nervorum have been hypothesized to occur in hypertensive uremic patients whose neuropathy was unresponsive until their hypertension abated following bilateral nephrectomy [255].

Electrophysiologic Investigations

Measuring the threshold to vibration [264] and recording sensory nerve action potentials [44] are sensitive tests for incipient uremic neuropathy. Single fiber electromyography with a small surface electrode enables noninvasive assessment of neuromuscular transmission, which may be impaired in some patients with renal failure at a time when nerve conduction velocity is normal [160]. Markedly decreased nerve conduction velocity with relative preservation of muscle action potentials—a pattern typical of segmental demyelination—occurs in some patients [106]. Whereas both sensory and motor nerve conduction velocities are decreased in flagrant neuropathy, they may be significantly reduced in patients without clinical evidence of a neuropathy [225,226]. Exploration of conduction velocity in the proximal portion of nerves can be accomplished by recording the latency of the monosynaptic H-reflex and late F-response [1a,38a,116]. With the addition of somatosensory evoked potential studies to measure central latencies [174,230,280], it is possible to localize pathology precisely in the peripheral or central pathways of patients with altered superficial or proprioceptive sensation.

In adults, both nerve conduction velocity and clinical evidence of a neuropathy are related to the duration and severity of the renal failure; when kidney function is reduced to about 10% of normal, slowing of nerve conduction velocity can be expected in half of the patients [225]. Close correlation with particular renal toxins is poor, with the possible exception of PTH [4,22,142,225,324]. This relationship appears to be less clear in children [2].

Management

Successful renal transplantation is the most effective treatment for the peripheral neuropathy of renal failure [233]. Recovery is said to occur within two to six months in adults [38,227] but may require one to three years in children [12]. Vigorous peritoneal dialysis and, to a lesser extent, hemodialysis may improve uremic neuropathy, especially in patients with a purely sensory neuropathy [76,77,177,269]. Not all patients improve, however; in some, the neuropathy may progress or even appear during the course of chronic hemodialysis [1,111,142,303]. Recovery is infrequent in patients with severe motor weakness and moderate-to-severe sensory loss.

Disorders of Muscle

Patients with mild-to-moderate renal failure often complain of muscle cramps, which occur predominantly at night. They are not correlated with specific serum electrolyte abnormalities, including hypocalcemia. Cramps also occur as a complication of dialysis [230]. Signs of muscle irritability, e.g., fasciculations and fascicular twitching, are frequent, especially around the mouth. Frank tetany and sustained tetanic muscle spasms occur but are uncommon [88].

Proximal muscle wasting and weakness, involving in particular the quadriceps, muscles of the pelvic girdle, and neck flexors, occur in some uremic patients [95,168, 180,335]. These findings cannot be ascribed to uremic neuropathy, which affects the distal portion of axons selectively. Cardiomyopathy has occurred in some dialyzed adults [80].

Myopathy is most often associated with the hypercalcemia and osteomalacia of secondary hyperparathyroidism and with aluminum intoxication [11,15,250,267,335]. Nutritional deficiency may contribute to the myopathy of some patients. Muscle pathology was present in 69% of uremic patients biopsied because of neuromuscular symptoms [168]; morphologic findings suggested a pure myopathy of mild intensity in 11%, a neuropathy in 29%, and both in 29%. Muscle fibers show disarray of the myofibrillar sarcoplasm, streaming of Z-band material, and hypertrophy of mitochondria; damage predominates at the periphery of the myofibril where amorphous remnants form a subsarcolemal ring [290]. Pathology in muscle tends to be more severe than expected clinically.

Rarely, acute muscle weakness or even paralysis has occurred as a manifestation of hypokalemia in adequately monitored dialysis patients or has followed the administration of toxic amounts of aminoglycoside antibiotics that produce a block at the neuromuscular junction (see Table 30-5) [335]. Ischemic myopathy has occurred as a result of widespread vascular calcinosis in secondary hyperparathyroidism [112]. Inflammatory myopathy (polymyositis), with its characteristic pathology and often elevated serum creatine kinase level, occurs occasionally in patients with renal grafts. Its favorable response to high dosage steroids suggests that it has an immunologic basis. Muscle biopsy may be required in order to make a logical therapeutic decision in transplanted patients with significant muscle weakness; those with polymyositis require an increase in their dose of steroids, while those with steroid or toxic (uremic) myopathy require a decrease.

Dialysis Dysequilibrium Syndrome
Clinical Features

Although peritoneal dialysis and hemodialysis are generally safe and effective means of treating renal failure, cerebral manifestations may occur during, toward the end of, or immediately after dialysis (Table 30-3). This encephalopathy may occur at a time when the clinical chemistries in blood appear to be greatly improved. For unexplained reasons, cerebral symptoms have been reported to occur occasionally as late as 8 to 48 hours after dialysis [334]. Patients with the dialysis dysequilibrium syndrome require careful evaluation in order to avoid missing more serious neurologic complications.

The major neurologic manifestations of the dialysis dy-

Table 30-3. *Dialysis dysequilibrium syndrome*

Conditions of Occurrence
With hemodialysis more often than peritoneal dialysis
Most common in the early phase of dialytic treatment
Usually toward the end or immediately following dialysis

Symptoms and Signs
Restlessness, headache, nausea, vomiting
Increasing agitation, confusion, hallucinations
Muscle twitching, fasciculations, asterixis
Seizure or series of seizures, coma

sequilibrium syndrome are (1) single or recurrent seizures, (2) toxic encephalopathy, and (3) psychosis [151,335]. These clinical occurrences are more common following hemodialysis than following peritoneal dialysis and more common in children than adults [253]. They tend to occur in the early weeks of treatment and in patients with acute renal failure, but they may also happen in patients who have had many uneventful dialyses.

Restlessness associated with headache, nausea, and vomiting are the usual initial complaints. If dialysis is continued, these symptoms may be followed by increasing agitation, confusion, hallucinations, twitching, fasciculations, and asterixis. A seizure or series of seizures followed by coma may occur. If appropriate measures are taken, a slow return to the predialysis status over a period of 24 to 36 hours can be expected.

Pathophysiology

Cerebral dysfunction during dialysis may be the consequence of several different mechanisms acting singly or in concert [151]. The dialysis dysequilibrium syndrome is most likely to occur in severely uremic patients at the onset of hemodialysis, especially if the procedure results in a rapid change in the concentration of low molecular weight constituents of plasma [17].

Acidemia and hyperphosphatemia cause hypocapnia and shift the hemoglobin-oxygen dissociation curve to the left [156]. The diminished availability of arterial oxygen may result in tissue hypoxia in the brain. There are no data on the effects of uremic metabolic acidemia upon the blood-brain barrier, cerebral blood flow, autoregulation of cerebral blood flow, or the tissue compartmentation of hydrogen ion; because autoregulation of cerebral blood flow is destabilized by hypoxia and hypocapnia [148], destabilization may occur in renal failure.

A persistent intracellular elevation of low molecular weight compounds, i.e., urea, creatinine, and as yet unidentified molecules (idiogenic osmoles), can lead to water shifts from plasma into cerebral parenchyma, with attendant brain swelling and increased intracranial pressure [124,149,161,224,354a]. Increased plasma osmolality may result in brain shrinkage which carries the risk of tearing of bridging veins and of development of subdural hemorrhage [169]. Compromise of cell membrane pumps, because of tissue hypoxia, further impairs the maintenance of a normal cellular volume; it also alters neuronal excitability. Altered excitability may give rise to myoclonus and seizures and to decreased brain function. Hypocalcemia in the course of dialysis may cause hyperirritability of muscles, cramps, tetany, and seizures. The capacity of the autonomic nervous system to maintain homeostatic regulation is impaired during renal failure [173]; this may limit adaptability to changes in blood volume during hemodialysis.

Compositional characteristics of the dialysate may contribute to the dialysis dysequilibrium syndrome [151]. Hyponatremia [340] and hypoglycemia can be avoided by the use of appropriate dialysis solutions. Adding glycerol to the dialysate may mitigate rapid osmolar shifts in the brain. Air embolism and inadvertent overheating of dialysates are avoidable complications.

Management

The most important goal is prevention of dialysis dysequilibrium. Timely institution of dialysis, thus avoiding rapid removal of low molecular weight compounds such as urea, moderates this complication and decreases the frequency of its occurrence (see Chap. 39).

When the child becomes restless during the course of hemodialysis, sedation with intravenous diazepam is usually helpful. It is advisable to terminate dialysis if seizures develop. Dialysis can be reinstituted after a few hours if it is critically needed.

Seizures that occur following rapid correction of blood chemistries are almost always self-limited, and the patient usually improves in 6 to 24 hours without any specific therapy. Nevertheless, it may be wise to administer appropriate anticonvulsants if seizures are severe (see the section on management of acute seizures) because of the danger of prolonged or recurrent seizures. Long-term anticonvulsant therapy is unnecessary unless the child has a preexisting convulsive disorder or has sustained an epileptogenic focal brain lesion.

The prophylactic use of phenytoin prior to the start of dialysis and during the first few sessions has been recommended [125], but no controlled study is available to evaluate its effectiveness.

Other Complications of Dialysis

Intracranial hemorrhage, more frequently subdural hematoma than subarachnoid hemorrhage and intracerebral hematoma, may complicate hemodialysis [31,169,303,335, 343]. Several factors predispose to its occurrence: (1) Use of anticoagulants; (2) the bleeding tendency that is common in advanced renal disease; (3) hypertension; (4) rapid shifts in water compartmentation, especially those likely to decrease intracranial pressure; and (5) trauma. Diagnosis is usually difficult, because intracranial bleeding tends to occur in patients who have other derangements of central nervous system function as a result of renal disease or of its treatment by hemodialysis. Prolonged or increasing headache, signs of meningeal irritation, the appearance of unilateral neurologic signs or of papilledema, or persistently impaired consciousness must alert the clinician to the possibility of this complication. Such symptoms indicate the need for appropriate neuroradiologic investigations, because surgical treatment may be required. The neuroimaging procedure of choice is CT, although subdural hemorrhage is occasionally missed by this technique.

Other rare complications have been reported in chronically ill dialyzed uremic patients with poor nutrition. They include Wernicke's encephalopathy [91] and central pontine myelinolysis [181].

Aluminum-Related Encephalopathies
Clinical Features

Progressive dialysis dementia was first recognized in the early 1970s in adult patients on long-term hemodialysis. It occurred in small epidemics in only some hemodialysis centers [6,7,8,14,15,80,234]. The presenting sign is a speech disorder with dysarthria and verbal apraxia. Speech is slow, slurred, hesitant, with stuttering-like pauses due to a word-finding problem; these manifestations may improve with intravenous diazepam [318]. The patient's personality is labile, with inappropriate mood swings. Eventually the patient becomes demented, develops severe myoclonus and seizures, and may be unable to swallow.

Some patients also suffer from proximal muscle weakness associated with osteomalacia and, occasionally, pathologic fractures [234,250]. Neurologic symptoms may be intermittent initially and worsen during dialysis, but the course is usually rapidly progressive, culminating in stupor and death within months. In some patients, symptoms may start subacutely at the time of an intercurrent illness that puts them to bed and causes mobilization of mineral from bone.

At first the EEG shows characteristic bilateral bursts of slow waves with a frontal preponderance against normal background rhythms. Later, the EEG becomes diffusely slow, and the CT reveals brain atrophy. Decreased levels of gamma-aminobutyric acid (GABA), an inhibitory neurotransmitter, are present in the CSF and, postmortem, in selected brain areas [318]. Potential participation of excitatory amino acids (EAA) and/or an altered intracellular $[Ca^{2+}]$ [291a] in causing these changes remains to be elucidated.

A chronic encephalopathy with similar features has been described in children whose renal failure started in infancy [26,96,103,281]. It appears to be more frequent in boys than in girls [253]. Most of the children were not on dialysis but had received aluminum hydroxide orally as a phosphate binder.

Pathology

Dialysis encephalopathy is characterized by severe loss of neurons, occasionally leading to a spongy appearance of layers 1 and 3 of the cortex [46], lipofuscin accumulation, and, in some but not all cases, the appearance of neurofibrillary tangles in neurons of the cortex, especially of the motor cortex, red nucleus, inferior olive, and dentate nucleus of the cerebellum [285]. Neurofibrillary changes have been produced in immature rabbits by intracisternal injection of aluminum salts [322,350]. In one child who died at six years of age, brain weight was reduced to less than half of normal; there was severe loss of cortical neurons, hypertrophy of astrocytes, and sponginess of the cortex [96].

Pathophysiology

The epidemic occurrence of this syndrome in hemodialyzed patients has been correlated with the aluminum content of the dialysate. New cases ceased to occur when appropriately deionized water was used. Affected patients had raised levels of aluminum in brain, muscle, and bone [7,14]. The contributory role of oral aluminum hydroxide, prescribed to avoid secondary hyperparathyroidism, is controversial, even though it is clearly implicated in a few adults and in many of the infants [11,26,96,103,253]. Elevated levels of PTH in renal failure foster gastrointestinal absorption of aluminum and its mobilization from stores in bone [199]. Aluminum intoxication may not cause all cases of dialysis dementia, however [15]. The progressive dementia of end-stage renal failure in very young children may result from both maldevelopment and damage, to which malnutrition, uremic toxins, and aluminum probably all contribute [36,103a,253].

Management

The use of water with less than 20 µg/L of aluminum prevents the occurrence of epidemic dialysis dementia. Substitution of deionized water and renal transplantation have not ameliorated severe dementia but have improved some milder cases [234,253]. Completely curtailing the use of aluminum hydroxide phosphate binders is not recommended [15] unless it is replaced by an effective substitute, such as calcium carbonate, because hyperphosphatemia will inevitably lead to secondary hyperparathyroidism; parathyroidectomy does not seem to be effective in preventing the dementia [234,253]. Aluminum chelation may be efficacious in some cases [8a,254].

Complications of Transplantation

Successful transplantation usually ameliorates the neurologic complications of renal failure. Few children who undergo renal transplantation develop neurologic complications attributable to this treatment [276]. Complications may occur, however, in the first few days or weeks following transplantation or may be delayed for months or years. Some evolve acutely, while others present as chronic problems (Table 30-4).

Renal failure, through a number of mechanisms, subverts normal immunologic defenses [53,272]. Cell-mediated functions as well as some humoral factors are altered. Autoantibody levels are increased; this increase may be greater

TABLE 30-4. *Neurologic complications of transplantation*

Early Phase
Associated with rejection:
   Hypertensive crisis with encephalopathy
   Toxic psychosis associated with kidney necrosis
Associated with a well-functioning transplanted kidney
   The phase of massive diuresis may precipitate a clinical picture analogous to the dialysis dysequilibrium syndrome
Early complications of immunosuppressive therapy

Chronic Phase
Associated with episodes of rejection: as above
Complications of immunosuppressive therapy:
   Intracranial bleeding due to thrombocytopenia
   Opportunistic infections: bacterial, fungal, or viral
Intracranial lymphomas
Corticosteroid-induced hypertensive crisis with encephalopathy
Corticosteroid-induced psychosis
Corticosteroid-induced myopathy

in patients who are treated by hemodialysis than in those who are treated by continuous ambulatory peritoneal dialysis [99]. Leukocyte phagocytic functions are depressed in renal failure, and the alternative complement pathway is activated in hemodialyzed patients [110,287]. Immunosuppression, required for successful transplantation, may potentiate these immunologic abnormalities, although availability of cyclosporin seems to have decreased the susceptibility of transplanted patients to central nervous system complications [202] (see Chap. 41).

Rejection Encephalopathy

In one study, half of the adult patients who underwent an acute rejection episode developed signs of an encephalopathy [114]. Occurrence of the encephalopathy seemed to be related to the severity of the rejection crisis. More than half of the patients developed it within three months of transplantation, although in one patient it was delayed by two years. The patients were being given steroids and had hypertension, decreased renal function, and fluid retention. These factors, however, were not clearly responsible for the encephalopathy; its characteristics suggested a toxic state.

The patients developed generalized seizures, confusion, fever, irritability, and headache. CSF pressure was greatly elevated in patients who underwent lumbar puncture; in some, CT revealed edema of the white matter. The prognosis was excellent with complete recovery.

The differential diagnosis of rejection encephalopathy includes central nervous system infection, intracranial hemorrhage, lymphoma, and drug intoxication. Once the diagnosis of rejection encephalopathy has been firmly established, the treatment of choice, in addition to managing hypertension, transient renal dysfunction, and fluid retention, is to increase, not decrease, steroids.

Infections of the Central Nervous System

Infection contributes to much of the morbidity and to more than half of the mortality in transplanted patients of all ages [249,276,342]. It probably contributes even more in children, who are at low risk for cardiovascular disease and late complications of diabetes. Administration of steroids, other immunosuppressive agents, and antibiotics to patients whose immune system has already been depressed by chronic renal failure and dialysis [53,272] is in large part responsible for the many opportunistic infections that occur. More than 80% of transplant recipients develop infections, 5% to 10% of them infections of the nervous system, which is an immunologically privileged site, less accessible to immunologic surveillance than other tissues. It is appropriate, therefore, to have a high degree of suspicion for intracranial infection in all transplant recipients, even in the face of systemic illness or rejection crisis, because infection may contribute to both of these problems [60]. If a patient exhibits unexplained neurologic symptoms, investigations such as CT scan and CSF examination are obligatory.

Rubin and colleagues [283a], as well as Bolton and

Young [38a] have tabulated the time of occurrence of various infections in renal graft recipients. These are helpful data, because they provide guidelines as to which infectious agent should be suspected in an individual patient. Infections of the nervous system are especially likely to occur during the second posttransplant month. Three fourths of intracranial infections after renal grafting are due to *Listeria monocytogenes*, *Cryptococcus*, and *Toxoplasma gondii* [283a].

Intracranial infections may be predominantly meningitic. Acute meningitis is usually due to *Listeria*, while subacute or chronic meningitis suggests *Cryptococcus* [251], *Histoplasma* [71], or, less frequently, *Candida* and typical or atypical mycobacteria [175,329]. Infections may be parenchymal and relatively diffuse (viral encephalitis) or focal and space occupying (abscess). *Aspergillus* is a more common cause of brain abscess than *Listeria*, *Toxoplasma*, or *Nocardia* [283a]. *Toxoplasma* tends to produce mixed meningitic and parenchymal infections [284]. Progressive multifocal leukoencephalitis, a fatal viral demyelinating disease, occurs in adults [102,190,358]. Precise and early diagnosis of the infectious agent is essential, because many of these infections are responsive to appropriate antibiotic therapy [19,32].

Cytomegalovirus (CMV) is the most frequent cause of systemic viral infection in transplant recipients [34,283a]. It may produce chronic progressive chorioretinitis [60] or, rarely, an encephalitis [25,178]. Many patients are infected simultaneously by CMV and another viral, bacterial, or fungal agent [248]. Varicella-zoster virus, herpes simplex virus (HSV) [60], and Epstein-Barr virus (EBV) [59,192] are also common infectious agents in patients with renal grafts, but they rarely produce an encephalitis. Many more allograft recipients shed EBV in their oropharyngeal secretions compared with the normal population (47%–87% versus 17%) [127]. Rise in antibody titers against EBV, indicating either a new infection or the reactivation of a latent infection, is much more common than are clinical signs of infection. It is as an oncogene that EBV poses its greatest threat to the carrier of a grafted kidney. Human immunodeficiency virus (HIV) may be acquired from an infected graft or from hemodialysis [38a,283]. All potential donors and recipients, as well as those with opportunistic infections, should be screened for HIV antibodies.

Lymphoma of the Central Nervous System

The incidence of cancer is markedly increased in transplant recipients [247]. Loss of DNA repair mechanisms [51] and viral-associated genetic transformation [165] are believed to be two fundamental processes in oncogenesis; the latter is strongly implicated in renal graft recipients. More than 30% of posttransplant cancers are reticulum cell sarcomas. These B-cell immunoblastic lymphomas, most of which arise from EBV-induced malignant transformation of B-lymphocytes, are 40 to 350 times more frequent in transplanted patients than in the general population [127]. Half or more of these tumors involve the brain [194], compared to less than 2% of lymphomas affecting the central nervous system in the nontransplanted population [323].

Lymphomas tend to occur earlier in the central nervous system following grafting than systemic lymphomas and carcinomas [300]. Teenage patients with this tumor usually become symptomatic within a few months of transplantation; older individuals may not develop this complication until several years later [127]. The patients exhibit serologic evidence of either primary or reactivated EBV infection, and they frequently shed the infectious agent. The tumor cells often exhibit hybridization evidence of EBV DNA, which is not present in surrounding neural tissue [135].

Viral-induced oncogenesis is thought to require at least two cooperating oncogenes [165]. EBV transforms (immortalizes) B-lymphocytes that presumably escape immune surveillance in renal allograft recipients [158]; however, the specific interaction of these immortalized cells with an oncogene or proto-oncogene to induce malignancy has not yet been identified [165].

Clinically, the tumor usually presents with rapidly evolving focal neurologic deficits, with or without increased intracranial pressure. It may be multicentric. Because it is prone to infiltrate the brain and spread into the subarachnoid space, it may present in some patients with signs of diffuse brain dysfunction, multiple cranial nerve signs, and stupor [292]. Primary lymphomas of the brain must be included in the differential diagnosis of subacute or chronic sterile meningitis and of brain abscess with CSF pleocytosis. A CT scan with contrast or MRI helps in making a diagnosis but does not differentiate lymphoma from a subacute or chronic infectious process. Prompt histologic diagnosis is essential, because the tumor is remarkably radiosensitive and responds to acyclovir as long as it remains polyclonal and contains replicating virus [126]. Multiple remissions and prolonged survival without evidence of tumor have been achieved in some patients with this therapy.

Complications of Drug Therapy

The effects of renal failure on absorption, albumin binding, metabolism, distribution, and excretion of drugs are complex [101,164,215] (see Chap. 42); furthermore, patients with renal failure are likely to be taking several drugs that may interact. Dialyzability of drugs must also be considered. Some of the drugs that are likely to produce undesirable effects on the central nervous system of uremic patients are listed in Table 30-5, and some relevant data concerning drugs prescribed for neurologic symptoms in renal patients are listed in Table 30-6. Information concerning choice and dosage of drugs in children with renal failure is incomplete [164]. The information provided in Tables 30-5 and 30-6 should be considered tentative; readers are referred to the original publications for details.

Drug dosage must be individualized in renal failure and close attention paid to the clinical state of the patient, as well as to blood levels. Many factors alter drug bioavailability, and in some cases, blood assays may yield unreliable results [238]. It is wise to obtain blood levels at frequent intervals over a span of time and to measure free, rather than total, drug level in planning dose adjustments of some chronic medications in renal patients.

The effective dose of phenytoin may be unchanged in

Table 30-5. *Neurotoxicity of drugs commonly used in patients with renal insufficiency*

Seizures-Myoclonus	Psychosis Hallucinations	Depression
Penicillin	Steroids	Methyldopa
Meperidine	Tricyclic antidepressants	Reserpine
Phenothiazines	Lithium	
Benzodiazepines	Reserpine	
Tricyclic antidepressants	Propranolol	
Nitroprusside	Cimetidine	
Diazoxide		
Cyclosporine		
Aluminum		
Somnolence	Stupor Coma	Dementia
Anticonvulsants	Sedatives	Aluminum
Benzodiazepines	Anticonvulsants	Methotrexate and radiation
Sedatives	Antipsychotics	
Antipsychotics	Lithium	

Table 30-6. *Metabolism of commonly used drugs*

Drug	Elimination by Kidney (%)	Protein binding (%)	Dialyzable	Adjustment
Phenobarbital	20–40	60	Yes	No
Phenytoin	No	90	No	No
Carbamazepine	No	75	—	—
Valproate	No	90	—	No
Ethosuximide	10–25	No	—	—
Diazepam	Partly	95	No	No
Clonazepam	No	80	—	—
Primidone	50	No	—	—
Phenothiazines	No	≥ 90	No	No
Haloperidol	No	90	No	No
Levodopa	Yes	5	—	—
Neostigmine	Yes	No	—	Slight*
Pyridostigmine				
Aspirin	Yes	90	Yes	Decrease or avoid
Methylphenidate	Yes	—	—	—
Propranalol	No	95	No	No
Penicillamine	Yes	—	—	Decrease or avoid
Prednisone	Some	50–80	No	No
Chloral hydrate	No	35–40	Yes	Avoid

* Blood levels, particularly of unbound drug, are required.
—, no data.

renal patients despite many differences in its bioavailability: The rate of its intestinal absorption may decrease; its half-life is decreased; its unbound fraction in plasma is increased twofold to threefold because of competition by 2-hydroxybenzoyl-glycine for albumin binding sites [176]. An effective therapeutic level of total phenytoin may be 4 to 8 μg/ml in renal failure, compared to the usual 10 to 20 μg/ml. Because of a shorter half-life and in order to maintain a steady state without undue fluctuations, doses may have to be spread out over the day rather than being given once a day.

For patients on dialysis, measuring drug levels before and after dialysis is helpful, but it is important to keep in mind that levels may rebound in the hours following dialysis as tissue stores re-equilibrate with the blood [105]. Nomograms have been prepared to assist in drug management of patients on dialysis [215].

Drugs should be used sparingly and for definite indications. This is particularly true of lipid-soluble drugs that may accumulate in the brain and cause delayed and long-lasting side effects. Many sedatives and psychotropic drugs are hazardous, especially because blood levels may not be reliable gauges of their tissue stores [215]; drugs may cause hallucinations, myoclonus, seizures, stupor, and a toxic psychosis that is difficult to distinguish from uremic encephalopathy. The penicillins, which are excreted in urine, accumulate in the brain and can produce myoclonus, seizures, and an encephalopathy [35,235]. The aminoglycosides may produce neuromuscular blockade, including respiratory failure [245,341], and irreversible ototoxicity. Cyclosporin is nephrotoxic and may produce hypertension and seizures [147]. The possibility of drug toxicity must therefore be considered in any patient with renal failure who presents with unexplained or bizarre neurologic symptoms, because toxicity is frequent and likely to be overlooked but is usually reversible [335].

Potential Neuroscience Correlates

Neuronal excitability is dependent on ionic concentrations and fluxes, intracellular transport processes, and cellular energetics; all of these may be modified as a consequence of chemical alterations associated with renal failure. Renal failure may also alter the concentrations and functional efficacy of neurohumors that mediate interneuronal communication. Compounds that accumulate in body fluids during renal failure include peptides, such as PTH. PTH may act as a neuromodulator as well as regulator of calcium homeostasis. While calcium's role on the excitability of cell membranes has been well recognized, it is only recently that its role as an intracellular regulator has become apparent. Studies of intracellular calcium in neural tissue hold the promise of illuminating how uremia interferes with the function of the nervous system.

Alterations of Hydrogen Ion Concentration, Electrolytes, and Water

Plasma hydrogen ion concentration, $[H^+]$, increases during renal failure. This increase is the result of an accumulation of acidic catabolites, which include phenolic acids [265, 266,304]. The biologic properties of some peptides and many cellular constituents are exquisitely sensitive to $[H^+]$. It is not known which of the many potential alterations induced by acidemia is responsible for particular neurologic symptoms of uremic patients.

$[H^+]$ is regulated, in part, by the zinc metalloenzyme, carbonic anhydrase. This enzyme participates in the transport of CO_2 and regulation of the bicarbonate buffering of protons, H^+, in brain cells, as well as in the production of CSF. Carbonic anhydrase activity and zinc content are increased in erythrocytes during renal failure [113]; zinc content and the activity of this enzyme in neural tissue during renal failure remain to be determined.

Translocation of H^+ in mitochondria and synaptic vesicles is catalyzed by H^+-ATPases [9,268]. Linkage of neurologic symptoms in uremic patients to changes in the activities of these enzymes, to the intracellular content and ultrastructural compartmentation of H^+, or to transmembrane H^+-flux in neural tissue has not been established to date.

Low molecular weight compounds, such as urea and creatinine, accumulate in extracellular fluids as a result of renal failure [63,118,176,210,265,266,304,307]. When these uremic toxins are administered experimentally, in an attempt to duplicate the neurologic manifestations of renal failure, none alone replicates such dysfunction.

The aggregate presence of low molecular weight uremic toxins during untreated chronic renal failure increases the plasma osmolality [309]. Some of the neurologic manifestations of renal failure and its treatment, as discussed in earlier sections, may be due to osmolal stress and resulting

alterations in brain function that are beyond the nervous system's adaptive capacity [170]. Potential relationships between extracellular fluid osmolality, cell volumes in neural tissues, the cytoskeletal protein constituents of neural cells, Ca^{2+} homeostasis, and neurologic manifestations of renal disease have not been documented yet. Some of the low molecular weight catabolites that accumulate in body fluids during renal failure, e.g., urea and the guanidines, also denature proteins [11a]. Occurrence of such chaotropic events in neural membrane or intracellular proteins as a cause of nervous system complications of acute and/or chronic kidney disease has not been published to date.

Neuronal activity is contingent upon the periodic occurrence of directionally oriented electrical currents. These minute currents are generated by the intermittent flow of elementary ions across the neuronal plasma membrane [54, 134]. This flow ensues through specific channels in the membrane and is driven by a transmembrane diffusional gradient. Maintenance of this electrochemical gradient, as well as intracellular osmolality, depends on the presence of a number of enzymes and carriers [268,306]; these include sodium-potassium ATPase, calcium ATPase, and sodium:calcium antiporter activities in the neuronal plasma membrane, along with calcium ATPase activities in the endoplasmic reticulum, synaptic vesicles, and mitochondrial inner membrane of neural cells.

Slowed nerve conduction velocity [116,226,335] and increased epileptogenicity during renal failure have been attributed to changes in sodium-potassium ATPase activity [212]. Sodium-potassium ATPase activity is reduced in erythrocytes [355] and increased in intestinal mucosa [21] during renal failure. The molecular species of this enzyme in neurons, however, may differ from that in other tissues [268].

"Resting" sodium-potassium ATPase activity in synaptosomal preparations of brain from acutely uremic rats is normal [96a], but stimulation to maximal activity by inactivating voltage-gated monovalent cation channels with veratridine or ouabain inhibition is deficient. Documentation of these findings in a test tube medium that was devoid of "uremic" toxins suggests that enduring changes in membrane proteins may have occurred. Synaptosomes from acutely uremic rats also exhibit an increase in calcium uptake [96b]. Measurements of the activities of more representative samples of neuronal cell plasma membrane and their functional relationships with voltage-gated cation channels during uremia are obviously indicated.

Alterations of ATP and Energy Metabolism

During the preschool years, the brain's caloric expenditure exceeds half of the body's basal oxygen consumption, a greater proportion than when brain development is completed [150,182]. If renal dysfunction alters neural energetics, this high proportion may explain, in part, the greater likelihood of significant neuropsychologic deficits in uremic children than adults [40,92,260,331]; it may also explain the occurrence of microcephaly and brain atrophy in children whose renal failure started in infancy and was not complicated by aluminum intoxication [253,254, 281,299].

The intact brain derives most of its caloric expenditure from blood glucose and molecular oxygen [312]. Anoxia, hypoglycemia, and inhibitors of glycolysis are known convulsants, as well as disrupters of normal cerebral function [330]. Clinically documentable hypoxia and hypoglycemia are seldom responsible for the seizures of children with renal failure.

Energy metabolism and conservation occur in mitochondria. Mitochondria transfer the energy derived from the aerobic oxidation of glucose to the high-energy phosphate bond of ATP. Synthesis of ATP by brain mitochondria is fundamental to macromolecular synthesis and to the maintenance of electrochemical and solute gradients across neural membranes. Mitochondria in neural tissue also participate in intracellular Ca^{2+} homeostasis by functioning as low-affinity, high-capacity calcium sinks that are linked with H^+ exchange [52]. Thus, dysfunction of neural mitochondria can be expected to alter brain activity profoundly.

Cerebral utilization of oxygen and glucose is variably decreased during renal failure [295]. The capacity for ATP synthesis in the brain probably is not altered, but ATP utilization is diminished [337]. These changes in cerebral energetics cannot be attributed to decreased cerebral circulation [133,295].

Binding of cytosolic hexokinase to the mitochondrial outer membrane by a hexokinase-binding protein diminishes enzyme-product inhibition of hexokinase [349]. Bound hexokinase may have preferential access to mitochondrially synthesized ATP. This preferential availability of ATP augments the capacity of hexokinase to phosphorylate glucose and thus increases the rate of glycolysis. Investigations of cerebral energetics related to potential changes in the reversible mitochondrial binding of hexokinase during renal failure have not been reported.

Aluminum ion is a potent inhibitor of hexokinase [341]. Aluminum intoxication, associated with hemodialysis [7,8] and oral phosphate binding therapies [11,253,254], is a known cause of dementia in end-stage renal disease [15,281]. Whether aluminum produces dementia by inhibiting hexokinase and how it causes generalized hypotonia, muscle weakness, and osteomalacia in infancy are unknown [11]. The causative role of aluminum intoxication for some of the other neurologic manifestations of renal failure has not been determined [14,15].

Acetate buffer derived from dialysis fluid enters the plasma and causes an increased plasma concentration of isocitric acid and other tricarboxylic acid cycle intermediates [354]. The lowered capacity to oxidize this acetate load probably reflects a diminished capacity for aerobic glycolysis during the course of renal failure but has not been specifically localized to mitochondria in neural tissue.

Carnitine is required for the transport of fatty acids into mitochondria, where they, as well as tricarboxylic acid cycle intermediary metabolites, drive ATP synthesis. Carnitine deficiency is a known cause of myopathy [87]. Decreased levels of serum carnitine in the course of hemodialysis [29] have been identified as a cause of dialysis-related cardiomyopathy in adults [37,80].

Some of the enzymes of the mitochondrial electron transfer chain, such as the a^+a_3-type cytochrome oxidase complex, transform oxidation-reduction potentials derived from aerobic glycolysis into H^+ gradients [346]. These enzymes of the mitochondrial membrane contain heme, nonheme iron, and copper prosthetic groups. Copper in erythrocytes, cells that do not contain mitochondria, is reduced during renal failure [328]. These organometallic enzymes and their prosthetic groups have not been studied in neural tissue during renal failure.

ATP synthesis occurs on the inside surface of the inner membrane of mitochondria [70]. This arrangement requires inward movement of adenosine diphosphate and inorganic phosphate, in concert with outward transport of ATP. Cooperative occurrence of these molecular translocations and the stoichiometry of H^+ produced per unit of ATP synthesized suggest that mitochondrial oxidative phosphorylation is driven by a H^+ electrochemical gradient. Nonneural mitochondria promptly lose adenosine diphosphate–stimulated respiration during renal failure [45]; there are no neural tissue studies of this process in uremia.

An arginyl guanidinium group has been assigned, tentatively, to the catalytic active site of protein F1 that participates in mitochondrial ATP synthesis [9,70]. Guanidino compounds, which could potentially compete with such a guanidinium group, are known disrupters of mitochondrial energy conservation in nonneural tissue [57,58,257] and accumulate in body fluids during renal failure [64,313]. Experimental methylguanidine intoxication is known to cause convulsions [107]. Neurochemical studies that indict guanidino compounds as specific disrupters of cerebral mitochondrial energetics during renal failure have not been reported. Dinitrophenol is a well-known uncoupler of oxidative phosphorylation in mitochondria [132]. Related phenolic compounds that accumulate in plasma during renal failure may have a similar effect in neural tissue; their potency would be increased by acidosis [131].

"Renal Toxins" (Small, Middle, and Large Molecules)

Intermittent hemodialysis usually prevents or improves the overt toxic encephalopathy of renal failure. This may be due to removal of constituents such as urea, creatinine, and 2-hydroxybenzoylglycine. 2-hydroxybenzoylglycine displaces ionized drugs, e.g., phenytoin, digitoxin, coumadin, and diazepam, from their albumin binding sites [176].

Patients with renal failure who are treated with peritoneal dialysis rather than hemodialysis are often less troubled by peripheral neuropathy [163,288], even though they generally have higher serum levels of creatinine and urea than patients on hemodialysis. Compounds with molecular weights that are greater than 0.5×10^3 daltons are removed more efficiently from plasma by peritoneal dialysis than by hemodialysis because of the larger membrane surface area and longer dialysate retention time of peritoneal dialysis. Patients on peritoneal dialysis have lower levels of "middle molecules," nitrogenous compounds with molecular weights in the 0.5 to 3.0×10^3 dalton range that also accumulate in plasma during renal failure [221]. These observations have suggested that middle molecules rather than low molecular weight compounds are toxic to peripheral nerves.

The causative role of middle molecules in the neurologic manifestations of renal failure is unproven [221]. Even larger molecules accumulate in plasma during renal failure [97]. Increased blood levels of PTH and other polypeptide hormones, including insulin [189], luteinizing hormone [191], luteinizing hormone-releasing hormone [193], somatomedin [18], prolactin [104,115], and calcitonin [90], result from decreased renal catabolism, metabolic adaptation, and diminished urinary excretion. Accumulation of these peptides and of neurophysin, the oxytocin and pitocin carrier [271], is lowered more efficiently by peritoneal dialysis than by hemodialysis. Some of these peptide hormones may function as neuromodulators [139] and could cause some of the neurologic symptoms of uremic patients.

Alterations in Function of Neuronal Membranes

The information-processing function of the nervous system is a reflection of its membranous expanse and geometry [5]. Neurons conduct impulses along their extensive membranous processes that contain voltage-gated ion channels and energy-dependent ionic pumps. They intercommunicate through membranous specializations called *synapses* [50].

Interneuronal communication relies upon neurotransmitters and peptide neuromodulators [100] (first messengers; see Fig. 30-1) that couple functionally associated neurons. Following their release from the presynaptic membrane, neurohumors diffuse across the synaptic cleft and bind to specific postsynaptic membrane receptors. Alterations of neuronal function can, in theory, result from changes in (1) neurotransmitter or neuromodulator metabolism, (2) the characteristics of postsynaptic membrane receptors, and (3) processing of a neurohumor-receptor ligand after binding.

Neurohumors

Information concerning alterations in neurotransmitter or peptide neuromodulator metabolism, distribution, and physiology during renal failure is sparse. A recent review [38a] critically examines reports of a wide variety of changes in the plasma and CSF concentrations of amino acids during renal failure. Many of the reviewed studies are stated to fail to document normal ranges of content of amino acids in body fluids as well as to control for potential nutritional, developmental, and chronobiologic confounders that might occur during renal failure. Thus, it is difficult to discern a specific causative role for amino acid precursors of neurohumors in determining nervous system dysfunction during renal failure.

EAA, e.g. glutamate, putatively initiate nerve cell death by increasing the intracellular $[Ca^{2+}]$ during cerebral ischemia and status epilepticus [306a]. Occurrence of a diminished extracellular $[Ca^{2+}]$ during renal failure suggests that intracellular changes in Ca^{2+} homeostasis also may

occur. If intraneuronal $[Ca^{2+}]$ increases are found and correlate with the presence of neurologic dysfunction during renal failure, investigations of EAA/Ca^{2+} interactions [291] during renal failure may provide clinicians new therapeutic opportunities [217a] for treating such complications.

GABA, an inhibitory neurotransmitter [200], is reported to be increased in the CSF and brain tissue of patients with dialysis dementia and myoclonus [318]. Experimental renal failure [208] and hyperosmolarity sans renal failure [56] increase the brain content of GABA. An increased brain level of the putative inhibitory amino acid neurotransmitter, taurine, also has been found in experimental chronic renal failure [208]. The increased neural content of taurine in chronic uremia does not occur in acute renal failure. This compositional difference correlates with the comparatively decreased occurrence of seizures [138a] in chronic uremia.

Plasma clearance of phenylalanine, the essential amino acid precursor of the catecholamine neurotransmitters dopamine, norepinephrine, and epinephrine is diminished in uremic patients [173,252]. Erythrocyte activity of dihydropteridine reductase (DHPR) is reduced in adult patients with renal failure who have subencephalopathic aluminum intoxication and are on hemodialysis [8a]. DHPR catalyzes the regeneration of the cofactor that is required for synthesis of tyrosine, Dopa, and norepinephrine in the synthetic pathway of catecholamine from phenylalanine, as well as the synthesis of 5-hydroxy tryptophan in the synthetic pathway from tryptophan to serotonin. Variable changes in the plasma level of catecholamine have been reported in adult patients with renal failure [173,252], some of whom have aberrant autonomic responses to infused norepinephrine. The H^+:catecholamine antiporter-coupled storage of catecholamine [268], catecholamine-receptor binding, and catecholamine-receptor ligand processing have not been studied in renal failure.

Increased plasma levels of low molecular weight polyamines, which are putative neurotransmitters [50], are present during uremia [321]. Plasma levels of polyamines and other neurotransmitters do not necessarily reflect their brain concentrations, however.

The platelet's content of the neurotransmitter serotonin [200] is decreased during renal failure [86]. There is no information concerning the neural content of serotonin during renal failure. The platelet's content of neurotransmitters and neurotransmitter storage granules has recommended it as a clinically accessible model for neurons, however.

As stated earlier, plasma levels of many peptides with potential neuromodulator characteristics [100] are altered during renal failure. Insulin has been implicated as a neuromodulator in the olfactory bulb and hypothalamus [28]. Processing of the insulin-receptor ligand [141] may be deficient, because Maloff et al. [189] have shown that insulin resistance with hyperinsulinemia occurs in nonneural cells during renal failure.

Increased serum PTH [120,262] and calcitonin [217] may be viewed as adaptive mechanisms that attempt to restore extracellular calcium homeostasis, which is perturbed by renal failure. The amino acid sequence in the midportion residues (15–25) of PTH occurs in other peptides with putative neuromodulator activity, e.g., ACTH (residues 4–10). Thus, aberrant agonist-neuroreceptor interactions may result from the PTH elevation that occurs during renal dysfunction.

The calcitonin gene is expressed in neural tissue as the calcitonin-gene related peptide, which is a putative neuromodulator [277]. Feeding behavior and gastrointestinal motility–induced changes are associated with the intracerebroventricular injection of calcitonin [90]. The calcitonin and calcitonin-gene related peptide systems have been implicated in nociception and cardiovascular homeostasis. A rational correlation has been found between the lowering of diastolic blood pressure and increased plasma concentrations of calcitonin-gene related peptide, post dialysis, in adults with renal disease [231a]. This system deserves study in children with renal failure.

Receptors

Alterations of neuronal receptor functions during renal failure remain to be investigated. The efficacy with which receptors bind neurohumors is dependent in part on membrane fluidity [308] and cell membrane protein/cytoskeletal interactions [121,297]. Membrane fluidity is determined by the type of fatty acid hydrocarbon tails that are packed within the membrane lipid bilayer. Membrane fluidity controls the diffusional mobility and some other properties of membrane proteins; reduced diffusional mobility can limit receptor binding efficacy. Erythrocyte membrane fatty acids, and consequent changes in membrane fluidity, are not altered by lipoperoxidation during renal failure [130]. Studies of neuronal lipoperoxides, other lipid constituents of the neuronal plasma membrane, and the diffusional mobilities of neural membrane proteins have not been published.

Nonenzymatic glycosylation of hemoglobin has been demonstrated in renal failure [219]. Nonenzymatic glycosylation of hemoglobin also occurs in diabetes mellitus; erythrocyte membrane proteins [42,211], and peripheral nerve [338] additionally are nonenzymatically glycosylated in diabetes. Some neuronal membrane proteins are known to contain polysaccharide groups. Nonenzymatic glycosylation of these and other proteins, including neurohumoral receptors, can be anticipated to alter their biologic characteristics. There are no reports of investigations concerning the nonenzymatic glycosylation of neural membrane receptors and other neural membrane-associated proteins during renal failure. Administration of theophylline to reverse postrenal transplantation erythrocytosis [24a] suggests that urema does not cause persistent dysfunction of purinergic A_2 receptors; theophylline normally diminishes erythropoietin production, whose elevation causes postrenal transplantation erythrocytosis through an A_2 receptor–linked mechanism.

THE PROCESSING OF NEUROHUMOR-RECEPTOR LIGANDS

First messengers, i.e., neurohumors, initiate neuronal responses after they diffuse across the synapse and bind to a postsynaptic receptor, forming a neurohumor-receptor ligand. Mediation of postsynaptic responses may be associated with intracellular translocation of the neurohumor-receptor ligand through endocytosis and coated vesicle transport to characteristic intracellular loci, e.g., the Golgi apparatus in the case of insulin [141] in hypatocytes. The mediation of postsynaptic responses also may be associated with the production of a second messenger cofactor, such as a cyclic nucleotide [301], or with changes in the intracellular activity and localized availability of Ca^{2+} [49,262].

The content of erythrocyte cGMP, a second messenger, is increased during renal failure; this change may reflect an alteration of membrane permeability [72]. In the brain, cGMP is important in mediating the effects of acetylcholine at muscarinic receptors and of histamine at H_1 receptors [220]. The neurotoxicity of cimetidine, prescribed in uremic patients subject to gastrointestinal bleeding, is thought to be due to its blocking of cerebral H_2 receptors [296]. The content and dynamics of cGMP content in the brain during renal failure have not been determined.

cAMP has recently been demonstrated to be a second messenger for PTH in brain (310], as well as in kidney. Biologic effects of PTH in renal brush border vesicles include an increased Ca^{2+} uptake, as well as increased phosphorylation of membrane components [123,153]. A PTH-stimulated increase of cAMP in red cells during renal failure results in autoagglutination and an accelerated sedimentation rate [82]. Study of possible correlations between altered brain function, PTH, and cAMP during uremia appears to be indicated.

Brain tissue contains five calcium-dependent protein kinases that couple the second messenger activities of Ca^{2+} to neuronal responses. Changes induced by renal failure, in the activities of these protein kinases that mediate the transduction of neuronal signals, have not been reported.

Three protein kinases and two calcium-dependent proteins, protein kinase C(PKC) and Ca/calmodulin PK I, catalyze the phosphorylation of a specific threonine residue (site 1) on synapsin I [222]. Synapsin I is a neuron-specific polypeptide that is present in the synaptic vesicles of all neurons. A third calcium-dependent protein kinase (Ca/calmodulin PK II) phosphorylates two additional threonine residues of synapsin I (sites 2 and 3). Phosphorylation of synapsin I, catalyzed by Ca/calmoduin PK II, diminished synapsin I's affinity for binding to synaptic vesicles. Depolarization of nerve impulses by pharmacologic agents initiates synapsin I phosphorylation at sites 1, 2, and 3. The neurotransmitters serotonin, dopamine, and norepinephrine initiate site 1 phosphorylation. Changes in content and the degree of phosphorylation of synapsin I, as well as the content of other phosphoproteins in neural tissue, deserve to be investigated in renal failure. An alteration of synapsin I phosphorylation might be fundamental to a probable defect in receptor-ligand processing that would explain the changed autonomic responsivity of uremic patients to catecholamine infusion [173]. Neural tissue studies of intracellular calcium distribution, flux, and PKC activation during renal failure have not been reported.

Neurotransmitter and hormonal first messengers that use intracellular calcium as a second messenger in the process of neuronal signal transduction activate phospholipase C. PTH signal transduction is coupled to phospholipase C [80a]. Phospholipase C and a phosphodiesterase (PDE) catalyze the hydrolysis of the membrane lipids phosphatidylinositol and phosphorylated phosphatidylinositol (PIP + PIP$_2$; see Fig 30-2) [337a]. Diacylglycerol and inositol polyphosphates are the products of this hydrolysis [209]. Inositol polyphosphate mobilizes intracellular Ca^{2+} from a nonmitochondrial cytoplasmic store [146]; diacylglycerol activates the calmodulin-insensitive calcium-dependent PKC (Fig. 30-1); [228,229]. The tyrosine-specific protein kinases that are encoded by *ras* [188] and *src* [315] oncogenes may participate in the resynthesis cycle of neural membrane polyphosphatides (Fig. 30-2).

Inositol, a constituent of the inositol phospholipids that are involved in neuronal signal transduction, has an increased plasma concentration during renal failure. Some investigators feel that inositol is one of the low molecular weight "toxins" of uremia and a cause of uremic peripheral neuropathy [62]. Acyl phosphate is rapidly incorporated into myelin normally and its turnover in myelin is stimulated by the presence of the neurohumor acetylcholine [147a]. The increased plasma level of inositol during uremia could be the result of a diminished synthesis of phosphatidyl inositides, an increased consecutive hydrolysis by phospholipase C and PDE, or decreased oxidative catabolism of ingested and metabolically derived inositol. The latter mechanism, which has a renal localization, has been suggested by investigators who find abnormal, granular cytoplasmic inclusions in fetal avian dorsal root ganglion cells that are cultured in inositol concentrations similar to those found in the plasma of patients with renal failure [179].

The curare-like response to high plasma levels of aminoglycoside antibiotics during renal failure [245,341] may be related to similarities in molecular structure as well as to charge affinities between inositol and the aminocyclitol nucleus of these antibiotics. Aminocyclitol avidly binds anionic lipids such as phosphatidylinositol, as well as Ca^{2+} [258]. Reversal of such reactions by calcium gluconate administration strengthens the hypothesis that calcium-mediated molecular events may be involved in the pathogenesis of this iatrogenic complication of uremia.

Diacylglycerol derived from phosphatidylinositol may be hydrolyzed by diacylglycerol lipase to yield arachidonic acid for prostaglandin synthesis [228,229] (Fig. 30-2). Though there are no nervous system studies of prostaglandins during renal failure, leukocyte and platelet production of prostacyclin has been found to be increased in children with chronic renal failure [73]. Excitatory as well as inhibitory effects on spinal cord and brain stem vegetative reflexes have been attributed to prostaglandins [352]. Prostaglandins are also involved in neurotransmitter release in the

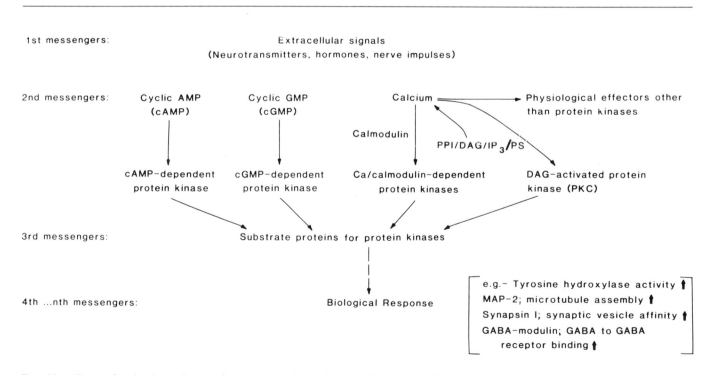

FIG. 30-1. *Proposed molecular pathways of neuronal signal-transduction. Abbreviations: Cyclic AMP = 3',5'-cyclic guanosine monophosphate; PPI = phosphatidylinositol polyphosphates (phosphatidylinositol-4-phosphate & phosphatidylinositol-4,5-biphosphate); IP$_3$ = inositol polyphosphate (inositol-1,4,5-trisphosphate); PS = phosphatidyl serine; DAG = 1,2-diacylglycerol; MAP-2 = high molecular weight microtubule associated protein; GABA = -aminobutyric acid; = increase. Modified from Morselli PL, Pippenger CE, Penry JK (eds): Nephrology: An approach to the Patient with Renal Disease. Philadelphia, JB Lippincott, 1982, p 608.*

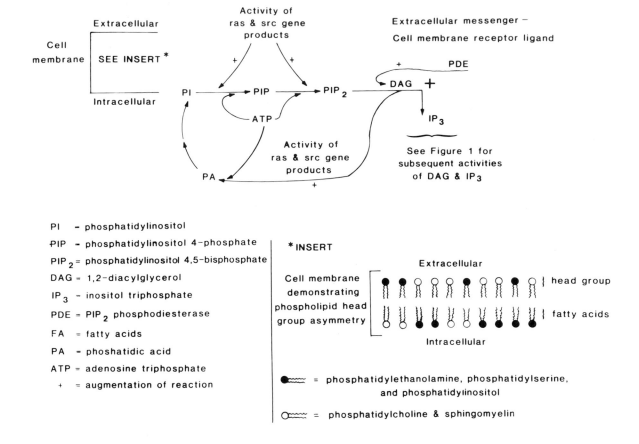

PI   – phosphatidylinositol

PIP   – phosphatidylinositol 4-phosphate

PIP$_2$ = phosphatidylinositol 4,5-bisphosphate

DAG = 1,2-diacylglycerol

IP$_3$ = inositol triphosphate

PDE = PIP$_2$ phosphodiesterase

FA   = fatty acids

PA   = phoshatidic acid

ATP = adenosine triphosphate

+   = augmentation of reaction

FIG. 30-2. *A proposed model for ras & src gene products' role in cell membrane signal transduction.* Modified from *Nestler EJ, Greengard P: Neuronal phosphoproteins: Physiological and clinical implications.* Science 225:1357, 1984.

brain and autonomic ganglia and in some thermoregulatory processes in the hypothalamus.

ALTERATIONS OF CELL STRUCTURE

Peripheral nerves in uremic neuropathy contain a decreased number of neurofilaments [24,81,335]. Intracellular calcium and cytoskeletal protein interactions are important determinants of axonal transport [231]. Neurofibrillary tangles have been found in the brains of some patients with aluminum dementia [285]. All three of the polypeptide units of neurofilaments are phosphorylated by a cAMP-dependent protein kinase [223]. PKC and other protein kinases phosphorylate the high molecular weight microtubule–associated protein (MAP-2 = HMW-2). A protein phosphorylation mechanism may regulate the dynamic state of association of these cytoskeletal components of neurons [311]. Appropriate investigations will be required to determine whether altered HMW-2 and neurofilamentous polypeptides play a role in the pathogenesis of neurofibrillary tangles, neuropathy, and potential alterations of axonal transport in uremia.

Cytoskeletal structures in endothelia of central nervous system blood vessels participate in maintaining the blood-brain barrier. Brain tissue and CSF concentrations of many water-soluble substances are maintained in spite of inward diffusional gradients from plasma [148]. Anatomic correlates of this blood-brain barrier are the tight junctions between contiguous capillary endothelial cells and a characteristic topology of some enzymes in these cells [339] in most parts of the brain. Brain capillary endothelial cells lack the fenestrations that occur between the capillary endothelial cells in many other organs and exhibit comparatively reduced pinocytosis. Enzymatic barriers and carrier-mediated transport mechanisms that are not found in other endothelial cells are present in brain capillary endothelia. A comparatively increased number of mitochondria in brain capillary endothelial cells provide the energy required for carrier-mediated transport into the brain.

Hyperosmolar solutions applied to capillary endothelial cells of cerebral vessels produce shrinkage of these cells, loosening of the tight junctions between them, and an increase in their pinocytic activity [148]. Loosening of tight junctions disrupts the blood-brain barrier and results in cerebral edema and/or focal vascular necrosis. The hypertensive encephalopathy of renal failure is associated with focal vascular necrosis and cerebral edema (see the section on pathology under Hypertensive Encephalopathy).

Alterations in the cytoskeleton of endothelial cells also might increase the permeability of cerebral vessels and threaten the integrity of the blood-brain barrier. Actin is a component of the cytoskeleton of neurons and endothelial cells [166]. In response to physical injury, actin in nonneural vascular endothelial cells changes their morphology as well as their sensitivity to plasma actin-destabilization factor [98]. Whether plasma actin-destabilization factor is responsible for altering cytoskeletal proteins of vascular endothelial cells in the uremic brain remains to be determined.

Calcium-Mediated Alterations

An association between tetanic contraction of muscle and an apparent absence of extracellular calcium was first recognized more than a century ago [274,275]. Hypocalcemic tetany has subsequently become a well-recognized though infrequent complication of renal failure. The very small solubility product constants of many biologically relevant calcium salts, such as the calcium phosphates [49], predict associated decrements in the normal extracellular Ca^{2+} content as a result of phosphate accumulation in plasma during renal failure. Elevations of plasma PTH and calcitonin levels may be viewed, teleologically, as an adaptive response that attempts to maintain Ca^{2+} homeostasis during renal failure [120,262].

Total brain calcium is increased in renal failure [69]. Some pathologic cells, such as the irreversibly sickled erythrocyte, are characterized by an excessive calcium content that is associated with the loss of normal cell properties [83,242]. An excessive increase of intracellular Ca^{2+} content is a well-known concomitant of cell death [291].

Normally, the intracellular Ca^{2+} concentration of excitable cells is approximately 10 to 100 nMol and is associated with an extracellular Ca^{2+} concentration of approximately 2 nMol. This concentration differential is several orders of magnitude greater than the gradient that is thermodynamically required to maintain the resting membrane potential of neurons and muscle cells. This gradient is produced by efflux through membrane Ca-Mg ATPase activity and Na^+-cotransport; these efflux mechanisms expend metabolic energy stored in ATP[49]. Neural tissue calcium content is increased in renal failure [13,16, 63,69,117], but intracellular Ca^{2+} content and calcium compartmentation have not been measured.

Though the Ca^{2+} gradient does not contribute greatly to the resting membrane potential of excitable cells, voltage-gated Ca^{2+}-channels [85] have been detected by measurements of calcium currents in vertebrate heart muscle, as well as in large invertebrate and vertebrate neurons during their depolarization [268]. Calcium-sensitive dye measurements of intracellular $[Ca^{2+}]$ document a transient increase in Ca^{2+} during such calcium currents. Voltage-gated Ca^{2+}-channels are most numerous in the presynaptic region of nerve terminals. Although there are no published studies of voltage-gated Ca^{2+}-channel function in neuromuscular tissues during renal failure, the known decrease in the extracellular Ca^{2+} concentration may lower the voltage-induced calcium current and its associated intracellular Ca^{2+} flow. Such a mechanism may contribute to the occurrence of hypocalcemic tetany, to some uremic seizures, and to other manifestations of neural dysfunction that complicate renal failure. Another potential calcium-mediated mechanism for neural dysfunction during renal failure is an alteration of Ca^{2+} regulated K^+-channels. These channels are required to reduce neuronal excitability and presynaptic exocytosis [268].

References

1. Abella R, Blondeel NJ, Rogusk J, et al: Periodic dialysis in terminal uremia. JAMA 199:362, 1967.
1a. Ackil AA, Shahari BT, Young RR: Sural nerve conduction studies and late responses in children undergoing hemodialysis. Arch Phys Med Rehabil 62:487, 1981.
2. Adams RD, Vander Eeken HM: Vascular diseases of the brain. Annu Rev Med 4:213, 1953.
3. Aicardi J, Chevrie JJ: Convulsive status epilepticus in infants and children: A study of 239 cases. Epilepsia 11:187, 1971.
4. Aiello I, Serra G, Gilli P, et al: Uremic neuropathy: Correlations between electroneurographic parameters and serum levels of parathyroid hormone and aluminum. Eur Neurol 21:396, 1982.
5. Albers RW: Biochemistry of cell membranes. In Siegel GJ, Albers RW, Agranoff BW (eds): Basic Neurochemistry (3rd ed). Boston, Little, Brown, 1981, p 49.
6. Alfrey AC: Dialysis encephalopathy syndrome. Ann Intern Med 29:93, 1978.
7. Alfrey AC, Legendre GR, Kaehny WD: The dialysis encephalopathy syndrome. N Engl J Med 294:184, 1976.
8. Alfrey AC, Mishell JM, Burks J, et al: Syndrome of dyspraxia and multifocal seizures with chronic hemodialysis. Trans Am Soc Artif Intern Organs 18:257, 1972.
8a. Altman P, Al-Sali F, Butter K, et al: Serum aluminum levels and erythrocyte dihydropteridine reductase activity in patients on hemodialysis. N Engl J Med 317:80, 1987.
9. Amzel L, Pedersen PL: Proton ATPases: Structure and mechanism. Annu Rev Biochem 52:801, 1983.
10. Anderson RJ, Schrier RW (eds): Clinical Use of Drugs in Patients with Kidney and Liver Disease. Philadelphia, WB Saunders, 1981.
11. Andreoli SP, Bergstein JM, Sherrard DJ: Aluminum intoxication from aluminum-containing phosphate binders in children with azotemia not undergoing dialysis. N Engl J Med 310:1079, 1984.
12. Arbus GS, Barnor N-A, Hsu AC, et al: Effect of chronic renal failure, dialysis and transplantation on motor nerve conduction velocity in children. Can Med Assoc J 113:517, 1975.
13. Arieff AI: Neurological complications of uremia. In Brenner BM, Recort FC Jr (eds): The Kidney (2nd ed). Philadelphia, WB Saunders, 1981, p 2306.
14. Arieff AI, Cooper JD, Armstrong D, et al: Dementia, renal failure and brain aluminum. Ann Intern Med 90:741, 1979.
15. Arieff AI, Mahoney CA: Pathogenesis of dialysis encephalopathy. Neurobehav Toxicol Teratol 5:641, 1983.
16. Arieff AI, Massry SG: Calcium metabolism of brain in

acute renal failure: Effects of uremia, hemodialysis, and parathyroid hormone. *J Clin Invest* 53:387, 1974.

17. Arieff AI, Massry SG, Barrientos SA, et al: Brain water and electrolyte metabolism in uremia: Effects of slow and rapid hemodialysis. *Kidney Int* 4:177, 1973.

18. Arnold WC, Uthne K, Spencer EM, et al: Somatomedin in children with chronic renal insufficiency—relationship to growth rate and energy intake. *Int J Pediatr Nephrol* 4:29, 1983.

19. Aronoff GR: Antimicrobial therapy in patients with impaired renal function. *Am J Kidney Dis* 3:106, 1983.

20. Asbury AK, Victor M, Adams RD: Uremic polyneuropathy. *Arch Neurol* 8:413, 1963.

21. Aviv A, Higashino H, Kobayashi T: The intestinal profile of Na-K-ATPase in two rat models of acute renal failure. *J Lab Clin Med* 100:533, 1982.

22. Avram MM, Feinfeld DA, Huatuco AH: Search for the uremic toxin: Decreased motor-nerve conduction velocity and elevated parathyroid hormone in uremia. *N Engl J Med* 298:1000, 1978.

23. Bach C, Iaina A, Eliahou EE: Autonomic nervous system disturbance in patients on chronic hemodialysis. *Isr J Med Sci* 15:761, 1979.

24. Bakke L: Uremic polyneuropathy. *Acta Neurol Scand* 46 (Suppl 44):205, 1970.

24a. Bakris GL, Sauter ER, Hussey JL, et al: Effects of theophylline on erythropoietin production in normal subjects and in patients with erythrocytosis after renal transplantation. *N Engl J Med* 323:86, 1990.

25. Bale JF: Human cytomegalovirus infection and disorders of the nervous system. *Arch Neurol* 41:310, 1984.

26. Baluarte HJ, Gruskin AB, Hiner LB, et al: Encephalopathy in children with chronic renal failure. *Proc Clin Dial Transplant Forum* 7:95, 1977.

27. Bar S, Savir H: Renal retinopathy—the renewed entity. *Metab Pediatr Syst Ophthalmol* 6:33, 1982.

28. Barbaccia ML, Chuang DM, Costa E: Is insulin a neuromodulator? *In* Costa E, Trabucchi M (eds): *Regulatory Peptides: From Molecular Biology to Function.* New York, Raven Press, 1982, p 511.

29. Bartel LL, Hussey JL, Shrago E: Effect of dialysis on serum carnitine, free fatty acids, and triglyceride levels in man and the rat. *Metabolism* 31:944, 1982.

30. Baum M, Powell D, Calvin S, et al: Continuous ambulatory peritoneal dialysis in children: Comparison with hemodialysis. *N Engl J Med* 307:1537, 1982.

31. Bechar M, Johannes PW, Lake F, et al: Subdural hematoma during long-term hemodialysis. *Arch Neurol* 26:513, 1972.

32. Bell WE, McCormick WF: *Neurologic Infections in Children* (2nd ed). Philadelphia, WB Saunders, 1981.

33. Bergstrom LV, Jenkins P, Sando I, et al: Hearing loss in renal disease: Clinical and pathological studies. *Ann Otol Rhinol Laryngol* 82:555, 1973.

34. Betts RF, Freeman RB, Douglas RG Jr, et al: Transmission of cytomegalovirus infection with renal allograft. *Kidney Int* 8:385, 1975.

35. Bloomer HA, Barton LJ, Maddock RK Jr: Penicillin-induced encephalopathy in uremic patients. *JAMA* 200:131, 1967.

35a. Bochner F, Hooper W, Sutherland JM, et al: Diphenylhydantoin concentrations in saliva. *Arch Neurol* 31:57, 1974.

36. Bock GH, Conners CK, Ruley J, et al: Disturbances of brain maturation and neurodevelopment during chronic renal failure in infancy. *J Pediatr* 114:231, 1989.

37. Bohmer T, Bergrem H, Eiklid K: Carnitine deficiency in-

duced during intermittent hemodialysis for renal failure. *Lancet* 3:126, 1978.

38. Bolton CF, Baltzan MA, Baltzan RB: Effects of renal transplantation on uremic neuropathy. A clinical and electrophysiological study. *N Engl J Med* 284:1170, 1971.

38a. Bolton CF, Young GB: *Neurological Complications of Renal Disease.* Boston, Butterworths, 1990.

39. Booker HE: Phenobarbital, mephobarbital and metharbital: Relation of plasma levels to clinical control. *In* Woodbury DM, Penry JK, Schmidt RP (eds): *Antiepileptic Drugs.* New York, Raven Press, 1972, p 329.

40. Brancaccio D, Damasso R, Spinnler H, et al: Does chronic kidney failure lead to mental failure? *Arch Neurol* 38:757, 1981.

41. Brodwall E, Stöa KF: A study of barbiturate clearance. *Acta Med Scand* 154:139, 1956.

42. Brownless M, Vlassara H, Cerami A: Nonenzymatic glycosylation and the pathogenesis of diabetic complications. *Ann Intern Med* 101:527, 1984.

43. Bruni J, Wang LH, Marbury TC, et al: Protein binding of valproic acid in uremic patients. *Neurology* 30:557, 1980.

44. Buchtal F: Electrophysiological abnormalities in metabolic myopathies and neuropathies. *Acta Neurol Scand* 46(Suppl 43):129, 1970.

45. Burke TJ, Wilson DR, Levi M, et al: Role of mitochondria in ischemic acute renal failure. *Clin Exp Dial Apheresis* 7:49, 1983.

46. Burks JS, Alfrey AC, Huddlestone JM: A fatal encephalopathy in chronic renal hemodialysis patients. *Lancet* 1:764, 1976.

47. Byrom FB: The pathogenesis of hypertensive encephalopathy and its relation to the malignant phase of hypertension: Experimental evidence from hypertensive rat. *Lancet* 2:202, 1954.

48. Callaghan N: Restless legs syndrome in uremic neuropathy. *Neurology* 16:359, 1966.

49. Cambell AK: *Intracellular Calcium: Its Universal Role as Regulator.* New York, John Wiley, 1983.

50. Carpenter DO, Reese TS: Chemistry and physiology of synaptic transmission. *In* Spiegel GJ, Albers RW, Agranoff BW (eds): *Basic Neurochemistry* (3rd ed). Boston, Little, Brown, 1981, p 162.

51. Carter DM: Human disease characterized by heritable DNA instability. *Birth Defects: Original Article Series* 17-2:117, 1981.

52. Carvalho AP: Calcium in the nerve cell. *In* Lajtha A (ed): *Handbook of Neurochemistry* (2nd ed), Vol I, *Chemical and Cellular Architecture.* London, Plenum Press, 1982, p 761.

53. Casciani CU, deSimone C, Bonini S, et al: Immunological aspects of chronic uremia. *Kidney Int* 13(Suppl 8):S49, 1978.

54. Catterall WA: The molecular basis of neuronal excitability. *Science* 223:653, 1984.

55. Chadwick D, French AT: Uraemic myoclonus: An example of reticular reflex myoclonus? *J Neurol Neurosurg Psychiatry* 42:52, 1979.

56. Chan PH, Fishman RA: Elevation of rat brain amino acids, ammonia and idiogenic osmoles induced by hyperosmolality. *Brain Res* 161:293, 1979.

57. Chance B, Hollunger G: Inhibition of electron and energy transfer in mitochondria. I. Effects of amytal, thiopental, progesterone and methylene glycol. *J Biol Chem* 238:418, 1963.

58. Chance B, Hollunger G: Inhibition of electron and energy transfer in mitochondria. II. The site and mechanism of guanidine action. *J Biol Chem* 238:432, 1963.

59. Cheeseman SH, Henle W, Rubin RH, et al: Epstein-Barr virus infections in renal transplant recipients. Effects of antithymocyte globulin and interferon. *Ann Intern Med* 93:39, 1980.

60. Cheeseman SH, Stewart JA, Winkle S, et al: Cytomegalovirus excretion 2–14 years after renal transplantation. *Transplant Proc* 11:71, 1979.

61. Clarke E, Murphy E: Neurological manifestations of malignant hypertension. *Br Med J* 2:1319, 1956.

62. Clements RS, DeJesus PV, Winegrad AI: Raised plasma-myoinositol levels in uremia and experimental neuropathy. *Lancet* 1:1137, 1973.

63. Cogan MG, Covey CM, Arieff AI, et al: Central nervous system manifestations of hyperparathyroidism. *Am J Med* 65:963, 1978.

64. Cohen BD: Guanidinosuccinic acid in uremia. *Arch Intern Med* 126:846, 1970.

65. Cohen SN, Syndulko K, Rever B, et al: Visual evoked potentials and long latency event-related potentials in chronic renal failure. *Neurology* 33:1219, 1983.

66. Cohen T, Brand-Auvaban A, Karshai C, et al: Familial infantile renal tubular acidosis and congenital nerve deafness: An autosomal recessive syndrome. *Clin Genet* 4:275, 1973.

67. Constantinides P: *Ultrastructural Pathobiology.* New York, Elsevier, 1984, p 282.

68. Coomes EN, Berlyne GM, Schaw AB: Incidence of neuropathy in nondialyzed chronic renal failure patients. *Proc Eur Dial Transplant Assoc* 2:133, 1965.

69. Cooper JD, Lazarowitz VC, Arieff AI: Neurodiagnostic abnormalities in patients with acute renal failure: Evidence for neurotoxicity of parathyroid hormone. *J Clin Invest* 61:1448, 1978.

70. Cross RL: The mechanism and regulation of ATP synthesis by F_1-ATPases. *Annu Rev Biochem* 50:681, 1981.

71. Davies SF, Sarosi GA, Peterson PK, et al: Disseminated histoplasmosis in renal transplant recipients. *Am J Surg* 137:686, 1979.

72. DeBari, VA, Bennun A: Cyclic GMP in the human erythrocyte. Intracellular levels and transport in normal subjects and chronic hemodialysis patients. *Clin Biochem* 15:219, 1982.

73. Deckmyn H, Proesmans W, Vermylen J: Prostacyclin production of whole blood from children: Impairment in the hemolytic uremic syndrome and excessive formation in chronic renal failure. *Thromb Res* 30:13, 1983.

74. DeMarchi S, Cecchin E, Camurri C, et al: Origin of glycosylated hemoglobin A1 in chronic renal failure. *Int J Artif Organs* 6:77, 1983.

75. Dettori P, LaGreca G, Biasioli S, et al: Changes of cerebral density in dialyzed patients. *Neuroradiology* 23:95, 1982.

76. Diaz-Buxo JA: Peritoneal dialysis—60 years later. *Mayo Clin Proc* 58:687, 1983.

77. Dinapoli RP, Johnson WJ, Lambert EH: Experience with combined hemodialysis-renal transplant program, neurologic aspects. *Mayo Clin Proc* 41:809, 1966.

78. Dinn JJ, Crane DL: Schwann cell dysfunction in uremia. *J Neurol Neurosurg Psychiatry* 33:605, 1970.

79. Donckerwolcke RA, Van Biervliet JP, Koorevaar G, et al: The syndrome of renal tubular acidosis with nerve deafness. *Acta Paediatr Scand* 65:100, 1976.

80. Drueke T, LePailleur C, Meilhac B, et al: Congestive cardiomyopathy in uremic patients on long term hemodialysis. *Br Med J* 1:350, 1977.

80a. Dunlay R, Hruska K: PTH receptor coupling to phospholipase C is an alternate pathway of signal transduction in bone and kidney. *Am J Physiol* 258:F223, 1990.

81. Dyck PJ, Johnson WJ, Lambert EH, et al: Segmental demyelination secondary to axonal degeneration in uremic neuropathy. *Mayo Clin Proc* 46:400, 1971.

82. Earon Y, Blum M, Bogin E: Effect of parathyroid hormone and uremic sera on the autoagglutination and sedimentation of human red blood cells. *Clin Chim Acta* 135:253, 1983.

83. Eaton JW, Skelton TD, Swofford HS, et al: Elevated erythrocyte calcium in sickle cell disease. *Nature* 246:105, 1973.

84. Egger J, Lake BD, Wilson J: Mitochondrial cytopathy: A multisystem disorder with ragged red fibers on muscle biopsy. *Arch Dis Child* 56:741, 1981.

85. Ehrlich BE, Finkelstein A, Forte M, et al: Voltage-dependent calcium channels from Paramecium cilia incorporated into planar lipid bilayers. *Science* 225:427, 1984.

86. Eknoyan G, Brown CH III: Biochemical abnormalities of platelets in renal failure. *Am J Nephrol* 1:17, 1981.

87. Engel AS, Angelini C: Carnitine deficiency of human skeletal muscle with associated lipid storage myopathy: A new syndrome. *Science* 179:899, 1973.

88. Ewer RW, Brissonette RP, Brakel FJ, et al: Tetanic neuromyopathy and renal failure: Diagnostic implications. *JAMA* 192:1117, 1965.

89. Fabre J, De Freudenreich J, Duckert A, et al: Influence of renal insufficiency on the excretion of chloroquine, phenobarbital, phenothiazines and methacycline. *Helv Med Acta* 33:307, 1966.

90. Fargeas MJ, Fioramonti J, Bueno L: Prostaglandin E_2: A neuromodulator in the central control of gastrointestinal motility and feeding behavior by calcitonin. *Science* 225:1050, 1984.

91. Faris A: Wernicke's encephalopathy in uremia. *Neurology* 22:1293, 1972.

92. Fennell RS III, Rasbury WC, Fennell EB, et al: Effects of kidney transplantation on cognitive performance in a pediatric population. *Pediatrics* 74:273, 1984.

93. Fishman RA: Permeability changes in experimental uremic encephalopathy. *Arch Intern Med* 126:835, 1970.

94. Fishman RA, Raskin NH: Experimental uremic encephalopathy: Permeability and electrolyte metabolism of brain and other tissues. *Arch Neurol* 17:10, 1967.

95. Floyd M, Ayyar DR, Barwick DD, et al: Myopathy in chronic renal failure. *Q J Med* 43:509, 1974.

96. Foley CM, Polinsky MS, Graskin AB, et al: Encephalopathy in infants and children with chronic renal disease. *Arch Neurol* 38:656, 1981.

96a. Fraser CL, Arieft AI: Nervous system complications in uremia. *Ann Int Med* 109:143, 1988.

97. Frohling PT, Kokot F, Cernacek P, et al: Relation between middle molecules and parathyroid hormone in patients with chronic renal failure. *Miner Electrolyte Metab* 7:48, 1982.

98. Gabbiani G, Babbiani F, Heimark RL, et al: Organization of actin cytoskeleton during early endothelial regeneration in vitro. *J Cell Sci* 66:39, 1984.

99. Gagnon RF, Shuster J, Kaye M: Auto-immunity in patients with end-stage renal disease maintained on haemodialysis and continuous ambulatory peritoneal dialysis. *J Clin Lab Immunol* 11:155, 1983.

100. Gainer H, Brownstein MJ: Neuropeptides. In Siegel GJ, Albers RW, Agranoff BW, et al (eds): *Basic Neurochemistry.* Boston, Little, Brown, 1981, p 269.

101. Gambertoglio J, Lauer RM: Use of neuropsychiatric drugs. In Anderson RJ, Schrier RW (eds): *Clinical Use of Drugs*

in Patients with Kidney and Liver Disease. Philadelphia, WB Saunders, 1981, p 276.

102. Gardner SD, Field AM, Coleman DV: New human papovavirus (B.K.) isolated from urine after renal transplantation. *Lancet* 1:1253, 1971.

103. Geary DF, Fennel RS III, Andriola M, et al: Encephalopathy in children with chronic renal failure. *J Pediatr* 97:41, 1980.

103a. Geary DF, Itaka-Ikse K: Neurodevelopment process in young children with chronic renal disease. *Pediatrics* 84:68, 1989.

104. Geffner ME, Kaplan SA, Lippe BM, et al: Precocious puberty and chronic renal failure. *Am J Dis Child* 137:956, 1983.

105. Gibson TP: Principles of drug dose adjustment during hemodialysis. *Am J Kidney Dis* 3:111, 1983.

106. Gilliatt RW: Nerve conduction in human and experimental neuropathies. *Proc R Soc Med* 59:989, 1966.

107. Giovannetti S, Biagini M, Balestri PL, et al: Uremia-like syndrome in dogs chronically intoxicated with methylguanidine and creatinine. *Clin Sci* 36:445, 1969.

108. Glaser GH: Diphenylhydantoin toxicity. *In* Woodbury DM, Penry JK, Schmidt RP (eds): *Antiepileptic Drugs.* New York, Raven Press, 1972, p 219.

109. Glaser GH: Brain dysfunction in uremia. *In* Plum F (ed): *Brain Dysfunction in Metabolic Disorders. Res Publ Assoc Nerv Ment Dis,* Vol 53. New York, Raven Press, 1974, p 173.

110. Goldblum SE, Reed WP: Host defenses and immunological alterations associated with chronic hemodialysis. *Ann Intern Med* 93:597, 1980.

111. Gonzales FM, Pabico RC, Brown HW, et al: Further experience with use of routine intermittent hemodialysis in chronic renal failure. *Trans Am Soc Artif Intern Organs* 9:11, 1963.

112. Goodhue WW, Davis JN, Porro RS: Ischemic myopathy in uremic hyperparathyroidism. *JAMA* 221:911, 1972.

113. Goriki K, Wada K, Hata J, et al: The relationship between carbonic anhydrases and zinc concentration of erythrocytes in patients under chronic hemodialysis. *Hiroshima J Med Sci* 31:123, 1982.

114. Gross MLP, Sweny P, Pearson RM, et al: Rejection encephalopathy: An acute neurological syndrome complicating renal transplantation. *J Neurol Sci* 56:23, 1982.

115. Grzeszczak W, Kokot F, Dulawa J: Prolactin secretion in patients with acute renal failure. *Arch Immunol Ther Exp (Warsz)* 30:413, 1982.

116. Guiheneuc P: Altered nerve conduction studied by reflex methods. *In* Busser PA, Cobb WA, Okuma T (eds): *Kyoto Symposia* [EEG Suppl No. 36]. Amsterdam, Elsevier, 1982, p 91.

117. Guisado R, Arieff AI, Massry SG: Changes in the electroencephalogram in acute uremia. Effects of parathyroid hormone and brain electrolytes. *J Clin Invest* 55:738, 1975.

118. Gulyassy PF, Peters JH, Lin SC: Hemodialysis and plasma aminoacid composition in chronic renal failure. *Am J Clin Nutr* 21:565, 1968.

119. Gutman RA, Burnell JM: Paraldehyde acidosis. *Am J Med* 42:435, 1967.

120. Habener JF, Rosenblatt M, Potts JT Jr: Parathyroid hormone: Biochemical aspects of biosynthesis, secretion, action, and metabolism. *Physiol Rev* 64:985, 984.

121. Haest CWM: Interactions between membrane skeleton proteins and the intrinsic domain of the erythrocyte membrane. *Biochim Biophys Acta* 694:331, 1982.

122. Halem B, Bourne JR, Ward JW, et al: Visually evoked cortical potentials in renal failure: Transient potentials. *Electroencephalogr Clin Neurophysiol* 44:606, 1978.

123. Hammerman MR, Cohn DE, Tamayo J, et al: Effect of parathyroid hormone on Na^+-dependent phosphate transport and cAMP-dependent ^{32}P phosphorylation in brush border vesicles from isolated perfused canine kidneys. *Arch Biochem Biophys* 227:91, 1983.

124. Hampers CL, Doak PM, Calaghan MN, et al: The electroencephalogram and spinal fluid during hemodialysis. *Arch Intern Med* 118:340, 1966.

125. Hampers CL, Schupak E: Neurological abnormalities. *In* Hampers CL, Schupak E (eds): *Long-term Hemodialysis* (2nd ed). New York, Grune & Stratton, 1973.

126. Hanto DW, Frizzera G, Gajl-Peczalska KJ, et al: Epstein-Barr virus-induced B-cell lymphoma after renal transplantation: Acyclovir therapy and transition from polyclonal to monoclonal B-cell proliferation. *N Engl J Med* 306:913, 1982.

127. Hanto DW, Frizzera G, Purtilo DT, et al: Clinical spectrum of lymphoproliferative disorders in renal transplant recipients and evidence for the role of Epstein-Barr virus. *Cancer Res* 41:4253, 1981.

128. Harris RD, Campbell JK, Howard FM, et al: Neurovascular complications of dialysis and transplantation. *Stroke* 5:725, 1974.

129. Hart RP, Pederson JA, Czerwinski AW, et al: Chronic renal failure, dialysis, and neuropsychological function. *J Clin Neuropsychol* 5:301, 1983.

130. Heldenberg D, Blum M, Levtow O, et al: Serum vitamin E and fatty acid composition of the red cell membrane phospholipids in patients with chronic renal failure treated by hemodialysis. *Clin Nephrol* 18:272, 1982.

131. Hemker HC: Lipid solubility as a factor influencing the activity of uncoupling phenol. *Biochim Biophys Acta* 63:46, 1962.

132. Hemker HC: The contribution of the various phosphorylating steps in the respiratory chain to the dinitropohenol-induced ATPase of rat liver mitochondria. *Biochim Biophys Acta* 73:311, 1963.

133. Heyman A, Patterson JL Jr, Jones RW Jr: Cerebral circulation and metabolism in uremia. *Circulation* 3:558, 1951.

134. Hille B: Excitability and ionic channels. *In* Siegel GJ, Albers RW, Agranoff BW, et al (eds): *Basic Neurochemistry* (3rd ed). Boston, Little, Brown, 1981, p 95.

135. Hochberg FH, Miller G, Schooley RT, et al: Central-nervous system lymphoma related to Epstein-Barr virus. *N Engl J Med* 309:745, 1983.

136. Hochman MS: Meperidine-associated myoclonus and seizures in long-term hemodialysis patients. *Ann Neurol* 14:593, 1983.

137. Hooper WD, Dubetz DK, Bocher F, et al: Plasma protein binding of carbamazepine. *Clin Pharmacol Ther* 17:433, 1975.

138. Hoyer JR, Michael AF, Fish AJ, et al: Acute poststreptococcal glomerulonephritis presenting as hypertensive encephalopathy with minimal urinary abnormalities. *Pediatrics* 39:412, 1967.

138a. Huxtable RJ: From heart to hypothesis: A mechanism for the calcium modulatory actions of taurine. *Adv Exp Med Biol* 217:371, 1987.

139. Iversen LL: Nonopioid neuropeptides in mammalian CNS. *Annu Rev Pharmacol Toxicol* 23:1, 1983.

140. Jacob JC, Gloor P, Elwan OH, et al: Encephalographic changes in chronic renal failure. *Neurology* 15:419, 1965.

141. Jacobs S, Cuatrescasas P: Insulin receptors. *Annu Rev Pharmacol Toxicol* 23:461, 1983.

142. Jebsen RH, Tenckhoff H, Honet JC: Natural history of uremic polyneuropathy and effect of dialysis. *N Engl J Med* 277:327, 1967.

143. Jellinek EH, Painter M, Prineas J, et al: Hypertensive encephalopathy with cortical disorders of vision. Q J Med 33:239, 1964.

144. Johansson B, Li CL, Olsson Y, et al: The effect of arterial hypertension on the blood-brain barrier to protein tracers. Acta Neuropathol (Berl) 16:117, 1970.

145. Johnson DW, Wathen RL, Mathog RH: Effects of hemodialysis on hearing threshold. Q R L 38:129, 1976.

146. Joseph SK, Thomas AP, Williams RJ, et al: Myo-inositol 1,4,5-triphosphate: A second messenger for the intracellular Ca^{2+} in liver. J Biol Chem 259:3077, 1984.

147. Joss DV, Barrett AJ, Kendra JR, et al: Hypertension and convulsions in children receiving cyclosporin A. Lancet 1:906, 1982.

147a. Kahn DW, Morell P: Phosphatidic acid and phosphoinositide turnover in myelin and its stimulation by acetylcholine. J Neurochem 50:1542, 1988.

148. Katzman R: Blood-brain-CSF barriers. In Siegel GJ, Albers RW, Agranoff BW, et al (eds): Basic Neurochemistry (3rd ed). Boston, Little, Brown, 1981, p 497.

149. Kennedy AC, Linton AL, Luke RG, et al: The pathogenesis and prevention of cerebral dysfunction during dialysis. Lancet 1:790, 1964.

150. Kennedy C, Sokoloff L: An adaptation of the nitrous oxide method to the study of the cerebral circulation in children; normal values for cerebral blood flow and cerebral metabolic rate in childhood. J Clin Invest 36:1130, 1957.

151. Kerr DNS: Clinical and pathophysiologic changes in patients on chronic dialysis: The central nervous system. Adv Nephrol 9:109, 1980.

152. Kersh ES, Kronfield SJ, Unger A, et al: Autonomic insufficiency in uremia as a cause of hemodialysis-induced hypotension. N Engl J Med 290:650, 1974.

153. Khalifa S, Mills S, Hruska A: Stimulation of calcium uptake by parathyroid hormone in renal brush-border membrane vesicles. J Biol Chem 158:14400, 1983.

154. Kiley J, Hines O: Electroencephalographic evaluation of uremia. Arch Intern Med 116:67, 1965.

155. Killam EK, Suria A: Benzodiazepines. In Glaser GH, Penry JK, Woodbury DM (eds): Antiepileptic Drugs: Mechanisms of Action. New York, Raven Press, 1980, p 597.

156. Kilmartin JV, Rossi-Bernardi L: Interaction of hemoglobin with hydrogen ions, carbon dioxide, and organic phosphates. Physiol Rev 53:836, 1973.

157. Klatzo I: Disturbances of the blood-brain barrier in cerebrovascular disorder. Acta Neuropathol (Berl) [Suppl VIII]:81, 1983.

158. Klein G, Purtilo D: Summary: Symposium on Epstein-Barr virus-induced lymphoproliferative diseases in immunodeficient patients. Cancer Res 41:4302, 1981.

159. Komsuoglu SS, Mehta R, Jones LA, et al: Brainstem auditory evoked potentials in chronic renal failure and maintenance hemodialysis. Neurology 35:419, 1985.

160. Konishi T, Nishitani H, Motomura S: Single fiber electromyography in chronic renal failure. Muscle Nerve 5:458, 1982.

161. Kretzschmar K, Nix W, Zschiedrich H, et al: Morphologic cerebral changes in patients undergoing dialysis for renal failure. AJNR 4:439, 1983.

162. Kuba M, Peragrin J, Vit F, et al: Pattern-reversal visual evoked potentials in patients with chronic renal insufficiency. Electroencephalogr Clin Neurophysiol 56:438, 1983.

163. Kurtz SB, Wong VH, Anderson CF, et al: Continuous ambulatory peritoneal dialysis: Three years experience at the Mayo Clinic. Mayo Clin Proc 58:633, 1983.

164. Kutt H: Effects of acute and chronic diseases on the disposition of antiepileptic drugs. In Morselli PL, Pippenger CE, Penry JK (eds): Antiepileptic Drug Therapy in Pediatrics. New York, Raven Press, 1983, p 293.

165. Land H, Parada LF, Weinberg RA: Tumorigenic conversion of primary embryo fibroblasts requires at least two cooperating oncogenes. Nature 304:596, 1983.

166. Lasek RJ: Cytoskeletons and cell motility in the nervous system. In Siegel GJ, Albers RW, Agranoff BW, et al (eds): Basic Neurochemistry (3rd ed). Boston, Little, Brown, 1981, p 403.

167. Lasker N, Harvey A, Baker H: Vitamin levels in hemodialysis and intermittent peritoneal dialysis. Trans Am Soc Artif Intern Organs 9:51, 1963.

168. Lazaro RP, Kirschner HS: Proximal muscle weakness in uremia. Arch Neurol 37:555, 1980.

169. Leonard A, Shapiro FL: Subdural hematoma in regularly dialyzed patients. Ann Intern Med 82:650, 1975.

170. Le Rudulier D, Strom AR, Dandekar AM, et al: Molecular biology of osmoregulation. Science 224:1064, 1984.

171. Letteri JM, Mellk H, Louis S, et al: Diphenylhydantoin metabolism in uremia. N Engl J Med 285:648, 1971.

172. Levene MI, Whitelaw A, Dubowitz V: Nuclear magnetic resonance (NMR) imaging of the brain in children. Br Med J 285:774, 1982.

173. Levitan D, Massry SG, Romoff MS, et al: Autonomic nervous system dysfunction in patients with acute renal failure. Am J Nephrol 2:213, 1982.

174. Lewis EG, Dustman RE, Beck EC: Visual and somatosensory evoked potential characteristics of patients undergoing hemodialysis and kidney transplantation. Electroencephalogr Clin Neurophysiol 44:223, 1978.

175. Lichtenstein IH, MacGregor RR: Mycobacterial infections in renal transplant recipients: Report of five cases and review of the literature. Rev Infect Dis 5:216, 1983.

176. Lichtenwalner DM, Byungse S: Isolation and chemical characterization of 2-hydroxybenzoylglycine as a drug binding inhibitor in uremia. J Clin Invest 71:1289, 1983.

177. Lindholm DD, Burnell JM, Murray JS: Experience in treatment of chronic uremia in an outpatient community hemodialysis center. Trans Am Soc Artif Intern Organs 9:3, 1963.

178. Linnemann CC Jr, Dunn CR, First MR, et al: Late onset of fatal cytomegalovirus infection after renal transplantation: Primary or reactivation infection? Arch Intern Med 138:1247, 1978.

179. Liveson JA, Gardner J, Bornstein MB: Tissue culture studies concerning myoinositol as a uremic neurotoxin. Einstein Quart J Biol Med 2:41, 1984.

180. Locke S, Merrill JP, Tyler HR: Neurological complications of acute uremia. Arch Intern Med 108:519, 1961.

181. Lopez RI, Collins GH: Wernicke's encephalopathy. A complication of chronic hemodialysis. Arch Neurol 18:248, 1968.

182. Lou HC: Perinatal hypoxic-ischemic brain damage and periventricular hemorrhage: The pathogenetic significance of arterial pressure changes. In Harel S, Anastasiow NJ (eds): The At-Risk Infant: Psycho/Socio/Medical Aspect. Baltimore, Paul H Brooks, 1985, p 153.

183. Lous P: Elimination of barbiturates. In Johansen SH (ed): Barbiturate Poisoning and Tetanus. Boston, Little, Brown, 1966.

184. Lubash GD, Stenzel KH, Rubin AL: Nitrogenous compounds in hemodialysate. Circulation 30:848, 1964.

185. Ludwig GD, Senesky D, Bluemle LW Jr, et al: Indoles in uremia. Identification by countercurrent distribution and paper chromatography. Am J Clin Nutr 21:436, 1968.

186. Lumsden CE: Glia and myelin in ischaemia, blood disorders and intoxications. In Vinken PJ, Bruyn GW (eds): Hand-

book of Clinical Neurology, Vol. 9. Amsterdam, North Holland Publishing Co, 1970, p 572.

187. Lund L: Anticonvulsant effect of diphenylhydantoin relative to plasma levels. *Arch Neurol* 31:289, 1974.

188. Macara IG, Marinetti GV, Balduzzi PC: Transforming protein of avian sarcoma virus UR2 is associated with phosphatidylinositol kinase activity: Possible role in tumorigenesis. *Proc Natl Acad Sci USA* 81:2728, 1984.

189. Maloff BL, McCaleb ML, Lockwood DH: Cellular basis of insulin resistance in chronic uremia. *Am J Physiol* 245:E178, 1983.

190. Manz HJ, Dinsdale HB, Morrin PA: Progressive multifocal leucoencephalopathy after renal transplantation. *Ann Intern Med* 75:77, 1971.

191. Marder HK, Srivastava LS, Burstein S: Hypergonadotropism in peripubertal boys with chronic renal failure. *Pediatrics* 72:384, 1983.

192. Marker SC, Ascher NL, Kalis JM, et al: Epstein-Barr virus antibody responses and clinical illness in renal transplant recipients. *Surgery* 85:433, 1979.

193. Maroteaux P, Humbel R, Strecker G, et al: Un nouveau type de sialidose avec atteinte renale: La nephrosialidose. *Arch Fr Pediatr* 35:819, 1978.

194. Matas AJ, Hertel BF, Rosai J, et al: Post-transplant malignant lymphoma. *Am J Med* 61:716, 1976.

195. Matsubara M, Nakagawa K, Nonomura K, et al: Plasma LRH levels in chronic renal failure before and during hemodialysis. *Acta Endocrinol (Copenh)* 103:145, 1983.

196. Mattson RH: The benzodiazepines. *In* Woodbury DM, Penry JK, Schmidt RP (eds): *Antiepileptic Drugs*. New York, Raven Press, 1972, p 497.

197. Maxwell RE, Long DM, French LA: The effects of glucosteroids on experimental cold-induced brain edema. *J Neurosurg* 34:477, 1971.

198. Maynert EW: Phenobarbital, mephobarbital and metharbital. Absorption, distribution and excretion. *In* Woodbury DM, Penry JK, Schmidt JP (eds): *Antiepileptic Drugs*. New York, Raven Press, 1972, p 303.

199. Mayor GH, Keiser JA, Makdani DS, et al: Aluminum absorption and distribution: Effect of parathyroid hormone. *Science* 197:1187, 1977.

199a. Maytal J, Shinnar S, Moshé SL, et al: Low morbidity and mortality of status epilepticus in children. *Pediatrics* 83:323, 1989.

199b. McEnery PT, Nathan J, Bates SR, et al: Convulsions in children undergoing renal transplantation. *J Pediatr* 115:532, 1989.

200. McGeer PL, McGeer EG: Amino acid neurotransmitters. *In* Siegel GJ, Albers RW, Agranoff BW, et al (eds): *Basic Neurochemistry* (3rd ed). Boston, Little, Brown, 1981, p 233.

201. McGraw ME, Haka-ikse K: Neurologic developmental sequelae of chronic renal failure in infancy. *J Pediatr* 106:579, 1975.

202. Merion RM, White DJG, Thiru S, et al: Cyclosporine: Five years' experience in cadaveric renal transplantation. *N Engl J Med* 310:148, 1984.

203. Merrill JP, Hampers CL: Uremia. *N Eng J Med* 282:953, 1014, 1970.

204. Mettier SR: Ocular defects associated with familial renal disease and deafness. *Arch Ophthalmol* 65:386, 1961.

205. Meyer JS, Charney JZ, Rivera VM, et al: Treatment with glycerol of cerebral oedema due to acute cerebral infarction. *Lancet* 2:993, 1971.

206. Meyer JS, Watz AG, Gotoh F: Pathogenesis of cerebral vasospasm in hypertensive encephalopathy. I. Effects of acute increases in intraluminal blood pressure on pial blood flow. *Neurology* 10:735, 1960.

207. Meyer JS, Watz AG, Gotoh F: Pathogenesis of cerebral vasospasm in hypertensive encephalopathy. II. Nature of increased irritability of smooth muscle of pial arteroles in renal hypertension. *Neurology* 10:859, 1960.

208. Michalk DV, Bohles HJ, Scharer K: Growth, taurine, and calcium metabolism in chronic renal failure: Effect of taurine and methionine deficiency. *Prog Clin Biol Res* 125:305, 1983.

209. Michell RH, Kirk CJ: Why is phosphatidylinositol degraded in response to stimulation of certain receptors? *TIPS* 2:86, 1984.

210. Mikami H, Orita Y, Ando A, et al: Metabolic pathway of guanidino compounds in chronic renal failure. *Adv Exp Med Biol* 153:449, 1982.

211. Miller JA, Gravallese E, Bunn HF: Nonenzymatic glycosylation of erythrocyte membrane proteins. *J Clin Invest* 65:896, 1980.

212. Minkoff L, Gaertner G, Darab M, et al: Inhibition of brain sodium-potassium ATPase in uremic rats. *J Lab Clin Med* 80:71, 1972.

213. Mitschke H, Schmidt P, Kopsa H, et al: Reversible uremic deafness after successful renal transplantation. *N Eng J Med* 292:1062, 1975.

214. Morgan RE, Morgan JM: Plasma levels of aromatic amines in renal failure. *Metabolism* 15:479, 1966.

215. Morrison G, Singer I: The use of drugs in renal failure. *In* Flomenbaum W, Hamburger RJ (eds): *Nephrology: An Approach to the Patient with Renal Disease*. Philadelphia, JB Lippincott, 1982, p 608.

216. Morselli PL, Pippenger CE, Penry JK (eds): *Epileptic Drug Therapy in Pediatrics*. New York, Raven Press, 1983.

217. Mulder H, Silberbusch J, Hackeng WHL, et al: Enchanced calcitonin release in chronic renal failure depending on the absence of severe secondary hyperparathyroidism. *Nephron* 32:123, 1982.

217a. Murphy SN, Miller RJ: Regulation of Ca^{++} in flux into striated neurons by kainic acid. *J Pharmacol Exp Ther* 249:184, 1989.

218. Myers GJ, Tyler HR: The etiology of deafness in Alport syndrome. *Arch Otolaryngol* 96:333, 1972.

219. Nath SS, Ramakrishna BR, Pattabiraman TN: Glycosylated haemoglobin in chronic renal failure. *Indian J Med Res* 75:846, 1982.

220. Nathanson JA, Greengard P: Cyclic nucleotides aid synpatic transmission. *In* Siegel GJ, Alberts RW, Agranoff BW, et al (eds): *Basic Neurochemistry* (3rd ed). Boston, Little, Brown, 1981, p 297.

221. Navarro P, Contreras P, Touraine JL, et al: Are "middle molecules" responsible for toxic henomena in chronic renal failure? *Nephron* 32:301, 1982.

222. Nestler EJ, Greengard P: Neuronal phosphoproteins: Physiological and clinical implications. *Science* 225:1357, 1984.

223. Nestler EJ, Walas SI, Greengard P: Protein phosphorylation in the brain. *Nature* 305:583, 1983.

224. Nielsen VK: The peripheral nerve function in chronic renal failure. I. Clinical symptoms and signs. *Acta Med Scand* 190:105, 1971.

225. Nielsen VK: The peripheral nerve function in chronic renal failure. V. Sensory and motor conduction velocity. *Acta Med Scand* 194:445, 1973.

226. Nielsen VK: The peripheral nerve function in chronic renal failure. VI. The relationship between sensory and motor nerve conduction and kidney function, azotemia, age, sex and clinical neuropathy. *Acta Med Scand* 194:455, 1973.

227. Nielsen VK: The peripheral nerve function in chronic renal failure. VIII. Recovery after renal transplantation. Clinical aspects. *Acta Med Scand* 195:163, 1974.

228. Nishizuka Y: The role of protein kinase C in cell surface

signal transduction and tumor promotion. *Nature* 308:693, 1984.

229. Nishizuka Y: Turnover of inositol phospholipids and signal transduction. *Science* 225:1365, 1984.

230. Nissenson AR, Levin ML, Klawans HL, et al: Neurological sequelae of end stage renal disease (ESRD). *J Chronic Dis* 30:705, 1977.

231. Ochs S: Axoplasmic transport. *In* Siegal GJ, Albers RW, Agranoff BW, et al (eds): *Basic Neurochemistry.* Boston, Little, Brown, 1981, p 425.

231a. Odar-Cederlof I, Theodorsson E, Eriksson C-G, et al: Plasma concentrations of calcitonin gene-related peptide increase during haemodialysis: relation to blood pressure. *J Internal Med* 226:177, 1990.

232. Oertel PJ, Lichtweld K, Hafner S, et al: Hypothalamo-pituitary-gonadal axis in children with chronic renal failure. *Kidney Int* (Suppl)15:834, 1983.

233. Oh SJ, Clements RS Jr, Lee YW, et al: Rapid improvement in nerve conduction velocity following renal transplantation. *Ann Neurol* 4:369, 1978.

234. O'Hare JA, Callaghan NM, Murnaghan DJ: Dialysis encephalopathy: Clinical, electroencephalographic and interventional aspects. *Medicine* 62:129, 1983.

235. Oldstone MBA, Nelson E: Central nervous system manifestations of penicillin toxicity in man. *Neurology* 16:693, 1966.

236. Olsen ST: The brain in uremia. *Acta Psychiatr Scand* 36 (Suppl 156):102, 1961.

237. O'Neill WM Jr, Atkins CL, Bloomer HA: Hereditary nephritis: A re-examination of its clinical and genetic features. *Ann Intern Med* 88:176, 1978.

238. Opheim KE, Ainardi V, Raisys VA: Increase in apparent theophylline concentration in the serum of two uremic patients as measured by some immunoassay methods (caused by 1,3-dimethyluric acid?) *Clin Chem* 29:1698, 1983.

239. Orr JM, Farrell K, Abbott FS, et al: The effects of peritoneal dialysis on the single dose and steady state pharmacokinetics of valproic acid in a uremic epileptic child. *Eur J Clin Pharmacol* 24:387, 1983.

240. Osberg JW, Meares GJ, McKee DC, et al: Intellectual functioning in renal failure and chronic dialysis. *J Chronic Dis* 35:445, 1982.

241. Painter MJ: How to use phenobarbital. *In* Morselli PL, Pippenger CE, Penny JK (eds): *Antiepileptic Drug Therapy in Pediatrics.* New York, Raven Press, 1981, p 245.

242. Palek J: Red cell calcium content and transmembrane calcium movements in sickle cell anemia. *J Lab Clin Med* 89:1365, 1977.

243. Papageorgiou C, Ziroyannis P, Vathylakis J, et al: A comparative study of brain atrophy by computerized tomography in chronic renal failure and chronic hemodialysis. *Acta Neurol Scand* 66:378, 1982.

244. Pappius HM: Water spaces. *In* Lajtha A (ed): *Handbook of Neurochemistry* (2nd ed), Vol 1, *Chemical and Cellular Architecture.* New York, Plenum Press, 1982, p 139.

245. Parisi AF, Kaplan MH: Apnea during treatment with sodium colistimethate. *JAMA* 194:298, 1965.

246. Passer JA: Cerebral atrophy in end-stage uremia. *Proc Dial Transplant Forum* 7:91, 1977.

247. Penn I: Tumor incidence in human allograft recipients. *Transplant Proc* 11:1047, 1979.

248. Peterson PK, Balfour HH Jr, Marker SC, et al: Cytomegalovirus disease in renal allograft recipients: A prospective study of the clinical features, risk factors, and impact on renal transplantation. *Medicine* 59:283, 1980.

249. Peterson PK, Ferguson R, Fryd DS, et al: Infectious diseases in hospitalized renal transplant recipients: A prospective

250. Pierides AM, Edwards WG, Cullum UX, et al: Hemodialysis encephalopathy with osteomalacia, fractures and muscle weakness. *Kidney Int* 18:115, 1980.

251. Pirson Y, Alexandre GPJ, van Ypersele de Strihou C: Neurologic disorders in uremia. *N Engl J Med* 294:1009, 1976.

252. Planz G, Haass H, Lamberts B: Plasma catecholamine concentration in hypertensive subjects with chronic renal failure before and during treatment with the beta-receptor blocking drug metipranolol. *Int J Clin Pharmacol Ther Toxicol* 20:469, 1982.

253. Polinsky MS: Neurologic complications of ESRD, dialysis, and transplantation. *In* Fine RN, Gruskin AB (eds): *End Stage Renal Disease in Children.* Philadelphia, WB Saunders, 1984, p 307.

254. Polinsky MS, Gruskin AB: Aluminum toxicity in children with chronic renal failure. *J Pediatr* 105:758, 1984.

255. Popovtzer MM, Rosenbaum BJ, Gordon A, et al: Relief of uremic polyneuropathy after bilateral nephrectomy. *N Engl J Med* 281:949, 1969.

256. Porter RJ, Penry JK: Phenobarbital: Biopharmacology. *In* Glaser GH, Penry JK, Woodbury DM (eds): *Antiepileptic Drugs: Mechanisms of Action.* New York, Raven Press, 1980, p 493.

257. Pressman BC: Specific inhibitors of energy. *In* Chance B (ed): *Energy-linked Functions of Mitochondria.* New York, Academic Press, 1963, p 181.

258. Putney JM Jr, Weiss SJ, Van de Walle CM, et al: Is phosphatidic acid a calcium ionophore under neurohumoral control? *Nature* 284:345, 1980.

259. Rapaport SI, Fredericks WR, Ohno K, et al: Quantitative aspects of reversible osmotic opening of the blood-brain barrier. *Am J Physiol* 238:421, 1980.

260. Rasbury WC, Fenneli RS III, Morris MK: Cognitive functioning of children with end-stage renal disease before and after successful transplantation. *J Pediatr* 102:589, 1983.

261. Raskin NH, Fishman RA: Neurological disorders in renal failure. *N Engl J Med* 294:143, 204, 1976.

262. Rasmussen H, Barrett PQ: Calcium messenger system: An integrated view. *Physiol Rev* 64:938, 1984.

263. Ratner DP, Adams KM, Levin NW, et al: Effects of hemodialysis on the cognitive and sensori-motor functioning of the adult chronic hemodialysis patient. *J Behav Med* 6:29, 1983.

264. Read DJ, Feest TG, Holman RH: Vibration sensory threshold: A guide to adequacy of dialysis? *Proc EDTA* 19:253, 1982.

265. Record NB, Gallagher BB, Glaser GH: Phenolic acids in experimental uremia. II. Relationship of phenolic acid structure to seizure threshold in uremia. *Arch Neurol* 21:395, 1969.

266. Record NB, Prichard JM, Gallagher BB, et al: Phenolic acids in experimental uremia. I. Potential role of phenolic acids in the neurological manifestations of uremia. *Arch Neurol* 21:387, 1969.

267. Reese GN, Appel SH: Neurologic complications of renal failure. *Semin Nephrol* 1:137, 1981.

268. Reichardt L, Kelly RB: A molecular description of nerve terminal function. *Annu Rev Biochem* 52:871, 1983.

269. Reichenmiller HE, Durr F, Bundschu HD: Neurological disorders in uremia. *In* Kluth R, Berylne G, Burton B (eds): *Uremia. An International Conference on Pathogenesis, Diagnosis and Therapy.* Stuttgart, Thieme, 1972, p 55.

270. Reidenberg MM, Odar-Cederlöf J, Von Bahr ML, et al: Protein binding of diphenylhydantoin and desmethylimi-

study of a complex and evolving problem. *Medicine* 61:360, 1982.

pramine in plasma from patients with poor renal function. *N Engl J Med* 285:264, 1971.

271. Reinharz AC, Favre H, Miller B, et al: Estrogen-stimulated neurophysin in chronic renal failure. *Nephron* 33:44, 1983.

272. Revillard JP: Immunologic alterations in chronic renal insufficiency. *Adv Nephrol* 8:365, 1979.

273. Richet G, Vaghon F: Neuropsychiatric disorders of chronic uremia. *Press Med* 74:1177, 1966.

274. Ringer S: An investigation regarding the action of strontium and barium salts compared with the action of lime in the ventricle of the frog's heart. *Practitioner* 31:81, 1983.

275. Ringer S: A third contribution regarding the influence of the inorganic constituents of the blood on the ventricular contraction. *J Physiol* 4:222, 1883.

276. Rosansky SJ, Sugimoto T: An analysis of the United States renal transplant patient population and organ survival characteristics: 1977–1980. *Kidney Int* 22:685, 1982.

277. Rosenfeld MG, Amara SG, Evans RM: Alternative RNA processing: Determining neuronal phenotype. *Science* 225:1315, 1984.

278. Rosenman E, Kobrin I, Cohen T: Kidney involvement in systemic lupus erythematosus and Fabry's disease. *Nephron* 34:180, 1983.

279. Rossini PM, Pirchio M, Treviso M, et al: Checkerboard reversal pattern and flash VEPs in dialyzed and nondialyzed subjects. *Electroencephalogr Clin Neurophysiol* 52:435, 1981.

280. Rossini PM, Treviso M, DiStefano E, et al: Nervous impulse propagation along peripheral and central fibers in patients with chronic renal failure. *Electroencephalogr Clin Neurophysiol* 56:293, 1983.

281. Rotundo A, Nevins TE, Lipton M, et al: Progressive encephalopathy in children with chronic renal deficiency in infancy. *Kidney Int* 21:486, 1982.

282. Rovit RL, Hagan R: Steroids and cerebral edema: The effects of glucocorticoids on abnormal capillary permeability following cerebral injury in cats. *J Neuropathol Exp Neurol* 27:277, 1968.

283. Rubin RH, Jenkins RL, Shaw BW, et al: The acquired immunodeficiency syndrome and transplantation. *Transplantation* 44:1, 1987.

283a. Rubin RH, Wolfson JS, Cosini AB, et al: Infections in the renal transplant recipient. *Am J Med* 70:405, 1981.

284. Ruskin J, Remington JS: Toxoplasmosis in the compromised host. *Ann Intern Med* 84:193, 1976.

285. Sabouraud O, Chatel M, Menault F, et al: L'encéphalopathie myoclonique progressive des dialyses (EMPD). Etude clinique, électroencéphalographique et neuropathologique. Discussion pathogénique. *Rev Neurol (Paris)* 134:575, 1978.

286. Salusky IB, Coburn JW, Paunier L, et al: Role of aluminum hydroxide in raising serum aluminum levels in children undergoing continuous ambulatory peritoneal dialysis. *J Pediatr* 105:717, 1984.

287. Sampol J: Factor VIII related antigen, coagulation tests and acute renal failure. *Proc Eur Dial Transplant Assoc* 19:325, 1983.

288. Savazzi GM, Buzio C, and Migone L: Lights and shadows in the pathogenesis of uremic polyneuropathy. *Clin Nephrol* 18:219, 1982.

289. Savazzi GM, Cambi V, Migone L, et al: The influence of uraemic neuropathy on muscle: EMG, histoenzymatic and ultrastructural correlations. *Proc Eur Dial Transplant Assoc* 17:312, 1980.

290. Savazzi GM, Govoni E, Bragaglia MM, et al: Ultrastructural findings of uraemic muscular damage: Functional implications. *Proc Eur Dial Transplant Assoc* 19:258, 1982.

291. Schanne FAX, Kane AB, Young EE, et al: Calcium dependence of toxic cell death. *Science* 206:700, 1979.

292. Schaumburg HH, Plank CR, Adams RD: The reticulum cell sarcoma-microglioma group of brain tumors: A consideration of their clinical features and therapy. *Brain* 95:199, 1972.

293. Schaumburg HH, Spencer PS, Thomas PK: *Disorders of Peripheral Nerves.* Philadelphia, FA Davis, 1983, p 69.

294. Scheie HG: Evaluation of ophthalmoscopic changes of hypertension and arteriolar sclerosis. *Arch Ophthalmol* 49:117, 1953.

295. Scheinberg P: Effects of uremia on cerebral blood flow and metabolism. *Neurology* 4:101, 1954.

296. Schentag JJ, Calleri G, Rose JQ, et al: Pharmacokinetic and clinical studies in patients with cimetidine-associated mental confusion. *Lancet* 1:177, 1979.

297. Schlessinger J: Mobilities of cell-membrane proteins: How are they modulated by the cytoskeleton? *TINS* 6:360, 1983.

298. Schmitz O, Moller J: Impaired prolactin response to arginine infusion and insulin hypoglycaemia in chronic renal failure. *Acta Endocrinol (Copenh)* 102:486, 1983.

299. Schnaper HW, Cole BR, Hodges FJ, et al: Cerebral cortical atrophy in pediatric patients with end-stage renal disease. *Am J Kidney Dis* 2:645, 1983.

300. Schneck SA, Penn I: De-novo brain tumours in renal-transplant recipients. *Lancet* 1:983, 1971.

301. Schramm M, Selinger Z: Message transmission: Receptor controlled adenylate cyclase system. *Science* 225:1350, 1984.

302. Schreiner G, Maher J: *Uremia: Biochemistry, Pathogenesis and Treatment.* Springfield, IL, Charles C. Thomas, 1961.

303. Schupak E, Merrill JP: Experience with long-term intermittent hemodialysis. *Ann Intern Med* 62:509, 1965.

304. Seligson DL, Bluemle LW Jr, Webster GD Jr, et al: Organic acids in body fluids of the uremic patient. *J Clin Invest* 38:1042, 1959.

305. Shapira E, Ben-Yoseph Y, Eyal G, et al: Enzymatically inactive red cell carbonic anhydrase B in a family with renal tubular acidosis. *J Clin Invest* 53:59, 1974.

306. Siegel GJ, Stahl WL, Swanson PD: Ion transport. In Siegel GJ, Albers RW, Agranoff RW, et al (eds): *Basic Neurochemistry* (3rd ed). Boston, Little, Brown, 1981, p 107.

306a. Siesjo BK: Calcium, ischemia and death of brain cells. *Ann NY Acad Sci* 522:638, 1988.

307. Simenhoff ML, Asatoor AM, Milne MD, et al: Retention of aliphatic amines in uremia. *Clin Sci* 25:65, 1963.

308. Singer SJ: The molecular organization of membranes. *Annu Rev Biochem* 43:805, 1974.

309. Sklar AH, Linas SL: The osmolal gap in renal failure. *Ann Intern Med* 98:481, 1983.

310. Smits MG, de Abreu RA, Froeling PGA, et al: Presence of cerebral parathyroid hormone-responsive adenylcyclase in humans. *Ann Neurol* 14:348, 1983.

311. Soifer D, Mack K: Microtubules in the nervous system. In Lajtha A (ed): *Handbook of Neurochemistry*, Vol 7. New York, Plenum, 1984, p 245.

312. Sokoloff L: Circulation and energy metabolism of the brain. In Siegel GJ, Albers RW, Agranoff BW, et al (eds): *Basic Neurochemistry* (3rd ed). Boston, Little, Brown, 1981, p 471.

313. Stein IM, Cohen BD, Kornhauser RS: Guanidinosuccinic acid in renal failure, experimental azotemia and inborn errors of the urea cycle. *N Engl J Med* 280:926, 1969.

314. Stenback A, Haapanen E: Azotemia and psychosis. *Acta Psychiatr Scand* (Suppl 197)43:1, 1967.

315. Sugimoto Y, Whitman M, Cantley LC, et al: Evidence that the Rous sarcoma virus transforming gene product phosphorylates phosphatidylinositol and diacylglycerol. *Proc Natl Acad Sci USA* 81:2117, 1984.

316. Swaiman KF: Neurologic complications of renal failure and

transplantation. *In* Swaiman KF, Wright FS (eds): *The Practice of Pediatric Neurology* (2nd ed). St. Louis, CV Mosby, 1982, p 793.

317. Swan JS, Kragten EY, Veening H: Liquid-chromatographic study of fluorescent materials in uremic fluids. *Clin Chem* 29:1082, 1983.

318. Sweeney VP, Perry TL: A biochemical basis for disorder of language? *Neurology* 34 (Suppl 1):249, 1984.

319. Szeto HH, Inturrisi CE, Houde R, et al: Accumulation of normeperidine, an active metabolite of meperidine, in patients with renal failure or cancer. *Ann Intern Med* 86:738, 1977.

320. Taclob L, Needle M: Drug-induced encephalopathy in patients on maintenance haemodialysis. *Lancet* 2:704, 1976.

321. Takagi T, Chung TG, Saito A: Determination of polyamines in hydrolysates of uremic plasma by high-performance cation-exchange column chromatography. *J Chromatogr* 272:279, 1983.

322. Takala J: Total plasma clearance of intravenous essential amino acids: Evidence of abnormal metabolism of amino acids in chronic renal failure. *J Parenteral Enteral Nutrit* 7:146, 1983.

323. Taylor CR, Russell R, Lukes RJ, Davis RL: An immunohistological study of the immunoglobulin content of primary central nervous system lymphomas. *Cancer* 41:2197, 1978.

324. Tenckhoff HA, Boen ST, Jepsen RH, et al: Polyneuropathy in chronic renal insufficiency. *JAMA* 192:1121, 1965.

325. Teschan PE, Ginn HE, Bourne JR, et al: Quantitative indices of clinical uremia. *Kidney Int* 15:676, 1979.

326. Thomas PK: Screening for peripheral neuropathy in patients treated by chronic hemodialysis. *Muscle Nerve* 1:396, 1979.

327. Thomas PK, Hollinrake K, Lascelles RG, et al: The polyneuropathy of chronic renal failure. *Brain* 94:761, 1971.

328. Thomson NM, Stevens BJ, Humphery TJ, et al: Comparison of trace elements in peritoneal dialysis, and uremia. *Kidney Int* 23:9, 1983.

329. Tilney NL, Kohler TR, Strom TB: Cerebromeningitis in immunosuppressed recipients of renal allografts. *Ann Surg* 195:104, 1982.

330. Tower DB: *Neurochemistry of Epilepsy*. Springfield, IL, Charles C. Thomas, 1960, p 24.

331. Trachtman H, Braden K, Scerra C, et al: Neuropsychological functioning in adolescents on chronic hemodialysis. *In* Brodhel J, Ehrich JHH (eds): Proceedings of the Sixth International Symposium of Pediatric Nephrology. Hannover, Federal Republic of Germany, August 29-September 2, 1983. Springer-Verlag, 1984.

332. Troncoso JC, Price DL, Griffin JW, et al: Neurofibrillary axonal pathology in aluminum intoxication. *Ann Neurol* 12:278, 1982.

333. Tyler HR: Studies in asterixis. *Arch Neurol* 10:360, 1964.

334. Tyler HR: Neurological disorders in renal failure. *Am J Med* 44:734, 1968.

335. Tyler HR: Neurological disorders seen in renal failure. *In* Vinkin PJ, Bruyn GW (eds): *Handbook of Clinical Neurology*, Vol 27. Amsterdam, North Holland, 1976, p 321.

336. Urizar RE, Largent JA, Gilboa N: *Pediatric Nephrology*. New Hyde Park, Medical Examiners Publishing Co, 1983.

337. van den Noort S, Eckel RE, Brine KL, et al: Brain metabolism in experimental uremia. *Arch Intern Med* 126:831, 1970.

337a. Varticouski L, Ling L: Signal transduction and phosphoinositide metabolism in the liver. *Prog Liver Dis* 9:181, 1990.

338. Vlassara H, Brownlee M, Cerami A: Nonenzymatic glycosylation of peripheral nerve protein in diabetes mellitus. *Proc Natl Acad Sci USA* 71:5190, 1981.

339. Vorbrodt AW, Lossinsky AS, Wisniewski HM: Enzyme cytochemistry of blood-brain barrier (BBB) disturbances. *Acta Neuropathol (Berl)* (Suppl VII):43, 1983.

340. Wakim KG: The pathophysiology of the dialysis disequilibrium syndrome. *Mayo Clin Proc* 44:406, 1969.

341. Warner WA, Sanders E: Neuromuscular blockade associated with gentamycin therapy. *JAMA* 215:1153, 1971.

342. Washer GF, Schröter GPJ, Starzl TE, et al: Causes of death after kidney transplantation. *JAMA* 250:49, 1983.

343. Weber DL, Reagan T, Leeds M: Intracerebral hemorrhage during hemodialysis. *NY State J Med* 72:1853, 1972.

344. Weiss RA, Edelmann CM Jr: Children on dialysis. *N Engl J Med* 307:1574, 1982.

345. Wigand ME, Meents O, Hennmann H, et al: Kochleovestibulare Störungen bei Urämie in Beziehung zum Electrolytstoffwechsel und Glomerulomfiltrat. *Schweiz Med Wochenschr* 102:477, 1972.

346. Wikstrom M, Krab K, Saraste M: Proton-translocating cytochrome complexes. *Annu Rev Biochem* 50:623, 1981.

347. Wilder BJ, Ramsay E, Wilmore LJ, et al: Efficacy of intravenous phenytoin in the treatment of status epilepticus: Kinetics of central nervous system penetration. *Ann Neurol* 1:511, 1977.

348. Wilensky AJ, Lowden JA: Inadequate serum levels after intramuscular administration of diphenylhydantoin. *Neurology* 23:318, 1973.

349. Wilson JE: Hexokinase. Enzymes in the nervous system. *In* Lajtha A (ed): *Handbook of Neurochemistry* (2nd ed), Vol 4. New York, Plenum Press, 1984, p 151.

350. Wisniewski HM, Sturman JA, Shek JW: Aluminum induced neurofibrillary changes in the developing rabbit: A chronic animal model. *Ann Neurol* 8:479, 1980.

351. Wisniewski KE, Kieras FJ, French JH, et al: Ultrastructural, neurological, and glycosaminoglycan abnormalities in Lowe's syndrome. *Ann Neurol* 16:40, 1984.

352. Wolfe LS: Prostaglandins and thromboxanes in the nervous system. In Siegel GJ, Albers AW, Agranoff RW, et al (eds): *Basic Neurochemistry* (3rd ed). Boston, Little, Brown, 1981, p 311.

353. Woodbury DM, Swinyard E: Diphenylhydantoin: Absorption, distribution and excretion. *In* Woodbury DM, Penry JK, Schmidt RP (eds): *Antiepileptic Drugs*. New York, Raven Press, 1972, p 113.

354. Yamakawa M, Yamamoto T, Kishimoto T, et al: Serum levels of acetate and TCA intermediates during hemodialysis in relation to symptoms. *Nephron* 32:155, 1982.

354a. Yoshida S, Tajika T, Yamasaki N, et al: Dialysis dysequilibrium syndrome in neurosurgical patients. *Neurosurgery* 20:716, 1987.

355. Zannad F, Royer RJ, Kessler M, et al: Cation transport in erythrocytes of patients with renal failure. *Nephron* 32:347, 1982.

356. Ziegler DK: Hypertensive vascular diseases of the brain. *In* Vinken PJ, Bruyn GW (eds): *Vascular Diseases of the Nervous System. Handbook of Clinical Neurology*, Vol 11. Amsterdam, North Holland, 1972, p 552.

357. Ziegler DK, Zosa A, Zileli T: Hypertensive encephalopathy. *Arch Neurol* 12:472, 1965.

358. ZuRhein GM, Varakis J: Progressive multifocal leukoencephalopathy in renal-allograft recipient. *N Engl J Med* 291:798, 1974.

MARTIN BLACK
STEVEN J. WIDZER

31
Disorders of the Gastrointestinal System

The gastrointestinal tract and associated organs are not commonly considered to be prime targets of the uremic syndrome. Accordingly, they rarely earn more than passing mention in many otherwise learned discussions of the clinical features and complications of chronic renal disease [23,266]. Nevertheless, the improved survival rate of many patients with chronic renal failure has led to an increased opportunity for recognition of the gastrointestinal complications of the uremic syndrome. In the following discussion of this subject, reference is made to relevant observations in both adults and children. It is assumed that most are applicable to uremic patients of all ages, even though the current literature includes few reports dealing specifically with children.

The Gastrointestinal Tract

Mucosal disease of the gastrointestinal (GI) tract complicating long-standing uremia has attracted the attention of physicians since the latter part of the nineteenth century [80,287] but has only recently become recognized as a significant clinical problem in the uremic patient. In a comprehensive survey of gastrointestinal changes occurring in 136 consecutive autopsied patients dying with uremia, Jaffe and Laing [132] ranked gastrointestinal ulceration as the third most common pathologic finding (following anhidrosis and fibrosis pericarditis, respectively), being present in nearly 20% of the patients examined. Mason [179] reviewed the protocols of 265 autopsied uremic patients at the Mayo Clinic and found a similar incidence of gastrointestinal complications. Furthermore, when he compared his findings in the uremic patients with those in 100 nonuremic patients autopsied over the same time period, he observed that gastrointestinal complications were twice as common in the esophagus, stomach, cecum, ascending colon, and rectum, with less frequent involvement of the ileum and jejunum. Interestingly, in view of recent observations, duodenal ulceration was not observed in either study.

The renewal of interest in this subject over the past few decades is attributable primarily to the development of GI bleeding or frank peptic ulceration in many uremic patients who are maintained for long periods of time on hemodialysis. Bleeding, ulceration, or perforation has been noted throughout the GI tract, although lesions in the esophagus, stomach, and duodenum remain the most common. With widespread use of endoscopy, erosions rather than ulcerations are more frequently documented, and attention has been focused in recent years on vascular malformations referred to as angiodysplasias. Although, gastric hypersecretion remains the most likely explanation for mucosal injury, other factors have been suggested. These include gastric atrophy, gastric hyperplasia, gastric inhibitory polypeptide effects, drug therapy, and pancreatic bicarbonate secretion. Additionally, McDermott and co-workers [184,185,186] have espoused the concept that uremia has an adverse effect on renewal of the gastrointestinal epithelium, which may be responsible for initiating or perpetuating ulcerative mucosal lesions.

Peptic Ulcer Disease

Peptic ulcer disease appears to be a common complication of both acute and chronic renal failure. Kleinknecht et al. [147] reported an incidence of 26% for gastrointestinal hemorrhage in 279 patients suffering from acute renal failure, and it was the second most common cause of death in that population of patients (responsible for 14% of the deaths as compared with 24% for septicemia). Institution of "prophylactic" hemodialysis reduced both its incidence and mortality. Lunding et al. [174] noted gastrointestinal hemorrhage in 12% of 154 patients with acute renal failure, and it was the cause of death in 6.5%. Nakayama [207] found gastrointestinal hemorrhage to be a major risk factor for death in 26 patients with acute renal failure.

Several groups have reported on the occurrence of peptic ulcer disease in patients with chronic renal failure [100,110,189,237,253,263,269,283]. Patients have often complained of typical dyspeptic symptoms and occasionally suffered hematemesis, but not infrequently the development of peptic mucosal disease has been clinically silent. It has been estimated that gastrointestinal hemorrhage secondary to peptic ulcer disease is responsible for 3% to 5% of all deaths in dialysis patients [100]. Endoscopic studies of patients with chronic renal failure on dialysis have demonstrated a high incidence of diffuse inflammation and erosions. Boyle and Johnston [30] found gastric mucosal lesions (in part secondary to drugs) to be the most common cause of significant acute upper GI bleeding in 20 patients with chronic renal failure. Margolis et al. [177] found gastritis, duodenitis, and esophagitis but no actual ulceration in a prospective study of 85 nonbleeding dialysis patients. In a similar investigation of 84 patients on hemodialysis, Tani et al. [273] showed hemorrhagic gastritis to be more common than erosive gastritis and both to be much more common than duodenal ulcer. Milito et al. [194] studied 75 patients on dialysis who were awaiting transplantation and found lesions by endoscopy in 49%. Superficial gastritis was more frequent than either duodenitis or atrophic gastritis. Franzin et al. [92] investigated 102 patients on dialysis and reported both gastric and duodenal hyperplasia, each associated with erosions and ulcers. Moorthy and Chesney [199] claimed an increased prevalence of peptic ulcer disease in children with uremia.

Peptic ulcer disease in uremia has been accompanied by gastric hypersecretion in many patients studied [110, 253,269], despite an earlier claim that gastric hyposecretion was the more common finding in uremic subjects [167]. A recent investigation by Shepherd et al. [253] demonstrated high overnight and basal acid secretion in several of the patients they studied. Goldstein and coworkers [110] investigated gastric acid secretion in seven dialysis patients (four with peptic ulcer disease) and noted that whereas basal acid output was in the normal range in these patients prior to dialysis, it increased considerably in several during dialysis—a phenomenon they attributed to rising serum calcium levels during dialysis secondary to the calcium content of the dialysate. Most recently, Sullivan and coworkers [269] observed markedly elevated basal acid secretion in three of 21 dialysis patients studied. All three groups [110,253,269], as well as Ventkateswaran and coworkers [283], also demonstrated increased peak acid outputs in response to betazole [110], pentagastrin [253,269], or a test meal [269] in the majority of patients studied. A contrary view has been presented by Ryabov and colleagues [243], who minimized the role of gastric hypersecretion in their patients and drew attention to the frequent presence of atrophic gastritis—a finding later supported by the study of Milito et al. [194].

The gastric hyperacidity of uremia has been attributed to increased fasting levels of serum gastrin [269], an observation that has been made repeatedly in uremic subjects [67,148,161,269]. Gastrin is removed or metabolized to a considerable extent by the normal kidney, and experimental studies in rats have shown that serum levels increase markedly following bilateral nephrectomy, but not at all following bilateral ureteral ligation [59]. Preliminary observations in human beings have indicated a return of elevated plasma gastrin levels to normal following renal transplantation [148]. The hypergastrinemic state in uremia differs from the Zollinger-Ellison syndrome in that a good response to exogenous pentagastrin is retained [253,269], and basal secretion is suppressed by infused se-

cretion [253]. On the other hand, Taylor et al. [274] observed a negative correlation between maximal acid output and basal serum gastrin concentrations and discounted an important role for gastrin in producing duodenal ulcer disease in chronic renal failure patients. Interestingly, Owyang and colleagues [217] found that cholecystokinin, glucagon, and gastric inhibitory polypeptide were also increased in chronic renal failure patients. An additional factor that may enhance the uremic subject's susceptibility to development of peptic ulcer disease is duodenogastric reflux, which has been demonstrated in some uremic patients [269]. Fisher and Cohen [88] and others [280] have implicated this entity in the production off gastric ulceration in nonuremic subjects, and Fisher and Cohen [88] have demonstrated that competency of the pyloric sphincter is adversely influenced by gastrin infusion, thus closely simulating the circumstances that prevail in many uremic patients. Boyle and Johnston [30] also considered that ulcerogenic drugs were an important factor in GI bleeding arising from gastric erosions or ulcers in chronic renal disease patients.

Gastric Angiodysplasias

In recent years, GI bleeding in patients with chronic renal failure has been attributed to gastric and duodenal angiodysplasias [30,50,56,305]. These vascular malformations have been recognized with increasing frequency in both the upper and lower intestinal tracts as endoscopy has been used more and the skills of the endoscopist improved (it is likely that such lesions were dismissed as mucosal hemorrhages in earlier times). In one series, the incidence of angiodysplasias was noted to be far higher in patients with chronic renal failure than those without [305], suggesting a particular susceptibility to their development in chronic renal failure. Other than this observation, angiodysplasia development in the GI tract has been most closely associated with aortic valve disease and advanced age [27, 165,191,292].

Angiodysplasias can be recognized at endoscopy [56,305] and through angiography [166]. They can be treated by procedures such as cautery [305], laser ablation, and surgical resection; interest is now emerging in medical therapies. Griffin et al. [114] have also reported angiomatous lesion in the mid-duodenum.

Ulcerative and Necrotic Lesions of the Small and Large Bowel

The differential diagnosis of gastrointestinal bleeding or acute abdomen in uremic patients includes conditions that appear to result from the uremic process. In 1959, Thoroughman and Peace [275] described 12 patients with chronic renal failure who presented as surgical emergencies because of the development of ulcerative or necrotic processes in various parts of the small or large bowel. Pathologic examination of the surgical specimens have demonstrated a necrotizing arteritis in some (probably secondary to malignant hypertension). Bounous [29] has claimed that pancreatic proteolytic enzyme digestion has a role in the pathogenesis of these lesions. Subsequent experience has not suggested that this is as common a complication of uremia as Thoroughman and Peace implied [275], but additional cases have been reported [21,103,121,168]. Clearly, the possibility of spontaneous ulceration or perforation of the small or large intestine has to be considered in any uremic patient presenting with an acute abdomen or gastrointestinal hemorrhage.

Other ulcerative processes affecting the small and large bowel have been reported in uremic patients. Bischel et al. [22] observed spontaneous perforation of the colon by a barium stercoraceous fecaloma two weeks after GI tract barium studies, and cytomegalovirus infection of the colon, perhaps arising as a result of compromised immune function, has also been noted [151]. Ischemic colitis occurring in three uremic patients was attributable by Aubia et al. [12] to accelerated arterial disease, and Scheff et al. [248] reported an increased incidence of diverticulosis and diverticulitis in patients with chronic renal failure resulting from polycystic kidney disease. Meshkinpour et al. [190], who observed gastrointestinal abnormalities in 20 of 23 consecutive patients with end-stage renal disease associated with spinal cord injury, found a high prevalence of secondary amyloidosis involving the gastrointestinal tract as well as cholelithiasis and inflammatory mucosal disease throughout the gastrointestinal tract.

Motility Disorders

Disorders of gastrointestinal motility have been reported in uremic patients. Intestinal pseudo-obstruction involving four patients was reported by Stephens in 1962 [265], and other cases have been contributed by Rubenstein et al. [240] and Adams et al. [1]. Whether these reports reflect an increased susceptibility of uremic patients to this condition is unclear. On the other hand, Wright et al. [298] failed to find evidence of altered gastric motility in uremic subjects, even in those with frequent symptoms of nausea and vomiting during hemodialysis.

Malignant Tumors

Although there appears to be an increased incidence of malignancy in the uremic patient [180,193] independent of the effects of long-term immunosuppressive therapy [193], the gastrointestinal tract has only rarely shared in its distribution. Miach et al. [193] reported the case of one patient with carcinoma of the stomach and another with carcinoid tumor of the small bowel out of six uremic (and nontherapeutically immunosuppressed) patients who were found to be suffering from a malignant tumor. Other groups [84] have not observed gastrointestinal malignancies.

Role of the Gastrointestinal Tract in Metabolic Disease Resulting from Uremia

The evidence favoring the evidence of malabsorptive phenomena of the intestine in the presence of uremia has been reviewed by Black and Arias [24]. Calcium and phosphate

malabsorption in uremic patients is well documented [113,143,212] and probably results from failure to form the 1,25-dihydroxy metabolite of vitamin D in such patients [32,33]. Intestinal absorption of the essential amino acid tryptophan is decreased [118], which probably accounts for the reduced blood levels of tryptophan observed in uremic patients [38,57,117]. Orally administered iron preparations are poorly absorbed by uremic patients [75,157], and Lawson et al. [157] showed that a minimum period of six months of uremia was required before the defect could be consistently demonstrated.

Absorption of certain drugs has also been shown to be deficient when appropriate studies have been performed [24]. However, in the absence of more extensive investigation, the scope of the problem cannot be adequately assessed. It seems unlikely, of course, that drug malabsorption would profoundly affect drug effectiveness in this group of patients, bearing in mind the more dramatic influence of decreased renal elimination on pharmacokinetic aspects of drug action.

Anemia is a major problem in patients with end-stage renal disease. Most patients have decreased erythropoiesis and decreased levels of serum erythropoietin. Brunois et al. [34] described increased erythropoiesis in 30 patients with hepatitis B, and Chan et al. [46] described increased erythropoiesis in one patient with viral hepatierythrocytosis and end-stage renal disease with increased erythropoietin levels in the absence of hepatitis. If hepatitis increases erythropoiesis, it may be by a mechanism other than increasing serum erythropoietin.

Patients with end-stage renal disease are commonly anemic and are expected to have greater than normal loss of blood through their GI tract or dialysis. Many centers have routinely given parenteral iron therapy. However, iron overload is frequently being reported. Aljama et al. [5] in adults and Ellis [74] in children report serum ferritin measurement to be the best noninvasive test for total body iron stores. Liver biopsy and bone marrow material stained for iron give the best indication of hemosiderosis. The effect of this iron overload on liver function is presently being determined.

Gokal [107] found 64 of 120 patients to have serum ferritin values greater than 1000 μg/L. In 22 patients autopsied, there was significant iron in the liver and spleen, and five also had iron deposition in the heart. Pitts and Barbour [223] and Kothari et al. [149] found hemosiderosis but no evidence of hemochromatosis. However, Ali et al. [4] reported findings in 50 autopsied patients in whom 18 had severe hepatosplenic siderosis with increased fibrous tissue and loss of cells apparent by special stains. Iron deposition was noted in adrenal glands, lymph nodes, and lungs, and there was sparse deposition in the heart, kidneys, and pancreas. Nineteen patients had scanty deposition in bone marrow, and the question of difference in availability of iron from different organs was raised as was the choice of which organ to sample for iron determination. Treatment with desferioxamine has been of some benefit [233b]. Therefore, the question of iron overload leading to hepatic dysfunction has not been answered and chelation therapy in patients with severe iron overload may be warranted.

The Liver

Autopsy examination of the livers of uremic patients and extensive clinical experience have not indicated that the uremic syndrome per se produces histopathologic changes in the liver. Nevertheless, as Black and Arias [24] concluded, a survey of certain metabolic manifestations of the uremic syndrome implies a functional alteration by the uremic liver. Experimentally, induction of uremia was found to be followed by ultrastructural changes in hepatocytes, reduction in some (but not all) hepatic microsomal enzymes, and impaired oxidative drug metabolism [11]. Shafritz and coworkers [115,251] have investigated molecular aspects of albumin synthesis in the livers of uremic rats in an attempt to explain the decreased levels of serum albumin observed consistently in uremic patients [51]. They demonstrated a significant reduction in the synthesis of albumin and other proteins by liver membrane-bound polysomes and an intercellular accumulation of albumin within the cytosol fraction. These changes were considered to result either from uremia-induced alterations in membrane properties or the presence of circulating toxic substances.

These experimental observations thus contribute to a growing literature that suggests that certain of the metabolic consequences of uremia and instances of drug toxicity [234] or therapeutic ineffectiveness can be directly attributed to subtle alterations in hepatic subcellular function. Evidently, even though the liver may have a relatively normal histopathologic appearance in uremic subjects, and the findings of conventional laboratory investigations of its "function" remain within normal limits, it shares in the profound metabolic disturbance produced by uremia. Failure to recognize this (which is implicit in the overly simplistic drug dosage guides for uremic patients [17,152] could have unforeseen and potentially deleterious consequences.

The Pancreas

Histopathologic and functional disorders of the pancreas (excluding endocrine disorders) are rarely listed among the recognized complications of uremia. However, pancreatitis has been reported in uremic patients, and its incidence in patients who have had transplantations has been estimated to be nearly 2% [133]. Gilboa et al. [105] reported pancreatitis in a child undergoing chronic hemodialysis. Factors considered to be important in its pathogenesis include corticosteroid therapy, other immunosuppressive regimens, surgical trauma, and "induced autoimmune pancreatic rejection" in the transplant recipient [133]. It is also a well-recognized complication of hyperparathyroidism [122], which is a frequent development in the uremic patient [3,45,188,239]. Avram and Iancu [14] reported a possible correlation between measured elevation of parathyroid hormone and histologic alterations in pancreatic histology in a retrospective autopsy study of 21 patients who died during maintenance hemodialysis.

Sachs [244] suggested a role for pancreatic exocrine hypofunction in the wasting syndrome of end-stage renal disease patients. Saris et al. [246] found low basal bicarbonate output in five patients on hemodialysis. Other than these observations, there is little evidence in the literature to suggest that pancreatic exocrine function is grossly affected by the uremic syndrome.

Idiopathic Ascites

Development of ascites in the uremic patient on long-term dialysis has been recognized as a clinical problem only in the last few years, but appears to be surprisingly common [11,49,54,82,119,128,235,255,287]. Accumulation of ascitic fluid occurs in the absence of detectable hepatic abnormality and without bacteriologic evidence of peritoneal inflammation. Some of the patients in whom this complication develops have been undergoing regular peritoneal dialysis, and others had been on peritoneal dialysis prior to being switched to hemodialysis. However, in other patients, both those on hemodialysis and those not on dialysis, ascites has occurred in the absence of a history of peritoneal dialysis, indicating that it is uremia and not peritoneal dialysis that is the important predisposing factor. Inspection of the peritoneum at laparotomy [49,235], laparoscopy [54], or autopsy [119,255] and histopathologic examination of peritoneal biopsy sections do not suggest an inflammatory cause. The ascitic fluid is generally high in protein (4–5 gm per deciliter), but values as low as 1.2 gm per deciliter have been reported [112]. Other findings such as specific gravity, lactic dehydrogenase, and amylase concentrations have not shown any consistent pattern, and the fluid is usually sterile and does not contain significant numbers of white cells. The pathogenesis of this type of ascites (sometimes referred to as "nephrogenic or nephrogenous ascites" [54,128] remains obscure, but increased fluid retention presumably plays an important role. It is, of course, necessary to exclude other causes of ascites before accepting this diagnosis [11].

Management of the ascites has generally been unsatisfactory. Hemodialysis does not have any dramatic effect, and diuretics are usually ineffective in the patient with end-stage renal disease. Repeated abdominal paracenteses may be successful in reducing the amount of fluid present, but this approach rarely eliminates the ascites altogether and introduces the potential for secondary infection. Several groups have noticed its disappearance after abdominal surgery [49,235], and one group has suggested that bilateral nephrectomy should be performed to control it [82]. The disorder generally resolves following renal transplantation [248,287].

Simultaneous Disorders of the Gastrointestinal System and Kidney
Polycystic Kidney Disease

Some disease processes that affect the kidney and impair renal function may also independently involve portions of the gastrointestinal system and vice versa. A typical example is polycystic disease of the kidney and liver (Chap. 47). Reported series of polycystic kidney disease have placed the incidence of liver cysts at somewhere between 19% and 33% [213,231], and Rall and Odell [231] observed involvement of the pancreas also in 9%. In other reports in which attention was directed to polycystic liver disease, concurrent renal involvement has been observed in more than 50% [51,156,200]. Clearly, therefore, there is a close relationship between development of cysts in the liver and kidney, but in many patients only one or the other may be involved.

The clinical and pathologic features of polycystic kidney disease are presented in Chap. 47, so that discussion here is limited to comments about hepatic aspects of the condition. Although cysts in the liver are not uncommon in patients presenting to the nephrologist with polycystic kidney disease, only rarely does such involvement become clinically significant. Symptoms such as pain or a dragging sensation in the upper abdomen may result from hepatic involvement, but these symptoms are not easily differentiated from those secondary to the renal disorder. The findings of laboratory studies of liver function are almost always within normal limits.

Sherlock [254] has divided polycystic disease of the liver into several categories—adult fibropolycystic disease and three forms of childhood fibropolycystic disease: perinatal, neonatal, and infantile. Congenital hepatic fibrosis and Caroli's disease (dilation of the intra- and extra-hepatic biliary tree) are regarded as closely related entities. Development of portal hypertension with hemorrhage from esophageal varices has been reported in a few patients with the adult form of fibropolycystic liver disease. In the case of a 54-year-old male patient with polycystic kidney disease (and an affected brother) reported by DelGuericio et al. [63], the renal disorder had progressed to the development of uremia at the time that radiologic studies demonstrated the presence of gastric varices. The authors presumed (but did not demonstrate) that polycystic liver disease was the basis for the portal hypertension. The same authors also described another patient, a 57-year-old woman, who had been diagnosed five years earlier as suffering from polycystic kidney and liver disease, who died following hemorrhage from esophageal varices. Autopsy disclosed only multiple cysts and fatty changes in the liver as the basis for the evident portal hypertension [63].

Adult cases of portal hypertension complicating polycystic kidney disease are clearly such a rarity that it has been concluded that the pathogenesis of the portal hypertension observed in young children with polycystic liver and kidneys involves hepatic changes other than the cysts. Liver biopsies or autopsy examinations in these children have regularly demonstrated that in addition to cysts, extensive fibrous bands containing bile ducts are present, closely simulating the appearances seen in congenital hepatic fibrosis (a developmental abnormality that commonly presents with bleeding esophageal varices) [141,142,183]. Since cystic changes are not infrequently observed in that condition, it has become generally accepted that polycystic liver disease and congenital hepatic fibrosis are closely related developmental disorders that may coexist in the same patient [26]. This concept is further supported by the frequent occurrences of renal abnormalities (including polycystic kidney disease [141,142,183], medullary sponge kidney, and nephronophthisis [26]) in patients diagnosed as having congenital hepatic fibrosis.

Caroli's Syndrome

Another related condition appears to be Caroli's syndrome, a disorder characterized by nonobstructive dilatation of the intrahepatic or extrahepatic biliary tree [41,42,202]. Murray-Lyon and coworkers, in a report on four patients and review of the world literature [204], suggested that congenital hepatic fibrosis and Caroli's syndrome were related entities and were occasionally present in the same individual. The occurrence of polycystic kidney disease or medullary sponge kidney (or renal tubular ectasia [175]) in the majority of the patients supported this concept and highlighted the complex interrelationships that exist between these relatively uncommon disorders of the liver and kidney.

Congenital Hepatic Fibrosis

Alvarez [6] reported 27 children with congenital hepatic fibrosis. Intravenous pyelography studies were abnormal in 24, ten had obvious polycystic kidney disease. Esophageal varices were present in 21, and three had cholangitis. Kerr [141] reviewed long-term prognosis in 30 patients with congenital hepatic fibrosis, 18 required shunt surgery. McGonigle [187] reported three patients with congenital hepatic fibrosis and childhood-type autosomal recessive polycystic kidney disease. He suggested prophylactic portacaval shunting prior to renal transplantation.

Hepatitis

Hepatitis B virus (HBV) infections are occasionally associated with extrahepatic manifestations, some involving the kidney. These are thought to be secondary to an immunologic response to hepatitis B surface antigen (HBsAg) or other antigens. Extra-hepatic syndromes include: (1) serum sickness-like reactions, (2) necrotizing vasculitis, (3) glomerulo-nephropathy, (4) "essential" mixed cryoglobulinemia, and (5) polymyalgia rheumatica. Pear [220] reported that necrotizing vasculitis (or polyarteritis) may result in severe renal disease as well as polyarthritis, peripheral neuropathy, gastrointestinal symptoms, and micro-aneurysms. Levy and Kleinknecht [163] reviewed the association of HBV infection with glomerulonephropathy. Evidence relating the two phenomena includes the detection within glomeruli of hepatitis B antigens and detection of circulating immune complexes.

Hemolytic-Uremic Syndrome

The hemolytic-uremic syndrome may involve both the kidney and the GI tract. It is defined as acute renal failure, hemolytic anemia, and thrombocytopenia (Chap. 60). There are a variety of causes, pathogenetic mechanisms, and subsets. Gastrointestinal symptoms, including abdominal pain and bloody diarrhea, frequently preceded the onset of renal failure [64]. In 20% of cases, hemolytic-uremic syndrome can mimic an acute abdomen. It is one cause of acute colitis with bloody diarrhea, ulcer, and friable mucosa in children and may mimic ulcerative colitis. Whitington et al. [294] reported bloody diarrhea in 12 consecutive patients. Kirks [146] reported radiologic features, including submucosal edema, spasm, and superficial ulcerations. There may be "thumprinting" as well as areas of narrowing and distention. Perforation, gangrene, intussusception, and colonic stricture have been reported. Vitamin E has been suggested [227] as a treatment for the syndrome.

There may be biochemical evidence of hepatitis as reported by Furginele [93]. Burns and Berman [36] reported hemorrhagic islet cell necrosis of the pancreas in one patient. A prodromal illness of gastroenteritis or upper respiratory infection is usual. Gastroenteritis may be due to shigella, campylobacter, or escherichia coli.

Other Conditions

Many other conditions may produce simultaneous injury to both liver and kidney. They include infections (bacterial sepsis, viral, or leptospirosis), Reye's syndrome, circulatory problems, collagen vascular diseases, Henoch-Schönlein purpura, and toxins. Abnormal renal function may occur as a consequence of many acute and chronic liver diseases. Renal failure occurs in patients with cirrhosis and is usually ascribed to hepatorenal syndrome or prerenal azotemia. It also may be induced by diuretic use or other drugs. Glomerulonephritis has been reported with chronic active hepatitis and other chronic liver diseases.

Gastrointestinal Disturbances Resulting from Therapeutic Regimens in the Uremic Patient

Dialysis

The evidence suggesting that hemodialysis, peritoneal dialysis, and drug administration may contribute to gastrointestinal complications such as peptic ulceration and idiopathic ascites has already been discussed. In those situations, an underlying predisposition to the complication due to the uremic process may be compounded by an additive effect of the therapeutic regimens employed. Krempien et al. [150] reported accumulation of foreign material in macrophages of lung, liver, and spleen in a patient on maintenance hemodialysis. Diethylphthalate from polyvinyl chloride tubing and silicone have both been implicated in cases of hepatic dysfunction ranging from mild fibrosis to granulomatous hepatitis and extensive fibrosis. A phasic inflammatory response followed by fibrogenesis and isolation of foreign material may be reflected in the fluctuation of serum hepatic enzymes levels seen in these patients. This is one possible explanation of liver abnormalities frequently seen in dialysis patients.

Fennell et al. [83] reported that liver dysfunction sometimes occurred in children and adolescents undergoing he-modialysis. He noted it in 12 patients in the End Stage Renal Diseases program at the University of Florida. Liver pathology was variable and the etiology was generally obscure. The occurrence of hepatitis or asymptomatic hepatitis B virus infection in the uremic patient can be identified more clearly with the treatment (namely, hemodialysis) than with the disease [233,233a]. Many hemodialysis centers have reported its frequent occurrence in their patients [109,130], and in some instances hepatitis B virus infection of both patients and staff has achieved epidemic proportions [170,296]. Use of markers other than HBsAg, particularly anti-hepatitis B core (anti-HBc), as reported by Gmelin et al. [106] and Kelly et al. [139], has resulted in documenting higher prevalence rates of infection in these populations. In recent times, however, the institution of careful public health measures [230,262], availability of protective globulin preparations [65,69, 228,271], the use of more completely disposable dialysis equipment, and the introduction of vaccination has progressively reduced its incidence [230].

Multiple use of dialyzers in the same patient does not seem to increase the risk of hepatitis B infection [79]. The suggestion has been made by Deane and Chalmers [60] to control Hepatitis B infection with close surveillance and geographically separate units for carriers. Peritoneal dialysis may carry a risk of spread of hepatitis B. Salo et al. [245] report the presence of HBsAg in peritoneal fluid of carriers even when there is no blood present.

Hepatitis B vaccination has been found effective in both children and adults on chronic hemodialysis [55]. The need for increased dose has been raised by Lelie et al. [158]. Consideration should be given to the need to immunize household contacts [95]. Most dialysis centers now routinely test candidate patients and new personnel and maintain a close surveillance of both throughout the duration of their contact with the center.

Hepatitis B virus infection in the uremic patient shows some important differences in its biologic profile from that observed in a nonuremic population [169,171]. Clinical hepatitis and the more severe forms of hepatic inflammatory disease appear to be less common following acquisition of the infection [98,130,232], but there is an increased likelihood of infected patients becoming chronic carriers [98,232]. Polyarteritis nodosa [100] and acute serositis [58] have been reported. Demonstration of "e" antigen (HBeAg), indicating the replicative phase of HBV infection, does not appear to be an indicator of progression of advanced chronic liver disease [53,293]. The diminished impact of HBV infection in uremic patients has been attributed to their altered immunologic status [98,232]. However, Walker and co-workers [286] believe that response to such an infection is also influenced by the sex of the patient, and the presence of human leukocytic antigens (HLA) phenotype BW35. Most importantly, recent studies [224] indicate that allograft survival is not significantly affected by chronic HBV infection (unless advanced liver disease is present). Thus, despite earlier suggestions to the contrary [123,145], renal transplantation should not be withheld in this group of patients.

Other viruses have been implicated in the production of hepatitis in hemodialysis patients. Acute, intermittent, and chronic forms were reported by Toussaint et al. [277]. Cytomegalovirus (CMV) infection was a possible etiology as indicated by seroconversion in his study. Antibody to hepatitis A has been found in high prevalence in dialysis patients [138]. Mayor et al. [182] found it to be related to increasing age, race, and underlying kidney disease and felt it was not associated with hemodialysis nor spread in the dialysis unit. Gmelin et al. [106] did find a high seroconversion rate in patients entering a dialysis unit.

Non-A non-B hepatitis has also been implicated as a cause for elevated liver enzymes in dialysis patients [288,289]. Avram et al. [13] reported five patients with elevated alanine aminotransferase (ALT) and associated fever, anorexia, nausea, hepatomegaly, and hypotension during dialysis with resolution in one to four months. Galbraith et al. [97,99] reviewed an outbreak of 29 cases of hepatitis in a dialysis center and found them to be non-A non-B; a relatively high percentage (28%) had a chronic course. Interestingly, early application of a test for hepatitis C virus (HCV) [153], the principle cause of non-A, non-B posttransfusion hepatitis, has demonstrated relatively low incidences of anti-HCV antibody positive patients in hemodialysis populations [76,236,304]. Whether this reflects infrequent HCV infection in dialysis patients, a methodological problem, or an abnormality in mounting an antibody response to the virus has not been determined.

Both continuous ambulatory and intermittent peritoneal dialysis are being used with increasing frequency in children. The major limitation is the risk of peritonitis. Powell et al. [226] reported 77 episodes of peritonitis in 30 children within a four-year period, an incidence of one episode per six patient-months. Risk was highest when aseptic technique was not maintained and in hospitalized patients. Special culture techniques were needed and organisms recovered were *Staphylococcus epidermidis*, *Staphylococcus aureus*, and fungi. Intraperitoneal administration of antibiotic was used, and most infections could be treated at home. Death and removal of catheters were complications.

In studies on adults, many different bacteria have been described as etiologic agents, although the two staphylococcus species are still most frequent. Suggestions for decreasing incidence and treating infection have been made. Gauntner et al. [101] suggests a separate unit for peritoneal dialysis, strict adherence to aseptic technique, replacement of manual with automated procedures, and antibiotic treatment for asymptomatic but culture-positive patients. Kerr et al. [140] state that for fungal peritonitis the treatment of choice is removal of the catheter. Kiddy et al. [144] advises antibiotic prophylaxis of oral lesions and dental surgery in these patients to prevent hematogenous spread of streptococcus viridans to the peritoneum. Buggy et al. [35] suggest adding rifampicin to manage patients with recurrent staphylococcus peritonitis on the basis of sequestration of viable staphylococcus within polymorphonuclear leukocytes. Goodship et al. [111] notes the possibility that viral infections predispose to peritonitis by altering host defense mechanisms.

Other complications secondary to peritoneal dialysis reported in adults include adhesions, protein losses, decreased ability to ultrafilter, and loss of peritoneal dialysis efficiency secondary to sclerosis and thickening of perito-

neum. Luciani et al. [172] reported multiple hepatic abscesses occurring in a patient with recurrent peritonitis.

Abdominal hernias are seen relatively frequently in patients with peritoneal dialysis, they may be inguinal, umbilical, ventral, or at the catheter insertion site. Incarcerations with small bowel obstruction have been reported. Dialysis ascites, a rare complication of hemodialysis in which no etiology is found, has been treated by peritoneal dialysis.

Renal Transplantation

Gastrointestinal complications following transplantation are fairly frequent and cause significant morbidity and mortality.

The common occurrence of peptic ulcer disease in the uremic patient poses considerable management problems when renal transplantation procedures are performed. Not only does such a patient have an increased likelihood of suffering from peptic ulcer disease prior to the operation, but the stress of operation [86] and the drugs employed in achieving immunosuppression [121,164] also favor ulcer development. The prolonged bleeding time and bleeding tendency of the uremic patient (associated with platelet and clotting factor abnormalities) [43,78,137] encourage hemorrhagic complications. Accordingly, gastrointestinal hemorrhage secondary to peptic ulcer disease is acknowledged to be one of the major life-threatening complications in the immediate posttransplantation period [48,121,164, 196,198,264]. Surgeons have attempted to reduce this threat by performing a prophylactic gastric operation in high-risk patients at the time of renal transplantation [196,264]. Thus, Spanos and coworkers [264] performed prophylactic vagotomy with pyloroplasty or antrectomy in 19 of 30 high-risk patients prior to transplantation and compared the results in this group with the 11 patients not subjected to this procedure. Only 3 of the 19 patients undergoing prophylactic gastric surgery suffered posttransplantation ulcer complications, whereas 9 of the 11 patients who were not subjected to a prophylactic operation had a gastrointestinal hemorrhage in the period before or after transplantation. Many centers now consider a pretransplantation assessment for evidence of peptic ulcer disease essential, and prophylactic gastric surgery is usually offered to the patient with evidence of such disease prior to transplantation [264]. The addition of cimetidine to antacid therapy postoperatively has also been associated with a decreased risk of bleeding. Feduska et al. [81] outlined further risk factors of rejection, sepsis, and hepatitis.

Colonic complications have been documented, including diverticulitis, ischemic colitis, and stercoral ulcers, which may lead to GI bleeding or perforation [116]. CMV inclusions have been seen at the base of cecal ulcers [270]. Primary intestinal tuberculosis has been reported [214] and pneumatosis intestinalis was reported by Polinsky et al. [225]. The role of steroids in all these complications has not been elucidated. Other reported complications include small bowel obstruction, pancreatitis, candida infection of the esophagus, and CMV infection of the stomach and duodenum.

Following transplantation, liver dysfunction is common. Severity ranges from biochemical abnormalities to fulminant hepatitis and death. Chronic hepatitis progressing to liver failure is also reported. Viral agents HBV, CMV, herpes, varicella, and non-A non-B have been implicated [201,288]. As reported by Aldrete et al. [2], Mozes et al. [201], and La Quaglia et al. [154] symptomatic acute hepatitis is associated with a high rate of death or progression to chronic disease. An immunosuppressive effect of hepatic disease has been suggested by La Quaglia et al. [154] and Yokoyama et al. [302], leading to increased graft survival but a higher incidence of life-threatening extra hepatic infection.

The effect of HBsAg-positive status at the time of transplantation has already been discussed. Shons et al. [256] believed that it led to increased rejection of cadaveric kidneys (but had no effect on living related kidneys), and Walker et al. [286] found that such patients had a poorer outcome, with infection or vascular compromise more likely. Berne et al. [19] reported no effect on graft or patient survival, while Vereerstraeten et al. [284] suggested that it was associated with improved patient and graft survival. In the most careful investigation of this issue performed to date, Pol et al. [224] showed that HBsAg status alone did not adversely affect outcome. However, the presence of significant liver disease (chronic hepatitis and or cirrhosis), whether due to HBV infection or other causes, was associated with reduced patient survival. Thus, selection of HBsAg-positive patients for kidney transplantation should include careful evaluation of the extent of concomitant liver disease (usually requiring liver biopsy) in addition to documentation of hepatitis B serologies.

Azathioprine has been linked to idiosyncratic mixed cholestatic-hepatocellular injury [68] and to hepatic venoocclusive disease [178], but in most cases of liver dysfunction, withdrawal of azathioprine is not associated with improvement.

References

1. Adams PL, Rutsky EA, Rostand SG, et al: Lower gastrointestinal tract dysfunction in patients receiving long-term hemodialysis. *Arch Intern Med* 142:303, 1982.
2. Aldrete JS, Sterling WA, Hathaway BM, et al: Gastrointestinal and hepatic complications affecting patients with renal allografts. *Am J Surg* 129:115, 1975.
3. Alfrey AC, Jenkins D, Groth CG, et al: Resolution of hyperparathyroidism, renal osteodystrophy and metastatic calcification after renal homotransplantation. *N Engl J Med* 279:1349, 1968.
4. Ali M, Fayemi A, Rigolosi R, et al: Hemosiderosis in hemodialysis patients. *JAMA* 244:343, 1980.
5. Aljama P, Ward M, Pierides A, et al: Serum ferritin concentration: A reliable guide to iron overload in uremic and hemodialyzed patients. *Clin Nephrol* 10:101, 1978.
6. Alvarez F, Bernard O, Brunelle F, et al: Congenital hepatic fibrosis in children. *J Pediatr* 99:370, 1981.
7. Amerio A, Campese V, Coratelli P, et al: Prognosis in acute renal failure accompanied by jaundice. *Nephron* 27:152, 1981.
8. Amir J, Dinari G, Zelikovic I, et al: Hepatorenal syndrome in neonates. *Helv Paediatr Acta* 39:167, 1983.
9. Anderson K, Kolmos H: Infectious peritonitis. The main complication of intermittent peritoneal dialysis. *The International Journal of Artificial Organs* 4:281, 1981.
10. Archibald S, Jirsch D, Bear R: Gastrointestinal complications of renal transplantation. 2. The colon. *CMA Journal* 119:1301, 1978.
11. Arismendi GS, Izard MW, Hampton WR, et al: The clinical spectrum of ascites associated with maintenance dialysis. *Am J Med* 60:46, 1976.
12. Aubia J, Lloveras J, Munne A, et al: Ischemic colitis in chronic uremia. *Nephron* 29:146, 1981.
13. Avram MM, Feinfeld D, Gan A: Non-A, Non-B hepatitis: A new syndrome in uraemic patients. *Proc EDTA* 16:141, 1979.
14. Avram R, Iancu M: Pancreatic disease in uremia and parathyroid hormone excess. *Nephron* 32:60, 1982.
15. Baker L, Barnett M, Brozovich B, et al: Hemosiderosis in a patient on regular hemodialysis: Treatment by desferrioxamine. *Clin Nephrol* 1:326, 1976.
16. Bartolomeo RS, Calabrese PR, Taubin HL: Spontaneous perforation of the colon. *Am J Dig Dis* 22:656, 1977.
17. Bennett WM, Singer I, Coggins CH: A practical guide to drug usage in adult patients with impaired renal function. *JAMA* 214:1468, 1970.
18. Berne T, Chatterjee S, Craig J, et al: Hepatic dysfunction in recipients of renal allografts. *Surg Gynecol Obstet* 141:171, 1975.
19. Berne T, Fitzgibbons T, Silberman H: The effect of hepatitis B antigenemia on long-term success and hepatic disease in renal transplant recipients. *Transplantation* 24:412, 1977.
20. Bergman L, Thomas W, Reddy C, et al: Nonviral hepatitis in patients maintained by long-term dialysis. *Arch Intern Med* 130:96, 1972.
21. Biggers JA, Remmers AR Jr, Lindley JD, et al: Femoral neuropathy and ischemic colitis associated with amyloidosis in hemodialysis patients. *Ann Surg* 182:161, 1975.
22. Bischel M, Reese T, Engel J: Spontaneous perforation of the colon in a hemodialysis patients. *Am J Gastroenterol* 74:182, 1980.
23. Black DAK (ed): *Renal Disease,* 2nd ed. Philadelphia, FA Davis, 1967.
24. Black M, Arias IM: Absorption, distribution, excretion and the response to the drug in the presence of chronic renal failure. *In* Eichler O, Farah A, Herken H, et al (eds): Handbook of Experimental Pharmacology, vol 28/3, New Series. New York, Springer, 1975, p 258.
25. Black M, Biempica L, Goldfischer S, et al: Effect of chronic renal failure in rats on structure and function of the hepatic endoplasmic reticulum. *Exp Mol Pathol* 27:377, 1977.
26. Boichis H, Passwell J, David R, et al: Congenital hepatic fibrosis and nephronophthisis. A family study. *Q J Med* 42:221, 1973.
27. Boley SJ, Sammartano R, Adams A, et al: On the nature and etiology of vascular ectasias of the colon. *Gastroenterology* 72:650, 1977.
28. Bommer J, Ritz E, Waldherr R: Silicone-induced splenomegaly. *Medical Intelligence* 18:1077, 1981.
29. Bounous G: Role of pancreatic secretions in uremic gastroenterocolitis. *Am J Surg* 119:264, 1970.
30. Boyle JM, Johnston B: Acute upper gastrointestinal hemorrhage in patients with chronic renal disease. *Am J Med* 75:409, 1983.
31. Bradford WD, Bradford JW, Porter FS, et al: Cystic disease of liver and kidney with portal hypertension. A cause of sudden unexpected hematemesis. *Clin Pediatr (Phila)* 7:299, 1968.

32. Brickman AS, Coburn JW, Massry SG, et al: 1,25-dihydroxy-vitamin D3 in normal man and patients with renal failure. *Ann Intern Med* 80:161, 1974.

33. Brickman AS, Coburn JW, Norman AW, et al: Short-term effects of 1,25-dihydroxycholecalciferol on disordered calcium metabolism of renal failure. *Am J Med* 57:28, 1974.

34. Brunois JP, Lavaud S, Melin JP, et al: Acute hepatitis and erythropoiesis in chronically haemodialyzed patients. *Nephron* 28:152, 1981.

35. Buggy B, Schaberg D, Swartz R: Intraleukocytic sequestration as a cause of persistent staphylococcus aureus peritonitis in continuous ambulatory peritoneal dialysis. *Am J Med* 76:1035, 1984.

36. Burns JC, Berman ER, Fagre JL, et al: Pancreatic islet cell necrosis: Association with hemolytic-uremic syndrome. *J Pediatr* 100:582, 1982.

37. Burzynski S: Bound amino acids in serum of patients with chronic renal insufficiency. *Clin Chim Acta* 25:231, 1969.

38. Callis L, Clanxet J, Fortuny G, et al: Hepatitis B virus infection and vaccination in children undergoing hemodialysis. *Acta Paediatr Scand* 74:213, 1985.

39. Campbell GS, Bick HD, Paulsen EP, et al: Bleeding esophageal varices with polycystic liver. Report of three cases. *N Engl J Med* 259:904, 1958.

40. Campion E, Wangel A, Lawrence J: Hepatitis B antigen, auto-antibodies and liver disease in a haemodialysis and transplantation unit. *Aust N Z J Med* 5:314, 1975.

41. Caroli J, Couinard C, Soupault R, et al: Une affection nouvelle, sans doute congenitale, des voies biliairies: La dilatation kystique unilobaire des canaux hepatiques. *Sem Hop Paris* 34:496, 1958.

42. Caroli J, Corcos V: La dilatation congenitale des voies biliairies intra-hepatiques. *Rev med-chir Mal Foie* 39:1, 1964.

43. Castaldi PA, Rozenberg MC, Stewart JH: The bleeding disorder of uremia. A qualitative platelet defect. *Lancet* 2:66, 1966.

44. Castleman B, Mallory TB: Parathyroid hyperplasia in chronic renal insufficiency. *Am J Pathol* 13:553, 1937.

45. Chamovitz B, Hartstein A, Alexander S, et al: Campylobacter jejuni-associated hemolytic-uremic syndrome in a mother and daughter. *Pediatrics* 71:253, 1983.

46. Chan N, Barton C, Mirahmadi M, et al: Erythropoiesis associated with viral hepatitis in end stage renal disease. *Am J Med Sci* 287:56, 1984.

47. Charpentier B, Salmon R, Arvis G, et al: Tuberculous acute colitis in kidney-transplant patient. *Lancet* 2:308, 1979.

48. Chisholm GD: Complications of renal transplantation. *Proc R Soc Med* 66:914, 1973.

49. Cinque TJ, Letteri J: Idiopathic ascites in chronic renal failure. *NY State J Med* 73:781, 1973.

50. Clouse RE, Costigen DJ, Mills BA, et al: Angiodysplasia as a cause of upper gastrointestinal bleeding. *Arch Intern Med* 145:458, 1985.

51. Coles GA, Peters DK, Jones JH: Albumin metabolism in chronic renal failure. *Clin Sci* 39:423, 1970.

52. Comfort MW, Gray HK, Dahlin DC, et al: Polycystic disease of the liver: A study of 24 cases. *Gastroenterology* 20:60, 1952.

53. Coughlin G, Van Deth A, Disney A, et al: Liver disease and the e antigen in HBsAg carriers with chronic renal failure. *Gut* 21:118, 1980.

54. Craig R, Sparberg M, Ivanovich P, et al: Nephrogenic ascites. *Arch Intern Med* 134:276, 1974.

55. Crosnier J: Hepatitis B in haemodialysis: Vaccination against HBS antigen. *Proc EDTA* 18:231, 1981.

56. Cunningham J: Gastric telangiectasias in chronic hemodialysis patients: A report of six cases. *Gastroenterology* 81:1131, 1981.

57. Czerniak Z, Burzynski S: Free amino acids in serum of patients with chronic renal insufficiency. *Clin Chim Acta* 24:367, 1969.

58. Dave MB, Choi YJ, Cohen BD: Hepatitis B virus: A possible cause of serositis in hemodialysis patients. *Nephron* 33:186, 1983.

59. Davidson WD, Moore TC, Shippey W, et al: Effect of bilateral nephrectomy and bilateral ureteral ligation on serum gastrin levels in the rat. *Gastroenterology* 66:522, 1974.

60. Deane N, Chalmers T: Hepatitis and hemodialysis revisited. *JAMA* 245:171, 1981.

61. DeGast G, Houwen B, Van Der Hem G: T-lymphocyte number and function and the course of hepatitis B in hemodialysis patients. *Infect Immun* 14:1138, 1976.

62. Degos F, Degott C, Bedrossian J, et al: Is renal transplantation involved in post-transplantation liver disease? A prospective study. *Transplantation* 29:100, 1980.

63. DelGuercio E, Greco J, Kim KE, et al: Esophageal varices in adult patients with polycystic kidney and liver disease. *N Engl J Med* 289:678, 1973.

64. Delans R, Biuso J, Saba S, et al: Hemolytic uremic syndrome after campylobacter-induced diarrhea in an adult. *Arch Intern Med* 144:1074, 1984.

65. Delons S, Kleinknecht D, Courouce AM: Hepatitis-B immunoglobulin in prevention of HBs antigenaemia in haemodialysis patients. *Lancet* 1:204, 1976.

66. Demling R, Salvatierra O, Belzer F: Intestinal necrosis and perforation after renal transplantation. *Arch Surg* 110:251, 1975.

67. Dent RI, Hirsch H, James JH, et al: Hypergastrinemia in patients with acute renal failure. *Surg Forum* 23:312, 1972.

68. DePinho R, Goldberg C, Lefkowitch J: Azathioprine and the liver. *Gastroenterology* 86:162, 1984.

69. Desmyter J, Bradburne AF, Vermylen C, et al: Hepatitis-B immunoglobulin in prevention of HBs antigenaemia in haemodialysis patients. *Lancet* 2:377, 1975.

70. Disler P, Meyers A, Kew M, et al: Hepatitis B virus-associated liver disease after renal transplantation. *S Afr Med J* 59:97, 1981.

71. Dobrin R, Hoyer J, Nevins T, et al: The association of familial liver disease, subepidermal immunoproteins, and membranoproliferative glomerulonephritis. *J Pediatr* 90:901, 1977.

72. Dusheiko G, Song E, Bowyer S, et al: Natural history of hepatitis B virus infection in renal transplant recipients— a fifteen-year follow-up. *Hepatology* 3:330, 1983.

73. Elliott W, Houghton D, Bryant R, et al: Herpes simplex type 1 hepatitis in renal transplantation. *Arch Intern Med* 140:1656, 1980.

74. Ellis D: Serum ferritin compared with other indices of iron status in children and teenagers undergoing maintenance hemodialysis. *Clin Chem* 25:741, 1979.

75. Eschback JW, Cook JD, Finch CA: Iron absorption in chronic renal disease. *Clin Sci* 38:191, 1970.

76. Esteban JI, Esteban R, Viladomiu L, et al: Hepatitis C virus antibodies among risk groups in Spain. *Lancet* 2:294, 1989.

77. Ettenger R, Tong M, Landing B, et al: Hepatitis B infection in pediatric dialysis and transplant patients: Significance of e antigen. *J Pediatr* 97:550, 1980.

78. Evans EP, Branch RA, Bloom AL: A clinical and experimental study of platelet function in chronic renal failure. *J Clin Pathol* 25:745, 1972.

79. Favero M, Deane N, Leger R, et al: Effect of multiple use of dialyzers on hepatitis B incidence in patients and staff. JAMA 245:166, 1981.

80. Fedou A: Contribution a l'etude des hemorragies intestinales au course de l'uremie. These de Toulouse, 1899. (Cited by Jaffe and Laing, reference 132.)

81. Feduska N, Amend W, Vincenti F, et al: Peptic ulcer disease in kidney transplant recipients. Am J Surg 148:51, 1984.

82. Feingold LN, Gutman RA, Walsh FX, et al: Control of cachexia and ascites in hemodialysis patients by binephrectomy. Arch Intern Med 134:989, 1974.

83. Fennell R, Andres J, Pfaff W, et al: Liver dysfunction in children and adolescents during hemodialysis and after renal transplantation. Pediatrics 67:855, 1981.

84. Fennell R, Garin E, Pfaff W, et al: Renal transplantation in children and adolescents. Clin Pediatr (Phila) 18:518, 1979.

85. Fine R, Malekzadeh M, Pennisi A, et al: HBs antigenemia in renal allograft recipients. Ann Surg 185:411, 1977.

86. Fisher R, Peter E, Mullane J: Experimental stress ulcers in acidotic and non-acidotic renal insufficiency. Arch Surg 109:409, 1974.

87. Fisher RS, Cohen S: Hormonal regulation of pyloric sphincter function. Clin Res 20:732, 1972.

88. Fisher RS, Cohen S: Pyloric sphincter dysfunction in patients with gastric ulcer. N Engl J Med 288:273, 1973.

89. Fong J, Chadarevian J, Kaplan B: Hemolytic-uremic syndrome. Pediatr Clin North Am 29:835, 1982.

90. Francis D, Schofield I, Veitch P: Abdominal hernias in patients treated with continuous ambulatory peritoneal dialysis. Br J Surg 69:409, 1982.

91. Franzin G, Musola R, Mencarelli R: Changes in the mucosa of the stomach and duodenum during immunosuppressive therapy after renal transplantation. Histopathology 6:439, 1982.

92. Franzin G, Musola R, Mencarelli R: Morphological changes of the gastroduodenal mucosa in regular dialysis uraemic patients. Histopathology 6:429, 1982.

93. Furgiuele T: Hemolytic uremic syndrome presenting as hepatitis. Tex Med 77:55, 1981.

94. Gabbert H, Wagner R, Hohn P, et al: Does uremic enterocolitis exist? A morphological and functional investigation of rat intestine in chronic renal insufficiency. Virchows Arch [B] 37:285, 1981.

95. Gahl G, Vogl E, Kraft D, et al: Hepatitis B virus markers among family contacts and medical personnel of 239 hemodialysis patients. Clin Nephrol 14:7, 1980.

96. Gaisford W, Bloor K: Congenital polycystic disease of kidneys and liver. Portal hypertension—portacaval anastomosis. Proc R Soc Med 2:61:304, 1968.

97. Galbraith R, Eddleston A, Portman B, et al: Chronic liver disease developing after outbreak of HBsAg-negative hepatitis in haemodialysis unit. Lancet 2:886, 1975.

98. Galbraith RM, Sheikh NE, Portmann B, et al: Immune response to HBsAg and the spectrum of liver lesions in HBsAg-positive patients with chronic renal disease. Br Med J 1:1495, 1976.

99. Galbraith R, Dienstag J, Purcell R, et al: Non-A non-B hepatitis associated with chronic liver disease in a haemodialysis unit. Lancet 1:951, 1979.

100. Garland HJ, Brunner FP, Von Dehn H, et al: Combined report on regular dialysis and transplantation in Europe, III, 1972. Proc Eur Dialysis Transplant Assoc 10:17, 1973.

101. Gauntner W, Feldman H, Puschett J: Peritonitis in chronic peritoneal dialysis patients. Clin Nephrol 13:255, 1980.

102. Gehr M, Chopra S, Chung T, et al: Polyarteritis nodosa

103. Ghose M, Sampliner J, Roza O: Spontaneous colonic perforation: A complication in a hemodialysis patient. JAMA 214:145, 1970.

104. Gibson PE: Antigen and antibody in outbreaks of hepatitis B in two renal dialysis units. J Clin Pathol 30:717, 1977.

105. Gilboa N, Largent J, Urizar R: Acute pancreatitis in an anephric child maintained in chronic hemodialysis. Int J Pediatr Nephrol 1:64, 1980.

106. Gmelin K, Ehrlich B, Kommerel B, et al: Viral hepatitis A and B in hemodialysed patients. Klin Wochenschr 58:365, 1980.

107. Gokal R, Milland P, Weatherall D, et al: Iron metabolism in haemodialysis patients. Q J Med 191:369, 1979.

108. Goldman R: Colon perforation in polycystic kidney disease. JAMA 233:137, 1975.

109. Goldsmith HJ: Viral hepatitis in dialysis units. Nephron 12:355, 1974.

110. Goldstein H, Murphy D, Sokol A, et al: Gastric acid secretion in patients undergoing chronic dialysis. Arch Intern Med 120:645, 1967.

111. Goodship THJ, Heaton A, Todger RSC, et al: Factors affecting development of peritonitis in continuous ambulatory peritoneal dialysis. Br Med J 289:1485, 1984.

112. Gore RM: Acute colitis and the hemolytic-uremic syndrome. American Society of Colon and Rectal Surgeons 25:589, 1982.

113. Gossman HH, Baltzer G, Helms H: Calciumstoffwechsel bei chronischer neireninsuffizienz. Klin Wochenschr 46:497, 1968.

114. Griffin PJA, Salaman JR, Lawrie BW: Mid-duodenal bleeding in chronic renal failure. Br Med J 1:1606, 1979.

115. Grossman SB, Yap SH, Shafritz DA: Influence of chronic renal failure on protein synthesis and albumin metabolism in rat liver. J Clin Invest 59:869, 1977.

116. Guice K, Rattazzi LC, Marchioro TL: Colon perforation in renal transplant patients. Am J Surg 138:43, 1979.

117. Gulyassy PF, Peters JH, Lin SC, et al: Hemodialysis and plasma amino acid composition in chronic renal failure. Am J Clin Nutr 21:565, 1968.

118. Gulyassy PF, de Torrente A: Tryptophan metabolism in uremia. Kidney International 7(Suppl 3):311, 1975.

119. Gutch CF, Mahony JF, Pingerra W, et al: Refractory ascites in chronic dialysis patients. Clin Nephrol 2:59, 1974.

120. Guttmann, RD: Renal transplantation. N Engl J Med 301:1038, 1979.

121. Hadjiyannakis EJ, Evans DB, Smellie DAB, et al: Gastrointestinal complications after renal transplantation. Lancet 2:781, 1971.

122. Haverback BJ, Dyce B, Bundy H, et al: Trypsin, trypsinogen and trypsin inhibitor in human pancreatic juice. Mechanism for pancreatitis associated with hyperparathyroidism. Am J Med 29:424, 1960.

123. Hillis WD, Hillis A, Walter WG: Hepatitis B surface antigenemia in renal transplant recipients. Increased mortality risk. JAMA 243:329, 1979.

124. Hricik D, Hussain R: Pancytopenia and hepatosplenomegaly in oxalosis Arch Intern Med 144:167, 1984.

125. Hubbard SG, Bivins BS, Lucas BA, et al: Acute abdomen in the transplant patients. Am Surg 46:116, 1980.

126. Huertas VE, Rosenzweig J, Weller JM: Starch peritonitis following peritoneal dialysis. Nephron 30:82, 1982.

127. Huges-Law G, DeGast GC, Houwen B, et al: Phytohemagglutinin-induced lymphocyte cytotoxicity in hemodialysis patients with hepatitis B virus infection. Hepato-Gastroenterol 28:93, 1981.

128. Hussey HH: Nephrogenous ascites. HAMA 229:1214, 1974.
129. Ing TS, Daugirdas JT, Popli S, et al: Treatment of refractory hemodialysis ascites with maintenance peritoneal dialysis. Clin Nephrol 15:198, 1981.
130. Ivey KJ, Clifton JA: Liver disease in patients treated with chronic hemodialysis. Gastroenterology 59:630, 1970.
131. Iwamura K, Itakura M: A case of polycystic disease of the liver and the kidney associated with cerebral aneurysm and fulminant hepatitis. Tokai J Exp Clin Med 5:339, 1980.
132. Jaffe RH, Laing DR: Changes of the digestive tract in uremia. A pathologic anatomic study. Arch Intern Med 53:851, 1934.
133. Johnson WC, Nabseth DC: Pancreatitis in renal transplantation. Ann Surg 171:309, 1970.
134. Jorkasky D, Goldfarb S: Abdominal wall hernia complicating chronic ambulatory peritoneal dialysis. Am J Nephrol 2:323, 1982.
135. Julien P, Goldberg H, Margulis A, et al: Gastrointestinal complications following renal transplantation. Diagnostic Radiology 117:37, 1975.
136. Kaiser L, Kelly T, Patterson M, et al: Hepatitis B surface antigen in urine of renal transplant recipients. Ann Intern Med 94:783, 1981.
137. Kazatchkine M, Sultan Y, Caen JP, et al: Bleeding in renal failure: a possible cause. Br Med J 2:612, 1976.
138. Kelly TJ, Patterson M, Hourani M, et al: Antibody to hepatitis A among Michigan hemodialysis patients. Proc Clin Dial Transplant Forum 9:174, 1979.
139. Kelly TJ, Sanchez T, Patterson M, et al: Hepatitis B markers among dialysis patients without hepatitis B surface antigen or antibody. Proc Clin Dial Transplant Forum 10:165, 1980.
140. Kerr C, Perfect J, Craven P, et al: Fungal peritonitis in patients in continuous ambulatory peritoneal dialysis. Ann Intern Med 99:334, 1983.
141. Kerr D, Okonkwo S, Choa A: Congenital hepatic fibrosis: The long-term prognosis. Gut 19:514, 1978.
142. Kerr DNS, Harrison CV, Sherlock S, et al: Congenital hepatic fibrosis. Q J Med 30:91, 1961.
143. Kessner DM, Epstein FH: The effect of uremia on the gastrointestinal transport of calcium. Clin Res 11:245, 1963.
144. Kiddy K, Brown P, Michael J, et al: Comparison of erythromycin and isoniazid in treatment of adverse reactions to BCG vaccination. Br Med J 290:969, 1985.
145. Kirkman RL, Strom TB, Weir MR, et al: Late mortality and morbidity in recipients of long-term renal allografts. Transplantation 34:347, 1982.
146. Kirks D: The radiology of enteritis due to hemolytic-uremic syndrome. Pediatr Radiol 12:179, 1982.
147. Kleinknecht D, Jungers P, Chanard J, et al: Uremic and non-uremic complications in acute renal failure: Evaluation of early and frequent dialysis on prognosis. Kidney Int 1:190, 1972.
148. Korman MG, Laver MC, Hansky J: Hypergastrinaemia in chronic renal failure. Br Med J 1:209, 1972.
149. Kothari J, Swamy A, Lee J, et al: Hepatic hemosiderosis in maintenance hemodialysis (MHD) patients. Dig Dis Sci 25:363, 1980.
150. Krempien B, Bommer J, Ritz D: Foreign body giant cell reaction in lungs, liver and spleen. A complication of long-term hemodialysis. Virchows Arch [A] Pathol Anal Histol 392:73, 1981.
151. Kumar R, Moretti LB, Jacobi K, et al: Hemorrhagic cytomegalovirus colitis in a patient with uremia. Tex Med 79:46, 1983.
152. Kunin CM: A guide to use of antibiotics in patients with renal disease. A table of recommended doses of factors governing serum levels. Ann Intern Med 67:151, 1967.
153. Kuo G, Choo Q-L, Alter HJ, et al: An assay for circulating antibodies to a major etiologic virus of human non-A, non-B hepatitis. Science 244:362, 1989.
154. LaQuaglia M, Tolkoff-Rubin N, Dienstag J, et al: Impact of hepatitis on renal transplantation. Transplantation 32:504, 181.
155. Last MD, Lavery IC: Major hemorrhage and perforation due to a solitary cecal ulcer in a patient with end-stage renal failure. Dis Col Rect 26:495, 1983.
156. Lathrop DB: Cystic disease of the liver and kidney. Pediatrics 24:215, 1959.
157. Lawson DH, Boddy K, King PC, et al: Iron metabolism in patients with chronic renal failure on regular dialysis treatment. Clin Sci 41:345, 1971.
158. Lelie P, Reesink H, Th. deJong-van Manen S, et al: Immune response to a heat-inactivated hepatitis B vaccine in patients undergoing hemodialysis. Arch Intern Med 145:305, 1985.
159. Leong A: Silicone—a possible iatrogenic cause of hepatic dysfunction in hemodialysis patients. Pathology 15:193, 1983.
160. Leong A, Path M, Disney A, et al: Spallation and migration of silicone from blood-pump tubing in patients on hemodialysis. N Engl J Med 306:135, 1982.
161. LeRoith D, Vinik AI, Epstein S, et al: Somatostatin and serum gastrin in normal subjects and in patients with pernicious anemia, chronic liver and renal disease. S Afr Med J 49:1601, 1975.
162. Levin M, Barratt T: Haemolytic uraemic syndrome. Arch Dis Child 59:397, 1984.
163. Levy M, Kleinknecht C: Membranous glomerulonephritis and hepatitis B virus infection. Nephron 26:259, 1980.
164. Lewicki AM, Saito S, Merrill JP: Gastrointestinal bleeding in the renal transplant patient. Radiology 102:533, 1972.
165. Lewis JW, Mason EE, Jochimsen PR: Vascular malformations of the stomach and duodenum. Surg Gynecol Obstet 153:225, 1981.
166. Lewis TD, Laufer I, Goodacre TL: Arteriovenous malformation of the stomach. Dig Dis 23:467, 1978.
167. Lieber CS, LeFevre A: Ammonia as a source of gastric hypoacidity in patients with uremia. J Clin Invest 38:1271, 1959.
168. Lipschutz DE, Easterling RE: Spontaneous perforation of the colon in chronic renal failure. Arch Intern Med 132:758, 1973.
169. London WT, Drew J: Sex differences in response to hepatitis B infection among patients receiving chronic dialysis treatment. Proc Natl Acad Sci USA 74:2561, 1977.
170. London WT, DiFiglia M, Sutnick AI, et al: An epidemic of hepatitis in a chronic-haemodialysis unit. Australia antigen and differences in host response. N Engl J Med 281:571, 1969.
171. London WT, Drew J, Lustbader E, et al: Host response to hepatitis B infection in patients in a chronic hemodialysis unit. Kidney International 12:51, 1977.
172. Luciani L, Gentile M, Scarduelli B, et al: Myxoedema coma induced by beta-adrenoreceptor-blocking agent. Br Med J 285:543, 1982.
173. Lunding M, Steiness I, Thaysen JH: Acute renal failure due to tubular necrosis: Immediate prognosis and complications. Acta Med Scand 176:103, 1964.
174. Madden M, Beirne G, Zimmerman S, et al: Acute bowel obstruction: An unusual complication of chronic peritoneal dialysis. Am J Kidney Dis, 1:219, 1982.

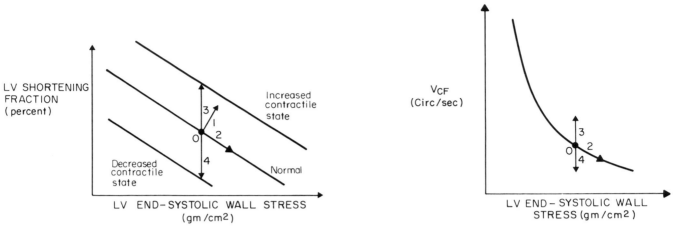

Fig. 32-4. Left panel. *Effect of several interventions on end-systolic stress-shortening relation of the left ventricle (LV). Changes in preload, unless extreme (1), have little effect on this relation. Increased afterload (2) leads to diminished LV shortening. Depression (4) or increase (3) in myocardial contractile state at a given afterload also affects LV shortening fraction.* Right panel. *Effect of several interventions on the end-systolic stress–VCF relation of the left ventricle. Preload changes have very little effect on this relation. Increased afterload (2) leads to diminished VCF. Depression (4) or increase (3) in myocardial contractile state at a given afterload also affects VCF.*

Hyperphosphatemia also occurs in ESRD and further lowers the serum calcium level by causing complexing of calcium and phosphate. Although calcium deposition (metastatic calcification) in adult ESRD patients occurs in blood vessels [26,155], the conduction system of the heart [80,155], the myocardium [10,26,80,155], and the mitral valve annulus and leaflets [42,120], its occurrence in the pediatric age group has not been reported. Calcification of the conduction system results most often in atrioventricular block. Restriction of dietary phosphate and use of phosphate-binding gels are helpful in reducing serum phosphate level; in order to avoid complexing calcium and phosphate, reduction of serum phosphate should precede the administration of calcium supplements or 1,25-dihydroxy vitamin D_3.

Acidemia [142], due to impaired ammonium excretion, has a direct negative effect on inotropic state [167] by blocking calcium influx through slow calcium channels [22].

HYPERMAGNESEMIA

Hypermagnesemia occurs commonly in ESRD [133], due to diminished excretion [32], and can be exacerbated by the ingestion of magnesium-containing antacids. Reports on whether the elevated serum magnesium reflects increased muscle content of this ion are conflicting [27,105]. Excess magnesium inhibits calcium-triggered calcium release [50]. The effects of hypermagnesemia on contractile state in vivo are probably not significant, provided that the calcium level is normal [27].

CARNITINE DEFICIENCY

Whether carnitine deficiency occurs in ESRD by itself [141] or whether it is merely a sequela of dialysis [16,17] is

controversial. Carnitine is a low-weight molecule that transports long-chain fatty acids into mitochondria, where they are oxidized to carbon dioxide and water. That systemic carnitine deficiency can present as cardiomyopathy [158] is not surprising, because under aerobic conditions, the heart's preferred substrate is long-chain fatty acids. Concomitant with a rise in free fatty acid levels [13], plasma carnitine level drops during hemodialysis [16,17]; it increases after dialysis, presumably by transfer from tissue stores. Plasma levels [3], skeletal (and presumably cardiac) muscle stores [3], and skeletal muscle performance [4] can be increased by oral administration of carnitine.

IRON OVERLOAD

Iron overload occurs in patients with ESRD as a result of blood transfusion therapy to correct the anemia of chronic renal failure. Perhaps this complication will be avoided by the use of recombinant erythropoietin. Iron deposition in the myocardium has been recognized in other conditions requiring transfusion therapy such as thalassemia major, and abnormalities in contractility have been detected noninvasively [21]. Whether reduction of body iron stores with iron-chelating agents [11] halts or reverses myocardial iron deposition remains to be seen.

UREMIC TOXINS

Finally, the existence of "uremic toxins" that directly reduce left ventricular contractility has been proposed. Most human studies have been inconclusive because they have used only *load-dependent* indices of contractile state such as systolic time intervals [103], shortening fraction [103], ejection fraction [28], and dp/dt [28]. Studies of the intact animal [121,145] or isolated animal heart [128,146] have also used load-dependent indices such as peak (dp/dt).

128. Hussey HH: Nephrogenous ascites. *HAMA* 229:1214, 1974.

129. Ing TS, Daugirdas JT, Popli S, et al: Treatment of refractory hemodialysis ascites with maintenance peritoneal dialysis. *Clin Nephrol* 15:198, 1981.

130. Ivey KJ, Clifton JA: Liver disease in patients treated with chronic hemodialysis. *Gastroenterology* 59:630, 1970.

131. Iwamura K, Itakura M: A case of polycystic disease of the liver and the kidney associated with cerebral aneurysm and fulminant hepatitis. *Tokai J Exp Clin Med* 5:339, 1980.

132. Jaffe RH, Laing DR: Changes of the digestive tract in uremia. A pathologic anatomic study. *Arch Intern Med* 53:851, 1934.

133. Johnson WC, Nabseth DC: Pancreatitis in renal transplantation. *Ann Surg* 171:309, 1970.

134. Jorkasky D, Goldfarb S: Abdominal wall hernia complicating chronic ambulatory peritoneal dialysis. *Am J Nephrol* 2:323, 1982.

135. Julien P, Goldberg H, Margulis A, et al: Gastrointestinal complications following renal transplantation. *Diagnostic Radiology* 117:37, 1975.

136. Kaiser L, Kelly T, Patterson M, et al: Hepatitis B surface antigen in urine of renal transplant recipients. *Ann Intern Med* 94:783, 1981.

137. Kazatchkine M, Sultan Y, Caen JP, et al: Bleeding in renal failure: a possible cause. *Br Med J* 2:612, 1976.

138. Kelly TJ, Patterson M, Hourani M, et al: Antibody to hepatitis A among Michigan hemodialysis patients. *Proc Clin Dial Transplant Forum* 9:174, 1979.

139. Kelly TJ, Sanchez T, Patterson M, et al: Hepatitis B markers among dialysis patients without hepatitis B surface antigen or antibody. *Proc Clin Dial Transplant Forum* 10:165, 1980.

140. Kerr C, Perfect J, Craven P, et al: Fungal peritonitis in patients in continuous ambulatory peritoneal dialysis. *Ann Intern Med* 99:334, 1983.

141. Kerr D, Okonkwo S, Choa A: Congenital hepatic fibrosis: The long-term prognosis. *Gut* 19:514, 1978.

142. Kerr DNS, Harrison CV, Sherlock S, et al: Congenital hepatic fibrosis. *Q J Med* 30:91, 1961.

143. Kessner DM, Epstein FH: The effect of uremia on the gastrointestinal transport of calcium. *Clin Res* 11:245, 1963.

144. Kiddy K, Brown P, Michael J, et al: Comparison of erythromycin and isoniazid in treatment of adverse reactions to BCG vaccination. *Br Med J* 290:969, 1985.

145. Kirkman RL, Strom TB, Weir MR, et al: Late mortality and morbidity in recipients of long-term renal allografts. *Transplantation* 34:347, 1982.

146. Kirks D: The radiology of enteritis due to hemolytic-uremic syndrome. *Pediatr Radiol* 12:179, 1982.

147. Kleinknecht D, Jungers P, Chanard J, et al: Uremic and non-uremic complications in acute renal failure: Evaluation of early and frequent dialysis on prognosis. *Kidney Int* 1:190, 1972.

148. Korman MG, Laver MC, Hansky J: Hypergastrinaemia in chronic renal failure. *Br Med J* 1:209, 1972.

149. Kothari J, Swamy A, Lee J, et al: Hepatic hemosiderosis in maintenance hemodialysis (MHD) patients. *Dig Dis Sci* 25:363, 1980.

150. Krempien B, Bommer J, Ritz D: Foreign body giant cell reaction in lungs, liver and spleen. A complication of long-term hemodialysis. *Virchows Arch [A] Pathol Anal Histol* 392:73, 1981.

151. Kumar R, Moretti LB, Jacobi K, et al: Hemorrhagic cytomegalovirus colitis in a patient with uremia. *Tex Med* 79:46, 1983.

152. Kunin CM: A guide to use of antibiotics in patients with renal disease. A table of recommended doses of factors governing serum levels. *Ann Intern Med* 67:151, 1967.

153. Kuo G, Choo Q-L, Alter HJ, et al: An assay for circulating antibodies to a major etiologic virus of human non-A, non-B hepatitis. *Science* 244:362, 1989.

154. LaQuaglia M, Tolkoff-Rubin N, Dienstag J, et al: Impact of hepatitis on renal transplantation. *Transplantation* 32:504, 181.

155. Last MD, Lavery IC: Major hemorrhage and perforation due to a solitary cecal ulcer in a patient with end-stage renal failure. *Dis Col Rect* 26:495, 1983.

156. Lathrop DB: Cystic disease of the liver and kidney. *Pediatrics* 24:215, 1959.

157. Lawson DH, Boddy K, King PC, et al: Iron metabolism in patients with chronic renal failure on regular dialysis treatment. *Clin Sci* 41:345, 1971.

158. Lelie P, Reesink H, Th. deJong-van Manen S, et al: Immune response to a heat-inactivated hepatitis B vaccine in patients undergoing hemodialysis. *Arch Intern Med* 145:305, 1985.

159. Leong A: Silicone—a possible iatrogenic cause of hepatic dysfunction in hemodialysis patients. *Pathology* 15:193, 1983.

160. Leong A, Path M, Disney A, et al: Spallation and migration of silicone from blood-pump tubing in patients on hemodialysis. *N Engl J Med* 306:135, 1982.

161. LeRoith D, Vinik AI, Epstein S, et al: Somatostatin and serum gastrin in normal subjects and in patients with pernicious anemia, chronic liver and renal disease. *S Afr Med J* 49:1601, 1975.

162. Levin M, Barratt T: Haemolytic uraemic syndrome. *Arch Dis Child* 59:397, 1984.

163. Levy M, Kleinknecht C: Membranous glomerulonephritis and hepatitis B virus infection. *Nephron* 26:259, 1980.

164. Lewicki AM, Saito S, Merrill JP: Gastrointestinal bleeding in the renal transplant patient. *Radiology* 102:533, 1972.

165. Lewis JW, Mason EE, Jochimsen PR: Vascular malformations of the stomach and duodenum. *Surg Gynecol Obstet* 153:225, 1981.

166. Lewis TD, Laufer I, Goodacre TL: Arteriovenous malformation of the stomach. *Dig Dis* 23:467, 1978.

167. Lieber CS, LeFevre A: Ammonia as a source of gastric hypoacidity in patients with uremia. *J Clin Invest* 38:1271, 1959.

168. Lipschutz DE, Easterling RE: Spontaneous perforation of the colon in chronic renal failure. *Arch Intern Med* 132:758, 1973.

169. London WT, Drew J: Sex differences in response to hepatitis B infection among patients receiving chronic dialysis treatment. *Proc Natl Acad Sci USA* 74:2561, 1977.

170. London WT, DiFiglia M, Sutnick AI, et al: An epidemic of hepatitis in a chronic-haemodialysis unit. Australia antigen and differences in host response. *N Engl J Med* 281:571, 1969.

171. London WT, Drew J, Lustbader E, et al: Host response to hepatitis B infection in patients in a chronic hemodialysis unit. *Kidney International* 12:51, 1977.

172. Luciani L, Gentile M, Scarduelli B, et al: Myxoedema coma induced by beta-adrenoreceptor-blocking agent. *Br Med J* 285:543, 1982.

173. Lunding M, Steiness I, Thaysen JH: Acute renal failure due to tubular necrosis: Immediate prognosis and complications. *Acta Med Scand* 176:103, 1964.

174. Madden M, Beirne G, Zimmerman S, et al: Acute bowel obstruction: An unusual complication of chronic peritoneal dialysis. *Am J Kidney Dis*, 1:219, 1982.

175. Mall JC, Gharhremani GG, Boyer JL: Caroli's disease associated with congenital hepatic fibrosis and renal tubular ectasia. *Gastroenterology* 66:1029, 1974.

176. Maggiore G, Martini A, Grifeo S, et al: Hepatitis B virus infection and Schönlein-Henoch purpura. *Am J Dis Child* 138:681, 1984.

177. Margolis D, Saylor J, Geisse G, et al: Upper gastrointestinal disease in chronic renal failure. *Arch Intern Med* 138:1214, 1978.

178. Marubbio AT, Danielson G: Hepatic veno-occlusive disease in a renal transplant patient receiving azathioprine. *Gastroenterology* 69:739, 1975.

179. Mason E: Gastrointestinal lesions occurring in uremia. *Ann Intern Med* 37:96, 1952.

180. Matas AJ, Simmons RL, Kjellstrand CM, et al: Increased incidence of malignancy during chronic renal failure. *Lancet* 1:883, 1975.

181. Mattenheimer R, Friedel F, Schwartz F: (abstracts of papers).

182. Mayor G, Klein A, Kelly T, et al: Antibody to hepatitis A and hemodialysis. *Am J Epidemiol* 116:821, 1982.

183. McCarthy LJ, Baggenstoss AH, Logan GB: Congenital hepatic fibrosis. *Gastroenterology* 49:27, 1965.

184. McDermott FT, Galbraith AJ, Corlett RJ: Inhibition of cell proliferation in renal failure and its significance to the uremic syndrome: A review. *Scott Med J* 20:317, 1975.

185. McDermott FT, Galbraith AJ, Dalton MK: Effects of acute renal failure on ileal epithelial cell kinetics: Autoradiographic studies in the mouse. *Gastroenterology* 66:235, 1974.

186. McDermott FT, Nayman J, DeBoer WGRM: Effect of acute renal failure upon cell division on the jejunum: Radioautographic and ultrastructural studies in the mouse. *Ann Surg* 174:274, 1971.

187. McGonigle R, Mowat A, Bewick M, et al: Congenital hepatic fibrosis and polycystic kidney disease; role of portacaval shunting and transplantation in three patients. *Q J Med* 50:269, 1981.

188. McIntosh DA, Peterson EW, McPhaul JJ Jr: Autonomy of parathyroid function after renal homotransplantation. *Ann Intern Med* 65:900, 1966.

189. McLeod L, Mandin H, Davidman M, et al: Intermittent hemodialysis in terminal chronic renal failure. *Can Med Assoc J* 94:318, 1966.

190. Meshkinpour H, Vaziri N, Gordon N: Gastrointestinal pathology in patients with chronic renal failure associated with spinal cord injury. *Am J Gastroenterol* 77:562, 1982.

191. Meyer CT, Troncale FJ, Galloway S, et al: Arteriovenous malformations of the bowel: An analysis of 22 cases and a review of the literature. *Medicine* 60:36, 1981.

192. Meyers W, Harris N, Stein S, et al: Alimentary tract complications after renal transplantation. *Ann Surg* 190:535, 1979.

193. Miach PJ, Dawborn JK, Zipell J: Neoplasia in patients with chronic renal failure on long-term dialysis. *Clin Nephrol* 5:101, 1976.

194. Milito G, Taccone-Gallucci M, Brancaleone F, et al: Assessment of upper gastrointestinal tract in hemodialysis patients awaiting renal transplantation. *Am J Gastroenterol* 78:328, 1983.

195. Miller D, Williams A, LeBouvier G, et al: Hepatitis B in hemodialysis patients: Significance of HBeAg. *Gastroenterology* 74:1208, 1978.

196. Miller J, Kyriakides G, Ma KW, et al: Factors influencing mortality of renal transplantation in a high risk population. *Surg Gynecol Obstet* 140:1, 1975.

197. Mills B, Zuckerman G, Sicard G: Discrete colon ulcers as a cause of lower gastrointestinal bleeding and perforation in end-stage renal disease. *Surgery* 89:548, 1981.

198. Moore TC, Hume DM: The period and nature of hazard in clinical renal transplantation. II. The hazard to transplant kidney function. *Ann Surg* 170:12, 1969.

199. Moorthy A, Chesney R: Peptic ulcer in uremic children. *J Pediatr* 92:420, 1978.

200. Moschowitz E: Non-parasitic cysts (congenital) of the liver, with a study of aberrant bile ducts. *Am J Soc Med* 31:674, 1906.

201. Mozes M, Ascher N, Balfour H, et al: Jaundice after renal allotransplantation. *Ann Surg* 188:783, 1977.

202. Mujahed Z, Glenn F, Evans JA: Communicating cavernous ectasia of the intrahepatic ducts (Caroli's disease). *Am J Roentgenol Radium Ther Nucl Med* 113:21, 1971.

203. Muolo A, Ghidini O, Ancona G, et al: Gastroduodenal mucosal changes, gastric acid secretion, and gastrin levels following successful kidney transplantation. *Transplantation Proceedings* 11:1277, 1979.

204. Murray-Lyon IM, Shilkin KB, Laws JW, et al: Non-obstructive dilatation of intrahepatic biliary tree with cholangitis. *Q J Med* 41:477, 1972.

205. Najem G, Louria D, Thind I, et al: Control of hepatitis B infection. *JAMA* 245:153, 1981.

206. Nakanuma Y, Terada T, Ohta G, et al: Caroli's disease in congenital hepatic fibrosis and infantile polycystic disease. *Liver* 2:346, 1982.

207. Nakayama M, Shinob T, Nakamura K, et al: Experience of 26 acute renal failure cases. *Tokai J Exp Clin Med* 7:101, 1982.

208. Neergard J, Nielsen B, Faurby V, et al: Plasticizers in PVC and the occurrence of hepatitis in a haemodialysis unit. *Scand J Urol Nephrol* 5:141, 1971.

209. Neergaard J, Nielsen B, Faurby V, et al: On the exudation of plasticizers from PVC haemodialysis tubings. *Nephron* 14:263, 1975.

210. Nielsen V, Clausen E, Ranek L: Liver impairment during chronic hemodialysis and after renal transplantation. *Acta Med Scand* 197:229, 1975.

211. Noland E: Acute renal failure and hepatitis in infectious mononucleosis. *Va Med* 107:563, 1980.

212. Ogg CS: The intestinal absorption of ^{47}Ca by patients in chronic renal failure. *Clin Sci* 34:467, 1968.

213. Oppenheimer GD: Polycystic disease of the kidney. *Ann Surg* 100:1136, 1934.

214. Ortuno J, Teruel J, Marcen R, et al: Primary intestinal tuberculosis following renal transplantation. *Nephron* 31:59, 1982.

215. Owens M, Passaro E, Wilson S, et al: Treatment of peptic ulcer disease in the renal transplant patient. *Ann Surg* 186:17, 1977.

216. Owens M, Wilson S, Saltzman R, et al: Gastrointestinal complications after renal transplantation. *Arch Surg* 111:467, 1976.

217. Owyang C, Miller LJ, DiMango EP, et al: Gastrointestinal hormone profile in renal insufficiency. *Mayo Clin Proc* 54:769, 1979.

218. Papper S: Hepatorenal syndrome. *Contrib Nephrol* 23:55, 1980.

219. Paus P, Larsen E, Sodal G, et al: Pancreatic affection after acute hypotonic hemodialysis. *Acta Med Scand* 212:83, 1982.

220. Pear B: Radiologic recognition of extrahepatic manifestations of hepatitis B antigenemia *AJR* 137:135, 1981.

221. Pendras JP, Erickson RV: Hemodialysis: A successful therapy for chronic uremia. *Ann Intern Med* 64:293, 1966.

222. Pineau M: Des hemorrhagies gastro-intestinales d'origine

uremique. These de Paris, 1899. (Cited by Jaffe and Laing, ref 132.)

223. Pitts T, Barbour G: Hemosiderosis secondary to chronic parenteral iron therapy in maintenance hemodialysis patients. Nephron 22:316, 1978.

224. Pol S, Debure A, Degott C, et al: Chronic hepatitis in kidney allograft recipients. Lancet 1:878, 1990.

225. Polinsky MS, Wolfson BJ, Gruskin AB, et al: Development of pneumatosis cystoides intestinalis following transplantation in a child. Am J Kidney Dis 111:414, 1984.

226. Powell D, Luis E, Calvin S, et al: Peritonitis in children undergoing continuous ambulatory peritoneal dialysis. Am J Dis Child 139:29, 1985.

227. Powell H, McCredie D, Taylor C, et al: Vitamin E treatment of haemolytic uraemic syndrome. Arch Dis Child 59:401, 1984.

228. Prince AM, Szmuness W, Mann WK, et al: Hepatitis B "immune" globulin: Effectivenss in prevention of dialysis-associated hepatitis. N Engl J Med 293:1063, 1975.

229. Prompt C, Lee D, Upham A, et al: Medical complications of renal transplantation. Urology 9(Suppl 6):32, 1977.

230. Public Health Laboratory Service Survey. Hepatitis B in retreat from dialysis units in United Kingdom in 1973. Br Med J 1:1579, 1976.

231. Rall JE, Odell HM: Congenital polycystic disease of the kidneys: Review of the literature and data on 207 cases. Am J Med Sci 218:399, 1949.

232. Rashid A, Sengar D, McLeisch W, et al: The effect of host immunity on hepatitis B antigen (HBAg) infection in hemodialysis patients. Trans Am Soc Artif Intern Organs 21:483, 1975.

233a. Rashid H, Morley AR, Ward MK, et al: Hepatitis B infection in glomerulonephritis. Br Med J 283:948, 1981.

233b. Rembold C, Krumlovsky F, Roxe D, et al: Treatment of hemodialysis hemosiderosis with desferrioxamine. Trans Am Soc Artif Intern Organs 28:621, 1982.

234. Richet G, Fabre J, DeFreundenreich J, et al: Drug intoxication and neurological episodes in chronic renal failure. Br Med J 1:394, 1970.

235. Rodriguez HJ, Walls J, Slatopolsky E, et al: Recurrent ascites following peritoneal dialysis. A new syndrome? Arch Intern Med 134:283, 1974.

236. Roggendorf M, Deinhardt F, Rasshofer R, et al: Antibodies to hepatitis C virus. Lancet 2:324, 1989.

237. Roguska J, Simon NM, Del Greco F, et al: Ten-year experience with maintenance hemodialysis for chronic uremia. Trans Am Soc Artif Intern Organs 20:579, 1974.

238. Rosenblatt SG, Drake S, Fadem S, et al: Gastrointestinal blood loss in patients with chronic renal failure. Am J Kidney Dis 1:232, 1982.

239. Rotter W, Roettger P: Comparative pathologic-anatomic study of cases of chronic global renal insufficiency with and without preceding hemodialysis. Clin Nephrol 1:257, 1973.

240. Rubenstein R, Lantz J, Stevens K, et al: Uremic ileus. NY State J Med 79:248, 1979.

241. Rubin J, Raju S, Teal N, et al: Abdominal hernia in patients undergoing continuous ambulatory peritoneal dialysis. Arch Intern Med 142:1453, 1982.

242. Rubin J, Ray R, Barnes T, et al: Peritoneal abnormalities during infectious episodes of continuous ambulatory peritoneal dialysis. Nephron 29:124, 1981.

243. Ryabov SI, Ryss ES, Prochukhanov RA, et al: Present day concepts on gastric pathology in patients with chronic renal failure. Int Urol Nephrol 12:189, 1980.

244. Sachs E, Pharm D, Hurwitz F, et al: Pancreatic exocrine hypofunction in the wasting syndrome of end-stage renal disease. Am J Gastroenterol 78:170, 1983.

245. Salo R, Salo A, Fahlberg W, et al: Hepatitis B surface antigen (HBsAg) in peritoneal fluid of HBsAg carriers undergoing peritoneal dialysis. J Med Virol 6:29, 1980.

246. Saris A, Clearfield H, Dinoso V, et al: Secretory, hormonal and enzymatic profile of renal patients. Gastroenterology 80:1270, 1981.

247. Sawyerr O, Garvin P, Codd J, et al: Colorectal complications of renal allograft transplantation. Arch Surg 113:84, 1978.

248. Scheff RT, Zuckerman G, Harter H, et al: Diverticular disease in patients with chronic renal failure due to polycystic kidney disease. Ann Intern Med 92:202, 1980.

249. Schiessel R, Starlinger M, Wolf A, et al: Failure of cimetidine to prevent gastroduodenal ulceration and bleeding after renal transplantation. Gastroenterology 80:1275, 1981.

250. Schnyder P, Brasch R, Salvatierra O: Gstrointestinal complications of renal transplantation in children. Pediatr Radiol 130:361, 1979.

251. Shafritz DA, Grossman SB, Yap SH: Influence of chronic uremia on hepatic protein synthesis (abstr). Gastroenterology 781:929, 1976.

252. Shalhoub RJ, Rajan U, Kim VV, et al: Erythrocytosis in patients on long-term hemodialysis. Ann Intern Med 97:686, 1982.

253. Shepherd AMM, Steward WK, Wormsley KG: Peptic ulceration in chronic renal failure. Lancet 1:1357, 1973.

254. Sherlock S: Cysts and congenital biliary abnormalities. In Sherlock S (ed): Diseases of the Liver and Biliary System, 7th ed. Boston, Blackwell Scientific Publications, 1985, p 429.

255. Singh S, Mitra S, Berman LB: Ascites in patients on maintenance hemodialysis. Nephron 12:114, 1974.

256. Shons AR, Simmons RL, Kjellstrand CM, et al: Renal transplantation in patients with Australia antigenemia. Am J Surg 128:699, 1974.

257. Siegler R, Eggert J, Udomkesmalee E: Diagnostic indices of zinc deficiency in children with renal diseases. Ann Clin Lab Sci 11:428, 1981.

258. Simon N, Mery J, Trepo C, et al: A non-A non-B hepatitis epidemic in a HB antigen free haemodialysis unit. Demonstration of serological markers of non-A non-B virus. Proc EDTA 17:173, 1980.

259. Skinhoj P, Steiness I: Radioimmunoassay of hepatitis B antigen and antibody in dialysis and transplant patients. Acta Path Microbiol Scand 83:125, 1975.

260. Slingeneyer A, Mion C, Beraud J, et al: Peritonitis, a frequently lethal complication of intermittent and continuous ambulatory peritoneal dialysis. Proc EDTA 18:212, 1981.

261. Smith C, Schuster S, Gruppe W, et al: Hemolytic-uremic syndrome: A diagnostic and therapeutic dilemma for the surgeon. J Pediatr Surg 13:597, 1978.

262. Snydman DR, Bryan JA, Dixon RE: Prevention of nosocomial viral hepatitis, type B (hepatitis B). Ann Intern Med 83:838, 1975.

263. Sokol A, Gral T, Edelbaum DN, et al: Correlation of autopsy findings and clinical experience in chronically dialysed patients. Trans Am Soc Artif Intern Organs 13:51, 1967.

264. Spanos PK, Simmons RL, Rattazzi LC, et al: Peptic ulcer disease in the transplant recipient. Arch Surg 109:193, 1974.

265. Stephens FO: The syndrome of intestinal pseudo-obstruction. Br Med J 1:1248, 1962.

266. Strauss MB, Welt LG (ed): Diseases of the Kidney, 2nd ed. Boston, Little, Brown, 1971.

267. Strife C, Hug G, Chuck G, et al: Membranoproliferative glomerulonephritis and α1-antitrypsin deficiency in children. *Pediatrics* 71:88, 1983.

268. Stuart F, Reckard C, Schulak J, et al: Gastroduodenal complications in kidney transplant recipients. *Ann Surg* 194:339, 1981.

269. Sullivan SN, Tustanoff E, Slaughter DN, et al: Hypergastrinemia and gastric acid hypersecretion in uremia. *Clin Nephrol* 5:25, 1976.

270. Sutherland D, Chan F, Foucar E, et al: The bleeding cecal ulcer in transplant patients. *Surgery* 86:386, 1979.

271. Szmuness W, Prince AM, Hoffnagle JH, et al: Effectiveness of hepatitis-B immune globulin in haemodialysis patients. *Lancet* 2:1512, 1974.

272. Sztriha L, Gyurkovits K, Ormos J, et al: Congenital hepatic fibrosis with polycystic disease of the kidneys, *Hepatogastroenterology* 29:259, 1982.

273. Tani N, Harasawa S, Suzuki S, et al: Lesions of the upper gastrointestinal tract in patients with chronic renal failure. *Gastroenterology* 15:480, 1980.

274. Taylor I, Sells R, McConnell R, et al: Serum gastrin in patients with chronic renal failure. *Gut* 21:1062, 1980.

275. Thoroughman JC, Peace RJ: Abdominal surgical emergencies caused by uremic enterocolitis: Report of twelve cases. *Am Surg* 25:533, 1959.

276. Tong M, Bischel M, Scoles B, et al: T and B lymphocytes in uremic patients with type B hepatitis infection. *Nephron* 18:162, 1977.

277. Toussaint C, Dupont E, Vanherweghem J, et al: Liver disease in patients undergoing hemodialysis and kidney transplantation. *Adv Nephrol* 8:269, 1979.

278. Udani R, Desai A, Joshi A, et al: Multiple cysts in the liver and infantile polycystic disease of kidneys. *J Postgrad Med* 28:109, 1982.

279. Ulreich S, Burrell M, Lowman R: Radiology of the gastrointestinal abnormalities seen in patients with adult hepatorenal polycystic disease. *Clin Radiol* 29:547, 1978.

280. Valenzuela JE, Defilippi C: Pyloric-sphincter studies in peptic ulcer patients. Pylorus in peptic ulcer. *Amer J Digest Dis* 21:229, 1976.

281. Van Roermund H, Tiggeler R, Berden J, et al: Cimetidine prophylaxis after renal transplantation. *Clin Nephrol* 18:39, 1982.

282. Van Siegmann G, Lilly J: Surgical lesions of the colon in the hemolytic uremic syndrome. *Surgery* 85:357, 1979.

283. Ventkateswaran PS, Jeffers A, Hocken A: Gastric acid secretion in chronic renal failure. *Br Med J* 4:22, 1972.

284. Vereerstraeten P, Dupont E, D'Orchimont R, et al: Factors influencing patient and graft survivals in kidney transplantation. *Proceedings of the European Dialysis of Transplant Association* 13:134, 1976.

285. Wall L, Michael D, Linshaw A, et al: Pneumatosis intestinalis in a pediatric renal transplant patient. *J Pediatr* 101:745, 1982.

286. Walker W, Hillis W, Hillis A: Hepatitis B infection in patients with end stage renal disease: Some characteristics and consequences. *Trans Am Clin Climatol Assoc* 92:142, 1980.

287. Wang F, Pillay V, Ing T, et al: Ascites in patients treated with maintenance hemodialysis. *Nephron* 12:105, 1974.

288. Ware A, Luby J, Eigenbrodt E, et al: Spectrum of liver disease in renal transplant recipients. *Gastroenterology* 68:755, 1975.

289. Ware A, Luby J, Hollinger B, et al: Etiology of liver disease in renal-transplant patients. *Ann Intern Med* 91:364, 1979.

290. Washer G, Schroter G, Starzi T, et al: Causes of death after kidney transplantation. *JAMA* 250:49, 1983.

291. Wasnich R, Puapongsakorn R, Seto D: Significance of antibody to hepatitis B core antigen in a hemodialysis unit. *West J Med* 132:279, 1980.

292. Weaver GA, Alpern HD, Davis JS, et al: Gastrointestinal angiodysplasia associated with aortic valve disease: Part of a spectrum of angiodysplasia of the gut. *Gastroenterology* 77:1, 1979.

293. Werner B, Blumberg B: e Antigen in hepatitis B virus infected dialysis patients: Assessment of its prognostic value. *Ann Intern Med* 89:310, 1978.

294. Whitington P, Friedman A, Chesney R: Gastrointestinal disease in the hemolytic-uremic syndrome. *Gastroenterology* 76:728, 1979.

295. Wilkinson SP: The kidney and liver diseases. *J Clin Pathol* 34:1241, 1981.

296. Williams S, Huff J, Feinglass E, et al: Epidemic viral hepatitis, type B, in hospital personnel. *Am J Med* 57:904, 1974.

297. Woodring J, Fried A, Lieber A: The gallbladder in polycystic liver disease. *JAMA* 246:864, 1981.

298. Wright R, Clemente R, Wathen R: Gastric emptying in patients with chronic renal failure receiving hemodialysis. *Arch Intern Med* 144:495, 1984.

299. Wright S, Huff J, Feinglass E, et al: Epidemic viral hepatitis, type B, in hospital personnel. *Am J Med* 57:904, 1974.

300. Wyke R, Williams R: Clinical aspects of non-A, non-B hepatitis infection. *J Virol Methods* 2:17, 1980.

301. Yates R, Osterholm R: Hemolytic-uremic syndrome colitis. *J Clin Gastroenterol* 2:359, 1980.

302. Yokoyama E, Endo T, Kumano K, et al: Is hepatic dysfunction beneficial to allograft function? *Transplant Proc* 11:1279, 1979.

303. Young R, Bryk D: Colonic intussusception in uremia. *Am J Gastroenterol* 71:229, 1979.

304. Zeldis JB, Depner TA, Kuramoto IK, et al: The prevalence of hepatitis C virus antibodies among hemodialysis patients. *Ann Intern Med* 112:958, 1990.

305. Zuckerman GR, Cornette GL, Clouse RE, et al: Upper gastrointestinal bleeding in patients with chronic renal failure. *Ann Intern Med* 102:588, 1985.

ALVIN J. CHIN
WILLIAM F. FRIEDMAN

32
Cardiovascular System and Dynamics

The heart's essential function is to deliver sufficient cardiac output to satisfy the metabolic requirements of the various tissues of the body (Table 32-1). The four determinants of cardiac performance (cardiac output) are preload, afterload, contractility (inotropic state), and heart rate (chronotropic state). The distinction between cardiac performance (Fig. 32-1) and inotropic state of the myocardium, one of its determinants, is important because there are circumstances in which abnormal mechanical loading conditions imposed upon the heart may result in poor cardiac performance, even though no depression of intrinsic myocardial contractility exists. Conversely, favorable loading conditions can normalize cardiac performance in the face of a depression in the inotropic state of the myocardium. This latter concept, for example, underlies the use of vasodilator therapy for congestive heart failure.

The kidney, in addition to its excretory function, has numerous endocrine functions, including the production of many vasoactive hormones and autacoids. Chronic renal failure results in widespread disturbances of both excretory and endocrine renal function. These derangements affect the loading conditions of the heart (preload, afterload) and may also alter the inotropic state of the heart. Chronotropic state (heart rate) may or may not be directly affected by chronic renal failure and will be discussed further.

Effects of Renal Failure on Determinants of Cardiac Performance

Preload

The capacity of a cardiac muscle cell (containing many sarcomeres) to vary its force of contraction on a beat-to-beat basis as a function of its initial (end-diastolic) length is known as the Frank-Starling phenomenon [151] (Fig. 32-2). In the intact heart, ventricular end-diastolic wall stress determines the initial length (preload) of the sarcomeres. In the patient with end-stage renal disease (ESRD), the resting sarcomere length is often greatly increased by hypervolemia, which results from an impaired ability to excrete water in proportion to sodium, and frequently also

by an arteriovenous fistula or external shunt inserted to facilitate vascular access for hemodialysis. The heart's response to chronic volume overload is ventricular dilatation [140].

The signs of hypervolemia are jugular venous distension, hepatomegaly, increase in weight, peripheral edema, and increase in rate and depth of breathing from pulmonary edema.

Palliative therapy consists of (1) regulation of sodium and water intake, (2) diuretics, and (3) dialysis.

Afterload

Afterload is defined as the stress (force per unit cross-sectional area) in the ventricular wall during contraction. Determinants of afterload include compliance of the blood vessels, radius of the small arteries, and blood viscosity. Therefore, both resistance (time-invariant) and capacitance components of vascular impedance need to be taken into account.

Possible causes of the systemic arterial hypertension experienced by nearly all chronic renal failure patients include an increase in blood volume [43,51,160] and alterations in vascular impedance caused by (1) an increase in plasma renin activity (PRA) [168], triggering the production of angiotensin II, a potent vasoconstrictor; (2) an imbalance between the sympathetic and parasympathetic neural control of vascular tone; and (3) a reduction or absence of vasodilator substances, such as some of the prostaglandins [49,172]. Moreover, any one of these disturbances may have complex effects because there are interactions between these three systems—the renin-angiotensin system, the autonomic nervous system, and the prostaglandin system (discussed later).

Excessive blood volume [160] is the most common mechanism of hypertension in patients with ESRD. Reduction of plasma volume should be the cornerstone of therapy in these patients. This implies dietary sodium restriction and the administration of diuretics. In cases in which the arterial pressure remains elevated despite these measures, vasodilator agents may be used (see Chap. 24).

High-renin hypertension is much less common than vol-

Table 32-1. *Pump function versus muscle function*

Pump function (cardiac performance)
  Ability of the heart to meet the peripheral demands of organ
  perfusion
Muscle function (myocardial performance)
  Ability of the heart muscle to develop force or shorten

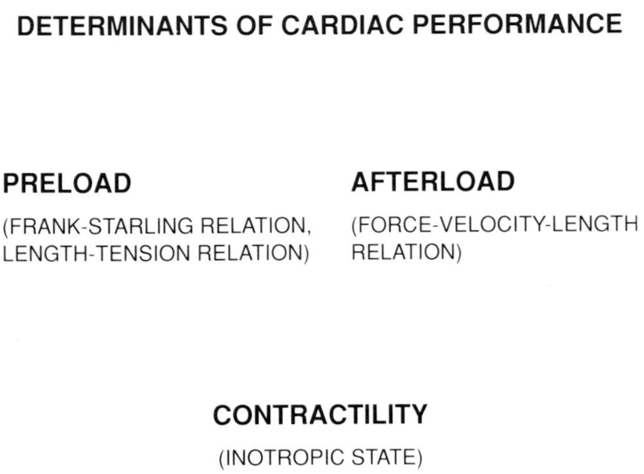

DETERMINANTS OF CARDIAC PERFORMANCE

PRELOAD

(FRANK-STARLING RELATION,
LENGTH-TENSION RELATION)

AFTERLOAD

(FORCE-VELOCITY-LENGTH
RELATION)

CONTRACTILITY

(INOTROPIC STATE)

Fig. 32-1. *Cardiac performance is assessed by measurement of cardiac output (stroke volume times heart rate). Preload, afterload, and contractility independently affect stroke volume.*

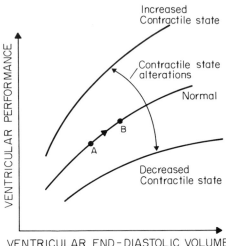

Fig. 32-2. *Within the physiologic range (normal), an increase in end-diastolic volume (preload) results in an increase in ventricular performance, characterized by moving from point A to point B. Alterations in contractile state produce a family of such ventricular performance curves.*

ume-dependent hypertension [99] and appears to occur most frequently in patients with primary arteriologlomerular disease (nephrosclerosis and glomerulonephritis) [163], in whom renal disease has apparently produced arteriolar disease analogous to the Goldblatt experimental preparation [74,160]. Captopril, which inhibits the enzymatic conversion of angiotensin I to angiotensin II, would appear to be a logical choice of therapy in high-renin hypertension [144]; however, it can produce nephrotic syndrome in patients with renal disease and can cause deterioration in glomerular filtration rate (GFR) [161]. Other medications that reduce PRA are α-methyldopa [115] and propranolol [83,106]; the latter appears to directly block intrarenal β-adrenoreceptor-controlled renin release [92,169]. The development of these drugs has virtually obviated the need for bilateral nephrectomy as a treatment for refractory hypertension in ESRD. The major disadvantage of bilateral nephrectomy is that it worsens the anemia of chronic renal failure [98] (see section on other complications).

Contractility (Inotropic State)

No question has elicited more controversy than the issue of whether ESRD has a direct effect on the inotropic state of the left ventricle. A *change in contractility* (inotropic state) is defined as a change in cardiac performance that is independent of changes in preload, afterload, and heart rate.

The effect of various factors such as hypocalcemia, hyperparathyroidism, acidemia, hypermagnesemia, carnitine deficiency, iron deposition (from transfusion therapy), "uremic toxins," or inappropriate autonomic neural activity on inotropic state can thus only be measured by using a load-independent index of contractility. For example, stroke volume, derived from calculations of left ventricular volume at end-diastole and end-systole, is by itself insufficient to characterize contractile state; in the presence of a fixed afterload and heart rate, a diminished stroke volume may reflect either a depression of contractility or a reduction in preload or both.

Ejection phase indices, such as left ventricular shortening fraction (percent dimension change) and ejection fraction, are dependent on both preload and afterload, whereas velocity of circumferential fiber shortening (VCF), although relatively insensitive to changes in preload, is still sensitive to changes in afterload. *Systolic time intervals* and *systolic ejection rate* (defined as cardiac index divided by systolic ejection time per minute) are also sensitive to both preload and afterload.

Isovolumetric phase indices such as *dp/dt* (the first derivative of left ventricular pressure with respect to time) and peak dp/dt are both afterload-sensitive and preload-sensitive.

In an effort to eliminate the preload and afterload dependence of the isovolumetric phase indices, several authors have proposed peak (dp/dt)/end-diastolic circumference [131] and (dp/dt)/DP_{40} [41,110] (the ratio of dp/dt to a DP of 40 mm Hg, where DP is developed left ventricular pressure minus end-diastolic pressure). Both indices are relatively insensitive to changes in afterload and only mildly sensitive to alterations of preload; however, the measurement of left ventricular dp/dt requires a high-fidelity catheter-tip micromanometer, limiting its clinical utility for long-term studies. In addition, there is a relatively wide normal range for these two indices.

Finally, functional mitral regurgitation (see section on valvular disease) is not uncommon in ESRD; isovolumetric phase indices are not useful in cases of mitral regurgitation, in which there is no isovolumetric period.

The most useful method for determining contractility involves determination of (1) the end-systolic pressure-volume relationship [143] (Fig. 32-3); (2) the end-systolic stress-shortening fraction relationship [19] (Fig. 32-4); or (3) the systolic wall stress–VCF relationship [68,77] (Fig. 32-4). Their limitation is the presence of regional rather than global dysfunction, which invalidates the assumption of ellipsoidal geometry of the left ventricle necessary for the calculation of wall stress. All three of these relationships can be measured noninvasively, although the first requires measurements at several different afterloads [20]. It should be recognized that although afterload manipulation can be achieved pharmacologically, this requirement limits the clinical utility of the end-systolic pressure-volume relationship for longitudinal studies. Therefore, the assessment of the end-systolic stress-shortening and stress–

VCF relationships may be the most promising noninvasive tools to confirm or refute the specific effect on inotropic state of each of the metabolic disturbances of ESRD that will now be discussed.

HYPOCALCEMIA AND HYPERPHOSPHATEMIA

Total serum calcium is usually reduced in ESRD because of diminished renal synthesis of 1,25-dihydroxy vitamin D_3, which is responsible for intestinal absorption of calcium. Hypocalcemia affects contractile state because the slow secondary inward current, which corresponds to the plateau phase of the myocardial action potential, results from opening of a slow channel that permits some cations to enter the cell. The influx of calcium ions causes a release of calcium stored in the terminal cisternae of the sarcoplasmic reticulum into the cytoplasm (calcium-triggered calcium release); there calcium binds to troponin, an inhibitor of the reaction between actin and myosin, the contractile proteins of the heart. Lang [102a] has reported that left ventricular contractile state varies directly with blood ionized calcium in adults with ESRD.

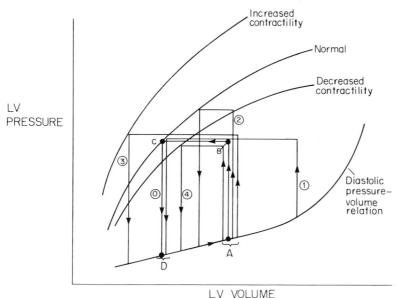

FIG. 32-3. *Effects of various interventions on the pressure-volume loop of the left ventricle (LV). Contraction 0 is characterized by a loop starting at end-diastole, A. Isovolumetric contraction occurs from A to B. Ejection occurs from B to C. End-systole occurs at point C and is followed by isovolumetric relaxation (C-D). Filling occurs along the diastolic pressure-volume relation (D-A). Increasing preload (1) results in end-diastolic volume being larger; however, note that after ejection the end-systolic volume is unchanged (point C). Increasing afterload (2) requires the generation of a higher LV pressure during isovolumetric contraction; after ejection the end-systolic volume is larger for a given end-diastolic volume, thus, compared to the normal (0) contraction or the contraction with increased preload (1), there is a reduction in LV stroke volume (end-diastolic volume minus end-systolic volume). Note that for any given contractile or inotropic state, all of the end-systolic pressure-volume points fall on the same line. To determine the end-systolic pressure-volume line, multiple points must be obtained, which necessitates pharmacologic manipulation of afterload. Depression (4) or increase (3) in myocardial contractility alters stroke volume at a given afterload and preload. Afterload reduction (proceeding from loop 2 to loop 0) increases stroke volume; this principle underlies the use of vasodilator therapy.*

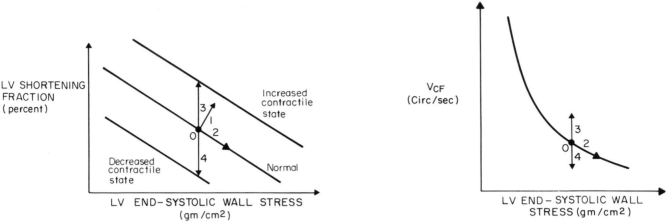

FIG. 32-4. Left panel. *Effect of several interventions on end-systolic stress-shortening relation of the left ventricle (LV). Changes in preload, unless extreme (1), have little effect on this relation. Increased afterload (2) leads to diminished LV shortening. Depression (4) or increase (3) in myocardial contractile state at a given afterload also affects LV shortening fraction.* Right panel. *Effect of several interventions on the end-systolic stress–VCF relation of the left ventricle. Preload changes have very little effect on this relation. Increased afterload (2) leads to diminished VCF. Depression (4) or increase (3) in myocardial contractile state at a given afterload also affects VCF.*

Hyperphosphatemia also occurs in ESRD and further lowers the serum calcium level by causing complexing of calcium and phosphate. Although calcium deposition (metastatic calcification) in adult ESRD patients occurs in blood vessels [26,155], the conduction system of the heart [80,155], the myocardium [10,26,80,155], and the mitral valve annulus and leaflets [42,120], its occurrence in the pediatric age group has not been reported. Calcification of the conduction system results most often in atrioventricular block. Restriction of dietary phosphate and use of phosphate-binding gels are helpful in reducing serum phosphate level; in order to avoid complexing calcium and phosphate, reduction of serum phosphate should precede the administration of calcium supplements or 1,25-dihydroxy vitamin D_3.

Acidemia [142], due to impaired ammonium excretion, has a direct negative effect on inotropic state [167] by blocking calcium influx through slow calcium channels [22].

HYPERMAGNESEMIA

Hypermagnesemia occurs commonly in ESRD [133], due to diminished excretion [32], and can be exacerbated by the ingestion of magnesium-containing antacids. Reports on whether the elevated serum magnesium reflects increased muscle content of this ion are conflicting [27,105]. Excess magnesium inhibits calcium-triggered calcium release [50]. The effects of hypermagnesemia on contractile state in vivo are probably not significant, provided that the calcium level is normal [27].

CARNITINE DEFICIENCY

Whether carnitine deficiency occurs in ESRD by itself [141] or whether it is merely a sequela of dialysis [16,17] is

controversial. Carnitine is a low-weight molecule that transports long-chain fatty acids into mitochondria, where they are oxidized to carbon dioxide and water. That systemic carnitine deficiency can present as cardiomyopathy [158] is not surprising, because under aerobic conditions, the heart's preferred substrate is long-chain fatty acids. Concomitant with a rise in free fatty acid levels [13], plasma carnitine level drops during hemodialysis [16,17]; it increases after dialysis, presumably by transfer from tissue stores. Plasma levels [3], skeletal (and presumably cardiac) muscle stores [3], and skeletal muscle performance [4] can be increased by oral administration of carnitine.

IRON OVERLOAD

Iron overload occurs in patients with ESRD as a result of blood transfusion therapy to correct the anemia of chronic renal failure. Perhaps this complication will be avoided by the use of recombinant erythropoietin. Iron deposition in the myocardium has been recognized in other conditions requiring transfusion therapy such as thalassemia major, and abnormalities in contractility have been detected noninvasively [21]. Whether reduction of body iron stores with iron-chelating agents [11] halts or reverses myocardial iron deposition remains to be seen.

UREMIC TOXINS

Finally, the existence of "uremic toxins" that directly reduce left ventricular contractility has been proposed. Most human studies have been inconclusive because they have used only *load-dependent* indices of contractile state such as systolic time intervals [103], shortening fraction [103], ejection fraction [28], and dp/dt [28]. Studies of the intact animal [121,145] or isolated animal heart [128,146] have also used load-dependent indices such as peak (dp/dt).

Recently, Colan [33a] has reported that contractile state is normal if a load-independent index is employed (see section on effect of hemodialysis and renal transplantation on cardiovascular system). Using pressure-volume loops, Kramer [100a] also denies that there is a primary cardiomyopathy due to uremic toxins in adults.

AUTONOMIC NERVOUS SYSTEM

Because contractility is also influenced by autonomic nervous activity (sympathetic and parasympathetic systems), autonomic imbalance or dysfunction could potentially affect inotropic state in ESRD (see the section on autonomic nervous system dysfunction).

Effects of Renal Failure on Diastolic Properties

Diastolic Ventricular Function

The assessment of diastolic performance is more difficult than the assessment of systolic performance. Whereas the latter has been characterized by four parameters (preload, afterload, contractility, and heart rate), diastolic performance is more complicated to describe. Diastole may be evaluated during the phases of relaxation and passive filling. Relaxation is a complex, energy-dependent process, whose behavior has been assessed by such indices as T, the time constant of the exponential decline in left ventricular pressure during early diastole [65], and peak negative (dp/dt) [113]. Both these indices are dependent on loading conditions, inotropic state (systolic function), or heart rate [54,65], however.

After relaxation and during passive filling, the diastolic behavior of the ventricle can be characterized by passive stress-strain relations [70], although the viscoelastic models [73,76,134] proposed are complex. A major factor limiting clinical use of diastolic stress-strain relations is that their calculation requires invasive measurement of left ventricular pressure, because the aortic valve is closed during diastole. Thus, detailed investigation of diastolic function in ESRD has not yet been attempted.

Pericardial Disease

An additional factor confounding studies of diastolic function in the intact ventricle is the effect of the pericardium [135], which is frequently abnormal in ESRD.

Pericarditis can occur in patients who have never been on dialysis as well as in those who have been on dialysis for variable lengths of time [111]. The precise mechanism is not known. The pericardial fluid is almost always hemorrhagic [101]; whether this results from the coagulation abnormalities present in ESRD [152] is unclear. Cases of fibrinous pericarditis, without hemorrhage, can occur [12].

The diagnosis of uremic pericarditis is made by the same clinical criteria used for other forms of pericarditis [111]: fever, chest pain ameliorated by sitting up and leaning forward, electrocardiographic changes of ST elevation without reciprocal ST depression, increases in cardiac silhouette on chest radiograph, and a pericardial friction rub.

Effusions can be most easily detected by echocardiography [85] (Fig. 32-5).

Pericardial effusions can be large enough to result in tamponade [12,118], which in turn may cause further deterioration of renal function by virtue of low cardiac output. Tamponade may be heralded by symptoms of fatigue, lethargy, dyspnea, and chest discomfort, as well as by signs of pulsus paradoxus (>10 mm Hg decrease in systolic pressure during inspiration) and Kussmaul's sign (an inspiratory increase in jugular venous distention); however, the patient with tamponade may be only minimally symptomatic. Dialysis can precipitate a sudden marked drop in arterial pressure in the tamponade patient by causing acute hypovolemia. Tamponade should be treated with immediate pericardiocentesis.

For recurrent large effusions, instillation of steroids such as triamcinolone [66] into the pericardial space, oral indomethacin [114], pericardial window creation [63], and partial pericardiectomy [37,111] have been suggested.

Finally, chronic constrictive pericarditis appears to develop only rarely in ESRD [138]. The symptoms of constriction are lethargy, weakness, and occasionally, mental confusion. Tachycardia, a reduced pulse pressure, peripheral edema, and ascites may be present; the hemodynamics simulate restrictive cardiomyopathy. Definitive diagnosis should be made by computed tomography [116] or magnetic resonance imaging [150]. Constrictive pericarditis should be treated by pericardial resection [129].

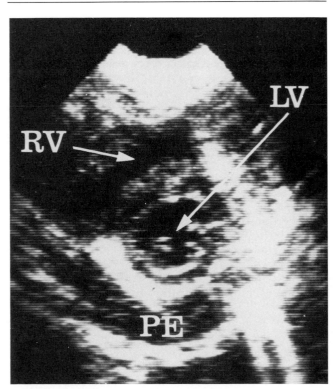

FIG. 32-5. *Two-dimensional echocardiogram, short axis view. Pericardial effusion (PE) is easily visualized. LV, Left ventricle; RV, right ventricle.*

Dysrhythmia

Life-threatening hyperkalemia can occur in acute oliguric or anuric renal failure and in ESRD. The earliest electrocardiographic abnormality is peaking of the T waves, followed by an increase in T-wave amplitude and a widening of the QRS complex.

The incidence of significant ventricular or supraventricular arrhythmias is low in the pediatric age group, which may be due to the absence of significant coronary artery disease or to an increasingly sparing use of digitalis glycosides. Supraventricular arrhythmias may occur in the setting of uremic pericarditis [35].

Correction of the underlying metabolic disorder is the first treatment priority in many patients. Among the mechanical and pharmacologic approaches to stop supraventricular tachyarrhythmias are induction of heightened vagal activity (Valsalva maneuver, diving reflex); digitalis; adenosine; and drugs fostering calcium channel blockade, such as verapamil.

Valvular Disease

Pansystolic apical murmurs have been described in patients with ESRD and are presumably due to mitral regurgitation. The mechanism is probably annular dilatation secondary to left ventricular distention.

Diastolic murmurs of aortic regurgitation have been noted in ESRD patients with poorly controlled hypertension [154]. Because pathologic examination has not revealed structural abnormalities, the aortic regurgitation is presumably secondary to dilatation of the aortic root from systemic hypertension [112,154].

Calcific mitral stenosis has been reported in a patient demonstrating rapidly progressive metastatic calcification [42].

Effect of Hemodialysis and Renal Transplantation on Cardiovascular System
Hemodialysis

Hemodialysis results in marked changes in both preload and afterload, two of the determinants of cardiac performance. Attempts at assessing the acute effect of hemodialysis on contractility (inotropic state) of the left ventricle have been made by measurement of load-dependent ejection phase indices (VCF) [18,30,33,81,86,87,89,109,122], left ventricular posterior wall velocity [33], ejection fraction [18,30,33,86,122], and shortening fraction [18,30, 87,89]. It is not surprising, therefore, that these have yielded disparate results. As discussed previously, Colan et al. [33a] claim that contractile state is normal when a load-independent index of contractility is employed.

Hemodialysis causes a fall in the partial pressure of arterial oxygen. This fall is usually on the order of 10 to 15 mg/dl, a level that would not be expected to greatly alter contractility. The mechanism of this arterial desaturation is unresolved but appears to be related to acetate influx [125,132], because substituting bicarbonate for acetate in the dialysate abolishes the phenomenon.

Renal Transplantation

Along with correction of metabolic disturbances and the anemia of ESRD, renal transplantation appears to decrease the left ventricular end-diastolic volume [88,117] and wall thickness [88]; Colan et al. [33a] states that this is a result of a change in loading conditions. Disparate results were reported previously when only load-dependent indices (shortening fraction [88,117,127], VCF [88,102,127], ejection fraction [102,127], and left ventricular posterior wall velocity [102]) were used. In adults, exercise capacity as assessed by maximal oxygen consumption measurement [127a] increases. Finally, plasma atrial natriuretic factor normalizes after renal transplantation [131a].

Hypertension can occur in renal transplant patients; causes include ureteral obstruction, graft rejection, recurrent disease in the graft, and stenosis of the transplanted renal artery, the last of which is associated with high PRA.

Autonomic Nervous System Dysfunction

Autonomic nervous system dysfunction occurs in many ESRD patients. Its most frequent clinical manifestation is severe hypotension, not associated with pericardial tamponade, during hemodialysis. Lilley et al. [104] studied the response to inhalation of the vasodilator amyl nitrite (an index of the entire baroreceptor reflex arc) and the early response to the cold pressor test (an index of efferent sympathetic nervous activity) in 20 uremic adults. Plasma dopamine β-hydroxylase, a long-lived enzyme released by sympathetic neural discharge, was measured as well. The patients who had previously demonstrated frequent episodes of hypotension during hemodialysis demonstrated a diminished response (change in R-R interval per change in arterial pressure) to amyl nitrite–induced vasodilatation but a normal response to the cold pressor test. They also had higher dopamine β-hydroxylase activity both predialysis and postdialysis. These data suggest that a subset of uremic patients exhibits a defect in baroreceptors or in visceral afferent autonomic nerves or both. A diminution in the afferent limb of the baroreceptor reflex arc would manifest in two ways: (1) inadequate increase in vascular impedance and heart rate after hypovolemic challenge, and (2) inadequate inhibitory influence on sympathetic efferent activity [104]. The latter is consistent with the finding of increased dopamine β-hydroxylase levels.

Chaignon et al. [29] showed a diminished response of total peripheral resistance to fluid depletion in patients who demonstrated significant hypotension during hemodialysis compared with those who did not. Mean heart rate, however, was relatively unchanged in both groups, illustrating that vascular impedance and heart rate are controlled independently.

Others have noted that uremic patients have subnormal heart rate responses to the Valsalva maneuver [58,96, 126,149]. Moreover, spontaneous R-R interval fluctuation is decreased compared with normal [25,55]. Beat-to-beat fluctuations in hemodynamic parameters such as heart rate and vascular impedance reflect the dynamic response of cardiovascular control systems to a variety of physiologic perturbations [2]. Assessment of the frequency-specific contributions of the three main rapidly reacting cardiovascular control systems—the sympathetic, parasympathetic, and renin-angiotensin systems—to the genesis of heart rate fluctuations can be done by power spectrum analysis [2,10a]. This technique should be a powerful quantitative, noninvasive means of evaluating cardiovascular regulation of ESRD.

Renin-Angiotensin System

The peripheral renin-angiotensin system, a variety of alterations of which can potentially occur in ESRD, plays a role in short-term cardiovascular control [78], just as do the sympathetic and parasympathetic nervous systems; the efferent limbs of these rapidly reacting control systems alter heart rate, atrioventricular conduction, contractile state, and vascular impedance [2].

Recently, the existence of a central renin-angiotensin system has been demonstrated. The role of this brain renin-angiotensin system in control of blood volume is currently under study. Angiotensin II, when injected intracranially in an animal model, induces a marked drinking response [61]. Bilaterally nephrectomized rats, unable to excrete volume, exhibit time-dependent increases in the level of angiotensinogen in the areas of the hypothalamus and the midbrain known to mediate angiotensin II-induced drinking [75] and demonstrate striking increases in angiotensin II-induced drinking. Gregory et al. proposes that the activity of angiotension II-responsive neurons is depressed after nephrectomy, which results in the build-up of angiotensinogen and a compensatory increase in sensitivity of postsynaptic angiotensin II-responsive neurons [75].

The precise interaction between the peripheral and the central renin-angiotensin systems has not been defined; it is hypothesized that steroid hormones, which readily cross the blood–brain barrier, may mediate this interaction [130].

Prostaglandins in Renal Failure

The prostaglandins, which are synthesized by many component cell types in the kidney, appear to have many important functions. For example, renin release is controlled by three mechanisms: (1) intrarenal baroreceptors, (2) the macula densa, and (3) intrarenal β-adrenergic receptors. Prostaglandins (probably PGI_2 and PGE_2) are an integral component in baroreceptor-mediated as well as macula densa–mediated renin release but appear not to participate in renin release induced by β-adrenergic receptors [90]. Because, as mentioned earlier, the renin-angiotensin system plays a major role in short-term regulation of vascular impedance, the prostaglandin system may prove to be just as important a cardiovascular control system.

As has been noted, a small subset of ESRD patients have high-renin, or renin-dependent, hypertension. Studies of a high-renin rat model, in which the aorta is ligated between the renal arteries, demonstrate that indomethacin, a cyclo-oxygenase inhibitor, lowers PRA and arterial pressure [91]. Whether similar results will be obtained in a subset of human subjects with ESRD and hyperreninemic hypertension remains to be seen.

Apart from its role in renin release, the prostaglandin system may also have other effects on systemic vascular impedance regulation, either by influencing autonomic neural control [24,79] or by local effects on various vascular beds [164]. For example, the interaction between angiotensin II and the major vascular prostaglandin, prostacyclin (PGI_2), may also be important. PGI_2 appears to blunt the vasoconstrictor activity of angiotensin II [40].

Although there is as yet no conclusive evidence defining whether these non–renin-dependent actions of the prostaglandin system play an important role in human ESRD, Benabe et al. [14] has shown in an animal model of acute renal failure that production is augmented of thromboxane A_2, a potent vasoconstrictor.

Finally, the prostaglandin system has an important role in the long-term maintenance of water balance (through its interaction with vasopressin [7,8,48,174]) and may also influence renal tubular sodium handling [48,69,153]. Further studies in this area may shed light on the majority of hypertensive ESRD patients, who manifest "volume-dependent" rather than renin-dependent hypertension.

Other Complications Affecting Cardiac Performance

Anemia

The normochronic normocytic anemia of chronic renal failure is caused by several factors: deficient production of erythropoietin [5,6,162], depression of erythropoiesis in bone marrow by "uremic toxins" [60], and shortened red cell survival [62,139,171]. Megaloblastic anemia in ESRD is less common and results from folate deficiency secondary to poor dietary intake, dialysis, or drugs [137].

Chronic anemia, by decreasing the oxygen-carrying capacity of the blood, evokes peripheral vasodilation and thus lowers afterload [47,159]. Diminished blood viscosity also contributes to afterload reduction [119]. The heart's response to chronic anemia is ventricular dilatation and hypertrophy appropriate to cavity dimension [148a]. Administration of recombinant erythropoietin corrects the anemia of ESRD.

Infective Endocarditis

With the advent of the subcutaneous arteriovenous fistula [23] for vascular access, the incidence of bacterial endocarditis [38,44,123] among hemodialysis patients has dramatically diminished. Reported septicemia rates are approximately 0.15 episodes per patient dialysis year [44]. Nsouli [123] reported a 3.6% incidence of bacterial endocarditis among bacteremic hemodialysis patients. The most frequent organism is *Staphylococcus aureus* [38]. The aortic and mitral valves are most frequently involved [38].

Pharmacology of Inotropic Agents, Antiarrhythmic Agents, Vasodilators, and Diuretics in Renal Failure

The general principles of drug therapy in renal failure have been extensively reviewed [15,67]. The four main pharmacokinetic parameters are the major route of drug elimination (renal excretion or hepatic biotransformation), the volume of distribution, the plasma half-life, and the extent of drug-binding to plasma proteins.

Drugs with large distribution volumes are not substantially dialyzed because very little of the drug is in the blood compartment from which dialysis takes place. Drugs with a high degree of protein binding are not dialyzable because only unbound drug can cross dialysis membranes.

To adjust drug dosage in patients with ESRD, the interdose interval can be lengthened, keeping the dosage size normal (interval extension method); alternatively, the dosage can be reduced, keeping the interdose interval the same (dosage reduction method).

Table 32-2 contains information to facilitate the use of cardioactive drugs in patients with renal disease. The table categorizes the pharmacokinetic properties of four groups of drugs: inotropic agents, antiarrhythmic agents, vasodilators, and diuretics.

TABLE 32-2. *Pharmacokinetic properties of cardioactive drugs*

Drug	Elimination and metabolism	Half-life in ESRD (hr)	Plasma protein binding (%)	V_D (L/kg)	Removed by dialysis	References
Inotropic agents						
Cardiac glycosides						
Digoxin*	Renal	80–120	20–30	5–8	NO	[1,15,59,100,165,166]
Digitoxin	Hepatic Renal	210	94	0.6	NO	[15]
Dopamine	Hepatic	0.03	?	?	?	
Dobutamine	Hepatic	0.03	?	0.2	?	[94]
Antiarrhythmic agents						
Procaineamide†	Renal 60% Hepatic 40%	10–19	15	1.5–2.0	YES	[71,72,97]
Quinidine	Hepatic 80% Renal 20%	4–14	70–95	2–3.5	NO	[15,36,45,107,170]
Disopyramide	Renal 50%	11–17	50–65	0.5–1.0	NO	[39,64,82,93]
Lidocaine	Hepatic	1.3–3.3	60–66	1.3–2.2	NO	[15,34,56,157]
Phenytoin	Hepatic	6–10	75–93	1–1.8	NO	[124,136]
Propranolol	Hepatic	2–4	90–96	3–4	NO	[15,57,108,156]
Verapamil	Hepatic 95% Renal 5%	3–7	90	3–6	NO	[53,95,147]
Amiodarone	Hepatic	13–107 days	?	18–150	NO	[84,148,173]
Vasodilators						
Hydralazine	Hepatic	7–16	85	0.5–0.9	NO	[15]
Nitroprusside‡	Hepatic	< 10 min	?	?	YES	[15]
Nitroglycerin (intravenous)	Hepatic	< 3 min	?	0.14	?	[9]
Prazosin	Hepatic	2.5–6	97	1.2–1.7	NO	[15,31]
Captopril	Renal	?	25–30	0.7	YES	[15,46]
Nifedipine	Hepatic	2	92–98	0.04–0.14	NO	[52]
Diuretics						
Chlorthiazide	Renal	4–6	20–80	?	?	[15]
Furosemide	Renal	2–4	95	0.07–0.21	NO	[15]
Spironolactone	Renal	10–35	98	?	?	[15]

* Dosage should reduce by 50% in patients on quinidine.
† N-acetyl procaineamide, an active metabolite, is excreted by the kidney.
‡ Metabolized to cyanide and then thiocyanate, which is excreted by the kidney.
ESRD, end-stage renal disease; V_D, volume of distribution.

References

1. Ackerman GL, Doherty JE, Flanigan WJ: Peritoneal dialysis and hemodialysis of tritiated digoxin. *Ann Int Med* 67:718, 1967.

2. Akselrod S, Gordon D, Ubel FA, et al: Power spectrum analysis of heart rate fluctuation: A quantitative probe of beat-to-beat cardiovascular control. *Science* 213:220, 1981.

3. Albertazzi A, Capelli P, DiPaolo B, et al: Endocrine-metabolic effects of L-carnitine in patients on regular dialysis treatment. *Proc Eur Dial Transpl Assoc* 19:302, 1982.

4. Albertazzi A, Spisni C, Del Rosso G, et al: Electromyographic changes induced by oral carnitine. *Proc Clin Dial Transpl Forum* 10:1, 1980.

5. Anagnostou A, Barone J, Kedo A, et al: Effect of erythropoietin therapy on the red cell volume of uraemic and non-uraemic rats. *Brit J Haematol* 37:85, 1977.

6. Anagnostou A, Vercellotti G, Barone J, et al: Factors which affect erythropoiesis in partially nephrectomized and sham-operated rats. *Blood* 48:425, 1976.

7. Anderson RJ, Berl T, McDonald KM, et al: Evidence for an in vivo antagonism between vasopressin and prostaglandin in the mammalian kidney. *J Clin Invest* 56:420, 1975.

8. Anderson RJ, Berl T, McDonald KM, et al: Prostaglandins: Effects on blood pressure, renal blood flow, sodium and water excretion. *Kidney Int* 10:205, 1976.

9. Armstrong PW, Armstrong JA, Marks GS: Pharmacokinetic-hemodynamic studies of intravenous nitroglycerin in congestive cardiac failure. *Circulation* 62:160, 1980.

10. Arora KK, Lacy JP, Schacht RA, et al: Calcific cardiomyopathy in advanced renal failure. *Arch Intern Med* 135:603, 1975.

10a. Axelrod S, Lishner M, Oz O, et al: Spectral analysis of fluctuations in heart rate: An objective evaluation of autonomic nervous control in chronic renal failure. *Nephron* 45:202, 1987.

11. Baker LRI, Barnett MD, Brozovic B, et al: Hemosiderosis in a patient on regular hemodialysis: treatment by desferrioxamine. *Clin Nephrol* 6:326, 1976.

12. Baldwin JJ, Edwards JE: Uremic pericarditis as a cause of cardiac tamponade. *Circulation* 53:896, 1976.

13. Bartel LL, Hussey JL, Shrago E: Effect of dialysis on serum carnitine, free fatty acids, and triglyceride levels in man and the rat. *Metabolism* 31:944, 1982.

14. Benabe JE, Klahr S, Hoffman MH, et al: Production of thromboxane A_2 by the kidney in glycerol-induced acute renal failure. *Prostaglandins* 19:33, 1980.

15. Bennett WM, Aronoff GR, Morrison G, et al: Drug prescribing in renal failure: Dosing guidelines for adults. *Am J Kidney Dis* 3:155, 1983.

16. Bertoli M, Battistella PA, Vergani L, et al: Carnitine deficiency induced during hemodialysis and hyperlipidemia: Effect of replacement therapy. *Am J Clin Nutr* 34:1496, 1981.

17. Bohmer T, Bergrem H, Eiklid K: Carnitine deficiency induced during intermittent haemodialysis for renal failure. *Lancet* 1:126, 1978.

18. Bornstein A, Gaasch WH, Harrington J: Assessment of the cardiac effects of hemodialysis with systolic time intervals and echocardiography. *Am J Cardiol* 51:332, 1983.

19. Borow KM, Green LH, Grossman W, et al: Left ventricular end-systolic stress-shortening and stress-length relations in humans. *Am J Cardiol* 50:1301, 1982.

20. Borow KM, Neumann A, Wynne J: Sensitivity of end-systolic pressure-dimension and pressure-volume relationship to the inotropic state in humans. *Circulation* 65:988, 1982.

21. Borow KM, Propper R, Bierman FZ, et al: The left ventricular end-systolic pressure-dimension relation in patients with thalassemia major. *Circulation* 66:980, 1982.

22. Braunwald E, Sonnenblick EH, Ross J: Contraction of the normal heart. *In* Braunwald E (ed): *Heart Disease.* Philadelphia, WB Saunders, 1980, p 413.

23. Brescia MJ, Cimino JE, Appel K, et al: Chronic hemodialysis using venipuncture and a surgically created arteriovenous fistula. *N Engl J Meds* 40275:1089, 1966.

24. Brody MJ, Kadowitz PJ: Prostaglandins as modulators of the autonomic nervous system. *Fed Proc* 33:48, 1974.

25. Burgess ED: Cardiac vagal denervation in hemodialysis patients. *Nephron* 30:228, 1982.

26. Bylsma F, Walmsley JBW: Metastatic myocardial calcification. *Can Anaesth Soc J* 28:167, 1981.

27. Cantigulia SR, Alfrey AC, Miller N, et al: Total body magnesium excess in chronic renal failure. *Lancet* 1:1300, 1972.

28. Capelli JP, Kasparian H: Cardiac work demands and left ventricular function in end-stage renal disease. *Ann Intern Med* 86:261, 1977.

29. Chaignon M, Chen W-T, Tarazi RC, et al: Blood pressure response to hemodialysis. *Hypertension* 3:333, 1981.

30. Chaignon M, Chen W-T, Tarazi RC, et al: Acute effects of hemodialysis on echographic-determined cardiac performance: Improved contractility resulting from serum increased calcium with reduced potassium despite hypovolemic-reduced cardiac output. *Am Heart J* 103:374, 1982.

31. Chatterjee K, Parmley WW: Vasodilator therapy for chronic heart failure. *Ann Rev Pharmacol Toxicol* 20:475, 1980.

32. Coburn JW, Popovtzer MM, Massry SG, et al: The physicochemical state and renal handling of divalent ions in chronic renal failure. *Arch Intern Med* 124:302, 1969.

33. Cohen MV, Diaz P, Scheuer J: Echocardiographic assessment of left ventricular function in patients with chronic uremia. *Clin Nephrol* 12:156, 1979.

33a. Colan SD, Sanders SP, Ingelfinger JR, et al: Left ventricular mechanics and contractile state in children and young adults with end-stage renal disease: Effect of dialysis and renal transplantation. *J Am Coll Cardiol* 10:1085, 1987.

34. Collingsworth KA, Strong JM, Atkinson AJ, et al: Pharmacokinetics and metabolism of lidocaine in patients with renal failure. *Clin Pharmacol Ther* 18:59, 1975.

35. Comty CM, Cohen SL, Shapiro FL: Pericarditis in chronic uremia and its sequels. *Ann Intern Med* 75:173, 1971.

36. Conn HL, Luchi RJ: Some quantitative aspects of the binding of quinidine and related quinoline compounds by human serum albumin. *J Clin Invest* 40:509, 1961.

37. Connors JP, Kleiger RE, Shaw RC, et al: The indications for pericardiectomy in the uremic pericardial effusion. *Surgery* 80:689, 1976.

38. Cross AS, Steigbigel RT: Infective endocarditis and access site infections in patients on hemodialysis. *Medicine* 55:453, 1976.

39. Cunningham JL, Shen DD, Shudo I, et al: The effects of urine pH and plasma protein binding on the renal clearance of disopyramide. *Clin Pharmacokinet* 2:373, 1977.

40. Currie MG, Needleman P: Renal arachidonic acid metabolism. *Annu Rev Physiol* 46:327, 1984.

41. Davidson DM, Covell JW, Malloch CI, et al: Factors influencing indices of left ventricular contractility in the conscious dog. *Cardiovasc Res* 8:299, 1974.

42. DePace NL, Rohrer AH, Kotler MN, et al: Rapidly progressing, massive mitral annular calcification. *Arch Intern Med* 141:1663, 1981.

43. DePlanque BA, Mulder E, Dorhout Mees EJ: The behavior

of blood and extracellular volume in hypertensive patients with renal insufficiency. *Acta Med Scand* 186:75, 1969.

44. Dobkin JF, Miller MH, Steigbigel NH: Septicemia in patients on chronic hemodialysis. *Ann Intern Med* 88:128, 1978.

45. Drayer DE, Lowenthal DT, Restivo KM, et al: Steady-state serum levels of quinidine and active metabolites in cardiac patients with varying degrees of renal function. *Clin Pharmacol Ther* 24:31, 1978.

46. Duchin KL, Singhvi SM, Willard DA, et al: Captopril kinetics. *Clin Pharmacol Ther* 31:452, 1982.

47. Duke M, Abelman WH: The hemodynamic response to chronic anemia. *Circulation* 39:503, 1969.

48. Dunn MJ: Renal prostaglandins. *In* Dunn MJ (ed): *Renal Endocrinology.* Baltimore, Williams and Wilkins, 1983, p 1.

49. Dunn MJ, Hood VL: Prostaglandins and the kidney. *Am J Physiol* 233:F169, 1977.

50. Dunnett J, Nayler WG: Calcium efflux from cardiac sarcoplasmic reticulum: Effects of calcium and magnesium. *J Mol Cell Cardiol* 10:487, 1978.

51. Dustan HP, Page IH: Some factors in renal and renoprival hypertension. *J Lab Clin Med* 64:948, 1964.

52. Eichelbaum M: Clinical pharmacokinetics of calcium ion antagonists. *Clin Invest Med* 3:13, 1980.

53. Eichelbaum M, Ende M, Remberg G, et al: The metabolism of ^{14}C-verapamil in man. *Drug Metab Dispos* 7:145, 1979.

54. Eichhorn P, Grimm J, Koch R, et al: Left ventricular relaxation in patients with left ventricular hypertrophy secondary to aortic valve disease. *Circulation* 65:1395, 1982.

55. Endre ZH, Perl SI, Kraegen EW, et al: Reduced cardiac beat-to-beat variation in chronic renal failure: A ubiquitous marker of autonomic neuropathy. *Clin Sci* 62:561, 1982.

56. Eriksson E, Granberg P-O, Ortengren B: Study of renal excretion of prilocaine and lidocaine. *Acta Chir Scand* [Suppl]358:55, 1966.

57. Evans GH, Nies AS, Shand DG: The disposition of propranolol. *J Pharmacol Exp Ther* 186:114, 1973.

58. Ewing DJ, Winney R: Autonomic function in patients with chronic renal failure on intermittent hemodialysis. *Nephron* 15:424, 1975.

59. Fenster PE, Hager WD, Perrier D, et al: Digoxin-quinidine interaction in patients with chronic renal failure. *Circulation* 66:1277, 1982.

60. Fisher JW, Nelson PK, Beckman B, et al: Kidney control of erythropoietin production. *In* Dunn MJ (ed): *Renal Endocrinology.* Baltimore, Williams and Wilkins, 1983, p 142.

61. Fitzsimons JT, Kucharczyk J: Drinking and haemodynamic changes induced in the dog by intracranial injection of components of the renin-angiotensin system. *J Physiol* 276:419, 1978.

62. Forman S, Bischel M, Hochstein P: Erythrocyte deformability in uremic hemodialyzed patients. *Ann Intern Med* 79:841, 1973.

63. Forst DH, O'Rourke RA: Cardiovascular complications of chronic renal failure. *In* Brenner BM, Stein JH (eds): *Chronic Renal Failure.* New York, Churchill Livingstone 1981, p 84.

64. Francois B, Mallein R, Rondelet J, et al: Pharmacokinetics of disopyramide in patients with chronic renal failure. *Eur J Drug Metab Pharmacokinet* 8:85, 1983.

65. Frederiksen JW, Weiss JL, Weisfeldt ML: Time constant of isovolumic pressure fall; determinants in the working left ventricle. *Am J Physiol* 235:H701, 1978.

66. Fuller TJ, Knochel JP, Brennan JP, et al: Reversal of

intractable uremic pericarditis by triamcinolone hexacetonide. *Arch Intern Med* 136:979, 1976.

67. Gambertoglio JG: Effects of renal disease: Altered pharmacokinetics. *In* Benet LZ, Massoud N, Gambertoglio JG (eds): *Pharmacokinetic Basis for Drug Treatment.* New York, Raven Press, 1984, p 149.

68. Gault JH, Ross J, Braunwald E: Contractile state of the left ventricle in man. *Circ Res* 22:451, 1968.

69. Gerber JG, Anderson RJ, Schrier RW, et al: Prostaglandins and the regulation of renal circulation and function. *Adv Prostaglandin Thromoxane Leukotriene Res* 10:227, 1982.

70. Gibson DG, Brown DJ: Relation between diastolic left ventricular wall stress and strain in man. *Br Heart J* 36:1066, 1974.

71. Gibson TP, Lowenthal DT, Nelson HA, et al: Elimination of procainamide in end-stage renal failure. *Clin Pharmacol Ther* 17:321, 1975.

72. Gibson TP, Matusik EJ, Briggs WA: N-acetylprocaineamide levels in patients with end-stage renal failure. *Clin Pharmacol Ther* 19:206, 1976.

73. Glantz SA, Parmley WW: Factors which affect the diastolic pressure-volume curve. *Circ Res* 42:171, 1978.

74. Goldblatt H, Lynch J, Hanzal RB, et al: Studies in experimental hypertension: I. The production of persistent elevation of systolic blood pressure by means of renal ischemia. *J Exp Med* 59:347, 1934.

75. Gregory TJ, Wallis CJ, Printz MP: Regional changes in rat brain angiotensinogen following bilateral nephrectomy. *Hypertension* 4:827, 1982.

76. Grossman W, McLaurin L: Diastolic properties of the left ventricle. *Ann Intern Med* 84:316, 1976.

77. Gunther S, Grossman W: Determinants of ventricular function in pressure overload hypertrophy in man. *Circulation* 59:679, 1979.

78. Gutman FD, Tagawa H, Haber E, et al: Renal arterial pressure, renin secretion, and blood pressure control in trained dogs. *Am J Physiol* 224:66, 1973.

79. Hedqvist P: Prostaglandin action on transmitter release at adrenergic neuroeffector junctions. *Adv Prostaglandin Thromboxane Leukotriene Res* 1:357, 1976.

80. Henderson RR, Santiago LM, Spring DA, et al: Metastatic myocardial calcification in chronic renal failure presenting as atrioventricular block. *N Engl J Med* 284:1252, 1971.

81. Henrich WL, Hunt JM, Nixon JV: Increased ionized calcium and left ventricular contractility during hemodialysis. *N Engl J Med* 310:19, 1984.

82. Hinderling PH, Garrett ER: Pharmacokinetics of the antiarrhythmic disopyramide in healthy humans. *J Pharmacokinet Biopharm* 4:199, 1976.

83. Hollifield JW, Sherman W, Vander Zwagg R, et al: Proposed mechanisms of propranolol's antihypertensive effect in essential hypertension. *N Engl J Med* 295:68, 1976.

84. Holt DW, Tucker CT, Jackson PR, et al: Amiodarone pharmacokinetics. *Am Heart J* 106:840, 1983.

85. Horowitz MS, Schultz CS, Stinson EB, et al: Sensitivity and specificity of echocardiographic diagnosis of pericardial effusion. *Circulation* 50:239, 1974.

86. Hung J, Harris PJ, Uren RF, et al: Uremic cardiomyopathy—effect of hemodialysis on left ventricular function in end-stage renal failure. *N Engl J Med* 302:547, 1980.

87. Ikaheimo M, Huttunen K, Takkunen J: Cardiac effects of chronic renal failure and haemodialysis treatment. *Br Heart J* 45:710, 1981.

88. Ikaheimo M, Linnaluoto M, Huttunen K, et al: Effects of renal transplantation on left ventricular size and function. *Br Heart J* 47:155, 1982.

89. Ireland MA, Mahta BR, Shiu MF: Acute effects of haemodialysis on left heart dimensions and left ventricular function: An echocardiographic study. *Nephron* 29:73, 1981.

90. Jackson EK, Branch RA, Oates JA: Participation of prostaglandins in the control of renin release. *Adv Prostaglandin Thromboxane Leukotriene Res* 10:255, 1982.

91. Jackson EK, Oates JA, Branch RA: Indomethacin decreases arterial blood pressure and plasma renin activity in rats with aortic ligation. *Circ Res* 49:180, 1981.

92. Johnson JA, Davis JO, Witty RT: Effects of catecholamines and renal nerve stimulation on renin release in the nonfiltering kidney. *Circ Res* 29:646, 1971.

93. Karim A: The pharmacokinetics of Norpace. *Angiology* (Suppl I)26:85, 1975.

94. Kates RE, Leier CV: Dobutamine pharmacokinetics in severe heart failure. *Clin Pharmacol Ther* 24:537, 1978.

95. Keefe DL, Yee Y-G, Kates RE: Verapamil protein binding in patients and in normal subjects. *Clin Pharmacol Ther* 29:21, 1981.

96. Kersh ES, Kronfield SJ, Unger A, et al: Autonomic insufficiency in uremia as a cause of hemodialysis induced hypotension. *N Engl J Med* 290:650, 1974.

97. Koch-Weser J, Klein SW: Procaineamide dosage schedules, plasma concentrations and clinical effects. *JAMA* 215:1454, 1971.

98. Kominami N, Lowrie EG, Ianhez LE, et al: The effects of total nephrectomy on hematopoiesis in patients undergoing chronic hemodialysis. *J Lab Clin Med* 78:524, 1971.

99. Kotchen TA, Roy MW: Renin-angiotensin. *In* Dunn MJ (ed): *Renal Endocrinology*. Baltimore, Williams and Wilkins, 1983, p 181.

100. Koup JR, Greenblatt DJ, Jusko WJ, et al: Pharmacokinetics of digoxin in normal subjects after intravenous bolus and infusion doses. *J Pharmacokinet Biopharm* 3:181, 1975.

100a. Kramer W, Wizemann V, Lammlein G, et al: Cardiac dysfunction in patients on maintenance hemodialysis. *Contrib Nephrol* 52:110, 1986.

101. Kumar S, Lesch M: Pericarditis in renal disease. *Prog Cardiovasc Dis* 22:357, 1980.

102. Lai KN, Barnden L, Mathew TH: Effect of renal transplantation on left ventricular function in hemodialysis patients. *Clin Nephrol* 18:74, 1982.

102a. Lang RM, Fellner SK, Neumann A, et al: Left ventricular contractility varies directly with blood ionized calcium. *Ann Intern Med* 108:524, 1988.

103. Lewis BS, Milne FJ, Goldberg B, et al: Left ventricular function in chronic renal failure. *Br Heart J* 38:1229, 1976.

104. Lilley JJ, Golden J, Stone RA: Adrenergic regulation of blood pressure in chronic renal failure. *J Clin Invest* 57:1190, 1976.

105. Lim P, Dong S, Khoo OT: Intracellular magnesium depletion in chronic renal failure. *N Engl J Med* 280:981, 1969.

106. Lindner A, Douglas SW, Adamson JW: Propranolol effects in long-term hemodialysis patients with renin-dependent hypertension. *Ann Intern Med* 88:457, 1978.

107. Lowenthal D: Pharmacokinetics of propranolol, quinidine, procaineamide and lidocaine in chronic renal disease. *Am J Med* 62:532, 1977.

108. Lowenthal DT, Briggs WA, Gibson TP: Propranolol kinetics in chronic renal disease (abstr). *Clin Res* 21:956, 1973.

109. Macdonald IL, Uldall R, Buda AJ: The effect of hemodialysis on cardiac rhythm and performance. *Clin Nephrol* 15:321, 1981.

110. Mahler F, Ross J, O'Rourke RA, et al: Effects of changes in preload, afterload, and inotropic state on ejection and isovolumic phase measures of contractility in the conscious dog. *Am J Cardiol* 35:626, 1975.

111. Marini P, Hull AR: Uremic pericarditis; a review of incidence and management. *Kidney Int* 7(Suppl 2):S163, 1975.

112. Matalon R, Moussalli ARJ, Nidus BD, et al: Functional aortic insufficiency; a feature of renal failure. *N Engl J Med* 285:1522, 1971.

113. Mathey D, Bleifeld W, Franken G: Left ventricular relaxation and diastolic stiffness in experimental myocardial infarction. *Cardiovasc Res* 8:583, 1974.

114. Minuth ANW, Nottebohm GA, Eknoyan G, et al: Indomethacin treatment of pericarditis in chronic hemodialysis patients. *Arch Intern Med* 135:807, 1975.

115. Mohammed S, Fasola AF, Privitera PJ, et al: Effect of methyldopa on plasma renin activity in man. *Circ Res* 25:543, 1969.

116. Moncada R, Baker M, Salinas M, et al: Diagnostic role of computed tomography in pericardial heart disease: Congenital defects, thickening, neoplasms, and effusions. *Am Heart J* 103:263, 1982.

117. Montague RJ, MacDonald RPR, Boutilier FE, et al: Cardiac function in end-stage renal disease. *Chest* 82:441, 1982.

118. Morin JE, Hollomby D, Gondu A, et al: Management of uremic pericarditis: A report of 11 patients with chronic tamponade and a review of the literature. *Ann Thorac Surg* 22:588, 1976.

119. Murray JF, Escobar E: Circulatory effects of blood viscosity; comparison of methemoglobinemia and anemia. *J Appl Physiol* 25:594, 1968.

120. Nestico PF, DePace NL, Kotler MN, et al: Calcium phosphorus metabolism in dialysis patients with and without mitral annular calcium. *Am J Cardiol* 51:497, 1983.

121. Nivatpumin T, Yipintsoi T, Penpargkul S, et al: Increased cardiac contractility in acute uremia: interrelationships with hypertension. *Am J Physiol* 229:501, 1975.

122. Nixon JV, Mitchell JH, McPhaul JJ, et al: Effect of hemodialysis on left ventricular function. *J Clin Invest* 71:377, 1983.

123. Nsouli KA, Lazarus JM, Schoenbaum SC, et al: Bacteremic infection in hemodialysis. *Arch Intern Med* 139:1255, 1979.

124. Odar-Cedelof I, Borga O: Kinetics of diphenylhydantoin in uraemic patients. Consequences of decreased plasma protein binding. *Eur J Clin Pharmacol* 7:31, 1974.

125. Oh MS, Uribarri JV, Del Monte ML, et al: Consumption of CO_2 in the metabolism of acetate as an explanation for hypoventilation and hypoxemia during hemodialysis. *Proc Clin Dial Transp Forum* 9:226, 1979.

126. Ono K: The cardiovascular response to the Valsalva maneuver and sustained handgrip test in patients on hemodialysis. *Proc Clin Dial Transpl Forum* 10:234, 1980.

127. O'Regan S, Douste-Blazy MY, Ducharme G, et al: Renal transplantation and cardiac function in pediatric patients. *Clin Nephrol* 17:237, 1982.

127a. Painter P, Messer-Rehak D, Hanson P, et al: Exercise capacity in hemodialysis, CAPD, and renal transplant patients. *Nephron* 42:47, 1986.

128. Penpargkul S, Scheuer J: Effect of uraemia upon the performance of the rat heart. *Cardiovasc Res* 6:702, 1972.

129. Pillay VKG, Sarpel SC, Kurtzman NA: Subacute constrictive uremia pericarditis: Survival after pericardiectomy. *JAMA* 235:1351, 1976.

130. Printz MP, Hawkins RL, Wallis CJ, et al: Steroid hormones as feedback regulators of brain angiotensinogen and catecholamines. *Chest* 83:308, 1983.

high amounts of protein does not improve the plasma protein concentration. The significance of the plasma decrease in individual cases is difficult to assess in the absence of pool measurements.

ALTERATION IN PROTEIN-BINDING

The binding of several metabolic compounds and drugs to plasma proteins is altered in uremia [60,61,102]. In uremic as in normal subjects, the major protein with binding properties is albumin [61]. It was suggested that potentially toxic compounds bind to albumin. Normally, the renal proximal tubule extracts the protein-bound metabolic compounds from the peritubular plasma and secretes them into the tubular lumen, preventing accumulation of protein-bound toxins [61]. When this extraction is impaired, binding sites of albumin may be saturated, and compounds or drugs that are normally bound will remain free if they compete for the same binding sites [61]. Other possible causes of impaired albumin binding are the presence of binding inhibitors and the alteration of albumin itself. The low plasma albumin level plays but a minor role.

The binding alteration is partially, but not fully, corrected by prolonged dialysis of uremic plasma and is not observed with normal plasma after addition of urea, creatinine, or uric acid, showing that other "toxins" cause binding inhibition.

The main albumin-bound substances are acidic drugs. Among the metabolic compounds are the free fatty acids (FFA), bilirubin, tryptophane, and thyroid hormone T3 [75]. The displacement of bound drugs in uremics results in alterations in volume of distribution; elimination rate; and local activity, which is correlated to the free plasma level of the drug; and finally, to enhanced or even toxic effects, demanding a modification of the doses used.

AMINO ACIDS

Disturbances of plasma amino acid (AA) levels have been reported by many authors. The plasma AA pattern has been considered as characteristic of CRF [78], notably low branched chain AA, particularly valine and not corrected by augmented valine intake; reduced essential AA (EAA) pool despite elevated phenylalanine; expanded nonessential AA (NEAA) pool with augmented glycine, citrulline, proline, and other NEAA levels; but reduced tyrosine concentration and decreased ratios such as EAA/NEAA, valine/glycine, and tyrosine/phenylalanine.

Plasma AA concentrations reported in several series of children are presented in [18–21,28,37,72,107] Table 33-1. The plasma values showed wide variations from one series of children with CRF to another. Particularly intriguing is the difference in EAA between two series of children on peritoneal dialysis, one showing no reduction of any EAA, including valine, and EAA pool enlargement [20], whereas in the other, all EAA were clearly decreased [107].

Another unexplained and surprising finding is the degree of reduction of most EAA in children with moderate CRF [19] as compared to the normal, or almost normal, level in children with more severe disease [20,37]. Table 33-1

shows that no change in any of the EAA is consistent, although a fall in valine is found in all series but one, and a fall in leucine is frequent. Phenylalanine and histidine, which have been reported as significantly altered, seem remarkably stable and normal when all available data are considered.

Plasma NEAA pool was expanded in most series, although the values for each NEAA vary. The only constant changes are the rise of citrulline, which is evident in moderate CRF and reaches very high values, and the rise of aspartic acid, which reaches impressively high levels in infants [18]. The rise of glycine and proline are less dramatic. The only NEAA showing a significant decrease is tyrosine. Plasma serine may be low or normal.

In adult series [4,26,45,79], the changes in plasma AA are comparable to those reported in children. Of the EAA, valine and leucine are low, whereas phenylalanine and histidine remain within the normal range. Of the NEAA, citrulline is consistently elevated, glycine and aspartic acid are frequently elevated, while serine and tyrosine may be reduced. The plasma levels of 1-methylhistidine and 3-methylhistidine, not shown in Table 33-1, were considerably elevated in all series.

In two series, an EAA-ketoanalogue mixture was added to a low [18] or to a moderately restricted [72] protein diet. All branched-chain AA remained low in both series; the other EAA were normal in one series [18] and low in the other, except for phenylalanine [72]. These diets, which resulted in a low blood urea level, did not influence the NEAA plasma levels.

Muscle AA have been less frequently measured [4,10,19, 37] (Table 33-2). Intracellular disturbances are less severe than plasma changes. The EAA pool is often enlarged, and valine concentration is the only EAA to be constantly low, even in children with moderate CRF who fared well and had normal nutrition. The NEAA pool is enlarged, particularly in patients requiring dialysis, with elevated levels of citrulline only in these patients.

Some of our experimental data are shown in Tables 33-3 and 33-4. Plasma and muscle AA concentrations were measured in rats who were either normal or in CRF (GFR from 5% to 30% that of controls) and who were fed four protein diets: 12 g/100 g casein, 6 g/100 g casein (insufficient in protein), and 6 g/100 g protein supplemented either with EAA or with an EAA-keto acid mixture.

In normal rats, the insufficient protein diet resulted in low EAA except for lysine and histidine. The plasma levels of branched-chain AA were not corrected by the administration of their keto analogues, but were corrected by the addition of the corresponding EAA. A rise of lysine and threonine was observed when they were administered in a synthetic form.

In rats with CRF, there was no decrease in any of the EAA as compared to normal rats fed the same diet, in spite of lower food intake. It is remarkable that with the insufficient protein diet, the plasma levels of all EAA except lysine and histidine were higher in rats with CRF than in controls who had a better appetite. Similarly, the branched-chain amino acids were higher in rats with CRF fed the EAA-keto acid diet than in controls fed the same diet. This finding, added to the poor relationship between

89. Ireland MA, Mahta BR, Shiu MF: Acute effects of hae-modialysis on left heart dimensions and left ventricular function: An echocardiographic study. *Nephron* 29:73, 1981.

90. Jackson EK, Branch RA, Oates JA: Participation of prostaglandins in the control of renin release. *Adv Prostaglandin Thromboxane Leukotriene Res* 10:255, 1982.

91. Jackson EK, Oates JA, Branch RA: Indomethacin decreases arterial blood pressure and plasma renin activity in rats with aortic ligation. *Circ Res* 49:180, 1981.

92. Johnson JA, Davis JO, Witty RT: Effects of catecholamines and renal nerve stimulation on renin release in the nonfiltering kidney. *Circ Res* 29:646, 1971.

93. Karim A: The pharmacokinetics of Norpace. *Angiology* (Suppl I)26:85, 1975.

94. Kates RE, Leier CV: Dobutamine pharmacokinetics in severe heart failure. *Clin Pharmacol Ther* 24:537, 1978.

95. Keefe DL, Yee Y-G, Kates RE: Verapamil protein binding in patients and in normal subjects. *Clin Pharmacol Ther* 29:21, 1981.

96. Kersh ES, Kronfield SJ, Unger A, et al: Autonomic insufficiency in uremia as a cause of hemodialysis induced hypotension. *N Engl J Med* 290:650, 1974.

97. Koch-Weser J, Klein SW: Procaineamide dosage schedules, plasma concentrations and clinical effects. *JAMA* 215:1454, 1971.

98. Kominami N, Lowrie EG, Ianhez LE, et al: The effects of total nephrectomy on hematopoiesis in patients undergoing chronic hemodialysis. *J Lab Clin Med* 78:524, 1971.

99. Kotchen TA, Roy MW: Renin-angiotensin. *In* Dunn MJ (ed): *Renal Endocrinology.* Baltimore, Williams and Wilkins, 1983, p 181.

100. Koup JR, Greenblatt DJ, Jusko WJ, et al: Pharmacokinetics of digoxin in normal subjects after intravenous bolus and infusion doses. *J Pharmacokinet Biopharm* 3:181, 1975.

100a. Kramer W, Wizemann V, Lammlein G, et al: Cardiac dysfunction in patients on maintenance hemodialysis. *Contrib Nephrol* 52:110, 1986.

101. Kumar S, Lesch M: Pericarditis in renal disease. *Prog Cardiovasc Dis* 22:357, 1980.

102. Lai KN, Barnden L, Mathew TH: Effect of renal transplantation on left ventricular function in hemodialysis patients. *Clin Nephrol* 18:74, 1982.

102a. Lang RM, Fellner SK, Neumann A, et al: Left ventricular contractility varies directly with blood ionized calcium. *Ann Intern Med* 108:524, 1988.

103. Lewis BS, Milne FJ, Goldberg B, et al: Left ventricular function in chronic renal failure. *Br Heart J* 38:1229, 1976.

104. Lilley JJ, Golden J, Stone RA: Adrenergic regulation of blood pressure in chronic renal failure. *J Clin Invest* 57:1190, 1976.

105. Lim P, Dong S, Khoo OT: Intracellular magnesium depletion in chronic renal failure. *N Engl J Med* 280:981, 1969.

106. Lindner A, Douglas SW, Adamson JW: Propranolol effects in long-term hemodialysis patients with renin-dependent hypertension. *Ann Intern Med* 88:457, 1978.

107. Lowenthal D: Pharmacokinetics of propranolol, quinidine, procaineamide and lidocaine in chronic renal disease. *Am J Med* 62:532, 1977.

108. Lowenthal DT, Briggs WA, Gibson TP: Propranolol kinetics in chronic renal disease (abstr). *Clin Res* 21:956, 1973.

109. Macdonald IL, Uldall R, Buda AJ: The effect of hemodialysis on cardiac rhythm and performance. *Clin Nephrol* 15:321, 1981.

110. Mahler F, Ross J, O'Rourke RA, et al: Effects of changes in preload, afterload, and inotropic state on ejection and isovolumic phase measures of contractility in the conscious dog. *Am J Cardiol* 35:626, 1975.

111. Marini P, Hull AR: Uremic pericarditis; a review of incidence and management. *Kidney Int* 7(Suppl 2):S163, 1975.

112. Matalon R, Moussalli ARJ, Nidus BD, et al: Functional aortic insufficiency; a feature of renal failure. *N Engl J Med* 285:1522, 1971.

113. Mathey D, Bleifeld W, Franken G: Left ventricular relaxation and diastolic stiffness in experimental myocardial infarction. *Cardiovasc Res* 8:583, 1974.

114. Minuth ANW, Nottebohm GA, Eknoyan G, et al: Indomethacin treatment of pericarditis in chronic hemodialysis patients. *Arch Intern Med* 135:807, 1975.

115. Mohammed S, Fasola AF, Privitera PJ, et al: Effect of methyldopa on plasma renin activity in man. *Circ Res* 25:543, 1969.

116. Moncada R, Baker M, Salinas M, et al: Diagnostic role of computed tomography in pericardial heart disease: Congenital defects, thickening, neoplasms, and effusions. *Am Heart J* 103:263, 1982.

117. Montague RJ, MacDonald RPR, Boutilier FE, et al: Cardiac function in end-stage renal disease. *Chest* 82:441, 1982.

118. Morin JE, Hollomby D, Gondu A, et al: Management of uremic pericarditis: A report of 11 patients with chronic tamponade and a review of the literature. *Ann Thorac Surg* 22:588, 1976.

119. Murray JF, Escobar E: Circulatory effects of blood viscosity; comparison of methemoglobinemia and anemia. *J Appl Physiol* 25:594, 1968.

120. Nestico PF, DePace NL, Kotler MN, et al: Calcium phosphorus metabolism in dialysis patients with and without mitral annular calcium. *Am J Cardiol* 51:497, 1983.

121. Nivatpumin T, Yipintsoi T, Penpargkul S, et al: Increased cardiac contractility in acute uremia: interrelationships with hypertension. *Am J Physiol* 229:501, 1975.

122. Nixon JV, Mitchell JH, McPhaul JJ, et al: Effect of hemodialysis on left ventricular function. *J Clin Invest* 71:377, 1983.

123. Nsouli KA, Lazarus JM, Schoenbaum SC, et al: Bacteremic infection in hemodialysis. *Arch Intern Med* 139:1255, 1979.

124. Odar-Cedelof I, Borga O: Kinetics of diphenylhydantoin in uraemic patients. Consequences of decreased plasma protein binding. *Eur J Clin Pharmacol* 7:31, 1974.

125. Oh MS, Uribarri JV, Del Monte ML, et al: Consumption of CO_2 in the metabolism of acetate as an explanation for hypoventilation and hypoxemia during hemodialysis. *Proc Clin Dial Transp Forum* 9:226, 1979.

126. Ono K: The cardiovascular response to the Valsalva maneuver and sustained handgrip test in patients on hemodialysis. *Proc Clin Dial Transpl Forum* 10:234, 1980.

127. O'Regan S, Douste-Blazy MY, Ducharme G, et al: Renal transplantation and cardiac function in pediatric patients. *Clin Nephrol* 17:237, 1982.

127a. Painter P, Messer-Rehak D, Hanson P, et al: Exercise capacity in hemodialysis, CAPD, and renal transplant patients. *Nephron* 42:47, 1986.

128. Penpargkul S, Scheuer J: Effect of uraemia upon the performance of the rat heart. *Cardiovasc Res* 6:702, 1972.

129. Pillay VKG, Sarpel SC, Kurtzman NA: Subacute constrictive uremia pericarditis: Survival after pericardiectomy. *JAMA* 235:1351, 1976.

130. Printz MP, Hawkins RL, Wallis CJ, et al: Steroid hormones as feedback regulators of brain angiotensinogen and catecholamines. *Chest* 83:308, 1983.

131. Quinones MA, Gaasch WH, Alexander JK: Influence of acute changes in preload, afterload, contractile state, and heart rate on ejection and isovolumic indices of myocardial contractility in man. *Circulation* 53:293, 1976.

131a. Raine AEG, Anderson JV, Bloom SR, et al: Plasma atrial natriuretic factor and graft function in renal transplant recipients. *Transplantation* 48:796, 1989.

132. Raja R, Kramer M, Rosenbaum JL, et al: Prevention of dialysis induces hypoxemia with bicarbonate dialysate—role of acetate in etiology. *Proc Clin Dial Transpl Forum* 10:7, 1980.

133. Randall RE, Cohen MD, Spray CC, et al: Hypermagnesemia in renal failure. *Ann Intern Med* 61:73, 1964.

134. Rankin JS, Arentzen CE, McHale PA, et al: Viscoelastic properties of the diastolic left ventricle in the conscious dog. *Circ Res* 41:37, 1977.

135. Refsum H, Juneman M, Lipton MJ, et al: Ventricular diastolic pressure-volume relations and the pericardium. *Circulation* 64:997, 1981.

136. Reidenberg MM, Odar-Cederlof I, VonBahr C, et al: Protein binding of diphenylhydantoin and desmethylimipramine in plasma from patients with poor renal function. *N Engl J Med* 285:264, 1971.

137. Retief FP, Heyns AD, Oosthuizen M, et al: Aspects of folate metabolism in renal failure. *Br J Haematol* 36:405, 1977.

138. Reyman TA: Subacute constrictive uremic pericarditis. *Am J Med* 46:972, 1969.

139. Rosenmund A, Binswanger U, Straub PW: Oxidative injury to erythrocytes, cell rigidity, and splenic hemolysis in hemodialyzed uremic patients. *Ann Intern Med* 82:460, 1975.

140. Ross J, Sonnenblock EH, Taylor RR, et al: Diastolic geometry and sarcomere lengths in the chronically dilated canine left ventricle. *Circ Res* 28:49, 1971.

141. Rumpf KW, Leschke M, Eisenhauer T, et al: Quantitative assessment of carnitine loss during haemodialysis and haemofiltration. *Proc Eur Dial Transpl Assoc* 19:298, 1982.

142. Sabatini S: The acidosis of chronic renal failure. *Med Clin North Am* 67:845, 1983.

143. Sagawa K: Editorial: The end-systolic pressure-volume relation of the ventricle; definition, modification, and clinical use. *Circulation* 63:1223, 1981.

144. Schalekamp MADH, Wenting GJ, DeBruyn JHB, et al: Hemodynamic effects of captopril in essential and renovascular hypertension: Correlations with plasma renin. *Cardiovasc Rev Report* 3:651, 1982.

145. Scheuer J, Nivatpumin T, Yipintsoi T: Effects of moderate uremia on cardiac contractile responses. *Proc Soc Exp Biol Med* 150:471, 1975.

146. Scheuer J, Stezoski SW: The effects of uremia compounds on cardiac function and metabolism. *J Mol Cell Cardiol* 5:287, 1973.

147. Schomerus M, Spiegelhalder B, Stieren B, et al: Physiological disposition of verapamil in man. *Cardiovasc Res* 10:605, 1976.

148. Siddoway LA, McAllister CB, Wilkinson GR, et al: Amiodarone dosing: A proposal based on its pharmacokinetics. *Am Heart J* 106:951, 1983.

148a. Silberberg JS, Rahal DP, Patton DR, et al: Role of anemia in the pathogenesis of left ventricular hypertrophy in end-stage renal disease. *Am J Cardiol* 64:222, 1989.

149. Soriano G, Eisinger RP: Abnormal responses to the Valsalva maneuver in patients on chronic hemodialysis. *Nephron* 9:251, 1972.

150. Stark DD, Higgins CB, Lanzer P, et al: Magnetic resonance imaging of the pericardium: Normal and pathologic findings. *Radiology* 150:469, 1984.

151. Starling EH: The Linacre Lecture on the Law of the Heart. Given at Cambridge, 1915. London, Longmans, Green, 1918.

152. Stockman JA: Hematologic manifestations of systemic diseases. *In* Nathan DG, Oski FA (eds): *Hematology of Infancy and Childhood.* Philadelphia, WB Saunders, 1981, p 1348.

153. Stokes JB, Kokko JP: Inhibition of sodium transport by prostaglandin E_2 across the isolated, perfused rabbit collecting tubule. *J Clin Invest* 59:1099, 1977.

154. Storstein O, Orjavik O: Aortic insufficiency in chronic renal failure. *Acta Med Scand* 203:175, 1978.

155. Terman DS, Alfrey AC, Hammond WS, et al: Cardiac calcification in uremia. A clinical, biochemical, and pathologic study. *Am J Med* 50:744, 1971.

156. Thompson FD, Joekes AM, Foulkes DM: Pharmacodynamics of propranolol in renal failure. *Br Med J* 2:434, 1972.

157. Thompson PD, Melmon KL, Richardson JA, et al: Lidocaine pharmacokinetics in advanced heart failure, liver disease, and renal failure in humans. *Ann Intern Med* 78:499, 1973.

158. Tripp ME, Katcher ML, Peters HA, et al: Systemic carnitine deficiency presenting as familial endocardial fibroelastosis. *N Engl J Med* 305:385, 1981.

159. Varat MA, Adolph RJ, Fowler NO: Cardiovascular effects of anemia. *Am Heart J* 83:415, 1972.

160. Vertes V, Cangiano JL, Berman LB, et al: Hypertension in end-stage renal disease. *N Engl J Med* 280:978, 1969.

161. Vidt DG, Bravo EL, Fouad FM: Captopril. *N Engl J Med* 306:214, 1982.

162. Walle AJ, Weiland E, Proppe D, et al: Is the erythropoietin-hematocrit feedback control operative in chronic renal failure? *Nephron* 31:229, 1982.

163. Weidmann P, Maxwell MH, Lupu AN, et al: Plasma renin activity and blood pressure in terminal renal failure. *N Engl J Med* 285:757, 1971.

164. Wennmalm A: Participation of prostaglandins in the regulation of peripheral vascular resistance. *Adv Prostaglandin Thromboxane Leukotriene Res* 10:303, 1982.

165. Wettrell G: Distribution and elimination of digoxin in infants. *Eur J Clin Pharmacol* 11:329, 1977.

166. Wettrell G, Andersson K-E: Clinical Pharmacokinetics of digoxin in infants. *Clin Pharmacokinet* 2:17, 1977.

167. Wildenthal K, Mierzuriak DS, Myers RM, et al: Effects of acute lactic acidosis on left ventricular performance. *Am J Physiol* 214:1352, 1968.

168. Wilkinson R, Scott DF, Uldall PR, et al: Plasma renin and exchangeable sodium in the hypertension of chronic renal failure. The effect of bilateral nephrectomy. *Q J Med* 39:377, 1970.

169. Witty RT, Davis JO, Johnson JA, et al: Effects of papaverine and hemorrhage on renin secretion in the nonfiltering kidney. *Am J Physiol* 221:1666, 1971.

170. Woie L, Oyri A: Quinidine intoxication treated with hemodialysis. *Acta Med Scand* 195:237, 1974.

171. Yawata Y, Jacob HS: Abnormal red cell metabolism in patients with chronic uremia. Nature of the defect and its persistence despite adequate hemodialysis. *Blood* 45:231, 1975.

172. Zins GR: Renal prostaglandins. *Am J Med* 58:14, 1975.

173. Zipes DP, Prystowsky EN, Heger JJ: Amiodarone: Electrophysiologic actions, pharmacokinetics and clinical effects. *J Am Coll Cardiol* 3:1059, 1984.

174. Zusman RM: Prostaglandins, vasopressin, and renal water reabsorption. *Med Clin North Am* 65:915, 1981.

Claire Kleinknecht
Denise Laouari
Michel Broyer

33
Disturbances of Carbohydrate, Lipid, and Nitrogen Metabolism

The metabolic abnormalities related to uremia are of special interest to pediatricians because they contribute to the growth retardation observed in uremic children. It is known that uremic children have insufficient food intake and that malnutrition and related metabolic disorders also interfere with the growth process. Thus, nutrition and metabolism are considered together in this chapter.

Many metabolic abnormalities have been described in uremia. They concern the three main biochemical compounds: carbohydrates, lipids, and nitrogen derivatives. Each will be considered separately, although this separation is made for practical purpose only, as there are many interactions between carbohydrates and lipids, for example, or between carbohydrates and nitrogen compounds.

Carbohydrates

Glucose intolerance is a well known feature of uremia. Blood glucose values often are elevated, but it must be stressed that substances that accumulate in uremia interfere with the measurement of glucose unless a specific method is used. Oral and intravenous glucose tolerance tests characteristically show a decrease in the rate of fall of blood glucose to baseline values. Plasma insulin levels are often abnormally high for a given level of blood glucose, possibly due to a decrease of proinsulin degradation in the kidney, leading to an increase of immuno-reactive insulin, which includes the biologically inactive proinsulin.

The main reason for hyperinsulinemia and glucose intolerance is the decrease of insulin activity in the peripheral tissues. Response to intravenous insulin is impaired in uremic patients [67], and forearm uptake of glucose is significantly lower in uremic patients during insulin infusion [117].

More recent investigations using the glucose clamp technique (blood glucose maintained at a given level after a priming dose, followed by a variable glucose infusion) allowed more precise study of the uptake of glucose metabolized by the cells (M), the secretion of insulin (I), and the sensitivity to insulin (expressed by the ratio M/I).

These studies showed a clear decrease of glucose metabolism by the cells, as well as a decrease in insulin secretion in uremic patients, but the most constant and most important abnormality was the decreased sensitivity to insulin observed in almost all subjects [33,34].

The site of insulin resistance seems to be in the peripheral tissues, as documented in several studies in humans [35] and in animals [92]. Hepatic glucose production and hepatic glucose uptake appear unchanged in uremic patients as compared to controls [35], but this remains controversial [32].

The nature of insulin resistance is not yet fully understood. It could concern the receptor or the post receptor step. Though insulin binding to red cells has been found to be decreased [22], binding to adipocytes appears normal [85]. More recent data on monocytes showed a normal number of insulin receptors per cell and a normal affinity of insulin for its receptor in uremics as compared to normal controls [35].

Thus, the reason for insulin resistance is probably related to postreceptor events. Glucose uptake or consumption [15,38] and oxidative phosphorylation [55] are inhibited by uremic sera. Abnormalities in glycolysis in leukocytes from uremic patients, including decrease in activity of pyruvate kinase [89], phosphofructokinase [15,43], and lactic dehydrogenase [42], have been described. Since insulin resistance could be reversed by dialysis [34] or by a low protein diet [111], it can be suggested that some more or less dialyzable toxins that accumulate in uremia are responsible for these metabolic abnormalities. Among these toxins, parathormone could play a critical role, since uremic children, studied by the hyperglycemic clamp technique before and after parathyroidectomy or medical treatment of hyperparathyroidism, showed a dramatic improvement of insulin secretion and glucose metabolism without change in sensitivity to insulin [84]. Excess parathyroid hormone in chronic renal failure seems to interfere with the ability of the beta cells to augment insulin secretion appropriately in response to the insulin resistant state [3].

Other factors could also impair glucose metabolism through cellular potassium deficiency. Although K deficiency may be a cause of insulin resistance, the ability of insulin to promote K penetration into the cells is maintained in uremic patients [35].

High plasma level of growth hormone in uremic patients, with a paradoxical rise after glucose infusion [104], may relate to poor glucose utilization by the cells in an attempt to mobilize fat as an alternative source of energy.

Finally, high glucagonemia, not suppressed by glucose infusion in uremic children [40], could also play a role in the disorders of glucose metabolism, since it promotes gluconeogenesis and glycogenolysis.

In conclusion, impairment of carbohydrate metabolism in uremia is related mainly to a loss of sensitivity of peripheral tissues to insulin, resulting in a lack of energy at the cellular level. This abnormality can be partially reversed by intense dialysis and suppression of hyperparathyroidism. In children with end-stage renal failure, these therapeutic measures are recommended in addition to physical exercise, which has been shown to improve glucose metabolism in adult uremic patients [64].

Glucose Metabolism in Children on CAPD

Glucose uptake from dialysate constitutes a considerable supplement of energy intake and must be taken into account in energy balance. Glucose absorption from dialysate appears to be more rapid in younger children, probably because of differences in peritoneal structure and consequently greater ultrafiltration. Blood glucose can remain in the normal range or be raised during peritoneal exchanges with standard bags, but it is always elevated, along with insulin levels, with hypertonic bags. The long term consequence of this permanent load of glucose is not yet fully appreciated, but glucose tolerance tests performed six months and one year after CAPD were not different from the initial test, even in young children [20].

Lipids

Disturbances of lipid metabolism in uremic patients have created great interest in recent years, since vascular complications are recognized to be the main cause of death in subjects on renal replacement therapy [82,119]. It seemed probable that these complications could also threaten uremic children after a longer interval, and this risk justified a number of studies in young uremic patients on treatment by dialysis or after transplantation [6,16,29, 39,69,96,97,105,118].

The level of reduction in GFR necessary to be associated with lipid abnormalities has been shown to be below 40 ml/min/1.73 m^2 [6,96]. The majority of patients on treatment by dialysis exhibit hyperlipidemia, due essentially to an increase of the triglycerides (TG) contained in serum, very low density lipid (VLDL), intermediary density lipid (IDL), and low density lipid (LDL). While the total serum lipoprotein profile of most uremic children corresponds to type IV hyperlipoproteinemia, according to the Frederickson classification (increased TG, no chylomicrons, normal cholesterol), there are also some patients whose lipid pattern resembles other types, especially type II.

In addition, parts of VLDL of uremic patients have been found to migrate more slowly than "normal" VLDL; they are called B VLDL and are considered to increase the risk for atherogenesis. HDL cholesterol is usually decreased in uremia. This decrease is associated with a diminished ability to form cholesterol-rich Apo E HDL involved in the atherogenic defense.

Important deviations from normal have been described for apolipoprotein distribution within lipoproteins: Total serum Apo A I and A II are decreased; total serum Apo A IV is increased and has been detected in LDL from which it is normally absent. Apo B is increased in LDL, and Apo B48, a marker of intestinal lipoprotein, has been found in serum VLDL from which it is also normally absent. Apo C II is decreased and Apo C III increased in VLDL and HDL, with a decrease of ratio Apo C II/Apo C III [94,101]. All these abnormalities are probably involved in the increased atherogenic risk observed in uremic patients, a risk that appears much higher than the moderate increase of TG usually reported in these patients would lead us to suppose.

Pathogenesis of Lipid Abnormalities

Hypertriglyceridemia can be the result of increased TG production, decreased TG removal, or both. Insulin resistance with hyperinsulinism was thought to play a role in hypertriglyceridemia by increasing TG synthesis [8], but the positive correlation between plasma insulin and plasma TG [7] does not necessarily imply increased TG synthesis. It could be related also to decreased removal as a result of insulin resistance. Despite a persistant controversy on this point, it is now generally accepted that defective removal plays the main role. A number of studies showed a decreased fractional clearance rate (K2) of exogenous chylomicrons (intralipid), with a negative correlation between plasma TG and K2 [23].

Normally the TG contained in VLDL and chylomicrons are rapidly hydrolyzed by lipoprotein lipase (LPL), an enzyme localized on the endothelial surface of blood vessels in extra-hepatic tissues. Under its action, IDL and remnants are formed, are subsequently hydrolyzed by the liver enzyme hepatic lipase (HL), and are transferred to HDL. Hepatic lipase also plays a role in the formation of HDL cholesterol.

In uremic patients, the activities of both LPL and HL were generally found to be decreased in adults [68] and in children [6]. Nevertheless there is still some controversy about the relative depression of the two enzymes [13] as they are difficult to measure indirectly after heparin administration. The synthesis of these enzymes could be impaired by uremia, but the decrease of activity can also be explained by the presence of inhibitors or the decrease of normal activators. As an example, Apo C II, which normally activates LPL, is reduced in uremia; this defect could contribute to the decreased removal of TG. Decrease of lecithin-cholesterol acyl transferase (LCAT) usually observed in uremic patients may also contribute to the defective TG removal [59].

The influence of diet could also have a major role. Since

the work of Simmons et al [110], who showed a relationship between growth velocity and energy intake in uremic children, high carbohydrate diets are prescribed for these patients. Some authors failed to find a relationship in children between lipid abnormalities and dietary carbohydrate [39], although others have [16,97], especially between saccharose and TG or VLDL. As a consequence, pediatricians must be very cautious when prescribing diets for uremic children, avoiding excess saccharose, and using starch preferentially for supplementation.

Decrease of TG has been reported after dietary manipulation, including very low carbohydrate intake [108], but such a diet is very difficult to apply in children. Another dietary recommendation could be the prescription of a high polyunsaturated/saturated fatty acid ratio, which has been shown to improve lipid abnormalities in uremic patients [56].

Role of Dialysis, Transplantation, and Other Iatrogenic Factors

Patients on CAPD have higher plasma TG and cholesterol than patients on hemodialysis [20,106], but it is uncertain to what extent this difference might increase the atherogenic risk. Intensive hemodialysis does not consistently improve TG removal, probably because the inhibitor(s) of lipase are poorly dialysable. In addition, acetate transfer during dialysis could contribute to hypertriglyceridemia [49]. Carnitine loss during dialysis has been considered as another possible factor for hypertriglyceridemia. Carnitine is involved in the transfer of long chain free fatty acids across mitochondrial membranes to the site of oxidation, and carnitine depletion, therefore, could theoretically result in hypertriglyceridemia. Carnitine supplementation has been found to improve hyperlipidemia of uremic patients [14], but its usefulness in uremic children remains to be shown. Carnitine depletion was not found in muscle of uremic children on dialysis, despite postdialysis decreased plasma carnitine levels (personal unpublished data).

Finally, the hyperlipemic action of some drugs currently prescribed in uremic patients must be considered. Thiazide diuretics and beta blockers are known to increase triglycerides, and long-term use of these drugs could probably increase the lipid abnormalities.

After transplantation, even when successful, 30% to 60% of children remain hyperlipidemic [6,17,69,97,105], but the lipid profile and the pathogenesis are not the same as in patients with normal renal function. Plasma cholesterol is more often elevated alone or in combination with TG, so that the lipid abnormalities are similar to type IIb or III at least as often as type IV. Steroid treatment is probably the main cause of these abnormalities, by promoting insulin resistance and increased TG production. The difficulty of correlating steroid dosage and lipid abnormalities could be related to the different individual response to steroid therapy [17].

Recently cyclosporin has been implicated in post–transplantation hyperlipidemia [62]. It is noteworthy that normal post heparin LPL and HL have been found in transplanted patients [29].

Since increased hepatic TG production is probably the main factor, transplanted patients can be rendered normotriglyceridemic by caloric restriction [99], which is recommended anyway in children on steroid therapy to limit their weight increase.

Finally, the question remains of the risk of accelerated atherosclerosis in transplanted patients with normal renal function who receive a low dose of corticosteroid. There may be positive risk factors, such as hypercholesterolemia and high Apo B; negative risk factors may include a high level of Apo AI and Apo AII in plasma and in HDL and a high ratio Apo AI/Apo B and Apo AII/Apo B [57].

Nitrogen Compounds
Nitrogen Retention and Its Relationship to Uremic Toxicity

The main activity of the kidney is to maintain water and electrolyte balance and to excrete the nitrogenous waste products resulting from endogenous and exogenous protein catabolism. Because of the "functional reserve" of the nephrons, i.e., their capacity to augment their filtration rate, there is no detectable retention of these products when the number of intact nephrons is only moderately impaired. Retention becomes apparent when nephron reduction reaches 60% to 70% of normal. The plasma level of the waste products begins to rise when GFR is reduced below a threshold level, which varies according to the production rate of the waste product.

Dialysis therapy has demonstrated that the most critical symptoms of chronic renal failure (CRF) result from the accumulation of substances that can be removed by dialysis. It is surprising, however, that so little is known regarding the toxicity of these substances and their contribution to the uremic syndrome. Many studies have been devoted to the so-called "uremic toxins" [11,51,70,73,109], and the number of substances considered possibly to be involved has progressively increased. Their enumeration, which would produce a vast catalogue, would be of little interest, because no definite effect can be defined for individual substances.

These uremic toxins may include (1) substances normally present in the body and excreted or destroyed by the kidney, hence accumulating when renal function is impaired; (2) substances resulting from an abnormal metabolic pathway due to the excessive level of the former products or to the lack of some enzymes or other material synthesized by the normal kidney; or (3) substances such as parathormone synthesized in response to derangements present in uremia. The interactions between these different mechanisms render any analysis regarding the role of each product difficult. Moreover, though the prominent role of dialyzable substances cannot be denied, it is established that dialysis therapy does not suppress all the uremic symptoms. Either dialysis is insufficient to remove all the toxins or deficiency of another renal function is the cause. Finally, the uremic syndrome is not well defined. In fact, except in the terminal phase, which is nowadays avoided in end-stage renal disease (ESRD), there are few clinical symptoms, even in the presence of marked biological abnormalities. Several in vitro tests have shown the toxic effects of uremic plasma. However, the role of each presumed uremic toxin is less well established, since they show toxicity only for levels higher than found in clinical practice.

UREA

The rise in blood urea was the first hallmark of CRF to be described, which led to the term "uremia." Urea readily diffuses throughout all body water and rises in cells as well as in the extra-cellular compartment. The responsibility of urea for uremic toxicity has been examined in a number of papers [11,70], but remains a challenge. Because of the rapid elimination of urea by the normal kidney, the amount of urea necessary to obtain elevated blood urea levels in normal subjects is very high and represents an osmotic load that could be the cause of the observed symptoms, including headache and vomiting. Most authors have concluded from studies in uremic dogs [58,88] and men—treated by dialysis while adding urea to the dialysate—that few symptoms develop. Merrill stressed that clinical improvement persisted despite urea administration in a dialyzed patient with acute renal failure [88]. However, other authors have observed the occurrence of abnormal symptoms in such patients when the blood urea level reached 30 mmol/l [71].

Although there is some evidence for a modest role of very high blood urea levels, such as those observed in end-stage renal failure, most authors consider that urea is not toxic by itself but is a marker of the accumulation of all nitrogen-containing waste products [73,86]. The blood urea level would then be a criterion of toxicity and therapy, particularly dietary prescription. Aims to decrease its level are sensible, assuming that the retention of other nitrogenous substances would parallel that of urea. Such an assumption is widely accepted and is discussed further below.

OTHER NITROGEN COMPOUNDS

As previously stated, nitrogenous compounds that have been found to be elevated in uremia are numerous. *Cyanate* can be formed from urea; its toxicity has been supported in uremic dogs [48], but its role in clinical conditions remains unknown. It may result in carbamylation of proteins and of hemoglobin; in uremia, the presence of carbamylated hemoglobin interferes with the measurement of glycosylated hemoglobin so that assessment of glucose metabolism from the A1C hemoglobin measurement by usual methods is not reliable [44].

Since liver function is preserved, *ammonia* is but moderately elevated in uremia, except in ESRD where the blood levels may rise abruptly.

Uric acid rises in uremia; symptoms of gout are rare, but the role of hyperuricemia in the development of pericarditis has been suggested [73].

The accumulation of *guanidines*, which seems greater in cells than in plasma [54,95], has been stressed by several authors and is influenced by dietary protein [5,95] and the blood urea level. The importance of guanidine compounds, particularly but not exclusively methylguanidine, has been

claimed. They caused symptoms when given in large amounts to normal dogs [53] and in vitro inhibited glucose utilization [9], platelet function, and DNA synthesis. Such results, however, were obtained by levels much higher than those observed in uremic sera. Thus, the actual toxicity of these compounds is not established [73].

Plasma *creatinine* level is used as an index of the severity of renal disease and frequently as an indicator for starting dialysis therapy. It is little influenced by protein ingestion, since creatinine is produced mainly by muscle metabolism. Other substances, such as 1-methylhistidine, 3-methylhistidine, and citrulline, are little influenced by nitrogen intake and accumulate in uremia. However, no evidence has been afforded for their direct toxicity.

Some authors have emphasized the rise of *amine derivatives* and their possible toxicity [73]. They include a number of substances, the toxicity of which is more or less established, including spermine, which seems to be involved in inhibition of erythropoiesis [100].

The substances referred to above have a small molecular weight and rapidly diffuse through the dialytic membrane. The role of molecules of molecular weight greater than 500 daltons ("middle molecules") has been questioned. They include a number of substances that are less easily dialyzed. Attempts to separate middle molecules in uremia have demonstrated that they represent a mixture of different compounds, most often peptides or glucuronides. Gel filtration and chromatography have separated several subfractions (such as fraction 7a, 7b, 7c, etc.) isolated by Bergström and Fürst [11] that do not correspond to pure molecules.

The middle molecules rise in proportion to the reduction of GFR. Their toxicity has been studied by many authors, with contradictory results. It is likely that they play a role in production of anemia, immunological disturbances, neuropathy, and possibly abnormalities in mitochondrial metabolism [11]. They include some inhibitors, the role of which can be important in uremic disturbances, such as the inhibitor(s) of insulin [87] and of somatomedin [98].

Many other substances have been incriminated as uremic toxins. For most of them, in vitro studies suggest a possible toxic effect on cellular metabolism [11,83], function, and proliferation, but for none has the toxicity been demonstrated in vivo. Whether the uremic syndrome is due to their interactions or to metabolic disturbances other than, or in addition to, nitrogen retention, remains a puzzle, despite more than one century of research.

Metabolism of Nitrogen Waste Products

MODIFICATIONS BY UREMIA

The production of urea is influenced by both nitrogen intake (positive correlation) [93] and energy intake (negative correlation) [1,2,79] in uremic and in normal subjects. It is generally admitted that urea levels are a good index of nitrogen intake and allow the calculation of "protein catabolic rate." Such an assumption considers that (1) fecal and other non-urinary nitrogen losses are negligible (although they are known to change with protein consumption); (2) the excretion on non-urea urinary nitrogen including ammonia is constant; and (3) the energy intake is high and similar in all patients. In some studies, urea production was shown to be unrelated to nitrogen intake but inversely related to energy intake [2]. Numerous reports stress the good overall relationship between urea production and nitrogen intake. This relationship is found, however, only in large scale studies of nitrogen intake; prediction in individuals remains poor, most likely because energy intake is not as constant as presumed. It must be kept in mind that because actual energy intake is extremely difficult to assess, nitrogen intake cannot be adequately estimated without the help of a trained dietitian.

Another aspect of urea metabolism that has created interest is the reuse of urea for protein synthesis after transformation to ammonia in the gut. Several authors found that [15]nitrogen, administered as urea or ammonia, was recovered in body proteins [50,52,103]. Giordano [50,52] improved the balance of uremic patients fed suboptimal amounts of proteins by adding urea to the diet. It was supposed that urea hydrolysis increased with blood urea levels so that significant amounts of endogenous nitrogen were available for protein synthesis in uremic patients. This hypothesis was the basis for using low-protein, semi-synthetic diets and particularly nitrogen-free analogues of essential amino-acids (EAA) [114]. Several findings, however, do not agree with this hypothesis: (1) urea hydrolysis is not substantially increased in uremia [113]; (2) no more than 6% total nitrogen is supplied by urea for albumin synthesis [113]; (3) oral antibiotics decrease urea production rate, suggesting that most urea degraded by the gut bacteria is directly transformed back into urea by the liver, without entering protein synthesis [91]; and (4) ketoanalogues do not increase the efficiency of urea utilization for protein synthesis [41].

Enrichment by ^{15}N of body protein after ^{15}N urea or NH_3 administration [52] could be due to exchange of [15]NH_3 in the hepatic pool. The possibility remains that some significant reuse of urea might occur in uremic patients receiving marginal amounts of essential aminoacids as their sole source of dietary nitrogen, but such diets have many practical and clinical disadvantages.

The urinary excretion of creatinine is low in CRF, compared to normal values for body weight, a finding that was at first considered to suggest loss in muscle mass or abnormal muscle metabolism. In fact, creatinine production is unchanged [90], but the fraction of creatinine metabolized, i.e., extra renal clearance, is increased. This degradation of creatinine was found to occur mainly in the gut, but to be little influenced by gut flora. With regard to urea, the gut degradation does not result in enhanced extrarenal nitrogen loss, but nitrogen recycling [90].

Uric acid production depends on nitrogen intake. The extrarenal clearance is also enhanced in uremia, accounting for as much as 30% to 70% of the uric acid produced. It is markedly influenced by gut bacteria and results in nitrogen recycling.

The production rate of some other nitrogen waste products is enhanced in uremia; the synthesis of guanidine compounds, for example, seems to be increased, presumably due to increased conversion of creatinine to creatine.

UREMIC TOXICITY AND DIETARY PROTEIN

Many nitrogenous compounds considered as potential toxins are derived from dietary protein, and their accumulation can be alleviated by lowering the protein intake. In severe CRF, lowering the amount of protein ingested lessens uremic symptoms. The aim of numerous studies has been to provide as little protein and nitrogen as is compatible with maintenance of nutrition, by using low protein diets supplemented with EAA or their keto-analogues [80] and defining the best EAA balance to promote protein synthesis. Such diets do reduce blood urea.

In an experiment in uremic rats [77], we concluded that high-protein diet supplied as a dry powder was deleterious for growth as well as for progression of renal lesions. However, normal to high protein diets have been allowed in many dialyzed patients without clear evidence of a harmful effect. In another experiment [76] uremic rats received casein in an agar-gel containing 80% water. Under these conditions, protein consumption was much higher than in the preceding study, resulting in extremely high blood urea levels (mean: 80 mmol/l) and severe acidosis; yet neither impairment of growth rate nor symptoms of poor health were observed, at least until ESRD was reached, which happened more rapidly than with lower protein intakes. Such a high protein intake seemed well tolerated, provided that large amounts of water were given at the same time.

Finally, it is not clear whether the nitrogen, osmotic, phosphorus, or other compounds of proteins are toxic. It is not even certain that protein excess causes uremic symptoms before ESRD is reached. There have been few attempts to control the consequent changes of toxicity of the uremic sera by using the numerous in vitro tests that measure effects on protein synthesis [36], for example, incorporation of amino acids or thymidine, and cell proliferation. So far, the benefit of semi-synthetic diets lacks positive evidence. Whether some toxins, probably produced by endogenous metabolism, such as 1-methylhistidine, 3-methylhistidine, creatinine, citrulline, or, more importantly, metabolic inhibitors, are modified by such diets remains doubtful.

Plasma and Muscle Protein and Free Amino Acid Concentrations

PROTEINS

In all human studies, plasma total proteins, albumin, and transferrin are lower in uremics than in normals [12,25, 65,107,116], although the differences are often small and the plasma concentrations are sometimes indicated as "within normal range." This slight decrease has been ascribed to protein depletion [12,116] because of the similarities between CRF and undernutrition, but few authors observed a rise in plasma proteins when nutrition was improved. The intravascular albumin pool was shown to be normal, the low plasma concentration resulting from expanded plasma volume, but total body albumin pool was reduced. Other proteins that are reduced in chronic undernutrition may be elevated in CRF, such as retinol binding protein and prealbumin [12,20]. Feeding uremic rats high amounts of protein does not improve the plasma protein concentration. The significance of the plasma decrease in individual cases is difficult to assess in the absence of pool measurements.

ALTERATION IN PROTEIN-BINDING

The binding of several metabolic compounds and drugs to plasma proteins is altered in uremia [60,61,102]. In uremic as in normal subjects, the major protein with binding properties is albumin [61]. It was suggested that potentially toxic compounds bind to albumin. Normally, the renal proximal tubule extracts the protein-bound metabolic compounds from the peritubular plasma and secretes them into the tubular lumen, preventing accumulation of protein-bound toxins [61]. When this extraction is impaired, binding sites of albumin may be saturated, and compounds or drugs that are normally bound will remain free if they compete for the same binding sites [61]. Other possible causes of impaired albumin binding are the presence of binding inhibitors and the alteration of albumin itself. The low plasma albumin level plays but a minor role.

The binding alteration is partially, but not fully, corrected by prolonged dialysis of uremic plasma and is not observed with normal plasma after addition of urea, creatinine, or uric acid, showing that other "toxins" cause binding inhibition.

The main albumin-bound substances are acidic drugs. Among the metabolic compounds are the free fatty acids (FFA), bilirubin, tryptophane, and thyroid hormone T3 [75]. The displacement of bound drugs in uremics results in alterations in volume of distribution; elimination rate; and local activity, which is correlated to the free plasma level of the drug; and finally, to enhanced or even toxic effects, demanding a modification of the doses used.

AMINO ACIDS

Disturbances of plasma amino acid (AA) levels have been reported by many authors. The plasma AA pattern has been considered as characteristic of CRF [78], notably low branched chain AA, particularly valine and not corrected by augmented valine intake; reduced essential AA (EAA) pool despite elevated phenylalanine; expanded nonessential AA (NEAA) pool with augmented glycine, citrulline, proline, and other NEAA levels; but reduced tyrosine concentration and decreased ratios such as EAA/NEAA, valine/glycine, and tyrosine/phenylalanine.

Plasma AA concentrations reported in several series of children are presented in [18–21,28,37,72,107] Table 33-1. The plasma values showed wide variations from one series of children with CRF to another. Particularly intriguing is the difference in EAA between two series of children on peritoneal dialysis, one showing no reduction of any EAA, including valine, and EAA pool enlargement [20], whereas in the other, all EAA were clearly decreased [107].

Another unexplained and surprising finding is the degree of reduction of most EAA in children with moderate CRF [19] as compared to the normal, or almost normal, level in children with more severe disease [20,37]. Table 33-1

shows that no change in any of the EAA is consistent, although a fall in valine is found in all series but one, and a fall in leucine is frequent. Phenylalanine and histidine, which have been reported as significantly altered, seem remarkably stable and normal when all available data are considered.

Plasma NEAA pool was expanded in most series, although the values for each NEAA vary. The only constant changes are the rise of citrulline, which is evident in moderate CRF and reaches very high values, and the rise of aspartic acid, which reaches impressively high levels in infants [18]. The rise of glycine and proline are less dramatic. The only NEAA showing a significant decrease is tyrosine. Plasma serine may be low or normal.

In adult series [4,26,45,79], the changes in plasma AA are comparable to those reported in children. Of the EAA, valine and leucine are low, whereas phenylalanine and histidine remain within the normal range. Of the NEAA, citrulline is consistently elevated, glycine and aspartic acid are frequently elevated, while serine and tyrosine may be reduced. The plasma levels of 1-methylhistidine and 3-methylhistidine, not shown in Table 33-1, were considerably elevated in all series.

In two series, an EAA-ketoanalogue mixture was added to a low [18] or to a moderately restricted [72] protein diet. All branched-chain AA remained low in both series; the other EAA were normal in one series [18] and low in the other, except for phenylalanine [72]. These diets, which resulted in a low blood urea level, did not influence the NEAA plasma levels.

Muscle AA have been less frequently measured [4,10,19,37] (Table 33-2). Intracellular disturbances are less severe than plasma changes. The EAA pool is often enlarged, and valine concentration is the only EAA to be constantly low, even in children with moderate CRF who fared well and had normal nutrition. The NEAA pool is enlarged, particularly in patients requiring dialysis, with elevated levels of citrulline only in these patients.

Some of our experimental data are shown in Tables 33-3 and 33-4. Plasma and muscle AA concentrations were measured in rats who were either normal or in CRF (GFR from 5% to 30% that of controls) and who were fed four protein diets: 12 g/100 g casein, 6 g/100 g casein (insufficient in protein), and 6 g/100 g protein supplemented either with EAA or with an EAA-keto acid mixture.

In normal rats, the insufficient protein diet resulted in low EAA except for lysine and histidine. The plasma levels of branched-chain AA were not corrected by the administration of their keto analogues, but were corrected by the addition of the corresponding EAA. A rise of lysine and threonine was observed when they were administered in a synthetic form.

In rats with CRF, there was no decrease in any of the EAA as compared to normal rats fed the same diet, in spite of lower food intake. It is remarkable that with the insufficient protein diet, the plasma levels of all EAA except lysine and histidine were higher in rats with CRF than in controls who had a better appetite. Similarly, the branched-chain amino acids were higher in rats with CRF fed the EAA-keto acid diet than in controls fed the same diet. This finding, added to the poor relationship between

TABLE 33-1. *Plasma amino acid concentrations in children with chronic renal insufficiency (% control values)*

Authors	Counahan et al (1976)	Delaporte et al (1978)	Broyer et al (1983)	Salusky et al (1983)	Broyer et al (1980)		Broyer et al (1983)		Jones et al (1983)		Bulla et al (1986)
Patients	HD	ESRD	PD	PD	Moderate CRF	Severe CRF	CRF (Infants) LP** + KA***		CRF	KA***	CRF
N° patients	16	8	15	10	10	5	5	6	7	7	11
Essential amino acids											
Valine	70	71	90	68	74	74	65	42	74	60	64
Leucine	68	93	94	51	75	86	72	46	74	74	62
Isoleucine	81	110	118	73	80	92	104	69	95	78	75
Methionine	82	147	110	86	76	114	156	156	90	71	70
Lysine	86	119	148	65	100	103	114	103	70	70	87
Threonine	—	130	137	65	58	68	87	91	65	53	78
Phenylalanine	98	100	110	81	77	97	147	145	111	109	92
Histidine	81	113	116	74	120	133	117	110	95	78	80
Non-essential amino acids											
Glycine	181	193	201	138	78	73	139	197	131	101	141
Serine	51	92	96	58	77	57	108	129	72	55	79
Citrulline	114	320	491	326	226	282	352	395	264	330	194
Tyrosine	58	75	100	46	70	61	98	—	80	56	62
Aspartic Acid	—	333	422	364	181	313	679	500	175	137	—
Alanine	—	131	136	88	57	71	139	128	107	74	144
Arginine	106	133	152	82	116	118	114	124	80	88	127
Asparagine	—	144	160	71	83	100	107	107	—	—	—
Glutamine	—	130	149	81	116	115	146	159	—	—	39
Glutamic Acid	—	105	133	87	87	87	198	150	—	—	—
Ornithine	105	150	167	97	119	125	155	120	98	109	125
Proline	174	177	206	121	100	140	221	172	184	132	—
Taurine	—	158	113	98	70	105	110	109	104	127	44
Cystine	160	91	169	90	66	164	108	96	89	84	105
E/NE amino acids											
Tyr/Phe	62	74	91	57	87	59					
Val/Gly	42	37	25	53	105	102					

** Low protein diet; *** Insufficient protein diet supplemented with an essential AA-keto acid mixture.
HD: hemodialysis patients; ESRD: end-stage renal disease; PD: peritoneal dialysis; CRF: chronic renal failure.

Table 33-2. *Muscle amino acid concentration in patients with chronic renal failure (% control values)*

Author	Delaporte et al (1976)	Children Broyer et al (1980)		Adults Bergstrom et al (1978)	Alvestrand et al (1978)
Patients	ESRD	Moderate CRF	Severe CRF	ESRD and PD	ESRD
N° patients	8	10	5	14	16
Essential amino acids					
Valine	89	56	80	46	58
Leucine	120	97	112	101	75
Isoleucine	108	108	108	118	68
Methionine	179	127	141	86	78
Lysine	150	135	121	76	110
Threonine	137	79	81	61	60
Phenylalanine	108	108	103	126	141
Histidine	104	112	110	73	109
Non-essential amino acids					
Glycine	161	83	75	113	144
Serine	144	95	89	85	92
Citrulline	366	59	67	192	158
Tyrosine	86	98	87	73	102
Aspartic Acid	147	73	126	164	304
Alanine	94	71	63	118	121
Arginine	244	144	125	112	139
Asparagine	163	90	95	133	100
Glutamine	158	140	154	90	113
Glutamic	135	107	141	195	90
Acid	256	166	178	51	126
Ornithine	127	110	88	100	82
Proline	158	108	157	116	118
Taurine	73	119	129	—	—
Cystine					

ESRD: end-stage renal disease. CRF: chronic renal failure. PD: peritoneal dialysis.

the intensity of plasma EAA changes and the severity of CRF, as shown on Table 33-1, emphasizes the difficulty of interpreting any "improvement" or "deterioration" of the plasma EAA pattern and casts doubt on its value as a nutritional index in CRF. Moreover, supplements of EAA or keto acids may result in imbalanced plasma levels, which may prove harmful in the long term.

Among the NEAA, plasma levels of glycine, citrulline, and aspartic acid were elevated, with little influence by the diet. A rise in taurine levels was observed in rats fed semisynthetic diets.

As in humans, the alterations of the AA pattern due to CRF were less evident in muscle than in plasma. There was a rise of the EAA in response to added synthetic EAA and a rise of the NEAA already elevated in plasma.

In addition to low branched-chain AA plasma levels, reduced branched-chain keto acid concentrations were found, with a ratio of AA to keto acids that was elevated for leucine and isoleucine but not for valine [30].

The disparities observed between series are difficult to explain. Different protein or energy intakes, mode of dialysis, and circumstances of sampling may create problems. Holliday et al [66] showed that plasma leucine levels rose more during fasting in rats with CRF than in controls. It can be imagined that plasma EAA is raised more in the fasting state in patients with severe CRF than in those with moderate CRF, accounting for the relatively high levels encountered in ESRD, compared to moderate uremia. Kopple et al [79] found that most EAA increased when energy intake was reduced. In fact, the different series are too small to draw definite conclusions, particularly for moderate CRF.

There is no satisfactory explanation for the alteration of muscle and plasma AA patterns except for 1-methylhistidine and 3-methylhistidine, which are normally excreted by the kidney and which accumulate when excretion is impaired. Low dietary intake plays some role, but its importance is not clear. Wang et al. found in rats that the EAA/NEAA varied with the dietary protein and not with the uremic state [115]. Kopple and Swendseid [78], comparing normal and uremic subjects receiving identical protein diets, also found that EAA/NEAA was influenced by the diet and not by uremia, whereas the valine/glycine ratio was influenced by both. Plasma valine was influenced by the valine content of the diet, and could be normal when crystalline EAA were administered; the low valine levels found in uremic patients fed restricted protein diets were associated with no alteration of valine metabolism.

Most authors do not find any correlation between plasma AA levels and protein or energy intake [19,21,37,60] or

Table 33-3. *Plasma amino acid concentrations in rats fed different protein diets (% of values found in normal rats fed a 12 g/100 g casein diet)*

Diet	Normal rats			Rats with chronic renal failure			
	6% CAS + EAA	6% CAS + EAA-KA	6% CAS	12% CAS	6% CAS + EAA	6% CAS + EAA-KA	6% CAS
Essential amino acids							
Valine	103	76	76	96	118	108	97
Leucine	124	69	65	89	128	95	97
Isoleucine	92	67	71	107	123	110	105
Methionine	102	104	55	95	120	115	79
Lysine	123	99	83	85	115	156	78
Threonine	181	220	32	104	202	277	49
Phenylalanine	105	87	60	110	120	109	98
Histidine	146	132	131	111	143	185	127
Non-essential amino acids							
Glycine	111	82	91	237	252	312	290
Serine	104	78	94	82	103	97	108
Citrulline	138	121	98	301	506	405	403
Tyrosine	102	113	51	72	77	56	53
Aspartic Acid	110	85	124	175	175	187	166
Alanine	110	118	95	117	138	201	117
Arginine	117	92	80	77	97	102	79
Asparagine	120	115	79	95	141	203	88
Glutamine	104	83	88	74	94	103	84
Glutamic Acid	124	102	107	77	81	77	62
Ornithine	141	120	102	98	120	143	131
Proline	134	143	77	122	164	147	115
Taurine	187	332	79	100	339	605	182
Cystine	87	112	32	68	86	143	32

CAS: casein; EAA: Essential amino acids; KA: Keto analogues; six rats per group were studied.

with plasma albumin and transferin [28,37]. However, Gulyassy and De Torente [60] reported an inverse correlation between tryptophane and energy intake, and Salusky et al [107] found that valine levels correlated directly and glycine levels correlated inversely with energy and protein intakes. By contrast, Kopple et al. found [78] an inverse correlation between several EAA, including valine, an energy intake.

The influence of exercise has been little studied. The plasma branched-chain AA decreased slightly during exercise but increased during the recovery period in one study, as did the keto acids [30].

It is possible that altered handling of AA by the diseased kidney directly affects the plasma AA levels [79a]. The normal kidney takes up and releases a large amount of AA. The low tyrosine plasma level and low plasma tyrosine/phenylalanine ratio could result from impaired conversion of phenylalanine to tyrosine in the kidney; this is supported by the low phenylalanine hydroxylase levels in the diseased kidney [112]. Similarly, the impaired uptake of glycine by the kidney could result in elevated glycine and decreased serine levels in plasma. Net production of serine and net use of glycine were found to correlate with renal function in uremic dogs [79a]. However, serine is not constantly decreased in uremic patients.

It is known that uremic plasma impairs the activity of many enzymes. The phenylalanine hydroxylase activity in the liver may also be inhibited in uremia and is lowered

by feeding an inadequate protein diet [120]. Finally, several separate causes may collectively modify the AA plasma levels.

Raised citrulline levels could be accounted for by deficient conversion of citrulline to arginine. The arginine synthetase activity was found to be reduced in the kidney of uremic rats [115], though the enzymes responsible for the conversion were normal in the liver. However, the citruline originating in the gut is essentially metabolized in the kidney. Similarly, the rise of aspartic acid could not be explained and was not associated with reduced levels of asparagine.

Protein Synthesis and Degradation

An important question is to what extent the numerous plasma and cellular alterations found in CRF, together with hormonal disturbances and decreased appetite, affect protein metabolism.

Several authors have stressed the "catabolic state" and wasting of patients with CRF. Wasting develops in ESRD and is avoided by early dialysis, provided it is started before weight loss and evident catabolism occurs. Children with CRF do grow, although at a reduced rate, when they are on dialysis; marked protein catabolism is not likely.

The question remains whether protein synthesis and catabolism are normal or altered in uremia, compared to

Table 33-4. *Muscle free amino acid concentrations in rats fed different protein diets (% of values found in normal rats fed a 12 g/100 g casein diet)*

Diet	Normal rats			Rats with chronic renal failure			
	6% CAS + EAA	6% CAS + EAA-KA	6% CAS	12% CAS	6% CAS + EAA	6% CAS + EAA-KA	6% CAS
Essential amino acids							
Valine	99	72	74	100	131	81	108
Leucine	158	112	119	175	216	167	189
Isoleucine	95	92	85	113	136	115	129
Methionine	85	98	67	104	124	80	110
Lysine	172	197	146	149	188	323	95
Threonine	132	264	54	119	222	235	50
Phenylalanine	105	107	81	109	185	133	124
Histidine	162	198	174	172	189	229	154
Non-essential amino acids							
Glycine	110	102	107	185	210	240	194
Serine	98	103	148	105	117	90	103
Citrulline	167	129	168	334	431	321	446
Tyrosine	90	120	92	119	132	136	77
Aspartic Acid	107	121	117	176	172	144	136
Alanine	123	142	102	135	175	156	96
Arginine	143	174	133	118	175	196	84
Asparagine	112	132	128	130	163	167	96
Glutamine	117	128	125	103	141	117	88
Glutamic Acid	103	94	150	164	133	123	163
Ornithine	141	140	137	125	143	189	137
Proline	—	152	—	161	217	186	—
Taurine	181	262	120	94	250	230	127
Cystine	100	111	52	52	111	89	43

CAS: casein; EAA: Essential amino acids; KA: Keto analogues; Six rats per group were studied.

normal people, and whether any change results from diminished food intake or from uremia itself. Experimental data are contradictory.

Several in vitro studies demonstrated enhanced protein catabolism in muscle taken from uremic rats compared to normals. Garber observed an increased release of alanine and glutamine that was related to muscle catabolism [46], and a decreased inhibition of amino acid release by epinephrine or serotonin. These disturbances were similar to those found in normal muscle in the presence of parathormone, whereas parathormone itself had no effect on uremic muscle, suggesting that the alterations of muscle metabolism in uremia could be accounted for by the chronically elevated level of parathormone [47].

Harter et al. [63] examined the release of phenylalanine and tyrosine, neither of which are synthesized or metabolized in muscle. In muscle from uremic rats, they found an enhanced release, indicating enhanced protein breakdown, which declined to control levels after the addition of insulin and 25-OH-D_3. Phenylalanine and tyrosine release was markedly influenced by the protein diet previously given to both the control and uremic experimental animals. In uremics, it was also influenced by exercise training, which reduced the enhanced catabolic rate. Davis et al. [31] confirmed the enhanced release of phenylalanine and tyrosine in uremic rats and its reduction by exercise training. In this study, protein synthesis was unaffected by either uremia or exercise.

Other models have yielded different conclusions. Holliday et al. [66] examined the in vivo incorporation of ^{14}C-leucine in muscle and found no difference between uremic and control rats who were fed, but a reduced incorporation in uremic studies after an 18- to 24-hour fast. Li and Wassner [81], studying the hemicorpus preparation and phenylalanine incorporation, found that neither synthesis nor degradation differed between uremic and controls who were fed; however, after a 24- or 48-hour fast, uremic rats showed decreased protein synthesis and enhanced protein catabolism. Their finding was in agreement with those of Holliday et al. [66]. D. Laouari (personal communication) found that fractional protein synthesis, estimated from in vivo incorporation of phenylalanine into muscle, was lower in uremic rats than in controls fed ad lib, but did not differ between uremic rats and pair-fed controls.

Some sequences of hepatic messenger ribonucleic acid were found to be markedly altered in uremic rats, but most of these changes were also present in pair-fed control rats, suggesting the prominent role of reduced food intake [75]. Since only some sequences were affected, it seems that the synthesis rate of the different proteins may be altered differentially. The possibility that uremia and undernutrition may result in a decrease of specific messenger ribonucleic acids coding for proteins not essential for maintaining life has been suggested [75].

Li and Wassner [81] suggested that the increased protein catabolism observed in fasting animals resulted from reduced amount of body fat in uremics and postulated that the isolated muscle preparation resembled fasting since it lacked extra energy reserves.

Studies in humans are few. In children, protein turnover, estimated from plasma ^{15}N-lysine enrichment, was found to be lower than normal and influenced by food intake [27]. It is clear that further studies, particularly in vivo and in clinical conditions, are needed.

References

1. Abitbol CL, Holliday MA: The effect of energy and nitrogen intake upon urea production in children with uremia and undernutrition. *Clin Nephrol* 10:9, 1978.
2. Abitbol CL, Jean G, Broyer M: Urea synthesis in moderate experimental uremia. *Kidney Int* 19:648, 1981.
3. Akmal M, Massry SG, Goldstein DA, et al: Role of parathyroid hormone in the glucose intolerance of chronic renal failure. *J Clin Invest* 75:1037, 1985.
4. Alvestrand A, Bergström J, Fürst P, et al: Effect of essential amino-acid supplementation on muscle and plasma free amino-acids in chronic uremia. *Kidney Int* 14:323, 1978.
5. Ando A, Orita Y, Nakata K, et al: Effect of low protein diet and surplus of essential amino acids on the serum concentration and the urinary excretion of methylguanidine and guanidosuccinic acid in chronic renal failure. *Nephron* 24:161, 1979.
6. Assayama K, Ito H, Nakahara C, et al: Lipid profile and lipase activities in children and adolescents with chronic renal failure treated conservatively or with hemodialysis or transplantation. *Pediatr Res* 18:783, 1984.
7. Attman PO, Gustafson A: Lipid and carbohydrate metabolism in uremia. *Eur J Clin Invest* 9:285, 1979.
8. Bagdade JD, Porte D Jr, Bierman EL: Hypertriglyceridemia. A metabolic consequence of chronic renal failure. *N Engl J Med* 279:181, 1968.
9. Balestri PL, Rindi P, Biagini M, et al: Effects of uraemic serum, urea, creatinine and methylguanidine on glucose metabolism. *Clin Sci* 42:395, 1972.
10. Bergström J, Fürst P, Norée LO, et al: Intracellular free amino acids in muscle tissue of patients with chronic uraemia: effect of peritoneal dialysis and infusion of essential amino-acids. *Clin Sci Molec Med (Lond)* 54:51, 1978.
11. Bergström J, Fürst P: Uraemic toxins. *In* Drukker W, Parsons FM, Maher JF (eds): *Replacement of Renal Function by Dialysis*. Boston, Martinus Nijhoff, 1983, p 340.
12. Blumenkrantz MJ, Kopple JD, Gutamn RA, et al: Methods for assessing nutritional status of patients with chronic renal failure. *Am J Clin Nutr* 33:1567, 1980.
13. Bolzano K, Krempler F, Sandhofer F: Hepatic and extrahepatic triglyceride lipase activity in uremic patients on chronic hemodialysis. *Eur J Clin Invest* 8:289, 1978.
14. Bougneres PF, Lacour B, Di Guiglo S, et al: Hypolipaemic effect of carnitine on uremic patients. *Lancet* 1:1401, 1979.
15. Briggs WA, Jillix DH, Mahagan S, et al: Leukocyte metabolism and function in uremia. *Kidney Int* (suppl 16)24:593, 1983.
16. Broyer M, Tete MJ, Laudat MH, et al: Plasma lipid abnormalities in children on chronic hemodialysis. Relationships to dietary intake. *Proc EDTA Pitman Medical* 13:385, 1976.
17. Broyer M, Tete MJ, Laudat MH, et al: Plasma lipids in transplanted children and adolescents. Influence of pubertal development, dietary intake and steroid therapy. *Eur J Clin Invest* 2:397, 1981.
18. Broyer M, Guillot M, Niaudet P, et al: Comparison of three low-nitrogen diets containing essential amino-acids and their alpha-analogues for severely uremic children. *Kidney Int* (suppl 16)24:S290, 1983.
19. Broyer M, Jean G, Dartois AM, et al: Plasma and muscle free amino acid in children at the early stages of renal failure. *Am J Clin Nutr* 33:1396, 1980.
20. Broyer M, Niaudet P, Champion G, et al: Nutritional and metabolic studies in children on continuous ambulatory peritonneal dialysis. *Kidney Int* (suppl 15)24:S106, 1983.
21. Bulla M, Bremer HJ, Ronda-Vildozola R, et al: The effect of oral essential amino-acids and their keto-analogues on children receiving regular haemodialysis. *Int J Pediatr Nephrol* 7:73, 1986.
22. Cambnir KK, Herurker SG, Cruz AC, et al: Insulin receptor defect in diabetic man with chronic renal failure. A comparison of erythrocyte insulin binding in diabetic and nondiabetic patients on maintenance hemodialysis. *Biochem Med* 25:62, 1981.
23. Chan MK, Varguepe Z, Moorhead JF: Lipid abnormalities in uremia dialysis and transplantation. *Kidney Int* 19:625, 1981.
24. Chapman GV, Ward RA, Farrell PC: Separation and quantification of the "middle molecules" in uremia. *Kidney Int* 17:82, 1980.
25. Coles GA, Peters DK, Jones JH: Albumin metabolism in chronic renal failure. *Clin Sci* 39:423, 1970.
26. Condon JR, Asatoor AM: Amino acid metabolism in uraemic patients. *Clin Chim Acta* 32:333, 1971.
27. Conley SB, Rose GM, Robson AM, et al: Effects of dietary intake and hemodialysis on protein turnover in uremic children. *Kidney Int* 17:837, 1980.
28. Counahan R, El-Bishti M, Cox BD, et al: Plasma amino acids in children and adolescents on hemodialysis. *Kidney Int* 10:471, 1976.
29. Crawford GA, Savdie E, Stewart JH: Heparin-released plasma lipases in chronic renal failure and after renal transplantation. *Clin Sci* 57:155, 1979.
30. Dalton RN, Chantler C: The relationship between branched-chain amino acids and alpha-keto acids in blood in uremia. *Kidney Int* (suppl 16)24:61, 1983.
31. Davis TA, Karl IE, Tegtmeyer ED, et al: Muscle protein turnover: effects of exercise training and renal insufficiency. *Am J Physiol* 248:E337, 1985.
32. Deferrari G, Garibotto G, Robaudo C, et al: Glucose interorgan exchange in chronic renal failure. *Kidney Int* (suppl 16)24:S115, 1983.
33. Defronzo RA, Alvestrand A: Glucose intolerance in uremia. Site and mechanism. *Am J Clin Nutr* 33:1438, 1980.
34. Defronzo RA, Tobin JD, Rowe JW, et al: Glucose intolerance in uremia. Quantification of pancreatic beta cell sensitivity to glucose and tissue sensitivity to insulin. *J Clin Invest* 62:425, 1978.
35. Defronzo RA, Smith D, Alvestrand A: Insulin action in uremia. *Kidney Int* (suppl 16)24:102, 1983.
36. Delaporte C, Gros F: In vitro inhibition of protein synthesis by dialysates of plasma from uraemic patients. *Eur J Clin Invest* 11:139, 1981.
37. Delaporte C, Jean G, Broyer M: Free plasma and muscle amino acids in uremic children. *Am J Clin Nutr* 31:1647, 1978.
38. Dzurik R, Valovicova E: Glucose utilization during uremia. In vitro study. *Clin Chim Act* 30:137, 1970.
39. El-Bishti M, Counahan R, Jarrett RS, et al: Hyperlipidemia in children on regular haemodialysis. *Arch Dis Child* 52:932, 1977.
40. El-Bishti M, Counahan R, Bloom S, et al: Hormonal and

metabolic response to intravenous glucose in children on regular hemodialysis. *Am J Clin Nutr* 31:1865, 1978.

41. Ell S, Fynn M, Richards P, et al: Metabolic studies with keto acid diets. *Am J Clin Nutr* 31:1776, 1978.

42. Emerson PM, Withycomby A, Wilkinson JH: Inhibition of lactate dehydrogenase by sera of uremic patients. *Lancet* 2:571, 1965.

43. Fiaschi E, Campanacci I, Guarmeri G, et al: Muscle glucose content and hexokinase activity in patients with chronic uremia. *Kidney Int* 7:S341, 1975.

44. Flückiger R, Harmon W, Meier W, et al: Hemoglobin carbamylation in uremia. *N Engl J Med* 304:823, 1981.

45. Flügel-Link RM, Jones MR, Kopple JD: Red cell and plasma amino acid concentrations in renal failure. *J Parenteral Enteral Nutr* 7:450, 1983.

46. Garber AJ: Skeletal muscle protein and amino acid metabolism in experimental chronic uremia in the rat. *J Clin Invest* 62:623, 1978.

47. Garber AJ: Effects of parathyroid hormone on skeletal muscle protein and amino acid metabolism in the rat. *J Clin Invest* 71:1806, 1983.

48. Gilboe DD, Javid MJ: Breakdown products of urea and uremic syndrome. *Proc Soc Exp Biol Med* 115, 1984.

49. Giorcelli G, Dalmasso F, Bruno M, et al: RDT with acetate-free bicarbonate buffered dialysis fluid: long-term effects on lipid pattern, acid-base balance and oxygen delivery. *Proc EDTA Pitman Medical* 16:115, 1979.

50. Giordano C: Use of exogenous and endogenous urea for protein synthesis in normal and ureamic subjects. *J Lab Clin Med* 63:231, 1963.

51. Giordano C: The biochemical basis of uremic toxity. *Int J Pediatr Nephrol* 3:239, 1982.

52. Giordano C, de Pascale C, Balestrieri C, et al: Incorporation of urea N^{15} in amino acids of patients with chronic renal failure on low nitrogen diet. *Am J Clin Nutr* 21:394, 1968.

53. Giovanneti S, Biagini M, Balestri PL, et al: Uraemia-like syndrome in dogs chronically intoxicated with methylguanidine and creatinine. *Clin Sci* 36:445, 1969.

54. Giovannetti S, Balestri TI, Barsotti G: Methylguanidine in uremia. *Arch Intern Med* 131:703, 1973.

55. Glaze RP, Morgan JM, Morgan RE: Uncoupling of oxidative phosphorylation by ultrafiltrates of uremic serum. *Proc Soc Exp Biol Med* 126:172, 1967.

56. Gokal R, Mann JL, Olliver DO, et al: Treatment of hyperlipidemia in patients on chronic haemodialysis. *Br Med J* 1:82, 1978.

57. Goldstein S, Duhamel G, Laudat MH, et al: Plasma lipids, lipoproteins and apolipoproteins AI, AII and B in renal transplanted children, what risk for accelerated atherosclerosis. *Nephron* 38:87, 1984.

58. Grollman EF, Grollman A: Toxicity of urea and its role in the pathogenesis of uremia. *J Clin Invest* 38:749, 1959.

59. Guarnieri GF, Moracchiello M, Campanacci L, et al: Lecithincholesterol acyl transferase (LCAT) activity in chronic uremia. *Kidney Int* (suppl 8)13:S26, 1978.

60. Gulyassy PF, Torrente de A: Tryptophan metabolism in uremia. *Kidney Int* 7:S311, 1975.

61. Gulyassy PF, Depner TA: Impaired binding of drugs and endogenous ligands in renal diseases. *Am J Kidney Dis* 11:578, 1983.

62. Harris KP, Russel GI, Parvins SD, et al: Alterations in lipid and carbohydrate metabolism attributable to cyclosporine A in renal transplant recipient. *Br Med J* 292:16, 1986.

63. Harter HR, Davis TA, Karl IE: Enhanced muscle protein catabolism in uremia. *Adv Exp Med Biol* 167:557, 1984.

64. Harter HR, Goldberg AP: Endurance exercise training an

effective therapeutic modality for hemodialysis patients. *Med Clin North Am* 69:159, 1985.

65. Heidland A, Kult J: Long term effects of essential amino acids supplementation in patients on regular dialysis. *Clin Nephrol* 3:234, 1975.

66. Holliday MA, Chantler C, Mac Donnel R, et al: Effect of uremia on nutritionally-induced variations in protein metabolism. *Kidney Int* 11:236, 1977.

67. Horton ES, Johnson C, Lebowitz HE: Carbohydrate metabolism in uremia. *Ann Intern Med* 68:63, 1968.

68. Ibels LS, Reardon MF, Nestel PJ: Plasma post-heparin lipolytic activity and triglyceride clearance in uremic and hemodialysis patients and allograft recipients. *J Lab Clin Med* 87:648, 1976.

69. Ibels LS, Alfrey AC, Weil R: Hyperlipidemia in adult, pediatric and diabetic renal transplant recipients. *Am J Med* 64:634, 1978.

70. Johnson WJ: Does elevated blood urea participate in the pathogenesis of the uremic syndrome. *Semin Nephrol* 3:265, 1983.

71. Johnson WJ, Hagge WW, Wagoner RD, et al: Effects of urea loading in patients with far-advanced renal facture. *Mayo Clin Proc* 47:21, 1972.

72. Jones R, Dalton N, Turner C, et al: Oral essential amino acid and keto acid supplements in children with chronic renal failure. *Kidney Int* 24:95, 1983.

73. Kelly RA, Mitch WE: Creatinine, uric acid, and other nitrogenous waste products: clinical implication of the imbalance between their production and elimination in uremia. *Semin Nephrol* 3:286, 1983.

74. Keshaviah P, Kjellstrand CM: Middle molecules: do they exist? Are they toxic? *Semin Nephrol* 3:295, 1983.

75. Kinlaw WB, Schwartz HL, Mariasch CN, et al: Hepatic messenger ribonucleic acid activity profiles in experimental azotemia in the rat. *J Clin Invest* 74:1934, 1984.

76. Kleinknecht C, Laouari D, Thorel D, et al: Protein diet and uremic toxicity: Myth or reality? Study with protein self selection. *Kidney Int* 32:(Suppl 22), S-62, 1987.

77. Kleinknecht C, Salusky I, Broyer M, et al: Effects of various protein diet on growth, renal junction, and survival of uremic rats. *Kidney Int* 15:534, 1979.

78. Kopple JD, Swendseid ME: Protein and amino acid metabolism in uremic patients undergoing maintenance dialysis. *Kidney Int* (suppl 2)7:64, 1975.

79. Kopple JD, Monteon FJ, Shaid JK: Effect of energy intake or nitrogen metabolism in non dialysed patients with chronic renal failure. *Kidney Int* 29:734, 1986.

79a. Kopple JD, Fukuda S: Effects of amino acid infusion and renal failure on the uptake and release of amino acids by the dog kidney. *Am J Clin Nutr* 33:1363, 1980.

80. Laouari D, Kleinknecht C, Broyer M: Utilisation des céto-analogues d'acides aminés dans l'insuffisance rénale chronique. *Néphrologie*, 1986.

81. Li JB, Wassner SJ: Protein synthesis and degradation in skeletal muscle of chronically uremic rats. *Kidney Int* 29:1136, 1986.

82. Lindner AL, Chara B, Sherrard DJ, et al: Accelerated atherosclerosis in prolonged maintenance hemodialysis. *N Engl J Med* 290:697, 1974.

83. Liveson JA, Gardner J, Bornstein MB: Tissue culture studies of possible uremic neurotoxin: myoinositol. *Kidney Int* 12:131, 1977.

84. Mak RHK, Bettinelli A, Turner C, et al: The influence of hyperparathyroidism on glucose metabolism in uremia. *J Clin Endocrinol Metab* 60:229, 1985.

85. Maloff B, Lockwood D: Cellular basis for insulin resistance in uremia. *Diabetes* (suppl 1)30:28, 1981.

86. Maroni BJ, Steinman TI, Mitch WE: A method for estimating nitrogen intake of patients with chronic renal failure. *Kidney Int* 27:58, 1985.

87. McCaleb ML, Izzo MS, Lockwood DH: Characterization and partial purification of a factor from uremic serum that induces insulin resistance. *J Clin Invest* 75:391, 1985.

88. Merrill JP, Legrain M, Hoigne R: Observations on the role of urea in uremic (abstr). *Am J Med* 14:519, 1953.

89. Metcoff J, Dutta S, Burns G, et al: Effects of amino-acid infusions on cell metabolism in hemodialysed patients with uremia. *Kidney Int* (suppl 16)24:S87, 1983.

90. Mitch WE, Collier VU, Walser M: Creatinine metabolism in chronic renal failure. *Clin Sci* 58:327, 1980.

91. Mitch WE, Lietman P, Walser M: Effect of neomycin or kanamycin in chronic uremic subjects. I. Urea metabolisms. *Kidney Int* 11:116, 1977.

92. Mondon C, Dolkas C, Reaven G: The site of insulin resistance in acute uremia. *Diabetes* 27:571, 1978.

93. Munro HM: Energy and protein intakes as determinants of nitrogen balance. *Kidney Int* 14:313, 1978.

94. Nestel PJ, Fidhe NH, Tan MH: Increased lipoprotein-remnant formation in chronic renal failure. *N Engl J Med* 307:329, 1982.

95. Orita Y, Ando A, Tsubakihara Y, et al: Tissue and blood cell concentration of methylguanidine in rats and patients with chronic renal failure. *Nephron* 27:35, 1981.

96. Papadopoulou Z, Sandler P, Tina L, et al: Hyperlipidemia in children with chronic renal insufficiency. *Pediatr Res* 15:887, 1981.

97. Pennisi AJ, Heuser ET, Mickey MR, et al: Hyperlipidemia in pediatric hemodialysis and renal transplant patients. *Am J Dis Child* 130:957, 1976.

98. Phillips LS, Fusco AC, Unterman TG, et al: Somatomedin inhibitor in uremia. *J Clin Endocrinol Metab* 59:764, 1984.

99. Ponticelli C, Barbi GL, Cantaluppi A, et al: Lipid disorders in renal transplant recipients. *Nephron* 20:189, 1978.

100. Radtke HW, Rege AB, Lamarche MB, et al: Identification of spermine as an inhibitor of erythropoiesis in patients with chronic renal failure. *J Clin Invest* 67:1623, 1981.

101. Rapaport J, Aviram M, Chaimovitz C, et al: Defective high-density lipoprotein composition in patients on chronic hemodialysis. *N Engl J Med* 299:1326, 1978.

102. Reidenberg MM, Drayer DE: Alteration of drug protein in renal disease. *Clin Pharmocokinetics* (suppl 1)9:18, 1984.

103. Richards P, Metcalfe-Gibson A, Ward EE, et al: utilisation of ammonia nitrogen for protein synthesis in man, and the effects of protein restriction in uremia. *Lancet* 2:845, 1967.

104. Roth D, Meade R, Barboriank J: Glucose insulin and free fatty acids in uremia. *Diabetes* 22S:111, 1973.

105. Saldanha LP, Hurst KS, Amend JC, et al: Hyperlipidemia after renal transplantation in children. *Am J Dis Child* 130:951, 1976.

106. Salusky I, Kopple J, Fine RN: Continuous ambulatory peritoneal dialysis in pediatric patients: a 20 months experience. *Kidney Int* (suppl 15)24:S101, 1983.

107. Salusky IB, Fine RN, Nelson P, et al: Nutritional status of children undergoing continuous ambulatory peritoneal dialysis. *Am J Clin Nutr* 38:599, 1983.

108. Sanfelippo ML, Swenson RS, Reaven GM: Reduction of plasma triglyceride by diet in subjects with chronic renal failure. *Kidney Int* 11:54, 1977.

109. Schreiner GE: The search for uremic toxins. *Kidney Int* 7:S270, 1975.

110. Simmons JM, Wilson CJ, Potter DE, et al: Relation of calorie deficiency to growth failure in children or hemodialysis and the growth response to caloric supplementation. *N Engl J Med* 285:653, 1971.

111. Snyder D, Pulido LB, Kagan A: Dietary reversal of the carbohydrate intolerance in uremia. *Proc EDTA Pitman Medical* 5:205, 1968.

112. Swendseid ME, Wang M, Vyhmeister I, et al: Amino acid metabolism in the chronically uremic rat. *Clin Nephrol* 3:240, 1977.

113. Varcoe R, Halliday D, Carson ER, et al: Efficiency of utilization of urea nitrogen for albumin synthesis by chronically uraemic and normal man. *Clin Sci Molec Med* 48:379, 1975.

114. Walser M: Urea metabolism in chronic renal failure. *J Clin Invest* 53:1385, 1974.

115. Wang M, Vyhmeister I, Kopple JD, et al: Effect of protein intake on weight gain and plasma amino acid levels in uremic rats. *Am J Physiol* 230:1455, 1976.

116. Wardle EN, Kerr DNS, Ellis HA: Serum proteins as indicators of poor dietary intake in patients with chronic renal failure. *Clin Nephrol* 2:114, 1975.

117. Westervelt FB: Uremia and insulin response. *Arch Intern Med* 126:865, 1970.

118. Widhalm K, Singer P, Balzar E: Serum lipoprotein in children with nephrotic syndrome and chronic renal failure. *Artery* 8:191, 1980.

119. Wing AJ, Brunner FP, Brynger H, et al: Cardiovascular-related causes of death and the fate of patients with renovascular disease. *In Contributions to Nephrology Karger, Basel* 41:306, 1984.

120. Young GA, Parsons FM: Impairment of phenylalanine hydroxylation in chronic renal insufficiency. *Clin Sci Mol Med* 45:89, 1973.

PAUL SAENGER
JOAN DiMARTINO-NARDI

34
Endocrine System in Uremia

Growth Failure in Uremia

Poor growth is common in uremic children. Potter and Greifer [160] reported that the heights of one third to two thirds of uremic children were below the third percentile for age. Moreover, height age was retarded more than bone age.

In chronic renal failure (CRF) a catabolic metabolic state may exist despite normal or even increased levels of insulin and growth hormone (GH) and somatomedin/insulin-like growth factor I (IFG I), suggesting either lack of sufficient nutrients for anabolism and growth or antagonism of hormone action [21,29,81,114,148,196,222]. Limited caloric intake may play a role [22,96,196], although studies of pair-fed rats revealed that anabolism was blunted in the uremic animals even when nutrition was kept constant [174,185]. Other factors contributing to poor growth include metabolic acidosis, infection, anemia, hypertension, and altered bone mineral metabolism [69] (Chap. 25).

Children receiving chronic ambulatory peritoneal dialysis (CAPD) have been reported to grow better than those not receiving dialysis and those receiving hemodialysis [62,199,217] although not all authors agree. However, children receiving peritoneal dialysis continue to grow poorly [217]. The growth response of transplant recipients is variable [62,199] and reflects the different postoperative regimens used, incidence of complicating infections, and function of the transplant. The impact of renal transplantation on the child's final height is also limited by the child's remaining growth potential as indicated by the bone age at the time of surgery [213]. Recent reports indicate accelerated and even catch-up growth is achieved when transplantation is performed at an early age, when low-dose prednisone is used, and if allograft function is excellent [23]. Attempts to improve growth with caloric supplementation in children can increase growth rate but do not lead to accelerated or compensatory growth [5].

The final height of children with CRF is also limited by the magnitude of the pubertal growth spurt. Normal pubertal growth can occur with conservative medical treatment [110]. Among children requiring dialysis, the pubertal growth spurt in children receiving CAPD is better than those receiving hemodialysis [199]. Renal allograft

recipients can also have a normal pubertal growth spurt, which can be arrested if chronic rejection intervenes [213]. Therefore, the interaction of multiple factors, which are not entirely corrected by optimal current medical and surgical management, results in a short child with renal failure.

GH, insulin, and somatomedins have been the subjects of intense investigation in the causes of poor growth in CRF. In order to understand the underlying pathophysiology, a brief review of hormonal regulation of normal growth is necessary.

Hormonal Regulation of Normal Growth

Classic regulators of growth include GH, somatomedins, insulin, and thyroid hormones.

GHs, somatomedins, insulin, and thyroxin have a major positive influence on growth rate; corticosteroids have a major negative influence. Parathyroid hormone and vitamin D affect skeletal development and ossification. Gonadal and adrenal steroids are of particular importance in skeletal maturation and the pubertal growth spurt. GH and sex steroids probably act synergistically in normal puberty [136].

Growth Hormone

Pituitary GH is the major stimulus for normal growth. Its secretion is regulated primarily by the interaction between two hypothalamic hormones: growth hormone–releasing factor (GRF), 44 amino acids long, and somatostatin. Somatostatin, a polypeptide with 14 amino acids, inhibits the secretion not only of GH but also of many other pituitary, pancreatic, and parathyroid hormones.

GH exists within the pituitary in several molecular forms that are separable by physiochemical means. In plasma the bulk of GH is monomeric (single chain, 191 amino acids, 22,000 daltons, 22 K), but small amounts of the dimer ("big" GH) and even larger aggregates ("big, big" GH) may also be found. The bioactivity of GH probably resides in fragments smaller than the complete 191 amino acid sequence [166,184]. The second most common form is the 20,000 daltons (20 K) GH coded for the same gene sequence as is the 22 K form. A segment of an exxon (expressed part of a gene) immediately following an intron (unexpressed part of the gene) in the GH gene is bypassed [93].

Physiologic stimuli for GRF and thus release of GH include intake of food, strenuous exercise, and early phases of sleep with a slow EEG pattern. Its secretion from the pituitary gland is episodic. About seven or eight discrete pulses are detected in peripheral blood during a 24-hour period, a pattern that is established by three months of age [176]. GH secretion is regulated by several factors including the stimulatory GRF from the hypothalamus and somatostatin (also called somatotropin-releasing inhibitory factor), which is inhibitory, and possibly also by IGF I/Somatomedin C. The hypothalamic-pituitary-peripheral axis is a closed loop system in which episodic GH release is a result of concomitant reduction in hypothalamic somatotropin-releasing inhibitory factor secretion and an increase in GRF secretion. The interplay of both hormones generates the ultradian rhythm of GH secretion [205].

The secretion of human GH is enhanced by sex hormones. Ambulatory levels of GH are higher in women than in men and may be increased by estrogen priming. Androgens also sensitize GH releasing mechanisms [136].

Insulin- and tolbutamide-induced hypoglycemia and infusion of the amino acid L-arginine, L-DOPA (the precursor of the GH releasing neurotransmitter dopamine), vasopressin, glucagon, beta-adrenergic blockers (such as propranolol), and alpha-adrenergic stimuli (such as clonidine) [70,75] have all been used to provoke GH release in testing procedures.

Inhibition of GH secretion occurs in part in response to somatomedin C, which may act by stimulating hypothalamic secretion of somatostatin and suppression of secretion of GH directly at the pituitary gland [17].

Inhibition of GH secretion also occurs during hyperglycemia, in obesity, after prior stress-induced GH secretion, during excessive administration of glucocorticoids, in hypothyroidism, and in psychosocial deprivation.

GH has profound effects on the metabolism of protein, fats, carbohydrates, and minerals. It does not affect skeletal growth directly but acts through production of somatomedins, which promote cartilage cell mitosis and sulfation and exert an insulin-like effect. However, a direct mitogenic action of GH on thymocytes, erythroid lines, and arterial media cells has been reported in vitro [79]. Furthermore, when GH is injected unilaterally near the rat tibial epiphysis, the injected side exhibits differentially accelerated growth [101]. Such local effects of GH offer strong arguments against the original endocrine somatomedin hypothesis, though these effects may be mediated through local somatomedin production [184] in a paracrine or autocrine fashion, rather than a classical endocrine fashion.

Somatomedins

The somatomedins are a group of polypeptides synthesized predominantly in the liver, but also in muscle and kidney, under the influence of GH. Somatomedins differ in their physicochemical properties. Somatomedin A is a neutral protein with a molecular weight of 2000 daltons; somatomedin B is an acidic peptide of 5000 daltons; and somatomedin C is a basic protein of 8000 daltons [29]. Purified somatomedins resemble proinsulin in amino acid sequence but have limited cross-reactivity with insulin in binding to receptors. Somatomedins A and C stimulate the incorporation of radiolabeled sulfate into cartilage (sulfation factor). Somatomedin B stimulates thymidine incorporation into DNA in glia-like cells in tissue culture. In serum, the somatomedins circulate bound to proteins. Unlike GH, somatomedin levels remain fairly constant throughout the day. Somatomedin C, which has recently been fully synthesized, is identical with IGF I [109,127,159].

Measurement of somatomedin in a single blood sample provides a rough integrated estimate of the functional GH status. Levels are age dependent, being much lower in children below six years of age. There is a distinct increase in somatomedins in boys and girls during adolescence, at a time when the maximum growth spurt occurs, although somatomedin levels fail to correlate with growth velocity [184]. Changing levels of carrier protein or altering end-organ sensitivity may explain these age-dependent changes. For example, somatomedin receptor sites in newborns are markedly increased while somatomedin levels are low [177].

The role of somatomedins in growth is suggested largely by correlations between somatomedin and growth velocity in children receiving GH therapy [86]. It should be stressed that only circumstantial evidence has accrued that somatomedin is the mediator of skeletal growth. Only a few in vivo assays with somatomedin preparations have been carried out [212].

The recent availability of recombinant IGF I has led to exciting new data: IGF I stimulates skeletal growth in rats and has distinct effects on weight of kidneys and spleen. Short-term administration of rh IGF I in humans caused increased insulin secretion in contrast to GH. This suggests that the therapeutic spectrum of IGF I is quite different from that of GH [82,83]. It seems likely, however, that much of the postnatal growth is due to stimulation of growth cartilage by somatomedins. Local (paracrine) secretion of somatomedin C as well as true "endocrine" secretion of somatomedin C may be important in promoting somatic growth [184].

Thyroid Hormones

Thyroid hormones do not appear to play a significant role in the early growth and development of the human fetus, since infants with congenital aplasia of the thyroid gland are of normal size at birth. Bone age and development of the CNS are retarded, however. The importance of thyroid hormone for postnatal somatic growth is exemplified by the severe growth failure that regularly accompanies thyroid hormone deficiency. Severe hypothyroidism causes nearly absolute growth arrest and the most pronounced retardation in development of bone maturation.

Insulin

Insulin is a stimulator of fetal growth, as evidenced by the oversized infants born to diabetic mothers. Postnatally, the role of insulin as a growth-promoting hormone is far from clear. Insulin levels may be markedly increased, and acceleration of linear growth occurs in some otherwise normal children with exogenous obesity and in hyperphagic children who have had surgery for craniopharyngioma [39].

Glucocorticoids

Glucorticoid excess appears to inhibit growth at the level of the chondrocyte. After prolonged exposure to daily, high-dose glucocorticoids, catch-up growth is often insufficient to normalize the patient's height. In one study, administration of high-dose glucocorticoids in growing rats resulted in permanent, profound biochemical and structural changes in the cartilage [149].

Definition of Short Stature

A child is small if standing height is two standard deviations or more below the mean for age. Growth velocity (centimeters per year) is another important calculation in the evaluation of growth. Although growth velocity is age dependent, a growth rate of less than 4 cm/yr denotes poor growth at any age.

Initial evaluation of growth in children with CRF should include calculation of growth velocity, documentation of glucocorticoid therapy, assessment of nutritional intake, and recordings of the heights of family members. A bone age determination of the wrist and hand is necessary for more precise classification. Appropriate height standards for calculation of standard deviation scores of height and growth velocity relative to bone age form the basis for clinical evaluation of growth disorders in children.

Endocrine Causes of Growth Failure in Uremia

Growth Hormone

In uremia, growth failure ensues despite the presence of levels of insulin and GH in blood that are normal or elevated [61]. Thus, poor growth is probably due to impaired GH action rather than low GH production. The degree of elevation tends to parallel the rise in serum creatinine [36,182,224]. An exaggerated rise of plasma GH after administration of thyroid-releasing hormone has been reported, the relevance and the mechanism of which are not understood [42,80]. GH response to various stimuli, such as insulin-induced hypoglycemia or the infusion of arginine, is increased in uremia [99]. A lack of suppression of GH has been noted during an oral glucose tolerance test [57,203].

GH is diabetogenic since it has an antagonistic effect on insulin-induced cellular uptake of glucose, but the degree of insulin resistance in uremia does not appear to correlate with the increased levels of GH.

The cause of GH increase in uremia is poorly understood. Decreased metabolic clearance may be one factor. Elevated arginine levels may stimulate GH secretion [34,58,102]. Normalization of GH levels has been reported after renal transplantation [24,99,181,224].

Recent studies have been performed to assess nocturnal GH secretory dynamics in children with CRF [112]. Included in the study were six children with a mean creatinine clearance of 24.9 ± 14.2 ml/min/1.73 m^2, five children treated with continuous peritoneal dialysis, and seven children who had received renal transplants, treated with corticosteroids and with a creatinine clearances of 40.3 ± 25.3 ml/min/m^2. Three patterns were seen: low amplitude and low frequency of GH peaks; a failure of elevated GH levels to return to baseline; and "normal" GH peaks. It is unlikely that the study of GH secretion pattern in CRF will aid in the understanding of their growth failure.

GRF is a peptide that has been used extensively to elucidate GH secretory dynamics. In children receiving CAPD, the GH response to GRF is more pronounced than the response in normal children [19]. The exaggerated GH response to GRF in uremic children may be due to abnormal regulation of GH secretion. It has been suggested that altered dopaminergic tone may contribute to the higher GH response to GRF as dopamine inhibits pituitary GH secretion [77].

PRELIMINARY STUDIES

Preliminary studies are being performed to assess the effect of recombinant human GH therapy in children with CRF [113]. Five boys with congenital renal disease with a mean age of 55.8 ± 21.4 months and creatinine clearance of 18.2 ± 6.3 ml/min/1.73 m^2 were treated with GH for 9 months. Their growth velocity improved from 4.9 ± 1.4 cm/yr before treatment to 9.06 ± 1.75 cm, with no deterioration of renal function during this period.

This same group administered GH for six months to 10 patients with varying degrees of renal failure [112,113]. The best response was seen in those children with a creatinine clearance of 24.9 ± 14.2 ml/min/1.73 m^2. In those children growth rates increased from 4.94 ± 1.4 cm/yr to 10.08 ± 1.97. Three children maintained on continuous cycling peritoneal dialysis demonstrated modest improvements from 2.37 ± 1.99 cm/yr to 4.13 ± 3.23 cm/yr. Successful GH therapy in children after transplantation has also been reported by others [104]. Three-year data published recently are encouraging, suggesting continued acceleration in growth [68]. The effect of chronic GH therapy on final height in these children remains to be determined. Questions of optimal dose of recombinant GH, effects on glomerular filtration, and possible perturbations of carbohydrate metabolism remain to be solved. Until such a time this therapy should be considered experimental. To date carbohydrate tolerance was not adversely affected by this treatment regimen, however [113].

Somatomedins

Since GH is thought to stimulate skeletal growth indirectly through generation of somatomedins, attention has focused the possibility that abnormal somatomedin generation or action or both may contribute to impaired growth in uremia.

Somatomedin production is decreased by a number of factors, including malnutrition, glucocorticoids, estrogens,

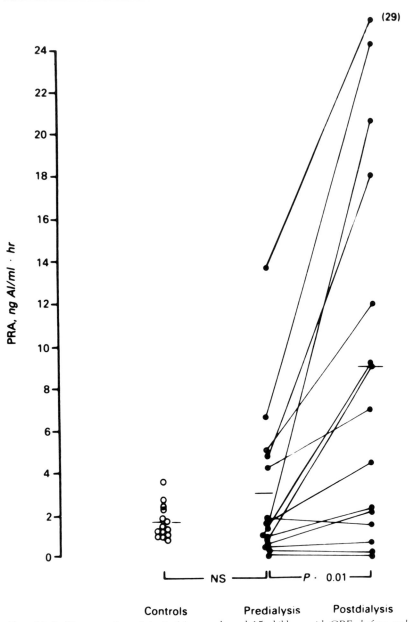

FIG. 34-6. *Plasma renin activity in 14 controls and 15 children with CRF, before and after hemodialysis. (From Rauh W, Hund E, Sohl G, et al: Vasoactive hormones in children with chronic renal failure. Kidney Int 24:S27, 1983, with permission.)*

Catecholamines

In uremic adults, increased plasma norepinephrine levels have been reported by several authors [27,91,120,143] while plasma epinephrine levels vary widely [27,91, 120,143]. Raised plasma catecholamines in uremia could be due to increased synthesis, diminished re-uptake at the nerve terminals, deficient enzyme inactivation, or decreased renal excretion [18,92,120]. In a recent study [168], dialysis and ultrafiltration caused a marked increase in catecholamines, indicating an adequate sympathetic re-

sponse to volume depletion and to the decrease in BP (see Table 34-1).

Vasopressin

Basal vasopressin concentrations are elevated in children and adults with CRF. Increased serum osmolality may play a role. Nonosmotic factors, including BP, blood volume, and stress, may also influence vasopressin release. The metabolic clearance rate of vasopressin is diminished in

role of insulin as a growth-promoting hormone is far from clear. Insulin levels may be markedly increased, and acceleration of linear growth occurs in some otherwise normal children with exogenous obesity and in hyperphagic children who have had surgery for craniopharyngioma [39].

Glucocorticoids

Glucorticoid excess appears to inhibit growth at the level of the chondrocyte. After prolonged exposure to daily, high-dose glucocorticoids, catch-up growth is often insufficient to normalize the patient's height. In one study, administration of high-dose glucocorticoids in growing rats resulted in permanent, profound biochemical and structural changes in the cartilage [149].

Definition of Short Stature

A child is small if standing height is two standard deviations or more below the mean for age. Growth velocity (centimeters per year) is another important calculation in the evaluation of growth. Although growth velocity is age dependent, a growth rate of less than 4 cm/yr denotes poor growth at any age.

Initial evaluation of growth in children with CRF should include calculation of growth velocity, documentation of glucocorticoid therapy, assessment of nutritional intake, and recordings of the heights of family members. A bone age determination of the wrist and hand is necessary for more precise classification. Appropriate height standards for calculation of standard deviation scores of height and growth velocity relative to bone age form the basis for clinical evaluation of growth disorders in children.

Endocrine Causes of Growth Failure in Uremia

Growth Hormone

In uremia, growth failure ensues despite the presence of levels of insulin and GH in blood that are normal or elevated [61]. Thus, poor growth is probably due to impaired GH action rather than low GH production. The degree of elevation tends to parallel the rise in serum creatinine [36,182,224]. An exaggerated rise of plasma GH after administration of thyroid-releasing hormone has been reported, the relevance and the mechanism of which are not understood [42,80]. GH response to various stimuli, such as insulin-induced hypoglycemia or the infusion of arginine, is increased in uremia [99]. A lack of suppression of GH has been noted during an oral glucose tolerance test [57,203].

GH is diabetogenic since it has an antagonistic effect on insulin-induced cellular uptake of glucose, but the degree of insulin resistance in uremia does not appear to correlate with the increased levels of GH.

The cause of GH increase in uremia is poorly understood. Decreased metabolic clearance may be one factor. Elevated arginine levels may stimulate GH secretion [34,58,102]. Normalization of GH levels has been reported after renal transplantation [24,99,181,224].

Recent studies have been performed to assess nocturnal GH secretory dynamics in children with CRF [112]. Included in the study were six children with a mean creatinine clearance of 24.9 ± 14.2 ml/min/1.73 m^2, five children treated with continuous peritoneal dialysis, and seven children who had received renal transplants, treated with corticosteroids and with a creatinine clearances of 40.3 ± 25.3 ml/min/m^2. Three patterns were seen: low amplitude and low frequency of GH peaks; a failure of elevated GH levels to return to baseline; and "normal" GH peaks. It is unlikely that the study of GH secretion pattern in CRF will aid in the understanding of their growth failure.

GRF is a peptide that has been used extensively to elucidate GH secretory dynamics. In children receiving CAPD, the GH response to GRF is more pronounced than the response in normal children [19]. The exaggerated GH response to GRF in uremic children may be due to abnormal regulation of GH secretion. It has been suggested that altered dopaminergic tone may contribute to the higher GH response to GRF as dopamine inhibits pituitary GH secretion [77].

PRELIMINARY STUDIES

Preliminary studies are being performed to assess the effect of recombinant human GH therapy in children with CRF [113]. Five boys with congenital renal disease with a mean age of 55.8 ± 21.4 months and creatinine clearance of 18.2 ± 6.3 ml/min/1.73 m^2 were treated with GH for 9 months. Their growth velocity improved from 4.9 ± 1.4 cm/yr before treatment to 9.06 ± 1.75 cm, with no deterioration of renal function during this period.

This same group administered GH for six months to 10 patients with varying degrees of renal failure [112,113]. The best response was seen in those children with a creatinine clearance of 24.9 ± 14.2 ml/min/1.73 m^2. In those children growth rates increased from 4.94 ± 1.4 cm/yr to 10.08 ± 1.97. Three children maintained on continuous cycling peritoneal dialysis demonstrated modest improvements from 2.37 ± 1.99 cm/yr to 4.13 ± 3.23 cm/yr. Successful GH therapy in children after transplantation has also been reported by others [104]. Three-year data published recently are encouraging, suggesting continued acceleration in growth [68]. The effect of chronic GH therapy on final height in these children remains to be determined. Questions of optimal dose of recombinant GH, effects on glomerular filtration, and possible perturbations of carbohydrate metabolism remain to be solved. Until such a time this therapy should be considered experimental. To date carbohydrate tolerance was not adversely affected by this treatment regimen, however [113].

Somatomedins

Since GH is thought to stimulate skeletal growth indirectly through generation of somatomedins, attention has focused the possibility that abnormal somatomedin generation or action or both may contribute to impaired growth in uremia.

Somatomedin production is decreased by a number of factors, including malnutrition, glucocorticoids, estrogens, systemic illness, and cirrhotic liver disease. GH, prolactin and insulin, increase somatomedins.

Dietary protein appears to be particularly important for the generation of somatomedins and their action on growth of cartilage. (See reference 159 for review.) Evidence is now emerging that indicates that the nutritional status is one of the major determinants of somatomedin concentration in serum. Serum levels are low in patients with protein calorie malnutrition, despite extremely high levels of GH. Even in well-nourished individuals, acute fasting causes a decline in serum concentrations within a few days. Suboptimal nutritional status may be an important mechanism whereby the somatomedin C concentration is reduced in children with a wide variety of chronic illnesses [41,46], including CRF.

Discrepancies in reports of mesurements of somatomedin levels in uremia are due to differences in assay techniques and differences in the compounds compared; some assays measure somatomedin C, others measure somatomedin A [197]. Since somatomedin levels respond to changes in caloric intake [41], the poor nutritional status of uremic children may also affect somatomedin levels. Most *bioassay* examinations using rib cartilage from hypophysectomized rats have indicated that the circulating somatomedin activity is decreased in uremia [11,156,157,192,201,206,223]. In adult uremic patients, bioassayable somatomedin levels were decreased in proportion to urea nitrogen or creatinine concentration [157].

Following hemodialysis, an increase of bioassayable somatomedin levels into the normal range has been reported [156,157]. This may be due to the removal of somatomedin inhibitors [157]. Heparinization during hemodialysis may be another contributing factor. After renal transplantation, bioassayable somatomedin levels are indistinguishable from healthy controls and correlate positively with growth velocity [181].

Examination of uremic patients using radioreceptor assay techniques indicated that somatomedin levels were elevated and increased with increasing serum creatinine [188,197,206], but were unchanged by hemodialysis [197]. Similarly, somatomedin levels measured by competitive protein binding assay were elevated [28,185]. It seems likely that somatomedins measured in these studies included a varying combination of both somatomedin C/IGF I and IGF II [158].

More recent studies with highly specific radioimmunoassays and radioreceptor assays revealed a 25% to 60% decrease in IGF I (somatomedin C) in uremia and an approximately 40% increase in IGF II [14,78,159]. Since the ability of IGF II to stimulate growing cartilage is about 50% that of IGF I, the findings to date suggest that the net circulating biologically active somatomedins (IGF I/somatomedin C + IGF II) are probably normal in renal failure [18].

The presence of low somatomedin activity in bioassay systems despite normal or even elevated somatomedin levels by radioimmunoassay suggests that somatomedin activity (and growth) might be decreased in renal failure due to a circulating, low molecular weight, and hence, dialysable inhibitor of somatomedin. Based on gel filtration studies, such an inhibitor with a molecular weight of about

940 daltons (range 800 to 1100) has now been reported [158]. The molecular weight should permit renal clearance. A decrease in inhibitory activity after exposure to proteolytic enzymes suggests that the uremic inhibitor is a peptide. Based on apparent size, it seems likely that this inhibitor is one of the circulating "middle molecules" that accumulate in renal failure [18,38] and may contribute to decreased insulin binding and insulin resistance [55,108,140,145], decreased bone marrow thymidine incorporation [85], inhibition of protein synthesis [52], cardiotoxicity, and cytotoxicity [53]. To the extent that middle molecules (500 to 5000 daltons) contribute to growth failure in uremia, their removal by improved dialytic methods, such as chronic ambulatory peritoneal dialysis, might enhance growth. Growth of children maintained with chronic ambulatory peritoneal dialysis, however, is only a little better than that of children treated by chronic hemodialysis, if improved at all [6,54,62,63,199].

The recent elucidation that IGF I binding protein is extremely high in uremia may explain the long known discrepancy between the low somatomedin bioactivity and the normal immunoreactive serum IGF I concentration. Unsaturated IGF I binding protein acts, as previously postulated by Powell et al. [161,162], as an inhibitor in uremia by reducing the serum concentration of unbound IGF I. During recently initiated recombinant GH treatment in uremia, serum IGF I concentration increased markedly, whereas the serum IGF I binding protein increased only slightly [211]. The excess of unbound IGF I results in normal somatomedin bioactivity. IGF I binding protein may indeed be the elusive inhibitor [158]. Unsaturated somatomedin carrier protein interferes with somatomedin assay systems unless it is separated from the somatomedin fraction by acid chromatography [161].

IGF I may also be the mediator of the well documented effects of GH on renal plasma flow and glomerular filtration rate (GFR). Patients with acromegaly have increased renal plasma flow as well as increased GFR. Injection of GH in humans causes the same alterations. The increases in renal plasma flow and GFR do not occur for several hours after the injection, suggesting the release of one or more mediators. IGF I may be one such mediator. Studies are now needed to resolve the question whether recombinant human GH induces kidney hyperfiltration in children with uremia and whether this adversely affects long-term renal function. In short-term studies no such effect has been seen to date [95,211]).

Gonadotrophins and Sex Hormones

Together with short stature, delayed pubertal development is among the most frequent endocrine disturbances in chronic renal disease. Delayed puberty has been attributed to defects at the hypothalamic and the gonadal levels [28,64].

GONADAL FUNCTION

In men, gynecomastia, impotence, and decreased sexual activity are frequently seen in uremia and are not signifi-

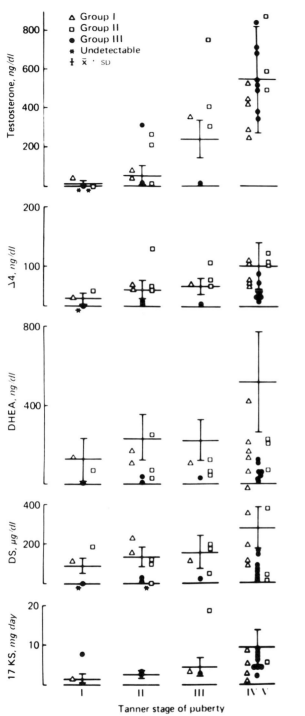

FIG. 34-1. *Serum testosterone (Δ4) Δ4-androstenedione dehydro-epiandrosterone (DHEA), dehydroepiandrosterone sulfate (DS), and urinary 17-ketosteroid (17KS) in progressive stages of puberty (Tanner stages). Mean ± SD depicts normal androgen and 17KS levels in boys (see refs. 115–118,125,154). Group I: 9 patients with chronic renal insufficiency not undergoing dialysis. Group II: 10 patients on chronic hemodialysis. Group III: 12 patients after renal transplantation. (From Ferraris J, Senger P, Levine L, et al: Delayed puberty in males with chronic renal failure. Kidney Int 18:344, 1980, with permission.)*

cantly altered by dialysis [67,84,89,128,164,200]. Plasma testosterone levels have been found to be low/normal (Fig. 34-1), and they respond rather poorly to stimulation with human chorionic gonadotrophin. Abnormalities in sperm motility are also seen frequently. Leydig cells, the source of testicular testosterone, are often atrophied.

The peripheral conversion of testosterone to its more potent metabolite 5-dihydrotestosterone (DHT) is reduced, suggesting impaired 5α-reductase activity. Since both testosterone and DHT are reduced, the testosterone to DHT ratio is normal [153] (Fig. 34-2). DHT is necessary for spermatogenesis and also stimulates beard and prostatic growth. Low DHT levels and increased plasma binding of androgens [64,67,128,164] may contribute to the impaired sexual function in uremic adults.

Our group [64] as well as others [175] reported low or low-normal plasma testosterone levels in pubertal and prepubertal boys with CRF (see Figs. 34-2 and 34-3). DHT levels are proportionately low, suggesting that in children the 5α-reductase activity is normal (see Fig. 34-2). Oertel et al. [153] found that free testosterone levels in CRF were not different from control, this would suggest that plasma protein binding of testosterone is normal in prepubertal boys with CRF (see Fig. 34-3). The testosterone response to human chorionic gonadotropin stimulation, on the other hand, is decreased in prepubertal as well as in pubertal boys, pointing to changes of Leydig cell functional reserve already present before puberty [187].

Zinc deficiency has been implicated in the etiology of Leydig cell damage in one study [131]. Treatment with

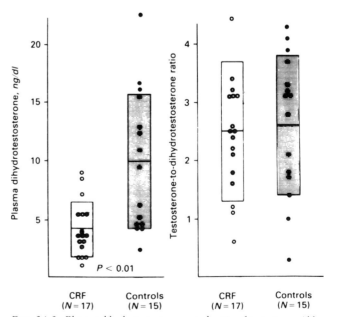

FIG. 34-2. *Plasma dihydrotestosterone and ratio of testosterone/dihydrotestosterone in prepubertal boys with CRF (N = 17) and in age-matched controls (N = 15). The columns represent means ± SD. (From Oertel PJ, Lichtwald K, Rauh W, et al: The hypothalamo pituitary-gonadal axis in prepubertal children with chronic renal failure (CRF). Kidney Int 24:S34, 1983, with permission.)*

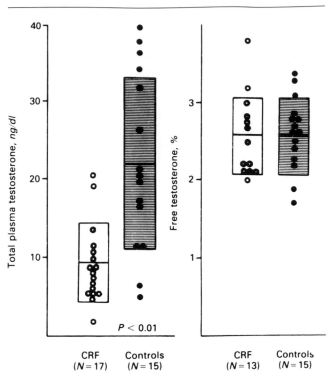

Fig. 34-3. *Total plasma testosterone and percent free testosterone in prepubertal boys with CRF (N = 17) and in age-matched controls (N = 15). The columns represent means ± SD. (From Oertel PJ, Lichtwald K, Rauh W, et al: The hypothalamo pituitary-gonadal axis in prepubertal children with chronic renal failure (CRF). Kidney Int 24:S34, 1983, with permission.)*

cyclophosphamide beyond a certain amount (>200 mg/kg) may damage the germinal epithelium and lead subsequently to elevated FSH levels. Treatment with testosterone injections at pharmacologic doses will lead to small reductions in FSH and LH, indicating some conservation of a negative feedback [13,73,107].

No data are available on ovarian function in prepubertal or pubertal girls with CRF. In women with end-stage renal disease sex hormones are often decreased [202,219]. Menstrual abnormalities, infertility, and diminished libido have been reported in uremic women [147,202,219].

HYPOTHALAMIC–PITUITARY FUNCTION

Although the data in the previous section point to functional impairment at the gonadal level, the gonadotrophin regulation at the hypothalamic and the pituitary level may also be altered.

In uremic adults, luteinizing hormone (LH) and follicle-stimulating hormone (FSH) levels are high [73,128]. In children, both low and high gonadotrophin levels have been reported. More recently LH levels have been found to be elevated in pubertal boys, whereas FSH levels were normal and showed elevations only in older teenagers [22]. Serum LH levels correlated with the severity of uremia [135] (Figs. 34-4 and 34-5). LH levels declined after successful transplantation [153,175,187,195].

It has been argued previously that in men with CRF the

absolute elevation of FSH and LH is in fact inadequate when contrasted to the reduced levels of gonadal hormones, indicating an additional defect at the hypothalamic pituitary level. The blunted response of LH and FSH to gonadotrophin releasing hormone (GnRH) in uremic children, both pubertal and prepubertal, supports this hypothesis and suggests inadequate compensation by the hypothalamus, the pituitary gland, or both [175]. This dampened response to GnRH is very much akin to the blunted TSH response described previously. Alternatively, there may also be an accumulation of an immunoreactive LH molecule that lacks bioactivity. In adults on the other hand gonadotrophins retain their responsiveness to GnRH [96].

Recent technological advances have permitted the measurement of GnRH levels in plasma. GnRH was elevated in adult uremic subjects of both sexes in the presence of high LH levels [138]. This again suggests decreased feedback inhibition by primary gonadal failure in uremia [207].

High serum prolactin levels and decreased responsiveness of prolactin to TRH stimulation have been reported in children and adults with uremia [40,42,100,150]. Long-term testosterone administration also did not affect the elevated mean prolactin levels [13,107]. Regulation of prolactin secretion may also be impaired due to a decrease in hypothalamic prolactin-inhibiting factor [150,183]. L-DOPA fails to suppress prolactin levels [155], suggesting

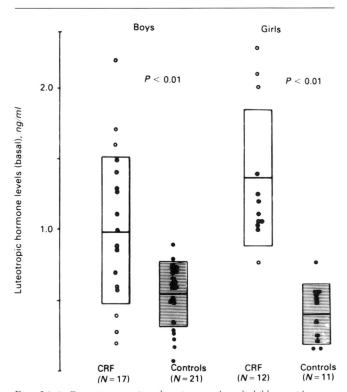

Fig. 34-4. *Basal luteotropic values in prepubertal children with CRF (N = 17 boys) and (N = 2 girls) and in controls (N = 21 boys) and (N = 11 girls). The columns represent means ± SD. (From Oertel PJ, Lichtwald K, Rauh W, et al: The hypothalamo pituitary-gonadal axis in prepubertal children with chronic renal failure (CRF). Kidney Int 24:S34, 1983, with permission.)*

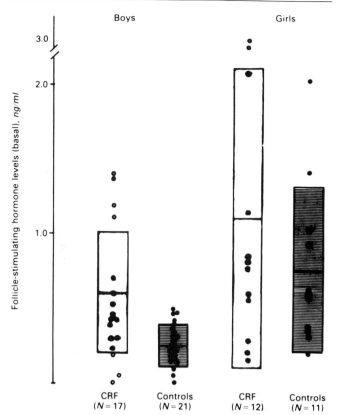

FIG. 34-5. *Basal follicle-stimulating hormone values in prepubertal children with CRF (N = 17 boys) and (N = 12 girls) and in controls (N = 21 boys) and (N = 11 girls). The columns represent means ± SD. (From Oertel PJ, Lichtwald K, Rauh W, et al: The hypothalamo pituitary-gonadal axis in prepubertal children with chronic renal failure (CRF). Kidney Int 24:S34, 1983, with permission.)*

an insensitivity of pituitary lactotrophs to suppression in uremia. The positive correlation between prolactin and creatinine and the normalization of prolactin after successful transplantation suggest that the kidney has an important role in prolactin metabolism.

Elevated prolactin levels may affect gonadal function and, consequently, the dopaminergic agonist bromocryptine has been used to decrease prolactin levels and to improve sexual activity in uremic men [26].

The advent of adrenarche, which precedes puberty by about 1 to 2 years, can also be disturbed in uremic patients. We found the levels of adrenal androgens (dehydroepiandrosterone, andrestenedione) to be normal or decreased in uremic boys, depending on whether they were related to height age, bone age, or chronologic age [64,175]. In patients after transplantation the customary glucocorticoid therapy will invariably lower adrenal androgens. Since adrenal androgens may possibly play a role in the pubertal growth spurt, this may explain the poor post-transplant growth velocity in some children [64]. (see Fig. 34-1).

Recent studies suggest that the administration of anabolic steroids might be beneficial to protein anabolism and growth in uremic children [103]. Oxandrolone, a powerful anabolic steroid with only weak androgenic properties, has been shown to improve growth in children with a variety of causes of short stature, although excessive skeletal maturation may occur. Jones et al. [103] report beneficial effects from up to 1.3 years of therapy with oxandrolone on growth velocity. No longitudinal data on pubertal growth and development in children with CRF are currently available. Observed salt and water retention after oxandrolone administration was controlled by a reduction in dosage. With the recent availability of recombinant human GH the interest in anabolic agents as sole therapy has diminished considerably.

In uremic men, Zumoff et al. measured decreased dehydroepiandrosterone and dehydroepiandrosterone sulfate in the face of elevated cortisol levels. This may suggest a biosynthetic block in the adrenal cortex at the $C_{17,20}$ lyase (cytochrome p450 C17α) step. If a similar defect were present in the testis, it could account for the diminished synthesis of testosterone [225]. These preliminary results await further study and confirmation.

Other Endocrine Disturbances
Carbohydrate Metabolism

CRF results in a variety of metabolic derangements that alter glucose homeostasis. These may result, in part, from the fact that the kidney plays a prominent role in the metabolism of insulin as well as a number of other low molecular weight peptide hormones (e.g., C-peptide) that affect carbohydrate metabolism [47,49]. Because of the altered renal tubular threshold for glucose, urine glucose cannot be used in monitoring blood glucose control. Glycosylated hemoglobin levels may be falsely low in uremia [43].

INSULIN

In uremic children and adults on chronic hemodialysis, increased blood glucose levels are associated with elevated insulin levels in the fasting state [49,57]. Plasma glucagon levels are also higher and fail to decrease normally after intravenous administration of glucose [57,121]. The pathogenesis of glucose intolerance in uremia is unclear. The most recent and cogent physiologic concept has been developed using hepatocytes from chronically uremic rats [35]. These studies showed that insulin resistance in uremic rat liver is not due to defects in insulin binding or internalization. Despite high levels of circulating immunoreactive insulin, there was neither "down-regulation" of insulin receptors nor an increased rate of insulin degradation [35]. In contrast, studies in uremic humans using the euglycemic clamp technique, showed that insulin-mediated glucose uptake by the liver is not impaired, although glucose uptake by nonhepatic tissue is. This tissue insensitivity to insulin is the primary cause of insulin resistance in uremia [47,48]. Surprisingly, insulin-mediated potassium uptake is not altered [3]. McCaleb et al. [141] identified a low molecular weight inhibitor of insulin action in vitro at the cellular level. The substance has a molecular weight of 1 kilodalton and can be removed with long-term dialysis. These observations suggest that the various actions of insulin are differentially impaired in uremia and that steps *distal* to the insulin receptor must be ultimately responsible for insulin resistance in uremia [3].

A molecule of C-peptide is released from each molecule of proinsulin. Since the kidney is the major organ for degradation of C-peptide, high C-peptide levels in uremia are not surprising [173].

GLUCAGON

Glucagon binding to hepatocytes is increased in uremic rats. Despite high levels of glucagon, hepatocytes do not show downregulation of their binding sites. This emphasizes again the primary role of postbinding events in the regulation of glucagon action [35,146,173].

GLUCOSE INTOLERANCE

Abnormally increased release of pancreatic polypeptide in uremia may also contribute to the impaired glucose tolerance in uremia [88]. In addition, a relative insensitivity of the pancreatic beta cells to glucose [47,51], altered insulin metabolism, and increased gluconeogenesis from alanine [179,180] may contribute to the disturbed carbohydrate metabolism.

An increase in gluconeogenesis, which is partially normalized by chronic hemodialysis, has been observed in uremic patients [179,180]. Hemodialysis appears also to reduce insulin requirements [66,190,197]. Furthermore, cortisol and catecholamines, all of which are elevated in uremia, may antagonize the action of insulin [57]. GH, which is also elevated, is not responsible for the glucose intolerance and insulin resistance [50].

Impaired peripheral utilization of glucose and cellular energy supply may affect protein metabolism and, therefore, contribute to the poor growth of children with uremia [57]. Hyperinsulinemia and hyperglycemia are also associated with hyperlipidemia [56], which may predispose to premature atherosclerosis [129].

The secondary hyperparathyroidism of uremia may also stimulate gluconeogenesis [133]. An improvement of glucose intolerance following treatment with high-dose phosphate binder was reported in children on chronic hemodialysis [133]. Mak et al. [132] used clamp studies to demonstrate convincingly that uremic children with hyperparathyroidism are both insulin resistant and glucose intolerant. Glucose intolerance resolved with successful control of the hyperparathyroidism due apparently to increased insulin levels, but insulin resistance remains. The authors [132] conclude that both insulin resistance and hyperparathyroidism contribute to glucose intolerance in chronic uremia in children.

In summary, impaired insulin action at a step distal to the insulin receptor appears to be the basis for the glucose intolerance of uremia. Chronic hemodialysis may partially correct some of the abnormal glucose kinetics [66,179, 180,197]. Although glucose intolerance is common, fasting hyperglycemia secondary to the uremic state is rare [148].

Thyroid Function

Thyroid hormone plays an important role in the maturation and development of the skeleton. Thyroid hormone influences endochondral calcification and the entire process of cartilage growth. In contrast to testosterone and estrogen, thyroid hormone is unique in that it stimulates the proliferation of cartilage as well as epiphyseal maturation [9].

Some of the clinical manifestations of chronic renal failure, such as dry skin, yellowish complexion, lethargy, fatigue, and cold intolerance, resemble the features of hypothyroidism [170]. The reported increased incidence of goiter in adult uremic patients has not been confirmed [195].

There are conflicting reports of diminished, exaggerated, or normal thyroid-stimulating hormone (TSH) responses to thyroid-releasing hormone (TRH). Degradation of both TRH and TSH may be impaired in the uremic state. However, in the few reported studies of thyroid function in uremic children, basal metabolic rate was normal [96].

TSH concentration in uremia is normal in the basal state. The time course of TSH response to TRH shows a lower and delayed peak response. No difference exists between patients on hemodialysis or peritoneal dialysis. The data in children and adults point to the existence of secondary or tertiary hypothyroidism [76].

The prolonged elevation of TSH after administration of TRH may be due to an increased half-life of TSH in renal failure [60]. TSH responsiveness and thyroid function are probably also influenced by the clinical status of uremic patients. Patients on regular hemodialysis who were clinically stable showed normal pituitary responsiveness to TRH and normal thyroidal response to endogenous TSH secretion [44].

Total T_4 and T_3 levels have been found to be low or low normal in uremia. In one study, T_3 was more decreased than T_4. Free T_4 may be normal or decreased. Free T_3 is reduced both before and during dialysis therapy. The concentration of thyroid-binding globulin is usually in the low normal range [1].

Recent studies suggest an abnormal peripheral as well as intrathyroidal metabolism of thyroid hormones in uremia. The conversion of T_4 to T_3 is decreased. Both free and bound reverse T_3 have been found to be increased [36,105,106,119]. Thus, CRF profoundly changes the kinetics of most iodothyronines [59]. Nuclear T_3 receptors are decreased in uremic rats [208] similar to states of starvation.

The alterations of thyroid hormone indices in renal failure are similar to those of other nonthyroidal illnesses. It is entirely possible that decreased T_3 levels provide a protective mechanism against the catabolic effects of chronic uremia [24]. After successful transplantation, thyroid parameters usually return to normal.

An elevated TSH level remains the most useful index of hypothyroidism. Only in certain diseases that lead to CRF, such as cystinosis and congenital nephrotic syndrome, has overt hypothyroidism been documented [32,144]. Cystine crystals in the thyroid lead to destruction of the gland and to frank hypothyroidism. Pituitary resistance to thyroid hormone treatment has been reported in cystinosis. In a recent study, 11 children with nephropathic cystinosis who were clinically and biochemically euthyroid had elevated basal TSH levels, with a response to TRH similar to that seen in children with primary hypothyroidism [16]. Serum TSH levels were suppressed to normal only after elevation of serum levels of thyroid hormone with high-dose thyroxine replacement therapy.

With these exceptions, it is unclear whether the changes in thyroid function described in uremic subjects suggest a mild hypothyroid state and whether these children should be treated with thyroid hormones. Therapeutic trials have led to inconclusive results [165,195]. Use of T_3 to treat the anemia of uremia cannot be recommended [65].

Until a clearer picture of the metabolic consequences of the diverse abnormalities of thyroid hormone levels is available, no general recommendation for thyroid hormone therapy in uremic children can be given.

Adrenal Function

ADRENOCORTICOTROPIC HORMONE

Basal ACTH levels may be increased, without an increase after metyrapone or suppression after dexamethasone administration. The feedback control of the hypothalamic-pituitary-adrenocortical axis appears to be altered. High autonomous ACTH excretion, akin to Cushing's syndrome, may lead to hypercortisolemia. It is conceivable that some of the complications of renal failure, such as osteopathy, negative nitrogen balance, and glucose intolerance, may be due at least in part to chronic hypercortisolemia caused by high ACTH levels [142].

CORTISOL

Although most investigators have found normal basal plasma concentrations of cortisol [20], elevated cortisol levels, both total and free (non-protein bound) have also been reported.

No correlation was found between circulating free cortisol levels and the degree of renal insufficiency, within a range of GFRs of 2 to 44 ml/min/1.73 m^2 [20]. Circadian rhythmicity of cortisol was normal, as evidenced by peak secretory activity and number of peaks per 24 hours [12,24,61,111,142,218]. Mean 24-hour plasma cortisol levels may be increased, however [218]. Prolongation of the cortisol half-life may contribute to the elevated serum cortisol [45].

Chronic hemodialysis produced a shift of secretory activity into the dialysis time period, possibly related to the stress of the procedure [218]. An increase of plasma cortisol has also been noted in adults and children during hemodialysis or hemofiltration [2,172].

Spurious overestimation of plasma cortisol in uremic serum may occur, possibly due to cross-reactivity of antisera with glucuronide conjugates that circulate at high concentrations in patients with renal failure [152].

The adrenocorticotropic hormone (ACTH) stimulation test demonstrates a normal increase in plasma cortisol

[2,142]. Both normal and incomplete suppression of cortisol have been reported in response to dexamethasone [12, 142,178,218].

Renin-Angiotensin-Aldosterone System

Over 70% of children with CRF become hypertensive before the onset of dialysis treatment [169]. Sodium and volume overload has been reported to play a major role in the pathogenesis [186]. The importance of the renin-angiotensin system in causing and maintaining arterial hypertension in uremic children and adults has recently been underscored by the antihypertensive effect of the angiotensin-converting enzyme inhibitor captopril [31,72].

RENIN

Adults and children with CRF show a wide range of value of basal plasma renin activity (PRA) [168,221]. Rauh et al. [168] found the highest PRA levels in children with sodium-losing nephropathies and nephronophthisis (Fig. 34-6, Table 34-1).

High PRA levels in uremic patients may be due to the renin secretory process responding only partially to the usual control mechanisms. Furthermore, normal or even low plasma PRA levels may be inappropriately high if they occur in the presence of volume expansion and hypertension. Without some knowledge of total body sodium and intravascular or extracellular volume, the renin levels in children with CRF remain difficult to interpret [142, 186,221].

Following hemodialysis, an increase in PRA has been reported by several authors [142,186,221]. The decrease in BP during hemodialysis may stimulate renin release either directly through a renal baroreceptor mechanism or indirectly through β-adrenergic stimulation. Salt and volume depletion and a decrease in serum potassium may also contribute to the increase in PRA. Conversely long-term administration of propranolol [30,91] may also contribute to renin suppression.

After renal transplantation high levels of renin originating from the patient's remaining kidney or from the graft (e.g., as a consequence of renal artery stenosis) may cause serious hypertension [72].

ALDOSTERONE

There is a significant correlation between PRA and plasma aldosterone levels in children with terminal renal failure. Elevated serum potassium levels may also be responsible for the increase in plasma aldosterone in CRF [4,74,221] (see Table 34-1).

During dialysis aldosterone secretion is high because of stress-related ACTH stimulation of the renin-angiotensin system. Although aldosterone increases tubular reabsorption of sodium, it is unlikely that it plays a role in the pathogenesis of hypertension when the excretory function of the kidney has ceased [168].

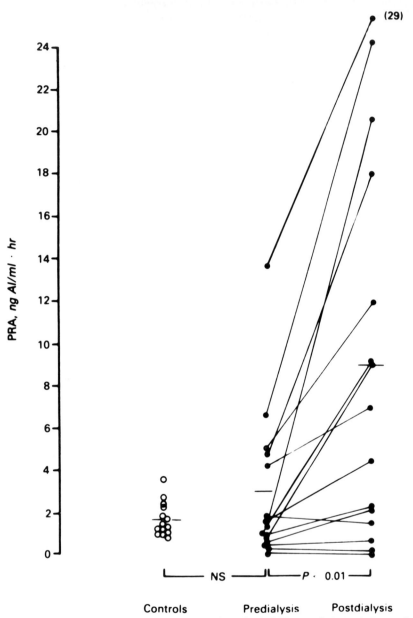

FIG. 34-6. *Plasma renin activity in 14 controls and 15 children with CRF, before and after hemodialysis. (From Rauh W, Hund E, Sohl G, et al: Vasoactive hormones in children with chronic renal failure. Kidney Int 24:S27, 1983, with permission.)*

Catecholamines

In uremic adults, increased plasma norepinephrine levels have been reported by several authors [27,91,120,143] while plasma epinephrine levels vary widely [27,91, 120,143]. Raised plasma catecholamines in uremia could be due to increased synthesis, diminished re-uptake at the nerve terminals, deficient enzyme inactivation, or decreased renal excretion [18,92,120]. In a recent study [168], dialysis and ultrafiltration caused a marked increase in catecholamines, indicating an adequate sympathetic re-

sponse to volume depletion and to the decrease in BP (see Table 34-1).

Vasopressin

Basal vasopressin concentrations are elevated in children and adults with CRF. Increased serum osmolality may play a role. Nonosmotic factors, including BP, blood volume, and stress, may also influence vasopressin release. The metabolic clearance rate of vasopressin is diminished in

TABLE 34-1. *Hormone activity in 15 control children and in 15 children with chronic renal failure before and after dialysis*

	PRA (ng AL/ml hr)	ALDO (ng/dl)	AVP (ng/liter)	NOR (ng/liter)	ADR (ng/liter)
Control children	1.7 ± 0.2	8.2 ± 1.1	3.2 ± 0.8	193.4 ± 18.6	28.4 ± 3.4
Children with CRF					
Predialysis	3.1 ± 0.9	40.0 ± 20.1	9.7 ± 2.5[b]	230.4 ± 42.1	39.2 ± 8.5
Postdialysis	9.0 ± 2.4[c]	96.6 ± 35.7	17.5 ± 6.2	462.3 ± 74.5[c]	196.9 ± 32.8[c]

[a] Values are SEM. Abbreviations: PRA = plasma renin activity; ALDO = aldosterone; AVP = vasopressin; NOR = noradrenalin; ADR = adrenalin.
[b] Significantly different from control values, $P < 0.01$.
[c] Significantly different from predialysis values, $P < 0.01$.
From Rauh W, Haud E, Sohl G, et al: Vasoactive hormones in children with chronic renal failure. *Kidney Int* 24:S27, 1983, with permission.

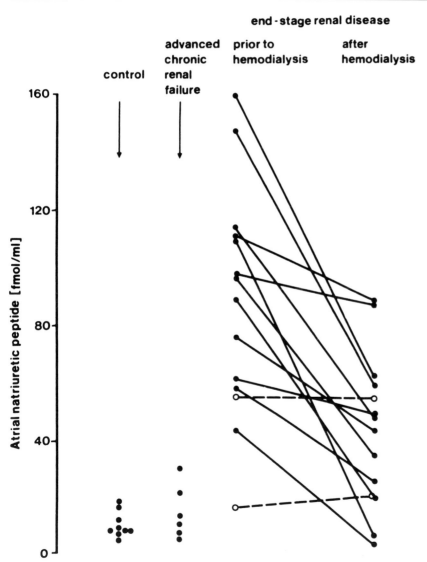

FIG. 34-7. *Plasma atrial natriuretic peptide in healthy children, in children with advanced renal failure, and in children with end-stage renal disease before and after hemodialysis. (From Rascher W, Tulassay T, Lang RE: Atrial naturiuretic peptide in plasma of volume overloaded children with chronic renal failure.* Lancet *2:303, 1985, with permission.)*

uremia, emphasizing the role of the kidney in vasopressin degradation [15]. The complex and divergent interplay of these factors probably explains why during hemodialysis, when osmolality decreases, vasopressin does not always fall [97,171,191] (see Table 34-1). It is not clear whether elevated vasopressin levels contribute to the development of hypertension in CRF.

Atrial Natriuretic Factor

Atrial natriuretic factor (ANF) is a peptide found in atrial muscle cells that has a critical role in the regulation of fluid volume as well as renal and cardiovascular function [7]. The release of ANF is stimulated by maneuvers that result in an increase in atrial wall tension as elicited by acute blood volume expansion, atrial tachyarrhythmias, and congestive heart failure [122,134,189,194,210].

ANF has several sites of action. The central effect of ANF is to induce a marked increase in the GFR and glomerular filtration pressure [33,71,94,98]. ANF produces an increase in the absolute and fractional excretion of sodium chloride, other solutes, and water [123]. ANF also

relaxes large arteries and other vascular beds through an increase in cyclic guanosine monophosphate [123].

In addition to inducing natriuresis and diuresis, ANF causes a marked reduction in BP in hypertensive animal models (including experimental renovascular hypertension and volume expanded hypertension) [193,215,216]. Infusions of atrial natriuretic factor result in a decrease in plasma renin levels—possibly mediated by the increased delivery of sodium to the macula densa [37,214]. ANF directly inhibits the secretion of aldosterone from the glomerulosa and blocks the angiotensin II stimulation of aldosterone [130]. Therefore, ANF exerts diuretic, natriuretic, and hypotensive effects in a volume overloaded state.

In uremic adult patients ANF levels are elevated but decrease with hemodialysis [130]. The expanded extracellular volume stimulates the secretion of ANF in CRF, and this increase reflects a compensatory mechanism in volume homeostasis. Because the kidney is the main site of ANF degradation [204], it has been suggested that elevated levels of ANF in CRF are due to impaired metabolism and excretion of ANF by the nonfunctioning kidneys. However, the lack of significant correlation between plasma ANF and serum creatinine concentration in both dialyzed and nondialyzed patients is not consistent with this hypothesis.

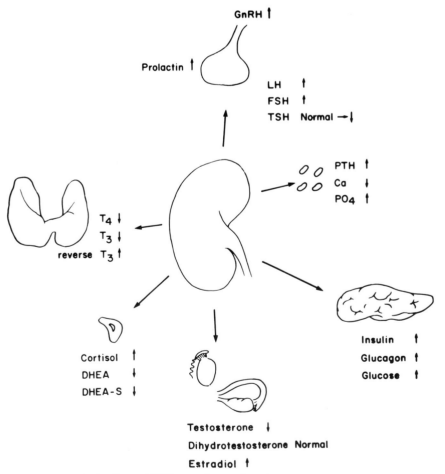

Fig. 34-8. *Multiple effects of CRF on endocrine function.*

Persistent volume overload despite elevated ANF implies the diseased kidney is resistant to the natriuretic and diuretic properties of ANF. However, the role of ANF in renal failure remains to be clarified.

Few reports have been published regarding the concentrations of ANF in children. Rascher [167] compared ANF levels in children with end-stage renal disease with that of healthy children and children with advanced renal failure without evidence of volume expansion (Fig. 34-7). Children with advanced CRF have predialysis ANF levels slightly higher than healthy children and children with advanced renal failure without evidence of volume expansion. Two children with CRF who received dialysis but who had a residual urine output of more than 1 liter/d did not have markedly elevated ANF levels. Again, the increase in ANF correlates with volume status; and its release represents an attempt by the heart to decrease its workload.

Summary

In summary, the kidney has a central role in the production and metabolism of hormones. The biochemical changes of CRF result in alterations in the internal milieu affecting synthesis and secretory rate of hormones and impeding hormonal effects on target tissues (Fig. 34-8).

Some adverse effects of CRF on the hormonal milieu are corrected by successful transplantation. In other instances inhibitors of hormonal action are present in uremia, as in the case of somatomedin.

The recent observation that treatment with recombinant human growth hormone can ameliorate the growth failure accompanying CRF holds particular promise for the young patients in our care.

References

1. Afrasiabi MA, Vaziri ND, Gwinup G, et al: Thyroid function studies in the nephrotic syndrome. *Ann Intern Med* 90:335, 1979.
2. Akmad M, Manzier AD: Simplified assessment of pituitary-adrenal axis in a stable group of chronic hemodialysis patients. *Trans Am Soc Artif Intern Organs* 23:703, 1977.
3. Alvestrand A, Wahren J, Smith D, et al: Insulin-mediated potassium uptake is normal in uremic and healthy subjects. *Am J Physiol* 246:E174, 1984.
4. Ammenti A, Muller-Wiefel DE, Schaerer K, et al: Mineralocorticoids in the nephrotic syndrome of children. *Clin Nephrol* 14:238, 1980.
5. Arnold WC, Danford D, Holliday MA: Effects of caloric supplementation on growth in children with uremia. *Kidney Int* 24:205, 1983.
6. Asaba H, Alvestrand A, Furst P, et al: Clinical implications of uremic middle molecules in regular hemodialysis patients. *Clin Nephrol* 19:179, 1983.
7. Atlas SA: Atrial natriuretic factor: A new hormone of cardiac origin. *Recent Prog Horm Res* 42:207, 1986.
8. Atuk NO, Bailey CJ, Turner S, et al: Red blood catecholamines and renin in renal failure. *Trans ASAIO* 22:195, 1976.
9. Avioli LV: Endocrine disturbances in uremia. In Edelmann CM (ed): *Pediatric Kidney Disease*. Boston, Little, Brown, Vol. 1, 443, 1978.
10. Bagdade JD: Disorders of glucose metabolism in uremia. *Adv Nephrol* 8:87, 1979.
11. Bala RM, Hankins C, Anderson D, et al: Serum somatomedin in health and disease. (abstr) *Clin Res* 22:188A, 1974.
12. Barbour GL, Sevier BR: Adrenal responsiveness in chronic hemodialysis. *N Engl J Med* 290:1258, 1974.
13. Barton CH, Mirahmade MK, Vaziri ND: Effects of long-term testosterone administration on pituitary-testicular axis in end-stage renal failure. *Nephron* 31:61, 1982.
14. Baxter RC, Brown AS, Turtle JR: Radioimmunoassay for somatomedin-C: comparison with radioreceptor assay in patients with growth-hormone disorders, hypothyroidism and renal failure. *Clin Chem* 28:488, 1982.
15. Benmansour M, Rainfray M, Paillard F, et al: Metabolic clearance rate of immunoreactive vasopressin in man. *Europ J Clin Invest* 12:475, 1982.
16. Bercu BB, Orloff S, Schulman JD: Pituitary resistance to thyroid hormone in cystinosis. *J Clin Endocrinol Metab* 5:1262, 1980.
17. Berelowitz M, Szabo M, Frohman LA, et al: Somatomedin-C mediates growth hormone negative feedback by effects on both the hypothalamus and the pituitary. *Science* 212:1279, 1981.
18. Bergstrom J, Furst P: Uremic middle molecules. *Clin Nephrol* 5:143, 1976.
19. Bessarione D, Perfumo F, Giusti M, et al: Growth hormone response to growth hormone-releasing hormone in normal and uraemic children. Comparison with hypoglycemia following insulin administration. *Acta Endocrinol* (Copenh) 114:5, 1987.
20. Betts PR, Hose PM, Morris R, et al: Serum cortisol concentrations in children with chronic renal insufficiency. *Arch Dis Child* 50:3, 1975.
21. Betts PR, Magrath G, White RHR: Role of dietary energy supplementation in growth of children with chronic renal insufficiency. *Br Med J* 1:416, 1977.
22. Betts PR, Magrath G: Growth pattern and dietary intake of children with chronic renal insufficiency. *Br Med J* 2:189, 1974.
23. Blifeld C, Ettenger RB, Nelson P, et al: Accelerated growth following successful renal transplantation. *Pediatr Res* (Copenh) 21:472A, 1987.
24. Bonomini V, Orgoni G, Stefoni S, et al: Hormonal changes in uremia. *Clin Nephrol* 11:275, 1979.
25. Blum WF, Ranke MB, Kietzmann K, et al: A specific radioimmunoassay for the growth hormone (GH)-dependent somatomedin-binding protein: Its use for diagnosis of GH deficiency. *J Clin Endocrinol Metab* 70:1272, 1990.
26. Bommer J, Ritz E, Del Pozo E, et al: Improved sexual function in male hemodialysis patients on bromocriptine. *Lancet* 2:496, 1979.
27. Brecht HM, Ernst W, Koch KM: Plasma noradrenaline levels in regular hemodialysis patients. *Proc Eur Dial Transplant Assoc* 12:218, 1976.
28. Broyer M, Kleinknecht C, Loirat C, et al: Maturation osseuse et development pubertaire chez l'enfant et l'adolescent en dialyse chronique. *Proc Eur Dial Transplant Assoc* 9:81, 1972.
29. Broyer M, Kleinknecht C, Loirat C, et al: Growth in children treated with long-term hemodialysis. *J Pediatr* 84:642, 1974.
30. Brunner HR, Baier L, Sealey JE, et al: The influence of potassium administration and potassium deprivation on plasma renin in normal and hypertensive subjects. *J Clin Invest* 49:2128, 1970.
31. Brunner HR, Weber B, Wauters JP, et al: Inappropriate

renin secretion unmasked by captopril (SQ) 14225 in hypertension of chronic renal failure. *Lancet* 2:704, 1978.

32. Burke JR, El-Bishti MM, Maisey MN, et al: Hypothyroidism in children with cystinosis. *Arch Dis Child* 53:947, 1978.

33. Camargo MJF, Kleinert HD, Atlas SA, et al: Calcium dependent hemodynamic and natriuretic effect on atrial extract in isolated rat kidney. *Am J Physiol* 264:F447, 1984.

34. Cameron DP, Burger HG, Catt KJ, et al: Metabolic clearance rate of human growth hormone in patients with hepatic and renal failure, and in the isolated perfused pig liver. *Metabolism* 21:895, 1972.

35. Caro JF, Lanza-Jacoby S: Insulin resistance in uremia. Characterization of lipid metabolism in freshly isolated and primary cultures of hepatocytes from chronic uremic rats. *J Clin Invest* 72:882, 1983.

36. Chopra IJ, Chopra U, Smith SR, et al: Reciprocal changes in serum concentrations of 3,3',5'-triiodothyronine (reverse T3) and 3,3',5'-triiodothyronine (T3) in systemic illness. *J Clin Endocrinol Metab* 41:1043, 1975.

37. Cody RJ, Covit AB, Laragh JH, et al: Atrial natriuretic factors (ANF) in normal men: Renal hemodynamic/hormonal responses. *Hypertension* 7:845, 1985.

38. Contreras P, Later R, Navarro J, et al: Molecules in the middle molecular weight range. *Nephron* 32:193, 1982.

39. Costin G, Kogut MD, Phillips LS: Craniopharyngeoma: The role of insulin in promoting postoperative growth. *J Clin Endocrinol Metab* 42:370, 1976.

40. Cowden EA, Ratcliffe WA, Ratcliffe JG, et al; Hyperprolactinemia in renal disease. *Clin Endocrinol* 9:241, 1978.

41. Crawford JD: Meat, potatoes and growth hormone. *N Engl J Med* 305:163, 1981.

42. Czernichow, H, Dauzet MC Broyer M, et al: Abnormal TSH, PRL, and GRH response to TSH releasing factor in chronic renal failure. *J Clin Endocrinol Metab* 43:630, 1976.

43. Dandona P, Freedman D, Moorhead JF: Glycosylated haemoglobin in chronic renal failure. *Br Med J* 1:1183, 1979.

44. Davis FB, Spector DA, Davis PJ, et al: Comparison of pituitary-thyroid function in patients with end-stage renal disease and in age- and sex-matched controls. *Kidney Int* 21:362, 1982.

45. Deck KA, Baur P, Hillen H: Plasma clearance of cortisol as a function of plasma cortisol levels in normal and obese persons and in patients with uremia or cirrhosis of the liver. *Acta Endocrinol (Copenh)* 91:122, 1979.

46. D'Ercole JD: Use of the RIA for somatomedin-C estimation. *J Peds* 99:735, 1981.

47. DeFronzo RA: Pathogenesis of glucose intolerance in uremia. *Metabolism* 27:1866, 1978.

48. DeFronzo RA, Alvestrand A, Smith D, et al: Insulin resistance in uremia. *J Clin Invest* 67:563, 1981.

49. DeFronzo RA, Andres R, Edgar P, et al: Carbohydrate metabolism in uremia: A review. *Medicine* 52;469, 1973.

50. DeFronzo RA, Tobin J, Boden G, et al: The role of growth hormone in the glucose intolerance of uremia. *Acta Diabetol Lat* 16:279, 1979.

51. DeFronzo RA, Tobin JD, Row JW, et al: Glucose intolerance in uremia. Quantification of pancreatic beta, cell sensitivity to glucose and tissue sensitivity to insulin. *J Clin Invest* 62:425, 1978.

52. Delaporte C, Gros F: In vitro inhibition of protein synthesis by dialysates of plasma from uremic patients. *Eur J Clin Invest* 11:139, 1981.

53. Delaporte C, Gros F: In vitro inhibition of protein synthesis by dialysates of plasma from uremic patients. *Eur J Clin Invest* 11:139, 1981.

54. DeSanto NG, Gilli G, Capasso G, et al: Growth during

55. Dzurik R, Hupkova V, Cernacek P, et al: The isolation of an inhibitor of glucose utilization from the serum of uraemic subjects. *Clin Chim Acta* 46:77, 1973.

56. El-Bishti MM, Counahan R, Jarrett RJ, et al: Hyperlipidaemia in children on regular haemodialysis. *Arch Dis Child* 52:932, 1977.

57. El-Bishti MM, Counahan R, Bloom SR, et al: Hormonal and metabolic responses to intravenous glucose in children on regular hemodialysis. *Am J Clin Nutr* 31:1865, 1978.

58. Emmanouel DS, Lindheimer MD, Katz AI: Pathogenesis of endocrine abnormalities in uremia. *Endocr Rev* 1:28, 1980.

59. Faber J, Heaf J, Kirkegaard C, et al: Simultaneous turnover studies of thyroxine, 3,5,3' and 3,3',5'-triiodothyronine, 3.5-. 3,3'-, and 3',5'-diiodothyronine and 3'-monoiodothyronine in chronic renal failure. *J Clin Endocrinol Metab* 56:211, 1983.

60. Fang VS, Refetoff S: Sustained thyrotropin elevation in patients with renal failure. Studies of mechanisms in azotemic rats. *American Thyroid Association*, Abstract T6, 1976.

61. Feldman HA, Singer I: Endocrinology and metabolism in uremia and dialysis: A clinical study: *Medicine* 54:345, 1974.

62. Fennell RS, Orak JK, Hudson T, et al: Growth in children with various therapies for end-stage renal disease. *Amer J Dis Child* 138:28, 1984.

63. Fennell RS, Orak JK, Garin EH, et al; Continuous ambulatory peritoneal dialysis in a pediatric population. *Am J Dis Child* 137:388, 1983.

64. Ferraris J, Saenger P, Levine L, et al: Delayed puberty in males with chronic renal failure. *Kidney Int* 18:344, 1980.

65. Ferrer J, Diaz-Ewald M, Garcia R, et al: Effects of triiodothyronine on the anemia of chronic renal failure. *Am J Hematol* 5:139, 1978.

66. Ferrinnini E, Pilo A, Navalesi R, et al: Insulin kinetics and glucose-induced insulin delivery in chronically dialyzed subjects: Acute effects of dialysis. *J Clin Endocrinol Metab* 49:15, 1979.

67. Fichman MP: Pituitary, gonadal and thyroid function. In Massry SG, Sellers AL (eds): *Clinical Aspects of Uremia and Dialysis.* Springfield, Illinois, Charles C Thomas, Publisher, 1976, p 273.

68. Fine RN, Yadin O, Pyke-Grimm KA, et al: Recombinant human growth hormone (rhGH) treatment of growth retarded children with chronic renal failure—3 years experience (abstr). *Pediatr Res* 27:328A, 1990.

69. Foreman JM, Chan JCM: Chronic renal failure in infants and children. *J Pediatr* 113:793, 1988.

70. Fraser SD: A review of growth hormone stimulation tests in children. *Pediatrics* 53:929, 1974.

71. Fried TA, McCoy RN, Osgood RW, et al: The effect of atrial natriuretic peptide on glomerular hemodynamics. *Clin Res* 33:584A, 1985.

72. Friedman A, Chesney RW, Ball D, et al: Effective use of captopril (angiotensin I-converting enzyme inhibitor) in severe childhood hypertension. *J Pediatr* 97:664, 1980.

73. Geisthovel W, von zur Muhlen A, Bahlmann J: Studies on the pituitary-testicular axis in male patients with chronic renal failure with different glomerular filtration. *Klin Wochenschr* 54:1027, 1976.

74. Ghione S, Fommei E, Clerico A, et al: Major determinants of plasma aldosterone levels in chronic uremia on dialytic treatment. *Nephron* 30:110, 1982.

75. Gil-Ad I, Topper E, Laron Z: Oral clonidine as a growth hormone stimulation test. *Lancet* 2:278, 1979.

76. Giordano C, De-Santo NG, Carella C, et al: TSH response

to TRH in hemodialysis and CAPD patients. *Int J Artif Organs* 7:7, 1984.

77. Giusti M, Mazzocchi G, Sessarego P, et al: Effects of GRF (1-40) and domperidone on GH secretion in normal man. *Clin Endocrinol* 21:339, 1984.

78. Goldberg AC, Trivedi B, Delmez JA, et al: Uremia reduces serum insulin-like growth factor I, increases insulin-like growth factor II, and modifies their serum protein binding. *J Clin Endocrinol Metab* 55:1040, 1982.

79. Golde DW: Growth factors. *Ann Intern Med* 92:650, 1980.

80. Gonzalez-Barcena D, Kastin AJ, Schalch DS, et al: Responses to thyrotropin releasing hormone in patients with renal failure and after infusion in normal men. *J Clin Endocrinol Metab* 36:117, 1973.

81. Grodstein GD, Blumenkrantz MJ, Kopple JD: Nutritional and metabolic response to catabolic stress in uremia. *Am J Clin Nutr* 33:1411, 1980.

82. Guler HP, Zapf J, Scheiwiller E, et al: Recombinant insulin-like growth factor I stimulates growth and has distinct effects on organ size in hypophysectomized rats. *Proc Natl Acad Sci USA* 85:4889, 1988.

83. Guler HP, Schmid C, Zapf J, et al: Effects of recombinant insulin-like growth factor I on insulin secretion and renal function in normal human subjects. *Proc Natl Acad Sci USA* 86:2868, 1989.

84. Gupta D, Bundschu HD: Testosterone and its binding in the plasma of male subjects with chronic renal failure. *Clin Chim Acta* 36:479, 1972.

85. Gutman RA, Huang AT: Inhibitor of marrow thymidine incorporation from sera of patients with uremia. *Kidney Int* 18:715, 1980.

86. Hall K, Filipsson R: Correlation between somatomedin A in serum and body height development in healthy children and children with certain growth disturbances. *Acta Endocrinol (Kbh)* 78:239, 1975.

87. Hall K, Sara VR, Enberg G, et al: Somatomedins and postnatal growth. *In* Ritzen EM, Hall K, Zetterberg A, et al (eds): *The Biology of Human Growth.* New York, Raven Press, 1981, p 275.

88. Hallgren R, Fjellstrom KE, Lundquist G: Abnormal pancreatic polypeptide response to intravenous glucose in uraemics. A possible mechanisms behind impaired glucose tolerance in uraemia. *Clin Endocrinol (Oxf)* 17:165, 1982.

89. Handelsman DJ: Hypothalamic-pituitary gonadal dysfunction in renal failure dialysis and renal transplantation. *Endocr Rev* 6:151, 1985.

90. Hasegawa K, Matsushita Y, Inoue T, et al: Plasma levels of atrial natriuretic peptide in patients with chronic renal failure. *J Clin Endocrinol Metab* 63:819, 1986.

91. Heinrich WL, Katz FH, Molinoff PB, et al: Competitive effects of hyperkalemia and volume depletion on plasma renin activity, aldosterone and catecholamine concentrations in hemodialysed patients. *Kidney Int* 12:297, 1977.

92. Hennemann H, Havendehl G, Rebel B, et al: Untersuchungen zur urämischen Sympathikopathie in vitro und in vivo. *Dtsch Med Wochenschr* 98:1630, 1973.

93. Hintz RL: The physiologic basis of growth. *In* Hintz RL, Rosenfeld RG (eds): *Growth Abnormalities.* New York, Churchill-Livingstone, 1987, p 1.

94. Hintze TH, Currie MG, Needleman P: Atriopeptin: Renal specific vasodilators in conscious dogs. *Am J Physiol* 248:H587, 1985.

95. Hirschberg R, Kopple JD: Evidence that insulin-like-growth factor I increases renal plasma flow and glomerular filtration rate in fasted rats. *J Clin Invest* 83:326, 1989.

96. Holliday MA, Chantler C: Metabolic and nutritional factors in children with renal insufficiency. *Kidney Int* 14:306, 1978.

97. Horky K, Sramkova J, Lachmanova J, et al: Plasma concentration of antidiruetic hormone in patients with chronic renal insufficiency on maintenance dialysis. *Horm Metab Res* 11:241, 1979.

98. Ichikawa I, Dunn BR, Troy JL, et al: Influence of atrial natriuretic peptide on glomerular microcirculation in vivo (abstr). *Clin Res* 33:487A, 1985.

99. Ijaiya K: Pattern of growth hormone response to insulin, arginine and hemodialysis in uremic children. *Eur J Pediatr* 131:185, 1979.

100. Ijaiya K, Roth B, Schwenk A: Serum prolactin levels in renal insufficiency in children. *Acta Paediatr Scand* 69:299, 1980.

101. Isalesson OG, Janssen TO, Gause IAM: Growth hormone stimulates bone growth directly. *Science* 216:1237, 1982.

102. Johnson V, Maack T: Renal extraction, filtration, absorption, and catabolism of growth hormone. *Am J Physiol* 233:F185, 1977.

103. Jones RWA, El Bishti MM, Bloom SR, et al: The effects of anabolic steroids on growth, body composition and metabolism in boys with chronic renal failure on regular hemodialysis. *J Pediatr* 97:559, 1980.

104. Kamil ES, Yadin O, Pyke-Grimm KA, et al: Recombinant human growth hormone treatment following renal transplantation (abstr). *Pediatr Res* 27:332A, 1990.

105. Kaptein EM, Feinstein EI, Massry SG: Thyroid hormone metabolism in renal disease. *Contrib Nephrol* 33:122, 1982.

106. Kaptein EM, Levitan D, Feinstein EI, et al: Alterations of thyroid hormone indices in acute renal failure and in acute critical illness with and without acute renal failure. *Am J Nephrol* 1:138, 1981.

107. Katz AL, Emmanouel DS: Metabolism of polypeptide hormones by the normal kidney and in uremia. *Nephron* 22:69, 1978.

108. Kauffman JM, Caro JF: Insulin resistance in uremia. Characterization of insulin action, binding, and processing in isolated hepatocytes from chronic uremic rats. *J Clin Invest* 71:698, 1983.

109. Klapper DG, Svoboda ME, Van Wyk JJ: Sequence analysis of somatomedin-C: Confirmation of identity with insulin-like growth factor I. *Endocrinology* 112:2215, 1983.

110. Kleinknecht C, Broyer M, Huot D, et al: Growth and development of non-dialyzed children with chronic renal failure. *Kidney Int* 24:S40, 1983.

111. Klett M, Gilli G, Scharer K, et al: Plasma-HGH-TSH and cortisol in children with chronic renal failure (CRF), *Pediatr Res* 10:897, 1976.

112. Koch VB, Lippe B, Sherman BM, et al: Integrated growth hormone determinations in children with chronic renal failure (abstr). *Pediatr Res* 23:541A, 1988.

113. Koch VH, Lippe B, Nelson PA, et al: Accelerated growth after recombinant human growth hormone treatment of children with chronic renal failure. *J Pediatr* 115:365, 1989.

114. Kopple JD: Abnormal amino acid metabolism in uremia. *Kidney Int* 14:340, 1978.

115. Korth-Schutz S, Levine LS, New MI: Serum androgens in normal prepubertal and pubertal children with precocious adrenarche. *J Clin Endocrinol Metab* 42:117, 1976.

116. Korth-Schutz S, Levine LS, New MI: Dehydroepiandrosterone sulfate (DS) levels, a rapid test for abnormal adrenal androgen secretion. *J Clin Endocrinol Metab* 42:1005, 1976.

117. Korth-Schutz S, Levine LS, New MI: Evidence for the adrenal source of androgens in precocious adrenarche. *Acta Endocrinol* 82:342, 1976.

118. Korth-Schutz S, Virdis R, Saenger P, et al: Serum androgens as a continuing index of adequacy of treatment of congenital adrenal hyperplasia. *J Clin Endocrinol Metab* 46:452, 1978.

119. Kosowicz J, Malczewska B, Czekalski C: Serum reverse triiodothyronine (3,3'5'-L-triiodothyronine) in chronic renal failure. *Nephron* 26:85, 1980.

120. Ksiazek A: Beta dopamine hydroxylase activity and catecholamine levels in the plasma of patients with renal failure. *Nephron* 24:170, 1979.

121. Kuku SF, Jaspan JB, Emmanouel DS, et al: Heterogeneity of plasma glucagon. Circulating components in normal subjects and patients with chronic renal failure. *J Clin Invest* 58:742, 1976.

122. Lang RE, Tholken H, Ganten D, et al: Atrial natriuretic factor—a circulating hormone stimulated by volume loading. *Nature* 314:264, 1985.

123. Laragh JH: Atrial natriuretic hormone, the renin-aldosterone axis and blood-pressure-electrolyte homeostasis. *N Engl J Med* 313:1330, 1985.

124. LeRoith D, Danovitz G, Trestian S, et al: Dissociation of pituitary glycoprotein response to releasing hormones in chronic renal failure. *Acta Endocrinol* (Copenh) 93:277, 1980.

125. Levine LS, Rauh W, Gottesdiener K, et al: New studies of the 11-hydroxylase and 18-hydroxylase enzymes in the hypertensive form of congenital adrenal hyperplasia. *J Clin Endocrinol Metab* 50:259, 1980.

126. Lewy JE, New MI: Growth in children with renal failure. *Am J Med* 58:65, 1975.

127. Li CH, Yamashiro D, Gospodarowicz D, et al: Total synthesis of insulin-like growth factor I (somatomedin-C). *Proc Natl Acad Sci USA* 80:2216, 1983.

128. Lim VS, Fang VS: Gonadal dysfunction in uremic men. A study of the hypothalamo-pituitary-testosterone axis before and after renal transplantation. *Am J Med* 58:655, 1975.

129. Lindler A, Charra B, Sherrard DJ, et al: Accelerated atherosclerosis in prolonged maintenance haemodialysis. *N Engl J Med* 290:697, 1974.

130. Maack T, Marion DN, Camargo MJF, et al: Effects of auriculin (atrial natriuretic factor) on blood pressure, renal function, and the renin-aldosterone system in dogs. *Am J Med* 77:1069, 1984.

131. Mahajan SK, Abbasi AA, Prasad AS, et al: Effect of oral zinc therapy on gonadal function in hemodialysis patients. A double blind study. *Ann Intern Med* 97:357, 1982.

132. Mak RHK, Turner C, Haycock CB, et al: Secondary hyperparathyroidism and glucose intolerance in children with uremia. *Kidney Int* (suppl 16)24:S128, 1983.

133. Mak RHK, Bettinelli A, Turner C, et al: The influence of hyperparathyroidism on glucose metabolism in uremia. *J Clin Endocrinol Metab* 60:229, 1985.

134. Manning PT, Schwartz D, Katsube HC, et al: Vasopressin-stimulated release of atriopeptins endocrine antagonists in fluid homeostasis. *Science* 229:395, 1985.

135. Marder HK, Srivastava LS, Burstein S: Hypergonadotropism in peripubertal boys with chronic renal failure. *Pediatrics* 72:384, 1983.

136. Martin LG, Clark SW, Connor TB: Growth hormone secretion enhanced by androgens. *J Clin Endocrinol Metab* 28:425, 1968.

137. Marti-Henneberg C, Domenech JM, Montoya E: Thyrotropin-releasing hormone responsiveness and degradation in children with chronic renal failure: Effect of time of evolution. *Acta Endocrinol* 99:508, 1982.

138. Matsubara M, Nakagawa K, Nonomura K, et al: Plasma LRH levels in chronic renal failure before and during haemodialysis. *Acta Endocrinol* (Copenh). 103:145, 1983.

139. Maxwell MH, Weidman P: The renin-angiotensin system in parenchymal renal disease. *In* Hamburger J, Crosnier J, Maxwell MH (eds): *Advances in Nephrology*, Vol 5, Chicago, Year Book Medical Publishers, 1975, p 301.

140. McCaleb ML, Lockwood DH: Insulin-resistance in uremia caused by low molecular weight peptide. *Diabetes* (Suppl 1) 432:33A (Abstr), 1983.

141. McCaleb ML, Izzo MS, Lockwood DH: Characterization and purification of a factor from uremic human serum that induces insulin resistance. *J Clin Invest* 75:391, 1985.

142. McDonald WJ, Golper TA, Mass RD, et al: Adrenocorticotropin-cortisol axis abnormalities in hemodialysis patients. *J Clin Endocrinol Metab* 48:92, 1979.

143. McGrath BP, Ledingham JGG, Benedict CR: Catecholamines in peripheral venous plasma in patients on chronic hemodialysis. *Clin Sci Mol Med* 55:89, 1978.

144. McLean RH, Kennedy TL, Rosoulpour M, et al: Hypothyroidism in the congenital nephrotic syndrome. *J Pediatr* 101:72, 1982.

145. Milutinovic S, Breyer D, Jankovic N, et al: Inhibitor of insulin binding to erythrocytes in plasma of uremic patients. *Nephron* 34:99, 1983.

146. Mondon CS, Marcus R, Reaven GM: Role of glucogon as a contributor to glucose intolerance in acute and chronic uremia. *Metabolism* 31:374, 1982.

147. Morley JE, Distiller LA, Epstein S, et al: Menstrual disturbances in chronic renal failure. *Horm Metab Res* 11:68, 1979.

148. Mooradian AD, Morley JE: Endocrine dysfunction in chronic renal failure. *Arch Intern Med* 144:351, 1984.

149. Mosier HD Jr, Jansons RA, Hill RR, et al: Cartilage sulfation and serum somatomedin in rats during and after cortison-induced growth arrest. *Endocrinology* 99:580, 1976.

150. Nagel TC, Freinkel N, Bell RH, et al: Gynecomastia, prolactin and other peptide hormones in patients undergoing chronic hemodialysis. *J Clin Endocrinol Metab* 36:428, 1973.

151. New MI, Levine LS, Pang S: Adrenal androgens and growth. *In* Ritzen M, Hall K, Zetterberg A, et al (eds): *The Biology of Normal Human Growth.* New York, Raven Press, 1981.

152. Nolan GE, Smith JB, Chavre VJ, et al: Spurious overestimation of plasma cortisol in patients with chronic renal failure. *J Clin Endocrinol Metab* 52:1242, 1981.

153. Oertel PJ, Lichtwald K, Rauh W, et al: The hypothalamo-pituitary-gonadal axis in prepubertal children with chronic renal failure (CRF). *Kidney Int* 24:515, 1983.

154. Pang S, Levine LS, Saenger P, et al: Dihydrotestosterone and its relationship to testosterone in infancy and childhood. *J Clin Endocrinol Metab* 48:821, 1979.

155. Peces R, Horcajada C, Lopez-Novoa JM, et al: Hyperprolactinemia in chronic renal failure: Impaired responsiveness to stimulation and suppression. Normalization after transplantation. *Nephron* 28:11, 1981.

156. Phillips LS, Kopple JD: Circulating somatomedin activity and sulfate levels in adults with normal and impaired kidney function. *Metabolism* 30:1091, 1981.

157. Phillips LS, Pennisi AJ, Belosky DC, et al: Somatomedin activity and inorganic sulfate in children undergoing dialysis. *J Clin Endocrinol Metab* 46:165, 1978.

158. Phillips LS, Fusco AC, Unterman TG, et al: Somatomedin inhibitor in uremia. *J Clin Endocrinol Metab* 59:764, 1984.

159. Phillips LS, Vassilopoulou-Sellin R: Somatomedins, *New Engl J Med* 302:371, 1980, and 302:438, 1980.

160. Potter DC, Greifer I: Statural growth of children with renal disease. *Kidney Int* 14;334, 1978.

161. Powell DR, Rosenfeld RG, Baker BK, et al: Serum somatomedin levels in adults with chronic renal failure: The

importance of measuring insulin-like growth factor (IGF-I) and IGF-II in acid chromatographed uremic serum. *J Clin Endocrinol Metab* 63:1186, 1986.

162. Powell DR, Rosenfeld RG, Sperry JB, et al: Serum concentration of insulin-like growth factor (IGF)-I, IGF II and unsaturated somatomedin carrier proteins in children with chronic renal failure. *Am J Kidney Dis* 10:287, 1987.

163. Quellhorst E, Schuenemann B, Hildebrand U, et al: Response of the vascular system to different modifications of hemofiltration and hemodialysis. *Proc Eur Dial Transplant Assoc* 17:197, 1980.

164. Rager K, Bundschu HD, Gupta D: The effect of HCG on testicular androgen production in adult men with chronic renal failure. *J Reprod Fertil* 42:113, 1975.

165. Ramirez G, Juviz W, Gutch CF, et al: Thyroid abnormalities in renal failure. A study of 53 patients on chronic hemodialysis. *Ann Intern Med* 79:500, 1973.

166. Raiti S: Ed. Advances in human growth hormone research *DHEW Publication* No. (NIH) 74-612, 1974 p 321.

167. Rascher W, Tulassay T, Lang RE: Atrial natriuretic peptide in plasma of volume overloaded children with chronic renal failure. *Lancet* 2:303, 1985.

168. Rauh W, Hund E, Sohl G, et al: Vasoactive hormones in children with chronic renal failure. *Kidney Int* 24:S-27, 1983.

169. Rauh W, Muller-Wiefel DE, Heide B, et al: Hypertension bei chronischer Niereninsuffizienz im Kindsalter. *Monatsschr Klinderheilk* 125:1375, 1977.

170. Rauh W, Oertel PJ: Endocrine function in children with end stage renal disease. *In* Fine RN, Gruskin AB (eds): *End Stage Renal Disease in Children.* Philadelphia, WB Saunders, 1984, p 296.

171. Rauh W, Rascher W, Huber KH, et al: Nonosmotic factors in the regulation of antidiuretic hormone (ADH) in childhood (abstr) *Eur J Pediatr* 38:98, 1982.

172. Rauh W, Steels P, Klare B, et al: Plasma catecholamines, renin and aldosterone during hemodialysis and hemofiltration in children. *In* Bulla M (ed): *Renal Insufficiency in Children,* 3rd International Symposium, Cologne, May 2–3, 1981, Berlin, Heidelberg, New York, Springer verlag, 1982, p 110.

173. Regeur L, Faber OK, Binder C: Plasma C-peptide in uraemic patients. *Scand J Clin Lab Invest* 38:771, 1978.

174. Ritz E, Mehls O, Krempien B, et al: Skeletal growth in uremia. *In* Massry SG, Ritz E (eds): *Phosphate Metabolism.* New York, Plenum Press, 1977, p 515.

175. Roger M, Royer M, Scharer K, et al: Gonadotropines et androgenes plasmatiques chez les garcons traites pour insuffiance renale chronique. *Pathol Biol* 29:378, 1981.

176. Root A, Reiter E: Human perinatal endocrinology. *In* Quilligan E, Kretchmer N (eds): *Fetal and Maternal Medicine.* New York, John Wiley & Sons, 1980, p 15.

177. Rosenfeld R, Thorsson AV, Hintz RL: Increased somatomedin receptor sites in newborn circulating mononuclear cells. *J Clin Endocrinol Metab* 48:456, 1979.

178. Rosman PM, Faray A, Peckham R, et al: Pituitary-adrenocortical function in chronic renal failure: Blunted suppression and early escape of plasma cortisol levels after intravenous dexamethasone. *J Clin Endocrinol Metab* 54:528, 1982.

179. Rubenfeld S, Garber AJ: Abnormal carbohydrate in chronic renal failure. The potential role of accelerated production, increased gluconeogenesis, and impaired glucose disposal. *J Clin Invest* 62:20, 1978.

180. Rubenfeld S, Garber AJ: Impact of hemodialysis on the abnormal glucose and alanine kinetics of chronic azotemia. *Metabolism* 28:934, 1979.

181. Saenger P, Wiedemann E, Schwartz E, et al: Somatomedin and growth after renal transplantation. *Pediatr Res* 8:163, 1974.

182. Samaan NA, Freeman RM: Growth hormone levels in severe renal failure. *Metabolism* 19:102, 1970.

183. Sawin CT, Longcope GW, Ryan RJ: Blood levels of gonadotropins and gonadal hormones in gynecomastia associated with chronic hemodialysis. *J Clin Endocrinol Metab* 36:988, 1973.

184. Schaff-Blass E, Burstein S, Rosenfield RL: Advances in diagnosis and treatment of short stature, with special reference to the role of growth hormone. *J Pediatr* 104:801, 1984.

185. Schalch DS, Burstein PJ, Tewel SJ, et al: The effect of renal impairment on growth in the rat: Relationship to malnutrition and serum somatomedin levels. *Endocrinology* 108:1683, 1981.

186. Schalekamp MADH, Schalekamp-Kuyken MPA, De Moor-Friutier M, et al: Interrelationship between blood pressure, renin, renin substrate and blood volume in terminal renal failure. *Clin Sci Mol Med* 45:417, 1973.

187. Scharer K, Broyer M, Vescei P, et al: Damage to testicular function in chronic renal failure of children. *Proc EDTA* 17:725, 1980.

188. Schiffrin A, Guyda H, Robitaille P, et al: Increased plasma somatomedin reactivity in chronic renal failure as determined by acid gel filtration and radioreceptor assay. *J Clin Endocrinol Metab* 46:511, 1977.

189. Schiffrin EL, Gutkowska J, Kuchel O, et al: Plasma concentrations of atrial natriuretic factor in a patient with paroxysmal atrial tachycardia. *N Engl J Med* 312:1196, 1985.

190. Schmitz O: Effect of haemodialysis on insulin requirements in uraemic diabetic patients. Studies with the artificial beta-cell. *Proc Eur Dial Transplant Assoc* 19:769, 1983.

191. Schrier RW, Berl T, Anderson RJ: Osmotic and nonosmotic control of vasopressin release. *Am J Physiol* 236:F321, 1979.

192. Schwalbe SL, Betts PR, Rayner PHW, et al: Somatomedin in growth disorders and chronic renal insufficiency in children. *Br Med J* 1:679, 1977.

193. Seymour AA, Marsh EA, Mazack EK, et al: Synthetic atrial natriuretic factor in conscious normotensive and hypertensive rats. *Hypertension* 7:1, 1985.

194. Shenker Y, Sider RS, Ostafin EA, et al: Plasma levels of immunoreactive atrial natriuretic factor in healthy subjects and in patients with edema. *J Clin Invest* 76:1684, 1985.

195. Silverberg DS, Ulan RA, Fawcett DM, et al: Effects of chronic hemodialysis on thyroid function in chronic renal failure. *Can Med Asso J* 109:282, 1973.

196. Simmons JM, Wilson CJ, Potter DE, et al: Relation of calorie deficiency to growth failure in children on hemodialysis and the growth response to calorie supplementation. *New Engl J Med* 285:653, 1971.

197. Smith D, DeFronzo RA: Insulin resistance in uremia: evidence for receptor and post receptor deficits. *Kidney Int* 19:229, 1981.

198. Spencer EM, Uthne KO, Arnold WC: Growth impairment with elevated somatomedin levels in children with chronic renal insufficiency. *Acta Endocrinol* (Copenh) 91:36, 1979.

199. Stefanidis CJ, Hewitt IK, Balfe JW: Growth in children receiving continuous ambulatory peritoneal dialysis. *J Pediatr* 102:681, 1983.

200. Stewart-Bently M, Gans D, Horton R: Regulation of gonadal function in uremia. *Metabolism* 23:1065, 1974.

201. Stuart M, Lazarus L, Hayes J: Serum somatomedin in growth hormone levels in chronic renal failure. *IRCS* (Research on Endocrine System; Kidneys and Urinary System; Physiology) 2:1102, 1974.

202. Swamy AP, Woolf PD, Cestero RVM: Hypothalamic-pituitary-ovarian axis in uremic women. *J Lab Clin Med* 93:1967, 1979.

203. Swenson RS, Weisinge JR, Reaven GM: Effect of chronic uremia and hemodialysis on carbohydrate metabolism. *Clin Res* 22:209A, 1974.

204. Tang J, Weber RJ, Chang JK, et al: Depressor and natriuretic activities of several atrial peptides. *Regul Pept* 9:53, 1984.

205. Tannenbaum S, Ling N: The interrelationship of growth hormone (GH)-releasing factor and somatostatin in generation of the ultradian rhythm of GH secretion. *Endocrinology* 115:1952, 1984.

206. Takano K, Hall K, Kastrup KW, et al: Serum somatomedin A in crhonic renal failure. *J Clin Endocrinol Metab* 48:371, 1979.

207. Textor SC, Gavras H, Tifft CP, et al: Norepinephrine and renin activity in chronic renal failure: Evidence for interacting roles in hemodialysis hypertension. *Hypertension* 3:3, 1981.

208. Thompson P, Burman KD, Lukes YG, et al: Uremia decreases nuclear 3,5,3'-triodothyronine receptors in rats. *Endocrinology* 107:1081, 1980.

209. Thorner MO, Vance ML: Growth hormone, 1988. *J Clin Invest* 82:745, 1988.

210. Tikkanen I, Fyhrquist R, Metsarine K, et al: Plasma atrial natriuretic peptide in cardiac disease and during infusion in healthy volunteers. *Lancet* 2:66, 1985.

211. Toenshoff B, Mehls O, Heinrich U, et al: Growth stimulating effects of recombinant human growth hormone in children with end-stage renal disease. *J Pediatr* 116:561, 1990.

212. Van Buul-Offers S, Vanden Brande L: Effects of growth hormone and peptide fractions containing somatomedin activity on growth and cartilage metabolism of Snell dwarf mice. *Acta Endocrinol* 92:242, 1979.

213. van Diemen-Steenvoorde R, Donckerwolcke RA, Brackel H, et al: Growth and sexual maturation in children after kidney transplantation. *J Pediatr* 110:351, 1987.

214. Villarreal D, Freeman RH, Davis JO, et al: Renal mechanisms for suppression of renin secretion by atrial natriuretic factor. *Hypertension* 8:1128, 1986.

215. Volpe M, Odell G, Kleinert HD, et al: Effect of atrial natriuretic factor on blood pressure, renin, and aldosterone in Goldblatt hypertension. *Hypertension* 7:143, 1985.

216. Volpe M, Sosa RE, Muller FB, et al: Differing hemodynamic responses to atrial natriuretic factor in two models of hypertension. *Am J Physiol* 250:H871, 1986.

217. Von Lihen T, Salusky TB, Boechat I, et al: Five year experience with continuous ambulatory or continuous cycling peritonel dialysis in children. *J Pediatr* 111:513, 1987.

218. Wallace EZ, Rosman P, Toshav N, et al: Pituitary-adrenocorticol function in chronic renal failure: Studies of episodic secretion of cortisol and dexamethasone suppressibility. *J Clin Endocrinol Metab* 50:46, 1980.

219. Wass VJ, Wass JAH, Rees L, et al: Sex hormone changes underlying menstrual disturbances on haemodialysis. *Proc Eur Dial Transplant Assoc* 15:178, 1978.

220. Wehrenberg WB, Brazeau P, Luben R, et al: Inhibition of the pulsatile secretion of growth hormone by monoclonal antibodies to the hypothalamic growth hormone releasing factor (GRF). *Endocrinology* 111:2197, 1982.

221. Weidman P, Beretta-Piccoli C, Steffen F, et al: Hypertension in terminal renal failure. *Kidney Int* 9:294, 1976.

222. West CD, Smith WC: An attempt to elucidate the cause of growth retardation in renal disease. *Amer J Dis Child* 91:460, 1956.

223. Wiedemann E, Ackad AS, Lewy JE, et al: Bioassayable serum somatomedin activity (SMA) in chronic renal failure: Age dependence and role of dialysis and heparin. *Clin Res* 25:403A, 1977.

224. Wright AD, Lowy D, Fraser TR: Serum growth hormone and glucose intolerance in renal failure. *Lancet* 2:798, 1968.

225. Zumoff B, Walter L, Rosenfeld RS, et al: Subnormal plasma adrenal androgen levels in men with uremia. *J Clin Endocrinol Metab* 51:801, 1980.

Mark Benfield
Alfred F. Michael

35
Immunology of Uremia

Many lines of evidence have led physicians to believe that uremia has profound effects on the human immune system. Clinical studies during World War II and the Korean War stressed the association of renal failure and infection [120]. During that time, other studies demonstrated that renal and skin transplants survived longer in uremic patients and animals than in normal controls [41–43,45,75,108, 121,162,169,171]. Because of these early findings, many subsequent systematic studies have been carried out.

Infection

Early studies of infection in uremia revealed that up to 60% of patients had serious infections, and in 38% of these patients infection contributed to their death [120]. With the advent of modern antibiotic therapy, these percentages have improved, but infection continues to be a leading cause of death [86,132,164]. The infections seen are caused by bacterial, viral, and fungal agents. For example, the incidence of tuberculosis has been shown to be increased by 6-fold to 16-fold [16,24,152,155], and a much higher incidence of hepatitis B followed by chronic antigenemia has been demonstrated [8,104,147,160,177].

Although an increased incidence of infection in uremia is established, it has been difficult to support these observations experimentally. Animals made uremic by a five-sixths nephrectomy demonstrate little difference in their response to a variety of infections [39,114].

Malignancies

Evidence has also accumulated suggesting that malignancies are more common in the uremic patient. Various forms of cancer have developed in approximately 2% to 6% of these patients, representing a 7-fold to 10-fold increase in incidence over the general population [76,89,103, 108,112,131,176]. These findings have been supported by animal studies in which surgically induced uremia, followed by subcutaneous injections of malignant tumors, revealed a marked increase in local and metastatic tumor invasion, compared with sham-operated controls [170].

Granulocytes

Studies evaluating the number of granulocytes in uremia have been confusing, likely related to the way in which measurements are performed. These cells exist in several different "pools"—bone marrow, marginated, tissue, and circulating. Of these, the measured circulating pool is vastly smaller than the others and poorly reflects the total granulocyte count [66,171]. Nonetheless, existing data suggest that uremic patients have a normal to slightly elevated number of granulocytes [58,78,148,159,180]. The exchange of granulocytes between pools is difficult to study because determinants, which affect this movement, are altered in chronically ill patients. However, a slight decrease in the movement of cells from the marrow pool has been demonstrated, whereas demargination appears normal [28,139]. Functional assessment of uremic granulocytes has shown mild abnormalities, including decreased migration of cells into skin windows, and the demonstration of serum factors that block chemoxtaxis. Phagocytosis, however, has usually been shown to be normal [6,23,32,38,64,70,126–128,140,153,167].

Lymphocytes

A number of investigators have found differing degrees of lymphopenia in uremic patients, varying from patient to patient and with the duration of uremia (Table 35-1). In contrast, other studies demonstrated no changes in lymphocyte number [95,105]. Furthermore, little correlation has been shown between lymphocyte number and function. In one study [95], before transplantation patients had normal lymphocyte numbers with decreased response to mitogens, whereas after transplant they developed decreased numbers of lymphocytes and normal responses to mitogenic stimulation.

Table 35-1. *Studies of cellular immunity in patients with uremia*

Cell or function		Response	References
Lymphocyte	Total	Decreased	2,35,43,72,73,78,81,85, 95,105,142,143,148,149, 154,157,168,179,184
		No change	95,105
	T4	Decreased	2,96,106,143,181
	T8	Decreased	96
		No change	106
	T4:T8	Reversed	143,181
		No change	2,95,96
Natural killer cells		Decreased	20
		No change	102,143,166,181
T-cell function	E-rosette	Decreased	5,35,118,119
	Skin test	Decreased	31,33,35,43,56,57,67, 74,88,94,117,154,157, 158,179,185
		No change	181
	Mitogen response	Decreased	1,3,4,44,72,81,84,95,96, 99,100,102,109,123, 134,142,143,160
		No change	28,116,161,182,186
		Increased	33,85,158,179
	Alloantigen stimulation	Decreased	28,46,48,69,74,82,95,96, 143,179
		No change	161
	Soluble antigen stimulate	Decreased	10,110,123
		Present	16,30,44,48,51,59,60,71, 72,74,81,84,87,98,100, 129,142,159,161,165, 179
Inhibitory effect of serum		Absent	101
Monocyte/macrophage function	Suppressor cell activity	Increased	7,9,65,97,134,145,159 183
		Decreased	10,106,116

Evaluation of T-cell subsets has also given mixed results. Most studies demonstrate a decrease in both CD4$^+$ and CD8$^+$ T cells with normal ratios [96,105,106], whereas one study showed no change in the total number or ratio [106].

Humoral Immunity

Measurement of serum immunoglobins in uremic patients has revealed normal levels of IgG, IgA, and IgM [29,35,109]. Specific antibody levels to tenanus and diphtheria toxoids are normal [22,175]. The seroconversion rate after hepatitis B vaccination in high-risk populations has been shown to be approximately 95% [178], whereas in hemodialysis patients, this rate is variably reported to be 50% to 70% [26,31,93,172,173]. In one study, patients with renal failure, but not on dialysis, had a better response than those on dialysis [156]. Pneumovax immunization similarly has been shown to result in a decreased response in both the percentage of patients showing sero-

conversion and antibody titer [40,53,62]. Studies evaluating the response to influenza vaccine have been conflicting, with some showing no difference between uremic and normal patients, whereas others show a decrease in seroconversion and antibody titer [34,79,131,133,135,136].

Cellular Immunity

Measurements of T-cell function have been variable, although most show impaired function. Early studies demonstrated decreased E-rosette forming ability and delayed hypersensitivity to skin testing. (For specific references see Table 35-1). The majority of investigations have shown a significant decrease in T-cell proliferative response to mitogens, alloantigens, and soluble antigens. However, these findings are far from uniform. Closer inspection of this impaired response has suggested involvement of multiple aspects of cellular immunity.

For some time it was thought that renal failure might allow the accumulation of a toxin in the serum that inhib-

Table 35-2. *Studies of cellular immunity in experimental uremia*

Cell or function		Response	References
T-cell function	Proliferative response	Decreased	9,13,55,77,144
		No change	174
		Increased	54,55
Monocyte/macrophage function	Suppressor cell activity	Increased	10,13,14,111,144,146
Inhibitory effect of serum		Present	54,55,122,144,145,174
		Absent	175

ited the immune response. This was supported by findings that removal of uremic serum improves the proliferative response of uremic T cells, whereas addition of uremic serum to normal T cells inhibits it; in vitro dialysis only partially restores this response. In other studies, a "middle molecule" was isolated from the serum and dialysate of uremic patients and shown to have an inhibitory effect on the proliferative response of normal T cells [15,21,27,54, 59,68,113,125,130,146,150,174].

An increased suppressor cell activity and/or an intrinsic monocyte/macrophage dysfunction, has also been demonstrated in uremic patients. Assays for this activity involve purifying T cells by plastic adherence and passage over nylon wool. The response of these purified T cells is suppressed by the addition of autologous adherent cells (monocyte/macrophage). Several investigators have shown an increased suppression in uremic patients (see Table 35-1). Furthermore, isolated T cells from uremic patients combined with nonuremic adherent cells have normal proliferative responses to mitogenic stimulation, whereas uremic adherent cells inhibit the proliferative response to nonuremic T cells. Uremic serum has also been shown to induce "suppressor cell" activity in normal lymphocytes [182].

Others have shown evidence to suggest that abnormal production of interleukin-2 (IL-2) is involved in the impaired immune response seen in uremia. These studies demonstrated decreased IL-2 production and restoration of the proliferative response with the addition of IL-2 [96,99,110]. However, other studies on a variety of lymphokines have not supported this finding [186].

In a variety of systems of experimentally induced uremia, the proliferative response to mitogens, alloantigen, or soluble antigen is reduced; uremic serum inhibits the response of normal cells; and increased suppressor cell activity is demonstrated (Table 35-2). However, even under controlled circumstances, the results have been inconsistent. Some studies have shown no difference, whereas others have shown an increased response in uremia. In one study [77], thymocytes from uremic animals enhanced the response of both uremic and control lymph node cells. In a recent study [144], uremic rats were compared with sham-operated and control animals with respect to skin allograft survival, mixed lymphocyte response, suppressor cell activity, inhibitory effect of serum, resistance to tumor induction, and induction of cytolytic T cells. No differences

between study populations were observed initially, but after 20 to 22 weeks of uremia, each of these tests became significantly abnormal in the uremic group.

Finally, specimens from patients with renal failure were found to have marked thymic atrophy at autopsy, with decreased lymphoid elements, fatty infiltration, and absence of germinal centers [184]. Similar specimens from patients who died as a result of trauma were normal. This led many investigators to believe that the lack of thymic influence may play some role in the impaired cellular immunity seen in uremic patients. Subsequent studies demonstrated a thymic factor that could restore normal lymphocyte [2], sheep E-rosette formation [1,3–5], and proliferative response to mitogens [1,4,161] in uremic patients and T cells.

Associated Factors

It is well accepted that malnutrition and its associated vitamin and mineral deficits have profound effects on the immune system [47], and most uremic patients have at least some degree of malnutrition. Furthermore, several investigators have shown that replacement of these vitamin and minerals restores normal immune responses [17,18]. In addition, some patients with end-stage renal disease have been treated for prolonged periods with immunosuppressive drugs that are known to have effects on immunity.

The issue is further confused in view of the fact that hemodialysis has been demonstrated to affect the immune system, including lymphocyte number, suppressor cell activity, and complement levels [19,25,36,37,61,63, 83,138,163]. Further, blood transfusions, which frequently are given to uremic patients, are variables in the immunologic adaptation of these patients [49,50,52,80,90–92,124,141,151].

Summary

Although it has been demonstrated that uremic patients have an increased incidence of infections and malignancies and show poor responses to a variety of provocative tests of the immune system, it remains difficult to prove that these findings are solely a consequence of the uremic state. The pathogenetic mechanisms involved are likely multifactorial.

References

1. Abiko T, Sekino H: Synthesis of calf thymosin β-4 fragment 16-38 and its effect on the impaired blastogenic response of T-lymphocytes of a uremic patient with pneumonia. Chem Pharm Bull (Tokyo) 35:3757, 1987.

2. Abiko T, Sekino H: Synthesis of deacetyl-thymosin β10 and examination of its immunological effect on T-cell subpopulations of a uremic patient with tuberculosis. Chem Pharm Bull (Tokyo) 34:4708, 1986.

3. Abiko T, Sekino H: Synthesis of the nonatetracontapeptide corresponding to the entire amino acid sequence of thymopoietin I and its effect on the low E-rosette-forming cells of a uremic patient. Chem Pharm Bull (Tokyo) 33:1583, 1985.

4. Abiko T, Sekino H: Synthesis of the revised amino acid sequence of thymopoietin II and examination of its immunological effect on the impaired T-lymphocyte transformation of a uremic patient with pneumonia. Chem Pharm Bull (Tokyo) 35:2016, 1987.

5. Abiko T, Sekino H: The effect of ubiquitin hexadecapeptide fragment on E-rosette forming cells of a uremic patient. Chem Pharm Bull (Tokyo) 29:2949, 1981.

6. Abrutyn E, Solomons NW, St. Clair L, et al: Granulocyte function in patients with chronic renal failure: Surface adherence, phagocytosis and bactericidal activity in vitro. J Infect Dis 135:1, 1977.

7. Agostino GJ, Kahan BD, Kerman RH: Suppression of mixed leukocyte culture using leukocytes from normal individuals, uremic patients and allograft recipients. Transplantation 34:367, 1982.

8. Albert FW, Brisam A, Traut G, et al: Antigen in the serum of HB antigen-positive patients on maintenance dialysis and after transplantation. Proc Eur Dial Transplant Assoc 15:306, 1978.

9. Alevy Y, Slavin R: Immune response in experimentally induced uremia. II. Suppression of PHA response in uremia is mediated by an adherent Ia negative and indomethacin insensitive suppressor cell. J Immunol 126:2007, 1981.

10. Alevy YG, Mueller KR, Anderson JR, et al: The role of monocytes and responder cells in suppression of antigen-specific T cell proliferation in chronic renal failure. Int Arch Allergy Appl Immunol 73:97, 1984.

11. Alevy YG, Mueller KR, Slavin RG: Immune response in experimentally induced uremia. IV. Characterization of suppressor peritoneal macrophages in the uremic rat. J Lab Clin Med 100:735, 1982.

12. Alevy YG, Mueller KR, Slavin RG: Immune response in experimentally induced uremia. VI. Uremic macrophages are defective in their ability to present antigen to T cells. Clin Immunol Immunopathol 29:433, 1983.

13. Alevy YG, Slavin RG, Hutcheson P: Immune response in experimentally induced uremia. I. Suppression of mitogen responses by adherent cells in chronic uremia. Clin Immunol Immunopathol 19:8, 1981.

14. Alevy YG, Slavin RG: Immune response in experimentally induced uremia. III. Uremic adherent spleen cells are defective in their ability to act as stimulators in mixed-leukocyte culture. Clin Immunol Immunopathol 24:227, 1982.

15. Alomran A, Shenton BK, Donnelly PK, et al: A possible mechanism of immunoregulation produced by alpha 2-macroglobulin. Ann NY Acad Sci 421:394, 1983.

16. Andrew OT, Schoenfeld PY, Hopewell PC, et al: Tuberculosis in patients with end-stage renal disease. Am J Med 68:59, 1980.

17. Antoniou LD, Shalhoub RJ, Schechter GP: The effect of zinc on cellular immunity in chronic uremia. Am J Clin Nutr 34:1912, 1981.

18. Antoniou LD, Shalhoub RJ: Zinc-induced enhancement of lymphocyte function and viability in chronic uremia. Nephron 40:13, 1985.

19. Atkins RC, Holdsworth SR, Fitzgerald MG, et al: The effect of maintenance dialysis on lymphocyte function. II. Peritoneal dialysis. Clin Exp Immunol 33:102, 1978.

20. Badger AM, Bernard DB, Idelson BA, et al: Depressed spontaneous cellular cytotoxicity associated with normal or enhanced antibody-dependent cellular cytoxicity in patients on chronic haemodialysis. Clin Exp Immunol 45:568, 1981.

21. Baker RI, Marshall RD: A reinvestigation of methylguanidine concentrations in sera from normal and uremic subjects. Clin Sci 41:563, 1971.

22. Balch HH: The effect of severe battle injury and of posttraumatic renal failure on resistance to infection. Ann Surg 142:145, 1955.

23. Baum J, Cestero VM, Freeman RB: Chemotaxis of polymorphonuclear leukocyte and delayed hypersensivity in uremia. Kidney Int (suppl 2)7:147, 1975.

24. Belcon MC, Smith EKM, Kahana LM, et al: Tuberculosis in dialysis patients. Clin Nephrol 17:14, 1982.

25. Bender BS, Curtis JL, Nagel JE, et al: Analysis of immune status of hemodialyzed adults. Association with poor transfusions. Kidney Int 4:436, 1984.

26. Benhaumou E, Courouce A-M, Jungers P, et al: Hepatitis B vaccine: Randomized trial of immunogenicity in hemodialysis patients. Clin Nephrol 21:143, 1984.

27. Bergström J, Fürst P, Zimmerman L: Uremic middle molecules exist and are biologically active. Clin Nephrol 11:229, 1979.

28. Birkeland SA: Uremia as a state of immune deficiency. Scand Immunol 5:107, 1976.

29. Bishop CR, Athens JW, Boggs DR, et al: Leukokinetic studies. XIII. A non-steady state kinetic evaluation of the mechanism of cortisone-induced granulocytosis. J Clin Invest 47:249, 1968.

30. Boulton-Jones JM, Vick R, Cameron JS, et al: Immune response in uraemia. Clin Nephrol 1:351, 1973.

31. Bramwell SP, Briggs JD, Stewart J, et al: Dinitrochlorobenzene skin testing predicts response to hepatitis B vaccine in dialysis patients. Lancet 1:1412, 1985.

32. Buchanan WW, Klinenberg JR, Seegmiller JE: The inflammatory response to injected microcrystalline monosodium urate in normal, hyperuricemic, gouty and uremic subjects. Arthritis Rheum 8:361, 1965.

33. Byron PR, Mallick NP, Taylor G: Immune potential in human uraemia. 1. Relationship of glomerular filtration rate to depression of immune potential. J Clin Pathol 29:765, 1976.

34. Cappel R, Van Beers D, Liesnard C, et al: Impaired humoral and cell-mediated immune responses in dialyzed patients after influenza vaccination. Nephron 33:21, 1983.

35. Casciani CU, DeSimone C, Bonini S, et al: Immunological aspects of chronic uremia. Kidney Int (suppl 8)13:S49, 1978.

36. Chandy KG, Pahl M, Vaziri ND, et al: Acute effects of dialysis on T lymphocytes in patients with end-stage renal disease. J Clin Lab Immunol 17:119, 1985.

37. Charpentier B, Lang PH, Martin B, et al: Depressed polymorphonuclear leukocyte functions associated with normal cytotoxic functions of T and natural killer cells during chronic hemodialysis. Clin Nephrol 19:228, 1983.

38. Clark RA, Hamory BH, Ford GH, et al: Chemotaxis in acute renal failure. *J Infect Dis* 126:460, 1972.

39. Clarke IA, Ormrod DJ, Miller TE: Host immune status in uremia. V. Effect or uremia on resistance to bacterial infection. *Kidney Int* 24:66, 1983.

40. Cosio FG, Giebink GS, Le CT, et al: Pneumococcal vaccination in patients with chronic renal disease and renal allograft recipients. *Kidney Int* 20:254, 1981.

41. Couch NP, Murray JE, Dammin GJ, et al: The fate of the skin homograft in the chronically uremic patient. *Surg Forum* 7:626, 1957.

42. Dammin GJ, Couch NP, Murray JE: Prolonged survival of skin homografts in uremic patients. *Ann NY Acad Sci* 64:967, 1957.

43. Daniels JC, Sakai H, Remmers AR Jr, et al: In vitro reactivity of human lymphocytes in chronic uraemia: Analysis and interpretation. *Clin Exp Immunol* 8:213, 1971.

44. De Gast GC, Houwen B, van der Hem GK: T-lymphocyte number and function and the course of hepatitis B in hemodialysis patients. *Infection and Immunity* 14:1138, 1976.

45. Dobbelstein H: Immune system in uraemia. *Nephron* 17:409, 1976.

46. Dobbelstein H, Korner WF, Mempel W, et al: Vitamin B6 deficiency in uremia and its implication for the depression of immune responses. *Kidney Int* 5:233, 1974.

47. Dowd P, Keatley R: The influence of undernutrition on immunity. *Clin Sci* 66:241, 1984.

48. Elves MW, Israels MCG, Collinge M: An assessment of the mixed leucocyte reaction in renal failure. *Lancet* 1:682, 1966.

49. Fehrman I, Groth CG, Lundgren G, et al: Improved renal graft survival in transfused uremics. *Transplantation* 30:324, 1980.

50. Fehrman I, Ringden O: Reduced immunologic responsiveness in multitransfused anemic nonuremic patients. *Transplant Proc* 14:341, 1982.

51. Fehrman I, Ringden O, Bergstrom J: MLC-blocking factors in uremic serum. *Clin Nephrol* 14:183, 1980.

52. Fehrman I, Ringden O: Lymphocytes from multitransfused uremic patients have poor MLC reactivity. *Tissue Antigens* 17:386, 1981.

53. Friedman EA, Beyer MM, Hirsch SR, et al: Intact antibody response to pneumococcal capsular polysaccharides in uremia and diabetes. *JAMA* 244:2310, 1980.

54. Fromtling RA: Chemiluminescence and lymphocyte transformation of immune cells in experimental uremia. *Nephron* 43:78, 1986.

55. Fromtling RA, Fromtling AM, Staib F, et al: Effect of uremia on lymphocyte transformation and chemiluminescence by spleen cells of normal and cryptococcus neoformans-infected mice. *Infect Immunol* 32:1073, 1981.

56. Gagnon RF: Delayed-type hypersensitivity skin reaction in the chronically uremic mouse: Influence of severity and duration of uremia on the development of response. *Nephron* 43:16, 1986.

57. Gagnon RF, Gold J, Gerstein W: A mouse model for delayed-type hypersensitivity skin changes in chronic renal failure. *Uremia Invest* 8:121, 1985.

58. Gallen IR, Limarzi LR: Blood and bone marrow studies in renal disease. *Am J Clin Pathol* 20:3, 1950.

59. Giacchino F, Quarello F, Pellerey M, et al: Continuous ambulatory peritoneal dialysis improves immunodeficiency in uremic patients. *Nephron* 35:209, 1983.

60. Gibbs JH, Robertson AJ, Brown RA, et al: Mitogen-stimulated lymphocyte growth and chronic uraemia. *J Clin Lab Immunol* 9:19, 1982.

61. Goldblum SE, Reed WP: Host defenses and immunologic alterations associated with chronic hemodialysis. *Ann Intern Med* 93:597, 1980.

62. Goldblum SE, Reed WP: Host defenses and immunological alterations associated with chronic hemodialysis. *Ann Intern Med* 93:597, 1980.

63. Goldblum SE, Van Epps DE, Reed WP: Serum inhibitor of C5 fragment-mediated polymorphonuclear leukocyte chemotaxis associated with chronic hemodialysis. *J Clin Invest* 64:255, 1979.

64. Greene WH, Ray C, Mauer SM, et al: The effect of hemodialysis on neutrophil chemotactic responsiveness. *J Lab Clin Med* 88:971, 1976.

65. Guillou PJ, Woodhouse LF, Davison AM, et al: Suppressor cell activity of peripheral mononuclear cells from patients undergoing chronic haemodialysis. *Biomedicine* 32:11, 1980.

66. Hammerschmidt DE, Goldberg R, Raij L, et al: Leukocyte abnormalities in renal failure and hemodialysis. *Semin Nephrol* 5:91, 1985.

67. Hanicki Z, Cichocki T, Komorowska Z, et al: Some aspects of cellular immunity in untreated and maintenance hemodialysis patients. *Nephron* 23:273, 1979.

68. Hanicki Z, Cichocki T, Sarwecka-Keller M, et al: Influence of middle-sized molecule aggregates from dialysate of uremic patients on lymphocyte transformation in vitro. *Nephron* 17:73, 1976.

69. Harris JE, Page D, Posen G, et al: Suppression of in vitro lymphocyte function by uremic toxins. *J Urol* 108:312, 1972.

70. Hassner A, Kleter J, Peresecenschi G, et al: Phagocytosis and candidacidal activity of polymorphonuclear luekocytes in uremia. *Isr J Med Sci* 16:162, 1980.

71. Holdsworth SR, Fitzgerald MG, Hosking CS, et al: The effect of maintenance dialysis on lymphocyte function. I. Haemodialysis. *Clin Exp Immunol* 33:95, 1978.

72. Hosking CS, Atkins RC, Scott DF, et al: Immune and phagocytic functions in patients on maintenance dialysis and post-transplantation. *Clin Nephrol* 6:501, 1976.

73. Hoy WE, Cestero RVM, Freeman RB: Deficiency of T and B lymphocytes in uremic subjects and partial improvement with maintenance hemodialysis. *Nephron* 20:182, 1978.

74. Huber H, Pastner D, Dittrich P, et al: In vitro reactivity of human lymphocytes in uraemia—a comparison with the impairment of delayed hypersensitivity. *Clin Exp Immunol* 5:75, 1969.

75. Hume DM, Merrill JP, Miller BF, et al: Experiences with renal homotransplantation in humans: Report of nine cases. *J Clin Invest* 34:327, 1955.

76. Jacobs C, Reach I, Degoulet P: Cancer in patients on hemodialysis. *N Engl J Med* 300:1279, 1979.

77. Jatoi I, Slavin RG, Alevy YG: Immune response in experimentally induced uremia. VII. Uremic thymocytes amplify the response of control lymph node cells to alloantigens. *Clin Immunol Immunopathol* 30:80, 1984.

78. Jensson O: Observations on the leucocyte blood picture in acute uraemia. *Br J Haematol* 4:422, 1958.

79. Jordan MC, Rousseau WE, Tegtmeier GE, et al: Immunogenicity of inactivated influenza virus vaccine in chronic renal failure. *Ann Intern Med* 79:790, 1973.

80. Kahan BD: Effects of transfusion on recipient immune status: Relationship to transplantation. *Prog Clin Biol Res* 182:345, 1985.

81. Kamata K, Okubo M: Derangement of humoral immune system in nondialyzed uremic patients. *Jpn J Med* 23:9, 1984.

82. Kamata K, Okubo M, Sada M: Immunosuppressive factors

in uraemic sera are composed of both dialysable and non-dialysable components. *Clin Exp Immunol* 54:277, 1983.

83. Kaplow LS, Goffinet LA: Profound neutropenia during the early phase of hemodialysis. *JAMA* 203:1135, 1968.

84. Kasakura S, Lowenstein L: The effect of uremic blood on mixed leukocyte reactions and on cultures of leukocytes with phytohemagglutinin. *Transplantation* 5:283, 1967.

85. Kauffman CA, Manzler AD, Phair JP: Cell-mediated immunity in patients on long-term haemodialysis. *Clin Exp Immunol* 22:54, 1975.

86. Keane WF, Raij L: Host defenses and infectious complications in maintenance hemodialysis patients, in Drukker W, Parsons FN, Maher JF (eds): *Replacement of Renal Function by Dialysis*. Boston, Martinus Nijoff, 1983, p 646.

87. Kerman RH, Ing TS, Hano JE, et al: Prognostic significance of the active thymus-derived rosette-forming cells in renal allograft survival. *Surgery* 82:607, 1977.

88. Kirkpatrick CH, Wilson WEC, Talmage DW: Immunologic studies in human organ transplantation. I. Observation and characterization of suppressed cutaneous reactivity in uremia. *J Exp Med* 119:727, 1964.

89. Kjellstrand CM: Are malignancies increased in uremia? *Nephron* 23:159, 1979.

90. Klatzmann D, Bensussan A, Gluckman JC, et al: Blood transfusions suppress lymphocyte reactivity in uremic patients. II. Evidence for soluble suppressor factors. *Transplantation* 36:337, 1983.

91. Klatzmann D, Gluckman JC, Foucault C, et al: Suppression of lymphocyte reactivity by blood transfusions in uremic patients. I. Proliferative responses. *Transplantation* 35:332, 1983.

92. Klatzmann D, Gluckman JC, Foucault C, et al: Suppression of lymphocyte reactivity by blood transfusions in uremic patients. III. Regulation of cell-mediated lympholysis. *Transplantation* 38:222, 1984.

93. Kohler H, Arnold W, Renschin G, et al: Active hepatitis B vaccination of dialysis patients and medical staff. *Kidney Int* 25:124, 1984.

94. Kroe DJ, Vazquez JJ: Hypersensitivity reactions in experimental uremia. *Am J Pathol* 50:401, 1967.

95. Kunori T, Fehrman I, Ringden O, et al: In vitro characterization of immunological responsiveness of uremic patients. *Nephron* 26:234, 1980.

96. Kurz P, Kohler H, Meuer S, et al: Impaired cellular immune responses in chronic renal failure: Evidence for a T cell defect. *Kidney Int* 29:1209, 1986.

97. Lamperi S, Carozzi S: Suppressor resident peritoneal macrophages and peritonitis incidence in continuous ambulatory peritoneal dialysis. *Nephron* 44:219, 1986.

98. Lang I, Taraba I, Hering A, et al: Effect of haemodialysis on the antibody-dependent and spontaneous cell-mediated cytotoxicity of patients with chronic renal failure. *Immunology* 5:55, 1982.

99. Langhoff E, Hofmann B, Odum N, et al: Kinetic analysis of interleukin 2 (IL-2) production and expression of IL-2 receptors by uraemic and normal lymphocytes. *Scand J Immunol* 25:29, 1987.

100. Langhoff E, Ladefoged J: Cellular immunity in renal failure: Depression of lymphocyte transformation of uraemia and methylprednisolone. *Int Arch Allergy Appl Immunol* 74:241, 1984.

101. Langhoff E, Ladefoged J: In vitro natural killer and killer cell functions in uremia. *Int Arch Allergy Appl Immunol* 78:218, 1985.

102. Langhoff E, Ladefoged J, Odum N: Effect of interleukin-2

and methylprednisolone on in vitro transformation of uremic lymphocytes. *Int Arch Allergy Appl Immunol* 81:5, 1986.

103. Lindner A, Farewell VT, Sharrard DJ: High incidence of neoplasia in uremic patients receiving long-term dialysis. *Nephron* 27:292, 1981.

104. London WT, Drew JS, Lustbader ED, et al: Host responses in hepatitis B infection in patients in a chronic hemodialysis unit. *Kidney Int* 12:51, 1977.

105. Lopez C, Simmons RL, Touraine JL, et al: Discrepancy between PHA responsiveness and quantitative estimates of T-cell numbers in human peripheral blood during chronic renal failure and immunosuppression after transplantation. *Clin Immunol Immunopathol* 4:135, 1975.

106. Lortan JE, Kiepiela P, Coovadia HM, et al: Suppressor cells assayed by numerical and functional tests in chronic renal failure. *Kidney Int* 22:192, 1982.

107. Mannick JA, Powers JH, Mithoefer J, et al: Renal transplantation in azotemic dogs. *Surgery* 47:340, 1960.

108. Matas AJ, Simmons RL, Kjellstrand CM, et al: Incidence of malignancy during chronic renal failure. *Lancet* 2:883, 1975.

109. McIntosh J, Hansen P, Ziegler J, et al: Defective immune and phagocytic functions in uraemia and renal transplantation. *Int Arch Allergy Appl Immunol* 51:544, 1976.

110. Meuer SC, Hauer M, Kurz P, et al: Selective blockade of the antigen-receptor-mediated pathway of T cell activation in patients with impaired primary immune responses. *J Clin Invest* 80:743, 1987.

111. Mezzano S, Pesce A, Peters T Jr, et al: Antibody production and antigenic specific suppression to bovine serum albumin in uremic rats. *Clin Exp Immunol* 48:111, 1982.

112. Miach PJ, Dawborn JK, Xippel J: Neoplasia in patients with chronic renal failure on long-term dialysis. *Clin Nephrol* 5:101, 1976.

113. Migowe L, Dall'aglio P, Buzio C: Middle molecules in uremic serum, urine and dialysis fluid. *Clin Nephrol* 3:82, 1975.

114. Miller TE, Findon G: Host resistance to *Candida albicans* in uraemia. *J Med Microbiol* 17:181, 1984.

115. Miller TE, Stewart E: Host immune status in uraemia. I. Cell-mediated immune mechanisms. *Clin Exp Immunol* 41:115, 1980.

116. Mirapeix E, Montoliu J, Suarez C, et al: Defective radioresistant suppressor cell activity in hemodialysis patients. *Nephron* 41:184, 1985.

117. Modai D, Bar Sagi D, Maor J: Effect of levamisole on skin reactions to DNCB in chronically dialyzed patients. *Nephron* 25:280, 1979.

118. Modai D, Peller S, Weissgarten J, et al: Effect of uremic serum on E-rosette formation of normal lymphocytes modulated by levamisole. *Isr J Med Sci* 17:1115, 1981.

119. Modai D, Weissgarten J, Peller S, et al: The effect of levamisole on E-rosette formation in the uremic state. *Thymus* 4:309, 1982.

120. Montgomerie JZ, Kalmanson GM, Guze LB: Renal failure and infection. *Medicine* 47:1, 1968.

121. Morrison AB, Maness K, Tawes R: Skin homograft survival in chronic renal insufficiency. *Arch Pathol* 75:139, 1963.

122. Munster AM, Leary AG, Wilson RA, et al: Cell-mediated immunity in the uremic rat. *Int Arch Allergy Appl Immunol* 48:294, 1975.

123. Nakhla LS, Goggin MJ: Lymphocyte transformation in chronic renal failure. *Immunology* 24:229, 1973.

124. Nanishi F, Inenaga T, Onoyama K, et al: Immune alterations in hemodialyzed patients. I. Effect of blood transfusion

on T-lymphocyte subpopulations in hemodiayzed patients. *J Clin Lab Immunol* 19:167, 1986.

125. Navarro J, Grossetete MC, Defrasne A, et al: Isolation of an immunosuppressive fraction in ultrafiltrate from uremic sera. *Nephron* 40:396, 1985.

126. Nelson J, Ormrod DJ, Miller TE: Host immune status in uraemia. VI. Leucocytic response to bacterial infection in chronic renal failure. *Nephron* 39:21, 1985.

127. Nelson J, Ormrod DJ, Miller TE: Host immune system in uremia. IV. Phagocytosis and inflammatory response in vivo. *Kidney Int* 23:312, 1983.

128. Nelson J, Ormrod DJ, Wilson D, et al: Host immune status in uraemia. III. Humoral response to selected antigens in the rat. *Clin Exp Immunol* 42:234, 1980.

129. Newberry WM, Sanford JP: Defective cellular immunity in renal failure: Depression of reactivity of lymphocytes to phytohemagglutinin by renal failure serum. *J Clin Invest* 50:1262, 1971.

130. Niese D, Gilsdorf K, Hiester E, et al: Immunomodulating properties of the uremic pentapeptide H-Asp-Leu-Trp-Glu-Lys-OH in vitro. *Klin Wochenschr* 64:642, 1986.

131. Nikoskelainen J, Vaananen P, Forsstrom J, et al: Influenza vaccination in patients with chronic renal failure. *Scand J Infect Dis* 14:245, 1982.

132. Nsouli KA, Lazarus J, Schoenbaum SC, et al: Bacteremic infection in hemodialysis. *Arch Intern Med* 139:1255, 1979.

133. Ortbals DW, Marks ES, Liebhaber H: Influenza immunization in patients with chronic renal disease. *JAMA* 239:2562, 1978.

134. Osaki K, Otsuka H, Uomizu K, et al: Monocyte-mediated suppression of mitogen responses of lymphocytes in uremic patients. *Nephron* 34:87, 1983.

135. Osanloo EO, Berlin BS, Popli S, et al: Antibody responses to influenza vaccination in patients with chronic renal failure. *Kidney Int* 14:614, 1978.

136. Pabico RC, Douglas RG, Betts RF, et al: Influenza vaccination of patients with glomerular diseases. *Ann Intern Med* 81:171, 1974.

137. Penn I: Tumors arising in organ transplant recipients. *Adv Cancer Res* 28:31, 1978.

138. Peresecenschi G, Blum M, Aviram A, et al: Impaired neutrophil response to acute bacterial infection in dialyzed patients. *Arch Intern Med* 141:1301, 1981.

139. Peresecenschi G, Zakouth V, Spirer Z, et al: Leukocyte mobilization by epinephrine and hydrocortisone in patients with chronic renal failure. *Experientia* 33:1529, 1977.

140. Perillie PE, Nolan JP, Finch SC: Studies of the resistance to infection in diabetes mellitus: Local exudative cellular response. *J Lab Clin Med* 59:1008, 1962.

141. Pollak R, Blanchard JM, Lazda VA, et al: The influence of pretransplant blood transfusions and uremia on cardiac allograft survival in histoincompatible rats. *Transplantation* 43:445, 1987.

142. Quadracci LJ, Ringden O, Kryzmanski M: The effect of uraemia and transplantation on lymphocyte subpopulations. *Kidney Int* 10:179, 1976.

143. Raska K, Raskova J, Shea SM, et al: T cell subsets and cellular immunity in end-stage renal disease. *Am J Med* 75:734, 1983.

144. Raskova J, Czerwinski DK, Shea SM, et al: Cellular immunity and lymphocyte populations in developing uremia in the rat. *J Exp Pathol* 2:229, 1986.

145. Raskova J, Morrison AB: A decrease in cell-mediated immunity in uremia associated with an increase in activity of suppressor cells. *Am J Pathol* 84:1, 1976.

146. Raskova J, Raska K: Humoral inhibitors of the immune response in uremia. IV. Effects on serum and of isolated serum very low density lipoprotein from uremic rats on cellular immune reactions in vitro. *Lab Invest* 45:410, 1981.

147. Ribot S, Rothstein M, Goldblat M, et al: Duration of hepatitis B surface antigenemia (HBsAg) in hemodialysis patients. *Arch Intern Med* 139:178, 1979.

148. Riis P, Stougaard J: The peripheral blood leukocytes in acute uremia. *Dan Med Bull* 6:90, 1959.

149. Riis P, Stougaard J: The peripheral blood leukocytes in chronic renal insufficiency. *Dan Med Bull* 6:85, 1959.

150. Rola-Pleszczynski M, Bolduc D, Forand S, et al: Cellular immune function in uremia: Altered cytotoxic and suppressor cell responses to an immunomodulating heptapeptide. *Clin Immunol Immunopathol* 28:177, 1983.

151. Roy R, Beaudoin R, Roberge F, et al: Blood transfusion in renal dialysis patients. *Tissue Antigens* 23:203, 1984.

152. Rutsky EA, Rostand SG: Mycobacteriosis in patients with chronic renal failure. *Arch Intern Med* 140:57, 1980.

153. Salant D, Glover AM, Anderson R, et al: Depressed neutrophil chemotaxis in patients with chronic renal failure and after transplantation. *J Lab Clin Med* 88:536, 1976.

154. Samra SA, Mudawwar F, Shehadeh I, et al: Immunologic patterns in hemodialysis patients with and without HBV infection. *Nephron* 33:248, 1983.

155. Sasaki S, Akiba T, Suenaga M, et al: Ten years' survey of dialysis-associated tuberculosis. *Nephron* 24:141, 1979.

156. Seaworth B, Drucker J, Starling J, et al: Hepatitis B vaccines in patients with chronic renal failure before dialysis. *J Infect Dis* 157:332, 1988.

157. Selroos O, Pasternack A, Virolainen M: Skin test sensitivity and antigen-induced lymphocyte transformation in uraemia. *Clin Exp Immunol* 14:365, 1973.

158. Sengar DPS, Rashid A, Harris JE: In vitro cellular immunity and in vivo delayed hypersensitivity in uremic patients maintained on hemodialysis. *Int Arch Allergy* 47:829, 1974.

159. Sengar DPS, Rashid A, Perelmutter L, et al: Lymphocytotoxins and mixed leucocyte culture blocking factor activity in the plasma of uraemic patients undergoing haemodialysis. *Clin Exp Immunol* 20:249, 1975.

160. Sengar DPS, Rashid A, McLeish WA, et al: Hepatitis B surface antigen infection in a hemodialysis unit. II. Factors affecting host immune response to HBsAg. *CMA J* 113:945, 1975.

161. Sengar DPS, Rashid A, Harris JE: In vitro reactivity of lymphocytes obtained from uraemic patients maintained by haemodialysis. *Clin Exp Immunol* 21:298, 1975.

162. Shackmen R, Castro JE: Prelusive skin grafts in live-donor kidney transplantation. *Lancet* 2:521, 1975.

163. Shohat B, Boner G, Waller A, et al: Cell-mediated immunity in uremic patients prior to and after 6 months treatment with continuous ambulatory peritoneal dialysis. *Isr J Med Sci* 22:551, 1986.

164. Siddiqui JY, Fitz AE, Lawton RL, et al: Causes of death in patients receiving long-term hemodialysis. *JAMA* 212:1350, 1970.

165. Silk MR: The effect of uremic plasma on lymphocyte transformation. *Invest Urol* 5:195, 1967.

166. Silvennoinen-Kassinen S, Karttunen R, Tiilikainen A, et al: Isoprinosine enhances PHA responses and has potential effect on natural killer cell (NK) activity of uremic patients in vitro. *Nephron* 46:243, 1987.

167. Siriwatratananonta P, Sinsakul V, Stern K, et al: Defective chemotaxis in uremia. *J Lab Clin Med* 92:402, 1978.

168. Slavin RG, Kelly JF, Garrett JJ: Lymphocyte response in acute experimental renal failure. *J Immunol* 104:1424, 1970.

169. Smiddy FG, Burwell RG, Parsons FM: The effect of acute

uraemia upon the survival of skin homografts. *Br J Surg* 48:328, 1960.

170. Soubrane C, Jacobs C, Jacquellat C, et al: Influence of the uremic state on the development of malignancy. An experimental study in the rat. *Am J Nephrol* 6:363, 1986.

171. Souhami RL, Smith J, Bradfield JWB: The effect of uraemia on organ graft survival in the rat. *Br J Exp Pathol* 54:183, 1973.

172. Stevens CE: Hepatitis B vaccine in patients receiving hemodialysis. Immunogenicity and efficacy. *N Engl J Med* 311:496, 1984.

173. Stevens CE, Szmuness W, Goodman AI, et al: Hepatitis B vaccine: Immune responses in haemodialysis patients. *Lancet* 2:1211, 1980.

174. Stewart E, Miller TE: Host immune status in uraemia. II. Serum factors and lymphocyte transformation. *Clin Exp Immunol* 41:123, 1980.

175. Stoloff IL, Stout R, Myerson RM, et al: Production of antibody in patients with uremia. *N Engl J Med* 259:320, 1958.

176. Sutherland GA, Glass J, Gabriel R: Increased incidence of malignancy in chronic renal failure. *Nephron* 18:182, 1977.

177. Szmuness W, Prince AM, Grady GF, et al: Hepatitis B infection: A point-prevalence study in 15 U.S. hemodialysis centers. *JAMA* 227:901, 1974.

178. Szmuness W, Stevens CE, Harley EJ, et al: Hepatitis B vaccine. Demonstration of efficacy in a controlled clinical trial in a high risk population in the United States. *N Engl J Med* 303:833, 1980.

179. Touraine JL, Touraine F, Revillard JP, et al: T-lymphocytes and serum inhibitors of cell-mediated immunity in renal insufficiency. *Nephron* 14:195, 1975.

180. Vincent PC, Sutherland R, Morris TCM, et al: Inhibitor of in vitro granulopoiesis in plasma of patients with renal failure. *Lancet* 2:864, 1978.

181. Webel ML, Ritts RE, Briggs WA, et al: Lymphocyte blastogenesis in patients receiving hemodialysis. *Arch Intern Med* 136:682, 1976.

182. Weissgarten J, Modai D, Cohen N, et al: Induction of suppressor cells in normal lymphocytes by uremic serum. *Int Arch Allergy Appl Immunol* 81:180, 1986.

183. Wierusz-Wysocka B, Wysocki H, Michta G, et al: Phagocytosis and neutrophil bactericidal capacity in patients with uremia. *Folia Haematol (Leipz)* 111:589, 1984.

184. Wilson WEC, Kirkpatrick CH, Talmage DW: Suppression of immunologic responsiveness of uremia. *Ann Intern Med* 62:1, 1965.

185. Yousefi S, Vaziri ND, Carandang G, et al: Evaluation of the in vitro production of inteferon γ and other lymphokines in uremic patients (42464). *Proc Soc Exp Biol Med* 184:179, 1987.

Roberto A. Jodorkovsky
Robert A. Weiss
Esther H. Wender

36
Psychological Disturbances in Pediatric Patients with End-Stage Renal Disease

End-stage renal disease (ESRD) invariably has a stressful and often lifelong impact on children and their families. Frequently, renal replacement therapy, either dialysis or transplantation, is necessary to sustain life. Few other chronic illnesses of childhood are comparable in their dependence on medical technology. As in other chronic illnesses in childhood, the impact of ESRD varies with the age of the child, since each developmental period is associated with different psychological issues. Additional unique features of ESRD in childhood include the effect of uremia on the CNS and, therefore, on behavior and alterations in body image resulting from growth retardation, cushingoid features, external devices for collection of urine, and multiple surgical procedures.

The complexity of these biopsychosocial factors and their important contribution to the success or failure of overall treatment require the involvement of a coordinated health care team including several different disciplines. In addition to biomedical care, the pediatric ESRD team should anticipate, assess, and attempt to ameliorate the often devastating impact of ESRD on the psychological and emotional development of the patient and its effect on the family.

ESRD and Developmental Considerations

The psychological consequences that ESRD shares with other chronic illnesses is best understood within a developmental framework that considers the child's specific age-related developmental tasks. The goals of the pediatric ESRD team are to recognize the needs of children and families at different developmental stages and to counsel the child and family to minimize the impact of chronic illness and medical care on normal psychological maturation.

According to Erikson [20,21], *infants* face the task of achieving a basic sense of trust that depends on the availability and constancy of the nurturance given by parents or other primary caretakers. The development of a strong sense of trust serves as a lifelong basis for an adequate sense of self-esteem. Erikson asserts that in the next stage of psychosocial development, *toddlers* and young preschoolers achieve self-esteem through a mastery of locomotor activities, which allows them to start feeling control over the environment and their body. When these tasks are accomplished, the child achieves what Erikson has called "autonomy." Conversely, when these tasks are not accomplished, the child is left with a sense of shame and self-doubt that can impede the successful resolution of conflicts typical of this age.

Similar to other chronic illness, ESRD often results in a need for repeated hospitalizations and extensive, painful, and frightening diagnostic or therapeutic procedures. These are accompanied by some degree of separation and often immobilization and restraint. Therefore, these chronically ill infants and toddlers must deal with issues of separation and abandonment, often leading ultimately to mistrust and loss of autonomy and control. Common reactions of the child to these factors include sleeping and eating problems, anxiety, regressed behavior, and apathy or depression [8,12,30,37,46,49,50,60,61]. The disruptive effect of separation can be ameliorated by providing home-like environments in hospitals, arranging flexible visiting hours, and providing for rooming-in facilities for parents.

According to Erikson, *preschool children* face the conflict of initiative versus guilt [20,21]. By "initiative," Erikson means the normal eagerness and curiosity to learn experienced by the child in a world that he or she gradually understands. By "guilt," he means the reluctance and hesitation experienced by the child who is uncertain of his or her ability and range. Children of this age do not understand cause and effect and, therefore, misinterpret the reason for events [43,44]. They are easily threatened by procedures and by other aspects of the medical care atmosphere that seem strange and threatening [31]. They frequently respond with fears of mutilation and loss of control over body parts. Thus, it is common for preschoolers to misinterpret their illness as punishment brought about by parents or health professionals, in response to previous misdeeds, such as minor dietary transgressions or common misbehavior. Children who imagine such punishment may react with anger or submission, withdrawal, and depression. Moreover, preschoolers view parents and physicians as omnipotent beings. Therefore, they fantasize that such all-powerful people punish them by not wishing to cure their condition [25,41,42,56,58]. Health care providers who are aware of children's usual misinterpretations about disease and environment can help to reassure them about the nature of procedures, the reason for the illness, and the need for hospitalization and immobilization. Child-life specialists employing playroom facilities have the potential to foster the child's mastery of fears and anxiety that are related to hospitalization and frightening procedures.

In *school-aged* children, cognitive capacities change substantially. Children become less self-centered and begin using elementary logic that enables them to see order and relationships that follow rules and principles. The concept of time transcends the here and now. The child's interpretation of illness becomes more sophisticated. Therefore, different symptoms can be correlated with different organs, and illness causality becomes less magical and more realistic, albeit quite simple, concrete, and related to concepts with which the child has had some experience [9,43,44]. This age group faces that task of what Erikson calls "industry" [20,21]. Children of this age are largely involved in acquiring knowledge and skill. Because these tasks are accomplished in groups, self-comparison with peers is an important issue at this age. When the child feels that he or she has not accomplished these goals, inferiority and low self-esteem ensue. At this stage, peers, teachers and other adult leaders become crucial in determining how the child evaluates his or her own worth [21]. The school experience provides an important setting in which to develop social skills and incorporate peer values. It is also a place where role models are perceived and where the child begins to identify with adults who do not belong to the nuclear family, hence, laying ground for the child's eventual independence and separation from the family [67].

Like other chronic conditions, ESRD places the child at a great disadvantage to pursue these school-aged developmental tasks. School absenteeism is frequent because of illness, repeated hospitalizations, and regular in-center dialysis treatment. The child may become reluctant to attend school, stemming from the realization that he or she has moved outside of the mainstream of academic and social pursuits, which contributes to academic underachievement and alienation from the peer group. The child's sense of being "different" is at times exacerbated by the teacher's attitude toward the chronically ill child. There are some teachers who, because of their own anxiety, impose unnecessary, overprotective restrictions on the child and foster dependence. Attempts to conceal the child's disease create feelings of shame, guilt, vulnerability, and inadequacy [67].

Several of the emotional reactions described are clearly influenced by the attitudes of teachers and peers. However, the child's premorbid personality and the nature of the family interaction play a major role in determining the type of behavior and emotional response that will emerge. Patients whose premorbid personalities were characterized by independence and confidence and whose families,

teachers, and health care providers tend to foster realistically based feelings of independence and autonomy are likely to accept their differences, while at the same time retaining optimism about the opportunities available to them. These children tolerate their disease and disability by intellectualizing, by becoming interested in learning more about their disorder, and by pursuing special hobbies and skills in which they become competent and successful [25,56,58]. On the other hand, less confident children have more difficulty adjusting, especially when parents and teachers are critical and overly anxious. They may continue to show regressive and dependent behavior, often suffering from anxiety, loneliness, isolation, guilt, and depression. A knowledgeable health care practitioner could provide empathy and support, crucial factors that may also facilitate better adjustment. He or she should also educate teachers and parents to understand the factors that promote normal development, which, in turn, may help shift a pathologic child-family-school relationship into a healthier one.

The long-range task of *adolescence* is to develop a personal identity [21]. Success involves the gradual confrontation and resolution of several age-related tasks, summarized as follows [23]: establishing independence, becoming comfortable with bodily changes, building new and meaningful relationships, seeking social and economic stability, developing a workable value system, and verbalizing conceptually. The latter is related to the maturation of cognitive abilities. Even more than the school-aged child, adolescents need to feel that they belong to a peer group and that they conform to its norms and values. The group can help the individual adolescent through temporary stages of indecision and confusion, thus allowing time to search for ways to achieve a sense of self. When adolescents cling to each other within a clan, they feel freer to verbalize their feelings and concerns and to compare issues such as bodily changes, value systems, and idols [9,21,42,58].

The chronically ill adolescent is usually deprived of this crucial support system. He or she may feel different, alienated, and rejected by peers, which generally leads to withdrawal, depression, and poor development of meaningful social relationships. Adolescents with ESRD face special difficulty in establishing independence, due to the forced submission to and dependence on health professionals, medications, restrictive dietary regimens, and rigorous and time-consuming dialysis treatments. They realize, often subconsciously, that their dependence on treatment modalities and those that administer them is mandatory, thus leaving little room for personal control and autonomy over the disease and its management. Those patients who were able to meet earlier developmental tasks adaptively and whose families and medical staff supported and fostered their autonomy may eventually overcome the obstacles imposed by their condition and enter adulthood with realistic expectations, independence, and dignity. Unfortunately, however, it is common to observe patients who succumb to the stress produced by their illness and either regress toward dependence, or rebel against medical and social authorities. This rebelliousness is often expressed as medical noncompliance or acting-out behavior in the school, the hospital, the dialysis unit, or within the family. Another maladaptive response is to deny completely the existence of the disease, resulting in obvious self-destructive behavior such as noncompliance with diet, medications, or even dialysis treatment [56]. The adolescent's cognitive maturation allows him or her to have better insight into concepts of causality and prognosis. Because the long-term outcome of ESRD and the risk of complications are often unpredictable, adolescents may experience overwhelming anxiety and helplessness. Also, fears of death are common, since adolescents understand death as a real and irreversible event. The demise of a fellow ESRD patient often provokes such emotions. These feelings are devastating when teenagers sense that they might die before future wishes have been fulfilled [55].

Dealing with adolescents with ESRD can be frustrating and arduous. The health delivery team should help the adolescent and family identify the patient's sources of anxiety, helplessness, and maladaptive behavior. Concerted efforts should be made to provide warmth, emotional support, appropriate limit setting, and empathy toward the patient's concerns. Skill in providing support and remediation comes, in part, by acquiring an understanding of normal adolescent development and by channeling these preventive efforts through a multidisciplinary health team.

ESRD and the Family Environment

The pediatric patient with ESRD invariably has a significant impact on the family system and produces changes in the parent-child relationship that are important in determining the child's adjustment to illness. When confronted with a child affected by a serious medical condition, parents mourn the loss of the longed-for, idealized, and healthy child [48,57]. After the diagnosis is first made, there is usually a stage of denial. This stage may be brief or continue indefinitely. However, most parents are able to perform the initial chores imposed by the illness, such as arranging follow-up visits to the physician, complying with treatment, and restructuring daily activities at home. In situations in which the diagnosis of ESRD is made without forewarning, necessitating prompt and sometimes heroic treatment, the family may not be ready to make appropriate decisions at the pace that the medical circumstances demand. In other cases, the initial state of shock may be so devastating that families respond with a prolonged and profound sense of disbelief, leading to changes of physicians or hospitals and interfering with the implementation of adequate diagnostic and therapeutic strategies. Congenital disease almost invariably results in intense parental feelings of guilt and inadequacy. Denial is often followed by fear, guilt, and depression [57].

Some parents respond to these stresses by devoting themselves full-time to their child's care, sacrificing their marital lives, neglecting their other children, and giving up their own personal fulfillment as a way to "expiate for their sins." The affected child may then become overprotected and overindulged and hence deprived of the opportunity to cultivate and pursue his or her normal drive toward independence. Conversely, some parents respond to this guilt by mobilizing more adaptive coping mechanisms, for example, channeling their energies into lobbying for ESRD legislation, organizing fund-raising activities, or forming parent groups. The guilt is likely to be less overwhelming in acquired renal failure. However, the family may have a greater sense of loss because their experience with a child who previously was normal produces mourning for that child, and expectations for the future must be drastically altered. If these new expectations are compatible with the child's actual potential, a better chance for adaptive adjustment and appropriate development exists [58].

Parents of ESRD children often suffer from anger and frustration. A frequent consequence of these emotions is to blame the health care providers. Occasionally such feelings become generalized as chronic bitterness directed toward hospitals, other institutions, or society at large, which may result in social isolation. In some families, severe and prolonged parental depression may result, with marital discord and eventual separation or neglect of the healthy siblings. Rejection of the child with ESRD may ensue. This reaction should be suspected when there is inconsistent care, unnecessary demands for hospitalization, avoidance of child care responsibilities by one or both parents, or excessive and harsh punishment. When the medical staff is oblivious to such events and reacts with hostility and defensiveness in return, the potentially supportive relationship between health care providers and the family may be seriously impaired. The uncertain long-term prognosis and lack of specific, reliable, curative treatment place the family with an ESRD child at especially high risk for such complications. Family function in families that were disturbed prior to the advent of the disease is likely to worsen [22,36]. All of these possible patterns of family dysfunction are influenced by cultural factors [51,56], and the medical staff must be able to adjust their assessment and place their recommendations in an appropriate cultural context.

If the family is provided with compassionate support and empathy based on an understanding of these patterns of reaction to stress, "acceptance" of the disease can be reached. This stage is characterized by rational planning, intellectualization, and a realistic acceptance of the child's illness and its effect on the family. Adaptive acceptance is more likely to occur when the premorbid family structure is cohesive and stable and when there has been consistent support available from the health system and the social environment [22,51,56,58,63].

Siblings pose special problems. When the child with ESRD receives a large share of the parental attention and protection, siblings may be neglected. Their care may be left to the extended family or other providers, sometimes distorting and impairing the relationship with their parents. Siblings often feel envious of the excessive attention that the child with ESRD receives, giving rise to guilt. The latter is aggravated by the relief experienced at not having been stricken by the disease. In some families, the responsibility for the care of the ESRD child is given to older siblings. This creates anger and resentment and interferes with the older sibling's development of independence and the formation of an active social life with peers. These factors may explain the higher incidence of behavioral problems, school underachievement, and social problems reported in older siblings of chronically ill children

[13,51,63]. The health care provider should explore these issues to detect problems that may be relieved by anticipatory guidance and counseling. However, when such intervention fails or when the family problems are severe, referral for mental health services should be considered.

Specific Features of ESRD

Neuropsychologic Disturbances in the Uremic Syndrome

Symptoms such as apathy, irritability, somnolence, distractibility, restlessness, diminished attention span, impaired memory, and difficulties in visual-motor coordination and nonverbal abstraction have been described in advanced uremia (see chap. 30). Sensory disturbances may even reach the proportions of a psychotic syndrome. These physiologically based symptoms increase vulnerability to psychosocial maladjustment [29,45,54,59]. Studies based on EEG recordings have been used to assess the effect of uremia on neurologic function. The EEG abnormalities are directly proportional to the degree of renal failure, improve with dialysis, and resolve following successful transplantation [59].

Adult patients with chronic renal failure have been found to have low-performance IQ scores as well as defects in short-term visual and auditory memory, sustained and selective attention, and speed of decision making. These difficulties improve after the onset of dialysis treatment [39]. Studies of neuropsychological function in adolescents on long-term hemodialysis have revealed poor scores on memory tasks and arithmetic tests; IQ scores are significantly below the level of a matched control group of chronically ill, asthmatic children. Moreover, children in whom hemodialysis was initiated prior to 12 years of age score much lower on tests of intelligence, auditory and visual memory skills, and school achievement than their counterparts who began dialysis after age 12 and a comparison group of children with chronic asthma [62].

Research information on the effects of kidney transplantation on cognitive performance in younger patients is limited. Some data suggest that successful kidney transplantation improves cognitive functioning in children with ESRD [16,47]. However, it appears that the cognitive performance is not always completely rectified by successful transplantation, especially when the ESRD has begun at an early age or its duration has been prolonged [24]. One may speculate that there is an increased vulnerability of the developing nervous system to the effect of uremia in early childhood, which may result in irreversible cognitive deficits. These findings indicate the need for developing early intervention strategies aimed at preventing or ameliorating these cognitive impairments and their accompanying psychosocial disturbances.

Parents and teachers attempting to respond effectively to the child's behavior may fail to recognize the role of altered physiology on that behavior. The ESRD team should remain alert to the possibility that the reported behavioral problems are produced or exacerbated by uremia. Likewise, deterioration in school performance may be due largely, or in part, to these neuropsychological factors that may appear insidiously as children survive with ESRD over longer periods of time. Further research is needed to determine the specific changes and the degree of impairment that can be expected.

Body Image

Although negative changes in body image are seen in many chronic illnesses, their presence in patients with ESRD is almost universal. Children with chronic renal failure often suffer from growth retardation and bone deformities due to osteodystrophy. Stigmata of hemodialysis therapy include multiple scars, needle puncture marks, and disfiguring fistulas or arteriovenous shunts. The presence of peritoneal dialysis catheters, external urine collection devices (often accompanied by a characteristic odor), and believed or real genital abnormalities is particularly devastating. Even successful transplantation requires the price of cushingoid features. These bodily changes may exacerbate the child's feelings of being different and result in alienation from the peer group. They may also restrict the school-aged child from normal engagement in athletic activities, since events that require body exposure within the group, such as changing clothes at swimming pools and undressing for gymnasium showers, create anxiety and shame. Children whose condition affects the appearance of the genitalia are prone to have fantasies of loss of function of the organs involved, which may be accompanied by sadness and despair [25,41,55,56,63,67]. These physical changes are particularly stigmatizing in adolescents, who normally are preoccupied with their dramatic and rapidly occurring physical changes. These problems are often exacerbated by the delay in the emergence of secondary sexual characteristics that accompanies uremia. For these reasons, adolescents affected by ESRD feel unattractive and rejected and often experience anxiety, depression, and low self-esteem [39,41,42,45,55,58].

The effect of these bodily changes are among the most difficult psychological issues to ameliorate. Frequently the important adults in the child's environment dismiss the importance of these issues, thus inhibiting open communication by the child or adolescent. To the patient, such issues may seem more important than life and death. The patient with ESRD may be helped by the opportunity to ventilate his or her feelings and fears. Peer support groups attended by others of the same age with similar problems provide the best possibility for self-expression.

Dialysis

Dialysis makes possible the prolongation of life in the majority of ESRD patients. However, this technologically advanced treatment may have exceeded the capacity of individuals and society to adjust, as indicated by the many maladaptive patterns exhibited by dialysis patients [18,38].

More than a decade ago, many adult patients placed on dialysis were described during the early, post-treatment phase as manifesting a "Lazarus phenomenon," during which patients behaved as if they were "returning from the dead." It was not uncommon to observe psychotic symptoms, characterized by feelings of depersonalization accompanied by perceptual distortions of the dialysis machine, such as the latter being bestowed with human or animal properties [1,2,4]. These reactions were, in part, due to the imperfections of the early machines and to the prevailing practice of starting treatment under conditions of advanced uremia, in which patients were usually obtunded and often moribund. The advent of more efficient machines, beginning dialysis at an earlier stage of uremia, and a more psychologically sophisticated approach have made these earlier, dramatic observations less common.

Studies of preschool children on dialysis are few in number and lack detailed observations of behavioral or emotional response. Available information on school-aged children and adolescents [33,34,52] depicts two types of reactions to hemodialysis. Some children show initial withdrawal and depression, during which denial and regression are common. After a period of a few weeks or months, continued contact with the staff appears to facilitate a freer communication of feelings in these children. The feelings include fears produced by altered body image, pain, and dependency conflicts toward the machine and caretakers. In adolescents, the partial regression on dialysis [64], which is said to be a necessary prerequisite to achieving good adjustment to maintenance dialysis treatment, may seem intolerable because of the adolescent's struggle with dependence-independence. Some adolescent patients respond to this conflict by adopting a bravado attitude, fighting the staff, becoming noncompliant with dialysis treatments and dietary regimens, or sometimes even attempting suicide. Alternatively, some children tend to show an engaging behavior from the outset of treatment. These patients easily regress and become dependent on the staff, enjoying the increased attention. Both coping styles retard the completion and resolution of crucial developmental tasks. School and extracurricular activities may be drastically curtailed because of the time-consuming nature of dialysis procedures. These reactions increase school underachievement, social isolation, and alienation from peers.

Depression becomes a way of life for many patients. This response to long-term hemodialysis is what Abram [1] has called "the problem of living rather than dying." It reflects the response to persistent fears of death, which are poignantly heightened every time a machine-related technical problem or a medical complication arises. This is combined with the patient's painful realization of his or her total dependence on dialysis and its extensions, namely, the health professionals [4,7].

The psychodynamic mechanisms that characterize the child's adaptation to dialysis are difficult to assess because of the child's difficulty expressing his or her concern [19]. Sampson [53] has studied this issue by eliciting fantasy productions of children with ESRD. He found that the fantasy themes were constricted and consistent. Themes of aggression were frequently seen and were usually linked to the child's perception that the disease is a punishment for some act the child may have committed. Furthermore, these children's perceptions of the world were confusing,

hostile, threatening, and fearful. They viewed the environment with mistrust and suspicion. The second major fantasy was related to dependency conflicts. These fantasies were thought to have a problem-solving quality and were, therefore, likely to be in the service of adjustment. Additional studies of socially deprived children and adolescents on dialysis have used free drawings and storytelling techniques. It was found that most children experienced great depression and fears of suffering further losses in the form of bodily damage. Their fantasies were frequently persecutory in nature. Analysis of storytellings revealed the need for protection and closeness as well as submissiveness and fears of abandonment and death. Depression, sadness, and low self-esteem were common [11]. Long-term psychosocial observations are difficult to obtain because the current tendency in most pediatric dialysis units is to consider hemodialysis as a temporary stage, while arrangements for kidney transplantation are made in the hope that a functioning graft would permit a better quality of life.

The advent of continuous ambulatory peritoneal dialysis (CAPD) has created an attractice alternative to hospital-based dialysis. It has been hoped that issues of dependency on the machine and staff and school absenteeism would be minimized with this treatment modality. It has been suggested by some that many CAPD patients who have started this type of treatment with optimism gradually become disenchanted because of repeated episodes of peritonitis, catheter obstructions, and disturbances of body and sexual image caused by the presence of catheters and dialysate fluid in the abdomen. The psychological impact of this approach, however, requires further study.

REACTION OF DIALYSIS STAFF

Children and adolescents with ESRD spend a considerable part of their lives in hospital settings, and many of them become dependent on the dialysis machine and its operators. Children's developmental growth is strongly influenced by the adults in their world. Therefore, like family reactions, the reactions of the dialysis staff influence the patient's adjustment. The staff's ability to understand the psychological experience of patients and their families is crucial in determining their response. This ability, in turn, is affected by the stresses that patients, families, and the medical care system exert on the staff. ESRD is incurable, and the patient's quality of life is generally suboptimal.

Many staff physicians and nurses are unable to tolerate their limitations in providing effective treatment for patients with ESRD, leading to feelings of helplessness, hopelessness, and guilt. Research in adult dialysis units [10,17] has revealed the following common sources of stress: intra-team and team-patient tensions; patients' setbacks, such as acute deterioration or death; and doubts about the effectiveness of dialysis for improving the quality of life for patients. Furthermore, nearly 50% of the staff reported feeling greater stress on the dialysis unit than on other medical wards. In addition, the majority of the staff expressed the desire for more frequent discussion of patients' problems with team members. It is likely that in the pediatric setting these sources of stress are compounded by involvement with the children's parents with whom staff tend to identify [40].

Kaplan De Nour [32] has suggested that patients' maladaptive behavior and attitudes frustrate the high expectations of skilled and devoted dialysis staff, producing angry feelings. Because anger toward patients is unacceptable in our culture, defense mechanisms and coping styles are often employed by staff to deal with such hostility [3,32]. They may use denial to avoid the frustration of patients not living up to expected behavior. Obviously the exaggerated use of this mechanism may lead to the underdiagnosis of psychosocial disturbances, hence precluding early therapeutic interventions. Alternatively, they may develop excessive concern and overidentification with the patient's plight. This attitude, a common one in pediatric settings, seems to reflect arousal of the staff's own parental instinct and anxieties. This is usually accompanied by overprotectiveness and the fostering of dependency. In this age group, dependency wards off the threat of potential rebelliousness, thus maintaining the staff member's feelings of control. Finally, staff may become irritated with patients and resentful of their parents, especially when cooperation is poor.

For these reasons, the staffs of pediatric dialysis units are likely to function more effectively if given the opportunity to meet together as a team, with consultation from a mental health expert. Team discussions also serve the purpose of helping the staff to understand and to tolerate the behavior of particularly disturbed families and patients. If, instead, referrals are made to mental health services outside the renal unit, these consultants should periodically be invited to team meetings. The professional who facilitates team meetings should, preferably, not provide direct patient service as a member of that team.

Transplantation

The emotional responses to kidney transplantation may be described in three stages: (1) preoperative period, (2) early postoperative stage, and (3) late postoperative stage [26,34,52,68].

PREOPERATIVE PERIOD

If cognitive ability is sufficient, the anxious and depressed mood that characterizes many children on long-term dialysis turns into hope and confidence with the prospect of successful kidney transplantation. However, because most grafts derive from cadaveric donors, the waiting time can be quite prolonged, creating uncertainty, impatience, and anxiety in recipients and their families. Some patients respond by planning for the future. However, it has been observed that the dialysis patients awaiting a transplant often adapt better to treatment than those who have no hope of receiving a transplant. As time passes, anxiety reactions and ambivalence toward the procedure seem to increase. These feelings appear to be caused by the conflict created by fantasies of "becoming a new person" and having better health versus the progressive acknowledgment of realistic medical-surgical complications such as pain, prolonged hospitalization, possibility of rejection, and return to dialysis.

EARLY POSTOPERATIVE STAGE

As long as the allograft functions satisfactorily and there are no medical or surgical complications, patients are elated, appreciating the new freedom given by absence of dialysis. These feelings may suddenly reverse, should an episode of rejection occur, during which depression, emotional liability, and anxiety ensue. The rejection episode reinforces the potential for allograft loss. Anxiety and uncertainty are associated with thoughts of future rejection episodes. In the event that irreversible rejection or another surgical complication requires a transplant nephrectomy, severe depression may develop. It is important to emphasize that although the nephrectomy is reasonable and justifiable medically, from the patient's perspective it usually represents a major and permanent sense of loss; it invariably is accompanied by mourning and grief.

LATE POSTOPERATIVE STAGE

Approximately 3 to 4 weeks postsurgery and usually within the outpatient setting, children and adolescents may feel unhappy and mildly depressed, once they realize that the transplant did not transform them into a new person. Frequent hospital visits and rigorous medication and dietary regimens may contribute to this depression. Likewise, many patients respond with apprehension and anxiety to the side effects from steroids and other immunosuppressive agents. The return to school, usually feasible by 3 months after surgery, almost always proves to be quite difficult, as a result of the altered body image and feelings of inferiority. During this stage, preoccupations with the new kidney and possibility of rejection are ever present, leading to persistent feelings of vulnerability. These feelings are reinforced whenever medical complications actually occur.

Grushkin et al. [28] have reported that a significant number of transplanted adolescents have an excellent psychosocial recovery one year postsurgery, provided that the new graft is functioning well and that a comprehensive team approach is available. The same study showed that the most important predictors of maladjustment are the presence of severe personality disturbances prior to transplantation and lack of supportive figures within the family system.

The psychodynamic issues associated with organ transplantation have been studied extensively [5,6,14,15, 65,66]. The incorporation of a foreign organ into the patient's body schema may be associated with the illusion that life has been extended. This has been called the "rebirth phenomenon" and often produces elation. The new organ may be perceived as psychologically active because it comes from another human being. It is not uncommon to observe patients who identify themselves with the psychological and physical traits of the donor (if known), which they fantasize have been conferred by the transplanted organ. These traits are more or less acceptable to the recipient depending on how compatible they are with his or her own personality structure. For example, it has been shown that receiving an organ from a person of the opposite sex can be quite distressing if the recipient has unresolved conflicts surrounding sexual identity [65]. Some information suggests that the quality of the relationship of recipient to donor seems to influence the occurrence of rejection, hence affecting the outcome of the graft [6,14,65,66]. These psychodynamic considerations provide an explanation for some unusual observations in families of transplanted children in which one of its members has been the donor. Some families characteristically respond to the recipient child with an attitude of overprotection, fostering dependence and hypochrondriacal symptoms, which may disrupt the emotional lives of remaining family members [34,52,68]. Dependency conflicts, hostility, guilt, and fantasies of retaliation have been found to be experienced by some recipients toward their donors [15,19, 34,68].

Conclusions

The vicissitudes experienced by patients affected by ESRD and their families exert a formidable challenge on the professionals that participate in their health care. However, a multidisciplinary and comprehensive approach by a team consisting of nephrologists, nurses, social workers, dietitians, and a behavioral-oriented pediatrician or a child psychiatrist can provide a sound program, geared toward detecting and preventing emotional and social problems as well as providing or facilitating therapeutic interventions. Such teams can improve the patients' abilities to cope by applying their knowledge of age-appropriate developmental and cognitive issues and by providing empathy and support, especially during times of crisis [27,33,35]. In addition, regular team meetings, during which the patients' problems are discussed within a developmental framework, may help to clarify and improve some of the staff's reactions and attitudes, thus reducing patient-staff conflicts. The implementation of such a holistic program brings the promise of turning arduous and potentially frustrating work into a rewarding and fulfilling experience.

References

1. Abram HS: The psychiatrist, the treatment of chronic renal failure, and the prolongation of life, Part I. *Am J Psychiatry* 124:10, 1968.
2. Abram HS: Idem, Part II. *Am J Psychiatry* 126:2, 1969.
3. Abram HS: The psychology of chronic illness (editorial). *J Chronic Dis* 25:659, 1972.
4. Abram HS: Psychiatric reflections on adaptation to repetitive dialysis. *Kidney Int* 6:67, 1974.
5. Abram HS, Buchanan DC: The gift of life: A review of the psychological aspects of kidney transplantation. *Int J Psychiatry Med* 7:153, 1976–1977.
6. Bash SH: The intrapsychic integration of a new organ: A clinical study of kidney transplantation. *Psychoanal Q* 42:364, 1973.
7. Beard BH: Fear of death and fear of life: The dilemma in chronic renal failure, hemodialysis and kidney transplantation. *Arch Gen Psych* 21:373, 1969.
8. Bergmann T, Freud A: *Children in the Hospital.* New York, International Univ Press, 1965.
9. Bibace R, Walsh MD: Development of children's concept of illness. *Pediatrics* 66:912, 1980.
10. Black FB, Dvorak M, Speidel H, et al: Staff's problems and staff's affective reactions to dialysis patients' problems. *In* Levy NB (ed): *Psychonephrology*, 2nd ed. New York, Plenum Publishing, 1983, p 15.
11. Blum-Gordillo B, Gordillo-Paniagua G, Eustace R, et al: The psychological impact of uremia on social handicapped children. *In* Brodhel J, Ehrich JHH (eds): *Proceedings of the Sixth International Symposium of Pediatric Nephrology.* Springer-Verlag, 1984.
12. Bowlby J: Maternal care and maternal health. *In* Lehman PR (ed): 2nd ed. Geneva, Switzerland, World Health Organization, 1952, p 179.
13. Breslau N, Weitzman M, Messenger K: Psychological functioning of siblings of disabled children. *Pediatrics* 67:344, 1981.
14. Castelnuova-Tedesco P: Ego vicissitudes in response to replacement or loss of body parts: Certain analogies to events during psychoanalytic treatment. *Psychoanal Q* 47:381, 1978.
15. Castelnuovo-Tedesco P: Transplantation-psychological implications of changes in body image. *In* Levy NB (ed): *Psychonephrology*, 1st ed. New York, Plenum Publishing, 1981, p 219.
16. Critlendeen M, Holliday M, Potter D, et al: I.Q. in children with renal failure. *Pediatric Res* 14:617, 1980.
17. Czaczkes JW, Kaplan De Nour A: *Chronic Hemodialysis as a Way of Life.* New York, Brunner/Mazel, 1978.
18. Drees AD, Gallagher EB: Hemodialysis, rehabilitation and psychological support. *In* Levy NB (ed): *Psychonephrology*, 1st ed. New York, Plenum Publishing, 1981, p 133.
19. Epstein S: Toward a unified theory of anxiety. *In* Mahler BA (ed): *Progress in Experimental Personality Research.* Vol 4. New York, Academic, 1967.
20. Erikson, EH: *Adulthood.* New York, WW Norton, 1976.
21. Erikson EH: *Childhood and Society.* New York, WW Norton, 1963.
22. Gherin PJ (ed): *Family Therapy: Theory and Practice.* New York, Gardner Press, 1976.
23. Felice M, Friedman SB: The adolescent as a patient. *Journal of Continuing Education Pediatrics* 20:15, 1978.
24. Fenell RS III, Rasbury WC, Fennell EB, et al: Effects of kidney transplantation on cognitive performance in a pediatric population. *Pediatrics* 74:273, 1984.
25. Freud A: The role of bodily illness in the mental life of children. *Psychoanal Study Child* 7:42, 1952.
26. Freyberger H: The renal transplant patient: Three state model and psychiatric therapeutic strategies. *In* Levy NB (ed): *Psychonephrology*, 2nd ed. New York, Plenum Press, 1983, p 259.
27. Ganofsky MA, Drotar D: Growing up with renal failure: Problems and perspectives. *In* Levy NB (ed): *Psychonephrology*, 2nd ed. New York, Plenum Press, 1983, p 195.
28. Grushkin CM, Korsch BM, Fine RN: The outlook for adolescents with chronic renal failure. *Pediatr Clin North Am* 29(4):953, 1973.
29. Hagberg B: A prospective study of patients in chronic hemodialysis/III predictive value of intelligence, cognitive deficit and ego defense structures in rehabilitation. *J Psychosom Res* 18(3):151, 1974.
30. Jackson K, Winkley R, Faust OA, et al: Problems of emotional trauma in hospital treatment of children. *JAMA* 149:1536, 1952.
31. Jessner L, Blom GE, Waldfogel S: Emotional implications of tonsillectomy and adenoidectomy in children. *Psychoanal Study Child* 7:448, 1952.
32. Kaplan De Nour A: Staff-patient interaction. *In* Levy NB (ed): *Psychonephrology*, 2nd ed. New York, Plenum Publishing, 1983.

33. Kemph JP: End stage renal disease-dialysis. *Psychiatr Clin North Am* 5(3):407, 1982.
34. Korsch BM, Fine RN, Grushkin CM, et al: Experiences with children and their families during extended hemodialysis and kidney transplantation. *Pediatr Clin North Am* 18(2):625, 1971.
35. Korsch BM: Psychological complications of renal disease in childhood. *In* Edelman CM (ed): *Pediatric Kidney Disease.* Vol 1. Boston, Little Brown, 1978, p 342.
36. Liebman R, Minuchin S, Baker L: The use of structural family therapy in the treatment of asthma. *Am J Psychiatry* 131:535, 1974.
37. Mahler MS: On human symbiosis and the vicissitudes of individuation. *In* Aronson J (ed): *Infantile Psychosis.* Vol 1. *The Selected Papers of Margaret S. Mahler, MD.* Vol 2. New York, International Universities Press, 1979.
38. Ogburn WF: *Social Change.* New York, Viking Press, 1930.
39. Osberg JW, Meares GJ, McKee DC, et al: Intellectual functioning in renal failure and chronic dialysis. *J Chronic Dis* 35:445, 1982.
40. Pakes EH: Child psychiatry and pediatric practice: How disciplines work together. *Ontario Med Review* 41:69, 1974.
41. Perrin EC, Gerrity PS: There is a demon in your belly: Children's understanding of illness. *Pediatrics* 67:841, 1981.
42. Perrin EC, Gerrity PS: Development of children with a chronic illness. *Pediatr Clin North Am* 31(1):19, 1984.
43. Piaget J: *The Child's Conception of the World.* New York, Harcourt Brace, 1920.
44. Piaget, J: *The Child's Conception of Physical Causality.* New York, Littlefield, Adams, 1960.
45. Pless IB: Clinical assessment: Physical and psychological functioning. *Pediatr Clin North Am* 31:33, 1984.
46. Prugh DG, Staub EM, Sands HH, et al: A study of emotional reactions of children and families to hospitalization and illness. *Am J Orthopsychiatry* 23:70, 1953.
47. Rasbury W, Fennell RS III, Morris MK: Cognitive functioning of children with end stage renal disease pre- and post-successful transplantation. *J Pediatr* 102:589, 1984.
48. Richmond JB: The pediatric patient in illness. *In* Hollander MH (ed): *The Psychology of Medical Practice.* Philadelphia, WB Saunders, 1958, p 195.
49. Robertson J: *Two Year Old Goes to the Hospital.* New York, Library Film Library, 1953.
50. Robertson J: *Young Children in Hospitals.* New York, Basic Books, 1958.
51. Sabbeth B: Understanding the impact of chronic childhood illness on families. *Pediatr Clin North Am* 31(1):47, 1984.
52. Sampson TF: The child in renal failure: Emotional impact of treatment on the child and his family. *J Am Acad Child Psychoanal* 14(3):462, 1975.
53. Sampson TF: Use of fantasy for conflict resolution in the pediatric hemodialysis patient. *In* Levy NB (ed): *Psychonephrology,* 1st ed. New York, Plenum Publishing, 1981, p 177.
54. Schneire GE: Mental and personality changes in the uremic syndrome. *Med Ann of the District of Columbia* 28:316, 1959.
55. Schowalter JE: Psychological reactions to physical illness and hospitalization in adolescence. *J Am Acad Child Adolesc Psychiatry* 16:500, 1977.
56. Schowalter JE: The chronically ill child. *In* Noshpitz JN (ed): *Basic Handbook of Child Psychiatry.* Vol 1. Basic Books, 1979, p 432.
57. Solnit AJ, Stark MM: Mourning and the birth of defective child. *Psychoanal Study Child* 16:523, 1961.
58. Steinhaurer PD, Mushin DN, Grant QR: Psychological aspects of chronic illness. *Pediatr Clin North Am* 11:825, 1974.
59. Teschan PE: Measurements of neurobehavioral responses to renal failure, dialysis, and transplantation. *In* Levy NB (ed): *Psychonephrology.* Plenum Press, 1981, p 13.
60. Thomas A, Chess S: *The Dynamics of Psychological Development.* New York, Brunner Mazel Publications, 1980.
61. Through the looking glass: Nursery school pupils preview hospital routines. *Hospitals* 34:47, 1960.
62. Trachtman H, Braden K, Scerra C, et al: Neuropsychological functioning in adolescents on chronic hemodialysis. *In* Brodhel J, Ehrich JHH (eds): *Proceedings of the Sixth International Symposium of Pediatric Nephrology.* Hannover, Federal Republic of Germany, August 29-September 2, 1983. Springer-Verlag, 1984.
63. Vance J, Frazan L, Satterwhite B, et al: Effects of nephrotic syndrome on the family: A controlled study. *Pediatrics* 65:948, 1980.
64. Viederman M: Adaptive and maladaptive regression in hemodialysis. *Psychiatry* 37:283, 1974.
65. Viederman M: The search for meaning in renal transplantation. *Psychiatry* 37:283, 1974.
66. Viederman M: Psychogenic factors in kidney transplant rejection: A case study. *Am J Psychiatry* 132:967, 1975.
67. Weitzman M: School and peers relations. *Pediatr Clin North Am* 31(1):59, 1984.
68. Zarinsky I: Psychological problems of kidney transplanted adolescents. *Adolescence* 10(37):101, 1975.

V
Treatment of
Renal Insufficiency

SCOTT LONG
KAREN M. GAUDIO
NORMAN J. SIEGEL

37
Nondialytic Treatment of Acute Renal Failure

In this chapter we describe therapies, both established and experimental, of acute renal failure in infants and children. Incidence and etiologies of acute renal failure (ARF) in pediatric populations vary. For example, ARF in developing countries is associated more frequently with gastroenteritis than in Western Europe and North America [21,56], and both the incidence and mortality are higher in the Third World. Since this discussion is restricted to data from economically advantaged countries, we refer the reader to Cameron's excellent and provocative review for consideration of renal disease in other parts of the world [21]. We begin with a presentation of standard supportive treatment for patients with ARF, followed by a discussion of therapy specific to particular underlying causes of ARF. The final section deals with experimental approaches to therapy for ARF, in most cases developed from the perspective of active intervention.

Supportive Therapy in Acute Renal Failure

The most common generic problems encountered in patients with ARF and their treatments are discussed here. Following the example of Arbus and Farine [5], each problem is divided into an emergent and a nonacute category.

Water Balance

EMERGENT CARE

The child with fluid depletion, regardless of an oliguric or anuric state, needs replacement with isotonic fluids such as saline or lactated Ringer's, to be infused at rates of 20 ml/kg body wt over 30 to 60 minutes. If blood loss accounts for circulatory insufficiency, blood should be used. For children with fluid depletion and edema, one may need to infuse albumin; this will rarely be emergent and needs a careful diagnostic evaluation. In the child whose only cause of anuria or oliguria is fluid depletion, resuscitation with fluid or blood or both should restore urine flow in a few

hours, generally less than six. If resuscitation has not occurred by that time, the patient may require central venous monitoring to assess volume status.

Patients with fluid overload, on the other hand, especially those with pulmonary edema, require diuresis or, failing that, dialysis. A loop diuretic given intravenously, e.g., furosemide or ethacrynic acid, may be used in escalating doses up to a maximum of 10 mg/kg before considering dialysis. It is wise to limit the rate of infusion of furosemide to 10–15 mg/min to avoid ototoxicity [49,80].

Although not truly emergent, the question of converting oliguric to nonoliguric ARF arises early in the care of the patient. The efficacy of this conversion using mannitol and diuretics has been investigated primarily in adult patients. Many nephrologists agree that prophylactic use of mannitol and diuretics (as well as fluid challenges and in some cases calcium channel blockers) is probably helpful in avoiding acute renal shut-down in potentially nephrotoxic situations [11,26,95]. The literature is not encouraging with regard to their use after ARF is established [34]. Twenty percent mannitol given soon after the renal insult is associated in some, but not all, patients with abbreviation of the period of oliguria and improved tubular function. In these studies, however, the responding patients appear to have had less serious renal compromise prior to therapy relative to nonresponders [74]. Mannitol given at the time of cardiovascular surgery improves urine flow postoperatively [26, 65,91]. Animal studies show that renal blood flow and glomerular filtration rate also appear to be protected with mannitol infusion [19]. Intravenous furosemide has been shown to promote blood flow to the renal cortex during bypass surgery [70].

Even when successful conversion of oliguric ARF to nonoliguric ARF occurs, there may be no demonstrable benefit in terms of survival or need for dialysis. In a prospective study, Brown and colleagues demonstrated abbreviation of oliguria in patients with postsurgical or post-traumatic ARF; however, they did not show significant differences in time for return of creatinine toward baseline, days of dialysis, or mortality [16]. Similar results had been obtained in a controlled study by Kleinknecht and colleagues using ethacrynic acid, although that study showed that patients who had converted to nonoliguric ARF had less need for dialysis [67].

It has been reported that furosemide combined with dopamine promoted urine flow in oliguric ARF [72]; however, no controlled studies have appeared. Interestingly, newborns receiving indomethacin to promote closure of a patent ductus arteriosus showed fewer renal side-effects if given furosemide shortly after indomethacin administration than those treated without furosemide [116].

In a recent review of the use of drugs in managing ARF, Cronin concludes that in such patients routine use of mannitol, diuretics, and dopamine is "without scientific support of efficacy" and "increases the complexity and cost of care with little tangible evidence of benefit to the patient or the physician" [34]. The greater facility of volume control and of providing nutrition in nonoliguric renal failure does not appear to change the course of patients.

NONEMERGENT CARE

Fluid management in anuric or oliguric children requires careful monitoring of blood pressure, weight, and fluid intake and output (two or three times daily) as well as serum chemistries. Input must be limited to insensible pulmonary and cutaneous losses, estimated at one-third of daily maintenance fluid requirements in afebrile children, and increasing by approximately 12% per degree centigrade elevation in body temperature. Neonates, especially those who are preterm, have increased insensible losses due to greater surface/volume ratios and less keratinization of skin. Great care is necessary to achieve adequate fluid and salt balance in these patients since the glomerular filtration rate in preterm infants is low. The renal tubules are immature and unprepared to handle either salt deprivation or excesses, in part due to immaturity in both the renin-angiotensin-aldosterone system and distal tubular response to aldosterone [32]. The use of phototherapy, warming lights, and humidified oxygen affects losses in premature infants. These factors must be included in approximating daily fluid balance and consequent replacement.

Overall estimation of fluid status depends, to a large extent, on physical examination in addition to quantifying input and output and evaluation of laboratory data. Synthesis of all this information allows the physician to choose the appropriate composition and amount of replacement fluid, including possible use of parenteral nutrition. If an appropriate volume of fluids is being given, the patient's serum sodium stabilizes and body weight decreases 0.5% to 1.0% per day. If serum sodium falls and body weight increases, excess fluids are being given; if serum sodium rises and weight falls, insufficient fluids have been administered.

Children in the diuretic phase of recovery from ARF or postobstructive diuresis need special attention to volume and electrolyte losses, which may be considerable. Our preference, especially in younger children, is quantitative replacement (i.e., fluid given for each milliliter excreted) in patients not previously fluid overloaded. Replacement fluids can be progressively decreased as renal function returns to normal.

Hyperkalemia

The physician must be particularly alert to causes of ARF associated with ongoing release of potassium from intracellular stores, such as rhabdomyolysis, sepsis, postoperative states, trauma, and tumor-lysis syndrome.

EMERGENT CARE

Immediate therapy for verified hyperkalemia simply shifts potassium from extracellular to intracellular spaces and usually precedes definitive correction of potassium overload, which can be accomplished with ion exchange resins or dialysis. The electrocardiogram (ECG) may be particularly helpful in assessing the pathophysiologic impact of an elevated serum potassium ([K]).

Figure 37-1 shows changes in ECG tracings associated with various degrees of hyperkalemia: (a) widening of the QRS complex, (b) ST wave depression, and (c) peaked T waves. These findings are not found in every patient with hyperkalemia, and the [K] at which they occur may also vary.

Immediate therapy for hyperkalemia, which is usually initiated when either [K] exceeds 6 mEq/L or ECG changes are noted, involves intravenous infusion of calcium gluconate, sodium bicarbonate ($NaHCO_3$), or glucose and insulin. Table 37-1 lists the dosages, with onset, duration, and mechanisms of action. Intravenous calcium is reserved primarily for patients with ECG changes and acts more quickly than the other therapies. Because of its action on the myocardium, ECG monitoring should be used when calcium is infused. Despite its brief duration, $NaHCO_3$ is an appropriate agent in patients whose ARF is complicated by acidosis that may exaggerate the hyperkalemia. However, $NaHCO_3$ must be given with caution because it contributes to volume overload and hypertension and it also favors a decrease in free calcium concentration through the effect of pH on protein charge and increased calcium binding.

In some patients, the use of an ion exchange resin suffices to remove excess potassium from the body. Kayexelate (sodium polystyrene sulfonate) is given in a dose of 1 gm/kg body wt, suspended in sorbitol and 5% dextrose, administered orally or rectally. This is appropriate treatment for [K] greater than 6 mEq/L without concomitant ECG changes. Dosing schedules depend on the individual case, but generally, the exchange resin must be given every 4 to 6 hours. It should be noted that children are even less successful than adults at retaining the resin rectally. Sometimes inflating the balloon on a urinary catheter inserted into the rectum aids in retention. In all cases, the resin contributes to volume load since it exchanges 2 to 3 milliequivalents of sodium for each milliequivalent of potassium.

NONEMERGENT CARE

Hyperkalemia of less striking proportions can often be treated with dietary restrictions or even daily use of an oral ion exchange resin. In the severely hyperglycemic diabetic

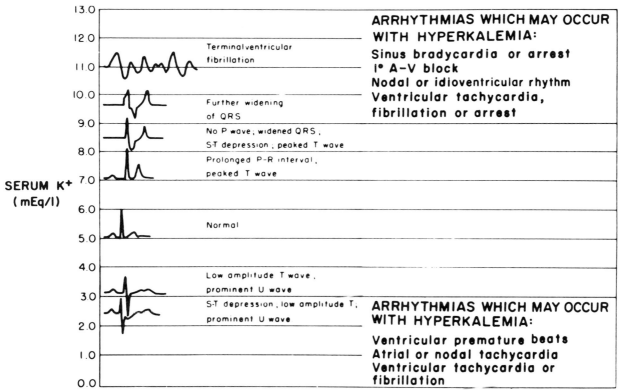

FIG. 37-1. *Approximate relationship between plasma potassium concentration and electrocardiographic abnormalities. Adapted from Williams GS, et al: Acute renal failure in pediatrics. In Winters RW (ed): The Body Fluids in Pediatrics, Boston, Little, Brown & Co., 1973.*

TABLE 37-1. *Treatment of hyperkalemia*

Drug	Action	Dose	Complications
Calcium	Stabilizes plasma membrane	Calcium gluconate 10%, 0.5 ml/kg IV over 2–4 min	Bradycardia; hypercalcemia
Bicarbonate	Intracellular shift of K^+	2–3 mEq/kg over 30–60 min	Hypernatremia; fluid overload with HTN; alkalosis
Glucose and insulin	Increased active uptake of K^+	Glucose 0.5 g/kg with insulin 0.1 U/kg over 30 min	Hyper- or hypoglycemia
Sodium polystyrene sulfonate		1 g/kg PO or rectally with 1–2 ml/kg 70% sorbitol or 5% dextose	Constipation; risk of hypernatremia and fluid overload with hypertension

HTN = Hypertension.
Modified from Gauthier B, Edelmann CM: *Nephrology and Urology for the Pediatrician.* Boston, Little, Brown, 1982.

patient, correction of the blood sugar may also correct the hyperkalemia.

Hyponatremia

EMERGENT CARE

Manifestations of hyponatremia are related to the central nervous system, including change of mental status, loss of consciousness, and seizures. These symptoms occur when the serum sodium concentration ([Na]) falls precipitously and are usually not found unless the serum sodium is below 120 mEq/L. In such cases hypertonic saline (3% NaCl), which is approximately 0.5 mEq/ml, can be given cautiously to increase the [Na] by approximately 10 mEq/L.

Patients with adequate urine output can be treated with isotonic saline supplemented by a diuretic. This diminishes the threat of volume overload while helping to restore the [Na] to normal levels. The speed at which sodium concentrations may safely be corrected is controversial. Those favoring a slower rate do so to avoid the danger of central pontine myelinosis and the risk of permanent CNS damage, while others maintain that correction of symptomatic hyponatremia outweighs the risk of this rare disorder [7].

NONEMERGENT CARE

Usually hyponatremia is mild and results from continued intake of dilute fluid without adequate amounts of sodium. It can often be treated successfully with fluid restriction.

In some cases of nonoliguric renal failure, as well as in the diuretic phase during recovery from ARF, sodium wasting may occur. In all cases, one must follow serum electrolytes carefully. The measurement of urinary sodium concentrations and the fractional excretion of sodium may be particularly misleading in neonates and preterm infants in whom tubular immaturity may result in higher values than those expected in older children.

Hypocalcemia and Hyperphosphatemia

EMERGENT CARE

In ARF, hypocalcemia is usually the result of hyperphosphatemia and does not produce symptoms, although it can be associated with convulsions, tetany, and cardiac arrhythmias. When patients are symptomatic and hypocalcemia is a significant part of the differential diagnosis, calcium can be administered as a constant intravenous infusion. In children, 10% calcium gluconate solutions are diluted to 2% for better control of the rate and the amount infused. Values of ionized calcium should be monitored every 4 to 6 hours.

When acidosis is being corrected concomitantly, hypocalcemia may correct more slowly or actually worsen, since alkalinization of blood pH promotes binding of calcium to proteins. Tapering of the infusion rate as normocalcemia is approached allows better control of the patient's levels and symptoms, especially when acidosis is also being corrected.

NONEMERGENT CARE

Oral phosphate binders with or without oral calcium supplements, as well as control of acid-base balance, may be sufficient to achieve normocalcemia. The oral dose of calcium is 50 mg/kg body wt/day. The risk of metastatic calcification with phosphate salts is reduced when oral rather than intravenous calcium is given to hyperphosphatemic, hypocalcemic patients and explains why control of serum phosphate without oral calcium supplementation is preferable. In some cases, one may later need vitamin D supplements to promote calcium absorption from the gut and mobilization from bone. In patients with residual renal function, vitamin D promotes phosphate excretion. In the majority of children with short-term ARF, vitamin D supplementation is not required.

Metabolic Acidosis

EMERGENT CARE

Arterial blood gases should be obtained in all patients presenting with ARF; those with blood pH less than 7.25 and bicarbonate concentration less than 12 mEq/L should receive bicarbonate therapy. Administration of NaHCO$_3$ should be done *only* in situations in which (a) there is maximal respiratory compensation, i.e., carbon dioxide tension (PCO$_2$) less than 25 torr and (b) the acidosis is contributing to other abnormalities, e.g., hyperkalemia. The bicarbonate deficit can be calculated in milliequivalents as (24 − observed [HCO$_3$]) × 0.5 body wt in kg). Half of this amount is given intravenously over 2 to 4 hours, followed by a reevaluation of acid-base status. The infusion is continued at the same rate until pH is greater than 7.25 and bicarbonate is greater than 12 to 13 mEq/L.

NONEMERGENT CARE

Patients receiving food (see below) have ongoing endogenous production of acid, which may be limited by use of a low protein diet. The physician should be alert to those conditions in which acid production may require continued intravenous therapy, in particular hypercatabolic states such as sepsis, postsurgery, and trauma. Provision of nutrition may help to limit acid production (as does treatment of underlying complications, such as the use of antibiotics) but may accelerate the need for dialysis.

Hypertension

EMERGENT CARE

Hypertension in patients with ARF is frequently due to volume overload. In symptomatic patients or patients with persistently elevated diastolic pressures (> 95th percentile for age), antihypertensive agents are necessary. Hydralazine is often used in doses of 0.2–0.5 mg/kg/dose (not more than 15 mg) IV or IM every 4 to 8 hours. For extreme cases, one can use intravenous nitroprusside at 0.5 μg/kg/min or diazoxide at 2–3 mg/kg. In some patients sublingual nifedipine (0.3 mg/kg/dose) may be helpful. For patients with residual renal function, diuresis can be attempted.

NONEMERGENT CARE

In most instances, control of blood pressure is directly linked to volume status and salt intake. If hypertension persists, despite these measures, dialysis may be required for fluid removal.

Convulsions

Many of the underlying imbalances in patients with ARF may produce seizures, including hyponatremia, hypocalcemia, and hypertension. Correction of these potential causes is important in prevention of seizures.

Intravenous diazepam is used for seizures at a dose of 0.2 mg/kg body wt, given slowly; it can be repeated at 15 minute intervals. Phenytoin and phenobarbital are alternative agents. Because protein binding of these agents, especially phenytoin and phenobarbital, is often diminished in uremia, patients may suffer adverse side effects at lower doses than expected unless drug levels, including free concentrations of the agents, are monitored. In many cases, seizures associated with a metabolic disturbance do not remit until the underlying abnormality is corrected.

Medications

In patients with ARF, one must avoid medications that may increase renal damage. In the pediatric population, these include aminoglycosides, non-steroidal anti-inflammatory agents, and radiocontrast media.

Many medications may need adjustment of either dose or dosing intervals. Recently, Trompeter has provided a comprehensive review of drug prescribing in children with renal insufficiency [110]. In using the tables included in this review, it must be remembered that pediatric patients with ARF have a glomerular filtration rate less than 10 ml/min. The serum creatinine in patients with ARF increases by 0.5–1.5 mg/dl/day. Therefore, with the onset of an acute renal insult, the serum creatinine does not rise abruptly from normal values to renal failure levels (> 6 mg/dl). Consequently, during the first few days after the onset of ARF the serum creatinine may be minimally elevated (2–3 mg/dl) despite a filtration rate that is very low.

Nutrition

It must be recognized that much of the critical work on nutrition in ARF has been carried out in adult patients. Infants and children with serious illnesses, including ARF, are at even greater risk of malnutrition than are adults; their metabolic rate per unit body weight is higher, and their body stores of nutrients are lower.

Although all agree that dialysis enhances implementation of nutritional support in ARF, there is little consensus on the efficacy of various regimens in restoration of renal function and in impact on overall morbidity and mortality. Abel and colleagues reported that infusion of hypertonic glucose and essential amino acids (EAA) slowed the rise in urea and decreased serum levels of potassium, phosphate, and magnesium [1]. A subsequent double-blind, controlled study by the same group showed faster return of renal function, but no difference in mortality, among patients receiving hypertonic glucose and EAA compared to those receiving only glucose [2]. Others [46] have not shown clear improvement with EAA in either renal function or survival. A variety of animal and patient studies of biochemical response to nutrition, however, support the idea that nutritional supplementation in hypercatabolic patients improves survival and the likelihood of restoring renal function. The data supporting this contention are conflicting, as are those concerning which mix of nutrients might be most helpful. (Indeed no controlled trials exist to show that nutritional supplementation in fact is beneficial). Nonetheless, whatever combination of oral and parenteral modes best approximates the required calories, nitrogen, carbohydrate, fat, vitamins, and trace elements needed by the individual patient is usually implemented.

Oral or enteral feeding is less invasive and more physiologic and, therefore, preferable [48]. Oral intake allows less tailoring of intake to patients' needs, although a variety of supplements with protein of high biologic value is available. Diets for patients fed by nasogastric tube or tubes designed for delivery into the small intestine can be tailored more specifically and may use elemental diets, i.e., ami-noacid mixtures or protein hydrolysates rather than protein; glucose rather than sucrose; medium chain triglycerides rather than a mix of fats. Gastric feedings may be used intermittently or continuously, but use of the small intestine (including jejunostomy tubes) requires continuous feeding rather than a bolus or intermittent schedule. Both should begin with small amounts of diluted solutions, gradually increased to meet the estimated needs, and may be limited by development of cramps, abdominal distention, and diarrhea. If enteral feeding is inadequate for delivery of needed nutrients, it can be combined with parenteral methods. Some authors recommend that, wherever possible, some portion of the daily nutrition, however small, should be delivered into the gut to maintain induction of mucosal enzymes for ready resumption when oral feedings resume.

Peripheral venous feeding is generally better tolerated by infants than children, primarily because of better tolerance of repeated needle sticks. Many of the same solutions used for other forms of parenteral feeding can be used, including lipids (but not hypertonic glucose solutions) [47].

Finally, many of the most seriously ill and hypercatabolic patients need to be fed through a central line, in conjunction with dialysis, in order to receive adequate calories and nitrogen delivered in hyperosmolar solutions. Filler and Wesson [47] have described in general terms the composition of fluids providing nitrogen, glucose, and fat peripherally, enterally, or by central lines. However, there are no recipes that relieve the necessity for assessment and adaptation of approaches to the individual patient, both initially and afterward, by frequent monitoring of body weight, input and output, and blood and urine chemistries.

Many metabolic perturbations occur in patients with ARF and contribute to complications observed during nutritional supplementation. Glucose intolerance and hyperglycemia may require insulin therapy. Metabolic acidosis and hyperammonemia are more likely to occur in the smallest, often premature infants. Hypomagnesemia, changes in serum calcium and phosphate, as well as deficits of copper and zinc, can generally be controlled by adjustment of the composition of infusate. Essential fatty acids are maintained by intermittent use of lipid solutions. Caution should be used in providing lipids to patients with sepsis since the compounds are taken up by the reticuloendothelial system and may compromise the activity of this system. Likewise, lipids displace albumin-bound bilirubin and may cause congestion of smaller vessels in the lung, thereby complicating the course of hyperbilirubinemia and producing respiratory distress syndrome, respectively [48].

It is clear that adequate nutritional supplementation for patients with acute renal failure in general is desirable. On the other hand, a careful assessment of attempts to provide *unrestricted* alimentation yields conflicting results. One possible explanation is that the beneficial effects of this therapy may be obscured in the more severely ill patients who have a limited ability to use excess calories. Because of the limited and conflicting clinical experience, definitive indications for the initiation of supplemental alimentation in patients with acute renal failure cannot be established. The potentially beneficial effects of increased intake of calories and nutrients must be carefully evaluated in the context of each patient's clinical setting, with consideration of the local expertise for the administration of parenteral nutrition and recognition of the risk of these procedures. Future investigations must be directed toward optimal composition of nutritional solutions, the role of nonessential and branched chain amino acids, and other sources of calories. Direct application of nutritional support for patients with acute renal failure requires a more detailed understanding of the mechanisms that underly the processes of repair and regeneration of the renal epithelium.

Therapies for Specific Conditions Producing ARF in Children

Acute Tubular Injury and Necrosis

Table 37-2 presents the etiologies assigned as causes of acute renal failure in pediatric patients (exclusive of neonates) in three tertiary care centers. Many, but not all, the patients received dialysis [17,33,71].

In this category, we include all those conditions producing acute tubular necrosis (ATN), including prolonged hypoperfusion, hypovolemia associated with uncorrected hemorrhage or GI losses, direct tubular toxins, various hemodynamic consequences of sepsis, as well as tubulointerstitial disease. In individual patients, ARF may have multiple causes, and ATN is frequently multifactorial.

Iatrogenic nephrotoxicity is frequently associated with:

1. aminoglycosides,
2. amphotericin B
3. antineoplastic drugs
4. cyclosporine A
5. radiocontrast dyes
6. the nonsteroidal anti-inflammatory drugs (NSAIDs)

TABLE 37-2. *Etiologies of acute renal failure for 210 pediatric patients in three tertiary care centers 1955-1973**

Hemolytic uremic syndrome	31.0%
Acute glomerulonephritis	13.0
Toxins including antibiotics	8.0
Postsurgical causes	7.0
Cortical necrosis	5.0
Neoplasma and chemotherapy	2.0
Sepsis	3.5
Obstructive uropathy	3.0
Stone disease	3.0
Gastroenteritis	3.0
Acute and chronic renal failure	2.5
Dehydration	2.5
Renal venous thrombosis	2.0
Nephrotic syndrome	2.0
Trauma	1.5
Congenital malformations	1.0
Other	10.0

*Hopital des Enfants Malade, Paris: 1955–1971 (130 neonates) [17]
Childrens Hospital, Los Angeles: 1973 (30 neonates, 2 neonates omitted) [71]
Guy's Hospital, London: 1971–1975 (56 episodes of acute renal failure in 53 patients, 2 infants < 1 omitted) [33]

The best approach to renal problems with these agents is prophylactic, i.e., their substitution by less noxious medications. For example, several antibiotics such as the synthetic beta-lactams or the so-called monobactams, e.g., aztreonam [43], may cover the same range of bacteria as the aminoglycosides as well as the compendious third-generation cephalosporins.

Amphotericin B, rifampin, and EDTA infrequently give rise to ATN; treatment consists of substitution with another agent where possible. Of interest, is the development of triazole antifungal agents that can be given intravenously or orally [41].

The antineoplastic agents methotrexate and cisplatin are both associated with renal insufficiency at high doses and may cause ARF [88]. In methotrexate toxicity, proximal tubular necrosis has been found, although intratubular obstruction is considered the primary etiology. Vigorous hydration and alkalinization of the urine before and during its administration, in addition to leucovorin rescue, will significantly reduce the renal toxicity. In combination with leucovorin rescue, alkalinization of urine and diuresis produced marked reduction of nephrotoxicity in children receiving methotrexate for osteosarcoma [85]. Pretreatment is important since methotrexate and its numerous metabolites are poorly cleared by either peritoneal dialysis or hemodialysis. Concomitant use of cisplatin worsens methotrexate nephrotoxicity [57].

Cisplatin is used in testicular and ovarian tumors, Wilms' tumor, and neuroblastoma. Pretreatment with hydration and the use of saline rather than dextrose and water for infusion of cisplatin are reported to reduce renal damage. Hypocalcemia and tetany associated with magnesium wasting are additional complications of cisplatin administration [14].

Cyclosporin A, which is a potent immunosuppressant, has been associated with ARF secondary to direct tubular damage, glomerular thrombosis, and interstitial nephritis [78]. Its nephrotoxicity appears exacerbated by concomitant use of aminoglycosides, acyclovir, amphotericin B, and ketoconazole, as well as renal ischemia from any cause. Dose adjustment and, in some cases, use of other immunosuppressive regimens, must be considered.

Radiocontrast materials with osmolalities in excess of 1000 mOsm/L can produce vasoconstriction, erythrocyte aggregation in glomerular capillaries, and intratubular precipitation of Tamm-Horsfall protein. To prevent these complications, Berkseth and Kjellstrand [11] recommend a mannitol/furosemide infusion for all patients with plasma creatinine greater than 2 mg/dl, in addition to careful hydration and use of the smallest possible volume of contrast agent. Several studies show that 50% of patients with serum creatinine values greater than 1.5–2 mg/dl will experience exacerbation of renal insufficiency. The risk is greatest in diabetics, the aged, and those with previous radiocontrast damage. Lower osmolality agents have been developed in an effort to circumvent nephrotoxicity [12,45]. The great expense of these new agents suggests that they should be reserved for patients at the greatest risk for renal damage.

Acute renal failure is only one aspect of renal damage associated with the use of NSAIDs [28]. Patients with low extracellular fluid volume of any cause, such as dehydration, nephrotic syndrome, and diuretic-induced hypovolemia, and patients with systemic lupus erythematosus, are particularly susceptible to renal toxicity. Once again, prophylactic avoidance is the best approach; if ARF develops, discontinuation of the drug and provision of supportive care are essential.

Allergic interstitial nephritis (AIN), which may present as ARF, can be caused by NSAIDs, as well as a variety of commonly used medications, including penicillin derivatives (e.g., methicillin, ampicillin), cephalosporins, sulfonamide antibiotics, and diuretics (furosemide, thiazides), phenytoin, allopurinol, carbamazepine, cimetidine, and clofibrate [44,68]. The most obvious therapy is stopping the suspected medication. Administration of steroids appeared to be beneficial in an uncontrolled, but often quoted, study of 14 patients with AIN associated with methicillin [50]. Serum creatinine returned to baseline in six of eight patients treated for 10 days, compared to only two of six treated conservatively. Reports of the use of intravenous methylprednisolone are conflicting.

In the report of Ellis and coworkers of 47 children with AIN, medications were thought to be causative in two-thirds, infections in nearly one-third, and only two cases were considered idiopathic [44]. Nine of their original thirteen cases had serum creatinine levels of 2–11 mg/dl and an average creatinine clearance less than 50 ml/min/1.73m^2. Supportive care, withdrawal of suspected agents, and treatment of infection were used in all but the two cases of idiopathic interstitial nephritis, who were treated with immunosuppression. Complete recovery of renal function and clearing of the urinary sediment occurred within one to three months from onset of symptoms, and all 13 patients had normal renal function and urine sediments at follow-up one to one and a half years later.

Acute renal failure occurs after cardiac surgery, with an incidence of 8% in one study [26]. In another report, 5% of children subjected to cardiopulmonary bypass surgery required peritoneal dialysis for postoperative ARF, and nearly 40% of those patients died during dialysis [90]. In a randomized study, mean serum creatinine was significantly lower in 20 children receiving prophylactic infusion of mannitol (0.5 gm/kg) compared to 20 children receiving the same supportive care but without mannitol infusions preoperatively; however, no patient in either group experienced acute renal failure [91].

Noniatrogenic causes of tubular damage leading to ARF are frequently related to intravascular hemolysis and rhabdomyolysis. Tubular damage is attributed to heme-related breakdown products, but vasoconstriction and tubular obstruction with casts contribute to ARF in these conditions. Hydration, to maintain extracellular volume and to promote urine flow, appears decisive [69,92]. Isotonic or half isotonic saline is used and should be supplemented with mannitol if urine output diminishes. The advisability of alkalinizing the urine with a bicarbonate infusion to prevent intratubular precipitation has been questioned [69]. Many patients have hypocalcemia secondary to hyperphosphatemia. Therefore, alkalinization of plasma may promote further binding of calcium to proteins and exacerbate the hypocalcemia. Calcium replacement is generally

not necessary or advisable since serum calcium, presumably released from precipitated stores, returns to normal or near normal levels with correction of the other metabolic abnormalities, in particular acid-base balance and hyperphosphatemia.

ARF is frequently seen in patients with sepsis, although the underlying mechanisms have not been fully elucidated [40]. Treatment of the underlying disease is obviously of major importance in limiting the extent of renal damage. It should be recognized that patients with sepsis may develop ATN without a period of hypotension and tubular injury due to direct tubular injury from bacterial endotoxins.

Hemolytic-Uremic Syndrome

As shown in Table 37-2, hemolytic-uremic syndrome (HUS) is the most frequent cause of ARF in children. Treatment of this disorder begins with the general supportive measures outlined above, since patients may present with fulminant ARF. In addition, packed red blood cells may be needed to bolster the rapid hemolysis. Packed RBC (10 cc/kg) are given to maintain the hematocrit above 15% to 20%, especially if hemolysis does not seem to be abating. Thrombocytopenia does not usually require platelet replacement since counts generally exceed 10,000/µl. However, if invasive procedures are planned for patients with less than 50,000 platelets/µl or if a child is actively bleeding, platelets can be administered. However, platelet transfusions should be avoided if possible because of potential aggravation or extension of microthrombi in capillary loops. Infusion of platelets and red cells may, of course, precipitate pulmonary edema, and in children with inadequate urine output, the concomitant volume overload may hasten the need for dialysis.

Several investigational therapies have been tried to halt the intravascular thrombus formation [66,99]. None of these has been convincingly demonstrated to be of substantial benefit.

Glomerular Disease

Among children, acute postinfectious glomerulonephritis (APGN) and the various causes of crescentic or rapidly progressive glomerulonephritis (RPGN) [4,15] are the glomerulopathies most commonly associated with ARF at presentation. Renal therapy is primarily supportive, with control of hypertension and fluid overload. Antibiotics do not affect the glomerular disease but may control local disease and prevent the spread to other susceptible persons. Dialysis is usually not necessary since these patients generally retain enough function to respond to diuretics and do not become uncontrollably uremic.

IgA nephropathy and Henoch-Schönlein purpura lack clearly defined and effective treatment options despite investigation of many drugs, including steroids, cytotoxic agents, anticoagulants, plasmapheresis, and the use of phenytoin to lower IgA levels [77,112].

Lupus nephritis presenting as RPGN is an uncommon but dramatic presentation of ARF. Intravenous methylprednisolone and/or plasmapheresis has been used in patients with acute decompensation in renal function [23,87,113].

The three major approaches to treatment of RPGN are steroids with immunosuppressive agents, anticoagulants with antiplatelet drugs, and plasmapheresis [4,38,73,89, 100]. The benefits of these therapies, however, are unproved.

Urolithiasis

The association of urolithiasis and ARF in North America is uncommon. Prevalence for pediatric stone disease has ranged from one of 1100 to one of 7600 hospital admissions. Only patients with bilateral obstruction, unilateral obstruction of a solitary kidney, or obstruction of the urethral outlet, develops ARF. In such patients, supportive care, as described in the first section of this chapter, is indicated. Specific therapy is directed toward removal of the stone. Surgical therapy is often needed [13]. From 1957 to 1983, 57% and 92% of pediatric patients with urolithiasis in North America and Europe, respectively, required surgical intervention. Recently, extracorporeal shock wave lithotripsy has been used in pediatric patients [86].

Neoplasia

ARF may be the clinical presentation of neoplasia of the urinary tract, but this is distinctly unusual. The most common pediatric genitourinary neoplasm is the nephroblastoma or Wilms' tumor [39,64].

Rhabdomyosarcoma, the most common tumor of the lower genitourinary tract, occurs in 0.5 to 1 child per million, about one-tenth the incidence of Wilms' tumor. In a series of 14 patients from the Mayo Clinic, two patients presented with renal dysfunction [102].

Acute renal failure in neoplasia affecting non-genitourinary tissues has many etiologies [75]. For example, renal hypoperfusion can be precipitated by hypovolemia secondary to unreplaced gastrointestinal losses related to the primary disease or its therapy, from third space losses, or from pericardial tamponade compromising renal perfusion. Postrenal factors such as retroperitoneal fibrosis and ureteral or vascular compression by lymph nodes generally produces a slower onset of renal failure. Glomerulopathies related to neoplasia, such as minimal change nephrotic syndrome in Hodgkin's disease and membranous glomerulonephritis in lymphoma, appear to be less frequent in children than in adults [101]. Rarely, direct invasion of the kidney may present with azotemia or frank renal failure [29].

Tumor lysis syndrome associated with rapidly growing tumors, especially non-Hodgkin's lymphomas and leukemias or with aggressive chemotherapy may cause ARF [20,30,88]. Tsokos and his colleagues describe 33 patients (not all children) of whom nine presented with azotemia before therapy and an additional five developed renal insufficiency or failure within a week of initial therapy [111]. All patients except two with azotemia had advanced disease (stage C with abdominal tumor, stage D with abdominal and extra-abdominal disease); excisional reduction of abdominal tumor bulk was associated with decreased incidence of ARF and metabolic abnormalities after therapy. Prior to chemotherapy, allopurinol was given and a diuresis was induced. If uric acid was greater than 7 mg/dl, NaHCO$_3$ was added to the infusion in order to raise urinary pH above 7. This was done to minimize calcium phosphate deposits in the renal tubules and the associated risk of acute anuric nephrocalcinosis. Even with these precautions, five patients developed renal failure with peak creatinines of 1.5–4.5 mg/dl.

Therapy of Underlying Disease in Acute Renal Failure in Neonates

Table 37-3 presents data from neonatal intensive care units in two tertiary care centers [27,81]; ARF occurred in 1% to 6% of patients. Overall mortality was 36%; it is noteworthy that no patient with non-oliguric ARF died.

Transient Renal Dysfunction

Hijazi and colleagues [62] observed three neonates with transient oliguric renal failure characterized by a period of oliguria associated with a rise in serum creatinine that did not appear to be predominantly hemodynamically related. All three infants had identical renal sonographic findings that included mild bilateral renal enlargement with abnormal echogenicity of the apices of all renal medullary pyramids. All infants recovered, and follow-up sonograms showed a normal kidney within three to six months. This characteristic pattern of changes on ultrasonography may be of importance in identifying those infants whose renal function will resolve spontaneously and may be an important predictor of a good outcome for the neonate with oliguria.

Sepsis

The leading cause of death in the two series presented in Table 37-3 was sepsis, which occurs in many settings, most often with necrotizing enterocolitis, urinary tract infection, pneumonia, or intravenous line infection. Disseminated intravascular coagulation, a dreaded complication, is associated most often with gram negative organisms. Suspi-

TABLE 37-3. *Etiologies of acute renal failure in 36 neonates in two tertiary care centers**

Disseminated intravascular coagulation	21.4%
Sepsis	21.4
Asphyxia	21.4
Congenital genitourinary abnormalities	16.7
Congenital cardiovascular abnormalities	9.5
Renal venous thrombosis	4.8
Renal arterial emboli	4.8

*University of Virginia, Charlottesville: 1978–1983 (16 neonates) [27]
Children's Hospital, Philadelphia: 1976–1977 (20 neonates) [81]

cion of sepsis prompts most physicians to start antibiotic therapy while waiting for culture results to guide more specific therapy.

Asphyxia

Asphyxia may be associated with respiratory distress syndrome (RDS) or meconium aspiration. While RDS is associated with reduced renal function, meconium aspiration may result in ATN or cortical necrosis. Respiratory therapy to correct oxygenation and acid-base deficits can also contribute to ARF. Both positive expiratory end pressure and continuous positive airway pressure, applied to optimize gas exchange, have been shown to decrease glomerular filtration rate and urine output, by decreasing venous return [59,60].

The volume status of an infant with asphyxiation may be difficult to evaluate, and central pressure monitoring may be necessary. Signs of hypovolemia include vasoconstriction, tachycardia greater than 180 beats per minute, acidosis with pH less than 7.20, and hypotension. Infusion of blood, plasma, or isotonic saline at 5–15 ml/kg body wt over 30 to 60 minutes is the first step toward restoration of intravascular volume. The infusion should proceed cautiously, especially in preterm infants who are at increased risk for intraventricular hemorrhage. Some physicians use only saline and/or packed cells for volume restoration since plasma proteins, and albumin in particular, may cross leaky pulmonary capillaries and exacerbate RDS.

Cardiovascular Disturbances

Seventy-five percent of renal venous thrombosis (RVT) occurs in neonatal kidneys, which are thought to be particularly susceptible because of high renal vascular resistance and low renal perfusion in the perinatal period. The risk of RVT is increased with severe dehydration, blood loss, administration of radiocontrast material, polycythemia associated with cardiac failure, sepsis, and disseminated intravascular coagulation (DIC), as well as in infants of diabetic mothers [8,10]. RVT originates in intrarenal veins. It was bilateral in 16% of 45 cases in one series [6]. Therefore, the association of ATN and cortical and medullary necrosis with RVT is not surprising. Heparin is used routinely in adult cases of RVT [93], but it has not been studied in a controlled series in infants and is not recommended (see Chap. 88). In general, thrombectomy for bilateral RVT is less popular than it was in the past [8,82]. Thrombolytic therapy for RVT in adults has been used but without great success [37].

Renal artery thrombosis is most commonly associated with catheterization of the umbilical artery, in particular with placement of the catheter above the origin of the renal arteries. The risk of renal artery thrombosis is increased when infusions are given through an umbilical artery, especially the delivery of radiocontrast materials. Complete occlusion leads to loss of renal function on the affected side unless collateral circulation to the capsule or pelvic structures exists. Hypertension may result, often resistant to pharmacologic control, and may require nephrectomy [3].

Congenital Anomalies With and Without Obstruction

Congenital cardiac malformations presenting in the neonatal period may be accompanied by ARF, either as a result of congenital syndromes involving both cardiovascular and genitourinary systems [55] or as a result of renal hypoperfusion. Correction of the cardiac abnormality is crucial to maintenance of renal function, especially when the renal dysfunction is hemodynamic. In one series of 16 patients with neonatal ARF, four had primary cardiovascular anomalies [27].

Congenital syndromes "with a renal component" [55] are legion, and their treatment, ranging from supportive care to dialysis and transplantation, is beyond the scope of this chapter [58].

Experimental Approaches to Treatment

Although conservative therapy, dialysis, and transplantation have proved helpful in mitigating the dire outcome of ARF in children, the morbidity and mortality from this syndrome remains high. In 70 children treated from 1971 to 1975 at Guy's Hospital, Counahan and colleagues [33] noted that mortality fell from 33% in 1972 to 20% in later years, which they attribute solely to the availability of maintenance dialysis. In the three series in Table 37-2, the mortality ranged from 23% to 34%. Much of the mortality was related to concomitant illnesses and to the survival of the more seriously ill patients who eventually succumbed to nonrenal causes. Although isolated ARF may be associated with a mortality rate less than 10%, its superimposition on pre-existing trauma, for example, was associated with a five-fold increase in mortality rate compared to patients with comparable trauma but free of ARF [31].

There has been an increased intensity of research into the causes of ARF, both clinically and experimentally, in attempts to define therapy more effectively tailored to the underlying pathophysiology. The thrust of these studies has been to define therapies that can be initiated *after* the insult that produces the acute renal failure.

Adenine Nucleotides

The adenine nucleotide system (adenosine triphosphate, ATP; adenosine diphosphate, ADP; adenosine monophosphate, AMP; inorganic phosphate, P_i; magnesium, Mg) is vital to the maintenance of critical cellular functions, including carbohydrate metabolism, muscle contraction, protein synthesis, lipogenesis, the maintenance of cell structure, the regulation of cell volume, and electrolyte transport. Chaudry et al. [25] demonstrated that the intravenous infusion of ATP-magnesium chloride ($MgCl_2$) before, during, or immediately after hemorrhagic hypotension reduced the mortality in conscious rats. Our laboratory has carried out a large number of investigations concerning the infusion of adenine nucleotides combined with magnesium chloride in several different forms of experimental acute renal failure, including ischemic, toxic, and obstructive renal injury [52,53]. These studies have demonstrated that:

1. postischemic infusion of any of the adenine nucleotides combined with magnesium chloride resulted in significant improvement in renal function
2. these compounds were effective when given after either 30, 45, or 60 minutes of ischemia but were ineffective when the ischemic interval was extended to 90 minutes
3. there was a direct dose response relationship between the quantity of ATP-MgCl$_2$ infused and the extent of improvement in renal function
4. the infusion of these compounds resulted in marked improvement in the histomorphologic changes that occur in association with ischemia
5. the infusion of these compounds could be delayed for as much as 24 hours but would still be effective in ameliorating the ischemic insult
6. the initial salutary effect of these compounds was sustained and resulted in an enhanced recovery to normal levels of renal function. The beneficial effect of the ATP-MgCl$_2$ infusion is related to the restoration of cellular ATP levels, the most likely being the provision of precursors for the resynthesis of cellular ATP

At the present time, there are only limited reports of the use of adenine nucleotides in patients [24,82], and very little information is available concerning the safety and efficacy of these compounds.

Thyroxine

In 1971, Straub published the first of a series of papers demonstrating protective effects of thyroxine administered to rabbits and mice with mercuric chloride-induced ARF [103,104,105]. Straub and co-workers [96] later showed that daily administration of thyroxine in rats for one to two weeks after exposure to corrosive mercuric chloride (HgCl$_2$) enhanced the recovery of alkaline phosphatase (found in proximal tubular brush border), acid phosphatase (apical cytoplasm), adenosinetriphosphatase (ATPase) (basolateral membranes), and leucine aminopeptides (cytoplasm).

Cronin and Newman have likewise shown in two models of nephrotoxic ARF that thyroxine, administered for 10 days before exposure to gentamicin [34] or uranyl nitrate [35] and for several days thereafter, was associated with significant improvement in creatinine clearance, urine osmolality, and renal cortical sodium, potassium-ATPase activity. When examined five days after the exposure to uranyl nitrate, cells of the inner and outer cortex showed less damage and more regeneration in rats receiving thyroxine than in rats given only the nephrotoxin.

Siegel and coworkers [98] investigated similar questions, but administered thyroxine as a single dose (4-20 μg/100 mg birth wt) at the time of maximal renal injury (as established in earlier studies). Using both nephrotoxic (potassium dichromate) [98] and ischemic [108] models of ARF, they observed better preservation of inulin clearance, urinary concentration, and fractional sodium reabsorption in animals given thyroxine compared to the controls. These effects were observed in isolated perfused kidneys exposed to dichromate and appear, therefore, not to be due to extrarenal hemodynamic changes. Histologic comparison of kidneys from rats receiving thyroxine showed less patchy necrosis in S$_2$ and S$_3$ segments of the proximal tubule, no loss of cells from the basement membranes, and better preservation of cellular architecture. The accelerated improvement of renal function in thyroxine-treated rats was sustained. In the ischemic model, recovery of intracellular ATP as determined by ^{31}P nuclear magnetic resonance spectroscopy in vivo was accelerated.

Only a single report of clinical use of thyroxine in ARF exists. Straub reported an uncontrolled study of oral thyroxine (5–6 μg/kg/day in divided doses) administered to eight children eight weeks to 11 years of age, who were anuric for three to five days, with serum creatinines in the range of 3–6 mg/dl [106]. All begin to produce urine within 36 to 48 hours after the first dose of thyroxine. By the sixteenth day, creatinine and urea had returned to normal levels in every patient except one who died of complications of the underlying disease. Straub [107] subsequently reported that another six patients had been treated successfully with thyroxine.

Reactive Oxygen Species and Their Scavengers

In recent years, evidence has accumulated to indicate reactive oxygen species (ROS), like hydrogen peroxide and the hydroxy and superoxide radicals, as major contributors to tissue damage in a wide variety of diseases, including diseases of the kidney [9]. Specific scavengers of several ROS have been used in animal experiments to delineate their effects and to investigate potential therapeutic uses. Allopurinol, which inhibits xanthine oxidase, a central component of ROS production, has been used in a clinical trial.

Paller and colleagues examined modulation of ischemic ARF in uninephrectomized rats by the enzyme superoxide dismutase (SOD), a scavenger of the superoxide radical [83]. When compared to control rats, those exposed to SOD just before and during ischemia showed lower serum creatinines, higher inulin clearances, and less tubular injury. Dimethylthiourea (DMTU), a scavenger of the hydroxy radical, and allopurinol, both given before ischemia, also produced lower serum creatinines at one, two, and three days postischemia. The authors concluded that reflow after release of RAO provided oxygen to the ischemic kidney with subsequent production of ROS, which in turn produced renal injury by lipid peroxidation. Others would include damage to proteins and nucleic acids as well. Administration of scavengers of ROS appeared to prevent this.

Gamelin and Zager [51] suggested that the ischemic model of these experiments had two major artifactual problems as a result of severe blood trapping in the outer medulla. Other investigators found no structural or functional protection by pretreatment with allopurinol, SOD, DMTU, catalase, or glutathione [117].

Therapeutic use of ROS scavengers in clinical settings has been limited. At this point there is no evidence to suggest that scavengers might be helpful when used after the onset of ARF. One can imagine their use as prophylaxis or immediately after the known onset of ARF, e.g., surgical trauma. Allopurinol has been used to protect isolated canine kidneys from ischemic damage in transit from donors to recipients. Initial promising studies were not substantiated in clinical trials with human kidneys, in which no difference in post-transplant renal performance was associated with the presence of allopurinol in the perfusion solutions [109].

Atrial Natriuretic Factor

Atrial natriuretic factor (ANF) has been examined as therapy in several animal models of ARF, since it produces dilatation of the afferent glomerular arteriole and constriction in the efferent arteriole; even without a change in renal blood flow, the glomerular filtration rate rises. There may also be tubular effects contributing to the diuresis and natriuresis that follows administration of ANF [115].

Higher inulin clearances were found in rats receiving ANF infusion for one to four hours after release of renal artery occlusion than in rats infused with saline vehicle only. One study [97] using a 1 to 4-hour infusion showed histologic protection against ischemic damage and improved inulin clearance, urine flow, net tubular reabsorption of sodium, and increased intracellular ATP. Nakamoto and collaborators [79] also found that recovery of intracellular ATP concentrations in the two hours after ischemia was significantly more rapid in rats receiving ANF than in those getting only saline. Similar results have been reported in ARF induced with norepinephrine, cisplatin, and glycerol [22,61,94].

In terms of clinical studies, some investigators report significant hypotension with infusion of ANF in volunteers. They suggest that intrarenal infusion of ANF might promote the desired renal effects without systemic hypotension; alternatively, one might combine infusions of dopamine and ANF [52]. Careful studies need to be conducted in controlled populations of patients who are appropriately monitored.

Calcium Channel Blockers

Burke and colleagues [19] demonstrated that the infusion of verapamil either prior to or following the induction of acute renal failure by norepinephrine infusion resulted in improvement in renal function one and 24 hours after the insult. Other investigators [84] have also reported that the infusion of verapamil prior to 60 minutes of renal artery clamping in the dog resulted in better initial renal function. However, other groups have studied the effects of other calcium channel blockers and the effect of verapamil in other species, with conflicting results [76,114]. Clinical studies concerning the use of calcium channel blockers have not produced consistent results [42,63].

References

1. Abel RM, Abbott WM, Fischer JE: Intravenous essential L-amino acids and hypertonic dextrose in patients with acute renal failure. *Am J Surg* 123:632, 1972.
2. Abel RM, Beck CH Jr, Abbott WM, et al: Improved survival from acute renal failure after treatment with intravenous essential L-amino acids and glucose. Results of a prospective, double-blind study. *New Engl J Med* 288:695, 1973.
3. Adelman RD: Non-surgical management of renoovascular hypertension in the neonate. *Pediatr* 62:71, 1978.
4. Anand SK, Trygstad CW, Sharma HM, et al: Extracapillary proliferative glomerulonephritis in children. *Pediatr* 56:434, 1974.
5. Arbus GS, Farine M: Acute renal failure. *In* Postlethwaite RJ (ed): *Clinical Paediatric Nephrology*. Bristol, Wright, 1986, p 197.
6. Arneil GC, MacDonald AM, Murphy AV, et al: Renal venous thrombosis. *Clin Nephrol* 1:119, 1973.
7. Ayus JC, Krothapalli RK, Arieff AI: Changing concepts in treatment of severe symptomatic hyponatremia. *Am J Med* 78:897, 1985.
8. Barratt TM, Rigden SPA: Acute renal failure. *In* Williams DI, Johnston JH (eds): *Paediatric Urology*, 2nd ed. London, Butterworths, 1982, p 27.
9. Baud L, Ardaillou R: Reactive oxygen species: Production and role in the kidney. *Am J Physiol* 251:F765, 1988.
10. Belman AB: Renal venous thrombosis in infancy and childhood. *Clin Pediatr (Phila)* 15:1033, 1976.
11. Berkseth RO, Kjellstrand CM: Radiologic contrast-induced nephropathy. *Med Clin North Am* 68:351, 1984.
12. Bettmann MA: Radiographic contrast agents—a perspective. *N Engl J Med* 317:891, 1987.
13. Bianchi A: Common urological problems. *In* Postlethwaite RJ (ed): *Clinical Paediatric Nephrology*. Bristol, Wright, 1986, p 270.
14. Blachley JD, Hill JB: Renal and electrolyte disturbances associated with cisplatin. *Ann Intern Med* 95:628, 1981.
15. Bock GH, Ruley EJ: Crescentic glomerulonephritis. *In* Holliday MA, Barratt TM, Vernier RL (eds): *Pediatric Nephrology*, 2nd ed. Baltimore, Williams & Wilkins, 1986, p 431.
16. Brown CB, Ogg CS, Cameron JS: High dose furosemide in acute renal failure. A controlled trial. *Clin Nephrol* 15:90, 1981.
17. Broyer M: Acute renal failure. *In* Royer P, Habib R, Mathieu H, et al (eds): *Pediatric Nephrology*, vol 11, *Major Problems in Clinical Pediatrics*. Baltimore, Williams & Wilkins, 1974, p 343.
18. Burke TJ, Arnold PE, Gordon JA, et al: Protective effect of intrarenal calcium membrane blockers before or after renal ischemia. Functional, morphological, and mitochondrial studies. *J Clin Invest* 74:1830, 1984.
19. Burke TJ, Cronin RE, Duchin KL, et al: Ischemia and tubular obstruction during acute renal failure in dogs: Mannitol in protection. *Am J Physiol* 238:F305, 1980.
20. Cadman E, Lundberg WB, Bertino JR: Hyperphosphatemia and hypocalcemia accompanying rapid cell lysis in a patient with Burkitt's lymphoma and Burkitt cell leukemia. *Am J Med* 62:283, 1977.
21. Cameron JS: Historical, social, and geographic factors: Pediatric nephrology in an unfair world. *In* Holliday MA, Barratt TM, Vernier RL (eds): *Pediatric Nephrology*, 2nd ed. Baltimore, Williams & Wilkins, 1986, p 341.
22. Capasso G, Anastasio P, Giordano D, et al: Beneficial effects of atrial natriuretic factor on cisplatin-induced acute renal failure in the rat. *Am J Nephrol* 7:228, 1987.

23. Cathcart ES, Scheinberg MA, Idelson BA, et al: Beneficial effects of methylprednisolone "pulse" therapy in diffuse proliferative lupus nephritis. Lancet 1:163, 1976.

24. Chaudry IH, Keefer JR, Barash P, et al: ATP-MgCl₂ infusion in man: Increased cardiac output without adverse systemic hemodynamic effects. Surg Forum 35:14, 1984.

25. Chaudry IH, Sayeed MM, Baue AE: Effects of adenosine triphosphate-magnesium chloride administration in shock. Surgery 75:220, 1974.

26. Chesney RW, Kaplan BS, Freedom RM, et al: Acute renal failure: An important complication of cardiac surgery in infants. J Pediatr 87:381, 1976.

27. Chevalier RL, Campbell F, Brenbridge ANAG: Prognostic factors in neonatal acute renal failure. Pediatrics 74:265, 1984.

28. Clive DM, Stoff JS: Renal syndromes associated with nonsteroidal antiinflammatory drugs. N Engl J Med 310:563, 1984.

29. Coggins CH: Renal failure in lymphoma. Kidney Int 17:847, 1980.

30. Cohen LF, Balow JE, Magrath IT, et al: Acute tumor lysis syndrome: A review of 37 patients with Burkitt's lymphoma. Am J Med 68:486, 1980.

31. Conger JD: How can the high mortality of acute renal failure be reduced? Seminars in Dialysis 1:128, 1988.

32. Costarino A, Baumgart S: Modern fluid and electrolyte management of the critically ill premature infant. Pediatr Clin North Am 33:153, 1986.

33. Counahan R, Cameron JS, Ogg CS, et al: Presentation, management, complications, and outcome of acute renal failure in childhood: Five years' experience. Br Med J 1:599, 1977.

34. Cronin RE: Drug therapy in the management of acute renal failure. Am J Med Sci 292:112, 1986.

35. Cronin RE, Newman JA: Protective effect of thyroxin but not parathyroidectomy on gentamicin nephrotoxicity. Am J Physiol 248:F332, 1985.

36. Cronin RE, Brown DM, Simonsen R: Protection by thyroxin in nephrotoxic acute renal failure. Am J Physiol 251:F408, 1986.

37. Crowley JP, Matarese RA, Quevedo SF, et al: Fibrinolytic therapy for bilateral renal vein thrombi. Arch Intern Med 144:159, 1984.

38. Cunningham RJ III, Gilfoil M, Cavallo T, et al: Rapidly progressive glomuleronephritis in children: A report of thirteen cases and a review of the literature. Pediatr Res 14:128, 1980.

39. D'Angio GJ, Duckett JW, Belasco JB: Tumors: Upper urinary tract. In Williams DI, Johnston JH (eds): Clinical Pediatric Urology, 2nd ed. London, Butterworths, 1985, p 1157.

40. DeCamp M, Demling RH: Post-traumatic multisystem organ failure. JAMA 260:530, 1988.

41. Dismukes WE: Azole antifungal drugs: Old and new. Ann Intern Med 109:177, 1988.

42. Duggan KA, Macdonald GJ, Charlesworth JA, et al: Verapamil prevents post-transplant oliguric renal failure. Clin Nephrol 24:289, 1985.

43. Duma RJ: Aztreonam the first monobactam. Ann Intern Med 106:766, 1987.

44. Ellis D, Fried WA, Yunis EJ, et al: Acute interstitial nephritis in children: A report of 13 cases and a review of the literature. Pediatrics 67:862, 1981.

45. Evans RJ, Shankel SW, Cutler RE: Low osmolar contrast agents and nephrotoxicity. Ann Intern Med 107:116, 1987.

46. Feinstein EI, Blumenkrantz MJ, Healy M, et al: Clinical and metabolic responses to parenteral nutrition in acute renal failure. Medicine 60:124, 1981.

47. Filler RM, Wesson DE: The pediatric surgical patient. In Deitel M (ed): Nutrition in Clinical Surgery. Baltimore, Williams & Wilkins, 1985, p 185.

48. Freund HR: Acute renal failure. In Deitel M (ed): Nutrition in Clinical Surgery. Baltimore, Williams & Wilkins, 1985, p 348.

49. Gallagher L, Jones JK: Furosemide-induced ototoxicity. Ann Intern Med 744, 1979.

50. Galpin JP, Shinaberger JH, Stanley TM, et al: Acute interstitial nephritis due to methicillin. Am J Med 65:756, 1978.

51. Gamelin LM, Zager RA: Evidence against oxidant injury as a critical mediator of postischemic acute renal failure. Am J Physiol 2255:F450, 1988.

52. Gaudio KM, Siegel NJ: New approaches to the treatment of acute renal failure. Pediatr Nephrol 1:339, 1987.

53. Gaudio KM, Siegel NJ: Pathogenesis and treatment of acute renal failure. Pediatr Clin North Am 34:771, 1987.

54. Gauthier B, Edelman CM: Nephrology and Urology for the Pediatrician. Boston, Little, Brown, 1982.

55. Gilli G, Berry AC, Chantler C: Congenital disease. Syndromes with a renal component. In Holliday MA, Barratt TM, Vernier RL (eds): Pediatric Nephrology. Baltimore, Williams & Wilkins, 1986, p 384.

56. Gordillo-Paniagua G, Velasquez-Jones L: Acute renal failure. Pediatr Clin North Am 23:817, 1976.

57. Goren MP, Wright RK, Horowitz ME, et al: Enhancement of methotrexate nephrotoxicity after cisplatin therapy. Cancer 58:2617, 1986.

58. Grupe WE: The dilemma of intrauterine diagnosis of congenital renal disease. Pediatr Clin North Am 34:629, 1987.

59. Guignard JP: Renal function in the newborn infant. Pediatr Clin North Am 29:777, 1982.

60. Guignard JP: Neonatal nephrology. In Holliday MA, Barratt TM, Vernier RL (eds): Pediatric Nephrology. Baltimore, Williams & Wilkins, 1986, p 921.

61. Heidbreder E, Schafferhans K, Schramm D, et al: Toxic renal failure in the rat: Beneficial effects of atrial natriuretic factor. Klin Wochenschr 64:78, 1986.

62. Hijazi Z, Keller MS, Gaudio KM, et al: Transient renal dysfunction of the neonate. Pediatrics 82:929, 1988.

63. Hull RW, Hasbargen JA: No clinical evidence for protective effects of calcium-channel blockers against acute renal failure (letter). N Engl J Med 313:1477, 1985.

64. Williams DI, Martin J: Renal tumors. In Williams DI, Johnston JH (eds): Clinical Pediatric Urology, 2nd ed. London, Butterworths, 1982, p 381.

65. John EG, Levitsky S, Hastreiter AR: Management of acute renal failure complicating cardiac surgery in infants and children. Crit Care Med 8:562, 1980.

66. Jones RWA, Morris M, Maisey MN, et al: Endarterial urokinase in childhood hemolytic uremic syndrome. Kidney Int 20:723, 1981.

67. Kleinknecht D, Ganeval D, Gonzalez-Duque LA, et al: Furosemide in acute oliguric renal failure: A controlled trial. Nephron 15:51, 1976.

68. Kleinknecht D, Vanhille P, Morel-Maroger L, et al: Acute interstitial nephritis due to drug hypersensitivity. An up-to-date review with a report of 19 cases. Adv Nephrol 12:277, 1983.

69. Knochel JP: Rhabdomyolysis and myoglobinuria. In Suki WN, Eknoyan G (eds): The Kidney in Systemic Disease. New York, Wiley, 1981, p 263.

70. Kron IL, Joob AW, VanMeter C: Acute renal failure in the

cardiovascular surgical patient. *Ann Thorac Surg* 39:590, 1985.

71. Lieberman E: Management of acute renal failure. *Nephron* 2:193, 1973.

72. Lindner A: Synergism of dopamine and furosemide in diuretic-resistant, oliguric acute renal failure. *Nephron* 33:121, 1983.

73. Lockwood CM, Rees A, Pinching A, et al: Plasma exchange and immunosuppression in treatment of fulminating immune complex crescentic nephritis. *Lancet* 1:63, 1977.

74. Luke RG, Briggs JD, Allison ME, et al: Factors determining response to mannitol in acute renal failure. *Am J Med Sci* 259:168, 1970.

75. Martinez-Maldonado M, Baez-Diez L, Benabe JE: Nonrenal neoplasms and the kidney. *In* Schrier RW, Gottschalk CV (eds): *Diseases of the Kidney.* Boston, Little, Brown, 1988, p 2511.

76. Malis CD, Cheung JY, Leaf A, et al: Effects of verapamil in models of ischemic acute renal failure in the rat. *Am J Physiol* 245:F735, 1983.

77. Melvin T, Kim Y: Isolated glomerular diseases. D. IgA nephropathy. *In* Holliday MA, Barratt TM, Vernier RL (eds): *Pediatric Nephrology,* 2nd ed. Baltimore, Williams & Wilkins, 1986, p 437.

78. Myers BD: Cyclosporin nephrotoxicity. *Kidney Int* 30:964, 1986.

79. Nakamoto M, Shapiro JI, Shanley PF, et al: In vitro and in vivo protective effect of atriopeptin III on ischemic acute renal failure. *J Clin Invest* 80:698, 1987.

80. Nierenberg DW: Furosemide and ethyacrynic acid in acute tubular necrosis. *West J Med* 133:163, 1980.

81. Norman ME, Asadi FK: A prospective study of acute renal failure in the newborn infant. *Pediatrics* 63:475, 1979.

82. Odaka M, Hirasawa H, Tabata Y, et al: A new treatment of acute renal failure with direct hemoperfusion, enhancement of reticuloendothelial system and ATP-MgCl₂. *In* Eliahou HE (ed): *Acute Renal Failure.* London, John Libbey, 1982, p 168.

83. Paller MS, Hoidal JR, Ferris TF: Oxygen free radicals in ischemic acute renal failure in the rat. *J Clin Invest* 74:1156, 1984.

84. Papadimitriou M, Alexopoulos E, Vargemezis V, et al: The effect of preventive administration of verapamil on acute ischaemic renal failure in dogs. *Proc Eur Dial Transplant Assoc* 20:650, 1983.

85. Pitman SW, Frei E III: Weekly methotrexate-calcium leucovorin rescue: Effect of alkalinization on nephrotoxicity; pharmacokinetics in the CNS; and use of CNS non-Hodgkin's lymphoma. *Cancer Treat Rep* 61:695, 1977.

86. Polinsky MS, Kaiser BA, Baluarte HJ: Urolithiasis in childhood. *Pediatr Clin North Am* 34:683, 1987.

87. Ponticelli C, Zucchelli P, Banfi G, et al: Treatment of diffuse proliferative lupus nephritis by intravenous high dose methylprednisolone. *Q J Med* 51:16, 1982.

88. Rieselbach RE, Garnick MB: Renal diseases induced by antineoplastic agents. *In* Schrier RW, Gottschalk CV (eds): *Diseases of the Kidney.* Boston, Little, Brown, 1988, p 1275.

89. Rifle G: Therapy of idiopathic acute crescentic glomerulonephritis by immunosuppression and plasma exchange. *Eur Dial Transpl Assoc* 18:493, 1980.

90. Rigden SP, Barratt TM, Dillon MJ, et al: Acute renal failure complicating cardiopulmonary bypass surgery. *Arch Dis Child* 57:425, 1982.

91. Rigden SP, Barratt TM, Dillon MJ, et al: The beneficial effect of mannitol on post-operative renal function in chil-

dren undergoing cardiopulmonary bypass surgery. *Clin Nephrol* 21:148, 1984.

92. Ron D, Taitelman U, Michaelson M, et al: Prevention of acute renal failure in traumatic rhabdomyolysis. *Arch Intern Med* 144:277, 1984.

93. Salant DJ, Ader S, Bernard DB, et al: Acute renal failure associated with renal vascular disease, vasculitis, glomerulonephritis and nephrotic syndrome. *In* Brenner BM, Lazarus JM (eds): *Acute Renal Failure.* Boston, Little, Brown, 1988, p 371.

94. Schafferhans K, Heidbreder E, Grimm D, et al: Norepinephrine-induced acute renal failure: Beneficial effects of atrial natriuretic factor. *Nephron* 44:240, 1986.

95. Schilsky RL: Renal and metabolic toxicities of cancer chemotherapy. *Semin Oncol* 9:75, 1982.

96. Schulte-Wisserman H, Straub E, Funke P: Influence of L-thyroxin upon enzymatic reactivity in the renal tubular epithelia of the rat under normal conditions and in mercuryinduced lesions. *Virchows Arch [B]* 23:163, 1977.

97. Shaw SG, Weidmann P, Hodler J, et al: Atrial natriuretic peptide protects against acute ischemic renal failure in the rat. *J Clin Invest* 80:1232, 1987.

98. Siegel NJ, Gaudio KM, Katz LA, et al: Beneficial effect of thyroxin on recovery from toxic acute renal failure. *Kidney Int* 25:906, 1984.

99. Siegler RL: Management of hemolytic-uremic syndrome. *J Pediatr* 112:1014, 1988.

100. Siegler RL, Bond RE, Morris AH: Treatment of Goodpasture's syndrome with plasma exchange and immunosuppression. *Clin Pediatr* 19:488, 1980.

101. Silva FG: Overview of pediatric nephropathology. *Kidney Int* 33:1016, 1988.

102. Smithson WA, Benson RC: Tumors: Lower genitourinary tract. *In* Williams DI, Johnston JH (eds): *Clinical Pediatric Urology.* London, Butterworths, 1985, p 1189.

103. Straub E: Einfluss von Thyroxin auf den Verlauf des akuten Nierenversagen. I. Einfluss der L-Thyroxin-Applikation auf die Letalität von Kaninchen und Mausen mit manifestem akutem Nierenversagen. *Z Ges Exp Med* 154:177, 1971.

104. Straub E II: Einfluss der L-Thyroxin-Applikation auf Plasmaspiegel und renale Ausscheidung verschiedener Substanzen bei Kaninchen mit manifestem akutem Nierenversagen. *Z Ges Exp Med* 154:32, 1971.

105. Straub E III: Einfluss der L-Thyroxin-Applikation auf die Glomerulumfiltration, den effektiven Nierenplasmastrom und die tubulare Sekretions-und Rückresportions-Kapazität von Kaninchen mit toxischem Nierenschaden. *Z Ges Exp Med* 155:56, 1971.

106. Straub E: Effects of L-thyroxin in acute renal failure. *Res Exp Med (Berl)* 168:81, 1976.

107. Straub E: Influences of thyroid hormones on kidney function. *In* Hesch RD (ed): *The Low T₃ Syndrome.* London, Academic, 1981, p 153.

108. Sutter PM, Thulin G, Stromski M, et al: Beneficial effect of thyroxin in the treatment of ischemic acute renal failure. *Pediatr Nephr* 2:1, 1988.

109. Toledo-Peyrera LH, Simmons RL, Najarian JS: Clinical effect of allopurinol on preserved kidneys: A randomized double-blind study. *Ann Surg* 185:128, 1977.

110. Trompeter RS: A review of drug prescribing in children with end-stage renal failure. *Pediat Nephrol* 1:183, 1987.

111. Tsokos GC, Balow JE, Spiegel RJ, et al: Renal and metabolic complications of undifferentiated and lymphoblastic lymphomas. *Med* 60:218, 1981.

112. VanEs LA, Kauffmann RH, Valentijn RM: Renal manifestations of systemic disease. A. Henoch-Schönlein Purpura.

In Holliday MA, Barratt TM, Vernier RL (eds): *Pediatric Nephrology,* 2nd ed. Baltimore, Williams & Wilkins, p 492, 1986.

113. Verrier Jones J, Cummings RH, Bacon PA, et al: Evidence for a therapeutic effect of plasmapheresis in patients with serum lupus erythematosus. *Q J Med* 48:555, 1979.

114. Wait RB, White G, Davis JH: Beneficial effects of verapamil on postischemic renal failure. *Surg* 94:276, 1983.

115. Weidmann P, Saxenhofer H, Ferrier C, et al: Atrial natriuretic peptide in man. *Am J Nephrol* 8:1, 1988.

116. Yeh TF, Wilks A, Singh J, et al: Furosemide prevents the renal side-effects of indomethacin therapy in preterm infants with patent ductus arteriosus. *J Pediatr* 101:433, 1982.

117. Zager RA: Hypoperfusion-induced acute renal failure in the rat: An evaluation of oxidant tissue injury. *Circ Res* 62:430, 1988.

Robert A. Weiss

38
Dietary and Pharmacologic Treatment of Chronic Renal Failure

Chronic renal failure (CRF) is defined as a permanent reduction in glomerular filtration rate (GFR) of at least two standard deviations below normal for age. The biological implications of a progressive decline in GFR involve virtually all organ systems, often in a geometric fashion as the patient approaches end-stage renal disease (ESRD). The complications of progressive renal failure in infants and children, such as anorexia and metabolic bone disease, produce unique problems in terms of growth and development. Maintenance of solute, water, hydrogen ion, and mineral homeostasis, as well as proper nutrition, require specialized expertise to minimize the deleterious and predictable consequences of CRF, especially when its onset is during infancy. Astute conservative management during this critical period of infancy and early childhood has implications that may profoundly affect the quality as well as the quantity of life for the affected child.

It is the aim of this chapter to outline the principles of management of these disturbances in homeostasis and to provide specific recommendations regarding the nature and timing of therapeutic interventions. Special attention is directed toward new developments in nutritional therapy to maximize linear growth in infants with CRF, alteration in the rate of progressive renal insufficiency by dietary modification (experimental and clinical), prevention of neurodevelopmental deficits, and prophylactic therapy for renal osteodystrophy.

Nutrition

There is little doubt that the growth retardation seen in many infants and children with CRF, even in the presence of obvious renal osteodystrophy [39], may be minimized by proper, aggressive nutritional management. While Betts and McGrath [10] concluded that growth velocity declines when the GFR falls below 25 ml/min/1.73m^2, further work by Betts and White [11] established that delay in skeletal maturation and, thus, growth retardation is most marked in those whose CRF had its onset during infancy, unrelated to the magnitude of reduction in GFR. In a series of 47 patients with GFR less than 80 ml/min/1.73m^2, Hodson et

al. [39] found only four children whose height was less than minus two standard deviations (SD) relative to bone age. These authors demonstrated that there was no significant difference in the percentage of patients with bone histopathology between those with height less than 2 SD below the mean and those with height greater than 2 SD above the mean. This evidence suggests that renal osteodystrophy does not play a significant role in growth retardation of CRF, at least when the GFR is less than 20 ml/min/1.73m^2.

Kleinknecht et al. [49] and Rizzoni et al. [68] demonstrated that while linear height or length was often below normal at the time of diagnosis of CRF, growth velocity during the follow-up period was usually normal. These observations, as well as those summarized by Wassner et al [84], have directed the thrust of medical management toward nutrition in infants and young children with CRF, including the use of nasogastric tube feeding to deliver sufficient nutrients.

While there is evidence that the energy and/or protein cost of growth is increased in experimental uremia [59], it appers that only the recommended daily allowance (RDA) for calories is required to sustain a normal growth velocity in infants with CRF [68]. Therefore, the limiting factor in the achievement of normal growth may be the delivery and absorption of adequate calories. This can be a formidable task in infants and young children with CRF whose spontaneous intake is usually below the RDA, presumably due to the anorectic effect of uremia, although gastroesophageal reflux recently has been shown to be a common feature of feeding problems in these infants [71]. The salutary effect of caloric supplementation on growth velocity in children on dialysis was clearly demonstrated by Simmons et al [78]. More recently, Arnold et al [5] have shown in a crossover study that caloric supplementation resulted in an increase in energy intake from 73% to 103% of normal, commensurate with an increase in growth velocity from 59% to 90% of that expected. Catch-up growth was not seen.

Given the role of proper nutrition in the management of the infant or child with CRF, one must possess the tools to assess nutritional status, both initially and sequentially, such that therapeutic interventions may be appropriately interpreted. A renal dietitian with pediatric experience is invaluable in this regard. Dietary intake should be recorded prospectively by the parents or caretakers for a minimum of three days. Use of standard tables of food comparison or the appropriate computer program [67] will yield exact nutrient intake, both in absolute terms and as a percentage of RDA (Table 38-1). Only in this manner can a proper diagnosis be made regarding possible deficit of nutrients.

Anthropometric measurements such as skin fold thickness at the triceps and subscapular sites, mid-arm muscle circumferences, and weight-for-height index are often useful in guiding nutritional therapy. Biochemical measures, such as serum transferrin and serum albumin [43], rarely provide additional information regarding the adequacy of protein intake.

Energy

Approximately 10% to 15% of total caloric intake is directed toward growth; thus, the greater the energy intake in excess of that required for maintenance metabolism, the less the risk of insufficient energy for growth. The concept of RDA is merely a crude guide to mean energy and nutrient intake among the healthy pediatric population. There is no evidence that one can achieve supranormal growth velocity by exceeding RDA for energy and, in fact, obesity may result [17]. However, the supply of sufficient energy to meet RDA may present a difficult challenge.

During infancy and the preschool years, the diet is almost exclusively controlled by the parent, and the physician can presribe precisely its volume and composition. Anorexia can be circumvented by nasogastric tube feeding, either on an intermittent (overnight) or 24-hour schedule through an infusion pump. This should not be considered a technique of last resort, but should be employed as soon as it is established that conventional feeding methods are unable to meet energy and nutrient needs for the infant or child with CRF. While provision of RDA energy intake will not guarantee normal linear growth [5], energy intake of less than 70% to 80% RDA will almost certainly be associated with growth regardation [10].

The distribution of energy may be calculated by prescribing protein intake for height age, but no more than 10% to 11% of total energy intake [82]. The remaining calories comprise carbohydrate (50% to 75%) and fat (at least 20%). In addition, 3% of total energy should be in the form of essential polyunsaturated fatty acids.

Caloric supplementation is most easily accomplished with the use of high caloric density carbohydrate preparations (Table 38-2). These products have the advantage of relatively low osmolality, thus reducing the risk of osmotic diarrhea. To supplement fat intake, one may prescribe MCT oil with a caloric density of 7.7 kcal/ml. Corn or safflower oil contains 8 kcal/ml. Butter may be added liberally to all foodstuffs. However, excessive fat intake may be associated with hyperlipidemia. Caloric density of infant formulas may be gradually increased to 24 or even 30 kcal/oz according to gastrointestinal tolerance. Volume is rarely a limiting factor with GFR above 10 ml/min/1.73m². Beyond infancy, caloric supplements may be added in powder form to table foods.

Protein

Protein malnutrition may occur during the course of CRF, especially when total energy intake is insufficient due to anorexia or persistent nephrotic syndrome [49]. Supplemental protein may be supplied from a choice of several commercially available products (see Table 38-2).

TABLE 38-1. *Recommended daily allowances for children with chronic renal insufficiency**

Age	Height (cm)	Energy (kcals)	Minimal Protein (gm)	Calcium (gm)	Phosphorus (gm)
0–2 months	55	120/kg	2.2/kg	0.4	0.2
2–6 months	63	110/kg	2.0/kg	0.5	0.4
6–12 months	72	100/kg	1.8/kg	0.6	0.5
1–2 years	81	1100	18	0.7	0.7
2–4 years	96	1300	22	0.8	0.8
4–6 years	110	1600	29	0.9	0.9
6–8 years	121	2000	29	0.9	0.9
8–10 years	131	2200	31	1.0	1.0
10–12 years	141	2450	36	1.2	1.2
12–14 years M	151	2700	40	1.4	1.4
12–14 years F	154	2300	34	1.3	1.3
14–18 years M	170	3000	45	1.4	1.4
14–18 years F	159	2350	35	1.3	1.3
18–22 years M	175	2800	42	0.8	0.8
18–22 years F	163	2200	33	0.8	0.8

* At least 25% of total energy should be provided by carbohydrate (normal children take about 50% total energy as carbohydrate), and at least 3% of total energy should be in the form of essential polyunsaturated fatty acids. An adequate vitamin and trace element intake must be given. Sodium and potassium intake will depend on renal function but, for normal children, an intake of 1.5 to 2.5 mmol/kg body weight per day (2 mg to 3 mg) is recommended. Chantler C: Nutritional assessment and management of children with renal insufficiency. *In* Fine R, Gruskin AB (eds): *End Stage Renal Disease in Children.* Philadelphia, WB Saunders, 1984, p 198.

Table 38-2. *Infant formulas and nutritional supplements*

	kcal/ml	Osmolality mOsm/kg H_2O	Protein gm/L	Fat gm/L	CHO gm/L
Infant Formulas					
PM 60/40 (Ross)	0.68	260	16	38	69
SMA (Wyeth)	0.68	300	15	36	72
S 29 (Wyeth)	0.68	*	17	23	101
Milk, cow	0.65	288	35	35	48
Milk, human	0.73	300	11	45	71
Carbohydrate Modules					
Corn syrup	3.9	*	0	9	1008
Polycose (Ross)	2 (4/g)	850	0	0	500
Controlyte (Doyle)	2 (5/g)	598	0	96	286
Sumacal (Organon)	(4/g)	*	0	0	95/100 g
Protein Modules					
Casec (Mead-Johnson)	(4/g)	*	88/100 g	2/100 g	0
Pro-Mix (Nubro, Inc.)	(4/g)	*	85/100 g	0	9/100 g
Propac (Organon)	(4/g)	*	78/100 g	8/100 g	5/100 g
Electrodialyzed Whey (Wyeth)	(4/g)	*	35/100 g	3/100 g	56/100 g
Fat Modules					
MCT Oil (Mead-Johnson)	7.7	*	0	858	0
Vegetable oil, corn	8.0	*	0	898	0
Essential Amino Acid Supplements					
Aminaid (McGaw)	1.9	1095	19	46	366
Travasorb Renal (Travenol)	1.35	590	23	18	271
Calories/Protein Supplements					
Ensure (Ross)	1.0	450	37	37	145
Sustacal (Mead-Johnson)	1.0	625	61	23	140

Nelson P, Stover, J: Principles of nutritional assessment and management of the child with ESRD. *In* Fine R, Gruskin AB (eds): *End Stage Renal Disease in Children.* Philadelphia, WB Saunders, 1984, p 214.
* Information not available.

Total protein intake often exceeds RDA [31,43] and is well tolerated. Rarely does total protein intake require restriction because of gastrointestinal symptoms prior to the need for dialysis. The iatrogenic production of a state of protein malnutrition simply to delay the inevitable requirement for dialysis is to be discouraged. The role of restricted protein intake in the amelioration of progressive renal insufficiency is discussed below.

The protein provided to the infant or child with CRF should be at least 70% of high biological value (HBV), i.e., protein that contains all essential amino acids (including histidine, which is essential in uremia) in a concentration proportional to its RDA [3]. The highest biological value is found in egg protein. Milk, meat, fish, and fowl also contain HBV protein, with cereal and vegetable proteins having lower biological values. For adult males, the recommended minimum HBV protein intake is 37 g, with a protein to energy ratio of 1.9 g/100 kcal; for adult females, 29 g and 1.6 g/100 kcal, respectively [30]. In adults with uremia, whether on a diet of HBV protein or on low quality protein supplemented with essential amino acids [34], protein balance did not become negative even with a ratio of 1.5 g/100 kcal, providing that the total caloric intake was adequate. Such a diet, effectively eliminating

vegetables, pasta, rice, bread, cookies, and cake, is extremely difficult to sustain in chilren with CRF, due to anorexia and social and cultural factors. In seven children with CRF studied over a six-month interval, Jones et al. [43] were able to use a nutritional program composed of non-selected protein supplemented with essential amino acids, with a protein to energy ratio of 1.25 g/100 kcal. Blood urea concentration declined dramatically, nitrogen balance remained positive, plasma transferrin concentrations and weight for height ratios were maintained, but true catch-up linear growth was not demonstrated. Equally important was the observation that the dietary prescription could not be sustained, and the actual diet consumed at the end of the study period had a mean protein to energy ratio of 1.9 g/100 kcal. Similar results were observed by Sigstrom et al. [77] without formal nitrogen balance studies. Abitol and Holliday [1] examined urea nitrogen production in a series of uremic children receiving overnight intravenous infusions of dextrose and essential amino acids. They demonstrated that urea nitrogen production was inversely proportional to energy intake and that energy intakes of less than 60 kcal/kg/day were associated with negative nitrogen balance (nitrogen intake less than urea nitrogen production).

Recently, the Southwest Pediatric Nephrology Study Group proposed that to sustain a normal weight velocity of 3 g/kg/day to 4 g/kg/day, infants should receive 1.4 g/kg/day of dietary protein [82].

An alternative dietary approach has been the use of nitrogen-free alpha-keto acid and alpha hydroxy acid analogues. Jones et al. [43] studied seven children with a mean GFR of 9 ml/min/1.73m². They received the RDA of total protein intake for height age, with 20% administered as an essential amino acid/keto acid supplement. Total energy intake was maintained at RDA for height age by the use of a glucose polymer. The authors demonstrated that when such nutritional therapy was administered for periods of up to one year, growth velocity increased significantly (less so when compared to bone age, i.e., catch-up growth). However, no difference in body composition, as measured by total body water and extracellular volume, was noted. Nitrogen retention was demonstrated, and plasma urea and phosphate concentrations declined. Plasma calcium increased, and immunoreactive PTH concentrations fell. GFR did not change. The plasma amino acid profile was not altered significantly. These investigators concluded that nitrogen-free keto analogues of essential amino acids, when compared to essential amino acids alone, allowed a greater intake of nonessential amino acids and, thus, a more liberal, palatable diet. However, a study by Giordano et al. [35], using a more severe restriction of total protein intake, found negative nitrogen balance in six children with CRF, but improved nitrogen balance when keto analogues were removed from the formulation. Of greater interest was their observation in two uremic infants that growth was worse with keto acid compared to an essential amino acid supplement.

Broyer et al. [14] fed six infants with advanced CRF isocaloric diets with three different sources of protein intake: diet A, human milk only; diet B, human milk plus essential amino acids; diet C, human milk plus alpha keto and hydroxy analogues of essential amino acids. If analogues were not available for certain essential amino acids, the standard essential amino acid preparation was used. Total protein intake was equal in all three diets. Urea nitrogen appearance rate to nitrogen intake was used to estimate nitrogen balance. The salient findings were that diet C yielded the largest decrement in BUN and the lowest urea nitrogen appearance rate. However, the actual difference between urea nitrogen appearance rate and nitrogen intake was also lowest with this diet, and weight gain was least. The greatest weight gain was observed with diet B.

Thus, there is insufficient evidence to recommend the keto analogues of essential amino acids in the non-dialytic management of CRF in infants and children. In fact, there appears to be little reason to deviate from the historical dietary protein prescription of at least RDA [57,58], preferably with 70% derived from high biologic value protein.

Nutritional Intervention to Modify the Rate of Progressive Renal Insufficiency

Klahr et al. [48] summarized the experimental evidence that nutritional factors can affect the rate of progression of CRF. Numerous historical studies have demonstrated that high protein intakes—often uncorrected for the higher sodium, phosphorus, and calcium content of such diets—accelerate the progression of CRF of experimental nephritis, ablation, and aging. More recent investigations by Ichikawa et al. [42] have revealed that glomerular capillary plasma flow rate and the ultrafiltration coefficient (K_f) are inversely proportional to the protein intake. These findings have been extended by Brenner and co-workers [13] to a general hypothesis in which the progressive glomerular sclerosis observed in many forms of renal injury is secondary to glomerular hyperfiltration and intra-glomerular hypertension, conditions that can be ameliorated experimentally by reducing dietary protein intake. Ibels et al. [41], using the rat remnant kidney model of uremia, hypothesized that hyperphosphatemia results in calcification of the remnant renal parenchyma, thus accelerating further nephron loss. They demonstrated that both GFR, renal histology, and tissue calcium content were maintained when the experimental rats were given a diet depleted in phosphorus. Protein intake was identical to that of control rats. While this particular experimental model may not apply to human forms of progressive CRF, the results of this study must be noted when one interprets the findings of clinical trials of low protein diets, which are necessarily low in phosphorus.

In contrast, Laourie et al. [53], using a similar ablation model, found that rats fed a diet markedly deficient in phosphorus had severe anorexia, growth arrest, and hypophosphatemic rickets. They attributed the stabilization of declining GFR to decreased total nutrient intake and not phosphorus depletion alone. Karlinsky et al. [45] examined the role of PTH in the apparent protective effect of a low phosphorus diet. While thyroparathyroidectomy was successful in ameliorating the progressive fall in GFR of this ablation model, selective parathyroidectomy was not. Thyroid supplementation in the former group of rats was associated with progressive uremia.

Mitch et al. [64] reported treatment of 24 adults, of whom 17 had a well defined rate of progression of uremia, with a diet low in phosphorus (less than 600 mg) and low in protein (20g to 30 g, mixed quality), supplemented with essential amino acids and their keto analogues. Ten of these 17 patients had a significant decrement in the slope of time versus the reciprocal of serum creatinine [63]. Within this group, seven patients began this nutritional therapy with serum creatinine values of less than 8 mg/dl; six of these had a positive response. Nitrogen balance remained positive, and biochemical indices of nutrition remained normal. However, this important study lacked a control group, and the authors were unable to provide specific evidence for the beneficial role of keto analogues beyond that of the low phosphorus, low protein intake.

Alverstrand et al. [2] examined the effect of low protein diet supplemented with either essential amino acids (14 patients) or their keto analogues (3 patients) in a retrospective survey of their adult CRF patients, with sufficient observation time prior to and following institution of the diet. Protein intake was only 15g to 30 g and phosphorus intake was 300 mg to 400 mg. Similar to Mitch's study, the sample size was small, and there was no control group. The slope of the regression line describing the relationship between the reciprocal of serum creatinine and time decreased significantly.

Maschio et al. [56] used a diet containing 0.6 g/kg of protein (75 percent high biologic value), 700 mg phosphorus, and 40 kcal/kg energy intake in a series of 45 adults with serum creatinine values of 1.55 mg/dl to 5.4 mg/dl (mean 3.2). A control group of 30 patients, with a mean serum creatinine of 2.3 mg/dl, received no specific dietary regimen; their estimated intakes from dietary recall were 70 g of protein, 900 mg of phosphorus, and 35 kcal/kg. A similar proportion of patients in each group was hypertensive. The duration of follow-up averaged 48 months in the experimental group and 24 months in the control group. These investigators demonstrated that the rate of deterioration of GFR, as estimated by the slope of the regression line of the reciprocal of serum creatinine versus time, was twice as rapid in the control group. In an extension of this work [66], they examined the rate of progression among patients with chronic glomerulonephritis ($n = 33$), polycystic kidney disease ($n = 17$), and chronic pyelonephritis ($n = 28$). In all three groups, the rate of progression was less with the reduced intake of protein and phosphorus described above, when compared to controls within the same diagnostic group but without dietary manipulation. The mean duration of follow-up was 44, 42, and 41 months, respectively; 57%, 41%, and 68% of patients in each diagnostic group had no progression of functional deterioration during the period of observation.

Gretz et al. [38] prospectively evaluated the effect of low protein diet, supplemented with keto analogues of essential amino acids, on the rate of progression of serum creatinine from 6 mg/dl to 10 mg/dl in a population of 138 adults. The experimental group ($n = 31$) received 30 g of protein plus keto acids, while the control group received no dietary instruction. No details were provided by the authors as to selection criteria for the experimental versus control group. When patients with glomerulonephritis, polycystic kidney disease, and pyelonephritis/interstitial nephritis were examined separately, the delay in progression of CRF was apparent in each group.

An additional controlled trial of dietary protein restriction by Rosman et al. [70] included 228 adults with CRF. Stratification was undertaken for age, sex, and GFR (10 ml/min/1.73m^2 to 30 ml/min/1.73m^2, versus 31 ml/min/1.73m^2 to 60 ml/min/1.73m^2). Patients were randomly allocated to 0.4 g/kg/day protein intake in the lower GFR group, and 0.6 g/kg/day protein intake in the higher GFR group. A total of 149 patients had follow-up of at least 18 months. Dietary protein restriction reduced the median rate of progression by threefold to fivefold. No adverse effects, either clinical or biochemical, were observed in the low protein patients. However, acceptance of the diet was a frequent problem, and intensive nutritional counseling was considered an essential component of the program. While the term "low protein" diet suggests an abnormally low protein intake, the WHO has established 0.5 g/kg/day as a safe minimum intake for healthy adults, providing energy intake is adequate.

Giovanetti [36] reviewed the Italian experience with dietary therapy in patients with CRF. As with any form of medical management, he concluded that patient selection is of paramount importance. Contraindications include (1) uremia so far advanced that anorexia and vomiting preclude adequate energy intake; (2) extra-renal complications of uremia, such as pericarditis or peripheral neuropathy; (3) severe proteinuria; and (4) absence of motivation to delay renal replacement therapy and/or willingness to alter dietary habits.

In addition to slowing the progression of CRF, Barsotti et al. [7] claimed improvement in secondary hyperparathyroidism when dietary protein intake was reduced from 0.6 g/kg/day (primarily high biologic value) to 0.3 g/kg/day (all of vegetable origin) with supplemental essential amino acids and their keto analogues to meet nitrogen needs. The usual phosphorus intake of 10 mg/kg/day to 12 mg/kg/day in the former, can be further reduced to 6 mg/kg/day to 7 mg/kg/day with dialysis of dietary meat, fish, rice, and potatoes. Such a rigorous artificial diet has been demonstrated to reduce serum PTH concentrations, coincident with a rise in serum calcium and fall in serum phosphate. The inability to maintain serum phosphate in the normal range has been an indication for transfer from the conventional low protein-low phosphorus diet to the one described above. In addition, these same investigators have demonstrated that this diet is associated with a further decline in the rate of progression of renal failure.

Despite the rather impressive evidence that a low protein—and low phosphorus—diet will slow the rate of progression of CRF provided that energy intake is adequate, there has been little published support for this treatment modality in the United States. A multicenter controlled clinical trial [47] is now underway to test three primary hypotheses related to diet and progressive renal failure: (1) that a low protein-low phosphorus diet will retard the rate of progressive renal failure, (2) such a diet will not cause malnutrition, and (3) such a diet will be acceptable to patients over the long term. Patients with GRF 25 ml/min/1.73m^2 to 55 ml/min/1.73m^2 will be randomized into moderate versus low protein-low phosphorus with identical BP goals (study A). A second group of patients with GFR 13 ml/min/1.73m^2 to 24 ml/min/1.73m^2 will be randomized to either low protein-low phosphorus or very low protein and phosphorus with a supplemental mixture of essential amino acids and keto acid analogues. Preliminary observations from a pilot study have revealed substantial design flaws. Serum creatinine was demonstrated to correlate poorly with true GFR, casting doubt on its validity in slope calculations to assess the rate of progression of renal failure. Compliance with the diets has generally been poor. Blood pressure control has appeared as a dominant factor in preservation of GFR, while the effect of diet has not been detected in the pilot study.

Despite the generally impressive results of low protein-low phosphorus diets in Europe, Giovanetti notes that many physicians are reluctant to prescribe dramatic alterations in the dietary habits of their patients, and there is great pessimism concerning the palatability of and compliance with such a regimen. In addition, the physician's time and effort must be more intense than that required for maintenance dialysis, a nursing procedure. Finally, the reimbursement system in the United States provides economic incentive to initiate maintenance dialysis for more and more CRF patients, despite the fact that many of them can be appropriately managed with dietary therapy.

The optimal diet for infants and children that might preserve GFR must also allow for sufficient nutrients to sustain somatic and brain growth [33]. A two-year feasibility study has recently been completed by the members of the Southwest Pediatric Nephrology Study Group to address the proper design of a clinical trial to test the hypotheses that (1) a low protein diet in children 6 months to 18 months with GFR <50 ml/min/1.73 m^2 will slow the progression of renal insufficiency and (2) such a diet will support normal growth and development. The control group received 100% to 120% RDA calories for length with a protein composing 10.4% of total energy, compared to 5.6% in the experimental group. The preliminary results of the study failed to show significant decrement in GFR in either treatment group.

Vitamins and Trace Elements

Vitamin deficiency may develop consequent to the general decline in nutrient intake due to anorexia or dietary restrictions. Boiling of foodstuffs to dialyze out potassium and phosphorus may also deplete nutrients of water soluble vitamins of the B complex group.

Only vitamin B6 (pyridoxine) is recognized to be deficient in patients with CRF [80]. It contributes to immunological competence [25], amino acid and fatty acid metabolism, and neurologic function. All CRF patients should receive at least 10 mg/day of pyridoxine hydrochloride. Folic acid deficiency, as measured by serum or RBC folate concentration, even prior to the onset of dialysis, is described and can be prevented by daily supplementation with 1 mg [51]. Iron supplementation is not routinely indicated, as iron absorption is normal, and the anemia of CRF is not responsive. Zinc deficiency has been implicated in the etiology of the anorexia, impaired taste acuity, and poor growth associated with CRF. Measurement of zinc stores in various tissues were reported to be increased [73], while plasma zinc concentration was decreased in another study [81]. Zinc supplementation for children with CRF improved taste acuity and appetite, but did not improve growth velocity [26].

A well balanced diet, with adequate intake of essential nutrients, will obviate the need for routine supplementation of vitamins (except B6), iron, and zinc. However, for those infants and children with suboptimal intake due to anorexia, or those with drastic dietary restrictions, a standard commercially available multivitamin supplement with iron is appropriate.

Aluminum hydroxide has been used routinely to bind dietary phosphorus intake. Since infants derive much of their nutrition from milk, phosphorous intake is high, and correspondingly large doses of phosphorous binding antacids are required to prevent or treat hyperphosphatemia. The recognition of the toxic effects of aluminum in uremic patients has led to a severe restriction in their use.

A search for alternative phosphorous binding agents has not been particularly fruitful, although calcium carbonate in large doses, usually 4 g/day to 10 g/day, is effective [54,72]. Each 650-mg (10-grain) tablet contains 250 mg of elemental calcium, and at 40% is the most potent of the calcium supplements. In addition, each tablet binds 7.5 mEq of gastric HCl. The liquid preparation contains 1000 mg of calcium carbonate/5 ml (400 mg of elemental calcium).

The management of infants and young children with CRF should not include the use of aluminum-containing antacids. Dietary counselling should be available to eliminate sources of excessive dietary phosphorous, and the use of a low phosphorous milk, such as SMA, S29, or PM 60/40 should be encouraged. However, the latter has recently been found to have a high aluminum content and has been implicated in the etiology of encephalopathy in infants with CRF receiving this product [32].

Maintenance of Fluid and Electrolyte Homeostasis

As the population of functioning nephrons declines, their ability to regulate solute and water balance becomes more restricted (Chap. 26). External stresses, such as acute water or electrolyte loading or depletion, are poorly tolerated. Polydipsia and polyuria are common with advanced CRF of any etiology. However, when GFR is very low, water intoxication may occur from rapid infusion of solute free intravenous fluids.

Sodium

Sodium restriction to less than the usual maintenance requirement of 1 mEq/kg/day to 3 mEq/kg/day is indicated in the management of edema due to nephrotic syndrome or hypertension. In the adult, avoidance of table salt, prepared meats, and, obviously salty foods will reduce dietry sodium intake to approximately 2 g (80 mEq). Consultation with a renal dietitian is advised to ferret out more obscure sources of dietary sodium. Despite good intentions, such a regimen is difficult to maintain, and diuretic therapy may be needed to restore sodium balance (Table 38-3). Furosemide is almost always successful, providing the oral dose is high enough (up to 4 mg/kg/dose) [83]. Combination therapy using high doses of furosemide and usual doses of hydrochlorothiazide has recently been demonstrated to be effective in hypertensive, azotemic patients who are resistant to either drug alone [86]. Metalozone [23,27], 2.5 mg for pre-school-age children and 5 mg for school-age children, or bumetanide [85], 0.5 mg and 1.0 mg, respectively, may be added when a more dramatic natriuresis is necessary. As discussed above, the relationship between GFR and extracellular volume is maintained even in the patient with CRF, and contraction of the extracellular fluid space by diuretic therapy will uniformly result in an acute, but reversible fall in GFR.

During an acute illness, in which either intake is reduced or excessive electrolyte losses occur, extracellular volume contraction may develop rapidly, with a consequent albeit

Table 38-3. *Commonly used medications in the infant and child with CRF*

Indication	Therapy	Dose
ECF volume contraction ± hyponatremia	Na supplementation	up to 5–10 mEq/kg divided tid or qid
ECF volume expansion (edema)	dietary Na restriction + diuretic Rx	
—mild to moderate	hydrochlorothiazide	1–2 mg/kg/day divided bid
—moderate to severe	furosemide	up to 8 mg/kg/day divided bid
	metalazone	5 mg bid for school-age children
		2.5 mg bid for pre–school-age children
	bumetanide	1.0 mg bid for school-age children
		0.5 mg bid for pre–school-age children
Metabolic Acidosis	NaHCO₃	2–3 mg/kg/day divided tid or qid, increase until normal plsma HCO₃ concentration
	Bicitra	2–3 ml/kg/day divided tid or qid, increase until normal plasma HCO₃ concentration
Prevention or treatment of renal osteodystrophy	Vitamin D metabolites	
	− DHT (dihydrotachysterol)	15 μg/kg/day, given once daily as either Hytakerol (0.25 mg/ml) or DHT tablets of 0.1 or 0.2 mg
	− 25 OH vitamin D₃ (calcifediol)	1–2 μg/kg/day given once daily
	− 1,25 (OH₂) vitamin D₃ (calcitriol) (OH)₂	15 ng/kg/day given daily or divided bid

reversible fall in GFR. Tubulo-interstitial diseases are often characterized by defects in salt and water conservation out of proportion to the compromise in GFR. Congenital renal and urologic maldevelopment syndromes, such as hypoplasia, dysplasia, and obstructive uropathy, typically produce a "salt wasting" state. Infants with such diseases, who may not have the same free access to fluids as do older children, are often at risk for dehydration during an intercurrent illness. Such patients frequently require 5 mEq/kg/day to 10 mEq/kg/day of extra sodium and up to 150 ml/kg/day of fluids to maintain extracellular volume; in contrast to patients with acquired glomerulopathies, they are rarely hypertensive.

Potassium

Regulation of potassium homeostasis is usually preserved until CRF is far advanced. Measurement of total body potassium [62] has usually yielded normal or low values. Poor nutrition, especially protein depletion, may account for the latter [9,50]. Bilbrey et al [12] demonstrated that a state of intracellular potassium depletion exists in uremic patients, which improves with the onset of maintenance dialysis. Despite evidence of low total body potassium stores, some patients with CRF have hyperkalemia with a hyperchloremic metabolic acidosis out of proportion to the magnitude of their reduction in GFR. Initially described as hyporeninemic hypoaldosteronism in elderly patients with diabetes mellitus, it is now recognized in patients with CRF of diverse etiologies [76]. Administration of 2 mEq/kg/day to 5 mEq/kg/day of bicarbonate and 0.5 mg/day of

9-alpha fluorohydrocortisone is effective in normalizing plasma potassium and bicarbonate concentrations. One mg/kg/day to 2 mg/kg/day of furosemide will also normalize the electrolyte pattern.

The limitation of the end-stage kidney to excrete a potassium load is of great significance. Potassium intoxication can be produced by inadvertent administration of excess potassium in drugs or intravenous fluids. Treatment of acute hyperkalemia in the CRF patient is not different from that in acute renal failure (see Chapter 37).

Management of Metabolic Acidosis

The maintenance of hydrogen ion homeostasis, similar to that of electrolytes, becomes compromised as CRF progresses, and the nephron population diminishes (Chap. 27). The role of chronic metabolic acidosis in growth failure and development of bone disease in uremic patients is discussed in Chapters 25 and 28, respectively.

Correction of metabolic acidosis requires provision of enough alkali to buffer endogenous hydrogen ion production, plus replacement of bicarbonate lost in the urine. The customary initial therapy is 2 mEq/kg/day to 3 mEq/kg/day in divided doses, increased as necessary to bring the plasma bicarbonate concentration within the normal range. One 10-grain (650-mg) tablet of sodium bicarbonate provides 7.7 mEq of bicarbonate, while one teaspoon of baking soda supplies about 3.7 g or 44 mEq. Alternatively, citrate may be chosen as a bicarbonate precursor. Shohl's solution or its USP formulation, Bicitra, consists of 70 g citric acid (for palatability), plus 50 g sodium citrate, qs 500 ml water to provide an alkali concentration of 1 mEq/ml.

Management of Disordered Divalent Ion Homeostasis

During the development of progressive renal insufficiency, several pathophysiologic events ensue that result in defective bone mineralization and secondary hyperparathyroidism, collectively known as renal osteodystrophy. The details of the pathogenesis of this extremely common manifestation of CRF in infants and children are reviewed in Chapter 28. The purpose of this section is to provide the physician with rational guidelines for effective prevention and therapy of this disorder. The cornerstones of nondialytic management of CRF involve restoring the plasma concentrations of calcitriol, calcium, and phosphorous to normal. Achievement of these goals should result in the prevention of renal osteodystrophy.

Vitamin D therapy may take several forms. The administration of vitamin D_2 is to be discouraged, as the therapeutic window between the proper dose (one that produces normocalcemia) and the toxic dose (resulting in hypercalcemia) is small. In addition, since this preparation is highly lipophilic, it remains in adipose tissue for weeks to months [24]. Thus, when it is discontinued due to hypercalcemia, the effect is prolonged [15].

Dihydrotachysterol (DHT) has been available for several decades. While its use for the prevention and treatment of renal osteodystrophy is widespread, published experience with its use in infants and children with CRF is limited [55]. The biological activity of this compound resides in a 3-OH group that is free to rotate to form a pseudo 1-alpha-OH group. 25-hydroxylation in the liver results in 25-OH DHT [40], which increases calcium transport across intestinal epithelium. Renal 1-alpha hydroxylase is not necessary for its activity. The advantages of DHT over vitamin D_2 are its shorter duration of action and its greater potency. The recommended dosage is 15 μg/kg/day; 0.1 mg and 0.2 mg tablets are available, and a suspension of 0.25 mg/ml (Hytakerol oil) is especially attractive for use in infants and children unable to swallow tablets. A prospective randomized clinical trial is currently underway to compare DHT and calcitriol for the prevention of renal osteodystrophy and improvement of growth and nutrition in children between the ages of 1.5 years and 11.5 years, with GFR between 20 ml/min/1.73m^2 and 75 ml/min/1.73 m^2.

25-OH vitamin D_3, the immediate precursor of calcitriol, is present in normal concentrations in the plasma of North American children with CRF [20,52]. Despite this, therapeutic use of this agent has been successful in improving bone histology and ameliorating hyperparathyroidism. Langman et al. [52] reported a series of nine children, ages three to eight years, with a GFR of 30 ml/min/1.73m^2 to 60 ml/min/1.73 m^2. They received 25-OH vitamin D_3, 1 μg/kg/day to 2 μg/kg/day, with supplemental calcium carbonate to achieve a total oral calcium intake of 750 mg to 1500 mg daily. Aluminum hydroxide was administered as needed to maintain serum phosphate between 4 mg/dl and 6 mg/dl. Plasma concentrations of 25-OH vitamin D_3

increased sixfold during the therapy, and a positive correlation was demonstrated with growth velocity. Plasma concentration of iPTH declined, and bone histology returned to normal after two years in five of nine patients, all of whom had osteomalacic and/or osteitis fibrosa lesions prior to therapy. Plasma concentrations of calcitriol did not increase, suggesting a direct effect of 25-OH vitamin D_3.

Additional therapeutic uses of 25-OH vitamin D_3 include replacement of urinary losses of this metabolite, which are seen in patients with persistent nephrotic syndrome regardless of GFR [37,74]. CRF patients may also suffer from seizure disorders that require medications such as carbemazepine, phenobarbital, and diphenylhydantoin. All induce the ctyochrome p450 enzyme system in the endoplasmic reticulum of hepatocytes. Induction of this system accelerates the metabolism of 25-OH vitamin D_3, producing low plasma concentrations of this metabolite and, potentially, anti-convulsant rickets [44].

Therapeutic usage of calcitriol for children with CRF has increased dramatically since the initial description by Chesney et al. [21]. Several studies [16,69], albeit uncontrolled, have demonstrated its effectiveness in restoring plasma calcium concentration to normal, improving intestinal calcium absorption, and decreasing plasma concentration of iPTH (but not to normal). In addition, reduction of the plasma concentration of alkaline phosphatase and healing of the lesions of osteodystrophy by either radiographic or histological criteria are observed. Most dramatic is the improvement in uremic myopathy, gait disturbances, and bone pain, months in advance of radiographic healing. While serum calcium concentration increases within one week to two weeks of the onset of therapy, due to improved intestinal absorption of calcium, calcitriol has the same effect on phosphorous absorption. The dosage of binders often must be increased to prevent hyperphosphatemia.

Hypercalcemia, a potential untoward effect of any vitamin D analog, is commonly observed with calcitriol. However, it tends to be mild, and rapidly reversible due to the very short half-life (four hours to six hours) of this preparation [16,18]. While an early report of Christiansen [22] suggested that calcitriol therapy accelerated deterioration of GFR in patients with CRF, presumably through the mechanism of hypercalcemia and hypercalciuria, follow-up studies have failed to confirm this observation [16,18,19]. In fact, both Chesney [19] and Chan [16] have demonstrated that calcitriol therapy reduces urinary calcium excretion. Frequent monitoring of serum calcium is mandatory for children with CRF receiving treatment with this agent.

Bone histomorphometry in children treated with calcitriol [69] has demonstrated, similar to adults, that osteitis fibrosa lesions improve or heal completely. However, calcitriol therapy is less successful in the treatment of deficient mineralization (osteomalacia). The description of aluminum as an etiologic agent in the production of such lesions may explain the failure of calcitriol to remineralize such affected bone and the frequent observation of hypercalcemia in such patients.

Linear growth velocity has been examined in children with CRF receiving calcitriol. The majority of patients who demonstrate accelerated growth are pre-pubescent and pre-dialysis in their degree of CRF [16]. Few children have been treated in infancy, when the most severe loss of growth potential occurs, to determine whether or not calcitriol can completely prevent growth retardation (assuming proper nutrition). The question of whether or not true catch-up growth occurs must also await greater experience with this agent.

The practical use of calcitriol is frustrating in that the smallest available dosage unit is a capsule of 0.25 µg. The recommended starting dose is 15 µg/kg/day, which limits its use to children above 15 kg body weight and to those who can swallow capsules. However, innovative parents and their physicians can aspirate the capsule's contents with a tuberculin syringe and dilute the drug with corn or vegetable oil for doses less than 0.25 µg. Alternatively, the capsule can be perforated with a needle and the contents squirted directly into the child's mouth. Although a parenteral form of calcitriol (Calicijex) is now available, an oral suspension is still wanting. A second practical problem is the short half-life of the drug. This requires at least twice or even thrice daily dosing for sustained normalization of plasma calcitriol concentrations, thus increasing the risk of poor compliance.

Hypertension

Progressive renal insufficiency is commonly associated with hypertension, particularly when CRF is caused by chronic glomerulonephritis as opposed to congenital etiologies of CRF such as obstructive malformations of the urinary tract or dysplasia/hypoplasia. Current theories of the progressive nature of CRF implicate systemic as well as intraglomerular hypertension in the pathogenesis of the glomerulosclerosis that is the final common pathway of nephron loss [4]. In most experimental models of CRF associated with hypertension, effective treatment of elevated systemic blood pressure, particularly with angiotensin converting enzyme inhibitors, has been shown to slow the rate of progressive renal failure [6]. In addition, the dominant risk factor for the increased cardiovascular morbidity in chronic dialysis patients is hypertension. Presumably, proper antihypertensive therapy from the onset of hypertension during the course of CRF would impact positively on the outcome.

While a more comprehensive approach to the subject is presented in Chapter 87, the choice and dosage schedule of antihypertensive drugs must be carefully considered, as their metabolic clearance rate may be prolonged with reduced GFR. Also, control of blood pressure is commonly associated with a temporary reduction in GFR, often proportional to the severity of hypertension and the decrement brought on by effective treatment. In particular, diuretics must be used with caution, as reduction in extra-cellular volume will also produce further reduction in GFR.

Growth Failure

Despite adequate nutrient intake, preventive treatment of disordered mineral balance, and correction of metabolic acidosis, some infants and children suffer from progressive growth retardation. Anabolic steroids such as norethandrolone, nandrolone phenpropionate, and oxandrolone are not recommended for pediatric patients due to their virilizing effects and the risk of early epiphyseal closure.

The most exciting development in the field has been the use of human recombinant growth hormone (rhGH) for infants and children with CRF and reduced growth velocity. Experimental work by Mehls et al. [60] in the uremic rat model demonstrated significant increments in weight and length, independent of nutrient intake. Preliminary studies in children with CRF have shown marked increases in growth velocity when compared to pretreatment values [61]. Currently, a randomized, double-blinded, placebo-controlled trial is underway to determine the efficacy of safety of this preparation in infants and children with growth failure.

Anemia

The normochromic, normocytic anemia of CRF is due primarily to a deficiency in erythopoietin production by the renal parenchyma [28]. It is usually modest in degree and very rarely requires packed red cell transfusion for symptoms of fatigue or high output congestive heart failure. With the onset of maintenance hemodialysis, the severity of the anemia usually increases, often with the hemoglobin falling below 7 gm/dl. The magnitude of anemia in the dialysis-dependent infant or child, compared to the adult, may be more impressive due to the lack of androgen stimulation of erythrogenesis.

Until recently, many pediatric patients required packed red cell transfusions on a regular basis, placing them at risk for transfusion-acquired infectious diseases and iron overload [75]. Recombinant human erythropoietin (r-HuEPO) is now commercially available for treatment of anemia in the dialysis population. Its efficacy and relative safety have been established in both adults [28] and children [65,79] who are dependent on dialysis. Its utility in the pre-dialysis CRF adult patient has also been demonstrated [29].

Hyperuricemia

Increased plasma concentration of uric acid occurs routinely as glomerular filtration rate declines due to insufficient excretion. However, symptoms of gouty arthritis are very rare and generally hyperuricemia does not require treatment with the xanthine oxidase inhibitor, allopurinol. Untoward effects are common with CRF and include gastrointestinal disturbances, leukopenia, thrombocytopenia, hepatitis, and vasculitis [46]. However, when therapy is required, the dosage should be reduced from the usual adult value of 100 mg and the interval extended from 8 hours to 12 hours or 24 hours [8].

References

1. Abitol C, Holliday M: Total parenteral nutrition in uraemic children. *Clin Nephrol* 5:153, 1976.

2. Alverstrand A, Ahlberg M, Bergstrom J: Retardation of the progression of renal insufficiency in patients treated with low protein diets. *Kidney Int* (suppl 16)24:268, 1983.

3. Anderson C, Nelson R, Margie J, et al: Nutritional therapy for adults with renal disease. *JAMA* 223:68, 1973.

4. Anderson S: Progression of chronic renal disease: Role of systemic and glomerular hypertension. *Am J Kidney Dis* (suppl)13:8, 1989.

5. Arnold W, Danford D, Holliday M: Effects of caloric supplementation on growth in children with uremia. *Kidney Int* 24:205, 1983.

6. Baldwin D, Neugarten J: Blood pressure control and progression of renal insufficiency. *In* Mitch W, Brenner B, Stein J (eds): *The Progressive Nature of Renal Disease.* New York, Churchill-Livingstone, 1986, p 81.

7. Barsotti G, Morelli E, Giannoni A, et al: Restricted phosphorous and nitrogen intake to slow the progression of chronic renal failure: A controlled trial. *Kidney Int* (suppl 16)24:278, 1983.

8. Bennett W, Muther R, Parker M, et al: Drug therapy in renal failure: Dosing guidelines for adults. *Ann Intern Med* 93:312, 1980.

9. Berlyne G, van Laethem L, Ari J: Exchangeable potassium and renal potassium handling in advanced chronic renal failure in man. *Nephron* 8:264, 1971.

10. Betts P, Magrath G: Growth patterns and dietary intake of children with chronic renal insufficiency. *Br Med J* 2:189, 1974.

11. Betts P, White R: Growth potential and skeletal maturity in children with chronic renal insufficiency. *Nephron* 16:325, 1976.

12. Bilbrey G, Carter N, White M, et al: Potassium deficiency in chronic renal failure. *Kidney Int* 4:423, 1973.

13. Brenner B, Meyer T, Hostetter T: Dietary protein and the progressive nature of kidney disease: The role of hemodynamically mediated glomerular injury in the pathogenesis of progressive glomerular sclerosis in aging, renal ablation, and intrinsic renal disease. *N Engl J Med* 307:652, 1982.

14. Broyer M, Guillot M, Niaduet P, et al: Comparison of three low nitrogen diets containing essential amino acids and their alpha analogues for severely uremic children. *Kidney Int* (suppl 16)24:290, 1983.

15. Bulla M, Delling G, Offermann G, et al: Renal bone disorder in children: Therapy with Vitamin D3 or 1,25-dihydroxycholecalciferol (1,25-DHCC). *In Vitamin D: Basic Research and its Clinical Application.* Berlin, Walter de Gruyter & Co, 1979, p 853.

16. Chan J, Kodroff M, Landwehr D: Effects of 1,25 dihydroxyvitamin D3 on renal function, mineral balance and growth in children with severe chronic renal failure. *Pediatrics* 68:559, 1981.

17. Chantler C, El-Bishti M, Counahan R: Nutritional therapy in children with chronic renal failure. *Am J Clin Nutr* 33:1682, 1980.

18. Chesney R: 1,25-Dihydroxyvitamin D3 in the treatment of juvenile renal osteodystrophy. *In Pediatric Nephrology.* The Hague, Martin Nifhoff Publishers, 1980, p 209.

19. Chesney R, Hamstra A, Jax D, et al: Influence of long-term oral 1,25-dihydroxyvitamin D in childhood renal osteodystrophy. *Contrib Nephrol* 18:55, 1980.

20. Chesney R, Hamstra A, Mazess R, et al: Circulating vitamin D metabolite concentrations in childhood renal diseases. *Kidney Int* 21:65, 1982.

21. Chesney R, Moorthy A, Eisman J, et al: Increased growth after long term oral 1-alpha, 25-vitamin D3 in childhood renal osteodystrophy. *N Engl J Med* 298:238, 1978.

22. Christiansen C, Rodbro P, Christiansen M, et al: Deterioration of renal function during treatment of chronic renal failure with 1,25-dihydroxycholecalciferol. *Lancet* 2:700, 1978.

23. Dargie H, Allison M, Kennedy A, et al: High dosage metolazone in chronic renal failure. *Br Med J* 4:196, 1972.

24. DeLuca H: The vitamin D system in the regulation of calcium and phosphorous metabolism. WO Atwater Memorial Lecture. *Nutr Rev* 37:161, 1979.

25. Dobblestein H, Korner W, Melpel W, et al: Vitamin B6 deficiency in uremia and its implications for the depression of immune responses. *Kidney Int* 5:233, 1974.

26. Eggert J, Siegler R, Edamkesmalee E: Zinc supplementation in chronic renal failure. *Int J Pediatr Nephrol*

27. Epstein M, Lepp R, Hoffman R, et al: Potentiation of furosemide by metolazone in refractory edema. *Curr Ther Res* 21:656, 1977.

28. Eschbach J: The anemia of chronic renal failure: Pathophysiology and the effects of recombinant erythropoietin. *Kidney Int* 35:134, 1989.

29. Eschbach J, Kelly M, Haley N, et al: Treatment of the anemia of progressive renal failure with recombinant human erythropoietin. *N Engl J Med* 32:158, 1989.

30. FAO/WHO Expert Committee: Protein and energy requirements. *WHO Technical Bulletin* 522, Geneva, 1973. WHO Sales and Services, 1211, Geneva 17, Switzerland.

31. Foreman J, et al: Nutrient intake in children with renal insufficiency: A report of the GFRD study. Presented at the annual meeting of the GFRD study March 31-April 2, 1989.

32. Freundlich M, Abitol C, Zilleruelo G, et al: Infant formula as a cause of aluminum toxicity in neonatal uraemia. *Lancet* 2:527, 1985.

33. Friedman A: Dietary manipulation and progression of renal disease: strategies for the growing animal. *Semin Nephrol* 9(1):14, 1989.

34. Giordano C: Protein restriction in chronic renal failure. *Kidney Int* 22:401, 1982.

35. Giordano C, DeSanto N, DiToro R, et al: Amino acid and keto acid diet in uremic children and infants. *Kidney Int* (suppl 8)13:83, 1978.

36. Giovanetti S: Dietary treatment of chronic renal failure: Why is it not used more frequently? *Nephron* 40:1, 1985.

37. Goldstein D, Haldimann B, Sherman D, et al: Vitamin D metabolites and calcium metabolism in patients with nephrotic syndrome and normal renal function. *J Clin Endocrinol Metab* 52:116, 1981.

38. Gretz N, Korb E, Strauch M: Low protein diet supplemented by keto acids in chronic renal failure: a prospective controlled study. *Kidney Int* (suppl 16)24:263, 1983.

39. Hodson E, Shaw P, Evans R, et al: Growth retardation and renal osteodystrophy in children with chronic renal failure. *J Pediatr* 103:735, 1983.

40. Hollick R, DeLuca H: 25-Hydroxydihydrotachysterol: Biosynthesis in vivo and in vitro. *J Biol Chem* 246:5733, 1971.

41. Ibels L, Alfrey A, Haut L, et al: Preservation of function in experimental renal diesase by dietary restriction of phosphate. *N Engl J Med* 298:12, 1978.

42. Ichikawa I, Purkerson M, Klahr S, et al: Mechanism of reduced glomerular filtration rate in chronic malnutrition. *J Clin Invest* 65:982, 1980.

43. Jones R, Dalton N, Turner C, et al: Oral essential amino acid and keto acid supplements in children with chronic renal failure. *Kidney Int* 24:95, 1983.

44. Jubiz W, Haussler M, McCain T, et al: Plasma 1,25-dihydroxy vitamin D levels in patients receiving anticonvulsant drugs. *J Clin Endocrinol Metab* 44:617, 1977.

45. Karlinsky M, Haut L, Buddington B, et al: Preservation of renal function in experimental glomerulonephritis. *Kidney Int* 17:293, 1980.
46. Kelly W: Pharmacologic approach to maintenance of urate homeostasis. *Nephron* 14:99, 1975.
47. Klahr S: The modification of diet in renal disease study. *N Engl J Med* 320:864, 1989.
48. Klahr S, Buerkert J, Purkerson M: Role of dietary factors in the progression of chronic renal disease. *Kidney Int* 24:579, 1983.
49. Kleinknecht C, Broyer M, Huot D, et al: Growth and development of non-dialyzed children with chronic renal failure. *Kidney Int* (suppl 15)24:40, 1983.
50. Kopple J, Coburn J: Metabolic studies of low protein diets in uraemia. 1. Nitrogen and potassium. *Medicine* (Baltimore) 52:583, 1973.
51. Kopple J, Swendseid M: Vitamin nutrition in patients undergiong maintenance hemodialysis. *Kidney Int* 7:S-79, 1975.
52. Langman C, Mazur A, Baron R, et al: 25-Hydroxyvitamin D3 (calcifediol) therapy of juvenile renal osteodystrophy: Beneficial effect on linear growth velocity. *J Pediatr* 100:815, 1982.
53. Laouari D, Kleinknecht C, Cournot-Witmer G, et al: Beneficial effects of low phosphorous diet in uraemic rats: a reappraisal. *Clin Sci* 63:539, 1982.
54. Mak R, Turner C, Thompson T, et al: Suppression of secondary hyperparathyroidism in children with chronic renal failure by high dose phosphate binders: Calcium carbonate versus aluminum hydroxide. *Br Med J* 291:623, 1985.
55. Malekzadeh M, Stanley P, Ettinger R, et al: Treatment of renal osteodystrophy in children on hemodialysis with dihydrotachysterol. *In Vitamin D: Biochemical, Chemical and Clinical Aspects Related to Calcium Metabolism.* Berlin, Walter de Gruyter & Co, 1977, p 681.
56. Maschio G, Oldrizzi L, Tessitore N, et al: Effects of dietary protein and phosphorous restriction on the progression of early renal failure. *Kidney Int* 22:371, 1982.
57. Mehls O, Bonzel K, Strehlau J, et al: Low protein diet in children with chronic renal failure. *Contrib Nephrol* 53:31, 1986.
58. Mehls O, Wingen K, Bonzel K, et al: Protein restriction in children with chronic renal failure? *Blood Purif* 7:46, 1989.
59. Mehls O, Ritz E, Gilli G, et al: Nitrogen metabolism and growth in experimental uremia. *Int J Pediatr Nephol* 1:34, 1980.
60. Mehls O, Ritz E, Gilli G, et al: Growth in renal failure. *Nephron* 21:237, 1978.
61. Mehls O, Fine R: The use of recombinant growth hormone for treatment of growth failure in uremia. *Semin Nephrol* 9(1):43, 1989.
62. Mitch W, Wilcox C: Disorders of body fluids, sodium and potassium in chronic renal failure. *Am J Med* 72:536, 1982.
63. Mitch W, Walser M, Buffington G, et al: A simple method of estimating progression of chronic renal failure. *Lancet* 2:1326, 1976.
64. Mitch W, Walser M, Steinman T, et al: The effect of a keto acid diet supplement to a restricted diet on the progression of chronic renal failure. *N Engl J Med* 311:623, 1984.
65. Mueller-Wiefel D, Bosch A, Feist K, et al: Epo treatment in pediatric patients with renal anemia: Application forms, dosage, and response. *J Pediatr Nephrol* 3(4):C69, 1989.
66. Oldrizzi L, Ruguiu C, Valvo E, et al: Progression of renal failure in patients with renal disease of diverse etiology on protein restricted diet. *Kidney Int* 27:553, 1985.
67. Pennington JAT: *Dietary Nutrient Guide.* Westport, Conn, AVI Publishing Co, 1976.
68. Rizzoni G, Basso T, Setari M: Growth in children with chronic renal failure on conservative treatment. *Kidney Int* 26:52, 1984.
69. Robitaille P, Marie P, Delvin E, et al: Renal osteodystrophy in children treated with 1,25-dihydroxycholecalciferol: histologic bone studies. *Acta Paediatr Scand* 73(3):315, 1984.
70. Rosman J, Meijer S, Sluiter W, et al: Prospective randomised trial of early dietary protein restriction in chronic renal failure. *Lancet* 2:1291, 1984.
71. Ruley E, Bock G, Kerzner B, et al: Feeding disorders and gastroesophageal reflux in infants with chronic renal failure. *Pediatr Nephrol* 3:424, 1989.
72. Salusky I, Coburn J, Paunier L, et al: Aluminum containing phosphate binding agents and plasma aluminum levels in children undergiong CAPD: Preliminary results with the use of calcium carbonate. *In Fine R, Scharer K, Mehls O (eds): CAPD in Children.* Berlin, Springer-Verlag, 1985.
73. Sandstead H: Trace elements in uraemia and haemodialysis. *Am J Clin Nutr* 33:1501, 1980.
74. Sato K, Gray R, Lemann J Jr: Urinary excretion of 25-hydroxy vitamin D in health and in the nephrotic syndrome. *J Lab Clin Med* 99:325, 1982.
75. Schafer A, Cheron R, Dluhy R, et al: Clinical consequence of acquired transfusional iron overload in adults. *N Engl J Med* 304:319, 1981.
76. Schambelan M, Sebastian A: Hyporeninemic hypoaldosteronism. *Adv Intern Med* 24:385, 1978.
77. Sigstrom L, Altman P-O, Jodal U, et al: Growth during treatment with low protein diet in children with renal failure. *Clin Nephrol* 21:152, 1984.
78. Simmons J, Wilso C, Potter D, et al: Relation of calorie deficiency to growth failure in children on hemodialysis and the growth response to calorie supplementation. *N Engl J Med* 285:653, 1971.
79. Sinai-Treman L, Salusky I, Fine R: Use of subcutaneous recombinant human erythropoietin in children undergiong CCPD. *J Pediatr* 11:550.
80. Spannuth C, Wagner C, Warnock L, et al: Response of uremic patients to vitamin B6 (abstr). *Am Soc Nephrol* 38, 1975.
81. Tsukamoto Y, Iwanami S, Murumuno F: Disturbances of trace element concentrations in plasma of patients with chronic renal failure. *Nephron* 26:174, 1980.
82. Uauy R, Hogg R, Holliday M: Protein-energy requirements of children with chronic renal insufficiency: A report from the Southwest Pediatric Nephrology Study Group and the Infant Diet Protein Study Group. *Semin Nephrol* 9(1):24, 1989.
83. Vereerstraeten PJC, Dupuis F, Toussaint C: Effects of large doses of furosemide in end-stage chronic renal failure. *Nephron* 14:333, 1975.
84. Wassner S, Abitol C, Conley S, et al: Nutritional requirements for infants with renal failure. *Am J Kidney Dis* 7(4):300, 1986.
85. Witte M, et al: Dose ranging pharmacokinetics and pharmacodynamic evaluation of bumetanide in infants with volume overload. *Acta pharmaologica and toxicologica* (suppl 5)59:152, 1986.
86. Wollam G, Tarazi R, Bravo E, et al: Diuretic potency of combined hydrochlorothiazide and furosemide therapy in patients with azotemia. *Am J Med* 72:929, 1982.

ALAN B. GRUSKIN
H. JORGE BALUARTE
SHERMINE DABBAGH

39

Hemodialysis and Peritoneal Dialysis

Dialytic therapy, the process of separating crystalloid from colloid by using semipermeable membranes, has become an increasingly important component of pediatric nephrology. The principles and techniques of dialysis have been adapted and successfully applied to children of all ages. The consideration of the principles of dialysis, their clinical application to children experiencing renal failure, and the problems related to dialysis are the major thrust of this chapter. Although many aspects of dialysis are similar in patients of all sizes, optimal dialytic therapy for children requires a database that makes it possible to deal with problems related to providing safe and effective dialysis for children of widely differing body size. The impact of renal failure on growth always must be considered. Existing data defining unique pediatric approaches to dialytic therapy are emphasized.

Incidence and Etiology of Renal Failure

The number of children developing renal failure and requiring dialysis is relatively low in comparison to adult populations. In children, the incidence and etiology of renal failure are age dependent, vary according to geography and nationality, and reflect the changing nature of pediatric services.

The incidence of acute renal failure in neonates and young children, especially acute tubular necrosis, has increased with the widespread development of neonatal intensive care units, transportation services, and aggressive surgical approaches to critically ill children, for example, open heart surgery in infants [144]. Congenital and vascular disorders comprise most other diseases giving rise to acute or chronic renal failure in neonates [395]. Throughout the remainder of childhood, acute renal failure necessitating dialysis is usually due to acute tubular necrosis secondary to postoperative hypotension (acute extracellular volume depletion leading to renal hypoperfusion), sepsis, the hemolytic uremic syndrome, or rapidly progressive glomerulonephritis [479].

The reported annual incidence of new cases of renal insufficiency in children requiring long-term dialysis ranges

from 1.5 to 6 per million total population [133,652]. The largest database defining the etiology of end stage renal disease (ESRD) in children is that developed by the European Dialysis and Transplantation Association (EDTA) [111]. The incidence in children with ESRD increases with age. In early childhood, structural congenital abnormalities predominate, whereas the incidence of acquired renal disorders as a cause of ESRD increases progressively throughout childhood. Some changes have occurred during the past few years in the reported etiology of childhood ESRD: The percentage of cases due to glomerulopathies has fallen, whereas cases related to congenital defects have increased [110]. Regional and single center differences in ESRD have been reported. These differences reflect primarily the numbers of children afflicted with congenital disorders [110,139,242]. Such differences are due in part to the fact that young infants may not routinely receive ESRD care for technical or ethical reasons. This practice also helps explain the limited data defining incidence and etiology of ESRD in children less than 5 years of age. The causes of ESRD in children less than and greater than 5 years of age collected by the EDTA registry are summarized in Table 39-1.

Dialysis Membranes—An Overview

Dialysis involves the use of semipermeable membranes that permit the simultaneous passage of smaller molecular weight solutes and water while retarding or inhibiting the movement of larger sized particles. The basic principles controlling the transmembrane movement of solute and water are similar whether the membrane is manufactured (hemodialysis) or natural (peritoneal dialysis).

Solute transfer across semipermeable membranes occurs by two mechanisms: diffusion and convection. The magnitude of diffusive transport, which reflects the intrinsic molecular motion and activity of atoms and solute, is influenced by four factors: membrane permeability, surface area of the membrane, molecular weight and charge of the solute, and the transmembrane concentration gradient. Different semipermeable membranes have unique permea-

Table 39-1. *Nature of renal disease resulting in ESRD*

	Diagnosis in children less than 5 years of age			Diagnosis in all children at time of onset of dialysis		
Actual number	All 263	Before 1980 159	1980–81 104	All 3342	Before 1980 2541	1980–81 801
Disease	*Percentage of actual number affected*					
Glomerulonephritis	20.9	23.2	17.3	31.3	32.7	26.4
Pyelonephritis and malfunction of urinary tract	15.2	10	23	22.5	22	23.9
Renal hypoplasia	12.1	8.8	17	12.1	11.6	13.8
Hereditary diseases	13.7	15.7	10.5	16.2	15.9	16.6
Systemic diseases	13.5	16.7	10.4	7.0	6.9	7.6
Vascular diseases	4.2	3.7	4.8	1.5	1.51	1.6
Miscellaneous diagnoses	14.7	16.3	11.3	5.7	5.8	6.4
Diagnosis unknown	5.7	5.6	5.7	3.7	3.6	3.7
Total (%)	100%	100%	100%	100%	100%	100%

Adapted from Broyer M: Incidence and etiology in ESRD in children. *In* Fine RN, Gruskin AB (eds): *End Stage Renal Disease in Children.* Philadelphia, WB Saunders, 1984, p 9.

bility characteristics based on the number and size of "pores," the thickness of the membrane, and the resistance of the component parts. Transit of small molecular weight solutes occurs more rapidly across a membrane with a large number of small pores than a membrane with a fewer number of large pores. Solute diffusion is directly proportional to the amount of membrane surface area in contact with solution. Consequently, small surface area membranes are less efficient and vice versa.

Solute movement across semipermeable membranes is inversely related to molecular weight. Thus, a solute with a molecular weight of 400 daltons diffuses half as quickly as one weighing 200 daltons, even though the membrane is freely permeable to both solutes. The charge and molecular configuration of the solute also influences its rate of diffusion. For example, phosphate diffuses more slowly than would be expected considering its molecular weight. Most importantly, diffusive transport is directly proportional to the concentration gradient across the membrane. The degree to which concentration gradients persist over time depends on whether solute is continuously removed from the side of the membrane having the lower concentration of solute or whether the concentration of solute increases over time.

Convective transport of solute (solvent drag) refers to the transmembrane movement of solute due to the passage of solvent water. In the absence of any solute concentration gradient, the passive movement of solute entrained (dragged) by water is controlled by the transmembrane osmotic gradient. Convective transport is directly proportional to the magnitude of ultrafiltrate generated and to the concentration of solute contained in the transported solvent. Varying concentrations of solute occur in the transported solution because of the sieving properties of the membrane. Each membrane has its distinctive sieving coefficient for each solute. Sieving coefficients range in value from zero to one. A value of zero means that the

solute being examined is unable to move through the membrane; a value of 0.25 indicates that the pore size is sufficently large to permit 25% of the molecules to cross the membrane with 75% being unable to cross; a sieving coefficient of one would imply that the membrane does not prevent the movement of any solute. Molecular size, shape, and charge as well as the pore number, size, and shape influence sieving coefficients.

Ultrafiltration, the process by which water is moved across the membrane, is achieved by generating a transmembrane pressure gradient. In peritoneal dialysis, the pressure gradient is due to the development of osmotic gradients that are clinically accomplished by adding glucose to dialysate in varying concentrations. Solvent moves to solutions of high osmolality from those having a lower osmolality. In hemodialysis, pressure gradients are hydrostatically generated and are achieved either by applying negative pressure on the dialysate or by applying positive pressure to the blood compartment. The net rate of ultrafiltrate formed reflects the combined influence of surface area available for exchange, the unique ultrafiltration coefficient of the membrane, and the transmembrane pressure gradient, both hydrostatic and osmotic. The ultrafiltration coefficient depends on the intrinsic structure and thickness of the membrane.

Hemodialysis Equipment
Hemodialysis Machines

The processing of a patient's extracellular fluid by hemodialysis to achieve biochemical stability is accomplished by perfusing blood and dialysate simultaneously through two parallel fluid-filled systems, the blood and dialysate circuits, separated by the semipermeable membrane of the dialyzer. Two types of dialysis machines are currently used: (1) parallel flow machines for which dialysate can be prepared and delivered either centrally or by individual units and (2) recirculating single-pass machines.

Central delivery systems are rarely used in pediatric dialysis units because of the relatively few children dialyzed at one time. Individual machines allow the physician to vary the dialysate composition easily, thereby individualizing dialysis prescriptions. Also, machine malfunction affects only one patient. Dialysate for such machines is available as a concentrated solution. Currently available machines use 34 parts of water to 1 part of concentrate. One system pumps concentrate and treated water into separate chambers and empties the chambers together; another pumps treated water at a fixed rate with concentrate being added by a second pump. Varying the speed of the second pump enables the final concentration of solutes, primarily sodium and base, to be manipulated. Both systems monitor the conductivity of the effluent continuously to ensure that the final concentration of the dialysate is clinically acceptable.

Ultrafiltration rates are controlled by setting and varying the total transmembrane pressure (TMP) across the dialyzer membrane. The primary source of positive pressure is the blood pump. The magnitude of the transdialyzer pressure gradients within the blood compartment is set by varying the resistance on the venous side of the dialyzer. The TMP in most machines can be further modified by applying a negative pressure to the dialysate side of the membrane. This is done either by increasing the speed of the outlet pump draining dialysate or by altering the size of the entry port through which dialysate enters the dialyzer. Ultrafiltration rates are independent of blood flow rates.

The use of recirculating single-pass machines requires preparing a tank of dialysate, placing some dialysate in a reservoir, and pumping some through the coil. Concentrated dialysate is added to the reservoir and appropriately diluted by adding water. The appropriateness of the dialysate is verified by measuring the conductivity of the final solution. When coil dialyzers are used, dialysate is rapidly recirculated through the coil, while the dialysate in the reservoir and holding tank is exchanged at a much slower rate. The reservoir is drained and fresh dialysate added to the tank once or twice during the dialysis. When single-pass machines are used, dialysate is continuously made and added to the system. Sorbent dialysis systems offer portability. They should not be used to treat hyperammonemia or patients with a BUN less than 30 mg/dl.

Ongoing monitoring of the functioning of the component parts of hemodialysis equipment is an essential aspect of performing dialysis. Monitoring is automatically done when modern equipment is used. Variables to monitor include blood flow rates, dialysate composition and temperature, pressures in the dialysate and blood compartments, leakage of blood into dialysate, and the entry of air into the returning blood. Such systems function best when monitors and alarms are separated from control and adjustment sites.

The use of an arteriovenous fistula as a vascular access requires that a blood pump be used to perfuse the extracorporeal blood circuit, because the large pressure drop between the patient's arterial and venous circulations does not generate a large enough positive pressure to achieve adequate perfusion of the blood circuit. Most systems use a peristaltic roller pump that can accommodate a variety of sizes of blood tubing. Despite the repetitive occlusive action of the pump on the cells within the tubing [374], hemolysis is not a significant problem and red cell survival [832] approaches normal. It is the rate of blood flow through the dialyzer that is the predominant determinant for small solute in contrast to large solute movement across the dialyzing membrane. Precise blood flow rates are difficult to measure. Techniques used to measure rates of blood flow include the "bubble" transit time method, in vitro calibration of blood pumps [360], and ultrasonic or electromagnetic flow meters [493]. Most often, rates of blood flow are approximated by a meter that converts the armature voltage of the pump to a flow rate, the pump having been calibrated in vitro using an electrolyte solution. The package inserts of most dialyzers contain graphs displaying the anticipated small molecular weight solute clearance (urea and creatinine) for a given rate of blood flow.

Dialysate composition is automatically monitored by either inductive or impedance conductivity meters. Both not only measure the total ionic content of the dialysate as a reflection of dialysate composition, but also correct for the effect of temperature on conductivity. Most meters detect a 1% change, and system alarms are usually set at a 3% change. Many units have two conductivity meters: one that can be adjusted to vary dialysate composition and a second monitor that automatically switches the machine into a bypass mode should the conductivity exceed predescribed limits. Air bubbles, the accumulation of deposits on electrodes, or the elective bypassing of the meter can lead to problems including death from hypo-osmolality or hyperosmolality [702].

Dialysate temperature is maintained in the range of 36 to 42°C by thermostatically controlled immersion heating elements or heat exchangers. Most systems measure the temperature of the water before concentrate is added to reduce the development of corrosion on heat sensing elements. When the dialysate temperature reaches 40° C, properly functioning machines switch to a bypass mode. Underheating leads to chilling and discomfort. Clotting of the dialyzer by cold agglutinins has been reported [337]. Heating of dialysate produces a warm feeling. If the patient's temperature is allowed to increase to values above 40°C, protein denaturation, hemolysis, and death can occur. Failure of temperature [258] regulation in a central delivery system will affect many patients.

Pressure monitoring serves two functions: to control the rate of ultrafiltration and to detect obstruction within or disconnection of the blood containing system. Pressures are measured by electronic pressure transducers, mechanical manometers, and enclosed "pillow" pressure monitors. The latter measures the degree of negative pressure generated by the action of the blood pump in removing blood from the patient. The blood pump is the source of the positive pressure within the rest of the blood circuit. "Pillow" monitors cannot be used in single needle access systems. Pressure monitors are separated from direct contact with blood by disposable nonpermeable membranes or pore filters that close on contact with liquids.

Pressures within both the dialysate and the blood circuits

require continuous monitoring. It is possible to monitor both the inlet and the outlet pressures in the blood and dialysate compartments to measure precisely transcompartment pressure drops and thereby accurately measure the TMP available for ultrafiltration. In many clinical settings, only the pressure on the venous side of the dialyzer and either the inlet or the outlet pressure of the dialysate circuit are measured because the pressure drops across these compartments are usually only a few mm Hg. Most blood pressure monitors alarm when either a pressure change of 10 mmHg occurs at pressures less than 50 mmHg, or when a 10% change occurs at higher pressures. When blood circuit monitors are activated, they simultaneously set off audible signals and shut off the blood pump. Dialysate and TMP pressure monitors are accurate to ±20 mm Hg or ±10% of the readings. To control ultrafiltration rates more critically, some units provide servo-control of the TMP; others measure directly the amount of ultrafiltrate formed.

Membrane breaks and leaks occur frequently enough to require ongoing monitoring to detect the entry of blood into the dialysate circuit or the entry of air into the blood circuit. Modern hemodialyzers incorporate photo-optic cells to detect the presence of 0.25 to 0.35 ml blood per liter of dialysate. Blood leak curvettes need periodic testing to detect chemical deposits from dialysate, which can coat the lining of the cuvette.

Air embolism is a major risk associated with the use of blood pumps. Varying amounts of air have been reported to be clinically significant. As little as 5 ml [82] has been reported to cause death in an adult; others believe that 65 to 125 ml [857] or 1.0 ml/kg/minute of air can be fatal [844]. Air leaks developing in the system prior to the blood pump are the most hazardous because the negative pressure, suction, generated by the pump continuously sucks air into the blood path. Effective measures to reduce the incidence of air leaks include the avoidance of inserting intravenous lines into tubing prior to the blood pump and the use of tight-fitting connections between outflow needles and blood tubing. Air detectors, which are generally placed on the venous air trap, should recognize foam as well as free air. The most practical method uses an ultrasonic device that senses the movement of ultrasonic waves across the membrane within the bubble trap [572]. Such devices are able to detect small air bubbles. When air within the blood line is detected, an occlusive blood clamp is activated.

Hemodialysis Membranes

The semipermeable membranes used to perform clinical hemodialysis are made of different materials and configured differently. Most currently used hemodialyzers are made from Cuprophan, which is regenerated or twice-processed cellulose. Cuprophan membranes are made by solubilizing cellulose in an ammonia solution of cupric acid. The material is then extruded into an acid bath to yield a cellulose film, which is then made into flat sheets or hollow fibers. Other available dialyzers contain cellulose acetate or synthetic materials such as polyacrylonitrile, polymethylmethacrylate, or polysulfone membranes, which are more permeable to larger solutes and have higher ultrafiltration coefficients [822]. These membranes lack any charge, and transport across them is primarily through pores. Each type of membrane has different characteristics regarding their ability to clear solutes of different molecular weight and to ultrafilter. Noteworthy is the fact that drugs may be removed at different rates when different types of membranes are used, e.g., vancomycin removal rates are increased when polyacrylonitrile membranes [801a] or hollow fiber cellulose acetated membranes [732a] are used. Biocompatibility differences also exist [362].

Three different dialyzer configurations are available; each offers advantages and disadvantages (Table 39-2). Coil dialyzers are constructed by wrapping the semipermeable membrane around a cylinder and function by having dialysate forced between the coiled membrane and recirculated. Flat plate dialyzers consist of a number of physically separated rectangular membranes stacked on top of each other and enclosed in a rigid structure. The direction of dialysate flow can be either concurrent or countercurrent to that of blood. Not only can the total surface area of the dialyzer be altered by varying the number of individual plates, the thickness of the membrane itself can be varied during the manufacturing process. Parallel plate dialyzers, perhaps the most widely used type of hemodialyzer in pediatric patients, are available in a range of sizes that permit infants as well as adolescents to be dialyzed over a long-term period. The hollow fiber dialyzer is made of many thousands of capillary sized cellulose tubes bound together. The dialysate flows in a direction opposite that of blood.

The priming volume of the dialyzer together with the volume of the blood lines determines the amount of blood that will be removed from the body (extracorporeal blood volume) at the onset of dialysis. As a rule, it should not exceed 10% of the blood volume. When estimating the extracorporeal volume anticipated during dialysis, it is important to account for the changing volume within the dialyzer, i.e., compliance. This volume changes in the same direction as the TMP when it is altered to achieve ultrafiltration. On completing the dialysis, the extracorporeal blood is returned to the patient by flushing the system with saline or air. Transfusion requirements are determined by the residual blood volume of the dialyzer, the rate at which connection tubing separates from patients or dialyzers, hemolysis within the system, and the frequency with which dialyzers rupture (determined in part by the intrinsic thrombogenicity of the dialyzing membrane).

Cost

An important practical consideration in the clinical practice of dialysis is its cost. Despite the fact that the cost per dialysis has remained stable or even decreased in the past decade, the total cost for dialytic services continues to rise because of the increased number of patients receiving treatment. The cost per treatment in children has been shown to exceed that of adults for a number of reasons, including the need for more personnel and the inability to bulk purchase dialyzers [312]. The major source of the yearly high cost of dialysis is the recurring expense for disposable

Table 39-2. *Comparison of the features of similar size hemodialyzers*

Type	Coil	Hollow Fiber	Plate
Surface area per unit extracorporeal volume	Low	High	High
Solute clearance	Low	High	Medium
Ultrafiltration rate	Low	High	Medium
Prime volume	High	High	Low
Residual blood volume	High	High	Low
Compliance	High	Low	Medium
Reservoir	Yes	No	No
Cost	Low	High	Medium

supplies. Cost per treatment for hardware, solutions, blood lines, and dialyzers varies with the type, availability, quantity purchased, whether hardware is purchased or leased, and whether dialyzer reuse is practiced.

Dialyzer First Use Reactions

A number of clinical problems occur during dialysis when an unused and unreprocessed dialyzer is used for the first time [171], classified into major and minor reactions. The major type is characterized by signs and symptoms of anaphylaxis. Major manifestations include onset within 20 minutes, dyspnea, a burning sensation at the access site or throughout the body, and angioedema. Itching, abdominal cramping, rhinorrhea, lacrimation, urticaria, and repetitive symptoms during subsequent dialyses using the same dialyzer can occur. Minor reactions include mild back and chest pain. A trend toward an increased incidence of hypotension, nausea, cramps, and vomiting has been noted. The reported incidence of first use reactions has been 4 per 100,000 and 3 to 5 per 100 new dialyzers sold, for major and minor first use reactions, respectively [171]. Reactions occurred three times more often in patients under 30 years of age and in black as compared with white patients [172].

The etiology of first use reactions is multifactorial and includes exposure to limulus positive dialysate, presumably endotoxin [588], ethylene oxide and its breakdown products, other chemicals used in the manufacturing of dialyzers, contaminated dialysate, the entry of bacterial breakdown products, constituents of dialyzer membranes, interleukin-1, and acetate. First use reactions are reduced when reuse is practiced [176,489] or the cleansing process of reuse or a modification of the reuse process is performed prior to the first use of the dialyzer. Preventive steps include the flushing of the blood compartment with 1000 ml of saline and a second flush immediately prior to use. Formaldehyde pretreatment is also effective [141]. The dialysate compartment should also be rinsed with dialysate heated to 37°C. In patients with known hypersensitivity reactions, anithistamines may be helpful. Treatment of first use reactions depends on severity. When the reaction is severe, dialysis should be stopped immediately. Antihistamines, glucocorticoids, and epinephrine may be needed. If the dialyzer was sterilized with ethylene oxide, a dialyzer that is gamma-sterilized or autoclaved and made of materials other than cuprammonium cellulose should be used. The concomitant use of gamma-sterilized blood tubing is also indicated. Mild reactions may be treated by using the same dialyzer and pre-treating with antihistamines. Autoantibodies may develop with repetitive hemodialysis [739]. Continued hemodialysis may not be possible, and a switch to peritoneal dialysis may be required.

Dialyzer Reuse

Various techniques and procedures for reusing hemodialyzers, initially described for coil dialyzers in 1964 [741] and parallel plate dialyzers in 1967 [641], are available [554]. One center has reported on 22 years of reuse [738]. As of January 1983, 43% of 1015 hemodialysis centers surveyed in the United States practiced reuse [379]. Manual and automated techniques for reprocessing dialyzers are available. A few pediatric hemodialysis centers reuse hemodialyzers, although most reuse involves adults.

An overview of the steps involved in reuse follows [177]. First, the patient's blood is returned. The blood and dialysate compartments of the dialyzer are then flushed with water treated by reverse osmosis. The blood path is cleansed by perfusing it with one or various solutions that remove residual red cells; the most widely used chemical is sodium hypochlorite. The blood and dialysate compartments are filled with a sterilizing antimicrobial agent, most often 2% formaldehyde. The dialyzer is then stored until the next treatment. Prior to its next use, the dialysate compartment is first rinsed with dialysate, and while dialysate is still running, the blood compartment is flushed with sterile heparinized saline. The venous effluent is tested for any residual formaldehyde, the concentration of which should have been reduced to less than 2 μg/ml [553].

Ongoing controversy exists about the efficacy and safety of reuse. These concerns center on the toxic effects of agents used in the reuse process, the efficacy of sequential dialysis treatments, and the risk of introducing infection. Formaldehyde may be a carcinogen. The Occupational Safety and Health Administration (Federal Register: vol 52, no. 223, pp 46168–46312) requires that exposure to formaldehyde be limited to 1.0 ppm of air averaged over an 8-hour period. Peak exposure should not exceed 10 ppm for more than 30 minutes.

Mortality rates and the need for hospitalization [405] are unchanged with reuse. When formaldehyde is used properly, the risk of infection is not increased [416]. An increased incidence of anti-N antibodies in patients treated with reuse has been attributed to the use of formaldehyde [232,799]. However, when the effluent concentration of formaldehyde is less than 1 μg/dl, anti-N antibodies are not found [477]. Clinical effects attributed to these antibodies include more anemia, hemolysis [440], and perhaps early allograft rejection. Available data do not support an increased incidence of post-transplant rejection [477]. Some cleansing agents can cause neutropenia during the ensuing hemodialysis [268]. Acute allergic reactions have been reported when reprocessed hemodialyzers have been used [4a].

Water Supply

Because it is known that the nature and concentration of contaminants in the water used for preparing dialysate and performing dialysis may adversely affect dialysis equipment and patients, the current practice of hemodialysis routinely involves water purification. Depending on the nature of the local water supply, more than one process is often needed because no one system removes all contaminants. Available systems include water softening, filtration, reverse osmosis, and deionization.

Water softening removes calcium and magnesium ions in exchange for sodium. Regeneration of the ion exchanger is done by flushing it with sodium chloride. Patients may develop hypernatremia if the brine flush is not properly removed from the system [567]. Other ions, such as manganese and iron, which are also removed during the softening process, are less completely removed during the regeneration process and may reduce the efficiency of the softening procedure.

Filters function to absorb or obstruct the passage of particulate matter and chemicals. Activated carbon filters, charcoal filters with granular activated carbon, are used to remove chloramine, chlorine, pyrogens, endotoxins, and organic compounds. Sediment filters are available in varying sizes and are used to trap particulate matter. They are often used as prefilters close to the water spigot or downstream from charcoal filters and reverse osmosis equipment. Whenever the water system is altered, it is important to be sure that the filtration system is appropriately adjusted to handle any increase in chloramine. Two filters in series should be used, and the water should be regularly tested. Chloramine concentrations should be less than 0.1 ppm. When filters are replaced, the housing should be disinfected and thoroughly rinsed before installing the new filter.

Reverse osmosis, believed by most to be the method of choice for cleansing water, removes 85% to 95% of dissolved solutes in water [497]. It is accomplished by applying a hydrostatic pressure to one side of a semipermeable membrane forcing solvent across the membrane while leaving solute behind. Water should be pretreated to remove hardness, dissolved gasses, and particulate matter. Subsequent treatment using a deionizer will remove most of the remaining fluoride and nitrate.

Deionizers function like water softeners and work as ion exchangers. They remove both anions and cations in exchange for hydrogen and hydroxide ions depending on whether cationic or anionic resins are used. Deionizers alone should not be used to remove chloramine because the exposure of chloramine to organic nitrogen can generate nitrosamines, which are carcinogenic [756].

Each of the aforementioned water purification systems requires ongoing monitoring to ensure proper functioning. Deionizers and reverse osmosis can be monitored by the continuous measurement of electrical resistance. Commercial kits to test water hardness and chloramine as chlorine are available.

Four classes of water-borne contaminants exist: dissolved inorganic substances, dissolved organic substances, microbiologic contaminants, and particulates. Most municipal water supplies contain dissolved inorganic ions in concentrations exceeding the recommendations of the Association for the Advancement of Medical Instrumentation (AAMI) and the American Society for Artificial Internal Organs (ASAIO) [152]. Recommendations for permissible levels of water contaminants and their toxic effects are summarized in Table 39-3 [152,272]. Even though harmful effects from naturally occurring organic substances derived from plant material decomposition have not yet been documented, the potential exists for toxic effects from organic detergents, herbicides, pesticides, and polyelectrolytes used in farming, manufacturing, and water treatment.

Dialysis units need to operate programs of infection control and bacteriologic surveillance even though bacteria do not normally cross intact hemodialysis membranes. Bacteria can enter the blood stream through breaks in dialysis membranes and cause bacteremia. Also, endotoxin resulting from bacterial growth in dialysate can cross membranes and cause pyrogenic reactions. The incidence of pyrogenic reactions in adult units has been reported to be 5% to 6% [668,683]. It is recommended that the upper limits for bacteria be set at 2000 and 200 organisms per ml for dialysate and water, respectively [272]. Despite extensive treatment aimed at removing particulate matter from municipal water systems and the belief that particulate matter does not generally pose any health hazard, the removal of particles greater in size than 5 μm is indicated to prevent blockage of tubing and deterioration of water purification systems.

Hemodialysis Procedure
Hemodialysis Kinetics

The precise details of the physical principles involved in the movement of solute and water across artificial membranes are complex and beyond the scope of this chapter. A number of reviews of the biophysical principles involved in solute and water movement across semipermeable membranes are available [84,150,343,715]. A working knowledge of the principles allows for the appropriate choice of a dialyzer, the opportunity to anticipate the effects of therapy, and the ability to evaluate new dialyzers properly. The outcome of a hemodialysis treatment—the net transmem-

TABLE 39-3. *Standards for water used in hemodialysis and known toxic effects*

Contaminant	Suggested allowable level in mg/liter	Toxic effect
Aluminum	0.01	Encephalopathy, osteomalacia osteodystrophy
Arsenic	0.005	
Barium	0.1	
Cadmium	0.001	
Calcium	2–10	Hypercalcemia, hard water syndrome
Chloramines	0.1	Hemolytic anemia, methemoglobinemia
Chlorine	0.5	
Chromium	0.014	
Copper	0.1	Hemolysis, fever, chills, headache, liver damage
Fluoride	0.2	Bone disease
Iron	2.0	Damages equipment
Lead	0.005	
Magnesium	4.0	Hypermagnesemia, hard water syndrome
Manganese	2.0	Damages equipment
Mercury	0.002	
Nitrate	2.0	Methemoglobinemia
Potassium	8.0	Hyperpotassemia
Selenium	0.09	
Sodium	70.0	Hypernatremia, hypertension, seizures, pulmonary edema
Silver	0.005	
Sulfate	100.0	Vomiting, acidosis, catharsis
Zinc	0.1	Vomiting, hemolytic anemia

Adapted from references 17, 152 and 272.

brane movement of solute (mass transfer) and water (ultrafiltration)—reflects the intrinsic properties of the hemodialysis membrane. These two intrinsic properties of the hemodialysis membrane are controlled by the rate of blood flow through the dialyzer, the pressure drop across the membrane, and the compliance of the dialyzer. Each factor is individually considered.

Hemodialysis systems can be viewed as a two-compartment system with inlets and outlets attached to both compartments, which in turn are separated by a semipermeable membrane. One compartment contains blood, the other dialysate. Blood is continuously moving, while dialysate may either be continuously moving or remain within a confined space. Currently available hemodialyzers use different geometric relationships for exposing dialysate to blood. In single-pass systems, flat-plate and hollow-fiber dialyzers, dialysate flow can be in the same direction as that of blood (co-current) or in opposite directions (counter-current). When coil dialyzers are used, blood and dialysate flow at right angles (cross-flow) to each other.

In the twin coil system with a fixed dialysate volume and a cross-flow geometry, transfer of solute from blood to dialysate is most rapid at the beginning of dialysis, when the transmembrane concentration gradient for solute is greatest. Because the membrane is equally permeable to

solute movement in both directions, solute begins to move from dialysate to blood as soon as solute appears in the dialysate. When the concentration of solute in blood and dialysate equalize, no further net transfer occurs. The volume of the dialysate compartment, which is usually large, determines the rate at which its solute concentration rises with time and, therefore, becomes the limiting factor in determining net transfer of solute. The contents in the dialysate compartment are changed at least once during the dialysis procedure.

When parallel flat-plate or hollow-fiber dialyzers are used, dialysate is continuously pumped through the dialysate compartment. A major advantage of these systems is that large fluid reservoirs are not needed. In concurrent flow systems the net rate of transfer of solute is greatest at the site where initial contact occurs between the two compartments and decreases as the dialysate reaches the end of its path. In fact, the concentration gradient may be quite small over a significant portion of the dialysate pathway. In countercurrent flow systems, greater rates of exchange of solute occur because a larger concentration gradient is maintained as solute free dialysate is continuously exposed to solute remaining in the blood compartment.

In addition to the transmembrane concentration or diffuse gradient, the net rate at which solute crosses artificial membranes is determined by the permeability and surface area of the membrane in contact with dialysate and blood and the delivery of solute (blood flow) to the exchange site. The above factors acting together determine the mass transfer or diffusion of solute in the absence of any ultrafiltration. Because permeability and surface area of hemodialyzers differ, and because dialysate flow rates for individual dialyzers are set in a given patient, the major variable determining solute transfer is delivery (blood flow rate) to the exchange site. Expressed in mathematical terms, $J = P [C_1 - C_2]/L$, where J is the mass flux of solute across the membrane, P is the membrane permeability factor, C_1 and C_2 are the concentrations of solute on the two sides of the membrane, and L is the thickness of membrane through which the solute must pass. The membrane permeability, P, is determined by the diffusion coefficient of the solute within the membrane. The diffusion coefficient of solute, which is influenced by the molecular radius, charge, temperature, and viscosity, cannot be measured directly in hemodialysis systems.

The most widely used expression to characterize transmembrane solute movement is clearance. Dialyzer clearance can be viewed similarly to the classic measurement of renal clearance and adequately describes what happens to patients. The formula for dialyzer clearance, a virtual number, is $Cl (ml/min) = F \times (C_A - C_V)/C_V$, where F is equal to the blood flow rate through the dialyzer in ml/minute, and C_A and C_V equal the arterial and venous solute concentrations, respectively.

Because the dialysate concentration of solute increases with time, especially in coil dialysis, diffusion slows, $C_A - C_V$ falls, and the clearance is reduced. Thus, even though clearance reflects what transpires in patients, the measurement of clearance is not capable of defining the "pure" or intrinsic diffusion characteristics of a given membrane. The measurement of dialysance, which is consistent for any given membrane, accounts for the changing blood to dialysate solute concentration during dialysis [869]. This measurement more precisely defines the intrinsic characteristics of an artificial membrane controlling solute diffusion. The formula for dialysance follows:

$$D = F(C_A - C_V)/(C_A - C_B),$$

where D = dialysance in ml/min, C_A, C_V, and C_B are the solute concentrations in mg/dl in artery, vein, and bath, respectively. When the solute concentration in the dialysate is zero, a situation seen in most single-pass dialysate systems, clearance and dialysance become equal. In coil systems, where a large reservoir is used, clearance changes throughout dialysis, yet dialysance is constant.

A second, less important, aspect of transmembrane solute movement during dialysis is the quantity of solute transported by solvent drag or convective transport. Solvent drag may be viewed as the entrainment of solute within a solvent stream. In turn, the quantity of solute so transported during a dialysis treatment reflects the quantity of water ultrafiltered. Two major factors, hydraulic permeability and the reflection coefficient, limit the transport of solute by convective transport through artificial membranes. Hydraulic permeability can operationally be defined

as the rate of movement of solute per second per mm Hg driving force per square centimeter of membrane. The Staverman reflection coefficient refers to the amount of solute rejected by a membrane when solvent flow through the membrane is generated solely by hydrostatic pressure. In clinical practice, convective movement of solute is relatively unimportant because Cuprophan membranes have a low hydraulic permeability. For example, only 2% to 3% of urea is transported by convective transport during a conventional hemodialysis; the remaining solute transport in such systems is by diffusive transport. The contribution of convective transport to net solute movement is much greater in some of the newer, more water permeable, high flux membranes [343].

In summary, the net solute transport in hemodialysis sytems can be mathematically expressed as [413]:

$$J_S = C_S(1 - \sigma)J_V + w \times \Delta OP,$$

where J_S = net solute flux, C_S = mean solute concentration, σ = Staverman reflection coefficient, J_V = solvent flux, w = solute diffusive permeability coefficient, and ΔOp = the osmotic pressure across the dialyzing membrane.

Water removal in hemodialysis systems is determined by a combination of hydrostatic and osmotic pressure gradients across the dialysis membrane. The net hydrostatic pressure equals the sum of the positive pressure generated within the blood compartment by the blood pump and the negative pressure applied to the dialysate side of the membrane. The osmotic gradient is equal to the difference between the oncotic pressure difference between the blood and dialysate compartment. This pressure is generated primarily by the quantity of glucose added to the dialysate. In reality the osmotic pressure in a solution equals the sum of pressures developed by each individual solute. The osmotic pressure generated by a dissolved solute can be expressed by the equation $OP = CRT$, where OP = osmotic pressure, C = solute concentration in g.moles/L, R = gas constant, and T = absolute temperature. The relative contribution to water movement of these two simultaneously operating pressures can be expressed as follows:

$$J_V = k_1(\Delta P/t - k_2) \Delta OP/t$$

where J_V = solvent flux, P and OP are the hydrostatic and osmotic pressure gradients across the semipermeability dialysis membrane, t = time, and k_1 and k_2 are constants that include the combined influence of hydraulic permeability, solute diffusive permability coefficient, and the Staverman reflection coefficient.

Other factors influencing solute and water movement in dialysis systems are the viscosity of solutions, blood rheology, differences between stagnant and flowing fluid layers, the impact on flow through series or parallel circuits or tubes versus flat ducts conduits, and whether flow is laminar or turbulent. A detailed discussion of these factors can be found elsewhere [150,343]. These factors are important considerations in the design and ultimate function of hemodialysis machines and, as such, define the operational limits of hemodialysis systems. Their contribution, however, is fixed when applied to clinical dialysis.

Initiation and Termination of Hemodialysis

The techniques used to begin and complete dialysis treatments vary in accordance with the child's clinical condition and size. Dialyzer and blood lines are usually primed with isotonic saline in normovolemic and asymptomatic hypervolemic children. In symptomatic, hypovolemic, or hypoalbuminemic patients, 5% albumin can be used. When the extracorporeal volume is anticipated to exceed 10% of blood volume because size appropriate equipment is not available, the system can be primed with compatible whole blood, which also may be used as a primary solution in symptomatic anemic children. In most hypervolemic or normovolemic anemic children who are not severely symptomatic, it is usually sufficient to prime with saline and transfuse with packed red cells with a hemoglobin concentration in the range of 18 to 22 g/dl during dialysis. A useful formula to calculate the quantity of packed red cells to raise the hemoglobin concentration, if needed, is:

$$4 \times (\text{desired Hgb g/dl} - \text{observed Hgb g/dl}) \times \text{wt}_{kg} \text{ [309]}$$

When children have pulmonary edema, have gained excessive weight between treatments, or have severe hypertension because of volume overload, the child can be "bled" into the system and the venous blood line connected to the child when the tubing and dialyzer are full if the priming volume of the system is equal to or less than 10% of blood volume.

At the end of a treatment, the blood in the system is usually returned to the patient by flushing the tubing and dialyzer with saline or air. The thoroughness with which this is done determines the child's residual blood volume and ultimately the frequency of blood transfusions. In children with volume dependent hypertension, options available at the end of a dialysis treatment include continuing dialysis with ultrafiltration for an additional period of time, performing "dry" dialysis (ultrafiltration alone), not returning the blood within the extracorporeal circuit if the child can tolerate the blood loss, and performing a partial exchange transfusion using packed red cells. In bilaterally nephrectomized children given vasodilator antihypertensive agents during dialysis, retransfusing extracorporeal blood may be associated with severe hypertension when the pharmacologic effect of the drug wears off [515]. The precise factors contributing to hypertension at the end of the dialysis are more difficult to recognize and treat in patients with intact kidneys. In some, volume expansion may be responsible. Hypertension, however, can also worsen toward the end of dialysis in acutely volume depleted, renin dependent, hypertensive end stage patients because of volume mediated acute renin release [830,854] or noncompliant vasculature. In such patients, antihypertensive agents, vasodilators, may be needed to lower blood pressure and increase intravascular volume so that sufficient extracorporeal volume can be transfused to reverse the cycle. Noteworthy is the observation that in patients with

end stage kidneys in situ, compared with those who have had a bilateral nephrectomy, the blood pressure is higher at a given plasma volume and presumably is renin mediated [423,424].

Choosing a Hemodialyzer

A number of factors require consideration when selecting a hemodialyzer, including extracorporeal blood volume, rate of solute removal (dialyzer efficiency), blood flow rates, rates of ultrafiltration, and length of treatment per session and per week [649,747].

EXTRACORPOREAL BLOOD VOLUME

Extracorporeal blood volume, including the volume in the blood lines and the dialyzer, should not exceed 10% of a child's blood volume [430] of 80 ml/kg body weight [200]. Extracorporeal volume usually ranges from 2% to 5% of blood volume in adults undergoing maintenance hemodialysis. Various sized blood lines are available; adult lines contain 150 ml [200]; and neonatal and pediatric blood lines hold 15 ml [460] and 35–75 ml [200], respectively. A dialyzer with as low a compliance as possible should be used to avoid progressive volume accumulation in the extracorporeal circuit. It is possible to account for any additional extracorporeal volume that develops because of dialyzer compliance. The packet insert accompanying most hemodialyzers contains data on compliance.

DETERMINATION OF DIALYSIS TIME

Several guidelines can be used to select a dialyzer and the time required for adequate dialysis. Each dialyzer has a characteristic curve describing its solute clearance, usually urea, in relation to the blood flow rate. The initial choice of dialyzer size (surface area) depends on the patient's body size and is estimated as 75% of the child's body surface area in square meters (Fig. 39-1) [200]. When highly permeable dialyzers are used, this ratio should be reduced.

The most widely used approach for initially selecting the magnitude of dialyzer clearance during dialysis is to choose a blood flow rate that clears urea at a rate of 3 ml/min/kg [427]. A dialyzer operated at a blood flow rate that meets this criterion should decrease the child's blood urea nitrogen (BUN) by approximately 65% in 4 hours [430]. Performing dialysis at this rate three times a week should maintain the predialysis BUN at levels less than 100 mg/dl. Studies performed on dialyzers in vitro have established a predictive relationship between the fractional change in either BUN or creatinine and a constant derived as the product of the dialyzer clearance expressed as ml/min/kg times the number of hours on dialysis (Fig. 39-2) [515].

In many pediatric dialysis centers, the total amount of time spent per week on hemodialysis is determined empirically by measuring predialysis and postdialysis levels of BUN, creatinine, or both. The concepts of a dialysis index (square meter hypothesis) and urea kinetic modeling have been applied to pediatric populations as ways of improving hemodialysis prescriptions.

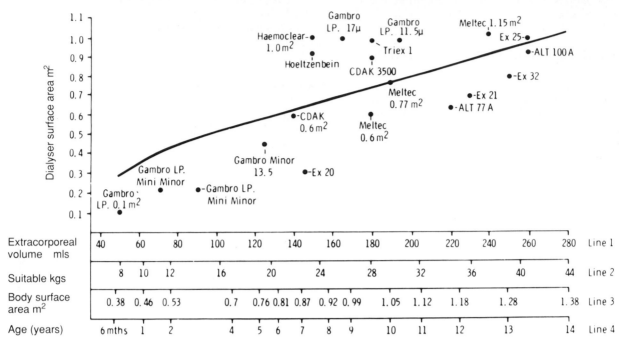

FIG. 39-1. *Available dialyzers according to surface area for use in children of varying age, weight, and body surface area. To select a dialyzer, first locate the patient's dry weight (suitable kg) or surface area on the appropriate abscissa (X) axis. The dialyzer and extra-corporeal volume to use are then located on the corresponding ordinate (Y) axis.* (From Gardiner AOP, Sawyer AN, Donckerwolcke RA, et al: Assessment of dialysis requirement for children on regular haemodialysis. Dial Transpl 11:754, 1982, with permission.)

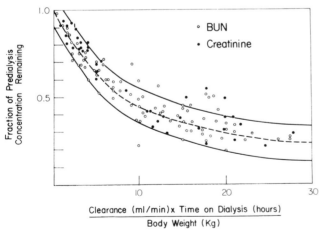

FIG. 39-2. *Predicted fractional decrease in BUN and creatinine in children as a function of dialyzer clearance, time, and body weight.* (From Kjellstrand CM, Mauer SM, Busemeier TJ, et al: Hemodialysis of premature and newborn babies. Proc Eur Dial Transplant Assoc 10:349, 1973, with permission.)

Kinetic Modeling

The dialysis index assumes that the limiting factor in achieving adequate dialysis is the quantity of middle molecules (substances with molecular weights 500 to 2000 daltons) removed during dialysis, and that the transport of middle molecules depends on the duration of dialysis and the surface area permeability product of the membrane [40,41,83]. In addition to the dialyzer clearance of middle molecules, the dialysis index accounts for the quantity of renal clearance of these solutes. In children, the total number of hours of dialysis required per week to achieve a dialysis index in the range of 13 to 18 can be calculated as dialyzer surface area (DSA) in square meters/body surface area (BSA) in square meters times the dialysis index. When a group of children was evaluated using this index assuming the DSA/BSA to be 0.75, a significant correlation between the dialysis index and plasma urate, but not BUN or creatinine, was observed [273]. Once dialysis was begun and the initial number of hours of treatment per week estimated using this formula, subsequent individualized schedules of dialysis time were based on predialysis urate levels [273].

The square meter hypothesis has been tested by using protocols that alter the dialysis prescription by varying blood flow, dialysate flow, dialyzer size, and total dialysis time. It has not been unequivocably established that the use of the dialysis index to determine total weekly dialysis time improves the clinical well-being of patients. Some studies suggest that the degree of peripheral neuropathy, which is believed by some to be a reliable indicator of the overall clinical adequacy of dialysis, is inversely related to this index [282]. Others have failed to find positive correlations between the dialysis index and serum middle molecule levels (e.g., vitamin B_{12}), nerve conduction velocity, or other outcome criteria [432,670]. The removal of smaller molecular weight solutes is believed by some to be equally important. Small molecular weight solute clearance (e.g., urea) parallels changes in middle molecular weight solute clearance. Thus, a dialysis prescription based on the control of small molecular weight solutes such as urea ought to provide adequate control of uremia [294].

The solute with the most intensively studied clearance as an indicator of the efficacy of dialysis is urea. During the past few years, the concept of urea kinetic modeling has been applied to pediatric populations as a method of determining an individual dialysis prescription [333, 334]. The rationale for using urea kinetic modeling is based on a number of factors. The uremic state is related to the end products of protein metabolism; consequently blood urea levels can be related to these effects [147,394]. Also, hydrogen ion production [295] and the dietary intake of potassium and phosphorus directly parallel protein intake [717].

The principles of urea kinetic modeling follow. Urea is generated at a constant rate, proportional to the protein catabolic rate; is distributed throughout body water; and is eliminated at a rate equal to the sum of any residual renal function and the dialyzer urea clearance. The relationship between these three variables, generation, removal, and accumulation—the overall mass balance—can be expressed as $d(VC)/dt = G - KC$.

In the absence of changes, the volume of distribution of urea during hemodialysis becomes:

$$C_T = C_O e^{-Kt/V} + G/K[1 - e^{-Kt/V}]$$

where C_T and C_O are urea concentrations at times T and O, respectively, K equals the sum of the residual renal and dialyzer clearance, t equals the time between T and O, V equals the volume of distribution of urea, and G is the urea generation rate. G and V are calculated by an iterative computer technique using known values for K and t and the repetitive measurements of urea at C_T and C_O. The volume (V) cleared is calculated from the change in urea concentration that occurs during dialysis, the duration of treatment, and the overall clearance. The interdialytic change in urea concentration and V are then used to calculate the urea generation rate (G). Subsequently, this value for G is used to recalculate a more precise value for V, and the process is continuously repeated until the best solution for G and V is obtained [333,491,716].

The results of a multicenter study of the clinical outcome of different adult dialysis regimens using urea kinetic modeling demonstrate the usefulness of this approach [490]. Four groups were studied, shorter (2.5 to 3.5 hours) and longer (4.5 to 5 hours) treatment times, and time average BUN concentrations (average BUN level between dialysis treatments) of 50 and 100 mg/dl. To maintain the BUN within these boundaries, the dialyzer clearance was adjusted. Mean concentrations of BUN were 52 and 89 mg/dl in the two groups. Treatment time did not affect patient morbidity. The morbidity in the low and high BUN groups differed, with the low BUN group experiencing less anorexia and pericarditis and fewer days of hospitalization. Many, however, believe that the factors determining the adequacy of dialysis are more complex [83].

As regards the application of urea kinetic modeling to pediatric hemodialysis prescriptions, a number of factors should be considered. The terms of the formula that describe the relationship between urea generation and protein catabolism are different in children than in adults. Also, accurate predictions of dialysis time in individual children require that a patient's specific volume of distribution of urea be determined. In a group of 26 children, the mean volume of distribution of urea (V)-to-body weight ratio varied from 0.50 to 0.70. Also, the mean volume-weight ratio was 0.57, and the individual patient coefficient of variation was 6% [333]. In children, it has been shown that the protein catabolic rate derived from urea kinetics appropriately reflects changes in their dietary intake of protein.

It is possible to estimate the time required to reduce the BUN by a given fraction of the predialysis BUN once a dialyzer clearance is selected, if the contribution of the residual renal clearance and urea generation rate during the dialysis treatment is ignored. During hemodialysis, the rate of change of BUN is that of a first order equation, $\log_e$ versus time [404]. The equation defining this curve is:

$$C_T/C_O = e^{-Kt/V}$$

where C_T/C_O is the desired fractional decrease in BUN, K is the dialyzer clearance to be used, t is the duration of the dialysis procedure, and V is the volume of distribution of urea assumed to be 60% of body weight.

Using the above formula, tables can be developed to list the desired fractional decrease in BUN and a term K × t/Wt_{kg}. This expression can be used either to calculate the desired length of treatment using a dialyzer set at a known BUN clearance or to determine the dialyzer clearance necessary to lower the BUN by a certain fraction in a fixed period of time. Its use in determining dialysis parameters requires that either K or t be held constant (Table 39-4).

An example of solving for t when K is fixed follows. The therapeutic goal of the treatment in a 10-kg child is to lower the BUN by 70%, and the dialyzer arbitrarily

TABLE 39-4. *Treatment variable to use in computing the time necessary to lower BUN by a given degree when performing dialysis with the dialyzer clearance set at 36 ml/min.*

Desired fraction of BUN at end of dialysis C_T/C_O	Treatment variable K × t/Wt_{kg}
0.9	63
0.8	134
0.7	214
0.6	306
0.5	415
0.4	549
0.3	722
0.2	965
0.1	1381

Terms are as defined in the text. C_T and C_0 = concentrations at time T and time zero; K = dialyzer clearance; t = time.

selected is a Gambro Mini Minor, which at a blood flow rate of 50 ml/minute has a clearance (K) of 36 ml/minute. The dialysis time required is calculated by using the above formula, as follows: fraction of predialysis BUN desired = $0.30 = C_T/C_O$ and $K \times t/Wt_{kg} = 722$ ml/kg (see Table 39-4); upon entering the child's weight, 10 kg, the expression becomes $K \times t = (10 \times 722)$ ml. The duration of treatment, t, is determined after introducing the value for the dialyzer clearance, $K = 36$ ml/min: $t = (10 \times 722) \div 36 = 200$ minutes.

This approach is most useful in acute hemodialysis or in determining individual treatment changes in BUN in children on long-term dialysis. Kinetic modeling is believed by some to offer better control of the uremic state than other approaches used to prescribe dialysis treatments. In practice, kinetic modeling is done using either a computer or a programmable calculator.

The most widely practiced clinical approach for selecting dialysis parameters is to evaluate dialysis efficiency by measuring BUN predialysis and postdialysis. The therapeutic objective is to maintain predialysis values for BUN in the range of 100 to 120 mg/dl and to lower the BUN during dialysis by 60% to 75%. If careful attention is paid to the child's nutritional status, such an approach is often acceptable. The shortcoming of such an approach, however, is that it fails to account for any residual renal function, the ongoing urea generation, the precise volume of distribution of urea, and the impact on BUN of changes in dietary protein intake.

Ultrafiltration

Because blood flow rates and treatment times can be easily manipulated to achieve the desired dialyzer clearance, a major consideration in choosing a dialyzer is its ultrafiltration characteristics. Each membrane has a unique ultrafiltration coefficient. Ultrafiltration rates are inversely related to the thickness of the membrane and also depend on its size, structure, and composition. In practice, dialyzer ultrafiltration rates are obtained by continuously measuring weight loss with a bed or chair scale in patients dialyzed for 30 to 90 minutes at a fixed transmembrane pressure. The correlation between ultrafiltration rate and the TMP used in clinical dialysis is linear. Ultrafiltration characteristics for pediatric dialyzers are summarized in Table 39-5. Although each dialyzer comes with a graph or table describing the TMP needed to achieve a desired amount of ultrafiltration (standard ultrafiltration coefficient, SUFC), most patients do not respond as predicted. The TMP used during the first dialysis treatment is selected on the basis of ultrafiltration information provided by manufacturers. In the event that satisfactory ultrafiltration does not occur, it is possible to compute an individual patient ultrafiltration coefficient (IPUFC) [623] (Table 39-6).

Two clinical situations suggest that the ultrafiltration coefficient ought to be individualized: first, the child loses the desired amount of weight but becomes symptomatic before completing treatment and requires intravascular fluid expansion; second, the child fails to lose the predetermined amount of weight during dialysis. A scheme for calculating an IPUFC follows. Assume a child gained 1 kg since the last dialysis, which used a 0.54-m² dialyzer. During the first 2 hours of treatment, when TMP is set at 365 mm Hg, the child requires 50 ml of mannitol and 200 ml of saline to treat repeated episodes of hypotension. The child's postdialysis weight is 1 kg less than predialysis weight. By the end of the treatment, even though the child lost the desired amount of fluid, 1000 ml, the treatment cannot be considered ideal because of hypotensive episodes.

What happens to water balance during dialysis? The water loss during the treatment is in fact greater than that suggested by changes in predialysis versus postdialysis weights. The child's total weight loss (water) during the procedure, in addition to that indicated by the difference in predialysis and postdialysis weights, includes the fluid contained in the blood lines and the dialyzer (priming and compliance volumes) and fluid given orally or intravenously. The weight loss contributed by each of these factors as well as the anticipated weight loss based on the SUFC provided by the manufacturer is summarized in Table 39-5. The child, however, actually lost 498 ml more than the amount originally calculated (1528 ml − 1030 ml = 498 ml). The formula for calculating the child's IPUFC is:

Actual weight loss/calculated weight loss = IPUFC/SUFC or 1528/1030 = IPUFC/1, and IPUFC = 1.5.

Once an IPUFC is determined, the TMP for the same dialyzer in subsequent treatments is calculated by first choosing the total amount of fluid that needs to be ultrafiltered, dividing this volume by the hours of dialysis to ascertain the ultrafiltration rate per hour, and dividing this value by the IPUFC. IPUFC adjustments may be calculated for each dialysis treatment or readjusted at monthly intervals in stable patients. The IPUFC should be recalculated whenever a different sized dialyzer is used or a new batch of dialyzers arrives.

The amount of ultrafiltration planned for a dialysis treatment needs to account for the child's interdialytic weight gain and degree of volume related hypertension. It is reasonable to try to limit the interdialytic sodium intake, the major factor controlling water intake, so that interdialytic weight gain does not exceed 5% of "dry" weight. A fluid loss of 5% to 6% of body weight from ultrafiltration is usually well tolerated; volume removal in excess of this amount often leads to acute hypotension, although edematous hypertensive children may tolerate ultrafiltration volumes of 10% of body weight [515]. In problem patients and in small infants, the accurate and continuous weighing of patients throughout dialysis permits the quality of ultrafiltrate formed to be determined [431,560]. Recently developed equipment contains monitoring devices that are capable of continuously and accurately determining the amount of ultrafiltrate formed. Two problems may develop unless the compliance characteristics of the dialyzer are considered when deciding which size surface area dialyzer will achieve specific ultrafiltration objectives. First, hypotension can occur because of the accumulation of too much blood in the extracorporeal circuit when the transmembrane pressure is increased. Second, hypertension can occur because of the reinfusion of too much blood when the transmembrane pressure is lowered.

Two techniques, dry dialysis and sequential ultrafiltra-

Table 39-5. *Characteristics of pediatric hemodialyzers arranged by size*

Dialyzer	Effective surface area m^2	Type of dialyzer	Priming volume ml	Ultrafiltration	
				Compliance ml/100 mm Hg	Coefficient ml/hr mm Hg TMP
Mini Minor-Gambro	0.20	Plate	20	6	0.4–0.6
ExCel 0.3p-Extracorporeal	0.30	Capillary	30	0	1.4
Lundia Minor-Gambro	0.41	Plate	33	10	1.2–1.6
Travenol CA-50	0.5	Capillary	38	0	2.4
TAF 0.6-Terumo	0.60	Capillary	48	0	2.3–2.4
HPF 50-Erika	0.60	Capillary	45	0	1.7
LENTO-Organon Teknika	0.70	Capillary	65	0	2.8
HF 70-Cobe	0.70	Capillary	52	0	2.3
HF 100-Cobe	0.77	Capillary	54	0	3.3
Travenol CA-70	0.7	Capillary	51	0	2.5
TAF 0.8-Terumo	0.80	Capillary	56	0	3.3–3.6
DISSAP 0.8-Hospal	0.80	Capillary	52	0	2.7
L-Travenol	0.80	Capillary	59	0	2.7
PPD 0.8-Cobe	0.80	Plate	45	25	2.0
EX P 200-Extracorporeal	0.85	Plate	65	11	2.0
SEC 70-Cordis	0.90	Capillary	71	0	1.8–2
HPF 100-Erika	0.90	Capillary	67	0	3.2

* Data supplied by manufacturers.

Table 39-6. *Stepwise ultrafiltration calculation (SUFC) of individual patient ultrafiltration coefficient (IPUFC)*

1. Calculate anticipated weight loss using SUFC provided with dialyzer. SUFC = 1.0

Time	TMP	Ultrafiltration volume
2 hrs	365	730 ml
2 hrs	150	300 ml
Totals 4 hrs		1030 ml predicted weight loss

2. Calculate total fluid (actual weight loss) removed from the body

Measured weight loss (pre-post dialysis weight)	1000 ml
Priming volume dialyzer	43 ml
Volume of blood lines	85 ml
Oral intake of fluid during dialysis	150 ml
Mannitol	50 ml
Saline	200 ml
Total fluid ultrafiltrated	1528 ml

3. Determine IPUFC

   Actual weight loss/calculated weight loss = IPUFC/SUFC 1528 ml/1030 ml; IPUFC = 1.50

4. Calculate TMP to use in subsequent treatments

   Determine total fluid to lose during the treatment. Add:

volume of blood lines	_____ ml
prime volume of dialyzer	_____ ml
anticipated fluid intake during dialysis	_____ ml
fluid to remove during dialysis	_____ ml
total fluid to ultrafiltrate	_____ ml
Divide amount of ultrafiltration needed by the number of hours of treatment	_____ ml/hr
Divide ultrafiltration rate ml/hr by IPUFC to ascertain TMP to use	_____ mmHg

tion dialysis, can be used to reduce extracellular volume. Dry dialysis is done by perfusing blood through a dialyzer with the dialysate pump turned off. This procedure can be used either at the beginning or at the end of a dialysis treatment. Large amounts of iso-osmotic extracellular fluid can be quickly removed without significantly affecting the chemical composition of blood. Sequential ultrafiltration dialysis involves performing diffusion dialysis alone. The

TMP is set at zero for the usual length of time and is either preceded or followed by pure ultrafiltration for 1 to 2 hours so that ultrafiltration goals are met [71]. Cartridges used for continuous arteriovenous hemofiltration can be used alone or in series with hemodialyzers to remove excess edema.

Vascular Access

Vascular access, a necessary condition for performing hemodialysis, remains its most frustrating aspect [220,745]. A number of shunts fail to function immediately, and their long-term use continues to be associated with clotting problems, infection, and mechanically related problems. Historically, the external Scribner arteriovenous Silastic shunt was the first angioaccess used in children. This shunt, which is rarely used now in children because of the many technical, infectious, and clotting problems associated with its use, has been replaced by newer devices and techniques for cannulating large vessels.

Acute hemodialysis can be performed after inserting either single-lumen or double-lumen catheters. Using the Seldinger percutaneous technique [335,740], catheters are placed in both femoral veins with one of the catheters advanced to the inferior vena cava. The inferior vena cava catheter serves as the return conduit, while the catheter left in the external iliac vein functions as the "arterial" blood line. A more practical approach in children is to place a single catheter in the inferior vena cava and connect it to a single needle device that allows blood to be intermittently withdrawn and returned to the patient. The use of single-lumen catheters results in blood being recirculated and a reduced solute clearance. Another technique is to withdraw blood from the femoral venous catheter and return it to a vein in the upper extremity. Double lumen catheters available in pediatric and neonatal sizes are preferred.

Femoral vein catheters cannot be left in place between dialysis treatments unless the extremity is immobilized. When the catheter is removed, pressure needs to be applied over the puncture site for 15 to 30 minutes so that adequate hemostasis occurs and hematoma formation is avoided. Complications associated with this procedure include thrombosis, hematoma, local and systemic infection, and femoral vein–artery fistula [742]. Small vessels and the need for repeated femoral vein puncture tend to restrict the use of femoral catheters in small children.

The use of the subclavian vein for hemodialysis access avoids the aforementioned problems [819]. Even though subclavian catheters can be inserted in the patient's room, most prefer to have these catheters inserted in the operating room, where meticulous attention can be paid to sterile technique and patient cooperation is not needed. Two general types of catheters are currently used: catheters available with either a single or a double lumen [810,811] or the Silastic right atrial single or double lumen Hickman catheter. The latter has been successfully used in infants [499] and is clearly superior to the external Scribner shunt for acute access in children [280]. The double lumen catheter has also been successfully used in older children for

months. A detailed review of the types of hemodialysis catheters and access devices is available [357].

The technique for placement of catheters in the neck is as follows. An incision is made, the external or internal jugular vein is identified, and a venotomy is performed. The catheter is tunneled through a skin exit site on the anterior chest and passed through the venotomy to the desired location. The position of its tip is verified by x-ray and its patency demonstrated. The lumen of the catheter, whose volume is approximately 1 ml, is filled with 5000 U/ml of heparin and the external opening of the catheter capped. Finally, the exit site is covered with a sterile dressing.

Some leave the catheter alone between dialysis treatments; others prefer to flush the lumen with a heparin solution once or twice a day. Acute complications following insertion of these catheters include hemothorax and pneumothorax, hemomediastinum and pneumomediastinum, and bleeding at the exit site. In some centers, the catheters are changed every week by passing a guidewire through the existing system, withdrawing the catheter and reinserting a new catheter over the guideline. Others change catheters only when chronic problems with clotting or infection develop. These catheters, especially the Hickman catheter in neonates and infants, have been successfully used for a number of months as access for chronic dialysis.

An alternative to the Hickman catheter that has been used in children for central vein access is a single hole silicone rubber catheter that does not have a Dacron cuff and can be readjusted at the bedside [847]. Grommets are placed on the catheter to insert it into the venous system and to fix it to the sternomastoid muscle.

Complications related to the use of subclavian catheters include local pain, local hematoma, thrombosis within the catheter, sepsis, thrombosis of the subclavian vein and vena cava, ipsilateral and contralateral hemothorax, pneumothorax, mediastinal hematoma, and pericardial tamponade [819]. Vascular perforation may result in death. Vessel perforation and right atrial perforation can occur either at the time of initial insertion or after repeated hemodialyses. Reasons for dysfunction include the to and fro movement of catheters during dialysis as well as the direct contact of rigid materials against vascular endothelium.

Long-term angioaccess is achieved by direct arteriovenous anastomosis with either autologous or homologous vessels or by connecting an artery to a vein with synthetic materials. The external Silastic-teflon Scribner shunt or one of its modifications, the Ramirez, Thomas, Allen-Brown, or Buselmeier shunts, is rarely used anymore for long-term vascular access for many reasons, including the separation of teflon tubes used to connect the arterial and venous tubing, the sacrifice of the distal segment of the artery as part of the surgical procedure, the risk of developing bacteremia and infection at exposed exit sites, the erosion of either tubing or stabilizing attachments through the skin, and the frequent development of thrombosis, the major limiting factor affecting shunt survival. The long-term patency rate of external shunts is in the range of 2.2 to 15.6 months [256]. The technical details of external shunt surgery can be found elsewhere [565,745].

The internal arteriovenous fistula is now the most widely used vascular access for long-term hemodialysis in older children. Major advantages include long survival, low rates of infection, and the ability to use the extremity freely between dialysis treatments. The Cimino-Brescia internal arteriovenous shunt, initially described in 1966 [105], requires a single incision through which either the radial artery and cephalic vein in the wrist or the brachial artery and basilic or cephalic vein at the elbow are anastomosed. The creation of a similar type fistula within the anatomic snuffbox has been described [525]. An arteriovenous fistula can be constructed within the antecubital fossa [425]. Four anastomotic variations of connecting an artery to a vein are possible: side to side, artery side to vein, artery end to vein, or end to end. The use of the end of the artery avoids the potential problem of developing a steal (ischemic) syndrome with blood being shunted through the palmer arch from the ulnar artery. When the artery is sewn into the side of the vein, varicosities of the veins in the hand may develop. If the diameter of the anastomosis exceeds 69% of the arterial diameter, adequate fistula function should occur [611].

Internal arteriovenous fistulae are not used for 5 to 6 weeks after creation so that arterialization of the anastomosed vein can occur. Otherwise, excessive leakage after removal of the dialysis needle, with the associated risk of thrombosis, tends to occur. Blood pressures should not routinely be taken in the arm with the fistula because of the risk of thrombosis. Also, the routine administration of intravenous fluids and phlebotomies should not involve the fistula. Complications associated with the use of such access include failure of the fistula to mature, development of aneurysms at the anastomotic lines, hematoma, and both local and systemic infection.

Immediate success of forearm fistulas in children weighing over 20 kg ranges from 70% [267] to 80% [750]. Long-term patency has been reported in one study to be 84% and 78% at 1 year for forearm and elbow fistulas, respectively [267]. A 3-year patency rate of 80% has been reported [529]. In a report of 434 angioaccesses in 380 children (74 weighing less than 10 kg), 85% and 60% of distal radial cephalic fistula were patent after two and four years, respectively [99a]. The failure rate for the ulnar basilic fistula was 41% and was attributed to a lower ulnar artery blood flow rate. Fistula in children weighing less than 10 kg did not last as long as those in larger children.

Because of the small size of blood vessels in younger children, many believe that a synthetic bridge graft placed subcutaneously is the preferred method for gaining access. The development of expanded polytetrafluorethylene (PTFE) grafts, Impra and Gore-Tex, has to a large extent replaced the use of bovine carotid artery, human umbilical vein, and autologous basilic or saphenous vein grafts, which all have high failure rates [96,529], cannot be used in small children, require more surgery, tend to thrombose and form aneurysms, and often result in the loss of a vein. Limited experience with the use of saphenous vein [626] and bovine carotid artery grafts [167] in older children has been reported.

PTFE grafts, available since 1975, are preferably implanted in the upper extremity. A number of anastomotic connections can be made: a straight graft between the brachial artery and the axillary vein, a straight graft between the radial artery and the basilic vein, or a loop graft between the brachial artery and the basilic vein. When necessary, shunts can be implanted between the superficial or deep femoral artery and saphenous vein. Infectious complications and thrombosis of patent vessels, however, are greater when the lower extremity is used [745]. Shunts placed in the lower extremity are not desirable because of the possibility of distal embolization secondary to thrombus formation. Such grafts can be placed from artery to artery as a last resort [565]. An elevated basilic vein arteriovenous fistula has been used as an alternative to a PTFE graft [175]. In a series involving 66 patients, the 2-year patency rate was 83.3%, and no infections occurred.

The graft material is cut at a 30° to 45° angle, sutured first end-to-side to the artery, with the size of the lumen of the anastomosis being 1.5 to 2.0 times that of the diameter of the graft, drawn through a previously prepared subcutaneous tunnel, and finally anastomosed end-to-side to the vein. It is recommended that at least 2 to 4 weeks be allowed for a pseudointima to form in artificial conduits. Otherwise, bleeding may occur from puncture sites after removing dialysis needles, with the attendant risk for developing thrombosis from the compression required to secure hemostasis. Also, infection is more prone to develop when a hematoma forms. The patency rate for Gortex grafts in adults is 70% at 2 years [529]. Varying results have been reported in children [267,745]. A dose of vancomycin, approximately 15 mg/kg infused every 2 weeks through the venous sleeve during the last 90 minutes of dialysis, has been shown to reduce the incidence of graft infection in children [253].

It is generally believed that vascular access for hemodialysis with two needles is preferred to using a single needle system, which may not allow high enough blood flow rates and results in recirculation. Clinical experience, however, using a single needle system has been acceptable. Urea kinetic modeling, hematocrit, nerve conduction velocity, hospital admission rate, and cumulative patient survival rates in adults being dialyzed with a single needle system have been shown to be similar to that observed in patients undergoing dual needle dialysis [820]. Most importantly the 5-year fistula survival rate was 74% with single needle systems, exceeding rates published for dual needle access systems. Blood pump systems for single needle access can achieve blood flow rates of 288 ± 33 ml/minute, rates equal to those observed with dual needle access [361]. Also, dual needle access systems are associated with recirculation, especially when increased venous resistance is present. A recirculation rate of 14% reduces dialyzer urea clearance by 8.2%. Overall urea clearance still remains within the range of values obtained with dual needle systems. The percent recirculation is calculated as follows:

$$\% \text{ Recirculation} = (C_{Bv} - C_{Bi})/(C_{Bv} - C_{Bo})$$

where C_B equals the blood urea concentration in samples obtained from v, venous blood; o and i, outlet and inlet dialyzer lines.

The major complications of vascular access are infection,

clotting, and venous stenosis [790a]. Most often clotting and stenosis in children are treated surgically. Urokinase flushes have been used to declot clotted subclavian catheters. Percutaneous angioplasty techniques have been used to treat venous stenosis. Intravascular ultrasound as well as angiography have been used to evaluate the anatomy of involved vessels [173a]. Infection is most commonly caused by S. aureus or S. epidermidis. Local cellulitis, abscess, and tunnel infections can occur. The infected vein of a Cimino fistula usually must be excised and the subcutaneous tunnel drained. In synthetic grafts a jump graft may be tried. The incidence of infections is higher in synthetic compared to native grafts. Bacteremia leading to bacterial endocarditis, osteomyelitis, meningitis, septic arthritis, and empyema may develop. Ischemic symptomatology distal to the graft can occur.

Anticoagulation

Heparin, which is the most widely used anticoagulant to prevent clotting within blood lines and dialyzers, is most often obtained from beef lung. It is also available from other sources (porcine heparin) when heparin allergy develops. The half-life of heparin, which is similar in uremic and non-uremic individuals, is approximately 1 hour. Its disappearance follows first order elimination kinetics. In practice, the dose of heparin is individualized for each child because the response, or degree of anticoagulation observed, and the rate of elimination of heparin display a large degree of individual variability.

The Lee-White clotting time and the activated whole blood coagulation time (ACT) are used to monitor anticoagulation. The Lee-White whole blood clotting time is performed by adding 1 ml of blood to several small test tubes and measuring the time required for a visible clot to form. Preferably, the blood should be kept at 37°C, but, in practice, clotting times are usually done at room temperature. The tubes are tilted at 30-second intervals until clotting occurs to the degree that the tubes can be inverted without spilling. The clotting time, measured with a stop watch, is taken as the average of the clotting times of the individual tubes. Once the pattern of heparinization has been established, some use only one tube to reduce blood loss.

Although often used without major problems, the Lee-White whole blood clotting technique has some shortcomings. The end point tends to be imprecise, and rapid adjustments in anticoagulation are not possible because of the long time required for clotting in already heparinized patients. More precise monitoring and control of anticoagulation, used either systemically or regionally, can be accomplished by measuring the ACT, which has replaced the Lee-White whole blood clotting time in most dialysis centers.

The ACT is performed by adding whole blood to tubes containing a substance such as ground glass, kaolin, or earth. These substances quickly activate the early steps in the coagulation process and lead to the rapid clotting of blood. A machine that automatically performs and provides values for the ACT is available. At room temperature, the

ACT in normals has a range of 90 to 140 seconds. In uncomplicated patients undergoing dialysis, the ACT should be maintained in the range of 180 to 240 seconds. The ACT in patients with bleeding problems should be kept between 150 and 180 seconds by administering heparin either as a continuous infusion or by giving boluses of heparin intermittently [821]. Outlined in Table 39-7 is a scheme to determine the required quantity of heparin based on increases in ACT per unit of heparin administered, heparin sensitivity, and the fractional elimination of heparin (heparin elimination constant) [231,821]. A detailed description of this technique is provided elsewhere [485].

Anticoagulation can be either systemic or regional. When systemic heparinization is used, it is given as a bolus dose followed by either a continuous infusion or additional boluses at a lower dose. In children who do not have bleeding problems, heparin at a loading dose of 50 units per kg body weight is followed either by a continuous infusion of 50 U/kg/hour [200] or an additional bolus of heparin at a dose of 25 U/kg 2 hours into the treatment. In both situations, the dose of heparin is adjusted to keep the Lee-White clotting time in the range of 20 to 30 minutes, the normal clotting time being 8 to 12 minutes.

In children who are to have surgery within 24 hours after undergoing dialysis, who have had surgery within the past 5 days, or who otherwise are at risk for bleeding, lower doses of heparin should be considered. This is done by initially giving a loading dose of 25 U/kg, followed by intermittent doses of 25 U/kg, with the Lee-White clotting time kept at 12 to 15 minutes. Protamine infused over a few minutes at the end of dialysis, in the amount of 1 mg per 100 U of heparin given during the last 2 hours of dialysis, will counteract 50% of the administered heparin. Side effects associated with too much protamine include anaphylactic reactions and anticoagulation. Another method to achieve low dose heparinization is not to give a loading dose to the patient but to give a continuous infusion of heparin and maintain the ACT at less than 180 seconds. Usually 250–500 units of heparin per hour is infused using a pump with a syringe containing 1000 units of heparin per ml.

Regional heparinization can also be used. It requires the simultaneous infusion of heparin into the arterial blood line and protamine into the venous side of the dialyzer. It also requires frequent measurements of clotting times and

Table 39-7. *Scheme to determine loading and replacement doses of heparin using whole blood activated clotting times (ACT)*

Heparin sensitivity (HS)	=	[ACT immediately after loading dose of heparin − ACT base line] / units of heparin given
Heparin elimination (HE)	=	[ACT 1 hr after giving heparin − ACT baseline] / [ACT immediately after loading dose − ACT baseline]
Loading dose (LD)	=	ACT desired time − ACT baseline / HS

Units of heparin to give every 2 hrs = LD × E

Units of heparin required hourly as a continuous infusion =
$$[LD \times E] + [LD \times E^2]$$

repeated adjustments of the infusion rates of heparin or protamine or both. The use of regional heparinization is difficult and often does not work as expected. Dialyzers tend to clot, and rebound heparinization may occur 2 to 3 hours after dialysis is completed [328]. Rebound heparinization occurs because protamine is metabolized faster than heparin. Thus, when regional heparinization is used, the clotting time should be checked 3 to 4 hours after completing the dialysis. Finally, it is important that the same vial of heparin be used throughout a given dialysis because the heparin content between bottles may vary by as much as 10%. Heparin vials may become contaminated with bacteria and bacterial endotoxin and cause pyrogenic reactions [406].

Another application of anticoagulation agents in dialysis patients involves the use of antiplatelet drugs to prevent platelet initiated clotting in patients with arteriovenous fistula or Silastic catheters. Acetylsalicylic acid [338], sulfinpyrazone [400], and dipyridamole are believed by some to prolong shunt life. Although anticoagulation with warfarin (Coumadin) also enhances shunt life, its use is contraindicated because of the increased risk of hemorrhagic complications [866]. In adult sized individuals, the doses of these drugs are aspirin, 325 to 625 mg daily; dipyridamole, 100 mg two to three times daily; and sulfinpyrazone, 200 mg four times a day. Some believe that a combination of two antiplatelet agents given at a lower dose may be more effective than a single agent. Prospective controlled trials demonstrating the relative effectiveness of antiplatelet agents are unavailable. In most pediatric dialysis units, the use of these agents is reserved for patients who experience problems with the patency of their shunts.

Additional anticoagulants that have been used with limited success include citrate and prostacyclin. The use of prostacyclin as an anticoagulant is associated with a high rate of complications, including hypotension and chest pain [878]. Regionally delivered citrate anticoagulation has been used without significant problems in patients with bleeding problems [864]. Its use requires that calcium be continuously provided in the venous return. One recommended approach is to infuse a 0.1 M solution of citrate at a mean flow rate of 4.3% of the dialyzer blood flow rate [149a]. The excessive volume may become a problem.

Infant Hemodialysis

The past decade has seen the application of hemodialysis to infants in only a limited number of pediatric centers. Premature infants weighing as little as 1500 g have been hemodialyzed for several weeks [560]. Some systems have been modified to perform simultaneously exchange transfusion [560] or hemoperfusion [142] in addition to hemodialysis. Long-term hemodialysis is used predominantly to prepare infants with advanced renal insufficiency for transplantation. Acute hemodialysis has also been used in infants to treat inborn errors of metabolism [862], poisoning, electrolyte imbalance, and volume overload.

The principles of hemodialysis and the machines used in infants are similar to those used in older children. However, a small body size imposes differences related to access,

blood lines, dialyzers, and monitoring. In infants, most forms of vascular access have been used with varying degrees of success. Umbilical vessels can be used in neonates. Although prone to clotting and infection, Scribner shunts in appropriate size can be placed into the superficial femoral artery and saphenous vein or the brachial artery and cephalic or basilic vein [121]. Arteriovenous fistula [100,259], polytetrafluoroethylene grafts [25], and polyethylene tubing (size 190 or 240 inserted using the Seldinger technique) [560] have also been successfully used. Standard Shaldon femoral vein catheters are too large to use in infants. The access most widely used is the right atrial Hickman catheter [356,499]. Dialysis is done with a unipuncture system if a single lumen catheter is used. Advantages include ease of insertion, immediate usability, and long-term survival when the catheter is cared for properly. Patency between dialysis is achieved by instilling a heparin solution and capping the catheters between treatment. Some prefer to flush the catheter with a heparin saline solution daily or every other day.

The hemodialyzer most often used in children weighing less than 10 kg is the Gambro Mini-Minor, which has a surface area of 0.23 m^2, priming volume of 19 ml, and a compliance of 6% (6 ml/100 mm Hg TMP). In those infants needing greater clearances or ultrafiltration rates, the Gambro Lundia Minor, with a priming volume of 29 ml and a 10% compliance, can be used if the system is primed with either 5% albumin or whole blood. Neonatal blood lines, 15 or 25 ml, should be used in neonates; pediatric lines, 52 or 65 ml, can be used in children weighing more than 5 kg. In practice, the system is primed with blood for the initial few treatments in infants weighing less than 5 kg. In stable patients, 5% albumin is used in subsequent treatments, but blood should be available.

It is the painstaking attention to the details of monitoring infants that makes hemodialysis possible in this age range. Equipment that is not routinely used in performing dialysis in older children is needed. Monitoring of vital signs is most effectively done using a cardiac monitor for determining pulse rate, an intra-arterial blood pressure line or a Doppler blood pressure apparatus to measure blood pressure, and a rectal probe to measure core body temperature. Neonates are especially at risk for developing hypothermia related to transport to the dialysis unit or related to the failure to preheat and maintain dialysate at body temperature and are best dialyzed under an external infrared heater. Most importantly, weight needs to be continuously and accurately measured to ensure that neither volume overload nor hypovolemia occurs. Scales accurate to 5 to 10 g should be used. All equipment to be used during the dialysis should be placed in the crib, and the lines connected to ventilators, monitors, and the dialysis machine should be taped to the side of the crib. These lines are taped a second time to a platform adjacent to the crib so that traction will not be applied to the crib and the weight of the crib altered. The bed scale, which now supports the infant and all of the tubing, is set at zero. Any weight changes that occur during dialysis are assumed to be changes in water balance.

Dialysis is begun with the lowest possible blood flow rate and TMP. Adjustments can be made every 10 to 15 minutes until the desired, predetermined dialysis parameters are reached. Heparinization is usually done starting with an infusion rate of 0.6 to 0.8 U/kg/minute for the first 30 minutes and then adjusted to keep the Lee-White clotting time at 150% of predialysis values [428]. Sequential ultrafiltration dialysis can be done in infants; however, such infants are prone to becoming hypothermic because there is no warm dialysate in contact with the dialyzing membrane. Also, the TMP should be kept at values less than 400 mm Hg to minimize the risk of membrane rupture [560].

Hemofiltration

Hemofiltration is the process of convective solute removal from uremic whole blood [343,349] (Fig. 39-3). Blood is diluted either before or after being exposed to a high flux membrane and reconstituted before being returned to the patient. Hemofiltration can be performed alone or can be done simultaneously with hemodialysis, a process labeled as diafiltration or hemodiafiltration. Vascular access for hemofiltration is similar to that of hemodialysis.

The characteristics of membranes used for hemofiltration differ from those used in hemodialysis in that solutes of low and middle molecular weight readily pass through the membrane, whereas neither formed cellular elements nor macrosolutes such as albumin are able to traverse the membrane. Different hemofiltration membranes (hemofilters) constructed from triacetate, polysulfone, polyamide, or polyacrylonitrile permit the passage of solutes with molecular weights of 15,000–50,000 daltons [663,664].

The site at which the diluting fluid is added affects the hemofiltration process. In comparison to post-dilution, pre-dilution necessitates up to 30% more substitution fluid, permits the filtrate flow to be increased, and enables more solute with a molecular weight greater than 5000 to be removed [782]. The concentration of solute in the ultrafiltrate is less. The major problem with predilution is the cost involved in preparing increased amounts of diluting fluid. Recommended concentrations of solutes to add to the diluting fluid are variable. Reported ranges include sodium, 130 to 150 mEq/liter; potassium, 0 to 4 mEq/liter; calcium, 4.0 to 8.0 mg/dl; magnesium, 1.4 to 1.6 mg/dl; lactate, acetate, or bicarbonate, 35 to 40 mmol/liter; and chloride, 105 to 115 mEq/liter. Dextrose is added in concentrations ranging from 0 to 100 mg/dl. Attempts to produce the required amount of sterile diluting fluid by regenerating filtrate by oxidation techniques [663,665] or by sorbent regeneration [349] have met with limited success as a means of reducing cost. The total amount of diluting fluid used during a single treatment in adults varies from 20 to 40 liters; in one report involving children, the quantity of diluent used averaged 57% of body weight with a range of 28% to 92% [548].

The large quantity of fluid that is rapidly removed and reinfused during the hemofiltration process requires that the fluid balance of the patient be carefully monitored. This is done by continuously weighing the substitution fluid and filtrate and adjusting the speed of the filtrate and substitution fluid pumps. Fluid removal and its replacement need to be done at a constant continuous rate so as to avoid abrupt fluid shifts in the patient.

Current indications for hemofiltration are limited to the long-term control of uremia and the removal of large quantities of edema in patients with acute renal failure, ne-

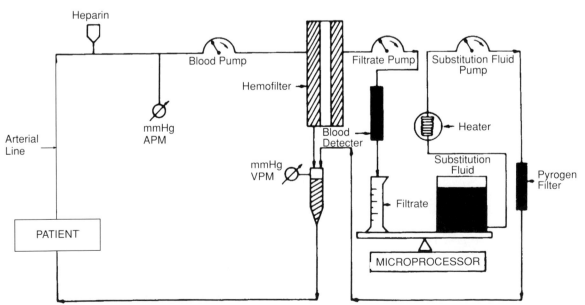

FIG. 39-3. *Schematic drawing of an automated hemofiltration system. (From Pascual JF, Lopez JD, Molina M : Hemofiltration in children with renal failure. Pediatr Clin North Am 34:803, 1987, with permission.)*

phrotic syndrome [860], and diuretic resistant congestive heart failure [664]. Other applications of hemofiltration include removal of drugs and the treatment of hepatic coma. Improved technology within the past few years has made it possible to expand the application of hemofiltration [331].

The clinical effects of hemofiltration differ from those of hemodialysis. Compared with hemodialysis and peritoneal dialysis (in which the occurrence of headache, nausea, and muscle cramps is related to the fractional reduction of body weight during the treatment), the incidence of similar symptoms at similar degrees of weight loss is considerably less with hemofiltration. Also, in a controlled prospective study, peripheral neuropathy improved when patients were switched from hemodialysis to hemofiltration [664].

Compared with hemodialysis, hemofiltration affects the cardiovascular system differently. Post-treatment blood pressures are higher, the number of hypotensive episodes is lower [46,71], peripheral resistance either increases or does not change [46], and serum catecholamine levels remain stable [46]. These findings are best explained by a rapid refilling of the extracellular space with fluid derived from the intracellular space [692]. Hemofiltration is believed by some to improve the long-term control of hypertension in both volume and renin dependent hypertensive patients [347,665]; others have not had similar experiences [46]. Data on the long-term development of cardiovascular complications are not yet available. Cholesterol levels are reported to be unchanged. Some suggest that plasma triglyceride levels can be favorably influenced by hemofiltration [352].

In adults followed for 8 years, survival rates were similar in groups undergoing hemodialysis or hemofiltration [331]. Morbidity, however, was higher in the group receiving hemodialysis. Also, higher long-term survival rates were obtained when hemofiltration rather than hemodialysis was used in patients over 60 years of age [721]. Long-term morbidity and mortality data in children treated with hemofiltration are not available.

Hemofiltration does not materially affect calcium balance and may enable a reduction in the dose of phosphate binders. Hypercalcemia is not a characteristic of hemofiltration. Hemofiltration is more efficient than hemodialysis in lowering serum concentrations of phosphate. Serum phosphate levels may remain reduced over a long-term period with hemofiltration therapy [265]; others have not had a similar experience [46]. Parathormone levels are reported to remain unchanged or to fall [664]. In 10 children treated for 6 months with hemofiltration and $1,25(OH)_2D_3$ to maintain serum calcium concentrations between 9.5 and 11.0 mg/dl, N-terminal iPTH levels did not change, whereas C-terminal levels fell [76]. Discontinuation of therapy in five children was associated with worsening of hyperparathyroidism.

Long-term studies of the impact of hemofiltration on most endocrine systems are lacking. Available data indicate that T_3, T_4, and thyroid-stimulating hormone (TSH) decrease, but hypothyroidism does not develop [732]. TSH, testosterone, cortisone, gastrin, and somatomedin B levels do not change during the course of single treatments. Growth hormone levels are reported to fall during hemo-

filtration treatments, but this finding may have reflected the ingestion of food during the treatment [454].

Limited data on the use of hemofiltration in children are available. One report from a single center involved 182 treatments, 10 for acute and 172 for chronic renal failure in 18 children, ages 2 to 21 years, and weighing 9.6 to 65.5 kg [548,549]. A positive linear correlation was demonstrated between the filtration flow rate of the Sartorius Haemoprocessor (Sartorius Wesbury, NY) and blood flow rate when the mean filtration flow rate was set at 55 ml/minute, blood flow rate was set at 224 ml/minute, and the TMP was set at 500 mmHg. The postdilution volume of substitution fluid averaged 75% of body weight (range 28% to 92%). In 87 treatments, percentile weight loss ranged from 1.5% to 11.8%. The larger the filtered volume, the greater the loss of amino acids and glucose. The latter was not added to the diluting fluid in these studies. Amino acid losses exceed those of conventional hemodialysis.

Side effects of treatment occurred primarily in patients whose weight loss exceeded 1% of body weight per hour. In 100 consecutive treatments, side effects developed in 22 patients. Complications included back pain (1), cramps (2), headaches (9), paresthesia (1), shivers (6), and vomiting (3). When children undergoing hemofiltration were compared with children undergoing hemodialysis and experiencing similar losses of weight, the children treated by hemofiltration had neither as great a rise in their pulse rate nor as great a decline in blood pressure.

In another center in which hemodialysis was discontinued and hemofiltration started in four children because of symptomatic hypotension, the frequency of hypotensive episodes fell from 40% to 20%. Also, the incidence of dizziness decreased from 72% with hemodialysis to 8% with hemofiltration [620]. In a third report involving six children placed on hemofiltration after being on hemodialysis for 12 months, hemofiltration was associated with fewer dialysis related complications (3% compared with 24%) such as hypotension, headaches, and cramps (which disappeared) [252].

Continuous Arteriovenous Hemofiltration

Continuous arteriovenous hemofiltration (CAVH) is a useful technique for treating edematous states in children, particularly neonates [686,687]. Pumpless or spontaneous arteriovenous hemofiltration was first described in 1977 as a way of removing excess iso-osmotic fluid [455]. A catheter is placed into an artery and connected to a hemofiltration filter, and the venous effluent is returned to a vein. The factors impacting on solute and fluid transfer across hemofilters are outlined in Figure 39-4. Infusion sites within the system include ports to infuse heparin into the arterial line and a balanced electrolyte solution into the venous line. In most situations the infusate is a solution such as Ringer's lactate; saline and bicarbonate containing solutions are also used. The driving energy for blood flow is derived from the blood pressure generated from the patient's contracting heart.

CAVH has been used in children to treat edema secondary to the nephrotic syndrome, cardiac failure, and

$$TMP = \frac{P_i + P_o}{2} + Pf - \frac{\pi_i + \pi_o}{2}$$

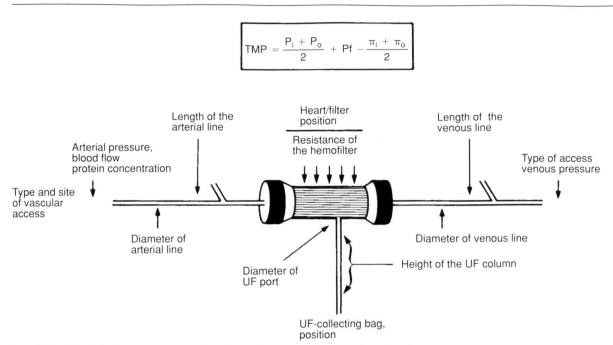

FIG. 39-4. *Detailed schematic representation of a continuous arteriovenous hemofiltration system outlining the factors that determine the rate of formation of ultrafiltrate. TMP equals the transmembrane pressure. P_i, P_o, and π_i and π_o are the hydrostatic and oncotic pressures, respectively, of the arterial and venous segments of the circuit. (From Ronco C: Continuous arteriovenous hemofiltration in infants. In Paganini EP (ed): Acute Continuous Renal Replacement Therapy. Boston, Martinus Nijhoff, 1986, p 201, with permission.)*

renal failure. Other indications for its use include electrolyte and acid–base derangements and controlled parenteral nutrition. CAVH has also been used successfully to treat neonatal branched chain aminoacidemia (maple sugar urine disease) [877]. Hypervolemia can usually be corrected in 6 to 72 hours after which parenteral nutrition, if needed, can be instituted. Although effective in removing fluid, CAVH is limited in its capacity to remove solute.

The use of a standard Amicon Diafilter results in ultrafiltration rates of 5 to 20 ml/minute. Miniature hemofilters (Amicon Diafilters with 25 polysulphone fibers, Gambro FH22 hemofilter) can be used to treat renal failure and volume overload states in neonates and infants [686,687,877]. Umbilical, brachial, and femoral vessels can be used in neonates [481] (Fig. 39-5); in older children femoral vessels are commonly used. In neonates and infants, blood flow rates of 1.25 to 31.3 ml/minute and ultrafiltration rates of 0.23 to 2.5 ml/minute have been reported using CAVH. The total extracorporeal volume needed to perform CAVH ranges from 15 to 22 ml [686]. Anticoagulation for neonates can be achieved by a bolus loading dose of heparin of 10 to 40 U/kg followed by a continuous infusion of 5 to 10 U/kg/hour [480]. A negative suction of 100 mm Hg can be used with neonatal hemofilters to maximize ultrafiltration rates. The predicted urea clearance and ultrafiltration rates of 4 hours of hemodialysis, 24 hours of peritoneal dialysis, or 24 hours of CAVH are urea clearances, 2100, 2400, and 1600 ml/24 hours and ultrafiltration volumes, 200, 600 and 1600 ml/24 hours [480].

CAVH as originally described has been modified to perform continuous arteriovenous hemodiafiltration, predilution CAVH, and slow continuous ultrafiltration [342]. Experience with each of these techniques is limited; minimal data are available in children. The technique of continuous arteriovenous hemodialysis (CAVHD), accomplished by circulating dialysate in a countercurrent fashion through the ultrafiltrate compartment, has been successfully applied to infants [36]. CAVHD combines both convective and diffuse transfer of solute. Solute clearance in CAVHD is not critically determined by blood flow but rather by the rates of ultrafiltration and dialysate flow. Overall, small solute clearance (urea) in CAVHD is approximately three times higher than that obtained with CAVH. Satisfactory control of BUN can be achieved with CAVHD in patients with acute renal failure. CAVHD has been performed using flat plate polyacrylonitrile commercially available dialyzers [753] (Fig. 39-6) and hollow-fiber dialyzers [621] and circulating a solution similar to that of peritoneal fluid through the dialysate compartment. Patients with central venous lines can be treated with continuous venous hemofiltration by applying a blood pump to the "arterial" line.

Reports of significant numbers of children treated with CAVH in a single center are limited. In one report involving 15 neonates, CAVH provided acceptable therapy in 11 [480]. Eight recovered satisfactory renal function; 10 of the infants died from nonrenal causes. Two of four neonates survived in another center [686]. CAVH has been used in conjunction with extracorporeal membrane oxy-

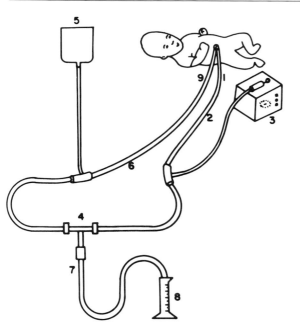

FIG. 39-5. *Continuous arteriovenous hemofiltration (CAVH) circuit in a neonate. The numbers identify the components of the system. (1) umbilical artery catheter; (2) arterial line; (3) heparin infusion pump; (4) neonate mini hemofilter; (5) replacement infusate; (6) venous line; (7) ultrafiltrate outlet; (8) drainage line and ultrafiltrate volumetric collecting device; (9) umbilical vein catheter. (From Pascual JF, Lopez JD, Molina M: Hemofiltration in children with renal failure. Pediatr Clin North Am 34:803, 1987, with permission.)*

genation (ECMO) to treat simultaneously renal and pulmonary failure [736]. CAVH can also be used to treat the tumor lysis syndrome [350a]. CAVH and CAVHD are widely used in pediatric intensive care units to treat resistant edema, electrolyte abnormalities, and acute renal failure. The mortality rates in this patient population are related primarily to the nature of the underlying disorder.

Short Time Dialysis

A number of dialytic techniques that reduce dialysis time to 3 hours or less are available. Available techniques result in significantly higher clearances and ultrafiltration rates. They are best used in stable patients whose interdialytic chemistries do not vary too greatly; water retention should not exceed 2.5% to 3% of dry weight [561]. Rapid dialysis techniques are best avoided if the patient experiences hypotension during 25% to 30% of their dialyses. In adult size patients, blood flow rates of at least 325 to 400 ml/ minute are needed. Recirculation should be less than 10% to 15%.

High flux dialysis uses membranes that have ultrafiltration coefficients greater than 9 ml/hour/mm Hg. High flux dialyzers, which are made of n-polyacrylonitrile, polymethylmethacrylate, or polysulfone, have large pores and enable more solute and water to be transported. Their use requires precise control of ultrafiltration. Acetate or bicarbonate can be used; bicarbonate is preferred.

Rapid high efficiency dialysis is performed using a dialyzer with a surface area 50% to 75% greater than usual.

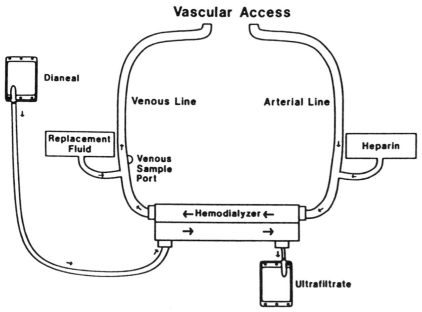

FIG. 39-6. *Schematic circuit of a continuous arteriovenous hemofiltration dialysis system. The Dianel solution used is a 1.5% glucose containing solution to which potassium chloride is added in a concentration of 1 to 3 mEq/liter. (From Pattison ME, Lee SM, Ogden DA: Continuous arteriovenous hemofiltration: An aggressive approach to the management of acute renal failure. Am J Kidney Dis 11(1):43, 1988, with permission.)*

Higher blood flow and dialysate flow rates are used; bicarbonate is the base usually used.

Hemodiafiltration uses a high flux membrane as a hemodiafilter, a delivery system with volumetric ultrafiltration control and bicarbonate dialysis. Treatment times have been reduced to as low as 90 minutes. Some data suggest that long-term survival is reduced when short-time dialysis is used [339a].

Data on the use of these techniques in children are limited.

Hemoperfusion

Hemoperfusion is performed by passing blood through adsorbent materials to remove toxic compounds from the circulation (Fig. 39-7) (Table 39-8). Hemoperfusion, which is easily adaptable for use in children [298], is most effective in removing substances that are tightly protein bound, poorly distributed in plasma water, and lipid soluble. A large number of drugs can be removed by hemoperfusion [615,865]. Those that are removed more rapidly by hemoperfusion than by hemodialysis at similar blood flow rates include acetaminophen, glutethimide, and short and medium acting barbiturates. Additional clinical applications for hemoperfusion have included hepatic encephalopathy, uremia, thyroid storm, removal of anti-cancer drugs such as methotrexate and adriamycin, and the removal of antibody [615,865].

The most widely used adsorbent in hemoperfusion is polymer activated charcoal, either as individually coated particles or fixed within a thin film of chlorosulfonated polyethylene. Solutes ranging in mass from 60 to 21,500 daltons can be removed by hemoperfusion. At higher molecular weights, however, solute adsorption is significantly reduced. Ion exchange resins made of uncharged or charged polysterene resins (Amberlite) are also available. The material is sterilized and placed in cartridges with inlet and outlet ports. Prior to connecting the patient to regular dialysis lines with an arterial blood pump, the detoxifier needs to be rinsed with saline to remove any remaining particulate matter. Pressure monitors are placed on both sides of the cartridge. A pressure gradient of more than 100 mm Hg is indicative of increasing clotting within the column and the need to stop treatment to avoid particulate embolization. The system is primed with either heparinized saline or heparinized whole blood. Dextrose rinsing reduces glucose adsorption. The patient should be systemically heparinized. As with hemodialysis, the extracorporeal volume should not exceed 10% of the child's blood volume. Most devices require priming volumes of 200 to 300 ml; some cartridges with priming volumes of 100 to 150 ml are also available. The patient is connected to the system and blood pumped in an antigravity direction through the column at a rate of 2.5 to 5.0 ml/kg/minute.

Hemoperfusion has been successfully used in children [614] and neonates [142] without significant complications. Ammonia clearance across a charcoal hemoperfusion device was found to be negligible in a neonate [142]. Problems associated with hemoperfusion include clotting of columns, thrombocytopenia, particulate embolization, decreased toxin clearance over time, hypotension, hypothermia, and hypocalcemia. Careful, continuous monitoring is needed to avoid complications.

Plasmapheresis

Plasmapheresis is a technique in which plasma is separated from blood using automated techniques [678,850]. The plasma is separated using either filtration or centrifugation through large pore membranes. Three types of filter systems are available: plasmapheresis, cryopheresis, and cascade plasmapheresis. In simple plasmapheresis a single synthetic

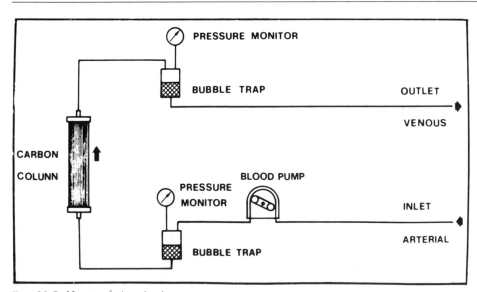

Fig. 39-7. Hemoperfusion circuit.

Table 39-8. *Compounds removed by charcoal or resin hemoperfusion*

Antidepressants	Uric acid*	Nonbarbiturate hypnotics, sedatives,
Amitriptyline	Creatinine*	and tranquilizers
Clomipramine	Cholic acid	Ethchlorvynol*
Desipramine	Polyamino acids	Glutethimide*
Nortriptyline	Polypeptides	Methyprylon*
Alcohols	Uremic toxins*	Methaqualone*
Ethyl alcohol	Indicans*	Diazepam
Analgesics	Phenolic compounds*	Chloral hydrate
Acetylsalicylic acid*	Organic acids*	Carbromal
Methyl salicylate*	Middle molecules*	Chlorpromazine
Acetaminophen*	Insulin*	Phenytoin*
Antimicrobials/anticancer agents	Throxine*	Promazine
Adriamycin*	Triiodothyronine*	Promethazine
Ampicillin	Immune proteins	Meprobamate
Chloroquine*	Miscellaneous	Plant/animal toxins,
Erythromycin	Angiotensin II	herbicides/insecticides
Gentamicin	Epinephrine	*Amanita phalloides**
Methotrexate*	Norepinephrine	Amanitin
Barbiturates*	L-Dopamine	Phalloidin
Amobarbital	Methoxamine	Chlorinated insecticides
Butabarbital	Theophylline*	Polychlorinated biphenyls
Heptabarbital	Diphenhydramine	Methyl parathion
Phenobarbital	Serotonin	Demeton-S-methyl sulfoxide*
Quinalbital	Nucleotides	Dimethoate*
Secobarbital	Cholic acid	Nitrostigmine
Cardiovascular agents	Vitamin B_{12}	Paraquat*
Digoxin*	Folic acid	Solvents/gases
Procainamide	Bromosulphthalein	Carbon tetrachloride
N-acetyloprocainamide	Inulin	Ethylene oxide
Endogenous compounds	Sucrose dilaurate	
Amino acids		

* Studied in vivo.
Adapted from Winchester J, MacKay J, Forbes C, et al: Hemostatic changes induced in vitro by hemoperfusion over activated charcoal. *Artif Organs* 2(3):293, 1978.

membrane with a high molecular weight cutoff is used. Blood is pumped into a centrifuge bowl and plasma separated from cells. As with hemodialysis, the extracorporeal blood volume should be less than 10% of blood volume. Some systems, such as the Haemonetics 30-S (Haemonetics Braintree, MA) discontinuous centrifuge system, are available with different sizes of bowls, 125 ml and 225 ml [850]. The cells, together with a replacement solution, fresh frozen plasma, 5% albumin in 0.9% saline, or plasma protein fraction, are returned to the patient. Calcium salts are either added to the replacement solution to avoid acute depletion of these solutes or given if patients become symptomatic. As with hemodialysis, the patient must be heparinized. Vascular access is similar to that of hemodialysis; vein to vein access can be used.

Cryopheresis is performed as a three step process. Routine plasma separation is performed. The separated plasma is chilled to 4°C. The chilled plasma is passed through a second membrane, which inhibits the passage of precipitated cryoglobulins.

In cascade plasmapheresis, a double filter system is used. The first and second filters have high and low molecular weight cutoffs, respectively. The low molecular weight fraction can be returned to the patient and reduces the need for replacement solutions. Such a system can be used

to remove specific weight proteins, e.g., anti–basement membrane antibodies. The second filter can also be modified to function as an immunoadsorption filter to remove antibodies against a specific protein, such as acetylcholinesterase inhibitor antibody.

A system for performing neonatal hemodialysis, hemofiltration, and plasmapheresis using a miniaturized blood pump unit and plasma filters of 0.09 to 0.14 m² and priming volumes of 10 to 15 ml has been described [57].

Plasmapheresis is used as a means of removing immunologically active components within plasma such as immunoglobulins, complement, and antigen-antibody complexes. Its use is often accompanied by the simultaneous administration of drugs known to alter immunologic processes. The precise therapeutic role for plasmapheresis is still evolving. Most therapeutic reports involve small numbers of patients. Diseases in which plasmapheresis has been shown to be clinically effective include anti-glomerular basement membrane antibody disorder [102], cryoglobulinemia, hyperviscosity syndrome, homozygous type II hypercholesterolemia [868], Guillain-Barré syndrome [850], myasthenia gravis [678,764], immune hemolytic anemia [20], Refsum disease, and factor VIII AB hemophilia. Plasmapheresis has been reported to be effective in improving the glomerulonephritis of systemic lupus erythematosus in pediatric patients [397], but larger series in adults have not found plasmapheresis to be effective. Other pediatric disorders in which plasmapheresis has been used include dermatomyositis [170], rapidly progressive glomerulonephritis [532], Henoch-Schönlein purpura [364], transplant rejection [850], juvenile rheumatoid arthritis [106], and Rh-erythroblastosis [57]. Plasmapheresis has been used to treat pregnant women with known Rh-incompatibility [682].

Complications of plasmapheresis included allergic reactions, fever, chills, hypocalcemia, hypertension, thrombocytopenia, cardiac arrhythmia, and decreased concentrations of fibrinogen and immunoglobulins. In 431 procedures in 61 children ages 1.7 to 19 years, the complications included bowel malfunction, cardiac arrest, chills, clotted shunt, numbness and paresthesia, syncope, and urticaria [850]. The infusion of solutions of albumin during plasmapheresis, which often contain high concentrations of aluminum, has been shown to elevate blood aluminum levels [534].

Complications of Hemodialysis

Each form of dialysis is associated with acute and chronic complications. The unique problems of hemodialysis and peritoneal dialysis are treated separately. In another section, dialysis related complications common to both modes of dialysis are discussed. It is worth remembering that many symptoms associated with dialysis related problems are similar to those of nonrenal or nondialysis related illness. Also, children may present with new disease at any time. Consequently, when symptoms develop, a complete differential diagnosis should be considered prior to reaching a decision as to the etiology of the problem. Not only can the presentation of nonrenal disease be modified by one or more ESRD related problems, ESRD related symptoms may be inappropriately attributed to a nonrenal related disorder.

Hypotension

The most frequently encountered complication of hemodialysis is dialysis related hypotension [341]. It ranges in severity from mild and transient to severe requiring major resuscitative steps. Between 20% and 30% of hemodialysis treatments are associated with hypotension [699], which may result from blood loss, excessive or too rapid ultrafiltration, autonomic nervous system dysfunction [638], or acetate usage. Each cause may occur alone, or more than one factor may be operative.

BLOOD LOSS

Blood loss may be either internal and due to hemorrhage or external and reflect a mechanical problem. Internal bleeding is considered in a subsequent section. External blood loss is usually due to breaks in the dialyzing membrane, manufacturing defects, formation of blood clots, or the use of a high TMP. Major membrane leaks (rupture of a dialysis membrane) require clamping of the arterial and venous blood lines and the simultaneous discontinuation of dialysis. This causes loss of blood within the blood lines

and dialyzer. Less severe leaks can be treated by clamping the arterial line and returning as much blood as possible to the patient. Decisions regarding transfusion are based on the magnitude of blood loss, clinical onset of symptoms of blood loss, and the pre-dialysis hemoglobin level. Another cause of acute blood loss is the separation of blood lines. When this occurs, reconnection and continuation of the dialysis treatment is usually possible. Many patients can safely tolerate the blood loss without incident and can be transfused, when indicated, during the next dialysis treatment. A third cause of acute blood loss is due to "bleeding" into the extracorporeal circuit at the onset of dialysis. Children at increased risk for experiencing this form of hypotension include those with pre-existing extracellular–vascular volume depletion due to recent onset gastroenteritis, diminished oral intake with obligate high urinary flow rates, increased insensible water loss, or the chronic ingestion of a low sodium diet.

EXCESSIVE ULTRAFILTRATION

Excessive ultrafiltration, either absolute or relative to the extracellular fluid volume (ECF), is the most common factor leading to hypotension. During the process of ultrafiltration, fluid is initially removed from the plasma volume compartment and then replaced with fluid from the interstitial space [450]. The etiology of this form of hypotension is multifactorial; there is a finite rate at which fluid can move from the interstitial to the plasma compartment; obstruction to venous flow may lead to an increase in the TMP; and the peripheral vascular resistance, which is the hemodynamic variable primarily involved in responding to acutely diminished blood volume, may not appropriately increase, owing to the presence of intrinsic vascular disease, autonomic dysfunction [415,638], or an acetate effect [299]. Two postulated mechanisms by which excessive acetate exposure leads to hypotension are the direct depression of myocardial function and peripheral vasodilation [8,426]. Patients who cannot convert acetate to bicarbonate as rapidly as others may be at increased risk [196,837]. The use of large surface area dialyzers, especially when combined with a high blood flow rate, predisposes the patient to both an excessive rate of ultrafiltration and an increased rate of absorption of acetate. The substitution of bicarbonate for acetate has been shown to increase peripheral vascular resistance [382] and improve tolerance to ultrafiltration in hypotension-prone patients [299]. The presence of hyponatremia because of concurrent disease or the use of dialysate with a low sodium content (132 mEq/liter) also increases the risk of developing hypotension by altering the usual ratio of extracellular to intracellular water [309,315]. Some of the differences in response to rapid ultrafiltration can be explained by the predialysis volume of the interstitial space [450]. Impaired myocardial responsivity and unresponsiveness of the renin angiotensin system may also contribute to hemodialysis related hypotension [552].

The treatment of ultrafiltration induced hypotension includes reducing additional ultrafiltration and acutely expanding intravascular volume. Maneuvers that diminish continuing fluid loss include reducing the TMP, blood flow rate, and negative dialysate pressure. A number of different solutions can be infused to expand intravascular volume, including albumin, NaCl, and mannitol. By virtue of remaining within the vascular space and driving fluid from interstitial to plasma compartments, albumin, at a dose of 0.5 g/kg, effectively reverses hypotension. Because of its expense, its use should be reserved for patients who are known to be either hypoalbuminemic or unresponsive to other forms of therapy. Also, expansion with too much albumin may lead to intravascular overload with its attendant consequences. Most hypotensive children respond to infusions of 0.9% NaCl, 3% NaCl, or 20% mannitol by increasing their blood pressure. The rapid infusion of 1.5 to 3.0 ml/kg of 0.9% NaCl in conjunction with the transient lowering of the TMP usually results in the blood pressure and pulse rate returning to acceptable values. Because the volume of saline infused often needs to be removed to achieve ultrafiltration objectives, some prefer to administer a smaller volume of a more hyperosmotic solution. This will expand intravascular volume by initially increasing intravascular and extracellular osmolality and subsequently redistributing fluid between the intracellular and extracellular spaces. The infusion of 0.15 to 0.30 ml/kg of 3% NaCl or 0.5 g/kg of 20% mannitol generally increases the blood pressure to an acceptable degree without significantly increasing total body water. If dialysis is able to be continued, most of these solutes will again be dialyzed.

The excessive use of mannitol presents some risk. In normal adults, 80% of mannitol is excreted by the kidney with the remainder either being excreted in bile or metabolically converted [197,722]. Four mannitol related problems may develop: hyponatremia secondary to water movement into the extracellular compartment, hyperosmolality with its effect on CNS function, redevelopment of hypotension as mannitol is removed by diffusion during subsequent dialysis and as water moves back into cells, and development of a dialysis dysequilibrium syndrome as a result of rapidly lowering an elevated serum osmolality due to mannitol persisting in the patient between dialysis treatments. The periodic determination of serum osmolality is useful in monitoring patients who receive multiple doses of mannitol during either a single treatment or over the course of a number of treatments. Mannitol intoxication has been reported in patients with renal failure receiving large doses of mannitol. Problems include lethargy disproportionate to the degree of uremia, confusion, hyponatremia, volume overload, cataracts, hyperosmolality, and death [38,99].

PREVENTION

Dialysis related hypotension can be prevented or reduced in frequency in most hemodialysis patients. Because most episodes of ultrafiltration related hypotension occur in patients whose intradialytic weights exceed 5% of body weight, keeping the intradialytic weight gain less than that by limiting sodium and water intake should be encouraged. The use of a dialysate sodium concentration equal to or greater than that of the patient's serum helps prevent rapid intracompartmental fluid shifts. Also, maintenance of a stable plasma osmolality may improve cardiovascular stability and reduce the incidence of cramping, nausea, and vomiting. Symptomatic improvement and increased hemodynamic stability has been associated with the use of a dialysate sodium concentration of 150 mEq/liter. Use of the higher sodium containing dialysate was associated with a greater loss of intracellular volume, while decreases in plasma and extracellular volumes were less [669]. A higher interdialytic weight gain did occur; however, the extra water could be removed during the next dialysis. Additional problems with hypertension did not develop [353]. Finally, the use during dialysis of vasopressors such as dopamine or norepinephrine or the long-term administration of drugs containing sympathomimetic agents such as phenylephrine or ephedrine may be effective in either increasing or preventing the drop in blood pressure in patients with autonomic dysfunction who experience symptomatic hypotension during dialysis.

Air Embolism

Air in the hemodialysis system can lead to air embolism and death [82]. Routes of air entry include leakage around the hub of needles connected to the arterial lines (the blood pump creates a negative pressure), breaks in syringes used to infuse drugs, defects in arterial and venous drip chambers, vented bottles or bags, and leaks in the dialysate delivery systems and during the return of blood to the patient at the end of the treatment particularly when air is used to flush the system. Infusions should be delivered into arterial lines beyond the blood pump, where the infusate is given against a positive pressure. Photocell air detectors placed on venous lines may not detect microbubbles; clots may also mask the photocell. Conductance activated detectors are more likely to detect small quantities of air.

Air entering veins can take a number of routes. If the patient is upright, air moves retrograde up the jugular vein to reach the brain. If the patient is lying flat, air will enter the right atrium, right ventricle, and lung. Foam detectable by x-ray film is generated within the heart and may cause mechanical cardiac dysfunction. Auscultation of a heart containing foam reveals a churning sound. Air can pass through the lungs and enter the systemic circulation. Air can travel to the legs if the patient is in the Trendelenburg position.

Symptoms of air embolism are those of acute cardiac and pulmonary distress or neurologic dysfunction. The amount of air entering the blood stream and the localization of the air together determine the clinical course. Treatment involves the immediate clamping of the venous line and placing the patient on the left side. Foam that can be aspirated from the heart should be removed before starting cardiopulmonary resuscitation. Decompression chambers have been used to treat air embolism [62].

Dialysis Dysequilibrium Syndrome

Dialysis dysequilibrium syndrome (DDS) is a symptom complex that initially includes irritability, restlessness, lethargy, nausea, vomiting, and headache and that subsequently includes muscle twitching, myoclonic asterixis, hypertension, disorientation, and visual disturbances. If treatment is not provided, life-threatening complications such as seizures, coma, and cardiac arrhythmias may occur [633,675,809]. The acute onset of headaches during dialysis, in addition to being related to DDS, may occur in patients who become hypotensive from excessive ultrafiltration [58,630]. Such headaches may be related to changes in the binding of oxygen to hemoglobin following the abrupt correction of acidemia or hyperphosphatemia.

In patients with DDS, characteristic EEG features include increased slow wave activity, increased spike wave activity, loss of alpha waves, and bursts of delta wave activity [29]. Cerebrospinal fluid pressure rises during dialysis, and post mortem studies in patients dying during dialysis have shown brain swelling and tentorial herniation [143]. CT studies in patients undergoing dialysis are compatible with intracerebral fluid accumulation [458].

The pathophysiology of DDS remains unclear; however, its onset is clearly related to the rapid correction of uremia. It is more likely to develop during the first few dialysis procedures in newly diagnosed patients in whom high dialysis clearances are used. In the past, DDS has been reported to occur more frequently in children than in adults [307]. This is due in part to the use of dialyzers with a disproportionately high surface area relative to the child's surface area or a high blood flow rate or both. Large surface area dialyzers and high blood flow rates result in a high dialyzer clearance. Symptoms tend to occur toward the end of a treatment but may begin any time within the next 24 hours.

DDS results from the acute onset of cerebral edema. Experimental studies suggest that the cerebral edema most probably occurs because of the development of intracellular "idiogenic osmoles" [29]. Other suggested mechanisms include acute decreases in the serum sodium concentration [839], acute changes in pH [28,838], dialysis against a low glucose containing dialysate [329], and the disproportionate rate of removal of urea from blood versus that of brain [414].

Prevention of DDS is more readily achieved than its treatment. In patients beginning dialysis with high serum concentrations of urea, the onset of symptoms usually can be avoided by performing shorter treatments, with the dialyzer BUN clearance adjusted to 1.0 to 1.5 ml/minute/kg and by infusing 1.0 g/kg of 25% mannitol over the course of the treatment [430,684]. The first three hemodialysis treatments are best performed on three consecutive days with the length of the initial treatment being 2 hours and each succeeding treatment being increased by 1 hour. Prophylactic treatment with mannitol should also be considered in stable children undergoing long-term dialysis whenever the BUN suddenly increases above pre-existing levels because of the onset of a hypercatabolic state or excessive protein ingestion. The onset of mild symptoms during dialysis can be treated with a mannitol infusion. When major symptoms develop, dialysis should be discontinued, and a diagnostic evaluation should be done to rule out other problems. Intravenous diazepam (Valium) or parenteral barbiturates can be used to treat seizures. The value of long-term therapy with anticonvulsant medication in children who sustain seizures related to DDS is unclear. In five adolescents monitored by continuous EEG during hemodialysis, significant subclinical seizure activity was noted in children dialyzed against an acetate containing solution [257]. Children with known seizures were at increased risk for developing further subclinical seizure activity. Less seizure activity was noted when a bicarbonate bath was used [257].

Muscle Cramps

Isolated painful muscle cramps commonly occur during and between hemodialysis treatments. They develop more frequently in patients from whom either extracellular fluid is rapidly removed or in whom the serum sodium concentration is acutely lowered. Muscle cramps occur twice as frequently in patients dialyzed against a solution containing a sodium concentration of 132 versus 145 mEq/liter [778]. Whether such cramps are a pathologically distinct problem or part of the spectrum of DDS remains undecided.

Treatment consists of volume expansion with isotonic saline (5 to 10 ml/kg) or the intravenous infusion of 0.15 to 0.25 ml/kg of hypertonic saline (17.5% or 3 mol/liter [384] or 50% glucose [555]. Patients with recurrent severe cramps may benefit from the use of dialysate with a sodium concentration of 140 mEq/liter or sequential ultrafiltration hemodialysis. Quinine sulfate has been shown in a double blind study to reduce both the frequency and severity of cramps [402]. The dose given to adults prior to each dialysis was 320 mg. Data are unavailable in children.

Fever

Febrile responses during hemodialysis are most often due to pyrogenic reactions but may also be due to infection or a defect in the machine's temperature control system. Pyrogen reactions are characterized by fever, often accompanied by chills, developing during the middle third of dialysis. The demonstration of circulating endotoxins, endotoxins in dialysate [668], and antibodies to dialysate bacterial endotoxins [277] in dialysis patients developing febrile reactions suggests that endotoxin in dialysate enters the blood stream through small breaks in the dialysis membrane and is the principle mechanism by which pyrogenic reactions occur.

Infection-related fever should be suspected in patients who are febrile prior to initiating dialysis and in those who develop fever shortly after terminating dialysis. Other causes of fever include the improper handling of dialyzers that are being reused, shunt infection, and malfunctioning temperature regulating devices. Whenever a patient becomes febrile, the temperature regulating devices of the hemodialysis system must be checked. Malfunctioning central delivery systems can cause fever in more than one patient simultaneously. Deaths have been associated with dialysis related blood warming. Overheating of dialysate causes hemolysis and acute hyperkalemia; the onset of hemolysis may be delayed for 48 hours [72]. Even though pyrogenic reactions are the major cause of dialysis related fever, all febrile reactions should be evaluated on the assumption that a bacterial infection has occurred and blood cultures should be obtained. An individual decision can be made as to whether antibiotic therapy should be initiated [449].

Acute Biochemical Changes

Hemodialysis can lead to acute problems as a result of rapid changes in both monovalent and divalent ions, primarily sodium, potassium, calcium, and magnesium. The failure to check conductivity to ensure that the proper amount of water and concentrate have been added in batch systems or the failure of proportioning systems to dilute dialysate appropriately can lead to the development of acute hypernatremia [483] or hyponatremia.

Acute hypernatremia results in extracellular hyperosmolality and intracellular volume contraction. Symptoms include thirst, vomiting, headache, seizure, and coma. Treatment includes symptomatic support, discontinuation of dialysis, and infusion of 5% dextrose to reduce extracellular osmolality rapidly. Once the nature of the problem is identified and treated, dialysis should be restarted using appropriate dialysate so that the excessive sodium and water used as therapy can be removed.

Acute hypo-osmolality causes hemolysis, potentially fatal hyperkalemia, and the acute dilution of all extracellular constituents. Subsequently, there is an internal rearrangement of total body water giving rise to the symptom complex of acute water intoxication. Symptoms include pain along the path of the vein receiving the hypotonic infusion, severe abdominal cramps, and chest pain. Signs include a change in the rate and quality of pulse, neck vein distention, altered neurologic function including seizures and coma, cold extremities, and hypotension. If acute hypo-osmolality is suspected, dialysis should be discontinued and symptomatic support initiated. Oxygen should be administered, and intravascular volume expansion with saline, colloid, or blood should be undertaken to replace that lost. A blood count and the measurement of serum electrolytes, osmolality, creatinine phosphokinase, and transaminases, to establish whether hypoxic tissue damage has occurred, are indicated.

Hypokalemia (a serum potassium less than 3.0 mEq/liter) commonly occurs when children are dialyzed with potassium free dialysate. Although this is not usually a problem, the rapid lowering of potassium predisposes to the development of cardiac arrhythmias in adult patients with left ventricular hypertrophy receiving digitalis [545]. Using potassium free dialysate, the mean potassium removal during dialysis is 1.22 ± 0.2 mEq/kg [233]. Rates of removal correlate with the predialysis serum concentration of potassium. Potassium levels rebound after hemodialysis at a rate of 0.47 mEq/liter and 0.20 mEq/liter for the initial and subsequent 2 hours. Also, hypokalemia has been described to occur during hemodialysis because of the correction of acidemia and the shift of potassium from the extracellular to intracellular space [861]. The development of hypokalemia can be avoided in most patients if potassium containing dialysate is used; most nephrologists recommend

that dialysate potassium concentration should be at least 1 mEq/liter. Most hemodialysis is done using a dialysate potassium concentration of 2 to 4 mEq/liter. Hyperkalemia may persist in already hyperkalemic individuals in whom a high degree of recirculation occurs when single needle dialysis is used.

In children during acetate hemodialysis, plasma acetate levels rise, pCO_2 falls, pH increases, and blood bicarbonate remains unchanged [401]. After dialysis is stopped, there is a rapid increase in bicarbonate as the acetate is metabolized. Bicarbonate dialysis offers improved control in acid–base metabolism [823], but the degree to which bicarbonate hemodialysis offers improvement over acetate hemodialysis remains controversial [185,196].

Prior to the widespread routine use of water purification systems, some patients experienced a "hard water syndrome" [261] secondary to the acute transfer from bath to patient of calcium and magnesium. After the first hour of dialysis, affected patients developed nausea, vomiting, headaches, lethargy, muscle weakness, hypertension (presumably calcium mediated), a feeling of burning in the skin (perhaps due to hypermagnesemia), and on occasion, pancreatitis [227]. Treatment consists of terminating dialysis, arranging to have the water treated, and reinstituting dialysis.

A number of acute problems related to trace metals and exposure to organic compounds have been described. They include intoxication with chloramines [207], copper [434], nickel [852], nitrates [126], and zinc [270]. Clinical problems related to such exposure are considered in the section on water.

Acute Hemorrhage

Spontaneous bleeding either during dialysis or in the peridialysis period occurs more often in patients receiving hemodialysis than in those on peritoneal dialysis because of the required use of anticoagulation. Acute bleeding develops most often when the clinical setting predisposes to bleeding. Problems have included petechial skin hemorrhages, bleeding around skin puncture sites, subungual splinter hemorrhage, subcapsular liver hematoma [98], retroperitoneal [78] and perirenal [804] hemorrhage, bleeding into the pleural [269] and pericardial [509] space, gastrointestinal bleeding (aggravation of a bleeding ulcer), and subdural hematoma [470]. An increased incidence of subdural hematomas has been reported in hemodialysis populations. Symptoms and signs, in addition to those of acute blood loss superimposed on an already anemic base, are those of a space occupying lesion.

Treatment consists of supportive therapy, provision of blood, support of intravascular volume, and, in those situations in which life-threatening complications may develop, evacuation of the blood collection. Consideration should be given to altering the patient's heparinization prescription, i.e., low dose, intermittent, or regional heparinization, or to switching to peritoneal dialysis. Patients have been restarted on hemodialysis after 6 to 8 weeks of peritoneal dialysis after having developed a hemodialysis associated subdural hematoma [801]. Although data are unavailable in pediatric populations, in adults hemodialysis without anticoagulation during the perioperative period is reported as being 95% successful, i.e., without coil clotting or other coagulative problems [714], and compares favorably with the incidence of bleeding problems of 19% and 10% when regional and low dose heparinization is used [785].

Pulmonary Dysfunction, Leukopenia, and Other Complications

Hemodialysis is associated with leukopenia, decreased carbon monoxide diffusion, and hypoxemia. These changes occur during the initial 15 to 45 minutes of dialysis; by 1 hour, there is a return to baseline of the white count, but the defect in pulmonary function persists throughout dialysis. Dialysis leads to sequestration of leukocytes within both the dialyzer and the pulmonary capillaries by a complement mediated process [165]. The diffusion defect may, in part, be related to the white cell sequestration but also has been shown to occur independently. The degree of sequestration is related to the composition of the dialyzing membrane; sequestration is minimal, intermediate, or most severe in patients dialyzed with polyacrylonitrile, cellulose acetate, Cuprophan or regenerated cellulose membranes, respectively [383,850a].

Some studies suggest that dialysis related hypoventilation is due to the diffusion of CO_2 from blood to dialysate and a decreased CO_2 effect on the respiratory center [196]. Others have suggested that the respiratory drive is decreased by the dialysis related correction of acidosis and the tendency toward becoming alkalemic. Dialysis hypoxemia, however, can occur in the absence of any changes in systemic pH [178]. If bicarbonate rather than acetate dialysate is used, these changes are usually mitigated [211]. Others have not been able to document a positive effect of bicarbonate dialysis on pulmonary function. Acetate infusion in patients between dialyses does not increase ventilation [178]. The type of hemodialyzing membrane used may explain some of the differences reported, because some membranes do not cause leukostasis. In a study comparing acid–base parameters in 10 adults dialyzed against either an acetate or bicarbonate dialysate, similar degrees of hypoxemia and hypoventilation were noted [2]. In summary, hemodialysis related changes in oxygenation and ventilation are most likely a two-step phenomenon: leukostasis, which is influenced by the type of membrane, and dialyzer losses of CO_2, which can be mitigated by using HCO_3 dialysate. Decreases in PO_2 of 26.2% and in pCO_2 have been reported during hemodialysis in eight children using the technique of continuous transcutaneous monitoring [733].

Anaphylaxis secondary to ethylene oxide used to sterilize a hollow fiber kidney has been reported in a 10-year-old boy undergoing his first hemodialysis [373]. Also, it has been shown that children increase their minute ventilation after dialysis as a consequence of developing an increased tidal volume [727,728].

Acute respiratory distress, sometimes accompanied by wheezing, chills, fever, and chest pain, occasionally de-velops when dialysis is begun using a new dialyzer [588,640]. This first use syndrome, although usually mild, may require treatment with antihistamines, adrenaline, antipyretics, and analgesics. Etiologic significance has been attributed to 2-chloroethanol production subsequent to the use of ethylene oxide gas to sterilize dialyzers [326].

Metastatic pulmonary calcifications, both symptomatic and asymptomatic, have occurred in children on dialysis. Four of 18 children without chest film evidence of pulmonary calcification had a positive technetium 99m hydroxymethylene diphosphate scan [202]. Compared with those without pulmonary calcifications, the four affected children had been on dialysis longer and had higher blood concentrations of aluminum. Metastatic calcification involving multiple organs (76% incidence) has been described in children undergoing dialysis [534a].

Peritoneal Dialysis

The proportion of children with end stage renal disease treated primarily with peritoneal dialysis varies among pediatric centers. The modality of treatment depends on the experience and enthusiasm of the nephrology team and the availability of kidneys for transplantation. During the past decade, there has been a progressive increase in the number of children beginning some form of long-term peritoneal dialysis. Some programs offer families and children a choice between hemodialysis and peritoneal dialysis; others tend to encourage one form of dialysis.

Prior to considering the topic of peritoneal dialysis in chronic renal failure, the factors influencing the transperitoneal movement of solute water, the basis for developing peritoneal dialysis prescriptions, and its use in acute renal failure and in the neonate are discussed.

Transperitoneal Movement of Solute and Water

SOLUTE TRANSPORT

Solute transport across the peritoneal membrane [193a] occurs by both diffusion and convective transport [254a]. Three kinetic terms, peritoneal clearance, peritoneal dialysance, and the mass transfer area coefficient (MTAC), are used to describe this movement and to characterize the intrinsic properties of the peritoneal membrane. All three measurements have been used to describe the transperitoneal movement of solute in children. The clinical implication of each term is considered, and the data developed in pediatric populations are discussed.

The most precise term for defining solute movement is the MTAC, which is defined as the instantaneous diffusive clearance in milliliters per minute—the maximum clearance—at time zero of an exchange when the transperitoneal gradient for solute is greatest [643,647]. The MTAC is determined by instilling dialysate containing a marker such as inulin or radiolabeled albumin to measure the changing volume of dialysate over time while simultaneously obtaining a number of samples of dialysate and blood to measure the changing concentration ratio of solute.

Using the reflection coefficient of the solute being studied, the quantity of solute transported by convection is calculated. This value is subtracted from the overall amount of solute moving across the peritoneal membrane (mass transfer) to ascertain the quantity of solute transported by pure diffusion. The diffusive transport is determined for each of the samples obtained for measuring the dialysate and blood concentrations of solute; each of these clearance values is different. A curvilinear plot of peritoneal clearance versus time is developed, and the clearance at time zero, the MTAC, is derived by extrapolation. Because the mathematics are complex, they are done using an iterative least-squares computer program [662]. The MTAC most accurately describes the intrinsic properties of the peritoneal membrane. It is believed to be independent of changing dialysate to blood solute concentration gradients, dwell time, and perhaps the volume of exchange used in clinical practice. It is also believed to obviate the effect of changing spatial relationships between dialysate and peritoneal membrane that occur during the instillation and drainage phases of an exchange.

The most widely used descriptor of peritoneal solute movement is the measurement of peritoneal clearance, which conceptually is similar to a classical renal clearance. The formula for peritoneal clearance is:

$$C = (S_D)/(S_P) \times Q_D$$

where C is equal to the peritoneal clearance in ml/min; S_D and S_P equal the concentration of solute in dialysate and plasma, respectively; and Q_D equals the dialysate flow rate expressed in ml per min, determined as the measured volume (V) of dialysate drained divided by the elapsed time (T) from the initiation of inflow to the end of outflow of an exchange.

The peritoneal clearance differs from the MTAC of dialysance in that the former defines a mean or average quantity of plasma cleared of solute per unit time, whereas the latter measurement reflects the instantaneous rate of solute movement occurring at time zero of an exchange. Peritoneal clearance varies as the transmembrane solute concentration gradient changes during the time the abdomen is filled with fluid. Thus, if the peritoneal cavity were infused with 40 ml/kg of dialysate, the clearance of BUN would be different if dialysate were to be drained after 30, 60, or 240 minutes. Most importantly, the measurement of a peritoneal clearance does not distinguish between the contribution of diffusive and convective transport [344].

The formula for peritoneal clearance contains two discrete terms. One term, Q_D, reflects dialysis mechanics, factors under the precise control of the nephrologist. These factors are the volume of dialysate to be used per exchange and the time allotted to the three phrases of an exchange: inflow, dwell, and outflow. The second term, S_D/S_P, reflects the combined contribution of the peritoneal surface area able to participate in exchange and its intrinsic permeability.

Theoretical consideration of the peritoneal clearance formula provides practical insights into the dialytic process (Table 39-9). Changes in any of the values that determine the contribution of dialysis mechanics, dialysate volume, or dwell times markedly influence the peritoneal clearance of solute. These changes are independent of any changes in the properties of the dialyzing membrane. Any such changes have significant impact on attempts to correct peritoneal clearances for body size. If dialysis mechanics are held constant when performing either a number of sequential exchanges or comparative studies in different subjects, any changes found in peritoneal clearances can then be attributed to differences occurring in the intrinsic properties of the peritoneal membrane, surface area, or permeability. When compared with control, such changes

TABLE 39-9. *Theoretical impact of altering factors, extrinsic and intrinsic, on peritoneal clearance in a child weighing 10 kg, having a surface area of 0.47 m², and a pre-exchange BUN of 100 mg/dl*

Example	Dialysate BUN mg/dl	Ratio S_D/S_B	Dialysate flow (V = ml/kg)	T minutes
Control	60	0.6	40	60
Time	60	0.6	40	30
Volume	60	0.6	20	60
Permeability and/or surface area change (decrease)	40	0.4	40	60
Above plus time	40	0.4	40	30

	BUN Clearance in ml/min per		
	kg	70 kg	1.73 m²
Control	0.4	28.0	14.7
Time	0.8	55.9	29.2
Volume	0.2	13.3	7.4
Permeability and/or surface area change (decrease)	0.3	18.6	9.8
Above plus time	0.5	37.3	19.6

S_D and S_B = solute concentration in dialysate and blood.

will be reflected by altered values in the term S_D/S_P. The finding of a difference in the dialysate-to-blood concentration ratio by itself does not permit any conclusion as to whether the change is due to an alteration in peritoneal permeability or to the surface area available for exchange.

The peritoneal clearance index, a measurement of the relative contribution of the membrane's surface area and permeability to the exchange process, is determined by simultaneously obtaining the peritoneal clearance of two different molecular weight solutes. For example, one can measure urea (60 daltons) and creatinine (112 daltons) or inulin (5200 daltons) and divide the clearance of the smaller by the larger molecular weight solute [584,586]. Changes in the peritoneal clearance index indicate a change in peritoneal permeability with or without a simultaneous change in the participating peritoneal surface area; changes in peritoneal clearance in the absence of any change in the peritoneal clearance index reflect an alteration in the amount of peritoneal surface area participating in the exchange process. These interpretations apply best when exchanges are done in the absence of high dialysate concentrations of glucose. When rapid rates of ultrafiltration occur in response to hypertonic glucose in the dialysate, observed increases in peritoneal clearance in the absence of any change in the peritoneal clearance index may reflect the impact of convective transport on the transperitoneal movement of solute [345].

With dialysis mechanics held constant, the performance of a series of peritoneal clearances approaches those concepts that serve as the basis for evaluating peritoneal solute transport by measuring peritoneal dialysance. The measurement of peritoneal dialysance is theoretically done without adding glucose to the dialysate to eliminate any contribution of convective transport to solute transport. In addressing clinical questions, peritoneal dialysance has been done with dialysate containing 1.5% dextrose. A number of variables are assumed to remain constant during the exchanges used to measure dialysance: peritoneal blood flow, the size of the body compartments in which solute is distributed, and the use of similar dialysis mechanics if comparative data are sought. It is not possible to compare dialysance values that are obtained by performing exchanges using different dwell times [348]. Indeed, the time allotted to inflow, dwell, and outflow should be similar.

Transport of solute from the capillary lumen to the fluid-filled peritoneal cavity, or vice versa, occurs by movement through a number of membranes. Each has a different composition [576] and offers varible degrees of resistance to the movement of both solute and water. Movement may be intercellular, transcellular, or by vesicles. Resistance sites include stagnant fluid films lining capillaries and the peritoneal cavity, capillary endothelium and mesothelium, capillary basement membrane, and interstitium. In vitro studies have shown that the stagnant fluid film lining the peritoneal cavity significantly limits small solute transport [521]. For solutes whose molecular weight is 30,000 daltons or less, the predominant site of solute transport occurs in the mesothelium and mesenteric capillaries [160,409] through intercellular channels. Studies in isolated mesentery indicate that the functional pore size is 500 Å [551,674]. Mesentery and mesothelial cell thickness is approximately 13.1 and 0.67 μm, respectively [297]. In isolated mesentery transport studies, the flux of larger molecular weight solutes, such as albumin, is similar in both directions, whereas the flux of smaller molecular weight solutes, e.g., rubidium (85.5 daltons), is greater in the direction from mesothelium to the vascular side of the membrane [103]. The intercellular gaps in capillary sized venules appear to be the site through which large molecules such as proteins move [851]. Unless the membrane is damaged, movement of protein through the mesothelium occurs by intracellular vesicles [238,296]. The intact mesothelial layer is not as permeable as isolated mesentery. Injury such as peritonitis produced by destroying cells or by increasing intercellular gaps leads to an increased protein loss and a more rapid absorption of glucose. This results in a dissipation of the transmembrane [696,828] osmotic gradient and loss of ultrafiltration capacity.

WATER TRANSPORT

The driving force for water movement across the peritoneum during peritoneal dialysis is the glucose generated osmotic gradient. An osmotic gradient of 1 mOsm of glucose generates a hydrostatic gradient [346] of 19 mm Hg. Assuming the plasma glucose concentration to be 100 mg/dl, the maximum transperitoneal hydrostatic gradient for ultrafiltration generated by 1.5% or 4.25% glucose containing dialysate would be 1481 mm Hg (78 mOsm) and 4391 mm Hg (231 mOsm), respectively.

Ultrafiltration mechanisms operative during peritoneal dialysis are incompletely understood [409]. One hypothesis [574] is that permeability to water increases from the afferent to the efferent segments of the capillary. The proximal portion of the capillary has a tight membrane and a higher hydraulic than osmotic pressure. This combination inhibits glucose uptake while permitting hydrostatic driven ultrafiltration to occur. The more distal segments are more permeable and have a lower hydraulic pressure. Although glucose moves into the capillary lumen at distal sites, the high glucose concentration within the interstitium offsets the intraluminal to interstitial osmotic gradient by exerting an osmotic pressure and enables distal capillary ultrafiltration to occur. However, neither the extent nor rate of glucose accumulation in the interstitium is known.

The kinetics of water movement across the peritoneal membrane have been studied three ways: first, by measuring drainage volumes after leaving instilled dialysate in the peritoneal cavity for varying periods of time; second, by sequentially measuring the intraperitoneal volume after adding nonpermeable solutes to the infusate (e.g., radiolabeled albumin) (Fig. 39-8); and third, by sequentially determining the dialysate and blood concentrations of osmoles, glucose, or both. In adult populations undergoing 1-hour, 2000-ml exchanges containing 4.25% or 1.5% glucose, the average drainage volume exceeds infused volume by 10% to 20% and 5% to 10%, respectively. In six children, measured drainage volumes following 30-minute sequential 1.5%, 4.25%, and 1.5% glucose exchanges exceeded input volumes by 6%, 16.5%, and 13%, respectively [321]. The latter value reflects the persistent effect of hypertonic exchanges. In another group of eight chil-

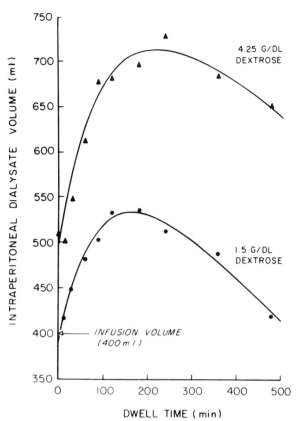

FIG. 39-8. *Changes in intraperitoneal volume over time after instill-ing dialysate with different concentrations of glucose into the perito-neal cavity of a 14.7 kg child. (From Popovich RP, Pyle WK, Moncrief JW: Kinetics of peritoneal transport. In Nolph KD (ed): Peritoneal Dialysis. Development in Nephrology 2. The Hague, Martinus Nijhoff, 1981, p 79, with permission.)*

is the entrainment of solute within a solvent stream. The concentration ratio of solute within the solvent stream to that of its blood concentration is determined by the in-trinsic properties of the peritoneal membrane (reflection coefficient). Because the sodium concentrations of com-mercially available dialysate usually exceed 130 mEq/liter, most sodium removed during dialysis is the result of con-vective transport. Convective transport adds sodium to the dialysate, dilutes the dialysate concentration of sodium, creates an increased concentration gradient for sodium across the peritoneal membrane, and allows for additional transperitoneal movement of sodium by diffusive transport.

PERITONEAL LYMPHATICS

The peritoneal lymphatic system has been shown to play an important role in the absorption of solute and water [494,495]. The formula for calculating the peritoneal lym-phatic absorption rate follows:

$$F_L = (IPV_0 \times C_0) - (IPV_t \times C_t)/C_P,$$

where F_L = total peritoneal lymph flow rate over time; IPV_0 and IPV_t = intraperitoneal fluid volumes at times 0 and t; C_0 and C_t = intraperitoneal tracer concentration at times 0 and t; and C_P = the geometric mean intraperi-toneal concentration of tracer.

Radiolabeled albumin, colloid, and red blood cells have been used as tracers to measure lymphatic flow. In animals, factors shown to increase peritoneal lymphatic flow rates include hyperventilation, increased intraperitoneal hydro-static pressure, peritonitis, and the supine position.

The range of values reported for peritoneal flow rates in humans is quite large. In one study involving 10 patients on continuous ambulatory peritoneal dialysis (CAPD), the mean peritoneal lymphatic flow rate was 11 to 12 ml/hour. In another study, the mean lymphatic flow rate following peak ultrafiltration was found to be 87 ml/hour and to reduce the net transcapillary ultrafiltration rate by 51% [495]. In rats, net ultrafiltration is reduced by lymphatic drainage; also, the peak intraperitoneal volume did not occur at osmotic equilibrium but when the lymphatic ab-sorption rate equaled the transcapillary ultrafiltration rate [580]. Transport by lymphatics can be decreased by aspirin and indomethacin and increased by leukotrienes and some prostaglandins [390]. As the latter agents are increased in the presence of peritonitis [774], an increased rate of lymph absorption may in part explain the reduced ultrafiltration observed when peritonitis exists [496].

In six children aged 2 to 13 years on CAPD or contin-uous cycle peritoneal dialysis (CCPD), cumulative lym-phatic absorption during 4-hour exchanges using 40 ml/kg of 2.5% dialysate averaged 10.4 ± 1.6 ml/kg per exchange [494] (Fig. 39-9). During the exchange, the peak intra-peritoneal volume occurred before osmolar equilibrium was reached. The calculated impact of lymphatic drainage on the daily rates of ultrafiltration and peritoneal clearance was to reduce mean ultrafiltration by 27% and peritoneal clearances of creatinine and urea by 22% and 24%, re-spectively. Compared with 2-liter exchanges in adults (a value closer to 30 ml/kg), the children were found to have

dren, similar time related changes were found when changes in intraperitoneal volume were evaluated by in-traperitoneal radioalbumin dilution studies using 1.5%, 2.5%, and 4.25% glucose dialysate [544]. Older children, when compared with adults, have a similar shaped curve of dialysate glucose or osmolar concentration versus time after introducing 1.5% and 4.25% dextrose containing dialysate [447]. These findings support the conclusion that in older children and adults glucose moves into the body at the same rate that water moves into the peritoneal cavity. Limited data suggest that the intraperitoneal vol-ume versus time curve, when scaled for body size, including its component parts (initial slope, apogee, and disappear-ance segments), is similar. Thus, in children beyond in-fancy, maximal ultrafiltration rates, maximum intraperi-toneal volumes, and the subsequent rate of absorption of fluid are similar when scaled for body size [447,647]. Re-flection coefficients in children for BUN, creatinine, urate, and glucose are similar to adult values, while that of total protein is less [544]. Prolonging dwell times decreases the ultrafiltration coefficient [500]. Thus, the most effective way to obtain maximal ultrafiltration is to use dwell times of 30 to 90 minutes.

Osmotic forces determine convective transport, which

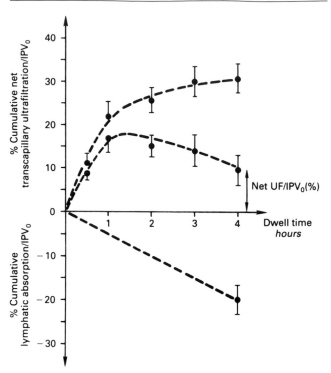

FIG. 39-9. *Cumulative net lymphatic absorption, net ultrafiltration rate, and net transcapillary ultrafiltration rate (mean ± SEM) over 4 hours in six children ages 2 to 13 years undergoing CAPD or CCPD. Dialysate volume used was 40 ml/kg of 2.5% dextrose containing dialysate. Values are expressed as the percentage change in comparison with values at the beginning of the exchange. (From Mactier RA, Khanna R, Moore H, et al: Kinetics of peritoneal dialysis in children: Role of lymphatics. Kidney Int 34:82, 1988, with permission.)*

more rapid absorption of dialysate glucose and more rapid equilibration of urea. A lower net transcapillary ultrafiltration rate was obtained when values were scaled for body surface area, intraperitoneal volume, and dialysate glucose load; higher values were obtained when the values were scaled for body weight. Higher lymphatic absorption was noted when values were corrected for body weight but not for values scaled for body surface area, intraperitoneal volume, or dialysate glucose load.

FACTORS INFLUENCING PERITONEAL TRANSPORT

The transperitoneal movement of solute and water is related, in part, to factors under the direct control of the physician, including the volume of dialysate infused and the duration of the inflow, dwell, and drain segments of the exchange cycle. Manipulating dialysate flow rates primarily affects small solutes. Clearances of small solutes can be increased by shortening cycle length. When exchanges are done in the usual fashion, progressive shortening of the time in which dialysate comes in contact with the exchange membrane leads to a progressive increase in the proportion of cycle length occupied by the inflow and outflow segments and to a net reduction in solute transport.

Also, peritoneal clearances are influenced by the ratio of peritoneal surface area to intraperitoneal volume. For example, when a constant time for inflow, dwell, and drain is used, the peritoneal clearance of BUN decreases after dialysate flow rates exceed 3.5 liters/hour [90,92,625].

Although increasing dialysate volume increases peritoneal clearances [694], the change is not directly proportional to the change in volume. Changes in intraperitoneal volume alter transperitoneal solute movement by changing the usual relationship of volume to peritoneal surface area and permeability [289]. Various maneuvers can be used to alter these relationships and increase peritoneal clearances. It is possible to increase peritoneal clearances by increasing the dialysate flow rate by using two catheters or double-lumen catheters. Channeling, the streaming of dialysate from inflow to outflow without intraperitoneal mixing and contact with the exchange membrane, can limit such increases [575,775]. Another technique used to increase dialysate flow rate is reciprocating peritoneal dialysis. This is accomplished by using in and out 2-minute cycles containing 5% to 10% of the standard exchange volume after initially filling the peritoneal cavity with the usual quantity of dialysate [248,845].

Two of the more important factors that play a significant role in the clinical care of patients are the temperature and glucose content of dialysate. Increasing the temperature of dialysis solutions from room to body temperature raises peritoneal clearances 30% to 35% and makes the patient more comfortable [305]. In adults and children, increasing the dialysate concentration of glucose enhances peritoneal dialysance and clearances [321,345,348]. The mechanisms involved include a combination of solvent drag and hyperosmotic induced vasodilation. The effect persists when the osmolality of the dialysate is lowered, but its duration has not been clearly defined.

A few additional factors can influence transperitoneal transport. Dialysate pH, which in commercially available dialysate ranges from 5.0 to 5.8, has a minimal effect on peritoneal clearances [577]. A high dialysate pH can increase the transperitoneal transfer of weak acids such as barbiturates [124] and urate [438] by converting the transported acid to a less diffusable anionic salt. The addition of albumin to dialysate has been shown to "trap" salicylate and copper [149]. Lipid added to dialysate improves salicylate [514] and glutethimide [748] transport.

DEVELOPMENTAL ASPECTS OF PERITONEAL DIALYSIS KINETICS

Two major issues face pediatric nephrologists when dialyzing children of varying age and body size. First, do the intrinsic properties of the peritoneal membrane change with age? Second, how can the measurements that characterize the transperitoneal movement of solute and water be compared in children of different size and age? A number of studies support the hypothesis that the intrinsic properties of the peritoneal membrane are different during the neonatal period. Insofar as anatomic studies measure the segment of the peritoneal membrane that participates in the exchange process, the surface area of the peritoneal membrane scaled for weight is larger in newly born animals

[226] and humans [661]. Noteworthy is the observation that adequate peritoneal dialysis could be performed in a 2-week-old infant who had 93% of her small intestine resected, leaving her with only 44% of the normal peritoneal surface area [16]. Peritoneal dialysance in dogs during the first few weeks of life is greater than similarly obtained values in adult dogs [215,216,219]. The cause may be attributed to the participation of a larger functioning and a more permeable peritoneal membrane. In the few human neonates evaluated after installing similar weight scaled volumes of dialysate, a higher S_D-S_P solute ratio was found than in older children. This finding offers indirect support that the peritoneal membrane in the human neonate is more permeable than the membrane in the older child [318] (Table 39-10). Finally, some studies of the movement of glucose into the blood stream from the peritoneal cavity have shown that glucose is absorbed more readily in the neonate and infant compared with adults [447].

There is no agreement concerning the best way to compare data obtained in children of varying body size from kinetic studies of the transperitoneal movement of solute. Support for scaling values for both weight and surface area has been developed by the same group of investigators [319,321,543,544]. Theoretical considerations of the formulas for peritoneal dialysance and clearance as well as empirical data from studies in dogs and children lead to the conclusion that when the quantity of dialysate infused was weight scaled, the resulting values were most comparable after they too were weight scaled [215,217,218, 310,316,319,321]. Although the initial report of four MTAC measurements in children supported the use of weight rather than surface area scaled values [608], more recent studies in eight children indicate that values for MTAC scaled for surface area provided better comparisons despite the installation of weight scaled volumes [543]. A recent re-evaluation of MTAC data suggests that its measurement fits best when height rather than surface area or weight is used as a correction factor [662]. This finding may reflect the fact that height is the most important determinant of both surface area and average body mass.

A number of studies in neonates of peritoneal clearance of BUN or creatinine suggest that the peritoneal clearance of these solutes is increased [64,226,235,316,317,751]. However, most studies do not permit meaningful age-related comparisons because dialysis mechanics were not similar. Measurements of peritoneal dialysance and the dialysance index (ratio of dialysance of urea to inulin) in

puppies and adult dogs clearly document that the peritoneal membrane functions differently in the neonate [215,319]. High dialysate-to-blood ratios of urea and creatinine also occur in human neonates [318]. Studies performed so that meaningful comparisons could be made indicate that differences in both peritoneal permeability and functional surface area exist in the neonate. Measurements of the peritoneal clearance and the MTAC of a number of solutes suggest that the rate of movement of smaller molecular weight solutes across the peritoneal membrane in children after the first year of life is similar to that observed in adults. Weight scaled values [321,578,648] for both measurements are within the range of values reported in adults (see Table 39-9) [319,321,648].

Ultrafiltration rates appear to be reduced in neonates. This may be explained by an increased rate of disappearance of dialysate glucose. In neonates, it has been found that dialysate glucose falls quickly with dialysate being reabsorbed after as short a dwell time as 60 minutes [447]. During CAPD, daily absorption of dextrose in children less than 2 years, older than 6 years, and in adults occurred at rates of 2.74 ± 1.06, 1.79 ± 0.87 [48], and 2.3 g/kg/day, respectively [303]. After a 5-hour dwell containing either 2.5% or 4.25% glucose, the mean dialysate glucose concentration in six children less than 2 years old compared with 12 older children was 407 ± 170 mg/dl and 677 ± 192 mg/dl, respectively [49]. Mechanisms to explain the rapid intraperitoneal drop in glucose concentration in neonates include an increased peritoneal permeability or functional surface area and the existence of a greater transperitoneal glucose concentration gradient because glucose utilization in the young is more rapid. Glucose utilization in neonates is approximately three times greater than that of adults (5 to 7 compared with 1.8 to 2.2 mg/kg/minute).

Pediatric Peritoneal Dialysis Prescriptions

Six issues require consideration when developing the initial peritoneal dialysis prescription [311]. (1) What is the contribution of diffusive transport to solute transport across the peritoneal membrane? (2) How much do convective transport and ultrafiltration contribute to solute removal? (3) What does residual renal function contribute? (4) How much ultrafiltration is required? (5) What ought to be the glucose concentration of each exchange? (6) What if any solutes and drugs should be added to the dialysate? The last question is addressed in the section on dialysis solutions.

TABLE 39-10. *Comparison of reflection coefficients in children and adults*

Solute	Pediatric	Adult	P value
Urea	0.14 ± 0.08	0.22 ± 0.06	NS
Creatinine	0.28 ± 0.01	0.31 ± 0.13	NS
Glucose	0.49 ± 0.17	0.59 ± 0.24	NS
Total protein	0.95 ± 0.03	0.99 ± 0.004	< 0.01
Uric acid	0.44 ± 0.16	0.41 ± 0.29	NS

Modified from Morgenstern BZ, Pyle WK, Gruskin AB, et al: Convective characteristics of pediatric peritoneal dialysis. *Perit Dial Bull* 4:S155, 1984.

THEORETICAL PRESCRIPTION FOR CONTINUOUS AMBULATORY PERITONEAL DIALYSIS

The theoretical construct for CAPD is based on being able to maintain water balance and stable concentrations of solutes simultaneously within the body [51,311,403,647]. Solute can be cleared through the peritoneum and by the kidneys. The persistence of a steady state requires that the combined clearance equals the generation rate of the solute being removed. Assume that the BUN is an adequate indicator of uremic control, that the therapeutic goal of CAPD is to maintain the BUN at 60 mg/dl (0.6 mg/ml), and that a child weighing 35 kg has a urea generation rate of 7.7 mg/min (BUN generation rate of 3.6 mg/min; BUN = 28/60 × urea). Children undergoing dialysis have been shown to have urea generation rates of 1.4 to 5.25 mg/min [333,336] and adult sized individuals may have urea generation rates as high as 9.0 mg/min. The renal contribution is assumed to be an actual (uncorrected) BUN clearance of 2 ml/min. The daily urine output is 200 ml/min.

When in balance, the child's urea generation rate (G) equals the concentration of urea in plasma (S_P) times the quantity of plasma cleared by both the kidney (K_R) and peritoneum (K_D), i.e., total clearance (K_T). The formula is:

$$G = S_P \times K_T = S_P \times (K_R + S_P) \times K_D$$

To maintain the BUN at 0.6 mg/ml (60 mg/dl), the total clearance needed becomes $0.6 K_T = 3.6$ mg of BUN/minute or 6 ml/minute. In an anephric child, the required daily BUN clearance would be 8640 ml/day (K_T times 1440).

After a dwell of 4 hours, the dialysate concentration of urea, initially zero, rises to equal the plasma concentration of urea. In such exchanges, typical of CAPD, the formula for peritoneal clearance, $V_D/t \times (S_D/S_P)$ (where $S_D/S_P = 1$), reduces to V_D/t. T equals the exchange time in minutes and V_D the volume of dialysate drained. In short, the daily peritoneal clearance of BUN equals the daily dialysate flow rate when 3- to 4-hour exchanges are used. In this example, 8640 ml/day of dialysis effluent are needed to maintain the patient's BUN at 60 mg/dl.

The estimated volume of dialysate can be reduced by the clearance of BUN contributed by any residual renal function. The residual renal BUN clearance is estimated by obtaining a 24-hour urine collection, measuring BUN in urine and plasma, and calculating an uncorrected renal clearance, K_R in ml/minute = UV/P. A child with an actual BUN clearance of 1.0, 2.0, 5.0, and 10.0 ml/minute would have a BUN clearance of 1440, 2880, 7400, and 14400 ml/day, respectively. The urine volume in which this amount of solute is excreted varies. In theory, the 8640 ml/day of peritoneal clearance required for CAPD can be reduced by the solute cleared and the volume contributed by the remaining renal function. The child with a residual renal BUN clearance of 10 ml/minute would not require dialysis to control azotemia. The important contribution to the dialysis prescription of any residual GFR is obvious, as is the impact of further reductions in GFR once dialysis is begun. In this example of the child with an actual BUN clearance of 2 ml/minute, the total amount of peritoneal clearance required falls to 5760 ml (8640 − 2880).

The estimated total daily volume of dialysate required in patients undergoing CAPD can also be reduced by the amount of volume formed by ultrafiltration since the clearance calculation uses the drained volume. Peritoneal volumes following instillation of 1.5% or 4.25% dextrose peak at 120 and 180 minutes, respectively, and subsequently fall as fluid is absorbed. After a 4-hour exchange in older children, drainage volumes exceed infused volumes of dialysate containing glucose in concentrations of 1.5% or 4.25% by approximately 15% to 25%, and 30% to 40%, respectively [12,447].

The amount of body water that needs to be ultrafiltered is often unclear when dialysis is initiated. Unless there is a pressing need to ultrafilter large amounts of water because of the presence of severe hypertension or volume overload, one might start by assuming that an amount of water corresponding to 4% to 5% of body weight should be removed. Ultrafiltration may not be needed in children with large urine outputs. If visible edema is present, as when non-malnourished children gain 7% to 8% of body weight, the amount of water needing removal should be increased. Net dialysate drainage and measured weights should be followed and a "dry weight" established. Subsequent ultrafiltration requirements are based on this weight.

In the 35-kg child, assuming insensible water losses of 850 ml/day and a urine output of 200 ml/day, the net water balance per day is derived as 1800 (calculated maintenance) − 850 (insensible loss) − 200 (urine output). Assuming the average amount of ultrafiltrate (formed using 1.5% glucose containing dialysate) exceeds input by 15% to 20%, 5 exchanges per day of 1000 ml of 1.5% glucose should return an additional 750 to 1000 ml (150 to 200 ml per exchange) and meet the requirements for both solute clearance and water removal. A 1000-ml exchange (40 ml/kg) is clinically tolerated by most chidren.

By eliminating the remaining renal function, bilateral nephrectomy increases the requirements for peritoneal clearance of solute and has significant impact on ultrafiltration requirements. The water formerly excreted by the kidney must be removed by dialysis, necessitating either greater concentrations of glucose or larger volumes of dialysate to maintain balance.

THEORETICAL PRESCRIPTION FOR INTERMITTENT PERITONEAL DIALYSIS

The objective of intermittent peritoneal dialysis (IPD) is to remove metabolites and water accumulated between dialyses by performing a number of sequential dialysis exchanges, usually 30 to 90 minutes in duration. IPD is performed at intervals ranging from every night to twice or three times weekly, depending on the child's clinical status and remaining degree of renal function [535]. The process by which an initial dialysis precription can be developed is illustrated by providing an example. Assume that the goal of IPD in a 25-kg child gaining 1 kg between each dialysis is to maintain the BUN at 60 mg/dl and reach "dry weight" at the end of dialysis; that the interdialytic interval is 36 hours; that the urea space is equivalent to that occupied by total body water, 60% of body weight (25 × 0.6 = 15 liters); that the BUN generation rate is 3.6 mg/minute; and that the residual renal BUN clearance is 1.0 ml/min.

During the interdialytic period, total body water increases from 15 to 16 liters (1-kg weight gain); by the end of the next dialysis (48 hours after completing the last dialysis), body metabolic processes generate 10,368 mg of BUN at a rate of 3.6 mg/minute for 2880 minutes. In the absence of renal function, the anticipated increase in BUN is 65 mg/dl (10,368/16 = 648 mg/liter = 64.8 mg/dl); and the child's BUN at the beginning of the next dialysis would be 60 mg/dl + 65 mg/dl or 125 mg/dl. With more residual GFR, the BUN would be lower.

Based on first order diffusion kinetics, a formula estimates the serum concentration of urea, S_{pt}, after a defined time of peritoneal dialysis [403]:

$$S_{pt} = S_{po}e^{-kt/V}$$

where S_{po} and S_{pt} equal the solute concentration at the onset (125 mg/dl) and the end of dialysis (60 mg/dl), respectively, e equals the base of natural logarithm, k equals the maximum peritoneal clearance during an exchange and is assumed to be 30 ml/min, t equals the duration of dialysis in minutes (720 minutes or 12 hours), and V equals the volume of dialysate.

Rearranging the formula to solve for V, the quantity of dialysate needed to lower the BUN from 125 mg/dl to 60 mg/dl, the formula becomes:

$$V = \frac{-kt}{\ln(S_{pt}/S_{pO})}$$

$$V = -30 \times \frac{(720)}{\ln(60/125)}$$

$$V = -30 \times \frac{(720)}{0.73}$$

Provided in Table 39-11 is a set of values for various postdialysis-to-predialysis ratios for BUN with corresponding values that can be used in the denominator of this formula.

Depending on whether 30- or 60-minute exchange cycles are desired, and assuming a total time for dialysis of 12 hours, a dialysis prescription providing 30,000 ml divided by 12 (hourly exchanges) or 24 (half-hourly exchanges) would require 2500 ml (100 ml/kg) or 1250 ml (50 ml/kg)

TABLE 39-11. *Values for the natural log of the ratio of the postdialysis to predialysis BUN*

Ratio S_D/S_P	Value
ln 0.60	−0.51
ln 0.55	−0.60
ln 0.50	−0.69
ln 0.45	−0.79
ln 0.40	−0.91

exchanges, respectively. The former value is not technically feasible because of the large intraperitoneal volume required. Peritoneal volumes in the range of 25 to 50 ml/kg are satisfactorily tolerated by most children.

The estimated dialysate volume needed for solute removal can be reduced by the contribution of residual renal function, because of convective solute transport and the anticipated amount of ultrafiltration. Thirty-minute exchanges in a group of children using 30 ml/kg of dialysate containing 1.5% or 4.25% glucose are associated with drainage volumes that exceed infused volumes of dialysate by 4% to 8% and 12% to 18%, respectively [321]. In adults, drainage volumes associated with hourly exchanges containing 1.5% or 4.25% glucose are reported to exceed infused volumes of 10% to 15% and 20% to 30%, respectively [344].

As discussed, 30 liters of dialysate volume would be needed were the child anephric. Because this child has some residual renal function (GFR = 1 ml/minute), the BUN would not actually reach 125 mg/dl. In practical terms, this issue is addressed by assuming what the maximal BUN would have been in an anephric child and subsequently removing from this value the contribution made by the remaining renal function. In this example, the estimated volume needed to achieve the desired peritoneal clearance can be reduced by the contribution of the residual renal function. One ml/minute of actual BUN clearance reduces the requirement for peritoneal clearance by 60 ml/hour, 2 ml by 120 ml/hr, and so forth. If the time on IPD plus the interdialytic period is 48 hours, the required volume to achieve the desired peritoneal clearance can be reduced 2880 ml (48 hours × 60 ml/hour). Because the S_D/S_P ratio for BUN during short dwell exchanges is less than 1.0, the amount of solute clearance obtained per exchange does not equal the dialysate flow rate as it does in CAPD. Because the expected S_D/S_P ratio for a 30-minute dwell is 0.4, 1 ml/minute of renal clearance reduces the required volume of dialysate by 2.5 ml/minute. Residual renal clearance = $(SD/SP) \times (Vdialysate/T)$. V, the dialysate volume corresponding to the contribution of renal function, would be 1800 ml in a 12-hour treatment. The clearance is derived as follows:

Dialysate volume = *Residual renal function* ÷ (S_D/S_P)
= 1 ÷ (0.4) × 720 = 1800 ml

The impact of residual renal function is to reduce the amount of dialysate required to 28,200 ml (30,000 ml − 1800 ml).

If the quantity of water accumulated by the child prior to dialysis is 5%, 1.25 liters (25 kg × 0.05) need to be removed by ultrafiltration. It is assumed that there is no further contribution of residual renal function to water balance during the dialysis treatment and that the excess water present at the onset of dialysis is determined by either physical examination or weight gain between subsequent dialysis treatments.

Because of the contribution of ultrafiltration provided by convective solute transport, the value of 28,200 ml of dialysate necessary to clear urea can be reduced by multiplying the solute sieving coefficient for urea, 0.8 times the ultrafiltered volume of 1250 ml, i.e., 1000 ml. Twenty-three exchanges of 1250 ml would be needed were no additional ultrafiltration to occur during dialysis. Twenty-one exchanges of 1250 ml (50 ml/kg), or 26 exchanges of 1000 ml (40 ml/kg), each lasting 30 minutes, would provide 26,000 to 26,250 ml; if 5% (1300 to 1350 ml) were ultrafiltered, approximately 27,500 ml would be drained. This volume meets the solute clearance and ultrafiltration requirements. In patients undergoing CCPD, a similar approach can be used to estimate the dialysis parameters. In summary, the factors to consider in developing intermittent peritoneal dialysis prescriptions are the impact of dwell time on the S_D/S_P ratio, the inherent diffusive and sieving characteristics of the solute involved, and amount of ultrafiltrate formed.

Peritoneal Dialysis in Acute Renal Failure

INDICATIONS AND PROGNOSIS

Children, especially infants and neonates with acute renal failure, are usually critically ill. Because the metabolic aberrations are rapid in onset, investigation and treatment should proceed simultaneously. The increased metabolic rates and energy demands of younger children result in earlier and more frequent dialysis [162,486]. Indications for immediate dialysis in children with acute renal failure include severe or persistent hyperkalemia, intractable hypertension, congestive heart failure, pulmonary edema from volume overload, severe and persistent acidosis, and neurologic complications of uremia [752]. The decision to initiate dialysis should also anticipate the natural history of acute renal failure in various pediatric clinical settings (see Chapter 90).

Both hemodialysis and peritoneal dialysis are comparably effective in managing acute renal failure. The choice of a specific modality depends on patient size, availability of vascular access, integrity of the peritoneal membrane and abdominal cavity, and, perhaps most importantly, clinical experience and expertise [200,463,752]. Although hemodialysis is technically possible in infants and neonates [433,516,560], peritoneal dialysis is the method usually chosen because of its simplicity, availability, effectiveness and relative safety. Low volume exchanges, 10 ml/kg per exchange, can be used to ultrafiltrate infants on mechanical ventilation without significantly affecting respiration [869a]. Minor ventilatory changes may be needed. Return volumes using 1.5% to 4.25% glucose average 125% to 140% of that infused. CAVH and CAVHD are increasingly being used to manage infants with acute renal failure. The prognosis of acute renal failure due to primary kidney disease is relatively good [134], with the majority of children recovering. Survival is poor when acute renal failure is secondary to infectious diseases or major operations (e.g., open heart surgery) [429].

DIALYSIS TECHNIQUE

Premedication is recommended before inserting the peritoneal catheter. One premedication scheme uses meperidine HCl, 2 mg/kg; promethazine HCl, 1 to 2 mg/kg; and chlorpromazine, 1 mg/kg, intramuscularly 30 to 60 minutes before beginning to introduce the catheter into the abdo-

men, to reduce anxiety and make the child more comfortable. After local anesthesia and lidocaine (Xylocaine), the abdomen is filled with 15 to 20 ml/kg body weight of dialysate delivered through a soft angiocath or small bore needle. This will distend the anterior abdominal wall and help avoid puncturing an intra-abdominal organ, bowel, or a major blood vessel. A stylet catheter is inserted through a small incision along the linea alba at a point approximately one-third of the distance from the umbilicus to the pubis symphysis. If a midline insertion is not possible, the catheter can be inserted in the flank area outside the line of the inferior epigastric artery. After the peritoneum is entered, the stylet is partially withdrawn and the catheter advanced to the right or left (preferred) side of the pelvis. All the catheter perforations must be within the peritoneal cavity to avoid subcutaneous fluid infiltration of the abdominal wall. The dialysis solution should be kept warm at 37 to 38°C in a water bath. Heparin (500 to 1000 U/liter) can be added to the dialysis solution for the first three cycles and should be continued as long as the dialysis effluent is bloody. Bloody effluent from the first exchange occurs in approximately one-third of dialyses [816]. Because hyperkalemia is often present, potassium is omitted from the dialysis solution for the first three to six cycles. KCl is then added at a concentration of 3.0 mEq/liter unless the serum potassium exceeds 5.5 mEq/liter. The selection of a glucose concentration (1.5%, 2.5%, 4.25%) depends on the fluid balance of the patient. Dialysis solutions containing 7% dextrose should be avoided in pediatric dialysis because of the risk of hyperglycemia and excessive ultrafiltration. When hyperglycemia occurs (>300 mg/dl), regular insulin, 0.1 to 0.2 units/kg, can be given intravenously. Alternatively, 1.0 units of regular insulin can be added to each 5.0 gm of glucose in the dialysate. Blood sugar levels should be monitored. In newborns and infants, replacement of acetate or lactate by bicarbonate in the dialysis solution has been advocated, especially if lactic acidosis is to be treated. Most pharmacies can make up a sterile solution containing bicarbonate at 30 to 40 mmol/liter with appropriate concentrations of sodium, potassium, chloride, calcium, magnesium, and glucose.

The dialysis solution initially is delivered into the abdomen in amounts of 15 to 20 ml/kg and gradually increased to 40 to 50 ml/kg in infants and small children and 30 to 40 ml/kg in older children; 2000 ml per cycle is not usually exceeded. The first exchange can be immediately drained to check catheter function. Dialysate is infused by gravity flow over a period of 5 to 10 minutes and allowed to equilibrate for at least 30 minutes before beginning the outflow phase. Although equilibration at 30 minutes is less than complete [90], the bulk of exchange occurs during this time, and the most efficient acute dialysis results from exploiting this fact [403]. Drainage should take 10 to 20 minutes. Once biochemical and volume overload problems are stabilized, exchange times can be lengthened. The total dialysis time is usually limited to 36 to 48 hours. If renal failure continues, the procedure is repeated 48 hours later [200]. The patient is begun on a regular routine of IPD, CAPD, or CCPD if a protracted course is anticipated.

Volumetric fluid balance measurements are essential whenever acute dialysis is performed. If a manual system is used, an accurate record of fluid balance should be kept, and the volume of the spent dialysis solution should be measured. Commercially prepared bottles or bags are often overfilled; many 1000-ml bottles or bags contain 1040 to 1060 ml. Monitoring of weight during dialysis (two or three times a day) is imperative even if accurate records of fluid balance are kept, especially if semiautomatic cycler machines are used. In acutely ill patients, ongoing fluid losses from vomiting and diarrhea should be continuously replaced. Also, a progressive daily loss of 1.0% to 1.5% of weight should be anticipated as a result of a reduction of lean body mass. Vital signs (temperature, pulse and blood pressure recumbent and upright) should initially be recorded at the end of each exchange or more often if needed. Measuring vital signs can be done less frequently after stabilization has occurred.

A CBC and serum urea, creatinine, electrolytes, calcium, phosphorus, magnesium, glucose, and total protein levels should be obtained prior to and at regular intervals throughout dialysis therapy to assess therapy and prevent complications. Dialysate is cultured daily by aseptically aspirating effluent fluid through the side-arm injection site. Whenever cloudy fluid appears or undue abdominal pain or fever develops, blood and dialysate should be cultured. Antibiotic therapy, administered systemically, intraperitoneally, or both, should be considered.

Neonatal Peritoneal Dialysis

Many neonates with acute renal failure can be managed conservatively. If renal failure is prolonged beyond 7 to 10 days or uremic complications arise, peritoneal dialysis should be performed. Relatively few reports describe the use of peritoneal dialysis in premature and term newborn infants [19,486,506]. No ideal dialysate volume per exchange has been agreed on. Larger dialysate volumes (50 to 70 compared with 30 to 40 ml/kg per exchange) if tolerated, are more likely to result in greater ultrafiltration rates with 4-hour dwells [446]. Interference with diaphragmatic movement and cyclic changes in PO_2 and PCO_2 using continuous transcutaneous monitoring when dialyzing low-birth-weight infants have been observed [385].

In some premature and full-term infants, the intraperitoneal space is too small to accommodate all the drainage holes of a standard pediatric catheter, and a number of different approaches have been developed [842]. The drainage holes in the standard size pediatric peritoneal dialysis catheter are limited to its distal 4.2 cm. It must be placed well into the peritoneal cavity. An infant peritoneal dialysis catheter is available (Trocath, infant size, McGaw Laboratories, Los Angeles, California) that has the same diameter as the standard pediatric dialysis catheter but has drainage holes limited to the distal 2.1 cm [19]. A pediatric Tenckhoff catheter can be used in infants weighing more than 2.5 kg body weight; however, it cannot be used in children weighing less than 2.5 kg because its dacron cuffs are too thick to fit within the abdominal wall. The pediatric and neonatal Tenckhoff catheters have perforations occupying the distal 7.0 and 5.0 cm, respectively. Both sets of perforations begin 5.0 cm from the cuff. A homemade catheter constructed from silastic lines used for cor-

onary artery perfusion has been used successfully by some centers for dialysing very small children [368]. Catheters modified from neonatal chest tubes [540], No. 14 angiocaths with side holes made with a No. 22 gauge needle [771], have been used. A neonatal peritoneal dialysis catheter (Pendlebury, Medcomp, Harleysville, PA) incorporating these features is commercially available. A double lumen peritoneal dialysis catheter is the basic element of the BODA pediatric peritoneal dialysis system (Medcomp, Harleysville, PA) that allows continuous peritoneal dialysis to be performed in neonates.

Long-Term Maintenance Peritoneal Dialysis

INDICATIONS

Long-term peritoneal dialysis is extensively used in the treatment of end-stage renal disease (ESRD) in children and is as effective as regular hemodialysis for controlling uremia and its complications [52,64,107,164]. The choice of a dialysis modality is rarely straight-forward and is best decided by children and their families after discussing alternatives with the pediatric nephrologist and the dialysis nurses.

Reasons for choosing long-term peritoneal dialysis in pediatric patients include the technical difficulties of hemodialysis in small children, a need for prolonged dialysis prior to renal transplantation such as with a malignancy or high cytotoxic antibody titers, failure of vascular access, a long travel time to a hemodialysis or pediatric nephrology center, and patient or parent preference for this modality of treatment [52,134]. The few relative contraindications for initiating peritoneal dialysis in children include multiple abdominal surgeries with subsequent adhesions resulting in a loss of peritoneal surface area, the presence of a ventriculoperitoneal shunt (VP), and the presence of urinary diversions (ileal conduits or cutaneous ureterostomies) because the constant exposure of the catheter to moisture and infected secretions increases the risk for developing exit site and tunnel infections and peritonitis. VP shunts can be converted to ventriculo, atrial, or pleural shunts and peritoneal dialysis used.

A number of factors influence patients and families in choosing or changing a peritoneal dialysis modality, including the unwillingness of older children to perform dialysis exchanges at school, the feeling of impaired level of activity with a full abdomen, and the greater incidence of peritonitis with CAPD. Family demands and parental burnout also may lead to requests for changing dialysis modalities.

Patient and family preference is obviously important when selecting peritoneal dialysis modalities, but definite criteria do not exist. One approach is to offer all who request home peritoneal dialysis an opportunity to do so unless specific contraindicating factors are present. Children and families are best considered unsuitable for peritoneal dialysis if they are unwilling to accept responsibility for performing the dialysis procedure and to change their lifestyle to do so. Poor socioeconomic background and poor personal hygiene are relative contraindications to home peritoneal dialysis because of the greater risk of infection.

In-center overnight peritoneal dialysis can be used as an alternative.

DIALYSIS SOLUTIONS

There are a variety of commercially available solutions despite recommendations for limiting their formulation [792]. The range of values for concentrations of dialysate solutes in mEq/liter are sodium, 130 to 140; chloride, 98 to 108; acetate or lactate, 35 to 45; calcium, 3 to 4 (6 to 8 mg/dl); magnesium, 0.5 to 1.5 (1.8 md/dl); and dextrose monohydrate, 1.5, 2.5, 4.25 g/dl. Potassium is usually not included and is added only when medically necessary. Small quantities of sodium bisulfite are added to dialysate to minimize caramelization of dextrose during autoclaving. The final pH of sterile apyrogenic solutions is in the range of 5.2 to 5.8. The aluminum concentration of dialysate should not exceed 10 μg/liter.

Dialysate Sodium

The sodium concentration of dialysate affects the amount of sodium and the postdialysis serum sodium level. The most commonly used dialysate sodium concentration is 132 mEq/liter, which provides satisfactory sodium removal and blood pressure control in most patients. The availability of dialysis solutions with two different sodium concentrations (130 and 140 mEq/liter) offers sufficient flexibility for regulating sodium removal. When dialysis is performed in patients with hypernatremia, a dialysis solution with a sodium concentration of 130 mEq/liter is recommended [582]. In certain circumstances, a lower sodium concentration (118 mEq/liter) may be necessary to remove more sodium and to avoid thirst after osmotic ultrafiltration [743]. When excessive ultrafiltration occurs [669], hypernatremia may develop because the sodium concentration in ultrafiltrate is in the range of 120 to 126 mEq/liter, reflective of the fact that the net sieving coefficient of sodium is considerably less than 1.0 [578,695]. Noteworthy is the fact that a variation of 5% in the dialysate sodium concentration, because of the manufacturing process, can result in a dialysate sodium concentration that ranges from 132 to 148 mEq/liter [783].

Dialysate Potassium

Because severe dietary potassium restriction is difficult to achieve and because of its low peritoneal clearance [108], potassium-free dialysate is used in the dialysis of most patients with renal failure. The addition of potassium chloride may be necessary in patients treated with digitalis, in cases of hypokalemia due to intestinal losses and inadequate intake, in patients with peritonitis, and in those undergoing frequent exchanges [538,601]. Hypokalemia has been reported in 10% of patients on CAPD when potassium-free dialysate was used [601].

Dialysate Buffers

Acetate and lactate are the usual buffers in dialysis solutions because insoluble calcium and magnesium salts will form in the presence of bicarbonate. Optimal concentrations of these buffers are in the range of 38 to 40 mEq/liter [792]. The frequently used concentration of 35 mEq/liter

of acetate or lactate does not compensate for the obligatory bicarbonate loss during dialysis [791]. The use of a peritoneal dialysis solution (Dianeal PD-2, Travenol, Chicago, IL) with higher lactate levels (40 mEq/liter) results in more normal levels of bicarbonate in patients on IPD but can lead to metabolic alkalosis in those on CAPD [504]. Theoretical advantages for using acetate instead of lactate exist: acetate solutions have a higher final pH (5.8 to 6.2) than do lactate solutions (5.4); acetate is a more effective source of bicarbonate [459]; and finally, acetate has been shown to be bacteriostatic under certain experimental conditions [681]. Lactate is often chosen by manufacturers because dextrose caramelization during autoclaving is less marked with this anion because of its pK of 3.9. Acetate may decrease ultrafiltration [581,601]. In one study involving adults from France, 15.2% of 295 patients had to be switched from CAPD to hemodialysis because of permanent reductions in or the loss of ultrafiltration; they had received acetate dialysate [761]. Patients using lactate dialysate may also lose their ultrafiltration capacity [579]. When lactate is not converted to bicarbonate in patients with lactic acidosis, a bicarbonate dialysate can be prepared by sterilely mixing solutions of hypertonic bicarbonate, glucose water, potassium chloride, and physiologic saline. Final concentrations of electrolytes should be: HCO_3^-, 30 to 35 mEq/liter; sodium, 140 mEq/liter; potassium, 0 to 4 mEq/liter; chloride, 105 to 110 mEq/liter; and glucose, 1500 to 4500 mg/dl. Calcium and magnesium salts cannot be added because they will form a precipitate.

Dialysate Calcium

Calcium in dialysis solutions exists as ionized calcium. When the calcium concentration of the dialysis solution is 6.5 to 7 mg/dl, a positive calcium balance occurs during dialysis [393]. The calcium concentration in hypertonic dialysis solutions should be 0.5 to 1 mEq/liter higher than that in isotonic solutions. This is because calcium transfer from dialysate to blood is impeded by ultrafiltration and results in a negative calcium balance [607,619]. Low calcium (3.5 mg/dl) dialysate solutions are available for use in patients with hypercalcemia. Aggravation of renal osteodystrophy has been observed when a low calcium concentration (3 mEq/liter) is used [117,603].

Dialysate Magnesium

Most peritoneal dialysis solutions contain magnesium at a concentration of 1.5 mEq/liter. Because hypermagnesemia has been a problem for some patients on CAPD [582,601], it has been suggested that the magnesium concentration be routinely lowered to 0.5 mEq/liter to allow for better control of the serum magnesium concentration [504]. Hypomagnesemia can occur when dialysate containing low concentrations of magnesium is used, especially in malnourished patients [601].

Osmotic Agents

Dextrose remains the osmotic agent of choice and is available as dextrose monohydrate in concentrations of 1.5, 2.5, and 4.25 g/dl. Dialysate with 1.5% dextrose monohydrate contains 1.36 g/dl of anhydrous dextrose or 75.6 mmol/liter. The higher the concentration of dextrose, the greater the rate and amount of ultrafiltration. Ultrafiltration in peritoneal dialysis is a self-limited process because dextrose diffuses readily across the peritoneal capillary wall into the blood stream and is metabolized [90,303]. Ultrafiltration rates that are maximal immediately after an infusion of dialysate decrease proportionally as the dextrose concentration falls [585]. To avoid dextrose loading during dialysis, several alternative osmotically active agents have been tried, including gelatin, glycerol [169], glucose polymers [284a], dextran, fructose, sorbitol, and xylitol. The lack of a definitive advantage for any of these substances precludes their routine use [538]. A polymer containing 3 to 8 glucose molecules per osmotically active unit has been shown to provide adequate ultrafiltration while simultaneously diminishing the glucose load presented to the body [359,805]. Dialysate containing a mixture of amino acids at concentrations of 1 to 2 g/dl has been proposed as an alternative to glucose. Such a solution can also provide a source of nutrients for patients with malnutrition [184, 421,597]. The long-term use of amino acids remains to be evaluated for efficacy and safety. The net amino acid absorption of amino acids added to dialysate is proportional to their concentration in dialysate [332]. As currently formulated, their use in dialysate often results in undesirable elevations of serum amino acids.

INTERMITTENT PERITONEAL DIALYSIS

Although manual IPD can be used as an alternative form of long-term peritoneal dialysis [235], automatic or semiautomatic cycling machines are more convenient and efficient. Two forms of automated peritoneal dialysis machines, automatic proportioning and cycler machines, are available [92,464,796]. Automatic proportioning machines are not widely used because of their complexity and frequent need for repair.

The original cycling device (AMP 80/2 peritoneal dialysis system, American Medical Products Corporation, Freehold, New Jersey) used premixed, commercially available dialysis solutions and a series of valves that constricted dialysis tubing at preset intervals (drain timer/fill-dwell timer) for peritoneal filling and drainage. The cycler is operated by gravity and retains the simplicity of the manual peritoneal dialysis technique. Available inflow volumes range from 240 to 750 ml in the pediatric model and from 1000 to 2000 ml in the standard model. Dialysate leaves its plastic container to enter the heater bag, where it stays for the period preset by the drain timer and is warmed to body temperature. Next, fluid empties into the peritoneal cavity, where it stays for a period controlled by the fill-dwell timer. At the end of this period, the fluid drains out into the weigh bag. It sounds an alarm and automatically stops the dialysis if the patient has not drained 75% of the preset volume in 75% of the preset drain time. Finally, fluid drains from the weigh bag into the final drainage bag.

Newer automated cyclers are now available. Pediatric cycler machines (Pac-Xtra, Baxter, Deerfield, IL; Amperosol, Abbott, Chicago, IL) capable of infusing dialysate volumes as low as 50 ml are available. These machines offer a wide range of settings to control dialysate volume and

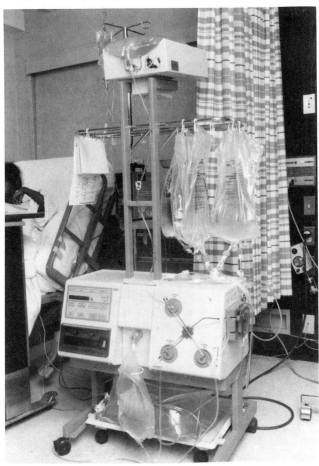

FIG. 39-10. *The Baxter Pac-Xtra (Deerfield, IL) peritoneal dialysis automatic cycler.*

dwell times. Multiple types of dialysis prescriptions, IPD, CCPD, and tidal dialysis, can be easily programmed. Commercially available dialysate solutions are available.

Catheter Break-In

After inserting the catheter, dialysis is started immediately with small volumes of dialysate (10 ml/kg). It is continued without interruption for 2 to 3 days to avoid early catheter obstruction by blood clots or fibrin plugs and to enable satisfactory healing to occur. Some attach a CAPD bag containing heparin and flush the catheter every 20 to 60 minutes for the first few hours, after which hourly exchanges are begun. The dialysate volume can either be gradually increased over the next 3 to 4 days or low volume exchanges continued for this period of time and then increased. Low volume exchanges for the first few days may help avoid pericatheter hernia formation or dialysate leak. The aforementioned technique can be used for all forms of peritoneal dialysis. Adequate dialysis is generally achieved with an exchange volume in the range of 35 to 50 ml/kg (maximum is usually 2–3 liters). Dialysis cycles of 30 to 60 minutes with three-quarters of the cycle length for fill and dwell and one-quarter for drainage are commonly used. The final exchange volume, which usually parallels the weight of the patient, also depends on the patient's ability to tolerate intraperitoneal fluids, the delivery range of the cycler model, and the contribution of residual renal function.

Each IPD treatment lasts 10 to 12 hours; it is performed three or more times a week, with the total dialysis time ranging from 40 to 60 hours per week, adjusted according to blood chemistries and fluid balance. The home training of cycler dialysis takes 10 to 12 dialysis days. Home peritoneal dialysis using the cycler is usually performed at night while the patient is asleep and unattended. Performing dialysis in this fashion offsets the major disadvantage of the long dialysis time required to perform IPD.

CONTINUOUS AMBULATORY PERITONEAL DIALYSIS

The basic principle of CAPD is to enable a stable biochemical internal milieu to exist by a continuous bathing of the peritoneal cavity by dialysis solutions exchanged every 4 to 10 hours [644]. It was the introduction of dialysate in varying volumes in plastic bags that made this procedure possible [599]. The long dwell times allow maximal equilibration of solutes between plasma and dialysate. When CAPD was first introduced, five exchanges per day were done [605]. It was subsequently found that some adults could be successfully dialyzed with three exchanges of 3 liters/day [422,808]. Similar volumes of dialysate per unit of body weight (30 to 50 ml/kg) and similar frequencies of exchange (3 to 5) can be used in children. Infants usually require 5 or more exchanges per day.

Bags of dialysate are connected to a permanent peritoneal catheter by a short connecting tube. After inflow, the empty dialysate bag still attached to the connecting tube is carried rolled up in a waist purse under the patient's clothing until it is unrolled for outflow. At the end of the diffusion period, the dialysate is drained into the same bag, which is then discarded. A fresh bag is attached to the same connecting line, which is usually changed once a month by a nurse to decrease the risk of peritonitis. It is reportedly safe to change transfer set lines bimonthly to twice yearly [387]. During and after the manipulations associated with transfer set changes, some children experience pain or redness at the exit site. Holding the peritoneal catheter tightly with a sterile gauze during the disconnect-reconnect procedure may prevent these problems [829]. Advantages of CAPD over cycler peritoneal dialysis are that no machine, electrical outlet, or water source are needed and the method is portable [645]. A major advantage attributed to CAPD is that the chemical composition of the internal milieu is constant [442,708,709].

CONTINUOUS CYCLE PERITONEAL DIALYSIS

CCPD is an evolutionary offshoot of CAPD and IPD developed to retain the physiologic advantages of continuous equilibration dialysis (CAPD) while reducing the incidence of infection. CCPD also improves convenience to the patient and parent by avoiding dialysate exchanges during the day. Patients treated with CCPD perform three to five dialysis exchanges with a dialysis cycling machine for approximately 2 hours during the night and a single daytime dwell at half the nocturnal cycle volume, using the same dialysis solution as for CAPD [191] (Nocturnal cycling peritoneal dialysis). Occasionally the abdomen is not filled during the day. Although the reported experience with CCPD in children is limited, it has been shown to be an effective, well-tolerated dialysis modality for children similar to that of CAPD except for a small difference in serum creatinine levels [104,157]. Peritonitis rates are also similar or less than those seen in patients on CAPD [15,710]. In one pediatric center, 24 of 63 children were switched from CAPD to CCPD for medical (42%) and psychosocial (58%) reasons.

RECIRCULATING PERITONEAL DIALYSIS

Recirculating peritoneal dialysis in neonates has been reported [842]. A single 2.0-liter bag of dialysate was connected to the dialysis catheter and 10 to 40 ml/kg was infused, allowed to dwell for 30 to 60 minutes, and drained into the same bag. The procedure was continued for 8 hours. A bag change after 4 hours improved overall peritoneal clearances of urea and creatinine. A satisfactory clinical course was observed. Tidal peritoneal dialysis has been used overnight in older children with limited success [253a]. Adequate peritoneal clearance required tidal dialysate flow rates exceeding 50 ml/kg per hour.

LONG-TERM PERITONEAL DIALYSIS

The long-term effects of various peritoneal dialysis modalities differ. In adults on IPD, complications that develop over time include acidosis, anemia, overhydration, and malnutrition. A need to switch to hemodialysis or another form of peritoneal dialysis begins after 2 years. Such deterioration tends to parallel decreases in residual renal function [190]. Only 40% of adults remain on IPD more than 2 years [6].

Limited data suggest that CAPD or CCPD may be associated with an improved long-term control of the uremic state. An overview of the first few years' experience of CAPD is provided by data developed by the NIH CAPD registry [773]. Approximately 50% of patients in the United States (of which 5% are less than 20 years of age) are included. The probability of developing a CAPD related complication is summarized in Table 39-12. A change in dialysis modality occurred in 22.6% and 31.2% of patients after 12 and 18 months, respectively. Reasons include medical problems, excessive episodes of peritonitis, failure to control chemistries or fluid balance, loss of membrane function, patient choice, and socioeconomic problems.

Long-term experience with various peritoneal dialysis modalities in children is limited because most children receive renal transplants. After 36 months of dialysis, continued use of CAPD or CCPD was 20% and 93%, respectively, in 93 children [834]. Thirty of 70 children who started on CAPD switched to CCPD. Six children were switched to hemodialysis. In a review of 226 children on peritoneal dialysis, 14 had to discontinue peritoneal dialysis because of peritoneal membrane failure [146]. Other available data reveal that long-term peritoneal dialysis in children, as in adults, is associated with an increasing morbidity, especially bone and neurologic problems.

TABLE 39-12. *Percentage of patients of developing a CAPD-related complication during successive 6-month intervals in 6656 patients (5% less than 20 years) after starting treatment*

	Months on CAPD		
	0–6	6–12	12–18
Catheter replacement	12.3	20.9	28.7
Exit site and/or tunnel infection	26.8	40.4	51.5
Peritonitis	45.6	68.4	78.5
First hospitalization related to complication	38.4	57.7	71.0
Changed modality	11.1	22.6	31.2
Died while on CAPD	7.4	14.5	20.8

Modified from Steinberg SM, Cutler SJ, Nolph KD, et al: A comprehensive report on the experience of patients on continuous ambulatory peritoneal dialysis for the treatment of end-stage renal disease. *Am J Kidney Dis* 4:233, 1984.

In one study, when the clinical course of 29 children treated with IPD was compared with 17 children treated with CAPD, the children treated with CAPD did better [313]. They had lower blood concentrations of urea and phosphate and tended to grow better, although they had higher rates of peritonitis.

In another study of 51 children treated with CAPD compared with 25 children treated with hemodialysis, complications were more frequent in the CAPD group [64,656]. Five CAPD children died; seven transferred to hemodialysis. One child on hemodialysis died; four transferred to CAPD. There were 46 failures of peritoneal catheters; hemodialysis access failed in 12. Linear growth was better in CAPD patients when examined one way but not by another method. The CAPD patients experienced better blood pressure control and required fewer medications. CAPD patients had higher blood concentrations of hematocrit, CO_2 content, and cholesterol; they had lower concentrations of BUN and albumin. Compared with patients on hemodialysis, patients undergoing chronic peritoneal dialysis lose a large number of serum proteins, including hormones, enzymes, carrier proteins, immunoglobulins, and proteins involved in the coagulation process [205]. The long-term significance of such losses needs to be more clearly defined.

CATHETERS

The disposable stylet catheter (Trocath peritoneal dialysis catheter, McGaw Laboratories) [858] is used only in acute situations. Indications for using disposable catheters include acute poisoning when only one dialysis session is anticipated, severe extracellular volume overload and hyperkalemia, the need for prompt drainage of the peritoneal cavity because of marked abdominal distention from an obstructed Silastic catheter, and temporary use during antibiotic treatment of skin infections of the abdominal wall before inserting a permanent Silastic catheter [538].

The permanent Silastic catheter is commercially available [797] and is used for both short-term and long-term dialysis. The introduction of the permanent Silastic catheter by Tenckhoff eliminated the need for repeated painful peritoneal punctures, reduced the risk of organ perforation, allowed high dialysate flow rates independent of position, permitted relatively infection-free, long-term access to the peritoneal cavity with few restrictions in physical or recreational activities [794,797], and allowed home peritoneal dialysis to develop [795].

Catheter choice and function are influenced by the material used in its construction, the nature of the external seal, and its intraperitoneal shape. Most peritoneal catheters used in long-term dialysis are made of siliconized rubber. Some are impregnated with barium sulfate (shadow stripe by Quinton Instrument Co., Seattle, WA), making the catheter radiopaque and easy to localize radiographically. The permanent catheter is fitted with one or two bonded dacron felt cuffs (Fig. 39-11). They fix the catheter within the abdominal wall and act as a barrier against bacterial invasion of the peritoneum along the outside of the catheter [797]. Many centers prefer the double cuff catheter; others use only the single cuff catheter because it is simpler to implant and to remove, avoids the complications of extrusion of the subcutaneous (distal) cuff from the exit site, and avoids exit site redness and infection [52, 473,600,831]. In a study involving 374 single-cuff and 60 double-cuff catheters, no difference in catheter survival occurred in patients on IPD; catheter survival of the double-cuff catheter exceeded that of single-cuff catheters in patients on CAPD [189].

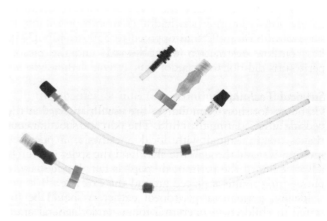

FIG. 39-11. *Single-cuff and double-cuff catheters and connecting devices including rubber cap, beta cap system, and titanium adapter.*

fluid. Patients with pancreatitis, bowel perforation, or gall bladder disease will have marked elevations of amylase in both serum and peritoneal fluid [129].

BLEEDING AND THROMBOSIS

Bloody effluent occurs as a result of the surgical trauma of implantation in about 30% of patients [606]. Although the bleeding subsides spontaneously in most cases, blood clots can cause obstruction of the catheter. It is common practice to add heparin, 1000 U/liter, to the dialysate and to perform more frequent exchanges until bleeding ceases. When a major vessel is penetrated, an organ lacerated, or a clot lysed by constant bathing with dialysate, major bleeding can occur. Transfusions and surgical repair may be required. Bleeding is seen more commonly in patients undergoing partial omentectomy and in patients with a history of previous abdominal operations, frequent episodes of peritonitis, and adhesions [473]. Occasionally, bloody dialysate may appear at the time of ovulation or menses [159], during defecation or bouts of severe diarrhea, during strenuous exercise, during coughing, and following abdominal trauma. Infection and trauma account for most cases of bleeding. Splenic rupture secondary to trauma or erosion from a displaced Tenckhoff catheter has been reported [182]. Bleeding can occur from the rupture of any intra-abdominal organ. Anemia has been described secondary to prolonged intraperitoneal bleeding, presumably as a result of catheter irritation of omental vessels [457]. When catheters are removed, patients need to be monitored for occult intraperitoneal bleeding.

Major thrombotic episodes occasionally develop in patients on CAPD [75]. Clotting factor abnormalities similar to those observed in patients with the nephrotic syndrome have been noted in patients on CAPD. The hypercoagulable state is secondary to losses of protein, high levels of fibrinogen and factor VIII, and a reduced half-life for fibrinogen.

DIALYSATE LEAKS

The incidence of dialysate leakage varies from as few as 5% to as high as 25% of patients [473]. The risk of leakage is greater in patients who have had previous abdominal surgery, including previous catheter insertions [60,533, 535,734], in debilitated patients with lax abdominal walls, in those receiving corticosteroids, and in obese patients. If early leakage at the catheter exit site occurs during the initial cycle performed in the operating room, the problem should be surgically corrected. Problems caused by early leakage predispose patients to infection because of persistent moisture at the exit site and in the subcutaneous tunnel; subcutaneous collections of dialysate result in delays in patient training. Leakage does not usually require catheter removal since it will cease and the wound will heal if smaller volumes of dialysate are used. Sometimes it is necessary to stop dialysis for a few days to allow an adequate tissue seal to form around the cuff [600]. Late leakage as a result of peritoneal tears leads to fluid dissecting into the abdominal wall. The leak may spread into the scrotum, vagina, thighs, or up to the chest wall. These leaks cause discomfort and necessitate discontinuation of dialysis to allow the tear in the peritoneal tissue to heal. It is recommended that peritoneal tears be given 8 to 10 days to heal [420]. Such patients may benefit from hemodialysis for a few days through a short-term subclavian vascular access [810] when a long-term vascular access is unavailable. Although not very common, dialysate can enter the pleural cavity through a congenital defect in the diaphragm [73,208,250,366,700]. In cases of acute hydrothorax (reported incidence of 2%), peritoneal dialysis is usually discontinued and the patient switched to hemodialysis therapy [208]. Peritoneal dialysis can be successfully restarted in some patients. In some children, acute hydrothorax has been treated by thoracotomy and repair of the diaphragmatic eventration, followed by an immediate resumption of peritoneal dialysis [80a].

OUTFLOW OBSTRUCTION

A most important mechanical complication of peritoneal dialysis is the failure of dialysate to drain. This problem often requires removal of the catheter. A major cause of outflow obstruction is fibrin clots, which usually form as a result of bleeding soon after catheter implantation or during or after an episode of peritonitis. Large amounts of heparin (2500 to 5000 U) in a small volume of dialysis can be used to irrigate the catheter in an attempt to expel the fibrin or clot. Another approach is to add 5 U of heparin to each milliliter of dialysate, infuse the dialysate, and wait 4 to 12 hours to see whether dialysate begins to drain better. Subsequently, exchanges are done for a few days with 1 U of heparin added to each milliliter of dialysate. Mechanical manipulations may also be attempted [327], but passage of a Fogarty catheter is considered safer [52].

Combined inflow-outflow obstruction is usually due to twisted catheters and entanglement of the catheter in the omental tissue; it usually develops a few days after implantation. The patient may experience localized or diffuse abdominal discomfort. Fluoroscopy after dye injection can help define the nature of the problem [606]. Catheter replacement is necessary when attempts to reposition the catheter prove ineffective.

Catheter migration is a frequent cause of permanent drainage failure, leading to removal of the catheter in 90% of affected patients [473]. Constipation may be associated with inflow problems and catheter tip migration. Bowel evacuation results in the catheter returning to its original position. Some suggest using less mobile catheters such as the Toronto Western Hospital catheter for these problems [288,604,642]. In recurrent cases of catheter migration, the tip of the catheter can be sutured with nonreabsorbable material to the pelvic peritoneum [734]. Intra-abdominal catastrophes (e.g., ruptured viscus) may cause catheter malfunction.

CUFF PROBLEMS

Catheter cuff erosion and prolapse are usually late complications and are due to pressure necrosis of the skin by the distal cuff at the catheter exit site. These complications are best prevented by making the subcutaneous catheter tunnel appropriately long or, as recommended by some, by using a single-cuff Tenckhoff catheter. Cuff erosion is usu-

ally an indolent process unless accompanied by an exit site infection or subcutaneous tunnel abscess. If the extrusion of the cuff is incomplete, surgical exposure is necessary. The cuff may be "shaved," or a cuff splicing technique may be performed using a ridged connector [566,685]. Catheter replacement is often required [793].

EXIT SITE AND TUNNEL INFECTIONS

Appropriate care of the exit site is essential to minimize the risk of developing infection. It involves the daily cleansing of the exit site using an aseptic technique. The exit site is cleansed with water and an antibacterial soap. If crusting is present, the crusts are loosened with applicators impregnated with hydrogen peroxide. The site is then dried. Subsequently, beginning at the catheter, povidone-iodine is painted around the exit site and allowed to dry. If redness, crusting, or draining is visible, povidone-iodine ointment is put onto a sterile applicator and worked around the site, which is left open or covered by sterile gauze taped in place.

Care of the exit site remains controversial. Available data in children suggest that covering the exit site in children may prevent infection [849], although in adults no differences in infection of the exit site were found with or without a dressing. The application of soap or povidone-iodine to the exit site in children gave equivalent results [841], in comparison to a prospective trial in adults, in which cleansing with soap and water gave better results than the use of a combination of water and povidone-iodine or hydrogen peroxide and povidone-iodine. Lotions, powders and ointments should not be applied to exit sites. If clothing irritates the exit site or the adaptor irritates the skin, a loose gauze pad should be placed over the exit site and the adaptor should be wrapped in gauze. Showering is the preferred method of personal hygiene and should be done prior to performing daily catheter care. The bag tube connection or adapter should be kept dry when showering or bathing.

Exit site infections present initially as continued moisture at the exit site followed by a colorless or cloudy discharge. Subsequently, bleeding, malodorous discharge, pain, and tenderness develop. A yellowish serum with associated crusting at the exit site is not itself indicative of an infectious process. External cuff infections are usually associated with the discharge of pus. When the cuff is palpated, tenderness is elicited. Ultrasound examination of the catheter tunnel and exit site may be helpful in determining the extent of an infectious process and may help in deciding whether a catheter needs to be removed [364a].

Four types of catheter infection occur: localized skin inflammation, cellulitis of tissues surrounding the exit site and tunnel, catheter cuff infection, and tunnel infection [158]. Exit site infections are potentially serious because they lead to tunnel infection and peritonitis. Stratified squamous epithelium grows inward along the periluminal surface of the catheter to the cuff, which, after becoming embedded with collagen fibers, retards further epithelialization and forms a sinus tract. If the barrier is disrupted by mechanical trauma or excessive trauma on the cuff, or if poor drainage exists, bacteria can migrate periluminally

and cause cuff, tunnel, and peritoneal infections. External contamination is the other major cause of exit site infection. Families and patients should be trained to inspect the exit site carefully for redness, sloughing of the skin, discharge, or tenderness and to notify the appropriate member of the health care team immediately.

When infection is suspected, cultures are taken, aggressive local treatment with povidone-iodine is begun, and systemic antibiotics are given for 10 to 15 days. Noteworthy, however, is the observation that the bactericidal activity of povidone-iodine is inhibited by pus, blood, and glove powder [873]. Exit site infection is most commonly due to *Staphylococcus aureus* or *Staphylococcus epidermidis* and occurs in 15% to 60% of patients [52,538,604,793]. The wide variation in the incidence of infection clearly relates to the care exercised in maintaining aseptic technique when manipulating the catheter. Exposure of the exit site to contaminated water, e.g., bathing and swimming in highly contaminated lakes and rivers, can lead to peritonitis [824]. Swimming can be allowed if the exit site is healthy. Care of the exit site should be given immediately after swimming, which is best done in chlorinated pools. Ocean and clean fresh lake swimming may be allowed.

Nasal carriage of S. aureus has been shown to increase the rate of peritoneal catheter related infections [493a]. Rifampin prophylaxis [pediatric dosage 10–20 mg/kg/day) for five days every three months reduces the rate of catheter related infections and possibly peritonitis rates [876a]. Parents should be advised that the peritoneal fluid and urine will become orange in color. The nasal carriage of S. aureus may or may not be eradicated.

Tunnel infection presents as swelling, pain, and fever. These infections, which can occur in the absence of an exit site infection, may also extend deeply into the abdominal wall, causing a cellulitis. They may give rise to persisting or recurrent peritonitis by intraperitoneal seeding with bacteria. Tunnel infections are difficult to cure; in addition to antibiotic treatment and surgical drainage, removal of an otherwise functioning catheter is almost always necessary. An unroofing technique has been successfully used in a few adolescents. The distal cuff is removed if present, and the catheter bed is surgically drained, irrigated, and packed with a gauze impregnated with povidone-iodine for 24 hours. A new exit site and tunnel can then be created [23,566]. The infection should be controlled before implanting a new permanent catheter. During this time, the patient may need to be maintained on hemodialysis. The use of the Y-set is associated with reduced numbers of catheter infections [628a].

PERITONITIS

Peritonitis remains the predominant medical problem of long-term peritoneal dialysis [91,246,773]. The routes of peritoneal contamination are through the lumen of the peritoneal catheter, through the sinus tract around the catheter, across the wall of an intraperitoneal hollow viscus, from the blood stream or peritoneal lymphatics, and from the female genital tract. Contamination of the peritoneal cavity occurs primarily through the catheter as a result of a break in sterile technique during connection and disconnection of the dialysate delivery circuit. The diagnosis of peritonitis is difficult in patients treated with peritoneal dialysis because the usual symptoms and signs of acute peritoneal inflammation are often masked by peritoneal irrigation. Patients with pancreatitis and other forms of intra-abdominal pathology will have an elevated peritoneal fluid amylase level [119a]. Serum amylase levels may or may not be elevated. The differential diagnosis of peritonitis includes many intra-abdominal processes [773a]. Evidence of peritonitis includes abdominal pain, fever, nausea, vomiting, cloudy dialysate drainage, a WBC count in dialysate effluent of more than 100 cells/ml with a neutrophil count exceeding 50% of the total, and a positive culture of peritoneal fluid [228]. Some believe that the finding of more than 50% neutrophils is a more sensitive indicator of peritonitis than the absolute WBC count [254]. Noninfected dialysate contains 3 to 25 WBC/ml [698]. Because Coulter-counters do not detect all of the white cells in dialysate, peritoneal cell counts are best done using a hemocytometer.

Microbiologic examination of the peritoneal fluid is essential to diagnose and manage peritonitis. Although peritoneal WBC counts with differential evaluation and Gram staining provide supportive evidence for diagnosing peritonitis, peritoneal fluid cultures are the keystone of the diagnostic process. Methodology for culturing peritoneal fluid varies and ranges from direct culturing of peritoneal fluid to the use of complex concentrating techniques [825]. Infection is caused by Gram positive cocci (S. epidermidis, S. aureus, Streptococcus viridans) in 60% to 70% of cases. Although in adults the ratio of S. epidermidis to S. aureus approximates 2:1 to 3:1, S. aureus isolates in children are equal [657] or higher [780]. This difference may be due to a higher incidence of exit site infections in children [780]. S. aureus is more commonly associated with catheter related infections. Gram-negative bacteria (Enterobacter, Pseudomonas sp., Acetobacter sp.) account for 15% to 40% of infections [52,538,825,840]. Fungal peritonitis occurs primarily in patients who have been treated repeatedly with antibiotics; Candida species account for 1% to 4% of infections. Anaerobic peritonitis is rare, and its occurrence should be considered a sign of bowel leakage [825].

Most series of peritonitis in children are small in number. When eight series totaling 646 episodes of peritonitis in children were reviewed, 44% of cases were due to gram-positive organisms, 21% had gram-negative organisms, 2% had fungal peritonitis, 25% had no growth, and 8% had a variety of uncommon organisms [146]. Tuberculous peritonitis presents as a sterile peritonitis that does not respond to treatment. Peritoneal biopsy is required for its early diagnosis since stains for acid-fast bacilli are often negative [5a]. A list of the organisms associated with peritonitis is provided in Table 39-13. A number of cases of non-tubercular mycobacterial peritonitis have occurred in patients on various forms of chronic peritoneal dialysis [205a]. Treatment with intraperitoneal deferoxamine has been reported to be associated with the development of mucormycosis septicemia and peritonitis [552a].

Sterile peritonitis may represent the failure to identify an infecting organism and should be considered only after

TABLE 39-13. Organisms causing peritonitis

Bacterial	
Acinetobacter sp.	Listeria monocytogenes
Actinomyces israelii	Micrococcus sp.
Bacteroides sp.	Neisseria sp.
Bordetella bronchiseptica	Nocardia asteroides
Campylobacter jejuni	Pasteurella multocida
Citrobacter sp.	Propionibacterium sp.
Clostridium sp.	Proteus sp.
Corynebacterium sp.	Pseudomonas aeruginosa
Enterobacter sp.	Pseudomonas sp.
Enterococci	Serratia sp.
Escherichia coli	Staphylococcus aureus
Flavobacterium sp.	Staphylococcus epidermidis
Fusobacterium sp.	Streptococcal sp.
Haemophilus influenzae	Vibrio alginolyticus
Klebsiella sp.	

Fungal	Mycobacterial
Aspergillus sp.	Mycobacterium avium, intracellularae
Candida albicans	
Candida parapsilosis	Mycobacterium chelonei
Cephalosporium acremonium	Mycobacterium chelonei-like
	Mycobacterium fortuitum
Coccidiodes immitis [18]	Mycobacterium tuberculosis
Dreschlera spicifera	
Exophialia jeanselmei	
Fusarium sp.	
Mucor sp.	
Penicillium sp.	
Rhodotorula rubra	
Trichoderma viride	
Trichosporon sp.	

Modified from Everett ED: Diagnosis, prevention and treatment of peritonitis. Perit Dial Bull 4:S139, 1984.

carefully excluding a microbiologic etiology. The etiology of this condition remains obscure, although irritation of the peritoneum by the high osmolality and the low pH of dialysis solutions has been suggested as a possible cause [538,722]. Criteria for diagnosing sterile eosinophilic peritonitis include cloudy fluid, an increased peritoneal WBC count with more than 10% eosinophils, and the absence of identifiable organisms. Some patients develop a peripheral eosinophilia. In a prospective study of 23 patients on CAPD followed for a mean duration of 7.9 months, peritoneal eosinophilia developed in 14 [137]. Thirteen of these patients had peripheral blood eosinophilia and had higher initial levels of IgE prior to and during dialysis.

Etiologic significance has been attributed to the effect of the instilled dialysate on the peritoneal inflammatory response and the possibility that peritoneal lymphocytes release an eosinophilic stimulating factor. The injection of 100 to 500 ml of sterile air intraperitoneally in five patients resulted in all developing a peritoneal cell count that ranged from 23 to 335 cells/mm^3 [173]. In a few patients, monocytes and eosinophils predominated. The pleocytosis lasted from 4 to 49 days. Most cases of eosinophilic peritonitis occur soon after inserting peritoneal catheters. Late onset eosinophilic peritonitis may result from fungal infection or as a reaction to intraperitoneal drugs [369]. The usual course of this condition is benign; antibiotics are not indicated [285,376,538]. In one series involving 61 patients, the mean percentage of peritoneal eosinophils after catheter insertion fell from 18% at 2 months to 3% at 6 months [629]. Children have been reported to develop eosinophilic peritonitis [657].

The incidence of peritonitis in children undergoing IPD, CAPD, or CCPD is one case per 3.3 to 46 patient-months [15,52,54,146,168a,538,654,840] (Fig. 39-13). A relatively small group of patients (30%) accounts for the majority of the episodes of peritonitis (65%) [657,848]. Over a ten-year period, 67% of children in a single center developed peritonitis [558a]. Home treatment was successful in 72% of the cases. Reasons for such a high rate of peritonitis among these patients include poor socioeconomic background [772], need for more frequent exchanges because of the loss of ultrafiltration, an open urogenital sinus [840], lack of motivation, severe depression after loss of allograft, poor manual dexterity due to crippling bone deformities, and overlooked episodes of tunnel infection. Aggressive nutritional regimens may lower peritonitis rates [168a]. Others have suggested that hypogammaglobulinemia [410a], chemicals contained in dialysate [681], and host factors including alterations in chemotaxis, opsonization, phagocytosis, and intracellular destruction may explain frequent episodes of peritonitis. The phagocytic and bactericidal activity of macrophages in unaffected dialysate is similar to that of circulating polymorphonuclear cells [827]. A 10-fold increase in the peritonitis rate has been attributed to differences in the opsonic activity of dialysis fluid in different patients [412]. Children with nephrostomies experience a high rate of peritonitis, and the etiology

is often gram-negative. Peritonitis in such children tends to occur shortly after transfer set changes [840].

Advances in catheter and equipment design have led to reductions in the frequency of peritoneal infections. One such modification of the peritoneal dialysate delivery system for all forms of peritoneal dialysis involves in-line bacterial filters. A Millipore filter is attached at the spike-bag junction, and as fluid flows through the filter, bacterial contaminants are filtered out and retained. Clinical trials using this filter demonstrate reduced episodes of peritonitis [34,718,762,763]. The incidence in an unselected adult population on CAPD was halved. Its use can be recommended in patients with recurrent episodes of peritonitis in the absence of predisposing factors. The use of the Y-set has been shown to be associated with a reduced rate of peritonitis [146a].

A germicidal system based on ultraviolet radiation is available (Travenol Laboratories, Inc., Deerfield, Illinois) to reduce the touch and airborne contamination that occur from spike contamination. The system consists of an enclosed box protecting the junction where the spike is inserted into a new peritoneal dialysis bag. The germicidal chamber is fully automatic, is readily transportable, compensates electronically for variations in environmental conditions, and can be operated using ordinary electrical current or a rechargeable battery [212,367,388,646]. The system is reported to be 75% to 100% effective in eliminating microorganisms introduced by touch. The system more effectively removes organisms from the external than the lumenal surface of the spike. It should be used as adjunct therapy without any reduction in aseptic efforts. A knife splicing technique that is fully automatic and eliminates any finger contact has been developed by the DuPont Corporation (Wilmington, DE). Both devices have been shown to decrease peritonitis rates [865a]. Fi-

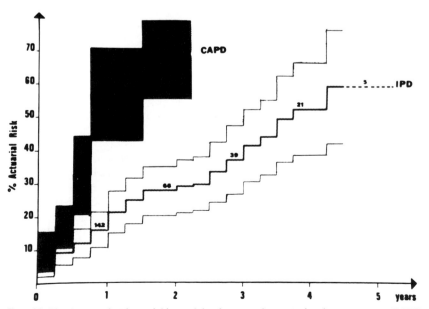

FIG. 39-13. *Actuarial risk in children of developing a first episode of peritonitis on CAPD or IPD.*

nally, the use of a non-disconnect Y-set has been shown to reduce peritonitis rates, compared to the disconnect Y-set.

Treatment

The treatment of peritonitis includes eradicating the peritoneal infection, preserving the integrity of the peritoneal membrane, and sustaining the child's general condition during the acute phase of the disease. Early recognition of infection and prompt initiation of therapy increase the ease of bacterial cure and the continued availability of a functional peritoneal membrane. The accepted therapeutic regimen consists of peritoneal lavage and antibiotic administration [389,600,793,825]. A number of antibiotic regimens can be used. The combination of cephalothin and tobramycin has a broad antibacterial spectrum, which is effective against most bacteria. However, the ultimate choice of antibiotic(s) is modified according to the in vitro sensitivity of the isolated organism. Data concerning appropriate concentrations of antibiotics in dialysis solutions for initial loading and sustaining exchanges are summarized in Table 39-14. Most antibiotics, with the exception of penicillin G, retain at least 75% of their bioactivity in routinely used dialysate solutions [737]. Of interest is the fact that the bioactivity of some antibiotics drops significantly in 30% to 50% glucose dialysate [879].

CAPD

1. Perform three rapid in and out exchanges with 1.5% dialysis solution without antibiotics or heparin.
2. Add cephalothin, 10 to 15 mg/kg; tobramycin, 1.7 mg/

TABLE 39-14. *Recommended loading and maintenance dosages for treating peritonitis complicating dialysis. When possible blood drug levels should be monitored.*

Drug	Loading dose intravenously or intraperitoneal mg/kg	Maintenance dose dialysate concentration mg/L
Amikacin	7.5	25
Amphotericin	unavailable	5
Ampicillin	50	125
Carbenicillin	unavailable	200
Cefazolin	20	125
Cefotaxime	20	250
Cefuroxime	20	125
Ceftazidime	20	125
Cephalothin	20	250
Clindamycin	unavailable	1–2
Cloxacillin	50	125
5-Fluorocytosine	unavailable	50
Gentamicin	1.7	4–8
Miconazole	unavailable	20
Netilmicin	2.5	4–8
Penicillin G	unavailable	50,000 units
Septra (SMZ, TMP)	unavailable	25, 5
Ticarcillin	50	250
Tobramycin	1.7	4–8
Vancomycin	20	15–25

Adapted from Blint AJ: Diagnosis and management of peritonitis in continuous ambulatory peritoneal dialysis. Report of a working party of the British Society for antimicrobial chemotherapy. *Lancet* 1:845, 1987.

kg; and heparin, 500–1000 U/liter to the dialysate as a loading dose and perform an exchange with a dwell time of 4 hours.
3. Add cephalothin, 250 mg/liter; tobramycin, 4–8 mg/liter; and 500–1000 U/liter heparin to the dialysate as a maintenance dose and proceed with exchanges every 4 hours for the next 24 hours.
4. Resume the usual dialysis schedule, continuing with the above-noted intraperitoneal antibiotic therapy until the results of culture and sensitivities are known. Select the most appropriate antibiotic to complete a 10- to 14-day course of treatment. If no organism is identified, continue cephalothin for 14 days and tobramycin for 7 days.
5. Assuming an appropriate clinical response, repeat the peritoneal cell count and culture of the peritoneal fluid 2 days after stopping antibiotics.

Treatment with five rapid exchanges of cephalothin, 250 mg/liter, and heparin, 250 U/liter, followed by resumption of the usual CAPD or CCPD regimen with added cephalothin for 10 to 14 days is also known to be effective therapy for peritonitis in most children [840].

CCPD

1. Perform three rapid in and out exchanges with 1.5% dialysis solution without antibiotics or heparin.
2. Add cephalothin, 10 to 15 mg/kg; tobramycin, 1.7 mg/kg; and heparin, 500–1000 U/liter to the dialysate as a loading dose and perform an exchange with a dwell time of 4 hours.
3. After completing the 4-hour dwell, IPD is started with the dialysate containing 4–8 mg/liter of tobramycin and cephalothin 250 mg/liter for 48–72 hours. IPD is discontinued when the peritoneal fluid WBC count falls to less than 100 cells per ml and the percentage of neutrophils falls to less than 50%.
4. CCPD is resumed, with antibiotics added, for 10–14 days. The peritoneal cavity should have a daytime dwell of at least 20–50% of the volume used at night if the patient is on nocturnal peritoneal dialysis.

IPD

1. Start IPD for 48 hours after adding cephalothin, 250 mg/liter; tobramycin, 5 mg/liter; and heparin, 1000 U/liter to the dialysis solution.
2. After 48 hours of continuous peritoneal dialysis, change to nightly dialysis for 3 days, then resume the usual schedule.
3. Patients remain on the same intraperitoneal antibiotic therapy until the results of culture and sensitivities are known, after which the most appropriate antibiotic is given to complete a 10- to 14-day course of treatment.
4. If the usual dialysis schedule is every other day, tobramycin is prescribed every 48 hours, and oral cephalexin, 25 to 50 mg/kg/day (four divided doses), is given until the completion of the treatment course.

Alternative therapeutic schemes not yet formally evaluated in pediatric populations exist. Recommended approaches include a single dose of vancomycin intravenously weekly for 4 weeks [456] or the intraperitoneal instillation of trimethoprim, 40 μg/ml, and sulfamethoxazole, 200 μg/ml [283]. Symptoms should diminish within the first 12 to 24 hours of treatment and usually disappear within 48 hours. The patients should be hospitalized if the clinical condition worsens during the early phases of therapy. Over 90% of the episodes of peritonitis are home acquired, and two-thirds of the episodes can be successfully treated on an outpatient basis [55]. Supportive treatment is helpful in ensuring the ultimate success of peritonitis therapy. The oral intake of protein should be increased to compensate for the greater protein losses during peritonitis. Total parenteral nutrition may be required in anorectic patients to maintain a good nutritional state. Extracorporeal ultrafiltration can be used as an adjunct to peritoneal dialysis when control of extracellular volume becomes difficult. Examples would include a reduced peritoneal ability to ultrafilter and the intravenous infusion of liberal amounts of fluid during hyperalimentation to increase caloric intake. Sometimes hemodialysis is the only alternative for satisfactorily controlling uremia, electrolyte, and water balance. Catheter removal during the course of peritonitis should be considered when peritoneal fluid cultures remain positive for more than 4 to 5 days. In 439 episodes of peritonitis involving children on CAPD and CCPD, 55 episodes (13%) led to catheter being removed [146]. Removal is often indicated when the use of appropriate antibiotics fails, in the presence of a tunnel abscess or perforated intra-abdominal viscous, and in cases of tuberculous or fungal peritonitis [825]. An eightfold increased risk for initial nonfunction (40% versus 5%) exists when peritoneal catheters are placed in patients who have had previous peritoneal infection or major intra-abdominal surgery [474].

Most patients with fungal peritonitis will have to have their catheters removed to achieve a cure. However, successful management with systemic and intraperitoneal antifungal agents occurs [505]. In any event, treatment of fungal peritonitis with intraperitoneal antifungal agents and irrigation until the dialysate is free of particulate matter may help avoid the subsequent development of peritoneal adhesions [229]. Examination of catheters from patients with fungal peritonitis shows that they are usually heavily colonized with fungi and contain amorphous material with imbedded fungi [510]. The most widely used antibiotic is amphotericin B. Treatment with intravenous miconazole, fluconazole [178a], oral and intraperitoneal 5-flucytosine [210], and oral ketoconazole alone or in various combinations in adults produced varying rates of clinical cure. Most children reported to have fungal peritonitis have not responded to antifungal treatment [590]. Some children have responded to therapy and have been able to remain on peritoneal dialysis [7,219a].

The outcome and prognosis of peritonitis associated with peritoneal dialysis are favorable in the majority of affected children. A summary of six reports on peritonitis in children revealed that 55 of 439 (13%) episodes of peritonitis necessitated catheter removal, that 14 of 226 (6%) lost peritoneal membrane function, and that 1 of 299 (0.4%) resulted in death from peritonitis [146]. Few deaths have been directly attributable to this complication. As discussed elsewhere, there is evidence that peritonitis can reduce peritoneal clearances [322,695,793,794]. Peritonitis

can also be followed by an abdominal abscess, by a permanent or temporary loss of ultrafiltration [238], and by the development of sclerosing peritonitis.

EXCESSIVE DIALYSATE VOLUME

Raised intra-abdominal volume and pressure can cause a number of problems [59a]. An excessive volume of intraperitoneal fluid may cause abdominal pain or dyspnea. The effect of excessive volume initially occurs in the supine position. In adults, each liter increase in intraperitoneal volume increases intra-abdominal pressure by 2 to 3 cm of water and abdominal girth by 2.0 cm. Forced vital capacity is decreased in the supine and sitting positions when intraperitoneal volumes exceed 3.0 liters [808]. Arterial PO_2 falls by 3 to 26 mm Hg and returns to baseline when the abdomen is filled and drained with 2.0 liters of dialysate [304]. Basal atelectasis, bronchitis, pneumonia, and pleural effusions can occur as a consequence of too large an intraperitoneal volume, especially if used over a prolonged period of time [73]. Most cases of hydrothorax involve the right side. Seven of 64 children in one pediatric center developed hydrothorax; five were undergoing acute peritoneal dialysis [119]. Three were asymptomatic. The demonstration of a high glucose and low protein content in pleural fluid confirms its origin. Pleuroperitoneal connections can be demonstrated by isotopic techniques [768] or the injection of methylene blue into the peritoneal cavity. Treatment strategies include the use of smaller volumes of dialysate over shorter periods of time, performing dialysis in a more upright position, and the temporary or permanent discontinuation of peritoneal dialysis. Talc and tetracycline pleurodesis have been used to prevent recurring effusions [68,700].

Too large an intraperitoneal volume may lead to hernia formation. Children may develop unilateral or bilateral hydroceles due to dialysate accumulation; this may necessitate the ligation of a patent processus vaginalis. Abdominal hernias (inguinal, periumbilical, and incisional) become more prominent and symptomatic owing to the increased intra-abdominal pressure from the dialysis fluid and may require surgical correction. Children undergoing peritoneal dialysis may experience a higher incidence of hernias than adults. In adults on CAPD and CCPD, the incidence of hernias ranges from 2.5% to 26.7% [192,836]. Hernias occurred in 19 of 68 (28%) of children receiving CAPD or CCPD; 56% related to the catheter, 22% umbilical, and 22% inguinal [468]. When this series was extended to include 93 children, 37 (40%) developed 60 hernias [836]. An inverse correlation between age and hernia occurrence was found. The incidence was similar in children on either form of continuous dialysis. Fifty percent of hernias appear during the first 6 months of dialysis.

Some recommend that a peritoneogram be done at the time of catheter insertion to identify hernias that can be corrected at the same time [10,608,789]. Because of the mechanical problems in obtaining intraoperative peritoneograms, others prefer to evaluate patients only after a clinically apparent hernia develops. Treatment of the aforementioned 37 children included surgical repair in 75% of cases. It is recommended that a formal Cooper ligament repair be performed to avoid recurrence [421a]. The remaining patients were managed by reduction in dialysate volume, conversion from CAPD to CCPD, or discontinuation of the daytime dwell in patients on CCPD. One of three management approaches can be used during the postoperative period to control uremia. Dialysis can be discontinued and conservative management used, hemodialysis can be substituted, or low volume peritoneal dialysis can be continued.

Another cause of genital swelling related to peritoneal dialysis is skin edema secondary to the dissection of peritoneal fluid from breaks in the peritoneum [758]. CT scanning can be useful in determining the origin of genital swellings. Hemorrhoids may also develop in patients on peritoneal dialysis.

DURABILITY OF THE PERITONEAL MEMBRANE

Relatively little is known about factors influencing the durability of the peritoneal membrane [186,380]. Functional and anatomic changes have been described. Exposure to dialysate affects mesothelial cells. In addition to intercellular edema, there is loss of microvilli and varying degrees of degeneration and disruption of cytoplasmic structures [194]. Most prospective studies of peritoneal clearances involving large numbers of adult patients do not demonstrate a progressive loss of function over 6 to 72 months in significant numbers of patients [88,187,230, 697,766]. Persistence of the responsiveness of the peritoneal membrane to nitroprusside stimulation occurs in most patients [697]. Others have noted decreases in peritoneal clearances in a significant proportion of their patient population [249,673].

Limited data indicate that most children on long-term peritoneal dialysis preserve peritoneal clearances of lower molecular weight solutes [230,237]. In a group of eight children, weight scaled peritoneal clearances of inulin, but not urea, were lower after 6 months of long-term peritoneal dialysis [321,322]. Others have reported an increase in inulin clearance in children after 4 to 8 months on CAPD [97]. It has been suggested that intermittent peritoneal dialysis may be superior to continuous forms of dialysis in maintaining the ultrafiltration capacity of the peritoneal membrane [203]. Peritoneal kinetic studies consisting of peritoneal clearances, peritoneal dialysance, and the dialysate-to-plasma ratio in 47 children on CAPD/CCPD (18 had repeated studies performed over 55 months using the same dialysate inflow volume) are available [835]. Significant changes did not occur over time, and they were not permanently altered by episodes of peritonitis. However, in 18 children evaluated repetitively, creatinine clearance decreased in five and urea clearance increased in three. Such changes may suggest early membrane failure. In 11 children dialyzed in France with lactate containing dialysate, ultrafiltration rates fell in all after 1.5 to 25 months [562].

The development of severe secondary hyperparathyroidism after starting peritoneal dialysis is reported to decrease peritoneal clearances. An improvement in clearances follows correction of the hyperparathyroidism [188]. The development of peritoneal sclerosis, first described in 1979

[271], is a major factor leading over time to decreases in peritoneal solute clearances and ultrafiltration rates in some patients [453,579]. It occurs in children [203,563,564, 690]. Factors thought to contribute to its etiology are summarized in Table 39-15. The two most likely etiologies are peritoneal membrane exposure to acetate or chlorhexidine in alcohol [399]. Most cases occur in patients who have had multiple bouts of peritonitis. The peritoneum becomes covered by a thick, leathery white tissue, which eventually alters the intrinsic transport characteristics of the membrane. Affected patients experience weight loss, pain, fever, ascites, and occasionally intestinal obstruction and bowel perforation. Mortality rates have been high because of bowel related surgical problems, sepsis, and malnutrition. Diagnosis is best made by laparotomy and biopsy [194]; CT can be used to diagnose a thickened peritoneum [399]. No effective therapy is known, and peritoneal dialysis may need to be discontinued. Improvement in the function of the peritoneal membrane has been described when the early stage of membrane failure characterized by peritoneal membrane hyperpermeability was treated by not using the peritoneal membrane for a month and instilling heparin into the peritoneal cavity every 3–4 days [538a].

Ultrafiltration capacity of the peritoneal membrane may be lost together with or develop independently of solute movement. Contributing factors include peritonitis, peritoneal sclerosis, loss of surface area, hyperpermeability of the membrane, and rapid absorption of glucose. The loss of ultrafiltration may be transient or permanent. Many cases have had no explanation [419]. It has been shown that the rate of peritoneal lymphatic reabsorption may exceed transcapillary ultrafiltration and lead to a net negative ultrafiltration rate [495].

A peritoneal equilibration test can be used to evaluate the transperitoneal movement of solute and water [807]. Three patterns of ultrafiltration can be recognized: normal, alterations because of increased membrane permeability, and reduced permeability because of the loss of surface area. Measurements of the drained dialysate volume; dialysate concentrations of protein; and the dialysate-to-blood ratio of glucose, urea, and creatinine over a 4-hour period can differentiate the two types of abnormalities [419]. Ex-

TABLE 39-15. *Factors potentially contributing to peritoneal sclerosis*

Acetate
Acidity
Acids, lactic, glucuronic
Antihypertensive agents, propranolol [508]
Antibiotics
Antiseptics, chlorhexidine
Catheter irritation
Endotoxin
Dextrose
Formaldehyde
Peritonitis
Plasticyzers
Silica
Talc

cessive permeability loss of ultrafiltration is characterized by excessive protein losses, rapid drops in the dialysate-to-plasma ratio for glucose, a rise in intraperitoneal volume followed by a drop, and normal to increased dialysate-to-plasma ratios for urea and creatinine. Ultrafiltration loss because of loss of surface area is characterized by reduced losses of protein, a slow drop toward normal values for the dialysate-to-plasma ratio of glucose, failure of the intra-peritoneal volume to increase significantly over time, and failure of the dialysate-to-plasma ratio for urea and creatinine to rise to normal over time. A dialysate-to-plasma ratio for creatinine after a 4-hour dwell of less than 0.45 suggests that an inadequate exchange of solute has occurred. Because dialysate to blood ratios for various solutes are different in young children than those in adults, it has been recommended that different ratios be used when performing peritoneal equilibration tests in children [214a].

ASCITES

Recurrent problems with ascites may develop after discontinuing peritoneal dialysis. Etiologic significance has been attributed to hypertonic and acidic dialysis. Repetitive paracentesis may be required. Spontaneous resolution occurs in some but not in others.

METABOLIC COMPLICATIONS

Oxalate stones have been described in adults on CAPD with residual renal function. Stone formation is thought to be due to higher serum oxalate levels in patients on peritoneal dialysis compared with those on hemodialysis [598].

Complications of Dialysis Related to the Uremic State

Long-term dialysis leads to multiple problems as a result of the impact of the dialysis procedure and the natural history of prolonging the uremic milieu. With prolonged survival on dialysis, many of the problems seen in advanced renal failure continue to progress. This section addresses dialysis related long-term complications affecting children undergoing all forms of long-term dialysis and emphasizes findings attributable to different dialysis modalities.

Growth Retardation

No issue so uniquely distinguishes the problem of ESRD in children as that of growth [260] (see Chap. 25). More than one-third of children beginning dialysis are growth retarded [724,725]. No form of long-term dialysis routinely restores normal rates of growth. Children with congenital anomalies or tubulopathies are particularly prone to growth retardation [111]; this effect is most pronounced during the first year of life [436]. The degree of growth retardation reflects not only the age of onset of renal failure but, as importantly, its duration [77,527]. Children need to be on dialysis for at least 6 and preferably 12 months prior to drawing conclusions about the effect of dialysis on their

growth [650]. An outline of the variables useful in assessing growth in children undergoing long-term dialysis is provided in [711] Table 39-16. Most long-term data on the subject of growth in dialyzed children is from the collaborating members of the EDTA Registry. Growth is best monitored by simultaneously evaluating statural height and bone age [302,790].

In prepubertal children, the hemodialysis prescription in terms of type of dialyzer, dialyzer efficiency, hours per session as well as the degree of residual renal function [435] does not seem to influence growth, with the exception of two versus three hemodialysis sessions per week [140]. Growth velocity in more than two-thirds of children undergoing maintenance hemodialysis is below the third percentile for both chronologic [435] and bone age [199]. In 17 children starting hemodialysis between the ages of 9 and 17 years and remaining on hemodialysis for longer than 1 year, the mean linear growth was 2.0 cm/year, which corresponded to a change in the standard deviation score of 0.36 [803].

During puberty, height gain averages 3 cm/year, with boys experiencing less growth than girls [201]. Growth often continues into the early twenties; however, catch-up

TABLE 39-16. *Monitoring of growth in children undergoing long-term dialysis*

Item	Frequency
Serum chemistries	
Urea	Monthly, appearance rate
Creatinine	Monthly, appearance rate
Total protein and albumin:	
hemodialysis	Every 3 months
peritoneal dialysis	Bimonthly
Immunoglobulins	Twice yearly
Transferrin	Twice yearly
Complement, C3, C4	Twice yearly
Dietary intake	
Diet records	Monthly, bimonthly
Anthropometry	
Height	Monthly
Weight	Monthly
Mid-arm thickness	Bimonthly
Skinfold thickness	Bimonthly
Head circumference	
< 2.5 yrs	Monthly
> 2.5 yrs	Twice yearly
Body proportions	
rump-feet, rump-crown	
< 2.5 yrs	Monthly
> 2.5 yrs	Twice yearly
Bone age	
left wrist, knees	Yearly
Sexual maturity	
Tanner staging	Twice yearly
Testicular size	Twice yearly

Modified from Salusky IB, Fine RN: Nutritional recommendations for children undergoing continuous peritoneal dialysis. *Perspect Perit Dial* 2:18, 1984.

growth rarely occurs. While on dialysis, the increase in bone age is delayed 0.5 to 0.6 standard deviation units per chronologic year [199,435]. Prepubertal children on hemodialysis for 3 years grew an average of 2.8 cm/year. In another study, equal percentages of prepubertal children on long-term hemodialysis, when compared with normal, grew normally, experienced moderate growth retardation, or suffered severe growth retardation [435]. Some centers report a progressive fall in growth velocity in children after 3 to 5 years on hemodialysis [140]; others do not [435]. The limited growth data on children less than 3 years of age who undergo long-term hemodialysis indicate that these children experience severe growth retardation [435].

Long-term peritoneal dialysis is also associated with growth retardation. In three series of children receiving intermittent peritoneal dialysis, linear growth averaged 0.31 cm/month respectively [52,164,654]. Another center reported that growth rates in their children averaged 37% of expected rates [107].

Although an improved internal milieu probably exists in children on CAPD, and a potential for an improved nutritional setting is present, growth is not as good as that originally anticipated. Some believe that growth in children on CAPD [47] exceeds that observed in hemodialyzed children; others do not agree [708]. In infants, statural growth has ranged from 42% to 108% [9,77,155,443]. Catch-up growth has been observed infrequently. In an analysis of 46 children from three centers, the growth velocity index (the ratio as a percentage of the observed to expected height increment) was greater than 100% in 10%, greater than 80% in 23%, between 50% and 80% in 11%, and less than 50% in 2% [50]. In a Paris study involving eight children ages 3 to 13 on CAPD, the growth data were similar [325]. Growth rates in children less than 1 year of age started on CAPD [448] or CCPD [713] usually decrease with time.

Growth potential in children on dialysis is influenced by a number of factors. Improved growth rates in patients on CAPD have been positively correlated with energy intakes greater than 80% of the recommended daily allowance (RDA), adequate protein intake, control of acidosis, and suppression of hyperparathyroidism [444,445,448]. An intake of protein and calories of less than 80% of the RDA is known to be associated with poor growth in children with ESRD [324,757]. Nasogastric tube feeding [155,324] and the addition of amino acids [602] to dialysate have been used to improve the nutritional intake of children on CAPD, but the potential of this approach to influence growth positively over time remains to be established. A significant fraction of infants (16 of 22 patients) with chronic renal insufficiency have gastroesophageal reflux as demonstrated by 24-hour esophageal pH monitoring [700a]. Although acidosis [156], anemia [410], and uremia [651] are believed to influence growth negatively in children, these factors are not different in children on CAPD who do or do not grow satisfactorily [50]. An important determinant of growth is the presence of renal osteodystrophy [372] and the degree to which it can be controlled [443].

Recombinant human growth hormone may increase growth velocity in children undergoing chronic dialysis [239a]. A doubling of height velocity from 4.4 to 8.0 cm/

year has been observed in some children without any acceleration in bone age. An increased growth velocity has been observed for up to three years in children with progressive renal insufficiency not requiring dialysis. It can be given intraperitoneally. The most appropriate dosage as well as its long term effect in this patient population remains unclear.

Renal Osteodystrophy

Disorders of mineral metabolism in children undergoing maintenance dialysis continue to be an important complication of long-term dialysis despite improved management in the past few years (see Chap. 28). The incidence of renal osteodystrophy in children is significantly greater than that reported in adults [251,655]. Its etiology is multifactorial and is related to changes in calcium and phosphorus during and between dialyses, alterations in vitamin D, and changes in parathormone regulation. Other factors impacting on the development of renal osteodystrophy are the prolongation of the uremic state, food intake, and aluminum exposure.

In children, the degree of crippling bone disease increases with the duration of long-term dialysis [140]. Of interest is the observation that the frequency of slipped epiphysis diminishes in children after starting dialysis; this may be due to an improved state of divalent ion metabolism [526,528].

To be considered are four forms of renal osteodystrophy found in children receiving maintenance dialysis: osteitis fibrosa cystica or hyperparathyroid bone disease, osteomalacia or rickets, osteopenia [617], and aluminum related osteomalacia. Although most children tend to have more than one form of renal osteodystrophy, one type often predominates. Although the onset of renal osteodystrophy often predates the beginning of dialysis, dialysis may be associated with the onset, stabilization, improvement, or worsening of bone disease. Such changes reflect the degree of compliance with diet, drug therapy, and growth rate, as well as the natural history of the uremic process.

The most prevalent form of renal osteodystrophy seen in children with ESRD is a combination of osteitis and osteomalacia or rickets. Osteitis fibrosa cystica is characterized by elevated concentrations of iPTH and radiographically by subperiosteal erosions in the long bones and phalanges. Bone biopsy reveals increased numbers of osteoblasts and osteoclasts, endosteal fibrosis, and excessive woven osteoid. Osteomalacia or rickets is characterized radiographically by coarsening of trabecular bone and fraying of the radiolucent zone of growth plates in the long bones. Because similar changes in the growth zone occur in patients with hyperparathyroidism, osteomalacia cannot always be easily differentiated [526]. Histologically, rickets is characterized by an increase in cartilage and osteoid, loss of the usual longitudinal columns of cartilage cells, and defective mineralization of the zone of provisional calcification.

Treatment of the aforementioned forms of renal osteodystrophy involves optimizing nutrition, providing adequate amounts of calcium, maintaining serum phosphate levels within normal limits, suppressing parathyroid hormone release, providing a vitamin D analog, and correcting acidosis.

A major source of calcium loss can be the dialysis treatment itself. Calcium balance during both peritoneal dialysis and hemodialysis depends on the dialysate calcium concentration. When it exceeds 7.0 mg/dl, a positive calcium balance occurs during dialysis and serum concentrations of calcium rise. Conversely, when the dialysate calcium is less than 6.0 mg/dl, a negative balance occurs [619]. In children undergoing a single hemodialysis, immunoreactive PTH levels fall as serum calcium levels rise; PTH levels increase again within a few hours of completing hemodialysis as serum calcium levels again fall [320].

The postdialysis increase in total calcium levels is in part due to increases in serum concentrations of proteins secondary to dialysis related volume contraction and accounts for half of the increase in serum calcium levels [127]. The dialysate loss of phosphorus also causes hypercalcemia [127]. When blood phosphorus falls, blood concentrations of calcium increase secondary to the efflux of calcium from bone. Infusion of phosphorus during hemodialysis prevents hypercalcemia. These data suggest that a portion of the calcium added to blood during hemodialysis is derived from bone rather than the dialysate. Such changes during repetitive dialyses may contribute to the development of osteomalacia.

Control of hyperparathyroidism is improved by the use of a dialysate calcium concentration of 7.0 mg/dl and by maintaining serum phosphorus at age-appropriate levels. This can be accomplished by the judicious use of diet, oral calcium preparations to provide additional dietary calcium, and vitamin D analogs to improve absorption of dietary calcium. Aluminum-containing phosphate binders are best avoided because of the risk of developing aluminum toxicity. The long-term use of dialysate calcium concentrations greater than 7.0 mg/dl (not commercially available) has been shown to reduce iPTH levels, maintain metacarpal bone thickness [95], and improve osteitis fibrosa cystica [391]. It has been suggested that the long-term maintenance of serum calcium levels above 10.8 mg/dl in children undergoing maintenance dialysis is a level above which PTH release is suppressed [622,713]. The degree of secondary hyperparathyroidism may also be reduced by the loss of iPTH in the dialysate [181]. The iatrogenic maintenance of too low a serum phosphate can lead to hypophosphatemic rickets.

Phosphate binders have been historically used to help control hyperparathyroidism. They function by lowering serum phosphate levels and thereby elevate serum calcium levels. Although once thought not to be absorbed, aluminum, which is contained in most phosphate binders, has been implicated as a cause of bone and neurologic disease [636]. A safe dose for aluminum-containing binder has not been established. During the decade of the 1980s recommendations ranged from an initial dose of 40 to 50 mg/kg/day when needed with a maximum dose not to exceed 100 to 150 mg/kg/day. Serum aluminum levels should be monitored if possible, and serious consideration given to lowering or discontinuing aluminum-containing binders when serum levels exceed 100 pg/dl. Available data in children indicate that aluminum toxicity occurs when serum levels exceed this value [308]. Some recommend using magnesium-containing binders and monitoring serum magnesium levels. Calcium carbonate is being increasingly used as a phosphate binder [706].

Current recommendations are that calcium salts, calcium carbonate or acetate, should be used for the chronic management of hyperphosphatemia. Aluminum-containing phosphate binders should be reserved for the acute treatment of hyperphosphatemia and used only for short periods of time. Calcium carbonate therapy in children undergoing chronic peritoneal dialysis has been shown to improve the skeletal lesions of hyperparathyroidism; these lesions did not improve or worsened in children given aluminum-containing phosphate binders [707a]. Calcium carbonate in a dosage of 47–595 mg/kg per day in combination with low doses of vitamin D or $1,25(OH)_2D_3$ has been shown to increase serum levels of calcium and to control secondary hyperparathyroidism [398a]. Its use may result in hypercalcemia and diarrhea.

When the combination of medical management and dialysis fails to control secondary hyperparathyroidism, parathyroidectomy should be considered [251]. Indications for parathyroidectomy include severe bone pain, calciphylaxis, epiphyseal slipping, fractures, metastatic calcifications, symptomatic hypercalcemia, and pruritus unresponsive to treatment, in addition to elevated levels of iPTH, progressive bony erosions, and osteitis fibrosa cystica on bone biopsy [168]. Before undertaking parathyroidectomy, sufficient quantities of vitamin D metabolites and oral calcium to raise the serum concentration of calcium to 10.5 or 11.0 mg/dl should be tried because the "set point" for PTH suppression by serum calcium is increased in uremic children [707]. Remineralization in seven children on CAPD was associated with a serum C-terminal iPTH decline of more than 40% [262]. Current surgical recommendations include either a $3\frac{3}{4}$ resection of the four parathyroid glands or a total parathyroidectomy with autotransplantation of functioning glandular tissue into a forearm muscle [547,787]. Oral calcium preparations—or more likely intravenous infusions of calcium—may be needed to prevent symptomatic hypocalcemia in the perioperative period. When needed, intravenous calcium may be started at a rate of 4 mg/kg/hour and progressively increased until the serum calcium level is raised to a low normal value. Large amounts of calcium may be needed for a prolonged time because the infused calcium may be taken up by calcium-depleted "hungry" bones. Calcitriol, $1,25(OH)_2D_3$, in doses as high as 2 μg per day usually leads to involution of the parathyroid glands. It can be given orally, intravenously, or intraperitoneally [707b].

Treatment of osteomalacia requires various combinations of calcium and some form of vitamin D. Elemental calcium can be started at a dose of 20 mg/kg/day. It is usually not possible to provide the required amount of calcium in a child's diet while on hemodialysis because of the need to limit the intake of protein and dairy products. However, sufficient dietary calcium may be provided in the diets of children who are on frequent peritoneal dialysis. Some of the calcium compounds, such as calcium carbonate, calcium acetate, and calcium citrate, also provide base and can reduce the need for other agents to treat acidosis. The dose of calcium is increased at intervals until the serum calcium reaches normal levels or until parathormone production is reduced. Gut calcium absorption is increased when some form of vitamin D is given simultaneously [461,867]. The use of vitamin D analogs has been reported to improve growth [135,145], although others have not had a similar experience [118,503]. Both $25(OH)D_3$, which is 98% protein bound, and $1,25(OH)_2D_3$, which is 62% protein bound, are removed by peritoneal dialysis [262]. Approximately 1% of the daily oral intake of $1,25(OH)_2D_3$ is removed by CAPD. Improvement in muscle strength usually occurs after starting treatment with a vitamin D metabolite [350]. The most widely used vitamin D metabolite to treat renal osteodystrophy in children is $1,25(OH)_2D_3$ [707], but which agent(s) is most effective remains under investigation.

Dialysis osteopenia [526] is characterized by a disproportionate reduction in the bone calcium content expected for the degree of existing secondary hyperparathyroidism and osteomalacia. It is associated with an increased incidence of bone pain and fractures, has been observed in a few children, and does not respond to the current therapy for renal osteodystrophy. Its etiology remains unclear; a role for aluminum ingestion has been suggested.

The clinical and histologic features of aluminum osteomalacia osteodystrophy [636] have been observed in children with progressive renal insufficiency and, recently, in increasing numbers of children on dialysis. There is reason to suspect that it occurs in many dialyzed children, even though it has been documented by bone biopsy in relatively few children [705]. Aluminum bone disease in both adults and children is characterized by myopathy, bone pain, multiple fractures, normal serum levels of calcium, phosphorus, alkaline phosphatase, and iPTH and unresponsiveness to vitamin D analogs [308,610], which tend to produce hypercalcemia [13,22]. These clinical features were initially described in children in the absence of serum aluminum measurements or bone biopsies [56]. Serum aluminum levels are usually elevated in affected patients but do not necessarily correlate with the findings on bone biopsy. Bone histomorphometry reveals aluminum accumulation, usually osteomalacia, and occasionally osteitis fibrosa [22,610]. The aluminum is localized predominately at the junction of osteoid and mineralized bone. Double tetracycline labeling studies have shown that the bone-apposition rate is reduced when the biopsy contains high concentrations of aluminum [610]. Thus, affected children would be expected to experience reduced rates of growth. Body burdens of aluminum can be reduced in children on hemodialysis by administering intravenous deferoxamine (dose 8.3–14 mg/kg) at the end of dialysis and allowing it to circulate until the next dialysis [588a]. Deferoxamine can also be added to peritoneal dialysate [308].

Descriptions of histologic features of renal osteodystrophy in 44 children undergoing CAPD and CCPD while receiving oral calcitriol are available [704]. The distribution included normal histology in 16%, mild changes in 25%, osteitis fibrosa in 39%, osteomalacia in 9%, and aplastic lesions in 11%. Bone surface aluminum was found in 10 of 20 children given aluminum-containing binders and none of 24 treated with calcium carbonate. Plasma aluminum levels and bone aluminum content were highest in those with osteomalacia. Neither blood chemistries nor the response of plasma aluminum levels to intravenous deferoxamine were predictive of the type of bone histology found. Bone formation rates were inversely correlated with the bone aluminum content. Surface aluminum staining exceeding 30%, a major criterion for diagnosing aluminum bone disease, was found in six children and distributed as follows: two had normal histology; one had aplastic bone disease; and three had osteomalacia. In another study of seven children on long-term dialysis, a significant correlation between serum aluminum levels and bone aluminum content was found [688]. The intravenous deferoxamine challenge offered no diagnostic advantage. However, the value of the deferoxamine challenge test remains controversial.

In children, serum levels of aluminum correlate positively with the intake of aluminum and inversely with age [22,705]. Most children on dialysis have elevated levels. The sources of aluminum are variable and include [308] transfer of aluminum from dialysate, the ingestion of aluminum-containing phosphate binders, the consumption of infant formula containing aluminum, the administration of pharmacologic and intravenous preparations containing aluminum, and, perhaps, increased gut absorption related to hyperparathyroidism [517,637]. Until recently, treatment of aluminum osteomalacia osteodystrophy has been inadequate. Healing may occur after discontinuing aluminum binders, and some initial success has been reported with the use of deferoxamine to chelate aluminum [4]. Chelation therapy has been helpful in patients on hemodialysis [109] and peritoneal dialysis. In children, deferoxamine, in a dose of 40 mg/kg, either intravenously or intraperitoneally, chelates significant amounts of aluminum and, if used over time, lowers the body burden of aluminum [354]. Also, intramuscular deferoxamine is equally effective in chelating aluminum [541]. The relationship between aluminum and neurologic dysfunction is considered in the following section on neurologic complications.

Chronic long-term dialysis can be associated with increased oxalate retention and oxalate deposits in bones. Because blood levels of oxalate are increased in the presence of renal failure, the best way to diagnose Type I oxalosis is to measure glycolate levels, which will be increased 250-fold [507a]. Dental abnormalities are commonly seen in children on dialysis. Caries may be reduced but discoloration and enamel hypocalcification are often observed, particularly in children with congenital forms of ESRD. Etiologic significance has been attributed to fluoride accumulation [841a].

Neurologic Complications

A significant proportion of the chronic morbidity in children undergoing maintenance dialysis is due to neurologic complications [386,633] (see Chap. 30). The neurologic problems associated with dialysis treatments are considered in the section on acute complications of dialysis. To be considered here are peripheral and cranial neuropathies, the dialysis encephalopathy syndrome (DES), and acquired encephalopathies related to hypertension and drugs.

Peripheral neuropathy occurs primarily in hemodialysis populations and rarely develops in patients on long-term peritoneal dialysis [798]. It initially manifests itself as lower motor neuron or sensory neuron dysfunction affecting the lower extremities first. Symptoms include muscle cramps, restless legs [122], burning feet, and paresthesias. The restless leg syndrome, which may originate centrally rather than peripherally, may respond to treatment with clonazepam [93]. Paresthesias involving the toes, bottom of the feet, and fingers are often the major manifestations of peripheral neuropathy in children [243]. Objective findings include loss of vibratory sensation and the loss of the ankle jerk. More than 90% of affected patients can be identified if both signs are sought [501]. The incidence of clinically apparent peripheral neuropathy in adult populations ranges from 11% to 75% [569]. Peripheral neuropathy occurs less frequently in children, especially younger children, with most affected children being above 10 years of age.

Electrophysiologic studies of peripheral nerves by means of testing nerve conduction velocities (NCV) reveal asymptomatic defects in most children prior to the onset of dialysis [530]. Such defects involve the lower more often than the upper extremity. In a group of 31 children, no correlation was found between the motor NCV and serum creatinine levels [26]. Once dialysis is begun, the NCV in most children remains stable and generally neither improves nor worsens [26,136,530]. Once believed to be an indicator of the adequacy of dialysis, serial measurements of NCV are no longer used for this purpose. Serial determinations of vibratory perception, which has not been well studied in children, are believed to be a better measurement of changing nerve function than the NCV in adults [568,569,570]. Because successful transplantation is usually accompanied by a marked improvement in peripheral neuropathy [386,589], demonstrating that such defects are in part functional, they cannot be totally explained by reports of structural changes and demyelination in axons and myelin sheaths [206]. Also, such histopathologic changes can occur in the absence of clinical symptoms. The pathophysiology of peripheral neuropathy remains incompletely understood. Etiologic significance has been attributed to vitamin B_1 and B_6 [193] deficiency, increased parathormone activity [290], enzyme dysfunction, transketolase [523], and the presence of middle molecules such as myoinositol [85] and methylguanidine [45].

Cranial nerve dysfunction observed in dialyzed patients includes amaurosis, sensorineural hearing loss, and decreased taste acuity. High frequency sensorineural hearing loss is often present in adults beginning dialysis; except for the impact of ototoxic drugs such as loop diuretics and aminoglycosides, hearing loss is apparently not influenced by dialysis [351]. Also, hypogeusia, which may in part reflect zinc deficiency, does not improve with long-term dialysis [498].

One of the most severe complications seen in dialysis populations is the *dialysis encephalopathy syndrome* (DES). Its clinical features (Table 39-17), initially described in adults [14], were first reported in pediatric populations in 1977 in a group of children not yet on dialysis [53]. In addition to their neurologic dysfunction [255], all had early onset chronic renal failure due to congenital renal defects,

TABLE 39-17. *Clinical features of the dialysis encephalopathy syndrome*

Motor abnormalities	*Speech difficulties*
Myoclonus, muscle spasm	Dysphagia
Asterixis, tremors	Dyspraxia-partial loss of
Seizures; focal, grand mal	coordinated movements
	Stuttering
Dementia	*Electroencephalogram*
Altered mood, depression	Diffuse slowing
Diminished alertness	Bursts of slow and high
Lethargy, coma	voltage activity

advanced renal osteodystrophy, characteristic EEG changes, and had been ingesting large quantities of aluminum [633]. Subsequently, similar changes were reported in children on hemodialysis and peritoneal dialysis and after transplantation [639]. Most affected adults have been on hemodialysis.

Although controversy regarding the etiology of DES still exists, most believe it is related to a toxic effect of aluminum. Etiologic significance has also been attributed to altered cerebrospinal fluid dynamics, slow virus infection, and the accumulation of calcium or tin by the cerebral cortex [633]. The most important sources of aluminum are the ingestion of aluminum-containing phosphate binders and the water used to prepare dialysate [636,637]. DES has occurred both sporadically and epidemically, with a temporal relationship between the patients' aluminum burden and their exposure to aluminum. The exposure in the epidemic form usually comes from aluminum rich dialysate [27,637]. The transmembrane movement of aluminum depends on the existing transmembrane free aluminum gradient, pH gradient, and the quantity of aluminum bound to protein. Aluminum is amphoteric and therefore more soluble when the dialysate pH is less than 6.50 or more than 7.60. Raising the dialysate pH with bicarbonate may enable more aluminum to traverse either the peritoneum or the hemodialyzing membrane [266]. The usual pH of commercial peritoneal dialysate favors the transfer of aluminum across the peritoneal membrane. An aluminum dialysate concentration of less than 0.30 μmoles/liter has been suggested as being nontoxic [689]. Because aluminum is deposited in intracellular sites, serum levels do not correlate directly with clinical symptoms and fail to reflect accurately a slow but progressive increase in total body aluminum. Aluminum absorption may be increased when secondary hyperparathyroidism is present.

Initial attempts at treating the DES were not successful in reversing or even stabilizing the neurologic symptoms; some success has been noted in response to discontinuing the use of aluminum-containing binders [512] and in response to the chelation of aluminum by deferoxamine [31,631]. To limit the exposure to aluminum, nonaluminum-containing binders, such as calcium carbonate or magnesium hydroxide, have been recommended. Serum magnesium levels should be measured in patients given magnesium-containing compounds. Switching from hemodialysis to CAPD lowers serum aluminum levels [689]. However, patients begun on CAPD and given aluminum

the use of oxygen, morphine, phlebotomy, rotating tourniquets, and the acute lowering of blood pressure. The onset of arrhythmias or an infectious process may lead to heart failure. If treatment for the aforementioned problems fails, digitalization should be considered. An evaluation of myocardial function by echocardiography is helpful in making such a decision.

Digoxin is the most widely used cardiac glycoside to treat heart failure in children. In uremic patients, its absorption is reduced, tissue binding is reduced, plasma levels may change in an unexplained fashion, and its functioning half-life is increased from a norm of 42 up to 120 hours [247,856]. Therapeutic serum levels range between 0.5 and 2.0 ng/ml; the incidence of toxicity increases when levels exceed 3.0 ng/ml [195] or when hypercalcemia or hypokalemia is present. Digitalis toxicity may occur in dialyzed populations at lower serum levels because of its altered metabolism in uremia. The dose of digoxin does not require modification in patients on hemodialysis or CAPD because it is poorly dialyzed [3,613]. The lowering of serum levels of potassium through dialysis may precipitate digoxin toxicity [818]. When initially digitalizing patients on dialysis, it is recommended that one use the lower end of the suggested range of digoxin dose. Long-term maintenance doses of digoxin may need to be reduced by up to 86% of the maintenance dose because of its reduced renal elimination [276,817]. Data are not yet available on the use of either aminophylline or vasodilator drug therapy to treat heart failure in children with ESRD.

Hyperlipidemia has been reported to occur in one-third of patients receiving maintenance hemodialysis [116] and peritoneal dialysis [418]. Hypertriglyceridemia, hypercholesterolemia, increased low density and very low density lipoproteins, and decreased high density lipoproteins have been noted in children on dialysis [70,114,214,616,624, 665a]. The apolipoprotein patterns in children on hemodialysis when combined with changes in plasma triglycerides and cholesterol are similar to those observed in adults as constituting a risk for developing cardiovascular disease [591]. Low levels of serum carnitine or its dialytic removal may contribute to the hypertriglyceridemia [61,875,876]. Administering L-carnitine in a dose of 100 mg/kg per day to children on CAPD has not caused significant changes in their serum triglyceride levels [839a]. The low levels of carnitine have been related to relative malnutrition [549a]. Although it is widely believed that atherosclerosis is accelerated in patients on dialysis, some believe that the incidence of ischemic heart disease in such patients has a better correlation with the presence of predialysis cardiovascular risk factors [42]. An increased incidence of collagenization of the intima of coronary arteries without plaque formation has been noted in children [624]. Clofibrate has been used to treat hyperlipidemia in adults; data in children are lacking [286]. Also, in adults receiving maintenance dialysis, controlled exercise positively influenced lipid abnormalities [287].

Additional cardiovascular complications include *arrhythmias* and *bacterial endocarditis* [469] secondary to fistula and cannula infection. The former may occur secondary to hypoxia, hyperkalemia, hypokalemia, hypocalcemia, hypomagnesemia, acidosis, and alkalosis and when pericar-

dial, myocardial, or endocardial disease is present [151]. An evaluation of the heart rhythm is indicated in any dialysis patient who develops cardiac problems.

Hematologic Complications

ANEMIA

The anemia of chronic renal failure usually worsens after children start dialysis. Mechanisms include further decreases in erythropoietin production, uremic toxin suppression of hemoglobin or erythroid synthesis, shortened red cell survival, blood loss, hemolysis, disordered iron metabolism, and folate deficiency. A database consisting of a white count and differential, platelet count, red blood cell indices, hematocrit and hemoglobin, reticulocyte count, peripheral smear examination, and serum ferritin level are indicated when dialysis is begun.

The classic anemia of renal failure is normocytic, normochromic, and hypoproliferative, with an inappropriately low erythropoietin level (Chap. 29). In fact, most patients with renal insufficiency have absolute concentrations of serum erythropoietin that are normal or elevated [128,472]. Inhibitors of red cell precursors also play a role in the development of anemia associated with ESRD. Polyamines, specifically spermine [667], and perhaps PTH or one of its fragments [667] have been shown to inhibit erythropoiesis. Various androgen preparations can be used to stimulate renal and hepatic erythropoietin production. In a controlled trial of intramuscular and oral androgens, anephric patients failed to respond to either. In adults, intramuscular nandrolone decanoate (3 mg/kg/week) and testosterone enanthate (4 mg/kg/week) were effective in increasing the red cell mass [557]. Their use, however, was associated with a 25% drop-out rate because of unacceptable side effects. Even though such agents are generally contraindicated in pediatric populations because of their negative effect on growth due to their accelerating epiphyseal fusion, their use may be helpful in children whose growth is completed or in those whose religious beliefs contraindicate blood transfusions.

The availability of recombinant erythropoietin (rHuEPO), which virtually cures the uncomplicated anemia of chronic renal failure, has altered the approach to the chronic anemia of all dialysis patients [223,224]. A dose of 37.5 to 300 units/kg given intravenously three times a week after hemodialysis will increase and maintain the hematocrit at 35% to 40%. In patients with excessive iron stores, serum ferritin levels fall; iron deficiency may occur if iron stores are low prior to starting therapy. Cardiomegaly decreases and exercise tolerance increases. No significant toxicity has been noted, and antibodies to the preparation have not been observed. Problems that have developed with its use include the development or acceleration of hypertension, occasionally complicated by seizures; increased predialysis concentrations of creatinine, urea, and potassium; and increased clotting of dialyzers. Osteitis fibrosa, aluminum intoxication, and inflammation interfere with the action of recombinant erythropoietin. Children on hemodialysis treated thrice weekly with rHuEPO at a dose of 100–150 units/kg responded within 9–13 weeks by

Peripheral neuropathy occurs primarily in hemodialysis populations and rarely develops in patients on long-term peritoneal dialysis [798]. It initially manifests itself as lower motor neuron or sensory neuron dysfunction affecting the lower extremities first. Symptoms include muscle cramps, restless legs [122], burning feet, and paresthesias. The restless leg syndrome, which may originate centrally rather than peripherally, may respond to treatment with clonazepam [93]. Paresthesias involving the toes, bottom of the feet, and fingers are often the major manifestations of peripheral neuropathy in children [243]. Objective findings include loss of vibratory sensation and the loss of the ankle jerk. More than 90% of affected patients can be identified if both signs are sought [501]. The incidence of clinically apparent peripheral neuropathy in adult populations ranges from 11% to 75% [569]. Peripheral neuropathy occurs less frequently in children, especially younger children, with most affected children being above 10 years of age.

Electrophysiologic studies of peripheral nerves by means of testing nerve conduction velocities (NCV) reveal asymptomatic defects in most children prior to the onset of dialysis [530]. Such defects involve the lower more often than the upper extremity. In a group of 31 children, no correlation was found between the motor NCV and serum creatinine levels [26]. Once dialysis is begun, the NCV in most children remains stable and generally neither improves nor worsens [26,136,530]. Once believed to be an indicator of the adequacy of dialysis, serial measurements of NCV are no longer used for this purpose. Serial determinations of vibratory perception, which has not been well studied in children, are believed to be a better measurement of changing nerve function than the NCV in adults [568,569,570]. Because successful transplantation is usually accompanied by a marked improvement in peripheral neuropathy [386,589], demonstrating that such defects are in part functional, they cannot be totally explained by reports of structural changes and demyelination in axons and myelin sheaths [206]. Also, such histopathologic changes can occur in the absence of clinical symptoms. The pathophysiology of peripheral neuropathy remains incompletely understood. Etiologic significance has been attributed to vitamin B_1 and B_6 [193] deficiency, increased parathormone activity [290], enzyme dysfunction, transketolase [523], and the presence of middle molecules such as myoinositol [85] and methylguanidine [45].

Cranial nerve dysfunction observed in dialyzed patients includes amaurosis, sensorineural hearing loss, and decreased taste acuity. High frequency sensorineural hearing loss is often present in adults beginning dialysis; except for the impact of ototoxic drugs such as loop diuretics and aminoglycosides, hearing loss is apparently not influenced by dialysis [351]. Also, hypogeusia, which may in part reflect zinc deficiency, does not improve with long-term dialysis [498].

One of the most severe complications seen in dialysis populations is the *dialysis encephalopathy syndrome* (DES). Its clinical features (Table 39-17), initially described in adults [14], were first reported in pediatric populations in 1977 in a group of children not yet on dialysis [53]. In addition to their neurologic dysfunction [255], all had early onset chronic renal failure due to congenital renal defects,

TABLE 39-17. *Clinical features of the dialysis encephalopathy syndrome*

Motor abnormalities	*Speech difficulties*
Myoclonus, muscle spasm	Dysphagia
Asterixis, tremors	Dyspraxia-partial loss of
Seizures; focal, grand mal	coordinated movements
	Stuttering
Dementia	*Electroencephalogram*
Altered mood, depression	Diffuse slowing
Diminished alertness	Bursts of slow and high
Lethargy, coma	voltage activity

advanced renal osteodystrophy, characteristic EEG changes, and had been ingesting large quantities of aluminum [633]. Subsequently, similar changes were reported in children on hemodialysis and peritoneal dialysis and after transplantation [639]. Most affected adults have been on hemodialysis.

Although controversy regarding the etiology of DES still exists, most believe it is related to a toxic effect of aluminum. Etiologic significance has also been attributed to altered cerebrospinal fluid dynamics, slow virus infection, and the accumulation of calcium or tin by the cerebral cortex [633]. The most important sources of aluminum are the ingestion of aluminum-containing phosphate binders and the water used to prepare dialysate [636,637]. DES has occurred both sporadically and epidemically, with a temporal relationship between the patients' aluminum burden and their exposure to aluminum. The exposure in the epidemic form usually comes from aluminum rich dialysate [27,637]. The transmembrane movement of aluminum depends on the existing transmembrane free aluminum gradient, pH gradient, and the quantity of aluminum bound to protein. Aluminum is amphoteric and therefore more soluble when the dialysate pH is less than 6.50 or more than 7.60. Raising the dialysate pH with bicarbonate may enable more aluminum to traverse either the peritoneum or the hemodialyzing membrane [266]. The usual pH of commercial peritoneal dialysate favors the transfer of aluminum across the peritoneal membrane. An aluminum dialysate concentration of less than 0.30 μmoles/liter has been suggested as being nontoxic [689]. Because aluminum is deposited in intracellular sites, serum levels do not correlate directly with clinical symptoms and fail to reflect accurately a slow but progressive increase in total body aluminum. Aluminum absorption may be increased when secondary hyperparathyroidism is present.

Initial attempts at treating the DES were not successful in reversing or even stabilizing the neurologic symptoms; some success has been noted in response to discontinuing the use of aluminum-containing binders [512] and in response to the chelation of aluminum by deferoxamine [31,631]. To limit the exposure to aluminum, nonaluminum-containing binders, such as calcium carbonate or magnesium hydroxide, have been recommended. Serum magnesium levels should be measured in patients given magnesium-containing compounds. Switching from hemodialysis to CAPD lowers serum aluminum levels [689]. However, patients begun on CAPD and given aluminum containing phosphate binders will develop increased serum levels of aluminum.

Cognitive function improves in adults and children [307] during the first few months following initiation of dialysis. Differences between peritoneal and hemodialysis have not been found [87]. Insofar as changes in brain electrical activity reflect improved CNS function once dialysis is begun, computer assisted analysis of EEGs in adults [799,800] has shown improvement, whereas neurometric analysis in eight children has not [634,635].

The most common cause of *acquired encephalopathy* is some form of neurovascular disease. Intracranial hemorrhage, including subdural hematoma, has occurred in a few children [66,244,307]. Such episodes are usually related to coagulation defects, excessive heparinization, infections, acute or chronic hypertension, and thromboembolization from arteriovenous shunts or declotting procedures. The nature and extent of these lesions are best evaluated by CT. Hypertension as a cause of encephalopathy is most easily recognized by the rapid disappearance of symptoms when blood pressure is lowered. Children undergoing dialysis may experience transient attacks of ischemia and a thrombotic or hemorrhagic stroke.

Encephalopathic symptoms have been described in dialysis populations following the administration of a number of drugs [633] including penicillins, aminoglycosides, barbiturates, antihistamines, and phenothiazines. The presenting clinical features are usually seizures, alterations of consciousness, or delirium. Treatment is supportive after discontinuation of the involved agent. In patients with neurologic damage, hemodialysis but not peritoneal dialysis is associated with an increase in intracranial pressure [455a]. The continuous addition of mannitol to the dialysate or a continuous intravascular infusion of mannitol can prevent or control this problem.

Musculoskeletal Complications

A unilateral or bilateral carpal tunnel syndrome (CTS) occurs in 2% to 31% of the adult dialysis population. Data in children are not available. Originally thought to affect only hemodialysis patients, the CTS has been shown to occur at equal rates in patients undergoing peritoneal dialysis [69]. The incidence of CTS in dialytic populations is similar in males and females, and differing from the 3:1 female-to-male ratio of CTS in nondialytic populations. The CTS may develop as early as the third to fifth month after starting dialysis. Electrical criteria for diagnosing CTS have been published [69].

Amyloid fibrils containing beta$_2$-microglobulin have been found in nodules removed from the perineurium of the median nerve and the synovium inside the carpal tunnel [278]. Both hemodialysis and peritoneal dialysis patients have increased blood levels of beta-2 microglobulin. Clinical features of beta-2 microglobulin-associated amyloidosis in addition to the CTS include dialysis-associated arthropathy (DAA), pathological fractures, lytic bone lesions, tendonitis, and soft tissue swellings [780a]. It is diagnosed by biopsy. Some data support the suggestion that the incidence of CTS and DAA is reduced when

polyacrylonitrile dialyzers are used; other data do not [416a].

Cardiovascular Complications

Long-term dialysis is associated with changes in blood pressure, myocardial function, and accelerated atherogenesis [617a]. The construction of a vascular access for hemodialysis, by virtue of creating a direct arteriovenous communication, alters cardiovascular hemodynamics. To maintain blood pressure, the decrease in peripheral resistance is compensated by an increase in cardiac output. The presence of a Brescia-Cimino fistula in most children does not usually depress myocardial function at the clinical level, even though postocclusion changes in systemic vascular resistance and cardiac index can be demonstrated [679]. Others have noted deterioration of myocardial function [595] and exercise tolerance [813] in children after insertion of arteriovenous shunts. Isolated cases of heart failure following the creation of arteriovenous shunts for hemodialysis have been noted in adults [5,21] and children [653]. Fistula flow rates in children [594] are similar to those in adults, in whom flow rates range from 300 to 800 ml/minute. The finding of normal myocontractility indices after transplantation in the presence of a functioning shunt suggests that many of the changes attributed to the shunt may have been due to the simultaneous presence of anemia.

A number of studies in adults and children [125,592,593] have reported *depressed left ventricular function* as assessed by cardiac catheterization [114], echocardiography [531], and systolic time intervals [814]. Others have not found similar changes in stable adult populations receiving long-term dialysis [492]; some studies note an improvement in myocardial performance with long-term dialysis [37]. In children, short-term hemodialysis, independent of changes in either intravascular volume or blood pressure, improves myocardial function as reflected by changes in the mean velocity of circumferential fiber shortening, and the pre-ejection period to left ventricular ejection time ratio [596,812].

The etiology of the depressed myocardial function in dialyzed patients is multifactorial and includes changes related to intravascular volume, congestive heart failure, anemia, persistent hypertension, electrolyte imbalance, anemia, possibly uremic toxins including PTH, and the coexistence of ischemic heart disease. Treatment of these problems as well as successful transplantation improves myocardial function. Myocardial function in children after transplantation may initially be depressed but usually returns to normal within a year [814].

Pericarditis, which may predate the onset of dialysis, has been reported to develop in 5% to 18% of patients stabilized on dialysis [151,154,754]. The difference in incidence can be explained by the use of echocardiography to identify small asymptomatic effusions [291,370]. Although usually seen in the first 3 months of dialysis, pericarditis may occur at any time [509].

In symptomatic patients, the more commonly observed clinical features of pericarditis include chest pain in 60% to 70%, a friction rub in more than 90%, fever (which may predate other manifestations) in 76% to 96% [153,204,680], congestive heart failure, elevated venous pressure, and a gallop rhythm [592]. Less commonly observed are hypotension, intolerance to ultrafiltration, arrhythmias, cardiomegaly, mental confusion, and pleural effusion. Effusions, which are usually serous, may become hemorrhagic because of uremic related dysfunctional hemostasis or the repetitive use of heparin. A reduced incidence of tamponade is claimed for peritoneal dialysis [148]. Constrictive pericarditis, which necessitates diagnostic catheterization and angiography, can occur [484,509]. Myocarditis and reversible cardiomyopathy have been described in uremic patients who have been under long-term protein restriction [462].

Therapy for pericarditis includes a number of steps. Most recommend that the frequency of dialysis be increased; intensive dialysis alone will control pericarditis in approximately 40% of cases [509, 870]. Also, intensive dialysis simultaneously improves the uremic milieu and helps control salt and water balance. In patients who cannot tolerate the acute hemodynamic changes associated with frequent hemodialysis, peritoneal dialysis may be helpful. Regional heparinization and the discontinuation of oral anticoagulants should be considered. Analysis of 55 variables in 97 patients found several that correlated with the failure of intensive dialysis to cure uremic pericarditis. These included fever above 39°C, diminished systolic blood pressure, rales, jugular venous distention, hemodynamic instability, a WBC count over 15,000/mm^3, left shift, the presence of both an anterior and posterior effusion by echocardiography, and a large effusion [183].

Anti-inflammatory agents may be helpful. Systemic corticosteroids and possibly indomethacin [537,769] can rapidly reverse symptoms and reduce the size of an effusion. One-third to one-half of patients do not respond or recur when treated systemically. Pericardiocentesis is indicated as a diagnostic procedure if an infectious etiology is suspected or as an acute therapy for treating tamponade. Some believe that a high mortality is associated with pericardial taps or catheter insertion [339]; others believe it to be low [43,204]. The best success, combined with the lowest mortality and recurrence rate, follows the intrapericardial infusion of triamcinolone [120,524]. An open surgical procedure, such as a subxiphoid or anterior pericardial window or total or partial pericardectomy, needs consideration in the presence of purulent pericarditis; hemorrhagic effusion; constrictive pericarditis; or in the failure of simple pericardial aspiration, intensive dialysis, or drug therapy [759]. Charcoal hemoperfusion has been used to treat pericardial effusions [511]; its efficacy remains unclear.

Extracellular volume expansion is the cause of most dialysis related *hypertension*. The majority of children with ESRD are hypertensive when starting dialysis. After successful dietary and dialytic management of sodium and water balance are accomplished, blood pressure is usually controllable; volume overload syndromes do not occur. A few weeks of dialysis is often required before blood pressure is chronically lowered. The maximum reduction in drug requirements occurs in CAPD patients [872]. In adult populations, 80% to 90% of dialysis patients who achieve their "dry" weight become normotensive [701]. Antihyperten-

sive medication is indicated in those whose blood pressure cannot be maintained within age-related limits [314,381]. In children beginning dialysis, an ECG and echocardiogram are indicated to establish the degree of myocardial change due to chronic hypertension and should be repeated to monitor changes over time.

Long-term control of hypertension is more readily achieved in children receiving daily peritoneal dialysis (CAPD, CCPD) [50,240] as compared with long-term hemodialysis. Hemodialysis may be more effective than IPD in controlling hypertension in children [726]. It is possible either to reduce the amount of antihypertensive medication or to eliminate its use in the majority of children undergoing CAPD.

Some hypertensive patients fail to lower their blood pressure in response to fluid removal. Most patients with this finding have high levels of plasma renin activity in relation to their volume status and may respond to the fluid depletion of dialysis by an increased renal release of renin [826] and by worsening of their hypertension [465]. The use of an angiotensin converting enzyme inhibitor has been advocated to ascertain whether a hyperreninemic state is present [482]. Bilateral nephrectomy [465,855], which needs to be considered when medical management fails, usually is successful in converting most patients to a volume-dependent hypertensive state. Bilateral nephrectomy is associated with increased problems related to nutritional intake and further impairment of vitamin D metabolism. An occasional patient will continue to remain hypertensive despite bilateral nephrectomy and adequate control of volume. The etiology of the persistent hypertension has been attributed to autonomic nervous system dysfunction [519] or the failure of vascular changes to reverse [466].

Congestive heart failure develops in dialyzed children in a number of settings. Most important is the combined impact of extracellular volume expansion, hypertension, and anemia. An increased risk for developing heart failure exists in the nonuremic patient whose hemoglobin is less than 5.0 g/dl [300]. Heart failure is hemodynamically related to decreased peripheral resistance. The increased cardiac output associated with anemia [101] can be reduced to normal in dialysis patients when the hemoglobin is raised to 10.0 g/dl. Because peripheral resistance rises as the hemoglobin is increased [558], hypertension may first appear or worsen if already present. The appearance of pulmonary edema may reflect, in part, renal failure related changes in permeability characteristics of pulmonary capillaries [279]. Other contributory factors include "uremic toxins," peripheral arteriovenous shunts, metastatic calcifications, atherosclerotic changes, vitamin deficiency (beri-beri), and endocrine dysfunction (hyperparathyroidism).

Approaches to controlling heart disease in children involve its prevention as well as therapy for acute and chronic congestive failure. Preventive steps involve control of extracellular volume by dietary and dialytic means, use of antihypertensive medications, selective bilateral nephrectomy, and control of anemia. In most children experiencing cardiac decompensation, a volume overload state is usually a contributing factor, and an acute ultrafiltration dialysis will be needed. Consideration needs to be given to the use of oxygen, morphine, phlebotomy, rotating tourniquets, and the acute lowering of blood pressure. The onset of arrhythmias or an infectious process may lead to heart failure. If treatment for the aforementioned problems fails, digitalization should be considered. An evaluation of myocardial function by echocardiography is helpful in making such a decision.

Digoxin is the most widely used cardiac glycoside to treat heart failure in children. In uremic patients, its absorption is reduced, tissue binding is reduced, plasma levels may change in an unexplained fashion, and its functioning half-life is increased from a norm of 42 up to 120 hours [247,856]. Therapeutic serum levels range between 0.5 and 2.0 ng/ml; the incidence of toxicity increases when levels exceed 3.0 ng/ml [195] or when hypercalcemia or hypokalemia is present. Digitalis toxicity may occur in dialyzed populations at lower serum levels because of its altered metabolism in uremia. The dose of digoxin does not require modification in patients on hemodialysis or CAPD because it is poorly dialyzed [3,613]. The lowering of serum levels of potassium through dialysis may precipitate digoxin toxicity [818]. When initially digitalizing patients on dialysis, it is recommended that one use the lower end of the suggested range of digoxin dose. Long-term maintenance doses of digoxin may need to be reduced by up to 86% of the maintenance dose because of its reduced renal elimination [276,817]. Data are not yet available on the use of either aminophylline or vasodilator drug therapy to treat heart failure in children with ESRD.

Hyperlipidemia has been reported to occur in one-third of patients receiving maintenance hemodialysis [116] and peritoneal dialysis [418]. Hypertriglyceridemia, hypercholesterolemia, increased low density and very low density lipoproteins, and decreased high density lipoproteins have been noted in children on dialysis [70,114,214,616,624, 665a]. The apolipoprotein patterns in children on hemodialysis when combined with changes in plasma triglycerides and cholesterol are similar to those observed in adults as constituting a risk for developing cardiovascular disease [591]. Low levels of serum carnitine or its dialytic removal may contribute to the hypertriglyceridemia [61,875,876]. Administering L-carnitine in a dose of 100 mg/kg per day to children on CAPD has not caused significant changes in their serum triglyceride levels [839a]. The low levels of carnitine have been related to relative malnutrition [549a]. Although it is widely believed that atherosclerosis is accelerated in patients on dialysis, some believe that the incidence of ischemic heart disease in such patients has a better correlation with the presence of predialysis cardiovascular risk factors [42]. An increased incidence of collagenization of the intima of coronary arteries without plaque formation has been noted in children [624]. Clofibrate has been used to treat hyperlipidemia in adults; data in children are lacking [286]. Also, in adults receiving maintenance dialysis, controlled exercise positively influenced lipid abnormalities [287].

Additional cardiovascular complications include *arrhythmias* and *bacterial endocarditis* [469] secondary to fistula and cannula infection. The former may occur secondary to hypoxia, hyperkalemia, hypokalemia, hypocalcemia, hypomagnesemia, acidosis, and alkalosis and when pericardial, myocardial, or endocardial disease is present [151]. An evaluation of the heart rhythm is indicated in any dialysis patient who develops cardiac problems.

Hematologic Complications

ANEMIA

The anemia of chronic renal failure usually worsens after children start dialysis. Mechanisms include further decreases in erythropoietin production, uremic toxin suppression of hemoglobin or erythroid synthesis, shortened red cell survival, blood loss, hemolysis, disordered iron metabolism, and folate deficiency. A database consisting of a white count and differential, platelet count, red blood cell indices, hematocrit and hemoglobin, reticulocyte count, peripheral smear examination, and serum ferritin level are indicated when dialysis is begun.

The classic anemia of renal failure is normocytic, normochromic, and hypoproliferative, with an inappropriately low erythropoietin level (Chap. 29). In fact, most patients with renal insufficiency have absolute concentrations of serum erythropoietin that are normal or elevated [128,472]. Inhibitors of red cell precursors also play a role in the development of anemia associated with ESRD. Polyamines, specifically spermine [667], and perhaps PTH or one of its fragments [667] have been shown to inhibit erythropoiesis. Various androgen preparations can be used to stimulate renal and hepatic erythropoietin production. In a controlled trial of intramuscular and oral androgens, anephric patients failed to respond to either. In adults, intramuscular nandrolone decanoate (3 mg/kg/week) and testosterone enanthate (4 mg/kg/week) were effective in increasing the red cell mass [557]. Their use, however, was associated with a 25% drop-out rate because of unacceptable side effects. Even though such agents are generally contraindicated in pediatric populations because of their negative effect on growth due to their accelerating epiphyseal fusion, their use may be helpful in children whose growth is completed or in those whose religious beliefs contraindicate blood transfusions.

The availability of recombinant erythropoietin (rHuEPO), which virtually cures the uncomplicated anemia of chronic renal failure, has altered the approach to the chronic anemia of all dialysis patients [223,224]. A dose of 37.5 to 300 units/kg given intravenously three times a week after hemodialysis will increase and maintain the hematocrit at 35% to 40%. In patients with excessive iron stores, serum ferritin levels fall; iron deficiency may occur if iron stores are low prior to starting therapy. Cardiomegaly decreases and exercise tolerance increases. No significant toxicity has been noted, and antibodies to the preparation have not been observed. Problems that have developed with its use include the development or acceleration of hypertension, occasionally complicated by seizures; increased predialysis concentrations of creatinine, urea, and potassium; and increased clotting of dialyzers. Osteitis fibrosa, aluminum intoxication, and inflammation interfere with the action of recombinant erythropoietin. Children on hemodialysis treated thrice weekly with rHuEPO at a dose of 100–150 units/kg responded within 9–13 weeks by increasing their mean hemoglobin to 10.9 g/dl [681a]. The hemoglobin level was maintained with a rHuEPO dose of 40 to 100 units/kg. Multiple dosage regimens and routes of administration of rHuEPO have been used. Children on CCPD treated with subcutaneous rHuEPO need only 50% of the weekly dose (101 versus 204 units/kg of rHuEPO per week) given intravenously to children on hemodialysis to increase and sustain their hemoglobin levels above 10 g/dl [167a]. Intravenous weekly rHuEPO in a dose of 300 units/kg in children undergoing CAPD or CCPD increased their hct from 18.5% to 27.5% within a month [587a]. After three months the weekly average dose to maintain the hct at 30% could be reduced to 100 units/kg per week. Adult studies have shown that treatment with rHuEPO also increases exercise tolerance [58a,123a], leads to regression of left ventricular hypertrophy [619a], improves nutrition [58b] and improves cognitive function [510a]. The antibody response to hepatitis B vaccine is increased [736a] and, in the absence of additional blood transfusions, lymphocytotoxic antibody levels fall by 33% over 36 weeks [168b]. Although the use of rHuEPO in children increases their sense of well being, clear cut improvements in their nutritional status and growth rates could not be attributed to rHuEPO.

Instituting long-term dialysis may improve anemia. Hemodialysis three times a week in adults increased their mean hematocrit from 22% to 29% [666]. In adults, CAPD is also associated with an increased hemoglobin [583,874]. The mean hematocrit in children on CAPD is higher than that in those on hemodialysis [64]. Some of the dialysis related improvement in anemia may reflect reductions in extracellular volume.

A shortened red cell survival is characteristic of patients starting hemodialysis. Its etiology is unknown. Long-term dialysis generally leads to a partial correction of this defect [441]. Improvement in red cell survival has been attributed to the removal with dialysis of an erythropoietic inhibitor. Red cells from patients with ESRD transfused into normal subjects have a normal life span; conversely, red cells from normals transfused into uremic patients have a shortened life span [94].

Blood loss as a cause of dialysis related anemia can occur from the failure to return all of the blood in hemodialysis tubing, venipuncture or phlebotomy for diagnostic tests, epistaxis, occult gastrointestinal bleeding from an ulcer, uremia, or defects in platelet function. Indications for transfusion are variable and include fatigue, anorexia, reduced exercise tolerance, incipient heart failure, chest pain, and a hemoglobin in the range of 5.0 to 6.0 g/dl. The required amount of packed red cells to raise the hemoglobin can be estimated by the formula: number of milliliters of packed red cells required equals four times the weight in kilograms times the desired minus the observed hemoglobin [309]. Transfusion requirements are less in children undergoing peritoneal dialysis compared with hemodialysis and in those children who have not had bilateral nephrectomies. This is presumably because of differences in the availability of erythropoietin. Transfusion requirements vary considerably in children on dialysis. Children who are anephric on hemodialysis and peritoneal dialysis tend to require 1 unit of blood monthly and bimonthly,

respectively. Nephric children need transfusions half as often [468].

Hemolysis leading to an increased need for transfusion may develop following exposure to chloramine, hydrogen peroxide [293a], or nitrates in the water supply, leaching of copper from copper tubing, the use of formaldehyde in reuse procedures, hyponatremia from hypotonic dialysate, overheated dialysate, or folic acid deficiency. A Coombs positive hemolytic anemia occasionally develops in patients exposed to alpha methyldopa, penicillin, or cephalosporins. Hemolysis due to hypersplenism secondary to myelofibrosis has been described in children [729]. Additional etiologies for hypersplenism include transfusion induced hemochromatosis and chronic hepatitis.

Both iron overload and deficiency occur in dialyzed populations. Iron overload leading to hemochromatosis occurs in dialyzed populations given excessive iron as oral supplements, as intravenous iron dextran, or in blood transfusions [720]. One unit of packed red cells contains one-sixth to one-seventh of the amount of iron stored in the body. The reason that overt hemochromatosis does not develop more quickly is best explained by the small amounts of blood lost with repetitive hemodialysis and the volume of blood lost with laboratory tests. Iron intoxication is best prevented by withholding iron supplementation unless body iron stores are depleted. Chelation therapy with intravenous deferoxamine has been used to treat iron overload in dialyzed patients. It can be given intraperitoneally to children on CAPD [292] at a dose of 10.0 to 17.5 mg/kg in the overnight exchange for 3 to 6 months [22a]. The use of rHuEPO reduces body stores of iron [167a]. Ferritin levels in children treated with rHuEPO may fall by 50% over 6 months.

In 18 children, 5.0 to 20.6 years, treated with hemodialysis for 4 to 90 months and evaluated for iron overload, six had serum ferritin levels above 400 ng/dl and eight had biochemical evidence of hepatocellular damage [209]. A positive correlation was found between serum ferritin levels and stainable iron in bone marrow and liver tissue. Treatment with 25 mg/kg of deferoxamine thrice weekly for 10 to 27 months was ineffective. Documented decreases in iron stores did occur in those who received fewer blood transfusions. Children who developed secondary hemosiderosis were younger and had been given more transfusions. Significant reductions in liver stores of iron have been demonstrated using a nuclear resonance scattering technique after giving 40 mg/kg of deferoxamine with each dialysis without significant changes in the usual clinical laboratory tests used to measure iron overload [546].

Iron deficiency, which can develop in hemodialysis patients because of a repetitive loss of small amounts of blood, rarely occurs in patients on peritoneal dialysis unless a nonrenal cause is present. In patients starting dialysis with normal iron stores, 6 to 24 months may pass before iron deficiency develops [222]. When it occurs, oral iron preparations are as effective as parenteral iron, the use of which is associated with a significant number of systemic reactions [618]. Iron absorption in dialyzed patients is similar to that found in normals [225]. Iron supplementation should again be withheld once iron stores have been repleted. Bone marrow iron stores in dialyzed adults correlate best with serum ferritin levels rather than serum iron, red cell volume, hematocrit, or transferrin saturation [67]. Iron stores should be monitored by measuring serum ferritin levels every 4 to 6 months. Normal values range from 10 to 300 µg/dl.

Chronic folate deficiency, which can lead to a megaloblastic anemia [330,340], occurs in three circumstances. Serum levels fall during hemodialysis [859] but not during peritoneal dialysis [340]; unless the dialyzed folate is replaced in hemodialyzed patients, a megaloblastic anemia can develop. Providing 1.0 mg/day of folate prevents the development of folate deficiency in most children receiving hemodialysis. A reduced protein intake increases the risk for developing folate deficiency. Finally, the use of drugs such as diphenylhydantoin can lead to a megaloblastic anemia by interfering with folate metabolism. Red cell levels are a better indicator of folate stores than are serum levels.

CLOTTING FACTORS

Thrombocytopenia and platelet dysfunction are improved by dialysis in most patients [130,398,777]. Improvement in "uremic" bleeding occurs when platelet rich plasma [833], factor VIII cryoprecipitate, or L-arginine vasopressin (DDAVP) is given [507]. The dose of DDAVP is 0.3 µg/kg in 50 ml D5W given over 15 to 30 minutes. The functional defect is similar to that observed in von Willebrand's disease. Platelet dysfunction may be improved by bicarbonate dialysis [804a]. Clotting abnormalities similar to those seen in children with the nephrotic syndrome occur in children undergoing chronic peritoneal dialysis [395a]. Abnormalities include increased activities of factors VII, VIII, von Willebrand factor, fibrinogen, factor XIIIA, and factor XIIIS. The activated partial thromboplastin time is increased and the thrombin clotting time is decreased. The relative contribution of chronic renal failure or dialysis in causing these abnormalities remains unclear.

LEUKOCYTES

Transient leukopenia commonly occurs during the first hour of hemodialysis [863]. Concentrations of C5a increase as a result of dialyzer membrane induced complement activation. Also, a role for neutrophil C3b receptors has been documented. Leukopenia is independent of bath composition and occurs to a greater extent when cuprophane as compared with cellulose acetate membranes are used. The use of heparin or citrate as an anticoagulant is associated with similar decreases in the WBC count. Leukopenia is avoided when polyacrylonitrile or methyl methacrylate membranes are used and is reduced by reusing membranes.

A number of abnormalities in circulating granulocyte and monocyte cells occur in patients on long-term dialysis [478]. Patients undergoing long-term hemodialysis have reduced oxidative responses of both cell lines to chemotactic stimuli and have decreased numbers of C5a receptors. A decreased in vitro chemotactic granulocyte response also occurs. Patients on long-term peritoneal dialysis have similar defects in receptors and oxidative responses. These defects may in part contribute to the high rate of infectious complications. The high osmolality but not the low pH of dialysate adversely affects granulocyte and monocyte function. Fresh dialysate kills 99% of lymphocytes after 3 hours of incubation in a 4.25% glucose solution and reduces the chemiluminescence response of peripheral leukocytes by 98.8%.

Infectious Complications

HEPATITIS

Viral hepatitis historically has been the most serious infectious disease occurring in hemodialysis units [749]. Not only does it affect patients with ESRD, but it also often involves support staff, hospital personnel, friends, family, and other patients being followed by the nephrology service. Viruses known to cause hepatitis in dialyzed patients include hepatitis viruses A, B(HBV), and C, formerly known as non-A non-B; herpes simplex type I; cytomegalovirus; varicella-zoster; and Epstein-Barr virus. The diagnosis, epidemiology, treatment, and incidence of infectious forms of hepatitis, other than HBV, is the same as in nondialyzed patients and will not be considered further. Dialysis populations are also known to develop liver dysfunction from silicone [471], polyvinyl chloride [556], and from a number of pharmacologic agents including furosemide, isoniazide, methyldopa, nitrofurantoin, and sulfonamide. Transplant patients who have returned to dialysis may have developed hepatotoxicity from azathioprine or cyclosporine A.

When hemodialysis units initially began to test patients routinely for serologic evidence of HBV, 10% of patients were found to be positive. Some centers reported 90% of their patients as having serologic evidence of hepatitis [236]. One pediatric dialysis unit reported that 58% of their children developed serologic evidence of HBV after starting dialysis [245]. In another study of 54 children, ages 2 to 18 years, undergoing hemodialysis, the prevalence of HBV markers was 66.7% and that of HBsAg (hepatitis surface antigen) was 13.0% [123]. Sixteen of 18 given twice the usually recommended dose of hepatitis B vaccine developed antibody responses; one response was low.

The source of the HBV is usually infected blood or cross contamination. HBV can cross dialyzer membranes [765] and has been transmitted in peritoneal fluid [703]. Although patients undergoing long-term dialysis who develop hepatitis may develop either fulminant [571,744] or chronic liver disease [802], most tend to have relatively mild symptoms [767] compared with the general population. Chronic active hepatitis may lead to cirrhosis. The natural history of chronic active hepatitis is that of exacerbations and remissions in some and continuous progression in some, whereas others remain asymptomatic. Chronic active hepatitis or the carrier state is considered to be present when the elevated HBsAg persists for more than 6 months [786]. In some patients, hepatitis may persist for a long time only to resolve completely eventually. Staff and others who become infected with HBV are at risk for developing serious liver disease [487].

In addition to the direct effect of HBV infection on morbidity and mortality in dialysis patients, some evidence suggests that transplanted patients with HBV antigenemia are at increased risk. Transplantation is best delayed until elevated levels return to normal in HBsAg positive patients as well as those with elevated liver enzymes from other causes.

Prevention of hepatitis involves three interrelated approaches: prevention of spread of virus, use of gamma globulin, and vaccine administration. Hepatitis surveillance and infection control programs are routine in dialysis units. Recommendations for controlling the spread of hepatitis virus include the routine use of gloves and disposable equipment, appropriate labeling of blood samples, consistent machine assignment, dialysis of HBsAg positive patients on a patient specific machine in isolation, switching of patients to home dialysis, and the screening of blood for hepatitis virus. Hyperimmune gamma globulin prepared from the blood of patients recovering from HBV virus infection provides transient passive immunity. It can be used to prevent the onset of an outbreak or control an epidemic of HBV infection in patients and staff [659]. It can also be used to treat individuals directly exposed to blood contaminated with HBV [735]. The vaccine against HBV infection [786] unfortunately fails to protect all dialysis patients. In one study of 10 hemodialyzed children immunized with HBV vaccine, all developed protective levels of antibody [573]. In a randomized, double blind, placebo-controlled study of three doses of HBV vaccine (Heptavax-B) in 1311 patients on hemodialysis, only 50% of the recipients developed an appropriate antibody response. The incidence of HBV infection during the 25-month trial was similar in both groups [776]. Some patients thought to have had an antibody response also developed HBV infection. Others have noted a higher conversion rate in dialysis populations. The reasons for such differences are not clear, but they may reflect population differences or the use of different lots or sources of vaccine.

AIDS

Increasingly, children have developed AIDS secondary to infection with T-lymphotropic virus type III. Children acquire the virus as a consequence of receiving blood products. Newborns can acquire HIV transplacentally. Cases of AIDS have been reported in dialyzed children. Since the virus is transmitted in blood, it is possible that some children with renal failure who have received blood transfusion will develop AIDS. Guidelines for monitoring blood donors and patients at risk are available [131,132,132a].

Screening for human immunodeficiency virus (HIV) by enzyme immunoassay (EIA) done in early 1986 suggested that false-positive results may be higher in patients undergoing long-term dialysis [30]. Repeat testing with an improved EIA kit that has a specificity of 99.8% was negative [843]. Western blot testing should be used to confirm positive EIA tests. The risk of transmission of HIV between dialysis patients is low [507b]. In a prospective study of 2 years duration in a long-term dialysis unit with a prevalence rate for HIV of 11%, only 1 of 45 HIV-negative patients seroconverted [627].

The risk for transmitting HIV in dialysis units is less than that of hepatitis for two reasons: the concentration of virus in blood is one million times less for HIV, and the environmental routes for transmission are absent. The CDC recommendations for universal blood and body fluid precautions are sufficient to prevent HIV transmission [131,132]. Periodic screening for HIV similar to that of hepatitis appears to be a reasonable practice. A patient found to be positive while on hemodialysis should be dialyzed in a separate room on a separate machine and dialyzers should not be reused. Machines should be cleaned with hypochlorite after each run and weekly to monthly with formaldehyde.

Endocrine Complications

Patients receiving maintenance dialysis display a variety of endocrine abnormalities [234]. These may be associated with clinical disease or with false-positive tests in the absence of any recognizable clinical features. Many of the findings noted in dialyzed populations are present in patients with advanced renal failure (Chap. 34). To be emphasized here are those findings found in patients undergoing dialysis. Abnormalities in PTH and vitamin D metabolism, excessive renin release, erythropoietin regulation, growth hormone, and somatomedin dysfunction are described in other sections.

ADRENAL DYSFUNCTION

Adrenocorticotropin hormone (ACTH) activity is variable in ESRD patients, with normal, low, and high concentration reported [281]. When measured in patients being dialyzed, cortisol levels are usually normal but occasionally high. The response to ACTH infusion is normal [59], plasma half-life is elevated [539], and the suppressive response to dexamethasone may be normal [59] or incomplete [520]. A single dialysis treatment in children can increase cortisol levels twofold [677]. Cortisol levels fall during the first hour of hemodialysis and then rise [378]. The total amount of cortisol removal by hemodialysis is minimal and not of clinical significance [539].

Aldosterone, which is loosely bound to albumin, is dialyzable, but the amount removed is not clinically significant [437]. In some patients, the metabolic clearance of aldosterone is increased. In patients who undergo bilateral nephrectomies, plasma aldosterone levels fall and do not increase in response to volume depletion [853]; but the levels do change when plasma potassium levels are altered [518]. Although heparin diminishes aldosterone production in normal subjects, the effect of smaller doses of heparin used in hemodialysis patients is not known [44]. In children, plasma aldosterone levels rise 1.5- to 2.0-fold following a single hemodialysis treatment [676]. Although the degree of this rise may be blunted by the dialysis related concomitant fall in serum potassium, the significant correlation between peripheral renin activity and plasma aldosterone in children on long-term hemodialysis demonstrates that the renin angiotensin system is the principal determinant of aldosterone secretion in these patients.

Plasma catecholamine levels range from normal to elevated in patients on dialysis and do not increase after dialysis [439]. After adults are supine for approximately 1 hour, norepinephrine and epinephrine levels are reported as being elevated and reduced, respectively [522]. In children, both hemodialysis and hemofiltration are associated with a twofold to fourfold increase in both epinephrine and norepinephrine levels above normal predialysis values [677].

THYROID DYSFUNCTION

Measurements of thyroid function are often altered in patients with renal disease [166]. A decreased response of thyroid stimulating hormone (TSH) to thyrotropin releasing hormone has been reported in children on maintenance hemodialysis [377]. Some have noted a normal response in chronically dialyzed patients [174]. TSH is not dialyzable. Iodine uptake in patients on IPD or hemodialysis may be normal or reduced [587,672]. Normal levels of serum thyroxine are reported in patients on peritoneal dialysis [587]. Triiodothyronine (T_3) and thyroxine (T_4) have been found to be either normal or low in patients on long-term dialysis, with a tendency toward normalization with increased dialysis time [672,719]. These differences may, in part, be due to the general health status of the patient or to the use of intravenous heparin [355], which can cause an increase in T_4 levels. Concentrations of thyroid binding globulin and free T_4 are usually normal; free T_3 levels are often low. The low T_3 levels are secondary to an impaired peripheral conversion of T_4 to T_3. Criteria for the diagnosis of hypothyroidism include a TSH level above 20 μU/ml. In those whose TSH is 10 to 20 μU/ml, the diagnosis is made by the finding of a low free T_4 and an exaggerated response to thyrotropin releasing hormone [788].

In eight of 20 children undergoing hemodialysis, one or more thyroid studies were abnormal. The abnormalities were attributed in part to stool losses [846]. Thyroid function has been examined in two studies evaluating 133 and 115 patients who had been dialyzed for less than and more than 1 year, respectively [408]. Goiter, which was found in 42.8% of the total population (control group 6.5%), was more frequent (49.6%) in those dialyzed for more than 1 year. The increased incidence of goiter was postulated to be due to increased serum iodine levels or a parathormone effect. Compared with a control group, the incidence of primary hypothyroidism was increased by a factor of 2.5; the incidence of primary hyperthyroidism was not increased.

Therapeutic trials of thyroid hormone replacement have not proved the functional presence of a hypothyroid state [755], and it is suggested that patients on dialysis should be assumed to be euthyroid [407] unless the diagnostic criteria for hypothyroidism are met. Successful transplantation leads to a normalization of thyroid hormone levels in most patients [377]. Hypothyroidism has occurred as a result of the absorption of iodine from the sealing caps of dialysis catheters [837a].

PANCREATIC DYSFUNCTION

The abnormal glucose metabolism commonly seen in dialyzed patients is contributed to by factors that include insulin resistance, a postbinding defect in insulin action, altered gluconeogeneses, and nonpancreatic endocrine abnormalities. In patients receiving long-term hemodialysis, fasting insulin levels as well as blood glucose levels are elevated [213]. Insulin binding to monocytes is unaltered [179]. The increased gluconeogenesis from alanine [693] seen in patients with advanced renal failure is improved by hemodialysis. Also, parathyroidectomy in children undergoing long-term hemodialysis improves glucose intolerance by reducing gluconeogenesis [371,502]. The action of other hormones, catecholamines, cortisol, and growth hormone, may antagonize the action of the insulin [365]. In some patients on long-term dialysis, the correction of chronic potassium deficiency improves carbohydrate metabolism, even though their peak insulin response to hyperglycemia is reduced [79]. A defined role for glucagon in the abnormal carbohydrate metabolism of dialyzed patients is not yet described. Glucagon levels, which are high in advanced renal failure, remain elevated in dialyzed patients [80]. The elevation may be explained by the retention of a large, inactive component. Amylase levels are often elevated in patients on dialysis because of reduced renal excretion. In pancreatitis they become markedly elevated [63].

REPRODUCTIVE HORMONE DYSFUNCTION

Disturbances of sexual hormone regulation at the level of the hypothalamic-pituitary axis and abnormalities in sex organ systems commonly occur in dialyzed patients. Many of the observed defects are already present when patients with progressive renal insufficiency are started on dialysis. Gonadal function does not usually return to normal in dialyzed patients. In adults on maintenance hemodialysis, levels of follicle stimulating hormone (FSH) and leuteinizing hormone (LH) are reported as being either normal or high [784]. Plasma estrogen and progesterone levels were decreased, and the expected ovulatory cyclic changes were not observed.

Limited data on ovarian function in children on dialysis are available. In a comparative study involving groups of prepubertal normal children, children with renal insufficiency, and children on dialysis, each group had similar levels of FSH. The children on dialysis had higher levels of LH, with a similar percentage of each group increasing their levels of FSH and LH following the administration of thyrotropin releasing hormone [628]. The elevated LH levels, which may increase with the onset of long-term dialysis, may account for the onset of gynecomastia and testicular enlargement in males [730,731]. In adolescent sexually mature females, menstruation and ovulation occasionally occur, although when dialysis is begun amenorrhea is commonly present. Conception rarely occurs in females on maintenance dialysis; when it does, spontaneous abortion usually occurs. However, a limited number of successful pregnancies have been reported in dialyzed females [5b,115]. Twenty to 25% of pregnancies in women on chronic dialysis result in viable offspring.

Elevated prolactin levels have been reported in approximately two-thirds and one-fourth of chronically hemodialyzed adult females and males, respectively [293]. The hyperprolactinemia in males is not thought to explain the onset of gynecomastia [437]. Dialyzed patients receiving alpha-methyldopa increase their prolactin levels and can experience galactorrhea [293]. Unstimulated levels of prolactin were higher in children on long-term dialysis than in children not yet on dialysis. Prolactin levels in normals compared with children with renal insufficiency did not increase following an infusion with thyrotropin releasing hormone [628]. Hemodialysis does not lower prolactin levels in adults or children [378].

Impotence, decreased spermatogenesis, and reduced libido, characteristics of advanced renal failure, may or may not be improved by long-term dialysis. In pubertal males with chronic renal failure, both normal and low levels of plasma testosterone and a diminished response to stimulation with HCG have been reported [723]. Delayed puberty also occurs [239]. Testosterone responsiveness improves in adults on long-term dialysis. Controversy still exists as to the role of zinc deficiency in the hypogonadism of uremia [24]. The significance of Leydig cell atrophy in uremic adults in unclear as applied to children [779].

Priapism was reported to develop 2 to 7 hours after hemodialysis in 17 of 3377 males [760]. Eleven had received androgens; two had sickle cell trait. No patients on peritoneal dialysis developed priapism.

Gastrointestinal Hormone Dysfunction

Plasma gastrin levels, which are high in dialyzed patients, may or may not be lowered by dialysis [612]. Elevated gastrin levels do not correlate with the increased gastric hyperacidity or peptic ulcer disease in patients undergoing long-term dialysis [437]. Hemodialysis, which does not lower cholecystokinin activity, decreases gastric inhibitory polypeptide levels [612].

Ophthalmologic Complications

Conjunctival and corneal deposition of calcium crystals, usually asymptomatic, may give rise to the "red eye" syndrome [74] in dialyzed patients. Such calcifications are among the earliest symptoms seen when metastatic calcifications develop. They indicate a need to lower the calcium-phosphorus product. Conjunctival hemorrhage can occur in overheparinized patients. Hemodialysis may be associated with an increase in intraocular pressure because accumulated urea is slowly removed from the aqueous [275]. A choroidal perfusion defect has been reported in a few dialyzed patients [632]. Retinal vascular changes of acute and chronic hypertension as well as arteriosclerotic changes are similar in dialyzed patients and those who do not have ESRD. Diabetic retinopathy may worsen in hemodialyzed patients. When peritoneal dialysis is used in diabetics, the avoidance of heparin may inhibit the progression of diabetic retinopathy. Cytomegalic retinitis may initially develop in children who are restarted on regular dialysis after a kidney transplant has failed.

Acquired Cystic Kidney Disease

Cystic degeneration occurs frequently in the native kidneys of patients with ESRD whose primary disease is other than cystic disease [411]. Acquired cystic kidney disease (ACKD) has been documented in patients with advanced renal failure and in those on hemodialysis and peritoneal dialysis. In adults the incidence of ACKD is approximately 44%, with a range from 8% to 95% [301]. In 15 children ages 7.3 to 21.6 years evaluated by ultrasonography and MRI, 80% had cysts. Five had multiple cysts in both kidneys, five had solitary cysts in one kidney and two had solitary cysts in both kidneys [467]. Complications of ACKD include bleeding into cysts, gross hematuria, retroperitoneal bleeding, and malignant degeneration [300a]. One of the aforementioned children had tubular neoplasia.

Mortality Rate

Mortality data for children on dialysis are limited. Actuarial survival in Europe for children on CAPD was 90% and 87% at 1 and 2 years, respectively [113]. Survival on dialysis has improved over the past decade. The 1990 Annual Report of the US Renal Data System reported on children starting on dialysis in 1987 after having been on dialysis for 90 days [622a]. Two year survival rates for children ages 0 to 4, 5 to 9, 10 to 14, and 15 to 19 were 75.3%, 97.7%, 97.9% and 90.0% respectively. In a multicenter study in the United States, nine of 82 children on CAPD and CCPD for a mean time of 10.2 months died [157]. In a single center experience, two of 27 children died over a 5-year period [11]. In another single center comparing their experience of children on CAPD with hemodialysis over 5.5 years, 5 of 51 on CAPD and 1 of 25 on hemodialysis died [656]. Overall mortality of 66 children on hemodialysis for up to 11 years was 9% [803].

Nutrition

The successful management of the nutritional needs of children on maintenance dialysis is necessary if they are to maintain an acceptable body mass and habitus and if they are to grow and avoid the consequences of crippling bone disease. In dialysis populations, adequate dietary management helps prevent uremic symptoms such as pericarditis, malnutrition, secondary hyperparathyroidism, volume overload syndromes, and life-threatening electrolyte imbalance. Nutritional objectives are most readily accomplished by sharing the responsibility for the overall nutritional management of dialyzed children with a pediatric renal nutritionist. Three aspects of nutritional management are discussed: assessment, compliance, and the dietary prescription.

Assessment

Each child beginning dialysis needs a structured nutritional assessment. The child ideally will have had the benefit of an ongoing relationship with a renal nutritionist prior to starting dialysis and will, therefore, be prepared for the additional nutritional guidance and limitations that will be necessary once dialysis is started. The nutritional assessment should include a set of anthropometric measurements; an estimate of energy intake; an evaluation of protein stores; evaluation of the impact of prescribed medications; a current dietary history; and review of lipid, mineral, and trace metal metabolism and water balance. Once an initial database is obtained, individual issues can be addressed at intervals ranging in frequency from almost daily to every 3 to 6 months. The younger the child and the closer the time to beginning dialysis, the greater the need to reassess the child's nutritional status frequently. Temporary or permanent modifications are needed whenever the dialysis prescription or modality is changed, medications are changed, intercurrent illness develops, or a further reduction in the level of native kidney function occurs. It is recommended that a formal re-evaluation of each child's total nutritional status be undertaken twice a year if further growth is not anticipated and three to four times a year if significant growth is anticipated.

ANTHROPOMETRY

Monthly anthropometric measurements, especially over periods exceeding 1 year, are indicated in children on maintenance dialysis. Height, weight, and head circumference in children below 2 to 3 years of age and their changes while on dialysis are good indicators of the degree of nutritional management and dietary compliance. Such data, when combined with a yearly measurement of skeletal maturation (bone age), enable growth velocity indices to be calculated and compared with established norms. The weight for height index can be used as a gross measurement of adipose and muscle mass. A better delineation is obtained when quarterly measurements are done of the non-dominant mid-arm circumference and the triceps skinfold thickness and the mid-arm muscle circumference is calculated and compared with established norms [263,264]. A positive correlation exists between muscle thickness and between total body muscle mass and between subcutaneous fat thickness and total body fat [89]. More meaningful information will be obtained if the skinfold thickness of the thoracic, subscapular and suprailiac areas are simultaneously obtained. Edema may alter these measurements [86]. Because renal insufficiency is associated with a retarded bone age, the evaluation of linear growth needs to account for differences between expected and observed growth. This is done by comparing height measurements to either height age or bone age. Protein and fat stores are best evaluated by comparing the affected child's measurements with those corresponding to children of similar height or bone age. Weight for height percentiles can be assumed to be independent of height or bone age. Finally, pubertal status and its impact on growth potential needs to be evaluated at yearly intervals.

ENERGY

An adequate caloric intake, at least 75% of the RDA, is essential if body mass is to be maintained and body protein stores kept intact. Additional calories are probably needed if sustained growth is to occur. In practice, these objectives are difficult to achieve in dialyzed children, who may be anorectic and protein, electrolyte and fluid restricted and who have absorbed large amounts of glucose or have lost large amounts of protein through the peritoneum [712]. Concentrated sources of calories used to increase caloric content include both manufactured supplements and natural foodstuffs containing high concentrations of fats or carbohydrates. Most manufactured supplements and oils are poorly tolerated by older children but are usually readily accepted by neonates and infants. Excessive intake of carbohydrates may initiate or sustain elevated triglyceride levels. The use of polyunsaturated fats should be encouraged.

Energy intake is usually assessed by estimating the dietary intake of calories. The impact of changes in caloric intake are reflected by gains or losses of appetite and by both the magnitude and the rate of change of weight, height, and skinfold measurements.

PROTEIN

In addition to a dietary estimate of protein intake and an evaluation of the same variables used to assess energy, the measurement of a number of serum protein moieties are helpful in evaluating body protein stores. Because of their shorter half-lives, changes in serum albumin and complement levels and plasma transferrin levels are useful indicators of body protein stores [396]. A sudden decrease in the concentration of these proteins may reflect a dilution effect; it is a gradual change over time that is indicative of decreasing body protein stores. There is no correlation between serum proteins and the duration of dialysis [323]. Serum amino acid patterns and muscle cell proteins are altered in children on hemodialysis and peritoneal dialysis [163,180]. Dialysance of amino acids varies inversely with molecular weight [1]. Amino acids added to the dialysate has been shown to improve blood levels of essential amino acids without significantly altering blood levels of nonessential amino acids. Another indicator of protein intake is the evaluation of the immunologic response by lymphocyte counts, measurement of immunoglobulins, and the determination of cellular immunity by skin testing with antigens such as candida.

SALTS

Although the process of potassium adaptation in patients with advanced renal failure improves potassium balance, it is not sufficient to prevent hyperkalemia from occurring in patients on long-term hemodialysis or intermittent peritoneal dialysis unless dietary restrictions are imposed and followed. Noteworthy is the fact that many sodium substitutes contain potassium salts. Appropriate control of sodium intake determines to a large extent the magnitude of water ingested and, consequently, the degree of edema formation and volume dependent hypertension. The degree to which residual renal function enables sodium and potassium to be excreted should be periodically evaluated. This is done by measuring the daily excretory rate of these minerals. Children with a salt losing nephropathy may need salt supplementations to promote their growth. The need for calcium, phosphorus, iron and trace metals is discussed elsewhere in this chapter.

VITAMINS

Supplementation in dialysis populations is generally recommended for those vitamins that are removed by dialysis or for those that are ingested in insufficient quantities because of dietary restrictions. Vitamin A levels are high in dialysis patients, in part as a result of being protein bound to an elevated retinol binding protein [550]. Ascorbic acid supplementation is often needed because it is readily dialyzable and high potassium containing foods, which often are restricted, contain most of the dietary source of ascorbic acid [550]. Vitamin B_6 deficiency has been found in some dialysis patients [451]. The need for folate is discussed in the section on anemia. In a group of 15 adults evaluated over a 1-year period and not given any vitamin supplements, most did not develop measurably low blood concentration of vitamins B_6, B_{12}, niacin, thiamine, folate, and ascorbic acid [671]. Others have reported variable values ranging from normal to low; high concentrations of blood vitamin levels have not been reported. Blood levels of vitamin A, thiamine, riboflavin, pyridoxal phosphate, and folic acid have been reported to be elevated in children undergoing chronic peritoneal dialysis [455b]. The primary cause was thought to be excessive intake.

WATER

Acute changes in body weight associated with dialysis treatments are assumed to reflect changes in body water. Changes in true body mass need to be differentiated from those related to changes in body water. An interdialytic weight gain of less than 5% of estimated dry weight is an acceptable degree of water retention. Additional help can be obtained by a physical examination directed toward detecting evidence of peripheral and central edema and changes in blood pressure. In children undergoing peritoneal dialysis, it is often helpful to ascertain an individual patient's profile of the degree of ultrafiltration that occurs with different concentrations of glucose and dwell times.

MEDICATIONS

Nutritional needs are altered by many of the medications used to treat children on dialysis. Examples include the potassium content of various penicillin preparations, sodium and calcium containing salts, and sodium polystyrene sulfonate (Kayexalate), which contains 100 mg of sodium per gram.

Compliance

Compliance with dietary recommendations may be evident on the basis of improved growth, more normal blood chemistries, or the need for fewer medications. Most often, evidence of dietary compliance is sought by obtaining a dietary history. The most useful approach is to record all foods ingested for 3 to 4 days and to analyze the content of ingested foods. Less precise is an evaluation of a 1-day intake of food. An evaluation of food preference, level of appetite, ethnic influences, social environment, family dynamics, and economic resources is necessary to predict compliance and a plan for an acceptable dietary prescription. Previous lifestyle patterns [871], the ability to function normally while on dialysis [660], and the length of time on dialysis [81] all have impact on the degree of compliance. Emphasizing positive accomplishments, as opposed to reinforcing noncompliance, may be helpful.

Dietary Prescription

The content of foodstuffs and their usage and manipulation in the dietary management of the child undergoing long-term dialysis exceed the intent of this chapter. An overview of the idealized nutritional requirements for dialyzed children is summarized in [559] Table 39-18. Insofar as possible, diets ought to include readily available foods rather than special foods, diet substitutes, or supplements. Reward systems [770] as well as cooking classes for parents and children [781] can positively influence both knowledge and compliance. To follow are a number of dietary management issues that relate to the dialysis modalities used. The diet can often be made more liberal once dialysis is begun.

In patients on hemodialysis, too low a potassium diet combined with low dialysate potassium may increase the risk for developing digitalis intoxication. The potassium allowance is best ingested throughout the course of the day so as to avoid acute elevations in serum potassium. Some permit children to increase their intake of sodium and potassium 8 to 9 hours prior to being dialyzed—a period of time that allows most minerals to be absorbed [274]—or to eat "forbidden" foods during dialysis. Such a practice usually leads to more problems and is best avoided. In patients undergoing peritoneal dialysis, the dietary prescription needs to account for protein losses through the peritoneum and for excessive glucose absorption [112]. Because of the excessive load of carbohydrate needing to be metabolized during peritoneal dialysis, hyperlipidemia, with its potential risk, commonly occurs. In children on CAPD or CCPD, especially those with excessive urinary outputs, extra sodium and potassium may be needed because of dialytic losses.

In neonates and infants, nasogastric feedings may be helpful in providing additional nutrition to compensate for a decreased appetite and to provide sufficient energy and protein so that linear growth can occur. Amino acid supplementation provided either orally or in the dialysate has been used to increase protein intake. Its role in sustaining or improving nutrition and growth in children over a long-term period on dialysis remains unclear. Gastrostomy tube feeding can be used to treat poor growth associated with suboptimal protein caloric uptake [475]. CAPD was able to be continued without incident. Fundal plication for gastroesophageal reflux, a common occurrence in dialyzed infants, may be needed. The incidence of peritonitis does not increase after the gastrostomy tube is surgically implanted, and further abdominal surgery can be undertaken without additional complications developing. Aggressive nutritional management may lower rates of peritonitis in children on peritoneal dialysis [168a]. The dietary prescription varies with the frequency of dialysis [476].

Dialysis Team

Optimal functioning of a dialysis and transplant program for children requires a health care team. Team agreement and a common philosophy are essential. Fundamental to its success is the recognition of different functions, roles, professional languages, and styles of intervention [392].

Table 39-18. *Daily dietary recommendations for children on dialysis*

	Energy	Protein	Sodium	Potassium	Calcium	Phosphorus	Vitamins	Trace minerals	Fluid
Hemodialysis									
Infants	Min. of RDA for statural age	RDA for statural age	1–3 mEq/kg if necessary	1–3 mEq/kg	Supplement as necessary	Restrict high content foods Use low content foods	1 ml multivit. drops, 1 mg folic acid + Vit. D metabolite if needed	Suppl. zinc, iron or copper	Insensible + ultrafiltration + urinary output
Children/ adolescents	Min. of RDA for height age	RDA for height age	1–3 mEq/100 kcal expended if necessary	25–50 mEq/day when necessary	Supplement as necessary	500–1000 mg/ day	1 mg folic acid, 50–100 mg vit. C, B-complex + vit. D metabolite as needed	Same as above	Same as above
Peritoneal Dialysis (IPD)									
Infants	Min. of RDA for statural age	2.5–3 g/kg	1–3 mEq/kg if necessary	1–3 mEq/kg	Supplement as necessary	Same as for hemodialysis	Same as for hemodialysis	Same as above	Same as above
Children Adolescents	Min. of RDA for height age	Usually midway between hemodialysis and CAPD recommendations	1–3 mEq/100 kcal expended if necessary	25–50 mEq/day when necessary	Supplement as necessary	Same as for hemodialysis	Same as for hemodialysis	Same as above	Same as above
Peritoneal Dialysis (CAPD)									
Infants	Min. of RDA for statural age	3–4 g/kg	3 mEq/kg based on edema, BP	3 mEq/kg and possibly not necessary	Supplement as necessary	May be liberalized based on serum levels	Same as for hemodialysis	Same as above	Same as above
Children Adolescents	Min. of RDA for height age	3.0 g/kg-ht age 2–5 yr; 2.5 g/ kg-ht age 5–10 yr; 2.0 g/kg-ht age 10–12 yr; 1.5 g/kg-ht age >12 yr	Usually unlimited, 85–174 mEq/day if necessary	Usually unlimited, 25–50 mEq/day if necessary	Supplement as necessary or equiv. in milk products	Generally 240 ml milk/day	Same as for hemodialysis	Same as above	Usually not necessary

Adapted from Nelson P, Stover J: Principles of nutritional assessment and management of the child with ESRD. *In* Fine RN, Gruskin AB (eds): *End Stage Renal Disease in Children.* Philadelphia, WB Saunders, 1984, p 209.

The team leader should be a pediatric nephrologist who is aware and comfortable with all aspects of dialysis and can be readily available to team members when problems arise. A primary nurse with technical and medical knowledge can function as the central link between the team and the patient and family [161,306]. The social worker is a valuable support to the patient and family and advises the team of how well the patient is coping with the stress of dialysis [54]. The social worker is also in a position to facilitate the work of the team and encourage their strengths through the judicious use of group and process skills. The nutritionist, in addition to counseling families on nutritional issues, often develops useful insights into family psychodynamics.

The interactional model supports the conclusion that such teams gain their satisfaction from both medical and psychosocial responses of the child and family to the services provided [392]. Regular team discussions place problems in perspective, develop holistic approaches to patient care, and also allow team members to support each other at times of stress [200]. A team value base evolves from mutual respect for each other and is most readily gained when members recognize the professional strengths and talents of each other and have appropriate and realistic expectations for colleagues and themselves [392]. The demands of meeting emotional needs of patients and their families (family centered care), however, can extend beyond the capacity of the team members. This can lead to reactions of withdrawal by members of the team and a disruption of meaningful communication within the group. The input of a pediatric psychiatrist, psychologist, or a clergyman can help resolve such crisis situations.

Psychosocial Issues

Well-organized pediatric dialysis programs are team efforts involving physicians, nurses, nutritionists, teachers, play therapists, social workers, and psychologists. They need to be available over time to cope with the multitude of psychosocial problems related to the child and family as well as those related to the disease. Optimal care of children with chronic renal failure necessitates not only appropriate medical and technical knowledge but also requires simultaneous attention to the emotional and social impact of the treatment on the patients and their families (Chap. 36) [200,392,452]. The psychological challenges of a long-standing disease, dialysis treatments, and renal transplantation differ for children from those facing adult patients. Children need to become mature individuals despite the miseries of their illness [513]. For children with chronic renal failure, the dialysis unit and hospital often become home for long periods of time. Team members and hospital staff need to share responsibility with parents for raising such children. Children naturally resent having their lives full of unpleasant restrictions. Dialysis adds stress, and successful adaptation is often difficult in the beginning. Characteristic behavior includes withdrawal from social contacts and increased dependence on parents, team members, and hospital staff. Some children react with excessive dependence, whereas others react with aggressive behavior.

Anxiety, either obvious or repressed, influences the adaptation process [200]. Despite everything that is done to support and comfort pediatric patients, sick children may experience anorexia or develop behavioral habits such as hair twirling or skin picking. These and other problems are signs of distress resulting from unavoidable life-threatening illness.

Separation from home and family during prolonged dialysis and hospitalization causes major setbacks in development. The number of people children must relate to is increased from two to many. Often, children are exposed to a lack of consistency in the shared parenting. The dialysis patient must follow a rather rigid regimen in dialysis units and hospitals, limiting freedom and privacy. The child's environment changes from home, school, or neighborhood to a hospital and treatment room.

As a child's health improves in response to adequate dialysis and successful treatment, drastic positive changes in attitude and behavior frequently occur. The child becomes more active and less frightened. One must be aware that recurrent patterns of maladjustment will emerge in the weeks and months following the initiation of dialysis. These children face necessary but painful surgical procedures, complications related to their underlying chronic illness, and dialysis related complications [200]. It is important to allow the child to make choices and decisions whenever possible [513].

Pediatric medicine has long recognized that to treat children outside the context of the family is to do a grave disservice to each other [392]. Families are powerful systems, and what happens to a child resonates throughout the family system and vice versa [536]. The initial pressure on parents of children requiring dialysis is in coming to terms with the need for treatment. Subsequently, parents often have excessive expectations of the beneficial effect of dialysis; if problems increase or even persist, certain predictable reactions occur. The negative reactions of parents and patients include aggressive behavior toward the staff, lack of cooperation, and unreasonable demands on the medical team. Early in the course of dialysis or prior to initiating dialysis, time spent by physicians and other team members in developing meaningful relationships with families and children is well invested, considering the cooperation subsequently needed [513]. The problems of repetitive dialysis, whether performed in hospital or at home, create a series of stresses and demands that influence relationships both within and beyond the family [200]. Daily family dynamics are disturbed by the demanding program of dialysis, diet, and medication; restriction of activity; and hospitalization of the child. When a child is first starting dialysis, parents should be encouraged to spend as much time as possible with the child. The maternal, paternal, sibling, and family bonding is of utmost importance. Once adaptation occurs, steps should be taken to encourage independence and psychosocial growth. Because mothers spend considerable time at the dialysis unit or hospital, other children in the family miss her care and attention. Siblings tend to express this deprivation by being demanding, hostile, or withdrawn. Parents should be encouraged to bring their other children to visit the sibling on dialysis, visit the hospital, and join in trips to shows, parties, summer picnics, and the like. The stresses and burdens that long-term dialysis places on the family often accentuate personal problems of members of the family: psychosomatic diseases, danger of divorce, and problems between parents and their friends and co-workers [200].

Rehabilitation

The outlook for children with ESRD has improved during the past decade as a result of technical and medical advances in dialysis and transplantation. It is commonly accepted that the most effective long-term therapy for ESRD is a good working renal transplant because it offers the best hope to children for full rehabilitation and a normal life [39,198,241]. Hemodialysis and peritoneal dialysis are most often viewed as offering only interim, supportive therapy. However, increasing numbers of children require open ended long-term dialysis. Neither form of dialysis is optimal when performed in medical facilities. Home dialysis, especially peritoneal dialysis, offers certain psychological [392,417] and medical advantages [64,198]. The aim of pediatric dialysis should be not only to prolong life but also to provide a solid foundation for normal life, including physical, social, and intellectual development [200].

Early involvement by a pediatric ESRD team during the conservative phase of treatment of a child with chronic renal failure helps educate and guide patients, families, and relatives. Good support lowers the anxiety of children and their families; later, it provides the basis for an acceptable lifestyle. Once dialysis is required, successful rehabilitation during dialysis depends on early team participation and support. Adequate anticipatory guidance is best given by a well-organized and harmonious team. A teacher should be part of the dialysis team, to provide tutoring during dialysis and establish ongoing communication between the hospital and the school system to develop the best possible educational program for each child. Proper school facilities should be provided and a normal school program should be sought whenever possible. Home dialysis facilitates school attendance. The selective assistance of relatives, friends, and the clergy can be most helpful in dealing with both acute and chronic psychosocial problems.

Rehabilitation of children undergoing long-term dialysis is difficult to assess because most surveys include a combination of dialyzed and transplant patients [138]. Psychosocial rehabilitation may be defined as being able to partake in age appropriate activities and educational programs. Of the 34 children who have undergone home peritoneal dialysis for more than 6 months in our program, five infants were engaged in appropriate preschool activities, 27 older children attended regular school, and two children required home tutoring. Rehabilitation, defined as being engaged in a full school educational program, was achieved in 51 of 58 children undergoing long-term hemodialysis [803].

References

1. Abitol CL, Mrozinska K, Mandel S, et al: Effects of amino acid additives during hemodialysis of children. *J Parenter Enter Nutrition* 8(1):25, 1984.

2. Abu-Hamdan DK, Desai SG, Mahajan SK, et al: Hypoxemia during hemodialysis using acetate versus bicarbonate dialysate. *Am J Nephrol* 4:248, 1984.

3. Ackerman GL, Doherty JE, Flanigan WJ: Peritoneal dialysis and hemodialysis of tritiated digoxin. *Ann Intern Med* 67:718, 1967.

4. Ackrill P, Ralston AJ, Day JP, et al: Successful removal of aluminum from patient with dialysis encephalopathy. *Lancet* 2:692, 1980.

4a. Acute allergic reactions associated with reprocessed hemodialyzers—United States, 1989–1990. From the CDC. *JAMA* 265:1511, 1991.

5. Ahearn DJ, Maher JF: Heart failure as a complication of hemodialysis arteriovenous fistula. *Ann Intern Med* 77:201, 1972.

5a. Ahijado F, Luno J, Soto I, et al: Tuberculous peritonitis. *Contr Neph* 89:79, 1991.

5b. Ahlstrom NG, Allen SR, Tisher CC: Successful pregnancy in a patient receiving hemodialysis. *South Med J* 84:276, 1991.

6. Ahmad S, Gallagher N, Shen F: Intermittent peritoneal dialysis: Status reassessed. *Trans Am Soc Artif Organs* 25:86, 1979.

7. Akl K, Milder JE: Ketoconazole treatment of candida peritonitis during continuous peritoneal dialysis. *Pediatr Infect Dis* 3:487, 1984.

8. Aizawa Y, Ohmori T, Imai K, et al: Depressant action of acetate upon the human cardiovascular system. *Clin Nephrol* 8:477, 1977.

9. Alexander SR: CAPD in infants less than one year of age. In Fine RN, Gruskin AB (eds): *End Stage Renal Disease in Children.* Philadelphia, WB Saunders, 1984, p 149.

10. Alexander SR, Tank ES: Surgical aspects of continuous ambulatory peritoneal dialysis in infants, children and adolescents. *J Urol* 127:501, 1982.

11. Alexander SR, Tank ES, Corneil AT: Five years' experience with CAPD/CCPD catheters in infants and children. In Fine RN, Scharer K, Mehls O (eds): *CAPD in Children.* Berlin, Springer-Verlag, 1985, p 174.

12. Alexander SR, Tseng H, Maksym KA, et al: Clinical Parameters in Continuous Ambulatory Peritoneal Dialysis for Infants and Children. In Moncrief JW, Popovich RP (eds): *CAPD Update.* New York, Masson, 1981, p 195.

13. Alfrey AC: Aluminum. *Adv Clin Chem* 23:69, 1983.

14. Alfrey AC, Mishell JM, Burks JM, et al: Syndrome of dyspraxia and multifocal seizures associated with chronic dialysis. *Trans Am Soc Artif Intern Organs* 18:257, 1972.

15. Alliapoulos JC, Salusky IB, Hall T, et al: Comparison of continuous cycling peritoneal dialysis with continuous ambulatory peritoneal dialysis in children. *J Pediatr* 105:721, 1984.

16. Alon U, Bar-Maor JA, Bar-Joseph G: Effective peritoneal dialysis in an infant with extensive resection of the small intestine. *Am J Nephrol* 8:65, 1988.

17. American National Standard for Hemodialysis Systems. Association for the Advancement of Medical Instrumentation. Arlington, VA, 1978, p 3.

18. Ampel NM, White JD, Varanasi UR, et al: Coccidioidal peritonitis associated with continuous ambulatory peritoneal dialysis. *Am J Kid Dis* 11(6):512, 1988.

19. Anand SK, Northway JD, Gresham E: Peritoneal dialysis catheter for newborn and small infants. *J Pediatr* 86:985, 1975.

20. Andersen A, Taaning E, Rosenkvist J, et al: Autoimmune haemolytic anaemia treated with multiple transfusions, immunosuppressive therapy, plasma exchange, and deferrioxamine. *Acta Paediatr Scand* 73:145, 1984.

21. Anderson CB, Codd JR, Craff GM, et al: Cardiac failure and upper extremity arteriovenous dialysis fistulas. *Arch Intern Med* 136:292, 1976.

22. Andreoli SP, Bergstein JM, Sherrard DJ: Aluminum intoxication from aluminum-containing phosphate binders in children with azotemia not undergoing dialysis. *N Engl J Med* 310:1079, 1984.

22a. Andreoli SP, Cohen M: Intraperitoneal deferoxamine therapy for iron overload in children undergoing CAPD. *Kid Int* 35(6):1330, 1989.

23. Andreoli SP, West KW, Grosfeld JL, et al: A technique to eradicate tunnel infection without peritoneal dialysis catheter removal. *Perit Dial Bull* 4:156, 1984.

24. Antoniou LD, Shalhoub RJ: Zinc in the treatment of impotence in chronic renal failure. *Dial Transpl* 7:912, 1978.

25. Applebaum H, Shashikumar VL, Somers LA, et al: Improved hemodialysis access in children. *J Pediatr Surg* 15:764, 1980.

26. Arbus GS, Barnor NA, Hsu AC, et al: Effect of chronic renal failure dialysis, and transplantation on motor nerve conduction velocity in children. *Can Med Assoc J* 113:517, 1975.

27. Arieff AI: Neurological complications of uremia. *In* Brenner BM, Rector FC (eds): *The Kidney,* 2nd ed. Philadelphia, WB Saunders, 1981, p 2320.

28. Arieff AI, Guisado R, Massry SG, et al: Central nervous system pH in uremia and the effects of hemodialysis. *J Clin Invest* 58:306, 1976.

29. Arieff AI, Massry SG: Dialysis dysequilibrium syndrome. *In* Massry SG, Sellers AL (eds): *Clinical Aspects of Uremia in Dialysis.* Springfield, IL, Charles C. Thomas, 1976, p 34.

30. Arnow PM, Fellner S, Harrington R, et al: False-positive results of screening for antibodies to human immunodeficiency virus in chronic hemodialysis patients. *Am J Kid Dis* 11(5):383, 1988.

31. Arze RS, Parkinson IS, Cartlidge NEF, et al: Reversal of aluminum dialysis encephalopathy after desferrioxamine treatment. *Lancet* 2:1116, 1981.

32. Ash SR: The Lifecath peritoneal implant: study of 46 consecutive patients (abstr). *Kidney Int* 23:142, 1983.

33. Ash SR, Handt AE, Bloch R: Peritoneoscopic placement of the Tenckhoff catheter: Further clinical experience. *Perit Dial Bull* 3:8, 1983.

34. Ash SR, Winchester JF: Effect of the Peridex filter on peritonitis rates in an unselected CAPD population. *Perit Dial Bull* 4(3):S118, 1984.

35. Ash SR, Wolf GC, Bloch R: Placement of the Tenckhoff peritoneal dialysis catheter under peritoneoscopic visualization. *Dial Transplant* 10:383, 1981.

36. Assadi FK: Treatment of acute renal failure in an infant by continuous arteriovenous hemodialysis. Brief Report. *Pediatr Nephrol* 2:320, 1988.

37. Astorri E, Cambi V, Assanelli D, et al: Comparison of the left ventricular function after 1 year in 67 patients under periodical hemodialysis for renal insufficiency. *Bull Soc Ital Cardiol* 23:505, 1978.

38. Aviram A, Pfau A, Czackes JW, et al: Hyperosmolality with hyponatremia, caused by inappropriate administration of mannitol. *Am J Med* 42:648, 1967.

39. Avner ED, Harmon WE, Grupe WE, et al: Mortality of chronic hemodialysis and renal transplantation in pediatric end stage renal disease. *Pediatrics* 67:412, 1981.

40. Babb AL, Popovich RP, Christopher TG, et al: The genesis of the square meter-hour hypothesis. *Trans Am Soc Artif Int Organs* 17:81, 1971.

41. Babb AL, Strand MJ, Uvelli DA, et al: Quantitative description of dialysis treatment: A dialysis index. *Kidney Int* 7(S2):S23, 1975.

42. Bagdade JD: Hyperlipidemia and atherosclerosis in chronic dialysis patients. *In* Drukker W, Parsons FM, Maher JF (eds): *Replacement of Renal Function by Dialysis.* Boston, Martinus Nijhoff, 1983, p 588.

43. Bailey GL, Hampers CL, Hager EB, et al: Uremic pericarditis, clinical features and management. *Circulation* 38:582, 1968.

44. Bailey RE, Ford GC: The effect of heparin on sodium conservation and on the plasma concentration, the metabolic clearance and the secretion and excretion rates of aldosterone in normal subjects. *Acta Endocrinol* 60:249, 1969.

45. Baker LRI, Marshall RD: A reinvestigation of methylguandine concentration in sera from normal and uraemic subjects. *Clin Sci* 41:563, 1971.

46. Baldamus CA, Schoeppe W, Koch KM: Comparison of haemodialysis (HD) and post dilution haemofiltration (HF) on an unselected dialysis population. *Proc Eur Dial Transpl Assoc* 15:228, 1978.

47. Balfe JW: Metabolic effects of CAPD in the child. *Perit Dial Bull* 3:21, 1983.

48. Balfe JW, Irwin MA, Oreopoulos DG: An assessment of continuous ambulatory peritoneal dialysis in children. *In* Moncrief JW, Popovich RP (eds): *CAPD Update.* New York, Masson, New York, 1981, p 211.

49. Balfe JW, Hanning RM, Vigneaux A, et al: A comparison of peritoneal water and solute movement in young and older children on CAPD. *In* Fine RN, Scharer K, Mehls O (eds): *CAPD in Children.* Berlin, Springer-Verlag, 1985, p 14.

50. Balfe JW, Stefanidis CJ, Steele BT, et al: Continuous ambulatory peritoneal dialysis: Clinical aspects. *In* Fine RN, Gruskin AB (eds): *End Stage Renal Disease in Children.* Philadelphia, WB Saunders, 1984, p 135.

51. Balfe JW, Vigneux A, Willumsen J, et al: The use of CAPD in the treatment of children with end stage renal disease. *Perit Dial Bull* 1:35, 1981.

52. Baluarte HJ: Intermittent peritoneal dialysis: Technical and clinical aspects. *In* Fine RN, Gruskin AB (eds): *End Stage Renal Disease in Children.* Philadelphia, WB Saunders, 1984, p 118.

53. Baluarte JH, Gruskin AB, Hiner LB, et al: Encephalopathy in children with chronic renal failure. *Proc Clin Dial Transplant Forum* 7:95, 1977.

54. Baluarte JH, Morgenstern BZ, Kaiser BA, et al: Clinical aspects of continuous ambulatory peritoneal dialysis in children. *Dial and Transplant* 14(1):18, 1985.

55. Baluarte JH, Morgenstern BZ, Polinsky MS, et al: Peritonitis in children undergoing IPD and CAPD. *Kid Int* 27:177, 1985.

56. Baluarte JH, Polinsky MS, Prebis JW, et al: Osteomalacia of dialysis without hyperparathyroidism in children on hemodialysis. *Am J Kidney Dis Prog Abstr.* CDT Forum, p 5, 1981.

57. Bambauer R, Jutzler GA, Philippi H, et al: Hemofiltration and plasmapheresis in premature infants and newborns. *Artif Organs* 12(1):20, 1988.

58. Bana DS, Graham JR: Renin response during hemodialysis headache. *Headache* 16:168, 1976.

58a. Baraldi E, Montini G, Zanconato S, et al: Exercise tolerance after anaemia correction with recombinant human erythropoietin in end-stage renal disease. *Pediatr Nephrol* 4(6):623, 1990.

58b. Barany P, Petterson E, Ahlberg M, et al: Nutritional assessment in anemic hemodialysis patients treated with

140. Chantler C, Donckerwolcke RA, Brunner FP, et al: Combined report on regular dialysis and transplantation of children in Europe, 1978. *Proc Eur Dial Transplant Assoc* 16:74, 1979.

141. Charoenpanich R, Pollak VE, Kant KS, et al: Effect of first and subsequent use of hemodialyzers on patient well-being: The rise and fall of a syndrome associated with new dialyzer use. *Artif Organs* 11:123, 1987.

142. Chavers BM, Kjellstrand CM, Wiegand C, et al: Techniques for use of charcoal hemoperfusion in infants: Experience in two patients. *Kidney Int* 18:386, 1980.

143. Chazan BI, Rees SB, Balodimos MC, et al: Dialysis in diabetics. *JAMA* 209:2026, 1969.

144. Chesney RW, Kaplan BS, Freedom RM, et al: Acute renal failure: An important complication of cardiac surgery in infants. *J Pediat* 87:381, 1975.

145. Chesney RW, Moorthy AV, Eisman JA, et al: Increased growth after long-term oral 1,25-vitamin D435 in childhood renal osteodystrophy. *N Engl J Med* 298:238, 1978.

146. Chesney RW, Zelikovic I: Peritonitis in childhood renal disease. *Am J Nephrol* 8:147, 1988.

146a. Churchill DN: Randomized clinical trial comparing peritonitis rates among new patients using the Y-set disinfection system to standard system. *Kid Int* 35:268, 1989.

147. Cohen BD, Handlesman DG, Pai, BN: Toxicity arising from the urea cycle. *Kidney Int* 7(3):S285, 1975.

148. Cohen GF, Burgess JH, Kaye M: Peritoneal dialysis for the treatment of pericarditis in patients on chronic hemodialysis. *Can Med Assoc J* 102:1365, 1970.

149. Cole DEC, Lirenman D: Role of albumin enriched peritoneal dialysate in acute copper poisoning. *J Pediatr* 92:955, 1978.

149a. Collart FE, Tielemans CL, Wens R, et al: Citrate anticoagulation for hemodialysis patients at risk of bleeding. *Am J Nephrol* 9:236, 1989.

150. Colton CK Lowrie EG: Hemodialysis: Physical Principles and Technical Considerations. *In* Brenner BM, Rector FC Jr (eds): *The Kidney.* Philadelphia, WB Saunders, 1981, p 2425.

151. Comty CM, Shapiro FL: Cardiac complications of regular dialysis therapy. *In* Drukker W, Parsons FM, Maher JF (eds): *Replacement of Renal Function by Dialysis.* The Hague, Martinus Nijhoff, 1983, p 595.

152. Comty CM, Shapiro FL: Pretreatment and preparation of city water for hemodialysis. *In* Drukker W, Parsons FM, Maher JF (eds): *Replacement of Renal Function by Dialysis.* The Hague, Martinus Nijhoff, 1983, p 142.

153. Comty CM, Wathen R, Shapiro FL: Pericarditis in chronic uremia and its sequels. *Ann Intern Med* 75:173, 1971.

154. Comty CM, Wathen RL, Shapiro FL: Uremic pericarditis. *Cardiovasc Clin* 7:219, 1976.

155. Conley SB, Brewer ED, Gandy S, et al: Chronic continuous peritoneal dialysis in infancy; successful treatment of end-stage renal disease with achievement of normal growth rates. *Am J Kidney Dis* 1:9, 1981.

156. Cooke RE, Boyden DG, Haller EH: The relationship of acidosis and growth retardation. *J Pediatr* 57:326, 1960.

157. Continuous ambulatory and continuous cycling peritoneal dialysis in children. A report of the Southwest Pediatric Nephrology Study Group. *Kidney Intern* 27:558, 1985.

158. Copley JB, FACP, COL, MC: Prevention of peritoneal dialysis catheter-related infections. *Am J of Kid Dis* 10(6):401, 1987.

159. Coronel F, Maranjo P, Torrente J, et al: The risk of retrograde menstruation in CAPD patients. *Perit Dial Bull* 4:191, 1984.

160. Cotran RS: The fine structure of the microvasculature in relation to normal and altered permeability. *In* Reeve EB, Guyton AC (eds): *Physical Bases of Circulatory Transport: Regulation and Exchange.* Philadelphia, WB Saunders, 1967, p 249.

161. Corea AL: Review of pediatric hemodialysis nursing and technical skills. *Dial Transplant* 13:573, 1984.

162. Counahan R, Cameron JS, Ogg C, et al: The presentation, management, complications and outcome of acute renal failure in childhood. *Br Med J* 1:599, 1977.

163. Counahan R, El-Bishti M, Cox, BD, et al: Plasma amino acids in children and adolescents on hemodialysis. *Kidney Int* 10:471, 1976.

164. Counts S, Hickman R, Garbaccio A, et al: Chronic home peritoneal dialysis in children. *Trans Am Soc Artif Intern Organs* 19:157, 1973.

165. Craddock PR, Fehr J, Brigham KL, et al: Complement and leukocyte-mediated pulmonary dysfunction in hemodialysis. *N Engl J Med* 296:769, 1977.

166. Cutler RE, Pettis JL: Thyroid function in renal disease. *Dialysis Transplant* 16:566, 1987.

167. D'Apuzzo VG, Grushkin CM, Brennan LP, et al: Saphenous vein autograft arteriovenous fistula for extended hemodialysis in children. *Acta Pediatr Scand* 62:28, 1973.

167a. Dabbagh S, Clement K, Ryckaert A, et al: One year later: A prospective study of the efficacy and safety of recombinant human erythropoietin in children undergoing hemo and continuous cycling peritoneal dialysis. *Pediatr Res* 29:340A, 1991.

168. Dabbagh S, Chesney RW: Treatment of renal osteodystrophy during childhood. *In* Fine RN, Gruskin AB (eds): *End Stage Renal Disease in Children.* Philadelphia, WB Saunders, 1984, p 251.

168a. Dabbagh S, Fassinger N, Clement K, et al: The effect of aggressive nutrition on infection rates in patients maintained on peritoneal dialysis. Advances in *Peritoneal Dialysis* 7:161, 1991.

168b. Dabbagh S, McWilliams D, Gruskin A, et al: Effect of recombinant human erythropoietin on circulating lymphocytotoxic antibody levels in pediatric patients undergoing hemo and continuous cycling peritoneal dialysis. *Pediatr Res* 29:340A, 1991.

169. Daniels FH, Leonard EF, Cortell S: Glucose and glycerol compared as osmotic agents for peritoneal dialysis. *Kidney Int* 25:20, 1984.

170. Dau PC, Bennington JL: Plasmapheresis in childhood dermatomyositis. *J Pediatr* 98:237, 1981.

171. Daugirdas JT, Ing TS: First-used reactions during hemodialysis: A definition of subtypes. *Kidney Int* 33(24):S37, 1988.

172. Daugirdas JT, Ing TS, Roxe DM, et al: Severe anaphylactoid reactions to cuprammonium cellulose dialyzers. *Arch Intern Med* 145:489, 1985.

173. Daugirdas JT, Leehey DJ, Popli S, et al: Induction of peritoneal fluid eosinophilia and/or monocytosis by intraperitoneal air injection. *Am J Nephrol* 7:116, 1987.

173a. Davidson CJ, Newman GE, Sheikh KH, et al: Mechanisms of angioplasty in hemodialysis fistula stenoses evaluated by intravascular ultrasound. *Kid Int* 40:91, 1991.

174. Davis FB, Spector DA, Davis PJ, et al: Comparison of pituitary-thyroid function in patients with end-stage renal disease and in age and sex-matched controls. *Kidney Int* 21:362, 1982.

175. Davis JB Jr, Howell CG, Humphries AL Jr: Hemodialysis access: Elevated basilic vein arteriovenous fistula. *J Pediatr Surg* 21(12):1182, 1986.

21. Anderson CB, Codd JR, Craff GM, et al: Cardiac failure and upper extremity arteriovenous dialysis fistulas. *Arch Intern Med* 136:292, 1976.

22. Andreoli SP, Bergstein JM, Sherrard DJ: Aluminum intoxication from aluminum-containing phosphate binders in children with azotemia not undergoing dialysis. *N Engl J Med* 310:1079, 1984.

22a. Andreoli SP, Cohen M: Intraperitoneal deferoxamine therapy for iron overload in children undergoing CAPD. *Kid Int* 35(6):1330, 1989.

23. Andreoli SP, West KW, Grosfeld JL, et al: A technique to eradicate tunnel infection without peritoneal dialysis catheter removal. *Perit Dial Bull* 4:156, 1984.

24. Antoniou LD, Shalhoub RJ: Zinc in the treatment of impotence in chronic renal failure. *Dial Transpl* 7:912, 1978.

25. Applebaum H, Shashikumar VL, Somers LA, et al: Improved hemodialysis access in children. *J Pediatr Surg* 15:764, 1980.

26. Arbus GS, Barnor NA, Hsu AC, et al: Effect of chronic renal failure dialysis, and transplantation on motor nerve conduction velocity in children. *Can Med Assoc J* 113:517, 1975.

27. Arieff AI: Neurological complications of uremia. *In* Brenner BM, Rector FC (eds): *The Kidney*, 2nd ed. Philadelphia, WB Saunders, 1981, p 2320.

28. Arieff AI, Guisado R, Massry SG, et al: Central nervous system pH in uremia and the effects of hemodialysis. *J Clin Invest* 58:306, 1976.

29. Arieff AI, Massry SG: Dialysis dysequilibrium syndrome. *In* Massry SG, Sellers AL (eds): *Clinical Aspects of Uremia in Dialysis*. Springfield, IL, Charles C. Thomas, 1976, p 34.

30. Arnow PM, Fellner S, Harrington R, et al: False-positive results of screening for antibodies to human immunodeficiency virus in chronic hemodialysis patients. *Am J Kid Dis* 11(5):383, 1988.

31. Arze RS, Parkinson IS, Cartlidge NEF, et al: Reversal of aluminum dialysis encephalopathy after desferrioxamine treatment. *Lancet* 2:1116, 1981.

32. Ash SR: The Lifecath peritoneal implant: study of 46 consecutive patients (abstr). *Kidney Int* 23:142, 1983.

33. Ash SR, Handt AE, Bloch R: Peritoneoscopic placement of the Tenckhoff catheter: Further clinical experience. *Perit Dial Bull* 3:8, 1983.

34. Ash SR, Winchester JF: Effect of the Peridex filter on peritonitis rates in an unselected CAPD population. *Perit Dial Bull* 4(3):S118, 1984.

35. Ash SR, Wolf GC, Bloch R: Placement of the Tenckhoff peritoneal dialysis catheter under peritoneoscopic visualization. *Dial Transplant* 10:383, 1981.

36. Assadi FK: Treatment of acute renal failure in an infant by continuous arteriovenous hemodialysis. Brief Report. *Pediatr Nephrol* 2:320, 1988.

37. Astorri E, Cambi V, Assanelli D, et al: Comparison of the left ventricular function after 1 year in 67 patients under periodical hemodialysis for renal insufficiency. *Bull Soc Ital Cardiol* 23:505, 1978.

38. Aviram A, Pfau A, Czackes JW, et al: Hyperosmolality with hyponatremia, caused by inappropriate administration of mannitol. *Am J Med* 42:648, 1967.

39. Avner ED, Harmon WE, Grupe WE, et al: Mortality of chronic hemodialysis and renal transplantation in pediatric end stage renal disease. *Pediatrics* 67:412, 1981.

40. Babb AL, Popovich RP, Christopher TG, et al: The genesis of the square meter-hour hypothesis. *Trans Am Soc Artif Int Organs* 17:81, 1971.

41. Babb AL, Strand MJ, Uvelli DA, et al: Quantitative description of dialysis treatment: A dialysis index. *Kidney Int* 7(S2):S23, 1975.

42. Bagdade JD: Hyperlipidemia and atherosclerosis in chronic dialysis patients. *In* Drukker W, Parsons FM, Maher JF (eds): *Replacement of Renal Function by Dialysis*. Boston, Martinus Nijhoff, 1983, p 588.

43. Bailey GL, Hampers CL, Hager EB, et al: Uremic pericarditis, clinical features and management. *Circulation* 38:582, 1968.

44. Bailey RE, Ford GC: The effect of heparin on sodium conservation and on the plasma concentration, the metabolic clearance and the secretion and excretion rates of aldosterone in normal subjects. *Acta Endocrinol* 60:249, 1969.

45. Baker LRI, Marshall RD: A reinvestigation of methylguandine concentration in sera from normal and uraemic subjects. *Clin Sci* 41:563, 1971.

46. Baldamus CA, Schoeppe W, Koch KM: Comparison of haemodialysis (HD) and post dilution haemofiltration (HF) on an unselected dialysis population. *Proc Eur Dial Transpl Assoc* 15:228, 1978.

47. Balfe JW: Metabolic effects of CAPD in the child. *Perit Dial Bull* 3:21, 1983.

48. Balfe JW, Irwin MA, Oreopoulos DG: An assessment of continuous ambulatory peritoneal dialysis in children. *In* Moncrief JW, Popovich RP (eds): *CAPD Update*. New York, Masson, New York, 1981, p 211.

49. Balfe JW, Hanning RM, Vigneaux A, et al: A comparison of peritoneal water and solute movement in young and older children on CAPD. *In* Fine RN, Scharer K, Mehls O (eds): *CAPD in Children*. Berlin, Springer-Verlag, 1985, p 14.

50. Balfe JW, Stefanidis CJ, Steele BT, et al: Continuous ambulatory peritoneal dialysis: Clinical aspects. *In* Fine RN, Gruskin AB (eds): *End Stage Renal Disease in Children*. Philadelphia, WB Saunders, 1984, p 135.

51. Balfe JW, Vigneux A, Willumsen J, et al: The use of CAPD in the treatment of children with end stage renal disease. *Perit Dial Bull* 1:35, 1981.

52. Baluarte HJ: Intermittent peritoneal dialysis: Technical and clinical aspects. *In* Fine RN, Gruskin AB (eds): *End Stage Renal Disease in Children*. Philadelphia, WB Saunders, 1984, p 118.

53. Baluarte JH, Gruskin AB, Hiner LB, et al: Encephalopathy in children with chronic renal failure. *Proc Clin Dial Transplant Forum* 7:95, 1977.

54. Baluarte JH, Morgenstern BZ, Kaiser BA, et al: Clinical aspects of continuous ambulatory peritoneal dialysis in children. *Dial and Transplant* 14(1):18, 1985.

55. Baluarte JH, Morgenstern BZ, Polinsky MS, et al: Peritonitis in children undergoing IPD and CAPD. *Kid Int* 27:177, 1985.

56. Baluarte JH, Polinsky MS, Prebis JW, et al: Osteomalacia of dialysis without hyperparathyroidism in children on hemodialysis. *Am J Kidney Dis Prog Abstr*. CDT Forum, p 5, 1981.

57. Bambauer R, Jutzler GA, Philippi H, et al: Hemofiltration and plasmapheresis in premature infants and newborns. *Artif Organs* 12(1):20, 1988.

58. Bana DS, Graham JR: Renin response during hemodialysis headache. *Headache* 16:168, 1976.

58a. Baraldi E, Montini G, Zanconato S, et al: Exercise tolerance after anaemia correction with recombinant human erythropoietin in end-stage renal disease. *Pediatr Nephrol* 4(6):623, 1990.

58b. Barany P, Petterson E, Ahlberg M, et al: Nutritional assessment in anemic hemodialysis patients treated with recombinant human erythropoietin. *Clin Neph* 35:270, 1991.

59. Barbour GL, Sevier BR: Adrenal responsiveness of chronic hemodialysis. *N Engl J Med* 290:1258, 1974.

59a. Bargman JM: Complications of peritoneal dialysis related to raised intra-abdominal pressure. *Dial Trans* 19:70, 1990.

60. Barry KG, Swartz FD: Peritoneal dialysis: Current status and future applications. *Pediat Clin North Am* 11:593, 1964.

61. Bartel U, et al: Effect of dialysis on serum carnitine, free fatty acids, and triglyceride levels in man and the rat. *Metabolism* 31:944, 1982.

62. Baskin SE, Wozniak RF: Hyperbaric oxygenation in the treatment of hemodialysis associated air embolism. *N Engl J Med* 293:184, 1975.

63. Bastani B, Mifflin TE, Lovell MA, et al: Serum amylases in chronic and end-stage renal failure: Effects of mode of therapy, race, diabetes and peritonitis. *Am J Nephrol* 7:292, 1987.

64. Baum M, Powell D, Calvin S, et al: Continuous ambulatory peritoneal dialysis in children: Comparison with hemodialysis. *N Engl J Med* 307:1537, 1982.

65. Bay WH, Cerilli GJ, Erlich L, et al: Analysis of a new technique to establish the chronic peritoneal dialysis catheter. *Am J Kidney Dis* 3:133, 1983.

66. Bechar M, Lakke JPWF, van der Hem GK, et al: Subdural hematoma during long-term dialysis. *Arch Neurol* 26:513, 1972.

67. Bell JD, Kincaid WR, Morgan RG, et al: Serum ferritin assay and bone-marrow iron stores in patients on maintenance hemodialysis. *Kidney Int* 17:242, 1980.

68. Benz RL, Schleifer CR: Hydrothorax in continuous ambulatory peritoneal dialysis: Successful treatment with intrapleural Tetracycline and a review of the literature. *Am J Kid Dis* 5:136, 1985.

69. Benz RL, Siegfried JW, Teehan BP: Carpal tunnel syndrome in dialysis patients: Comparison between continous ambulatory peritoneal dialysis and hemodialysis populations. *Am J Kid Dis* 11(6):473, 1988.

70. Berger M, James GP, Davis ER, et al: Hyperlipidemia in uremic children: Response to peritoneal dialysis and hemodialysis. *Clin Nephrol* 9:19, 1978.

71. Bergstrom H, Asaba H, Furst P, et al: Dialysis, ultrafiltration and blood pressure. *Proc Eur Dial Transpl Assoc* 13:293, 1976.

72. Berkes SL, Kahn SI, Chazan JA, et al: Prolonged hemolysis from overheated dialysate. *Ann Intern Med* 83:363, 1975.

73. Berlyne GM, Lee HA, Ralston AJ, et al: Pulmonary complications of peritoneal dialysis. *Lancet* 2:75, 1966.

74. Berlyne GM, Shaw AB: Red eyes in renal failure. *Lancet* 1:4, 1967.

75. Bertoli M, Gasparotto ML, Vertolli U, et al: Does hypercoagulability exist in CAPD patients? *Perit Dial Bull* 4:237, 1984.

76. Bettinelli A, Bianchi ML, Aimini E, et al: Effects of 1,25-dihydroxyvitamin-D$_3$ treatment on mineral balance in children with end stage renal disease undergoing chronic hemofiltration. *Pediatr Res* 20(1):5, 1986.

77. Betts PR, Magrath G: Growth pattern and dietary intake of children with chronic renal insufficiency. *Br Med J* 2:189, 1974.

78. Bhasin HK, Dana CL: Spontaneous retroperitoneal hemorrhage in chronically hemodialyzed patients. *Nephron* 22:322, 1978.

79. Bilbrey GL, Carter NW, White MG, et al: Potassium deficiency in chronic renal failure. *Kidney Int* 4:423, 1973.

80. Bilbrey GL, Faloona GR, White MG, et al: Hyperglucagonemia of renal failure. *J Clin Invest* 53:841, 1974.

80a. Bjerke HS, Adkins ES, Foglia RP: Surgical correction of hydrothorax from diaphragmatic eventration in children on peritoneal dialysis. *Surgery* 109:550, 1991.

81. Blackburn SL: Dietary compliance of chronic hemodialysis patients. *J Am Diet Assoc* 70:31, 1977.

82. Blagg CR: Acute complications associated with hemodialysis: *In* Drukker W, Parsons FM, Maher JF (eds): *Replacement of Renal Function by Dialysis*. Boston, Martinus Nijhoff, 1978, p 611.

83. Blagg CR: Adequacy of dialysis. *Am J Kidney Dis* 4(3):218, 1984.

84. Blaufox MD: Physical concepts of hemodialysis. *In* Hampers CL, Schupak ES (eds): *Long-Term Hemodialysis*. New York, Grune & Stratton, 1967, p 13.

85. Blumberg A, Esslen E, Burgi W: Myoinositol—a uremic neurotoxin. *Nephron* 21:186, 1978.

86. Blumenkrantz MJ, Kopple JD, Gutman RA, et al: Methods for assessing nutritional status of patients with renal failure. *Am J Clin Nutr* 33:1567, 1980.

87. Blumenkrantz MJ, Lindsay RM: Comparisons of hemodialysis and peritoneal dialysis: A review of the literature. *Contrib Nephrol* 17:20, 1979.

88. Blumenkrantz MK, Moran JK, Coburn JW: Peritoneal clearances during prolonged maintenance peritoneal dialysis in diabetic and non-diabetic patients. *Kidney Int* 14:671, 1978.

89. Blumenkrantz MJ, Schmidt RW: Managing the nutritional concerns of the patient undergoing peritoneal dialysis. *In* Nolph KD (ed): *Peritoneal Dialysis*. Boston, Martinus Nijhoff, 1981, p 281.

90. Boen ST: Kinetics of peritoneal dialysis: A comparison with the artificial kidney. *Medicine (Baltimore)* 40:243, 1961.

91. Boen ST: Overview and history of peritoneal dialysis. *Dial Transplant* 6(2):14, 1977.

92. Boen ST, Mulinari AS, Dillard DH, et al: Periodic peritoneal dialysis in the management of chronic uremia. *Trans Am Soc Artif Intern Organs* 8:256, 1962.

93. Boghen D: Successful treatment of restless legs with clonazepam. *Ann Neurol* 6:341, 1979.

94. Boineau FG, Fisher JW, Lewy JE: Anemia in children with ESRD. *In* Fine RN, Gruskin AB (eds): *End Stage Renal Disease in Children*. Philadelphia, WB Saunders, 1984, p 375.

95. Bone JM, Davison AM, Robson JS: Role of dialysate calcium concentration in osteoporosis in patients on hemodialysis. *Lancet* 1:1047, 1972.

96. Bone GE, Pomajel MJ: Prospective comparison of polytetrafluoroethylene and bovine grafts for dialysis. *J Surg Res* 29:223, 1980.

97. Bonzel KE, Mehls O, Graning M, et al: Transperitoneal movements of solutes of different molecular size in children on CAPD. *In* Fine RN, Schärer K, Mehls O (eds): *CAPD in Children*. Berlin, Springer-Verlag, 1985, p 20.

98. Bora S, Kleinfeld M: Subcapsular liver hematomas in a patient on chronic hemodialysis. *Ann Intern Med* 93:574, 1980.

99. Borges HF, Hocks J, Kjellstrand CM: Mannitol intoxication in patients with renal failure. *Arch Intern Med* 142:63, 1982.

99a. Bourquelot P, Cussenot O, Corbi P, et al: Microsurgical creation and follow-up arteriovenous fistulae for chronic haemodialysis in children. *Pediatr Nephrol* 4:156, 1990.

100. Bourquelot P, Wolfeler L, Lamy L: Microsurgery for haemodialysis distal arteriovenous fistulae in children weigh-

ing less than 10 kg. *Proc Eur Dial Transplant Assoc* 18:537, 1981.

101. Bower JD, Coleman TG: Circulatory function during chronic hemodialysis. *Trans Am Soc Artif Intern Organs* 15:373, 1969.

102. Brandis M, Offner G, Krohn HP, et al: Plasmapheresis in a 13-year-old girl with Goodpasture-like syndrome. *In* Bulla M (ed): *Dialysis and Kidney Transplantation in Children.* Melsungen, Bibliomed, 1979, p 171.

103. Breborowicz A, Knapowski J: Studies on the resistance of the peritoneal mesothelium to solute transport. *Perit Dial Bull* 4:37, 1984.

104. Brem AS, Toscano AM: Continuous cycling peritoneal dialysis for children: An alternative to hemodialysis treatment. *Pediatrics* 74:254, 1984.

105. Brescia MJ, Cimino JE, Appel K, et al: Chronic hemodialysis using venipuncture and a surgically created arteriovenous fistula. *N Engl J Med* 275:1089, 1966.

106. Brewer EJ, Nickeson RW Jr, Rossen RD, et al: Plasma exchange in selected patients with juvenile rheumatoid arthritis. *J Paediatr* 98:194, 1981.

107. Brouhard GH, Berger M, Cunningham RJ, et al: Home peritoneal dialysis in children. *Trans Am Soc Artif Intern Organs* 25:90, 1979.

108. Brown ST, Ahearn DJ, Nolph KD: Potassium removal with peritoneal dialysis. *Kidney Int* 4:67, 1983.

109. Brown DJ, Dawborn JK, Ham KN, et al: Treatment of dialysis osteomalacia with desferrioxamine. *Lancet* 2:343, 1982.

110. Broyer M: Incidence and etiology in ESRD in children. *In* Fine RN, Gruskin AB (eds): *End Stage Renal Disease in Children.* Philadelphia, WB Saunders, 1984, p 9.

111. Broyer M, Donckerwolcke R, Brunner F, et al: Combined report on regular dialysis and transplantation in Europe, 1980. *Proc Eur Dial Transplant Assoc* 18:59, 1981.

112. Broyer M, Niaudet P, Champion G, et al: Nutritional and metabolic studies in children on continuous ambulatory peritoneal dialysis. *Kidney Inter* 24:S106, 1983.

113. Broyer M, Rizzoni G, Donckerwolcke R, et al: CAPD in children: Data from the European Dialysis and Transplant Association (EDTA) Registry. *In* Fine RN, Scharer K, Mehls O (eds): *CAPD in Children.* Berlin, Springer-Verlag, 1985, p 30.

114. Broyer M, Tete MJ, Laudat MH, et al: Plasma lipid abnormalities in children on chronic hemodialysis: Relationship to dietary intake. *Proc Eur Dial Transplant Assoc* 13:385, 1976.

115. Brunner FP, Brynger H, Chantler C, et al: Combined report on regular dialysis and tranplantation in Europe, IX, 1978. *Proc Eur Dial Transpl Assoc* 16:43, 1979.

116. Brunzell JD, Albers JJ, Haas LB, et al: Prevalence of serum lipid abnormalities in chronic hemodialysis. *Metabolism* 26:903, 1977.

117. Bucciant G, Bianch ML, Valenti G: Progress of renal osteodystrophy during continuous ambulatory peritoneal dialysis. *Clin Nephrol* 22:279, 1984.

118. Bulla M, Delling G, Offermann G, et al: Renal bone disorder in children: Therapy with vitamin D3 or 1,25-dihydroxycholecalciferol (1,25-DHCC). *In* Norman AW (ed): *Vitamin D: Basic Research and Its Clinical Application.* Berlin, Walter de Gruyter, 1979, p 853.

119. Bunchman TE, Wood EG, Lynch RE: Hydrothorax as a complication of pediatric peritoneal dialysis. *Perit Dial Bull* 7(4):237, 1987.

119a. Burkart JB, Haigler S, Carunana R, et al: Usefulness of peritoneal fluid amylase levels in the differential diagnosis of peritonitis in peritoneal dialysis patients. *J Am Soc Neph* 1:1186, 1991.

120. Buselmeier TJ, Davin TD, Simmons RL et al: Treatment of intractable uremic pericardial effusion. Avoidance of pericardiectomy with local steroid installation. *JAMA* 240:1358, 1978.

121. Buselmeier TJ, Santiago EA, Simmons RL, et al: Arteriovenous shunts for pediatric hemodialysis. *Surgery* 70:638, 1971.

122. Callaghan N: Restless legs syndrome in uremic neuropathy. *Neurology* 16:359, 1961.

123. Callis LM, Clanxet J, Fortuny G, et al: Hepatitis B virus infection and vaccination in children undergoing hemodialysis. *Acta Paediatr Scand* 74:213, 1985.

123a. Canadian Erythropoietin Study Group: Association between recombinant human erythropoietin and quality of life and exercise capacity of patients receiving haemodialysis. *Br Med J* 300(6724):573, 1990.

124. Campion DS, North JP: Effect of protein binding of barbiturates on their rate of removal during peritoneal dialysis. *J Lab Clin Med* 66:549, 1965.

125. Capelli JP, Kasparian H: Cardiac work demands and left ventricular function in end-stage renal disease. *Ann Intern Med* 86:261, 1977.

126. Carlson DJ, Shapiro GL: Methemoglobinemia from well water nitrates: a complication of home dialysis. *Ann Intern Med* 73:757, 1970.

127. Carney SL, Alastair HB, Gillies MB: Acute dialysis hypercalcemia and dialysis phosphate loss. *Am J Kid Dis* 11(5):377, 1988.

128. Caro J, Brown S, Miller O, et al: Erythropoietin levels in uremic, nephric and anephric patients. *J Lab Clin Med* 93:449, 1979.

129. Caruana RJ, Burkart J, Segraves D, et al: Serum and peritoneal fluid amylase levels in CAPD. Clinical Studies. *Am J Nephrol* 7:169, 1987.

130. Castaldi PA, Rozenberg MC, Steward JH: The bleeding disorder of uraemia. *Lancet* 2:66, 1966.

131. Centers for Disease Control: Recommendations for providing dialysis treatment to patients infected with human T-lymphotropic virus type III/lymphadenopathy-associated virus. *MMWR* 35:376, 383, 1986.

132. Centers for Disease Control: Recommendations for prevention of HIV transmission in health-care settings. *MMWR* 36:(Suppl 2):3, 1987.

132a. Centers for Disease Control: Recommendations for preventing transmission of human immuno-deficiency virus and hepatitis B virus to patients during exposure-prone invasive procedures. *MMWR* 40:1, 1991.

133. Chan JCM: Hemodialysis in children: A 12 months experience. *Virg Med J* 107:141, 1980.

134. Chan JCM, Campbell RA: Peritoneal dialysis in children: a survey of its indications and applications. *Clin Pediatrics* 12:131, 1973.

135. Chan JCM, DeLuca HF: Growth velocity in a child on prolonged hemodialysis: Beneficial effect of 1-hydroxyvitamin D435. *JAMA* 238:2053, 1977.

136. Chan JCM, Eng G: Long-term hemodialysis and nerve conduction in children. *Pediatr Res* 13:591, 1979.

137. Chan MK, Chow L, Lam SS, et al: Peritoneal eosinophilia in patients on continuous ambulatory peritoneal dialysis: A prospective study. *Am J Kid Dis* 11(2):180, 1988.

138. Chantler C, Broyer M, Donckerwolcke RA, et al: Growth and rehabilitation of long term survivors of treatment of end stage renal failure in childhood. *Proc Eur Dial Transpl Assoc* 18:329, 1981.

139. Chantler C, Donckerwolcke RA, Broyer MJC: Pediatric dialysis. *In* Drukker W, Parsons F, Maher J (eds): *Replacement of Renal Function by Dialysis,* 2nd ed. The Hague, Martinus Nijhoff, 1982, p 514.

140. Chantler C, Donckerwolcke RA, Brunner FP, et al: Combined report on regular dialysis and transplantation of children in Europe, 1978. *Proc Eur Dial Transplant Assoc* 16:74, 1979.

141. Charoenpanich R, Pollak VE, Kant KS, et al: Effect of first and subsequent use of hemodialyzers on patient well-being: The rise and fall of a syndrome associated with new dialyzer use. *Artif Organs* 11:123, 1987.

142. Chavers BM, Kjellstrand CM, Wiegand C, et al: Techniques for use of charcoal hemoperfusion in infants: Experience in two patients. *Kidney Int* 18:386, 1980.

143. Chazan BI, Rees SB, Balodimos MC, et al: Dialysis in diabetics. *JAMA* 209:2026, 1969.

144. Chesney RW, Kaplan BS, Freedom RM, et al: Acute renal failure: An important complication of cardiac surgery in infants. *J Pediat* 87:381, 1975.

145. Chesney RW, Moorthy AV, Eisman JA, et al: Increased growth after long-term oral 1,25-vitamin D435 in childhood renal osteodystrophy. *N Engl J Med* 298:238, 1978.

146. Chesney RW, Zelikovic I: Peritonitis in childhood renal disease. *Am J Nephrol* 8:147, 1988.

146a. Churchill DN: Randomized clinical trial comparing peritonitis rates among new patients using the Y-set disinfection system to standard system. *Kid Int* 35:268, 1989.

147. Cohen BD, Handlesman DG, Pai, BN: Toxicity arising from the urea cycle. *Kidney Int* 7(3):S285, 1975.

148. Cohen GF, Burgess JH, Kaye M: Peritoneal dialysis for the treatment of pericarditis in patients on chronic hemodialysis. *Can Med Assoc J* 102:1365, 1970.

149. Cole DEC, Lirenman D: Role of albumin enriched peritoneal dialysate in acute copper poisoning. *J Pediatr* 92:955, 1978.

149a. Collart FE, Tielemans CL, Wens R, et al: Citrate anticoagulation for hemodialysis patients at risk of bleeding. *Am J Nephrol* 9:236, 1989.

150. Colton CK Lowrie EG: Hemodialysis: Physical Principles and Technical Considerations. *In* Brenner BM, Rector FC Jr (eds): *The Kidney.* Philadelphia, WB Saunders, 1981, p 2425.

151. Comty CM, Shapiro FL: Cardiac complications of regular dialysis therapy. *In* Drukker W, Parsons FM, Maher JF (eds): *Replacement of Renal Function by Dialysis.* The Hague, Martinus Nijhoff, 1983, p 595.

152. Comty CM, Shapiro FL: Pretreatment and preparation of city water for hemodialysis. *In* Drukker W, Parsons FM, Maher JF (eds): *Replacement of Renal Function by Dialysis.* The Hague, Martinus Nijhoff, 1983, p 142.

153. Comty CM, Wathen R, Shapiro FL: Pericarditis in chronic uremia and its sequels. *Ann Intern Med* 75:173, 1971.

154. Comty CM, Wathen RL, Shapiro FL: Uremic pericarditis. *Cardiovasc Clin* 7:219, 1976.

155. Conley SB, Brewer ED, Gandy S, et al: Chronic continuous peritoneal dialysis in infancy; successful treatment of end-stage renal disease with achievement of normal growth rates. *Am J Kidney Dis* 1:9, 1981.

156. Cooke RE, Boyden DG, Haller EH: The relationship of acidosis and growth retardation. *J Pediatr* 57:326, 1960.

157. Continuous ambulatory and continuous cycling peritoneal dialysis in children. A report of the Southwest Pediatric Nephrology Study Group. *Kidney Intern* 27:558, 1985.

158. Copley JB, FACP, COL, MC: Prevention of peritoneal dialysis catheter-related infections. *Am J of Kid Dis* 10(6):401, 1987.

159. Coronel F, Maranjo P, Torrente J, et al: The risk of retrograde menstruation in CAPD patients. *Perit Dial Bull* 4:191, 1984.

160. Cotran RS: The fine structure of the microvasculature in relation to normal and altered permeability. *In* Reeve EB, Guyton AC (eds): *Physical Bases of Circulatory Transport: Regulation and Exchange.* Philadelphia, WB Saunders, 1967, p 249.

161. Corea AL: Review of pediatric hemodialysis nursing and technical skills. *Dial Transplant* 13:573, 1984.

162. Counahan R, Cameron JS, Ogg C, et al: The presentation, management, complications and outcome of acute renal failure in childhood. *Br Med J* 1:599, 1977.

163. Counahan R, El-Bishti M, Cox, BD, et al: Plasma amino acids in children and adolescents on hemodialysis. *Kidney Int* 10:471, 1976.

164. Counts S, Hickman R, Garbaccio A, et al: Chronic home peritoneal dialysis in children. *Trans Am Soc Artif Intern Organs* 19:157, 1973.

165. Craddock PR, Fehr J, Brigham KL, et al: Complement and leukocyte-mediated pulmonary dysfunction in hemodialysis. *N Engl J Med* 296:769, 1977.

166. Cutler RE, Pettis JL: Thyroid function in renal disease. *Dialysis Transplant* 16:566, 1987.

167. D'Apuzzo VG, Grushkin CM, Brennan LP, et al: Saphenous vein autograft arteriovenous fistula for extended hemodialysis in children. *Acta Pediatr Scand* 62:28, 1973.

167a. Dabbagh S, Clement K, Ryckaert A, et al: One year later: A prospective study of the efficacy and safety of recombinant human erythropoietin in children undergoing hemo and continuous cycling peritoneal dialysis. *Pediatr Res* 29:340A, 1991.

168. Dabbagh S, Chesney RW: Treatment of renal osteodystrophy during childhood. *In* Fine RN, Gruskin AB (eds): *End Stage Renal Disease in Children.* Philadelphia, WB Saunders, 1984, p 251.

168a. Dabbagh S, Fassinger N, Clement K, et al: The effect of aggressive nutrition on infection rates in patients maintained on peritoneal dialysis. Advances in *Peritoneal Dialysis* 7:161, 1991.

168b. Dabbagh S, McWilliams D, Gruskin A, et al: Effect of recombinant human erythropoietin on circulating lymphocytotoxic antibody levels in pediatric patients undergoing hemo and continuous cycling peritoneal dialysis. *Pediatr Res* 29:340A, 1991.

169. Daniels FH, Leonard EF, Cortell S: Glucose and glycerol compared as osmotic agents for peritoneal dialysis. *Kidney Int* 25:20, 1984.

170. Dau PC, Bennington JL: Plasmapheresis in childhood dermatomyositis. *J Pediatr* 98:237, 1981.

171. Daugirdas JT, Ing TS: First-used reactions during hemodialysis: A definition of subtypes. *Kidney Int* 33(24):S37, 1988.

172. Daugirdas JT, Ing TS, Roxe DM, et al: Severe anaphylactoid reactions to cuprammonium cellulose dialyzers. *Arch Intern Med* 145:489, 1985.

173. Daugirdas JT, Leehey DJ, Popli S, et al: Induction of peritoneal fluid eosinophilia and/or monocytosis by intraperitoneal air injection. *Am J Nephrol* 7:116, 1987.

173a. Davidson CJ, Newman GE, Sheikh KH, et al: Mechanisms of angioplasty in hemodialysis fistula stenoses evaluated by intravascular ultrasound. *Kid Int* 40:91, 1991.

174. Davis FB, Spector DA, Davis PJ, et al: Comparison of pituitary-thyroid function in patients with end-stage renal disease and in age and sex-matched controls. *Kidney Int* 21:362, 1982.

175. Davis JB Jr, Howell CG, Humphries AL Jr: Hemodialysis access: Elevated basilic vein arteriovenous fistula. *J Pediatr Surg* 21(12):1182, 1986.

176. Deane N: Dialyzer reuse and therapeutic effect. *Contemp Dial* 5:40, 1984.

177. Deane N, Bemis JA: Multiple use of hemodialyzers. *In* Drukker W, Parsons FM, Maher JF, (eds): *Replacement of Renal Function by Dialysis.* The Hague, Martinus Nijhoff, 1983, p 286.

178. DeBroe ME, Heyrman RM, Debacker WA, et al: Pathogenesis of dialysis-induced hypoxemia: A short overview. *Kidney Int* 33(24):S57, 1988.

178a. Debruyne D, Ryckelynck J-P, Moulin M, et al: Pharmacokinetics of fluconazole in patients undergoing continuous ambulatory peritoneal dialysis. *Clin Pharmacokinet* 18:491, 1990.

179. De Fronzo RA: Pathogenesis of glucose intolerance in uremia. *Metabolism* 27:1866, 1978.

180. Delaporte C, Bergstrom J, Broyer M: Variations in muscle cell protein of severely uremic children. *Kidney Int* 10:239, 1976.

181. Delmez JA, Slatopolsky E, Martin KJ, et al: Minerals, vitamin D, and parathyroid hormone in continuous ambulatory peritoneal dialysis. *Kidney Int* 21:862, 1982.

182. De los Santos CA, von Eye O, d'Avila D, et al: Rupture of the spleen: A complication of continuous ambulatory peritoneal dialysis. *Perit Dial Bull* 6(4):203, 1986.

183. De Pace NL, Nestico PF, Schwartz AB, et al: Predicting success of intensive dialysis in the treatment of uremic pericarditis. *Am J Med* 76:38, 1984.

184. De Santo NG, Capodicasa G, Dileo VA, et al: Kinetics of amino acids equilibration in the dialysate during CAPD. *Int J Art Organs* 4:23, 1981.

185. Diamond SM, Henrich WL: Acetate dialysate versus bicarbonate dialysate: A continuing controversy. In-Depth Review. *Am J Kid Dis* 9(1):3, 1987.

186. Diaz-Buxo JA: Anatomy and Physiology: The durability of the peritoneal membrane. *Perit Dial Bull* 4:85, 1984.

187. Diaz-Buxo JA, Chandler JT, Farmer CD, et al: Long-term observation of peritoneal clearances in patients undergoing peritoneal dialysis. *ASAIO J* 5:21, 1983.

188. Diaz-Buxo JA, Farmer CD, Walker PJ, et al: Effects of hyperparathyroidism on peritoneal clearances. *Trans Am Soc Artif Intern Organs* 28:276, 1982.

189. Diaz-Buxo JA, Geissinger WT: Single cuff versus double cuff Tenckhoff catheter. *Perit Dial Bull* 4:S100, 1984.

190. Diaz-Buxo JA, Walker PJ, Chandler JT, et al: Experience with intermittent peritoneal dialysis and continuous cyclic peritoneal dialysis. *Am J Kidney Dis* 4:242, 1984.

191. Diaz-Buxo J, Walker P, Farmer C, et al: Continuous cycling peritoneal dialysis (CCPD). *Kidney Int* 19:145, 1981.

192. Digenis GE, Khanna R, Mathews R, et al: Abdominal hernias in patients undergoing continuous ambulatory peritoneal dialysis. *Perit Dial Bull* 2:115, 1982.

193. Dobbelstein H, Korner WF, Mempel W, et al: Vitamin B6 deficiency in uremia and its application for the depression of immune responses. *Kidney Int* 5:233, 1974.

193a. Dobbie JW: New concepts in molecular biology and ultrastructural pathology of the peritoneum: their significance for peritoneal dialysis. *Am J Kid Dis* 15:97, 1990.

194. Dobbie JW, Zaki M, Wilson L: Ultrastructural studies on the peritoneum with special reference to chronic ambulatory peritoneal dialysis. *Scott Med J* 26:213, 1981.

195. Doherty JE: Digitalis glycosides. Pharmacokinetics and their clinical implications. *Ann Intern Med* 79:229, 1973.

196. Dolan MJ, Whipp BJ, Davidson WD, et al: Hypopnea associated with acetate hemodialysis carbon dioxide—flow dependent ventilation. *N Engl J Med* 305:72, 1981.

197. Dominguez R, Coreoran AC, Page IH: Mannitol: Kinetics of distributions, excretion and utilization in human beings. *J Lab Clin Med* 32:1192, 1947.

198. Donckerwolcke RA: Survival on renal replacement therapy. *In* Fine RN, Gruskin AB (eds): *End Stage Renal Disease in Children.* Philadelphia, WB Saunders, 1984, p 541.

199. Donckerwolcke RA, Chantler C, Broyer M, et al: Combined report on regular dialysis and transplantation of children in Europe, 1979. *Proc Eur Dial Transplant Assoc* 17:87, 1980.

200. Donckerwolcke RA, Chantler C, Broyer MJC: Paediatric Dialysis. *In* Drukker W, Parsons FM, Maher JF (eds): *Replacement of Renal Function by Dialysis.* The Hague, Martinus Nijhoff, 1983, p 514.

201. Donckerwolcke RA, Chantler C, Brunner FP, et al: Combined report on regular dialysis and transplantation of children in Europe, 1977. *Proc Eur Dial Transplant Assoc* 15:77, 1978.

202. Drachman R, Baillet G, Gagnadoux M-F, et al: Pulmonary calcifications in children on dialysis. *Nephron* 44:46, 1986.

203. Drachman R, Niaudet P, Gagnadoux M-F, et al: Modification of peritoneal ultrafiltration capacity in children undergoing peritoneal dialysis. *J Ped Neph* 6:35, 1985.

204. Drueke T, Le Pailleur C, Zingraff J, et al: Uremic cardiomyopathy and pericarditis. *Adv Nephrol* 9:33, 1980.

205. Dulaney JT, Hatch FE Jr: Peritoneal dialysis and loss of proteins: A Review. *Kidney Int* 26:253, 1984.

205a. Dunmire RB, Breyer JA: Nontuberculous mycobacterial peritonitis during continuous ambulatory peritoneal dialysis; case report and review of diagnostic and therapeutic strategies. *Am J Kid Dis* 17:126, 1991.

206. Dyck PJ, Johnson WJ, Lambert EH, et al: Segmental demyelination secondary to axonal degeneration in uremic neuropathy. *Mayo Clin Proc* 46:400, 1971.

207. Eaton JW, Kolpin CF, Swofford HS, et al: Chlorinated water: a cause of dialysis-induced hemolytic anemia. *Science* 181:463, 1973.

208. Edward SR, Unger AM: Acute hydrothorax: a new complication of peritoneal dialysis. *JAMA* 199:853, 1967.

209. Eijgenraam FJ, Donckerwolck RA, van Dijken PJ: Diagnosis and treatment of iron overload in paediatric patients on chronic haemodialysis. *Pediatr Nephrol* 2:303, 1988.

210. Eisenberg ES: Intraperitoneal flucytosine in the management of fungal peritonitis in patients on continuous ambulatory peritoneal dialysis. *Am J Kid Dis* 11(6):465, 1988.

211. Eiser AR, Jayamanne D, Kokseng C, et al: Contrasting alterations in pulmonary gas exchange during acetate and bicarbonate hemodialysis. *Am J Nephrol* 2:123, 1982.

212. Eisinger AJ, Bending MP, Goodwin SW: Ultraviolet light sterilization in CAPD: Preliminary experience in the U.K. *Perit Dial Bull* 4:S21, 1984.

213. El-Bishti MM, Counahan R, Bloom SR, et al: Hormonal and metabolic responses to intravenous glucose in children on regular hemodialysis. *Am J Clin Nutr* 31:1865, 1978.

214. El-Bishti M, Counahan R, Jarrett RJ, et al: Hyperlipidemia in children on regular haemodialysis. *Arch Dis Child* 52:932, 1977.

214a. Ellis EN, Watts K, Wells TG, et al: Use of peritoneal equilibration test in pediatric dialysis patients. *Advances in Peritoneal Dialysis* 7:259, 1991.

215. Elzouki AY, Gruskin AB, Baluarte HJ, et al: Developmental changes in peritoneal dialysis kinetics in dogs. *Pediatr Res* 15:853, 1981.

216. Elzouki A, Gruskin A, Baluarte HJ, et al: Age-related changes in urea-C5144 peritoneal dialysance. *Clin Dial Trans Forum* 9:102, 1974.

217. Elzouki AY, Gruskin AB, Baluarte HJ, et al: Age-related changes in peritoneal dialysis (PD) kinetics. *Pediatr Res* 14:618, 1980.

218. Elzouki A, Gruskin A, Prebis J, et al: Age related changes in peritoneal dialysance. *Proceedings National Kidney Foundation, 9th Annual Clinical Dialysis & Transplant Forum,* November 16, 1979, p 37.

219. Elzouki AY, Gruskin AB, Baluarte HJ, et al: Developmental aspects of peritoneal dialysis. *In* Gruskin AB, Norman ME (eds): *Developments in Nephrology 3, Proc. Fifth Int Ped Neph Symp.* The Hague, Martinus Nijhoff, 1981, p 517.

219a. Enriquez JL, Kalia A, Travis LB: Fungal peritonitis in children on peritoneal dialysis. *J Pediatr* 117:830, 1990.

220. Erasmi H, Horsch S, Bodon P, et al: Shunt surgery in childhood. *In* Bulla M (ed): *Renal Insufficiency in Children.* Berlin, Springer-Verlag, 1982, p 169.

221. Erlich L, Powell SL: Care of the patient with a Gore-tex peritoneal dialysis catheter. *Dial Transplant* 12(8):572, 1983.

222. Eschbach JW: Hematologic problems of dialysis patients. *In* Drukker W, Parsons FM, Maher JF (eds): *Replacement of Renal Function by Dialysis.* The Hague, Martinus Nijhoff, 1983, p 630.

223. Eschbach JW, Adamson JW: Recombinant human erythropoietin: Implications for nephrology. In-Depth review. *Am J Kid Dis* 11(3):203, 1988.

224. Eschbach JW, Egrie JC, Downing MR, et al: Correction of the anemia of end-stage renal disease with recombinant human erythropoietin: Result of the Phase I and II clinical trial. *N Engl J Med* 316:73, 1987.

225. Eschbach JW, Cook JD, Scribner BH, et al: Iron balance in hemodialysis patients. *Ann Intern Med* 87:710, 1977.

226. Esperance MJ, Collins DL: Peritoneal dialysis efficiency in relation to body weight. *J Pediatr Surg* 1:162, 1966.

227. Evans DB, Slapak M: Pancreatitis in the hard water syndrome. *Br Med J* 3:748, 1975.

228. Everett ED: Diagnosis, prevention and treatment of peritonitis. *Perit Dial Bull* 4:S139, 1984.

229. Fabris A, Biasioli S, Borin D, et al: Fungal peritonitis in peritoneal dialysis: Our experience and review of treatments. *Perit Dial Bull* 4:75, 1984.

230. Farrell PC, Randerson DJ: Membrane permeability changes in longterm CAPD. *Trans Am Soc Artif Intern Organs* 26:197, 1980.

231. Farrell PC, Ward RA, Schindhelm K, et al: Precise anticoagulation for routine hemodialysis. *J Lab Clin Med* 92:164, 1978.

232. Fassbinder W, Pilar J, Scheuermann E, et al: Formaldehyde and the occurrence of anti-N-like cold agglutinins in RDT patients. *Proc Eur Dial Transpl Assoc* 13:333, 1976.

233. Feig PU, Shook A, Stearns RH: Effect of potassium removal during hemodialysis on the plasma potassium concentration. *Nephron* 27:24, 1981.

234. Feldman HA, Singer I: Endocrinology and metabolism in uremia and dialysis: A clinical review. *Medicine* 54:345, 1975.

235. Feldman W, Baliah T, Drummond KN: Intermittent peritoneal dialysis in the management of chronic renal failure in children. *Am J Dis Child* 116:30, 1968.

236. Fennell RS, Andres JM, Garin EH, et al: Liver problems associated with ESRD in children. *In* Fine RN, Gruskin AB (eds): *End Stage Renal Disease in Children.* Philadelphia, WB Saunders, 1984, p 389.

237. Fennell RS, Orak JK, Garin EH, et al: Continuous ambulatory peritoneal dialysis in a pediatric population. *Am J Dis Child* 137:388, 1983.

238. Feriani M, Biasioli S, Chiaramonte S, et al: Anatomical basis of peritoneal permeability. A reappraisal. Anatomy of peritonitis. *Int J Art Organ* 5:345, 1982.

239. Ferraris J, Saenger P, Levine L, et al: Delayed puberty in males with chronic renal failure. *Kidney Int* 18:344, 1980.

239a. Fine RN: Growth hormone and the kidney: The use of recombinant growth hormone in growth retarded children with chronic renal insufficiency. *J Am Soc Neph* 1:1128, 1991.

240. Fine RN: Metabolism and growth in pediatric CAPD. *Proceedings of 2nd Annual National Conference on CAPD.* 1982, p. 349.

241. Fine RN: Renal transplantation in children. *Proc Eur Dial Transplant Assoc* 18:321, 1981.

242. Fine RN: Renal transplantation in children. *In* Chaterjee SN (ed): *Organ Transplantation.* Boston, John Wright, 1982, p 243.

243. Fine RN, Korsch BM, Grushkin CM, et al: Hemodialysis in children. *Am J Dis Child* 119:498, 1970.

244. Fine RN, Malekzadeh MH, Pennisi, AJ, et al: Long term results of transplantation in children. *Pediatrics* 61:641, 1978.

245. Fine RN, Malekzadeh MH, Wright HT: Hepatitis B in a pediatric hemodialysis unit. *J Pediatr* 86:355, 1975.

246. Fine RN, Salusky IB, Hall T, et al: Peritonitis in children undergoing continuous ambulatory peritoneal dialysis. *J Pediatr* 71:806, 1983.

247. Finkelstein FO, Goffinet JA, Hendler ED, et al: Pharmacokinetics of digoxin and digitoxin in patients undergoing hemodialysis. *Am J Med* 58:525, 1975.

248. Finkelstein FO, Kliger AS: Enhanced efficiency of peritoneal dialysis using rapid, small-volume exchanges. *Trans Am Soc Artif Intern Organs* 2:103, 1979.

249. Finkelstein FO, Kliger AS, Bastl C, et al: Sequential clearance and dialysance measurements in chronic peritoneal dialysis patients. *Nephron* 18:342, 1977.

250. Finn R, Jowett EW: Acute hydrothorax: complication of peritoneal dialysis. *Br Med J* 2:94, 1970.

251. Firor HV, Moore ES, Levitsky LL, et al: Parathyroidectomy in children with chronic renal failure. *J Pediatr Surg* 7:565, 1972.

252. Fischbach M, Attal Y, Geisert J: Hemodiafiltration versus hemodialysis in children. *Int J Pediatr Nephrol* 5(3):151, 1984.

253. Fivush BA, Bock GH, Guzzetta PC, et al: Vancomycin prevents polytetrafluoroethylene graft infections in pediatric patients receiving chronic hemodialysis. *Am J Kid Dis* 5:120, 1985.

253a. Flanigan MJ, Doyle C, Miller L: Tidal peritoneal dialysis: A pediatric experience. *Advances in Peritoneal Dialysis* 7:275, 1991.

254. Flanigan MJ, Freeman RM, Lim US: Cellular response to peritonitis among peritoneal dialysis patients. *Am J Kidney Dis* 6:420, 1985.

254a. Flessner MF: Peritoneal transport physiology: Insights from basic research. *J Am Soc Nephrol* 2:122, 1991.

255. Foley CM, Polinsky MS, Gruskin AB, et al: Encephalopathy in infants and children with chronic renal disease. *Arch Neurol* 38:656, 1981.

256. Foran RF, Golding AL, Treiman RL, et al: Quinton Scribner cannulas for hemodialysis. Review of four years experience. *Calif Med* 112:18, 1970.

257. Ford DM, Portman RJ, Hurst DL, et al: Unexpected seizures during hemodialysis. Original Article. *Pediatr Nephrol* 1:597, 1987.

258. Fortner RW, Nowakowski A, Carter CB, et al: Death due to overheated dialysate during dialysis. *Ann Intern Med* 73:443, 1970.

259. Frazone AJ, Tucker BL, Brennan LP, et al: Hemodialysis in children: Experience with arteriovenous shunts. *Arch Surg* 102:592, 1971.

260. Freidman J, Lewy JE: Failure to thrive associated with renal disease. *Pediatr Ann* 7:11, 1978.

261. Freedman RM, Lawton RL, Chambertain MA: Hardwater syndrome. *N Engl J Med* 276:1113, 1967.

262. Freundlich M, Zilleruelo G, Abitbol C, et al: Minerals and bone-modulating hormones in children on continuous ambulatory peritoneal dialysis. *Nephron* 41:267, 1985.

263. Frisancho RA: New norms of upper limb fat and muscle areas for assessment of nutritional status. *Am J Clin Nutr* 34:2540, 1981.

264. Frisancho RA: Triceps skin fold and upper arm muscle size norms for assessment of nutritional status. *Am J Clin Nutr* 27:1052, 1974.

265. Fuchs C, Doht B, Dorn D, et al: Parathyroid hormone, calcium and phosphate balance in hemofiltration. *J Dial* 1:631, 1977.

266. Gacek EM, Babb AL, Urelli DA, et al: Dialysis dementia: the role of dialysate pH in altering the dialyzability of aluminum. *Trans Soc Artif Intern Organs* 25:409, 1979.

267. Gagnodoux MF, Pascal B, Bronstein M, et al: Arteriovenous fistulae in small children. *Dial Transplant* 9:318, 1980.

268. Gagnon RF, Kaye M: Hemodialysis neutropenia and dialyzer reuse: Role of the cleansing agent. *Uremia Invest* 8:17, 1984.

269. Galen MA, Steinberg SM, Lowrie EG, et al: Hemorrhagic pleural effusion in patients undergoing chronic hemodialysis. *Ann Intern Med* 82:359, 1975.

270. Gallery EDM, Blomfield J, Dixon SR: Acute zinc toxicity in haemodialysis. *Br Med J* 4:331, 1973.

271. Gandhi VC, Ing TS, Jablokow VR, et al: Thickened peritoneal dialysis membranes in maintenance peritoneal dialysis patients. *Kidney Int* 14:675, 1979.

272. Ganzi GC, Tice JE: Water treatment for home dialysis. Part I. *Dial Transplant* 13:222, 1984.

273. Gardiner AOP, Sawyer AN, Donckerwolcke RA, et al: Assessment of dialysis requirement for children on regular haemodialysis. *Dial Transpl* 11:754, 1982.

274. Gardner J: The GI lag and its significance to the dialysis patient. *Dial Transplant* 8:132, 1979.

275. Gardner Watson A, Greenwood WR: Studies on the intraocular pressure during hemodialysis. *Can J Ophthalmol* 1:4, 1966.

276. Gault MH, Jeffrey JR, Chirito E, et al: Studies of digoxin dosage, kinetics and serum concentrations in renal failure and review of the literature. *Nephron* 17:161, 1976.

277. Gazenfield-Gazit E, Eliahou HE: Endotoxin antibodies in patients on maintenance hemodialysis. *Israel J Med Sci* 5:1032, 1969.

278. Gejyo G, Odani S, Yamada T, et al: B$_2$ microglobulin: A new form of amyloid protein associated with chronic hemodialysis. *Kidney Int* 30:385, 1986.

279. Gibson DG: Haemodynamic factors in the development of acute pulmonary edema in renal failure. *Lancet* 2:1217, 1966.

280. Gibson TC, Dyer DP, Postlethwaite RJ, et al: Vascular access for acute haemodialysis. *Arch Dis Child* 62:141, 1987.

281. Gilkes JJH, Eady RAJ, Rees LH, et al: Plasma immunoreactive melanotrophic hormones in patients on maintenance haemodialysis. *Br Med J* 1:656, 1975.

282. Ginn HE, Bugel HJ, James L, et al: Clinical experience with small surface area dialyzers. *Proc Dial Transplant Forum* 1:53, 1971.

283. Glasson P, Favre H: Treatment of peritonitis in continuous ambulatory peritoneal dialysis patients with cotrinoxazole. *Nephron* 36:65, 1984.

284. Gloor HJ, Nichols K, Sorkin MI, et al: Peritoneal access and related complications in CAPD. *Am J Med* 74:593, 1983.

284a. Gokal R: Osmotic agents in peritoneal dialysis. *Contrb Nephrol* 85:126, 1990.

285. Gokal R, Ramos M, Ward MK, et al: "Eosinophilic" peritonitis in continuous ambulatory peritoneal dialysis. *Clin Neph* 15:328, 1981.

286. Goldberg AP, Applebaum-Bowden DM, Bierman EL, et al: Increase in lipoprotein lipase during clofibrate treatment of hypertriglyceridemia in patients on hemodialysis. *N Engl J Med* 301:1073, 1979.

287. Goldberg AP, Hagberg J, Delmez JA, et al: Metabolic effects of exercise training in hemodialysis patients. *Kidney Int* 18:754, 1980.

288. Goldberg EM, Hill W: A new peritoneal access prosthesis. *Proc Dial Trans Form* 3:122, 1973.

289. Goldschmidt ZH, Pote HH, Katz MA, et al: Effect of dialysate volume on peritoneal dialysis kinetics. *Kidney Int* 5:240, 1974.

290. Goldstein DA, Chui LA, Massry SG: Effects of parathyroid hormone and uremia on peripheral nerve calcium and motor nerve conduction velocity. *J Clin Invest* 62:88, 1978.

291. Goldstein DH, Nagar C, Srivastava N, et al: Clinically silent pericardial effusions in patients on long-term hemodialysis. *Chest* 72:744, 1977.

292. Gomez RA, Campbell F, Savory J, et al: Deferoxamine for the treatment of hemosiderosis during CAPD. *Int J Pediatr Nephrol* 8(1):21, 1987.

293. Gomez F, De La Cueva R, Wauters J, et al: Endocrine abnormalities in patients undergoing long-term hemodialysis. *Am J Med* 68:522, 1980.

293a. Gordon SM, Bland LA, Alexander SR, et al: Hemolysis associated with hydrogen peroxide at a pediatric dialysis center. *Am J Nephrol* 10:123, 1990.

294. Gotch FA: A quantitative evaluation of small and middle molecule toxicity in therapy of uremia. *Dial Transplant* 9:183, 1980.

295. Gotch F, Sargent JA: Measurement of H$^+$ balance during acetate and bicarbonate dialysis therapy (abstr). *Kidney Int* 16:887, 1979.

296. Gotloib L, Digenis GE, Rabinovich S, et al: Ultrastructure of normal rabbit mesentery. *Nephron* 34:248, 1983.

297. Gotloib L, Rabinovich S, Rodella H, et al: Ultrastructure of the rabbit mesentry. In Gahl GM, Kessel M, Nolph KD (eds): *Advances in Peritoneal Dialysis*. Amsterdam, Excerpta Medica, 1981, p 27.

298. Graben N, Sohn J, Pistor K: Treatment of life intoxications in infants and children by combination of hemoperfusion through charcoal or resin and hemodialysis. In Bulla M (ed): *Dialysis and Kidney Transplantation in Children*. Melsungen, Bibliomed, 1979, p 197.

299. Graefe U, Milutinovic J, Follette WC, et al: Less dialysis morbidity and vascular irritability with bicarbonate in dialysate. *Ann Intern Med* 88:332, 1978.

300. Graettinger JS, Parsons RL, Campbell JA: Correlations of clinical and hemodynamic studies in patients with mild and severe anemia with and without congestive failure. *Ann Intern Med* 58:617, 1963.

300a. Grantham JJ: Acquired cystic kidney disease. *Kid Int* 40:143, 1991.

301. Grantham JJ, Levine E: Acquired cystic disease: Replacing one kidney disease with another. *Kidney Int* 28:99, 1985.

302. Greulich WW, et al: *Radiographic Atlas of Skeletal Development of the Hand and Wrist,* 2nd ed. Stanford, CA, Stanford University Press, 1959, p 107.

303. Grodstein GP, Blumenkrantz J, Kopple JD, et al: Glucose absorption during CAPD. *Kidney Int* 19:564, 1981.

304. Groggin MJ, Joekes AM: II Pulmonary gas exchange during peritoneal dialysis. *Br Med J* 2:247, 1971.

305. Gross M, McDonald HP: Effect of dialysate temperature and flow rate on peritoneal clearance. *JAMA* 202:363, 1967.

306. Grossman MB: The role of the pediatric nephrology nurse in the dialysis unit. *In* Fine RN, Gruskin AB (eds): *End Stage Renal Disease in Children.* Philadelphia, WB Saunders, 1984, p 67.

307. Grushkin CM, Korsch B, Fine RN: Hemodialysis in small children. *JAMA* 221:869, 1972.

308. Gruskin AB: Aluminum: A pediatric overview. *In* Barness LA, DeVivo DC, Morrow G III, et al (eds): *Advances in Pediatrics,* vol 35. Chicago, Year Book, 1988, p 281.

309. Gruskin AB: Parenteral fluid therapy and treatment for electrolyte disorders for children. *In* Kendall AR, Karafin L (eds): *Practice of Surgery-Urology.* Hagerstown, MD, Harper & Row, 1981.

310. Gruskin AB: The kinetics of peritoneal dialysis in children. *Perspect Perit Dial* 1:9, 1983.

311. Gruskin AB: The peritoneal dialysis prescription in children. *Perspect Perit Dial* 3:42, 1985.

312. Gruskin AB: *Statement of the National Association of Children's Oversight of the Committee on Ways and Means of the Proposed Prospective Reimbursement Rates for the End Stage Renal Disease Program.* Washington, DC, Congressional Records, April 22, 1982.

313. Gruskin AB, Alexander SR Jr, Baluarte HJ, et al: Issues in pediatric dialysis. *Am J Kid Dis* 7(4):306, 1986.

314. Gruskin AB, Baluarte HJ, Polinsky MS, et al: Treatment of Severe Hypertension in Children With Renal Disease. *In* Strauss J (ed): *Acute Renal Disorders and Renal Emergencies.* The Hague, Martinus Nijhoff, 1984, p 143.

315. Gruskin AB, Baluarte HJ, Prebis JW, et al: Serum sodium abnormalities. An overview. *Ped Clin N Amer* 29:207, 1982.

316. Gruskin AB, Cote ML, Baluarte HJ: Peritoneal diffusion curves, peritoneal clearances and scaline factors in children of differing age. *Int J Ped Neph* 3:271, 1983.

317. Gruskin AB, Elzouki AY, Baluarte HJ, et al: Peritoneal dialysis kinetics: A pediatric perspective. *In* Strauss J (ed): *Pediatric Nephrology.* New York, Plenum Press, 1981, p 439.

318. Gruskin AB, Elzouki AY, Baluarte HJ, et al: Peritoneal dialysis kinetics. Developmental considerations perspective. *In* Spitzer A (ed): *The Kidney During Development. Morphology and Function.* New York, Masson, 1984, p 315.

319. Gruskin AB, Morgenstern BZ, Perlman SA: Kinetics of peritoneal dialysis in children. *In* Fine RN, Gruskin AB (eds): *End Stage Renal Disease in Children.* Philadelphia, WB Saunders, 1984, p 95.

320. Gruskin AB, Root AW, Duckett GE, et al: Parathyroid function in uremic children during the periods of renal insufficiency, hemodialysis and transplantation. *J Pediatr* 89:755, 1976.

321. Gruskin AB, Rosenblum H, Baluarte HJ, et al: Transper-

itoneal solute movement in children. *Kidney Int* 24:S95, 1983.

322. Gruskin A, Rosenblum H, Morgenstern BZ, et al: Changes in peritoneal clearances over time in children on maintenance peritoneal dialysis. *Pediatr Res* 17:350A, 1983.

323. Guarnieri G, Faccini L, Lipartiti T, et al: Simple methods for nutritional assessment in hemodialysis patients. *Am J Clin Nutr* 33:1598, 1980.

324. Guillot M, Broyer M, Chatelineau L: Continuous enteral feeding in pediatric nephrology. Long term results in children with congenital nephrotic syndrome, severe cystinosis and renal failure. *Arch Fr Pediatr* 37:497, 1980.

325. Guillot MG, Clermont MJ, Gagnadoux MF, et al: Nineteen months' experience with CAPD in children: main clinical and biological results. *In* Gahl GM, Kessel M, Nolph KD (eds): *Advances in Peritoneal Dialysis.* Amsterdam, *Excerpta Medica,* 1981, p 203.
Symposium on Peritoneal Dialysis. Berlin, 1981, p 203.

326. Gutch CF, Eskelson CD, Ziegler E, et al: 2-Chloroethanol as a toxic residue in dialysis supplies sterilized with ethylene oxide. *Dial Transpl* 5:21, 1976.

327. Haberstrob PB, Uniyal B, Trivedi H: A clot screw. *Dial Transpl* 3:27, 1974.

328. Hampers CL, Blaufox MD, Merril JP: Anticoagulation rebound after hemodialysis. *N Engl J Med* 275:776, 1966.

329. Hampers CL, Doak PB, Callaghan MN, et al: The electroencephalogram and spinal fluid during hemodialysis. *Arch Intern Med* 118:340, 1966.

330. Hampers CL, Streiff R, Nathan DG, et al: Megaloblastic hematopoiesis in uremia and in patients on long-term hemodialysis. *N Engl J Med* 276:551, 1967.

331. Handelsman H, Carter E: Hemofiltration as a substitute for hemodialysis in the treatment of end-stage renal disease (ESRD). *National Center for Health Services Research and Health Care Technology Assessment.* Rockville, MD, Health Technology Assessment Reports, #4, 1986.

332. Hanning RM, Balfe JW, Zlotkin SH: Effect of amino acid containing dialysis solutions on plasma amino acid profiles in children with chronic renal failure. *J Pediatr Gastroenterol Nutr* 6:942, 1987.

333. Harmon WE, Grupe WE: Urea kinetics in clinical management of children on chronic hemodialysis. *In* Fine RN, Gruskin AB (eds): *End Stage Renal Disease in Children.* Philadelphia, WB Saunders, 1984, p 54.

334. Harmon WE, Ingelfinger JR: Dialytic management of end-stage renal disease. *In* Brenner BM, Stein JH (eds): *Contemporary Issues in Nephrology 12. Pediatric Nephrology.* New York, Churchill-Livingstone, 1984, p 343.

335. Harmon WE, Meyer A, Grupe WE: Substitution of a percutaneous vascular access for repeated hemodialysis in children. *In* Bulla M (ed): *Renal Insufficiency in Children.* Berlin, Springer-Verlag, 1982, p 173.

336. Harmon WE, Spinozzi N, Meyer A, et al: Use of protein catabolic rate to monitor pediatric hemodialysis. *Dial Transplant* 10:324, 1981.

337. Harrison PB, Jansson K, Kronenberg H, et al: Cold agglutinin formation in patients undergoing hameodialysis. A possible relationship to dialyser re-use. *Aust NZ J Med* 5:195, 1975.

338. Harter HR, Burch JW, Majerus PW, et al: Prevention of thrombosis in patients on hemodialysis by low dose aspirin. *N Engl J Med* 301:577, 1979.

339. Hatcher CR, Logue RB, Logan WD, et al: Pericardiectomy for recurrent pericarditis. *J Thorac Cardiovasc Surg* 62:371, 1971.

339a. Held PJ, Levin NW, Bovbjerg RR, et al: Mortality and duration of dialysis treatment. *JAMA* 265:871, 1991.

340. Hemmeloff Andersen KE: Folic acid status of patients with chronic renal failure maintained by dialysis. *Clin Nephrol* 8:510, 1977.

341. Henderson L: Symptomatic hypotension during hemodialysis: Editorial review. *Kidney Int* 17:571, 1980.

342. Henderson LW: Dialysis. *In* Klahr S, Massry SG (eds): *Contemporary Nephrology*, New York, Plenum, vol 4. 1987, p 621.

343. Henderson LW: Biophysics of ultrafiltration and hemofiltration. *In* Drukker W, Parsons FM, Maher JF (eds): *Replacement of Renal Function by Dialysis*. The Hague, Martinus Nijhoff, 1983, p 242.

344. Henderson LW: Peritoneal dialysis. *In* Massry SG, Sellers AL, Thomas CC (eds): *Clinical Aspects of Uremia and Dialysis*. Springfield, IL, Charles C Thomas, 1976, p 555.

345. Henderson LW: Peritoneal ultrafiltration dialysis: Enhanced urea transfer using hypertonic peritoneal dialysis fluid. *J Clin Invest* 45:950, 1966.

346. Henderson LW: Ultrafiltration with peritoneal dialysis. *In* Nolph KD (ed): *Peritoneal Dialysis. Developments in Nephrology 2*. The Hague. Martinus Nijhoff, Hague, 1981, p 124.

347. Henderson LW, Ford CA, Lysaght MJ, et al: Preliminary observations on blood pressure response with maintenance diafiltration. *Kidney Int* 7:S413, 1975.

348. Henderson LW, Nolph KD: Altered permeability of the peritoneal membrane after using hypertonic peritoneal dialysis fluid. *J Clin Invest* 48:992, 1969.

349. Henderson LW, Parker HR, Schroeder JP, et al: Continuous low flow hemofiltration with sorbent regeneration of ultrafiltrate. *Trans Am Soc Artif Intern Organs* 24:178, 1978.

350. Henderson RG, Russel RGG, Ledingham JGG, et al: Effects of 1,25-dihydroxycholecalciferol on calcium absorption, muscle weakness and bone disease in chronic renal failure. *Lancet* 1:379, 1974.

350a. Heney D, Essex-Cater A, Brocklebank JT, et al: Continuous arteriovenous haemofiltration in the treatment of tumour lysis syndrome. *Pediatr Nephrol* 4:245, 1990.

351. Henich WI, Thompson P, Bergstrom L, et al: Effect of dialysis on hearing activity. *Nephron* 18:348, 1977.

352. Henning HV, Balusek E: Lipid metabolism in uremia: effect of regular hemofiltration and hemodialysis treatment. *J Dial* 1:595, 1977.

353. Henrich WL, Woodward TD, McPhaul JJ Jr: The chronic efficacy and safety of high sodium dialysate: Double-blind, crossover study. *Am J Kidney Dis* 3:349, 1982.

354. Hercz G, Salusky IB, Norris KC, et al: Aluminum removal by peritoneal dialysis: Intravenous vs. intraperitoneal deferoxamine. *Kidney Int* 30:944, 1986.

355. Hershman JM, Jones CM, Bailey AL: Reciprocal changes in serum thyrotropin and free thyroxine produced by heparin. *J Clin Endocrinol Metab* 34:574, 1972.

356. Hickman RO, Buckner CD, Clift RA, et al: A modified right atrial catheter for access to the venous system in marrow transplant recipients. *Surg Gynecol Obstet* 148:871, 1979.

357. Hickman RO, Watkins S: A review of hemodialysis catheters and access devices. *Dialysis & Transplant* 16(9):481, 1987.

358. Hickman RO, Watkins S: Peritoneal dialysis access: An introduction. *Dial Transplant* 17(1):10, 1988.

359. Higgins JT Jr, Gross ML, Somani P: Patient tolerance and dialysis effectiveness of a glucose polymer-containing peritoneal dialysis solution. *Perit Dial Bull* 4:S131, 1984.

360. Hoenich NA, Kerr DNS: Dialysers. *In* Drukker W, Parsons FM, Maher JF (eds): *Replacement of Renal Function by Dialysis*. The Hague, Martinus Nijhoff, 1983, p 106.

361. Hoenich NA, Pearson S, Downing N, et al: A clinical appraisal and comparison of double pump single needle dialysis systems. *Int J Artif Organs* 8:89, 1985.

362. Hoenich NA, Stenton SC, Woffindin C, et al: Comparison of membranes used in the treatment of end-stage renal failure. *Kidney Int* 33(24):S44, 1988.

363. Hogg RJ, Coln D, Chang J, et al: The Toronto Western Hospital catheter in Pediatric Dialysis Program. *Am J Kidney Dis* 3:219, 1983.

364. Holland PC, Dillon MJ, Welsh A, et al: Plasma exchange in renal disease in children. *Eur J Pediatr* 141:180, 1983.

364a. Holley JL, Foulks CJ, Moss AH, et al: Ultrasound as a tool in the diagnosis and management of exit-site infection in patients undergoing continuous ambulatory peritoneal dialysis. *Am J Kid Dis* 14:211, 1989.

365. Holliday MA, Chantler C: Metabolic nutritional factors in children with renal insufficiency. *Kidney Int* 14:306, 1978.

366. Holm J, Lieden B, Lindqrist B: Unilateral pleural effusion—a rare complication of peritoneal dialysis. *Scand J Urol Nephrol* 5:84, 1971.

367. Holmes CJ, Miyake C, Kubey W: In-vitro evaluation of an ultraviolet germicidal connection system for CAPD. *Perit Dial Bull* 4:215, 1984.

368. Hooghe L, Bouton JM, Hall M, et al: Peritoneal catheters for very small children. *Perit Dial Bull* 3(1):42, 1983.

369. Horisberger J-D, Bille J, Wauters J-P: Fungal eosinophilic peritonitis due to alternaria in a patient on continuous ambulatory peritoneal dialysis. *Perit Dial Bull* 4:255, 1984.

370. Horton JD, Gelfand MC, Sherber HS: Natural history of asymptomatic pericardial effusions in patients on maintenance hemodialysis. *Proc Clin Dial Transplant Forum* 7:76, 1977.

371. Hruska KA, Blondin J, Bass R, et al: Effect of intact parathyroid hormone on hepatic glucose release in the dog. *J Clin Invest* 64:1016, 1979.

372. Hsu AC, Kooh SW, Fraser D, et al: Renal osteodystrophy in children with chronic renal failure. An unexpectedly common and incapacitating complication. *Pediatrics* 70:742, 1982.

373. Hurley RM: Anaphylaxis during hemodialysis. *Inter J Pediatr Nephrol* 5(1):53, 1984.

374. Hyde SE III, Sadler JH: Red blood cell destruction in hemodialysis. *Trans Am Soc Artif Intern Organs* 15:50, 1969.

375. Hymes LC, Clowers B, Mitchell C, et al: Peritoneal catheter survival in children. *Perit Dial Bull* 6:185, 1986.

376. Humayun HM, Ing TS, Daugirdas JT, et al: Peritoneal fluid eosinophilic in patients undergoing maintenance peritoneal dialysis. *Arch Int Med* 141:1172, 1981.

377. Ijaiya K: TSH and PRL response to thyrotropin releasing hormone in children with chronic renal failure undergoing hemodialysis. *Arch Dis Child* 54:937, 1979.

378. Ijaiya K, Bulla M, Roth B, et al: The secretion of human growth hormone, cortisol, prolactin and thyrotropin during hemodialysis. *In* Bulla M (ed): *Renal Insufficiency in Children*. Berlin, Springer-Verlag, 1982, p 133.

379. Incidence of dialyzer reuse compared for 33 countries. *Contemp Dial* 5:17, 1984.

380. Ing TS, Daugirdas JT, Gandhi VC: Peritoneal sclerosis in peritoneal dialysis patients. *Am J Nephrol* 4:173, 1984.

381. Ingelfinger JR: Hypertension in children with ESRD. *In* Fine RN, Gruskin AB (eds): *End Stage Renal Disease in Children*. Philadelphia, WB Saunders, 1984, p 340.

382. Iseki K, Onoyama K, Maeda T, et al: Comparison of hemodynamics induced by conventional acetate hemodialysis to bicarbonate dialysis, and ultrafiltration. *Clin Nephrol* 14:294, 1980.

383. Jacob AI, Gavellas G, Zarco R, et al: Leukopenia, hypoxia and complement function with different hemodialysis membranes. *Kidney Int* 18:505, 1980.

384. Jenkins P, Dreher WH: Dialysis-induced muscle cramps: treatment with hypertonic saline and theory as to etiology. *Trans Am Soc Artif Intern Organs* 21:579, 1975.

385. Jenkins JG, Lim JHK, Bell A, et al: Transcutaneous blood gas monitoring during peritoneal dialysis in the neonate. *Int J Pediatr Nephrol* 7(2):85, 1986.

386. Jennekens FGR, Jennekens-Schinkel, Aagje: Neurological aspects of dialysis patients. *In* Drukker W, Parsons FM, Maher JF (eds): *Replacement of Renal Function by Dialysis*. The Hague, Martinus Nijhoff, 1983, p 724.

387. Jensen S, Davidson M, Durnell T, et al: An evaluation of monthly versus bi-monthly CAPD solution transfer set changes. *Perit Dial Bull* 4:213, 1984.

388. Jensen WM, Ahmad S: Evaluation of a germicidal device for peritoneal dialysis connectors. *Perit Dial Bull* 4:219, 1984.

389. Johnson CA, Zimmerman SW, Rogge M: The pharmacokinetics of antibiotics used to treat peritoneal dialysis-associated peritonitis. *Am J Kidney Dis* 4:3, 1984.

390. Johnston MG: Involvement of lymphatic collecting ducts in the physiology and pathophysiology of lymph flow. *In* Johnson MG (ed): *Experimental Biology of the Lymphatic Circulation*. Amsterdam, Elsevier, 1985, p 81.

391. Johnson JW, Hattner RS, Hampers CL, et al: Effects of hemodialysis on secondary hyperparathyroidism in patients with chronic renal failure. *Metabolism* 21:18, 1972.

392. Johnson RS: The role of the social worker in the management of the child with ESRD. *In* Fine RN, Gruskin AB (eds): *End Stage Renal Disease in Children*. Philadelphia, WB Saunders, 1984, p 560.

393. Johnson WJ: Optimum dialysate calcium concentration during maintenance hemodialysis. *Nephron* 17:241, 1976.

394. Johnson WJ, Hagge WW, Wagoner RD, et al: Toxicity arising from urea. *Kidney Int* 7:S285, 1975.

395. Jones AS, James E, Bland H, et al: Renal failure in the newborn. *Clin Pediat* 18:286, 1979.

395a. Jones CL, Andrew M, Eddy A, et al: Coagulation abnormalities in chronic peritoneal dialysis. *Pediatr Nephrol* 4:152, 1990.

396. Jones RWA, Rigdon SP, Barratt, TM, et al: The effects of chronic renal failure in infancy on growth, nutritional status and body composition. *Pediatr Res* 16:784, 1982.

397. Jordan SC, Ho W, Ettenger R, et al: Plasma exchange improves the glomerulonephritis of systemic lupus erythematosus in selected pediatric patients. *Pediatr Nephrol* 1:276, 1987.

398. Jubelirer SJ: Hemostatic abnormalities in renal disease. In-depth review. *Am J Kid Dis* 5:219, 1985.

398a. Juppner H, Hoyer PF, Latta K, et al: Efficacy of calcium carbonate and low-dose vitamin D/1,25(OH)$_2$D$_3$ in reducing the risk of developing renal osteodystrophy in children on continuous ambulatory peritoneal dialysis. *Pediatr Nephrol* 4:614, 1990.

399. Junor BJR, Briggs JD, Forwell MA, et al: Sclerosing peritonitis: The contribution of chlorhexidine in alcohol. *Perit Dial Bull* 5:101, 1985.

400. Kaedi A, Pinio GF, Shimizu A, et al: Arteriovenous shunt

401. Kaiser BA, Potter DE, Bryant RE, et al: Acid base changes and acetate metabolism during routine and high-efficiency hemodialysis in children. *Kidney Int* 19:70, 1981.

402. Kaji DM, Ackad A, Nottage WG, et al: Prevention of muscle cramps in haemodialysis patients by quinine sulphate. *Lancet* 2:66, 1976.

403. Kallen RJ: A method for approximating the efficacy of peritoneal dialysis for uremia. *Am J Dis Child* 111:156, 1966.

404. Kallen RJ, Zaltzman S, Coe FL, et al: Hemodialysis in children: Technique, kinetics aspects. Related to varying body size, and application to salicylate intoxication, acute renal failure and some other disorders. *Medicine* 45:1, 1966.

405. Kant KS, Pollak VE: Dialyzer reuse: safety and efficacy. *Chronic Renal Disease Conference NIAMDD* (abstr), 1980, p 33.

406. Kantor RJ, Carson LA, Graham DR, et al: Outbreak of pyrogenic reactions at a dialysis center. *Am J Med* 74:449, 1983.

407. Kaptein EM, Feinstein EI, Massry SG: Thyroid hormone metabolism in renal disease. *Contrib Nephrol* 33:122, 1982.

408. Kaptein EM, Quion-Verde H, Chooljian CJ, et al: The thyroid in end-stage renal disease. *Medicine* 67(3):187, 1988.

409. Karnovsky MJ: The ultrastructural basis of capillary permeability studied with peroxodes as a tracer. *J Cell Biol* 3:213, 1967.

410. Kattamis C, Touliatos N, Haidas S: Matsaniotis in growth of children with thalassemia: Effect of different transfusion regimens. *Arch Dis Child* 45:502, 1970.

410a. Katz A, Kashtan CE, Greenberg LJ, et al: Hypogammaglobulinemia in uremic infants receiving peritoneal dialysis. *J Pediatr* 117(2 Pt 1):258, 1990.

411. Katz A, Sombolos K, Oreopoulos DG: Acquired cystic disease of the kidney in association with chronic ambulatory peritoneal dialysis. *Am J Kid Dis* 9(5):426, 1987.

412. Keane WF, Comty CM, Verbrugh HA, et al: Opsonic deficiency of peritoneal dialysis effluent in continuous ambulatory peritoneal dialysis. *Kidney Int* 25:539, 1984.

413. Kedem O, Katchalsky A: Thermodynamic analysis of the permeability of biological membranes to nonelectrolytes. *Biochem Biophys Acta* 27:229, 1958.

414. Kennedy AC, Linton AL, Luke RG, et al: Electroencephalographic changes during haemodialysis. *Lancet* 1:408, 1963.

415. Kersh ES, Kronfield SJ, Unger A, et al: Autonomic insufficiency in uremia as a cause of hemodialysis-induced hypotension. *N Engl J Med* 290:650, 1974.

416. Keshaviah P: *Investigation of the Risks and Hazards Associated with Hemodialysis Devices*. Washington, DC, FDA, DHEW contract 223-78-5046, 1980, p 350.

416a. Kessler M, Netter P, Maheut H, et al: Highly permeable and biocompatible membranes and prevalence of dialysis-associated arthropathy (letter). *Lancet* 337:1092, 1991.

417. Khan AV, Herndon CH, Ahmadian SY: Social and emotional adaptations of children with transplanted kidneys and chronic hemodialysis. *Am J Psych* 128:1194, 1971.

418. Khanna R, et al: Lipid abnormalities in patients undergoing CAPD: Endocrine and metabolic implications of CAPD. *Perit Dial Bull* 3:513, 1983.

419. Khanna R, Nolph KD: Ultrafiltration failure and sclerosing peritonitis in peritoneal dialysis patients. *In* Nissenson

thrombosis: Prevention by sulfinpyrazone. *N Engl J Med* 290:304, 1974.

AR, Fine RN (eds): *Dialysis Therapy*. Philadelphia, Hanley & Belfus, 1986, p 122.

420. Khanna R, Oreopoulos DG: Complications of peritoneal dialysis other than peritonitis. *In* Nolph KD (ed): *Peritoneal Dialysis*. The Hague, Martinus Nijhoff, 1985, p 441.

421. Khanna R, Wu G, Rodella H, et al: Use of amino acid containing solution in CAPD patients. *Perit Dial Bull* 4(3):S121, 1984.

421a. Khoury AE, Charendoff J, Balfe JW, et al: Hernias associated with CAPD in children. *Advances in Peritoneal Dialysis* 7:279, 1991.

422. Kim D, Khanna R, Wu G, et al: Continuous ambulatory peritoneal dialysis with three-liter exchanges: A prospective study. *Perit Dial Bull* 4:82, 1984.

423. Kim KE, Onesti G, Schwartz AB, et al: Hemodynamics of hypertension in chronic end-stage renal disease. *Circulation* 45:410, 1972.

424. Kim KE, Onesti G, Swartz CD: Hemodynamics of hypertension in uremia. *Kidney Int* 7:S155, 1975.

425. Kinnaert P, Janssen F, Hall M: Elbow arteriovenous fistula (EAVF) for chronic hemodialysis in small children. *J Pediatr Surg* 18(2):116, 1983.

426. Kirkendol PL, Devia CJ, Bower JD, et al: A comparison of the cardiovascular effects of sodium acetate, sodium bicarbonate and other potential sources of fixed base in hemodialysate solutions. *Trans Am Soc Artif Intern Organs* 23:399, 1977.

427. Kjellstrand CM: Hemodialysis for Children. *In* Freidman EA (ed): *Strategy in Renal Failure*. New York, Wiley, 1978, p 149.

428. Kjellstrand CM, Buselmeier TJ: A simple method for anticoagulation during pre- and post-operative hemodialysis, avoiding rebound phenomenon. *Surgery* 72:630, 1972.

429. Kjellstrand CM, Lynch RE, Mauer SM, et al: Acute renal failure in children: conservative and dialysis management. *In* Strauss J (ed): *Pediatric Nephrology*, vol 4. New York, Garland, STP, 1978, p 89.

430. Kjellstrand CM, Mauer SM, Buselmeier TJ, et al: Hemodialysis of premature and newborn babies. *Proc Eur Dial Transplant Assoc* 10:349, 1973.

431. Kjellstrand CM, Mauer SM, Shideman JR, et al: Accurate weight monitoring during periatric hemodialysis. *Nephron* 10:302, 1973.

432. Kjellstrand CM, Petersen RJ, Evans RL, et al: Considerations of the middle molecule hypothesis. II: Neuropathy in nephrectomized patients. *Trans Am Soc Artif Intern Organs* 19:325, 1973.

433. Kjellstrand CM, Shideman JR, Santiago EA, et al: Technical advances in hemodialysis of very small pediatric patients. *Proc Clin Dial Transplant Forum* 1:124, 1971.

434. Klein WJ Jr, Metz EN, Price AR: Acute copper intoxication: a hazard of hemodialysis. *Arch Intern Med* 129:578, 1972.

435. Kleinknecht C, Broyer M, Gagnadoux MF, et al: Growth in children treated with long-term dialysis. A study of 76 patients. *Adv Nephrol* 9:133, 1980.

436. Kleinknecht C, Broyer M, Huot D, et al: Growth and development on non-dialysed children with chronic renal failure. *Kidney Int* 24(S15):40, 1983.

437. Knochel JP: Endocrine changes in patients on chronic dialysis. *In* Drukker W, Parsons FM, Maher JF (eds): *Replacement of Renal Function by Dialysis*. The Hague, Martinus Nijhoff, 1983, p 712.

438. Knochel JP, Mason AD: Effect of alkalinization on peritoneal diffusion of uric acid. *Am J Physiol* 210:1160, 1966.

439. Koch KM, Ernst W, Baldamus CA, et al: Sympathetic activity (SA) and hemodynamics in hemodialysis (HD), ultrafiltration (UF) and hemofiltration (HF). *Kidney Int* 16:891, 1979.

440. Koch KM, Frei U, Fassbinder W: Hemolysis and anemia in anti-N-like antibody positive hemodialysis patients. *Trans Am Soc Artif Intern Organs* 24:709, 1978.

441. Koch KM, Patya WD, Shaldon S, et al: Anemia of the regular hemodialysis patient and its treatment. *Nephron* 12:405, 1974.

442. Kohaut EC: Continuous ambulatory peritoneal dialysis. A preliminary pediatric experience. *Am J Dis Child* 135:270, 1981.

443. Kohaut EC: Growth in children with end-stage renal disease treated with CAPD for at least one year. *Perit Dial Bull* 2:159, 1982.

444. Kohaut EC: Growth of the patient on CAPD. *In* Fine RN, Sharer K, Mehls O (eds): *CAPD in Children*. Berlin, Springer-Verlag, 1985, p 106.

445. Kohaut EC: Growth in children treated with continuous ambulatory peritoneal dialysis. *Int J Pediatr Nephrol* 4(2):93, 1983.

446. Kohaut EC: The effect of dialysate volume on ultrafiltration in young patients treated with CAPD. *Int J Pediatr Nephrol* 7(4):13, 1985.

447. Kohaut EC, Alexander S: Ultrafiltration in the young patient on CAPD. *In* Moncrief JW, Popovich RP (eds): *CAPD Update*. New York, Masson, 1981, p 221.

448. Kohaut EC, Welchel J, Waldo FB, et al: Aggressive therapy of infants with renal failure. *Pediatr Nephrol* 1:150, 1987.

449. Kolmos JH, Moller S: The epidemiology of febrile reactions in haemodialysis. *Acta Med Scand* 203:345, 1978.

450. Koomans HA, Geers AB, Mees EJD: Plasma volume recovery after ultrafiltration in patients with chronic renal failure. *Kidney Int* 26:848, 1984.

451. Kopple JD, Mercurio K, Blumenkrantz MJ, et al: Daily requirement for pyridoxine supplements in chronic renal failuire. *Kidney Int* 19:694, 1981.

452. Korsch BM, Fine RN, Grushkin CM, et al: Experience with children and their families during extended hemodialysis and kidney transplantation. *Pediatr Clin N Am* 18:625, 1971.

453. Korzets A, Korzets Z, Peer G, et al: Sclerosing Peritonitis. *Am J Neprhol* 8:143, 1988.

454. Kramer P, Matthaei D, Arnold R, et al: Changes of plasma concentration and elimination of various hormones by haemofiltration. *Proc Eur Dial Transpl Assoc* 14:144, 1977.

455. Kramer P, Wigger W, Rieger J, et al: Arteriovenous hemofiltration. A new and simple method for treatment of overhydrated patients resistant to diuretics. *Klin Wochenschr* 55:1121, 1977.

455a. Krane NK: Intracranial pressure measurement in a patient undergoing hemodialysis and peritoneal dialysis. *Am J Kidney Dis* 13:336, 1989.

455b. Kriley M, Warady BA: Vitamin status of pediatric patients receiving long-term peritoneal dialysis. *Am J Clin Nutr* 53:1476, 1991.

456. Krothapalli RK, Senekjian HO, Ayns JC: Efficacy of intravenous vancomycin in the treatment of Gram positive peritonitis in long-term peritoneal dialysis. *Am J Med* 75:345, 1983.

457. Kwong MBL: Anemia in a child on CAPD caused by continuous minor intraperitoneal bleeding. Letter. *Perit Dial Bull* 4:111, 1984.

458. LaGreca G, Dettori P, Biasioli S, et al: Brain density studies during dialysis. *Lancet* 2:582, 1980.

459. LaGreca G, Biasioli S, Chiaramonte S, et al: Acid-base balance in peritoneal dialysis. *Clin Nephrol* 16:1, 1981.

460. Langfield BM, Meyer RM, Shideman JR, et al: Hemodialysis of children less than 10 kilograms. *Dial Trans* 10:789, 1981.

461. Langman CG, Mazur AT, Baron R, et al: 25-Hydroxyvitamin D435 (calcifediol) therapy of juvenile renal osteodystrophy: Beneficial effect on linear growth velocity. *J Pediatr* 100:815, 1982.

462. Lanhez LE, Lowen J, Sabbaga E: Uremic myocardiopathy. *Nephron* 15:17, 1975.

463. Lasker N: Chronic peritoneal dialysis. *Pa Med* 74:67, 1971.

464. Lasker N, et al: Management of end-stage kidney disease with intermittent peritoneal dialysis. *Ann Intern Med* 62:1147, 1963.

465. Lazarus JM, Hampers CL, Bennet AH, et al: Urgent bilateral nephrectomy for severe hypertension. *Ann Intern Med* 76:733, 1972.

466. Lazarus JM, Hampers C, Merril JP: Hypertension in chronic renal failure: Treatment with hemodialysis and nephrectomy. *Arch Intern Med* 133:1059, 1974.

467. Leichter HE, Deitrich R, Salusky IB, et al: Acquired cystic kidney disease in children undergoing long-term dialysis. *Pediatr Nephrol* 2:8, 1988.

468. Leichter HE, Salusky IB, Alliapoulos JC, et al: CAPD and CCPD in children: An experience of 31 years. *Dial Transplant* 13:382, 1984.

469. Leonard A, Raij L, Shapiro FL: Bacterial endocarditis in regularly dialyzed patients. *Kidney Int* 4:407, 1973.

470. Leonard A, Shapiro FL: Subdural hematoma in regularly hemodialyzed patients. *Ann Intern Med* 82:650, 1975.

471. Leong AS-Y, Disney APS, Gove DW: Spallation and migration of silicone from blood-pump tubing in patients on hemodialysis. *N Engl J Med* 306:135, 1982.

472. Lertora J, Dargon JL, Rege AB, et al: Studies on a radioimmunoassay for human erythropoietin. *J Lab Clin Med* 86:140, 1975.

473. Levey AS, Harrington JT: Continuous peritoneal dialysis for chronic renal failure. *Medicine* 61:330, 1982.

474. Levey AS, Simon GM, McCauley J, et al: Outcome of peritoneal catheter placement in the high-risk patient. *Perit Dial Bull* 4:S112, 1984.

475. Levin L, Balfe JW, Geary D, et al: Gastrostomy tube feeding in children on CAPD. *Perit Dial Bull* 7(4):223, 1987.

476. Levin S, Winkelstein JD: Diet and infrequent peritoneal dialysis in chronic anuric uremia. *N Engl J Med* 277:619, 1967.

477. Lewis KJ, Dewar PJ, Ward MK, et al: Formation of anti-N-like antibodies in dialysis patients: Effect of different methods of dialyzer rinsing to remove formaldehyde. *Clin Nephrol* 15:39, 1981.

478. Lewis SL, Van Epps DE: Neutrophil and monocyte alterations in chronic dialysis patients: In-depth review. *Am J Kid Dis* 9(5):381, 1987.

479. Lieberman E: Management of acute renal failure in infants and children. *Nephron* 11:193, 1973.

480. Lieberman KV: Continuous arteriovenous hemofiltration in children. Practical pediatric nephrology. *Pediatr Nephrol* 1:330, 1987.

481. Lieberman KV, Nardi L, Bosch JP: Treatment of an infant with acute renal failure using continuous arteriovenous hemofiltration. *J Pediatr* 106:646, 1985.

482. Lifschitz MD, Kirschenbaum MA, Rosenblatt SG, et al: Effect of saralasin in hypertension patients on chronic hemodialysis. *Ann Intern Med* 88:23, 1978.

483. Linder A, Moskovtchenko JF, Traeger J: Accidental mass hypernatremia during hemodialysis. *Nephron* 9:99, 1972.

484. Lindsay J Jr, Crawley IS, Callaway GM: Chronic constrictive pericarditis following uremic hemopericardium. *Am J Heart* 79:390, 1970.

485. Lindsay RM: Practical use of anticoagulants. *In* Drukker W, Parsons FM, Maher JF (eds): *Placement of Renal Function by Dialysis.* The Hague, Martinus Nijhoff, 1983, p 201.

486. Lloyd-Still JD, Atwell JD: Renal failure in infants with special reference to the use of peritoneal dialysis. *J Pediatr Surg* 1:466, 1966.

487. London WT, DeFiglia M, Sutnick AI, et al: An epidemic of hepatitis in a chronic-hemodialysis unit. Australia antigen and differences in host response. *N Engl J Med* 281:571, 1969.

488. Lovinggood JP: Peritoneal catheter implantation for CAPD. *Perit Dial Bull* 4:S106, 1984.

489. Lowrie EG, Hakim RM: The effect on patient health of using reprocessed artificial kidneys. *Proc Clin Dial Transpl Forum* 10:86, 1980.

490. Lowrie EG, Laird NM: Kidney International. *Cooperative Dialysis Study* (suppl 13). Berlin, Springer-Verlag, 1983.

491. Lowrie EG, Sargent JA: Clinical example of pharmacokinetic and metabolic modeling: Quantitative and individualized prescription of dialysis therapy. *Kidney Int* 18(S10):S11, 1980.

492. Lundin AP, Stein RA, Frank F, et al: Cardiovascular status in long-term hemodialysis patients: An exercise and echocardiographic study. *Nephron* 28:234, 1981.

493. Lunt MJ, Powell RJ, Cattell WR: Evaluation of an ultrasonic doppler flowmeter for measurement of extracorporeal blood flow during renal dialysis. *In* Frost TH (ed): *Technical Aspects of Renal Dialysis.* Tunbride Wells, Pitman Medical, 1977, p 210.

493a. Luzar MA, Coles GA, Fallar B, et al: Staphylococcus aureus nasal carriage and infection in patients on continuous ambulatory peritoneal dialysis. *N Eng J Med* 322:505, 1990.

494. Mactier RA, Khanna R, Moore H, et al: Kinetics of peritoneal dialysis in children: Role of lymphatics. *Kidney Int* 34:82, 1988.

495. Mactier RA, Khanna R, Twardowski ZJ, et al: Ultrafiltration failure in continuous ambulatory peritoneal dialysis due to excessive peritoneal cavity lymphatic absorption. *Am J Kid Dis* 10(6):461, 1987.

496. Mactier RA, Khanna R, Twardowski ZJ, et al: Role of peritoneal cavity lymphatic absorption in peritoneal dialysis. An editorial review. *Kidney Int* 32:165, 1987.

497. Madsen RF, Nielson B, Olsen OJ, et al: Reverse osmosis as a method of preparing dialysis water. *Nephron* 7:545, 1970.

498. Mahajan SK, Gardiner WH, Abbasi AA, et al: Hypoguesia in patients on hemodialysis. *Proc Dial Transplant Forum* 8:20, 1978.

499. Mahan JD, Mauer SM, Nevins TE: The Hickman catheter: A new hemodialysis access device for infants and small children. *Kidney Int* 24:694, 1983.

500. Maher JF, Hirszel P, Shostak A, et al: Prolonged intraperitoneal dwell decreases ultrafiltration coefficient in rabbits. *Am J Kid Dis* 12(1):62, 1988.

501. Maher JF, Scheiher GE: Hazards and complications of dialysis. *N Engl J Med* 273:370, 1965.

502. Mak RHK, Turner C, Bosque M, et al: Metabolic and hormonal responses to constant hyperglycemia in children with chronic renal failure (CRF). Abstracts of the *International Workshop on Recent Advances in Diagnosis and*

Treatment of Children with Chronic Renal Failure. Heidelberg, May 21–22, 1982.

503. Malekzadeh MH, Ettenger RB, Pennisi AJ, et al: Treatment of renal osteodystrophy in children with 1,25(OH)425D435. *In Fourth Workshop on Vitamin D,* Berlin, Kongresshalle, 1979, p 200.

504. Mandelbaum JM, Heistand ML, Schardin KE: Six months' experience with PD-2 solution. *Dial Transplant* 12(4):259, 1983.

505. Mandell IN, Ahern MH, Kliger AS, et al: Candida peritonitis complicating peritoneal dialysis: Successful treatment with low dose amphotericin B therapy. *Clin Nephrol* 6:492, 1976.

506. Manley GL, Collipp PD: Renal failure in the newborn: Treatment with peritoneal dialysis. *Am J Dis Child* 115:107, 1968.

507. Mannucci PM, Remuzzi G, Pusineri F, et al: Deamino-8-D-arginine vasopressin shortens the bleeding time in uremia. *N Engl J Med* 308:8, 1983.

507a. Marangella M, Petrarulo M, Bianco O, et al: Glycolate determination detects type I primary hyperoxaluria in dialysis patients. *Kid Int* 39(1):149, 1991.

507b. Marcus R, Favero MS, Banerjee S, et al: Prevalence and incidence of human immunodeficiency virus among patients undergoing long term hemodialysis. The Cooperative Dialysis Study Group. *Am J Med* 90:614, 1991.

508. Marigold JH, Pounder RE, Pemberton J, et al: Propranolol, oxprenolol and sclerosing peritonitis. *Br Med J* 284:870, 1982.

509. Marini PV, Hull AR: Uremic pericarditis: A review of incidence and management. *Kidney Int* 7(S2):163, 1975.

510. Marrie TJ, Noble MA, Costerton JW: Examination of the morphology of bacteria adhering to peritoneal dialysis catheters by scanning and transmission electron microscopy. *J Clin Microbiol* 18:1388, 1983.

510a. Marsh JT, Brown WS, Wolcott D, et al: rHuEPO treatment improves brain and cognitive function of anemic dialysis patients. *Kid Int* 39:155, 1991.

511. Martin AM, Gibbons JK, Kimmitt J, et al: Hemodialysis and hemoperfusion in the treatment of uremic pericarditis. A study of 13 cases. *Dial Transplant* 8:135, 1979.

512. Masselot JP, Adhemar JP, Jaudon MC, et al: Reversible dialysis encephalopathy: Role for aluminum-containing gels. *Lancet* 2:1386, 1978.

513. Matthews D, Van Leeuwen JJ, Christensen L: Psychosocial problems of young children and their families in a dialysis/transplant program. *Dial Transplant* 10(1):73, 1981.

514. Mattocks AM: Accelerated removal of salicylate by additive in peritoneal dialysis fluid. *J Pharm Sci* 58:595, 1969.

515. Mauer SM: Pediatric Renal Dialysis. *In* Edelmann CM Jr (ed): *Pediatric Kidney Disease.* Boston, Little, Brown, 1978, p 487.

516. Mauer SM, Lynch RE: Hemodialysis techniques in infants and children. *Pediatr Clin North Am* 23:843, 1976.

517. Mayor GH, Keiser JA, Makdani D, et al: Aluminum absorption and distribution: Effect of parathyroid hormone. *Science* 197:1187, 1977.

518. McCaa RE, McCaa CS, Read VH, et al: Influence of hemodialysis on plasma aldosterone concentration in nephrectomized patients. *Trans Am Soc Artif Intern Organs* 18:239, 1973.

519. McCubbin JW, Green JH, Page IH: Baroreceptor function in chronic renal hypertension. *Circ Res* 4:204, 1956.

520. McDonald WJ, Golper TA, Mass RD, et al: Adrenocor-

ticotropin-cortisol axis abnormalities in hemodialysis patients. *J Clin Endocrinol Metab* 48:92, 1979.

521. McGary TJ, Nolph KD, Rubin J: In vitro simulation of peritoneal dialysis: A technique for demonstrating limitations on solute clearance. *J Lab Clin Med* 96:148, 1980.

522. McGrath BP, Ledingham JGG, Benedict CR: Catecholamines in peripheral venous plasma in patients on chronic haemodialysis. *Clin Sci Mol Med* 55:89, 1978.

523. McVicar M, Gauthier B, Goodman CT: Uremic neuropathy: Monitoring of transketolase activity inhibition in a child. *Am J Dis Child* 125:263, 1973.

524. Medani CR, Ringel RE: Intrapericardial triamcinolone hexacetonide in the treatment of intractable uremic pericarditis in a child. Brief report. *Pediatr Nephrol* 2:32, 1988.

525. Mehigan JT, McAlexander RA: Snuffbox arteriovenous fistula for hemodialysis. *Am J Surg* 143:252, 1982.

526. Mehls O: Renal osteodystrophy in children: Etiology and clinical aspects. *In* Fine RN, Gruskin AB (eds): *End Stage Renal Disease in Children.* Philadelphia, WB Saunders, 1984, p 227.

527. Mehls O, Ritz E, Gilli G, et al: Growth in renal failure? *Nephron* 21:237, 1978.

528. Mehls O, Krempien B, Ritz E, et al: Renal osteodystrophy in children on maintenance hemodialysis. *Proc Eur Dial Transplant Assoc* 10:197, 1973.

529. Mehta S: *A Statistical Summary of the Results of Vascular Access Procedures for Hemodialysis Published 1966–1980.* Technical publication No. 236. Newark, DE, WL Gore, 1981.

530. Menster MI, Thy S, Malekzadeh MH, et al: Peripheral motor nerve conduction velocities in children undergoing chronic hemodialysis. *Nephron* 22:337, 1978.

531. Miach PJ, Dawborn JK, Louis WJ, et al: Left ventricular function in uremia: Echocardiographic assessment in patients on maintenance dialysis. *Clin Nephr* 15:259, 1981.

532. Michalk DV, Scharf J, Stehr K: The role of plasmapheresis in the treatment of autoimmune diseases (AID) and rapidly progressive glomerulonephritis (RPGN). *Eur J Pediatr* 141:179, 1983.

533. Miller RB, Tassistro CR: Peritoneal dialysis. *N Engl J Med* 281:945, 1969.

534. Milliner DS, Schinaberger JH, Shuman P, et al: Inadvertent aluminum administration during plasma exchange due to aluminum contamination of albumin-replacement solutions. *N Engl J Med* 312(3):165, 1985.

534a. Milliner DS, Zinsmeister AR, Lieberman E, et al: Soft tissue calcification in pediatric patients with ESRD. *Kid Int* 38:931, 1990.

535. Milutinovich J, Strand M, Casaretto A, et al: Clinical impact of residual glomerulifiltration rate on dialysis time. *Trans Am Soc Artif Int Organs* 20:410, 1974.

536. Minuchin S: *Families and Family Therapy.* Cambridge, Harvard University Press, 1974.

537. Minuth ANW, Nottebohm GA, Eknoyan G, et al: Indomethacin treatment of pericarditis in chronic hemodialysis patients. *Arch Intern Med* 135:807, 1975.

538. Mion CM: Practical use of peritoneal dialysis. *In* Drukker W, Parsons FM, Maher JF (eds): *Replacement of Renal Function by Dialysis.* The Hague, Martinus Nijhoff, 1983, p 457.

538a. Miranda B, Selgas R, Celadilla O, et al: Peritoneal resting and heparinization as an effective treatment for ultrafiltration failure in peritoneal hyperpermeability patients on CAPD. *Contr Neph* 89:199, 1991.

539. Mishkin MS, Hsu JH, Walker WG, et al: Studies on the

episodic secretion of cortisol in uremic patients on hemodialysis. *Johns Hopkins Med J* 131:160, 1972.

540. Mizrahi S, Barak M, Lunski I: Simple technique for bedside peritoneal dialysis in neonates. *Nephron* 48:258, 1988.

541. Molitoris BA, Alfrey PS, Miller NL, et al: Efficacy of intramuscular and intraperitoneal deferoxamine for aluminum chelation. *Kidney Int* 31:986, 1987.

542. Moncrief JW, Popovich RP: Continuous ambulatory peritoneal dialysis. *In* Nolph KD (ed): *Peritoneal Dialysis.* The Hague, Martinus Nijhoff, 1985, p 209.

543. Morgenstern BZ, Pyle WK, Gruskin AB, et al: Transport characteristics of the pediatric peritoneal membrane. *Kid Int* 25:259, 1984.

544. Morgenstern BZ, Pyle WK, Gruskin AB, et al: Convective characteristics of pediatric peritoneal dialysis. *Perit Dial Bull* 4:S155, 1984.

545. Morrison G, Michelson EL, Brown S, et al: Mechanism and prevention of cardiac arrhythmias in chronic hemodialysis patients. *Kidney Int* 17:811, 1980.

546. Mossey RT, Wielopolski L, Bellucci AG, et al: Reduction in liver iron in hemodialysis patients with transfusional iron overload by deferoxamine mesylate. *Am J Kid Dis* 12(1):40, 1988.

547. Mozes MF, Soper WD, Jonasson O, et al: Total secondary hyperparathyroidism. *Arch Surg* 115:378, 1980.

548. Muller-Wiefel DE, Klare B, Querfeld U, et al: Hemofiltration in childhood. *In* Bulla M (ed): *Renal Insufficiency in Children.* Berlin, Springer-Verlag, 1982, p 217.

549. Muller-Wiefel DE, Rauh W, Wingen A-M, et al: Hemofiltration in children. *Contr Nephrol* 32:128, 1982.

549a. Murakami R, Momota T, Yoshiya K, et al: Serum carnitine and nutritional status in children treated with continuous ambulatory peritoneal dialysis. *J Gastroenterol Nutr* 11(3):371, 1990.

550. Murray MA: Vitamin and mineral needs of chronic hemodialysis patient. *Dial Transplant* 9:921, 1979.

551. Nagel W, Kuschinsky W: Study of the permeability of isolated dog resentery. *Eur J Clin Invest* 1:149, 1970.

552. Naik RB, Mathias CJ, Reid JL, et al: Effect of haemodialysis on the control of the circulation in patients with chronic renal failure. *Am J Nephrol* 5:96, 1985.

552a. Nakamura M, Weil WB, Kaufman DB: Fatal fungal peritonitis in an adolescent on continuous ambulatory peritoneal dialysis: Association with deferoxamine. *Pediatr Nephrol* 3:80, 1989.

553. Nash T: The colorimetric estimation of formaldehyde by means of the Hantzsch reaction. *Biochem J* 55:416, 1953.

554. National Kidney Foundation Report on Dialyzer Reuse. A special report. *Am J Kid Dis* 11(1):1, 1988.

555. Neal CR, Resnikoff E, Unger AM: Treatment of dialysis related muscle cramps with hypertonic dextrose. *Arch Intern Med* 141:171, 1981.

556. Neergaard J, Nielsen B, Faurby V, et al: On the exudation of plasticizers from PVC haemodialysis tubings. *Nephron* 14:263, 1975.

557. Neff MS, Goldbeer J, Slifkin RF, et al: A comparison of androgens for anemia in patients on hemodialysis. *N Engl J Med* 304:871, 1981.

558. Neff MS, Kim KE, Persoff M, et al: Hemodynamics of uremic anemia. *Circulation* 43:876, 1971.

558a. Neiberger R, Aboushaar MH, Tawan H, et al: Peritonitis in children on chronic peritoneal dialysis: Analysis at 10 years. *Advances in Peritoneal Dialysis* 7:272, 1991.

559. Nelson P, Stover J: Principles of nutritional assessment and management of the child with ESRD. *In* Fine RN,

Gruskin AB (eds): *End Stage Renal Disease in Children.* Philadelphia, WB Saunders, 1984, p 209.

560. Nevins TE, Mauer SM: Infant hemodialysis. *In* Fine RN, Gruskin AB (eds): *End Stage Renal Disease in Children.* Philadelphia, WB Saunders, 1984, p 39.

561. Newton S: Rapid dialysis: Implications for nurses and patients. *Contemp Dial Nephrol* 1988, p 17.

562. Niaudet P, Drachman R, Broyer M: Loss of ultrafiltration in children undergoing CAPD. *International Symposium,* Heidelberg, May 14–15, 1984, p 39.

563. Niaudet P, Berard E, Revillon Y, et al: Sclerosing encapsulating peritonitis inchidren. *Constr Nephrol* 57:230, 1987.

564. Niaudet P, Drachman R, Gubler M-C, et al: Loss of ultrafiltration and peritoneal membrane alterations in children on CAPD. *In* Fine RN, Scharer K, Mehls O (eds): *CAPD in Children.* Berlin, Springer-Verlag, 1985, p 158.

565. Nichols WK: Vascular access. *In* Van Stone JC (ed): *Dialysis and the Treatment of Renal Insufficiency.* New York, Grune & Stratton, 1983, p 143.

566. Nichols WK, Nolph KD: A technique for managing exit site and cuff infection in Tenckhoff catheters. *Perit Dial Bull* 3:S54, 1983.

567. Nickey WA, Chinitz VL, Kim KE, et al: Hypernatreia from water softener malfunction during home dialysis. *JAMA* 214:915, 1970.

568. Nielsen VK: The peripheral nerve function in chronic renal failure. A survey. *Acta Med Scand Suppl* 573:8, 1975.

569. Nielsen VK: The peripheral nerve function in chronic renal failure: I. Clinical signs and symptoms. *Acta Med Scand* 190:105, 1971.

570. Nielsen VK: The peripheral nerve function in uremia. II. Intercorrelation of clinical symptoms and signs and clinical grading of neuropathy. *Acta Med Scand* 190:113, 1971.

571. Nielsen V, Clausen E, Ranek L: Liver impairment during chronic hemodialysis and after renal transplantation. *Acta Med Scand* 197:229, 1975.

572. Nishi RY: Ultrasonic detection of bubbles with doppler flow transducers. *Ultrasonics* 10:173, 1972.

573. Nivet H, Drucker J, Dubois F, et al: Vaccine against hepatitis B in children: Prevention of hepatitis in a pediatric hemodialysis unit. *Int J Pediatr Nephrol* 3:25, 1982.

574. Nolph KD: An hypothesis to explain the ultrafiltration characteristics of peritoneal dialysis. *Kidney Int* 20:543, 1981.

575. Nolph KD: Peritoneal anatomy and transport physiology. *In* Drukker W, Parsons FM, Maher JF (eds): *Replacement of Renal Function by Dialysis.* The Hague, Martinus Nijhoff, 1983, p 440.

576. Nolph KD: Solute and water transport during peritoneal dialysis. *Perspective in Peritoneal Dialysis* 1:4, 1983.

577. Nolph KD, Ghods AJ, Brown PA: Effects of intraperitoneal nitroprusside on peritoneal clearances in man with variations of dose frequency of administration and dwell times. *Nephron* 24:114, 1979.

578. Nolph KD, Hano JE, Teschan PE: Peritoneal sodium transport during hypertonic peritoneal dialysis. *Ann Intern Med* 70:931, 1969.

579. Nolph K, Legrain M, Mion C: A survey of ultrafiltration in continuous ambulatory peritoneal dialysis. An international cooperative study—second report, 29 participating centers. *Perit Dial Bull* 4:137, 1984.

580. Nolph KD, Mactier R, Khanna R, et al: The kinetics of ultrafiltration during peritoneal dialysis: The role of lymphatics. *Kidney Int* 32:219, 1987.

581. Nolph KD, Ryan L, Moore H: Factors affecting ultrafiltration in continuous ambulatory peritoneal dialysis. *Perit Dial Bull* 4:14, 1984.

582. Nolph KD, Sorkin MI, Gloor HJ: Considerations for dialysis solutions modifications. *In* Atkins RE, Thompson NM, Farrell PC (eds): *Peritoneal Dialysis.* Edinburgh, NY, Churchill Livingstone, 1981, p 236.

583. Nolph K, Sorkin M, Rubin J, et al: Continuous ambulatory peritoneal dialysis: three-year experience at one center. *Ann Intern Med* 92:609, 1980.

584. Nolph KD, Stoltz M, Maher JF: Altered peritoneal permeability in patients with systemic vasculitis. *Ann Intern Med* 75:753, 1971.

585. Nolph KD, Twardowski ZJ, Popovich RP, et al: Equilibration of peritoneal dialysis solutions during long-dwell exchanges. *J Lab Clin Med* 92:246, 1979.

586. Nolph KD, Whitcomb ME, Schrier RW: Mechanisms for inefficient peritoneal dialysis in acute renal failure associated with heat stress and exercise. *Ann Int Med* 71:317, 1969.

587. Oddie TH, Flanigan WJ, Fisher DA: Iodine and thyroxine metabolism in anephric patients receiving chronic peritoneal dialysis. *J Clin Endocrinol Metab* 31:277, 1970.

587a. Offner G, Hoyer PF, Latta K, et al: One year's experience with recombinant erythropoietin in children undergoing continuous ambulatory or cycling peritoneal dialysis. *Pediatr Nephrol* 4(5):498, 1990.

588. Ogden DA: New-dialyzer syndrome. *N Engl J Med* 302:1262, 1980.

588a. Ogborn MR, Dorcas VC, Crocker JFS: Deferoxamine and aluminum clearance in pediatric hemodialysis patients. *Pediatr Nephrol* 5:62, 1991.

589. Oh SJ, Clements RS, Lee YW, et al: Rapid improvement in nerve conduction velocity following renal transplantation. *Ann Neurol* 4:369, 1978.

590. Oh SH, Conley SB, Rose GM, et al: Fungal peritonitis in children undergoing peritoneal dialysis. *Pediatr Infect Dis* 4:62, 1985.

591. Ohta T, Matsuda I: Apolipoprotein and lipid abnormalities in uremic children on hemodialysis. *Clin Chim Acta* 147:145, 1985.

592. O'Regan S: Cardiovascular abnormalities in pediatric patients with ESRD. *In* Fine RN, Gruskin AB (eds): *End Stage Renal Disease in Children.* Philadelphia, WB Saunders, 1984, p 359.

593. O'Regan S, Matina D, Ducharme G, et al: Recent advances in diagnosis and treatment of children with chronic renal failure. *International Workshop,* Heidelberg, May 21–22, 1982.

594. O'Regan S, Robitaille PO, Davignon A, et al: Assessment of Brescia-Cimino fistula blood flow rates in pediatric patients. *Nephron* 24:138, 1979.

595. O'Regan S, Villemand D, Ducharme G, et al: Effects of Brescia-Cimino fistulae on myocardial function in pediatric patients. *Dial Transplant* 10:202, 1981.

596. O'Regan S, Villemand D, Revillon L, et al: Effects of hemodialysis on myocardial function in pediatric patients. *Nephron* 25:214, 1980.

597. Oren A, Wu G, Anderson GH, et al: Effective use of amino acid dialysate over 4 weeks in CAPD patients. *Trans Am Soc Artif Intern Organs* 29:604, 1983.

598. Oren A, Husdan H, Cheng P-T, et al: Calcium oxalate kidney stones in patients on continuous ambulatory peritoneal dialysis. *Kidney Int* 25:534, 1984.

599. Oreopoulos DG: Chronic peritoneal dialysis. *Clin Nephrol* 9:165, 1978.

600. Oreopoulos DG: Maintenance Peritoneal Dialysis. *In* Friedman EA (ed): *Strategy in Renal Failure.* New York, Wiley, 1978, p 393.

601. Oreopoulos DG: Peritoneal dialysis solutions. *Perit Dial Bull* 4(2):70, 1984.

602. Oreopoulos DG, Balfe JW, Khanna R, et al: Further experience with the use of amino acid containing dialysate in peritoneal dialysis. *In* Moncrief JW, Popovich RP (eds): *CAPD Update.* New York, Masson, 1981, p 109.

603. Oreopoulos DG, DeVeber GA: Peritoneal dialysis and blood chemical changes. *Ann Intern Med* 72:781, 1973.

604. Oreopoulos DG, Izatt S, Zellerman G, et al: A prospective study of the effectiveness of three permanent catheters. *Proc Dial Transpl Forum* 6:96, 1976.

605. Oreopoulos DG, Robson M, Izatt S, et al: A simple and safe technique for continuous ambulatory peritoneal dialysis (CAPD). *Trans Am Soc Artif Intern Organs* 24:484, 1978.

606. Oreopoulos DG, Khanna R: Complications of Peritoneal Dialysis other than Peritonitis. *In* Nolph KD (ed): *Developments in Nephrology: Peritoneal Dialysis.* The Hague, Martinus Nijhoff, 1981, p 309.

607. Oreopoulos DG: Peritoneal dialysis solutions. *Perit Dial Bull* 4:70, 1984.

608. Orfet R, Seybold K, Blumberg A: Genital edema in patients undergoing continuous ambulatory peritoneal dialysis (CAPD). *Perit Dial Bull* 4:251, 1984.

609. Ott S, Haas L, Scollard D, et al: Long term results in patients using a povidone-iodine connection device in peritoneal dialysis. *Dial Transplant* 11(4):275, 1982.

610. Ott SM, Maloney NA, Coburn JW, et al: The prevalence of bone aluminum deposition in renal osteodystrophy and its relation to the response to calcitriol therapy. *N Engl J Med* 307:709, 1982.

611. Owens ML, Boyer RW: Physiology of arteriovenous fistula in vascular access surgery. *In* Wilson SE, Owens ML (eds): *Vascular Access Surgery.* Chicago, Year Book, 1980, p 101.

612. Owyang C, Miller LJ, DiMagno EP, et al: Gastrointestinal hormone profile in renal insufficiency. *Mayo Clin Proc* 54:769, 1979.

613. Pancorbo S, Comty C: Digoxin pharmacokinetics in continuous peritoneal dialysis. *Ann Intern Med* 93:639, 1980.

614. Papadopoulou ZL, Novello AC, Gelfand MC, et al: The use of charcoal hemoperfusion in children. *Int J Pediatr Nephrol* 1:187, 1980.

615. Papadopoulou ZL, Novello AC: The use of hemoperfusion in children. *Pediatr Clin N Am* 29(4):1039, 1982.

616. Papadopoulou ZL, Sandler P, Tina LU, et al: Hyperlipidemia in children with chronic renal insufficiency. *Pediatr Res* 15:887, 1981.

617. Parfitt AM: Clinical and radiographic manifestations of renal osteodystrophy. *In* David DS (ed): *Calcium and Metabolism in Renal Failure and Nephrolithiasis.* New York, Wiley, 1977, p 145.

617a. Parfrey PS, Harnett JD, Barre PE: The natural history of myocardial disease in dialysis patients. *J Am Soc Neph* 2:2, 1991.

618. Parker PA, Izard MW, Maher JF: Therapy of iron deficiency anemia in patients on maintenance dialysis. *Nephron* 23:181, 1979.

619. Parker A, Nolph KD: Magnesium and calcium mass transfer during continuous ambulatory peritoneal dialysis. *Trans Am Soc Artif Intern Organs* 26:194, 1980.

619a. Pascual J, Teruel JL, Moya JL, et al: Regression of left ventricular hypertrophy after partial correction of anemia with erythropoietin in patients on hemodialysis: A prospective study. *Clin Neph* 35:280, 1991.

620. Pascual JF, Lopez JD, Molina M: Hemofiltration in chil-

dren with renal failure. *Pediatr Clin North Am* 34:803, 1987.

621. Pattison ME, Lee SM, Ogden DA: Continuous arteriovenous hemodiafiltration: An aggressive approach to the management of acute renal failure. *Am J Kid Dis* 11(1):43, 1988.

622. Paunier L, Salusky IB, Slatopolsky E, et al: Renal osteodystrophy in children undergoing continuous ambulatory peritoneal dialysis. *Pediatr Res* 18(8):742, 1984.

622a. Pediatric ESRD. U.S. Renal Data System, USRDS 1990 Annual Data Report. *Am J Kid Dis*. Philadelphia, WB Saunders, Vol 16, No 6(suppl 2), 1990, p 65.

623. Pedicino MJ, Baluarte HJ, Gruskin AB: Targeting fluid loss: Individualizing ultrafiltration rates for children. (Personal observations.)

624. Pennisi AJ, Heuser ET, Mickey MR, et al: Hyperlipidemia in pediatric hemodialysis and renal transplant patients. *Am J Dis Child* 130:975, 1976.

625. Penzotti SC, Mattocks AM: Effects of dwell time, volume of dialysis fluid, and added accelerators on peritoneal dialysis of urea. *J Pharm Sci* 60:1520, 1971.

626. Perez-Alvarez JJ, Vargas-Rosendo R, Gutierrez-Bosque R, et al: A new type of subcutaneous arteriovenous fistula for chronic hemodialysis in children. *Surgery* 67:355, 1970.

627. Perez GO, Ortiz C, De Medina M et al: Lack of Transmission of Human Immunodeficiency Virus in Chronic Hemodialysis Patients. *Am J Nephrol* 8:123, 1988.

628. Perfumo F, Guisti M, Gusmano R, et al: Study of pituitary secretion using the thyrothophin-releasing hormone test in uremic prepubertal children. *In* Bulla M (ed): *Renal Insufficiency in Children*. Berlin, Springer-Verlag, 1982, p 121.

628a. Piraino B, Bernardini J, Sorkin MI: The effect of the Y-set on catheter infection rates in continuous ambulatory peritoneal dialysis patients. *Am J Kid Dis* 16:46, 1990.

629. Piraino BM, Silver MR, Dominguez JH, et al: Peritoneal eosinophils during intermittent peritoneal dialysis. *Am J Nephrol* 4:152, 1984.

630. Plum F, Posner JE (eds): *The Diagnosis of Stupor and Coma*, 2nd edition. Philadelphia, Davis, 1972, p 142.

631. Pogglitsch H, Peter W, Wawschenek O, et al: Treatment of early stage of dialysis encephalopathy by aluminum depletion. *Lancet* 2:1344, 1981.

632. Polak BCP: Ophthalmological complications associated with haemodialysis. *In* Drukker W, Parsons FM, Maher JF (eds): *Replacement of Renal Function by Dialysis*. The Hague, Martinus Nijhoff, 1983, p 742.

633. Polinsky MS: Neurologic complications of ESRD, dialysis and transplantation. *In* Fine RN, Gruskin AB (eds): *End Stage Renal Disease in Children*. Philadelphia, WB Saunders, 1984, p 307.

634. Polinsky MS, Baird HW, Gruskin AB, et al: Evaluation of neurologic dysfunction in children with chronic renal failure (CRF) by neurometrics (NM). *Clin Dial Trans Forum* 10:299, 1980.

635. Polinsky MS, Baird HW, Gruskin AB, et al: Evaluation of neurologic dysfunction in children with chronic renal failure (CRF) by neurometrics (NM). *Pediatr Res* 15(4):698, 1981.

636. Polinsky MS, Gruskin AB: Aluminum toxicity in children with chronic renal failure. *J Pediatr* 105:758, 1984.

637. Polinsky MS, Gruskin AB, Baluarte JH, et al: Aluminum in chronic renal failure: A pediatric perspective. *In* Strauss J (ed): *Pediatric Nephrology, Vol 6: Current Concepts in Diagnosis and Management*. New York, Plenum, 1981, p 315.

638. Polinsky MS, Morgenstern BZ, Baluarte HJ, et al: Autonomic nervous system dysfunction in children with end stage renal disease: Comparison of hemo and peritoneal dialysis. *Pediatr Res* 18:367A, 1984.

639. Polinsky MS, Prebis JW, Elzouki AY, et al: A dialysis-encephalopathy-like syndrome in children: results of a survey to determine incidence and geographic distribution of cases. *Pediatr Res* 14:1017, 1980.

640. Pollak VE, Charoenpanich R, Robson M, et al: Dialyzer membranes: Syndromes associated with first use and effects of multiple use. *Kidney Int* 33(24):S49, 1988.

641. Pollard TL, Barnett BM, Eschbach JW, et al: A technique for storage and multiple reuse of the Kiil dialyzer and blood tubing. *Trans Am Soc Artif Intern Organs* 13:24, 1967.

642. Ponce SP, Pierratos A, Izatt S, et al: Comparison of the survival and complications of three permanent peritoneal dialysis catheters. *Perit Dial Bull* 2(2):82, 1982.

643. Popovich RP, Moncrief JW: Transport kinetics. *In* Nolph KD (ed): *Peritoneal Dialysis*. The Hague, Martinus Nijhoff, 1985, p 115.

644. Popovich RP, Moncrief JW, Decherd JB, et al: The definition of a novel portable/wearable equilibrium peritoneal dialysis technique. *Abstr Trans Am Soc Artif Intern Organs* 5:64, 1976.

645. Popovich RP, Moncrief JW, Nolph KD, et al: Continuous ambulatory peritoneal dialysis. *Ann Intern Med* 88:449, 1978.

646. Popovich RP, Moncrief JW, Sorrel S-Akar, et al: The ultraviolet germicidal system: The elimination of distal contamination in CAPD. *Perit Dial Bull* 4:S51, 1984.

647. Popovich RP, Pyle WK, Moncrief JW: Kinetics of peritoneal transport. *In* Nolph KD (ed): *Peritoneal Dialysis. Developments in Nephrology 2*. The Hague, Martinus Nijhoff, 1981, p 79.

648. Popovich RP, Pyle WK, Rosenthal DA, et al: Kinetics of peritoneal dialysis in children. *In* Moncrief JW, Popovich RP (eds): *CAPD Update*. New York, Masson, 1981, p 227.

649. Potter DE: Hemodialysis in children with ESRD: Technical Aspects. *In* Fine RN, Gruskin AB (eds): *End Stage Renal Disease in Children*. Philadelphia, WB Saunders, 1984, p 30.

650. Potter DE, Broyer M, Chantler C, et al: Measurement of growth in children with renal insufficiency. *Kidney Int* 14:378, 1978.

651. Potter DE, Greifer I: Statural growth of children with renal disease. *Kidney Int* 14:334, 1978.

652. Potter DE, Holliday MA, Piel CF, et al: Treatment of end-stage renal disease in children: A 15 year experience. *Kidney Int* 18:103, 1980.

653. Potter D, Larsen D, Leumann E, et al: Treatment of chronic uremia in childhood. II. Hemodialysis. *Pediatrics* 46:678, 1970.

654. Potter DE, McDaid TK, Ramirez JA: Peritoneal dialysis in children. *In* Atkins RC, Thompson NM, Farrell PC (eds): *Peritoneal Dialysis*. Edinburgh, NY, Churchill Livingstone, 1981, p 356.

655. Potter DE, Wilson CJ, Ozonoff MB: Hyperparathyroid bone disease in children undergoing long-term hemodialysis: Treatment with vitamin D. *J Pediatr* 85:60, 1974.

656. Potter DE, San Luis E, Wipfler JE, et al: Comparison of continuous ambulatory peritoneal dialysis and hemodialysis in children. *Kidney Int* 30:S11, 1986.

657. Powell D, San Luis E, Calvin S, et al: Peritonitis in children undergoing continuous ambulatory peritoneal dialysis. *Am J Dis Child* 139:29, 1985.

658. Primack WA, Harmon W: Incompatibility of CAPD equipment provided by two major manufacturers in the USA. *Perit Dial Bull* 4:183, 1984.

659. Prince AM, Szmuness W, Mann MK, et al: Hepatitis B immune globulin: Final report of a controlled multicenter trial of efficacy in prevention of dialysis-associated hepatitis. *J Infect Dis* 137:131, 1978.

660. Procci WR: Dietary abuse in maintenance hemodialysis patients. *Psychosomatics* 19:16, 1978.

661. Putiloff PV: Materials for the study of the laws of growth of the human body in relation to the surface areas of different systems; the trial on Russian subjects of planigraphic anatomy as a means for exact anthropometryone of the problems of anthropology. Presented at the Meeting of the Siberian Branch of the Russian Geographic Society, October 29, 1884, Omsk, 1886.

662. Pyle WK, Hiatt MP, Morgenstern BZ, et al: Physical characteristics correlated to peritoneal transport parameters. *Perit Dial Bull* 4:(S51), 1984.

663. Quellhorst E, Schuenemann B, Borghardt J: Haemofiltration: Current clinical applications and revolution of techniques. *Renal Physicians Assoc Proc* 2:1, 1978.

664. Quellhorst EA: Ultrafiltration and haemofiltration practical applications. *In* Drukker W, Parsons FM, Maher JF (eds): *Replacement of Renal Function by Dialysis.* The Hague, Martinus Nijhoff, 1983, p 265.

665. Quellhorst E, Schuenemann B, Doht B: Treatment of severe hypertension in chronic renal failure by haemofiltration. *Proc Eur Dial Transpl Assoc* 14:129, 1977.

665a. Querfeld U, LeBoeuf RC, Salusky I, et al: Lipoproteins in children treated with continuous peritoneal dialysis. *Pediatr Res* 29:155, 1991.

666. Radtke HW, Frei U, Erbes PM, et al: Improving anemia by hemodialysis: Effect on serum erythropoietin. *Kidney Int* 17:382, 1980.

667. Radtke HW, Rege AB, LaMarche MB, et al: Identification of spermine as an inhibitor of erythropoiesis in patients with chronic renal failure. *J Clin Invest* 67:1623, 1981.

668. Raij L, Shapiro FL, Michael AF: Endotoxemia in febrile reactions during hemodialysis. *Kidney Int* 4:57, 1973.

669. Raja RM, Cantor RE, Boreyko C, et al: Sodium transport during ultrafiltration peritoneal dialysis. *Trans ASAIO* 18:429, 1972.

670. Raja RM, Kramer MS, Rosenbaum JL: Long-term short hemodialysis. Implications to dialysis index. *Trans Am Soc Artif Intern Organs* 24:367, 1978.

671. Ramirez G, Chen M, Boyce HW Jr, et al: Longitudinal follow-up of chronic hemodialysis patients without vitamin supplementation. *Kidney Int* 30:99, 1986.

672. Ramirez G, Jubiz W, Gutch CF, et al: Thyroid abnormalities in renal failure. A study of 53 patients on chronic hemodialysis. *Ann Intern Med* 79:500, 1975.

673. Randerson DH, Farrell PC: Long-term peritoneal clearance in CAPD. *In* Atkins RC, Thomson NM, Farrell PC (eds): *Peritoneal Dialysis.* Edinburgh, NY, Churchill Livingstone, 1981, p 22.

674. Rasio EA: Metabolic control of permeability in isolated mesentery. *Am J Physiol* 276:962, 1974.

675. Raskin NJ, Fishman RA: Neurologic disorders in renal failure (Part II). *N Engl J Med* 294:204, 1976.

676. Rauh W, Oertel PJ: Endocrine function in children with ESRD. *In* Fine RN, Gruskin AB (eds): *End Stage Renal Disease in Children.* Philadelphia, WB Saunders, 1984, p 296.

677. Rauh W, Steels P, Klare B, et al: Plasma catecholamines, renin and aldosterone during hemodialyis and hemofiltration in children. *In* Bulla M (ed): *Renal Insufficiency in Children.* Berlin, Springer-Verlag, 1982, p 110.

678. Rees AJ: Plasma exchange: Principles and practice. *In* Drukker W, Parsons FM, Maher JF (eds): *Replacement of Renal Function by Dialysis.* The Hague, Martinus Nijhoff, 1983, p 872.

679. Revillon L, O'Regan S, Robitaille P, et al: The effects of Brescia-Cimino fistulas on cardiac function in transplanted pediatric patients. *Clin Nephrol* 12:26, 1979.

680. Ribot S, Frankel HJ, Gielchinsky I, et al: Treatment of uremic pericarditis. *Clin Nephrol* 2:127, 1974.

681. Richardson JA, Borchardt KA: Adverse effect on bacteria of peritoneal dialysis solutions that contain acetate. *Br Med J* 3:749, 1969.

681a. Rigden SPA, Montini G, Morris M, et al: Recombinant human erythropoietin therapy in children maintained by haemodialysis. *Pediatr Nephrol* 4:618, 1990.

682. Robinson EAE: Principles and practice of plasma exchange in the management of hemolytic disease of the newborns. *Plasma Ther Transfus Technol* 5:7, 1984.

683. Robinson PJA, Rosen SM: Pyrexial reactions during haemodialysis. *Br Med J* 1:528, 1971.

684. Rodrigo F, Shideman JR, McHugh R, et al: Osmolality changes during hemodialysis: Natural history, clinical correlations and influence of glucose and mannitol. *Ann Intern Med* 86:554, 1977.

685. Roman J, Gonzalez AR: Tenckhoff catheter repair by the splicing technique. *Perit Dial Bull* 4:89, 1984.

686. Ronco C: Continuous arteriovenous hemofiltration in infants. *In* Paganini EP (ed): *Acute Continous Renal Replacement Therapy.* Boston, Martinus Nijhoff, 1986, p 201.

687. Ronco C, Brendolan A, Bragantini L: Treatment of acute renal failure in newborns by continuous arterio-venous hemofiltration. *Kidney Int* 29:908, 1986.

688. Roodhooft AM, van De Vyver FL, D'Haese PC, et al: Aluminum accumulation in children on chronic dialysis: Predictive value of serum aluminum levels and deferrioxamine infusion test. *Clin Nephrol* 28(3):125, 1987.

689. Rottembourg J, Gallego JL, et al: Serum concentration and peritoneal transfer of aluminum during treatment by continuous ambulatory peritoneal analysis. *Kidney Int* 25:919, 1984.

690. Rottembourg J, Issad B, Langlois P, et al: Sclerosing peritonitis in patients treated by CAPD. *In* Fine RN, Scharer K, Mehls O (eds): *CAPD in Children.* Berlin, Springer-Verlag, 1985, p 167.

691. Rottembourg J, Jacq D, Vonlanthen M, et al: Straight or curled Tenckhoff peritoneal catheter for CAPD. *Perit Dial Bull* 1:151, 1981.

692. Rouby JJ, Rottembourg J, Durande JP, et al: Importance of the refilling rate in the genesis of hypovolaemic hypotension during regular dialysis and controlled sequential ultrafiltration haemodialysis. *Proc Eur Dial Transpl Assoc* 15:239, 1972.

693. Rubenfeld S, Garber AJ: Abnormal carbohydrate in chronic renal failure. The potential role of accelerated production, increased gluconeogenesis, and impaired glucose disposal. *J Clin Invest* 62:20, 1978.

694. Rubin J, Adair C, Barnes T, et al: Dialysate flow rate and peritoneal clearance. *Am J Kid Dis* 4:260, 1984.

695. Rubin J, Kirchner K, Barnes T, et al: Evaluation of continuous ambulatory peritoneal dialysis. *Am J Kid Dis* 3:199, 1983.

696. Rubin J, McFarland S, Hellems EW, et al: Peritoneal dialysis during peritonitis. *Kidney Int* 19:460, 1981.

697. Rubin J, Nolph K, Arfania D, et al: Follow up of peri-

toneal clearances in patients undergoing continuous ambulatory peritoneal dialysis. *Kidney Int* 16:619, 1979.

698. Rubin J, Rogers WA, Taylor HM, et al: Peritonitis during continuous ambulatory peritoneal dialysis. *Ann Intern Med* 92:7, 1980.

699. Rubin LJ, Gutman RA: Hypotension during hemodialysis. *Kidney* 11:21, 1978.

700. Rudnick MR, Coyle JF, Beck LH, et al: Acute massive hydrothorax complicating peritoneal dialysis, report of two cases and a review of the literature. *Clin Nephrol* 12:38, 1979.

700a. Ruley EJ, Bock GH, Kerzner B, et al: Feeding disorders and gastroesophageal reflux in infants with chronic renal failure. *Pediatr Nephrol* 3:424, 1989.

701. Russell RP, Whelton PK: Hypertension in chronic renal failure. *Am J Neph* 3:185, 1983.

702. Said R, Quintanilla A, Levin N, et al: Acute hemolysis due to profound hypo-osmolality. A complication of hemodialysis. *J Dial* 1:447, 1977.

703. Salo RJ, Salo AA, Fahlberg WJ, et al: Hepatitis B surface antigen (HB$_s$Ag) in peritoneal fluid in HG$_s$Ag carriers undergoing peritoneal dialysis. *J Med Virol* 6:29, 1980.

704. Salusky IB, Coburn JW, Brill J, et al: Bone disease in pediatric patients undergoing dialysis with CAPD or CCPD. *Kidney Int* 33:975, 1988.

705. Salusky IB, Coburn JW, Paunier L, et al: Role of aluminum hydroxide in raising serum aluminum levels in children undergoing continuous ambulatory peritoneal dialysis (CAPD). *J Pediatr* 105:717, 1984.

706. Salusky IB, Coburn JW, Paunier L, et al: Aluminum-containing phosphate binding agents and plasma aluminum levels in children undergoing CAPD: Preliminary results with the use of calcium carbonate. *In* Fine RN, Scharer K, Mehls O (eds): *CAPD in Children.* Berlin, Springer-Verlag, 1985, p 138.

707. Salusky IB, Fine RN, Kangarloo H, et al: "High-dose" calcitriol for control of renal osteodystrophy in children on CAPD. *Kidney Int* 32:89, 1987.

707a. Salusky IB, Foley J, Nelson P, et al: Aluminum accumulation during treatment with aluminum hydroxide and dialysis in children and young adults with chronic renal disease. *N Engl J Med* 324(8):527, 1991.

707b. Salusky IB, Goodman WG, Horst R, et al: Pharmacokinetics of calcitriol in continuous ambulatory and cycling peritoneal dialysis patients. *Am J Kid Dis* 16:126, 1990.

708. Salusky IB, Kopple JD, Fine RN: Continuous ambulatory peritoneal dialysis (CAPD) in pediatric patients—20 month experience. *Kidney Int* 24(S15):101, 1983.

709. Salusky IB, Lucullo L, Nelson P, et al: Continuous ambulatory peritoneal dialysis in children. *Pediatr Clin North Am* 29:1005, 1982.

710. Salusky IB, Davidson D, Wilson M, et al: Peritoneal dialysis in children: CAPD/CCPD in children: Update. *Perit Dial Bull* 4:S152, 1984.

711. Salusky IB, Fine RN: Nutritional recommendations for children undergoing continuous peritoneal dialysis. *Perspect in Perit Dial* 2:18, 1984.

712. Salusky IB, Fine R, Nelson P, et al: Nutritional status of children undergoing continuous ambulatory peritoneal dialysis. *Am J Clin Nutr* 38:599, 1983.

713. Salusky IB, von Lilien T, Anchondo M, et al: Experience with continuous cycling peritoneal dialysis during the first year of life. Original Article. *Pediatr Nephrol* 1:172, 1987.

714. Sanders PW, Taylor H, Curtis JJ: Hemodialysis without anticoagulation. *Am J Kid Dis* 5:32, 1985.

715. Sargent JA, Gotch FA: Principles and biophysics of dialysis. *In* Drukker W, Parsons FM, Maher JF (eds): *Re-*placement of Renal Function by Dialysis. Boston, Martinus Nijhoff, 1983, p 53.

716. Sargent JA, Gotch FA: The analysis of concentration dependence of uremic lesions in clinical studies. *Kidney Int* 7(S2):S35, 1975.

717. Sargent JA, Lowrie EG: Which mathematical model to study uremic toxicity? *Clin Nephrol* 17:303, 1982.

718. Sarles HE, Lindley JD, Fish JC, et al: Peritoneal dialysis using a Millipore filter. *Kidney Int* 9:54, 1976.

719. Savdie E, Stewart JH, Mahony JF, et al: Circulating thyroid hormone levels and adequacy of dialysis. *Clin Nephrol* 9:68, 1978.

720. Schaefer AI, Cheron RC, Robert C, et al: Clinical consequences of acquired transfusional iron overload in adults. *N Engl J Med* 304:319, 1981.

721. Schaefer K, Asmus G, Quellhorst E: Optimum dialysis treatment for patients over 60 years with primary renal disease. Survival data and clinical results from 242 patients treated with either haemodialysis or haemofiltration. *Proc EDTA-ERA* 21:510, 1984.

722. Schanker LS, Hogben AM: Biliary excretion of insulin, sucrose and mannitol: Analysis of bile formation. *J Physiol* 200:1087, 1961.

723. Scharer K, Broyer M, Vecsei P, et al: Damage to testicular function in chronic renal failure of children. *Proc Eur Dial Transplant Assoc* 17:725, 1980.

724. Scharer K, Chantler C, Brunner FP, et al: Combined report on regular dialysis and transplantation of children in Europe, 1975. *Proc Eur Dial Transplant Assoc* 13:59, 1976.

725. Scharer K, Giulio G: Growth in children with chronic renal insufficiency. *In* Fine RN, Gruskin AB (ed): *End Stage Renal Disease in Children.* Philadelphia, WB Saunders, 1984, p 271.

726. Scharer K, Rauh K, Ulmer HE: The management of hypertension in children with chronic renal failure. *In* Giovanelli G, New MI, Gorini S (eds): *Hypertension in Children and Adolescents.* New York, Raven Press, 1981, p 239.

727. Schidlow DV: Pulmonary function in ESRD. *In* Fine RN, Gruskin AB (eds): *End Stage Renal Disease in Children.* Philadelphia, WB Saunders, 1984, p 383.

728. Schidlow DV, Morgenstern BZ, Haas JM, et al: Ventilatory and acid-base changes following hemodialysis in adolescents. *Pediatr Res* 17:389(A), 1983.

729. Schlackman N, Green A, Naiman JL: Myelofibrosis in children with chronic renal insufficiency. *J Pediatr* 87:720, 1975.

730. Schmitt GW, Shehadeh I, Sawin CT: Chronic renal failure during chronic intermittent hemodialysis. *Ann Intern Med* 69:73, 1968.

731. Schmitt GW, Shehadeh I, Sawin CT: Transient gynecomastia in chronic renal failure during chronic intermittent hemodialysis. *Ann Intern Med* 69:73, 1968.

732. Schneider H, Streicher E: Thyroid function in long-term haemofiltration. *Proc Eur Dial Transpl Assoc* 15:187, 1978.

732a. Schoumacher R, Chevalier RL, Gomez RA, et al: Enhanced clearance of vancomycin by hemodialysis in a child. *Pediatr Nephrol* 3:83, 1989.

733. Schurr D, Pomeranz A, Drukker A: Dialysis-induced hypoxemia: Continuous monitoring of blood oxygen and carbon dioxide tension in children. *Nephron* 37:105, 1984.

734. Scott DF, Marshall VC: Insertion and complications of Tenckhoff catheters—surgical aspects. *In* Atkins RC, Thomson NM, Farrell PC (eds): *Peritoneal Dialysis.* Edinburgh, NY, Churchill Livingstone, 1981, p 61.

PAUL C. GRIMM
JOSEF LAUFER
ROBERT B. ETTENGER

40

The Immunobiology of Renal Transplantation

Renal Transplantation Immunobiology

Kidney transplantation is the optimal therapy for children with end-stage renal disease (ESRD). A well-functioning renal transplant confers a degree of physical, psychological, and social rehabilitation that is unmatched by any form of dialysis. The immunobiologic barriers to successful long-term engraftment, however, are quite formidable and only incompletely understood. The major barrier to successful transplantation is rejection. The traditional approach to avoiding rejection has been to optimize histocompatibility matching, while using nonspecific immunosuppression to attenuate immunologically mediated organ damage. Although short-term allograft survival rates continue to improve with newer immunosuppressive agents and histocompatibility matching strategies, the long-term attrition of renal allograft survival rates serves to remind us that this is an imperfect approach. The goal of much transplantation immunobiology research is the development of a strategy to attain specific immunologic unresponsiveness to the transplanted organ, a state wherein long-term nonspecific immunosuppression is unnecessary. Unfortunately, efforts toward this goal have fallen far short, in large part because of the complexity and imperfect understanding of allograft rejection.

In this chapter, we examine the current principles that make up our knowledge of transplantation immunobiology. Because transplantation immunobiology encompasses so many areas of investigation, we focus on the specific areas of histocompatibility, the molecular basis of alloreactivity, the immunologic aspects of rejection, and methods of modifying the immunologic reaction to the graft, including immunosuppressive agents.

Molecular Basis of Alloreactivity

The Human Leukocyte Antigen System

An allograft is a transplant of tissue from one member of a species to another genetically distinct member of that same species. Histocompatibility antigens are those moieties present on cells that are capable of eliciting an immune response in the allograft recipient, resulting in the rejection of the allograft.

Experimental models of transplantation led to the discovery of gene products (i.e., antigens) in the mouse, known as H2 antigens, which allow animals both to immunologically discriminate self from nonself and to influence allograft survival [74]. In every mammalian species studied since then, a single genetic complex has been located that encodes a series of polymorphic histocompatibility antigens. As these antigens provide the major barrier to transplantation, the gene complex encoding them is termed the major histocompatibility complex (MHC). In humans, the MHC is called the human leukocyte antigen (HLA) system. The understanding of the HLA system allowed the exploration of the role of tissue matching, the concept of anti-HLA sensitization, the pretransplant cross-match, and the concept of HLA-dependent immune reactivity (see following).

The human MHC is located on the short arm of chromosome 6. There are two major structurally different classes of glycosylated protein molecules coded for by this region: class I and class II. Both are members of the immunoglobulin gene superfamily of molecules involved in cell surface recognition and therefore have structural homology to immunoglobulins, the T-cell receptor, CD4, and CD8 antigens on lymphocytes, and other cell surface molecules [216]. Additional genes in this region control the structure of three complement components (so-called class III antigens)

The genetic organization of the HLA locus is shown schematically in Fig. 40-1. As can be seen from the diagram, class I genes are dispersed throughout the 1800 to 2000 kilobases that make up the class I region, whereas class II genes are clustered in the centromeric half of the remaining 920-kilobase fragment [113].

CLASS I

Class I molecules have two polypeptide chains. The heavy (44 Kd) chain has three immunoglobulin-like loops known

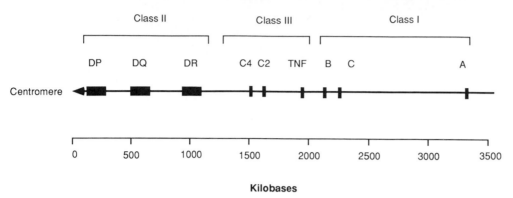

Human HLA Region on Chromosome #6

FIG. 40-1. *Organization of HLA region of chromosome 6. The loci for HLA-A, -B, and -C are found in the class I region. The loci encoding DR, DQ, and DP are found in the class II region, centrometric to class I. In between class I and II are the so-called class III genes. These include genes for some of the complement proteins as well as some cytokines.*

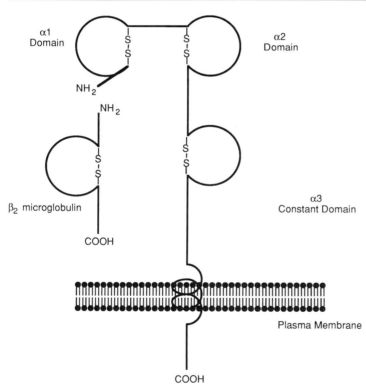

FIG. 40-2. *Organization of HLA class I molecule. The HLA class I molecule consists of a heavy chain with a membrane-spanning portion, constant alpha₃ domain and two variable alpha₂ and alpha₃ domains. The invariant chain beta₂ microglobulin is noncovalently associated.*

as alpha domains. Two alpha domains, $alpha_1$ and $alpha_2$, have variable antigenic regions, whereas the inner $alpha_3$ domain is constant. The other polypeptide chain is $beta_2$-microglobulin and is invariant (Fig. 40-2). Only the heavy chain is inserted into the cell membrane.

Class I molecules are constitutively expressed on the surface of most cells, although expression may be upregu-lated during inflammation [31]. Three sets of class I HLA antigens—A, B, and C—have been well characterized. Three others have been recently recognized but their func-tion is as yet unknown [14]. Each protein is coded for by a different although closely linked locus. Each locus has numerous antigenic products (alleles). HLA gene products are expressed in a codominant manner; both alleles at a given locus are expressed on the cell surface. Thus, an individual inherits one antigen at each locus from each parent. The term haplotype is given to the segment of each chromosome encoding the HLA antigens of the different loci; each person therefore has two haplotypes that together represent the HLA profile.

In 1988 there were 23 recognized A locus, 47 B locus, and 8 C locus alleles [44] (Table 40-1). Since that time numerous A and B alleles have been defined on the basis of differences in their nucleotide sequence. The signifi-

cance of these variably subtle differences is not yet known [14].

CLASS II

Class II antigens also consist of two glycosylated polypeptide chains that are noncovalently associated. Each peptide chain has a membrane spanning portion at its carboxy terminal end. The larger (34 Kd) chain is termed alpha and the smaller (28 Kd) is termed beta. Each chain is

Table 40-1. *Listing of HLA Specificities*

A	B	C	D	DR	DQ	DP
A1	B5	Cw1	Dw1	DR1	DQw1	DPw1
A2	B7	Cw2	Dw2	DR2	DQw2	DPw2
A3	B8	Cw3	Dw3	DR3	DQw3	DPw3
A9	B12	Cw4	Dw4	DR4		DPw4
A10	B13	Cw5	Dw5	DR5		DPw5
A11	B14	Cw6	Dw6	DRw6		DPw6
Aw19	B15	Cw7	Dw7	DR7		
A23(9)	B16	Cw8	Dw8	DRw8		
A24(9)	B17		Dw9	DRw9		
A25(10)	B18		Dw10	DRw10		
A26(10)	B21		Dw11(w7)	DRw11(5)		
A28	Bw22		Dw12	DRw12(5)		
A29(w19)	B27		Dw13	DRw13(w6)		
A30(w19)	B35		Dw14	DRw14(w6)		
A31(w19)	B37		Dw15			
A32(w19)	B38(16)		Dw16	DRw52(MT2)		
Aw33(w19)	B39(16)		Dw17(w7)	DRw53(MT3)		
Aw34(10)	B40		Dw18(w6)			
Aw36	Bw41		Dw19(w6)			
Aw43	Bw42					
AW66(10)	B44(12)					
Aw68(28)	B45(12)					
Aw69(28)	Bw46					
	Bw47					
	Bw48					
	B49(21)					
	Bw50(21)					
	B51(5)					
	Bw52(5)					
	Bw53					
	Bw54(w22)					
	Bw55(w22)					
	Bw56(w22)					
	Bw57(17)					
	Bw58(17)					
	Bw59					
	Bw60(40)					
	Bw61(40)					
	Bw62(15)					
	Bw63(15)					
	Bw64(14)					
	Bw65(14)					
	Bw67					
	Bw70					
	Bw71(w70)					
	Bw72(w70)					
	Bw73					
	(Bw4)					
	(Bw6)					

encoded by the MHC and has two domains. The amino terminal domain of each chain lies farthest from the cell membrane and demonstrates polymorphism.

The MHC codes for at least three sets of class II antigens: HLA-DR, DP, and DQ—and these are quite homologous. Their constitutive cellular expression is more restricted than class I antigens and includes B-lymphocytes, monocytes, macrophages, dendritic cells, and activated T-lymphocytes. During inflammation and under the control of interferon-gamma (IFN-γ), class II antigen expression is increased on these cells and can be induced on other tissues such as vascular endothelium and renal tubular epithelial cells [111].

STRUCTURE AND FUNCTION OF HLA ANTIGENS

A significant advance in the understanding of the HLA products and their involvement in antigen presentation occurred when Bjorkman and colleagues [12] solved the crystalline structure of HLA-A2. The alpha$_1$ and alpha$_2$ domains form a peptide antigen-binding groove directly opposite the membrane spanning portion of the molecule. The walls of this groove are made up of two alpha helices, whereas the floor of the groove is made up of a series of beta-pleated sheets. The surfaces of this peptide-binding groove that face inward and are able to physically interact with a peptide antigen are termed the desetopic surfaces. The surfaces of the molecule that face outward and could

therefore interact directly with apposing T-cell receptors are termed the histotopic surfaces (Fig. 40-3).

Studies of the association of free antigen to isolated HLA molecules suggest that all HLA molecules have antigen bound in the groove. Indeed, it is hypothesized that HLA molecules may be required to form from nascent chains by folding and associating around antigenic peptides and are unlikely to be found "empty" in nature [19]. Class I MHC molecules on a given cell tend to carry antigen originating from that cell. Class II MHC on a given cell tend to carry antigen that has been phagocytosed from the environment of that cell. Regardless of the source of the peptides displayed by MHC molecules (i.e., from inside the cell or from the outside environment), most of these peptides are believed to derive ultimately from endogenous sources [82].

T Cell Recognition

THE T CELL RECEPTOR FOR ANTIGEN

The function of the T cell is to recognize target antigen and initiate an appropriate immune response. It has been known for years that most T cells are restricted in their ability to recognize antigen; recognition will occur only when T cells see foreign antigen presented with some self component [222]. This self component is now believed to be the HLA molecules on antigen presenting cells. The T cell receptor (TCR) is believed to bind selectively to the complex of the HLA class I or II molecule and its

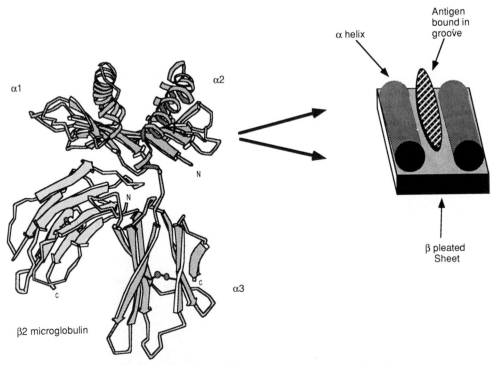

FIG. 40-3. *Structure of HLA class I molecule. The crystal structure of an HLA class I molecule is shown on the left. The alpha$_1$ and alpha$_2$ domains together form the antigen-binding groove shown schematically on the right with antigen in situ. (Modified from Bjorkman PJ, Saper MA, Samraoui B, et al: Structure of the human class I histocompatibility antigen, HLA-A2. Nature 329:506, 1987.)*

associated antigen contained in the peptide-binding groove [13] (Fig. 40-4).

The TCR is present in two forms. The alpha-beta-TCR is the most common and is made up of two subunits (alpha and beta). A minority of cells carry TCRs composed of γ and δ subunits, and their role in allogeneic responses is still unclear. The diversity and specificity of the TCR is generated in a manner similar to that of immunoglobulin molecules. The alpha gene is encoded on chromosome 14 and contains numerous V, J, and C segments; the beta gene is encoded on chromosome 6 and is comprised of V, D, J, and C segments. Different germline segments are selected, spliced, and, along with the insertion of a few random nucleotides, produce the finished alpha or beta gene [190]. A T cell produces only one type of finished TCR.

The areas of the finished TCR that contact the MHC molecule are called the complement determining regions. These are located on the outer surface of the TCR and are coded for by hypervariable V regions. The area that seems important for antigen binding is coded for by VDJ junctional regions.

CD3—T CELL—RECEPTOR COMPLEX

The TCR has a close physical association with five membrane proteins that together make up the CD3 receptor complex (Fig. 40-4). These invariant proteins are called γ, δ, ε, ζ, and η, and are important for transduction of the TCR-mediated signal to the interior of the cell. The first three are members of the immunoglobulin gene superfamily and have a high degree of sequence and structural homology [71]. They serve unknown functions but may be important in assembly of the TCR complex. The last two are different. Protein ζ exists as a nonglycosylated homodimer in most TCRs and as a heterodimer with η in a small number of TCRs. Protein ζ is the molecule that transduces the signal from the TCR alpha-beta subunit to the interior of the cell [67].

THYMIC SELECTION OF CELLS BEARING APPROPRIATE T CELL RECEPTORS

Less than 1% of all T cells generated actually survive long enough to be functional [190]. A number of selection events occur in the thymus, with the result that only appropriately functional T lymphocytes are released to the periphery. First, if the germline genes undergo rearrangement leading to a nonfunctional TCR, the cell will die. Next, T cells with functional TCRs that can interact with self-MHC go through a positive selection step in the thymic cortex; if they have insufficient affinity for the self-MHC restriction elements they will not survive [206].

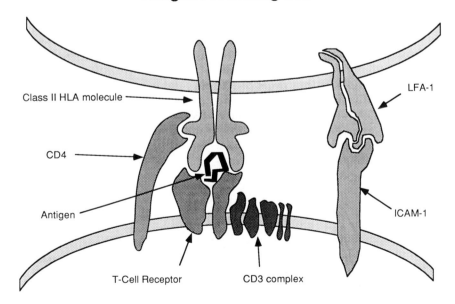

Antigen Presenting Cell

Class II HLA molecule

LFA-1

CD4

Antigen

ICAM-1

T-Cell Receptor

CD3 complex

Host T-lymphocyte

FIG. 40-4. Molecular interactions in antigen presentation. The antigen-presenting cell (top) presents antigen bound in the antigen-binding groove of an HLA molecule. The complex of antigen and HLA are "seen" by the T-cell receptor and the signal generated is transduced into the T cell through the CD3 complex. The interaction of HLA antigen and the T-cell receptor is strengthened by the interaction of CD4 or CD8 molecules. At the same time adhesion molecules such as LFA-1 interact with receptors on the T cell such as ICAM-1 to strengthen the cellular interaction and possibly transduce signals.

Finally, if the TCR has *too high* an affinity for self, and a consequent risk of generating autoimmune phenomena, the cell will be deleted in the thymic medulla (negative selection) [103]. The precise mechanisms by which these selection phenomena are accomplished are still incompletely understood. Nevertheless, the result of this intricate process is that surviving T cells released to the periphery are able to interact with self-MHC but do not have a high enough affinity to self-MHC (and self-antigen) to be autoreactive.

ALLOANTIGEN RECOGNITION

The manner by which antigens of the foreign graft (alloantigens) are recognized by the recipient is incompletely understood. Donor alloantigens may be recognized in a manner similar to other nominal antigens (such as viral antigens). This would involve a process whereby small peptide fragments of alloantigen are picked up and presented in the context of self-MHC antigens by recipient antigen-presenting cells. However, multiple lines of evidence indicate that alloantigen is also presented by *donor* antigen-presenting cells in the context of *donor* MHC [94,205]. How can this be reconciled with the self-restricted nature of TCR-MHC-antigen interactions? The answer appears to lie in the geometry of the TCR-MHC interaction and the differences between alloreactive MHC-antigen structures.

Many MHC molecules initiate a strong allogeneic response, although they differ from responder MHC only by amino acid substitutions that are predicted to lie deep within the interior of the peptide-binding cleft [164]. Current theory now predicts that these altered residues do not change the part of the MHC molecule that the TCR "sees" (the "histotopic surface") but rather affect the peptide antigens that are presented. An endogenous protein antigen that the responder is normally tolerant of when presented by self-MHC may be presented by the foreign MHC from a different angle or different geometry; this could initiate a T-cell response to this foreign antigen.

This scenario does not explain the allogeneic MHC combinations that *do* have significant differences in their histotopic surfaces. Here, one must return for a moment to the thymic education of T cells. TCRs with intermediate affinity for self-MHC are selected, whereas those with inadequate affinity are not, and those with too much affinity, potentially autoreactive, are deleted [190]. If the three-dimensional structure of the allo MHC molecule, by chance, has a high affinity for a responder TCR that is programmed for some other antigen in the context of self-MHC, then that T cell will be stimulated to initiate an allogeneic response. Indeed, Sharrock [174] found that circulating alloreactive precursors are present in normal recipients in a much higher frequency than are nominal antigen reactive precursors. Moreover, there are many T-cell clones described that are reactive to both a specific antigen presented in the context of self-MHC as well as to donor alloantigen [94]. These two scenarios, taken together, appear to provide a rational basis for the molecular events involved in allorecognition.

T Cell Activation

ACCESSORY SIGNALS

Engagement of the TCR by the specific antigen-MHC complex is the primary signal leading to T cell activation. Other (second) signals from antigen-presenting cells are required for full activation. In intact cells, stimulation of the TCR is not sufficient to initiate T cell activation. In fact, T cell receptor stimulation without accompanying second signals may lead to the inability of the T cell to respond to this antigen and instead, paradoxically, to a state of antigenic tolerance. The necessary second signal is provided by accessory cells; most typically these signals are provided by antigen-presenting cells (APC) [210].

INTERLEUKIN-1

One of the important accessory signals is interleukin-1 (IL-1). IL-1 is elaborated by monocytes/macrophages and is present in two forms, alpha and beta, sharing only 25% sequence homology but virtually identical in activity, binding, and function [132]. IL-1 is found in soluble form and in addition the alpha form is also present as a membrane-bound form on activated antigen-presenting cells [28]. One receptor for IL-1 has been cloned, and there is evidence that there is at least one other [125].

The actions of IL-1 are multiple and diverse [40]. It appears, for example, that IL-1 mediates pyrogenic systemic reactions to a number of stimuli [41]. In the context of T cell signaling, IL-1 has been considered one important accessory signal for T cell activation [140]. The exact way in which it facilitates T cell activation is unclear, but the binding of IL-1 to its receptor affects both phospholipid and AMP metabolism [40].

Recent data suggest that IL-1 may not be necessary or sufficient in providing the "accessory signal" for T cell activation. Some reports [135a] show that human dendritic cells stimulate a strong allogeneic response with no contribution from IL-1. Other work [88] suggests that the cytokine IL-6 is an important intermediate in IL-1 induced T-cell activation.

INTERLEUKIN-6

IL-6 is a very important cytokine involved in numerous cellular interactions including B- and T-cell activation [217]. IL-6 is produced by accessory cells and fibroblasts after stimulation by IL-1, and IL-6 is an intermediate in IL-1 driven T-cell proliferation. IL-1 increases the sensitivity of T cells to IL-6 [88] and IL-1 and 6 interact synergistically to stimulate T-cell proliferation [90]. Expression of mRNA for IL-6 is reduced by glucocorticosteroids [221] and actually increased by cyclosporine (CsA) [208].

CELL SURFACE MOLECULES

There are numerous other cell surface molecules that have a role in either or both cellular adhesion and signal transduction. They are important because they augment the binding between the T cell and the potential antigen-presenting cell. Alone, the TCR-antigen/HLA interaction is rather weak; furthermore, the initial adhesion between T cells and potential antigen-presenting cells must overcome a mutual net negative electrostatic repulsion. This initial adhesion is antigen nonspecific and mediated by interactions between one or more of a ubiquitous series of cell surface adhesion antigens and their receptors on the target cells (e.g., LFA-1 and ICAM-1). Other cell surface antigens on T cells (e.g., CD4 and CD8) are intimately involved in the interaction of the TCR to histocompatibility antigens of a specific class (see Fig. 40-4) (see following).

After approximately 30 to 60 minutes, if the TCR does not interact with antigen-MHC complexes on the surface of the APC with a high enough affinity, the cells disengage. If, however, the affinity of the TCR-antigen interaction is high enough, cellular activation initiated by the CD3 complex causes the adhesion to persist and strengthen. T-cell effector function will then occur [187].

CD4 AND CD8

CD4 and CD8 molecules are important surface markers used to differentiate T helper/inducer (CD4) from suppressor/cytotoxic (CD8) cells. They are expressed simultaneously on the surface of juvenile T cells in the thymus, but peripheral T cells express only one or the other [184]. They increase the strength of binding of the TCR to the MHC-antigen complex of the antigen-presenting cell. CD4 binds to a nonpolymorphic portion of the class II molecule (see Fig. 40-4), whereas the CD8 molecule binds to a similar region on the class I MHC molecule. This specific interaction raises the overall affinity of TCR binding to the respective histocompatibility antigen [157]. Both CD4 and CD8 have cytoplasmic tails that may transduce an intracellular signal, probably through tyrosine kinase activity [204]. In the situation of CD4, this protein tyrosine kinase activity is optimally stimulated when CD4 is crosslinked with the CD3 receptor complex [114].

LYMPHOCYTE FUNCTION-ASSOCIATED ANTIGEN AND INTERCELLULAR ADHESION MOLECULE

In nature, a series of cell surface adhesion molecules exist that promote cell-cell interactions by virtue of their binding to specific ligands. The lymphocyte function-associated antigen (LFA) family is one group of such adhesion molecules. The LFA system is composed of three structurally similar glycoproteins: LFA-1, CR3, and p150,95. They are each heterodimers of two polypeptide chains; each has a unique alpha subunit (CD11a,b, or c) and a common beta subunit-CD18 [129]. LFA-1 is a member of the integrin group of cell surface molecules and present only on lymphoid cells. The ligands for LFA-1 are intercellular adhesion molecules (ICAM): ICAM-1 and ICAM-2 (see Fig. 40-4). These molecules are expressed on a wide range of cells and can be upregulated by mediators of inflammation that include IL-1, tumor necrosis factor alpha (TNF alpha), and IFN-γ [45]. ICAM-1 expression is markedly increased on renal tubular epithelial cells during allograft rejection, and this may be important to increasing adhesion of leu-

kocytes to renal tubular cells and to initiation and effector phases of allograft rejection [11]. LFA-1 is normally present on leukocyte membranes but does not induce significant clumping without a stimulus. When T cells are stimulated (e.g., by stimulation through the TCR), LFA-1's binding affinity for its ligands rapidly increases [46] and the cells remain in contact. This is probably due to a conformational change that occurs when the cytoplasmic tail of the β chain is phosphorylated by protein kinase C [64]. At this stage the T cell expresses effector functions. In the case of CD4 + helper T cells, this involves the elaboration of certain cytokines, whereas with CD8 + cytotoxic cells, this entails the lysis of target cells bearing the triggering class I histocompatibility antigen. Detachment is probably mediated by a decrease in phosphorylation of LFA-1 after TCR signal transduction is downregulated by autoregulatory pathways [130].

CD2 AND LYMPHOCYTE FUNCTION-ASSOCIATED ANTIGEN 3

CD2 is a molecule expressed on most T cells. It is a single chain with at least three important epitopes termed $T11_1$, $T11_2$, and $T11_3$. The $T11_1$ epitope is the sheep red cell receptor, the classic receptor by which T cells were first identified. Different CD2-mediated functions are induced by monoclonal antibodies to various epitopes. For example, antibody to $T11_1$ inhibits T-cell responses, whereas antibodies directed against $T11_2$ and $T11_3$ together induce T-cell activation by a non-CD3 dependent mechanism [89]. CD2's natural ligand LFA-3 is widespread in tissue distribution. CD2 is important in thymic development of the T cell. Even more important in the context of alloreactivity, the CD2/LFA3 system is implicated as an accessory pathway of T-cell activation [101]. Work by Suthanthiran [191] has recently suggested that crosslinking of CD2 with CD3 is an important pathway of antigen-dependent T-cell activation. The binding of CD2 to LFA-3 may be the second signal necessary for the alloactivation of T cells in vivo.

CD28

CD28, is another T-cell surface antigen that appears to regulate T-cell activation. It is a cell surface 44 Kd glycosylated homodimer, a member of the immunoglobulin gene superfamily that is present on most CD4 + cells and approximately 50% of CD8 + cells. Stimulation of the CD28 receptor increases the transcription [100] and inhibits the degradation [119] of normally evanescent mRNA transcripts for cytokines, including IL-2, INF-γ, tumor necrosis factor, and lymphotoxin. This results in increased amount of cytokine message and consequent augmented synthesis and release of cytokines by the T cell. This in turn has profound implications for T-cell activation and effector cell function (see following).

OTHER MOLECULES

Other members of the integrin family of adhesion molecules include VLA-4 and VLA-5, receptors for fibronectin

IL-1, IL-6, and TNF. The B cell becomes activated when its cell surface antigen receptor (membrane Ig) is bound by antigen. The B cell's immunoglobulin specificity is produced by a mechanism of germline *VDJ* rearrangements as have been described previously for the T cell. During the process of antigen-stimulated proliferation, the immunoglobulin gene also undergoes a series of tiny mutations in a process known as somatic mutation. This generates increasing diversity and provides a mechanism for selection of the clones that produce antibody with the most avidity [77]. With the help of cytokines the B cell proliferates and differentiates.

Secreted antibody causes injury to allogeneic cells by a number of mechanisms. Antibody in sufficient density may fix complement if it is of the appropriate isotype, and such complement fixation initiates a series of cytotoxic steps. Cell-bound antibody causes recruitment of inflammatory cells by virtue of the antibody's Fc portion. Finally, cell-bound antibody with intact Fc receptors can generate antibody-dependent cell mediated cytotoxicity (ADCC). In this process, certain lymphoid killer cells with Fc receptors bind the antibody's Fc region and mediate cytotoxicity.

Allograft Rejection

Rejection of organ allografts has been somewhat artificially divided into two forms, so-called cellularly mediated rejection and antibody-mediated rejection. In fact, in most clinically apparent instances of rejection, both cellular and humoral mechanisms are operational, with one or the other predominating. In acute rejection episodes, cell-mediated rejection predominates, whereas in hyperacute or other accelerated forms of rejection, antibody-mediated rejection is the major pathogenic process. From a theoretical standpoint, HLA-antigen matching is helpful in ameliorating both cellular and antibody-mediated rejection. Nonspecific maintenance immunosuppression is aimed mostly at retarding cellular rejection processes; there is little in our clinical armamentarium that can ameliorate established humorally mediated rejection.

Cellular Rejection

Cellular rejection is the well-described sequence of events whereby the allograft is destroyed by a process that is characterized by infiltration of the allograft by mononuclear cells of host origin. These cells can include T helper and cytotoxic lymphocytes, B lymphocytes, plasma cells, monocytes, and macrophages. The accumulation of these metabolically active cells and their cytokine products can lead to tissue edema, hemorrhage, and recruitment of polymorphonuclear cells as well as platelets and the coagulation cascade. The processes of acceptance of the graft and downregulation of histocompatibility antigen expression are opposed by the processes that result in graft rejection. The process that nephrologists define as a rejection is the clinical manifestation of the summation of these processes taking place in the graft, with the balance tilted toward graft destruction. The immunologic events that occur are

divided into initiation (afferent) and effector (efferent) phases of the allograft response.

Afferent Phase

The initial interaction involves allogeneic MHC molecules carried by the graft on residual blood, lymphocytes, the graft tissue itself, and passenger dendritic cells. Recipient cells may recognize allogeneic MHC molecules that are presented directly by donor APCs or after processing and presentation by self-APCs (in the context of self-MHC molecules) [205]. The incompatible alloantigens must be recognized by recipient TCR-bearing lymphocytes to initiate the effector phase of the response.

The recipient lymphoid system can be sensitized within the graft by interaction of circulating recipient T cells that are reactive to donor antigens (peripheral route). The other sensitization route is through antigen or antigenic cells released from the donor that are picked up by recipient lymphoid structures. After renal transplantation in dogs, venous outflow contains detectable donor alloantigens for at least three days [145]. Probably both mechanisms come into play as traffic of cellular elements exhibits a striking increase during allograft rejection [87]; conversely, transplant of draining lymph nodes from graft-bearing animals to unsensitized animals results in an adoptive immune state [139].

T helper cells (usually CD4 bearing) produce numerous lymphokines that provide activation signals to the source T cell, other local T cells, B cells, natural killer (NK) cells, and cells of the monocyte/macrophage series. Only 4% of the cells in a rejection infiltrate are believed to be targeted specifically against the transplantation antigens [159]. The bulk of the cells in the infiltrate are nonspecifically recruited by the action of inflammatory mediators. Important inflammatory mediators include lymphocyte growth and differentiation factors such as IL 2, as well as IFNγ, and macrophage inhibitory factor (MIF). IFNγ upregulates MHC class II molecules on grafted and autologous tissue [138] and increases binding of leukocytes to endothelial cells [117]; MIF recruits macrophages. An important part of the recruitment of the infiltrating cellular elements is activation and upregulation of adhesion molecules on the cells of the graft. These molecules (such as CD44 [8]) cause circulating lymphoid cells to bind to vascular endothelium and migrate to the site of inflammation. Arachidonic acid metabolites are important in the events of leukocyte recruitment. PGE$_2$ produced by endothelial cells can oppose the effect IFNγ has on increasing surface class II MHC expression. Products of the 5-lipoxygenase pathway such as LTB-4 as well as platelet activation factor (PAF) increase leukocyte binding and increase capillary permeability, enhancing cellular penetration to the area [86].

EFFERENT PHASE

The cascade of the interconnecting pathways of the rejection process that are initiated by the initial interaction of antigen-specific T helper cells culminates in the destruction of the allograft. The destruction is mediated by antigen-specific mechanisms that include cell-mediated cytotoxicity. Cells of both the CD8 and the CD4 lineage are able to perform this effector function [136]. There is blurring of the distinction between T helper and T cytotoxic cells as clones of a single T cell can have functions that include both secretion of cytokines and cytotoxicity [39]. The mechanism of the cell killing of cytotoxic T cells has been discussed previously. Expression of granzyme B mRNA has been used as a marker of CTL activation in the graft [26]. The relative importance of the CTL to allograft rejection is the subject of some debate and probably depends on the experimental model and degree of MHC mismatch (class I or II) [124,134].

Other antigen-specific mechanisms use immunoglobulin produced by antigen-specific B cells that are stimulated by the T cell derived cytokines in the local milieu. In spite of their abundance in allograft infiltrates, only 10% of plasma cells actually export immunoglobulin [87]. Much of the B-cell proliferation may be nonspecifically induced by the abundance of cytokine help. Immunoglobulin that is directed against cell surface antigens of the graft serves to focus a number of processes. One process is ADCC, which is mediated by cells with Fc receptors such as NK cells and macrophages. Immunoglobulin may activate complement to cause cellular destruction. Vascular endothelial cells are likely targets of circulating antibody and complement as they are immediately exposed to these components in hyperacute rejection. In cellular rejection the intense edema, increased capillary permeability, and hemorrhage may deliver more complement proteins to the graft interstitium to interact with any specific antibody bound to allograft cells.

Antigen-nonspecific mechanisms may be of great importance in the cellular rejection process. The intense cellular infiltrate is made up of only a minority of antigen-specific cells (see above). The bulk are made up of lymphocytes and monocytes/macrophages nonspecifically recruited by the process of inflammation. NK cells (large granular lymphocytes) are important components in some models of rejection [131], but their contribution in human renal allograft rejection is uncertain [162]. An important component of the cellular inflammation is the macrophage. These are activated by macrophage-activating factor and concentrated in the area of inflammation by MIF; both are produced by T cells. Macrophages produce a number of substances that damage the allograft such as oxygen radicals and TNF [38]. Macrophages also produce procoagulant, which stimulates the clotting cascade [47] and eicosanoid products such as thromboxane A_2, which mediate vasoconstriction and platelet aggregation.

The cytokine components liberated by T cells that mediate delayed hypersensitivity serve to activate cellular mechanisms such as macrophages. The cytokines also induce direct cytotoxicity. The cytokine lymphotoxin may directly induce renal tissue damage [126] as can the combination of IL-1 with IFNγ [128].

Rejection Suppression

In 1970 it was demonstrated that a population of cells exist that could, when transferred to a syngeneic animal, suppress in an antigen-specific manner the immune response of the adoptive animal [70]. Since that time the answer to the questions does the suppressor cell actually exist, is this population phenotypically distinct, and what is the mechanism that induces suppression remain elusive. Numerous studies suggest the presence of one or more populations of lymphoid cells that suppress experimental immune responses. Cells that have been identified as having suppressor activity include, but are not limited to T cells with a CD 8 phenotype, NK cells and monocytes. However, the clinical importance of such mechanisms has not been conclusively established. In some models presentation of a class I antigen mismatch alone or antigen without accessory signals may lead to a suppression or tolerant state. Poor production of IL-2 has been identified in some of these models [218]. In animal experiments cyclosporine A has been demonstrated to spare suppressor pathways [95].

The presence or development of anti-idiotype antibodies has also been postulated to be involved in the process of allograft acceptance [17].

Hyperacute Rejection

Hyperacute rejection has fortunately become a rare occurrence with the routine use of pretransplant crossmatching to detect preformed antidonor antibodies. When it does occur it is often dramatically soon after revascularization, with the kidney turning soft and cyanotic immediately; however, cessation of urine output may be delayed as much as 48 hours [15]. On biopsy there is diffuse coagulation in the glomeruli and peritubular capillaries. Hyperacute rejection is initiated by the binding of preformed anti-HLA antibody to vascular endothelium, with activation of the complement cascade causing endothelial damage [66]. Complement products attract neutrophils and macrophages. Platelets attracted and aggregated by the damaged endothelium activate the clotting cascade, leading to deposits of fibrin and cessation of blood flow.

Cellular events may also induce an early aggressive rejection within the first 48 hours. In animal models hyperacute rejections have been produced by adoptive transfer of sensitized T cells alone [48]. There is recent data that use of aggressive immunosuppression directed against T cells decreases the rate of early rejection and initial nonfunction in sensitized recipients [69].

Chronic Rejection

Chronic rejection is a slow process that causes progressive graft deterioration and ultimate graft loss. The exact components of this process are not known. The primary focus of damage is graft vasculature. Obliterative fibrous lesions develop in the intima of small arteries and arterioles. There is interstitial fibrosis and tubular atrophy, presumably due to ischemia because of the obliterative vascular lesions. The glomerular basement membrane is thickened. Antibody to vascular endothelial antigens is believed to play a role as donor-directed antibody is directly related to the severity of the vascular lesions [97]. Localized infiltrates of monocytes, mural immunoglobulin, and complement deposits [160] are regularly seen in chronic rejection and believed to lead to intimal proliferation and fibrosis [18]. Macrophages and monocytes can produce procoagulant, which leads to local fibrin deposition [47] and IL-1, which can stimulate fibroblast proliferation [170]. There also may be a nonimmunologic component involving a hemodynamically mediated injury initiated by depleted nephron mass in a fashion similar to that seen in other models of partial renal injury [59].

Prevention and Treatment of Rejection

Pretransplant Strategy to Minimize Immune Response to the Graft: HLA Matching

Prior to the use of cyclosporine A (CsA), it was generally accepted that optimal matching of HLA antigens improved both living related and cadaveric graft outcome [63]. The relative importance of HLA matching has been questioned in the CsA era. Initially, reports appeared showing no difference between well- and poorly matched patients. Most of these reports came from single centers with relatively small patient populations. Thus, the statistical power to detect even a moderate matching effect was low. More recent reports coming from larger databases such as that of the Collaborative Transplant Study (CTS) with over 10,000 first cadaver grafts show statistically and clinically significant matching effects. Opelz and the CTS [153] demonstrated a 17% one-year actuarial graft survival advantage when grafts fully matched at the B and DR loci were compared with totally mismatched grafts (88% versus 71%). In 1987 Cook reported long-term first cadaver graft survival with different levels of HLA and B-DR matching using extrapolated 10-year graft survival half-lives. The group of completely mismatched grafts had a half-life of 5.8 years, whereas the completely matched group had a 14-year half-life. Thus, for first cadaver-donor grafts HLA matching appears important for both short- and long-term graft success.

The data for repeat grafts show an even stronger matching influence. The CTS showed a 23% one-year survival advantage for grafts completely matched at the HLA-B and -DR loci when compared with those completely mismatched. They also showed that matching for HLA-A as well as HLA-B and -DR was important, contrary to the experience in primary grafts; fully matched grafts had a two-year cumulative survival of 82%, whereas totally mismatched transplants had a two-year outcome of only 49% [154].

In spite of this, the value of matching continues to be controversial because of the concern that the advantages of better matching may be outweighed by the disadvantages associated with the extra storage time required to transport organs that are shared over long distances to optimize matching. Evidence from the Southeastern Organ Procurement Foundation showed locally used, poorly matched grafts did as well as better matched grafts, shared over a long distance [1]. In contrast, a recent report [197] on six HLA antigen–matched, cadaveric kidneys shared between 56 distant centers showed that the one-year survival of these organs was 90%. This is superior to the 79% one-year graft survival rate observed in a control group that was not well matched, but not transported over long distances. Optimal matching also seemed to neutralize the

deleterious effect of high levels of anti-HLA antibodies, with one-year graft survival of 87% in highly presensitized patients.

The quality of the HLA match has implications for the transplant recipient, even if the graft is subsequently rejected. Sanfilippo et al. [169] showed that patients rejecting a first renal transplant were more likely to subsequently develop high levels of antibodies to HLA antigens if the kidney had been poorly matched. As would be expected from their data, the patients in their study who received first allografts with a better histocompatibility match experienced significantly shorter waiting times for retransplantation. Most children with ESRD will require multiple transplants over their lifetime. Thus, when considering transplantation in children, it is prudent to optimize histocompatibility matching, both to prolong long-term graft function as well as to maintain the best prospects for future retransplantation.

Immunosuppression

CYCLOSPORINE

CsA is a cyclic 11 amino acid peptide isolated by Borel from the fungus *Tolypocladium inflatum Gams*. This hydrophobic molecule has emerged as the major advance in rejection immunoprophylaxis in the 1980s. The immunosuppressive effect of CsA is mediated at least in part by blocking transcription of lymphokine genes (e.g., IL 2 and gamma interferon) involved in early T-cell activation [49]. Early events of T-cell activation are not affected by CsA. Initial increases in cytosolic Ca^{2+} and changes in IP_3 and PKC metabolism still occur. However, the cytosolic messages are not transduced to the nucleus to initiate transcription of mRNA for lymphokines. This mechanism of action may be dependent on binding to and inhibiting the action of peptidyl-prolyl *cis-trans* isomerase (PPI), a protein that catalyses refolding of proteins that are necessary for activation of transcription of these lymphokine genes [195]. Quesniaux et al. [163] have shown a strong relationship between immunosuppressive potency and the strength of PPI binding of CsA metabolites. Alternatively, others [107] believe that a CsA-sensitive cytoplasmic activator of DNA replication (ADR) unrelated to PPI is more important to the mechanism of action of CsA. Ultimately, lymphokine genes are not transcribed. CsA has been shown to inhibit the development of DNA binding activity by NF-AT, AP-3, and NF-kappa B [49]. Because binding of these DNA-binding proteins to their sites on the control region of the gene for IL-2 is necessary for gene transcription, CsA blocks IL-2 transcription. Responsiveness to the immunosuppressive drug CsA is lost in certain mutants with deletions of the IL-2 mRNA transcription control region, suggesting that CsA action in some way is mediated through this control region [49].

In addition to the well-known effects of CsA in blocking T-cell activation, there is evidence implicating a direct CsA effect of blockade of alloantigen presentation to T cells by macrophages pulsed with CsA [121]. In addition, there is evidence that CsA may block an early event in B-lymphocyte activation by crosslinking of surface immunoglobulin [42].

When CsA first came into use, children did not have the same rapid gains in graft survival that were seen early on in adults [54]. Reasons for this may include the shorter small intestine of children, leading to diminished oral absorption of CsA [214], and more rapid equilibration, metabolism, and elimination of CsA in the young child [146]. As a result, CsA levels are often inadequate when using conventional adult dosing schedules. Offner and Hoyer [151] made an important contribution to CsA dosing by relating the dose to body surface area rather than weight in young children. Their protocol specifies a starting dose of 500 mg/m^2, tapered by 50 mg/m^2 weekly to a maintenance dose of 300 mg/m^2. According to this formula an infant may require initial doses in excess of 30 mg/kg. Even when these larger doses are used, it is often necessary to administer CsA to young children three times a day. This regimen has led to excellent graft survival of 84% at two years and 78% at three years [151].

There are wide variations in results between pediatric centers using CsA [54]. Differences in graft survival at different centers may be related to the proportion of living related and cadaveric transplants reported and the age mix of the recipients. At UCLA a sequential [186] immunosuppressive regimen tailored specifically for children is employed. Under this protocol, CsA and its accompanying nephrotoxic potential is not introduced until good allograft function is established. In the meantime, an anti-lymphocyte preparation (see following) provides baseline immunosuppression until CsA can be started. When good urine output ensues and the creatinine decreases to less than 2 mg/dl, oral CsA is started, using 500 mg/m^2 for children younger than age 5 or 12 to 14 mg/kg/d in older children, divided into two or three doses daily. In the perioperative period we seek target CsA serum 12-hour trough levels of 500 to 700 ng/ml using a polyclonal whole blood antibody assay; over the first six post-transplant months we gradually lower the CsA dosage so that target levels of 250 to 350 ng/ml are reached by four to six months [53].

Polyclonal antibody assays measure both CsA parent compound and numerous CsA metabolites; monoclonal antibody and high pressure liquid chromatograpy assays (HPLC) detect only parent compound. We have found that HPLC values may vary from 30% to 70% of the values obtained with a polyclonal antibody assay. In patients with abnormal CsA metabolic profiles (e.g., patients with hepatic disease or receiving drugs that alter CsA metabolism) we follow parent compound levels. We seek target parent compound levels 50% of those obtained with the polyclonal assay.

CsA is recognized as a major advance in transplantation. Showstack et al. [181] have demonstrated that the use of CsA has led to a striking reduction in the costs of transplantation, including length of hospital stay, use of ancillary diagnostic services, treatment of complications, and overall hospital costs.

CsA used in the context of a sequential immunosuppressive strategy has been quite effective in improving transplant outcome. In 67 recipients of first cadaveric allografts at UCLA, the use of CsA with sequential immunosuppression was associated with improved allograft outcome at one, two, and three years after transplantation

[55]. At one year the cumulative graft survival rate was 92%, at two years it was 87%, and at three years it was 84%. Similarly, in recipients of cadaveric retransplants, the results again were significantly better in those 25 patients who received CsA in a sequential therapy fashion than in those who received either AZA and prednisone or CsA/prednisone from the outset of transplantation. The cumulative graft survival rate for the retransplant recipients receiving sequential therapy was 84% at one year and 74% at two years.

Cyclosporine A–Related Complications

In spite of its demonstrated efficacy, CsA is difficult to use because of its toxic effects. Clearly, the most significant of these is nephrotoxicity. There are three clinical pictures of nephrotoxicity: (1) synergism with ischemic damage accompanying early graft dysfunction; (2) reversible impairment of GFR induced by high CsA levels; and (3) indolent chronic renal impairment. Renal vasoconstriction, especially involving the afferent renal arteriole [198], has been strongly implicated as a primary etiologic factor in acute and reversible CsA nephrotoxicity. The chronic tubulointerstitial injury has been related to the ischemia attendant on chronic renal vasoconstriction.

CsA induces a striking increase in renal vascular resistance in animal models [142] and in human transplant recipients receiving oral CsA [33,106]. Possible mechanisms underlying the increased afferent arteriolar resistance include increased renal sympathetic tone, increased catecholamines [143], an activated renin-angiotensin system [96], and an increased ratio of vasoconstrictor thromboxanes to vasodilatory prostaglandins [211]. Endothelin release leading to profound intrarenal vasoconstriction has recently been demonstrated in an animal model of acute CsA-induced nephrotoxicity [109]. Alpha-adrenergic blockade [156] and calcium-channel blockade with either verapamil [36,167] or nifedipine [106] ameliorate both the vasospasm and impairment of renal function that accompany CsA administration [108]. Cyclosporine-induced vasospasm has been shown to augment and delay resolution of ischemic damage in animals [188] and humans [81]. This may explain the relatively poor graft survival rate when CsA is used from the outset in patients whose grafts had long reanastomosis times and initial nonfunction [21].

When CsA was first introduced into practice, it was administered in doses much higher than are used at present. Myers et al. [144] observed an ominous progressive nephropathy in the native kidneys of cardiac transplant recipients, frequently leading to end-stage renal failure. Studies disagree as to whether chronic CsA nephrotoxicity is progressive. Some groups have shown progressive renal impairment [202], whereas others have found impaired but stable GFR [213]. Methods of measuring GFR that use serum or urinary creatinine are unreliable for this purpose as they may substantially overestimate the true GFR [168]. However, using a DTPA clearance technique that accurately measures true GFR, Slomowitz et al. [182] have found that renal transplant recipients receiving CsA maintain stable albeit reduced GFRs. In this study, the only recipients who progressed to allograft failure had GFRs of less than 40 ml/min/1.73 m² in the early post-transplant period.

CsA has other adverse side effects that can complicate post-transplant clinical management. Hypertension is seen in more than 80% of CsA-treated renal allograft recipients [127]. It appears to be due in large part to an increased renal sodium reabsorption [34]. We have favored treatment of the hypertension with calcium-entry blockers, because, as noted previously, these agents may relax some of the CsA-induced afferent arteriolar vasoconstriction.

Hepatotoxicity occasionally manifests as a mild cholestasis; elevated transaminases are seen in 19% of treated patients and may be dose related [123]. Renal wasting of phosphate and/or magnesium often occurs soon after transplant and may become clinically significant requiring supplementation. The early renal phosphate loss appears to be secondary to preexisting hyperparathyroidism and tends to decrease over time after transplantation. Hypomagnesemia is due, at least in part, to a CsA-induced renal magnesium loss [5].

Seizures have been noted as a sign of CsA-associated neurotoxicity, and this may be aggravated by hypomagnesemia. The features of CsA neurotoxicity include seizures, cortical blindness, structural CNS changes, and coma. This form of neurotoxicity has been linked to the presence of low cholesterol levels and is seen more frequently in liver than in kidney transplantation [37]. CsA has been hypothesized to be transported largely in the low density lipoprotein (LDL) fraction of the serum and enters cells through the LDL receptor. In conditions characterized by low LDL cholesterol levels such as liver disease, the neural and peripheral LDL receptors may be upregulated, thus leading to increased CNS uptake by the LDL receptor and consequent neurotoxicity [37].

Cosmetic side effects include hypertrichosis, tremor, and gingival hyperplasia. The latter is also a side effect of the commonly used calcium-entry blocker nifedipine, and children treated with CsA alone or in combination should have close periodontal follow-up. Some pediatric patients may develop changes in facial appearance during treatment with CsA. There is a thickening of the lips, cheeks, and nares, along with mandibular prognathism and prominent supraorbital ridges [166].

Cutler [35] has summarized the numerous drug interactions that increase or decrease CsA levels and risks of nephrotoxicity. Drugs that increase CsA levels frequently used by pediatric patients include erythromycin, certain calcium-channel blocking antihypertensive agents, and metoclopramide. Agents that decrease CsA levels include phenytoin, carbamazepine, phenobarbital, and rifampin.

GLUCOCORTICOSTEROIDS

Glucocorticosteroids (GSs) are used by most transplant centers both to prevent rejection and to treat rejection episodes when they occur. At relatively low doses (0.2 to 2 mg/kg/d) prednisone, the most commonly used GS, serves to protect against rejection; at higher doses (3 mg to ≥10 mg/kg/d) oral prednisone or parenteral methylprednisolone remains the mainstay of rejection episode reversal. GSs have multiple immunosuppressive effects that

are believed to be mediated through glucocorticoid response elements. These are short segments of DNA with some similar sequences that can bind to the glucocorticoid receptor. GSs may inhibit gene transcription by causing GS receptors or GS-induced proteins to bind to DNA in the area of the response elements [6]. GSs decrease macrophage production of IL-1 by decreasing both transcription and the stability (survival time) of the IL-1 mRNA. GSs also inhibit transcription of message for IL-6 by peripheral blood mononuclear cells [221]. They secondarily inhibit alloactivation of the T cell and depress IL-2 release. In antirejection doses GSs also cause lympholysis.

Long-term GS therapy in pediatric patients causes numerous side effects. More than 8.5 mg/d will stunt growth [161]. Some pediatric transplant centers attempt to wean their patients from GSs by 3 to 6 months post-transplant [196], whereas others continue GSs on an alternate-day basis [135]. Still other centers continue daily low-dose GS indefinitely [53]. It has been noted that alternate-day steroid use may be accompanied by decreased compliance and impaired allograft function [60]. Though some studies in adults show no difference between outcome with or without low-dose prednisone [76,79], there is a consensus based on clinical observation that GSs augment CsA-mediated immunosupression [54,189]. There is a question whether the present studies of high- or low-dose prednisone have the statistical power to recognize a clinically significant difference [73]. Attempts to slowly wean pediatric patients off of prednisone have been met with unacceptable rates of acute rejection (56%); half of these acute rejection episodes lead to permanent allograft impairment or return to dialysis [165]. Improvement in statural growth is one of the most important reasons for attempting to minimize or discontinue GSs in children. However, optimal growth is dependent on more than just a low GS dose; the best growth is obtained in young (<9 years of age) renal transplant recipients with nearly normal renal function (calculated creatinine clearance of ≥89 ml/min/1.73 m²) [50]. In patients who have renal allografts, the increased height gain obtained by omitting GSs from the regimen must be weighed against increased risk of rejection and consequent impairment in growth and renal function that may occur.

AZATHIOPRINE

AZA in combination with prednisone was the mainstay of maintenance immunosupression in renal transplantation for more than 20 years. Its active metabolites include 6-mercaptopurine and 6-thioinosinic acid. These can impair synthesis of DNA and RNA by blocking synthesis of adenine and guanine nucleic acids. 6-Thioinosinic acid can be incorporated into nucleic acids and lead to chromosome breaks. Initial stages in AZA metabolism are mediated by xanthine oxidase. Xanthine oxidase inhibitors (e.g., allopurinol) used concurrently with AZA may be dangerous as they can lead to markedly elevated immunosuppressive and hematologic effects. AZA is used to prevent rejection and is not useful in treating established rejection. It is generally used in combination with CsA and prednisone (so-called triple immunosuppression) and its use is thought to permit lower dosages of the other two agents. AZA is used alone with prednisone when CsA nephrotoxicity becomes intractable [122] or in the situation of a living-related fully matched allograft. Other groups have electively converted recipients from CsA to AZA to prevent CsA toxicity or because of the financial burden of CsA therapy. However, these patients may have a high incidence of peri- or post-conversion graft rejection [65].

ANTILYMPHOCYTE PREPARATIONS

Antilymphocyte preparations can be divided into polyclonal and monoclonal reagents. Polyclonal reagents may target a number of antigens on the lymphocytes; the precise antibody(s) that cause the therapeutic effect are not identified. Polyclonal preparations include heterologous antisera against lymphocytes, or the globulin fraction of these antisera against thymocytes (ATG) or lymphoblasts (ALG).

Polyclonal

ALG and ATG have been used for both prophylaxis against rejection and the treatment of rejection episodes. The efficacy of ATG and ALG on rejection prophylaxis has been variable. Although some studies show improvement in one-year graft outcome [110], others did not find that prophylactic ATG improved allograft survival [203]. However, there is nearly unanimous agreement that the use of ATG or ALG significantly delays the onset of first rejection episodes. It is this property, and the risk of CsA use during the period of early renal dysfunction (see previous discussion), that has led to the recent increased and successful use of ATG or ALG prophylaxis during the early post-transplant course [186]. Both ATG and ALG have been successfully used to reverse acute rejection episodes [115,176] and even those that are steroid resistant [84].

Monoclonal

A major drawback to the use of the polyclonal preparations is the lack of standardization of potency and purity of different preparations and lots of the same preparation. This has led to the emergence of immunosuppressive monoclonal antibodies. Unlike the relatively nonspecific polyclonal preparations, monoclonal antibodies can be targeted against subsets of lymphocytes and unique cell surface antigens. Because the monoclonal hybridomas from which monoclonal antibodies are produced are clones originating from single cells, there are no lot-to-lot variations in composition, purity, or potency.

The first of the monoclonal antibodies to be used in clinical transplantation is OKT3. OKT3 is a mouse monoclonal antibody directed against the CD3 T cell–receptor complex. Initial treatment with this antibody causes disappearance of all T cells from the circulation. With continued treatment, T-lymphocytes devoid of the CD3 complex appear in the circulation. This modulation of CD3 antigen from the T cell surface renders the circulating T-lymphocyte functionally "blind" to antigen and unable to engage in the process of allograft rejection. After treatment is stopped, CD3 is reexpressed on the T cell surface. Cells already resident in tissue may be affected to a lesser extent than those in the circulation, as Kerr and Atkins

[105] have shown persistence of CD3+ cells in allografts on the fifth day of effective rejection treatment with OKT3. This suggests that OKT3 blocks antigenic targeting of circulating lymphocytes, preventing importation of new alloreactive cells into the graft. By the tenth treatment day most grafts demonstrate no CD3+ cells [20].

OKT3 is quite effective in reversing allograft rejection. In a randomized, prospective, multicenter trial, renal allograft rejection episodes were reversed significantly more often with OKT3 (94%) than with high-dose steroids (75%) [155]. Others have reported similar results, both in using OKT3 as primary antirejection therapy as well as rescue therapy for rejection episodes that fail to respond to high-dose corticosteroid treatment [102,149,199]. OKT3 is effective for rejection reversal in children [149], with the reversal of steroid-resistant rejection in more than 90% of children treated [51]. After the course of OKT3 is completed, rebound rejection has been noted in up to two-thirds of the patients [155]. This has led to a consensus that resumption of basal immunosuppression should overlap the conclusion of OKT3 administration. Indeed, we noted that increasing maintenance CsA immunosuppression at the conclusion of OKT3 administration resulted in virtually no rebound rejection [51].

OKT3 has also been successfully used as rejection prophylaxis in the early post-transplant period. Light et al. [118] have found that the use of a sequential protocol starting with prophylactic OKT3 (followed by CsA, AZA, and prednisone) led to renal allograft outcome superior to that observed when Minnesota antilymphocyte globulin was used from the outset. The data of Shield et al. [178] suggest that prophylactic OKT3 leads to improved long-term allograft outcome when compared with standard triple therapy.

OKT3 SIDE EFFECTS. OKT3 also has significant adverse side effects. The most dramatic and serious of these are seen with the first few doses of OKT3, hence the term "first-dose" effect. This first-dose effect is thought to be due to synthesis and release of cytokines, particularly TNF alpha, by T cells after they are activated by their interaction with OKT3. Once circulating CD3+ cells are no longer present, the cytokine-related effects subside. Noncardiogenic pulmonary edema is the most serious of the first-dose effects and may be life-threatening in fluid overloaded patients [155]. Other first-dose effects include fever, chills, bronchospasm, diarrhea, headache, and vomiting. Cytokine release may also be implicated in the transient worsening of graft function commonly seen during treatment; in addition it may be implicated in the development of aseptic meningitis, which may at times be quite severe with development of cerebral edema (personal observation).

Suthanthiran et al. [192] have postulated that some of the adverse effects of OKT3 administration are secondary to OKT3-induced transient T-cell activation. Following this line of reasoning, they suggest that the use of concomitant CsA and/or corticosteroids may abrogate this reaction in vivo as it does in vitro.

Another strategy is to use smaller initial doses (two) of OKT3 (1 mg). This is just as effective at removing circulating CD3+ cells and is associated with a decreased incidence of delayed graft function (a possible cytokine associated event) [148]. Finally, one group has demonstrated that anti-TNF antibody abrogates a large portion of OKT3 side effects without impairing immunosuppression [62]. Two pediatric studies reported that typical OKT3 first-dose effects include fever, diarrhea, and headache. Rashes, conjunctivitis, and seizures can occur but are less common [51,116]. A later side effect attributable to OKT3 is propensity to infection, especially viral, which increases with prolonged or recurrent use [200].

Appropriate immunologic monitoring is crucial to the optimal use of OKT3. Monitoring the circulating levels of CD3-bearing lymphocytes during the course of therapy helps assess the effectiveness of OKT3. In many protocols, the target level for the absolute number of circulating CD3+ cells during OKT3 therapy is less than 20/mm^3. A failure to reach this goal or a secondary rise after transiently reaching this goal suggests that the administered dose is ineffective or inadequate [177]. OKT3 serum levels should remain above 800 to 1000 ng/ml [72]. If these monitoring techniques suggest inadequate dosing, increased dosages may be beneficial [177].

The major reason for a suboptimal response to OKT3 is the generation of anti-OKT3 antibody. These antibodies may be directed against the CD3 combining site of the OKT3 molecule, so-called anti-idiotype antibodies, or they may be directed against species-specific determinants on the OKT3 molecule, anti-murine antibody. These antibodies are usually measured using an enzyme-linked immunosorbent assay technique, and the anti-idiotypic antibodies are generally present in a low titer (<1:100), whereas the anti-mouse antibodies are often present at high titer levels (≥1:1000). These antibodies appear after one week, with up to 85% of patients having detectable titers [72]. Leone et al. [116] found anti-OKT3 antibody in 90% of tested children following OKT3 administered for rejection, whereas Ettenger et al. [51] found their presence in only 27% of the children treated. These differences may be due to different levels of concomitant immunosuppression during OKT3 treatment or, alternatively, to different assay methods for the anti-OKT3 antibody. Some centers have continued prednisone and low-dose CsA and/or AZA throughout the duration of OKT3 treatment to prevent the development of anti-OKT3 antibodies. Schroeder et al. [172] have suggested that the amount of anti-OKT3 antibody formed varies inversely with the amount of immunosuppression used during the OKT3 treatment. Anti-OKT3 antibodies should be sought 3 to 4 weeks after cessation of exposure to OKT3. Negative or low titre (<1:100) antibodies predict a good response to OKT3 retreatment, although the OKT3 dose may have to be raised if monitoring parameters suggest an inadequate response (see previous discussion). Higher titer antibodies predict failure of repeat treatment [64a].

New Immunosuppressive Medications

There are a group of new immunosuppressive medications in various stages of development. These include mono-clonal antibodies directed against a plethora of cell surface molecules. Recombinant DNA technology has been used to make soluble receptors for specific cytokines. In addition, engineered fusion proteins have been formed from ligands for cell surface receptors and toxins, and these can produce directed toxicity for a specific subpopulation of cells. As well, a concerted effort at discovery and synthesis of new immunosuppressive molecules has produced a new generation of powerful immunosuppressive agents that are being introduced into the clinic.

PHARMACOLOGIC AGENTS
FK-506

FK-506 was the product of an effort to find chemicals that impair IL-2 production by lymphocytes. It is an immunosuppressive macrolide antibiotic that is nearly insoluble in water. It is 100 times as potent as CsA at inhibiting the mixed lymphocyte reaction (1 ng/ml versus 100 ng/ml for CsA) [150]. Besides IL-2, production of other cytokines such as IFN-γ and IL-3 is also inhibited. Like CsA, FK-506 blocks expression of a population of genes involved in T-cell activation [201]. Preformed cytotoxic T cells or previously activated T cell clones are not affected by FK-506 [133]. FK-506 may not spare certain suppressor cell pathways as does CsA [220]. FK-506 has an inhibitory effect on a peptidyl-prolyl cis-trans isomerase that is distinct from the one affected by CsA [83]. FK-506 inhibits B cell function by blocking T cell–derived helping factors [193]. FK-506 has shown good results in preliminary trials of renal transplantation in primary cadaveric recipients, but sensitized retransplant recipients still have poorer outcomes under FK-506 than do first transplant recipients. Importantly, gingival hypertrophy and hirsutism have not been observed in these patients. FK 506 has some neprotoxicity, but the extent of this nephrotoxicity remains to be determined. Full knowledge of the spectrum of side effects induced by FK-506 awaits introduction of FK-506 into multicenter trials.

Rapamycin

Rapamycin is an antibiotic with some structural similarity to FK-506. In addition to being a powerful anticandidal drug, it has immunosuppressive properties. Its effects occur later in the T cell activation cycle than those of CSA or FK-506, Thus, it inhibits T cell proliferation in response to stimulation from allogeneic cells as well as mitogens. It has synergistic in vitro activity with CsA. Its primary mode of action is to suppress IL-2 driven and IL-4 driven proliferation of T cells [43]. Rapamycin has no effect on macrophage release of IL-1 or TNF [173]. It has shown promise in many laboratory models of allograft rejection, and human trials are pending.

Deoxyspergualin

15-Deoxyspergualin (DSG) is another antibiotic that has recently been noted to have immunosuppressive effects. It appears to block responsiveness to IL-2. In addition, it may decrease generation of CTL by decreasing activity of IFN-γ [147]. The exact immunologic mechanism is not clear, but there is evidence that DSG blocks the allogeneic mixed lymphocyte culture as well as mitogen-stimulated responses [104]. Because it induces significant nausea and vomiting in some animal models long-term administration has been problematic; however, short-term treatment, such as treatment of rejection, has been successful. DSG has been used in a multicenter study of 30 renal transplant recipients in combination with methylprednisolone ± OKT3 to treat rejection; there were few side effects [2]. Its efficacy is equal to pulse methylprednisolone alone (72% and 73% rejection reversal, respectively). DSG appears to have additive efficacy when used in combination with methylprednisolone [2].

RS-61443

RS-61443 is a prodrug that when hydrolyzed in vivo, forms mycophenolic acid, its active metabolite. This antipurine agent effectively blocks proliferative responses of both T- and B-lymphocytes. It decreases formation of CTL, activity of memory B cells, generation of antibody, and expression of adhesion molecules. Initial experimental and clinical studies suggest that RS-61443 is highly effective in preventing and reversing acute allograft rejection. Preliminary studies also suggest that toxicity from this agent is minimal.

Antibodies

There are a number of monoclonal antibodies directed at various cell surface antigens that are in various stages of development. Antibody to the IL-2 receptor holds much promise as it selectively targets only those T cells that are actively engaged in an immune-activated process. Human trials have been reported with good preliminary results when used for prophylaxis [22,25]. Use of monoclonal antibody against the IL-2 receptor may not be effective in treatment of ongoing graft rejection [22]. Targeting T helper cells by designing monoclonal antibodies against CD4 is also promising. Targeting the CD4 T cell while leaving the CD8 T cell undisturbed has the potential to lead to tolerance induction [80]. There is promising preliminary work in primate models [30] as well as in humans [141]. Other targets include the T cell receptor itself [207] and intercellular adhesion molecules [27] such as ICAM-1 [29].

An interesting target for future study is specific T cell receptor gene rearrangement products. In analysis of clones propagated from rejecting allografts, a fairly limited number of TCR beta chains were detected. This suggests that alloresponsive cells may share a small number of TCR beta chains, in which case they may be suitable for targeting with monoclonal antibodies specific for those beta chains [68,137].

A problem with monoclonal antibodies of nonhuman origin is the high incidence of development of antibodies against the species of origin of the antibody, e.g., anti-mouse antibodies developing during OKT3 therapy. These antibodies render therapy ineffective and potentially exclude the patient from benefiting from other monoclonal antibodies derived from the same animal species. In order to minimize immunogenicity but maintain the targeting of the antibody, the techniques of genetic engineering have been used to graft the antigen-binding portion of the molecule onto a human constant region. This group of *chimeric* monoclonal antibodies has just entered clinical trials [194].

Another strategy that is being studied is to use monoclonal antibodies to minimize immunogenicity of the donor organ before implantation into the recipient. In a recent study, renal allografts were perfused with an anti-CD45 monoclonal antibody of rat origin. CD45 is a "common leukocyte antigen" present on most if not all T cells. The anti-CD45 antibody was expected to coat passenger leukocytes including dendritic cells (believed to be strong allostimulators) and residual lymphocytes. This was believed to lead to destruction or neutralization of these donor cells. In this double-blinded randomized study, treated organs had significantly fewer rejection episodes than controls (18% versus 63%). The treated group also had significantly superior renal function at 3 and 12 months [16].

FUSION PROTEINS

Some monoclonal antibodies coat their target but may inefficiently fix complement, leading to limited effectiveness. To get around this problem attempts have been made to fuse monoclonal antibodies to toxin molecules, with some success. The monoclonal anti-CD5 fused to the toxin ricin (zomazyme) is a case in point. Along this same line a genetically engineered IL-2-diphtheria toxin fusion protein has been fashioned. The IL-2 molecule provides targeting to high affinity IL-2 receptors (on the surface of antigen-activated T cells) and the diphtheria toxin provides highly selective killing once the molecule is bound and internalized by the activated T cell. This fusion protein has yielded promising results in both in vitro and in vivo models [189].

SOLUBLE CYTOKINE RECEPTORS

Because the cytokines are such powerful molecules pivotal to the immune response, efforts have been made to adsorb these cytokines from the circulation and the graft milieu and thereby prevent transduction of their message to target cells. This is being accomplished by infusions of soluble receptors for the target cytokine. Soluble IL-1 receptor has been used with some efficacy in delaying graft rejection of a rat heterotopic heart graft [58]. Similarly, soluble IL-4 receptor has been used with moderate success in an animal model.

Conclusion

The past few years have seen a dramatic increase in our level of understanding of the immunobiologic principles that underlie successful solid organ transplantation. This understanding has, in turn, yielded important therapeutic breakthroughs. However, although short-term renal transplant success rates are improved, chronic rejection and graft loss continue inexorably in virtually all grafts. The principles outlined in this chapter must be extended if we are to be able to succeed one day in providing long-term successful care for all children with ESRD.

References

1. Alexander JW, Vaughn WK, Pfaff WW: Local use of kidneys with poor HLA matches is as good as shared use with good matches in the cyclosporine era: An analysis at one and two years. *Transplant Proc* 19:672, 1987.

2. Amemiya H, Dohi K, Otsubo O, et al: Markedly enhanced therapeutic effect of deoxyspergualin on acute rejection when combined with methylprednisolone in kidney transplant patients. *Transplant Proc* 23:1087, 1991.

3. Amemiya H, Suzuki S, Ota K, et al: A novel rescue drug, 15-deoxyspergualin. First clinical trials for recurrent graft rejection in renal recipients. *Transplantation* 49:337, 1990.

4. Balkwill FR, Burke F: The cytokine network. *Immunol Today* 10:299, 1989.

5. Barton CH, Vaziri ND, Martin DC, et al: Hypomagnesemia and renal magnesium wasting in renal transplant recipients receiving cyclosporine. *Am J Med* 83:693, 1987.

6. Beato M: Gene regulation by steroid hormones. *Cell* 56:335, 1989.

7. Bendtzen K, Svenson M, Jønsson V, et al: Autoantibodies to cytokines—friends or foes? *Immunol Today* 11:167, 1990.

8. Berg EL, Goldstein LA, Jutila MA, et al: Homing receptors and vascular adressins: Cell adhesion molecules that direct lymphocyte traffic. *Immunol Rev* 108:5, 1989.

9. Berridge MJ, Irvine RF: Inositol trisphosphate, a novel second messenger in cellular signal transduction. *Nature* 312:315, 1984.

10. Bevilacqua MP, Pober JS, Wheeler ME, et al: Interleukin-1 acts on cultured human vascular endothelial cells to increase the adhesion of polymorphonuclear leukocytes, monocytes, and related cell lines. *J Clin Invest* 76:2003, 1985.

11. Bishop GA, Hall BM: Expression of leucocyte and lymphocyte adhesion molecules in the human kidney. *Kidney Int* 36:1078, 1989.

12. Bjorkman PJ, Saper MA, Samraoui B, et al: Structure of the human class I histocompatibility antigen, HLA-A2. *Nature* 329:506, 1987a.

13. Bjorkman PJ, Saper MA, Samraou B, et al: The foreign antigen binding site and T cell recognition regions of class I histocompatibility antigens. *Nature* 329:512, 1987b.

14. Bodmer JG, Marsh SGE, Albert E: Nomenclature for factors of the HLA system, 1989. *Immunol Today* 11:3, 1990.

15. Braun WE: The immunobiology of different types of renal allograft rejection. *In* Milford EL (ed): *Renal Transplantation Contemporary Issues in Nephrology.* Vol 19. New York: Churchill-Livingstone, 1989.

16. Brewer Y, Palmer A, Taube D, et al: Effect of graft perfusion with two CD45 monoclonal antibodies on incidence of kidney allograft rejection. *Lancet* 2:935, 1989.

17. Burlingham WI, Grailer A, Sparks-Markety EMG, et al: Improved renal allograft survival following donor-specific transfusions. II. In vitro correlates of early (DST-type) rejection episodes. *Transplantation* 43:41, 1987.

18. Busch GJ, Garovoy MR, Tilney NL: Variant forms of arteritis in human renal allografts. *Transplant Proc* 11:100, 1979.

19. Buus S, Sette A, Colon S, et al: Isolation and characterization of antigen-Ia complexes involved in T cell recognition. *Cell* 47:1071, 1986.

20. Caillat-Zucman S, Blumenfeld N, Legendre C, et al: The OKT3 immunosuppressive effect. In situ antigenic modulation of human graft-infiltrating T cells. *Transplantation* 49:156, 1990.

21. Canadian Multicenter Transplant Study Group : A randomized clinical trial of cyclosporine in cadaveric renal transplantation. *N Engl J Med* 309:809, 1989.

22. Cantarovich D, Le Mauff B, Hourmant J, et al: Anti-IL-2 receptor monoclonal antibody (33B3.1) in prophylaxis of early kidney rejection in humans: A randomized trial versus rabbit antithymocyte globulin. *Transplant Proc* 21:1017, 1989.

23. Cantarovich D, Le Mauff B, Hourmant J, et al: Anti-IL-2 receptor monoclonal antibody in the treatment of ongoing acute rejection episodes of human kidney graft—a pilot study. *Transplantation* 47:454, 1989.

24. Cantrell DA, Davis AA, Crumpton MJ: Activators of protein kinase C down-regulate and phosphorylate the T3/T-cell antigen receptor complex of human T lymphocytes. *Proc Natl Acad Sci USA* 82:8158, 1985.

25. Carpenter CB, Kirkman RL, Shapiro ME, et al: Prophylactic use of monoclonal anti-IL-2 receptor antibody in cadaveric transplantation. *Am J Kidney Dis* (suppl 2)14:54, 1989.

26. Clément M-V, Haddad P, Ring GH, et al: Granzyme B-gene expression: A marker of human lymphocytes "activated" in vitro or in renal allografts. *Hum Immunol* 28:159, 1990.

27. SL Wee, Cosimi AB, Preffer FI, et al: Functional consequences of anti-ICAM-1 (CD54) in cynomolgus monkeys with renal allografts, *Transplant Proc* 23:279, 1991.

28. Conlon PJ, Grabstein KH, Alpert A, et al: Localization of human mononuclear cell interleukin-1. *J Immunol* 139:98, 1987.

29. Cosimi AB, Conti D, Delmonico FL, et al: In vivo effects of monoclonal antibody to ICAM-1 (CD54) in nonhuman primates with renal allografts. *J Immunol* 144:4604, 1990.

30. Cosimi AB, Delmonico FL, Wright JK, et al: Prolonged survival of nonhuman primate renal allograft recipients treated only with anti-CD4 monoclonal antibody. *Surgery* 108:406, 1990.

31. Cotran RS, Pober JS: Effects of cytokines on vascular endothelium: Their role in vascular and immune injury. *Kidney Int* 35:969, 1989.

32. Crabtree GR: Contingent genetic regulatory events in T lymphocyte activation. *Science* 243:355, 1989.

33. Curtis JJ, Dubovsky E, Whelchel JD, et al: Cyclosporin in therapeutic doses increases renal allograft vascular resistance. *Lancet* 1: 477, 1986.

34. Curtis JJ, Luke RG, Jones P, et al: Hypertension in cyclosporine-treated renal transplant recipients is sodium dependent. *Am J Med* 85:134, 1988.

35. Cutler RE: Cyclosporine drug interactions. *Dial Transplant* 17:139, 1988.

36. Dawidson I, Rooth P, Fry WR, et al: Prevention of acute cyclosporine-induced renal blood flow inhibition and improved immunosuppression with verapamil. *Transplantation* 48:575, 1989.

37. de Groen PC: Cyclosporine, low-density lipoprotein, and cholesterol. *Mayo Clin Proc* 63:1012, 1988.

38. Decker T, Lohmann-Matthes ML, Gifford GE: Cell-associated tumor necrosis factor (TNF) as a killing mechanism of activated cytotoxic macrophages. *J Immunol* 138:957, 1987.

39. Dennert G, Weiss S, Warner JF: T cells may express multiple activities: Specific allohelp, cytolysis, and delayed type hypersensitivity are expressed by a cloned T cell line. *Proc Natl Acad Sci* 78:4540, 1981.

40. di Giovine FS, Duff GW: Interleukin 1: the first interleukin. *Immunol Today* 11:13, 1990.

41. Dinarello CA, Marnoy SO, Rosenwasser LJ: Role of arachidonate metabolism in the immunoregulatory function of human leukocyte pyrogen/lymphocyte-activating factor/interleukin 1. *J Immunol* 130:890, 1983.

42. Dongworth DR, Klaus GGB: Effects of cyclosporin A on the immune system of the mouse. I. Evidence for a direct selective effect of cyclosporin A on B-cells responding to anti-immunoglobulin antibodies. *Eur J Immunol* 12:1018, 1982.

43. Dumont FJ, Melino MR, Staruch MJ, et al: The immunosuppressive macrolides FK-506 and rapamycin act as reciprocal antagonists in murine T cells. *J Immunol* 140:1418, 1990.

44. Duquesnoy RJ, Trucco M: Genetic basis of cell surface polymorphisms encoded by the major histocompatibility complex in humans. *Crit Rev Immunol* 8:103, 1988.

45. Dustin ML, Springer TA: Lymphocyte function-associated antigen-1 (LFA-1) interaction with intercellular adhesion molecule-1 (ICAM-1) is one of at least three mechanisms for lymphocyte adhesion to cultured endothelial cells. *J Cell Biol* 107:321, 1988.

46. Dustin ML, Springer TA: T-cell receptor cross-linking transiently stimulates adhesiveness through LFA-1. *Nature* 341:619, 1989.

47. Edwards RL, Rickles FR: The role of monocyte tissue factor in the immune response. *Lymphokine Reports* 1:181, 1980.

48. Eichwald EJ, Jorgenson C, Graves G: Cell-mediated hyperacute rejection. IV. Lyt markers and adoptive transfer. *J Immunol* 128:2373, 1982.

49. Emmel EA, Verweij CL, Durand DB, et al: Cyclosporin A specifically inhibits function of nuclear proteins involved in T cell activation. *Science* 246:1617, 1989.

50. Ettenger RB, Blifeld C, Prince H, et al: The pediatric nephrologists' dilemma: Growth after transplantation and its interaction with age as a possible immunologic variable. *J Pediatr* 111:1022, 1987.

51. Ettenger RB, Marik J, Rosenthal JT, et al: OKT3 for rejection reversal in pediatric renal transplantation. *Clin Transplantation* 2:180, 1988.

52. Ettenger RB, Rosenthal JT, Marik J, et al: Cadaver renal transplantation in children: The long-term impact of new immunosuppressive strategies. *Clin Transplantation* (in press).

53. Ettenger RB, Rosenthal JT, Marik J, et al: Cadaver renal transplantation in children: Results with long-term cyclosporine immunosuppression. *Clin Transplantation* 4:329, 1990.

54. Ettenger RB, Rosenthal JT, Marik J, et al: Factors influencing the improvement in cadaveric renal transplant survival in pediatric recipients. *Transplant Proc* 21:1693, 1989.

55. Ettenger RB, Rosenthal JT, Marik J, et al: Long term results with cyclosporine immune suppression in pediatric cadaver renal transplantation. *Transplant Proc* 23:1011, 1991.

56. Ettenger RB, Tiwari J, Gaston RS, et al: Clinical transplantation. *Curr Nephrol* 12:397, 1989.

57. Fanslow W, Clifford K, Beckmann M, Widmer M: Regulation of in vivo alloreactivity by interleukin-4 and the soluble interleukin-4 receptor. XIII International Congress of the Transplantation Society, August 19–24, 1990, San Francisco, CA (abstr).

58. Fanslow WC, Sims JE, Sassenfeld H, et al: Regulation of alloreactivity in vivo by a soluble form of the interleukin-1 receptor. *Science* 248:739, 1990.

59. Feehally J, Harris KPG, Bennett SE, Walls J: Is chronic renal transplant rejection a non-immunological phenomenon? *Lancet* 1: 486, 1986.

60. Feldhoff C, Goldman AI, Najarian JS, et al: A comparison of alternative day and daily steroid therapy on children following renal transplantation. *Int J Pediatr Nephrol* 5:11, 1984.

61. Ferguson WS, Verret CR, Reilly EB, et al: Serine esterase and hemolytic activity in human cloned cytotoxic T lymphocytes. *J Exp Med* 167:528, 1988.

62. Ferran C, Sheehan K, Schreiber R, et al: Anti-TNF monoclonal antibody significantly abrogates the anti-CD3 induced reaction. *Transplant Proc* 23:849, 1991.

63. Festenstein H, Doyle P, Holmes J: Long-term follow-up in London transplant group recipients of cadaver renal allografts: The influence of HLA matching on transplant outcome. *N Engl J Med* 314:7, 1985.

64. Figdor CG, van Kooyk Y, Keizer GD: On the mode of action of LFA-1. *Immunol Today* 11:277, 1990.

64a. First MR, Schroeder TJ, Hurtubise PE, et al: Successful retreatment of allograft rejection with OKT3. *Transplantation* 47:88, 1989.

65. Flechner SM, Lorber M, Van Buren CT, et al: The case against conversion to azathioprine in cyclosporine-treated renal recipients. *Transplant Proc* (suppl 1)17:276, 1985.

66. Forbes RDC, Guttmann RD: Pathogenetic studies of cardiac allograft rejection using inbred rat models. *Immunol Rev* 77:5, 1984.

67. Frank SJ, Samelson LE, Klausner RD: The structure and signalling functions of the invariant T cell receptor components. *Seminars in Immunology* 2:89, 1990.

68. Frisman DM, Hurwitz A, Bennett WT, et al: Clonal analysis of graft-infiltrating lymphocytes from renal and cardiac biopsies. Dominant rearrangements of TcRβ genes and persistence of dominant rearrangements in serial biopsies. *Hum Immunol* 28:208, 1990.

69. Galishof M, Lipkowitz G, Germain M.J. et al.: The fate of paired kidneys: Recipient immunologic risk factors profoundly influence immediate post-transplant renal function. *Transplant Proc* 23:1325, 1991.

70. Gershon RK, Kondo K: Cell interactions in the induction of tolerance: The role of thymic lymphocytes. *Immunology* 18:723, 1970.

71. Gold DP, Clevers H, Alarcon B, et al: Evolutionary relationship between the T3 chains of the T-cell receptor complex and the immunoglobulin supergene family. *Proc Natl Acad Sci USA* 84:7649, 1987.

72. Goldstein G, Fuccello AJ, Norman DJ, et al: OKT3 monoclonal antibody plasma levels during therapy and the subsequent development of host antibodies to OKT3. *Transplantation* 42:507, 1986.

73. Gore SM, Oldham JA: Randomized trials of high-versus-low-dose steroids in renal transplantation. *Transplantation* 41:319, 1986.

74. Gorer PA, Lyman S, Snell GD: Studies on the genetic and antigenic basis of tumour transplantation. Linkage between a histocompatibility gene and "fused" mice. *Proc R Soc Lond [Biol]* 135:499, 1948.

75. Gray PW, Aggarwal BB, Benton CV, et al: Cloning and expression of cDNA for human lymphotoxin, a lymphokine with tumor necrosis activity. *Nature* 312:721, 1984.

76. Griffin PJA, Gomes Da Costa CA, Salamon JR: A controlled trial of steroids in cyclosporine-treated renal transplant recipients. *Transplantation* 43:505, 1987.

77. Griffiths GM, Berek C, Kaartinen M, et al: Somatic mutation and the maturation of immune response to 2-phenyl oxazolone. *Nature* 312:271, 1984.

78. Groux H, Huet S, Valentin H, et al: Suppressor effects

and cyclic AMP accumulation by the CD29 molecule of CD4 + lymphocytes. *Nature* 339:152, 1989.

79. Gulanikar A, MacDonald A, Belitsky P, et al: Randomized controlled trial of steroids vs. no steroids in stable CYA treated renal graft recipients. *Transplant Proc* 23:990, 1991.

80. Hall BM: Therapy with monoclonal antibodies to CD4: Potential not appreciated? *Am J Kidney Dis* (suppl 2)14:71, 1989.

81. Hall BM, Tiller DJ, Duggin GG, et al: Post-transplant acute renal failure in cadaver renal recipients treated with cyclosporine. *Kidney Int* 28:178, 1985.

82. Hämmerling G, Moreno J: The function of the invariant chain in antigen presentation by MHC class II molecules. *Immunol Today* 11:337, 1990.

83. Harding MW, Galat A, Uehling DE, et al: A receptor for the immunosuppressant FK506 is a cis-trans peptidyl-prolyl isomerase. *Nature* 341:758, 1989.

84. Hardy MA, Nowygrad R, Elberg A, et al: Use of ATG in treatment of steroid-resistant rejection. *Transplantation* 29:162, 1980.

85. Haynes BF, Denning SM, Singer KH, et al: Ontogeny of T-cell precursors: A model for the initial stages of human T-cell development. *Immunol Today* 10:423, 1989.

86. Hayry P, Renkonen R, Leszczynski D, et al. Local events in graft rejection. *Transplantation Proc* 21:3716, 1989.

87. Hayry P, von Willebrand E, Parthenais E, et al: The inflammatory mechanisms of allograft rejection. *Immunol Rev* 77:85, 1984.

88. Helle M, Boeije L, Aarden LA: IL-6 is an intermediate in IL-1 induced thymocyte proliferation. *J Immunol* 142:4335, 1989.

89. Holter W, Fischer GF, Majdic O, et al: T cell stimulation via the erythrocyte receptor. *J Exp Med* 163:654, 1986.

90. Houssiau FA, Coulie PG, Olive D, et al: Synergistic activation of human T cells by interleukin 1 and interleukin 6. *Eur J Immunol* 18:653, 1988.

91. Howard M, Farrar J, Hilliker M, et al: Identification of a T-cell derived B-cell growth factor distinct from interleukin-2. *J Exp Med* 155:914, 1982.

92. Howard M, Matris L, Malek TR, et al: Interleukin-2 induces antigen-reactive T cell lines to secrete BCGF-1. *J Exp Med* 158:2024, 1983.

93. Howell DM, Martz E. Nuclear disintegration induced by cytotoxic T lymphocytes: Evidence against damage to the nuclear envelope of the target cell. *J Immunol* 140:689, 1988.

94. Hünig T, Bevin MJ: Specificity of T-cell clones illustrates altered self hypothesis. *Nature* 294:460, 1981.

95. Hutchinson IV, Shadur CA, Duarte JSA, et al: Cyclosporin A spares selectively lymphocytes with donor-specific suppressor characteristics. *Transplantation* 32:210, 1981.

96. Jao S, Waltzer W, Arbeit LA: Acute cyclosporine induced decrease in GFR is mediated by changes in renal blood flow and renal vascular resistance. *Kidney Int* 29:431(A), 1986.

97. Jeannet N, Pinn V, Flax N, et al: Humoral antibodies and renal allotransplantation in man. *N Engl J Med* 282:111, 1970.

98. Jellnick DF, Lipinsky PE: Inhibitory influence of IL-4 on B cell responsiveness. *J Immunol* 141:164, 1988.

99. June CH, Ledbetter JA, Gillespie MM, et al: T-cell proliferation involving the CD28 pathway is associated with cyclosporine-resistant interleukin 2 gene expression. *Mol Cell Biol* 7:4472, 1987.

100. June CH, Ledbetter JA, Linsley PS, Thompson CB: Role of the CD28 receptor in T-cell activation. *Immunol Today* 11:211, 1990.

101. Kabelitz D: Do CD2 and CD3-TCR T-cell activation pathways function independently? *Immunol Today* 11:44, 1990.

102. Kahana L, Baxter J: OKT3 rescue in refractory rejection. *Nephron* (suppl 1)46:34, 1987.

103. Kappler JW, Roehm N, Marrack P: T cell tolerance by clonal elimination in the thymus. *Cell* 49:273, 1987.

104. Kerr PG, Atkins RC: The effects of deoxyspergualin on lymphocytes and monocytes in vivo and in vitro. *Transplantation* 48:1048, 1989.

105. Kerr PG, Atkins RC: The effects of OKT3 therapy on infiltrating lymphocytes in rejecting renal allografts. *Transplantation* 48:33, 1989.

106. Kiberd BA: Cyclosporine-induced renal dysfunction in human renal allograft recipients. *Transplantation* 48:965, 1989.

107. Kimball PM, Kerman RH, Kahan BD: Cyclosporine suppression of intracellular activation signal generation is not mediated by prolyl-peptidyl isomerase. 9th Annual Meeting of the American Society of Transplant Physicians, Chicago, 1990 (abstr).

108. Kirk AJB, Omar I, Bateman DN, et al: Cyclosporine-associated hypertension in cardiopulmonary transplantation: The beneficial effect of nifedipine on renal function. *Transplantation* 48:428, 1989.

109. Kon V, Sugiura M, Inagami T, et al: Role of endothelin in cyclosporine-induced glomerular dysfunction. *Kidney Int* 37:1487, 1990.

110. Kreis H, Mansouri R, Descamps JM, et al: Antithymocyte globulin in cadaver kidney transplant ion: A randomized trial based on T-cell monitoring. *Kidney Int* 19:438, 1981.

111. Krensky AM, Weiss A, Crabtree G, et al: T-lymphocyte-antigen interactions in transplant rejection. *N Engl J Med* 322:510, 1990.

112. Kuno M, Gardner P: Ion channels activated by inositol 1,4,5-triphosphate in plasma membrane of human T-lymphocytes. *Nature* 326:301, 1987.

113. Lawrence SK, Smith CL, Srivastava R, et al: Megabase-scale mapping of the HLA gene complex by pulsed field gel electrophoresis. *Science* 235:1387, 1987.

114. Ledbetter JA, Gilliland LK, Schieven GL: The interaction of CD4 with CD3/Ti regulates tyrosine phosphorylation of substrates during T cell activation. *Seminars in Immunology* 2:99, 1990.

115. Leichter HE, Ettenger RB, Jordan SC, et al: Short-course antithymocyte globulin for treatment of renal transplant rejection in children. *Transplantation* 41:133, 1986.

116. Leone MR, Alexander SR, Barry JM, et al: OKT3 monoclonal antibody in pediatric kidney transplant recipients with recurrent and resistant allograft rejection. *J Pediatr* 111:45, 1987.

117. Leszczynski D, Hayry P: Eicosanoids are regulatory molecules in gamma-interferon-induced endothelial antigenicity and adherence for leucocytes. *FEBS Lett* 242:383, 1989.

118. Light JA, Khawand N, Aquino A, et al: Quadruple immunosuppression: Comparison of OKT3 and Minnesota Antilymphocyte globulin. *Am J Kidney Dis* (suppl 2)14:10, 1989.

119. Lindsten T, June CH, Ledbetter JA, et al: Regulation of lymphokine messenger RNA stability by a surface-mediated T cell activation pathway. *Science* 224:339, 1989.

120. Linsley P, Clark EA, Ledbetter JA: T-cell antigen CD28 mediates adhesion with B cells by interacting with activation antigen B7/BB-1. *Proc Natl Acad Sci USA* 87:5031, 1990.

121. Little RG, Evertowski LA, David CS: Inhibition of alloantigen presentation by cyclosporine. *Transplantation* 49:937, 1990.

122. Lorber MI, Flechner SM, Van Buren CT, et al: Cyclosporine toxicity: The effect of combined therapy using cyclosporine, azathioprine and prednisone. *Am J Kidney Dis* 9:476, 1987.

123. Lorber MJ, van Buren CT, Flechner SM, et al: Hepatobiliary and pancreatic complications of CsA therapy in 466 renal transplant recipients. *Transplantation* 43:35, 1987.

124. Loveland BE, McKenzie IFC: Which T cells cause graft rejection? *Transplantation* 33:217, 1982.

125. Lowenthal JW, MacDonald HR: Binding and internalization of interleukin 1 by T cells. Direct evidence for high- and low-affinity classes of interleukin 1 receptor. *J Exp Med* 164:1060, 1986.

126. Lowry RP, Marghesco DM, Blackburn JH: Immune mechanisms in organ allograft rejection. *Transplantation* 40:183, 1985.

127. Luke RE: Hypertension in renal transplant recipients. *Kidney Int* 31:1024, 1987.

128. Maessen JG, Buurman WA, Kootstra G: Direct cytotoxic effect of cytokines in kidney parenchyma: A possible mechanism of allograft destruction. *Transplant Proc* 21:309, 1989.

129. Makgoba MW, Sanders ME, Shaw S: The CD2-LFA-3 and LFA-1-ICAM pathways: Relevance to T-cell recognition. *Immunol Today* 10:417, 1989.

130. Marano N, Holowka D, Baird D: Bivalent binding of an anti-CD3 antibody to Jurkat cells induces association of the T cell receptor complex with the cytoskeleton. *J Immunol* 143:931, 1989.

131. Marboe CC, Knowles DM, Ches L, et al: The immunologic and ultrastructural characterization of the cellular infiltrate in acute cardiac allograft rejection: Prevalence of cells with the natural killer (NK) phenotype. *Clin Immunol Immunopathol* 27:141, 1983.

132. March CJ, Mosley B, Larsen A, et al: Cloning, sequence and expression of two distinct human interleukin-1 complementary DNAs. *Nature* 315:641, 1985.

133. Maruyama M, Suzuki H, Yamashita N, et al: Effect of FK506 treatment on allocytolytic T lymphocyte induction in vivo: Differential effects of FK506 on L3T4 + and LY2 + cells. *Transplantation* 50:272, 1990.

134. Mayer TG, Fuller AA, Fuller TC, et al: Characterization of in vivo-activated allospecific T lymphocytes propagated from human renal allograft biopsies undergoing rejection. *J Immunol* 134:258, 1985.

135. McEnery PT, Fine R, Ascher N, et al: Renal transplant immunity and immunosupression. *Am J Kidney Dis* 7:312, 1986.

135a. McKenzie, Prickett T, Hart D. Human dendritic cells stimulate allogeneic T cells in the absence of IL-1. *Immunology* 67:290, 1989.

136. Meuer SC, Schlossman SF, Reinerz EL: Clonal analysis of human cytotoxic T lymphocytes: T4+ and T8+ effector T cells recognize products of different major histocompatibility complex regions. *Proc Natl Acad Sci* 79:4395, 1982.

137. Miceli MC, Finn OJ: T cell receptor β-chain selection in human allograft rejection. *J Immunol* 142:81, 1989.

138. Miller SM, Gupta R, Lee SHS, et al: Renal allograft rejection induces MHC class II upregulation in autologous kidney and liver of the recipient. *Transplant Proc* 21:328, 1989.

139. Mitchison NA, Phil D: Studies on the immunological response to foreign tumor transplants in the mouse. *J Exp Med* 102:157, 1955.

140. Mizel SB, Ben-Zvi A: Studies on the role of lymphocyte activating factor (interleukin 1) in antigen-induced lymph node proliferation. *Cell Immunol* 54:382, 1980.

141. Morel P, Vincent C, Cordier G, et al: Anti CD4 monoclonal antibody administration in renal transplanted patients. *Clin Immunol and Immunopathol* 56:311, 1990.

142. Murray BM, Paller MS, Ferris TF: Effect of cyclosporine administration on renal hemodynamics in conscious rats. *Kidney Int* 28:767, 1985.

143. Murray BM, Paller MS: Beneficial effects of renal denervation and prazosin on GFR and renal blood flow after cyclosporine in rats. *Clin Nephrol* 25:537, 1986.

144. Myers BD, Ross J, Newton L, et al: Cyclosporine-associated chronic nephropathy. *N Engl J Med* 311:699, 1984.

145. Najarian JS, May J, Cochrum KC, et al: Mechanisms of antigen release from canine kidney homotransplants. *Ann NY Acad Sci* 129:76, 1966.

146. Neiberger R, Weiss R, Gomez M, et al: Elimination kinetics of cyclosporine following oral administration to children with renal transplants. *Transplant Proc* 19:1525, 1987.

147. Nishimura K, Tokunaga T: Effects of 15-deoxyspergualin on the induction of cytotoxic T lymphocytes and bone marrow suppression. *Transplant Proc* 21:1104, 1989.

148. Norman DJ, Barry J, Munson J, et al: OKT3 for renal allograft induction immunosuppression: A comparison of three protocols. 9th Annual Meeting of the American Society of Transplant Physicians, Chicago, 1990 (abstr).

149. Norman DJ, Shield CF III: Orthoclone OKT3: First line therapy or last option? *Transplant Proc* 18:949, 1986.

150. Ochiai T, Nakajima K, Sakamoto K, et al: Comparative studies on the immunosuppressive activity of FK506, 15-deoxyspergualin, and cyclosporine. *Transplant Proc* 21:829, 1989.

151. Offner G, Hoyer PF, Brodehy J, et al: Cyclosporin in kidney transplantation. *Pediatr Nephrol* 1:125, 1987.

152. O'Garra A: Peptide regulatory factors. Interleukins and the immune system 2. *Lancet* 2: 1003, 1989.

153. Opelz G, for the Collaborative Transplant Study: Effect of HLA matching in 10,000 cyclosporine-treated cadaver kidney transplants. *Transplant Proc* 19:641, 1987.

154. Opelz G: Influence of HLA matching on survival of second kidney transplants in cyclosporine-treated recipients. *Transplantation* 47:823, 1989.

155. Ortho Multicenter Transplant Study Group: A randomized clinical trial of OKT3 monoclonal antibody for acute rejection of cadaveric renal transplants. *N Engl J Med* 313:337, 1985.

156. Paller MS, Murray BM: Renal dysfunction in animal models of cyclosporine nephrotoxicity. *Transplant Proc* (suppl 1)17:155, 1985.

157. Parnes JR: Molecular biology and function of CD4 and CD8. *Adv Immunol* 44:265, 1989.

158. Peters PJ, Geuze HJ, Van der Dong HA, et al: Molecules relevant for T cell-target cell interaction are present in cytolytic granules of human T lymphocytes. *Eur J Immunol* 19:1469, 1989.

159. Porter KA, Joseph NH, Randall JM, et al: The role of lymphocytes in the rejection of canine renal homotransplants. *Lab Invest* 18:1080, 1964.

160. Porter KA: Renal transplantation. *In* Heptinstall RH (ed): *Pathology of the Kidney*, 3rd ed. Boston, Little, Brown, 1983, p 1455.

161. Potter D, Belzer FO, Rames L, et al: The treatment of chronic uremia in childhood. I. Transplantation. *Pediatrics* 45:432, 1970.

162. Preffer FI, Colvin RB, Leary CP, et al: Two-color flow cytometry and functional analysis of lymphocytes cultured from human renal allografts: Identification of a *Leu-2+3+* subpopulation. *J Immunol* 137:2823, 1986.

163. Quesniaux VF, Schreier MH, Wenger RM, et al: Molecular

characteristics of cyclophilin-cyclosporine interaction. *Transplantation* 46:23S, 1988.

164. Reinsmoen NL, Bach FH: Structural model for T-cell recognition of HLA class II-associated alloepitopes. *Hum Immunol* 27:51, 1990.

165. Reisman L, Lieberman KV, Burrows L, et al: Follow-up of cyclosporine-treated pediatric renal allograft recipients after cessation of prednisone. *Transplantation* 49:76, 1990.

166. Reznik VM, Durham BL, Jones KL: Changes in facial appearance during cyclosporin treatment. *Lancet* 1:1405, 1987.

167. Rooth P, Dawidson I, Diller K, et al: Protection against cyclosporine-induced impairment of renal microcirculation by verapamil in mice. *Transplantation* 45:433, 1988.

168. Ross EA, Wilkinson A, Hawkins RA, et al: The plasma creatinine concentration is not an accurate reflection of the GFR in stable renal transplant patients receiving cyclosporine. *Am J Kidney Dis* 10:113, 1987.

169. Sanfilippo F, Goeken N, Niblack G, et al: The effect of first cadaver renal transplant HLA-A,B match on sensitization levels and retransplant rates following graft failure. *Transplantation* 43:240, 1987.

170. Schmidt JA, Mizel SB, Cohen D, et al: Interleukin-1, a potential regulator of fibroblast proliferation. *J Immunol* 128:2177, 1982.

171. Schrezenmeier H, Ahnert-Hilger G, Fleischer B: A T cell receptor-associated GTP-binding protein triggers TCR-mediated granule exocytosis in cytotoxic T lymphocytes. *J Immunol* 141:3785, 1988.

172. Schroeder TJ, First MR, Mansour ME, et al: Antimurine antibody formation following OKT3 therapy. *Transplantation* 49:48, 1990.

173. Sehgal SN, Chang JY: Rapamycin: A new immunosuppressive macrolide. *Transplantation and Immunology Letter* 7:12, 1990.

174. Sharrock CEM, Kaminski E, Man S: Limiting dilution analysis of human T cells: A useful clinical tool. *Immunol Today* 11:281, 1990.

175. Shaw J-P, Utz PJ, Durand DB, et al: Identification of a putative regulator of early T cell activation genes. *Science* 241:202, 1988.

176. Shield CF III, Cosimi AG, Tolkoff-Rubin N, et al: Use of antithymocyte globulin for reversal of acute allograft rejection. *Transplantation* 28:461, 1979.

177. Shield CF III, Norman DJ: Immunologic monitoring during and after OKT3 therapy. *Am J Kidney Dis* 11:120, 1988.

178. Shield CF: OKT3 induction therapy for cadaver renal transplantation. 9th Annual Meeting of the American Society of Transplant Physicians, Chicago, 1990 (abstr).

179. Shimizu Y, Van Seventer GA, Horgan KJ, et al: Regulated expression and binding of 3 VLA (beta-1) integrin receptors on T-cells. *Nature* (in press).

180. Shinkai Y, Takio K, Okumura K: Homology of perforin to the ninth component of complement. *Nature* 334:525, 1988.

181. Showstack J, Katz J, Amend W, et al: The effect of cyclosporine on the use of hospital resources for kidney transplantation. *N Engl J Med* 321:1086, 1989.

182. Slomowitz LA, Wilkinson A, Hawkins R, et al: Evaluation of kidney function in renal transplant patients receiving long-term cyclosporine. *Am J Kidney Dis* 15:530, 1990.

183. Smith KA: Interleukin-2: Inception, impact, and implications. *Science* 240:1169, 1988.

184. Smith L: CD4+ murine T cells develop from CD8+ precursors in vivo. *Nature* 326:798, 1987.

185. Snapper CM, Finkelman FD, Paul WE: Regulation of IgG$_1$

and IgE production by interleukin 4. *Immunol Rev* 102:29, 1988.

186. Sommer B, Ferguson R: Three immediate post renal transplant adjunct protocols combined with maintenance cyclosporine. *Transplant Proc* 17:1235, 1985.

187. Spits H, Van Schooten W, Keizer H, et al: Alloantigen recognition is preceded by nonspecific adhesion of cytotoxic T cells and target cells. *Science* 232:403, 1986.

188. Steinmuller DR, Kanazi G, Stowe N, et al: The enhancement of cyclosporine nephrotoxicity by renal ischemia in a rat model. *Kidney Int* 29:287A, 1986 (abstr).

189. Strom TB, Kelley VE: Toward more selective therapies to block undesired immune responses. *Kidney Int* 35:1026, 1989.

190. Strominger JL: Developmental biology of T cell receptors. *Science* 244:943, 1989.

191. Suthanthiran M: A novel model for antigen-dependent activation of normal human T cells. Transmembrane signaling by crosslinkage of the CD3/T cell receptor-alpha/beta complex with the cluster determinant 2 antigen. *J Exp Med* 171:1965, 1990.

192. Suthanthiran M, Wiebe ME, Stenzel KH: Effect of immunosuppressants on OKT3 associated T cell activation: clinical implications. *Kidney Int* 32:362, 1987.

193. Suzuki N, Sakane T, Tsunematsu T: Effects of a novel immunosuppressive agent, FK-506, on human B cell activation. *Clin Exp Immunol* 79:240, 1990.

194. Sweny P, Amlot P, Fernando O, et al: Pilot study of a chimeric human/mouse CD7 monoclonal antibody (SDZ CHH 380) in renal transplantation. XIII International Congress of the Transplantation Society San Francisco, CA, August 19–24, 1990 (abstr).

195. Takahashi N, Hayano T, Suzuki M: Peptidyl-prolyl *cis-trans* isomerase is the cyclosporine A-binding cyclophilin. *Nature* 337:473, 1989.

196. Tejani A, Butt KMH, Khawar MR, et al: Cyclosporine experience in renal transplantation in children. *Kidney Int* 30:S35, 1986.

197. Terasaki PI, Takemoto S, Mickey MR: A report on 123 six-antigen matched cadaver kidney transplants. *Clin Transplantation* 3:301, 1989.

198. Thiel G: Experimental cyclosporine A nephrotoxicity: A summary of the International Workshop (Basel, April 24–26, 1985). *Clin Nephrol* (suppl 1)25:205, 1986.

199. Thistlethwaite JR Jr, Gaber AO, Haag BW, et al: OKT3 treatment of steroid-resistant renal allograft rejection. *Transplantation* 43:176, 1987.

200. Thistlethwaite JR Jr, Stuart JK, Mayes JT, et al: Complications and monitoring of OKT3 therapy. *Am J Kidney Dis* 11:112, 1988.

201. Tocci MJ, Matkovich DA, Collier KA, et al: The immunosuppressant FK-506 selectively inhibits expression of early T cell activation genes. *J Immunol* 143:718, 1989.

202. Tomlanovich S, Leutscher J, Perlroth M, et al: Nature of chronic glomerular injury induced by cyclosporine. *Clin Res* 33:589A, 1985 (abstr).

203. Uittenbogaart CH, Robinson BJ, Malekzadeh, MH et al: The use of antithymocyte globulin (dose by rosette protocol) in pediatric renal allograft recipients. *Transplantation* 28:291, 1979.

204. Veillette A, Bookman MA, Horak EM, et al: The CD4 and CD8 T cell surface antigens are associated with the internal membrane tyrosine protein kinase p56lck. *Cell* 55:301, 1988.

205. Via CS, Tsokos GC, Stocks NI, et al: Human in vitro allogeneic responses. Demonstration of three pathways of T helper activation. *J Immunol* 144:2524, 1990.

206. von Boehmer H, Teh HS, Kisielow P: The thymus selects the useful, neglects the useless and destroys the harmful. *Immunol Today* 10:57, 1989.

207. Waid T, Lucas B, Thompson J, et al: Treatment of acute rejection with anti T-cell antigen receptor complex αβ (T10B9.1A-31) or anti CD3 (OKT3) monoclonal antibody: Results of a prospective randomized double blind trial. *Transplant Proc* 23:1062, 1991.

208. Walz G, Zanker B, Melton LB et al: Possible association of the immunosuppressive and B cell lymphoma-promoting properties of cyclosporine. *Transplantation* 49:191, 1990.

209. Wang HM, Smith KA: The interleukin 2 receptor. Functional consequences of its bimolecular structure. *J Exp Med* 166:1055, 1987.

210. Weaver CT, Unanue ER: The costimulatory function of antigen-presenting cells. *Immunol Today* 11:49, 1990.

211. Weir MR, Klassen DK, Shen SY, et al: Acute effects of intravenous cyclosporine on blood pressure, renal hemodynamics, and urine prostaglandin production of healthy humans. *Transplantation* 49:41, 1990.

212. Weiss A, Imboden JB: Cell surface molecules and early events involved in human T lymphocyte activation. *Adv Immunol* 41:1, 1987.

213. Wheatly HC, Datzman M, Williams JW, et al: Long-term effects of cyclosporine on renal function in liver transplant recipients. *Transplantation* 43:641, 1987.

214. Whitington PF, Emond JC, Whitington SH, et al: Small-bowel length and the dose of cyclosporine in children after liver transplantation. *N Engl J Med* 322:733, 1990.

215. Widmer MB, Grabstein KH: B-cell stimulating factor regulates the generation of cytolytic T-lymphocytes. *Nature* 326:795, 1987.

216. Williams AF: A year in the life of the immunoglobulin superfamily. *Immunol Today* 8:298, 1987.

217. Wong GG, Clarke SC: Multiple actions of interleukin 6 within a cytokine network. *Immunol Today* 9:137, 1988.

218. Wood KJ, Dallman MJ, Morris PJ: Cytotoxic cells alone are not sufficient to mediate renal graft rejection. *Transpl Proc* 21:338, 1989.

219. Yanelli JR, Sullivan JA, Mandell GL, et al: Reorientation and fusion of cytotoxic T lymphocyte granules after interaction with target cells as determined by high resolution cinemicrography. *J Immunol* 136:377, 1986.

220. Yoshimura N, Matsui S, Hamashima T, et al: A new immunosuppressive agent, FK-506, inhibits the expression of alloantigen-activated suppressor cells as well as the induction of alloreactivity. *Transplant Proc* 21:1045, 1989.

221. Zanker B, Walz G, Wieder KJ: Evidence that glucocorticosteroids block expression of the human interleukin-6 gene by accessory cells. *Transplantation* 49:183, 1990

222. Zinkernagel RM, Doherty PC: Restriction of in vitro T cell-mediated cytotoxicity in lymphocytic choriomeningitis within a syngeneic or semiallogeneic system. *Nature* 248:701, 1974.

S. Michael Mauer
Thomas E. Nevins
Nancy Ascher

41
Renal Transplantation in Children

Renal transplantation is now an accepted form of therapy for patients with end-stage renal failure. Children requiring this dramatic and dangerous treatment present special problems that frequently are different from those encountered in adults. Technical considerations and problems of growth, sexual maturation, and psychosocial development make transplantation in children a therapy requiring highly specialized knowledge, not only of nephrology but also of pediatrics. Pediatric nephrologists, surgeons, nurses, social workers, neurologists, psychologists, and psychiatrists must all work closely together if the myriad challenges of pediatric renal transplantation are to be adequately met. The center concept, with the availability of a broad range of expertise in many pediatric subspecialty areas, offers great advantages for the care of these children. Despite some opinions that transplantation in children may be inappropriate [213,214], transplantation programs for these patients continue to grow in all medically developed nations, and increasing experience indicates that children are suitable candidates for renal transplantation. More recently, experience with renal transplantation in infancy has been expanding and, we believe, represents a future direction that will receive accelerating emphasis.

In this chapter aspects of transplantation that are particularly relevant to children are emphasized. Although basic concepts and problems related to the general field of renal transplantation are also discussed, the reader is referred to earlier texts [102,185,210] and to Chap. 40, which cover these areas in greater detail.

Indications

Although glomerulonephritis is the most common single category of renal disease necessitating transplantation in children (Fig. 41-1), its frequency is approximately one-half of that seen in adults with terminal uremia [1]. In younger children especially (Table 41-1), congenital renal disorders make a major contribution to pediatric renal failure. The age distribution of children undergoing renal transplantation at our institution is shown in Fig. 41-2.

Young children with uremia generally require therapeutic intervention with dialysis or transplantation at lower levels of serum creatinine than adults. The chronically uremic malnourished infant with reduced muscle mass often has symptoms of end-stage renal disease (ESRD) at levels of serum creatinine that are well tolerated in older children or adults. Thus, severe failure to thrive or clinical deterioration occurring despite optimal medical management should guide treatment, and somewhat less reliance should be placed on laboratory values. For example, we have considered it necessary to transplant some children with congenital nephrotic syndrome before laboratory evidence of serious renal insufficiency developed; in some instances such patients had serum creatinine levels less than 2 mg/dl. Similarly, patients with primary hyperoxaluria (oxalosis) should be considered for early transplantation because long periods of advanced uremia, even with adequate dialysis support, appear to be associated with increasing extrarenal oxalate stores, which may compromise the renal allograft [224]. The expected frequency of recurrence of original diseases in renal grafts and the status of bladder function influence decisions about transplantation, as discussed in a subsequent section. Children with bilateral Wilms' tumor maintained on dialysis for a period of time adequate to define the absence of metastatic disease (usually 1 year) have been considered as acceptable candidates for transplantation [17,204,262].

A major dilemma frequently arises concerning children with uremia who exhibit psychomotor retardation. During the last decade, pediatricians have been increasingly aware of the CNS effects of chronic uremia in childhood. As more children survive infancy with renal insufficiency, the CNS ravages of uremia have become increasingly evident [10,78,216]. A progressive encephalopathic syndrome has been described in uremic infants [217]. The etiology of this syndrome is unknown, and, to date, no therapy is recognized as effective. However, earlier, aggressive therapy including dialysis or transplantation may be capable of stabilizing or protecting the developing CNS. Presently no data support "early" transplantation, but the frequent occurrence of neurologic problems in uremic children does favor transplantation as soon as the surgical risk is minimal.

Future studies may demonstrate a role for renal trans-

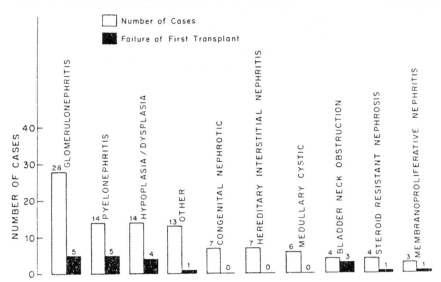

FIG. 41-1. Incidence of diseases leading to transplantation among 100 consecutive pediatric patients. The number of first transplants that ultimately failed is also shown. (From DeShazo CV, Simmons RL, Bernstein DM, et al: Results of renal transplantation in 100 children. Surgery 70:461, 1974.)

TABLE 41-1. Causes of renal disease in 42 children ages 1 to 5 years transplanted at the University of Minnesota

Hypoplastic dysplastic kidneys	16
Congenital nephrotic syndrome	12
Oxalosis	2
Hemolytic uremic syndrome	2
Infantile polycystic kidneys	1
Cystinosis	1
Rapidly progressive glomerulonephritis	1
Steroid-resistant nephrotic syndrome with focal segmental sclerosis	
Steroid-sensitive nephrotic syndrome and interstitial nephritis	1
Jeune's syndrome	1
X-Y gonadal dysgenesis (Drash syndrome)	1
Wilms' tumor	1
Birth asphyxia: cortical necrosis	1
Chronic glomerulonephritis; type unknown	1

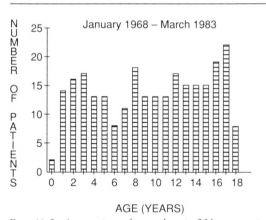

FIG. 41-2. Age at time of transplant in 231 consecutive pediatric patients at the University of Minnesota.

plantation in protecting the CNS of young uremic patients, thereby creating a new indication for the procedure. Ideally these studies will define prognostic or risk factors, allowing more aggressive therapy to be directed to a specific subpopulation of children with renal impairment and high CNS risk.

Selection and Evaluation of Patients for Renal Transplantation

Criteria for selecting suitable renal transplantation recipients have not been rigidly defined. The ideal candidates have been stated to be patients with end-stage renal disease between the ages of 15 and 45 years who have not had

other diseases. As knowledge and experience in renal transplantation has accumulated, however, the suitability of younger patients for transplantation has been demonstrated [188], and it is clear that, at this stage of our knowledge, rigid definitions of suitable patient populations are premature.

In 1968 Merrill [174] listed several factors he believed to be important in selecting recipients. Factors relevant to children included age, failure to respond to good conservative management, absence of reversible renal factors, normal lower urinary outflow tract, absence of major extrarenal complications, absence of prior sensitization, absence of infection, absence of malnutrition, absence of pancytopenia, and ABO compatibility. Some transplant centers have emphasized absence of a history of cancer and of severe socioeconomic problems and psychological disturbances in their selection criteria. Many of these limitations are arbitrary and unnecessarily restrictive; some, given experience during the intervening years, could even be considered unethical. *We suggest only one primary indication for renal transplantation: renal failure that cannot be corrected by conservative methods.* The only absolute contraindications to transplantation are ABO incompatibility, the presence of cytotoxic antibodies against donor lymphoid cells, high levels of circulating anti-glomerular basement membrane (GBM) antibodies, active infection, and malignancy that cannot be brought under control. One need place no arbitrary limitation on recipient selection. As greater clinical experience with transplantation among young children is gained, one learns to cope with the specific problems this special population presents. With rigid adherence to arbitrary criteria, many of the children presently undergoing transplantation at our unit would have been excluded. Under our liberalized acceptance criteria, approximately 97% of the patients evaluated are deemed suitable candidates for transplantation.

Age

Although transplantation is easier in patients between the ages of 15 and 45, our experience with more than 200 children less than 16 years of age has demonstrated that kidneys can be successfully transplanted in children over the age of 1 year. Successful transplantation in the first year of life has also been reported [38]. We now regularly accept infants of 5 to 6 months of age and 5 to 6 kg body weight as recipients of adult renal allografts. With advances in surgical technology and medical management, these acceptance criteria have not compromised patient or graft survival. These newer approaches have important implications for patient care strategies. In the past the commitment to dialysis support of the neonate or very young infant with the goals of achieving 1 year of age and 6 to 8 kg body weight was so formidable as to discourage all but the most aggressive and persistent physicians and families. With progress in infant peritoneal dialysis and hemodialysis (Chap. 39), with improved understanding of nutrition problems (Chap. 33) and renal osteodystrophy (Chap. 28) in small uremic children, and with the success of earlier transplantation, this undertaking is no longer unreasonable. However, the task of developing criteria based on estimated intellectual potential has become substantially more difficult in that prognostication in young infants is even less definite than in older infants and young children.

Psychomotor Development

Many children undergoing the transplant recipient evaluation are significantly retarded in their psychomotor development. The etiology of this delay is probably multifactorial since most small, uremic children have a long history of illness, hospitalizations, and surgery, in addition to progressive uremia. Anorexia, urinary protein loss, dietary restrictions, and anemia complicate their nutrition. These children also often manifest muscle weakness, peripheral neuropathy [7,172], and uremic bone disease. On careful

neurologic evaluation their developmental delay is somewhat uneven; that is, personal and social development is often better preserved, while major motor milestones are frequently markedly delayed. Thus, a 3-year old may be unable to walk owing to a combination of weakness, hypotonia, and perhaps pain from renal osteodystrophy, yet be verbal and socially relate well to adults and family members.

Younger children may demonstrate even more profound CNS dysfunction including seizures and dyskinesia. Despite the major impact of these problems, they should not per se exclude the patient from consideration for a transplantation. Seizures frequently are better controlled after transplantation, perhaps as a result of the more normal and stable biochemical milieu or because anticonvulsant therapy is more predictable with normal renal function. On the other hand, we have tended to exclude children with marked retardation due to a specific cause, such as birth asphyxia, structural abnormalities, and metabolic disorders. Fortunately (since refusal of treatment is painful for all concerned), children with these disorders rarely present as candidates for transplantation. However, if this situation presents itself and if the parents are eager that transplantation be carried out despite fixed and severe global CNS impairment, it is recommended that the issues be resolved at the level of the hospital's bioethics committee. This ensures that the elements involved in the decision-making process reflect a broader constituency than that of the individual physician or renal team.

An appreciation of these problems leads us to recommend a formal neurologic consultation and an EEG for each recipient, to document their status and detect subtle CNS problems. CT is performed as indicated, and we recognize that a number of children [225] will have findings of "cortical atrophy." Because the significance of these findings is unclear, we have not recommended against a renal transplant based on CT studies. Careful evaluation will help to avoid the error of excluding from transplantation a child with moderate developmental delay or a fixed neurologic lesion, owing to the mistaken impression that they have an unrelenting, progressive CNS disorder. Clearly, a comprehensive neurologic assessment fosters the early involvement of other physicians and therapists who can offer the child the best chance of having optimal posttransplant rehabilitation.

Growth

Generally we do not recommend transplantation for growth failure in uremic children. With attention to nutrition, including gavage feeding for infants with low caloric intake, slow but steady growth can usually be achieved, even in children with advanced uremia [131].

Urologic Disorders

Successful transplantation into ileal loops has been done in children with abnormal lower urinary tracts resulting from congenital anomalies or neurogenic bladders [154]. Currently serious consideration should be given to colonic loop diversion, since the colon can accommodate an antireflux ureteral implant tunnel [162].

Evaluation of the Potential Recipient

It is desirable that patients with renal disease be evaluated as potential transplant recipients before terminal renal failure is imminent and before dialysis becomes necessary, because complications of uremia can appear suddenly during the period of conservative management. Early evaluation allows time to deal with problems such as bladder outlet obstruction, bone deformities, and dental caries, before the development of terminal uremia. It also allows for early placement of an arteriovenous fistula as access for dialysis. Early referral for transplant evaluation can also permit adequate time for the development of planning that can ease the financial and social hardships associated with treatment of end-stage renal failure. It is important to use this time for family education and for exploring family structure and psychodynamics so that, whatever the outcome, all that is possible is done to ensure that the enormous stresses to be faced are not destructive to the family unit.

In general, the preoperative evaluation is quite simple. Most studies are used to assist with the management of the patient on hemodialysis or to serve as baseline examinations for comparisons following transplantation. Evaluation checklists such as those detailed by Merrill [174] and modified by Kjellstrand et al. [130] provide guidelines for ensuring complete evaluation (Table 41-2). The evaluation begins with a complete history and physical examination, chest radiographs, and hematologic profile. Kidney function is evaluated by levels of BUN, serum creatinine, and creatinine clearance.

Bladder Function

The lower urinary tract is examined for urethral patency and absence of vesicoureteral reflux and residual urine. In the majority of cases the voiding cystourethrogram provides enough information to ensure that there is no urethral obstruction, that the bladder empties normally, that there are no abnormalities of the bladder wall, and that ureteral reflux is absent. Outflow obstruction must be corrected before transplantation. However, males with complex urethral obstruction can be successfully transplanted into bladders drained through perineal urethrotomies with delay in surgical urethral reconstruction procedures until post-transplant stability and maintenance levels of immunosuppression have been achieved.

Patients with uremia who fail to empty their bladders completely should be re-evaluated after several weeks of dialysis, when the neuropathy due to uremia may have improved. The presence of residual urine is also difficult to evaluate in patients with vesicoureteral reflux. In such cases the bladder should be re-evaluated for complete emptying after bilateral nephrectomy and total ureterectomy. Vir-

tually every bladder that fails to empty completely due to neuropathy associated with uremia or disease can be rehabilitated, avoiding the need for an ileal loop. However, ileal loops are necessary in patients whose severe neurogenic bladders are due to serious spinal cord or nerve root dysfunction. The decision to use an ileal loop is made following complete evaluation of the lower urinary tract, which may include cystoscopy and cystometrogram with denervation supersensitivity testing. Bladders defunctionalized for extended periods of time by urinary diversion may have small capacities and poor function. However, even bladder wall biopsies demonstrating significant fibrosis cannot predict poor function of these organs after transplantation. We have successfully treated several children who have had complete urinary diversions for up to 12 years, with tiny bladder capacities; urinary continence was achieved within several weeks to a few months following successful undiversion [89] or transplantation. Thus, defunctionalized bladders should be used once outlet obstruction has been corrected.

Infection

A thorough search is made for sites of infection, because all infections must be eradicated before transplantation. Cultures of the urine are performed three times during this evaluation. Any required dental work is completed prior to transplantation. Although some studies did not document an increased risk to the allograft recipient who is carrying hepatitis B antigen, other studies have found that this carrier state is associated with a significantly greater death rate due to hepatic failure [106,201]. Active viral hepatitis should contraindicate transplantation, whereas chronic antigen carriers should be advised as to the potential hazards. Since serious deterioration in hepatic structure and function may become manifest only years after transplantation, hepatitis virus carriers should be followed carefully for the earliest warnings of activation of hepatic injury. If this develops, consideration should be given to reduction or withdrawal of immunosuppression.

Peritoneal fluid is cultured in patients with peritoneal dialysis catheters. Occasionally a child on peritoneal dialysis will have an elevated white blood count and no obvious infection. CT scan may localize an intra-abdominal source. Exploration is performed at the time of transplantation, with Gram stain of the peritoneal fluid if no source is located. With living related donor transplantations the donor operation should be delayed until it is assured that the abdomen of the recipient is free of contamination.

Gastrointestinal Abnormalities

A thorough search is made in all children for peptic ulcer disease and gastritis or esophagitis, including radiologic examination of the upper gastrointestinal tract, because both uremia and the drugs used after transplantation increase the susceptibility to these disorders. If there is a positive history or radiographic evidence of peptic ulcer

TABLE 41-2. *Pediatric kidney recipient evaluation*

1. History
2. Physical examination
3. Schedule appointment with Patient Education Service
4. Social Service consultation
5. Pneumococcal vaccine
6. Hepatitis B vaccine
7. Laboratory work:
   A. Blood bank
      1. ABO type
      2. Hepatitis profile
      3. Blood transfusions
   B. Immunology laboratory
      1. Tissue typing (HLA, A B, C, D/DR)
      2. Antileukocyte antibody screening
      3. Quantitative immunoglobulins
      4. FANA, complement, ASO, rheumatoid factor, anti-glomerular basement membrane antibodies, circulating immune complexes (if indicated)
   C. Hematology
      1. CBC, platelet count
      2. Coagulation battery (prothrombin time, partial thromboplastin time, thrombin time), fibrinogen, factor V
   D. Chemistry
      1. Na, K, Cl, HCO_3, BUN, creatinine
      2. Serum Ca, PO_4, Mg, alkaline phosphatase, SGOT, total protein, albumin, bilirubin, 2-hour glucose
   E. Urine
      1. Urinalysis × 3
      2. Twenty-four–hour creatinine clearance
      3. Twenty-four–hour protein excretion
   F. Microbiology
      1. Urine culture—catheter specimen
      2. Urine culture on the day following voiding cystourethrogram
   G. Virology
      1. Viral titers for cytomegalovirus, herpes simplex virus, herpes zoster virus and Epstein-Barr virus
      2. Throat and urine specimen for viral cultures
8. Roentgenograms
   A. Posteroanterior and lateral chest film
   B. Voiding cystourethrogram (before upper gastrointestinal series)
   C. Upper gastrointestinal series
   D. Cardiac echo as indicated for cardiac murmurs
   E. Bone age films
9. Pediatric neurology consultation
10. Psychology consultation (psychometric evaluation)
11. EEG (under age 3 years)
12. Record height, weight, and head circumference in chart
13. Dental consultation
14. Chickenpox history
15. Mantoux for Native American patients
16. Stool guiaic × 3

Modified from Kjellstrand CM, Simmons RL, Buselmeier TJ, et al: Kidney. Section 1. Recipient selection, medical management and dialysis. *In* Najarian JS, Simmons RL (eds): *Transplantation.* Philadelphia. Lea & Febiger, 1972, p 422.

disease, prophylactic vagotomy and pyloroplasty are performed, usually at the time of pretransplant nephrectomy. This approach has greatly reduced the incidence of hemorrhage from peptic ulceration after transplantation. Gastroesophageal reflux should be searched for in infants and small children. An increased incidence should be expected in patients with congenital nephrotic syndrome [147] as well as those with severe malnutrition. Surgical correction may be necessary to avoid the danger of aspiration pneumonitis in the immunocompromised host. Pyloric stenosis is not uncommon in congenital nephrotic syndrome [147].

Preparation of the Patient Before Transplantation

Splenectomy

Unlike most transplant centers, until recently we had continued to perform splenectomy prior to transplantation. This practice was begun because of the concern that leukopenia in nonsplenectomized patients often prevented the administration of adequate doses of azathioprine. However, a randomized prospective trial on the effects of splenectomy versus no splenectomy in approximately 300 patients (including very few children) documented a 12% to 14% increase in 2-year graft survival in all categories of patients treated with splenectomy, other than in HLA identical siblings, where no advantage was found [82]. The timing of splenectomy influenced the results, especially in recipients of related nonidentical kidneys, in that splenectomy before transplantation had a significantly greater positive effect than splenectomy simultaneous with the transplantation [82]. Five to 7 years post-transplantation it appears that the early graft survival advantages accruing to splenectomy may be diminishing, and further observation of this group of patients may qualify the indications for this procedure. Moreover, splenectomy may result in an increased risk of overwhelming bacterial sepsis (see Infectious Complications). Thus, splenectomy has been discontinued as a component of the protocol for pediatric transplantation at our institution.

Nephrectomy

Bilateral nephrectomy is performed if the patient's kidneys are a source of infection, if ureteral reflux is present, for hypertension not controlled by dialysis, in patients with anti-GBM antibodies (Goodpasture's syndrome), and in children with persistent nephrotic syndrome. In addition, children with X-Y gonadal dysgenesis and renal failure (Drash syndrome) should undergo bilateral nephrectomy because of the high risk of the development of Wilms' tumor [58]. Gonadectomy should also be carried out because of potential malignancy in these tissues [58,91].

Infections and Immunizations

Preparation of the patient for transplantation should include steps to prevent infectious complications. Hepatitis B vaccine should be administered as recommended, using higher doses for uremic and immunosuppressed patients. The series of immunizations is spread over 5 to 6 months but, in our experience, should not delay transplantation and can safely be administered following transplantation. Pneumococcal vaccination is warranted and may be particularly important for splenectomized patients. Impaired antibody synthesis should be anticipated in uremic and post-transplant patients, although the antibody response of patients on hemodialysis is normal [45]. Immunization for cytomegalovirus (CMV) [87,136] and chickenpox [96,121] is currently being tested and offers promising future options. If practicable, transplantation of a kidney from a CMV seropositive donor to a CMV seronegative recipient should be avoided since higher risks of clinical CMV infection, graft loss, and death have been associated with this circumstance (see Cytomegalovirus Infections). Routine immunizations are completed, if possible, prior to transplantation. We have avoided routine immunizations following transplantation fearing the theoretical adjuvant effect on graft-host immune balance and the risks of even attenuated live virus vaccines. Instead we have depended on herd immunity.

Blood Transfusion

It is reasonable to attempt to relate current information and controversies with regard to blood transfusion to the special needs of the child with terminal renal disease. If one accepts our premise that successful transplantation is the ultimate goal of treatment in children with ESRD and that long-term dialysis prior to transplantation is best avoided, then certain of the controversies can be placed in perspective. Although there is argument as to the number of blood transfusions required to achieve maximal benefit in terms of graft survival, it is our view that the risk of broadly reactive antibodies virtually dictating a life of dialysis for the child is unacceptable. Therefore, if possible, we restrict the number of pretransplant random donor transfusions to five [182]. Further support for a limited transfusion approach comes from evidence that the benefits of transfusion are less dramatic at centers with better than average success rates [191]. The excellent rate of success with donor-specific transfusions employed in situations of high mixed lymphocytic culture (MLC) reactivity with the prospective living related donor needs to be balanced against the 30% sensitization rate with this approach, which often precludes living related donor transplantation [222]. As enunciated by Kyriakides et al. [134], potent immunosuppressive regimens and post-transplant monitoring and treatment protocols may largely obliterate the strong association between MLC and graft survival reported from some centers. However, studies indicating much lower sensitization rates when donor-specific transfusions are administered under continuous azathioprine immunosuppression [5] may prove to support a significant shift in the risk-benefit ratio in favor of donor-specific transfusions. Along these lines it is important to remember that uremia diminishes immunologic responsiveness to transfusions, and multiple transfusions result in broad-spectrum antibodies in the majority of nonuremic patients [182]. In children to be transplanted with little or no uremia, blood transfusions should be avoided or administered with continuous azathioprine. Azathioprine may not prevent sensitization to blood from unrelated donors [209].

Selection of Donors

Approximately 68% of the kidneys transplanted in the United States come from cadaveric donors and 32% from related donors. Because of the willingness of parents to donate kidneys to their offspring, the percentage of living related donors in pediatric transplantation programs is significantly higher than among adult patients. At the University of Minnesota, 66% of all kidneys transplanted are from relatives, whereas among patients under 17 years of age approximately 80% are from related donors, usually one of the parents. We make no specific effort to search for pediatric cadaver donors for the smaller recipients, since such donors are rare and waiting for a well-matched pediatric cadaver donor would greatly prolong the time on dialysis. The approach is to treat the small child with aggressive medical and, if necessary, dialytic support until body size (5 to 6 kg) technically permits transplantation of an adult kidney [176].

Related Donors

Relatives who have ABO compatibility with the patient and who volunteer for kidney donation are tissue typed. An attempt is made to type as many relatives as possible to find the best possible tissue type match. The willing donor whose HLA-A,B,C and D/DR antigens most closely resemble those of the recipient is further evaluated. There exists a large and growing literature on the subject of living related donor selection, including the aspect of donor-specific transfusion touched on previously. There is universal acceptance that, short of the identical twin, the HLA-A,B,C and D/DR identical MLC nonstimulatory sibling donor provides the highest rate of success. In this circumstance donor-specific or nonspecific blood transfusions are not warranted, and post-transplant immunosuppression can be less aggressive (see Immunosuppressive Therapy). The one-haplotype mismatched sibling donor accords the next highest rate of success, but here controversy exists in how to choose between two or more of such donors in the same family. Albrechtsen et al. [3] have described an inverse relationship between MLC responsiveness and DR matching, whereas Salvatierra et al. [221] have argued that high MLC responsiveness confers increased risk of rejection; they recommend donor-specific transfusion in this situation. Others have suggested that the disadvantage of high MLC responsiveness can largely be overcome without donor-specific transfusions (see previously) and that the ability of recipients to generate in vitro donor-specific suppressor cells is the best available test for the prediction of graft acceptance without rejection episodes [134]. Our current policy in selecting between two or more equally well-matched siblings or parents (HLA-A,B,C and D/DR) is to attempt to discriminate on the basis of the MLC response. However, our experience suggests that in this situation the MLC test does not often provide a clear choice, and the decision is usually left to the family. Equally well-matched sibling donors may be more successful than parental donors.

Related donors should be in good health to minimize the risks inherent in any operation. Evaluation of related donors is shown in Table 41-3. If all the tests are normal, the donor undergoes a renal arteriogram to identify kidneys that have multiple or aberrant renal arteries, thus simplifying donor nephrectomy and recipient anastamosis. This evaluation of a prospective donor may detect previously unsuspected renal abnormalities [240].

The use of living related donors as a source of kidneys for transplantation has raised certain ethical questions. Kidney donation involves a major operative procedure, with the risks of harm or even death to the donor. The risks and benefits of kidney donation must be discussed very thoroughly with the potential donor. We have learned through psychological and sociologic studies of kidney donors that the act of donation usually has an important positive impact on the life of the donor [231].

We have limited the use of donors below the age of 18

Table 41-3. *Evaluation of potential related renal transplant donors*

General
History and physical examination
Repeated blood pressure determinations
Chest film
ECG
IVP

Laboratory Examinations
Hematocrit, hemoglobin, white blood cell, differentiatial, and platelet counts
Prothrombin, partial thromboplastin, and thrombin time
Serum sodium, potassium, chloride, bicarbonate, glutamic-oxalic transaminase, bilirubin, uric acid, calcium, phosphorus, urea, creatinine, and sugar
Urine culture, urinalysis
Twenty-four–hour creatinine clearance and albumin excretion
Cytomegalovirus, herpes simplex, and Epstein-Barr virus titers

Special Radiology
Renal arteriogram

years to circumstances in which no other donors were available. After expressing willingness, the underage donor is evaluated by a child psychologist to insure that a sufficient level of maturity has been attained. To help circumvent the possibility of parental pressure on the youthful donor, a court takes temporary custody of the teenager and gives permission for the kidney donation. No adverse psychological reactions have developed in our teenage donors, the youngest of whom was 16 years old. Donors as young as 7 years of age have been used, although this practice remains an area of intense controversy [81].

Although kidney donation has been a safe procedure, it is not without potential hazards. Among the approximately 10,000 relatives who have been used for kidney donation in the United States, there have been two recorded deaths. Although we have had no deaths in over 500 donor operations, we have reported a 28% incidence of major and minor complications in the donor [259].

More recently concern has been expressed that uninephrectomy performed in normal individuals may, after more than 10 years, be associated with an increased incidence of hypertension, proteinuria, and even renal insufficiency [51,88]. It has been argued that compensatory hypertrophy and glomerular hyperfunction resulting from uninephrectomy represents a maladaptive response that, presumably through alterations in glomerular hemodynamics, can be destructive to the residual nephron population [88]. However, centers, including our own, have not been able to confirm this level of risk [40,256]. It should be agreed, however, that the nephrology transplant community has a heavy obligation to resolve this question by careful and timely studies. Donors with hypertension, even if mild or labile, should not be used [40,256].

Cadaveric Donors

The ideal donor of a cadaveric kidney is young, has had normal vital signs until a short time before death, is free of transmissible infection and malignancy, and has died in the hospital after observation for a number of hours, during which time the blood group and tissue type have been determined and renal function has been assessed. However, insistence on these ideal criteria will result in failure to use many acceptable kidneys. It has been estimated that about 15,000 kidneys are needed in the United States each year to treat all patients who require transplantation. Each year approximately 60,000 people die as a result of automobile accidents, and a similar number die from other accidents and from strokes. Thus, only 5% to 10% of potential donors would be sufficient to supply kidneys for all patients with end stage disease. However, most of these patients never become donors, and a shortage of organs is constantly present. It should be clear that acquisition of cadaveric donors is largely dependent on the quality of the ongoing personal relationships established between the organ procurement team and the administration, nurses, and physicians in the hospitals in the service area of the transplant center.

DEFINITION OF DONOR DEATH

Procurement of cadaveric organs for transplantation has raised both ethical and legal problems about the definition of death. At our institution the diagnosis of death is primarily clinical and is made by a physician who is not a member of the transplant team. Clinical criteria of irreversible brain death have included fixed, dilated pupils; absence of response to external stimuli; absence of spontaneous respiration; negative caloric tests on repeated examination; and absence of reversible factors such as intoxication or hypothermia. More recent definitions of brain death include two isoelectric EEGs separated by an interval of 6 to 24 hours [244]. In addition or alternatively, an isotopic study indicating the absence of detectable cerebral blood flow can provide a useful evaluation that can be obtained at the bedside. It may be more difficult to diagnose brain death in a child, particularly if hypothermia or central nervous depressant chemicals complicate the clinical picture [43a].

MANAGEMENT OF THE DONOR PRIOR TO DEATH

The potential cadaveric donor is evaluated with a platelet count, coagulation parameters, serum electrolytes, BUN, and serum creatinine. A urinalysis is obtained and urine culture is sent. Although systemic infection, malignancy, and pre-existing kidney disease contraindicate donation, Reye's syndrome does not [77]. Marked hypotension with subsequent deterioration in renal function may be a relative contraindication depending on the potential for reversibility.

No special suggestions regarding management of the potential cadaveric donor are made until brain death has been declared, since up to that time all medical treatment is directed toward the donor's care. However, it is reasonable to take a sample of blood for ABO and tissue typing, thus allowing early determination of the best recipient prior to declaration of brain death and organ harvesting, to minimize the cold ischemia time. Blood group and tissue typing data on potential recipients from multiple centers are computerized to facilitate determination of the best potential recipient.

Potential donors frequently have marginal urine output as a result of attempts to minimize cerebral edema. Once brain death has been declared and permission for kidney donation has been obtained, we attempt to establish a large urine output by the administration of large quantities of saline, 12.5 to 25 g of mannitol, and up to 100 mg of furosemide. With adequate replacement of fluids, vasopressors frequently can be discontinued.

ORGAN HARVEST

Removal of the kidney is done under sterile conditions in the operating room. The ureters are transected close to the bladder and freed up to the kidneys. The renal veins are cleaned off, and the adrenal and gonadal veins are ligated and divided. The renal arteries are dissected free from the surrounding lymphatic and neural structures. Particular attention must be given to the renal arteries, since no arteriogram has been obtained and more than one renal artery may be present. We usually remove the kidneys separately, although some surgeons routinely remove both kidneys and aorta en bloc, claiming this technique allows easier arterial cannulation for perfusion. If more than one renal artery is encountered or if the donor is a child, the kidneys and aorta are removed en bloc so that both arteries can be perfused. Mesenteric lymph nodes are taken as a source of lymphocytes for tissue typing. Owing to the increased interest in transplantation of extrarenal organs, kidney harvest from a cadaveric donor must often be coordinated with the harvest of organs such as the heart, liver, and pancreas and may involve more than one surgical team.

ORGAN PRESERVATION

Preservation techniques have simplified the logistics of cadaveric transplantation and have allowed sharing organs among transplant centers. In general there are two types of preservation: simple hypothermic storage and pulsatile perfusion. For simple hypothermic storage the kidneys are first rapidly cooled by a combination of external cooling and flushing the kidney through the renal artery to reduce the core temperature as quickly as possible. Flushing solutions (i.e., Collins' or Sach's solution) with sodium and potassium concentrations similar to intracellular levels are widely used. These kidneys are stored in a sterile plastic container immersed in crushed ice (4°C). Hypothermic storage has the advantage of simplicity, low cost, and ease of transportation, but it is limited to approximately 36 hours of preservation [43].

Preservation machines, such as that designed by Belzer et al. [16] or the Gambro or the MOX 100 preservation machine [179], employ low perfusion pressures of approximately 60 mm Hg and generally have transport modules for shipment of kidneys to distant centers. Perfusion has been carried out with a variety of fluids, including cryoprecipitated plasma, albumin solution, Plasmanate, and a silica gel fraction of plasma. It has been suggested that pulsatile perfusion, which allows successful preservation for more than 48 hours, can lead to glomerular capillary obstruction. However, we have performed biopsies of more than 60 kidneys treated by the pulsatile perfusion techniques described here and have found no significant glomerular capillary abnormalities by light or electron microscopy [243]. Although it has been stated that pulsatile perfusion allows one to judge the quality of the kidney before its placement into the recipient, in practice we have not consistently found this to be the case. However, extremely poor pressure-flow characteristics should militate against use of the kidney. The major advantage of pulsatile perfusion, longer preservation time, needs to be balanced against the increased cost of the technology and the greater complexity of organ transplantation. Used appropriately, these preservation methods are not different in terms of the incidence, severity, or duration of postoperative acute tubular necrosis (ATN).

CROSSMATCH PROCEDURES

Regardless of the donor source, it is essential to determine whether the recipient has preformed antibodies against antigens present on the T lymphocytes of the donor. Patients may have been presensitized by blood or platelet transfusions, pregnancy, or previous transplantation. If these preformed antidonor leukocyte antibodies are present and the transplantation is carried out, an immediate (hyperacute) rejection usually ensues. The value of testing for anti-B cell antibodies has not been fully established, although there is some evidence that cold anti-B cell antibodies do not predict a poor graft outcome [3,49,63].

Because organ preservation techniques currently permit prolonged storage of kidneys, there is time for crossmatching, which takes several hours. At most transplant units, serum samples are drawn monthly from all patients awaiting transplantation to detect the formation of antidonor antibodies. Several of these sera should always be used for final crossmatching, including fresh serum from the patient. Antibodies may appear and disappear without apparent reason in a recipient. If a patient has previously made antibodies against the prospective donor, there is an increased risk of accelerated rejection at 2 to 7 days, so that this type of donor is only rarely used at our institution. However, significant success with cadaveric transplantation has been reported under these circumstances [33]. It has been suggested that preformed antibodies against graft endothelial antigens predicts a high incidence of graft loss and that screening of sera of prospective recipients against frozen sections of donor kidney could improve graft survival rates [194]. Wider application of this principle will probably await confirmatory studies and availability of simpler detection systems for circulating antibodies against donor kidney specific antigens.

Renal Transplantation
Anesthesia in the Anephric Patient

Certain precautions are necessary during surgery in the anephric or uremic patient. Anesthetics that are excreted almost exclusively by the kidney must not be used. Both curare and succinylcholine are metabolized by the liver but may result in prolonged paralysis in the postoperative period. Serum cholinesterase is broken down during hemodialysis so that succinylcholine would be expected to have prolonged action. Anesthesia, fluids, and potassium must be administered cautiously, with the assumption that the transplanted kidney will not function immediately. Hematocrit should be raised to 30% prior to transplantation; hypovolemia due to excessive ultrafiltration during hemodialysis prior to surgery should be avoided.

Intraoperative Management and Surgical Technique

Intraoperative management of infants and children requires meticulous attention to detail [176]. The risk of hypothermia is reduced by raising the ambient temperature to approximately 32°C and placing the patient on warming blankets. All solutions used for sterile preparation of the skin, irrigation solutions, and transfused blood products are warmed to above 32°C. The patient's core temperature is constantly monitored with a rectal probe. If hypothermia occurs (<36°C), warm saline abdominal lavage is instituted. At the time of revascularization, the kidney is warmed with saline prior to reperfusion.

Electrical cardiac activity is monitored with an ECG monitor. In small children, the arterial blood pressure is measured directly from an arterial catheter placed under direct vision or percutaneously or through the arterial limb of a Scribner shunt. These devices are used to draw periodic intraoperative blood specimens for arterial blood gases, hemoglobin, glucose, and electrolyte determinations. Central venous pressure is monitored. In smaller children, centrally located catheters are placed through the external or internal jugular vein. We prefer the Hickman catheter extending to the right atrium because it can also be used for dialysis blood access [146].

Light inhalation anesthesia consisting of halothane, nitrous oxide, and oxygen used with a muscle relaxant is recommended. At the time of induction, a prophylactic antibiotic (cephalosporin) is administered. A urethral catheter as large as possible, commensurate with safety, is placed after induction of anesthesia. A catheter specimen of urine is cultured, and the bladder is filled with 0.1% neomycin solution, left inside by clamping the catheter. The clamp is released at the time of ureteroneocystostomy. With the use of topical antibiotics in the irrigation solutions, in addition to systemic antibiotics, our incidence of superficial wound infections has decreased from 2.8% prior to 1975 to less than 0.5% currently. The transplant operation has been described in detail by Simmons et al [233]. In children weighing less than 15 to 20 kg, a transperitoneal approach through a long midline incision is used. Nephrectomy can also be performed through this approach. In children over 15 kg, the kidney allograft can be placed in the retroperitoneal iliac fossa as in adults. The right iliac fossa is preferred for placement of either a right or a left kidney because venous dissection of the right side is simpler. The right colon and small intestine are mobilized and reflected superiorly and to the left. Next, the distal aorta and vena cava and common iliac veins and arteries are dissected free. The two distal lumbar arteries and veins are ligated and divided. Perivascular lymphatics must be carefully ligated to avoid the formation of lymphoceles [212]. Revascularization of the kidney in children weighing more than 15 kg involves an end-to-side anastomosis between the renal artery and renal vein and the external iliac vessels. Alternatively, the renal artery may be anastomosed end-to-end using the distal hypogastric artery. The renal vein is first sutured to the side of the distal vena cava. Next the renal artery is sutured to the side of the distal aorta or proximal common iliac artery (Fig. 41-3). A donor kidney with two renal arteries may be preferred because such arteries can be of more suitable size for the very small aorta. Occasionally there is more than one renal vein and difficulty with multiple venous anastomoses to the inferior vena cava of the recipient. In this situation it appears that the smaller of the donor renal veins can be tied off with impunity. The ureter is brought into the opened bladder through a retroperitoneal tunnel, and a ureteroneocystostomy is performed. The kidney is placed in the right retroperitoneal space (Fig. 41-3); finally the right colon is replaced over the kidney, being sure that the lower pole is available for percutaneous renal biopsy, should this become necessary.

It is important to transfuse 75 to 100 ml of blood (acutely raising the central venous pressure to 10 to 12 cm H$_2$O) just prior to releasing the vascular clamps to compensate for the volume of blood required to fill the kidney. Also, approximately 1 mg/kg body weight of sodium bicarbonate is given before release of the aortic clamp to combat acidosis due to lactate accumulated in the lower body from aortic occlusion. Blood analysis should verify adequate correction of acidosis. Finally, it is critical to note that there is a tendency for diffuse intra-abdominal bleeding to complicate abdominal surgery in patients with large femoral artery–femoral vein shunts that result in venous hypertension. This bleeding can be rapidly controlled by clamping these shunts.

Post-Transplant Care

Patients are treated routinely with intravenous cephalosporin for 5 days as prophylaxis against wound infection. Mycostatin mouthwashes are given to prevent oral *Candida* infection, and sulfonamides are administered to prevent urinary tract infection. The patient also takes antacids to reduce the likelihood of gastrointestinal hemorrhage.

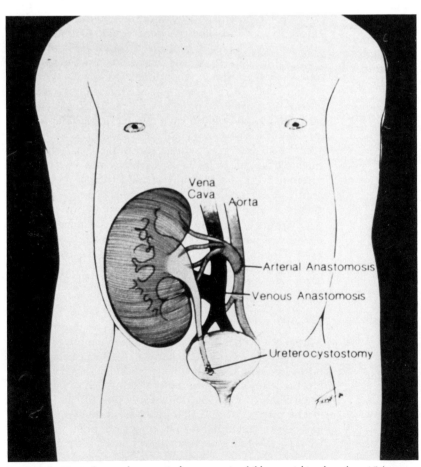

FIG. 41-3. *Typical transplant surgical anatomy in children weighing less than 15 kg.*

Fluids and Electrolytes

The main therapeutic aim in the immediate postoperative period is the maintenance of a high vascular volume to stimulate the kidney to produce large quantities of urine, which serves to prevent kidney shutdown and obstruction of the catheter due to blood clots. Catheter obstruction carries the risk of leakage of urine. A volume equivalent to 10 percent of the body weight may be lost as a result of third-space accumulation in the first postoperative day, especially in children who have also had nephrectomy and splenectomy. The third-space loss is replaced with colloid in the form of fresh frozen plasma (if coagulation studies are abnormal), Plasmanate, or packed red blood cells to maintain a moderately elevated blood pressure without producing tachycardia, cardiac gallop, pulmonary vascular congestion, or disturbed oxygenation reflecting pulmonary edema. It should be noted that pulmonary edema can be present in children with central venous pressure less than 5 cm H_2O. Once conditions are established as optimal for renal perfusion, however, the central venous pressure serves as a useful guide for further colloid administration.

Moderate hypertension is common in the early postoperative period and is treated vigorously with appropriate antihypertensive medications and diuretics; the onset of malignant hypertension can be sudden. Colloid should never be administered to the hypertensive child. If the hemoglobin is low, a partial volumetric exchange with packed cells is a safe strategy. Antihypertensive agents may be weaned as overhydration resolves and renal function returns to normal, but many children sensitive to prednisone require continued antihypertensive treatment. Our experience suggests that adult kidneys can be adequately perfused at blood pressure levels that are appropriate for the pediatric recipient. Thus, in our view, there is no justification for exposing the child to serious risks of hypertension with the rationalization that these pressures are necessary to avoid renal shutdown.

Crystalloid is administered in a volume equal to the urine volume. In small children with a large urine output, the urine volume should be measured at 15-minute intervals and replaced to prevent volume depletion. We use a solution containing 50 g glucose, 4.5 g sodium chloride, and 10 mEq sodium bicarbonate per liter. Potassium is added only when mild hypokalemia develops. Urinary potassium is measured and replaced accordingly. Serum calcium must be monitored closely in the early postoperative period because life-threatening hypocalcemia can develop rapidly. Insensible loss and nasogastric drainage ordinarily are not replaced.

In small children with a marked post-transplant diuresis, hyperglycemia may develop when 5% glucose is infused, creating a cycle of osmotic diuresis that results in the infusion of more glucose, which further aggravates the hyperglycemia. If more than 20 g of glucose/kg/day is infused or if significant glycosuria (checked hourly) or hyperglycemia develops, a solution containing 10 g glucose per liter is substituted. With a massive diuresis, crystalloid replacement less than the hourly urine volume may bring the urine volume down to a more manageable level. Urine output in the first few days in small children transplanted with adult kidneys appears to be dependent on fluid intake (Fig. 41-4). As postoperative fluid administration is relaxed, urine volume diminishes even though third-space fluid is being mobilized and body weight is falling. As oral intake is established after several days (Fig. 41-4), urine output again increases.

It is our experience that infants and small children, given a technically smooth transplantation, always perfuse the adult kidney adequately. However, we have repeatedly seen that infants and small children given adult kidneys may produce little urine in the first 6 to 8 hours post-transplantation. Overaggressive fluid pushes during this period are likely to produce pulmonary edema. Furosemide, 1 to 2 mg/kg given intravenously over 30 to 60 minutes, is administered for oliguria in the face of adequate vascular

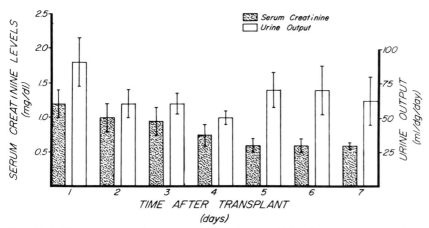

FIG. 41-4. Urine output and serum creatinine values in children between 5.4 and 8.8 kg in body weight at the time of transplantation from adult donors. (From Miller LC, Lum CT, Bock GH, et al: Transplantation of the adult kidney into the very small child: Technical considerations. Am J Surg 145:243, 1983.)

volume. More rapid administration risks ototoxicity. If volume and diuretics fail to increase urine output, further attempts at volume expansion are discontinued.

Other causes of oliguria in the early post-transplant period must be excluded. The bladder catheter should be checked for patency. A renogram and flow study are noninvasive methods of assessing adequacy of blood flow to the kidney. A flat renogram should be followed by arteriography to rule out technical problems with the renal artery anastomosis or renal artery thrombosis.

A 2-hour creatinine clearance is determined on the day of transplantation and daily thereafter for the first week. The hematocrit is measured every 4 hours for the first 24 hours, because a falling hematocrit is frequently the first indication of hemorrhage into the transplant wound. If the urine output is adequate, a ^{131}I-labeled iodohippurate sodium (Hippuran) renogram and scan are obtained the day following transplantation. Hemoglobin, white blood cell count, platelet count, and plasma sodium, potassium, chloride, calcium, bicarbonate, creatinine, urea nitrogen, and glucose are determined daily.

The Foley catheter is removed after 3 days for the first kidney transplantation. It is kept in for 7 days if the bladder has previously been opened. because of the increased risk of leakage from the cystotomy site.

Most patients receiving transplantations through a retroperitoneal approach can take oral fluids the day following transplantation. Small children who require an intraperitoneal procedure may have an ileus for 2 to 4 days and require continued nasogastric drainage. If ileus persists beyond this time, there should be no delay in instituting parenteral hyperalimentation. The combination of recent surgery and vigorous immunosuppression in the child already compromised by uremia can lead to rapid constitutional deterioration in the absence of adequate nutrition. Often in these small children abdominal distention develops on resumption of a regular diet. This distention apparently results from chylous ascites secondary to division of lymphatics during dissection of the aorta and vena cava. Temporary treatment with a medium-chain triglyceride diet can be helpful for this problem.

Immunosuppressive Therapy

Immunosuppressive therapy is aimed at modulating aspects of humoral and cellular immune mechanisms and nonspecific inflammation that are involved in immune destruction of the allograft (Chap. 40). The two immunosuppressive regimens currently used at the University of Minnesota (Table 41-4) include: conventional immunosuppresion using azathioprine, prednisone, and antilymphoblast globulin (ALG) along with donor-specific transfusion, and cyclosporine with prednisone. A third protocol using a combination of low dose azathioprine and cyclosporine along with prednisone is currently being developed and has had remarkable early success. In general, in the past, children receiving first transplantations other than HLA identical grafts have been treated with splenectomy, azathioprine, prednisone, and ALG. Children receiving second transplantations (after rapid rejection of the first transplanta-

TABLE 41-4. *Postoperative immunosuppression guidelines for kidney transplant recipients at the University of Minnesota*

Protocol I: Antilymphoblast Globulin (ALG) (Manufactured by the University of Minnesota), Azathioprine, Prednisone

Antilymphoblast Globulin

For mismatched cadaver and living related (other than A-match sibling)—30 mg/kg/day IV × 14 days

For HLA identical sibling 10 mg/kg/day IV × 14 days

Adjust dosage according to platelet count ($< 50,000/m^3$—hold dose; 50-$100,000/m^3$—$\frac{1}{2}$ ALG dose)

Azathioprine

For all recipients. Adjust dosage at all times with respect to WBC and platelets

Postop Day #	Mg/Kg/Day
0-2	5
3-5	4
6-8	3
9 and after	

Prednisone

For HLA identical sibling. Continue reducing dose every 1-2 months. Goal at 1 year (day 360) post-transplantation is 0.2-0.25 mg/kg/day

Postop Day #	Mg/Kg
0-2	1.0
3-5	0.75
6-8	0.6
9-11	0.5
12, and after	

For living related and cadaver (other than HLA-identical). Goal at 1 year (day 360) post-transplantation is:
a) Living related—0.25 mg/kg daily
b) Cadaver—0.25-0.3 mg/kg daily

Postop Day #	Mg/Kg
0-2	2.0
3-5	1.75
6-8	1.5
9-11	1.25
12-14	1.0
15-17	0.75
18	0.6

Protocol II: Cyclosporine and Prednisone
For all patients

Cyclosporine
14 mg/kg/day for 7 days
In 2 divided doses
12 mg/kg/day thereafter
Reduce dose for toxicity: usual dose at
1 year = 6-10 mg/kg/day

Prednisone
As in Protocol I: Faster reductions may be possible.

tion) were treated with cyclosporine and prednisone. Patients receiving HLA identical grafts did not undergo splenectomy but received azathioprine, prednisone, and antilymphoblast globulin (lower dose). However, as noted previously, these protocols are currently in flux, and it is likely that donor-specific transfusion and cyclosporine will be used more prominently, whereas splenectomy has been abandoned as a routine procedure.

AZATHIOPRINE

Azathioprine is an analog of 6-mercaptopurine; it is rapidly absorbed from the gastrointestinal tract and is metabolized in the liver to 6-mercaptopurine, which blocks the synthesis of purine ribonucleotides. Azathioprine can inhibit both humoral and cell-mediated immunity in humans and most laboratory animals, but it is more effective for primary than secondary immune responses. Inhibition of the primary immune response requires treatment with azathioprine during the inductive phase of antibody synthesis, that is, during the first 48 hours following exposure to the immunogen. Suppression of circulating IgG but not of IgM levels by azathioprine has been demonstrated in humans. Azathioprine is eliminated in the urine and metabolically degraded in the liver. Renal failure was initially thought to require reduction in the azathioprine dosage; however, our experience has been that this is not necessary unless dictated by leukopenia. Constant monitoring of the white blood cell count and adjustment of the azathioprine dose may be required in some patients. Azathioprine-induced hepatic injury is not dose-related, seems to be an idiosyncratic response to the drug, and may require substitution with the alkylating agent cyclophosphamide (Cytoxan).

CORTICOSTEROIDS

Prednisone is commonly used as the maintenance corticosteroid, whereas methyl-prednisone is frequently given in addition or instead of prednisone during rejection episodes. Steroids decrease the inflammatory response and produce destruction of thymus-dependent lymphocytes [265]. These lymphocytes disappear from the circulating pool, and histologically karyorrhexis and cytoplasmic shedding can be seen in lymphoid organs. Migration of polymorphonuclear leukocytes into experimentally induced inflammatory sites is remarkably reduced. However, precisely how steroids inhibit transplant rejection is still unknown.

Toxic effects of corticosteroids are widely known and include susceptibility to infection, poor wound healing, poor growth, truncal obesity, hypertension, cushingoid facies, osteoporosis, aseptic bone necrosis, myopathy, hyperglycemia and so-called steroid diabetes, pancreatitis, cataracts, personality changes, and pseudotumor cerebri.

ANTILYMPHOBLAST GLOBULIN

ALG has been shown to be a potent immunosuppressive agent in a variety of animals, including humans. The clinical use of ALG has been the subject of numerous articles, and its effectiveness in human renal transplantation has been questioned. However, Shiel et al. [227], Turcotte et al. [252], and Taylor et al. [246] have shown in prospective randomized studies that ALG increases survival of both cadaver and related kidney grafts.

ALG is produced by immunizing animals (horse, goat, rabbit) with blastic lymphoid cells from a variety of sources including thymus, lymph node, and cultured human lymphoblasts. ALG is separated from the animal serum by column chromatography. There is no standardization with respect to cell source, animal used, immunization schedules, and ALG separation.

The mechanism of ALG action is not completely known. It has been reported to act both peripherally and centrally [181]. More recently evidence has been presented from studies with monoclonal reagents directed against blast cells that the effectiveness of antilymphoid antibodies may be dependent on the elimination of cells capable of clonal proliferation to graft antigens [245]. These observations may help to explain variable results reported from different transplant centers using nonstandardized preparations of ALG. There is increasing evidence that ALG or monoclonal antilymphocyte (blast) antibodies may be even more effective for the reversal of rejection than for rejection prophylaxis [245]. However, it is our view that ALG has utility in both instances.

The direct toxicity of ALG is not great despite repeated intravenous administration of large amounts of foreign protein. Serum sickness has not been a major problem, nor has there been deposition of antigen-antibody complexes in glomerular structures. Thrombocytopenia or leukopenia may dictate temporary modification or reduction in dose, but it is our opinion that the total dose should be administered even if this prolongs hospitalization. In fact, we often allow patients to leave the hospital and to come in for a few hours each evening to complete the ALG schedule. Skin tests with horse gamma globulin have been negative in patients who receive horse ALG. However, occasionally fevers and rashes have been attributed to allergic manifestations of ALG. Some transplant centers administer ALG intramuscularly, which can cause pain and sterile abscesses at the injection site. As with any potent immunosuppressant, ALG may predispose to serious infection, and severe viral illness may be more common in centers using this agent.

CYCLOSPORINE

Cyclosporine is an undecapeptide, derived from a fungus, and discovered in 1976 by Borel [25] to have immunosuppressive effects in vitro and in vivo in a number of experimental animals. It suppresses helper T lymphocyte function most severely, with much less effect on T cytotoxic and B lymphocytes. Its mechanism of action relates to inhibition of production or release of interleukin-2 [70]. A number of clinical trials with cyclosporine in renal allografts have shown superior graft survival, with significantly lower incidence of infectious complications [242]. Cyclosporine is used with low dose prednisone and has resulted in 1-year kidney graft survival of 90% [242]. Complications of cyclosporine include nephrotoxicity, hypertension, hyperkalemia, neurologic complaints, and hirsutism. The long-term side effects of cyclosporine are not known. However, evidence from Stanford that long-term cyclosporine can cause irreversible uremia due to advanced tubulointerstitial injury in heart allograft recipients is disconcerting (Myers B: personal communication). Until more is known about the long-term effects of cyclosporine, we plan to use this agent sparingly in children. We are hopeful, however, based on preliminary observations, that the low dose azathioprine, cyclosporine, prednisone combination will obviate many of the current limitations of cyclosporine.

Given the current state of flux in renal allograft immunosuppressive protocols, it is suggested that changes in management at any center be based on data derived from carefully controlled studies done by experienced investigators and confirmed by others. Retrospective controls are largely inadequate because of improvements in results that occur because of experience. Finally, the risk-benefit ratio of any new approach must be viewed with long-term perspectives and goals in mind, especially in children.

Results

Center to center differences in protocols are increasing with the introduction of variables such as donor-specific transfusion with or without azathioprine, random donor transfusions, ALG, monoclonal antibodies, and cyclosporine. It is also difficult to judge protocols based on patient and graft survival alone, because experience and skill vary from center to center and cannot be easily measured. Furthermore, morbidity, time in the hospital, patient suffering, and expense are rarely carefully studied.

Present statistics indicate that approximately one-half to three-quarters of all transplanted children are alive with good renal function 3 to 5 years after transplantation (Fig. 41-5) [18,55,248]. For a 3-year-old child undergoing a renal transplantation today, however, the long-term outlook for a normal, relatively healthy life expectancy remains completely unknown. It may very well be that only 1 of 100 of these children will live "to see their grandchildren." Thus despite a growing experience in pediatric renal transplantation, the procedure must still be considered an adventure into the unknown.

In this section we discuss the results of renal transplantation in children, recognizing that the data are expressed in terms of only a small segment of the expected lifespan of these patients. The effects of variables such as the age of the patient, the donor source, and the type of immunosuppression employed are stressed.

Effect of Age on Outcome

Transplantation in infants in the first year of life has been successful but has been reported largely as anecdotal experiences. One pessimistic report has suggested a very poor outcome in patient and, especially, graft survival in infants and very young children treated largely by transplantation from pediatric cadaver donors. However, our current results in nine children ages 6 months to 1 year (5 to 7.7 kg) are much more promising. Eight patients received adult, living related donor (parental) grafts and 1 received a cadaver graft. There were no serious operative complications, and all grafts functioned initially. Eight are alive and 7 have functioning grafts 6 months to 5 years post-transplant. One infant with recurrent oxalosis was withdrawn by the parents from further active therapy and died. Another with oxalosis lost the graft at 2 years from chronic rejection. Thus, it appears that this group of patients represents an exciting evolution of pediatric renal transplant therapy, since preliminary results are comparable to those in older children and adults.

Several groups have reported their experience with children between the ages of 1 and 5 years [166]. These patients, who are frequently markedly dwarfed as a result of chronic renal disease, continue to present special challenges with regard to both dialysis support as well as surgical technique. However, based on current experience, these obstacles are much less formidable and are not as intimidating as in infants under 1 year of age.

Reviews of transplant registry statistics suggest that these small children do less well following transplantation than do older children. Our initial series included 53 children 5 years of age and younger who had received 65 kidney transplants, 53 from living related donors and 12 from cadaveric donors. After four years, 42 of these children

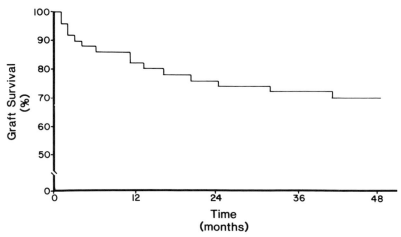

Fig. 41-5. *Cumulative graft survival of all first transplants in children ages 6 months to 18 years at the University of Minnesota from 1/68 to 12/83.*

were alive with functioning grafts, 8 had died, and 3 had returned to dialysis (Fig. 41-6). There are no differences in life-table patient or graft survival curves comparing these younger and smaller children to older children and adults. The list of renal diseases leading to transplantation in this younger group of children is dominated by disorders that do not recur in the transplanted kidney (see Table 41-1). Further, the growth and development of the large majority of young successful transplant recipients has been very satisfactory (see following). Thus, in our view the young child, despite the demand for highly specialized care, can be considered on a par with older children as a candidate for transplantation.

Source of Graft

We examined the outcome of first transplantations in 223 children from the inception of the current team in 1968 to the current era, for present purposes ending in 1983. The 100% 4-year patient and graft survival in the 14 recipients of HLA identical sibling grafts confirms other observations that this represents the premier treatment choice for renal failure. The results in this group are contrasted with 14 patients who received non-HLA identical living related donor grafts during the same period of time (Fig. 41-7). There appears to be a moderate advantage to living related as compared with cadaveric graft survival (Fig. 41-7), findings similar to those of the European Dialysis and Transplant Association [27] and the Los Angeles [71] and San Francisco [207] groups for children of approximately the same age as in the Minnesota experience. These results probably reflect the relatively privileged immunologic status of living related donor grafts. Nonetheless, we cannot explain why our results have recently improved for non-HLA identical related donor grafts (Fig. 41-8) while worsening slightly for cadaveric grafts over the

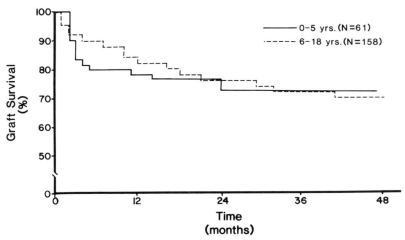

FIG. 41-6. *Effect of age or graft survival in all first transplants in children transplanted at the University of Minnesota from 1/68 to 12/83.*

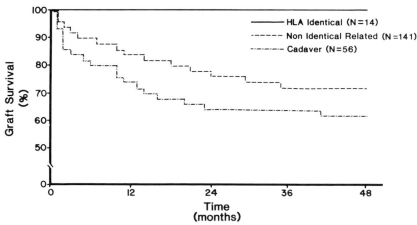

FIG. 41-7. *Effect of donor source on graft survival in all first transplants in children at the University of Minnesota from 1/68 to 12/83.*

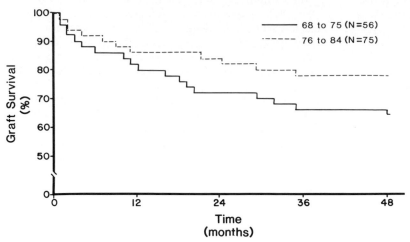

Fig. 41-8. *Effect of era on graft survival. All first transplants, non-identical living related donors.*

same time, despite identical treatment protocols for both groups. It may be that the results depicted in Fig. 41-8 reflect our improvement with experience and suggest that improvement is more difficult to obtain with cadaveric grafts. However, more recent results suggest that cadaveric transplantation is, again, catching up.

The slight advantage in patient survival for non-HLA identical related grafts as compared with cadaveric grafts has not been statistically significant in either the Minnesota or the combined European series [27]. Thus, the rationale for preferring living related non-HLA identical over cadaveric donors is based on advantages in graft survival (see Fig. 41-7) and on availability of the related donor kidney at the time when the recipient is medically prepared for the stress of transplantation surgery and immunosuppression. However, donor-specific transfusion protocols are likely to magnify the advantages of the living related donor.

We have shown that children age 6 to 13 years receiving maternal grafts have a much higher risk of rejection than those receiving paternal grafts [238]. These differences were not seen in older children or adults or in younger children [238]. It is difficult to understand these results, and it is recommended that these data not be used in decision making unless confirmed by other centers.

Starzl has argued that the excellent results with cyclosporine in cadaveric transplantation have so diminished the advantage of living related donor over cadaveric donor transplantation that the risks to the related donor are no longer warranted [80]. Indeed evidence for Starzl's warning comes from two separate centers reporting a high incidence of hypertension and proteinuria in donors 10 to 20 years after uninephrectomy, presumably based on damage to the remaining kidney from the hemodynamic stresses engendered by compensatory adaptations to the 50% reduction in nephron number [50,88]. Nevertheless, practice remains very different from Starzl's position that "living related donor transplantation is obsolete for me . . . I do not want to do it anymore" [80]. In an extensive review of more than 400 donors over a 12-year period, we have not found

any increased risk of hypertension or proteinuria [250]. In fact, even clinically undetectable microalbuminuria has been unusual [40]. What is clear from this work is the importance of eliminating individuals with mild or labile hypertension as donors, because these findings predict established hypertension in later years [40]. We also find that the substantial improvement in graft survival rates among HLA non-identical living related donors is not abrogated by the use of cyclosporine with CD. In fact, in our experience there has been no substantive difference in patient or graft survival results since using cyclosporine. In addition, we find that the wait for cadaveric kidneys exacts a heavy penalty from children requiring dialysis, and this translates to great family stress. The problem of organ availability is likely to become even more severe if living related donor transplantation is largely abandoned, as Starzl suggests. In addition, the small risk of development of broad cytotoxic antibodies, rendering children on dialysis virtually nontransplantable, is of tragic proportions. The development of improved protocols for donor-specific transfusions is likely to continue to influence positively the risk-benefit ratio of living related donor as compared with cadaveric transplantation [5]. Finally, one cannot, in our view, minimize the positive psychological and spiritual growth experienced by about 85% of living related donors [231]. Since this controversy cannot now be resolved, given current knowledge, technologies, and situations, it remains a personal decision for the responsible physician. In the last analysis, it is our opinion that families should be presented with the various options and viewpoints, even if some of these are not locally practiced.

Controversy exists as to the benefits derived from the selection of cadaveric donors based on histocompatibility with the recipients. Fine et al. [75] believe that their experience with children confirmed earlier data that typing in cadaveric transplantation has little influence on outcome. Hamburger et al. [102] concluded that "the evidence for the usefulness of typing is much more impressive with related living donors than in cadaveric renal transplantation." Although our experience with children is too limited for statistical comparisons, our overall results for cadaveric transplantations in all patients does suggest that HLA-A,B matching influences the outcome of cadaveric transplantation. An extensive study of 4998 cadaveric kidney transplantations by Opelz et al. [191] confirms this impression. More recently, studies have suggested that HLA-DR matching is important in cadaveric graft outcome and that this influence may be stronger than HLA-A,B matching [19]. However, these conclusions are not universally accepted [57]. Starzl et al. [242] have suggested that cyclosporine will diminish the role of tissue matching in future transplantation practices.

Antilymphocyte Globulin

Controversy persists as to the usefulness of ALG in preventing early rejection episodes and thus improving patient and graft survival [4]. In part, as mentioned previously, this controversy remains unresolved because of the paucity of controlled trials and the lack of uniformity in the antilymphocyte antibody preparations. Data for cadaveric transplantation and ALG [186] suggest that histocompatibility matching and ALG are independent variables influencing outcome. Well-matched cadaveric graft recipients receiving high doses of ALG had the best prognosis, whereas poorly matched recipients receiving little or no ALG had poor results.

No controlled studies of ALG treatment in children have been reported. However, our experience with children follows the trends noted previously. In addition, children appear to tolerate ALG treatment with fewer serious infectious complications than adults (see Infectious Complications).

Second Transplantations

Fine et al. [76] reviewed their experience with 59 children receiving second renal allografts from cadaveric donors. Half had functioning grafts 48 months following their second transplantations. These were excellent results when compared with the less favorable data of the combined European [27] and other reports.

Our results in children support the conclusion that second transplantations are usually warranted. Forty-eight of our children have received second renal allografts, 22 from cadaveric donors. Twenty-four of these retransplantations were performed between 1968 and 1975 and 24 between 1976 and 1982 (Table 41-5). The important improvement in patient and graft survival likely reflects accumulated experience as well as the changes in protocol discussed previously. The overall improvement in second graft survival resulted largely from better outcome in the cadaveric transplantation group.

It has been suggested that success is increased if the second transplantation is delayed more than 40 days after removal of the first graft [118], if the first graft was lost for reasons other than rejection [84], and if the recipient has undergone splenectomy [200]. We have not confirmed the findings of Opelz and Terasaki [192] that previous sensitization to more than 15% of the HLA-A,B antigens in a panel predicts a poor outcome. We had earlier reported that patients (including children) requiring second transplantations have excellent results with living related donor second grafts [84]. In this circumstance patient survival rate was 85% and graft function was 80% at 2 years posttransplantation, even though the first graft was lost from rejection; in contrast, patient and graft survivals were only 44% and 25%, respectively, in patients receiving two successive cadaveric transplantations [35,84]. The highest failure rate occurred in patients receiving a second cadaveric graft within a few months following the removal of the first graft and in patients rejecting a living related or cadaveric graft within 150 days of transplantation. More recent results suggest a more optimistic outlook, and the improvement in results of second transplantations with cadaveric donors has been particularly gratifying. However, the patients who rapidly reject their first graft continue to be at increased risk of rejection with the second graft. For these children we believe that the known and unknown

TABLE 41-5. *Second transplantations in children*

	Number of Patients	% Graft Function			% Patient Survival		
		1 yr	2 yr	4 yr	1 yr	2 yr	4 yr
1968-1975 (Cad & LRD)	24	67	58	38	83	79	79
1976-1982 (Cad & LRD)	24	79	70	70	92	92	87
1968-1975 (Cad)	10	40	30	—	—	—	—
1968-1975 (LRD)	10	86	79	—	—	—	—
1976-1982 (Cad)	12	75	65	—	—	—	—
1976-1982 (LRD, Non-HLA-ID)	10	90	80	—	—	—	—

Cad, cadaver; LRD, living related donor.
Data kindly provided by Dr. Sam So, Department of Surgery, University of Minnesota.

risks of cyclosporine are warranted. Patients with grafts that slowly lose function from chronic rejection need not have their rejected graft removed or retransplantation delayed [35].

Complications in the Postoperative Period
Urologic Complications

Urologic complications are frequent in transplant recipients. Malek et al. [150], in a literature review, found an incidence of urologic problems of 13.3% among 1301 recipients. Thirty-two percent of the patients with urologic complications died as a result of these events. A review at our institution revealed 102 urologic complications in 87 patients (5.7%) from 1965 to 1982 in 1780 renal transplantations. These complications include leaks from the bladder, ureter, and calyces; ureteral tip necrosis; total ureteral necrosis; pull out of the ureter from the bladder; ureteral reflux; and obstructive uropathy. These complications, formerly believed to be due to rejection, are almost always due to technical problems. A ureter that is too short and is implanted under tension may undergo retraction, resulting in ureter pull out and leakage of urine. Inadequate blood supply to the ureter from overly aggressive dissection may produce partial or total ureteral necrosis. With good surgical technique this complication can be avoided. Ureteral pull out and ureteral tip necrosis are difficult to distinguish and are manifest by a sudden decrease in urine output with or without wound drainage. Analysis of wound fluid revealing a BUN and creatinine level significantly higher than serum is helpful, but the absence of this diagnostic laboratory feature cannot rule out a urine leak. Either diagnosis may be missed in the patient with post-transplant acute tubular necrosis. An antegrade contrast study through the percutaneous approach frequently yields the diagnosis of a collecting system lesion and may be used to treat the pathology by placement of percutaneous nephrostomy tube. Exact localization of the leak frequently requires exploration. Both ureteral pull out and tip necrosis may be treated successfully with reimplantation. Necrosis of the renal pelvis or the proximal ureter is a devastating complication that is hard to distinguish from distal ureteral pathology. Occasionally it can be treated successfully with a capsular patch or ureterouretostomy. Often it is safer to perform nephrectomy in the face of pelvic or high ureteral necrosis. It is important to note that pelvic necrosis may not become clinically apparent for several weeks after transplantation. Occasionally high ureteral necrosis can be treated by direct anastomosis of the pelvis to the bladder or by pyeloureterostomy using the patient's own ureter.

Bladder breakdown and leak are often associated with suprapubic pain and diagnosed by cystogram. Half the patients in our series were treated successfully with a layered closure and Foley drainage. This diagnosis can be missed in children with intra-abdominal kidneys and must be suspected in children with abdominal discomfort and mild distention even in the absence of a rise in serum creatinine. It may be confused with prolonged ileus. If suspected, a low pressure cystogram should be obtained without delay. This complication is more frequent in situations in which early postoperative problems with a Foley catheter had been encountered. Urine leaks are serious complications that can result in death due to infection. Thus, transplant nephrectomy is preferable to a repair procedure that provides tenuous reconstruction of the urinary tract.

Obstructive ureteral complications result from improper ureteral reimplantation, ischemia of the distal ureter leading to stricture, or extrinsic compression. Ureteral stenosis is often associated with fluctuating serum creatinine levels. Diagnosis is best made by ultrasonography, which demonstrates dilated collecting systems, and is confirmed by intravenous pyelography. One-third of our patients who had ureteral stenosis had undergone previous repeat ureteral implantation. Careful observation of renal function and follow-up of the ureteral and upper tract dilatation by sequential studies with echography are essential. Progressive parenchymal atrophy, functional deterioration, or recurrent infection suggests that corrective surgery should be undertaken.

Mild ureteropelvic junction obstruction may be present in the donor and can become clinically manifest in the recipient because the total urine volume must be handled by the compromised pelvic system. Pyeloureterostomy or pyeloplasty may then be required. Occasionally ureteropelvic junction obstruction results from compression from vascular structures or from scar tissue.

Vesicoureteral reflux is an important complication because of its association with potentially serious urinary tract infections. All ureters that reflux prior to transplantation should be removed down to the bladder. Autogenous ureteral reflux with onset after transplantation is more frequent on the side of the graft, indicating surgical disturbance of the ureterovesical junction. If associated with recurring infections despite adequate antimicrobial therapy, or, in the case of transplanted ureters, if progressive dilatation of the upper tract occurs, operative intervention is indicated. It has been reported that transplant glomerulopathy with light microscopy of glomeruli resembling type 1 mesangiocapillary glomerulonephritis (MCGN) is a common consequence of ureteral reflux in the allograft [162]. We have been unable to confirm this observation.

Urologic complications are more frequent in kidneys transplanted into ileal conduits [154]. Any of the previously listed complications can occur, but reflux up the ureter implanted into the conduit is expected. Revision of the ureteral anastomosis because of stenosis is required frequently. Stasis and infection may lead to stone formation. Marchioro and Tremann [153] suggested that the kidney be placed "right side up" with vascular anastomoses to the aorta and vena cava rather than to the iliac vessels. This procedure allows the kidney to drain by gravity and may decrease the incidence of complications. Currently we prefer to attempt bladder and ureteral reconstruction and to turn to the ileal or colonic conduit only as a last resort. Newer urologic technologies have markedly diminished the need for extravesical drainage procedures. Intermittent bladder catheterization may be preferable to an ileal conduit for some patients with neurogenic bladders.

Vascular Complications

Arterial complications are more common than venous problems, and they include stenosis, thrombosis, and mycotic aneurysms. These problems are frequently due to technical errors made at the time of transplantation. Immediate isotopic renography, performed if anuria develops in the early post-transplant period, followed by arteriography, may permit diagnosis of arterial thrombosis early enough to allow operative correction. Late arterial thrombosis often involves small polar vessels and may present diagnostic problems. We have seen one child with late polar entry thrombosis presenting with acute abdominal pain, fever, hematuria, and serum creatinine elevation who was diagnosed by the fortuitous renal biopsy sampling of the infarcted area of kidney [156]. Rupture of the anastomosis with consequent hemorrhage is almost always due to mycotic aneurysm of the suture line.

Malekzadeh et al. [151] reported renal artery stenosis with hypertension and elevated plasma renin activity in four of 77 transplanted children. We have seen five cases in 300 transplantations in children, one occurring in the smaller of the two renal arteries in the donor kidney. Marked hypertension unexplained by vascular damage seen on transplant biopsy should be studied by arteriography. If the blood pressure is difficult to control medically, stenosis should be repaired.

Interest has developed in the treatment of allograft renal artery stenosis by percutaneous transluminal angioplasty. Faenza et al. [64] have classified this condition as follows: iliac artery stenosis (rare), stenosis of the suture line, angulation stenosis, and single segmental stenosis of the graft artery or the major branches. They suggest that surgical correction should be considered as the first choice for angulation stenosis. We would add that it is dangerous to treat anastomotic stenosis by transluminal angioplasty. We have lost three such kidneys (two in children) from renal artery rupture complicating this procedure. Because collagen fibrils represent the major structural strength at the suture line, it is our hypothesis that, in the absence of smooth muscle, stretching the vessel at this point leads to tearing of the anastomotic site, which lacks elasticity. These cases should be treated medically; if this fails, surgical correction should be attempted. Thus, although surgical correction is technically difficult because of scar tissue enveloping the renal hilus, this may be the procedure of choice for suture line stenosis.

Primary renal vein thrombosis is extremely rare and is probably due to technical errors. Venous thrombosis can also be caused by compression of the renal vein by lymphoceles, by the kidney, or by extravasated blood. Venous thrombosis can complicate the recurrence of nephrotic syndrome in the graft. Because collateral veins are absent, complete venous thrombosis leads to graft infarction.

Post-Transplant Renal Failure

One of the more serious complications of renal transplantation is the failure of the graft to initiate or maintain renal function. Although the causes of graft failure can be listed, differential diagnosis may be difficult. Functional failure of the kidney is best examined in relation to the time after transplantation. Therefore, the kidney may (1) never function, (2) have delayed onset of function, (3) fail to function after a brief or prolonged period of function, or (4) gradually lose function over a period of months or years. Within each phase, there are some general considerations, which include: (a) whether the kidney has undergone ischemic damage, (b) whether rejection is occurring, (c) technical complications or (d) development of new or recurrent primary renal disease, (e) drug toxicity, (f) systemic viral illness, and (g) combinations of these problems. The simplest, most direct assay for decreased renal function is frequent determinations of BUN and serum creatinine levels. In the differential diagnosis of renal malfunction, other tests that may be required include ultrasonography, renography, intravenous pyelography, cystography, retrograde pyelography, arteriography, measurement of blood levels of potentially nephrotoxic drugs, and renal biopsy. Technical problems can occur long after transplantation. Before a patient is treated for suspected rejection, other renal parenchymal disorders and arterial, venous, and urologic complications must be excluded [100]. We rely heavily on percutaneous renal biopsies to document ischemic or toxic damage to the kidney, rejection, and the development of new or recurrent disease.

Acute Tubular Necrosis

Acute tubular necrosis (acute post-transplant renal failure) in transplanted kidneys is usually due to ischemic injury secondary to prolonged hypotension of the donor prior to removal of the kidney, prolonged preservation, or hypovolemia in the recipient. Failure of graft function due to acute tubular necrosis may present with several patterns. The urine flow may be deficient or absent from the time of transplantation, or it may be good initially, only to be followed by oliguria. Frequently, following transplantation of adult kidneys into very small children, urine output is initially low. After insuring that vascular volume is adequate and that the Foley catheter is patent, patience is almost always rewarded by spontaneously increasing urine output over the next 3 to 6 hours [176]. The *dangerous* error here is to push unnecessary fluids, which can lead to hypertension, pulmonary edema, or congestive heart failure and further decline in renal function. There is no evidence that adult kidneys require "adult levels" of systemic arterial pressure for adequate perfusion [176].

Before attributing severe oliguria to acute tubular necrosis, other causes such as renal artery or vein occlusion, obstruction of urine flow at any level, and hyperacute rejection must be ruled out. Thus, immediate isotopic renography and ultrasonography may be indicated. The use of diuretics may reduce the severe oliguria of acute tubular necrosis. Diuretics should be administered while other diagnostic procedures are being carried out. The initial dose of furosemide we use is approximately 0.5 mg/kg, administered slowly over 20 to 30 minutes. More rapid administration may produce high peak blood levels, leading to permanent deafness. The dose of furosemide is increased every 2 hours to a maximum of 5 mg/kg. If this fails to increase the rate of urine flow, the diuretic treatment is abandoned. If a diuresis results, a mixture of 20% mannitol and furosemide (0.5 to 2 mg/kg/hour) can be administered slowly to help maintain the diuresis. If a diuresis cannot be established, the intravenous fluids and oral intake are reduced to an amount needed to replace losses only. Dialysis may have to be reinstituted for the duration of acute tubular necrosis, usually from 1 to 3 weeks. However, oliguria may persist as long as 6 weeks. The ^{131}I-labeled Hippuran renogram has been useful in following improvement in renal perfusion prior to a resumption of urine flow. A number of studies have shown that long-term function of renal transplantations is independent of the presence or absence of oliguria in the early post-transplant period. However, more recently, two groups have reported compromised graft survival in cadaveric transplantations with acute tubular necrosis [41,223]. Biopsy of the kidney with acute tubular necrosis after 2 to 3 weeks may be the only way that early rejection can be detected.

Cyclosporine may prolong acute tubular necrosis. In addition, the nephrotoxic effects of cyclosporine must be differentiated from acute tubular necrosis and rejection. The percutaneous renal biopsy is highly accurate in differentiating these disorders, but quantitation of lymphocyte subpopulations may be necessary for specific diagnosis (see following). Cyclosporine dose adjustment using blood levels is important especially during oliguric renal failure. An attempt is made to maintain the levels between 100 and 200 ng/1iter. Cyclosporine dosage is reduced in 1 mg/kg/day steps for 2 to 3 days to achieve an acceptable level and resumption of renal function. A strategy we currently employ is to use azathioprine, prednisone, and ALG in all patients with post-transplant acute tubular necrosis and begin cyclosporine only when graft function is well established.

General Surgical Complications

Transplant recipients are subject to all of the complications of any patient undergoing a major operative procedure.

Postoperative Bleeding

Tachycardia, hypotension and decreased central venous pressure, falling hemoglobin, abdominal distention and tenderness, and oliguria all indicate serious postoperative bleeding. Abdominal palpation usually reveals an expanding mass around retroperitoneal renal grafts, and echography may reveal a hematoma. However, this test may be difficult to interpret in small patients with intra-abdominal kidneys. Coagulation studies and platelet count may indicate the need for a blood product or vitamin K administration to control bleeding. After restoration of blood volume, some patients may require re-exploration to control the bleeding. If cross clamping of the kidney is required to effect repair of a bleeding anastomosis, acute oliguric renal

failure frequently results. However, if the period of compromised renal function has been brief and diuretics have been used, prompt restoration of renal function may occur after exploration. It is worth repeating that large femoral artery to vein shunts or grafts can lead to venous hypertension and diffuse intra-abdominal or retroperitoneal bleeding that cannot be controlled until this vascular access system is clamped. Most perinephric hematomas, unassociated with serious compromise of vascular volume or progressive oliguria from renal compression can be treated conservatively. However, it should be expected that subsequent biopsies of such kidneys will be difficult to perform by palpation alone, and biopsy under ultrasonographic or CT scan control is recommended.

Wound Infection

A deep perinephric wound infection is a tragedy in transplant recipients and frequently leads to death of the patient. These infections, which occurred at a rate of 1% in the first 1700 transplants performed at the University of Minnesota, are most common in diabetic recipients and are rare in children. All treatment short of transplant nephrectomy has been largely unsuccessful. Superficial wound infection not communicating with the perinephric space may be treated by open drainage and packing. Although the risk of contamination of the perinephric space is real, the superficial wound infection per se need not result in kidney loss.

Pancreatitis

Pancreatitis in transplant recipients occurs as a result of (1) splenectomy either prior to or simultaneous with the transplantation, resulting in pancreatic injury; (2) administration of large doses of steroids in the postoperative period; and (3) hyperparathyroidism and hypercalcemia. In most cases pancreatitis in transplant recipients is mild, and in children, if adequately treated with nasogastric suction, intravenous fluids, and antibiotics, only occasionally progresses to fulminant disease. The dose of prednisone should be reduced to low levels.

Lymphocele

A lymphocele is a perinephric fluid collection that presumably develops consequent to the cutting or tearing of allograft renal hilar lymphatics during donor surgery [212]. The fluid can collect weeks, months, or even years following transplantation. This complication does not occur with intra-abdominal kidneys, apparently because the lymph is reabsorbed transperitoneally. The lymphocele is often asymptomatic and is a frequent incidental finding on ultrasonography, where it is difficult to differentiate from a resolving hematoma, abscess, or urinoma. When this distinction is difficult, lymphangiography may be helpful. However, lymphoceles can present as a perinephric palpable mass with local discomfort. The largest lymphoceles may be associated with significant renal dysfunction requiring differentiation from rejection. In this situation renal biopsy may be indicated, but technically difficult, unless the fluid is first substantially drained. In these circumstances we have drained the fluid through the Vim-Silverman biopsy needle and proceeded with the biopsy when sufficient fluid has been removed to allow clear palpation of the outline of the kidney or access to the border of the kidney under ultrasonography. Large fluid collections that recur following needle aspiration and cause significant renal dysfunction or discomfort can be treated by surgically marsupializing the fluid cyst wall to the peritoneum. Infection in lymphoceles is rare but often causes loss of the graft or death. Fluid removed by aspiration can be sent for urea nitrogen and creatinine levels, and these values can be compared with those of serum. Substantially higher urea nitrogen and creatinine values in the perinephric fluid compared with serum is evidence of a urine leak, but values similar to serum do not rule out this possibility because equilibration with blood is not uncommon. Most lymphoceles can be treated conservatively and will spontaneously disappear.

Upper Gastrointestinal Hemorrhage

Upper gastrointestinal hemorrhage from duodenal ulcer, gastric ulcer, or gastric erosion is a severe complication in transplant recipients. The mortality is extremely high. Most patients at our institution who have required an operative procedure for relief of upper gastrointestinal hemorrhage in the post-transplant period have died. In our experience, this problem is rare in children. Prevention is the best policy, and, as mentioned previously, prophylactic vagotomy and pyloroplasty for patients with peptic ulcer disease has greatly diminished the incidence of upper gastrointestinal hemorrhage. Following transplantation all patients receive antacids hourly during the day and every 2 hours at night until the prednisone dosage is reduced to approximately 0.5 mg/kg/day. When the maintenance prednisone dose is reached, antacids are prescribed only at bedtime.

Bowel Obstruction

Six of our pediatric renal transplant patients have developed acute bowel obstruction; in one it was due to intussusception developing soon after bilateral nephrectomy and in five to adhesions presenting 3 months to 5 years after transplantation. As yet no child who has had transplantation through the transperitoneal approach has had intestinal obstruction in the immediate post-transplant period.

Infectious Complications

It is known that the immunosuppressed patient shows increased susceptibility to a wide variety of infectious agents. Viral infections seldom kill the patient outright, but they frequently set the scene for bacterial and fungal sepsis as the terminal event. Immunosuppressed patients often have unusual infections or common infections presenting in unusual ways. Only a high index of suspicion can overcome the diagnostic disadvantage of detecting infection in patients whose signs and symptoms are obscured by antiinflammatory drugs.

Three-quarters of the fevers that occur in renal allograft recipients are associated with infection, and in more than half of all febrile episodes viruses alone or in conjunction with other causes can be implicated [198]. Bacterial and fungal infections account for about 20% of fevers, and approximately 10% are due to allograft rejection alone. In approximately 15% of febrile illnesses rejection and viral infection, especially with cytomegalovirus (CMV), are concurrent. Less common causes of fevers include drug fever, intra-abdominal hematoma or tissue necrosis, and malignancy. Thus, fevers in transplant patients should lead to a thorough search for infection, recognizing that although viruses represent the most frequently diagnosed explanation, common and uncommon bacterial, fungal, and protozoal organisms must be considered. Further, it should be remembered that multiple infections including any combination of the above-listed classes of agents can be present in the same patient [198].

Viral Infections

As a general rule, viral infections other than those of the herpes group have not presented major threats to children with renal transplantations. It is our clinical impression, however, that routine viral illnesses may be associated with acute rejection episodes [144,236] as long as 4 years after transplantation. Thus, it is recommended that renal function studies be obtained within 1 week of even mild viral illnesses.

CYTOMEGALOVIRUS INFECTION

The most common viral infection with the greatest clinical impact in renal transplantation is caused by CMV. The infection can develop from reactivation of latent virus [218], passage through a latently infected kidney [107], or blood transfusion [203]. Reactivation of clinical infection occurs in one-quarter to one-third of seropositive recipients. Another high-risk group is seronegative recipients of kidneys from seropositive donors. Present evidence suggests that the effort to find a seronegative donor for the seronegative recipient is worthwhile, because risk of infection can be reduced by this strategy and because infection is associated with a significant decrease in both patient and graft survival [251]. Although the evidence is less developed, it seems that this approach is not helpful for the seropositive recipient.

The risk of acquiring primary CMV infection from a blood transfusion is from 2.7% to 12% [218]. It has been suggested that the incidence of overt CMV disease is decreased in patients receiving cyclosporin A compared with standard immunosuppression [187]. High dose ALG has been implicated in promoting overt CMV infection [187], whereas it has been suggested that monoclonal antilymphoblast antibody is less likely to impair cell-mediated immunity broadly and is, therefore, of lesser risk in diminishing resistance to CMV [245]. Clinical post-transplant CMV is less common in children than in adults.

Clinical CMV usually becomes evident 30 to 90 days after transplantation, although infections becoming manifest more than 1 year after transplantation are not rare. Three rather typical clinical courses can be described for CMV infections [197]. Approximately 40% to 50% are asymptomatic, 40% to 50% suffer self-limited infections, and 5% to 10% die of progressive unrelenting disease.

The self-limited and progressive, fatal CMV illnesses cannot be differentiated at onset. The disease initially has many of the following characteristics: high spiking fevers, rising serum creatinine levels, musculoskeletal aches, fatigue, anorexia and abdominal pain, leukopenia, lymphocytosis, neutropenia, atypical lymphocytosis, thrombocytopenia, anemia, and elevated hepatic enzymes. Respiratory symptoms or pulmonary infiltrates occur in one-third of these patients. CMV retinitis must be looked for repeatedly since this development demands immediate withdrawal of immunosuppressive therapy even if the CMV disease is otherwise not severe. Gastrointestinal ulceration and massive gastrointestinal bleeding may develop. Acute allograft rejection is frequent, although the pathogenesis of this association is unclear [236,251].

Our policy in children with CMV infection is to treat biopsy-proved rejection episodes (eliminating unnecessary immunosuppression of patients with viral-induced renal dysfunction) as long as leukopenia or significant major organ involvement (i.e., liver, lung, eye) is absent. If evidence of visceral involvement or clinical deterioration develops, immunosuppressive therapy is stopped. If rejection recurs or progresses, the kidney is removed. All patients should be studied for evidence of infection with herpes viruses before and with each febrile illness or rejection episode occurring within the first several months after transplantation.

The lethal CMV syndrome is unusual in children. The course begins as described but progresses to profound weakness and lethargy; worsening leukopenia, thrombocytopenia, and anemia; progressive hepatic and renal dysfunction; increasing confusion; pulmonary failure; and death from terminal superinfection with bacterial or fungal agents [197]. Coinfection with other herpes viruses may be present [197,198,218]. It may be difficult to sort out if this progression is primarily due to the underlying CMV infection or to superinfection. Thus, it is important to continue aggressive surveillance for other organisms, including bronchial washings or lung biopsy for more definite histologic and microbiologic diagnosis of pulmonary infiltrates.

Vaccine for seronegative patients [202], antiviral agents [178], transfer factor, and interferon [218] are being explored in the prevention and treatment of CMV disease. However, at present, management focuses on meticulous supportive care with attention to nutrition, treatment of fevers, pulmonary toilet, and decrease or withdrawal of immunosuppression if the clinical course indicates serious systemic disease. Again, if rejection progresses or recurs despite antirejection therapy in a patient with CMV disease, the kidney should be abandoned.

HERPES SIMPLEX VIRUS

Fulminant herpes simplex virus hepatitis and death have been reported in adult renal allograft recipients [218]. Acyclovir has proved to be safe and effective in the treatment of immunosuppressed patients infected with this virus [178]. However, scattered reports of viral resistance to this agent are beginning to emerge [42,47].

Herpesvirus hominis illness in transplanted children has usually occurred in association with CMV. In our experience, Herpesvirus hominis alone has caused serious illness in only one child in association with herpes progenitalis developing 2 years after transplantation at age 16. Herpes labialis has not been associated with serious consequences in children with kidney transplantations.

VARICELLA-ZOSTER VIRUS

Approximately 10% of our pediatric patients have developed severe varicella-zoster virus (VZV) infections following transplantation. In most instances this represented a primary chickenpox infection. However, at least one child developed chickenpox for the second time [67,114], following exposure to the virus 2 weeks prior to receiving her transplantation. In all but one child with primary chickenpox, azathioprine therapy was withheld on diagnosis, and several were treated with zoster-immune plasma.

Serious systemic illness in these children is manifested by high fevers for many days, recurrent crops of rash, marked mucosal involvement, hepatitis, neural involvement, including severe stabbing pains, bladder paralysis, and thrombocytopenia and leukopenia followed by relative and absolute lymphocytosis [67]. Death occurred in one child whose azathioprine therapy was continued after the illness developed. In addition, one child presented with chickenpox and acute abdominal pain. Bowel perforation was entertained, but abdominal exploration revealed only acute chickenpox hepatitis. Unfortunately, bowel perforation resulted from this surgery and ultimately led to the child's death. Because the bowel may be fragile in children with disseminated varicella infection, surgical exploration should be reserved for those with direct evidence of peritoneal contamination.

We recommend prophylactic zoster-immune plasma or globulin for all children exposed to chickenpox post-transplantation who have not had previous VZV infection or who are receiving high-dose immunosuppression therapy at the time of exposure [11,126]. If chickenpox develops, the child should be hospitalized and azathioprine therapy stopped. Prednisone dosage should be reduced to levels sufficient to prevent adrenal insufficiency in the stressed patient.

No controlled trials of zoster-immune globulin in established systemic VZV infection in immunosuppressed patients have been reported. We have administered this material to several children with serious illness without clear-cut benefit. Acyclovir has been used to treat immunocompromised children with VZV infection. However, the efficacy of this treatment is unproved. There is promise that effective immunization for varicella virus will soon be widely available [96]. Until then, it is recommended that children with renal diseases destined to develop renal failure should purposefully be exposed to chickenpox with a view to developing immunity before transplantation.

Children with zoster need not have immunosuppression withheld unless evidence of systemic spread of infection develops. Acyclovir may be useful for this condition [13].

HEPATITIS B

It has been suggested that the presence of hepatitis B antigen (HB$_s$) in renal transplant patients had no effect on patient survival [39,228] and might be associated with improved graft survival. However, these relatively short-term studies must be reinterpreted in view of a report [201] that 61 HB$_s$-positive transplant recipients followed for an average of more than 3 years had significantly reduced patient and graft survival. This group had a fivefold increase in mortality from liver disease. Death from liver disease occurred in 10 of these patients on an average of 3 years after transplantation.

One of more than 20 children in our series with circulating HB$_s$ died of chronic aggressive hepatitis 4 years after transplantation. Thus, persistent hepatitis B antigenemia provides a serious risk factor for the transplant patient. The effects of increasing or decreasing immunosuppressive medications on the outcome of patients with evidence of progressive liver disease from HB$_s$ after transplantation are unknown. Finally, it has been shown that nonidentical HLA kidneys transplanted into patients with previous hepatitis B infections are more frequently lost from rejection [143]. It is therefore worthwhile to immunize children approaching end-stage renal failure with hepatitis vaccine (Hepatovax). It should be remembered that the vaccine dose should be doubled for patients in renal failure and for patients receiving immunosuppressive medications [37]. Parenthetically, it should be remembered that the transplanted kidney can be the source of hepatitis B infection [264].

Although a majority of episodes of acute hepatitis in transplant recipients can be classified as hepatitis B, CMV, Epstein-Barr virus (EBV), adenovirus, herpesvirus, and azathioprine toxicity, the majority of cases of chronic hepatitis in transplant patients elude diagnosis. The hypothesis that these cases represent non-A, non-B hepatitis virus awaits microbiologic confirmation.

EPSTEIN-BARR VIRUS

The work of Hanto et al. [104] has done much to define the importance of EBV infections in renal transplant recipients. In fact, EBV now represents the leading cause of virus-related deaths in children at the University of Minnesota. Five children ages 11 to 16 years developed serious documented EBV infections, and four have died [104]. In young people (mean age 23 years) EBV infection manifested initially as a lymphoproliferative disease resembling infectious mononucleosis, with features within this group of fever, sore throat, lymphadenopathy, rash, disturbed liver function tests, and pulmonary nodular infiltrates presenting within a few weeks to 3 years post-transplantation. Concomitant CMV and herpes simplex virus infections were common. Two of these patients had received total lymphoid irradiation. In contrast, older patients with EBV

infections (mean age 46 years) presented with localized solid tumor masses 1 to 11 years post-transplantation, which followed an aggressive and lethal course [104].

In the young patients the natural history was that of a rapidly progressive disseminated lymphoproliferative disease, and only one patient survived following transplant nephrectomy and cessation of immunosuppression. More recently acyclovir has appeared to alter this course favorably in the younger patients but was ineffective in the older group [104].

The youngest to the oldest patients provide a spectrum of lymphoproliferative disease ranging from a "mono-like" polyclonal-B cell proliferation to a monoclonal B-cell lymphoma. The following tentative strategies have emerged. Patients with a "mono-like" illness and EBV-associated polymorphic diffuse B-cell hyperplasia are treated with acyclovir and reduction or cessation of immunosuppression, depending on severity and treatment response [104]. Those with polymorphic B-cell lymphoma and cytogenetic abnormalities are treated with acyclovir, cessation of immunosuppression, and if necessary, allograft nephrectomy. If serial biopsy indicates transition to monoclonal B-cell tumors or if these tumors are there at onset, conventional cancer therapy is instituted and the graft is abandoned [104].

Bacterial Infections

Bacterial infections are responsible for more than 25% of the deaths in children after transplantation. Frequently these serious bacterial infections result from technical complications, including urinary leak, wound infection, obstructive uropathy (especially in transplantations performed into ileal bladders), mycotic aneurysms arising from the performance of transplant nephrectomies in infected fields, infections in perinephric hematomas or lymphoceles, and peritoneal contamination from bowel contents spilled during surgical procedures. Every attempt should be made to prevent these infections by careful attention to surgical techniques and early removal of indwelling vascular and urinary catheters, which may cause bacteremia with secondary seeding of surgical areas. In addition, a brief course of prophylactic antistaphylococcal antibiotics should be given following surgery. A high index of suspicion is required to diagnose these infections, because specific signs and symptoms may be minimal.

Children who present with bacterial infections several months or years after transplantation and who are on maintenance immunosuppression often have typical clinical signs and symptoms and respond to appropriate antibiotic therapy. Thus, pharyngitis, otitis media, and urinary tract infection unassociated with urologic problems can be treated in a standard fashion.

The major exception to the principles outlined here occurs with pneumococcal infections in splenectomized children. McEnery et al. [167] have described six splenectomized patients (five of them children) who developed overwhelming pneumococcal sepsis while on maintenance dialysis and five who developed sepsis 6 to 16 months after transplantation. Five patients died. We have had seven serious pneumococcal infections, six occurring despite long-term sulfonamide prophylaxis and one despite penicillin prophylaxis. Two children developed meningitis, one had septic arthritis, and four had overwhelming pneumococcal sepsis ending fatally within 8 to 24 hours of onset. In addition, two splenectomized children on maintenance hemodialysis died from an overwhelming sepsis with *Escherichia coli* and *Haemophilus influenzae*, despite long-term penicillin prophylaxis. For this reason we have instituted both daily phenoxymethyl penicillin as well as trimethoprim-sulfamethoxazole prophylaxis for all splenectomized children who are on dialysis or have received transplantations. Further, routine splenectomy is no longer being performed. It may very well be that splenectomy should be considered only for children in whom persistent neutropenia precludes the administration of immunosuppressive medications in doses adequate to prevent rejection.

Renal transplant recipients have an increased incidence of *Mycobacterium* infections [142], thus providing the rationale for appropriate pretransplant skin testing and post-transplant vigilance. We have seen no overt tuberculosis in skin-test positive children treated with isoniazide for the first 1 or 2 years post-transplantation. It should be pointed out that *Mycobacterium* infections often involve atypical organisms. Atypical clinical presentations are common, including joint and subcutaneous tissue infections and lung inflammation resembling septic pulmonary emboli or bacterial pneumonia.

Since instituting the policy of prophylactic penicillin and trimethoprim-sulfamethoxazole in children we have seen only one serious infection with pneumococcus and none with *Listeria monocytogenes* [9], *Nocardia asteroides* [932], and *Legionella* species [249]. We have seen no significant complications from this approach, although others have reported serious bone marrow suppression and nephrotoxicity when trimethoprim-sulfamethoxazole has been given to renal allograft recipients.

Fungal Infection

Serious fungal infections may occur following transplantation [113,198,218], frequently associated with broad-spectrum antibiotic treatment or prolonged high-dose prednisone therapy. As mentioned previously, fungal infections may complicate systemic viral illness, especially if leukopenia is present.

Patients on high-dose prednisone therapy and patients on broad-spectrum antibiotics should receive oral nycostatin prophylaxis. *Candida* is a common surface contaminant in nose, throat, urine, and wounds of transplant patients. This is not a cause of great concern but should be carefully watched. However, pneumonia, esophagitis [125], peritonitis, pyelonephritis, and blood stream infection caused by *Candida* often result in death [113,125, 198,218].

Aspergillus infections are frequently clustered through air source contamination or hospital construction or renovation. Cavitary lung disease can respond to amphotericin B and excision of cavitary lesions [258]. However, diffuse pulmonary disease and CNS disease are usually fatal.

Transbronchial or open lung biopsy and covered brush bronchoscopy culture are important in diagnosis.

Cryptococcus CNS and disseminated infections require long-term amphotericin B therapy [113]. One of our patients died of this cause while on maintenance dialysis following the loss of his third renal graft. Histoplasmosis should also be considered with pulmonary or disseminated infections [113].

In the first 6 months after transplantation, when immunosuppression is heaviest, fungemia is almost always found in patients with concomitant infections. Because of slow growth the fungus may not be recognized in culture until too late. Thus, patients with life-threatening infections not responding to appropriate antibacterial treatment should be considered for systemic antifungal therapy. The second group of infections, in which fungus is the primary agent, occur later, often in patients having had multiple rejection episodes. Aggressive diagnostic procedures, including lumbar puncture and bronchoscopy, when indicated, should lead to appropriate diagnosis and treatment. Cryptococcal meningitis may occur years after transplantation. Lumbar puncture performed even for minor signs and symptoms of CNS infection should allow early diagnosis.

Parasitic Infections

Pneumocystis carinii pneumonitis has been reported in transplant recipients [109], rarely in the first 6 months following transplantation. When suspected, bronchoscopy with washing, brushing, and transbronchial biopsy or open lung biopsy should be immediately performed. We have not had a single case of *P. carinii* infection in a child since long-term sulfonamide treatment was instituted in 1969. This record has remained intact since trimethoprim-sulfamethoxazole was substituted for sulfisoxazole.

Rejection
Hyperacute Rejection

Hyperacute rejection is almost always due to preformed cytotoxic antibodies in the recipient that have developed consequent to exposure to foreign histocompatibility antigens through blood transfusions, pregnancies, or previous transplantations [34,241,261]. The application of sensitive assays for preformed cytotoxic antibodies against the donor has largely eliminated this problem.

In general, transplantation remains contraindicated following a positive crossmatch even if the crossmatch becomes negative several months later [247]. It has been reported that patients who have become seronegative and remained so for at least 6 months may be successfully transplanted with a kidney against which they were previously seropositive [33]. Although this report indicates a success rate of approximately 60%, it is our current position that transplantation under these circumstances should be reserved for patients who have or have had cytotoxic antibodies against a high percentage of the donor panel (predicting difficulty in finding a kidney to which the patient has never reacted) and who are poor candidates for long-term dialysis. Thus, all available recipient sera should be tested against the cells of the potential donor. Some authors recommend a search for antibodies using donor kidney cells as the target, since antibodies reacting with these cells and not with lymphocytes from the same donor have been described [53]. Ettinger et al. [63] reported false-positive crossmatches due to the presence of anti-B but not anti-T lymphocyte antibodies. Patients transplanted with only anti-B lymphocyte antibodies did not undergo hyperacute graft rejection. More recently, Feduska et al. [66] suggested that B-cold antibodies may be predictive of decreased graft loss from rejection. B-warm antibodies were associated with increased graft loss. False-positive crossmatches do occur, particularly in systemic lupus erythematosus. These may require extensive laboratory detective work to ferret out, including tests for destruction of autologous cells. Thus, standard crossmatch procedures need to be refined.

Hyperacute rejection frequently manifests as rapid intraoperative loss of renal perfusion producing the "soft blue kidney" [260]. Alternatively the kidney may appear to have normal perfusion intraoperatively but will have decreased blood flow within several hours of transplantation. At this point the kidney may be swollen, and fever, thrombocytopenia, consumption coagulopathy, and microangiopathic hemolytic anemia may develop [241]. Isotopic studies usually show little or no renal perfusion; renal angiography is compatible with cortical necrosis; and renal biopsy characteristically demonstrates [52] diffuse arteriolar and glomerular capillary fibrin thrombi, intense glomerular and peritubular capillary polymorphonuclear neutrophil infiltration, immunohistopathologic evidence of fibrin, immunoglobulins (most strikingly IgM), and C3 in arteriolar and glomerular capillary walls [157]. The final histologic picture in hyperacute rejection is that of cortical necrosis. Treatment with anticoagulation and immunosuppression invariably fails, and the kidney must be removed.

An attempt to replace a graft rejected hyperacutely during surgery with a second graft from the same cadaveric donor has also failed [260]. The theory that the first graft would "soak up the antibodies," thus protecting the second graft, is incorrect. Although plasmapheresis has been used in an attempt to remove preformed cytotoxic antibodies, clear evidence of efficacy is lacking [94].

Accelerated Rejection

Accelerated rejection should be suspected with the rapid development of oliguria, renal failure, graft swelling, and fever, possibly accompanied by leukopenia and thrombocytopenia, 2 to 7 days after transplantation [157,260]. As with hyperacute rejection, isotopic studies demonstrate markedly impaired renal blood flow. The severe graft swelling may lead to rupture of the graft, resulting in hemorrhage and shock [157]; this event was unrecognized in one of our pediatric patients and led to her death [157].

Accelerated rejection is associated with pathologic changes that vary from those resembling hyperacute rejection to those more typical of severe acute rejection. Many of our patients with this severe early rejection have had circulating cytotoxic antibodies against donor antigens at the time of rejection or shortly following removal of the rejecting kidney. Often immunopathologic evidence of humoral rejection is present.

These kidneys rarely respond to vigorous antirejection treatment. Plasmapheresis has been reported to be useful for the treatment of accelerated rejection but must still be considered as experimental treatment lacking rigorous proof for its efficacy [94]. Although functional recovery of early and severe cellular rejection may occur in response to antirejection treatment [157], the long-term outlook for graft survival is extremely poor [159], and these kidneys usually are best removed.

Acute Rejection

The term *acute rejection* is used to describe a rapidly developing, usually reversible decrease in renal function in which the dominant pathology is a tubulointerstitial inflammatory process [260]. In our pediatric series one or more acute rejection episodes, or "transplant crises" [102], have occurred in 50% of recipients of related kidneys and in 65% of cadaver recipients. These episodes may occur at any time after the first week following transplantation. In patients in whom ALG is used, acute rejection rarely occurs in the first 3 weeks after transplantation; when ALG is not employed, acute rejection frequently presents between the first and second week after transplantation. Although the risk of acute rejection diminishes after the first 3 to 6 months, we have seen vigorous, acute rejection occurring in patients with previously stable renal function for several years following transplantation.

CLINICAL FEATURES AND RENAL BIOPSY FINDINGS

When the patient presents with a rapid onset of fever, graft swelling and tenderness, oliguria, rapidly rising BUN and creatinine levels, fluid retention, hypertension, deterioration in the isotopic renogram, and a decrease in the graft bruit, there is little difficulty in concluding that acute rejection is present. The clinical and laboratory manifestations, however, may be far more subtle. This is particularly true in infants and small children in whom the functional reserve of the adult renal graft is so great that creatinine elevation may be a late finding, thus making fever, hypertension, and inordinate weight gain important early warning signals. Although there may be advantages to early diagnosis of acute rejection before overt renal functional deterioration occurs, to date there is no clear evidence that early cellular infiltrates in transplanted kidneys have the same diagnostic or prognostic importance as do similar findings in cardiac allografts [158].

We do not agree with the suggestion that unexplained fever per se is sufficient indication to begin antirejection treatment [6]. Fever in the absence of renal functional deterioration often represents a viral illness that can be adversely influenced by increased immunosuppressive therapy. Indeed, we have noted many instances of systemic viral illness associated with deterioration of renal function in the absence of any evidence of graft rejection on biopsy.

The renal function frequently improves as the viral illness subsides.

A number of tests have been developed with the aim of diagnosing early rejection. In addition to those listed in Table 41-6, Winchester et al. [263] have reviewed progress in immunologic predictions of rejection. However, none has proved entirely satisfactory, since they are too time-consuming to allow rapid decision making, they are not sufficiently specific, or they do not provide prediction of graft outcome; this latter point is of particular importance in considering fine needle aspiration of the kidney [60]. No test other than the kidney biopsy is as helpful in guiding therapy. One is much less likely to be very aggressive and to accept significant risks in treating rejection in a patient with severe acute vascular rejection than in one with moderate acute tubulointerstitial rejection (Table 41-7), yet these histologic types cannot be discriminated without a biopsy. Nonetheless, it should be noted that Miller et al.

TABLE 41-6. *Tests used for the diagnosis of rejection*

Lymphocyturia with pyroninophilic cells
Urinary and serum fibrin split products
Decreased serum IgG levels
Decreased serum complement levels
Lysozymuria
Urinary and serum β-2 microglobulin excretion
Tamm-Horsfall glycoproteinuria
Urinary lactic dehydrogenase
Blood leukocyte count
Presence of microangiopathic hemolytic anemia
Specific antibody consumption test
Mixed lymphocyte culture
Leukocyte migration test
Leukocyte DNA synthesis rate
Presence of hyperchloremic renal tubular acidosis
Ultrasonic detection of increased renal size

[175], monitoring mixed lymphocyte cultures, T-cell and B-cell quantitation, blast cell quantitation, and phytohemaglutinin responsiveness in a large group of adult transplant recipients, found these examinations to be useful guides in detecting and treating rejection. They suggested that such immunologic monitoring might favorably influence patient and graft survival. This approach has been expanded in studies of peripheral blood T-cell subsets defined and quantified using monoclonal antibodies [263]. For several years we have relied heavily on percutaneous renal biopsy to allow precise diagnosis in the setting of renal dysfunction, proteinuria, or fever of uncertain origin. Rapid processing of frozen sections or, even more useful, availability of permanent sections within 5 hours of biopsy permits accurate diagnosis and prognosis. Using techniques previously described [29], the incidence of significant biopsy complications has been less than 1%; no kidneys have been lost, and only one surgical procedure has been needed following more than 1600 such biopsies (in a patient with a severe coagulopathy).

Acute tubulointerstitial rejection is here defined by varying degrees of mononuclear interstitial infiltrate, interstitial edema, extravasation of erythrocytes, and tubular damage and varies from rare patches of this process (minimal) to diffuse involvement (severe) [159]. *Acute vascular rejection* is characterized by subendothelial infiltration of mononuclear cells with endothelial sloughing (endothelialitis). Minimal acute vascular rejection includes biopsies in which a few cells are found in one or two vessels while moderate acute vascular rejection involves larger numbers of vessels demonstrating a prominent endothelialitis [159]. Mild acute vascular rejection falls between minimal and moderate. Severe acute vascular rejection is defined by a necrotizing inflammatory process involving the media, fibrinoid necrosis of the vessel wall, or fibrin-platelet occlusion of the vessel lumen [159]. The value of this classification process is that it is predictive of graft survival (see Table 41-7) as determined in a retrospective study of more than two hundred biopsies [159]. Grafts with minimal or mild acute tubulointerstitial or vascular rejection have a 78%

TABLE 41-7. *Percent of allografts functioning 3 to 24 months following rejection; predictive value of renal biopsy*

Biopsy Interpretation	% Kidneys Functioning At:				
	3 mos	6 mos	12 mos	18 mos	24 mos
S CV (n = 10)	20	20	10	10	10
S AV (n = 14)	29	29	29	23	23
Mo CV (n = 30)	60	53	50	56	43
Mo AV (n = 23)	74	61	61	57	57
Min or Mi CV (n = 30)	83	83	80	77	77
SATI (n = 32)	59	53	50	47	47
Mo ATI (n = 53)	79	72	64	64	62
Only Min or Mi ATI, Min or Mi AV, CTI (n = 41)	83	80	78	78	78

A, acute; C, chronic; Min, minimal; Mi, mild, Mo; moderate; S, severe; TI, tubulo-interstitial rejection; and V, vascular rejection.
From Matas AJ, Sibley R, Mauer SM, et al: The value of the needle allograft biopsy. I. A retrospective study of biopsies performed during putative rejection episodes. *Ann Surg* 197:226, 1983.

2-year functional survival, whereas those with severe acute vascular rejection have only a 29% survival at 3 months and a 23% survival at 24 months. It is our experience that the biopsy changes little in the first few days of antirejection treatment and that biopsies performed after 10 to 14 days of treatment do reflect the effect of treatment on the rejection process.

Although it has been argued that indirect tests can be helpful in predicting rejection, there are no reports that indicate improved graft survival using these tests. Thus, it is unclear that antirejection treatment was initiated based on these tests alone. Furthermore, no direct test provides diagnostic as well as prognostic information.

In approximately 40% of our patients (a figure remarkably similar to that of Vangelista et al. [255]), biopsies led to a decision not to treat for rejection either because another diagnosis was made (such as normal kidney, ALG reaction, CMV infection with associated nephropathy, recurrent disease, de novo disease, acute tubular necrosis, bacterial or fungal infection of the kidney, or renal infarction) or because the acute rejection was considered irreversible. It is in the avoidance of unnecessary antirejection treatment that the allograft biopsy has its greatest value; however, it has also permitted early diagnosis of acute rejection in patients with subtle clinical and laboratory findings. Although we have had limited experience in children, the renal allograft biopsy has been very helpful in adult patients in differentiating cyclosporine nephrotoxicity from rejection [230] (Table 41-8).

Acute rejection must be differentiated from obstructive uropathy, pyelonephritis, recurrence of original disease in the transplant, arterial stenosis [234] or thrombosis, venous obstruction, renal dysfunction due to systemic infection, and perirenal lymph collections (lymphoceles) compressing renal structures [212].

RISK FACTORS

It is not known why, within similar tissue matching categories and immunosuppressive regimens, some patients have major problems with rejection, whereas others do not. It has been suggested that infection plays a role in triggering rejection [144]. Full discussion of the immunobiology of renal allograft rejection is beyond the scope of this chapter (see Chap. 40). However, patients at higher risk for rejection include those who have previously rejected a renal graft within the first posttransplant year [85], are high responders to the antibody-dependent cell-mediated cytotoxicity test [134], have received few or no pretransplant transfusions [191], or are HLA-DRW6-positive [105]. This latter risk factor is currently being disputed [54]. Patients at lower risk for rejection are those with HLA identical grafts, those with the ability to generate donor-specific suppressor cells in vitro to the LRD prior to transplantation [134], those who have received multiple donor-specific or donor nonspecific blood transfusions [191], and, possibly, those who have received kidneys from HLA-DRW6-positive donors [105]. There may be important differences between individuals in their pharmacokinetic handling of the immunosuppressive agents. Evidence that anticonvulsant drugs may increase the risk of rejection by altering liver metabolism of prednisone supports this possibility [257]. There may be individual differences in host response to foreign antigens. We have found no clear relationship between the presence of cytotoxic antibodies against a panel of leukocyte donors and rejection [30]. However, we continue to see patients who rapidly and repeatedly reject grafts for reasons that are not understood.

TREATMENT

Treatment of acute rejection varies greatly from center to center. Unfortunately very few controlled studies of the relative effectiveness and toxicity of different therapies are available. These modalities have included increased oral prednisone [233], intravenous methylprednisolone [253], ALG [111,112], antithymocyte globulin (ATG), monoclonal antiblast antibody [245], plasmapheresis [94], actinomyosin [173], anticoagulants [127,129], antiplatelet drugs [127,129], graft irradiation [124], and early graft removal with a view to retransplantation [133].

Based on controlled trials (unpublished observations), our mainstay of antirejection treatment is oral prednisone, increased to 2 mg/kg/day and tapered over 2 weeks to 0.5 to 0.75 mg/kg/day. Thereafter slow tapering to maintenance levels of prednisone is achieved over 1 to 2 months. We found parenteral methylprednisolone offered no advantage and resulted in increased toxicity when added to

TABLE 41-8. *Renal allograft biopsy in the differentiation of cyclosporine a nephrotoxicity from acute rejection*

		Cyclosporine A Nephrotoxicity	Rejection
Interstitial edema		−	+
Vasculitis		−	+
Glomerulitis (mononuclear exudation)		−	+
Ratio of interstitial to	≤1:3	+	−
intraperitubular capillary	≥3:1	−	+
mononuclear infiltrating cells			
Ratio of % interstitial	≤2.5:1	+	−
cells reactive with OKT8	≥2.5:1	−	+
to % reactive to OKT4			

the aforementioned treatment. By itself, methylprednisolone treatment was less effective. ALG treatment of rejection is, as mentioned, of proved benefit [111,112] and is
still used by us, although irregularly. There are uncontrolled observations that treatment with dipyridamole may
prevent the obliterative vascular reactions associated with
rejection, thus protecting against the development of hypertension [127,129].

Strategies for antirejection treatment must consider risk-
benefit factors. Obviously, if the patient has a serious underlying infection, the risks of treatment are high. Patients
with evidence of systemic viral illness, including fever,
leukopenia, elevated hepatic enzymes, or pulmonary involvement, should have their immunosuppression dosages
tapered. If rejection occurs or worsens in this setting, the
kidney should be abandoned. If treatment of repeated rejection episodes results in increasing steroid toxicity, especially if there is histologic deterioration of the kidney
[159] or if the episodes occur close together, strong consideration should be given to removal of the graft. On the
background of advanced small vessel disease, ischemic glomerular changes, and diffuse interstitial fibrosis, repeated
antirejection treatments are unlikely to procure satisfactory
long-term survival of grafts, and these findings should
weigh against the treatment of intermittent episodes of
acute rejection [159].

Chronic Rejection

Chronic rejection responds poorly if at all to increased
immunosuppressive therapy and frequently proceeds inexorably toward graft failure [159]. In general, two groups of
patients fall into the category of rejection. Some patients
with repeated episodes of "rejection crises" fail to return
to prerejection levels of renal function following treatment
and may develop progressive renal insufficiency, often associated with severe hypertension. The second group develops mild renal dysfunction that slowly worsens many
months or years after transplantation. Biopsy of these kidneys often reveals interstitial fibrosis, tubular atrophy, basement membrane thickening, and evidence of glomerular
ischemia with tuft shrinkage and basement membrane
wrinkling, thickening, and reduplication. There may be
mesangiocapillary glomerular pathology without striking
immunopathologic glomerular findings. Usually there is
striking arterial endothelial proliferation, medial thickening and fibrosis, so-called onion-skinning of small vessels,
and vascular luminal obliteration [110]. The inflammatory
infiltrate is generally in areas of interstitial scarring, is
mononuclear in type, and has few immunoblast-like cells.
This infiltrate often cannot be differentiated from that seen
in fibrous areas of the kidney approaching end stage from
any cause.

When biopsies are performed on a routine basis, it is
clear that many kidneys with excellent function have the
minor degrees of morphologic change described previously.
As Hamburger et al. [102] point out, these minor changes
"are never found in kidneys transplanted from an identical
twin" and indicate "a tenuous immunological tolerance of

the host for the graft." The significance of these minimal
changes for long-term graft function remains to be defined.

Recurrence of Original Disease in Transplanted Kidneys

Glomerulonephropathies

MESANGIOCAPILLARY GLOMERULONEPHRITIS

A high incidence (23% to 58%) of morphologic and clinical recurrence of mesangiocapillary glomerulonephritis
(MCGN) has been reported in transplanted kidneys
[161,170,254]. Although persistent post-transplant hypocomplementemia is said by some authors to predict recurrence, others find no clear relationship between complement levels and glomerular pathology [170]. Care must be
taken in evaluating recurrence of mesangiocapillary disease. From our unpublished observations, we concur with
the report of Mathew et al. [161] that pathology similar to
the subendothelial deposit type of nephritis may be found
several years after the transplantation in patients with excellent renal function whose original disease was not glomerulonephritis.

Recurrence of type I MCGN may be differentiated from
de novo transplant glomerulopathy by the paucity of immune reactant glomerular localization in the latter. Recurrence of this form of immune glomerular injury in the
graft results in serious renal dysfunction and graft loss in
only 10% of patients in the first several years post-transplantation [170], and thus transplantation is not contraindicated in patients with this form of glomerulonephritis.
With recurrence, however, problems such as proteinuria
and hypertension may develop.

The earliest and most frequently recurring type of
MCGN is dense deposit disease (type II). Although it has
been said that histologic recurrence is more often of scientific interest than of clinical import [32], it has recently
been suggested that 50% of grafts may fail because of
recurrent type II MCGN [59]. Although graft failure from
dense deposit disease may require many years to develop
and thus does not mitigate against transplantation, one
must be concerned about early graft failure in patients
whose original disease is characterized by a subacute clinical
course and crescentric-exudative glomerular pathology
[59]. In this situation a prolonged period of long-term
dialysis (1 or 2 years) and cadaveric transplantation may
be indicated.

STEROID-RESISTANT NEPHROTIC SYNDROME WITH FOCAL SEGMENTAL GLOMERULOSCLEROSIS

The original report by Hoyer et al. [116] of recurrence of
focal segmental glomerulosclerosis in transplanted kidneys
has been confirmed repeatedly [101,135]. However, recurrence is not inevitable [46]. Recurrence frequently presents
with massive proteinuria soon after transplantation, but
more gradual development of the nephrotic syndrome may
make difficult the differentiation from other entities, such
as the proteinuria of chronic rejection. In some instances
of recurrent steroid-resistant nephrotic syndrome, segmen-

tal sclerosis predominant at the corticomedullary junction has been noted [116].

It is difficult to determine the incidence of recurrence, but based on review of the literature, an estimate of 30% appears reasonable. Graft failure occurs within the first several years in about half of those affected. Recurrence in children with less virulent original disease has been less frequent [97], milder, and compatible with many years of useful graft function. Diminution of proteinuria with time with the first graft may indicate less serious recurrent disease in the second graft. Thus, patients' second or third grafts may escape recurrence. Children with rapid onset of renal failure and significant mesangial hypercellularity [149] are at particular risk, and in our experience severe recurrence with graft loss or death from infection has occurred in six of 24 cases. The clinical course of many of these children has been so devastating that we are at a loss to develop logical recommendations. It is suggested that, following the loss of the first graft, 1 or 2 years of dialysis precede a second transplantation, using a cadaveric kidney. Allograft nephrectomy should be considered if massive proteinuria redevelops and persists for more than 2 to 3 months.

ANAPHYLACTOID PURPURA GLOMERULONEPHRITIS AND IGA NEPHROPATHY (BERGER'S DISEASE)

Baliah et al. [12] reported that recurrence of anaphylactoid purpura glomerulonephritis may have contributed to the failure of a paternal renal allograft. However, we have had no evidence of recurrence in six children with this disorder, in agreement with the experience of others and suggesting that the risk is low.

Although recurrence of IgA nephropathy has been documented in children [20], it is difficult to determine whether this had any adverse influence on graft function.

RAPIDLY PROGRESSIVE GLOMERULONEPHRITIS

Goodpasture's syndrome, in which antiglomerular basement membrane antibody has fixed to the glomerular basement membrane of grafts and has injured or destroyed the kidney [15,56], is extremely rare in children. It appears reasonable to delay transplantation until circulating antiglomerular basement membrane antibody can no longer be detected. Sensitive radioimmunoassay techniques may be helpful in this regard [171].

Other types of rapidly progressive glomerulonephritis may redevelop with catastrophic consequences to the graft [139]. Strategies for the management of these patients, including bilateral nephrectomy, a prolonged period of dialysis, or immunosuppression prior to transplantation, are of unproved value [139]. Evidence has been presented that transplantation should not be carried out in these patients in the face of circulating cryoglobulins [169]. We have transplanted four children with rapidly progressive glomerulonephritis and none has had recurrence in the graft.

WEGENER'S GRANULOMATOSIS

Although uncommon in children, this disease may have unusual presentations in younger patients and may cause

ESRD. Two cases of serious systemic and renal recurrence have been documented in transplanted patients on azathioprine and prednisone [65,98]. For this reason cyclophosphamide is the drug of choice for long-term post-transplant immunosuppression, recognizing that permanent sterility is a likely outcome.

PRIMARY HYPEROXALURIA (OXALOSIS)

The high frequency of devastating damage to renal grafts from rapid oxalate deposition [99] has led some authors to conclude that this disorder represents an absolute contraindication to transplantation [139]. However, evidence suggests that successful transplantation is possible [123,184, 224]. Because extrarenal deposition of oxalate occurs only as renal failure develops and progresses despite dialysis treatment, and because these oxalate stores can deposit in the newly grafted kidney, it is our strong view that early transplantation, prior to the need for dialysis, is indicated [224]. We do not recommend transplantation for older children and adults after more than 2 to 3 years of dialysis, and just a few months of peritoneal dialysis may result in compromise to the allograft in infants with this disease. Long-term dialysis as a primary therapeutic choice has a gloomy outlook [122].

Transplantation is most likely to be successful if aggressive treatment with vitamin B_6, neutral phosphate, magnesium, thiazide diuretics, and high fluid intake is instituted immediately post-transplantation and maintained indefinitely [224] to increase the solubility of oxalate in urine. Because episodes of renal failure, including acute tubular necrosis and rejection, seriously compromise this medical management, transplantation with a well-matched LRD is recommended. Cyclosporine, which is frequently associated with renal functional impairment sufficient to restrict administration of neutral phosphate and magnesium, appears to be an unwise choice.

HEMOLYTIC UREMIC SYNDROME

Hemolytic uremic syndrome (HUS) is a heterogeneous disease that is not an uncommon cause of ESRD in young children. Folman et al. [79] and Cameron [31] have reported graft loss from recurrent HUS in a child and in two adults, respectively. We have observed that several forms of graft injury, especially acute rejection, ALG reactions, and hypertension, tend to produce more severe renal microangiopathy in HUS allograft recipients than in patients with other diseases. Thus, appropriate strategies to avoid these complications are indicated. Whether long-term prophylactic treatment with antiplatelet drugs or delay in transplantation following acute HUS is warranted in these patients is unclear. Cyclosporine, reported to cause microvascular glomerular thrombi in bone marrow transplant recipients [229], has been associated with rapid recurrence of HUS in the renal allograft [103,140], and we have encountered a parallel situation in which both the brain and the renal allograft were involved. Thus, given current knowledge, *cyclosporine should not be used in HUS patients.* Finally, it must be kept in mind that familial HUS with more than 1 year separating cases in the same family carries a high risk of serious renal destruction. The occurrence of

HUS ultimately leading to ESRD in a 21-year-old woman within days after donating a kidney to her HLA-identical 19-year-old sibling with HUS is cause for concern [21]. However, to our knowledge, no parental LRD to a young child with HUS has suffered a similar fate.

OTHER FORMS OF GLOMERULOPATHY

Congenital nephrotic syndrome does not recur in transplanted kidneys [115]. Chronic glomerulonephritis of unclassified type [86] and nephritis associated with systemic disorders such as systemic lupus erythematosus [28] and scleroderma (personal observation) usually do not recur in transplanted kidneys. Histologic recurrence with little or no impact on graft function may occur in membranous nephropathy and is the common pattern. However, the severity of glomerular involvement, influence on graft function, and production of proteinuria or hypertension have been variable. We have seen one graft lost owing to recurrence of this disorder.

DE NOVO GLOMERULONEPHRITIS IN THE TRANSPLANT

Mesangiocapillary glomerulopathy, characterized by expansion of the mesangium by hypercellularity and increased matrix and doubly contoured appearance of the glomerular basement membrane owing to mesangial interposition, is a relatively common histologic pattern observed several years after renal transplantation [117,190]. Although often associated with characteristic changes of chronic rejection, sometimes the glomerular changes are surprisingly disproportionate. De novo mesangiocapillary glomerulopathy has also been reported to be related to reflux into the graft. Immunohistochemical studies are often remarkably negative. Hypertension and proteinuria are frequently present, and loss of graft function, albeit slow, appears inexorable. Currently no proved therapy exists.

Membranous nephropathy also occurs as a de novo disease, possibly related to chronic infection in the immunosuppressed host [190]. The course is usually benign.

Males with hereditary nephritis may lack the Goodpasture antigen(s) in their native kidneys. Renal transplantation with a normal kidney thus results in exposure to a neoantigen that can stimulate antibody production. These antibodies can then mediate severe acute immune injury confined to the allograft and sparing the lungs, which apparently lack the target antigen(s) [177]. Although vigorous plasma exchange and prednisone therapy may salvage the situation, graft loss may occur despite these efforts. Strategies for retransplantation of these patients have not yet been delineated.

STRATEGIES IN TRANSPLANTATION OF CHILDREN WITH GLOMERULONEPHRITIS

Certain precautions should be taken to try to avoid the recurrence of serious immune glomerular injury in transplanted kidneys. Patients should not undergo transplantation in the presence of circulating antiglomerular basement membrane antibody or cryoglobulins. Nephrectomy is indicated in antiglomerular basement membrane antibody

disease to monitor continued antibody production accurately. Transplantation should not be performed when active systemic inflammatory disease such as systemic lupus erythematosus or vasculitis is present. Attempts should first be made to control these processes. In patients with systemic lupus erythematosus, serial serologic monitoring, including antinuclear antibody and complement studies, should be carried out. Immunosuppressive therapy should be aimed both at preventing rejection and at controlling the underlying disease. This principle includes the use of cyclophosphamide for patients with Wegener's granulomatosis. Patients with various forms of glomerulonephritis as their original disease should have renal biopsies performed if renal dysfunction develops in the graft. Otherwise, differentiation from rejection may be impossible, and unnecessary antirejection treatment may be given.

The problem of recurrent immune disease in transplanted kidneys is complicated by the de novo development of glomerulonephritic lesions in patients transplanted for nonimmune renal disorders [161]. Whether this "transplant nephritis" [119,161] represents chronic rejection, immune complex disease associated with chronic infection, or other pathogenetic factors is unknown. However, it is intellectually hazardous to assume recurrence if adequate controls are not available [31]. Only through prospective studies with matched controls followed with sequential biopsies can the true impact of recurrent disease be assessed. Thus, until clear information becomes available, except for the precautions mentioned previously, we do not consider any form of immune glomerulonephritis as an absolute contraindication to transplantation in children.

Cystinosis

Patients with cystinosis have done well following transplantation [148] in that the Fanconi syndrome has not recurred and hepatic and bone marrow involvement have not resulted in functional disturbances. Hypothyroidism may develop post-transplantation. Although cystine crystals may be seen in the grafted kidney, they are found in interstitial macrophages, not in the tubular epithelial cells. It is generally advantageous not to remove the original kidneys because their continued loss of salt helps prevent post-transplantation hypertension; at end stage, cystinotic kidneys do not produce significant bicarbonaturia, phosphaturia, or aminoaciduria. Idiopathic Fanconi syndrome [139] and hypophosphatemia with vitamin D–resistant rickets have recurred in grafts [183], indicating extrarenal causes for these disorders.

Other Complications
Growth

Many variables appear to influence linear growth following successful transplantation in children. We and others [120] have found that all children transplanted between ages 1 and 5 years who are growth retarded at the time of transplantation and who have no problems with repeated rejection episodes or serious infection begin to catch up in growth in the first year after transplantation [164,188]. Although growth thereafter is normal for age, catch-up usually ceases despite changing to alternate-day prednisone therapy. Thus, few of these growth-retarded children achieve a normal height for their age.

Grushkin and Fine [93] have emphasized the importance of bone age as a predictor of height potential in transplanted children. Normal growth rates may be achieved if the bone age at transplantation is less than 12 years but is poor if bone age is greater than 12 years. As uremia causes less retardation of bone age than height age, it appears that the longer the child is uremic prior to transplantation, the less the growth potential will be [24]. Pubescent growth spurts are muted in children with renal transplantations. Although secondary sexual characteristics usually develop, they are frequently delayed.

A prominent aspect of the progressive encephalopathy in uremic children (discussed previously) is acquired microcephaly. Following successful renal transplantation, young infants may experience a remarkable increase in their head size, even showing "catch-up" growth [180,239]. The impact of this growth is critical because head circumference is exponentially related to brain volume.

Prednisone has an important negative impact on growth. It is our policy to achieve by 12 months post-transplantation a maintenance dose of prednisone of 0.25 to 0.33 mg/kg administered once daily. If normal or catch-up growth occurs, this dose schedule is maintained. If growth is slow or becomes so and if renal function is stable, consideration is given to changing to alternate-day prednisone therapy over a period of 2 to 3 months, even though severe acute rejection and consequent graft loss have occurred in patients on alternate day prednisone as long as 5 to 8 years post-transplantation [68]. Rejection is rarely seen this late after transplantation in children on daily prednisone unless immunosuppressive therapy has been surreptitiously discontinued.

Improvement in growth in response to the change to alternate-day prednisone has been unpredictable and, in a matched pair retrospective analysis, did not achieve a statistically significant difference from controls [68]. Nonetheless greater improvement in growth than we have seen has been reported in other studies of alternate-day prednisone [108,168,205,215]. If graft function is impaired secondary to rejection or recurrent disease or if significant proteinuria develops, poor growth is to be expected. Thus, our current recommendations are that children who have not had early acute rejection episodes, do not have other growth impairing factors, and are growing poorly should be tried on alternate-day prednisone. This approach requires utmost vigilance for evidence of acute rejection.

Bone Disease

Prior to transplantation metabolic bone disease is present in most children (see Chap. 28). Parathyroid hormone (PTH) levels are markedly increased, and conversion of 25-hydroxycholecalciferol to 1,25-dihydroxycholecalciferol is impaired [199]. Following successful transplantation, these abnormalities tend to reverse [199]. Although several reports emphasize persistent hyperparathyroidism following transplantation in adults [83,137,226], there is little information on this problem in children. The disorder may present as asymptomatic hypercalcemia, renal insufficiency, pulmonary failure, progressive bone disease, renal lithiasis, emotional disorder, hypertension, electrolyte imbalance, or pancreatitis.

Routine follow-up of serum calcium levels is essential for early diagnosis of hyperparathyroidism. Geis et al. [83] have emphasized the importance of determining ionized calcium levels in patients with normal total serum calcium suspected of persistent hyperparathyroidism. We have seen several children with elevated total and ionized calcium and PTH levels following transplantation. Examples include a 2-year old with spontaneous fractures and progressive genu valgum requiring surgical correction, a $2\frac{1}{2}$-year old with personality changes, an asymptomatic 12-year old, a 4-year old with persistent microhematuria and recurrent gross hematuria, a 16-year old with persistent hypercalcemia with nephrocalcinosis documented $2\frac{1}{2}$ years post-transplantation, a 14-year old with severe persistent hypercalcemia developing after acute pancreatitis, and a 5-year old with mild renal failure complicated by the necessity for phosphate therapy because of primary hyperoxaluria developing osteitis fibrosa cystica. The conditions in most patients resolved spontaneously over several months with medical management including low calcium diet and oral furosemide. Thus, post-transplant hyperparathyroidism in children infrequently requires surgical intervention. Only the last three patients mentioned required subtotal parathyroidectomy. It is our impression that more careful and effective treatment of renal osteodystrophy in children with chronic renal insufficiency has resulted in a marked decrease in the incidence of significant post-transplant hyperparathyroidism.

Pre-existing bone deformities of renal osteodystrophy often heal with remarkable speed following successful transplantation. Occasionally genu valgum may progress, perhaps because rapid growth and weight gain as well as increased weight bearing and physical activity further stress the angular deformity. Femoral osteotomies are highly effective in these children.

The decision to perform corrective orthopedic procedures for bony deformities before as opposed to after transplantation needs to be individualized. On the one hand, pretransplant correction along with effective medical management of renal osteodystrophy is associated with excellent results and avoids the risk of bone surgery in the immunosuppressed patient. On the other hand, severe deformities may improve post-transplantation thus obviating the need for surgery. Orthopedic correction may prolong the time on dialysis. In the final analysis, factors such as convenience for the family and the child should be weighed in developing a treatment strategy.

Several children have developed aseptic necrosis (osteonecrosis) of bone following transplantation [90]. This complication most commonly involves the femoral head(s) or the knee(s) and often results from repeated assaults with high-dose steroid therapy for treatment of rejection or for repeated transplantation.

The 5% incidence of aseptic necrosis in our pediatric

series is much lower than that in our children treated with steroids for systemic lupus erythematosus [22] and may reflect the lower steroid dosage used in most transplant patients. Elmstedt [61,62] has confirmed that reduced steroid dose and use of non–phosphate binding antacids markedly reduce the incidence of post-transplant osteonecrosis. Bone pain generally precedes radiographic evidence of aseptic necrosis by several months, and bone scans may be helpful for early diagnosis [48]. Successful hip replacement has been performed in transplant recipients [26,90].

Other orthopedic complications include osteoporosis from steroid therapy, presenting as vertebral collapse or nontraumatic stress fractures, and slipped capital femoral epiphysis.

In most instances successful transplantation is associated with rapid healing of renal osteodystrophy. However, the patients with the most severe pre-existing bone disease should be followed carefully for calcium-phosphorus dysmetabolism and bone complications.

Steroid Diabetes

Fewer than 3% of transplanted children at our institution have developed steroid diabetes. Predisposing factors among patients with this complication have included female sex, patients with family histories of diabetes, obesity, and patients requiring multiple high-dosage corticosteroid treatments for transplant rejection [219]. Steroid-induced diabetes is usually mild; long-term insulin therapy may be unnecessary, although insulin may be required initially. One adult with long-standing post-transplant steroid diabetes developed diabetic vascular lesions in the transplanted kidney [163,165]. Thus, steroid diabetes that persists may have serious long-term implications. Patients with this complication should, if possible, be placed on alternate-day corticosteroid therapy.

Cataracts

Cataracts, a recognized complication of corticosteroid therapy, have been described in from 3.4% to 60% of children following transplantation [38,138,152]. Malekzadeh et al. [152], who reported the latter figure, found a significant correlation between the incidence and severity of these posterior lenticular opacities and corticosteroid dosage. Four of 69 patients in this report required cataract extraction. Although the incidence of this complication in our series is high (approximately 20%), most cataracts in children are minimal, and significant visual deterioration has not developed in our patients. Further, we found cataracts to be most closely associated with multiple antirejection treatments. In our experience, once a low-dose maintenance prednisone dose has been established for some months, progression is unusual.

It has been suggested that cataract development within the first year following transplantation may be an indication for alternate-day prednisone therapy [152]. However, we have found that significant cataracts develop mainly in patients treated repeatedly for rejection, i.e., in those pa-

tients with the greatest risk of rejection following reduction in steroid therapy.

Hypertension

Virtually every child undergoing transplantation at our institution has developed mild to moderate hypertension in the early post-transplant period. The only exceptions have been children with salt-losing nephropathies whose original kidneys were left in situ, thus indicating the important role of salt and water retention. Salt retention probably results from high-dose corticosteroids and elevated plasma renin activity [14], and salt restriction and diuretics are usually sufficient to control early hypertension. Most often hypertension relents spontaneously within the first few post-transplant months as maintenance levels of corticosteroids are achieved [151].

Although no consistent relationship between acute graft rejection, plasma renin activity, and hypertension has been found [14], it is well-known that hypertension frequently accompanies acute rejection. In fact, fluid retention and hypertension may become manifest prior to deterioration of renal function and thus may be the first indicator of rejection. With the institution of high-dose corticosteroid therapy for rejection, fluid retention and hypertension frequently worsen.

Causes of later or persistent hypertension after transplantation include chronic rejection, with its associated vascular damage; hypercalcemia; stenosis of the graft renal artery [237]; recurrent glomerulonephritis in the transplanted kidney; segmental ischemia of the graft caused by the surgical sacrifice of a polar artery [235]; and residual hypertension from diseased original kidneys or chronically rejected grafts left in situ. Further, we have seen hypertension associated with pseudotumor cerebri more than 1 year after transplantation in six children, two of whom have primary hyperoxaluria. Patients with persistent hypertension should be carefully evaluated and may require measures of plasma renin activity, intravenous pyelography, renal angiography, or renal biopsy for a full understanding of the disorder.

Potter et al. [206] have documented excellent responses to propranolol therapy in several children with high-renin hypertension after renal transplantation. In several of our patients with severe hypertension, however, vasodilator drugs such as hydralazine or minoxidil or the angiotensin converting enzyme inhibitor captopril had to be added to or substituted for propranalol and diuretic therapy before adequate blood pressure control could be achieved. In patients with chronic graft injury from rejection, captopril may induce an acute rise in serum creatinine similar to that seen when this agent is used in patients with graft renal artery stenosis; presumably the pathophysiology of this acute renal failure is similar in patients with main renal artery stenosis or with the multiple peripheral artery stenoses associated with chronic rejection.

The importance of aggressive efforts to control hypertension and its proximate causes (colloid administration, pain, corticosteroids) cannot be overemphasized. Small children *do not need* adult levels of blood pressure to perfuse the adult kidney adequately [176]. The consequences of inattention to the details of hypertensive management are all too often acute hypertensive encephalopathy and cerebrovascular accidents in the short run and acceleration of chronic vascular changes in the allograft in the longer term.

Hyperlipidemia

Hyperlipidemia has been documented in adults with renal transplantations [36]; cardiovascular disease is the second most common cause of death in these patients [145]. Hyperlipidemia has been documented in transplanted children [196,220]. Fifty percent of one group of transplanted children (ages 8 to 18) had abnormal lipoprotein electrophoresis, evenly divided between type II and type IV patterns [220]. In this study higher doses of corticosteroids were correlated positively with type II patterns and with elevated cholesterol and triglyceride levels. Pennisi et al. [196] documented elevated triglyceride levels in 31% and elevated cholesterol levels in 51% of children more than 1 year post-transplantation (mean 24.2 months). In this study 12 autopsied children treated with long-term hemodialysis or transplantation had an increased incidence of histologic lesions interpreted as early coronary artery disease. The pathogenesis of these lesions is unclear and may be related to the uremic state. Although documentation of premature clinical vascular disease in transplanted children is unavailable, evidence that alternate-day prednisone therapy is associated with significantly less hyperlipidemia in transplant recipients provides yet another rationale for this form of therapy.

Cancer

The incidence of malignancy is increased in transplant recipients. One review recorded 28 epithelial and 24 mesenchymal tumors in 5000 kidney and 170 heart graft recipients [195]. In patients followed for 4 months to 8 years, there was a 6% incidence of neoplasms. Perhaps the greatest relative increase has been in lymphoproliferative disorders with unusual anatomic distribution, affecting the brain and spinal cord in 46% of involved patients [155]. EBV-related lymphomas have been discussed previously.

Following renal transplantation we advise that adolescent girls receive gynecologic examinations every 6 months, including Pap smears, so that cervical cancer, which is increased in frequency in these patients, might be detected promptly [128]. Further, we advise avoidance of prolonged exposure to sunlight without a topical sunscreen because skin and lip cancers are a distinct risk.

Although the pathogenesis of the increased risk of malignancy in these patients is unknown, it has been suggested that immunosuppressive therapy, long-term antigenic stimulation, and chronic viral infections may play roles [160]. Only long-term follow-up of successfully transplanted children will delineate the seriousness of the cancer risk in these patients.

Psychological Considerations

The advances in scientific knowledge that have made successful kidney transplantation a commonplace reality have occurred with a relative paucity of tools to assess the psychological and social impact of this treatment [132] (see Chap. 36). Most authors indicate that serious psychological problems following successful transplantation are unusual [23,132,141]. Korsch et al. [132] reported good potential for psychosocial rehabilitation of the child and family. Surprisingly the number of children with obvious personality disturbance was no greater among transplanted children than in control groups of healthy children or children with other chronic illness [132]. These authors also showed that children with serious emotional problems manifesting at any time during their treatment had abnormalities previously detectable by the administration of simple personality tests.

Bernstein [23] found that in the early post-transplant period the most common parental reaction was one of overconcern in their care of the child. Return to school often represented a major stress to the child, particularly in the area of body image relating to cushingoid appearance, scars, and height. None of the children she studied spoke spontaneously to their peers about the transplantation.

In the middle post-transplant period (4 to 11 months), problems in relationships between related donors and recipients occasionally developed, manifested particularly by parental donors attempting to manipulate the behavior of the child based on their gift of the kidney. In the late post-transplant period, memory of the dialysis and surgical procedures had largely been suppressed. Loss of the transplanted kidney in the late stages often led to profound depression. Long after transplantation, adolescents often became negligent or rebellious in their self-care, omitting medications and avoiding follow-up blood studies and clinic visits [23,141,152]. Thus, it is particularly important to relate closely to adolescents who, for reasons of appearance, growth failure, or delayed sexual maturation, may discontinue their medication and risk rejection of the graft. With understanding of their feelings, they must be frequently warned against taking this step. Malekzadeh et al. [152] discussed 12 cases of noncompliance with immunosuppressive drugs. In most cases the noncompliance occurred among adolescent girls, especially those whose personality tests suggested high levels of neurotic anxiety. All these patients lost their grafts or developed chronic rejection.

Most young children adapt well following successful transplantation. Early involvement of all transplanted children with an interested child psychiatrist, psychologist, or social worker will allow earlier definition of the problems as they arise. Loss of the graft is a most stressful circumstance requiring support, understanding, and sometimes direct psychiatric intervention.

It is important to emphasize that successful transplantation most often has a salutary effect on psychosocial and intellectual development. Often this effect is nothing short of miraculous. Watching the withdrawn, depressed patient with chronic renal failure blossom into an outgoing, happy, and active new personality is a most rewarding experience.

With early graft failure in the young child, parental guilt, depression, and ambivalence frequently become manifest. A sense of hopelessness may lead to the abandonment of good medical and nutritional practices by the parents, leading to deterioration of the child now returned to dialysis. Under these circumstances, strong support of the family becomes critical.

It is the view of the authors that clearly identifiable staff physicians should maintain continued involvement with the child and family during the entire course of management. Only with consistent follow-up can difficulties in family dynamics be recognized and appropriately managed.

Rehabilitation

With the demonstration that renal transplantation in small children is feasible, the issues of rehabilitation and quality of life after transplantation have arisen [72]. As noted previously, the maturing nervous systems of younger uremic children seem especially at risk. It is unknown if this CNS vulnerability persists after initiating dialysis or even following transplantation.

Presently only minimal psychometric data exist for either short-term [211] or longer [69,188] follow-up in children following successful renal allografts. In the short term, children have a remarkable improvement in cognitive testing. It seems likely that this represents the immediate effect of an acute normalization of the brain's biochemical milieu. Later testing in young children following transplantation has also shown an improvement in developmental or IQ scores. Lacking is prospective data indicating whether these test improvements represent any more than the effect of improved biochemistry or even more importantly whether the age at transplantation or the duration of uremia or dialysis are factors that determine the long-term outcome [108,189].

We believe that uremic children should receive aggressive medical therapy. Nutritionally they should receive at least 100% to 120% of the recommended daily allowance of calories [8], adequate high-biologic value protein for growth [92], and multiple vitamin supplementation. Major fluid shifts secondary to dehydration or sodium depletion should be anticipated and avoided. Acidosis should be corrected. Because secondary hyperparathyroidism may initially be subtle, levels of active PTH molecule should be monitored and appropriate therapy with vitamin D analogs, low-phosphate diets, and phosphate binders should begin early (see Chap. 28).

With the potential for CNS problems, rickets, and growth failure, the possible benefits of earlier engrafting must be weighed against the increased complexity of transplantation in younger, smaller children. In our hands the risks of graft failure or patient death are no greater in children under 5 years of age than in young adults without diabetes (see Fig. 41-6). Therefore, we recommend early transplant surgery in the uremic child rather than accepting the complications and risks of chronic renal failure or dialysis therapy in addition to the risks of transplantation.

As noted previously, no prospective data support this approach but, based on our experiences, we believe this strategy offers children minimized risks and the best chance for optimal rehabilitation.

In the main, our transplanted children have been successful in returning to school and being accepted by their peers. However, problems have developed in the areas of training for and acquiring of jobs and professions commensurate with their abilities. As has been noted [152], there is strong bias against the hiring of these patients. Direct physician support of job applications has proved useful. However, further efforts in public education should be undertaken. We agree with the assertion that "science has given these patients new life, so we must now give them an opportunity to live it" [152].

Dialysis and Renal Transplantation as Primary Therapeutic Modalities for End-Stage Renal Disease in Infants and Children: A Perspective

The long-term implications of the decision to undertake aggressive treatment of the infant or child with ESRD remains shrouded in multiple uncertainties, because current approaches have a brief history relative to the normal lifespan. These uncertainties face both long-term dialysis and transplantation. It is known that both approaches are associated with increased risks of infection, malignancy, atherosclerosis, poor growth, bony complications, psychological and developmental problems, and difficulties in rehabilitation. Comparisons of the outcomes of these problems with the two treatment approaches for ESRD will undoubtedly continue to emerge. However, it is not an exaggeration to state that all the discussions that we have had with individuals in leadership positions in large and experienced pediatric dialysis-transplant programs in the United States and Europe support the view that transplantation is the treatment of preference. Thus, although there are many differences in approach between these centers, the dominant theme crosses regional, national, international, and cultural boundaries and can be summarized by the statement that the quality of life of the successful pediatric transplant recipient exceeds that attainable with long-term dialysis of any type. In our experience this is echoed by our patients who, having experienced both, almost universally opt for retransplantation rather than remaining on dialysis. With this unusual level of substantive agreement on such a complex issue and given the current state of the art of each form of treatment, it is difficult to recommend that large scale prospective studies be initiated in an attempt to quantify the assertions made here.

If one accepts the position enunciated here, the question arises as to the role of dialysis in ESRD in children. Clearly there are children awaiting cadaveric transplantation, possessing multiple cytoxic antibodies, and at very high risk for recurrent disease, for whom long-term dialysis is the only alternative to death. On the other hand, it is our view, once the decision is made for transplantation, that the time on dialysis should be minimized. As children approach ESRD, it is often possible to plan a course of action that obviates the need for dialysis, especially if a willing, living related donor is available. In fact, the relative ease of anticipatory planning is one of the major reasons why living related donor transplantation is emphasized in our program. In our view it does not make sense to suggest to the family that a trial of long-term dialysis be used in the decision about transplantation. Arguing that if the child does well on dialysis, transplantation should be postponed often results in the potentially dangerous decision to proceed with renal transplantation in the child not doing well on dialysis. The simplification of dialysis support with the advent of chronic ambulatory peritoneal dialysis (CAPD) represents a case in point. Because many more centers can initiate this treatment compared with hemodialysis or transplantation in small children, it is not infrequent that children are referred to transplant centers when CAPD is failing, frequently because of repeated technical problems requiring catheter replacement or because of multiple episodes of peritonitis. In both situations, especially in smaller children requiring intra-abdominal renal allograft placement, the resultant intraperitoneal adhesions and scarring and the risk of immunosuppression in the patient with potential occult intra-abdominal infection increase the hazards of transplantation.

Although the risks of transplantation may be influenced by the readiness of the infant in terms of age and body size, it should be re-emphasized that, in experienced centers, there are no currently measurable increased risks to transplantation once the patient is beyond 6 to 8 months of age and 5.5 to 6 kg body weight. Thus, efforts to provide dialysis support beyond these levels adds the inherent risks of dialysis to the inevitable risks of transplantation.

Finally, long periods of dialysis prior to transplantation substantially increase the costs of ESRD management. Monetary considerations must be placed in proper perspective in decision making that has life and death implications. On the other hand, it is increasingly the reality, especially in the United States, that the fiscal base for pediatric nephrology groups is becoming substantially dependent on dialysis-derived patient care dollars. It is hoped that this will play no role in the design of patient care strategies.

Helping the Helpers

Although common in medical practice, it is not an exaggeration to suggest that transplantation medicine places major stresses on the physicians, nurses, and others providing the care to children with ESRD. The issues raised here are perhaps crystallized by the enormous promise and the "magical" potential of successful organ transplantation. Medicine tends to attract perfectionistic, high achievers, and "action" fields exemplified by pediatric dialysis and transplantation may have more than their share of rugged individualists who measure their worth in terms of their success as battlers against death. In a letter written to one of the authors, a mother of a young renal transplant patient, herself dying of cancer, wrote "It must be tremen-

dously hard for you to say I've done all I can do when so much is at stake. The times when all you could do *was* enough, pale in the face of one failure." There are no easy answers to the dilemma that "If we care, we get hurt, and if we don't care, they get hurt." May we suggest that open sharing of our responsibilities and vulnerabilities can create an environment in which physicians, nurses, and others involved in the care of these children find needed support.

References

1. Advisory Committee to the Renal Transplant Registry. The tenth report of the Human Renal Transplant Registry. *JAMA* 221:1495, 1972.
2. Albrechtsen D: Serological typing of HLA-D: Predictive value in mixed lymphocyte cultures (MLC). *Immunogenetics* 6:91, 1978.
3. Albrechtsen D, Arnesen E, Solheim BG, et al: Significance of HLA-DR and B-cell cross match test in vitro and in cadaver renal transplantation. *Transpl Proc* 11:743, 1979.
4. ALG and transplantation (editorial). *Lancet* 1:521, 1976.
5. Anderson CB, Sicard GA, Etheredge EE: Pretreatment of renal allograft recipients with azathioprine and donor-specific blood products. *Surgery* 92:315, 1982.
6. Anthone S: Renal transplanting. *In* Ruben MI, Barratt TM (eds): *Pediatric Nephrology.* Baltimore, Williams & Wilkins, 1975, p 874.
7. Arbus GS, Barnor N-A, Hsu AC, et al: Effect of chronic renal failure, dialysis and transplantation on motor nerve conduction velocity in children. *Canad Med Assoc J* 113:517, 1975.
8. Arnold WC, Danford D, Holliday MA: Effects of caloric supplementation on growth in children with uremia. *Kidney Int* 24:205, 1983.
9. Ascher NL, Simmons RL, Manker S, et al: *Listeria* infection in transplant patients. Five cases and a review of the literature. *Arch Surg* 113:90, 1978.
10. Bale JF Jr, Siegler RL, Bray PF: Encephalopathy in young children with moderate chronic renal failure. *Am J Dis Child* 134:581, 1980.
11. Balfour HH Jr, McCullough JJ, Mauer SM, et al: Zoster immune plasma for the prevention or treatment of varicella-zoster infection in immunocompromised patients (abstr). *Clin Res* 24:545A, 1976.
12. Baliah T, Kim KH, Anthone S, et al: Recurrence of Henoch-Schonlein purpura (HSP) glomerulonephritis in transplanted kidneys. *Transplantation* 18:343, 1974.
13. Bean B, Braun C, Balfour HJ Jr: Acyclovir therapy for acute herpes zoster. *Lancet* 2:118, 1982.
14. Beckenhoff R, Uhlschmid G, Vetter W, et al: Plasma renin and aldosterone after renal transplantation. *Kidney Int* 5:39, 1974.
15. Beleil OM, Coburn JW, Shinaberger JH, et al: Recurrent glomerulonephritis due to anti-glomerular basement membrane-antibodies in two successive allografts. *Clin Nephrol* 1:377, 1973.
16. Belzer FO, Ashby BS, Dunphy JE: Twenty-four and seventy-two hour preservation of canine kidneys. *Lancet* 2:536, 1967.
17. Belzer FO, Schweitzer RT, Kountz SL, et al: Malignancy and immunosuppression. *Transplantation* 13:164, 1972.
18. Belzer FO, Schweitzer RT, Holliday M, et al: Renal homotransplantation in children. *Am J Surg* 124:270, 1972.
19. Berg B, Groth CG, Lundgren G, et al: Five-year experience

with DR matching in cadaveric transplantation. *Transpl Proc* 15:1137, 1983.

20. Berger J, Halina Y, Nabarra B, et al: Recurrence of mesangial deposition of IgA after renal transplantation. *Kidney Int* 7:232, 1975.

21. Bergstein J, Michael A Jr, Kjellstrand C, et al: Hemolytic-uremic syndrome in adult sisters. *Transplantation* 17:487, 1974.

22. Bergstein JM, Wiens C, Fish AJ, et al: Avascular necrosis of bone in systemic lupus erythematosus. *J Pediatr* 85:31, 1974.

23. Bernstein DM: After transplantation the child's emotional reactions. *Am J Psychiatry* 127:109, 1971.

24. Betts PR, White RHR: Growth potential and skeletal maturity in children with chronic renal insufficiency. *Nephron* 16:325, 1976.

25. Borel JF, Fuener C, Gubler HU, et al: Biological effects of cyclosporin A: A new antilymphocyte agent. *Agent Actions* 6:468, 1976.

26. Bradford DS: Bilateral hip arthroplasty after renal transplantation. *Minn Med* 56:44, 1973.

27. Broyer M, Donckerwolcke RA, Brunner FP, et al: Combined report on regular dialysis and transplantation of children in Europe, 1980. *Proc EDTA* 18:60, 1981.

28. Buda JA, Lattes CG, Grant JP, et al: Feasibility of renal transplantation in systemic lupus erythematosus. *Surg Forum* 21:252, 1970.

29. Buselmeier TJ, Schauer RM, Mauer SM, et al: A simplified method of percutaneous allograft biopsy. *Nephron* 16:318, 1976.

30. Callender CO, Simmons RL, Yunis EJ, et al: Anti-HLA antibodies: Failure to correlate with renal allograft rejection. *Surgery* 76:573, 1974.

31. Cameron JS: Effects of the recipient's disease on the results of transplantation (other than diabetes mellitus). *Kidney Int* 23(suppl 14):S-24, 1983.

32. Cameron JS, Turner DR, Heaton J, et al: Idiopathic mesangiocapillary glomerulonephritis. Comparison of Type I and II in children and adults and long-term progress. *Am J Med* 74:175, 1983.

33. Cardella CJ, Falk JA, Halloran P, et al: Renal transplantation in patients with donor specific T cell reactivity in non-current sera—long-term followup. *Transpl Proc* 1985

34. Carpenter CB, Winn HJ; Hyperacute rejection. *N Engl J Med* 280:47, 1969.

35. Casali R, Simmons RL, Ferguson RM, et al: Factors related to success or failure of second renal transplant. *Ann Surg* 184:145, 1976.

36. Casaretto A, Marchioro TL, Goldsmith R, et al: Hyperlipidemia after successful renal transplantation. *Lancet* 1:481, 1974.

37. Center for Disease Control. Inactivated hepatitis B virus vaccine. *MMWR* 31:317, 1982.

38. Cerilli J, Evans WE, Sotos JF: Renal transplantation in infants and children. *Transplant Proc* 4:633, 1972.

39. Chatterjee SN, Payne JE, Bischel MD, et al: Successful renal transplantation in patients positive for hepatitis B antigen. *N Engl J Med* 291:62, 1974.

40. Chavers BM, Michael AF, Weiland D, et al: Urinary albumin excretion in renal transplant donors. *Am J Surg* 1985

41. Cho SI, Azbreraitis BP, Bradley   : The influence of ATN on kidney transplant survival. *Transpl Proc* 1985

42. Coen DM: Acyclovir-resistant herpes simplex virus. *N Engl J Med* 307:681, 1982.

43. Collins GM, Jones AC, Halasz NA: Influence of preservation method on early transplant failure. Presented at the American Society of Transplant Surgeons, Chicago, IL, May 20, 1976.

43a. Committee on Brain Death. Determination of brain death. *J Pediatr* 110:15, 1987.

44. Cosimi AB, Colvin RB, Burton RC, et al: Use of monoclonal antibodies to T-cell subsets for immunologic monitoring and treatment in recipients of renal allografts. *N Engl J Med* 305:308, 1981.

45. Cosio FG, Giebink S, Than Le C, et al: Pneumococcal vaccination in patients with chronic renal disease and renal allograft recipients. *Kidney Int* 20:254, 1981.

46. Couser WG, Idelson BA, Stilmant MM, et al: Successful renal transplantation in focal glomerular sclerosis: Report of two cases. *Clin Nephrol* 4:62, 1975.

47. Crumpacker VS, Schnipper LE, Marlowe SI, et al: Resistance to antiviral drugs of herpes simplex virus isolated from a patient treated with acyclovir. *N Engl J Med* 306:343, 1982.

48. D'Ambrosia RD, Riggins RS, DeNardo SJ, et al: Fluoride-18 scintigraphy in avascular necrotic disorders of bone. *Clin Orthop* 107:146, 1975.

49. d'Apice AFJ, Tait DB: Improved survival and function of renal transplants with positive B-cell cross matches. *Transplantation* 27:324, 1978.

50. Delano BG, Lazar IL, Friedman EA: Hypertension and late consequence of renal donation. *Kidney Int* 23:168A, 1983.

51. Delano BB, Logan IL, Friedman EA: Hypertension, a late consequence of kidney donation. *Kidney Int* 23:168A, 1983.

52. Deodhar SD, Benjamin SP: Pathology of human allograft rejection. *Surg Clin North Am* 51:1141, 1971.

53. DePlanque B, Williams GM, Siegel A, et al: Comparative typing of human kidney cells and lymphocytes by immune adherence. *Transplantation* 8:852, 1969.

54. DeVerra V, Kerman RH: DRW6 phenotype, immune responder status and renal allograft outcome. *Transpl Proc* 1985 (in press).

55. DeShazo CV, Simmons RL, Bernstein DM, et al: Results of renal transplantation in 100 children. *Surgery* 76:461, 1974.

56. Dixon FJ, McPhaul JJ, Lerner RA: Recurrence of glomerulonephritis in the transplanted kidney. *Arch Intern Med* 123:554, 1969.

57. Dyer PA, Johnson RWG, Mallick NP, et al: A single center prospective study showing no benefit of HLA-DR matching between cadaver kidney donors and recipients. *Transpl Proc* 15:137, 1983.

58. Eddy AA, Mauer SM: Pseudohermaphroditism, glomerulopathy and Wilms' tumor (Drash syndrome): Frequency in end-stage renal failure. *J Pediatr* 1985 (in press).

59. Eddy A, Sibley R, Mauer SM, et al: Renal allograft failure due to recurrent dense intramembranous deposit disease. *Clin Nephrol* 21:305–313, 1984.

60. Egide F, deVecchi A, Bambi CT, et al: Comparison of renal biopsy and fine needle aspiration biopsy in renal transplant. *Transpl Proc* 1985 (in press).

61. Elmstedt E: Incidence of skeletal complications in renal graft recipients. Effect of changes in pharmacotherapy. *Acta Orthop Scand* 53:853, 1982.

62. Elmstedt E: Skeletal complications in the renal transplant recipient. A clinical study. *Acta Orthop Scand* 52(suppl 190):1, 1981.

63. Ettinger RB, Terasaki I, Opelz G, et al: Successful renal allografts across a positive cross-match for donor B-lymphocyte alloantigens. *Lancet* 2:56, 1976.

64. Faenza A, Spolaore R, Gilberto P, et al: Renal artery ste-

nosis artery transplantation. *Kidney Int* 23(suppl 14):S-54, 1983.

65. Fauci AS, Haynes BF, Katz P, et al: Wegener's granulomatosis: Prospective clinical and therapeutic experience with 85 patients for 21 years. *Ann Intern Med* 98:76, 1983.

66. Feduska NJ, Arnend WJ, Vincenti F, et al: Graft survival with high levels of cytotoxic antibodies. *Transpl Proc* 13:73, 1981.

67. Feldhoff CM, Balfour HH Jr, Simmons RL, et al: Varicella in children with renal transplants. *J Pediatr* 98:25, 1981.

68. Feldhoff C, Goldman AI, Najarian JS, et al: A comparison of alternate day and daily steroid therapy in children following renal transplantation. *Int J Ped Nephrol* 5:11, 1984.

69. Fennell RS, Rasbury WC, Fennell EB, et al: Effects of kidney transplantation on cognitive performance in a pediatric population. *Pediatrics* 74:273, 1984.

70. Filho MA, Kupiec-Weglensky JW, Araryo JL, et al: Interleukins and suppressor cells during cyclosporin A induced state of "tolerance." *Transpl Proc* 1985

71. Fine RN: Renal transplantation in children. *Proc EDTA* 18:321, 1981.

72. Fine RN: Historical perspectives of the treatment of ESRD in children. *In* Fine RN, Gruskin AB (eds): *End-Stage Renal Disease in Children.* Philadelphia, WB Saunders, 1984, p 1.

73. Fine RN, Grushkin CM, Anand S, et al: Cytomegalovirus in children post-renal transplantation. *Am J Dis Child* 120:197, 1970.

74. Fine RN, Korsch BM, Brennan LP, et al: Renal transplantation in young children. *Am J Surg* 125:559, 1973.

75. Fine RN, Korsch BM, Edelbrock HH, et al: Cadaveric renal transplantation in children. *Lancet* 1:1087, 1971.

76. Fine RN, Korsch BM, Riddell H, et al: Second renal transplants in children. *Surgery* 73:1, 1973.

77. Finlit CF, Jonasson O, Kahan BD, et al: Reye syndrome cadaveric kidneys. Their use in human transplantation. *Arch Surg* 109:797, 1974.

78. Foley CM, Polinsky MS, Gruskin AB, et al: Encephalopathy in infants and children with chronic renal disease. *Arch Neurol* 38:656, 1981.

79. Folman R, Arbus GS, Churchill B, et al: Recurrence of the hemolytic uremic syndrome in a $3\frac{1}{2}$-year-old, 4 months after second renal transplantation. *Clin Nephrol* 10:121, 1978.

80. Friedman EA, Najarian J, Starzl T, et al: Ethical aspects in renal transplantation. *Kidney Int* 23(suppl 14):S-90, 1983.

81. Frost N: Children as renal donors. *N Engl J Med* 296:363, 1977.

82. Fryd DS, Sutherland DER, Simmons RL, et al: Results of a prospective randomized study on the effect of splenectomy versus no splenectomy in renal transplant recipients. *Transplant Proc* 13:48, 1981.

83. Geis WP, Popovtzer MM, Carman JL, et al: The diagnosis and treatment of hyperparathyroidism after homotransplantation. *Surg Gynecol Obstet* 137:997, 1973.

84. Gifford RW, Doedhar SD, Stewart BHJ, et al: Retransplantation after failure of first renal homografts. *JAMA* 199:799, 1977.

85. Gifford RRM Sr, Sutherland DER, Fryd DS, et al: Duration of first renal allograft survival as an indicator of second allograft outcome. *Surgery* 88:611, 1980.

86. Glassock RJ, Feldman D, Reynolds ES, et al: Recurrent glomerulonephritis in human renal isograft recipients: A clinical and pathlogical study. *In* Dausset J, Hamburger J, Mathe G (eds): *Advances in Transplantation.* Copenhagen, Munksgaard, 1968, p 361.

87. Glazer JP, Friedman HM, Grossman RA, et al: Live cytomegalovirus vaccination of renal transplant recipients: A preliminary report. *Ann Intern Med* 91:676, 1979.

88. Goldszer RC, Hakim RM, Brenner BM: Long-term follow-up of renal function in kidney transplant donors. *Kidney Int* 23:124A, 1983.

89. Gonzalez R, LaPointe S, Sheldon CA, et al: Undiversion in children with renal failure. *J Ped Surg* 19:632, 1984.

90. Griffiths HJ, Ennis JT, Bailey G: Skeletal changes following renal transplantation. *Radiology* 113:621, 1974.

91. Grumbach MM, Conte RA: Disorders of sex differentiation. *In* Williams RH (ed): *Textbook of Endocrinology,* ed 6. Philadelphia, WB Saunders Co, 1981, p 448.

92. Grupe WE, Harmon WE, Spinozzi NS: Protein and energy requirements in children receiving chronic hemodialysis. *Kidney Int* 24:S6, 1983.

93. Grushkin CM, Fine RN: Growth in children following renal transplantation. *Am J Dis Child* 125:514, 1973.

94. Gurland HJ, Blumenstein M, Lysaght MJ, et al: Plasmaphoresis in renal transplantation. *Kidney Int* 23(suppl 14):S-82, 1983.

95. Gustaffson LA, Meyers MH, Berne TV: Total hip replacement in renal transplant recipients with aseptic necrosis of the femoral head. *Lancet* 2:606, 1976.

96. Ha K, Baba K, Ikeda T, et al: Application of live varicella vaccine to children with acute leukemia or other malignancies without suspension of anticancer therapy. *Pediatrics* 65:346, 1980.

97. Habib R, Hebert D, Gagnadoux MF, et al: Transplantation in idiopathic nephroses. *Transpl Proc* 14:489, 1982.

98. Hall SL, Miller LC, Duggan E, et al: Wegener's granulomatosis in pediatric patients. *J Ped* 1985 (in press).

99. Halverstadt DB, Wenzel JE: Primary hyperoxaluria and renal transplantation. *J Urol* 111:398, 1974.

100. Hamburger J: Immunologic follow-up of renal allograft recipients. *Transplant Proc* 4:669, 1972.

101. Hamburger J, Berger J, Hinglais N, et al: New insights into the pathogenesis of glomerulonephritis afforded by the study of renal allografts. *Clin Nephrol* 1:3, 1973.

102. Hamburger J, Crosnier J, Dormont J, et al: *Renal Transplantation: Theory and Practice.* Baltimore, Williams & Wilkins, 1972, p 37.

103. Hamilton DV, Calne RY, Evans DB: Hemolytic-uremic syndrome and cyclosporine A. *Lancet* 2:151, 1982.

104. Hanto DW, Gail-Peczalska KJ, Forzzera G, et al: Epstein-Barr diseases occurring after renal transplantation. *Ann Surg* 198:356, 1983.

105. Hendriks GFJ, Persijn GG, Lansbergen Q, et al: Excellent outcome after transplantation of renal allografts from HLA-DRW6-positive donors even in HLA-DR mismatches. *Lancet* 2:187, 1983.

106. Hillis WD, Hillils A, Walker G: Hepatitis B surface antigenemia in renal transplant recipients. Increased mortality risk. *JAMA* 242:329, 1979.

107. Ho M, Suwansirikul S, Doueleng JN, et al: The transplanted kidney as a source of cytomegalovirus infection. *N Engl J Med* 293:1109, 1975.

108. Hoda Q, Hasinoff DJ, and Arbus GS: Growth following renal transplantation in children and adolescents. *Clin Nephrol* 3:7, 1975.

109. Hodgkin JE, Anderson HA, Rosenow EC III: Diagnosis of *Pneumocystis carinii* pneumonia by transbronchoscopic lung biopsy. *Chest* 64:551, 1973.

110. Hou AC, Arbus GS, Noniega E, et al: Renal allograft biopsy: A satisfactory adjunct for predicting renal function after graft rejection. *Clin Nephrol* 5:260, 1976.

111. Howard RJ, Condie RM, Sutherland DER, et al: The use of antilymphoblast globulin in the treatment of renal allograft rejection. *Transpl Proc* 13:473, 1981.

112. Howard RJ, Condie M, Sutherland DER, et al: Use of

antilymphoblast globulin in the treatment of renal allograft rejection: A randomized study. *Transplantation* 24:419, 1977.

113. Howard RJ, Simmons RL, Najarian JS: Fungal infections in renal transplant recipients. *Ann Surg* 188:598, 1978.

114. Howarth CB: Recurrent varicella-like illness in a child with leukemia. *Lancet* 2:342, 1974.

115. Hoyer JR, Mauer SM, Kjellstrand CM, et al: Successful renal transplantation in 3 children with congenital nephrotic syndrome. *Lancet* 1:1410, 1973.

116. Hoyer JR, Raij L, Vernier RL, et al: Recurrence of idiopathic nephrotic syndrome after renal transplantation. *Lancet* 2:343, 1972.

117. Hsu H-C, Suzuki Y, Chung J, et al: Ultrastructure of transplant glomerulopathy. *Histopathology* 4:351, 1980.

118. Hume DM, Lee HM, Williams GM, et al: Comparative results of cadaver homografts in man and immunologic implications of the outcome of second and paired transplants. *Ann Surg* 164:352, 1966.

119. Hume DM, Sterling WA, Weymouth RJ, et al: Glomerulonephritis in human renal homotransplants. *Transplant Proc* 2:361, 1970.

120. Ingelfinger JR, Groupe WE, Harmon WE, et al: Growth acceleration following renal transplantation in children less than 7 years of age. *Pediatrics* 68:255, 1981.

121. Izawa T, Ihara T, Hattoni A, et al: Application of a live varicella vaccine in children with acute leukemia or other malignant diseases. *Pediatrics* 60:805, 1977.

122. Jacobs C, Broyer M, Brunner RP, et al: Combined report on regular dialysis and transplantation in Europe, XI, 1980. *Proc Eur Dial Transpl Assoc* 18:4, 1981.

123. Jacobs C, Rottenbourgh J, Reach L, et al: Terminal renal failure due to oaxlosis in 14 patients. *Proc Eur Dial Transplant Assoc* 11:359, 1974.

124. Johnson HK, Malcolm A, Al-Abdulla S, et al: The effect of local graft irradiation upon the reversal of renal allograft rejection. *Transpl Proc* 1985

125. Jones JM, Glass NR, Belzer RO: Fatal *Candida* esophagitis in two diabetics after renal transplantation. *Arch Surg* 117:499, 1982.

126. Judelsohn RG, Meyers JD, Ellis RJ, et al: Efficacy of zoster immune globulin. *Pediatrics* 53:476, 1974.

127. Kauffman HM, Sampson D, Fox PS, et al: Prevention of transplant renal artery stenosis. *Surgery* 81:161, 1977.

128. Kay S, Frable WJ, Hume DM: Cervical dysplasia and cancer developing in women on immunosuppression therapy for renal transplantation. *Cancer* 26:1048, 1970.

129. Kincaid-Smith P: Modification of the vascular lesions of graft rejection in cadaveric renal allografts by dipyridamole and anticoagulants. *Lancet* 2:920, 1979.

130. Kjellstrand CM, Simmons RL, Buselmeier TJ, et al: Kidney: Section I. Recipient selection, medical management, and dialysis. *In* Najarian JS, Simmons RL (eds): *Transplantation*. Philadelphia, Lea & Febiger, 1972, p 422.

131. Kleinknecht C, Broyer M, Huot D, et al: Growth and development of nondialyzed children with chronic renal failure. *Kidney Int* 24(suppl 15):S40–S47, 1983.

132. Korsch BM, Negrete VF, Gardner JE, et al: Kidney transplantation in children: Psychosocial follow-up study on child and family. *J Pediatr* 83:339, 1973.

133. Kountz SL, Belzer FO: The fate of patients after renal transplantation, graft rejection and retransplantation. *Ann Surg* 176:509, 1972.

134. Kyriakides GK, Severyn W, Fulber H, et al: Effects of histocompatibility testing versus immunoreactive predisposition on kidney transplant survival. *Surgery* 92:354, 1982.

135. Lameijer LDF. Schonherr-Scholtes YHCH, Westbrook DL,

et al: Recurrence of the nephrotic syndrome after renal transplantation (abstr). *Clin Nephrol* 1:49, 1973.

136. Lang DJ: Cytomegalovirus immunization. Status, prospects, and problems. *Rev Infect Dis* 2:449, 1980.

137. Latimer RG, Renning J, Stevens LE, et al: Tertiary hyperparathyroidism following successful renal allografting. *Ann Surg* 172:137, 1970.

138. Lawson RK, Campbell RA, Hodges CV: Renal transplantation in infants and small children. *Transplant Proc* 3:358, 1971.

139. Legrain M, Jacobs C, Kiiss R: Are there contraindications to transplantation? *In* Hamberger J, Crosnier J, Maxwell MH (eds): *Advances in Nephrology*. Chicago, Year Book, 1974, p 203.

140. Leithner C, Sinzinger H, Pahanka E, et al: Recurrence of haemolytic uraemic syndrome triggered by cyclosporin A after renal transplantation. *Lancet* 1:1470, 1982.

141. Lilly JR, Giles G, Hurwitz R, et al: Renal homotransplantation in pediatric patients. *Pediatrics* 47:548, 1971.

142. Lloveras J, Peterson B, Simmons RL, et al: Mycobacterial infections in renal transplant recipients. *Arch Intern Med* 142:888, 1982.

143. London WT, Drew JS, Blumberg BS, et al: Graft survival and host response to hepatitis B in kidney transplantation. *N Engl J Med* 296:241, 1976.

144. Lopez C, Simmons RL, Mauer SM, et al: Association of renal allograft rejection with viral infections. *Am J Med* 56:280, 1974.

145. Lowre EG, Lazarus JM, Mocelin AJ, et al: Survival of patients undergoing chronic hemodialysis and renal transplantation. *N Engl J Med* 288:863, 1973.

146. Mahan JD, Mauer SM, Nevins TE: The Hickman catheter: A new hemodialysis access device for infants and small children. *Kidney Int* 24:694, 1983.

147. Mahan JD, Mauer SM, Sibley RK, et al: Congenital nephrotic syndrome: The evolution of medical management and results of renal transplantation. *J Pediatr* 105:549, 1984.

148. Mahoney CP, Stricker GE, Heckman RO, et al: Renal transplantation for childhood cystinosis. *N Engl J Med* 283:397, 1970.

149. Maizell SE, Sibley RK, Horstman JB, et al: Incidence and significance of recurrent focal segmental glomerulosclerosis in renal allograft recipients. *Transplantation* 32:512, 1981.

150. Malek GH, Vehling DT, Daouk AA, et al: Urological complications of renal transplantation. *J Urol* 109:173, 1973.

151. Malekzadeh MH, Brenna LP, Payne VC Jr, et al: Hypertension in children after renal transplantation. *J Pediatr* 86:370, 1975.

152. Malekzadeh MHJ, Pennisi AJ, Vittenbogaart CH, et al: Current issues in pediatric renal transplantation. *Pediatr Clin North Am* 23:857, 1976.

153. Marchioro TL, Tremann JA: Ureteroileostomy in renal transplant patients: A modified technique. *Urology* 3:171, 1974.

154. Markland C, Kelly WD, Buselmeier T, et al: Renal transplantation into ileac urinary conduits. *Transpl Proc* 4:629, 1972.

155. Matas AJ, Hertel BF, Rosai J, et al: Post-transplant malignant lymphoma. *Am J Med* 61:716, 1976.

156. Matas AJ, Mauer SM, Sutherland DER, et al: Polar infarct of a kidney transplant simulating appendicitis. *Am J Surg* 131:363, 1976.

157. Matas AJ, Scheinman JI, Rattazzi LC, et al: Immunopathological studies of the ruptured human renal allograft. *Transplantation* 22:420, 1976.

158. Matas AJ, Sibley R, Mauer SM, et al: Pre-discharge, post-transplant kidney biopsy does not predict rejection. *J Surg Res* 32:269, 1982.

159. Matas AJ, Sibley R, Mauer SM, et al: The value of the needle allograft biopsy. I. A retrospective study of biopsies performed during putative rejection episodes. *Ann Surg* 197:226, 1983.

160. Matas AJ, Simmons RL, Najarian JS: Chronic antigenic stimulation, herpes virus infection and cancer in transplant recipients. *Lancet* 2:55, 1973.

161. Mathew TH, Mathews DC, Hobbs JB, et al: Glomerular lesions after renal transplantation. *Am J Med* 59:177, 1975.

162. Mathew TH, Kincaid-Smith P, Vikraman P: Risks of vesicoureteric reflux in the transplanted kidney. *N Engl J Med* 297:414, 1977.

163. Mauer SM, Barbosa J, Vernier RL, et al: Development of diabetic vascular lesions with diabetes mellitus. *N Engl J Med* 295:916, 1976.

164. Mauer SM, Kjellstrand CM, Buselmeier TJ, et al: Renal transplantation in the very young child. *Proc Eur Dial Transplant Assoc* 11:247, 1971.

165. Mauer SM, Miller K, Goetz FC, et al: Immunopathology of renal extracellular membranes in kidneys transplanted into patients with diabetes mellitus. *Diabetes* 25:709, 1976.

166. Mauer SM, Vernier RL, Nevins TE, et al: Renal transplantation in children ages 1–5 years. *In* Cummings N (ed): *Chronic Renal Disease: Unique Problems of the Child with Renal Failure.* New York, Plenum, 1984

167. McEnery PT, Flanagan J, First MR, et al: Fulminant pneumococcal sepsis in splenectomized renal allograft recipients. *Am Soc Nephrol Absts* 1975, p 103.

168. McEnery PT, Gonzalez LL, Manten LW, et al: Growth and development of children with renal transplants: Use of alternate-day steroid therapy. *Pediatrics* 8:806, 1973.

169. McIntosh RM, Gross M, LaPlante M, et al: Cryoproteins in immune complex disease: Role of nephrectomy and implications in recurrent glomerulonephritis in human transplants. *Exp Med Surg* 29:108, 1971.

170. McLean RH, Geiger H, Burke B, et al: Recurrence of membranoproliferative glomerulonephritis following kidney transplantation. *Am J Med* 60:60, 1976.

171. McPhaul JJ Jr, Mullins JD: Glomerulonephritis mediated by antibody to glomerular basement membrane. *J Clin Invest* 57:351, 1976.

172. Mentser MI, Clay S, Malekzadeh MH, et al: Peripheral motor nerve conduction velocities in children undergoing chronic hemodialysis. *Nephron* 22:337, 1978.

173. Merrill JP: Diagnosis and management of rejection in allografted kidneys. *Transplant Proc* 3:287, 1971.

174. Merrill JP: Medical management of the transplant patient. *In* Rapaport FT, Dausset I (eds): *Human Transplantation.* New York, Grune & Stratton, 1968, p 96.

175. Miller J, Lifton J, Dewoff WC, et al: The efficacy of immunological monitoring after renal transplantation. *Transplant Proc* 9:59, 1977.

176. Miller LC, Lum CT, Bock GH, et al: Transplantation of the adult kidney into the very small child: Technical considerations. *Am J Surg* 145:243, 1983.

177. Milliner DS, Pierides AM, Holley KE: Renal transplantation in Alport's syndrome: Antiglomerular basement membrane glomerulonephritis in the allograft. *Mayo Clin Proc* 57:35, 1982.

178. Mitchell CD, Bean B, Gentry SR, et al: Acyclovir therapy for mucocutaneous herpes simplex infections in immunocompromised patients. *Lancet* 1:1389, 1981.

179. Moberg AW, Mozes MF, Campos RA, et al: Simplified system of continued perfusion. *In* Hume DM, Rapaport FT (eds): *Clinical Transplantation.* New York, Grune & Stratton, 1973.

180. Moel D: The conservative management of uremia in childhood. *In* Friedman E (ed): *Strategy in Renal Failure.* New York, Wiley, 1978, p 126.

181. Monaco AP, Codish SD: Survey of the current status of the clinical use of antilymphocyte serum. *Surg Gynecol Obstet* 142:417, 1976.

182. Moorhead JF, Chan MK, El-Malik F, et al: Blood transfusion for renal transplantation: Benefits and risks. *Kidney Int* 23:S-20, 1983.

183. Morgan JM, Hamley WL, Chenoweth AI, et al: Renal transplantation in hypophosphatemia with vitamin D-resistant rickets. *Arch Intern Med* 134:549, 1974.

184. Morgan JM, Hartley MW, Miller AC Jr, et al: Successful renal transplantation in hyperoxaluria. *Arch Surg* 109:430, 1974.

185. Najarian JS, Simmons RL: *Transplantation.* Philadelphia, Lea & Febiger, 1972.

186. Najarian JS, Simmons RL, Condie RM, et al: Seven years' experience with antilymphoblast globulin for renal transplantation from cadaver donors. *Ann Surg* 184:352, 1976.

187. Najarian JS, Strand M, Fryd DS, et al: Comparison of cyclosporine versus azathioprine-antilymphocyte globulin in renal transplantation. *Transplant Proc* 15:2463, 1983.

188. Nevins T, Chang P-N, Mauer SM: Renal transplantation in the very young child. *In* Tune BM, Mendosa SA, Brenner BM, et al (eds): *Contemporary Issues in Nephrology,* Vol 12. New York, Churchill-Livingstone, 1984, p 381.

189. Newburger JW, Silbert AR, Buckley LP, et al: Cognitive function and age at repair of transposition of the great arteries in children. *N Engl J Med* 310:1495, 1984.

190. Olsen S, Bohman S-O, Potberg Peterson V: Ultrastructure of the glomerular basement membrane in long-term renal allografts with transplant glomerular disease. *Lab Invest* 30:176, 1974.

191. Opelz G, Mickey MR, Terasaki PI: Blood transfusions and kidney transplants: Remaining controversies. *Transplant Proc* 13:136, 1981.

192. Opelz G, Terasaki PI: Second kidney transplants and presensitization. *Transplant Proc* 4:743, 1972.

193. Palmer DL, Harvey RL, Wheeler JK: Diagnostic and therapeutic considerations in *Nocardia asteroides* infection. *Medicine* 53:391, 1974.

194. Paul LC, van Es LA, Van Rood JJ, et al: Antibodies directed against antigens on the endothelium of peritubular capillaries in patients with rejecting renal allografts. *Transplantation* 27:175, 1979.

195. Penn I: The incidence of malignancies in transplant recipients. *Transplant Proc* 7:323, 1975.

196. Pennisi AJ, Heuser ET, Mickey MR, et al: Hyperlipidemia in pediatric hemodialysis and renal transplant patients: Associated with coronary artery disease. *Am J Dis Child* 130:957, 1976.

197. Peterson PK, Balfour HA, Marker SC, et al: Cytomegalovirus disease in renal allograft recipients: A prospective study of the clinical features, risk factors, and impact on renal transplantation. *Medicine* 59:283, 1980.

198. Peterson PK, Ferguson D, Fryd DS, et al: Infectious diseases in hospitalized renal transplant recipients: Prospective study of a complex and evolving problem. *Medicine* 61:360, 1982.

199. Piel CF, Roob BS, Aviolli LV: Metabolism of tritiated 25-hydroxycholecalciferol in chronically uremic children before and after successful renal transplantation. *J Clin Endocrinol Metab* 37:944, 1973.

200. Pierce JC, Hume DM: The effects of splenectomy on the

survival of first and second renal homotransplant in man. *Surg Gynecol Obstet* 127:1300, 1968.

201. Pirson Y, Alexandre GPJ, von Ypersele de Strihou C: Long-term effect of HBS antigenemia on patient survival after renal transplantation. *N Engl J Med* 296:194, 1977.

202. Plotkin SA, Farquhar J, Hornberger E: Clinical trials of immunization with the Tocone 125 strain of human cytomegalovirus. *J Infect Dis* 134:470, 1976.

203. Pollard RP, Rand KH, Arvin AM, et al: Cell-mediated immunity to cytomegalovirus infection in normal subjects and cardiac transplant patients. *J Infect Dis* 137:541, 1978.

204. Potter DE, Belzer FO, Rames L, et al: The treatment of chronic uremia in childhood: I. Transplantation. *Pediatrics* 45:432, 1970.

205. Potter DE, Holliday MA, Wilson CJ, et al: Alternate-day steroids in children after renal transplantation. *Transplant Proc* 7:79, 1975.

206. Potter DE, Schamkelan M, Salvatierra O Jr, et al: Treatment of high renin hypertension with propranolol in children after renal transplantation. *J Pediatr* 90:307, 1977.

207. Potter DE, Holliday MA, Piel CF, et al: Treatment of end-stage renal disease in children: A 15-year experience. *Kidney Int* 18:103, 1980.

208. Prensky AL: Time—A fourth dimension for encephalopathies. *N Engl J Med* 310:1527, 1984.

209. Raftery MJ, Lang CJ, Schwarz G, et al: Failure of azathioprine to prevent sensitization due to third party donors. *Transpl Proc* 1985

210. Rapaport FT, Dausset J: *Human Transplantation.* New York, Grune & Stratton, 1968.

211. Rasbury WC, Fennell RS, Morris MK: Cognitive functioning of children with end-stage renal disease before and after successful transplantation. *J Pediatr* 102:589, 1983.

212. Rashed A, Posen G, Coutune R, et al: Accumulation of lymph around the transplanted kidney (lymphocele) mimicking renal allograft rejection. *J Urol* 111:145, 1974.

213. Reily CM: Thoughts about kidney transplantation. I. *Scand J Urol Nephrol* 8:37, 1974.

214. Reinhart JB: The doctor's dilemma. *J Pediatr* 77:505, 1970.

215. Reimold EW: Intermittent prednisone therapy in children and adolescents after renal transplantation. *Pediatrics* 52:235, 1973.

216. Roosen-Runge EC: Retardation of postnatal development of kidney in persons with early cerebral lesions. *Am J Dis Child* 77:185, 1949.

217. Rotundo A, Nevins TE, Lypton M, et al: Progressive encephalopathy in children with chronic renal insufficiency in infancy. *Kidney Int* 21:486, 1982.

218. Rubin RH, Cosimi AB: Infection in the immunocompromised host. *In* Simmons RL (ed): *Surgical Infectious Diseases.*

219. Ruiz JO, Simmons RL, Callender CO, et al: Steroid diabetes in renal transplant recipients: Pathogenetic factors and prognosis. *Surgery* 73:759, 1973.

220. Saldanha LF, Hurst KS, Amend WJC Jr, et al: Hyperlipidemia after renal transplantation in children. *Am J Dis Child* 130:951, 1976.

221. Salvatierra O, Amend W, Vincente F, et al: 1500 renal transplants at one center: Evolution of a strategy for optimal success. *Am J Surg* 142:14, 1981.

222. Salvatierra O Jr, Vincenti F, Amend W Jr, et al: Four-year experience with donor-specific transfusions. *Transpl Proc* 15(1):924, 1983.

223. Sanfillippo F, Vaughn WK, Spees   : The effects of delayed graft function on renal transplantation. *Transpl Proc* 1985

224. Scheinman JI, Najarian JS, Mauer SM: Successful strategies

225. Schnaper HW, Robson AM: Cerebral cortical atrophy in children receiving treatment for end-stage renal disease (ESRD). *Pediatric Res* 16:327A, 1982.

226. Schwartz GH, David DS, Riggio RR, et al: Hypercalcemia after renal transplantation. *Am J Med* 49:42, 1970.

227. Shiel AGR, Kelly GE, Mears D, et al: Antilymphocyte globulin in patients with renal allografts from cadaveric donors, late results of a controlled trial. *Lancet* 2:227, 1973.

228. Shons AR, Simmons RL, Kjellstrand CM, et al: Renal transplantation in patients with Australia antigenemia. *Am J Surg* 128:699, 1974.

229. Shulman H, Striker G, Deeg HJ, et al: Nephrotoxicity of cyclosporin A after allogeneic marrow transplantation. *N Engl J Med* 305:1392, 1981.

230. Sibley RK, Ferguson RM, Sutherland DER, et al: Morphology of cyclosporine nephrotoxicity and of acute rejection in cyclosporine-prednisone immunosuppressed renal allograft recipients. *Transplant Proc* 15(Suppl 1):2836, 1983.

231. Simmons RG: *The Gift of Life.* New York, Wiley, 1977.

232. Simmons RG, Klein SD: Family noncommunication: The search for kidney donors. *Am J Psychiatry* 129:63, 1972.

233. Simmons RL, Kjellstrand CM, Najarian JS: Kidney transplantation. *In* Najarian JS, Simmons RL (eds): *Transplantation.* Philadelphia, Lea & Febiger, 1972, p 445.

234. Simmons RL, Tallent MB, Kjellstrand CM, et al: Renal allograft rejection simulated by arterial stenosis. *Surgery* 68:800, 1970.

235. Simmons RL, Tallent MB, Kjellstrand CM, et al: Kidney transplantation from living donors with bilateral double renal arteries. *Surgery* 69:201, 1971.

236. Simmons RL, Weil R III, Tallent MB, et al: Do mild infections trigger the rejection of renal allografts? *Transplant Proc* 2:419, 1970.

237. Smellic WAB, Vinik M, Hume DM: Angiographic investigation of hypertension complicating human renal transplantation. *Surg Gynecol Obstet* 128:963, 1969.

238. So SKS, Mauer SM, Fryd DS, et al: The effect of donor relationship on renal allograft survival. *Kidney Int* 25:349A, 1984.

239. So SKS, Nevins TE, Chang P-N, et al: Preliminary results of renal transplantation in children under 1 year of age. *Transplant Proc* 1985

240. Spanos PK, Kjellstrand CM, Simmons RL, et al: Screening potential related transplant donors for unrelated disease. *Lancet* 1:645, 1974.

241. Starzl TE, Jerner RA, Dixon FJ, et al: Shwartzman reaction after human renal transplantation. *N Engl J Med* 278:642, 1968.

242. Starzl TE, Rosenthal JJ, Hakala TR, et al: Steps in immunosuppression for renal transplantation. *Kidney Int* 23(suppl 14):S-60, 1983.

243. Steffes MW, Barbosa J, Basgen JM, et al: Quantitative glomerular morphology of the normal human kidney. *Lab Invest* 49:82, 1983.

244. Stuart FP: Progress in legal definition of brain death. Presented at the American Society of Transplant Surgeons, Chicago, IL, May 20, 1976.

245. Takahashi H, Okazaki H, Trasaki PI, et al: Reversal of transplant rejection by monoclonal antilymphoblast antibody. *Lancet* 2:1155, 1983.

246. Taylor HE, Ackman CFD Jr, Horwitz F: Canadian clinical trial of antilymphocyte globulin in human cadaver renal transplantation. *Canad Med Assoc J* 115:1205, 1976.

247. Terasaki PI: Selection of organ donors (letter). *N Engl J Med* 280:1304, 1969.

248. The Twelfth Report of the Human Renal Transplant Registry. JAMA 233:787, 1975.

249. Tobin JO'H, Beane J, Dunnill MS, et al: Legionnaires' disease in a transplant unit: Isolation of the causative agent from shower baths. Lancet 2:18, 1980.

250. Toledo-Pereyra LH, Condre RM, Moberg AW, et al: Advantages of silica-gel-absorbed plasma perfusale for clinical renal preservation. Transplant Proc 7:573, 1975.

251. Tourkantonis A, Lazaridis A: Interaction between cytomegalovirus infection and renal transplant rejection. Kidney Int 23(suppl 14):S-46, 1983.

252. Turcotte JG, Feduska NJ, Haines RF, et al: Antithymocyte globulin in renal transplant recipients. Arch Surg 106:484, 1973.

253. Turcotte JG, Nicholas JF, Carpenter EW, et al: Rejection crises in human renal transplant recipients: Control with high dose methylprednisolone therapy. Arch Surg 105:230, 1972.

254. Turner DR, Cameron JS, Bewick M, et al: Transplantation in mesangiocapillary glomerulonephritis with intramembranous dense "deposits": Recurrence of disease. Kidney Int 9:439, 1976.

255. Vangelista A, Frasia GM, Stefoni S, et al: Graft biopsy in renal transplantation: Correlation with clinical, immunological, and virological investigations. Kidney Int 23(suppl 14):S-41, 1983.

256. Vincente F, Amend WJC Jr, Laysen G, et al: Long-term renal function in kidney donors. Sustained compensatory hyperfiltration with no adverse effects. Transplantation 36:626, 1983.

257. Wassner SJ, Pennisi AJ, Malekzadeh MH, et al: The adverse effect of anticonvulsant therapy on renal allograft survival. J Pediatr 88:134, 1976.

258. Weiland D, Ferguson RM, Peterson PK, et al: Aspergillosis in 25 renal transplant patients. Ann Surg 198:622, 1983.

259. Weiland D, Sutherland DER, Chavers BM, et al: Information on 628 living related kidney donors at a single institution with 1 to 19 years follow-up in 472 cases. Transplant Proc 1984

260. Williams GM: Clinical aspects of allograft rejection. In Lawrence W Jr, Pierce JE, Lee HM, et al (eds): The David M. Hume Memorial Symposium on Transplantation. New York, Grune & Stratton, 1974, p 71.

261. Williams GM, Hume DM, Hudson RP Jr, et al: "Hyperacute" renal homograft rejection in man. N Engl J Med 279:611, 1968.

262. Williams GM, Hume DM, Hudson RP Jr, et al: Renal transplantation in children. Transplant Proc 1:262, 1967.

263. Winchester JF, Gelfard MC, Foegh ML, et al: Early indications of renal allograft rejection. Kidney Int 25(suppl 14):S-34, 1983.

264. Woll JJ, Perkens HA, Schfeeder ML: The transplanted kidney as a source of hepatitis B infection. Ann Intern Med 91:412, 1979.

265. Yu DTY, Clements PJ, Paulus HE: Human lymphocyte subpopulations: Effect of corticosteroids. J Clin Invest 53:565, 1974.

Alan R. Sinaiko
Robert F. O'Dea

42
Use of Drugs in Renal Insufficiency

Effective use of pharmacologic agents in children with renal disease is complicated by a number of therapeutic problems that are unique to this patient population. Success or failure of therapy is dependent not only on an understanding of the usual complex interplay between biologic maturation, drug disposition, and pharmacodynamics, but also on an understanding of the mechanisms through which renal disease adversely influences each of these factors.

It is generally acknowledged that renal disease alters the disposition of drugs and drug metabolites dependent on the kidney for clearance from the body. What is not as well appreciated is that renal disease can exert an equally powerful influence on drug clearance by nonrenal mechanisms, such as hepatic metabolism, and can affect other determinants of drug distribution in body tissues and fluids, such as molecular binding to plasma proteins.

Compounding these basic issues of drug use in renal disease is the need to maintain competence with the explosive growth of biomedical technology in the areas of laboratory drug analysis and dialysis, i.e., hemodialysis and peritoneal dialysis. When integrated properly into the clinical care setting, new analytical methodologies (especially high performance liquid [HPLC] and gas chromatographic procedures) for measurement of drug concentrations in plasma and other body fluids are of inestimable benefit in treatment of the patient with renal disease. This is particularly true during periods of potentially rapid fluctuation in drug concentrations, such as are likely to occur with dialysis. Conversely, failure to follow established principles in collecting blood samples for measurement of drug levels or in interpreting results of those measurements can lead to costly overuse of plasma drug assays and cause drug-dosing errors.

The goal of this chapter is to provide an in-depth, practical approach to therapeutic decision-making in the child with renal disease. In addition to a comprehensive review of factors influencing the clearance of drugs from the body, special emphasis is placed on the interactions between renal disease and nonrenal mechanisms affecting drug distribution within body compartments. These principles can be applied to the large variety of agents employed in children with renal disease, so therefore, explicit dosing recommendations for individual drugs are not provided. The chapter concludes with a review of the pharmacology of diuretics and glucocorticoids. Because these agents are so widely used in the care of children with renal disease, a discussion of their pharmacologic and therapeutic properties is warranted.

Principles of Drug Clearance

The term *drug clearance* describes the relationship between drug concentration in the blood or plasma and rate of drug elimination from the body [154,227]:

Drug clearance (ml/min)
$$= \frac{\text{Rate of drug elimination (mg/min)}}{\text{Plasma drug concentration (mg/ml)}} \quad (1)$$

Drugs can be cleared from the body through excretion by the kidneys, lungs, or intestinal tract; through hepatic metabolism to active or inactive metabolites; and during hemodialysis or peritoneal dialysis.

Plasma drug concentration decreases in an exponential manner defined by an elimination rate constant (K_{el}). K_{el} is dependent on the characteristics of a given drug in combination with the individual characteristics of the patient. It is determined by the clearance of drug per unit time from the volume in which the drug is distributed within the body:

$$K_{el} = \frac{Cl}{Vd} \quad (2)$$

where Cl equals clearance and Vd equals volume of distribution.

In the clinical setting, the term *plasma half-life*, or $t\frac{1}{2}$, is more commonly used than *drug clearance*. $T\frac{1}{2}$ describes the duration of time required for drug elimination from the plasma and is related to the elimination rate constant:

$$t\frac{1}{2} = \frac{0.693}{K_{el}} \quad (3)$$

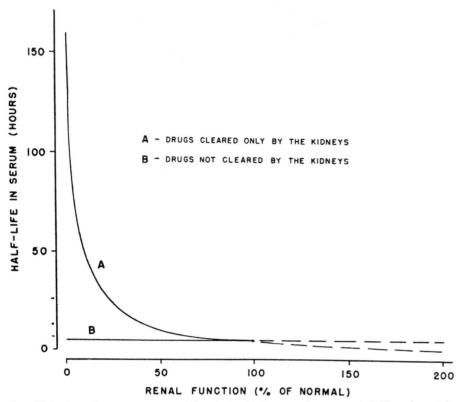

FIG. 42-1. *A graphic representation of the relationship between drug serum half-life and renal function.* (Reproduced from The Journal of Clinical Investigation, 1959, 38:1517, by copyright permission of the American Society for Clinical Investigation.)

When $t\frac{1}{2}$ is known, plasma drug concentrations can be anticipated by remembering that after a period of time equal to one half-life, the original plasma concentration will decline to 50%, after two half-lives to 25%, and after three half-lives to 12.5%.

Combining equations 2 and 3 by substituting for K_{el} in equation 3 as follows

$$t\frac{1}{2} = \frac{0.693 \times V_d}{Cl} \qquad (4)$$

shows that the elimination half-life of any drug is directly related to its volume of distribution and inversely related to its rate of clearance.

During chronic drug therapy, with administration of a uniform drug dose at regular dosing intervals, "steady-state" conditions are reached after a period of time equivalent to $t\frac{1}{2} \times 5$. Steady state implies that the amount of drug administered and the amount of drug eliminated are equal over a given period of time, so that plasma drug concentration is primarily dependent on and directly related to clearance, as expressed in the following equation:

$$C_{ss} \text{ (mg/ml)} = \frac{D \text{ (mg/min)}}{Cl \text{ (ml/min)}} \qquad (5)$$

where C_{ss} equals plasma drug concentration at steady state and D equals drug dose per unit time.

The relationship represented in equation 5 indicates that in the child with a reduction in renal function or in disease states associated with changing renal function, plasma drug concentrations should be more closely monitored, particularly for a drug with a narrow therapeutic index (i.e., plasma drug concentration associated with toxicity is very close to concentration needed for therapeutic success) [155]. Conversely, when using a drug with a wide therapeutic index, e.g., penicillin, whose fluctuations in plasma concentration have little potential adverse consequence, measurement of plasma drug concentrations makes little therapeutic or economic sense. For drugs dependent on the kidney for clearance, the rate of excretion is proportional to the glomerular filtration rate (GFR). Thus, drug dosage must be reduced according to the decrease in that rate [70].

The kidney plays a pivotal role in elimination of pharmacologic agents from the body through direct clearance of unchanged active drug or excretion of metabolites produced by drug biotransformation in other organs. Numerous strategies have been developed in response to the need to modify drug dosages and regimens in patients with renal insufficiency. These methodologies rely on nomograms for the calculation of adjustments in dosage and have provided a rapid and generally accurate approach for the design of

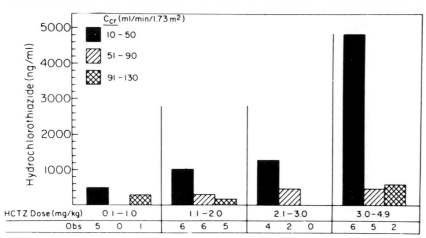

FIG. 42-2. *The effect of glomerular filtration rate on the plasma levels of hydrochlorthiazide in children, as a function of increasing dosage. (From Sinaiko AR, Green TP: Principles of drug therapy in children with ESRD. In Fine RN, Gruskin AB (eds): End Stage Renal Disease in Children. Philadelphia, WB Saunders, 1984, p 403, with permission.)*

therapeutic regimens. The use of nomograms, however, may have serious limitations in children with renal insufficiency: (1) Most do not consider the influence of age on creatinine clearance (C_{Cr}) (e.g., C_{Cr} in a normal full-term infant is only 20% to 35% of that in older children or young adults); (2) the nomogram method assumes that the elimination rate constant (K_{el}) is the only factor that changes as renal function deteriorates; (3) nomograms ignore the fact that pharmacologically active molecules are eliminated from the body through a variety of routes, such as the exocrine glands, the gastrointestinal tract, and the lungs [180]; and (4) other factors affecting drug disposition, including biotransformation pathways, plasma-protein binding, volume of drug distribution, and pharmacological effect can be significantly altered in renal insufficiency [178].

The fact that alternative, nonrenal pathways for drug elimination exist undoubtedly contributes to the observation that dosage modifications for drugs excreted by the kidneys are rarely necessary until GFR is reduced to 50% of normal renal function. Figure 42-1 illustrates a hypothetical curve relating plasma $t\frac{1}{2}$ and renal function for drugs dependent on the kidney for excretion [145]. As shown, progressive decrements in GFR result in a corresponding prolongation of plasma $t\frac{1}{2}$ and an increase in plasma drug concentrations unless dosing regimens are altered accordingly. A specific example of this relationship is depicted in Fig. 42-2. When GFR is greater than 50 ml/min/1.73 m^2, plasma levels of the diuretic hydrochlorothiazide are independent of drug dose over a wide dosage range; however, as glomerular filtration rate falls to less than 50 ml/min/1.73 m^2, hydrochlorothiazide excretion is significantly reduced, and drug accumulation becomes directly correlated with dose [240].

The nomogram in Fig. 42-3 takes into account nonrenal as well as renal clearance in calculating adjustments in drug dosing in patients with renal disease [23]. This is accomplished through incorporation of fractional elimination values (FE), i.e., the fraction of an absorbed dose of a given drug eliminated exclusively by the kidneys. Tables 42-1 and 42-2 contain a representative listing of FE values for a number of anti-infective and cardiovascular drugs and their elimination $t\frac{1}{2}$ in subjects with normal renal function [23]. To use the nomogram in Fig. 42-3, draw a line between the patient's kidney function (horizontal axis) and the appropriate FE for the drug in question. Next draw a horizontal line from the intersection point on the FE line to the dosage adjustment factor (Q) on the right vertical axis. To determine the decrease in maintenance drug dosage, multiply Q × dose. Alternatively, to lengthen the dosing interval, divide the usual interval used in children with normal renal function by Q.

Clearance and Tubular Transport Mechanisms

Renal tubular transport mechanisms, independent from glomerular clearance, also play a major role in drug excretion. Many drugs, especially those that are strong organic acids or bases (i.e., highly ionized at pH 7.4), function as substrates for energy-dependent organic acid and organic base transport systems localized to the proximal renal tubular cells [276]. The secretory capacity of each of these systems can be saturated at high drug concentrations and is competitively inhibited by organic anion and cation antagonists, respectively [274]. The mechanism regulating secretion of the organic anion para-aminohippurate (PAH) has been used as the prototype for renal tubular clearance. PAH secretion requires energy-dependent movement from interstitial fluid into a PAH-rich environment within the tubule intracellular space, a process that is saturable and inhibited by competitive antagonists [106,183]. This trans-

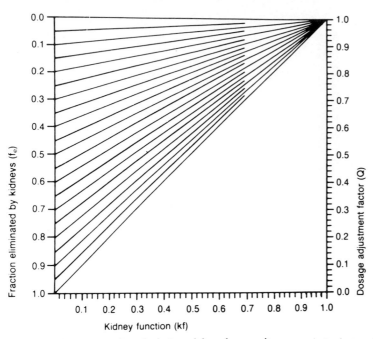

FIG. 42-3. *Nomogram for calculation of drug dosage adjustments in patients with renal disease, dependent on fraction of drug* (f_e) *undergoing renal elimination (see text). (From Bjornsson TD: Nomogram for drug dosage of adjustment in patients with renal failure. Clin Pharmacokinet 11:165, 1986, with permission.)*

port system is highly efficient, and the rate of tubular PAH secretion is dependent only upon the rate at which PAH is delivered to the peritubular membrane, justifying the use of PAH clearance as a measure of renal blood flow (RBF). Once concentrated in the tubular cell, PAH moves down its concentration gradient into the urine.

Agents excreted by the organic acid transport system include salicylate, penicillin, acetazolamide, ethacrynic acid, furosemide, and the glucuronide and sulfate conjugates of metabolized drugs [49]. The concurrent administration of more than one of these acidic drugs leads to competition for excretion at tubular sites. This phenomenon forms the basis for the well-known antagonism of penicillin secretion by the dicarboxylic anion probenecid with subsequent prolongation of the $t\frac{1}{2}$ for penicillin. Agents excreted by the organic base transport system include tolazoline, morphine, and numerous endogenous compounds such as histamine, catecholamines, thiamine, and choline [49].

The decrease in renal tubule-dependent drug clearance in renal disease is directly related to the degree of reduction in RBF. GFR can be used as an indicator of accumulation for drugs cleared through renal tubular secretion, however, because both GFR and RBF usually decrease proportionately with renal mass in severe kidney disease. Other factors may also influence tubular drug clearance in these patients. As azotemia progresses, there is an accumulation of endogenously produced organic acids. These endogenous products compete for clearance at tubular transport sites, thereby inhibiting drug excretion and further increasing plasma drug levels [140]. In contrast to organic acid trans-

port, there is little, if any, competition for organic base tubular transport sites by uremic substances [29].

Maturational Influence on Renal Drug Clearance

Drug excretion by the kidney is dependent on three interrelated factors: (1) glomerular filtration of unbound drug; (2) tubular secretion of drug by active transport mechanisms; and (3) passive reabsorption (nonionic diffusion) of lipid-soluble drugs from the tubular lumen back into the circulation [37]. In contrast to adults and older children, these fundamental processes of drug elimination are poorly developed at birth. Moreover, they have separate rates of maturation during postnatal life [37] with glomerular drug excretion reaching peak capacity prior to that of the tubular excretory mechanism [233]. These maturational changes affect not only drugs eliminated in their active form by the kidney, but also biologically active and inactive metabolites that are dependent upon mature renal excretory mechanisms for their elimination [264].

Glomerular Filtration

A detailed discussion of renal physiologic development can be found in other chapters in this textbook (Chaps. 3 and 4). Suffice it to say here, that the low rate of glomerular filtration during neonatal life dictates that toxic drugs dependent on glomerular filtration for clearance require a

TABLE 42-1. *Average fractional elimination values (FE) for selected anti-infective drugs*

Drug	FE	t½
Acyclovir	0.9	3
Aminoglycosides	>0.95	2
Amoxicillin	0.6	1
Amphotericin B	<0.05	360
Ampicillin	0.9	1.2
Benzylpenicillin	0.85	0.5
Carbenicillin	0.85	1
Cefaclor	0.7	0.8
Cefoperazone	0.2	2
Cefotaxime	0.6	1.2
Cefuroxime	>0.95	1
Cephalexin	0.95	1
Cephalothin	0.65	0.6
Chloramphenicol	0.05	2.5
Clindamycin	0.1	2.5
Cloxacillin	0.75	0.5
Erythromycin	0.15	1.5
Isoniazid	0.2	2
Methicillin	0.85	0.8
Nafcillin	0.3	0.8
Penicillin V	0.5	0.5
Piperacillin	0.7	1
Rifampin	0.2	2.5
Sulfamethoxazole	0.3	10
Ticarcillin	0.9	1.2
Trimethoprim	0.7	10
Vancomycin	>0.95	6

From Bjornsson TD: Nomogram for drug dosage adjustment in patients with renal failure. Clin Pharmacokinet 11:164, 1986, with permission.

TABLE 42-2. *Average fractional elimination values (FE) for selected cardiovascular drugs*

Drug	FE	t½
Acebutolol	0.4	3
Alprenolol	<0.05	3
Atenolol	0.85	6
Captopril	0.4	2
Clonidine	0.6	8
Diazoxide	0.2	20
Digoxin	0.7	40
Hydralazine	0.1	2.5
Labetalol	0.05	4
Methyldopa	0.6	2
Metoprolol	0.1	4
Minoxidil	0.1	4
Nadolol	0.7	16
Nifedipine	<0.05	4
Nitroprusside	<0.01	<0.15
Phenytoin	<0.05	20
Pindolol	0.4	3.5
Prazosin	<0.05	3
Procainamide	0.6	3
Propranolol	<0.05	4
Quinidine	0.2	6
Timolol	0.2	4

From Bjornsson TD: Nomogram for drug dosage adjustment in patients with renal failure. Clin Pharmacokinet 11:164, 1986, with permission.

reduction in drug dosage and/or an increase in drug-dosing intervals when used in this age group.

Tubular Secretion

As discussed earlier, drugs excreted through the tubular organic acid and base transport systems are subjected to active, directed, and energy-dependent processes (see Chap. 4) [37,274]. The age-dependent maturation of these processes is depicted in Fig. 42-4 using PAH [233]. Clearance increases to near-adult values in a near-linear fashion from birth by 14 days of age, followed by a slower rate of increase to normal adult rates by seven to eight weeks of age. Although the maturational sequence of organic base secretion is less well documented, a similar developmental process probably occurs. The pronounced delay in maturation of mechanisms for organic ion secretion in the newborn is poorly understood but has been suggested to be related to diminished tubular length and blood flow or immature transport carrier proteins [37].

Tubular Reabsorption

Drugs may be reabsorbed from the tubular lumen after filtration or active secretion depending on their chemical characteristics. Virtually all organic molecules have a degree of solubility in fat (i.e., they are lipophilic), and are subject to varying degrees of ionization depending upon the pH of the fluid in which they are dissolved. In general, un-ionized drug is substantially more lipophilic than the ionized form, enabling it to diffuse across lipid-rich cellular membranes. Accordingly, filtration or tubular secretion of un-ionized molecules into tubular urine would likely lead to an increase in drug reabsorption and reduce excretion.

In the newborn, two development-dependent processes tend to favor tubular reabsorption of drugs. First, nonrenal biotransformation of active drug molecules to their polar (i.e., ionized) metabolites is slower (see the following section), increasing the amount of lipophilic parent drug delivered to the tubular fluid. Second, the urine pH tends to be lower as a result of the relatively large excretion of organic acids in comparison to the excretion of organic bases [20]. Thus, the effect on organic acids such as sulfisoxazole, which are less ionized in an acid urine, is an increase in the t½, due to enhanced reabsorption from the tubular lumen [142]. Conversely, the urinary excretion rates of organic bases would be expected to be higher in the newborn, due to their predominantly ionized form present in acidic urine [275].

Effect of Renal Disease on Nonrenal Drug Elimination

Considerations regarding the effect of renal disease on drug clearance are usually restricted to the direct impact of the failing kidney on drug excretion. Renal disease adversely effects other organs and systems involved with drug clearance, however. Because the majority of drugs undergo nonrenal metabolic biotransformation and excretion

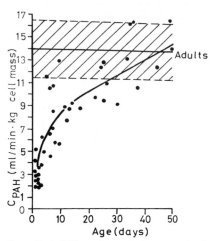

FIG. 42-4. *Effect of postnatal age on the development of tubular secretion of PAH by the kidney. (From Schreiter G: Neuere physiologische und klinische aspekte der nierenfunktion.* Dtsch Ges Wesen *21:433, 1966, with permission.)*

TABLE 42-3. *Drugs subject to extensive (>50%) hepatic first-pass elimination*

Codeine
Coumarin
Dihydroergotamine
5-Fluorouracil
Hydralazine
Imipramine
Labetalol
Lidocaine
Mercaptopurine
Metoprolol
Morphine
Naloxone
Nifedipine
Nortriptyline
Pentazocine
Propranolol
Quinidine
Ranitidine
Verapamil

through other pathways, in addition to renal pathways, these effects can profoundly influence drug therapy in patients with reduced renal function.

Effects on Drug Metabolism Pathways

Biotransformation of drugs by the liver follows four primary metabolic pathways: (1) oxidation (hydroxylation, demethylation); (2) reduction; (3) synthesis (glucuronidation, sulfation acetylation, glycine conjugation); and (4) hydrolysis (proteolysis, de-esterification). The effect of uremia on these pathways may be either enhanced or decreased. In many circumstances, however, it is variable, and few clinically apparent effects on any one specific metabolic pathway have been demonstrated [216].

Effects of renal disease on metabolic pathways for specific drugs cleared by the liver are difficult to predict. The actions of potential enzyme inducers, activators, and inhibitors may be compromised by availability of cofactors, which is dependent upon the nutritional status of uremic children.

Effects on Hepatic "First-pass" Metabolism

Certain drugs administered orally undergo substantial clearance by hepatic metabolizing systems after absorption from the gut and prior to reaching the systemic circulation. This phenomenon, known as *first-pass elimination*, has been reported to be decreased in patients with renal disease [162]. Using propranolol as the prototype for hepatic first-pass elimination, it was shown that plasma drug concentrations were increased threefold in patients with renal failure when compared to normal subjects.

If the fraction of drug usually cleared by the liver during the first pass is large, a reduction in first-pass elimination would likely have a significant clinical effect by increasing drug concentrations and potentiating the therapeutic response. More recent data suggest that the inhibition of first-pass elimination does not have a significant impact on patient care over the long term [283]. When propranolol plasma concentrations were measured in patients with renal failure under steady-state conditions, drug disposition was not found to differ in comparison to subjects with normal renal function. It is likely that this will also be true for other drugs subject to extensive (>50%) hepatic first-pass elimination [209] (Table 42-3). Nevertheless, until this issue is resolved, it is suggested that these drugs be closely monitored, particularly agents with a narrow therapeutic index.

Metabolite Excretion in Renal Disease

Renal disease may alter the disposition and clinical effects of a drug, even if that drug is extensively eliminated by nonrenal mechanisms [264]. There are three predominant consequences of altered metabolite excretion in renal disease: (1) accumulation of pharmacologically and/or toxicologically active metabolites; (2) regeneration of parent drug by metabolic transformation of the metabolite; and (3) a potential direct interaction between the metabolite and the parent drug.

Pharmacologically Active Metabolites in Renal Disease

Metabolic biotransformation of most drugs results in the enzymatic conversion of lipophilic, biologically active parent compounds into hydrophilic, inactive metabolites that are excreted in the urine. In some cases, however, the metabolites retain an equivalent or even enhanced pharmacologic activity [74,264] (Table 42-4) that becomes exaggerated during accumulation in renal failure.

TABLE 42-4. *Drug metabolites that accumulate in renal failure*

Parent drug	Metabolite
Allopurinol	Oxipurinol
Clofibrate	Clofibric acid
Digoxin	Digoxigenin-mono-digitoxoside
Meperidine	Normeperidine
Methyldopa	Methyldopa-O-sulfate
	α-Methyldopamine
Metoprolol	α-Hydroxymetoprolol
Procainamide	N-Acetylprocainamide
Propranolol	4-Hydroxypropranolol
Sodium nitroprusside	Thiocyanate
Sulfonamides	Acetylated metabolites

From Verbeeck RK, Branch RA, Wilkinson GR: Drug metabolites in renal failure: Pharmacokinetic and clinical implications. *Clin Pharmacokinet* 6:329, 1981, with permission.

Classic examples of metabolite toxicity have occurred during the use of α-methyldopa and sodium nitroprusside in children with renal disease and hypertension. Patients with renal failure are particularly sensitive to the hypotensive and adverse effects of α-methyldopa, despite serum concentrations of the unmetabolized α-methyldopa parent drug of as low as 25% of that found in hypertensive patients with normal renal function [52]. It has been shown that children with renal failure have significant elevations in serum concentrations of the 3-0-sulfate conjugate of α-methyldopa and the free and sulfated forms of α-methyldopamine [196]. The latter compound accumulates in rat brain after α-methyldopa treatment and may undergo further conversion to the centrally active α-methylnorepinephrine.

The primary metabolite of sodium nitroprusside is thiocyanate. Unlike the parent compound, this metabolite is eliminated very slowly in patients with renal failure [201]. Although the biologic effects of the thiocyanate ion are different from the parent compound, symptoms of nausea, muscle weakness, anoxia, and disorientation can occur during thiocyanate accumulation.

Regeneration of Parent Drug in Renal Disease

A prominent pathway for metabolism of many endogenous compounds and drugs is hepatic glucuronidation to form polar (i.e., ionized) conjugates that are pharmacologically inactive and excreted in the urine. These conjugated metabolites can also be secreted into bile, a process similar to the excretion of conjugated bilirubin. Although pharmacologically deactivated, the glucuronide conjugates are not chemically inert and can be hydrolytically converted by enteric flora to the lipophilic parent drug, which is then reabsorbed into the circulation. In patients with renal failure, biliary excretion increases, with a potential for accumulation of glucuronide metabolites [253]. As is the case with hepatic first-pass elimination, the clinical significance of this phenomenon has not been resolved [283]. Nevertheless, drug regeneration after systemic or gastrointestinal deglucuronidation has been reported after treatment with

the benzodiazepine anxiolytics oxazepam and lorazepam, the salicylate analgesic diflunisal, the cholesterol-lowering agent clofibrate, and the anti-inflammatory agent acetaminophen [264].

Parent Drug-Metabolite Interactions in Renal Disease

The accumulation of hydroxylated metabolites and glucuronide conjugates of commonly used drugs such as phenytoin and propranolol in patients with renal failure has led to the suggestion that these metabolites could alter the disposition or pharmacodynamics of their parent drugs or other therapeutic agents. The p-hydroxylated metabolite of phenytoin has been reported to displace native phenytoin from its binding sites on plasma proteins [26,152], although the presence of endogenous binding inhibitors in renal failure may complicate this apparent interaction [61]. At the present time there is little additional substantive data to directly implicate metabolites as initiators of drug interactions in man, either as competitors of plasma protein binding or as feedback inhibitors of hepatic enzyme systems [264].

Renal Disease and Drug-Protein Interactions

The magnitude of biologic response to a drug is directly proportional to the concentration of unbound (i.e., nonprotein bound) drug at its receptor site, and this active fraction is in direct equilibrium with the unbound drug in the vascular space. Conversely, drug bound to nonspecific tissue sites or plasma proteins is pharmacologically inactive. Almost all drug assay laboratories measure only the total concentration of drug in serum or plasma and do not distinguish between the unbound and bound fractions. Whereas this methodology is accurate enough to satisfy most clinical situations, alterations in drug-protein binding can affect total drug concentration in renal disease [217,227], and this effect will vary depending on a variety of factors, including the drug in question. Failure to recognize these changes will lead to excessive drug administration and consequent toxicity.

Organic acids in plasma are bound primarily to the albumin molecule at a site also responsible for the binding and transport of bilirubin [243]. The albumin molecule also contains accessory binding sites for basic drugs such as benzodiazepines and neutral agents such as digitoxin. The majority of these basic molecules bind to other serum macromolecules, however, including α_1-acid glycoprotein (orosomucoid), IgG, and various lipoproteins [208].

Age-Related Alterations in Drug-Protein Binding

Several drugs have been shown to have diminished protein binding in fetal and infant plasma [214] (Table 42-5). Various etiologies have been proposed to explain these differences, including the presence of competing endoge-

Table 42-5. *Drugs with decreased protein binding in newborn or infant serum*

Ampicillin
Desmethylimipramine
Diazepam
Digoxin
Lidocaine
Nafcillin
Phenobarbital
Phenytoin
Salicylates

From Rane A: Basic principles of drug disposition and action in infants and children. In Yaffe SJ (ed): Pediatric Pharmacology. New York, Grune & Stratton, 1980, p 7, with permission.

Table 42-6. *Drugs with decreased protein binding in patients with renal failure*

Cephalosporins
Diazoxide
Furosemide
Penicillins
Phenobarbital
Phenytoin
Salicylates
Sulfonamides
Theophylline
Valproic Acid
Warfarin

nous molecules (e.g., bilirubin and free fatty acids) and an altered configuration of the albumin-binding site in the newborn.

The Influence of Uremia on Drug-Protein Binding

Uremia adversely affects drug-protein binding between acidic drug molecules and albumin, with a wide spectrum of acidic drugs affected (Table 42-6). It is most likely that displacement of drug from protein-binding sites results from competition among drug and endogenous organic acids, fatty acids, or peptides [135,140,215] that are retained in high concentration in patients with renal failure. This hypothesis is supported by observations that drug-protein binding in patients with acute renal failure is improved after hemodialysis, that a dialyzable component in uremic plasma inhibits the binding of acidic drug to normal plasma proteins, and that nonspecific adsorption of uremic plasma onto activated charcoal can partially reverse the decreased binding of some acidic drugs [3,172,244].

It is also possible that the reduction in drug-protein binding in uremic patients is the result of alterations in the tertiary structure of albumin that affects the association constant between drug and binding site. The isoelectric point of albumin in uremic plasma differs significantly from that of normal plasma [238]. Moreover, chemical carbamylation of serum proteins, a process that may occur in the presence of high levels of urea, significantly diminishes the binding of acidic drugs to albumin [50,78]. Although the binding of acidic drugs to albumin is altered in renal failure, effects of uremia on the binding of basic and neutral drugs remains unchanged [197,217].

The anticonvulsant phenytoin represents a classic example of the adverse effect of renal failure on drug-protein binding. As the bound fraction of drug decreases from approximately 95% to 90% in renal failure, the total plasma drug concentration falls from 10 to 20 μg/ml to 5 to 10 μg/ml, while the unbound fraction remains unchanged at approximately 2 μg/ml [218]. Thus, attempts to maintain total drug at its usual plasma concentration in the face of reduced drug-protein binding would force the concentration of unbound drug to toxic levels.

As a result of alterations in drug-protein binding in renal failure, the plasma fraction of bound drug decreases and unbound drug increases. Under usual circumstances, this would potentiate the expected pharmacologic response associated with an increase in the unbound (or active) drug fraction; however, this is often not the case. In response to higher concentrations of unbound drug, there is a concomitant increase in hepatic metabolism, thereby restoring the unbound fraction to its normal level. The final outcome, as previously noted, is lower total plasma drug concentrations, unchanged concentrations of unbound drug, and an increased percentage of unbound drug:

$$\frac{\text{unbound drug}}{\text{total drug}} \times 100$$

Drug Clearance During Dialysis

Hemodialysis and peritoneal dialysis have added yet another dimension to the use of pharmacologic agents in children with renal failure. In Table 42-7, the primary route of drug clearance, the need for dosing adjustments in renal failure, and the expected clearance during dialysis are listed for a number of drugs. For specific details about dosing changes, the reader is referred to recent extensive reviews [17,150,166,203,262], with the caveat that very few studies have been performed specifically in children. The following discussion focuses on principles that can be expected to govern the use of drugs in dialysis patients.

Hemodialysis

The most critical variable in predicting drug dialyzability is volume of distribution (V_d). This parameter describes the extent to which a drug is distributed throughout the body and secondarily predicts the percentage of drug that is available within the plasma volume for dialysis. For example, lipophilic drugs with high capacity for transport across tissue membranes would be likely to have a larger V_d than hydrophilic agents that are confined to the extracellular fluid space and have a larger percentage of drug accessible to the dialyzer.

The pharmacokinetic parameter that is used to compare the dialyzability of drugs is referred to as the dialysis rate

Table 42-7. *Drug use in renal failure*

Drug	Primary drug clearance*	Dosing adjustment in renal failure	Significant clearance during dialysis‡
Antimicrobials			
Aminoglycosides [204]			
Amikacin			
Gentamicin [246]			
Kanamycin	R	Yes	He, P
Netilmicin			
Streptomycin			
Tobramycin [45]			
Cephalosporins [109,182,194]			
Cefaclor	R	Yes	He
Cefadroxil	R	Yes	He
Cefamandole [64]	R	Yes	He
Cefazolin [44,116]	R	Yes	He
Cefonicid [25]	R	Yes	
Cefoperazone [104]	B	No	
Ceforanide	R	Yes	He
Cefotaxime	R,H	Severe†	He
Cefoxitin	R	Yes	He
Ceftazidime	R	Yes	He
Ceftizoxime	R	Yes	He
Ceftriaxone	R,H	No	
Cefuroxime [266]	R	Yes	He
Cephalexin [44]	R	Yes	He
Cephalothin [224]	R,H	No	He
Cephapirin	R,H	No	He
Cephradine [245]	R	Yes	He
Moxalactam [132]	R	Yes	He
Cefpiramide	B	No	
Cefotetan	R	Yes	He
Cefmenoxime	R	Yes	He
Cefsulodin	R	Yes	He
Penicillins [12,281,284]			
Amoxicillin	R	Yes	He
Ampicillin [128]	R	Yes	He
Azlocillin	R,NR	Yes	He
Carbenicillin [147]	R	Yes	He
Cloxacillin	R,H	Severe	
Dicloxacillin	R,H	Severe	
Methicillin	R,H	Severe	
Mezlocillin [9]	NR	Yes	He
Nafcillin [71]	H	No	
Oxacillin	H,R	No	
Penicillin G	R,H	Severe	
Piperacillin [8]	R	Yes	
Ticarcillin [202]	R	Yes	He
Monobactam			
Aztreonam [256]	R	Yes	He,P
Carbapenem			
Imipenem [95]	R	Yes	He
Antifungal			
Amphotericin B [185]	H (?)	No	
Flucytosine	R	Yes	He,P

(continued)

TABLE 42-7. (continued)

Drug	Primary drug clearance*	Dosing adjustment in renal failure	Significant clearance during dialysis[‡]
Antimicrobials (continued)			
Antituberculous [81]			
Ethambutol	R	Yes	He,P
Isoniazid	H	Severe	He,P
Rifampin	H	No	
Antiviral			
Acyclovir [141,146]	R	Yes	He
Others			
Chloramphenicol	H	No	He
Clindamycin	H	No	
Erythromycin	H	No	
Nitrofurantoin	R,H	Yes	He
Sulfisoxazole	R,H	Severe	He
Sulfamethoxazole	R,H	Severe	He
Trimethoprim [119]	R,H	Yes	He
Vancomycin [46]	R	Yes	
Drugs Affecting Cardiovascular System			
Antihypertensives			
Beta Blockers			
Atenolol	R	Yes	He
Metoprolol	H	No	
Nadolol	R	Yes	He
Pindolol	H	No	
Propranolol [283]	H	No	
Timolol	H	No	
Acebutolol	H	Severe	He
Adrenergic Agents			
Clonidine	R,H		
Methyldopa [196]	R,H	Yes	He
Prazosin	H	No	
Guanabenz	NR	?	
Vasodilators			
Hydralazine	H	Severe	
Minoxidil	H	No	
Nitroprusside	NR	No	He
Calcium Channel Blockers			
Nifedipine [168]	H	No	
Diltiazem	H	No	
Verapamil	H	No	
Nitrendipine [7]	H	No	
Angiotensin Converting Enzyme Inhibitors			
Captopril [198,242]	R,H	Severe	He
Enalapril [164]	R,H	Yes	He
Other Cardiac Drugs			
Disopyramide [48]	H,R	Yes	He
Digoxin	R	Yes	He
Procainamide	H,R	Yes	He
Quinidine	H	No	He
Theophyilline	H	No	He

(continued)

TABLE 42-7. *(continued)*

Drug	Primary drug clearance*	Dosing adjustment in renal failure	Significant clearance during dialysis[‡]
Drugs Affecting Cardiovascular System (continued)			
Analgesics and Anti-inflammatory Drugs [93]			
Acetaminophen	H,	No	
Aspirin [154,163]	H,R	Yes	He
Indomethacin	H	No	
Sulindac	H	No	
Diflunisal	H,R	Severe	
Ibuprofen	H	No	
Fenoprofen	H	No	
Naproxen	H	No	
Tolmetin	H,R	No	
Piroxicam	H	No	
Other Drugs			
Benzodiazepines	H	No	
Chloral Hydrate	H		
Phenothiazines	H	No	
Tricyclic antidepressants			
Heparin [79]	H	No	
Warfarin [118]	R,H	Yes	
	H	No	
Anticonvulsants			
Phenobarbital	H,R	No	He
Carbamazepine	H	No	
Ethosuximide	H		He
Phenytoin	H	No	
Primidone	H		He
Valproic Acid	H	No	
Immunosuppresives			
Azathioprine	H	No	He
Cyclophosphamide [189]	H	Severe	He
Adriamycin	H	No	
Methotrexate [12]	R	Yes	
Vincristine	H	No	
Cyclosporin	H	No	
Glucocorticoids	H	No	
Cimetidine [232]	R,H	No	
Allopurinol [108]	R	Yes	He

* R, renal; H, hepatic; NR, non-renal
[†] Dosing adjustment only in severe renal failure
[‡] He, hemodialysis; P, peritoneal dialysis

constant (K_d), defined as the dialysis clearance rate (CL_{pl}) divided by the volume of distribution:

$$K_d = Cl_{pl}/V_d \text{ (6)} \qquad (6)$$

This equation provides a reasonable quantitation of the percentage of total body drug removed by the dialyzer over a fixed period of time. Its applicability is illustrated by comparing two drugs with different volumes of distribution but relatively similar dialysis clearance rates. Using readily accessible published data [150], the hemodialysis clearances of digoxin and gentamicin are compared in a 20-kg child. Digoxin has a V_d of 6.5 L/kg and a dialysis clearance rate of 10 ml/min, whereas gentamicin has a V_d of 0.25 L/kg and a dialysis clearance rate of 28 ml/min. Using equation 6, the calculated dialysis rate constants for digoxin and gentamicin are markedly different, 0.46%/hr and 35%/hr, respectively. The removal of digoxin by hemodialysis is negligible, whereas nearly one third of the total body load of gentamicin may be removed by the dialyzer each hour. In general, an agent with a V_d greater than 2 L/kg is poorly dialyzable, whereas an agent with a V_d less than 1 L/kg is likely to be cleared by hemodialysis [150].

In contrast to the V_d, the influence of other pharmacokinetic parameters on drug removal by hemodialysis are not as predictable. Drugs dependent on renal clearance for their primary route of elimination usually have high dialysis clearance rates. Drugs with a long $t\frac{1}{2}$ are not effectively dialyzed because of the relationship between $t\frac{1}{2}$ and V_d (see equation 4) and the fact that duration of dialysis is negligible in comparison to the $t\frac{1}{2}$ [18].

Hemodialysis does not effectively remove drugs that undergo high rates of endogenous clearance by organs other than the kidney. Tricyclic antidepressants are metabolized by the liver at endogenous clearance rates greater than 200 ml/min [21]. Because hemodialysis clearance rates for drugs seldom exceed 100 ml/min under the best of circumstances [150], the use of hemodialysis for the removal of tricyclic antidepressants following accidental overdose would not be expected to add greatly to the natural rate of clearance.

It is usually desirable to replace drugs removed during dialysis in order to maintain therapeutic plasma drug concentrations. The amount of drug removed by the dialyzer can be approximated:

$$D_{rep} = V_d (C_{pre} - C_{post}) \qquad (7)$$

where D_{rep} equals the replacement drug dose, C_{pre} equals the plasma drug concentration just prior to dialysis, and C_{post} equals the plasma drug concentration immediately after dialysis.

Drug clearance during hemodialysis can also be estimated by measuring drug concentrations during dialysis and applying these data to the individual flow characteristics of the dialyzer:

$$Cl_{HD} = Q\frac{A - V}{A} \qquad (8)$$

where Q is the dialyzer blood flow, A is the drug concentration in blood entering the dialyzer, and V is the drug concentration in blood leaving the dialyzer. It should be acknowledged that this equation presumes that drug does not accumulate.

Peritoneal Dialysis

Drug clearance is generally less efficient during peritoneal dialysis than during hemodialysis.

Unlike hemodialysis systems where clearance efficiencies are dependent on physical characteristics of the artificial membrane, geometry of the membrane supports, and blood flow, effective peritoneal clearance depends on the viability and surface area of tissue membranes. These membranes are regulated by endogenous factors working to maintain vascular and organ integrity, thus tending to limit clearance. Only a small percentage (less than 0.2%) of the peritoneal membrane contains physical "pores" that permit bulk transfer of solutes [42,177,195]. It is likely that small

molecules gaining access to the peritoneal cavity also traverse capillary endothelial cells as contents of membrane vesicles [42]. These factors limit the efficiency of peritoneal dialysis, even in those circumstances where the molecules are freely diffusible. For example, peritoneal clearances of urea and creatinine rarely exceed 30 to 40 ml/min, despite a rich blood flow through the splanchnic vasculature [260].

The pharmacokinetic system in peritoneal dialysis is best described by a two-compartment model, composed of the body and the volume of the peritoneal fluid exchanged during dialysis. In this system, drugs are capable of diffusing from one compartment to the other in a bidirectional manner, with the rate of diffusion determined by three variables: (1) the degree of protein binding in the plasma, (2) the volume of drug distribution in the body, and (3) the extent to which the drug is normally excreted by the kidney. The contributions of all three determine the net peritoneal clearance (Cl_{PD}):

$$Cl_{PD} = \frac{C_d \times V_{pf}}{C_p \times t} \qquad (9)$$

where C_d is the concentration of drug present in the dialysis fluid removed, V_{pf} is the volume of dialysis fluid removed, C_p is the plasma concentration of drug at the midpoint of the dialysis, and t is the duration of dialysis. Once the Cl_{PD} is determined, the peritoneal clearance rate constant (K_{PD}) can be calculated using the same equation employed for the hemodialysis rate constant:

$$K_{PD} = \frac{Cl_{PD}}{V_d} \qquad (10)$$

K_{PD} will then provide a quantitative estimate of that fraction (percentage) of drug eliminated by peritoneal dialysis from the body during a fixed period of time. In practical terms, it allows the pediatrician to establish a reasonable maintenance dosage regimen for a child on peritoneal dialysis. The Cl_{PD} and K_{PD} for numerous drugs used in uremic children have been published [203].

Drugs eliminated by peritoneal dialysis are usually those that are predominantly excreted by the kidneys, less bound to plasma proteins, and distributed within a relatively small body volume.

Glucocorticoids

Glucocorticoid therapy was introduced into the clinical practice of medicine in 1949 with the use of cortisone and ACTH to successfully treat patients with disabling rheumatoid arthritis [114]. During subsequent years, extensive medical experience with a variety of glucocorticoid drugs has defined the broad range of effects associated with this class of pharmacologic agents and refined the art of glucocorticoid therapy for inflammatory and other diseases in adults and children. Nevertheless, the basic mechanisms controlling the therapeutic effectiveness and many of the adverse consequences of glucocorticoids continue to be inadequately understood.

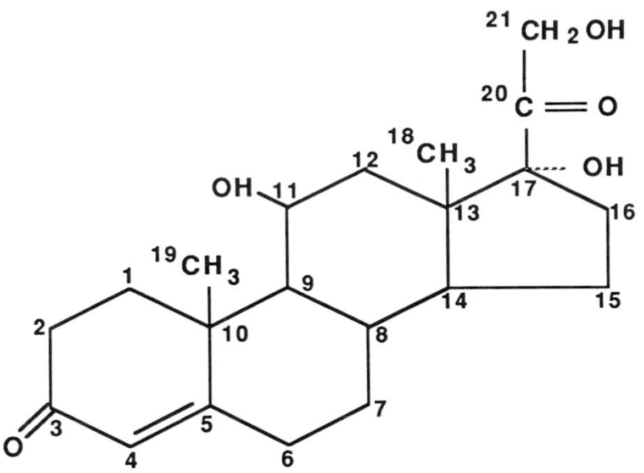

FIG. 42-5. *Molecular structure of hydrocortisone (cortisol) as an example of the basic glucocorticoid nucleus.*

Cortisol (also known as hydrocortisone) (Fig. 42-5), the naturally occurring glucocorticoid produced by the adrenal cortex, constitutes 90% of the daily adrenocortical steroid output [126]. Because little steroid is stored in the adrenal, production is virtually synonymous with secretion, and in humans this is equivalent to approximately 6 to 16 $mg/m^2/$ 24 hr (mean 12.1 ± 2.9) [134]. Glucocorticoids are synthesized from cholesterol and contain specific structural characteristics that are required for metabolic activity [210]. These include a double bond (Δ) between C4–5, a ketone at C3, and the presence of an oxygen, as either a ketone or hydroxyl group, at C11.

The metabolic consequences (gluconeogenesis, protein catabolism, reduced DNA synthesis, glycogenolysis, and lipolysis) and the sodium-retaining properties of the glucocorticoids result in a number of adverse effects that are familiar to all who use these drugs with any frequency. These adverse effects are inseparable from the anti-inflammatory and immunosuppressive activities that constitute the primary indications for glucocorticoid therapy. In an attempt to improve effectiveness while minimizing side effects, structural modifications have been introduced at specific loci in the steroid nucleus to exploit known structure-action relationships that influence glucocorticoid activity [210]. The addition of a double bond at C1–2 selectively increases glucocorticoid metabolic effects without increasing sodium retention; addition of a fluoride at the C9 position enhances all biologic activities; methylation at the C6 position alters activity but has an unpredictable outcome; and methylation or hydroxylation at the C16 position substantially reduces sodium retention while only slightly increasing metabolic and anti-inflammatory effects. These molecular modifications have been used to develop a variety of glucocorticoid analogues possessing varying degrees of anti-inflammatory, immunosuppressive, and sodium-retaining potency and duration of action (Table 42-8) [174,261].

Despite the availability of newer and more potent glu-cocorticoid drugs, prednisone continues to be used almost exclusively when glucocorticoid therapy is indicated for the specific diseases described in this textbook of pediatric nephrology. Although newer glucocorticoids have an enhanced metabolic effect and a lesser degree of sodium retention, other characteristics, such as their extended biologic half-life and duration of action, have greatly complicated the design of therapeutic regimens, particularly the use of alternate-day therapy. Thus, while prednisone does not provide any major advantages with regard to either therapeutic effectiveness or frequency of adverse effects, its intermediate potency and half-life, extensive clinical experience, and availability of accurate pharmacokinetic data in children [91,99] offer greater predictability for dosing, clinical response, and appearance of side effects in this age group.

After cortisol is released from the adrenal cortex, it circulates in the serum bound to a α_1-glycoprotein, corticosteroid-binding globulin. Other glucocorticoids bind to this protein in varying degrees [226], but the binding of prednisolone, the metabolically active form of prednisone, approximates that of cortisol [54]. At low serum concentrations, prednisolone is greater than 90% bound. At higher concentrations, however, such as those likely to be found in patients receiving prednisone for kidney-related diseases, the capacity for binding to corticosteroid-binding globulin is exceeded, and prednisolone circulates bound to albumin, which has a lower affinity but a high capacity for the drug [156].

The tissue effects of the glucocorticoids are initiated in sensitive cells by passage of the unbound fraction of circulating drug across the cell membrane and binding of the drug to specific intracytoplasmic protein receptors [15]. This glucocorticoid-receptor complex then penetrates the cell nucleus where it influences specific RNA in such a way as to alter coding for enzymes or other proteins that are responsible for the ultimate metabolic response. As might be expected because of the diverse biochemical and physiologic effects of the glucocorticoids, receptors have been identified in most tissues, including brain, heart, intestine, liver, kidney, lung, muscle, and lymphoid [15].

The metabolism of glucocorticoids occurs primarily in the liver, although some metabolism may also take place in other tissues [206]. Therefore, these drugs can be administered to patients with renal disease without dosage modification in cases of reduced renal function.

Alterations in glucocorticoid metabolism can be observed in patients treated concurrently with drugs that influence hepatic microsomal enzyme activity, and these may substantially affect therapeutic outcome. In adults, anticonvulsant drugs, which are known inducers of this enzyme system, have been reported to increase the metabolic clearance rate of prednisolone by 77%, while reducing its $t\frac{1}{2}$ by 45% [205], and to cause a deterioration in the clinical status of asthmatic patients previously controlled under steady-state conditions of prednisone dosing [40]. Similar effects have been observed in children treated with phenobarbital, phenytoin, or carbamazepine [12a]. The adverse impact of anticonvulsant therapy on renal allograft survival has also been documented in two separate pediatric

TABLE 42-8. *Biologic and pharmacologic properties of glucocorticoids using cortisol as the reference steroid*

Glucocorticoid	Equivalent dose (mg)	t½ (min)	Biologic half-life (hr)	Anti-inflammatory potency	Sodium-retaining potency
Cortisol (Hydrocortisone)	20	90	8–12	1	1
Cortisone (11-deoxycortisol)	25	90	8–12	0.8	0.8
Prednisolone (Δ1-cortisol)	5	200	12–36	4	0.8
Prednisone (Δ1-cortisone)	5	?*	12–36	4	0.8
6α-Methylprednisolone	4	200	12–36	5	0.5
Triamcinolone (9-fluoro-16-hydroxyprednisolone)	4	200	12–36	4	0
Dexamethasone (9-fluoro-16-methylprednisolone)	0.75	300	36–54	25	0
Betamethasone (9-fluoro-16-methylprednisolone)	0.75	300	36–54	25	0

* Rapidly metabolized to prednisolone

transplant programs [170,268]. Although this does not seem to be a universal finding among transplant centers, it has been recommended that transplant patients requiring anticonvulsant therapy be treated with drugs other than dilantin and phenobarbital [6].

An opposite effect on hepatic glucocorticoid metabolism, i.e., inhibition of enzyme activity and prolongation of t½, has not, as yet, been reported. The H-2 receptor inhibitor cimetidine, however, is known to interact with hepatic cytochrome P-450 and reduce the hepatic metabolic clearance of a number of drugs [236]. When this drug is used in conjunction with glucocorticoid therapy, patients should be carefully monitored for the early appearance of glucocorticoid toxicity.

An important potential modifier of glucocorticoid pharmacologic activity that may increase the risk of drug-related adverse reactions in patients with renal disease is hypoproteinemia. Because the glucocorticoid dose in most treatment regimens will result in serum concentrations that exceed the binding capacity of corticosteroid binding protein, serum glucocorticoid-protein binding becomes dependent on the serum concentration of albumin [226]. Theoretically, in hypoalbuminemic states, lower serum protein levels should result in a higher concentration of free (i.e., unbound) drug with greater pharmacologic activity and incidence of side effects. In fact, this relationship has been confirmed by the Boston Collaborative Drug Surveillance Program, in which the incidence of side effects in adults receiving prednisone was directly correlated with mean daily drug dose and inversely correlated with serum albumin concentration [226]. These findings were not confirmed when data from nephrotic children were evaluated, however. When prednisolone pharmacokinetics in the active phase of disease were compared with those in the remission phase [15], it was found that the reduction of prednisolone binding to albumin was modified by an upward accommodation of hepatic metabolism and clearance in response to the higher levels of free drug, and free drug prednisolone concentration was restored to usual therapeutic steady-state levels. Thus, the adverse effects of steroid therapy cannot be attributed solely to reduced glucocorticoid binding in children with nephrotic syndrome, and usual therapeutic regimens can be used regardless of degree of hypoalbuminemia and proteinuria.

Anti-inflammatory and Immunosuppressive Effects

Glucocorticoid therapy is used in clinical nephrology because of its anti-inflammatory and immunosuppressive properties. Although each of these effects has undergone extensive evaluation in animals and man, the mechanisms regulating this glucocorticoid action still have not been precisely established. Nevertheless, experimental studies have provided data supporting the conclusion that certain etiologic relationships play an active role in the glucocorticoid therapeutic response.

The glucocorticoid anti-inflammatory effect is multifaceted. It has been known for some time that glucocorticoids inhibit both chemotaxis and release of lysosomal enzymes from phagocytic cells [28]. More recently, it has been shown that a more direct effect on inflammation is mediated through inhibition of the prostaglandin (PG) pathway [121,267].

PGs are actively involved in the inflammatory response [143]. The PG biosynthetic pathway (Fig. 42-6) is initiated by the release of arachidonic acid from cellular phospholipid stores, directly through the activation of phospholipase A and indirectly through a diacylglyceride pathway activated by phospholipase C [220]. Arachidonic acid is then enzymatically converted through a cyclo-oxygenase pathway to a variety of PGs and thromboxane or through a lipoxygenase pathway to leukotrienes. The glucocorticoids have been shown to decrease phospholipase A activity by induction of a phospholipase A inhibitory protein [24,117]. Thus, unlike the nonsteroidal anti-inflammatory drugs that reduce PG production by inhibiting cyclo-oxygenase activity, glucocorticoids act at an earlier metabolic step to prevent arachidonic acid release and formation of both PGs and leukotrienes. This may have an additional impact on the inflammatory reaction, since leukotrienes also modulate inflammation through their role as chemotactic agents [143].

Glucocorticoids affect each of the human leukocyte populations, including neutrophils, lymphocytes, monocytes, and eosinophils [62]. The effect on circulating cells may be immediate in some cases or occur over a period of weeks. It is observed in patients receiving high-dose or low-dose therapy [239].

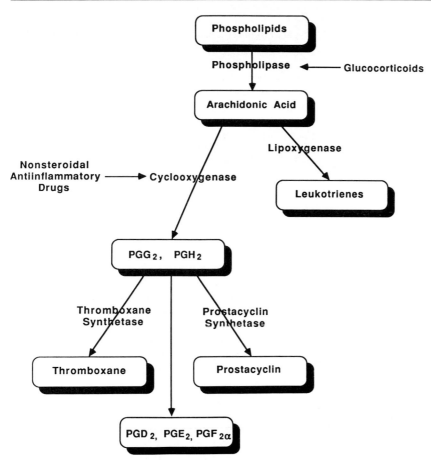

Fig. 42-6. *Prostaglandin biosynthetic pathway. Glucocorticoids have been shown to inhibit release of arachidonic acid from phospholipid stores through inhibition of phospholipase A.*

The blood neutrophil count increases within hours after the administration of glucocorticoid [235] as a result of recruitment of cells from the bone marrow [22,65], but these cells are retained within the vascular compartment [66]. Thus, despite normal neutrophil functional capacity [96], the increased total circulating cell count is misleading as an indicator of the degree of integrity of the patient's usual mechanism of defense [66].

In contrast to neutrophils, the number of circulating lymphocytes is decreased after glucocorticoid administration as a result of sequestration within the bone marrow [80]. Both B-cells and T-cells are decreased, although the effect on T-cells is significantly greater and accounts for most of the fall in the absolute lymphocyte count [107,286]. Whether there is a selective effect on specific T-lymphocyte populations is not clear. Earlier studies using the rosette technique demonstrated a decrease in the percentage and number of T-helper cells compared to T-suppressor cells [112]. More recently, however, in studies in which T-cell subtype was categorized with monoclonal antibody, the percentages of neither T4 nor T8 subtypes were altered in blood obtained from patients treated five hours previously with oral prednisone [235].

T-cell functional response to glucocorticoids has been reviewed and includes the well-recognized inhibition of mitogen and other stimulus-induced proliferation [62]. In particular, it appears that this inhibitory effect is dose-dependent [271] and varies according to the glucocorticoid administered [81].

Glucocorticoids cause a significant reduction in circulating monocytes, but this effect is transient and does not appear to last more than 12 to 24 hours, despite continued drug administration [223]. Monocyte chemotaxis is suppressed when cells from normal untreated subjects are incubated in vitro with prednisolone [222,258]; however, monocytes isolated from subjects receiving chronic steroid therapy do not demonstrate any inhibition of chemotactic activity, even after a period of in vitro steroid incubation [258]. In contrast, functional impairment (i.e., bactericidal and fungicidal activity) persists for up to 48 hours after glucocorticoid therapy has been discontinued [223].

Adverse Effects

The adverse effects of glucocorticoid therapy listed in Table 42-9 are well known to all who use these agents on a regular basis. They can occur with low dose [174] as well

TABLE 42-9. *Adverse effects of glucocorticoid therapy*

Cushingoid features
Hypertension
Peptic ulcers [56,175,250]
Growth retardation
Myopathy
Osteoporosis
Avascular necrosis [68,83]
Pancreatitis [221]
Infection
Cataracts [136]
Pseudotumor cerebri
Psychiatric disorders
Diabetes [167]
Secondary amenorrhea
Hypothalamic-pituitary-adrenal suppression

as high dose daily treatment and with topical [113], inhaled [118a,265,285], or systemic administration.

Systemic hypertension commonly occurs during chronic glucocorticoid therapy but rarely appears until after two or three weeks of drug treatment. It is highly variable in its severity. Occasionally, aggressive antihypertensive management is required.

The mechanisms underlying glucocorticoid-induced hypertension are not known. Studies in patients with Cushing's syndrome have shown that hypertension occurs in the absence of any laboratory evidence of mineralocorticoid excess [139]. Administration of glucocorticoids with little or no mineralocorticoid effect does not decrease urinary sodium excretion, increase body weight, or change plasma volume or hematocrit [277], and diuretics with specific antimineralocorticoid effects have not been particularly useful in treating glucocorticoid hypertension. It has been suggested that an increase in renin-angiotensin system activity may be related etiologically to the onset of hypertension, based on evidence that plasma renin substrate becomes elevated after the administration of glucocorticoid and in patients with Cushing's syndrome [139]. Therefore, patients with glucocorticoid hypertension may respond to antihypertensive therapy with angiotensin converting enzyme inhibitors. Animal studies have suggested a role for the adrenergic nervous system as well, however [137].

The association between glucocorticoid therapy and the development of peptic ulcers has been subjected to careful review during the past decade [56,175,250]. Although a small but finite increased incidence of peptic ulcer disease has been reported, routine antiulcer therapy is not used in conjunction with glucocorticoid administration in adults, and comparable data are not available for children. Antiulcer therapy has not been a routine component of glucocorticoid treatment regimens in pediatric patients, regardless of the dose of glucocorticoid administered or duration of therapy, and the incidence of peptic ulcer in these patients must be rare indeed. Rather than assuming too cavalier an attitude, however, the most prudent posture is to carefully observe those patients receiving high dose glucocorticoid therapy, particularly when other drugs known to have a high incidence of gastrointestinal side

effects, such as nonsteroidal anti-inflammatory agents, also are used.

Of particular concern is the effect of long-term glucocorticoid therapy on the hypothalamic-pituitary-adrenal axis because of the importance of endogenous glucocorticoid production once therapy has been discontinued. Activity within this axis is initiated with secretion by the hypothalamus of corticotropin-releasing factor (Fig. 42-7). This factor acts on the pituitary to release ACTH, which in turn directly stimulates the adrenal to release cortisol. Cortisol acts in a typical feedback fashion to inhibit secretion of corticotropin-releasing factor. Exogenously administered glucocorticoid acts in a fashion similar to endogenous cortisol. The ultimate result is inhibition of adrenal activity, and the degree and duration of this inhibition determines the integrity of the adrenal gland and its capacity to respond with production of cortisol once exogenous therapy is withdrawn.

In the normal individual, maximal secretion of ACTH and cortisol occurs in the early morning hours (6 a.m.–8 a.m.) and decreases gradually throughout the day to reach a nadir at approximately midnight [69,192] (Fig. 42-8). Because of this diurnal variation in normal adrenal function, the timing of glucocorticoid administration can have a substantial impact on endogenous cortisol release. As can be seen in Fig. 42-8a, administration of glucocorticoid shortly after the time of peak cortisol release reduces endogenous cortisol production during the day. It has little effect on the capacity of the adrenal to function as usual, however, because by the following morning, when maximal adrenal secretion of cortisol takes place, the pharmacokinetic characteristics of the glucocorticoid drugs have resulted in their virtual total clearance from the body and elimination of any feedback effect on the hypothalamus. In contrast, administration of glucocorticoid during the later afternoon (Fig. 42-8b) or evening (Fig. 42-8c) is likely to have a more profound inhibitory effect on cortisol release from the adrenal because circulating plasma drug levels will persist for a sufficient duration to maintain a negative feedback mechanism into the critical early morning hours.

The duration of glucocorticoid therapy associated with chronic adrenal suppression varies considerably between patients. Although it is clear that long-term daily use of steroids results in adrenal atrophy and/or a severely limited adrenal response to stress [84,157], even patients receiving glucocorticoids for one week or less and patients receiving "bursts" (less than seven days) of prednisone for acute therapy of asthma [72a] can show a reduction in adrenal function when therapy is discontinued. In most cases this suppression is short-lived and a return to normal function occurs within a few days [249,254], but suppression for up to a year has been reported [160].

After an extended period of glucocorticoid suppression of the hypothalamic-pituitary-adrenal axis, recovery of function is gradual and is completed within the hypothalamic-pituitary component before normal adrenal function returns [98]. Thus, secretion of ACTH from the pituitary may be observed in a diurnal rhythm at the same time that plasma cortisol continues to be depressed throughout the 24-hour period. This suggests that a period of adrenal

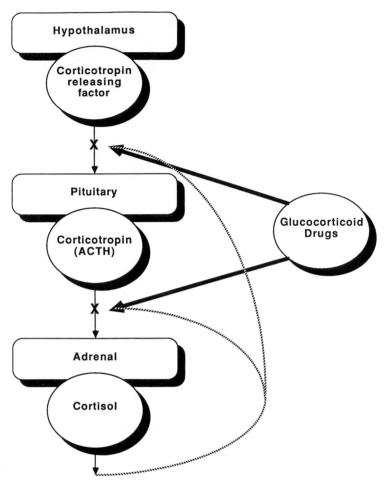

Fig. 42-7. *The hypothalamic-pituitary-adrenal axis. Cortisol produced by the adrenal gland, exerts a negative feedback effect on further cortisol production, as noted by the interrupted line. In a similar fashion, exogenously administered glucocorticoid acts at the same points in the axis to inhibit endogenous cortisol production (solid line).*

stimulation by ACTH is a necessary prerequisite to adrenal recovery, and it has been shown that a constant infusion of ACTH can accelerate adrenal recovery in the human [98]. The routine use of exogenous ACTH for this purpose is counterproductive to the overall therapeutic goal of restoration of the hypothalamic-pituitary-adrenal axis. Although ACTH may directly stimulate adrenal function, its use will perpetuate the negative feedback effect on the axis proximal to the adrenal. The result will be an ongoing suppression when ACTH is withdrawn. The major factor contraindicating ACTH administration in place of glucocorticoids is that its extended use not only is associated with the broad range of complications that accompany glucocorticoid therapy, but also includes those adverse effects associated with excessive adrenal secretion of mineralocorticoid and androgenic steroids.

In children, a gradual return of adrenal response occurs when prednisone doses are tapered, and one week following total discontinuation of drug therapy, early morning basal

cortisol levels and adrenal response to stress have been observed to return to normal [186]. The transition from high dose daily glucocorticoid therapy to alternate-day therapy is also associated with a gradual restoration of normal adrenal function. This may be extended over two months or more with the level of function ultimately achieved dependent on the maintenance dose of alternate-day therapy [188]. Alternate-day morning prednisone doses of 15 mg or less are associated with basal cortisol levels 24 hours after dosing only slightly lower than levels in untreated children, whereas alternate-day doses greater than 15 mg significantly depress basal cortisol production. Single morning prednisone doses as high as 60 mg only minimally reduce basal cortisol levels measured 48 hours after dosing.

It is virtually impossible to determine the degree of adrenal suppression in glucocorticoid treated patients without specific measurements of basal or poststress cortisol plasma concentrations, and even these may not be foolproof. Assuming that all patients treated with glucocorti-

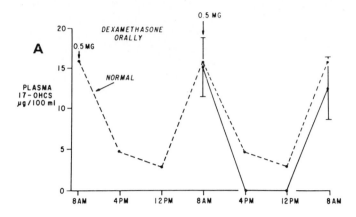

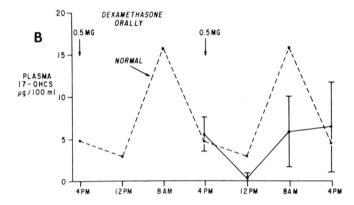

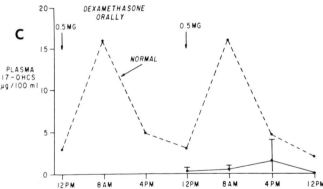

Fig. 42-8A-C. *Effect of administration of the glucocorticoid, dexamethasone on daily endogenous glucocorticoid production, determined by plasma levels of 17-hydroxycorticosteroid. Normal production is represented in each figure by the interrupted line showing maximal endogenous production in the early morning and reduced levels throughout the day. Early morning drug administration effectively eliminates endogenous glucocorticoid during the day, but does not significantly affect the usual adrenal response 24 hours later. Administration in late afternoon significantly affects adrenal function, but does not totally eliminate the early morning response. Administration in late evening severely affects adrenal function, including the early morning response. (From T Nichols, CA Nugent, FH Taylor: Diurnal variation in suppression of adrenal function by glucocorticoids. J. Clin Endocr 25:345–346. © by the Endocrine Society, 1965.)*

Table 42-10. *Principles of glucocorticoid withdrawal*

1. Glucocorticoid therapy of one-week duration or less can be discontinued abruptly without tapering or transition to alternate day therapy.
2. High dose daily glucocorticoid therapy must be converted to single dose daily therapy and then either gradually tapered over time or converted to alternate day therapy before the drug is discontinued.
3. Low dose alternate-day glucocorticoid therapy can be abruptly discontinued.
4. The above principles apply only to restoration of the hypothalamic-pituitary-adrenal axis. Rapid withdrawal of glucocorticoid therapy may precipitate
   • Nonspecific but characteristic withdrawal symptoms, including fever, malaise, arthralgia, and myalgia.
   • Exacerbation of symptoms and/or signs of a patient's basic inflammatory disease.

coid will have a measurable reduction in adrenal activity, the principles listed in Table 42-10 can be used as a guide to prevent adrenal insufficiency during glucocorticoid withdrawal.

Growth retardation is another important adverse effect of glucocorticoid therapy in children [14,161]. Linear growth is significantly reduced in patients receiving daily glucocorticoid therapy, with the degree of reduction dependent on dose and duration of therapy. Discontinuing therapy can restore growth patterns to normal, and use of alternate-day therapy does not appear to adversely effect growth, even during the use of high dose regimens.

The mechanism underlying glucocorticoid-induced growth retardation is unknown. It has been shown that glucocorticoids can inhibit cell replication and DNA synthesis [14,161]. A reduction in somatomedin levels has been reported to occur during glucocorticoid administration [77]; however, administration of growth hormone did not reverse the glucocorticoid effect on growth [187].

Diuretics

The number of diuretic agents available for clinical use has increased dramatically since the introduction of chlorothiazide in the 1950s. In many cases, these new diuretics represent congeners of the original chlorothiazide and have the same basic pharmacologic properties. Others represent the response to an expanded understanding of renal physiology, however, and, as such, have greatly improved therapeutic effectiveness. Whereas the primary pharmacologic effect of these drugs is an increase in urine volume and sodium excretion, the clinical indications for their use include conditions in which diuretic response is not necessarily the major therapeutic objective, such as hypertension or hypokalemia.

In this section the clinical pharmacology and antihypertensive effects of diuretics will be discussed. Because of their infrequent use and limited applicability to the pediatric nephrology patient, mercurial diuretics, osmotic diuretics, and carbonic anhydrase inhibitors will not be considered, and the reader is referred to other sources for information on those drugs [93,179].

Thiazides

The benzothiadiazide group of diuretics, referred to as the thiazide diuretics, constitutes a family of drugs with a common molecular structure but significantly different molar potencies (i.e., degree of effectiveness measured on a milligram basis). Other than differences in t½ noted in Table 42-11, the mechanisms and sites of action, disposition, therapeutic indications, and adverse effects for each of these drugs are virtually identical, so that data obtained in the earliest investigations with the initial thiazide, chlorothiazide, are applicable to the more recently developed thiazide derivatives. Chlorothalidone and metolazone are also included in the thiazide grouping because they incorporate the basic pharmacologic characteristics just noted.

The thiazide diuretics are rapidly absorbed after oral administration with a peak serum concentration occurring within two to four hours in children [16]. The drugs undergo very little metabolism prior to excretion, and almost all of the most commonly used thiazide, hydrochlorothiazide, is eliminated from the body within 12 hours [190]. If a satisfactory therapeutic response is not achieved with the usual dosages suggested in Table 42-11, additional increments in dosage are unlikely to improve thiazide effectiveness [191]; and for the shorter acting thiazides, increasing the dosing frequency to greater than every 12 hours only minimally increases the 24-hour excretion of water and electrolytes.

The kidney is the primary organ of drug clearance for the thiazides, with peak excretion occurring in four to six hours after drug dosing [16]. As a consequence, serum thiazide levels are dependent on renal function, and significant retention of thiazide and reduction in diuretic effect are noted when C_{Cr} falls below 50 ml/min [240]. An exception to this situation occurs in the newborn in whom diuretic effectiveness is undisturbed, even in the first few days of life, despite GFRs significantly lower than those in older children and adults [102].

Thiazide diuretics are secreted into the tubular lumen of the kidney through the proximal tubule organic acid transport system and must be present within the lumen to exert their diuretic effect. They act primarily at the thick ascending loop of Henle to block active reabsorption of chloride, although the cellular mechanisms through which this effect is mediated has not been isolated [47,125]. The consequent reversal of tubular transepithelial voltage inhibits passive sodium transport and results in a significant increase in natriuresis and diuresis. The thiazide diuretics also act in the proximal tubule to reduce chloride reabsorption [144,252], probably on the basis of carbonic anhydrase inhibition [125]. This is of relatively minor clinical importance, however, because the relatively small proximal diuretic effect is neutralized by compensatory reabsorption in the diluting segment of the tubule [47]; thus, the true impact of the thiazides on sodium and water balance is dependent on their distal tubular action [144].

A number of adverse effects have been observed during treatment with thiazide diuretics (Table 42-12). The most obvious of these, volume depletion and hyponatremia, are natural extensions of the primary pharmacologic effect of these drugs and are easily prevented by appropriate fluid and electrolyte replacement. The major adverse effect of potential concern in the treatment of children is hypokalemia. Urinary potassium excretion increases as the amount of sodium delivered distally to the tubular site of sodium-potassium exchange increases. Although excessive potassium losses usually can be corrected quite readily with oral potassium supplementation, this is not always necessary. Electrolyte balance can be maintained in many children by adjusting dietary intake to include foods rich in potas-

TABLE 42-11. *Diuretic drug dosing in children*

	Usual dosage (mg/kg/24 hr)	Frequency of administration
Thiazides		
Chlorothiazide	10–20	bid
Benzthiazide	2–4	bid
Hydrochlorothiazide	1–2	bid
Hydroflumethiazide	1–2	bid
Bendroflumethiazide	0.1–0.2	bid
Methyclothiazide	0.1–0.2	qd
Polythiazide	0.05–0.1	qd
Trichlormethiazide	0.05–0.1	qd
Loop diuretics		
Furosemide	0.5–2	bid
Bumetanide	0.01–0.05	bid
Potassium-sparing		
Spironolactone	1–2	bid
Triamterene	1–2	bid
Amiloride	0.1–0.2	qd

TABLE 42-12. *Adverse effects with thiazide diuretics*

Hyperglycemia
Hyperuricemia
Hyponatremia
Hypercalcemia
Hypokalemia
Volume depletion
Serum lipid abnormalities

sium. Even when potassium balance does not appear to be a problem during initiation of thiazide therapy, periodic monitoring of serum electrolytes remains an integral component in the medical management of patients on long-term diuretic therapy.

Hyperglycemia is rarely seen in children. Although hyperuricemia has been reported to occur in 55% of adult patients [51], it too is an uncommon finding in children. A statistically significant positive correlation between serum levels of hydrocholorthiazide and uric acid has been observed in the children [180], but concentrations of uric acid do not reach levels found in patients with adverse systemic reactions.

Thiazides have a positive effect on calcium balance as a result of reduced urinary calcium excretion [39,176], and in some patients receiving thiazides, this effect is profound enough to cause hypercalcemia [75]. The mechanism through which the hypocalciuric response to thiazides is mediated has not been identified. It appears that the presence of parathyroid tissue is a prerequisite, but there is no evidence that this ill-defined thiazide-parathyroid relationship is associated with induction of parathyroid activity [39,176]. Hypercalcemia rarely is observed in children, despite a similar effect of thiazides on urinary calcium excretion in this age group. This raises an important question about the ultimate disposition of the increased pool of total body calcium, and recent evidence suggests that thiazide use is associated with an increase in bone mineral content [269]. If this is confirmed, thiazides may prove to be of therapeutic value in patients with diseases complicated by osteoporosis.

Of more recent concern is the discovery that thiazide use is associated with an adjustment in serum lipid concentrations towards atherogenic serum lipid profiles [1]. Adults receiving these drugs for treatment of hypertension have an increase in serum cholesterol and triglycerides without a concomitant increase in high density lipoproteins to offset these changes. Although a number of investigators have reported a return of lipoprotein concentrations to baseline levels during long-term therapy [1a,86], studies incorporating placebo control groups have shown significantly lower lipoprotein levels in these subjects than thiazide-treated subjects, and others have shown significant reductions in lipoprotein levels after long-term thiazide therapy has been discontinued [1a,275].

Loop Diuretics

The most potent diuretic agents currently available for clinical use are the loop diuretics, so-named because of their major site of action at the ascending loop of Henle (see Table 42-11). Among the drugs in this class of diuretics, the use of ethacrynic acid has been severely limited by the purported greater incidence of drug-related ototoxicity [58], despite its equal effectiveness to other loop diuretics in adults and children [231]. The other loop diuretics, azosemide [30,32,35], piretanide [31], torasemide [35a], and bumetanide [53], are similar to furosemide, still the most popular agent in this group.

With the exception of bioavailability and potency, the loop diuretics have remarkably similar pharmacologic and pharmacokinetic characteristics. Azosemide has the lowest bioavailability (10%) but is as effective as furosemide, which has a bioavailability of approximately 40% [36], because the pharmacologic potency of azosemide is approximately seven times greater [35]. The bioavailability of bumetanide and piretanide is approximately 80%, but bumetamide has approximately 70 times greater potency than furosemide, whereas piretanide is only seven times more potent than furosemide [30,33]. Torasemide is four to five times more potent than furosemide [35a].

The loop diuretics are rapidly absorbed after oral administration. Their peak diuretic effect occurs within one to two hours, and they are rapidly excreted, with a t½ of approximately 0.5 to 1.5 hours. As is the case with the thiazide diuretics, the loop diuretics are cleared almost entirely through the proximal tubule organic acid transport system. In patients with reduced renal function, however, hepatic metabolism assumes a substantial role in clearance [2,63]. Concomitant use of other drugs that are dependent on the proximal tubule organic acid transport system for clearance, e.g., probenecid, causes a competitive inhibition of diuretic excretion and can reduce diuretic effectiveness [55,148].

Certain pathologic states alter the expected response to furosemide. In patients with congestive heart failure, the rate of excretion of furosemide by the kidney is reduced concomitant with a reduction in urinary volume and sodium excretion [4,34]. The total amount of furosemide excreted in the urine is not different from that in normal patients; however, the time course over which excretion takes place is extended, most likely on the basis of a reduction in RBF and extraction of drug at the proximal tubule. Because diuretic effect is correlated with delivery of furosemide to its site of action in the renal tubule, one might expect that the diuretic response would be prolonged but not quantitatively reduced. The hemodynamic response to heart failure and/or edema is known to alter renal tubular function, however, and contributes to the blunted response to diuretic therapy observed in these patients [122]. The response to furosemide in patients with hepatic disease and ascites is also less than normally expected, most likely on a basis similar to that proposed for patients with congestive heart failure [88,265].

The loop diuretics have had a dramatic impact on the clinical management of nephrotic syndrome in childhood. Yet it is clear that in patients with severe nephrosis there is a shift to the right in the dose-response curve (i.e., reduced diuretic response for a given diuretic dose), with the barest response noted in some cases. Although this is attributable, in part, to the hemodynamic considerations just noted and to alterations in intravascular and interstitial volumes, the increase in urinary protein concentration of itself influences diuretic effectiveness. Furosemide is highly protein bound (approximately 97% is bound to albumin) in the vascular space [211]. With an increase in the urinary concentration of albumin in nephrotic patients, it is likely that furosemide-protein binding in the lumen of the renal tubule also increases, as shown in experimental animal models [100]. The result is a decrease in tubular concentration of unbound furosemide. Because the unbound fraction represents the pharmacologically active form of the drug, diuretic effect also decreases.

As might be expected because of its dependence on renal function for elimination from the body, the rate of furosemide clearance is reduced in infancy, and the degree of reduction is dependent on gestational age [5,207,262]. In very low birth weight infants, $t\frac{1}{2}$ frequently exceeds 24 hours, and accumulation of furosemide to potentially ototoxic levels occurs with dosing every 12 hours [181]. Nevertheless, urine volume remains significantly above normal [102] because of the extended diuretic effect of furosemide corresponding to the prolonged duration of excretion [101].

The loop diuretics exert their principal effect at the thick ascending limb of the loop of Henle [124] by interfering with active chloride reabsorption [101,213]. In addition, the loop diuretics increase free water clearance [38,213,234] through an inhibition of carbonic anhydrase activity in the proximal tubule and/or by increasing urine flow rate through the collecting duct. This may account for the clinical usefulness of these agents in treating hyponatremic syndromes such as inappropriate secretion of antidiuretic hormone (ADH) [67,111] or edema [101].

Administration of the loop diuretics is associated with a number of hemodynamic responses that contribute to their primary diuretic action. Furosemide increases total renal vascular blood flow [94] and redistributes renal cortical blood flow [251], stimulates renin secretion from the juxtaglomerular cells of the kidney [199], and increases vascular capacitance while reducing peripheral vascular resistance in patients with congestive heart failure [72].

The regulatory mechanisms controlling each of these physiologic responses to furosemide are not well defined but appear to be mediated, in part, through the PG system, which is activated almost immediately after furosemide administration [272]. PGs are potent vasodilators in a variety of vascular beds [123] particularly the renal vasculature [159]. They are independent effectors of renin release from the kidney and participate in stimulation of renin secretion mediated through other physiologic systems [85]. Inhibition of PG biosynthesis by indomethacin not only prevents furosemide-induced vasodilatory and renin secretory effects but also reduces natriuresis and diuresis [193,257]. PGs also directly affect water balance through modification of (1) glomerular hemodynamics [237], (2) the renal tubular response to ADH hormone [105], and (3) sodium chloride transport in the distal tubule [138]. Thus, the entire spectrum of furosemide-related events may be intimately tied to activation of the PG system.

A number of side effects can occur during therapy with loop diuretics (Table 42-13). The most frequent of these are hypokalemia and alkalosis, which are almost always

TABLE 42-13. Adverse effects with loop diuretics

Hyponatremia
Hypokalemia
Alkalosis
Ototoxicity
Nephrocalcinosis
Interstitial nephritis

more pronounced with furosemide than with the thiazides. Hypokalemia is difficult to manage with an increase in dietary potassium alone and usually requires direct potassium chloride replacement throughout the course of therapy. Hypokalemia can be accentuated by the concurrent use of prednisone or other glucocorticoids.

Another serious but less frequent side effect is ototoxicity [229]. The degree of hearing impairment is correlated with blood levels of furosemide and can be either permanent or temporary [90]. The mechanism through which furosemide causes ototoxicity is not known. It appears, however, to be related to changes in endolymphatic electrical potential resulting from a furosemide-induced increase in sodium and decrease in potassium-endolymph concentration [127,228].

The routine use of furosemide in some neonatal intensive care units to treat respiratory disorders [102] has led to the development of nephrocalcinosis in a small percentage of infants and the recognition that furosemide is a potent hypercalciuric agent [120]. An increase in urinary calcium excretion is well documented in animals [76] and human adults and children [225,230,255] and is the rationale for its use as primary therapy for hypercalciuric states [255]. Other side effects such as interstitial nephritis [89] and leukopenia [270] have been reported but are far less common.

Potassium-Sparing Diuretics

Spironolactone, triamterene, and amiloride are considered together within the potassium-sparing diuretic class of drugs, despite their apparent diverse mechanisms of action and dissimilar chemical structures (see Table 42-11). They are relatively weak diuretic agents but have achieved wide clinical use because of their potassium-sparing properties. Each of these drugs exerts its primary inhibitory effect on sodium reabsorption in the collecting duct, with amiloride having an additional effect at the distal convoluted tubule [125]. Because most reabsorption of sodium in the nephron occurs proximal to these sites, a relatively small amount remains available for distal reabsorption; thus, the diuretic potency of the potassium-sparing diuretics is considerably reduced when compared to the thiazides and loop diuretics. The potassium-sparing agents are rarely indicated for primary diuretic therapy, with the exception of specific pathophysiologic conditions, such as nephrotic syndrome, congestive heart failure, and liver failure, in which aldosterone secretion is likely to be secondarily increased.

The potassium-sparing diuretics are widely used prophylactically in clinical practice to prevent potassium depletion or to re-establish potassium stores in patients receiving other diuretics for fluid retention and, in particular, for hypertension. Justification for their use under these conditions has been hotly debated during recent years. On the one hand are those who believe there is very little risk associated with moderate potassium deficiency and hypokalemia and conclude that the frequency with which potassium-sparing drugs are included in diuretic drug regimens far exceeds their proved utility and is not justified by their expense [110,133]. Others are equally as adamant in their contention that hypokalemia should be prevented in virtually all patients [130]. The truth probably lies somewhere between these two philosophies, so that the most prudent approach appears to be treatment only of those individuals with documented persistent hypokalemia.

The frequency of hypokalemia in pediatric patients treated with diuretics is poorly defined. While it seems clear that a high degree of urinary potassium loss can be expected during chronic therapy with loop diuretics, clinical experience also suggests that, as in adults, hypokalemia occurs far less frequently during therapy with thiazides [149,184,278].

Routine use of potassium-sparing agents is to be discouraged, and each patient should be managed individually. In many cases, nonpharmacologic strategies for increasing dietary potassium intake will be highly effective in maintaining electrolyte balance. In others, administration of potassium chloride should be attempted prior to adding additional pharmacologic agents to an already complex drug regimen. Newer wax matrix and microencapsulated extended-action formulations have eliminated many of the earlier compliance problems caused by the unpalatability of potassium chloride preparations. In particular, the microencapsulated "sprinkles" offer a feasible approach to potassium administration in very young children or those who have difficulty swallowing pills. Although these long-acting agents appear to be free from side effects, it has been suggested that the wax-matrix tablets may be associated with asymptomatic gastric lesions [171]. The clinical significance of these findings, if any, has not been determined.

SPIRONOLACTONE

The mechanisms of action of spironolactone have recently been reviewed [59]. It competitively inhibits the action of aldosterone by specific binding to intracellular receptor proteins [115]. It is similar in molecular structure to the naturally occurring mineralocorticoid, continuing the basic steroid nucleus, and is effective only when aldosterone is present [129,158].

Spironolactone is extensively metabolized to a number of active compounds, among which canrenone, a primary unconjugated metabolite found in high concentration, is presumed to be primarily responsible for its diuretic effect [97]. Recent studies incorporating more specific liquid chromatographic techniques have shown the parent compound to be present in higher concentration than previously recognized, in addition to a second major spironolactone metabolite, 7α-thiomethylspironolactone, which possesses a higher affinity for aldosterone receptors than canrenone and has a high degree of antialdosterone activity [200]. Despite the rapid metabolic conversion of spirono-

lactone, the half-life of its active metabolites is prolonged, permitting twice daily dosing schedules but requiring two or three days for a steady-state response to be realized.

An obvious potential side effect of spironolactone is the occurrence of hyperkalemia in patients with compromised renal function. Other serious adverse reactions are gynecomastia and menstrual irregularities, most commonly amenorrhea [41,103], that may be attributed to the antiandrogenic effect of the drug [60].

TRIAMTERENE AND AMILORIDE

Unlike spironolactone, the effect of triamterene and amiloride on the distal tubule is independent of aldosterone [10,11]. Triamterene was available for clinical use prior to amiloride, but it has not been studied as extensively. Consequently, the bulk of information about these similarly acting agents derives from primary investigation of amiloride [19].

Both drugs act on the distal tubule to inhibit sodium flux across the cellular membrane [11,19]. Triamterene exerts this effect from the peritubular side [92], whereas amiloride exerts its effect from the luminal side [19]. In either case, the result is an inhibition of sodium reabsorption and a consequent reduction in potassium and hydrogen ion excretion.

Triamterene undergoes rapid and extensive hepatic metabolism [212,247], with t½ of approximately three hours [212] and duration of action greater than six hours [10]. Amiloride is not metabolized prior to excretion through the kidney. It has a longer duration of action than triamterene, with a peak effect noted six to eight hours after administration [43].

Triamterene and amiloride are equally effective in clinical use when combined with a thiazide diuretic [169]. With certain formulations of triamterene and hydrochlorothiazide, however, bioavailability of each of these two drugs is reduced [27,280]. Newer combination tablets have eliminated these formulation problems while maintaining antihypertensive and potassium-sparing effectiveness [279, 280].

Use of Diuretics in Antihypertensive Therapy

Diuretics continue to be an important component of antihypertensive therapy in adults [261] and children [219], although the availability of newer agents with a variety of specific actions and increasing concern about plasma lipoprotein changes may ultimately reduce their popularity. In general, our basic understanding of the antihypertensive effect of diuretics is not any greater today than it was ten years ago [241].

The antihypertensive response to thiazides appears to be dependent on their diuretic action, despite the assertion that they also have a vasodilating effect based on the vascular response to the thiazide analogue diazoxide. The immediate response to diuretics in the hypertensive patient is an increase in urine volume and sodium excretion resulting in a decreased extracellular and plasma volume, body weight and cardiac output [87]. Compensatory homeostatic mechanisms are activated so that sodium loss if brought into balance with sodium intake, and plasma volume and extracellular fluid volume return toward their pretreatment levels over a 6- to 12-month period [57,282]. The ultimate effect of diuretic therapy, however, is a finite reduction in volume, a sustained decrease in peripheral vascular resistance, and a reduction in systemic blood pressure [151,259].

Spironolactone is indicated for the treatment of hypertension secondary to adrenal adenoma or hyperplasia. Its use in other forms of hypertension, including essential hypertension, has not been established. Although it was formerly recommended for patients with low-renin hypertension on the presumption that renin suppression is caused by excessive mineralocorticoid production [248], spironolactone has not been shown to be more effective in these patients than traditional diuretic therapy [73,82].

Triamterene and amiloride are not considered primary therapeutic agents for hypertension. If there is a role for these drugs in hypertensive patients, it is to reduce urinary potassium excretion during diuretic therapy when other strategies for maintaining serum potassium at normal levels fail. Despite the recent reawakening to the potential importance of potassium balance in blood pressure homeostasis [165] and evidence that potassium repletion in hypertensive patients with diuretic-induced hypokalemia can result in a significant reduction in blood pressure [131], the routine inclusion of potassium-sparing diuretics in antihypertensive regimens is to be discouraged.

References

1. Ames RP: Coronary heart disease and the treatment of hypertension: Impact of diuretics on serum lipids and glucose. *J Cardiovasc Pharmacol* 6:5466, 1984.
1a. Ames RP: Antihypertensive drugs and lipid profiles. *Am J Hypertens* 1:421, 1988.
2. Andreasen F, Hansen HE, Mikkelsen E: Pharmacokinetics of furosemide in anephric patients and in normal subjects. *Eur J Clin Pharmacol* 13:41, 1978.
3. Andreasen F, Jakobsen P: Determination of furosemide in blood plasma and its binding to proteins in normal plasma and in plasma from patients with acute renal failure. *Acta Pharmacol et Toxicol* (suppl 3)29:134, 1971.
4. Andreasen F, Mikkelsen E: Distribution, elimination and effect of furosemide in normal subjects and in patients with heart failure. *Eur J Clin Pharmacol* 12:15, 1977.
5. Aranda JV, Lambert C, Perez J, et al: Metabolism and renal elimination of furosemide in the newborn infant. *J Pediatr* 101:777, 1982.
6. Arbus GS, Hardy BE: Immunosuppressive therapy for pediatric renal allograft recipients. *In* Fine RN, Gruskin AB (eds): *End Stage Renal Disease in Children.* Philadelphia, WB Saunders, 1984, p 508.
7. Aronoff GR, Sloan RS: Nitrendipine kinetics in normal and impaired renal function. *Clin Pharmacol Ther* 38:212, 1985.
8. Aronoff GR, Sloan RS, Brier ME, et al: The effect of piperacillin dose on elimination kinetics in renal impairment. *Eur J Clin Pharmacol* 24:543, 1983.
9. Aronoff GR, Sloan RS, Stanish RA, et al: Mezlocillin dose dependent elimination kinetics in renal impairment. *Eur J Clin Pharmacol* 21:505, 1982.
10. Baba WI, Tudhope GR, Wilson GM: Triamterene, a new diuretic drug. *Br Med J* 2:756, 1962.
11. Baer JE, Beyer KH: Subcellular pharmacology of natriuretic and potassium-sparing drugs. *Prog Biochem Pharmacol* 7:59, 1972.
12. Balis FM, Savitch JL, Bleyer WA: Pharmacokinetics of oral methotrexate in children. *Cancer Res* 43:2342, 1983.
12a. Bartoszek M, Brenner AM, Szefler SJ: Prednisolone and methylprednisolone kinetics in children receiving anticonvulsant therapy. *Clin Pharmacol Ther* 42:424, 1987.
13. Barza M, Weinstein L: Pharmacokinetics of the penicillins in man. *Clin Pharmacokinet* 1:297, 1976.
14. Baxter JD: Mechanisms of glucocorticoid inhibition of growth. *Kidney Int* 14:330, 1978.
15. Baxter JD, Forsham PH: Tissue effects of glucocorticoids. *Am J Med* 53:573, 1972.
16. Beermann B, Groschinsky–Grind M, Rosen A: Absorption, metabolism and excretion of hydrochlorothiazide. *Clin Pharmacol Ther* 19:531, 1976.
17. Bennett WM, Aronoff GR, Morrison G, et al: Drug prescribing in renal failure: Dosing guidelines for adults. *Am J Kidney Dis* 3:155, 1983.
18. Bennett WM, Bagby SP, Golper TA, et al: Vancomycin therapy for difficult infections in hemodialysis patients. *Dialysis and Transplantation* 6:22, 1977.
19. Benos DJ: Amiloride: A molecular probe of sodium transport in tissues and cells. *Am J Physiol* 242:C131, 1982.
20. Berlin–Heimendahl SV: Bensoderheiten des wasser-mineral-und saurebassenstoff-wechsels in den ersten lebenstagen. *Dtsch Med Wochenschr* 89:2425, 1964.
21. Bickel MH: Poisoning by tricyclic antidepressant drugs: General and pharmacokinetic considerations. *Int J Clin Pharmacol and Biopharmacy* 11:145, 1975.
22. Bishop CR, Athens JW, Boggs DR, et al: Leukokinetic studies XIII. A non-steady state kinetic evaluation of the mechanism of cortisone-induced granulocytosis. *J Clin Invest* 47:249, 1968.
23. Bjornsson TD: Nomogram for drug dosage adjustment in patients with renal failure. *Clin Pharmacokinet* 11:164, 1986.
24. Blackwell GJ, Carnuccio R, DiRosa M, et al: Macrocortin: A polypeptide causing the anti-phospholipase effect of glucocorticoids. *Nature* 287:147, 1980.
25. Blair AD, Maxwell BM, Forland SC, et al: Cefonicid kinetics in subjects with normal and impaired renal function. *Clin Pharmacol Ther* 35:798, 1984.
26. Blum MR, Riegelman S, Becker CE: Altered protein binding of diphenylhydantoin in uremic plasma (letter). *N Engl J Med* 286:109, 1972.
27. Blume CD, Williams RL, Upton RA, et al: Bioequivalence study of a new tablet formulation of triamterene and hydrochlorothiazide. *Am J Med* 77(5A):59, 1984.
28. Bonney RJ, Wightman PD, Davies P, et al: Regulation of prostaglandin synthesis and of the selective release of lysosomal hydrolases by mouse peritoneal macrophages. *Biochem J* 176:433, 1978.
29. Bourke E, Frindt G, Preuss H, et al: Studies with uremic serum on the renal transport of hippurates and tetraethylammonium in the rabbit and rat. Effect of oral neomycin. *Clin Sci* 38:41, 1970.
30. Brater DC: Renal sites of action of azosemide. *Clin Pharmacol Ther* 25:428, 1979.
31. Brater DC, Anderson S, Baird B, et al: Effects of piretanide in normal subjects. *Clin Pharmacol Ther* 34:324, 1983.
32. Brater DC, Anderson SA, Strowig S: Azosemide; a loop diuretic and furosemide. *Clin Pharmacol Ther* 25:435, 1979.
33. Brater DC, Chennavasin P, Day B, et al: Bumetanide and furosemide. *Clin Pharmacol Ther* 34:207, 1983.

34. Brater DC, Chennavasin P, Seiwell R: Furosemide in patients with heart failure: Shift in dose-response curves. *Clin Pharmacol Ther* 28:182, 1980.

35. Brater DC, Day B, Anderson S, et al: Azosemide kinetics and dynamics. *Clin Pharmacol Ther* 34:454, 1983.

35a. Brater DC, Leinfelder J, Anderson SA: Clinical pharmacology of forasemide, a new loop diuretic. *Clin Pharmacol Ther* 42:187, 1987.

36. Brater DC, Seiwell R, Anderson S, et al: Absorption and disposition of furosemide in congestive heart failure. *Kidney Int* 22:171, 1982.

37. Braunlich H: Kidney development: Drug elimination mechanisms. *In* Morselli PL, (ed): *Drug Disposition During Development.* New York, Specrum Publications, 1977, p 89.

38. Brenner BM, Keimowitz RI, Wright FS, et al: An inhibitory effect of furosemide on sodium reabsorption by the proximal tubule of the rat nephron. *J Clin Invest* 48:290, 1969.

39. Brickman AS, Massey SG, Coburn JW: Changes in serum and urinary calcium during treatment with hydrochlorothiazide: Studies on mechanisms. *J Clin Invest* 51:945, 1972.

40. Brooks SM, Werk EE, Ackerman SJ, et al: Adverse effects of phenobarbital on corticosteroid metabolism in patients with bronchial asthma. *N Engl J Med* 286:1125, 1972.

41. Brown JJ, Ferriss JB, Fraser R: Spironolactone in the treatment of hypertension with aldosterone excess. *In: The Medical Uses of Spironolactone Symposium,* Excerpta Medica, 1970, p 27.

42. Bruns RR, Palade GE: Studies on blood capillaries. II. Transport of ferritin molecules across the wall of muscle capillaries. *J Cell Biol* 37:277, 1968.

43. Bull MB, Laragh JH: Amiloride: A potassium-sparing natriuretic agent. *Circulation* 37:45, 1968.

44. Bunke CM, Aronoff GR, Brier ME, et al: Cefazolin and cephalexin kinetics in continuous ambulatory peritoneal dialysis. *Clin Pharmacol Ther* 33:66, 1983.

45. Bunke CM, Aronoff GR, Brier ME, et al: Tobramycin kinetics during continuous ambulatory peritoneal dialysis. *Clin Pharmacol Ther* 34:110, 1983.

46. Bunke CM, Aronoff GR, Brier ME, et al: Vancomycin kinetics during continuous ambulatory peritoneal dialysis. *Clin Pharmacol Ther* 34:631, 1983.

47. Burg MB: Renal chloride transport and diuretics. *Circulation* 53:587, 1976.

48. Burk M, Peters U: Disopyramide kinetics in renal impairment: Determinants of interindividual variability. *Clin Pharmacol Ther* 34:331, 1983.

49. Cafruny EJ: Renal tubular handling of drugs. *Am J Med* 62:490, 1977.

50. Calvo R, Carlos R, Erill S: Effects of carbamylation on plasma proteins and competitive displacers on drug binding in uremia. *Pharmacology* 24:248, 1982.

51. Cannon PJ, Stason WB, Demartini FE, et al: Hyperuricemia in primary and renal hypertension. *N Engl J Med* 275:457, 1966.

52. Cannon PJ, Whitlock RT, Morris RC, et al: Effect of alpha-methyl DOPA in severe and malignant hypertension. *JAMA* 179:673, 1962.

53. Carriere S, Dandavino R: Bumetanide, a new loop diuretic. *Clin Pharmacol Ther* 20:424, 1976.

54. Chen PS, Mills IM, Bartter FC: Ultrafiltration studies of steroid-protein binding. *J Endocrinol* 23:129, 1961.

55. Chennavasin P, Seiwell R, Brater DC, et al: Pharmacodynamic analysis of the furosemide-probenecid interaction in man. *Kidney Int* 16:187, 1979.

56. Conn HO, Blitzer BI: Nonassociation of adrenocorticosteroid therapy and peptic ulcer. *N Engl J Med* 294:473, 1976.

57. Conway J, Lauwers P: Hemodynamic and hypotensive effects of long-term therapy with chlorothiazide. *Circulation* 21:21, 1960.

58. Cooperman LB, Rubin IL: Toxicity of ethacrynic acid and furosemide. *Am Heart J* 85:831, 1973.

59. Corvol P, Claire M, Oblin ME, et al: Mechanism of the antimineralocorticoid effect of spironolactones. *Kidney Int* 20:1, 1981.

60. Corvol P, Michaud A, Menard J, et al: Antiandrogenic effect of spironolactones: Mechanism of action. *Endocrinology* 97:52, 1975.

61. Craig WA, Evenson MA, Sawer PK, et al: Correction of protein binding defect in uremic sera by charcoal treatment. *J Lab Clin Med* 87:637, 1976.

62. Cupps TR, Fauci AS: Corticosteroid-mediated immunoregulation in man. *Immunol Rev* 65:133, 1982.

63. Cutter RE, Forrey AW, Christopher TG, et al: Pharmacokinetics of furosemide in normal subjects and functionally anephric patients. *Clin Pharmacol Ther* 15:588, 1974.

64. Czerwinski AW, Pederson JA: Pharmacokinetics of cefamandole in patients with renal impairment. *Antimicrob Agents Chemother* 15:161, 1979.

65. Dale DC, Fauci AS, Guerry D, et al: Comparison of agents producing a neutrophilic leukocytosis in man. *J Clin Invest* 56:808, 1975.

66. Dale DC, Fauci AS, Wolff SM: Alternate day prednisone: Leukocyte kinetics and susceptibility to infections. *N Engl J Med* 291:1154, 1974.

67. Decaux G, Waterlot Y, Genette F, et al: Treatment of the syndrome of inappropriate secretion of antidiuretic hormone with furosemide. *N Engl J Med* 304:329, 1981.

68. Deding A, Tougaard L, Jensen MK, et al: Bone changes during prednisone treatment. *Acta Med Scand* 202:253, 1977.

69. Demura H, West CD, Nugetn CA, et al: A sensitive radioimmunoassay for plasma ACTH levels. *J Clin Endocr* 26:1297, 1966.

70. Dettli L: Drug dose in renal disease. *Clin Pharmacokinet* 1:126, 1976.

71. Diaz CR, Kane JC, Perkin RH, et al: Pharmacokinetics of nafcillin in patients with renal failure. *Antimicrob Agents Chemother* 12:98, 1977.

72. Dikshit K, Vyden JK, Forrester JS, et al: Renal and extrarenal hemodynamic effects of furosemide in congestive heart failure after acute myocardial infarction. *N Engl J Med* 288:1098, 1973.

72a. Dolan LM, Kesarwala HH, Hoiroyoe JL, et al: Short-term high-dose, systemic steroids in children with asthma. The effect on the hypothalmic-pituitary-adrenal axis. *J Allergy Clin Immunol* 80:81, 1987.

73. Douglas JG, Hollifield JW, Liddle GW: Treatment of low-renin essential hypertension: Comparison of spironolactone and a hydrochlorothiazide-triamterene combination. *JAMA* 227:518, 1974.

74. Drayer DE: Active drug metabolites and renal failure. *Am J Med* 62:486, 1977.

75. Duarte CQ, Winnacker JL, Becker KL, et al: Thiazide-induced hypercalcemia. *N Engl J Med* 284:838, 1971.

76. Edwards BR, Baer PG, Sutton RAL, et al: Micropuncture study of diuretic effects on sodium and calcium reabsorption in the dog nephron. *J Clin Invest* 52:2418, 1973.

77. Elders MJ, Wingfield BS, McNatt ML, et al: Glucocorticoid therapy in children: Effect on somatomedin. *Am J Dis Child* 129:1393, 1975.

78. Erill S, Calvo R, Carlos R: Plasma protein carbamylation and decreased acidic drug protein binding in uremia. Clin Pharmacol Ther 27:612, 1980.

79. Estes JW: Clinical pharmacokinetics of heparin. Clin Pharmacokinet 5:204, 1980.

80. Fauci AS, Dale DC: The effect of hydrocortisone in the kinetics of normal human lymphocytes. Blood 46:235, 1975.

81. Fauci AS: Mechanisms of corticosteroid action on lymphocyte subpopulations. Clin Exp Immunol 24:54, 1976.

82. Ferguson RK, Turek DM, Rovner DR: Spironolactone and hydrochlorothiazide in normal-renin and low-renin essential hypertension. Clin Pharmacol Ther 21:62, 1977.

83. Fisher DE, Bickel WH: Corticosteroid-induced avascular necrosis. J Bone Joint Surg [Am] 53A:859, 1971.

84. Fraser CG, Preuss FS, Bigford WD: Adrenal atrophy and irreversible shock associated with cortisone therapy. JAMA 149:1542, 1952.

85. Freeman RH, Davis JO, Villarreal D: Role of renal prostaglandins in the control of renin release. Circ Res 54:1, 1984.

86. Fries ED: The cardiovascular risks of thiazide diuretics. Clin Pharmacol Ther 39:239, 1986.

87. Frolich ED, Thurman AE, Pfeffer MA: Altered vascular responsiveness: Initial hypotensive mechanism of thiazide diuretics. Proc Soc Exp Biol Med 140:1190, 1972.

88. Fuller R, Hoppel C, Ingalls ST: Furosemide kinetics in patients with hepatic cirrhosis with ascites. Clin Pharmacol Ther 30:461, 1981.

89. Fuller TJ, Barcenas CG, White MG: Diuretic-induced interstitial nephritis. JAMA 235:1998, 1976.

90. Gallagher KL, Jones JK: Furosemide-induced ototoxicity. Ann Intern Med 91:744, 1979.

91. Gatti G, Perucca E, Frigo GM, et al: Pharmacokinetics of prednisone and its metabolite prednisolone in children with nephrotic syndrome during the active phase and in remission. Br J Pharmacol 17:423, 1984.

92. Gatzy JT: The effect of K-sparing diuretics on ion transport across the excised toad bladder. J Pharmacol Exp Ther 176:580, 1971.

93. Gennari FJ, Kassirer JP: Osmotic diuresis. N Engl J Med 291:714, 1974.

94. Gerber JG, Nies AS: Furosemide-induced vasodilatation: Importance of the state of hydration and filtration. Kidney Int 18:454, 1980.

95. Gibson TP, Demetriades JC, Bland JA: Imipenem/cilastatin: Pharmacokinetic profile in renal insufficiency. Am J Med 78(6A):54, 1985.

95a. Gilman AG, Goodman LS, Rall TW, et al (eds): The Pharmacologic Basis of Therapeutics, 7th ed. New York, Macmillan, 1985.

96. Glasser L, Huestis DW, Jones JF: Functional capabilities of steroid-recruited neutrophils harvested for clinical transfusion. N Engl J Med 297:1033, 1977.

97. Gochman N, Gantt CL: A fluorimetric method for the determination of a major spironolactone (aldactone) metabolite in human plasma. J Pharmacol Exp Ther 135:312, 1962.

98. Graber AL, Ney RL, Nicholson WE, et al: Natural history of pituitary-adrenal recovery following long-term suppression with corticosteroids. J Clin Endocrinol 25:11, 1965.

99. Green OC, Winter RJ, Kawahara FS, et al: Pharmacokinetic studies of prednisolone in children. J Pediatr 93:299, 1978.

100. Green TP, Mirkin BL: Resistance of proteinuric rats to furosemide: Urinary drug protein binding as a determinant of drug effect. Life Sci 26:623, 1980.

101. Green TP, Mirkin BL: Determinants of the diuretic response to furosemide in infants with congestive heart failure. Pediatr Cardiol 3:47, 1982.

102. Green TP, Thompson TR, Johnson DE, et al: Furosemide promotes patent ductus arteriosus in premature infants with the respiratory-distress syndrome. N Engl J Med 308:743, 1983.

103. Greenblatt DJ, Koch–Wesen J: Gynecomastia and impotence. Complications of spironolactone therapy. JAMA 223:82, 1983.

104. Greenfield RA, Gerber AU, Craig WA: Pharmacokinetics of cefoperazone in patients with normal and impaired hepatic and renal function. Rev Infect Dis 5:S127, 1983.

105. Gross PA, Schrier RW, Anderson RJ: Prostaglandins and water metabolism: A review with emphasis on in vivo studies. Kidney Int 19:839, 1981.

106. Guggino SE, Morten GJ, Aronson PS: Specificity and modes of the anion exchangers in dog renal microvillus membranes. Am J Physiol 244:F612, 1983.

107. Gunn T, Reece ER, Metrakos K, et al: Depressed T-cells following neonatal steroid treatment. Pediatrics 67:61, 1981.

108. Hande KR, Noone RM, Stone WJ: Severe allopurinol toxicity. Description and guidelines for prevention in patient with renal insufficiency. Am J Med 76:47, 1984.

109. Harding SM: Pharmacokinetics of the third-generation cephalosporins. Am J Med (suppl 2A)79:21, 1985.

110. Harrington JT, Isuer JM, Kassirer JP: Our national obsession with potassium. Am J Med 73:155, 1982.

111. Hautman D, Rossier B, Zohlman R, et al: Rapid correction of hyponatremia in the syndrome of inappropriate secretion of antidiuretic hormone. Ann Intern Med 78:870, 1973.

112. Haynes BF, Fauci AS: The differetial effect of in vivo hydrocortisone on the kinetics of subpopulations of human peripheral blood thymus-derived lymphocytes. J Clin Invest 61:703, 1978.

113. Editorial: Hazards of potent topical corticosteroids. Lancet 1:870, 1973.

114. Hench PS, Kendall EC, Stocumb CH, et al: The effect of a hormone of the adrenal cortex (17-hydroxy-11-dehydrocorticosterone: Compound E) and of pituitary adrenocorticotropic hormone on rheumatoid arthritis: Preliminary report. Proc Mayo Clinic 24:181, 1949.

115. Herman TS, Fimognari GM, Edelman IS: Studies on renal aldosterone-binding proteins. J Biol Chem 14:3849, 1968.

116. Hiner LB, Balmarte HJ, Polinsky MS, et al: Cefazolin in children with renal insufficiency. J Pediatr 96:335, 1980.

117. Hirata F, Schiffmann E, Venkatasubramanian K, et al: A phospholipase A_2 inhibitory protein in rabbit neutrophils induced by glucocorticoids. Proc Natl Acad Sci USA 77:2533, 1980.

118. Holford NHG: Clinical pharmacokinetics and pharmacodynamics of warfarin. Clin Pharmacokinet 11:483, 1986.

118a. Hollman GA, Allen DB: Overt glucocorticoid excess due to inhaled corticosteroid therapy. Pediatrics 81:452, 1988.

119. Hoppu K, Koskimies O, Tuomisto J: Trimethoprim pharmacokinetics in children with renal insufficiency. Clin Pharmacol Ther 42:181, 1987.

120. Hufuagle KG, Khan SN, Penn D, et al: Renal calcifications: A complication of long-term furosemide therapy in preterm infants. Pediatrics 70:360, 1982.

121. Humes JL, Bonney RJ, Pelus L, et al: Macrophages synthesize and release prostaglandins in response to inflammatory stimuli. Nature 269:149, 1978.

122. Humphreys MH, Rector FC: Pathophysiology of edema formation. In Seldin DW, Giebisch G (eds): The Kidney:

Physiology and Pathophysiology. New York, Raven Press, 1985, p 1163.

123. Hyman AC, Kadowitz PJ: Pulmonary vasodilator activity of prostacyclin (PGI₂) in the cat. *Circ Res* 45:404, 1979.

124. Imai M: Effect of bumetanide and furosemide on the thick ascending limb of Henle's loop of rabbits and rats perfused in vitro. *Eur J Pharmacol* 41:409, 1977.

125. Jacobson HR, Kokko JP: Diuretics: Sites and mechanisms of action. *Annu Rev Pharmacol Toxicol* 16:201, 1976.

126. Jasani MK: Anti-inflammatory steroids: Mode of action in rheumatoid arthritis and homograft rejection. *In* Vane JR, Ferreira SH (eds): *Anti-inflammatory Drugs.* Vol 2. Springer-Verlag, 1979, p. 598.

127. Juhn SK, Rybak LP, Morizono T, et al: Pharmacokinetics of furosemide in relation to the alteration of endocochlear potential. *Scand Audiol* (Suppl)14:39, 1981.

128. Jusko WJ, Lewis GP, Schmitt GW: Ampicillin and hetacillin pharmacokinetics in normal and anephric subjects. *Clin Pharmacol Ther* 14:90, 1973.

129. Kagawa CM: Blocking the renal electrolyte effects of mineralocorticoids with an orally active steroidal spironolactone. *Endocrinology* 67:125, 1960.

130. Kaplan NM: Our appropriate concern about hypokalemia. *Am J Med* 77:1, 1984.

131. Kaplan NM, Carnegie A, Raskin P, et al: Potassium supplementation in hypertensive patients with diuretic-induced hypokalemia. *N Engl J Med* 312:746, 1985.

132. Kaplan SL, Berry PL, Mason EO, et al: Pharmacokinetics of moxalactam in anuric children and during hemodialysis. *Ped Pharmacol* 3:29, 1983.

133. Kassirer JP, Harrington JT: Fending off the potassium pushers. *N Engl J Med* 312:785, 1985.

134. Kenny FM, Preeyasombat C, Migeon CJ: Cortisol production rate. II. Normal infants, children and adults. *Pediatrics* 37:34, 1966.

135. Kinniburgh DW, Boyd ND: Isolation of peptides from uremic plasma that inhibit phenytoin binding to normal plasma proteins. *Clin Pharmacol Ther* 30:276, 1981.

136. Kobayashi Y, Akaishi K, Nishio T, et al: Posterior subcapsular cataract in nephrotic children receiving steroid therapy. *Am J Dis Child* 128:671, 1974.

137. Kohlmann O, Riberio AB, Larson O, et al: Methyl-prednisolone-induced hypertension. *Hypertension* (suppl II)3:II-107, 1981.

138. Kokko J: Effect of prostaglandins on renal epithelial electrolyte transport. *Kidney Int* 19:791, 1981.

139. Krakoff L, Nicolis G, Amsel B: Pathogenesis of hypertension in Cushing's Syndrome. *Am J Med* 58:216, 1975.

140. Kramer B, Seligson H, Baltrush H, et al: The isolation of several aromatic acids from the hemodialysis fluids of uremic patients. *Clin Chim Acta* 11:363, 1965.

141. Krasny HC, Liao SHT, de Miranda P, et al: Influence of hemodialysis on acyclovir pharmacokinetics in patient with chronic renal failure. *Am J Med* 73(1A):202, 1982.

142. Krauer B: The development of diurnal variation in drug kinetics in the human infant. *In* Morselli P, Garattini S, Sereni F (eds): *Basic and Therapeutic Aspects of Perinatal Pharmacology.* New York, Raven Press, 1975, p 347.

143. Kuehl FA, Egan RW: Prostaglandins, arachidonic acid and inflammation. *Science* 210:978, 1980.

143a. Kucers A, Bennett N McK (eds): *The Use of Antibiotics,* 3rd ed. London, William Heinemann, 1979.

144. Kunau RT, Weller DR, Webb HL: Clarification of the site of action of chlorothiazide in the rat nephron. *J Clin Invest* 56:401, 1975.

145. Kuin CM, Finland M: Persistence of antibiotics in blood of patients with acute renal failure. III. Penicillin, strep-

tomycin, erythromycin and kanamycin. *J Clin Invest* 38:1509, 1959.

146. Laskin OL, Longstreth JA, Whelton A, et al: Effect of renal failure on the pharmacokinetics of acyclovir. *Am J Med* 73(1A):197, 1982.

147. Latos DL, Bryan CS, Stone WJ: Carbenicillin therapy in patients with normal and impaired renal function. *Clin Pharmacol Ther* 17:692, 1975.

148. Lau HSH, Shih LJ, Smith DE: Effect of probenecid on the dose-response relationship of bumetanide at steady state. *J Pharmacol Exp Ther* 227:51, 1983.

149. Lawson DH, Boddy K, Gray JMB, et al: Potassium supplements in patients receiving long-term diuretics for edema. *Q J Med* 45:469, 1976.

150. Lee CS, Marbury TC: Drug therapy in patients undergoing hemodialysis. *Clin Pharmacokinet* 9:42, 1984.

151. Leth A: Changes in plasma and extracellular fluid volumes in patients with essential hypertension during long-term treatment with hydrochlorothiazide. *Circulation* 42:479, 1970.

152. Letteri JM, Mellk H, Louis S, et al: Diphenylhydantoin metabolism in uremia. *N Engl J Med* 285:648, 1971.

153. Levy G: Pharmacokinetics in renal disese. *Am J Med* 62:461, 1977.

154. Levy G, Tsuchiya T: Salicylate accumulation kinetics in man. *N Engl J Med* 287:430, 1972.

155. Levy RH, Moreland TA: Rationale for monitoring free drug levels. *Clin Pharmacokinet* (suppl 1)9:1, 1984.

156. Lewis GP, Jusko WJ, Burke CW, et al: Prednisone side-effects and serum protein levels: A collaborative study. *Lancet* 2:778, 1971.

157. Lewis L, Robinson RF, Yee J, et al: Fatal adrenal cortical insufficiency precipitated by surgery during prolonged continuous cortisone treatment. *Ann Intern Med* 39:116, 1953.

158. Liddle GW: Specific and non-specific inhibition of mineralocorticoid activity. *Metabolism* 10:1021, 1961.

159. Lifschitz MD: Prostaglandins and renal blood flow: In vivo studies. *Kidney Int* 19:781, 1981.

160. Livanou T, Ferriman D, James VHT: Recovery of hypothalamopituitary-adrenal function after corticosteroid therapy. *Lancet* 2:856, 1967.

161. Loeb JN: Corticosteroids and growth. *N Engl J Med* 295:547, 1976.

162. Lowenthal DT, Briggs WA, Gibson TP, et al: Pharmacokinetics of oral propranolol in chronic renal disease. *Clin Pharmacol Ther* 16:761, 1974.

163. Lowenthal DT, Briggs WA, Levy G: Kinetics of salicylate elimination by anephric patients. *J Clin Invest* 54:1221, 1974.

164. Lowenthal DT, Irvin JD, Morrill D, et al: The effect of renal function on enalapril kinetics. *Clin Pharmacol Ther* 38:661, 1985.

165. MacGregor GA: Sodium and potassium intake and blood pressure. *Hypertension* (suppl III)5:III-79, 1983.

166. Maher JF: Principles of dialysis and dialysis of drugs. *Am J Med* 62:475, 1977.

167. Marco J, Calle C, Roman D, et al: Hyperglucagonism induced by glucocorticoid treatment in man. *N Engl J Med* 288:128, 1973.

168. Martre H, Sari R, Taburet AM, et al: Haemodialysis does not affect the pharmacokinetics of nifedipine. *Br J Clin Pharmacol* 20:155, 1985.

169. Maxwell MH, Brachfeld J, Itskovitz H, et al: Blood pressure lowering and potassium conservation by triamterene-hydrochlorothiazide and amiloride-hydrochlorothiazide in hypertension. *Clin Pharmacol Ther* 37:61, 1985.

170. McEnery PT, Stempel DA: Commentary: Anticonvul-

sant therapy and renal allograft survival. *J Pediatr* 88:138, 1976.

171. McMahon FG, Ryan JR, Akdamar K, et al: Effect of potassium chloride supplements on upper gastrointestinal mucosa. *Clin Pharmacol Ther* 35:852, 1984.

172. McNamara PJ, Lalka D, Gibaldi M: Endogenous accumulation products and serum protein binding in uremia. *J Lab Clin Med* 98:730, 1981.

173. Meikle AW, Clarke DH, Tyler FH: Cushing syndrome from low doses of dexamethasone. *JAMA* 235:1592, 1976.

174. Melby JC: Systemic corticosteroid therapy: Pharmacology and endocrinologic considerations. *Ann Intern Med* 81:505, 1974.

175. Messer J, Reitman D, Sacks HS, et al: Association of adrenocorticosteroid therapy and peptic-ulcer disease. *N Engl J Med* 309:21, 1983.

176. Middler S, Pak CYC, Murad F, et al: Thiazide diuretics and calcium metabolism. *Metabolism* 22:139, 1973.

177. Miller FN: The peritoneal microcirculation. *In* Nolph KD (ed): *Peritoneal Dialysis.* The Hague, Martinus Nijhoff, 1981, p 42.

178. Mirkin BL, Green TP, O'Dea RF: Disposition and pharmacodynamics of diuretics and antihypertensive agents in renal disease. *Eur J Clin Pharmacol* 18:109, 1980.

179. Mirkin BL, Sinaiko AR: Clinical pharmacology and therapeutic utilization of antihypertensive agents in children. *In* New MI, Levine LS (eds): *Juvenile Hypertension.* New York, Raven Press, 1977, p 195.

180. Mirkin BL, Sinaiko AR, Cooper M: Hydrochlorothiazide therapy in hypertensive and renal insufficient children: Elimination kinetics and metabolic effects. *Pediatr Res* 11:418, 1977.

181. Mirochnick MH, Micell JJ, Kramer PA, et al: Furosemide pharmacokinetics in very low birth weight infants. *J Pediatr* 112:653, 1988.

182. Moellering RC, Swartz MN: The newer cephalosporins. *N Engl J Med* 294:24, 1976.

183. Moller JV, Sheikh MI: The renal organic anion transport system: Pharmacological, physiological and biochemical aspects. *Pharmacol Rev* 34:315, 1982.

184. Morgan DB, Davidson C: Hypokalemia and diuretics: An analysis of publications. *Br Med J* 1:905, 1980.

185. Morgan OJ, Ching MS, Raymond K, et al: Elimination of amphotericin B in impaired renal function. *Clin Pharmacol Ther* 34:248, 1983.

186. Morris HG, Jorgensen JR: Recovery of endogenous pituitary-adrenal function in corticosteroid-treated children. *J Pediatr* 79:480, 1971.

187. Morris HG, Jorgensen JR, Elrick H, et al: Metabolic effects of human growth hormone in corticosteroid treated children. *J Clin Invest* 47:436, 1968.

188. Morris HG, Neuman I, Ellis EF: Plasma steroid concentrations during alternate-day treatment with prednisone. *J Allergy Clin Immunol* 54:350, 1974.

189. Mouridsen HT, Jacobsen E: Pharmacokinetics of cyclophosphamide in renal failure. *Acta Pharmacol et Toxicol* 36:409, 1975.

190. Moyer JH, Fuchs M, Irie S, et al: Some observations on the pharmacology of hydrochlorothiazide. *Am J Cardiol* 3:113, 1959.

191. Murphy J, Casey W, Lasagna L: The effect of dosage regimen on the diuretic efficacy of chlorothiazide in human subjects. *J Pharmacol Exp Ther* 134:286, 1961.

192. Nichols T, Nugent CA, Tyler FH: Diurnal variation in suppression of adrenal function by glucocorticoids. *J Clin Endocrinol* 25:343, 1965.

193. Nies AS, Gal J, Fadul S, et al: Indomethacin-furosemide interaction: The importance of renal blood flow. *J Pharmacol Exp Ther* 226:27, 1983.

194. Nightingale CH, Greene OS, Quintiliani R: Pharmacokinetics and clinical use of cephalosporin antibiotics. *J Pharm Sci* 64:1899, 1975.

195. Nolph KD, Miller FN, Rubin J, et al: New dimensions in peritoneal dialysis concepts and applications. *Kidney Int* (suppl)18:S111, 1980.

196. O'Dea RF, Mirkin BL: Metabolic disposition of methyldopa in hypertensive and renal-insufficient children. *Clin Pharmacol Ther* 27:37, 1980.

197. Olsen GD, Bennett WM, Porter GA: Morphine and phenytoin binding to plasma proteins in renal and hepatic failure. *Clin Pharmacol Ther* 17:677, 1975.

198. Onoyama K, Hirakata H, Iseki K, et al: Blood concentration and urinary excretion of captopril in patients with chronic renal failure. *Hypertension* 3:456, 1981.

199. Osborn JL, Hook JB, Bailie MD: Control of renin release: Effects of D-propranolol and renal denervation on furosemide-induced renin release in the dog. *Circ Res* 41:481, 1977.

200. Overdiek HWPM, Hermens WAJJ, Merkus FWHM: New insights into the pharmacokinetics of spironolactone. *Clin Pharmacol Ther* 38:469, 1985.

201. Palmer RF, Lasseter KC: Sodium nitroprusside. *N Engl J Med* 292:294, 1975.

202. Parry MF, Neu HC: Pharmacokinetics of ticarcillin in patients with abnormal renal function. *J Infect Dis* 133:46, 1976.

203. Paton TW, Cornish WR, Manuel MA, et al: Drug therapy in patients undergoing peritoneal dialysis. Clinical pharmacokinetic considerations. *Clin Pharmacokinet* 10:404, 1985.

204. Pechere JC, Dugal R: Clinical pharmacokinetics of aminoglycoside antibiotics. *Clin Pharmacokinet* 4:170, 1979.

205. Petereit LB, Meikle AW: Effectiveness of prednisolone during phenytoin therapy. *Clin Pharmacol Ther* 22:912, 1977.

206. Peterson RE: Metabolism of adrenal cortical steroids. *In* Christy NP (ed): *The Human Adrenal Cortex.* New York, Harper & Row, 1971, p 87.

207. Peterson RG, Simmons MA, Rumack BH, et al: Pharmacology of furosemide in the premature newborn infant. *J Pediatr* 97:139, 1980.

208. Piafsky KM: Disease-induced changes in the plasma protein binding of basic drugs. *Clin Pharmacokinet* 5:246, 1980.

209. Pond SM, Tozer TN: First-pass elimination: Basic concepts and clinical consequences. *Clin Pharmacokinet* 9:1, 1984.

210. Popper TL, Watnick AS: Anti-inflammatory steroids. *In* Scherrer RA, Whitehouse MW (eds): *Anti-inflammatory Agents.* New York, Academic Press, 1974, p 245.

211. Prandota J, Pruitt AW: Furosemide binding to human albumin and plasma of nephrotic children. *Clin Pharmacol Ther* 17:159, 1975.

212. Pruitt AW, Winkel JS, Dayton PG: Variations in the fate of triamterene. *Clin Pharmacol Ther* 21:L610, 1977.

213. Puschett JB, Goldberg M: The acute effects of furosemide on acid and electrolyte excretion in man. *J Lab Clin Med* 71:666, 1968.

214. Rane A: Basic principles of drug disposition and action in infants and children. *In* Yaffe SJ (ed): *Pediatric Pharmacology.* New York, Grune and Stratton, 1980, p 7.

215. Reidenberg MM: The binding of drugs to plasma proteins from patients with poor renal function. *Clin Pharmacokinet* 1:121, 1976.

216. Reidenberg MM: The biotransformation of drugs in renal failure. *Am J Med* 62:482, 1977.

217. Reidenberg MM, Drayer DE: Alteration of drug-protein binding in renal disease. *Clin Pharmacokinet* (suppl 1)9:18, 1984.

218. Reidenberg MM, Odar–Cedarlof I, vonBahr C, et al: Protein binding of diphenylhydantoin and desmethylimipramine in plasma from patients with poor renal function. *N Engl J Med* 285:264, 1971.

219. Report of the Second Task Force on Blood Pressure Control in Children. *Pediatrics* 79:1, 1987.

220. Rettenhouse–Simmons S: Production of diglyceride from phosphatidylinositol in activated human platelets. *J Clin Invest* 63:580, 1979.

221. Riemenschneider TA, Wilson JF, Vernier RL: Glucocorticoid-induced pancreatitis in children. *Pediatrics* 41:428, 1968.

222. Rinehart JJ, Balcerzak SP, Sagone AVC, et al: Effects of corticosteroids on human monocyte function. *J Clin Invest* 54:1337, 1974.

223. Rinehart JJ, Sagone AC, Balcerzak SP, et al: Effects of corticosteroid therapy on human monocyte function. *N Engl J Med* 292:236, 1975.

224. Rolewicz TF, Mirkin BL, Cooper MD, et al: Metabolic disposition of cephalothin and deacetylcephalothin in children and adults: Comparison of high-performance liquid chromatographic and microbial assay procedures. *Clin Pharmacol Ther* 2:928, 1977.

225. Ross BS, Pollak A, Oh W: The pharmacologic effects of furosemide therapy in the low-birth-weight infant. *J Pediatr* 92:149, 1978.

226. Rousseau GG, Baxter JD, Tomkins GM: Glucocorticoid receptors: Relations between steroid binding and biological effects. *J Mol Biol* 67:99, 1972.

227. Rowland M: Protein binding and drug clearance. *Clin Pharmacokinet* (suppl 1)9:10, 1984.

228. Rybak LP, Green TP, Juhn SK, et al: Elimination kinetics of furosemide in perilymph and serum of the chinchilla. *Acta Otolaryngol* 88:382, 1979.

229. Rybak LR: Pathophysiology of furosemide ototoxicity. *J Otolaryngol* 11:127, 1982.

230. Savage MD, Wilkinson AR, Baum JD, et al: Furosemide in respiratory distress syndrome. *Arch Dis Child* 50:709, 1975.

231. Scalais E, Papageorgiou A, Aranda JV: Effects of ethacrynic acid in the newborn infant. *J Pediatr* 104:947, 1984.

232. Schentag JJ, Cerra FB, Calleri GM, et al: Age, disease, and cimetidine dispositon in healthy subjects and chronically ill patients. *Clin Pharmacol Ther* 29:737, 1981.

233. Schreiter G: Neuere physiologische und klinische aspekte der nierenfunktion. *Dtsch Ges Wesen* 21:433, 1966.

234. Schrier RW, Lehman D, Zacherle B, et al: Effect of furosemide on free water excretion in edematous patients with hyponatremia. *Kidney Int* 3:30, 1973.

235. Schuyler MR, Gerblich A, Urda G: Prednisone and T-cell subpopulations. *Arch Intern Med* 144:973, 1984.

236. Sedman AJ: Cimetidine—drug interactions. *Am J Med* 76:109, 1984.

237. Sehnermann J, Briggs JP: Participation of renal cortical prostaglandins in the regulation of glomerular filtration rate. *Kidney Int* 19:802, 1981.

238. Shoeman DW, Azarnoff DL: The alterations of plasma proteins in uremia as reflected by their ability to bind digitoxin and diphenylhydantoin. *Pharmacology* 7:169, 1972.

239. Shoenfeld Y, Gurewich Y, Gallant LA, et al: Prednisone-induced leukocytosis. *Am J Med* 71:773, 1981.

240. Sinaiko AR, Green TP: Principles of drug therapy in children with ESRD. *In* Fine RN, Gruskin AB (eds): *End Stage Renal Disease in Children.* Philadelphia, WB Saunders, 1984, p 403.

241. Sinaiko AR, Mirkin BL: Clinical pharmacology of antihypertensive drugs in children. *Pediatr Clin North Am* 25:137, 1978.

242. Sinaiko AR, Mirkin BL, Hendrick DA, et al: Antihypertensive effect and elimination kinetics of captopril in hypertensive children with renal disease. *J Pediatr* 103:799, 1983.

243. Sjoholm I: Binding of drugs to human serum albumin. *Proceedings of the 11th FEBS Meeting* 50:71, 1977.

244. Sjoholm I, Kober A, Odar–Cedarlof I, et al: Protein binding of drugs in uremic and normal serum. The role of endogenous binding inhibitors. *Biochem Pharmacol* 25:1205, 1976.

245. Solomon AE, Briggs JD, McGeachy R, et al: The administration of cephradine to patients in renal failure. *Br J Clin Pharmacol* 2:443, 1975.

246. Somani P, Shapiro RS, Stockard H, et al: Unidirectional absorption of gentamicin from the peritoneum during continuous ambulatory peritoneal dialysis. *Clin Pharmacol Ther* 32:113, 1982.

247. Sorgel F, Hasegawa J, Liu ET, et al: Oral triamterene disposition. *Clin Pharmacol Ther* 38:45, 1968.

248. Spark RF, O'Hare CM, Regan RM: Low-renin hypertension. Restoration of normotension and renin responsiveness. *Arch Intern Med* 133:205, 1974.

249. Spiegel RJ, Oliff AI, Bruton J, et al: Adrenal suppression after short-term corticosteroid therapy. *Lancet* 1:630, 1979.

250. Spiro HM: Is the steroid ulcer a myth? *N Engl J Med* 309:45, 1983.

251. Stein JH, Mauk RC, Broujarern S, et al: Differences in the effect of furosemide and chlorothiazide on the distribution of renal cortical blood flow in the dog. *J Lab Clin Med* 79:995, 1972.

252. Steinmuller SR, Puschett JB: Effects of metolazone in man: Comparison with chlorothiazide. *Kidney Int* 1:169, 1972.

253. Stone WJ, Walle T: Massive retention of propranolol metabolites in maintenance hemodialysis patients (abstr). *Clin Pharmacol Ther* 27:288, 1980.

254. Streck WF, Lockwood DH: Pituitary adrenal recovery following short-term suppression with corticosteroids. *Am J Med* 66:910, 1979.

255. Suki WN, Yium JJ, Von Minden M, et al: Acute treatment of hypercalcemia with furosemide. *N Engl J Med* 283:836, 1970.

256. Swabb EA: Review of the clinical pharmacology of the monobactam antibiotic aztreonam. *Am J Med* 78(2A):11, 1985.

257. Tan SY, Mulrow PJ: Inhibition of the renin-aldosterone response to furosemide by indomethacin. *J Clin Endocrinol Metab* 45:174, 1977.

258. Tanner AR, Halliday JW, Powell LW: Effect of long-term corticosteroid therapy on monocyte chemotaxis in man. *Scand J Immunol* 11:35, 1980.

259. Tarazi RC, Dustan HP, Frohlich ED: Long-term thiazide therapy in essential hypertension: Evidence for persistent alteration in plasma volume and renin activity. *Circulation* 41:709, 1970.

260. Tenckhoff H, Ward G, Boen ST: The influence of dialysate volume and flow rate on peritoneal clearance. *Proc Euro Dialysis and Transplant Assoc* 2:113, 1965.

261. Gilman AG, Goodman LS, Rall TW, et al: *The Pharmacologic Basis of Therapeutics,* 7th ed. New York, Macmillan, 1985.

261a. Kucers A and Bennett N McK (eds): *The Use of Antibiotics,* 3rd ed. London, William Heinemann, 1979.

262. The 1984 Report of the Joint National Committee on Detection, Evaluation and Treatment of High Blood Pressure. *Arch Intern Med* 144:1045, 1984.

262a. Tuck S, Morselli P, Broquaire M, et al: Plasma and urinary kinetics of furosemide in newborn infants. *J Pediatr* 103:481, 1983.

263. Vaz R, Senior B, Morris M, et al: Adrenal effects of beclomethasone inhalation therapy in asthmatic children. *J Pediatr* 100:660, 1982.

264. Verbeeck RK, Branch RA, Wilkinson GR: Drug metabolites in renal failure: Pharmacokinetic and clinical implications. *Clin Pharmacokinet* 6:329, 1981.

265. Verbeeck RK, Patwardhan RV, Villenenve JP, et al: Furosemide disposition in cirrhosis. *Clin Pharmacol Ther* 31:719, 1982.

266. Walstad RA, Nilsen OG, Berg KJ: Pharmacokinetics and clinical effects of cefuroxime in patients with severe renal insufficiency. *Eur J Clin Pharmacol* 24:391, 1983.

267. Ward PA: The chemosuppression of chemotaxis. *J Exp Med* 124:209, 1966.

268. Wassner SJ, Pennisi AJ, Malekzadeh MH, et al: The adverse effect of anticonvulsant therapy on renal allograft survival. *J Pediatr* 88:134, 1976.

269. Wasuich RD, Benfaute RJ, Yano K, et al: Thiazide effect on the mineral content of bone. *N Engl J Med* 309:344, 1983.

270. Wauters JP: Unusual complication of high-dose furosemide. *Br Med J* 4:624, 1975.

271. Webel MI, Donadio JV, Woods JE, et al: Effects of a large dose of methylprednisolone on renal function. *J Lab Clin Med* 80:765, 1972.

272. Weber PC, Seherer B, Larsson C: Increase of free arachidonic acid by furosemide in man as the cause of prostaglandin and renin release. *Eur J Pharmacol* 41:329, 1977.

273. Weinberger MH: Diuretics and their side effects. *Hypertension* (suppl II)11:16, 1988.

274. Weiner IM: Transport of weak acids and bases. *In* Beiliner RW, Orloff J (eds): *Handbook of Physiology, Renal Physiology.* Washington, DC, American Physiological Society, 1970, p 521.

275. Weiner IM, Mudge GH: Renal tubular mechanisms for excretion of organic acids and bases. *Am J Med* 36:743, 1964.

276. Weiner IM, Mudge GH: Inhibitors of tubular transport of organic compounds. *In* Gilman AG, Goodman LS, Rall TW, et al (eds): *The Pharmacologic Basis of Therapeutics.* New York, Macmillan, 1985, p 920.

277. Whitworth JA, Gordon D, Andrews J, et al: The hypertensive effect of synthetic glucocorticoids in man: Role of sodium and volume. *J Hypertens* 7:537, 1989.

278. Wilkinson PR, Hesp R, Issler H, et al: Total body and serum potassium during prolonged thiazide therapy for essential hypertension. *Lancet* 1:759, 1975.

279. Williams RL, Clark T, Blume CD: Clinical experience with a new combination formulation of triamterene and hydrochlorothiazide (Maxzide) in patients with mild to moderate hypertension. *Am J Med* 77(5A):62, 1984.

280. Williams RL, Thornhill MD, Upton RA, et al: Absorption and disposition of two combination formulations of hydrochlorothiazide and triamterene: Influence of age and renal function. *Clin Pharmacol Ther* 40:226, 1986.

281. Wilson CB, Koup JR: Clinical pharmacology of extended-spectrum penicillins in infants and children. *J Pediatr* 106:1049, 1985.

282. Wilson IM, Freis ED: Relationship between plasma and extracellular fluid volume depletion and the antihypertensive effect of chlorothiazide. *Circulation* 20:1028, 1959.

283. Wood AJJ, Vestal RE, Spannuth CL, et al: Propranolol disposition in patients with renal failure. *Br J Clin Pharmacol* 10:561, 1980.

284. Wright AJ, Wilkowske CJ: The penicillins. *Mayo Clin Proc* 58:21, 1983.

285. Wyatt R, Waschek J, Weinberger M, et al: Effects of inhaled beclomethasone dipropionate and alternate-day prednisone on pituitary-adrenal function in children with chronic asthma. *N Engl J Med* 299:1387, 1978.

286. Yu DTY, Clements PJ, Paulus HE, et al: Human lymphocyte subpopulations: Effect of corticosteroids. *J Clin Invest* 53:565, 1974.

Index

Index